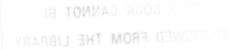

W. ALLAN WALKER, M.D.

Professor of Pediatrics, Harvard Medical School; Chief, Combined
Program in Pediatric Gastroenterology and Nutrition, Children's Hospital
and Massachusetts General Hospital, Boston, Massachusetts

PETER R. DURIE, B.SC., M.D., FRCPC

Associate Professor, University of Toronto Faculty of Medicine; Senior
Scientist, Research Institute, and Staff Physician, Division of
Gastroenterology, Department of Paediatrics, The Hospital for Sick
Children, Toronto, Ontario, Canada

J. RICHARD HAMILTON, M.D., FRCPC

Professor and Chairman, Department of Pediatrics, Faculty of Medicine,
McGill University; Physician-in-Chief, Montreal Children's Hospital,
Montreal, Quebec, Canada

JOHN A. WALKER-SMITH, M.D. (Syd.), F.R.C.P. (Lon., Edin.), F.R.A.C.P.

Professor of Paediatric Gastroenterology, The Medical College of St.
Bartholomew's Hospital; Consultant Paediatrician, Queen Elizabeth Hospital
for Children, London, England

JOHN B. WATKINS, M.D.

Professor of Pediatrics, University of Pennsylvania School of Medicine;
Director, Division of Gastroenterology and Nutrition, The Children's
Hospital of Philadelphia, Philadelphia, Pennsylvania

VOLUME ONE

Pediatric Gastrointestinal Disease

Pathophysiology • Diagnosis • Management

B.C. Decker Inc.
Philadelphia • Toronto

Publisher

B.C. Decker Inc
3228 South Service Road
Burlington, Ontario   L7N 3H8

B.C. Decker Inc
320 Walnut Street
Suite 400
Philadelphia, Pennsylvania   19106

Sales and Distribution

United States and Puerto Rico
Mosby-Year Book Inc.
11830 Westline Industrial Drive
Saint Louis, Missouri   63146

Canada
Mosby-Year Book Limited
5240 Finch Avenue E., Unit 1
Scarborough, Ontario   M1S 5A2

Australia
McGraw-Hill Book Company Australia Pty. Ltd.
4 Barcoo Street
Roseville East 2069
New South Wales, Australia

Brazil
Editora McGraw-Hill do Brasil, Ltda.
rua Tabapua, 1.105, Itaim-Bibi
Sao Paulo, S.P. Brasil

Colombia
Interamericana/McGraw-Hill de Colombia, S.A.
Carrera 17, No. 33-71
(Apartado Postal, A.A., 6131)
Bogota, D.E. Colombia

Europe
McGraw-Hill Book Company GmbH
Lademannbogen 136
D-2000 Hamburg 63
West Germany

France
MEDSI/McGraw-Hill
6, avenue Daniel Lesueur
75007 Paris, France

Hong Kong and China
McGraw-Hill Book Company
Suite 618, Ocean Centre
5 Canton Road
Tsimshatsui, Kowloon
Hong Kong

India
Tata McGraw-Hill Publishing Company, Ltd.
12/4 Asaf Ali Road, 3rd Floor
New Delhi 110002, India

Indonesia
Mr. Wong Fin Fah
P.O. Box 122/JAT
Jakarta, 1300 Indonesia

Italy
McGraw-Hill Libri Italia, s.r.l.
Piazza Emilia, 5
I-20129 Milano MI
Italy

Japan
Igaku-Shoin Ltd.
Tokyo International P.O. Box 5063
1-28-36 Hongo, Bunkyo-ku,
Tokyo 113, Japan

Korea
Mr. Don-Gap Choi
C.P.O. Box 10583
Seoul, Korea

Malaysia
Mr. Lim Tao Slong
No. 8 Jalan SS 7/6B
Kelana Jaya
47301 Petaling Jaya
Selangor, Malaysia

Mexico
Interamericana/McGraw-Hill de Mexico, S.A. de C.V.
Cedro 512, Colonia Atlampa
(Apartado Postal 26370)
06450 Mexico, D.F., Mexico

New Zealand
McGraw-Hill Book Co. New Zealand Ltd.
5 Joval Place, Wiri
Manukau City, New Zealand

Portugal
Editora McGraw-Hill de Portugal, Ltda.
Rua Rosa Damasceno 11A-B
1900 Lisboa, Portugal

South Africa
Libriger Book Distributors
Warehouse Number 8
"Die Ou Looiery"
Tannery Road
Hamilton, Bloemfontein 9300

Singapore and Southeast Asia
McGraw-Hill Book Co.
21 Neythal Road
Jurong, Singapore 2262

Spain
McGraw-Hill/Interamericana de Espana, S.A.
Manuel Ferrero, 13
28020 Madrid, Spain

Taiwan
Mr. George Lim
P.O. Box 87-601
Taipei, Taiwan

Thailand
Mr. Vitit Lim
632/5 Phaholyothin Road
Sapan Kwai
Bangkok 10400
Thailand

United Kingdom, Middle East and Africa
McGraw-Hill Book Company (U.K.) Ltd.
Shoppenhangers Road
Maidenhead, Berkshire
SL6 2QL England

Venezuela
Editorial Interamericana de Venezuela C.A.
2da. calle Bello Monte
Local G-2
Caracas, Venezuela

NOTICE

The authors and publisher have made every effort to ensure that the patient care recommended herein, including choice of drugs and drug dosages, is in accord with the accepted standards and practice at the time of publication. However, since research and regulation constantly change clinical standards, the reader is urged to check the product information sheet included in the package of each drug, which includes recommended doses, warnings, and contraindications. This is particularly important with new or infrequently used drugs.

Pediatric Gastrointestinal Disease

ISBN 1-55664-261-X (set)
1-55664-122-2 (Volume 1)
1-55664-209-1 (Volume 2)

Library of Congress catalog card number: 89-50930   10 9 8 7 6 5 4 3 2 1

Contributors

MARVIN E. AMENT, M.D.
Professor of Pediatrics, and Chief, Division of
Pediatric Gastroenterology and Nutrition, University
of California, Los Angeles, School of Medicine, Los
Angeles, California
Endoscopy: Fiberoptic Upper Intestinal Endoscopy
Nutritional Therapy: Home Total Parenteral Nutrition

JOEL M. ANDRES, M.D.
Associate Professor, University of Florida College of
Medicine, Gainesville, Florida
*The Liver and Biliary Tree: Congenital Infections of the
Liver*

MAGDALENA ARAYA, M.D.
Professor of Pediatrics, and Member, Gastroenterology
Unit, Institute of Nutrition and Food Technology,
University of Chile, Santiago, Chile
The Intestines: The Gut in Malnutrition

SALVATORE AURICCHIO, M.D.
Professor, Department of Pediatrics, II Faculty of
Medicine, University of Naples, Naples, Italy
*The Intestines: Genetically Determined Disaccharidase
Deficiencies*

**ALBERT AYNSLEY-GREEN, M.A., D. Phil.,
M.B., B.S., F.R.C.P. (Lon., Edin.)**
James Spence Professor of Child Health, University of
Newcastle-Upon-Tyne Medical School; Senior
Consultant Paediatrician, Royal Victoria Infirmary,
Newcastle-Upon-Tyne, England
Endocrine Function of the Gut in Early Life

PAUL BABYN, M.D.C.M.
Assistant Professor, University of Toronto Faculty of
Medicine; Staff Radiologist, The Hospital for Sick
Children, Toronto, Ontario, Canada
*Imaging: Radiography: Plain Film; Sonography; Computed
Tomography*

WILLIAM F. BALISTRERI, M.D.
Dorothy M.M. Kersten Professor of Pediatrics, and
Director, Division of Pediatric Gastroenterology and
Nutrition, University of Cincinnati College of
Medicine; Attending Physician, Children's Hospital
Medical Center, Cincinnati, Ohio
*The Liver and Biliary Tree: Prolonged Neonatal Obstructive
Jaundice*

GRAEME L. BARNES, M.D., Ch.B., F.R.A.C.P.
Director of Gastroenterology, Royal Children's
Hospital, Melbourne, Australia
The Intestines: Intestinal Viral Infections

LEWIS A. BARNESS, M.D.
Professor of Pediatrics, University of South Florida
College of Medicine, Tampa, Florida; Visiting
Professor of Pediatrics, University of Wisconsin
School of Medicine, Madison, Wisconsin
*Nutritional Therapy: Special Dietary Therapy for Specific
Disease States*

RONALD G. BARR, M.A., M.D.C.M., FRCPC
Associate Professor of Pediatrics, McGill University
Faculty of Medicine; Director, Child Development
Programme, Montreal Children's Hospital, Montreal,
Quebec, Canada
Colic and Gas

GERARD T. BERRY, M.D.
Associate Professor of Pediatrics, University of
Pennsylvania School of Medicine; Senior Physician,
The Children's Hospital of Philadelphia, Philadelphia,
Pennsylvania
*The Liver and Biliary Tree: Disorders of Amino Acid
Metabolism*

RAVI BERRY, M.D.
Former Fellow in Pediatric Gastroenterology, Mayo
Graduate School of Medicine, Rochester, Minnesota;
Pediatric Gastroenterologist, Riverside Medical Clinic,
Riverside, California
Gastrointestinal Bleeding

JULIE E. BINES, M.B.B.S.
Fellow, Harvard Medical School; Fellow, Combined
Program in Pediatric Gastroenterology and Nutrition,
The Children's Hospital and Massachusetts General
Hospital, Boston, Massachusetts
Endoscopy: Lower Endoscopy

ROBERT E. BLACK, M.D., M.P.H.
Professor and Chair, Department of International
Health, The Johns Hopkins University School of
Medicine, Baltimore, Maryland
The Intestines: Idiopathic Prolonged Diarrhea

EDGAR C. BOEDEKER, M.D.
Associate Professor, Department of Medicine,
Uniformed Services University of the Health Sciences,
Bethesda, Maryland; Chief, Department of
Gastroenterology, Walter Reed Army Institute of
Research, Washington, D.C.
Flora of the Gut and Protective Function

JOHN T. BOYLE, M.D.
Associate Professor of Pediatrics, Case Western
Reserve University School of Medicine; Chief,
Division of Gastroenterology and Nutrition, Rainbow
Babies and Children's Hospital, Cleveland, Ohio
Chronic Abdominal Pain

KENNETH H. BROWN, M.D.
Professor, Department of Nutrition, and Director,
Program in International Nutrition, University of
California, Davis, School of Medicine, Davis,
California
The Intestines: Idiopathic Prolonged Diarrhea

OSCAR BRUNSER, M.D.
Professor of Pediatrics, and Chief, Gastroenterology
Unit, Institute of Nutrition and Food Technology,
University of Chile, Santiago, Chile
The Intestines: The Gut in Malnutrition

PATRICIA E. BURROWS, M.D., FRCPC
Assistant Professor, University of Toronto Faculty of
Medicine; Staff Radiologist, The Hospital for Sick
Children, Toronto, Ontario, Canada
Imaging: Angiography

GEOFFREY J. CLEGHORN, M.B.B.S., F.R.A.C.P.
Senior Lecturer, Department of Child Health,
University of Queensland; Director of Paediatric
Gastroenterology, Mater Misericordiae Children's
Hospital; Visiting Gastroenterologist, Royal Children's
Hospital, Brisbane, Australia
*Drug Therapy: Pharmacologic Treatment of Exocrine
Pancreatic Insufficiency*

PAUL M. COATES, Ph.D.
Research Professor of Pediatrics, University of
Pennsylvania School of Medicine; Director, Fellowship
Research, and Director, Center for Mitochondrial
Biology, Division of Gastroenterology and Nutrition,
The Children's Hospital of Philadelphia, Philadelphia,
Pennsylvania
*The Liver and Biliary Tree: Lysosomal Acid Lipase
Deficiency: Cholesteryl Ester Storage Disease and Wolman's
Disease; Inherited Abnormalities in Mitochondrial Fatty Acid
Oxidation*

**MERVYN D. COHEN, M.B., Ch.B., M.D.,
F.R.C.R., M.R.C.P.**
Professor of Radiology, Indiana University School of
Medicine; Chief of Pediatric Radiology, James
Whitcomb Riley Hospital for Children, Indianapolis,
Indiana
*Imaging: Magnetic Resonance Imaging of the
Gastrointestinal Tract*

JEAN A. CORTNER, M.D.
Professor of Pediatrics, University of Pennsylvania
School of Medicine; Director, Lipid-Heart Research,
and Director, Nutrition Center, Division of
Gastroenterology and Nutrition, The Children's
Hospital of Philadelphia, Philadelphia, Pennsylvania
*The Liver and Biliary Tree: Lysosomal Acid Lipase
Deficiency: Cholesteryl Ester Storage Disease and Wolman's
Disease*

RICHARD COUPER, M.B., Ch.B., F.R.A.C.P.
Research Fellow in Gastroenterology, The Hospital for
Sick Children, Toronto, Ontario, Canada
Pancreatic Function Tests

GEOFFREY P. DAVIDSON, M.D., F.R.C.P.
Clinical Senior Lecturer, Department of Paediatrics,
University of Adelaide; Director, Gastroenterology
Unit, Adelaide Children's Hospital, North Adelaide,
South Australia, Australia
The Intestines: Idiopathic Villus Atrophy

MURRAY DAVIDSON, M.D.
Professor of Pediatrics, State University of New York
at Stony Brook School of Medicine, Stony Brook,
New York
The Intestines: Idiopathic Constipation

JEHAN-FRANÇOIS DESJEUX, M.D.
Director, Nutrition Research Center, Institut National
de la Santé et de la Recherchie Medicali (INSERM
U290); Consultant in Pediatric Gastroenterology,
Hôpital Saint-Lazare, Paris, France
*Transport of Water and Ions
The Intestines: Congenital Transport Defects*

MARTIN PETRIC, Ph.D.
Assistant Professor, University of Toronto Faculty of Medicine; Virologist, The Hospital for Sick Children, Toronto, Ontario, Canada
Laboratory Studies: Microbiologic Tests

MICHAEL J. PETTEI, M.D., Ph.D.
Assistant Professor of Pediatrics, State University of New York at Stony Brook School of Medicine, Stony Brook; Co-Chief, Division of Gastroenterology and Nutrition, Schneider Children's Hospital, New Hyde Park, New York
The Intestines: Idiopathic Constipation

ALAN D. PHILLIPS, B.A. (Hon.)
Principal Electron Microscopist, Queen Elizabeth Hospital for Children, London, England
Intestinal Biopsy

DAVID A. PICCOLI, M.D.
Assistant Professor of Pediatrics, University of Pennsylvania School of Medicine; Associate Physician, The Children's Hospital of Philadelphia, Philadelphia, Pennsylvania
The Liver and Biliary Tree: Neonatal Iron Storage Disease; Disorders of the Intrahepatic Bile Ducts; Disorders of the Extrahepatic Bile Ducts

C.S. PITCHUMONI, M.D., M.P.H., FRCPC, F.A.C.P.
Professor of Medicine and Professor of Community and Preventive Medicine, New York Medical College, Valhalla; Program Director, Internal Medicine, and Chief, Division of Gastroenterology, Our Lady of Mercy Medical Center, Bronx, New York
The Pancreas: Juvenile Tropical Pancreatitis

RANDI G. PLESKOW, M.D.
Assistant Professor, Tufts University School of Medicine; Pediatric Gastroenterologist, The Floating Hospital for Infants and Children, New England Medical Center, Boston, Massachusetts
The Liver and Biliary Tree: Wilson's Disease

DON W. POWELL, M.D.
Professor and Associate Chairman, Department of Medicine, Chief, Division of Digestive Diseases and Nutrition, and Director, Center for Gastrointestinal Biology and Disease, University of North Carolina at Chapel Hill School of Medicine, Chapel Hill, North Carolina
Diarrhea

ROY PROUJANSKY, M.D.
Associate Professor, Department of Pediatrics, Jefferson Medical College, Philadelphia, Pennsylvania; Chief, Division of Gastroenterology and Nutrition, Alfred I. DuPont Institute, Wilmington, Delaware
The Intestines: Protein-Losing Enteropathy

JENNIFER M. PUCK, M.D.
Assistant Professor of Pediatrics, University of Pennsylvania School of Medicine; Staff Physician, Division of Infectious Diseases, The Children's Hospital of Philadelphia, Philadelphia, Pennsylvania
The Liver and Biliary Tree: Bacterial, Parasitic, and Other Infections of the Liver

JON MARC RHOADS, M.D.
Assistant Professor of Pediatrics, University of North Carolina at Chapel Hill School of Medicine, Chapel Hill, North Carolina
Diarrhea

SUSAN E. RICHARDSON, B.Sc., M.D., C.M.
Assistant Professor, University of Toronto Faculty of Medicine; Medical Microbiologist, The Hospital for Sick Children, Toronto, Ontario, Canada
Laboratory Studies: Microbiologic Tests

PAUL I. RICHMAN, M.B.B.S., Ph.D., M.R.C.Path.
Senior Lecturer and Consultant in Histopathology, The Medical College of St. Bartholomew's Hospital, London, England
Intestinal Biopsy

CAROLINE A. RIELY, M.D.
Professor of Medicine and Pediatrics, University of Tennessee, Memphis, School of Medicine; Attending Physician, The William F. Bowld Hospital, The Regional Medical Center at Memphis, Le Bonheur Children's Medical Center, Memphis, Tennessee
The Liver and Biliary Tree: Familial Intrahepatic Cholestasis: An Overview

EVE A. ROBERTS, M.D., FRCPC
Assistant Professor of Paediatrics and Medicine, University of Toronto Faculty of Medicine; Staff Physician, Division of Gastroenterology, Department of Paediatrics, The Hospital for Sick Children, Toronto, Ontario, Canada
The Liver and Biliary Tree: Drug-induced Hepatotoxicity in Children
Drug Therapy: Treatment of Acid-Peptic Disease; Drug Therapy for Liver Disease

ARTHUR J. ROSS, III, M.D.
Assistant Professor of Pediatric Surgery, University of Pennsylvania School of Medicine; Attending Surgeon, The Children's Hospital of Philadelphia, Philadelphia, Pennsylvania
Acute Abdominal Pain
Abdominal Masses

DAVID C. RULE, B.D.S., F.D.S., D.Orth., M.C.C.D.
Honorary Senior Lecturer, Institute of Dental Surgery, University of London; Consultant, Department of Children's Dentistry, Eastman Dental Hospital, London, England
The Mouth: Disorders of the Oral Cavity

WILLIAM E. RUSSELL, M.D.
Assistant Professor of Pediatrics, Harvard Medical School; Assistant Pediatrician, Massachusetts General Hospital, Boston, Massachusetts
Growth Failure and Malnutrition

PATRICK J. ST. LOUIS, Ph.D., Dip.C.C.
Lecturer, Department of Clinical Biochemistry, University of Toronto Faculty of Medicine; Clinical Chemist, Department of Biochemistry, The Hospital for Sick Children, Toronto, Ontario, Canada
Laboratory Studies: Biochemical Studies: Liver and Intestine

RICHARD H. SANDLER, M.D.
Instructor, Harvard Medical School; Research Fellow in Gastroenterology, and Assistant in Nutrition, The Children's Hospital, Boston, Massachusetts
The Liver and Biliary Tree: Cholestasis Associated with Parenteral Nutrition

JACQUES SCHMITZ, M.D.
Professor of Pediatrics, Necker-Enfants Malades School of Medicine; Department of Pediatrics, Enfants Malades Hospital, Paris, France
Malabsorption
Digestive and Absorptive Function

BRENT SCOTT, M.D.C.M., FRCPC
Associate Professor of Paediatrics, University of Calgary Faculty of Medicine; Program Director, Division of Gastroenterology and Nutrition, Alberta Children's Hospital, Calgary, Alberta, Canada
The Intestines: Drug-Induced Bowel Injury; Motility Disorders
Motility Studies

ERNEST G. SEIDMAN, M.D.
Assistant Professor, Departments of Pediatrics and Nutrition, University of Montreal Faculty of Medicine; Director, Intestinal Immunology Lab, and Attending Physician, Division of Gastroenterology and Nutrition, Hôpital Ste. Justine, Montreal, Quebec, Canada
The Intestines: Gastrointestinal Manifestations of Immunodeficiency States

KENNETH D.R. SETCHELL, Ph.D.
Associate Professor of Pediatrics, University of Cincinnati College of Medicine; Director, Clinical Mass Spectrometry Laboratory, Children's Hospital Medical Center, Cincinnati, Ohio
The Liver and Biliary Tree: Disorders of Bile Acid Synthesis

ELDON A. SHAFFER, M.D., FRCPC, F.A.C.P., F.A.C.G.
Professor of Medicine, Head, Division of Gastroenterology, and Associate Dean (Clinical Services), University of Calgary Faculty of Medicine; Head, Division of Gastroenterology, Foothills Hospital, Calgary, Alberta, Canada
Hepatobiliary System: Structure and Function
The Liver and Biliary Tree: Gallbladder Disease

DAVID A. SHAFRITZ, M.D.
Professor of Medicine and Cell Biology, and Director, Marion Bessin Liver Research Center, Albert Einstein College of Medicine; Attending Physician, Weiler Hospital of Albert Einstein College of Medicine and Bronx Municipal Hospital Center, Bronx, New York
The Liver and Biliary Tree: Molecular Biology of Hepatitis B Virus

BARRY SHANDLING, M.B., Ch.B., F.R.C.S.(Eng.), FRCSC, F.A.C.S.
Associate Professor, Department of Surgery, University of Toronto Faculty of Medicine; Senior Staff Surgeon, The Hospital for Sick Children; Director, Bowel Clinic, The Hugh MacMillan Medical Centre; Consultant Surgeon, Sunnybrook Hospital and North York General Hospital, Toronto, Ontario, Canada
The Intestines: Peritonitis; Perianal Lesions; Appendicitis; Diverticular Disease

THOMAS A. SHAW-STIFFEL, M.D., C.M., FRCPC, F.A.C.G.
Assistant Professor of Gastroenterology and Clinical Pharmacology, University of Toronto Faculty of Medicine; Staff Physician, Sunnybrook Health Science Centre, Toronto, Ontario, Canada
Drug Therapy: Treatment of Acid-Peptic Disease

ROSS W. SHEPHERD, M.D., M.R.C.P., F.R.A.C.P.
Associate Professor of Child Health, University of Queensland; Director of Gastroenterology, Royal Children's Hospital, Brisbane, Australia
The Intestines: The Gut in Systemic Endocrinopathies

PHILIP SHERMAN, M.D., FRCPC
Associate Professor of Paediatrics and Microbiology, University of Toronto Faculty of Medicine; Staff Gastroenterologist, The Hospital for Sick Children, Toronto, Ontario, Canada
The Stomach and Duodenum: Gastritis in Childhood
The Intestines: Bacterial Overgrowth

ANA ABAD SINDEN, M.S., R.D.
Pediatric Nutrition Specialist, Department of Nutrition Services, University of Virginia Medical Center, Charlottesville, Virginia
Nutritional Therapy: Enteral Nutrition

JOHN D. SNYDER, M.D.
Assistant Professor of Pediatrics, Harvard Medical School; Associate in Gastroenterology, Children's Hospital, Boston, Massachusetts
The Intestines: Bacterial Infections

JUDITH M. SONDHEIMER, M.D.
Associate Professor of Pediatrics, and Chief of Pediatric Gastroenterology and Nutrition, University of Colorado School of Medicine; Chief of Gastroenterology, The Children's Hospital, Denver, Colorado
Esophageal pH Monitoring

STEPHEN P. SPIELBERG, M.D., Ph.D.
Professor of Paediatrics and Pharmacology, University of Toronto Faculty of Medicine; Director, Division of Clinical Pharmacology and Toxicology, The Hospital for Sick Children, Toronto, Ontario, Canada
The Liver and Biliary Tree: Drug-induced Hepatotoxicity in Children
Drug Therapy: Principles of Pediatric Therapeutics

MICHAEL SPINO, B.Sc.Phm., Pharm.D.
Associate Professor, University of Toronto Faculties of Pharmacy and Medicine; Senior Scientist, Division of Clinical Pharmacology and Toxicology, The Hospital for Sick Children, Toronto, Ontario, Canada
Drug Therapy: Pharmacologic Treatment of Gastrointestinal Motility

WILLIAM SPIVAK, M.D.
Associate Clinical Professor of Pediatrics, Albert Einstein College of Medicine, New York; Associate Attending Pediatrician, Montefiore Medical Center, Bronx, New York
The Liver and Biliary Tree: Disorders of Bilirubin Metabolism

CHARLES A. STANLEY, M.D.
Professor of Pediatrics, University of Pennsylvania School of Medicine; Associate Director, Clinical Research Committee, Endocrine/Diabetes Division, The Children's Hospital of Philadelphia, Pennsylvania
The Liver and Biliary Tree: Disorders of Carbohydrate Metabolism

MARTIN STERN, M.D.
Professor of Pediatrics, Universitaets-Kinderklinik, Tuebingen, West Germany
The Intestines: Gastrointestinal Allergy

DAVID A. STRINGER, B.Sc., M.B.B.S., F.R.C.R., FRCPC
Associate Professor, University of Toronto Faculty of Medicine; Head, Divisions of Ultrasound and Gastrointestinal Radiology, The Hospital for Sick Children, Toronto, Ontario, Canada
Imaging: Overview; Radiography: Plain Film; Radiography: Contrast Studies; Sonography; Computed Tomography; Interventional Radiology

JAMES L. SUTPHEN, M.D., Ph.D.
Associate Professor, University of Virginia School of Medicine; Chief, Division of Pediatric Gastroenterology and Nutrition, University of Virginia Children's Medical Center, Charlottesville, Virginia
Nutritional Therapy: Enteral Nutrition

LESLI A. TAYLOR, M.D.
Instructor in Pediatric Surgery, University of Pennsylvania School of Medicine; Fellow in Pediatric Surgery, The Children's Hospital of Philadelphia, Philadelphia, Pennsylvania
Abdominal Masses

M. MICHAEL THALER, M.D.
Professor of Pediatrics, University of California, San Francisco, School of Medicine; Attending Physician, University of California Medical Center, San Francisco, California
The Liver and Biliary Tree: Cirrhosis

WILLIAM R. TREEM, M.D.
Assistant Professor of Pediatrics, University of Connecticut School of Medicine; Associate Director, Division of Pediatric Gastroenterology and Nutrition, Hartford Hospital, Hartford, Connecticut
Hepatic Failure

GEORGE TRIADAFILOPOULOS, M.D., D.Sc., F.A.C.P., F.A.C.G.
Assistant Professor of Medicine, University of California, Davis, School of Medicine; Chief, Section of Gastroenterology, Martinez Veterans Administration Medical Center, Martinez, California
The Intestines: Pseudomembranous Colitis

DAVID N. TUCHMAN, M.D.
Assistant Professor of Pediatrics, The Johns Hopkins University School of Medicine, Baltimore, Maryland
The Mouth: Disorders of Deglutition

JOHN N. UDALL Jr., M.D., Ph.D.
Associate Professor of Pediatrics, University of Arizona School of Medicine; Chief, Pediatric Gastroenterology, University Medical Center, Tucson, Arizona
Development of Immune Function
Nutritional Therapy: Introduction

JAY P. VACANTI, M.D.
Assistant Professor of Surgery, Harvard Medical School; Assistant in Surgery, The Children's Hospital, Boston, Massachusetts
The Liver and Biliary Tree: Liver Transplantation

JORGE VARGAS, M.D.
Assistant Professor of Pediatrics, Division of Gastroenterology, University of California, Los Angeles, School of Medicine, Los Angeles, California
Endoscopy: Fiberoptic Upper Intestinal Endoscopy

FERNANDO E. VITERI, M.D., Sci.D.
Professor, Nutritional Sciences, University of California, Berkeley, California
Nutritional Therapy: Protein Energy Malnutrition

W. ALLAN WALKER, M.D.
Professor of Pediatrics, Harvard Medical School; Chief, Combined Program in Pediatric Gastroenterology and Nutrition, Children's Hospital and Massachusetts General Hospital, Boston, Massachusetts
Book Editor

JOHN A. WALKER-SMITH, M.D.(Syd.), F.R.C.P. (Lon., Edin.), F.R.A.C.P.
Professor of Paediatric Gastroenterology, The Medical College of St. Bartholomew's Hospital; Consultant Paediatrician, Queen Elizabeth Hospital for Children, London, England
The Intestines: Celiac Disease
Intestinal Biopsy
Book Editor

JOHN B. WATKINS, M.D.
Professor of Pediatrics, University of Pennsylvania School of Medicine; Director, Division of Gastroenterology and Nutrition, The Children's Hospital of Philadelphia, Philadelphia, Pennsylvania
The Liver and Biliary Tree: Neonatal Iron Storage Disease
Book Editor

RONALD R. WATSON, Ph.D.
Research Professor, Department of Family Community Medicine, University of Arizona School of Medicine, Tucson, Arizona
Development of Immune Function

LAWRENCE T. WEAVER, M.A., M.D., M.R.C.P., D.C.H.
Scientific Staff, MRC Dunn Nutrition Unit, University of Cambridge; Honorary Consultant Paediatrician, Department of Paediatrics, Addenbrooke's Hospital, Cambridge, England
Anatomy and Embryology

WILLIAM B. WEIL Jr., M.D.
Professor of Pediatrics and Human Development, Michigan State University College of Human Medicine, East Lansing, Michigan
Nutritional Therapy: Obesity

STEVEN L. WERLIN, M.D.
Professor of Pediatrics, Medical College of Wisconsin; Director of Gastroenterology, Children's Hospital of Wisconsin, Milwaukee, Wisconsin
Exocrine Pancreas: Structure and Function

BARRY K. WERSHIL, M.D.
Instructor, Harvard Medical School; Clinical Assistant in Gastroenterology, Combined Program in Pediatric Gastroenterology and Nutrition, Children's Hospital and Massachusetts General Hospital, Boston, Massachusetts
Gastric Function

DAVID WESSON, M.D.
Associate Professor, Department of Surgery, University of Toronto Faculty of Medicine; Staff Surgeon, The Hospital for Sick Children, Toronto, Ontario, Canada
The Intestines: Congenital Anomalies; Trauma and Foreign Bodies; Acute Intestinal Obstruction; Hernias

HARLAND S. WINTER, M.D.
Assistant Professor of Pediatrics, Harvard Medical School; Associate in Medicine, Combined Program in Pediatric Gastroenterology and Nutrition, Children's Hospital and Massachusetts General Hospital, Boston, Massachusetts
The Intestines: Intestinal Polyps
Endoscopy: Lower Endoscopy

CAMILLUS L. WITZLEBEN, M.D.
Professor of Pathology and Pediatrics, University of Pennsylvania School of Medicine; Pathologist-in-Chief, The Children's Hospital of Philadelphia, Philadelphia, Pennsylvania
The Liver and Biliary Tree: Neonatal Iron Storage Disease; Disorders of the Intrahepatic Bile Ducts; Disorders of the Extrahepatic Bile Ducts

BEATRICE WOOD, Ph.D.
Clinical Assistant Professor of Psychology in Psychiatry and Pediatrics, University of Pennsylvania; Director of Psychotherapy, Child Study Institute, Department of Human Development, Bryn Mawr College, Bryn Mawr, Pennsylvania
Biopsychosocial Care

VANESSA M. WRIGHT, M.B., B.S., F.R.C.S., F.R.A.C.S.
Consultant Paediatric Surgeon, Queen Elizabeth Hospital for Children, London University College Hospital, London, England
The Esophagus: Congenital Anomalies
The Stomach and Duodenum: Congenital Anomalies

ELI ZALZSTEIN, M.D.
Fellow in Clinical Pharmacology, The Hospital for Sick Children, Toronto, Ontario, Canada
Drug Therapy: Principles of Pediatric Therapeutics

W. ALLAN WALKER

*To Ted and Isabel Sattler
who are role models for life,
for their support and encouragement.*

PETER R. DURIE

*To Gordon Forstner,
whose insightful approach to research medicine and life
has provided continuing encouragement and direction.*

J. RICHARD HAMILTON

*To Andrew Sass-Kortsak and Jack French,
who stimulated my early interest in this fascinating field.*

JOHN A. WALKER-SMITH

*To Liz, Louise, Laura, and James Walker-Smith,
with appreciation for their patience.*

JOHN B. WATKINS

*To Mary, Sarah, and Leah Watkins and The Friendship Trust,
for their love, support, and encouragement.*

Preface

Over the last two decades, the field of pediatric gastroenterology has developed from an obscure subspecialty to an essential component of every major academic pediatric program throughout the world. Among the many pediatric texts available, none deals extensively with the pathophysiologic basis of gastrointestinal disease in children of all ages. Contributors to this text have been asked to undertake their writing with a plan to fill this void, extending pathophysiologic considerations to their coverage of diagnosis and management as well. In tandem with development of the subspecialty the literature of gastrointestinal and hepatic entities as they pertain to the pediatric patient has grown. Accordingly, we have prepared an approach to the subject that should provide a reference text for pediatricians, gastroenterologists, and pediatric gastroenterologists alike.

This new multivolume textbook is dedicated to establishing a comprehensive approach to pediatric gastroenterology. Each author was carefully selected to provide an authoritative, comprehensive, and complete account of his assigned topic. We have devised an approach to dealing with the families of children with gastrointestinal diseases, and a pathophysiologic section examines cardinal manifestations of gastrointestinal disease as well as the development of the gastrointestinal tract. These sections help to augment an in-depth approach to disease manifestations and management. A careful and unique approach to diagnosis of gastrointestinal diseases in children follows. Finally, the principles of therapy are explored. We hope and expect that this collective approach will be beneficial to all physicians dealing with gastrointestinal problems in children.

W. ALLAN WALKER, M.D.
PETER R. DURIE, B.SC., M.D., FRCPC
J. RICHARD HAMILTON, M.D., FRCPC
JOHN A. WALKER-SMITH, M.D., (SYD.),
    F.R.C.P. (LON., EDIN.), F.R.A.C.P.
JOHN B. WATKINS, M.D.

Acknowledgments

The editors wish to acknowledge the enormous and gracious efforts of our subsection editors. They include Dr. David A. Stringer (Imaging); Dr. John N. Udall Jr. (Nutrition); and Dr. Eve Roberts (Pharmacology). We would also like to thank Stacia Langenbahn for her editorial assistance. Finally we would like to thank Mary Mansor for her strong support in synthesizing the textbook and Leslie Fenton for her excellent editorial support and project management during final production.

Contents

VOLUME TWO

Pediatric Gastroenterology: An Emerging Specialty

J. Richard Hamilton, M.D., FRCPC

In the past 25 years, gastroenterology has evolved as a recognized pediatric subspecialty that has many of the trappings associated with professional status—a peer-reviewed journal, professional associations, task forces, and examinations to assess professional competence. From the time of the earliest pediatric texts, it has been clear that disorders of the digestive tract are central to any consideration of pediatric medicine or surgery. Over the years individual pediatricians and various groups have contributed tremendously to our understanding of many gastroenterologic disorders such as celiac disease, cystic fibrosis, hepatitis, and Wilson's disease. The recent rapid expansion of our understanding of the pathophysiologic basis of many gastrointestinal (GI) disorders, combined with the development of spectacular technology for observing hitherto mysterious events in the digestive tract organs, has provided the foundation for a higher level of professional expertise among physicians and other health care professionals in the field. Of particular importance is our more sophisticated understanding of the development and maturation of the digestive system during fetal and early postnatal life. Detailed controlled clinical studies of young patients with specific gastroenterologic defects have, in turn, contributed to our appreciation of normal developmental phenomena.

This text contributes to this relatively new, exciting discipline by bringing to its students a concise account of the relevant pathophysiologic, clinical, and technical knowledge. To provide a comprehensive, authoritative book, authors have been selected from within and without the field of pediatric gastroenterology.

The risk inherent in focusing on the new developments is that some time-honored, perhaps less exciting, facts and concepts might receive less attention. Although it is appropriate to reflect on the potential impact of modern advances in pediatric gastroenterology, from the standpoint of the patient and family we must consider whether there have been gains or losses from the emergence of this field. Clearly there have been both. From the all-important perspective of the patient and family, the powerful technology of modern pediatric gastroenterology at times can be highly beneficial, but sometimes it can be harmful.

In one form or another, cost-benefit issues always have been central to medical decision-making in all fields. For example, a decision to take blood for the measurement of serum electrolyte concentrations in a child with diarrhea takes account of a minimal risk to the patient of a venipuncture. However, in opting to do the test, has the physician considered its emotional impact on the child, its financial cost, and the likelihood of a laboratory error or misinterpretation of data leading to ill-advised management decisions? Venipuncture is simple and our laboratories handle a range of blood tests with great efficiency, but how often do these techniques really help the child?

More complex, glamorous, and expensive are the newer diagnostic techniques for biopsy, imaging, and endoscopy, many of which are invasive and unpleasant for the patient. The indications for each of these investigations are limited, and they are relatively definable. They do not pose a threat to life under normal circumstances, but in terms of possible misinterpretation and the patient's discomfort and anxiety, the negative "fallout" can be significant. Unfortunately, as new technology becomes more appealing and the public becomes more sophisticated medically, the pressure to test and to invade increases. Trainees want to perform a large number of procedures, manufacturers want to sell equipment, and parents want action taken. At times what parents may want done to their child is something they would not accept for themselves. The health care team, medical and nonmedical, must continue to develop rational indications and contraindications to govern the use of this technology. Nowhere is the need for sound, compassionate wisdom applied to these issues more apparent than in dealing with GI symptoms in children.

This book considers well-known common gastroenterologic problems and a range of more specialized disorders. It deals with precious, special patients—our children. The young of the human species have unique qualities, not the least of which are the endearment and fascination they hold for all who study them. They are not merely increasing in size with age, but they are maturing physically, metabolically, emotionally, and intellectually. From conception to birth and throughout childhood, they are extremely vulnerable and dependent on their care-givers. The approach to the young patient, therefore, cannot and should not always follow the models well established for the approach to adult patients with GI disorders. Nor is it safe to assume that management can be prescribed as for small adults.

As a background for the detailed content of subsequent sections, this chapter discusses some special features of young patients and their responses to gastroenterologic derangements.

CHILDHOOD: A PERIOD OF GROWTH AND MATURATION

From the moment of conception through fetal life, infancy, childhood, and adolescence, human life is a process not just of growth but also of integrated and complex maturation. Clinical pediatrics is based on the concept that children and therefore pediatric patients are not just miniature adults. Their susceptibility to disease processes and their responses to these diseases often are conditioned by the stage of maturation of a range of developmental processes. These considerations are particularly germane to the evolving field of pediatric gastroenterology. In fact, major stimuli to the emergence of the field have been the spectacular advances made in elucidating the normal developmental patterns of the organs of the digestive tract during fetal and postnatal life. The importance of these developmental observations to clinical practice is emphasized throughout this text.

Perhaps less apparent are the significant deficiencies that remain in our understanding of developmental events occurring in the digestive organs during early fetal life, regulation of these events, and their integration with the development of other organs. For example, little is known about the interaction of the central nervous system with the developing digestive tract. The patterns of absorption, metabolism, and excretion of drugs in young developing humans have received relatively little research attention. Significant scientific progress in these two areas alone should contribute enormously to the next era of progress in this young field.

SIGNS OF NORMAL GASTROENTEROLOGIC DEVELOPMENT IN YOUNG PATIENTS

If a middle-aged executive regurgitated after luncheon in the boardroom, she would be subjected to intense gastroenterologic or psychiatric evaluation. However, most babies who regurgitate large amounts after feedings during the first few months of life should receive a different type of attention, from a care-giver who appreciates the inadequacy of the infant's gastroesophageal apparatus. Assuming that the child is otherwise well, this situation requires the technical services of the laundry or the drycleaner, not the radiologist and endoscopist. Mild icterus, seen for a few postnatal days as the child's hepatic conjugating capacity matures, need not provoke the concern that visible jaundice would elicit in a cirrhotic adult. During infancy, as absorptive capacities and control of defecation mature, stool consistency and frequency differ greatly from those of the continent adult. During adolescence, that stage in our lives when we are preoccupied with ourselves and our bodies, the occurrence of a chronic disease, particularly one in which treatment alters appearance, has an effect on the psyche requiring special insight and expertise on the part of the care-giver.

For most babies carried to term, the function of the digestive tract organs is sufficiently mature to permit normal growth and development. However, in many cases there is little functional reserve at this early age and any disease process, even if it does not directly affect the digestive tract, may cause signs suggestive of gastroenterologic disease. For example, the stools may become watery or vomiting may develop in a baby with a urinary tract infection. If these signs can occur within the pattern of normal development, how does one recognize the abnormal? We hope that this text answers that important question in relation to specific disease states. Usually it is answered, at least in part, by determining the impact of the problem on the child's general health. Most critical to the assessment of that impact is evaluating the patient's weight gain, growth, and development compared with established normal patterns.

PROFILE OF GASTROENTEROLOGIC DISEASE IN YOUNG PATIENTS

Perhaps it is obvious that degenerative and neoplastic diseases that are of such great concern in adult patients are less frequent in children, except in cases in which there is genetic predisposition. Visible blood in stool, a legitimate signal of an intestinal tumor in a 60-year-old person, does not have the same alarming implication for most children unless a child has a genetic predisposition to one of the rare syndromes associated with intestinal neoplasia. It is during childhood that most anatomic anomalies and congenital defects surface. According to the same clinical example, blood in a child's stool could suggest the diagnosis of Meckel's diverticulum, a very unlikely concern in a 60-year-old patient. Since the immune system and mucosal barrier continue to mature after birth, the intestine of young infants is highly vulnerable to infection. In regions of the world where children are heavily exposed to enteric pathogens and where malnutrition may delay maturation of the immune system, the impact of this vulnerability can be devastating.

An understanding of the relative likelihood of various groups of diseases at different ages should have an important influence on one's clinical approach to the young patient and his family.

IMPACT OF GASTROENTEROLOGIC DISEASE ON YOUNG PATIENTS

Most young patients are extraordinarily resilient, in spite of their vulnerability and dependence. However, certain gastroenterologic diseases are particularly hazardous to infants and children. For example, systemic dehydration and electrolyte imbalance are much more likely to occur in the baby with acute diarrhea, than in an adult with diarrhea. The reasons for this difference include the relative lack of reserves of the immature gut, the immaturity of renal compensatory capacity, and the dependence of the baby on care-givers for adequate fluid intake. Disease that limits nutrient intake or causes excessive fecal nutrient losses will cause systemic undernutrition (poor weight gain, delayed growth and development) relatively early in young children, compared with older children, because of the relatively small nutritional reserves in babies. This impact on nutritional status is particularly noticeable in the periods of rapid growth and maturation, namely infancy and adolescence. Of course, as with any other significant health problem in a child, the impact on the parents and other family members must be recognized and managed in an informed, sensitive fashion.

Many gastroenterologic diseases are unpleasant enough for the young patient, but several modern diagnostic procedures used in pediatric gastroenterology also may be extremely unpleasant, since they involve the insertion of tubes, needles, or liquids into various orifices or organs. Most of our young patients handle these invasions with patience and courage. When used appropriately, biopsies, contrast radiographic studies, and endoscopy can be powerful, helpful diagnostic tools. Furthermore, complication rates for these procedures are low. With the fascination and excitement of new diagnostic technology goes the responsibility to use it appropriately and only when necessary. Inappropriate use of technology can impose unnecessary suffering on patients and carries the risk of a range of psychological or physical sequelae. If diagnostic studies like colonoscopy are to be used effectively and judiciously in children, one must be prepared in each case to determine whether the procedure actually will benefit the patient. A careful evaluation of these indications involves not only a knowledge of the new science of pediatric gastroenterology, but it also entails an understanding of children and respect for the time-honored tenets of pediatrics.

In a cost-benefit analysis of therapy for gastroenterologic problems in young patients, special considerations are advisable. For example, a range of special dietary products and techniques have been developed based on sound pathophysiologic principles. These new treatment strategies have greatly benefited many children. However, if the goal of such treatment is to improve the patient's nutritional status, but the diet is so unpalatable that it is rejected by the patient, this treatment may be deleterious or of little benefit. The technologies of nasogastric tube feeding or total parenteral nutrition have much to offer some patients with chronic intestinal disease and malnutrition. If this treatment strategy results in prolonged visits to hospital or confinement to home, the disadvantages to some teenagers attempting to conform and relate to peers could outweigh the advantages.

SUMMARY

The emergence of pediatric gastroenterology as a specialized medical field has been based on an impressive expansion of knowledge related to the developing GI tract and the evolution of new technology with which to evaluate young patients. As the field grows in size and scope, it will be important to continue to promote relevant science and technology while maintaining a close link with well-established tenets of clinical pediatrics. To achieve a harmonious and productive melding of new science with traditional clinical pediatric values and attitudes, we should consider with care the impact of gastroenterologic disease, its investigation, and its treatment on the young developing organisms we call our children.

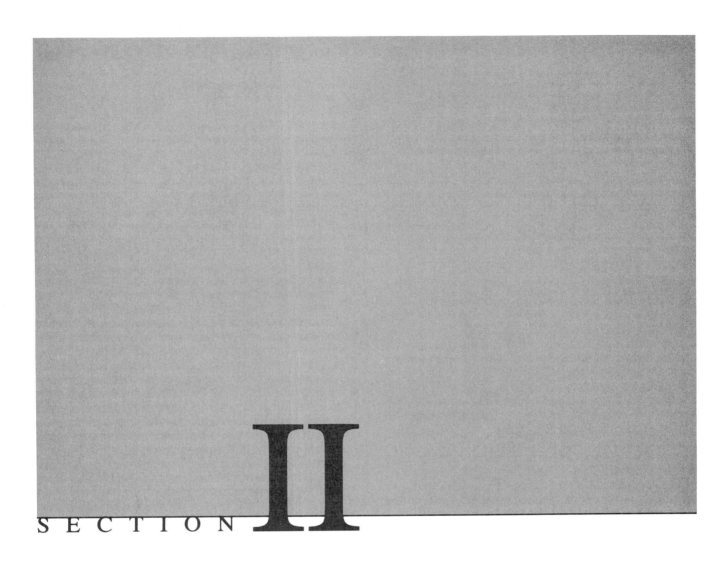

SECTION II

Cardinal Manifestations—Pathophysiology

Growth Failure and Malnutrition*

William E. Russell, M.D.

In affluent cultures, nutrition rarely limits growth in the absence of systemic disease. In developing cultures or among disadvantaged classes in generally well-fed populations, however, nutritional status is often a critical variable in determining the extent of somatic growth and the pace of development. In some extremes, it is the major determinant of survival.

The manifestations of malnutrition are often subtle, frequently masquerading as social, ethnic, or racial characteristics. In a study of ethnically homogeneous conscripts in the Polish army, Bielicki et al[1] documented that the young men who came from large families, from rural regions, and from lower socioeconomic classes were smaller than their counterparts from smaller, urban, and more privileged families. These authors concluded that the negative impact of these variables on stature could all be attributed to suboptimal nutrition. On a very large scale, the effect of malnutrition is often so striking as to produce major population differences in adult size that at first appear to be genetic. For instance, even though native Japanese were smaller than Americans of European ancestry and smaller than Japanese-Americans raised in the United States,[2] following World War II, with significant nutritional improvements in Japan, these differences vanished.[3]

The concept that "maximal growth" and "optimal growth" are synonymous with "normal growth" clearly reflects a value judgment and ignores the complex interactions of environment and growth that we observe in nature. Among animal populations, as among some human populations for whom climate and food supply are never optimal, smallness often holds the key to survival and to reproductive fitness.[4] A major theme to be illustrated in this review is that the endocrine changes seen in malnutrition are adaptive ones, meant to allow maximal benefit from less than maximal resources.

The prominent role played by hormones, growth factors, and other soluble substances in regulating growth and pubertal maturation suggests that a close scrutiny of the changes in these agents under different nutritional circumstances might elucidate the mechanisms by which nutrition impacts upon normal growth. Although growth is often loosely defined to include all aspects of somatic enlargement and maturation, this review is confined largely to issues of statural growth rather than weight gain. The principal impact of malnutrition on the growing child is to diminish or reverse weight gain; when malnutrition has been of long enough duration or intensity, statural growth is influenced eventually, although under some unusual circumstances, malnutrition may selectively impair linear growth without a preceding or concomitant loss in weight.[5]

In this review, we first examine several schemes whereby humoral agents regulate growth. The relationships between hormones and growth factors are outlined, and several of the major hormone systems that influence growth are systematically reviewed. We examine the interactions between nutritional surfeit and deficit on the growth of cells and tissues and the changes that over- and undernutrition effect on the hormonal milieu. Consideration is given to the use of hormones and growth factors to monitor and possibly to hasten the recovery from life-threatening catabolic states.

NUTRIENTS, HORMONES, AND GROWTH

Hormones and Growth Factors

Shortly after the turn of the century, when Starling[6] first proposed the concept of the "hormone," the intellectual domain of the endocrinologist began to shrink, as the definition of a hormone became limited to internal secretions that are produced only in glands and that require conveyance through the circulation to alter the function of distant tissues. Selectivity of response to hormones in an *endocrine* mode of regulation, therefore, depends upon the presence of receptors in the target organs and tissues. Regulation occurs not only through changes in the concentration of the hormone but also in the numbers of peripheral receptors, which can be independently regulated by developmental programs and by the local milieu of nutrients and other hormones.

The endocrine system, however, is also an integrating system that is superimposed upon multiple local systems of control of growth and function. In the 1930s, Feyrter,[7] among others, recognized endocrine-like cells in many tissues and postulated the presence of a peripheral endocrine system, which he named the "paracrine" system. As currently used, the term *paracrine* refers to the release by cells of soluble substances that act upon adjacent cells of another type. No circulatory system is required, since physical proximity and the presence of receptors are the major criteria for effect.

In 1980, Sporn and Todaro[8] added the concept of "autocrine" control to include the substances that cells in culture secrete to regulate their own growth. This was initially thought to be a mode of growth control for neoplastic cells exclusively, but it is now evident that autocrine control also characterizes the growth and function of many normal cells. In

* Supported in part by a grant from the Charles H. Hood Foundation and an Upjohn Scholars Award.

distinction to the classic hormones of the endocrine system, growth factors are the principal agents of the paracrine and autocrine systems.[9] The distinction between hormones and growth factors is generally a functional one, not based solely on structure, although growth factors are generally polypeptides whereas hormones have a greater structural diversity. There are instances in which a substance may be released from a gland into the circulation to act as a hormone at a distal site, while within a highly specialized tissue it may be secreted as a growth factor in very small amounts to influence the function of adjacent cells only. In conjunction with the neuroendocrine mode of regulation, which makes use of axons to direct regulatory neurotransmitters to their target cells, these systems provide a diversity of regulatory options. The characteristics of endocrine, paracrine, autocrine, and neuroendocrine modes of regulation are summarized in Table 1.

The origins of these various systems can be only speculative, but it is logical to assume that autocrine control was sufficient for identical single cells living in proximity to one another in a broth of nutrients. With the advent of cellular co-operativity, a paracrine mode of control provided some specialization of communication. Only with the complexity of specialized organ systems requiring a circulation to provide nutrients to the various tissues did the need for an endocrine system arise. In many instances, nature has retained the basic structure of successful regulatory molecules and through a divergent evolution has created new uses for them. The homology of insulin and the insulin-like growth factors, which are discussed below, illustrates how a substance with predominantly nutrient-transporting properties, which is found in even very primitive unicellular organisms, has taken on new functions that include regulation of highly differentiated function. Illustrations are provided of how, in many instances, hormones that circulate widely can produce highly individualized local effects by regulating tissue-specific production of local growth factors.

Nutrients and Cell Growth

Holley[10,11] was among the first to propose that the intracellular availability of nutrients is the ultimate regulator of cell growth. He postulated that when cellular nutrition is adequate, mammalian cells require no additional extrinsic growth-promoting substances, and that hormones and growth

factors regulate tissue growth ultimately by altering the availability of nutrients. In the laboratory, the growth of cells and tissues clearly requires the proper combinations of hormones and growth factors in addition to an adequate supply of nutrients. There is ample evidence that growth factors and hormones influence the transport and utilization of nutrients by cells.[12-16]

Hormones and nutrients interact in a delicate balance: Hormones alter the nutritional requirements of cells, and conversely, nutrients alter their hormonal requirements. For example, McKeehan and McKeehan[17,18] found that cultured human lung fibroblasts require lower concentrations of various minerals and substrates in the culture medium as the concentration of serum or growth factors is increased. Conversely, they found that adequate concentrations of nutrients reduce the need for growth factors. Sato and colleagues[19,20] have systematically probed the interactions of growth factors and nutrients for specific cell types by assessing the ability of defined combinations of hormones and nutrients to reduce or eliminate the need to supplement culture medium with serum or tissue extracts. This approach has helped identify those hormones and growth factors that regulate the growth of specific cell types and the role played by specific nutrients in the process.

While adequate supplies of nutrients are necessary to allow full manifestation of the effects signaled by hormones and growth factors, hormones influence cell growth by mechanisms other than changing cellular nutritional status. Thyroid and steroid hormones, for example, can change cell function by directly influencing the transcription of target genes in the nucleus, although, once again, adequate "nutrition" in the form of high-energy phosphates and other low molecular weight substrates is required for full manifestation of the signal. In contrast, most polypeptide hormones and growth factors bind to cell surface receptors, and their ability to influence the genome requires the initiation of a cascade of reactions and the induction of second messengers.

Nutrients and Tissue Growth

The study of cellular proliferation in the laboratory culture dish can provide information on the hormonal and nutritional needs of dividing cells, but the growth and development of the organism as a whole require that the enlargement and maturation of each tissue occur at the appropriate rate and in the proper sequence.[21] As they can influence nutrient requirements of individual cells, hormones can also affect the nutrient needs of complex tissues as well as the supply of nutrients in the fluid milieu in which they are bathed. The effects of a given hormone on its various target tissues can be quite different: catabolic in one tissue, anabolic in another (Table 2). These effects are generally not without coordination, as catabolism in one tissue can serve to increase the supply of nutrients to another tissue that is rendered anabolic by the same hormone.

The partitioning of nutrients to tissues in order to support growth or other physiologic activities, a process termed "homeorrhesis" by Bauman and Currie,[22] has received special attention in the fields of animal husbandry and dairy

TABLE 1
Modes of Humoral Regulation

Mode	Agent	Source	Vehicle	Target	Modulators
Endocrine	Hormone	Gland	Circulation	Heterologous	Neurons Growth factors
Paracrine	Growth factor	Local site	Diffusion	Heterologous	Hormones Growth factors
Autocrine	Growth factor	Local site	Diffusion	Autologous	Hormones Growth factors
Neuroendocrine	Neurotransmitter	Neuron	Axon	Heterologous/autologous	Hormones Growth factors Neurons

TABLE 2
Diversity of Hormone Actions on Nutrients in Target Tissues

Hormone	Protein	Carbohydrate	Fat
Glucocorticoid	Breakdown in muscle, synthesis in viscera	Permissive for gluconeogenesis, glycogen synthesis	Redistribution
Insulin	Synthesis in muscle and liver	Glycogen synthesis in liver, glycolysis	Lipogenesis; inhibits lipolysis
Growth hormone	Synthesis in muscle	Insulin-like (acutely), anti-insulin (chronically)	Lipolysis; inhibits lipogenesis
Thyroid	Synthesis in liver, breakdown in muscle	Glycogenolysis, gluconeogenesis	Lipolysis
Androgens	Synthesis in muscle, viscera		

From Russell WE, Underwood LE. Nutrition and the humoral regulation of growth. In: Walker WA, Watkins JB, eds. Nutrition in pediatrics: basic science and clinical application. Boston: Little, Brown, 1985.

science. While homeo*static* mechanisms serve to maintain the constancy of the internal environment, homeo*rrhetic* control mechanisms direct a flux of nutrients to processes such as growth and lactation and may even be deleterious to normal homeostatic mechanisms. For example, under normal circumstances, anabolic hormones serve to increase the protein content of both viscera and muscles.[23] In the nutrient-deficient state, however, anabolic agents such as growth hormone and androgens continue to preferentially support carcass protein (muscle) synthesis even at the expense of visceral protein. Androgens, for instance, will diminish the rate of muscle breakdown in fasted guinea pigs while accelerating the loss of protein from the liver.[24] Similarly, the weight loss of calorically deprived swine can be reduced by administration of growth hormone, but the effect is to preferentially retain muscle mass while depleting body fat.[25] An important adaptive response to longstanding malnutrition is a generalized turning off of anabolic systems, such as those involving growth hormone and androgens, in order to conserve essential body compartments.

Whereas anabolic hormones preferentially preserve muscle mass when nutrients are in short supply, catabolic hormones serve to protect the viscera. Brief exposure of rats to glucocorticoids or to thyroxine increases the protein and glycogen content of the liver, whereas the protein content of muscle is depleted.[23] These effects are direct ones on hepatic uptake and synthetic processes and not merely the result of increased substrate availability from the carcass.[26] Even a prolonged exposure to glucocorticoids, which depletes both viscera and muscle, reduces visceral mass proportionally less.

Critical Periods in Tissue Growth

The ability of tissues to recover from a nutritional insult varies greatly at different times during development. The study of normal tissue growth has provided a model of normal tissue development that has been used to analyze the variable effects of malnutrition at different developmental stages.

Based on the growth of rat tissues, Enesco and Leblond[27] proposed that tissue growth proceeds in three distinct phases (Fig. 1): During organogenesis, tissue growth is characterized primarily by cell proliferation; as the organ or tissue approaches its predetermined complement of cells, the organ grows by increasing both its cell number and the size of each cell; when the adult complement of cells is attained, cell division ceases and tissue growth results totally from enlargement of existing cells. In the growing rat, Enesco and Leblond found the strictly proliferative phase to last until the seventeenth postnatal day, while after 34 to 48 days of life, tissue growth resulted solely from increases in cell size without an

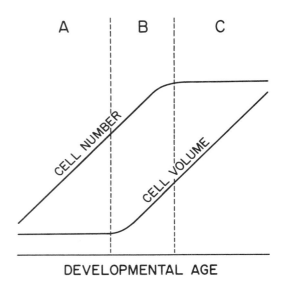

FIGURE 1 The phases of tissue growth as proposed by Enesco and Leblond. *A,* Growth by cellular proliferation. *B,* Growth by cellular proliferation and hypertrophy. *C,* Growth by cellular hypertrophy. (From Enesco and Leblond[27]; with permission of Company of Biologists Ltd.)

increase in new cells. Between these two periods tissue growth appeared to result from both cellular hyperplasia and hypertrophy.

Although this model has received validation from mathematic analysis of the growth patterns of multiple mammalian species,[28] it has not been universally accepted. In similar studies, Sands et al[29] found that rat tissues increased their cell size very early in development, while in many tissues proliferation continued as long as there was growth.

Widdowson and McCance performed studies on growing animals that clearly established the existence of critical periods of sensitivity to the effects of malnutrition.[30-32] They manipulated the litter size and therefore the milk supply of rat pups during suckling and observed their subsequent growth. Rats that were nutritionally deprived during this period were small, and their growth could not be restored by institution of normal food intake.[33] The mechanism for this runting appears to be an irreversible effect of undernutrition on the number of cells. Winick and Noble[34] provided further evidence that the nutritional state of the neonatal period influences cell proliferation and consequently determines the ultimate size of the animal and its organs. Food restriction in the first 21 days of life produced a subnormal complement of cells in most tissues; the size of the cells, however, was normal. Adequate nutrition after weaning could not restore normal growth, presumably because of an irreplaceable deficit of cells. Food restriction between 21 and 42 days resulted in a comparable stunting of growth in most tissues, but the brain and lung were able to resume normal growth with restoration of proper nourishment. In these tissues, the total adult cell number had already been attained, and malnutrition produced a reversible decrease in cell size. When malnutrition was induced between 65 and 86 days, almost all organs underwent a reversible decrease in cell size only.

Winick and Noble[35] also demonstrated that growing tissues are as sensitive to an excess of nutrients as to a shortage. When litter sizes were reduced to provide supranormal nutrition, the offspring were larger than normal and were found to have hypercellular organs.

As it has evolved from studies such as those described above, the critical-period hypothesis proposes that abnormal nutrition, either excessive or deficient, during the phase of tissue growth by cellular proliferation can increase or decrease the ultimate size of a tissue by enhancing or impairing cell division. These effects are irreversible, since they bring the tissue into the phase of growth by cellular hypertrophy with an abnormal number of cells. When nutritional surfeit or deficit occurs after establishment of the adult complement of cells, the net effect is a change in cell volume but not in cell number and is reversible by normalization of the nutrient supply. Because tissues mature at different rates, the long-term effects of nutritional variations occur most prominently in those tissues that are at a susceptible developmental period.[36]

Catch-Up Growth

At the complex level of organization that is required for statural growth, the ability of nutritionally deprived cells and tissues to be restored to functional health is reflected in the phenomenon of catch-up growth. It has long been documented that children have the capacity to accelerate their growth when recovering from a growth-impairing influence such as malnutrition or disease,[37] a phenomenon termed "catch-up" by Prader et al.[38] Subsequently, the term "catch-down" was used to refer to the slowing of growth that follows removal of growth-accelerating influences, such as occurs with suppression of precocious puberty, food restriction in obesity, or cessation of growth hormone therapy in hypopituitary children.

Even under the most favorable circumstances, the accretion of height in growing children does not occur at a fixed rate but is developmentally regulated, although gender-specific, nutritional, and, in some cultures, seasonal influences are superimposed. The changes in growth velocity during normal growth are illustrated in Figure 2. The period of most rapid growth occurs in the first months of life, when length increases by 14 to 22 cm per year. By the second birthday the mean growth velocity has slowed to about 8 cm per year and to about 5 cm per year just before puberty. Then, under the influence of sex steroids (but involving the coordinated actions of growth hormone, insulin-like growth factors (IGFs), thyroid hormones, and others), growth velocity nearly doubles before statural growth ceases, as the epiphyses close.

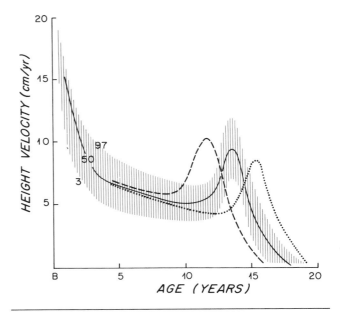

FIGURE 2 Normal height velocity in childhood. Growth velocity for age in boys. The third, fiftieth, and ninety-seventh percentiles are shown. The variation in height velocity during puberty is centered on the mean age for the attainment of peak height velocity. This method of depiction illustrates the differences in the timing of the pubertal growth spurt among the early (*dashed line*), normal (*solid line*), and late (*dotted line*) maturers. (Modified from Tanner JM, Davis PSW. Clinical longitudinal standards for height and height velocity for North American children. J Pediatr 1985; 107:317–329, to illustrate the early childhood deceleration in growth velocity.)

After the second year of life and continuing throughout childhood, growth velocity is modulated to maintain stature at a constant position relative to the general population. The percentile of height for age at about 2 years is maintained faithfully throughout childhood and correlates well with the height percentile in adulthood.[39] The course of statural growth along a predetermined percentile on a growth chart is often called "canalization." The influence of a pathologic growth-retarding or enhancing process pushes the child to a lower or higher channel. With amelioration of the abnormal condition, a compensatory acceleration or deceleration occurs to restore the original growth channel (Fig. 3).

Early in life, catch-up growth can be a normal phenomenon in children whose birth size is at variance with their genetic potential. Whereas statural growth from age 2 to adulthood is primarily controlled by genetic influences, the growth in body size during fetal life and consequently body size at birth are largely determined by maternal and nutritional influences. The interval between birth and roughly 2 years is a preprogrammed period of catch-up or catch-down growth and is characterized by a shift of growth channels as maternal influences recede and genetically determined forces prevail. It is essential for the clinician to be aware of the forces that compete during this critical period, since these normal physiologic changes in growth velocity could be misconstrued as a manifestation of disease.[40]

Inherent in the concept of catch-up or catch-down growth is an ability of the organism to actively modulate its growth velocity in order to maintain a channel, to monitor its size and determine the degree of deviation from the intended channel, to alter its velocity when unrestrained in order to quickly return to the channel, and finally to again modulate its altered velocity to prevent over- or undershooting the channel.[41-44] Possible mechanisms are discussed below.

From a practical standpoint, for catch-up growth to be complete the insult must be limited in duration and must not occur during certain vulnerable periods. Williams et al[45,46] found that the rate of catch-up growth is generally muted if it begins when normal growth is normally decelerating. Two disorders that have been considered to have great potential for essentially complete catch-up growth during treatment are growth hormone (GH) deficiency and hypothyroidism. However, recent studies by Rivkees et al[47] on the catch-up potential of children treated for hypothyroidism concluded that catch-up potential is diminished as the duration of hypothyroidism increases. Their subjects had been hypothyroid for approximately 5 years and had height deficits of 25 cm; however, at the conclusion of therapy an average deficit of 7 cm remained (Fig. 4). Similar conclusions have resulted from studies of children with late-treated GH deficiency.[48]

In addition to its duration, the specific nature of the insult may be important in determining the extent of catch-up, since some growth-arresting conditions appear to cause irreversible changes. Mosier[49] found that cortisone-treated rats failed to regain normal body size after cessation of treatment, whereas fasted rats that were comparably stunted resumed normal growth when refed. Cartilage from the cortisone-treated rats had increased numbers of dead and dying cells, altered cell morphology, and alterations in the ground substance.[50]

Ashworth[51] has suggested that the catch-up growth of recovery from malnutrition is associated with an increase in the efficiency of energy utilization. Studies in fasted rats have suggested that they are capable of a fivefold increase in efficiency of energy utilization for weight gain during recovery, perhaps by decreased thermogenesis.[52] Children recovering from malnutrition, however, generally have an increased appetite and increased caloric intake, suggesting to others that energy utilization is not efficient.[53] Some marasmic children do not begin to gain weight for 3 to 5 weeks, despite an intake of more than 130 kcal per kilogram per day.[54]

Several models have been put forward to explain the ability of the organism to monitor size. Tanner postulated the existence of a "sizostat" in the central nervous system.[55] An alternative, peripheral, model was suggested by Leibel,[56] who proposed that the concentration of a circulating hormone, such as insulin (or its ratio to other hormones or metabolites), could monitor the size of a body compartment, such as the adipose mass, by "reading" the number of insulin receptors on adipocytes.

Mosier and Jansons have confirmed the importance of the central nervous system for catch-up growth in their studies on head-irradiated rats.[57] Even though normal rats show increased secretion of GH in their recovery from fasting,[58] the head-irradiated rat is capable of accelerated growth without an increase in GH secretion.[59] Furthermore, during the recovery from a fast in normal rats, GH and insulin-like growth factors (IGFs) return to normal whether catch-up growth occurs or not.[60]

It is likely that both systemic (hormone) and local (growth factor) signals will be implicated as critical regulators of the

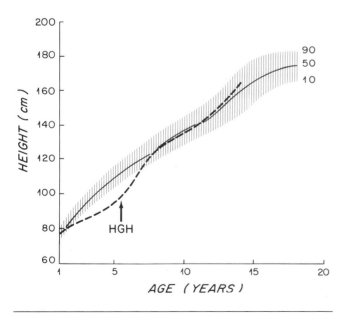

FIGURE 3 Catch-up growth in a 5½-year-old boy with growth hormone deficiency. Growth hormone therapy was instituted at age 5½ as indicated. The figure shows complete recovery to the fiftieth percentile, the approximate channel before growth deceleration began. (Data courtesy of Professor J.D. Crawford.)

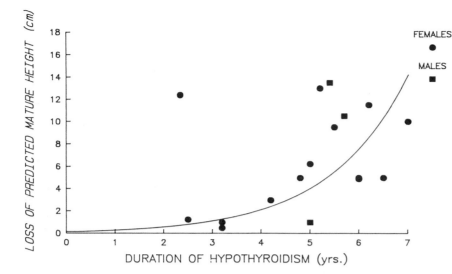

FIGURE 4 Loss of catch-up potential with longstanding hypothyroidism. Relationship of loss in adult height and duration of hypothyroidism at diagnosis in treated hypothyroid children. Loss of predicted height is predicted height at diagnosis minus actual mature height. Duration of hypothyroidism is chronologic age minus bone age at diagnosis. (From Rivkees et al[47]; with permission of the New England Journal of Medicine.)

proliferation that occurs during catch-up or catch-down growth, but solid evidence to suggest a mechanism is lacking. Growth acceleration must involve both a turning on and a subsequent turning off of growth-accelerating signals. A growing body of evidence in both normal and neoplastic tissues indicates that growth-stimulatory and growth-inhibitory influences are constantly in opposition. The tendency of a cell to proliferate or to remain quiescent is determined by the balance of these two forces, and in some instances, pathologic growth such as neoplasia results from disequilibrium of the two forces.[61] The past several years have seen the identification and molecular cloning of a number of very potent growth-inhibitory substances, among which the best characterized is transforming growth factor-beta and its homologues.[61] Some tissues, most notably the liver, have a remarkable capacity for self-regeneration without influencing the growth of other tissues when a portion of their mass has been ablated.[62] At the level of the whole organism, the catch-up process is certainly more complex than is the regeneration of a single tissue. This is demonstrated in the asynchronous return to normal of various tissues as they recover from a common insult.[63]

While most studies have focused on the serum concentrations of known growth factors and hormones such as insulin, GH, and IGFs, it is quite likely that locally regulated tissue growth will be shown to be critical, even when the overall process of catch-up or catch-down appears to be centrally co-ordinated. Bone, which is clearly a key component in the catch-up of statural growth, is rich in growth factors of both a stimulatory and an inhibitory nature, which are likely involved in controlling its growth.[64] As discussed below, the growth-promoting effects of GH probably result from IGFs that are produced at the growth plate itself. The co-ordinated action of the bone-derived stimulatory and inhibitory growth factors is certain to be critical for statural growth control under conditions of normal and compensatory growth.

GROWTH HORMONE, SOMATOMEDINS, AND INSULIN

Normal Growth

Growth Hormone in Normal Growth

It has been known for decades that pituitary GH (somatotropin) is essential for normal, balanced somatic growth from childhood to normal adult size. The mechanism by which this process is regulated, however, is poorly understood, especially in the fetus. In addition, it has only recently been appreciated that the GH-somatomedin axis is further entwined in a regulatory web that is modulated by nutritional signals.

Insulin-like Growth Factor and the Somatomedin Hypothesis. With the advent of techniques to culture cells and tissues in the laboratory in the 1950s, it was noted that many of the biochemical events that had been attributed to GH in vivo could not be reproduced on isolated tissues studied in the laboratory. These included effects on chondrocyte proliferation and sulfate incorporation into glycosaminoglycans by growth plate cartilage. These discrepancies led Salmon and Daughaday to propose that the growth-promoting effects of GH are not direct ones on its target tissues but result indirectly from the actions of a mediator substance that is under GH control. This substance was initially called "sulfation factor" or "thymidine factor" based on the assay system used to detect its presence. Later it was shown that these two activities actually resided in the same molecule, which was renamed "somatomedin."[65]

Although several crude isolates were initially deemed to be somatomedins, only somatomedin-C was ultimately shown to be a distinct substance. Somatomedins A and B were found to be impure or to derive their biologic properties from other growth factors. Two distinct somatomedins have been found

TABLE 3
Insulin-like Growth Factors*

Property	IGF-I	IGF-II
Synonyms	Somatomedin-C, basic somatomedin	Multiplication stimulating activity (MSA), neutral somatomedin
Chromosome location	12	11
Molecular weight	7,649	7,471
Serum concentration	193 ± 58 ng/ml	647 ± 126 ng/ml
GH dependence of serum concentration	+ + +	+
Insulin-like actions	+	+ + +
Mitogenicity in cultured cells	+ + +	+
Developmental role	Postnatal	Fetal
Sensitivity to undernutrition	+ + +	+/−

* A comparison of the two principal somatomedins: insulin-like growth factors I and II (IGF-I and IGF-II).

in most species studied and have a molecular structure and gene organization very similar to those of proinsulin. Somatomedins have insulin-like biologic actions in some tissues, and their initial biochemical purification was accomplished based upon their insulin-like activities.[66] Somatomedins and proinsulin are probably the biochemical descendents of primitive regulatory molecules with insulin-like biologic actions.

Current convention is to refer to the two major somatomedins as insulin-like growth factors (IGFs) I and II. Somatomedin-C (basic somatomedin) is identical to IGF-I, although a number of IGF-I assays available from clinical reference laboratories retain the name somatomedin-C. IGF-II had no counterpart in somatomedin terminology. The properties of IGF-I and IGF-II are contrasted in Table 3. Although the current nomenclature has the disadvantage of dissociating the IGFs from their regulatory link with growth hormone, it does more firmly root these substances in the realm of nutritional control.

Growth Hormone and Insulin-like Growth Factor Genes. In humans, GH is encoded within a cluster of five structurally similar genes on the long arm of chromosome 17.[67] These genes include the so-called normal GH gene (GH-N or GH-A), a "variant" GH gene (GH-V or GH-B), and three genes for placental lactogen (chorionic somatomammotropin). Only GH-N appears to be translated into GH in the pituitary, although two distinct forms of GH result from differential splicing of the mRNA that is transcribed from the gene. The predominant product of the GH-N gene is a single chain of 191 amino acids with a molecular weight of 22,000 (22 kDa). The product of alternate splicing of the GH-N gene is "20 kDa" GH, which results from a deletion of 15 amino acids and comprises about 10 percent of circulating GH. Clear evidence for a differential regulation of the secretion of these two GHs is lacking, although

they appear to differ in important ways in some of their "direct" biologic actions (see below).

The gene for IGF-I is located on the long arm of chromosome 12 in humans, while the gene for IGF-II is on the short arm of chromosome 11, downstream from the insulin gene.[68] A single gene encodes each of the IGFs, although alternative splicing of each of the genes and other post-transcriptional modifications result in multiple IGF mRNA species. The extent to which the modification of IGF gene transcripts is important in the regulation of IGF action is unclear.

Growth Hormone–Insulin-like Growth Factor Axis: Physiologic Regulation. GH release by the pituitary is regulated by two principal hypothalamic peptides, one stimulatory and one inhibitory: GH-releasing factor and somatostatin, respectively (Fig. 5). Blood concentrations and patterns of GH secretion result from an interplay between these two substances on the GH-producing cells of the anterior pituitary. The hypothalamus receives rich innervation from higher centers in the brain, providing a mechanism by which even emotional influences can alter GH secretion (see discussion of psychosocial dwarfism, below).

IGF concentrations, in turn, influence GH secretion by the pituitary. IGF-I has been shown to stimulate the secretion of somatostatin by the hypothalamus[69] and may directly inhibit GH synthesis.[70] Whether this results from a classic endocrine feedback of IGFs in the blood or from IGFs produced in the hypothalamus and pituitary has not yet been clarified. The changes in patterns of IGF and GH secretion that occur during fasting, however, suggest that circulating IGFs are important in the feedback process (see below).

In response to circulating GH but modified by other hormones and, most critically, nutritional status, multiple tis-

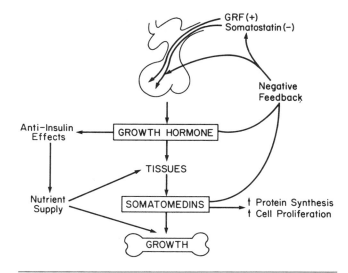

FIGURE 5 The growth hormone–insulin-like growth factor axis (growth hormone–somatomedin axis). GRF = growth hormone–releasing factor. (From Russell WE, Underwood LE. Nutrition and the humoral regulation of growth. In: Walker WA, Watkins JB. Nutrition and pediatrics: basic science and clinical application. Boston: Little, Brown, 1985.)

sues in the body synthesize and secrete IGFs. Although the liver was the first tissue to be shown to secrete IGFs and is the major producer of circulating IGFs, its primacy in the GH-IGF axis has been supplanted. Multiple cell types in virtually every tissue examined from both fetus and adult can synthesize IGFs. These data have shifted emphasis away from a primarily "endocrine" model of IGF action, which requires a circulatory system to bring IGFs from their "gland" (the liver, in initial formulations) to their sites of action (the growth plates of bones). Current concepts of IGF action emphasize a primarily "paracrine" model in which IGFs are produced practically everywhere and act upon target cells in the vicinity of the producing cells.

A paracrine model of IGF action predicts, first of all, that chondrocytes or other cells near the growth plates of bones are capable of IGF synthesis. Furthermore, since IGFs are ubiquitously produced, there are likely to be many other actions of the IGFs, many not yet identified, that have little or nothing to do with the growth of bones. Both of these predictions have received considerable experimental support. Studies have now shown an increase in both IGF-I mRNA and the actual peptide in the growth plates of GH-treated rats,[71] and a diversity of IGF actions relating to cell proliferation and differentiated regulatory functions has been identified.[91] Studies by Han et al[72] on human fetal tissues have detected the mRNA for IGF-I only in fibroblasts and other cells of mesenchymal origin: in the perichondrium of bone, in the perisinusoidal cells of liver, and in connective tissue layers in many other tissues. Mesenchymal cells are ideally situated to release IGFs for local action on neighboring cells.

Growth Hormone and Insulin-like Growth Factor Concentrations in Blood. Normal GH secretion in man is highly episodic. Blood concentrations are generally quite low or undetectable for much of the day and are interrupted by bursts of secretion that result in high concentrations for roughly 90 minutes before returning to the low baseline. This pattern is developmentally regulated.[73] The number and amplitude of secretory episodes are small in young children. Under the influence of gonadal steroids both the frequency and amplitude increase dramatically and reach their highest levels during puberty, especially during sleep; they then gradually decline over the ensuing decades. An additional but developmentally limited source of somatomedins is suggested by the detection of IGF-I and IGF-II as well as a truncated form of the IGF-I in colostrum.[74]

In contrast to GH, IGF secretion is relatively constant, and blood concentrations are maintained at relatively stable levels by the presence of serum-binding proteins that delay IGF clearance. The role of these binding proteins in IGF physiology is at this time unclear. They may keep the circulating IGFs in an inactive state after they have served their function at the site of origin, or they may serve to selectively present the IGFs to target tissues that are capable of liberating the free peptide from its binding proteins.

Although GH remains the predominant regulator of IGF production, a number of other hormones influence IGF-I concentrations in blood. This peptide is very low or nonexistent in fetal life, when IGF-II appears to be the predominant somatomedin. During fetal life, placental lactogen or the product of the GH-V gene is likely to be the major regulator of somatomedin production.[75] Prolactin, another GH-like hormone, can also stimulate the production of IGFs in cultured cells and probably in clinical conditions of prolactin excess. After birth, blood levels of the IGFs remain low during infancy and early childhood but rise dramatically at puberty in response to increases in GH secretory activity. In addition, IGF-I concentrations are low in patients with hypothyroidism.[76] Clinically, IGF-I concentrations in blood have been shown to reliably mirror the total GH secretory activity. Thus, in older children and adults who are well-nourished and do not have hypothyroidism, serum IGF-I measurements are more useful than random measurements of GH in diagnosing conditions of GH deficiency (hypopituitarism) and excess (gigantism or acromegaly). The marked influence of nutritional status on IGF production is discussed below.

Direct Versus Indirect Actions of Growth Hormone: A Unifying Hypothesis? GH initiates its physiologic actions by binding to specific receptors on the surface of target cells. The intracellular mechanism(s) by which this signal is transduced to influence cellular function is unclear, although elevations of intracellular cyclic AMP are not involved. Functional evidence accumulates for different forms of the GH receptor in different tissues, which would permit a functional diversity in GH action at its target organs.[77]

The actions of GH in vivo have been categorized as either indirect (IGF-mediated) or direct ones. The direct actions vary quite significantly depending on the duration of exposure. After short-term administration to GH-deficient individuals or to isolated GH-sensitive tissues in culture, GH has effects very much like those of insulin. These include the stimulation of glucose and amino acid transport and protein synthesis. GH also has inductive effects on a number of enzymes. However insulin-like they are, these actions are very rapid in onset, transient in duration, and *not* mediated through the actions of IGFs.

Chronic GH administration, in contrast, results in biochemical actions that appear antagonistic to insulin: Blood sugar rises and fat mobilization and fatty acid oxidation occur. In fact, rapid release of GH is one of the stress responses that the body uses to maintain a normal blood glucose. In 20 percent of individuals with GH-secreting tumors, frank diabetes mellitus occurs.

The origins of these paradoxical "direct" actions are not clear but may reside in the structure of the GH molecule itself. The 20-kDa variant has been reported to have only one-fifth the insulin-like activity of the 22-kDa GH molecule, while retaining normal growth-promoting and diabetogenic activity.[78]

The concept that IGFs can mediate the actions of GH in promoting linear growth has been validated by a number of studies that show that IGF-I injections increase tibial width and costal cartilage DNA synthesis in hypophysectomized rats to an extent that is comparable to that in GH-treated controls.[79] Isaakson and colleagues have maintained that the effects of the IGFs in promoting somatic growth in vivo are largely on weight gain and are not of the same magnitude as those of GH.[71] In an attempt to unify the direct and IGF-mediated effects of GH, those authors have suggested that GH renders undifferentiated prechondrocytes in the growth plate sensitive to the mitogenic effects of IGF-I while simultaneously inducing the local expression of the IGF-I gene. A similar model was proposed by Green to describe the actions of GH in promoting the differentiation of fetal fibroblasts to adipocytes.[80]

Insulin in Normal Growth

The prominent influence of insulin on normal growth is best illustrated in disorders at the extremes of altered insulin secretion. Especially in the fetus, hyperinsulinemia produces somatic overgrowth. Hyperinsulinemic infants born of poorly controlled diabetic mothers exhibit visceromegaly, increased body fat, and increased length, whereas the hypoinsulinemic infant born with severe insulin resistance or pancreatic agenesis is small and very depleted in body fat.[81] In postnatal life, poorly controlled diabetes mellitus can be associated with a striking growth failure, the so-called Mauriac syndrome.[82] The growth-promoting actions of insulin both in pre- and postnatal life are complex and are likely to result from both direct, largely metabolic, effects mediated through the insulin receptor and indirect, predominantly mitogenic, effects mediated through the structurally homologous IGF-I receptor.

Insulin Receptor-Mediated Actions. High-affinity insulin receptors mediate the rapid biologic actions of insulin in stimulating the cellular transport of substrates and in the induction of enzymes that promote glycogen and fat synthesis and that inhibit gluconeogenesis, lipolysis, and ketogenesis. The relative contribution of increased substrate availability in mediating the growth-promoting effects of insulin is not clear, but, as discussed previously, there is ample evidence from studies on isolated cells that enhanced "cellular nutrition" is important in regulating cell growth and function.

The insulin receptor is a "heterotetramer," consisting of two alpha and two beta subunits. Insulin binding to the two alpha subunits, which are paired on the extracellular surface of the cytoplasmic membrane, induces changes in the beta subunits, which extend into the cytoplasm. The exact nature of insulin signal transduction is unknown, but a prominent early event in insulin action is the phosphorylation of the beta subunit within the cell.[83]

An indirect consequence of insulin binding to insulin receptors appears to be a stimulation of IGF production. A number of clinical studies have shown that the depressed IGF concentrations associated with poorly controlled diabetes mellitus can be returned to normal with insulin therapy.[84] Insulin appears to directly stimulate IGF production in whole liver, liver slices, or cultured hepatocytes.[85] Additionally, insulin may regulate IGF production by influencing the number of GH receptors on important IGF-producing tissues. In poorly controlled diabetes mellitus, there is a dramatic reduction in the number of somatogenic GH binding sites in liver. These can be restored to normal with insulin therapy.[86]

Insulin-like Growth Factor Receptor–Mediated Insulin Actions. Some of the growth-promoting actions of insulin, at least in hyperinsulinemic states, can be attributed to insulin binding and activation of the IGF-I receptor. Given the structural homology between the IGFs and the proinsulin molecule, it should not be surprising that there is a comparable homology between the insulin receptor and IGF receptors. This is, in fact, the case with the receptor for IGF-I, the more mitogenic of the two IGFs. This receptor is also a heterotetramer composed of pairs of alpha and beta subunits.[87]

The mechanism by which insulin might mimic IGF effects in vivo is suggested by the binding characteristics of the insulin and IGF-I receptors. Although each receptor type binds both insulin and IGF-I, there is considerable specificity in terms of the concentration of each hormone required to achieve binding. On a molar basis it requires from 10 to 100 times as much insulin as IGF-I to activate IGF-I receptors, a condition achieved only in some states of hyperinsulinism, such as insulin-resistant states. Nonetheless, binding of insulin to IGF-I receptors is probably the mechanism by which insulin is mitogenic for a large number of cells in culture; the concentrations of insulin used in cell culture are generally well above those required to saturate insulin receptors. In a few cell types, however, insulin is mitogenic at physiologic concentrations. Thus, in hepatocytes, certain teratocarcinoma cells, mammary tumor cells, and others, insulin might be directly mitogenic by binding to its own receptor.

The IGF-II receptor, in contrast, is composed of a single, large protein with no structural similarity to the IGF-I or insulin receptors.[79] However, insulin at physiologic concentrations has been shown to dramatically increase the number of IGF-II receptors on adipocytes.[87] The function of the IGF-II cell surface receptor is, however, not known. An intriguing clue comes from the recent discovery that the IGF-II receptor is also (on another part of the molecule) the mannose-6-phosphate receptor, which plays a role in targeting glycosylated proteins to the lysosomes.[79]

Insulin Synergy with Other Growth Factors. One further mechanism by which insulin might influence cellular growth is to alter the cellular requirements for mitogenic signals from other growth factors. As discussed previously regarding the interactions of nutrients and hormones, growth factor signals frequently converge on common pathways within a cell so that low concentrations of two growth factors can amplify the actions of one another. In cultured hepatocytes insulin can potentiate the mitogenic signal of epidermal growth factor (EGF) or of vasopressin,[88] and in the well-studied BALB/c 3T3 fibroblast, the presence of insulin or IGF-I strongly modulates the mitogenic actions of EGF and platelet-derived growth factor (PDGF).

Malnutrition

Growth Hormone in Malnutrition

Growth Hormone Concentrations in Clinical and Experimental Malnutrition. In man, experimental fasting and malnutrition generally result in elevated serum concentrations of GH. Studies of malnourished populations in different parts of the world have often led to conflicting conclusions, in part from differing criteria for malnutrition, from the inaccuracies inherent in characterizing complex GH secretory patterns from a single blood sample, and perhaps to some extent from confounding features such as infection.[89] The normal physiology of nutrient regulation of GH secretion is also complex: Amino acids such as arginine stimulate GH release, whereas carbohydrates and fatty acids inhibit GH secretion. Clinical malnutrition results from a combination of dietary deficiencies that could be expected to have variable effects on GH release.

Recently, attention has turned to the effects of fasting on the pattern of GH release from the pituitary. As previously described, GH secretion in man is episodic, and measurement of GH concentrations on random blood samples, as is typical of field studies, might be expected to give inconsistent results. Ho et al[90] performed frequent blood sampling (every 20 minutes) of fasted volunteers and uncovered an inherent pulsatility in GH secretion in humans that appears to be suppressed in the fed state, perhaps by the negative feedback of IGFs. Over the course of a 5-day fast, those authors measured significant increases in GH pulse frequency, maximal pulse amplitude, and 24-hour integrated concentration (Table 4). These changes coincided with a decline in concentrations of IGF-I and glucose and a rise in those of free fatty acids and acetoacetate.

Serum GH concentrations are elevated in children with both kwashiorkor and marasmus[91-95] but do not allow distinction between the two. Becker et al[91] observed the magnitude of GH elevation to be inversely related to the severity of protein malnutrition, as judged by the serum albumin concentration. In their subjects, GH concentrations fell after feeding a protein-rich diet for 36 to 72 hours. The critical role of protein in the refeeding diet was also demonstrated by Pimstone et al,[95] who found that refeeding with a high-carbohydrate, protein-free diet does not normalize GH concentrations. When caloric deprivation predominates, the GH response appears to be variable; some groups have reported depressed GH concentrations and others have reported elevations.[96-98] In short-term malnutrition, the adaptive benefits of elevated GH concentrations are suggested by the known direct effects of GH to increase gluconeogenesis, lipolysis, and fatty acid oxidation. Elevated GH concentrations might be expected to increase glucose production initially, while shifting the organism to a lipolytic, protein-sparing state.

Whereas short-term protein-calorie malnutrition is associated with elevated GH concentrations, longstanding malnutrition results in depressed GH secretion. Beas et al[99]

TABLE 4
Enhanced Pulsatility of Growth Hormone Release in Fasting*

Measure of Pulsatility	Day 0	Day 1	Day 5
GH peaks (number/24 h)	5.8 ± 0.7	$7.3 \pm 0.6^{\ddagger}$	$9.9 \pm 0.7^{\ddagger}$
GH peak amplitude (ng/ml)	5.9 ± 1.1	$13.1 \pm 1.2^{\ddagger}$	$12.3 \pm 1.6^{\ddagger}$
24-h IGHC† (μg/ml/min)	2.8 ± 0.5	$7.8 \pm 1.1^{\S}$	$8.8 \pm 0.8^{\S}$

* Frequent venous sampling of six adult male subjects was performed during a control fed day (Day 0) and during the first (Day 1) and fifth (Day 5) days of a fast.
† IGHC = 24-hour integrated GH concentration.
‡ $P < 0.005$, compared with Day 0.
§ $P > 0.0009$.
From Ho et al[90]; with permission of the American Society for Clinical Investigation.

described a group of infants with low concentrations not only of GH but also of adrenal and thyroid hormones, suggesting generalized pituitary hypofunction. An adaptive function of a hypopituitary state in reducing metabolic activity had previously been proposed by Mulinos and Pomerantz,[100] who likened the malnourished state to a "pseudohypophysectomy."

Clinical Uses of Growth Hormone in Catabolic States. The adaptive changes in GH release that accompany malnutrition have prompted a number of studies on the possible uses of GH in promoting anabolism during the recovery from operation or injury. Clemmons et al[101] determined the effects of GH injections on obese individuals subjected to hypocaloric diets. Although dietary restriction produced comparable weight loss in subjects receiving GH and those receiving placebo, those treated with GH (0.1 mg per kilogram every 48 hr) had a significantly lower daily nitrogen deficit than controls. Similar findings were reported by Manson and Wilmore,[102] who administered GH to volunteers receiving hypocaloric parenteral nutrition (Fig. 6). GH therapy decreased the rate of weight loss and increased nitrogen retention. In parenterally nourished patients recovering from gastrointestinal (GI) surgery, GH administration has resulted in sustained nitrogen retention,[102,104] suggesting a possible role for this agent in promoting recovery from a variety of catabolic states.

Insulin-like Growth Factors in Malnutrition

IGF Bioactivity, IGF Inhibitors, and IGF-Binding Proteins. Despite elevated GH levels in fasting or short-term malnutrition, the production of IGF-I is dramatically reduced in malnutrition. Studies using somatomedin bioassays were the first to indicate that serum IGF bioactivity falls with malnutrition. More recent data using highly specific radioimmunoassays indicate that the depressed bioactivity of serum from fasted or malnourished individuals results from a dramatic fall in IGF-I concentrations, minimal if any change in IGF-II concentrations,[105] and a rise in serum IGF inhibitor proteins (Table 5).

Measuring serum somatomedin bioactivity in a sulfation factor assay, Grant et al[106] were among the first to show a nutritional influence on somatomedin activity when they found low levels in the serum of malnourished South African children despite elevated GH concentrations. Those authors found both hormones to return toward normal by the ninth day of refeeding. Similar results using somatomedin bioassays were forthcoming from other malnourished populations,[107] including malnourished Thai[108] and Nigerian[109] infants and children and patients with celiac disease[110] and anorexia nervosa.[111]

Bioassays of IGF activity in blood, although relatively nonspecific as to which of the two IGFs is being measured, allow the detection of physiologically important IGF inhibitors in serum. A number of physiologic substances, including fatty acids, glucocorticoids, and various peptides have been found to interfere with the IGF bioassays.[112] Increased concentrations of inhibitors have been found in the serum of malnourished children and hypopituitary adults[107,113,114] and in serum from starved, hypophysectomized, or diabetic rats.[115,116] Salmon and colleagues[117] partially purified a 27- to

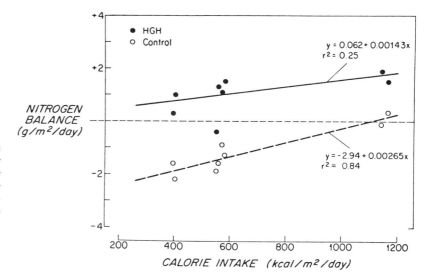

+4

● HGH
○ Control

$y = 0.062 + 0.00143x$
$r^2 = 0.25$

+2

NITROGEN
BALANCE
$(g/m^2/day)$

$y = -2.94 + 0.00265x$
$r^2 = 0.84$

−2

−4

200   400   600   800   1000   1200

CALORIE INTAKE $(kcal/m^2/day)$

FIGURE 6 Positive nitrogen balance in growth hormone–treated subjects at all levels of hypocaloric calorie provision. Eight male subjects were exposed to various levels of hypocaloric intravenous feeding. Only adequate energy intake resulted in positive nitrogen balance in the controls (*open circles*), whereas growth hormone–treated subjects (*closed circles*) were in positive nitrogen balance at all levels of energy intake. (From Manson and Wilmore.[102])

40-kDa, heat-labile inhibitor from fasted rat serum. A second, heat-stable inhibitor in the serum of starved and diabetic rats was shown to be corticosterone.[118] The liver appears to be the source of some of these inhibitors,[119] which can antagonize IGF (and insulin) actions in a variety of tissues.[120] Phillips et al[121] have recently shown that concurrent with the fasting-induced fall in IGF activity of rat serum, total IGF inhibitor activity rises. The IGF inhibitory activity of serum appears to be more nutritionally sensitive than the IGF activity itself. After 6 hours of refeeding, the IGF inhibitor activity had fallen significantly, but there was little change in IGF activity; both returned to normal with continued refeeding.

In addition to a nutritional influence on inhibitor proteins, recent evidence suggests that nutrition influences the concentration of an important serum IGF-I binding protein that has been shown to augment the cellular response to IGF-I. Busby et al[122] developed a radioimmunoassay for the 26-kDa serum IGF-I binding protein. They found that a 48-hour fast resulted in an almost twofold increase in serum concentrations of this protein, which returned to normal after 2 days of refeeding. They also documented a postprandial depression of the concentrations of this binding protein over the course of a 24-hour period of monitoring and concluded that it might serve to co-ordinate the cellular growth response to IGF-I with changes in nutrient intake.

IGF-I and IGF-II in Malnutrition. As measured by specific radioimmunoassays, IGF-I concentrations drop dra-

TABLE 5
Effects of Undernutrition on the GH-IGF Axis

Increased GH secretion

Decreased somatomedin bioactivity
    Decreased IGF-I production
    Normal IGF-II production
    Increased IGF inhibitor production
    Increased IGF-I binding protein production (26 kDa)

matically with fasting in adult volunteers,[123] while those of IGF-II do not.[105] Clemmons[123] found that fasting of overweight adult volunteers for 10 days produced a drop of IGF-I concentrations to hypopituitary levels; refeeding produced a return toward normal (Fig. 7). The decline in serum IGF-I correlated with nitrogen balance. In some physiologic circumstances, however, the fall in serum IGF-I concentrations becomes dissociated from the changes in nitrogen balance. Smith et al[124] studied six conditioned athletes and concluded that strenuous exercise, which produces negative caloric balance, causes as much of a fall in serum IGF-I but a much lower nitrogen loss than does comparable caloric restriction without exercise.

In contrast to the apparent insensitivity of serum IGF-II to fasting in adults,[105] Soliman et al[125] have documented depressed IGF-II concentrations in children with severe marasmus and marasmic kwashiorkor. These returned to normal with refeeding. The magnitude of IGF-II depression was not nearly as great as that of IGF-I, and the IGF-II concentrations in sera of children who were underweight or had only kwashiorkor were not depressed. Thus, severe or longlasting malnutrition in children may eventually depress IGF-II production, although IGF-I remains the more acutely sensitive to malnutrition.

Serum IGF-I Measurements as an Index of Nutritional Status. The striking correlation between (as yet unidentified) aspects of nutritional status and serum IGF-I concentrations has led some investigators to suggest that the latter might provide a highly sensitive and quantitative way of following nutritional status. Clemmons et al[126] found that IGF-I increased by 170 percent over 10 days in six malnourished patients with GI disorders that necessitated either total parenteral or tube feedings. All patients were in positive nitrogen balance when first measured on the second day of refeeding. Other commonly used indices of nutritional status fell much less dramatically and normalized much more slowly: prealbumin by 21 percent, retinol-binding protein by 18 percent, and transferrin by 10 percent (Fig. 8A). Unterman et al[127] came to similar conclusions when they compared IGF-I concentra-

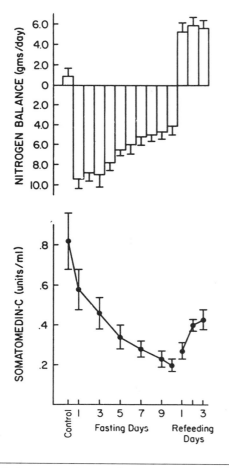

FIGURE 7 Somatomedin-C and nitrogen balance during starvation: the effects of fasting on plasma immunoreactive somatomedin-C (IGF-I) and nitrogen balance. The subjects were seven males 20 to 70 percent above ideal body weight. During the control period, they were fed a 1,500-calorie diet for 3 days. Between days 4 and 13, they fasted, receiving only water, vitamins, and potassium chloride. Refeeding consisted of resumption of the control diet. Each point is the mean ± SEM. (From Clemmons[123]; © by The Endocrine Society.)

tions with other indices in 37 generally elderly hospitalized patients with a variety of neoplastic, GI, and neurologic diseases. IGF-I was more depressed than albumin or transferrin in patients who had no reduction in either triceps skinfold thickness or mid-arm muscle circumference. In six patients given nutritional support, IGF-I concentrations rose by more than 70 percent in each patient, while the lymphocyte count and transferrin concentration rose in only four patients and albumin concentration in only one (Fig. 8B). Serum IGF-I measurements have also been suggested as a means to follow the progress of children and adolescents with chronic inflammatory bowel disease.[128]

Mechanisms of IGF Regulation by Nutrients. A number of studies have attempted to determine the specific components of the refeeding diet which regulate IGF-I production in recovery from an acute fast. When normal-weight human volunteers were fasted for 5 days and then refed with a normal diet, a diet that was isocaloric but protein deficient, or a diet deficient in both protein and calories, Isley et al[129] concluded that intake of adequate quantities of both protein and calories is critical for the restoration of IGF-I after a fast (Fig. 9). Animal studies have indicated that the roles played by protein and calorie intake in regulating serum IGF-I concentrations may be developmentally influenced. Prewitt et al[130] placed 3-week-old rats on diets in which the protein content was varied (5 percent, 10 percent, or 15 percent lactalbumin) at one of three levels of energy intake (100 percent, 75 percent, or 50 percent ad libitum). After 2 weeks, protein intake played the major role in regulating IGF-I concentrations, whereas after 9 weeks, both protein and caloric intake were important.

The mechanism by which nutrients influence IGF-I production is unclear. Since GH concentrations are generally elevated in fasting and malnutrition and the depressed IGF-I concentrations are unresponsive to GH administration,[131] it is evident that the IGF-I–producing tissues become refractory to the trophic actions of GH. Studies in fasted[132–134] and diabetic[86] rats have shown a striking correlation between the fall in serum IGF-I concentrations and the number of somatogenic GH binding sites in liver, suggesting that a primary effect of malnutrition, perhaps mediated through a drop in insulin concentrations, is to influence GH receptors and consequently IGF-I production. More recent studies by Maiter et al[135] showed that protein-deprived rats experience a drop in serum IGF-I concentrations well before GH binding sites are reduced. Those authors suggested the existence of a postreceptor defect in GH action which characterizes the early IGF response to protein deficiency.

Insulin in Malnutrition

With fasting or protein-calorie malnutrition, plasma insulin concentrations are reduced, although in some instances high and normal levels have been reported.[125] Some of these discrepancies might be explained by the observations of Lunn et al[93] that in kwashiorkor there is an early phase of hyperinsulinism that is followed by insulinopenia. Diminished insulin release results in impaired tolerance to glucose or an amino acid load.[136] Pimstone et al[137] noted that while the insulin response to oral glucose is abnormal in malnourished children, intravenous glucose elicits a normal response, suggesting that deficiencies of glucagon or other insulinotropic factors are important in determining the response to malnutrition. Those authors also demonstrated that the impaired insulin response to a glucose load in kwashiorkor could be ameliorated by the addition of potassium to the diet. The relationship of malnutrition and diabetes mellitus has recently been reviewed by Rao,[138] who concluded that a malnourished condition can influence the diabetogenicity of other agents, including dietary toxins, drugs, and viruses, but does not directly cause diabetes.

Psychosocial Growth Failure

The interactions of hormones and nutrients have been extensively studied in children with "psychosocial growth failure" or "deprivation dwarfism," terms used to describe

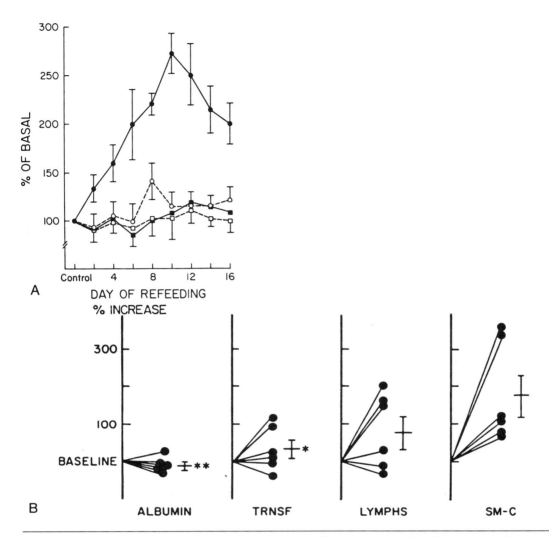

FIGURE 8 Changes in plasma IGF-I (Sm-C) and other indices during nutritional therapy. *A,* Plasma protein concentrations used as indices of nutritional therapy in six malnourished patients receiving nutritional support during the recovery from various GI disorders. The results are the percentage above basal value for each protein ± SEM. *Closed circles,* IGF-I; *open circles,* prealbumin; *closed squares,* retinol-binding protein; *open squares,* transferrin. (From Clemmons et al.[126]) *B,* Changes in nutritional indices in six patients tested during the course of nutritional support for GI disorders that resulted in kwashiorkor in one, marasmus in one, and a mixed pattern in four. For each index, values at the time of greatest protein and calorie intake are compared with values before therapy was begun. Values are mean ± SEM. *$P < 0.05$ versus somatomedin-C (Sm-C); **$P < 0.01$ versus somatomedin-C. TRNSF = transferrin; LYMPHS = lymphocyte count. (From Unterman et al.[127])

the growth failure that can accompany severe emotional deprivation. It was first described in institutionalized children; affected children were noted to have voracious appetites and bizarre behavior that included foraging, drinking from the toilet bowl, and gorging. Delayed speech, characteristic neurologic postures, and a protuberant abdomen have also been described.[139,140]

Considerable attention has been paid to whether the growth failure and hormonal changes of psychosocial dwarfism can result from emotional deprivation alone or require the presence of inadequate caloric intake. Speculation as to the mechanisms of the growth failure have included inadequate nutrition resulting either from underfeeding by the caregiver

or undereating as a result of emotionally induced anorexia, altered GI function, and changes in metabolism.[141] Psychological factors were invoked by Widdowson[142] to explain her observations on the growth of children in two German orphanages after World War II. Despite comparable food intake, children at the orphanage governed by a stern supervisor who disciplined them at meal times gained weight at about one-third the rate of children at a second orphanage. The pattern was reversed, however, when the first supervisor was transferred to another orphanage.

Considerable evidence suggests that a hypopituitary state has developed in some children with psychosocial growth failure. Talbot[143] studied a group of 51 children with growth failure of no clear etiology and postulated that they had developed a "functional hypopituitarism" as a means of adapting to limited caloric intake. A form of reversible hypopituitarism has, indeed, been documented in emotionally deprived children. Powell et al[144,145] documented abnormal reserves of ACTH and GH which were normalized when the affected children were removed from their adverse surroundings. Miller et al[146] demonstrated a loss of GH secretory peaks during a 6-hour period of blood sampling in four children with psychosocial deprivation. In one child, they documented a recovery of GH secretion after hospitalization and rehabilitation (Fig. 10). Despite the apparent state of GH deficiency, attempts to induce growth in such children with GH have been unsuccessful.[147,148]

A counter-theme to the hypothesis of a strictly emotional etiology of psychosocial growth failure has been the suggestion of Whitten et al[149] and others that underfeeding by caregivers is the primary cause of growth failure in these children. Those authors observed emotionally deprived infants between 3 and 24 months of age and documented dramatic weight gain in 11 of 13 when the infants were given adequate nutrition in a hospital setting designed to reproduce the deprived emotional ambience of their homes. Weight gain was no more rapid when these children were given equal amounts of food with a high level of mothering care. Biochemical studies have also supported a nutritional etiology for psychosocial dwarfism: Elevated fasting GH levels have been found in a number of infants with this disorder.[150]

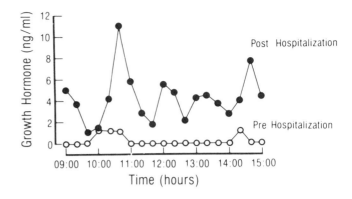

FIGURE 10 Return of pulsatile growth hormone secretory pattern during recovery from psychosocial deprivation. Six-hour growth hormone secretory profiles, prehospitalization and posthospitalization with rehabilitation, in a 5-year-old male with psychosocial dwarfism and a bone age of 5 years. (From Powell et al[145]; © by The Endocrine Society.)

Contemporary dietary and health misconceptions have created a modern-day version of the growth-retarded child from a turn-of-the-century foundling house or war orphanage. Pugliese et al[151] described a group of 14 adolescents who presented with short stature and malnutrition from self-imposed caloric restriction. These children showed no evidence of overt psychiatric disease or anorexia nervosa but had restricted their food intake from a fear of obesity. Similar findings were reported in a group of younger children, 7 to 22 months of age, who presented with nutritional failure to thrive secondary to parental restriction of food.[152] For a variety of reasons, including the fear that their children would develop obesity, cardiovascular disease, or unhealthy eating habits, the parents of these children had restricted their intake of fat, calories, or minerals below that required for normal growth. In both groups, nutritional and psychiatric counseling proved successful in restoring adequate food intake, linear growth, and sexual maturation.

It is probable that psychosocial growth failure results from both emotional and nutritional causes (Fig. 11). At one extreme are those children who either are not offered or for neurologic or psychiatric reasons will not consume adequate amounts of food or who have altered GI function. In these children, the endocrine changes that have been measured are probably adaptive ones in response to malnutrition. At the other extreme are those children whose emotional state has resulted in a direct inhibition of hypothalamic and pituitary function. It is likely that many of the children with clinical features of this condition combine features of both emotional and nutritional deprivation.

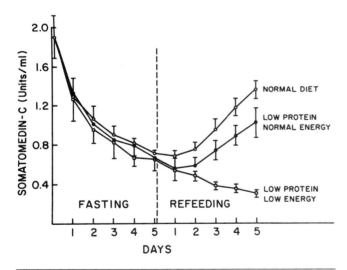

FIGURE 9 Effect of experimental fasting and refeeding on serum somatomedin-C. Subjects were two males and three females within 15 percent of ideal body weight. They fasted for 5 days and were then refed with one of three diets: normal diet (*open circles*), which consisted of 1.35 gm protein per kilogram of body weight and 35.3 kcal per kilogram of body weight; low-protein, isocaloric diet (*closed circles*), which contained comparable calories and 0.43 gm protein per kilogram of body weight; or low-protein, low-energy diet (*squares*), which contained 0.40 gm protein per kilogram of body weight and 10.8 kcal per kilogram of body weight. Each point is the mean ± SD for the five subjects. (From Isley et al[129]; with permission of the American Society for Clinical Investigation.)

Growth Hormone, Somatomedins, and Insulin in Overnutrition

Just as a deficiency of nutrients can retard growth, so can nutritional surfeit accelerate growth. This is perhaps most pronounced in fetal life, when excessive glucose and other nutrients from conditions such as mild maternal diabetes can

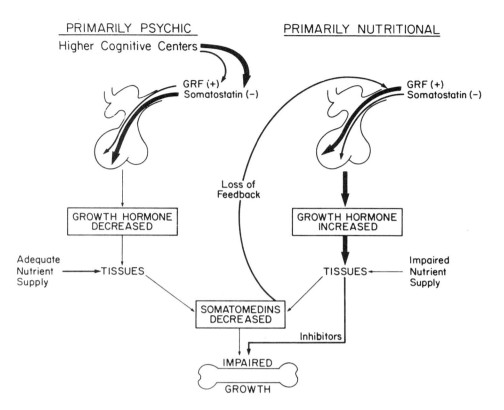

FIGURE 11 Psychosocial growth failure. There are two possible mechanisms of psychosocial growth failure: neuroendocrine (primarily psychic) and nutritional. *Left,* Under largely psychological influences, pituitary hormone secretion is diminished in the face of normal nutrition (see also Figure 10). *Right,* When undernutrition predominates, the endocrine changes observed are adaptive ones. Somatomedin production is reduced, inhibitor production is increased, and growth hormone secretion is increased (see also Table 4). (From Russell WE, Underwood LE. Nutrition and the humoral regulation of growth. In: Walker WA, Watkins JB. Nutrition and pediatrics: basic science and clinical application. Boston: Little, Brown, 1985.)

lead to significant overgrowth. A stimulatory influence of obesity on childhood growth appears to be the case as well. In the mid-1940s, Talbot[153] noted that obese children tend to be tall, to have advanced skeletal maturation, and to excrete more ketosteroids than nonobese children. Subsequent studies by Garn and others[154-156] have confirmed a correlation between obesity and height throughout childhood. In affluent societies socioeconomic factors influence obesity, making correlation of the latter with height difficult. However, a recent study by Garn et al[157] in Central America indicates that the augmented stature associated with obesity in childhood persists into adulthood.

In the fetus insulin appears to play a critical role in the more commonly recognized overgrowth syndromes. Although obesity is associated with elevated circulating insulin concentrations, it is unlikely that insulin plays a direct role in the facilitation of growth, since obese individuals are relatively insulin resistant and require high concentrations of insulin to maintain normal homeostasis.[158] A regulatory role for insulin in promoting growth, perhaps by stimulating appetite, has been suggested in a subgroup of children recovering from surgery for craniopharyngioma. These tumors compress the hypothalamus and often result in hypopituitarism, yet a significant number of patients are able to maintain normal growth velocities after surgery, despite a GH-deficient state. Bucher and colleagues[159] compared a group of rapidly growing children with groups of normal and slowly growing children after surgery for craniopharyngioma and found that those with supranormal growth rates were hyperphagic and had elevated insulin levels. Comparable findings of hyperphagia, obesity, and hyperinsulinism have been made in

animals with lesions in the ventromedial hypothalamus.[160]

Although IGF production is very sensitive to poor nutrition, there is no evidence that these growth factors are responsible for the stimulation of overgrowth in obese children. It has been noted that the fall of plasma IGF-I concentrations is slower in fasted obese individuals than in normal subjects.[161] Underwood and colleagues[162] studied the effects of overfeeding on IGF-I levels in GH-deficient subjects. After 10 days of an energy intake 50 percent above basal, those subjects experienced a significant increase in weight, nitrogen balance, fasting blood sugar, and insulin levels, but no significant change in IGF-I concentrations. GH secretion may be altered in obesity. GH release in response to pharmacologic stimuli is often blunted; however, pretreatment with beta-blocking drugs normalizes the secretory response, suggesting adequate GH reserves.[163]

THYROID HORMONES

Thyroid Hormones in Normal Growth

The actions of the thyroid hormones, like those of insulin, can be broadly separated into directly metabolic ones and those that result from thyroid induction of other genes that regulate cell growth and function. Increased oxygen consumption, heat production, and accelerated metabolism constitute the calorigenic effects of the thyroid hormones.[164] The mechanism by which thyroid hormones affect these actions is not clearly understood but probably does not involve an uncoupling of oxidative phosphorylation from respiration, as was originally postulated.[165] Unlike peptide hormones, which bind to cell membrane receptors and regulate cell function and gene transcription via second messengers, thyroid hormone receptors exist in the cytoplasm and directly regulate the transcription of other genes by binding to regulatory regions of DNA in the genome.[166] Many of the developmental effects of the thyroid hormones result from induction of the genes for other hormones and growth factors, such as epidermal and nerve growth factors.[167]

Thyroxine (T_4) is the major hormone secreted by the thyroid, but it is deiodinated at its outer ring to produce triiodothyronine (T_3), which is the metabolically active hormone. Deiodination occurs both in the thyroid gland and at peripheral sites such as liver, kidney, and brain. Thyroxine may also be deiodinated at its inner ring to form reverse T_3 (rT_3), which is metabolically inactive. Regulation of the relative activity of the inner and outer ring deiodinases to vary the concentrations of T_3 and rT_3 is a major control point in the thyroid economy. Thyroxine release from the thyroid is stimulated by thyroid-stimulating hormone (TSH, thyrotropin), which in turn is released from the anterior pituitary under the influence of the hypothalamic modulator, thyrotropin-releasing hormone (TRH). T_3, perhaps in conjunction with T_4, feeds back to inhibit TSH secretion.

The influence of thyroid hormones on growth occurs at many levels. Within the cell, they have profound effects on metabolic processes, including the induction of mitochondrial enzymes and an increase in Na,K-ATPase activity. Thyroid hormones influence the GH-IGF axis, as evidenced by the fact that hypothyroid rats have a diminished pituitary content of GH, low circulating GH levels, and depressed IGF

levels.[168–170] T_3 has been shown to stimulate transcription of the GH gene.[171] In contrast to animal models, hypothyroid children do not consistently demonstrate subnormal GH release.[76,172,173] Furthermore, the growth-retarding effects of hypothyroidism in rats are not reversed by GH treatment. In addition to a GH-mediated influence on IGF secretion, thyroid hormones augment IGF-I actions on cartilage growth,[174] and their absence is evident at the growth plate cartilage by altered morphology.[175] In addition, thyroid hormones directly accelerate cartilage maturation in the absence of IGFs.[176] The proliferative effects of thyroid hormones on growth plate chondrocytes appear to be IGF-mediated, as the mitogenic actions of T_3 on cartilage growth can be blocked with an antibody to IGF-I. In contrast, the effects of T_3 on cartilage morphology and functional maturation appear to be non–IGF-mediated, direct ones.[177]

Thyroid Hormones in Malnutrition

Fasting and malnutrition induce a hypothyroid-like state characterized by a diminished rate of T_3 production and, consequently, a depressed heart rate and basal metabolic rate as well as a diminished loss of nitrogen.[99,178,179] Concomitant with the fall in T_3 in malnutrition is a depression of sympathetic nervous system activity, as measured by norepinephrine secretion.[180] T_3 concentrations fall into the hypothyroid range within 48 hours of a fast, while concentrations of T_4 change little, and those of rT_3, the inactive metabolite of T_4, rise (Fig. 12). These changes result from a starvation-induced inhibition of the deiodination of T_4 to

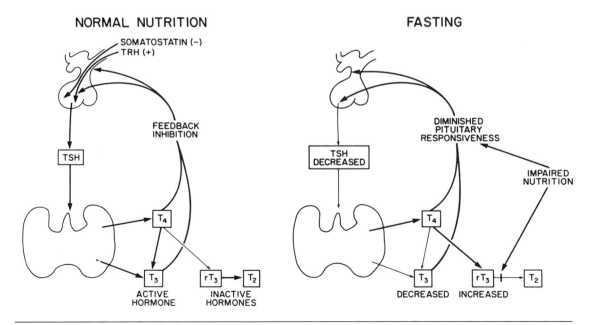

FIGURE 12 The pituitary-thyroid axis. When nutrition is normal, thyroxine (T_4) is converted primarily to the calorigenic hormone triiodothyronine (T_3). Concentrations of the inactive hormones, reverse T_3 (rT_3) and T_2 are low. During a fast, rT_3 concentrations rise, primarily because of decreased degradation to T_2 and to some extent because of preferential conversion of T_4 to rT_3 instead of T_3. Fasting also diminishes the pituitary responsiveness to hypothalamic factors, and thyroid-stimulating hormone levels do not rise. (From Russell WE, Underwood LE. Nutrition and the humoral regulation of growth. In: Walker WA, Watkins JB. Nutrition and pediatrics: basic science and clinical application. Boston: Little, Brown, 1985.)

T_3, while the serum half-life of rT_3 is prolonged by preventing its deiodination to T_2. In addition, malnutrition also results in a diminished synthesis of the plasma thyroid-binding proteins, which also results in depressed thyroid hormone levels.

The low levels of thyroid hormones in the undernourished state are likely to be an adaptive mechanism meant to diminish the extent of catabolism. Danforth and Burger[165] have shown that when T_3 is administered to fasting subjects sufficient to maintain T_3 levels in the normal range, nitrogen losses are accentuated. Despite a low serum T_3, TSH secretion is not increased in fasting, and the TSH response to TRH is either normal or somewhat blunted.[181,182] The condition of depressed levels of thyroid hormones without elevation in TSH in malnutrition or illness has often been called the "euthyroid sick syndrome."[183]

The depressed T_3 levels of the fasted state can be corrected by refeeding as little as 100 kcal of carbohydrate, whereas the protein or fat content of the diet does not significantly affect the recovery of T_3.[184] As little as 50 g of carbohydrate will prevent the effect of dietary restriction on serum T_3 levels.[185] As in those subjected to acute starvation, chronically malnourished children and adults have depressed serum T_3 and elevated rT_3 concentrations. However, the TSH concentrations are either normal or elevated in chronic malnutrition and the TSH response to TRH is exaggerated.[129,186,187]

Thyroid Hormones in Overnutrition

Overnutrition results in changes in thyroid hormone metabolism that are predictably opposite to those seen in undernutrition. The resting metabolic rate is increased, as are T_3 levels, while rT_3 levels are decreased.[188] The mechanism for the changes in T_3 and rT_3 appears to be increased outer ring deiodination of T_4, since overfeeding also results in an increased clearance of T_3. In contrast to the underfed state, it is not clear that the increased metabolic rate seen in overfeeding is associated with enhanced sympathetic nervous system activity, since beta-adrenergic blockade has no effect on the increased metabolic rate induced by overfeeding.[165]

The relationship between thyroid function and true obesity is minimal, despite popular opinion to the contrary. The weight gain seen in hypothyroidism is largely secondary to myxedema and fluid accumulation, and most of the metabolic effects of overfeeding on thyroid hormone levels occur independently of the degree of leanness or obesity of the subjects.

CORTISOL

Cortisol in Intestinal Maturation

There is a striking maturation of absorptive function of the intestine following birth, with ample evidence to suggest that glucocorticoids regulate the process. Most of the data on the regulation of gut maturation have been derived from studies in rats and other small mammals. Coincident with the period

of weaning and, consequently, a decreasing reliance on lactose and other milk sugars for nourishment, there is a fall in the high activity of lactase in the small intestine and a rise in the activity of intestinal sucrase, maltase, and pancreatic amylase. In addition, there is a loss in the abilities of the ileal and jejunal mucosae to take up macromolecules and to transport immunoglobulins. Delay of weaning has no significant effect on the timing of these changes. In contrast, deprivation in the pup of pituitary hormones by hypophysectomy in the newborn period elicits a marked delay.[189,190] These observations have led to studies of the role of pituitary-derived or pituitary-regulated hormones in the maturation of gut function.

The experimental data support roles for both glucocorticoids and thyroid hormones in intestinal maturation. Coincident with the enzymatic changes in the rat gut at the end of the second week of life, there is a prominent rise in circulating corticosterone. Breast milk might provide an additional source of glucocorticoids.[191] Glucocorticoid administration to preweanlings results in early maturation of intestinal enzymes such as sucrase[192] and of pancreatic amylase, of bile acid synthesis, and of transport phenomena such as bile salt absorption.[193] The dependence on glucocorticoids is not absolute, however, as adrenalectomy on day 9 of life does not prevent the appearance of sucrase. The absence of adrenals, however, does not delay the maturation of sucrose to adult levels of activity.[192] A comparable role for thyroid hormones has also been suggested, although it appears that the ability of thyroxine to induce maturation of the intestinal enzymes requires the presence of intact adrenal glands. Administration of thyroxine to rats results in increased blood concentrations of corticosterone. Thus, the observed effects of thyroxine may be through induction of glucocorticoids.[192]

Cortisol in Malnutrition

Reflecting the metabolic stress, malnutrition in humans and laboratory animals results in elevated cortisol concentrations, with an abolition of the normal diurnal rhythm and a slowed clearance of exogenous cortisol.[194] Fasting also depresses production of cortisol-binding proteins, resulting in a further elevation of levels of free glucocorticoids.[195] Despite the glucocorticoid excess induced by malnutrition, the adrenal glands remain suppressible with dexamethasone and responsive to ACTH.

A prominent metabolic effect of cortisol is the diversion of substrates to the liver for protein synthesis. Rao et al[196] have demonstrated that infants with marasmus have higher cortisol levels than do infants with kwashiorkor and that the response of cortisol to ACTH is better preserved in marasmus. Those authors postulated that the development of kwashiorkor is coincident with failure of the adrenal gland to secrete adequate cortisol to maintain normal protein levels. In rats, the biochemical manifestations of kwashiorkor resulting from a low-protein diet can be reversed by glucocorticoids.[197]

As previously indicated, glucocorticoids have a deleterious effect on cartilage growth and act as IGF antagonists in somatomedin bioassays. In his studies on malnourished

Nigerian children, Smith[109] postulated that elevated cortisol, acting as an inhibitor of IGF action at cartilage, was a major contributor to the poor growth of his subjects.

GONADAL STEROIDS

Reproductive Function in Malnutrition

The potent gonadal steroids testosterone and estradiol are primarily responsible for the establishment of reproductive fitness. Other, weaker androgenic hormones, however, that are produced by the gonads and adrenal glands of both sexes are important in the maintenance of normal anabolism. These include androstenedione, dehydroepiandrosterone (DHEA), and its metabolite DHEA-sulfate. Whereas reproductive function is expendable and potentially damaging during times of nutrient deficit, considerable attention has been paid to the importance of weaker androgenic hormones, or anabolic steroids, as possible therapeutic agents for the recovery from catabolic states.

In malnourished adults, hypogonadism often develops and the secretion of sex steroids by the gonads decreases; in malnourished children, the onset of puberty is delayed.[198] Men suffering from chronic protein-calorie malnutrition often experience gonadal failure. In adults, nutrients appear to influence reproduction at both the hypothalamic and gonadal levels. In a group of Indian men suffering from malnutrition, Smith et al[199] found low plasma testosterone and elevated gonadotropins, indicating impaired testicular function. During recovery, these men continued to have elevated levels of luteinizing hormone (LH) and a subnormal release of testosterone to chorionic gonadotropin (hCG). In contrast, Klibanski[200] found evidence for hypothalamic hypofunction in mildly obese men fasted for 10 days.

In addition to the effects of malnutrition in delaying puberty, a number of studies on young athletes have suggested a connection between body composition and reproductive fitness. In young female athletes and dancers who train extensively before puberty, menarche can be delayed by several years.[201] In some instances, the delay in menarche can be related directly to the duration of training prior to menarche: 5 months for every year of training.[202] These observations led Frisch and McArthur to propose that normal menstrual function depends upon attainment of at least 22 percent body fat.[203] This model, which has not been universally accepted,[204] assumes that some aspect of body fat content, presumably metabolic, signals permission for the secretion of gonadotropic hormones to trigger menstruation.

Anabolic Steroids as Therapeutic Agents in Catabolic Disease

Despite all attempts, it has been impossible to synthesize steroids with anabolic actions that are divorced from their androgenic (masculinizing) ones. Coupled with their anabolic effects, these hormones can have behavioral effects such as increased aggressiveness and an enhanced appetite. Like all androgens, they suppress gonadotropin production and result in a lipogenic profile of cholesterol metabolism. High doses can result in altered liver function and hepatocellular carcinoma. Anabolic agents have been shown to decrease nitrogen loss after minor surgery[205] but have had no consistent effect on weight gain in geriatric patients[206] or in patients with chronic renal failure.[207]

There has been considerable popular attention in recent years to the use of anabolic steroids to increase performance in body building and other sports. Well-controlled studies in adult male athletes are few, and the results are conflicting.[208] Individuals whose performance stands to benefit the most from increased androgenic activity are those who produce relatively low levels of androgens endogenously: females, prepubertal children, and adolescents. These are the groups in whom additional adverse effects such as virilization, balding, sexual precocity, and premature closure of the epiphyses would be the most damaging.

At this time, there appears to be no clear role for anabolic agents in the treatment of catabolic states; their use in male athletes is of uncertain benefit and entails significant medical risk; their use in female athletes is associated with equal risk and unacceptable side effects. The use of anabolic steroids to enhance athletic performance in children and adolescents is to be soundly condemned.

SUMMARY AND CONCLUSIONS

Whether in simple cells growing under carefully defined conditions in the laboratory or in populations of children growing under highly variable and unpredictable conditions of nutritional want or excess, nutrients and growth-regulating chemicals influence the actions of one another. The endocrine controls on growth are highly sensitive to aspects of both the quantity and the quality of the nutritional milieu and are programmed to alter and even abort the body's developmental scheme as required. The specific components of diet that are monitored by the various nutritionally sensitive endocrine systems, however, are not known. Nonetheless, a careful assessment of physical growth and maturation can serve as a sensitive and accurate index of nutritional status and disease, both for individuals and for whole populations.

The capacity of the growing organism to accommodate changes in the availability of nutrients by slowing or halting growth is a generally reversible process, designed to permit adaptation to a changing nutrient supply. However, the ability to resume normal growth after the correction of metabolic insults is highly dependent on the nature of the insult, its duration, and the developmental phase of the organism during which it occurred. The damage incurred during certain susceptible periods of growth may be irreversible, perhaps owing to a reduction in the number or critical organization of the cells that make up key tissues. The mechanisms by which the growing tissue or organism can monitor its own size and correct discrepancies between its actual size and its apparently preprogrammed "intended" size are unknown. However, they probably involve a co-ordination between mechanisms for "catch-up" that are extant in individual tissues and regulatory centers in the central nervous system; to date, hormones have not been shown to play a key regulatory role.

We have seen that in response to nutritional deficit, the survival strategy employed by living systems is to conserve energy and to preserve the integrity of essential biochemical functions. In individuals already in puberty, severe malnutrition results in cessation of reproductive function; in growing children, the onset of puberty is delayed. The inhibition of reproductive systems is complex, with evidence for nutritional control both in the central nervous system and in the periphery as well. Along with inhibition of the gonadal sex steroids and other anabolic hormones during periods of substrate deficit, there is also a down-regulation of the actions of the IGFs and other mitogenic agents. Once again, the influence of nutrients and nutritional signals is complex and occurs at many levels: Despite hypersecretion of GH, which under most circumstances is the primary regulator of IGF production, peripheral secretion of IGF-I is depressed, perhaps owing to interference with the GH-signaling mechanism. In addition, there is an increase in the production of IGF inhibitory proteins and significant alterations in the production of important serum-binding proteins. Acute rises in the concentrations of growth hormone and cortisol increase the resistance of many tissues to the actions of insulin, thereby facilitating the mobilization of substrates from tissue stores. Differential sensitivity of different body compartments to the changing hormonal environment ensures a shift of stored energy from structural proteins to the viscera. Concomitant with this flux of energy from stored forms is a shift in the thyroid hormones to noncalorigenic forms that help to conserve the available energy. The effects of overnutrition are generally opposite to those of undernutrition: increased anabolic and mitogenic activity and a shift in thyroid hormones to energy-expending forms.

At least from our current vantage point, the metabolic changes of undernutrition are adaptive ones, designed to ensure survival until adequate reserves exist to permit growth and reproduction once again. In some instances, however, morbidity may actually result from maladaptive endocrine changes. The development of kwashiorkor, for example, may result when the adrenal gland is no longer able to maintain adequate production of glucocorticoid hormones to facilitate withdrawal of proteins from structural stores such as muscle.

An understanding of the normal regulation and actions of hormones and growth factors in conditions of altered nutrition has suggested new diagnostic and therapeutic approaches. Plasma concentrations of IGF-I may provide a more sensitive means of assessing nutritional status than many other currently employed tests. GH administration to individuals in catabolic states may hasten their recovery, although this therapy may prove to be most useful in children with longstanding malnutrition or in the elderly, whose endogenous production of GH is diminished. Studies of anabolic steroid hormones in catabolic states have not been promising.

The challenge of the future is to better delineate the full spectrum of humoral changes that accompany nutritional alterations and to define those components of "nutrition" that are the actual signals that regulate the production and actions of hormones and growth factors. Are the nutritional signals themselves metabolites and elemental nutrients? Might these substances have direct effects on the expression of hormone and growth factor genes, or do they act through intermediates such as other hormones (the nutritionally regulated gut hormones, for example) and intracellular messengers? As best illustrated by the IGFs, the physiologic control of growth factors can be very difficult to study, since alterations in their production can be highly tissue specific and not reflected in their blood levels. Furthermore, specific tissues may vary in their sensitivity and responsiveness to growth factors and hormones that are ubiquitous and whose concentrations in blood may change little. At this time, the measurement of tissue concentrations of hormone receptors and growth factors is an invasive proposition, of little clinical practicality. When the physiology of these substances is better understood, the promise for therapeutic intervention will be great. Until we can learn to redirect the physiologic response to malnutrition, our ability to intervene therapeutically will, of necessity, be limited to augmenting the normal response.

REFERENCES

1. Bielicki T, Szczotka H, Charzewski J. The influence of three socioeconomic factors on body height in Polish military conscripts. Human Biol 1981; 53:543–555.
2. Greulich WW. A comparison of the physical growth and development of American-born and native Japanese children. Am J Phys Anthropol 1957; 15:489–515.
3. Greulich WW. Some secular changes in the growth of American-born and native Japanese children. Am J Phys Anthropol 1976; 45:553–568.
4. Thoday JM. Geneticism and environmentalism. In: Meade JE, Parker AS, eds. Biological aspects of social problems. London: Oliver & Boyd, 1965.
5. Trowbridge FL, Marks JS, deRomana GL, Madrid S, Boulton TW, Klein PD. Body composition of Peruvian children with short stature and high weight-for-height. II. Implications for the interpretation of weight-for-height as an indicator of nutritional status. Am J Clin Nutr 1987; 46:411–418.
6. Starling EH. The Croonian Lectures on the chemical correlation of the functions of the body. Lancet 1905; ii:579–583.
7. Feyrter F. Uber die peripheren endokrinen (parakrinen) Drusen des Menschen. Wien: W Maudrich 1953.
8. Sporn MB, Todaro GJ. Autocrine secretion and malignant transformation of cells. N Engl J Med 1980; 303:878–880.
9. Russell WE, Van Wyk JJ. Peptide growth factors. In: DeGroot LJ, ed. Endocrinology. 2nd ed. Orlando, FL: Grune & Stratton, 1988: 2504.
10. Holley RW. A unifying hypothesis concerning the nature of malignant growth. Proc Natl Acad Sci USA 1972; 69:2840–2841.
11. Holley RW. Control of growth of mammalian cells in culture. Nature 1975; 258:487–490.
12. Barnes D, Sato G. Serum free cell culture: a unifying approach. Cell 1980; 22:649–655.
13. Barsh GS, Cunningham DD. Nutrient uptake and control of animal cell proliferation. J Supramol Struct 1977; 7:61–77.
14. Eagle H. Metabolic controls in cultured mammalian cells. Science 1965; 148:42–51.
15. Gospodarowicz D, Moran JS. Growth factors in mammalian cell culture. Ann Rev Biochem 1976; 45:531–558.
16. Temin HM, Pierson HM, Dulak NC. The role of serum in the control of multiplication of avian and mammalian cells in culture. In: Rothblat GH, Cristofalo JJ, eds. Growth, nutrition, and metabolism of cells in culture. New York: Academic, 1972.
17. McKeehan WL, McKeehan KA. Serum factors modify the cellular requirement for Ca^{2+}, K^+, Mg^{2+}, phosphate ions, 2-oxycarboxylic acids for multiplication of normal human fibroblasts. Proc Natl Acad Sci USA 1980; 77:3417–3421.
18. McKeehan WL, McKeehan KA. Extracellular regulation of fibroblast multiplication: a direct kinetic approach to analysis of role of low molecular weight nutrients and serum growth factors. J Supramol Struct 1981; 15:83–110.
19. Rizzino A, Rizzino H, Sato G. Defined media and the determination of nutritional and hormonal requirements of mammalian cells in culture. Nutr Rev 1979; 37:369–378.

20. Wu R, Sato GH. Replacement of serum in cell culture by hormones: a study of hormonal regulation of cell growth and specific gene expression. J Toxicol Environ Health 1978; 4:427–448.
21. Palsson H. Conformation and body composition. In: Hammond J, ed. Progress in the physiology of farm animals, vol 2. London: Butterworths, 1955: 430.
22. Bauman DE, Currie WB. Partitioning of nutrients during pregnancy and lactation: a review of mechanisms involving homeostasis and homeorrhesis. J Dairy Sci 1980; 63:1514–1529.
23. Munro HN. General aspects of the regulation of protein metabolism by diet and by hormones. In: Munro HN, Allison JB, eds. Mammalian protein metabolism. New York: Academic, 1964; 1:381.
24. Kochakian CD, Tillotson C, Austin J. A comparison of the effect of inanition, castration and testosterone on the muscles of the male guinea pig. Endocrinology 1957; 60:144.
25. Machlin LJ. Effect of porcine growth hormone on growth and carcass composition of the pig. J Anim Sci 1972; 35:794–800.
26. Sokoloff L, Kauffman S. Thyroxine stimulation of amino acid incorporation into protein. J Biol Chem 1961; 236:795–803.
27. Enesco M, Leblond CP. Increase in cell number as a factor in the growth of the organs and tissues of the young male rat. J Embryol Exp Morphol 1962; 10:530–564.
28. Laird AK. Postnatal growth of birds and mammals. Growth 1966; 30:349–363.
29. Sands J, Dobbing J, Gratrix CA. Cell number and cell size: organ growth and development and the control of catch-up in rats. Lancet 1979; ii:503–505.
30. McCance RA. Critical periods of growth. Proc Nutr Soc 1976; 35:309–313.
31. Widdowson EM, McCance RA. Some effects of accelerating growth: I. General somatic development. Proc R Soc Lond [Biol] 1960; 152:188–206.
32. Widdowson EM, McCance RA. A review: new thoughts on growth. Pediatr Res 1975; 9:154–156.
33. Widdowson EM, McCance RA. The effect of finite periods of undernutrition at different ages on the composition and subsequent development of the rat. Proc R Soc Lond [Biol] 1963; 158:329–342.
34. Winick M, Noble A. Cellular response in rats during malnutrition at various ages. J Nutr 1966; 89:300–306.
35. Winick M, Noble A. Cellular response with increased feeding in neonatal rats. J Nutr 1967; 91:179–182.
36. Winick M, Brasel JA. Nutrition and cell growth. In: Goodhart RS, Shils ME, eds. Modern nutrition in health and disease. 6th ed. Philadelphia: Lea & Febiger, 1980:592.
37. Tanner JM. A note on the history of catch-up growth. Bull Mem Soc Anthropol 1979; 6:399–405.
38. Prader A, Tanner JM, von Harnack GA. Catch-up growth following illness or starvation: an example of developmental canalization in man. J Pediatr 1963; 62:646–659.
39. Tanner JM. Growth at adolescence, 2nd ed. Oxford: Blackwell Scientific, 1962.
40. Smith DW, Truog W, Rogers JE, Greitzer LJ, Skinner AL, McCann JJ. Shifting linear growth during infancy: illustrations of genetic factors in growth from fetal life through infancy. J Pediatr 1976; 89:225–230.
41. Forbes GB. A note on the mathematics of "catch-up" growth. Pediatr Res 1974; 8:929–931.
42. Mosier HD. Catch-up and proportionate growth. Med Clin North Am 1978; 62:337–350.
43. Tanner JM. Catch-up growth in man. Br Med Bull 1981; 37:233–238.
44. Williams JPG. Catch-up growth. J Embryol Exp Morphol 1981; 65:89–101.
45. Williams JPG, Hughes PCR. Catch-up growth in rats undernourished for different periods during the suckling period. Growth 1975; 39:179–193.
46. Williams JPG, Tanner JM, Hughes PCR. Catch-up growth in male rats after growth retardation during the suckling period. Pediatr Res 1974; 8:149–156.
47. Rivkees SA, Bode HH, Crawford JD. Long-term growth in juvenile acquired hypothyroidism. N Engl J Med 1988; 318:599–602.
48. Burns EC, Tanner JM, Preece MA, Cameron N. Final height and pubertal development in 155 children with idiopathic growth hormone deficiency treated for between 2 and 15 years with growth hormone. Eur J Pediatr 1981; 137:155–164.
49. Mosier HD. Failure of compensatory (catch-up) growth in the rat. Pediatr Res 1971; 5:59–63.
50. Dearden LC, Mosier HD. Longterm recovery of chondrocytes in the tibial epiphyseal plate in rats after cortisone treatment. Clin Orthop 1972; 87:322–331.
51. Ashworth A. Growth rates in children recovering from protein-calorie malnutrition. Br J Nutr 1969; 23:835–845.
52. Bjorntorp P, Yang M-U. Refeeding after fasting in the rat: effects on body composition and food efficiency. Am J Clin Nutr 1982; 36:444–449.
53. Krieger I, Whitten CF. Energy metabolism in infants with growth failure due to maternal deprivation, undernutrition or causes unknown. J Pediatr 1969; 75:374–379.
54. Maccioni A, Moenckeberg F, Donoso G, Contreas I. Correlation between weight increase and caloric intake in infants with severe marasmic malnutrition. Presented at the 26th Annual Meeting of the Society for Pediatric Research, Atlantic City, NJ, 1966.
55. Tanner JM. The regulation of human growth. Child Dev 1963; 34:817–847.
56. Leibel RL. A biologic radar system for the assessment of body mass: the model of a geometry sensitive endocrine system is presented. J Theor Biol 1977; 66:297–306.
57. Mosier HD, Jansons RA. Allometry of body weight and tail length after head X-irradiation in rats. Growth 1971; 35:23–31.
58. Mosier HD, Jansons RA, Swingle KF, Sondhaus CA, Dearden LC, Halsall LC. Growth hormone secretion in the stunted head-irradiated rat. Pediatr Res 1985; 19:543–548.
59. Mosier HD, Jansons RA, Swingle KF, Dearden LC. Dissociation of catch-up growth control and neural control of growth hormone secretion in the stunted head-irradiated rat. Pediatr Res 1986; 20:261–264.
60. Mosier HD, Dearden LC, Jansons RA, Hill RR. Growth hormone, somatomedin and cartilage sulfation: failure of catch-up growth after propylthiouracil-induced hypothyroidism in the rat. Endocrinology 1977; 100:1644–1651.
61. Sporn MB, Roberts AB. Peptide growth factors are multifunctional. Nature 1988; 332:217–219.
62. Russell WE, Coffey RJ, Ouellette AJ, Moses HL. Type beta transforming growth factor reversibly inhibits the early proliferative response to partial hepatectomy in the rat. Proc Natl Acad Sci USA 1988; 85:5126–5130.
63. Dickerson JWT, McAnulty PA. The response of hind-limb muscles of the weanling rat to undernutrition and subsequent rehabilitation. Br J Nutr 1975; 33:171–180.
64. Wozney JM, Rosen V, Celeste AJ, Mitsock LM, Whitters MJ, Kriz RN, Hewick RM, Wang EA. Novel regulators of bone formation: molecular cloning and activities. Science 1988; 242:1528–1534.
65. Daughaday WH, Hall K, Raben MS, Salmon WD Jr, Van den Brande JL, Van Wyk JJ. Somatomedin: proposed designation for sulphation factor. Nature 1972; 235:107.
66. Zapf J, Schmid CH, Froesch ER. Biological and immunological properties of insulin-like growth factors (IGF) I and II. In: Daughaday WH, ed. Clin Endocrinol Metab 1984; 13:3.
67. Miller WL, Eberhardt NL. Structure and evolution of the growth hormone gene family. Endocrinol Rev 1983; 4:97.
68. Brissenden JE, Ullrich A, Francke U. Human chromosomal mapping of genes for insulin-like growth factor I and II and epidermal growth factor. Nature 1984; 310:781–784.
69. Berelowitz M, Szabo M, Frohman LA, Firestone S, Chu L, Hintz RL. Somatomedin-C mediates growth hormone negative feedback by effects on both the hypothalamus and the pituitary. Science 1981; 212:1279.
70. Brazeau P, Guillemin R, Ling N, Van Wyk JJ, Humbel RE. Inhibition by somatomedin of growth hormone secretion stimulated by hypothalamic growth hormone releasing factor (somatocrinin, GRF), of the synthetic peptide hpGRF. C R Acad Sci 1982; iii:651–654.
71. Isaksson O, Lindahl A, Nilsson A, Isgaard J. Mechanism of the stimulatory effect of growth hormone on longitudinal bone growth. Endocr Rev 1987; 8:426–438.
72. Han VKM, D'Ercole AJ, Lund PK. Cellular localization of somatomedin (insulin-like growth factor) messenger RNA in the human fetus. Science 1987; 236:193–197.
73. Finklestein JW, Roffwarg HP, Boyar RM, Kream J, Hellman L. Age-related changes in the twenty-four hour spontaneous secretion of growth hormone. J Clin Endocrinol Metab 1972; 35:665–670.

74. Francis GL, Upton FM, Ballard FJ, McNeil KA, Wallace JC. Insulin-like growth factors 1 and 2 in bovine colostrum. Sequences and biological activities compared with those of a potent truncated form. Biochem J 1988; 251:95–103.
75. Frankenne F, Rentier-Delrue F, Scippo M-L, Martial J, Hennen G. Expression of the growth hormone variant gene in human placenta. J Clin Endocrinol Metab 1987; 64:635–637.
76. Chernausek SD, Underwood LE, Utiger RD, Van Wyk JJ. Growth hormone secretion and plasma somatomedin-C in primary hypothyroidism. Clin Endocrinol 1983; 19:337.
77. Smal J, Closset J, Hennen G, De Meyts P. The receptor binding properties of the 20K variant of human growth hormone explain its discrepant insulin-like and growth promoting activities. Biochem Biophys Res Commun 1986; 134:159–165.
78. Kostyo JL, Cameron DM, Olson KC, Jones AJS, Pai R-C. Biosynthetic 20-kilodalton methionyl-human growth hormone has diabetogenic and insulin-like activities. Proc Natl Acad Sci USA 1985; 82:4250–4253.
79. Roth RA. Structure of the receptor for insulin-like growth factor. II: The puzzle amplified. Science 1988; 239:1269–1271.
80. Green H, Morikawa M, Nixon T. A dual effector theory of growth hormone action. Differentiation 1985; 29:195–198.
81. Hill DJ, Milner RDG. Insulin as a growth factor. Pediatr Res 1985; 19:879–886.
82. Lee RGL, Bode HH. Stunted growth and hepatomegaly in diabetes mellitus. J Pediatr 1977; 91:82.
83. Cohen P. The role of protein phosphorylation in neural and hormonal control of cellular activity. Nature 1982; 296:613–620.
84. Amiel SA, Sherwin RS, Hintz RL, Gertner JM, Press CM, Tamborlane WV. Effect of diabetes and its control on insulin-like growth factors in the young subject with type I diabetes. Diabetes 1984; 33:1175–1179.
85. Binoux M, Lassarre C, Jardoudin N. Somatomedin production by rat liver in organ culture: III. Studies on the release of insulin-like growth factor and its carrier protein measured by radioligand assays. Acta Endocrinol 1982; 99:422–430.
86. Maes M, Ketelslegers J-M, Underwood LE. Low plasma somatomedin-C in streptozotocin-induced diabetes mellitus. Correlation with changes in somatogenic and lactogenic liver binding sites. Diabetes 1983; 32:1060–1069.
87. Rechler MM, Nissley SP. The nature and regulation of the receptors for insulin-like growth factors. Ann Rev Physiol 1985; 47:425–442.
88. McGowan JA, Strain AJ, Bucher NLR. DNA synthesis in primary cultures of adult rat hepatocytes in a defined medium: effects of epidermal growth factor, insulin, glucagon and cyclic-AMP. J Cell Physiol 1981; 108:353–363.
89. Whitehead RG, Rowland MGM, Cole TJ. Infection, nutrition and growth in a rural African environment. Proc Nutr Soc 1976; 35:369–375.
90. Ho KY, Veldhuis JD, Johnson ML, Furlanetto R, Evans WS, Alberti KGMM, Thorner MO. Fasting enhances growth hormone secretion and amplifies the complex rhythms of growth hormone secretion in man. J Clin Invest 1988; 81:968–975.
91. Becker DJ, Pimstone BL, Hansen JDL, Hendricks S. Serum albumin and growth hormone relationships in kwashiorkor and the nephrotic syndrome. J Lab Clin Med 1971; 78:865–871.
92. Coward WA, Lunn PG. The biochemistry and physiology of kwashiorkor and marasmus. Br Med Bull 1981; 37:19.
93. Lunn PG, Whitehead RG, May RW, Baker BA. Progressive changes in serum cortisol, insulin and growth hormone concentrations and their relationship to the distorted amino acid pattern during the development of kwashiorkor. Br J Nutr 1973; 29:399–422.
94. Parra A. Insulin-growth hormone adaptations in marasmus and kwashiorkor as seen in Mexico. In: Gardner LI, Amacher P, eds. Endocrine aspects of malnutrition. Santa Ynez, CA: The Kroc Foundation, 1973: 31.
95. Pimstone BL, Barbezat G, Jansen JDL, Murray P. Studies on growth hormone secretion in protein-calorie malnutrition. Clin Nutr 1973; 21:482–487.
96. Beas F, Contreras I, Maccioni A, Arenas S. Growth hormone in infant malnutrition: the arginine test in marasmus and kwashiorkor. Br J Nutr 1971; 26:169–175.
97. Beas F, Muzzo S. Growth hormone and malnutrition: the Chilean experience. Santa Ynez, CA: The Kroc Foundation, 1973.
98. Robinson H, Cocks T, Kerr D, Picou D. Fasting and postprandial levels of plasma insulin and growth hormone in malnourished Jamaican children, during catch-up growth and after complete recovery. In: Gardner LI, Amacher P, eds. Santa Ynez, CA: The Kroc Foundation, 1973: 45.
99. Beas F, Monckeberg F, Horwitz I, Figueroa M. The responses of the thyroid gland to thyroid-stimulating hormone (TSH) in infants with malnutrition. Pediatrics 1966; 38:1003.
100. Mulinos MG, Pomerantz L. Pseudo-hypophysectomy: a condition resembling hypophysectomy produced by malnutrition. J Nutr 1940; 19:493–504.
101. Clemmons DR, Snyder DK, Williams R, Underwood LE. Growth hormone administration conserves lean body mass during dietary restriction in obese subjects. J Clin Endocrinol Metab 1987; 64:878–883.
102. Manson JMcK, Wilmore DW. Positive nitrogen balance with human growth hormone and hypocaloric intravenous feeding. Surgery 1986; 100:188–197.
103. Ward HC, Halliday D, Sim AJW. Protein and energy metabolism with biosynthetic human growth hormone after gastrointestinal surgery. Ann Surg 1987; 206:56–61.
104. Zeigler TR, Young LS, Manson JMcK, Wilmore DW. Metabolic effects of recombinant human growth hormone in patients receiving parenteral nutrition. Ann Surg 1988; 208:6–16.
105. Davenport ML, Svoboda ME, Koerber KL, VanWyk JJ, Clemmons DR, Underwood LE. Serum concentrations of insulin-like growth factor II are not changed by short term fasting and refeeding. J Clin Endocrinol Metab 1988; 67:1231–1236.
106. Grant DB, Hambley J, Becker D, Primstone BL. Reduced sulphation factor in undernourished children. Arch Dis Child 1973; 48:596.
107. Van den Brande JL, Du Caju MVL. Plasma somatomedin activity in children with growth disturbance. In: Raiti S, ed. Advances in human growth hormone research. Washington, DC: U.S. Government Printing Office, 1974: 98.
108. Hintz RL. Plasma somatomedin and growth hormone values in children with protein-calorie malnutrition. J Pediatr 1978; 92:153.
109. Smith IF. Blood plasma levels of cortisol, insulin, growth hormone and somatomedin in children with marasmus, kwashiorkor and intermediate forms of protein-energy malnutrition. Proc Soc Exp Biol Med 1981; 167:607–611.
110. Lecornu M, David L, Francois R. Low somatomedin activity in celiac disease. Helv Paediatr Acta 1978; 33:509–516.
111. Rappaport R, Prevot C, Czernichow P. Somatomedin activity and growth hormone secretion I. Changes related to body weight in anorexia nervosa. Acta Paediatr Scand 1980; 69:37–41.
112. Salmon WD, Holladay LA, Burkhalter VJ. Inhibitors of somatomedin activity. In: Giordano G, Van Wyk JJ, Minuto F, eds. Somatomedins and growth. London: Academic Press, 1979.
113. Ashton IK, Franics MJO. An assay for plasma somatomedin: ^{3}H thymidine incorporation by isolated rabbit chondrocytes. J Endocrinol 1977; 74:205–212.
114. Van den Brande JL. Further observations on plasma somatomedin activity in children. Adv Metab Dis 1975; 8:171.
115. Phillips LS, Young HS. Nutrition and somatomedin: II. Serum somatomedin activity and cartilage growth activity in streptozotocin diabetic rats. Diabetes 1976; 25:516.
116. Salmon WD. Interaction of somatomedin and a peptide inhibitor of serum of hypophysectomized and starved rats. Adv Metab 1975; 8:183–199.
117. Salmon WD, Holladay LA, Burkhalter VJ. Partial characterization of somatomedin inhibitor in starved rat serum. Endocrinology 1983; 112:1360.
118. Bomboy JD Jr, Burkhalter J, Nicholson WE, Salmon WD. Similarity of somatomedin inhibitor in sera from starved, hypophysectomized and diabetic rats: distinction from a heat-stable inhibitor of rat cartilage metabolism. Endocrinology 1983; 112:371.
119. Vassilopoulou-Sellin R, Phillips LS, Reichard LA. Nutrition and somatomedin: VII. Regulation of somatomedin activity by the perfused rat liver. Endocrinology 1980; 106:260.
120. Phillips LS, Scholz TD. Nutrition and somatomedin. IX. Blunting of insulin-like activity by inhibitor in diabetic rat serum. Diabetes 1982; 31:97–106.
121. Phillips LS, Goldstein S, Gavin III JR. Nutrition and somatomedin XVI: Somatomedins and somatomedin inhibitors in fasted and refed rats. Metabolism 1988; 37:209–216.
122. Busby WH, Snyder DK, Clemmons DR. Radioimmunoassay of a

26,000-dalton plasma insulin-like growth factor-binding protein: control by nutritional variables. J Clin Endocrinol Metab 1988; 67:1225–1230.

123. Clemmons DR. Reduction of plasma immunoreactive somatomedin-C during fasting in humans. J Clin Endocrinol Metab 1981; 53:1247.

124. Smith AT, Clemmons DR, Underwood LE, Ben-Ezra V, McMurray R. The effect of exercise on plasma somatomedin-C/insulin-like growth factor I concentrations. Metabolism 1987; 36:533–537.

125. Soliman AT, Gassan AEHI, Aref MK, Hintz RL, Rosenfeld RG, Rogol AD. Serum insulin-like growth factors I and II: concentrations and growth hormone and insulin responses to arginine infusion in children with protein-calorie malnutrition before and after nutritional rehabilitation. Pediatr Res 1986; 20:1122–1130.

126. Clemmons DR, Underwood LE, Dickerson RN, et al. Use of plasma somatomedin-C/insulin-like growth factor I measurements to monitor the response to nutritional repletion in malnourished patients. Am J Clin Nutr 1985; 41:191–198.

127. Unterman TG, Vazquez RM, Slas AJ, Martyn PA, Phillips LS. Nutrition and somatomedin. XIII. Usefulness of somatomedin-C in nutritional assessment. Am J Med 1985; 78:228–234.

128. Kirschner BS, Sutton MM. Somatomedin-C levels in growth-impaired children and adolescents with chronic inflammatory bowel disease. Gastroenterology 1986; 91:830–836.

129. Isley WL, Underwood LE, Clemmons DR. Dietary components that regulate serum somatomedin-C concentrations in humans. J Clin Invest 1983; 71:175.

130. Prewitt TE, D'Ercole AJ, Switzer BR, Van Wyk JJ. Relationship of serum immunoreactive somatomedin-C to dietary protein and energy in growing rats. J Nutr 1982; 112:144.

131. Merimee TJ, Zapf J, Foresch ER. Insulin-like growth factors in the fed and fasted states. J Clin Endocrinol Metab 1982; 55:999.

132. Baxter RC, Bryson JM, Turtle JR. The effect of fasting on liver receptors for prolactin and growth hormone. Metabolism 1981; 30:1086–1090.

133. Postel-Vinay MC, Cohen-Tanugi E, Charrier J. Growth hormone receptors in rat liver membranes: effect of fasting and refeeding, and correlation with plasma somatomedin activity. Mol Cell Endocrinol 1982; 28:657–669.

134. Maes M, Underwood LE, Ketelslegers J-M. Plasma somatomedin-C in fasted and refed rats: close relationship with changes in liver somatogenic but not lactogenic binding sites. J Endocrinol 1983; 97:243–252.

135. Maiter D, Maes M, Underwood LE, Fliesen T, Gerard G, Ketelslegers J-M. Early changes in serum concentrations of somatomedin-C induced by dietary protein deprivation in rats: contributions of growth hormone receptor and post-receptor defects. J Endocrinol 1988; 118:113–120.

136. Cahill GF. Hormone fuel interrelationships during fasting. J Clin Invest 1966; 45:1751.

137. Pimstone B, Becker D, Weinkove C, Mann M. Insulin secretion in protein-calorie malnutrition. In: Gardner LI, Amacher P, eds. Endocrine aspects of malnutrition. Santa Ynez, CA: The Kroc Foundation, 1973: 289.

138. Rao RH. Diabetes in the undernourished: coincidence or consequence? Endocrinology 1988; 9:67–87.

139. Goldbloom RB. Failure to thrive. Pediatr Clin North Am 1982; 29:151–166.

140. Powell GF, Brasel JA, Blizzard RM. Emotional deprivation and growth retardation simulating idiopathic hypopituitarism: I. Clinical evaluation of the syndrome. N Engl J Med 1967; 276:1271–1287.

141. Patton RG, Gardner LI. Deprivation dwarfism (psychosocial deprivation): disordered family environment as a cause of so-called idiopathic hypopituitarism. In: Gardner LI, ed. Endocrine and genetic diseases of childhood and adolescence. 2nd ed. Philadelphia: WB Saunders, 1975: 85–98.

142. Widdowson EM. Mental contentment and physical growth. Lancet 1951: i:1316–1318.

143. Talbot NB. Dwarfism in healthy children: its possible relation to emotional, nutritional and endocrine disturbances. N Engl J Med 1947; 236:783–793.

144. Powell GR, Brasel JA, Raiti S, Blizzard RM. Emotional deprivation and growth retardation simulating idiopathic hypopituitarism: II. Endocrinologic evaluation of the syndrome. N Engl J Med 1967; 276:1279–1283.

145. Powell GF, Hopwood NJ, Barratt ES. Growth hormone studies before and during catch-up growth in a child with emotional deprivation and short stature. J Clin Endocrinol Metab 1973; 37:674–679.

146. Miller JD, Tannenbaum GS, Colle E, Guyda HJ. Daytome pulsatile growth hormone secretion during childhood and adolescence. J Clin Endocrinol Metab 1982; 55:989–993.

147. Fraiser SD, Rallisen ML. Growth retardation and emotional deprivation: relative resistance to treatment with human growth hormone. J Pediatr 1946; 80:603.

148. Tanner JM, Whitehouse RH, Hughes PCR, Vince FP. The effects of human growth hormone treatment for 1 to 7 years on growth of 100 children with growth hormone deficiency, low birth weight, inherited smallness, Turner's syndrome and other complaints. Arch Dis Child 1971; 46:745.

149. Whitten CR, Pettit MG, Fischoff J. Evidence that growth failure from maternal deprivation is secondary to undereating. JAMA 1969; 209:1675–1682.

150. Krieger I, Mellinger RC. Pituitary function in the deprivation syndrome. J Pediatr 1971; 79:216–225.

151. Pugliese MT, Lifshitz F, Grad G, Fort P, Marks-Katz M. Fear of obesity: a cause of short stature and delayed puberty. N Engl J Med 1983; 309:513–518.

152. Pugliese MT, Weyman-Daum M, Moses N, Lifshitz F. Parental health beliefs as a cause of nonorganic failure to thrive. Pediatrics 1987; 80:175–182.

153. Talbot NB. Obesity in children. Med Clin North Am 1945; 29:1217.

154. Forbes GB. Nutrition and growth. J Pediatr 1977; 91:40–42.

155. Garn SM, Haskell JA. Fat thickness and developmental status in childhood and adolescence. Am J Dis Child 1960; 99:746–751.

156. Johnston FE, Mack RW. Obesity, stature, and one year relative weight of 15-year-old youths. Hum Biol 1980; 52:35–41.

157. Garn SM, Rosenberg KR, Schaefer AE. Relationship between fatness level and size attainment in Central America. Ecol Food Nutr 1983; 13:157.

158. Paulsen EP, Richenderfer L, Ginsberg-Fellner F. Plasma glucose, free fatty acids, and immunoreactive insulin in sixty-six obese children. Diabetes 1968; 17:261–269.

159. Bucher H, Zapf J, Torresani T, Prader A, Froesch EF, Illig R. Insulin-like growth factors I and II, prolactin, and insulin in 19 growth hormone-deficient children with excessive, normal or decreased longitudinal growth after operation for craniopharyngioma. N Engl J Med 1983; 309:1142–1146.

160. Frohman LA, Bernardis LL. Growth hormone and insulin in weanling rats with ventromedial hypothalamic lesions. Endocrinology 1968; 82:1125–1132.

161. Caufriez A, Golstein J, Furlanetto RW, Copinschi G. Effect of fasting on immunoreactive somatomedin-C levels in obese subjects. Presented at the 64th Annual Meeting of the Endocrine Society, San Francisco, California, June 16–18, 1982.

162. Underwood LE, Smith EP, Clemmons DR, Maes M, Marter D, Ketelslegers J-M. The production and actions of insulin-like growth factors: their relationship to mutation and growth. In: Tanner M, ed. Auxology 88: perspectives in the science of growth and development. London: Smith-Gordon and Co Ltd, 1989:235.

163. Schneider BS, Hirsch J. Hypothalmic-pituitary function in obesity. In: Freinkel N, ed. New York: Plenum Press, 1982: 119.

164. Bernal J, Refetoff S. The action of thyroid hormone. Clin Endocrinol 1977; 7:227–249.

165. Danforth E Jr, Burger A. The role of thyroid hormones in the control of energy expenditure. Clin Endocrinol Metab 1984; 13:581–595.

166. Evans RM. The steroid and thyroid hormone receptor superfamily. Science 1988; 240:889–895.

167. Fisher DA, Hoath S, Lakshmanan J. The thyroid hormone effects on growth and development may be mediated by growth factors. Endocrinol Exp 1982; 16:259–271.

168. Burstein PJ, Draznin B, Johnson DJ, Schalch DS. The effect of hypothyroidism on growth, serum growth hormone, the growth hormone-dependent somatomedin, insulin-like growth factor, and its carrier protein in rats. Endocrinology 1979; 104:1107.

169. Coiro U. Effect of hypothyroidism and thyroxine replacement in growth hormone in the rat. Endocrinology 1979; 105:641.

170. Urist MR, DeLang RJ, Finerman GAM. Bone cell differentiation and growth factors. Science 1983; 220:680.

171. Wegnez M, Schachter BS, Baxter JD, Martial JA. Hormone regulation of growth hormone messenger RNA. DNA 1982; 1:145.

172. Katz HP, Youlton R, Kaplan SL, Grumbach MM. Growth and growth hormone: III. Growth hormone release in children with primary

hypothyroidism and thyrotoxicosis. J Clin Endocrinol Metab 1969; 29:346.

173. Root AW, Rosenfield RL, Bongiovanni AM, Eberlein WR. The plasma growth hormone response to insulin-induced hypoglycemia in children with retardation of growth. Pediatrics 1967; 39:844.

174. Froesch ER. Nonsuppressible insulin-like activity and thyroid hormones: major pituitary-dependent sulfation factors for chick embryo cartilage. Proc Natl Acad Sci USA 1976; 73:2904–2908.

175. Dearden LC, Espinosa T. Comparison of mineralization of the tibial epiphyseal plate in immature rats following treatment with cortisone, propylthiouracil or after fasting. Calcif Tissue Res 1974; 15:93–110.

176. Burch WM, Lebovitz HE. Triiodothyronine stimulates maturation of porcine growth-plate cartilage in vitro. J Clin Invest 1982; 70:496–504.

177. Burch WM, Van Wyk JJ. Triiodothyronine stimulates cartilage growth and maturation by different mechanisms. Am J Physiol (Endocrinol Metab 15) 1987; 252:E176–E182.

178. Jung RT, Shetty PS, James WPT. The effect of refeeding after semi-starvation on catecholamine and thyroid metabolism. Int J Obes 1980; 4:95–100.

179. Vagnati L, Finley RJ, Hagg S, Aoki TT. Protein conservation during prolonged fast: a function of triiodothyronine levels. Trans Assoc Am Phys 1978; 91:169–179.

180. O'Dea K, Esler M, Leonard P, et al. Noradrenaline turnover during under- and overeating in normal weight subjects. Metabolism 1982; 31:896–899.

181. O'Brian JT. Thyroid hormone homeostasis in states of relative caloric deprivation. Metabolism 1980; 29:721–729.

182. Vagnati L, Finley RJ, Hagg S, Aoki TT. Protein conservation during prolonged fast: a function of triiodothyronine levels. Trans Assoc Am Phys 1978; 91:169–179.

183. Wartofsky L, Burman D. Alterations in thyroid function in patients with systemic illness: the "euthyroid sick syndrome." Endocr Rev 1982; 3:164.

184. Azizi F. Effect of dietary composition on fasting-induced changes in serum thyroid hormones and thyrotropin. Metabolism 1978; 27:935–942.

185. Spaulding SW, Chopra IJ, Sherwin RS, Lyall SS. Effect of caloric restriction and dietary composition on serum T_3 and reverse T_3 in man. J Clin Endocrinol Metab 1976; 42:197–200.

186. Pimstone B, Becker D, Hendricks S. TSH response to synthetic thyrotropin-releasing hormone in human protein calorie malnutrition. J Clin Endocrinol Metab 1973; 36:779–783.

187. Rastogi GK, Sawhney RC, Panda NC, Tripathy BB. Thyroid hormone levels in adult protein calorie malnutrition (PCM). Horm Metab Res 1974; 6:528–529.

188. Danforth E. Dietary-induced alterations in thyroid hormone metabolism during overnutrition. J Clin Invest 1979; 64:1336–1347.

189. Yeh K-Y, Moog F. Development of the small intestine in the hypophysec-

tomized rat. II. Influence of cortisone, thyroxine, growth hormone, and prolactin. Dev Biol 1975; 47:173–184.

190. Moog F, Yeh K-Y. Pinocytosis persists in the ileum of hypophysectomized rats unless closure is induced by thyroxine or cortisone. Dev Biol 1979; 69:159–169.

191. Yeh K-Y. Corticosterone concentrations in the serum and milk of lactating rats: parallel changes after induced stress. Endocrinology 1984; 115:1364–1370.

192. Henning SJ. Ontogeny of enzymes in the small intestine. Ann Rev Physiol 1985; 47:231–245.

193. Little JM, Lester R. Ontogenesis of intestinal bile salt absorption in the neonatal rat. Am J Physiol (Gastrointest Liver Physiol) 1980; 239:G319–G323.

194. Alleyne GAO, Young VH. Adrenocortical function in children with severe protein-calorie malnutrition. Clin Sci 1967; 33:189.

195. Leonard PJ, MacWilliam KW. The binding of aldosterone in the serum in kwashiorkor. Am J Clin Nutr 1965; 16:360.

196. Rao KSJ, Srikantia SG, Gopalan C. Plasma cortisol levels in protein-calorie malnutrition. Arch Dis Child 1968; 43:365–367.

197. Lunn PG, Whitehead RG, Baker BA, Austin S. The effect of cortisone acetate on the course of development of experimental protein-energy malnutrition in rats. Br J Nutr 1976; 36:537–550.

198. Eveleth PB, Tanner JM. Worldwide variation in human growth. Cambridge: Cambridge University Press, 1976.

199. Smith SR, Chhetri MK, Johanson AJ, Radfar N, Migeon CJ. The pituitary-gonadal axis in men with protein-calorie malnutrition. J Clin Endocrinol Metab 1975; 41:60–69.

200. Klibanski A. Reproductive function during fasting in men. J Clin Endocrinol Metab 1981; 53:258–263.

201. Warren MP. The effects of exercise on pubertal progression and reproductive function in girls. J Clin Endocrinol Metab 1980; 51:1150.

202. Frisch RE, Gotz-Welbergen AV, McArthur JW, Albright J, Witschi J, Herman H. Delayed menarche and amenorrhea of college athletes in relation to age of onset of training. JAMA 1981; 246:1559.

203. Frisch RE, McArthur JW. Menstrual cycles: fatness as a determinant of minimum weight for height necessary for their maintenance or onset. Science 1974; 185:949.

204. Glass AR, Herbert DC, Anderson J. Fertility onset, spermatogenesis, and pubertal development in male rats: effect of graded underfeeding. Pediatr Res 1986; 20:1161–1167.

205. Tweedle D, Walton C, Johnston IDA. The effect of an anabolic steroid on postoperative nitrogen balance. Br J Clin Pract 1972; 27:130–132.

206. Watson RN, Bradley MH, Callahan R, et al. A six month evaluation of an anabolic drug, norethandrolone, in underweight persons. Am J Med 1959; 26:238–242.

207. Thaysen JH. Anabolic steroids in the treatment of renal failure. In: Gross F, ed. Protein metabolism. Berlin: Springer-Verlag, 1962: 450.

208. Wilson JD. Androgen abuse by athletes. Endocr Rev 1988; 9:181–199.

Vomiting and Regurgitation

John A. Dodge, M.D., F.R.C.P. (Lon., Edin., Ire.), D.C.H.

"Many times the stomake of ye child is so feble that it cannot retayne eyther meate or drynke."

Thomas Phaire, The Boke of Chyldren, 1553

Vomiting is such a familiar feature of early infancy that Shakespeare could describe the infant "mewling and puking in the nurse's arms" as the first of the seven ages of man. It is very difficult to define a clinical boundary between acceptable regurgitation and pathologic vomiting, and all pediatricians recognize the variations in threshold of concern among different mothers. The presence of failure to thrive in association with regurgitation, while helpful, is not in itself a reliable indicator of the need for further investigation, because sometimes an infant with a definite abnormality may have gained weight well in spite of his symptom.

Despite the clinical overlap of symptoms, vomiting is a well-defined, complex, co-ordinated process under central nervous system control, whereas regurgitation, which has not been subject to the same physiologic scrutiny, appears to be a simpler phenomenon. The presence of autonomic prodromal signs (nausea) and the muscular effort involved in true vomiting are helpful distinguishing features that are not always elicited in a standard medical history. Regurgitation ("spitting," posseting) is a frequent symptom of (but not synonymous with) gastroesophageal reflux.

PATHOPHYSIOLOGY OF VOMITING

Vomiting is a highly integrated, mainly somatic reflex response to a variety of stimuli. The muscular activity involved affects the respiratory muscles at least as much as the abdominal muscles. Many of the published studies of vomiting have been carried out in animals, and those in man focus on adults. The latter have mainly been observations made during radiographic examination. The early studies of Borison and Wang[1] are widely quoted. They defined vomiting as forceful expulsion of gastrointestinal (GI) contents through the mouth. It can be subdivided into three distinct phases: nausea, retching, and emesis.

Nausea

Nausea is a psychic sensation that may be induced by visceral, labyrinthine, or emotional stimuli and may not always progress to retching or vomiting. It is characterized by an imminent desire to vomit, which may be felt in the throat or abdomen. It is often associated with autonomic symptoms

and signs such as salivation, pallor, sweating, and tachycardia as well as anorexia. Vomiting caused by raised intracranial pressure or by mechanical obstruction is often not preceded by nausea. Active peristalsis ceases during nausea, and the lowest part of the greater curvature descends rather abruptly. In contrast to loss of tone in the fundus and body of the stomach, frequent contractions are seen in the gastric antrum (tachygastria), along with generalized contraction of the second part of the duodenum.[2] Tachygastria is also evoked by motion sickness in man and is closely related to the symptoms of nausea.[3,4] The duodenal bulb is distended, and reflux occurs from the bulb into the stomach.[5,6] Retrograde peristalsis has been shown to occur within the stomach and from as far as the upper jejunum.[7]

Retching

Retching may, of course, occur without vomiting. Retching involves a series of spasmodic and abortive respiratory movements with the glottis closed, during which an inspiratory effort of the chest muscles and diaphragm, creating a negative intrathoracic pressure, occurs simultaneously with an expiratory contraction of the abdominal muscles. The diaphragm moves downward violently with each retching movement, but the range of movement is initially small.

At the same time, movements of the stomach and its contents take place. The fundus dilates and remains flaccid, but the antrum and pylorus contract. Radiologic observations of pyloric contraction have been confirmed by gastroscopy, one of the earliest being the observation by Schindler, who noted that "retching usually interferes so much with the examination that it is not possible to observe the behavior of the stomach, but on two occasions it was possible to do so. Longitudinal folds appeared in a previously smooth antrum and rather quickly thickened, came together, and completely closed the antrum."[8]

Emesis

Retching culminates in a powerful sustained contraction of the abdominal muscles, accompanied by increased descent of the diaphragm. All of the diaphragm is seen to contract, apart from the hiatal portion, which relaxes.[9] For vomiting to occur the antireflux mechanism must be overcome, and this is not entirely explained by the increase in abdominal pressure, although sustained strong contractions of the abdominal muscles are an important component. The only portions of the stomach which contract during vomiting are the pylorus and antrum, the fundus and esophagus being relaxed and the mouth being open. The relaxation of the lower esophagus observed during vomiting is so marked that it has been described as funneling.[6,10]

Radiologic observations in animals and man show that vomiting and retching are accompanied by a temporary herniation above the diaphragm of the gastroesophageal sphincter and a loculus of stomach.[6,10] Displacement of the cardia into the thorax and elimination of the abdominal esophagus means that the lower esophageal sphincter cannot be augmented by the external pressure support it receives when normally placed within the abdomen. Increases in intra-abdominal pressure and contraction of the stomach transmitted through the lower esophagus can then easily overcome contraction of the relatively weak lower esophageal sphincter and its antireflux function. This is one reason why vomiting is often a prominent feature of anatomic hiatal hernias, particularly when they are small; a large hernia could to some extent act as a reservoir for contents regurgitated from the distal portion of the stomach.

McCarthy et al[11] studied the emetic process by correlating radiology, intrathoracic and intra-abdominal pressure changes, and electromyographic activity of the diaphragm during vomiting in the decerebrate cat. They showed that during a single emetic episode there were repeated negative thoracic and coincidental positive abdominal pressure pulses, which coincided radiographically with the rapid descent of the diaphragm to engulf the fundus of the stomach and abolish the intra-abdominal portion of the esophagus. With each repetition of this cycle there was reflux of gastric contents into the esophagus, with the formation of a sliding hiatal hernia. When expulsion occurred it was characterized by a positive thoracic pressure pulse, which distinguished the preceding retching from the vomiting that then occurred. At this point the diaphragm ascended rapidly without the stomach returning to the abdomen, and the compression of the herniated stomach was accompanied by expulsion of the vomitus.[11]

Projectile vomiting is preceded and accompanied by particularly vigorous and deep gastric peristaltic waves. It can be observed both clinically and radiologically. Projectile vomiting is typically associated with hypertrophic pyloric stenosis but may also be seen when there is a motor dysfunction of the pylorus (pylorospasm) and when there is an anatomic hiatal hernia. The combination of hiatal hernia and hypertrophic pyloric stenosis is known as the phrenopyloric or Roviralta syndrome.[12] This combination occurs 10 times more frequently than would be expected by chance[13] and underlines, but does not explain, the intimate association between lower esophageal and pyloric function. Hiatal hernia is a malformation present from birth, whereas infantile pyloric stenosis is almost always acquired postnatally.[14] Whatever may be the sequence of events giving rise to the phrenopyloric syndrome, there is no doubt that afferent signals arising from the lower esophagus are a potent stimulus to vomiting. There is also evidence that lower esophageal sphincter pressure is modified by gut regulatory peptides, particularly gastrin,[15] and this same peptide promotes contraction and, in young animals, actual hypertrophy of the pyloric circular muscle.[16,17] However, studies in healthy newborn infants have shown no correlation between serum gastrin levels and resting lower esophageal sphincter pressure,[18] although some relationships were observed following feeding.[19] A variant of the phrenopyloric syndrome has been described in neonates, in which incompetence and reflux through both the pylorus and the lower esophageal sphincter co-exist. It has been attributed to a deficiency of the gut hormone motilin.[20]

Nervous Control of Vomiting

The act of vomiting, including the physiologic correlates of nausea and retching, is under central nervous control, and two areas in the medulla are involved. A so-called *vomiting center* is found in the region of the medulla corresponding to the nucleus solitarius and an adjacent portion of the lateral reticular formation. It is close to other medullary centers concerned with respiration, inspiratory and expiratory centers, the vasomotor center, the salivatory nuclei, the vestibular nuclei, and the bulbofacilitatory and inhibitory systems.[1]

Although the concept of a vomiting center may be simplistic, it has received support by the observation of a family in which individuals with hereditary ataxia are unable to vomit. The failure to vomit is present from an early age, the gag reflux is absent, and there is no emetic response to intravenous apomorphine. The ataxia develops later. It is an autosomal dominant disorder, and the clinical features suggest that the neurologic lesion is situated in the medulla, involving the vomiting center.[21]

Despite this and much other evidence, the vomiting center cannot be precisely circumscribed, and recent studies[22,23] have cast doubt upon its existence as a single entity. An alternative model[24,25] proposes that instead of a single "vomiting" center that co-ordinates outputs from various sources, individual effector nuclei involved in the motor output of vomiting interact, so that the co-ordinated response is a result of these nuclei acting together. Local "paracrine" factors could be involved. This concept explains why all the motor components of vomiting have other important and regular main functions and do not produce vomiting in normal circumstances. This looser definition does not invalidate the basic fact that the motor control of vomiting lies in the medulla.

The center or centers concerned may be activated by afferent impulses arising from the posterior pharynx, the abdomen, or other parts of the brain. Taste sensation and gastric vagal afferent pathways converge in the medulla, and gastric afferents can modulate the gustatory pathway.[26] Nausea can be initiated via either of these closely associated pathways, either by unpleasant taste or, more commonly, by vagal sensations originating in the upper alimentary tract. These may be from mechanoreceptors (distention)[27] or mucosal chemoreceptors.[28] Local vagovagal reflexes explain the relaxation of the proximal stomach seen prior to emesis.[18] The medullary center is also activated by impulses from a second center that is known as the *chemoreceptive trigger zone*, which lies in the area postrema in the floor of the fourth ventricle. This region is sensitive to a variety of chemical agents, typified by apomorphine, but not to electrical stimulation. It is regarded as an afferent station for the vomiting center and cannot itself produce vomiting unless the medullary "vomiting center(s)" is intact.[1] This region can be activated to evoke emesis in two ways: directly by endogenous or exogenous agents, or by stimuli derived from the gut or elsewhere and transmitted by further vagal afferents. A wide variety of potential neurotransmitters, receptors, and enzymes have been demonstrated in the area postrema.[30] It is particularly rich in opiate receptors, enkephalins, and dopamine. Examples of agents acting directly on this "center" include exogenous opiates, ipecac, digoxin, and cytotoxic agents, and endogenous agents probably include enkephalins[31] and adrenaline[32] as well as high blood levels of urea, ammonia, ketone bodies, and other toxic metabolites. It is also believed that certain stimuli arising from the gut or elsewhere (e.g., radiation exposure) may release an endogenous "emetic" agent, possibly peptide YY, which can have a humoral effect on the area postrema.[33] The "parenteral" vomiting associated with acute febrile illnesses remote from the gut such as meningitis, tonsillitis, otitis media, pneumonia, and urinary tract infection is of uncertain pathophysiology but could utilize any of these afferent systems.

The main efferent fibers concerned with vomiting are carried in the phrenic nerves, spinal nerves, and special efferent fibers from the vagus to the voluntary muscles of the pharynx and larynx.

CLINICAL SIGNIFICANCE OF VOMITING

A recent and useful concept of vomiting regards it as one of the defense systems of the body, serving to identify and remove accidentally ingested toxins.[24] According to this view, the function of nausea, which has long been a mystery, can be explained as a protective reflex. The anorectic component of nausea prevents further ingestion of toxic material, while the unpleasant sensations aroused create a behavioral aversion response to the offending food or other stimulus. The reversed upper alimentary peristalsis seen during nausea, retching, and vomiting probably serves to protect the jejunum from diarrheagenic agents, including some (such as hyperosmolar solutions) that might overload its absorptive capacity.

The "side effect" of vomiting seen with a variety of drugs, particularly those such as cytotoxic agents and cardiac glycosides, can then be viewed as an appropriate physiologic protective response to a toxin. Similarly, the nausea and vomiting experienced in acute food allergy (e.g., to shellfish) or less spectacular food intolerances (e.g., some cases of cow's milk protein intolerance) are also easily understood.

The protective function of vomiting also goes some way to explain the true vomiting, often projectile, seen in some babies with gastroesophageal reflux. The rather leisurely regurgitation, apparently without nausea or discomfort, experienced by the majority of such infants is unlikely to be associated with esophagitis. When, however, esophageal afferents are stimulated by refluxed gastric acid on an inflamed or ulcerated mucosa, the response of the organism is to remove the offending agent as soon as possible, and coordinated vomiting results. This also explains why infants with pyloric stenosis may continue to vomit after surgery until coexisting esophagitis has healed.[34]

Finally, putative gut-derived "emetic" agents[33] explain the vomiting response to radiation and endogenous toxins, seen, for example, in some inborn metabolic errors, if the more "natural" trigger factor for such an agent's release is an ingested toxin. Such a humoral agent could function as a backup system of defense against toxins that have escaped recognition by taste and have failed to adequately activate the gastric chemoreceptor-vagal pathway.

REGURGITATION AND REFLUX

Almost all babies regurgitate from time to time. Such benign regurgitation occurs without apparent nausea and without retching. It is effortless and probably represents nothing more than the ultimate degree of gastroesophageal reflux. We know that a variable amount of reflux is universal in infancy and indeed occurs from time to time throughout life, so that infants who regurgitate may represent merely the end of a physiologic spectrum. Reflux often occurs without regurgitation, but it is self-evident that regurgitation cannot occur without reflux.

The important complications of frequent reflux are esophagitis and aspiration into the lungs of gastric contents. Both anatomic and physiologic factors appear to determine the severity of the reflux and the incidence of these complications.

Anatomic Factors

The lower esophageal sphincter is situated above the diaphragm in early infancy, perhaps until the age of 6 months.[35,36] Location of the sphincter above the diaphragm means that it is exposed to negative intrathoracic pressures during the respiratory cycle, and if a strong positive abdominal or intragastric pressure should happen to coincide with a negative pressure in the chest, contraction of the sphincter may be inadequate to prevent reflux.

Reflux was found to be much more benign when not associated with a hiatal hernia (partial thoracic stomach) in the large series studied by Carré over more than 30 years. None of more than 1,000 infants with radiologic evidence of reflux in the absence of a hiatal hernia developed a stricture, and none required surgery, whereas 5 percent of those with a partial thoracic stomach developed a stricture, and about 30 percent of untreated patients still had troublesome symptoms beyond 4 years of age.[37] The incidence of hiatal hernias in infancy seems to vary widely between centers, and there is evidence that this variation is related to clinical awareness and the techniques of investigation employed.[27,38] Eighty percent of infants with esophagitis in a series studied by Toccalino and his colleagues had an associated hiatal hernia.[39]

Physiologic Factors

The lower esophageal sphincter pressure is relatively low at birth but may reach "normal" levels within the first month.[40] In a series of 4,000 manometric studies on 680 apparently normal infants, Boix-Ochoa and Canals[41] showed that gradual maturation of lower esophageal sphincter pressure occurred by the age of 6 to 7 weeks regardless of gestational age or weight. Sphincter pressures may exceed adult values during the first year of life.[40] On the other hand, a study of 285 asymptomatic infants using the technique of 24-hour esophageal pH monitoring documented frequent gastroesophageal reflux in babies older than 4 months of age.[42] The authors suggested that buffering of gastric acid by milk would mask reflux when it was sought by this technique in younger infants.

These findings indicate that lower esophageal maturation as measured by pressure studies occurs within several weeks after birth, and therefore immaturity of lower esophageal sphincter strength cannot explain the observed frequency of reflux,[43] because sphincter pressure values in normals and refluxers overlap. However, sphincter pressure can vary with time, position, various circulating factors, the volume of gastric contents, and abdominal and thoracic pressures. Transient relaxations of the sphincter have been shown to occur with gastric distention in adults.[44] Thus, although reflux can be attributed to sphincter incompetence, a variety of factors may contribute, and the changing location of the sphincter from above to below the diaphragm during the first year appears to correlate well with the amelioration of reflux over the same period.

A connection between gastric emptying and gastroesophageal reflux has been suggested, but evidence is contradictory. Delayed gastric emptying is more likely to occur in older patients and in those with more severe degrees of reflux.[46] Studies in this department have also shown that patients fall into two groups, those in whom gastric emptying is normal and those in whom it is delayed.[47]

The multiplicity of investigations for reflux suggests that none is entirely satisfactory. What is quite clear is that the mere demonstration of reflux during upper alimentary radiology is not an indication for treatment unless it is of significant degree and accompanied by appropriate symptoms. The vomiting for which the child is being investigated may well have some other cause. When the examination is carried out by an experienced and interested radiologist, however, a useful impression of the degree of reflux may be obtained. More accurate measurement can be obtained either by scintigraphy (which tends to exaggerate the clinical significance of reflux) or by prolonged pH monitoring (which is more cumbersome). Although severe degrees of esophagitis may be detectable radiologically, and a reasonable correlation exists between the presence of esophagitis and the duration of esophageal exposure to a low pH, endoscopy and biopsy must be employed if the diagnosis of esophagitis is to be confirmed.

Such invasive investigations are not justified in the great majority of otherwise healthy refluxers, and the generally benign outlook in the absence of a hiatal hernia justifies a conservative attitude to both investigation and treatment.

Infants with reflux but no hiatal hernia or esophagitis usually respond well to simple thickening of the feeds, preferably with an agent such as carob seed flour (Nestargel, Carobel), which has little or no caloric value. Postural therapy can be added if there is no response. Documented esophagitis is an indication for gastric acid suppression with an H_2-receptor antagonist (ranitidine or cimetidine)[72] or a prokinetic agent (e.g., cisapride).[66] Re-examination at this stage may reveal a hiatal hernia in nonresponders, and even then the majority respond to postural therapy. However, continued symptoms (usually vomiting rather than regurgitation), particularly when there is bleeding or other evidence of active esophagitis, indicate that surgery should be considered.[37]

IMPORTANT CAUSES OF VOMITING IN CHILDREN

"How difficult it often is to appraise exactly the significance of vomiting in infancy...! How much and how little it may mean."

George Frederic Still,
Common Disorders and Diseases of
Childhood, 1927

Reference has already been made to the frequency of vomiting as a symptom in infancy. Mild degrees of gastroesophageal reflux and associated regurgitation are sufficiently common in the first few months of life to be considered physiologic. However, vomiting is also a prominent feature of many disorders of infancy and may be the presenting or perhaps the only complaint.

The clinical approach to vomiting in infants is determined to some extent by the age of the baby. During the first week, obstructive lesions of the alimentary tract must be considered, particularly when the vomitus is bile stained. Intrauterine vomiting of bile-stained fluid has been recorded in an infant with intestinal obstruction.[48] Persistent vomiting is also a feature of some inborn metabolic errors (see Table 2). Meningeal or urinary tract infection may also present as vomiting. The common, self-limiting vomiting of "mucus" during the first few days of life is rarely severe enough to require investigation and may denote acute gastritis associated with the relatively high acid secretion of the newborn. After the first week, congenital obstructive malformations are less likely to present for the first time, but pyloric stenosis needs to be considered more seriously, as does hiatal hernia (partial thoracic stomach) with associated esophagitis. A frequent and unsatisfactory diagnosis applied to vomiting babies in whom no cause can be elicited is that of "feeding problems." This description may be applied to infants whose vomiting stops on admission to hospital without special treatment and to those whose mother may be inexperienced, overanxious, rejecting, or incompetent. Vomiting and maternal anxiety in these cases form a vicious circle that can be broken by the intervention of sympathetic and supportive nursing staff.

Diagnoses to be considered in babies whose vomiting begins after the first month include infection, metabolic disturbances such as idiopathic hypercalcemia, food intolerance (particularly to cow's milk proteins), and subdural hematoma caused by nonaccidental injury.

In older children, except those with the unusual and puzzling condition of cyclic vomiting, other important symptoms are usually present, and these generally determine the lines of investigation that are most likely to be fruitful. Important causes of acute vomiting which must always be considered in the child include appendicitis and other acute surgical emergencies, including testicular torsion, gastroenteritis (including epidemic vomiting) and food poisoning, other ingested toxins, Henoch-Schönlein purpura, basal pneumonia, and diabetic ketoacidosis. Careful history-taking and examination should identify diagnostic features in most of these.

Persistent or recurrent vomiting occurs with raised intracranial pressure, metabolic derangements such as uremia (azotemia), and migraine. It is also a feature of peptic ulcer, whereas hiatal hernia occasionally presents for the first time in older children. Anorexia nervosa may be associated with vomiting, and other psychogenic problems are dealt with below (Table 1).

CLINICAL FEATURES

The following comments apply only to those children in whom vomiting is persistent and is the principal presenting symptom. Acute abdominal emergencies presenting with vomiting are dealt with elsewhere.

History

The relationship of vomiting to meals may sometimes be helpful, particularly when peptic ulcer or obstructive lesions are being considered, but is not usually of much diagnostic value. Of greater help is a description of the vomitus: Was the volume greater than the last meal; did it smell sour; did it contain blood or coffee grounds material, bile, or mucus? Projectile vomiting, described with the typical "pyloric gesture," strongly suggests pyloric stenosis but also occurs in some infants with hiatal hernia or adrenal hyperplasia. Nocturnal vomiting in infancy is characteristic of hiatal hernia, and vomiting accompanied by apparent pain strongly suggests esophagitis. The mother may have noticed that changes in the posture of an infant affect the frequency and severity of the vomiting, and this is important because it may also suggest hiatal hernia.

In older children, it may be apparent that they vomit only after particular foods, or that the vomiting is preceded by nausea or accompanied by headache, visual disturbances, or vertigo. The child's apparent appetite is important, including any features that suggest anorexia and/or bulimia nervosa. Other symptoms that should always be inquired about include diarrhea, constipation, and jaundice. The health of other family members and recent contacts is also relevant, as is awareness of current epidemics in the community. A family history of migraine is often a useful supporting factor if this diagnosis is suspected in the child, and a close family history of peptic ulcer increases the ulcer risk in children.[49]

Examination

During the standard clinical assessment of a vomiting baby, particular attention should be paid to examination of the mouth for candidiasis and for signs of dehydration. Jaundice in a vomiting infant should lead to a consideration of hepatitis, urinary tract infection, malformations of the biliary tract, and upper alimentary obstruction including pyloric stenosis. A tense fontanelle suggests meningitis, cerebral tumor, hydrocephalus, subdural hematoma, hypercalcemia, or vitamin A intoxication. Arterial hypertension occurs in some

renal and suprarenal disorders that may present with vomiting and in coarctation of the aorta—one of the causes of cardiac failure in infancy, which itself may produce vomiting as the result of visceral and venous engorgement. Sudden onset of vomiting is sometimes the presenting feature of acute cardiac failure, such as that caused by paroxysmal tachycardia.

In the abdomen, the presence and location of distention should be noted, as well as visible peristalsis and alterations in bowel sounds. The size of palpable organs, the presence of abnormal masses, and areas of tenderness or guarding are, of course, evident on routine examination. If the history suggests pyloric stenosis, a test feed, with palpation for a pyloric tumor, is required and is best performed after the stomach has been emptied either by vomiting or through a nasogastric tube. Intermittent aspiration during the course of the test feed prevents distention of the stomach and makes it easier to feel the pylorus. If the child is in hospital, nursing staff should be asked to record intake.

Examination of the older child concentrates on the evocation of tenderness and detection of enlarged abdominal organs or abdominal masses.

Investigation

Analysis of the urine for protein, blood, bile, acetone, and reducing substances should be routinely performed. Further analysis of the urine for amino acids is indicated if a metabolic cause is suspected, and the urine should be cultured and its deposit examined microscopically.

Blood samples should be analyzed for urea and electrolytes, calcium, phosphorus, and acid-base status. Metabolic acidosis may be the first indication of an error of organic acid metabolism. Blood amino acid analysis is needed if other features are suggestive of an inborn metabolic disorder. If the history suggests liver disease, liver function tests should be performed, and if Reye syndrome is suspected blood glucose and ammonia levels should be measured.

A *plain radiograph* of the abdomen, in supine and erect postures, is necessary if obstruction is considered, and unexpected intrathoracic lesions such as cardiac malformations or diaphragmatic hernia occur sufficiently often to justify a routine chest radiograph. *Contrast radiography* has been largely superseded as investigation of first choice by abdominal *ultrasound examination*, which is particularly useful for the diagnosis of infantile hypertrophic pyloric stenosis and intussusception. The value of a barium meal is considerably influenced by the experience and interest of the radiologist, particularly for the identification of significant degrees of reflux and/or hiatal hernia.[37,38] Initial imaging of the urinary tract, when indicated, should be by ultrasonography, but *intravenous urography* and/or a micturating cystogram is required for better definition of abnormalities such as pelvic-ureteric obstruction, whereas *isotope scans* (e.g., DMSA) provide information about renal function. *Computed tomography* (CT) scans and *magnetic resonance imaging*, although of great value in selected cases, are not indicated for the investigation of vomiting per se.

In infants suspected of esophagitis, particularly those who have vomited blood, *upper alimentary endoscopy* is a valuable diagnostic procedure. In these cases, small superficial *bi-*

TABLE 1
Causes of Vomiting in Infancy and Childhood

Digestive Tract Disorders		Infective Disorders	
Functional and Psychogenic		Gastroenteritis	1, 2, 3, 4
Idiopathic neonatal vomiting	1	Epidemic vomiting	3, 4
Idiopathic infantile vomiting ("pylorospasm")	(1), 2, 3	Food poisoning	3, 4
Feeding problems ("rumination," i.e., abnormal		Thrush	1, 2
mother-child relationship)	2, 3	Urinary tract infection (also hydronephrosis and	
Cyclic vomiting	4	renal calculi)	1, 2, 3, 4
Self-induced vomiting	4	Respiratory tract infection (including otitis)	1, 2, 3, 4
		Appendicitis (and other surgical emergencies)	3, 4
Malformations and Obstructions		**Neurologic Disorders**	
Hiatal hernia and gastroesophageal reflux	1, 2, 3, 4	Meningitis and encephalitis	1, 2, 3, 4
Gastric outlet malformation	1, (2), 3, 4	Intracranial birth injury	1
Acquired gastric outlet obstructions, e.g.,		Migraine	4
corrosive gastritis, chronic granulomatous		Motion sickness	4
disease	(3), 4		
Hypertrophic pyloric stenosis	(1), 2, 3	*Increased Intracranial Pressure*	
Volvulus: gastric or intestinal	1, 2, 3, (4)	Hydrocephalus	1, 2, 3, 4
Malrotation and partial obstructions	1, 2, 3, (4)	Subdural hematoma	(1), 2, 3, 4
Atresias	1	Tumor, including diencephalic syndrome	3, 4
Meconium ileus	1	Hypertension, including renal causes	(2), 3, 4
Ménétrier's disease	4	Kernicterus	1, 2
Distal intestinal obstruction syndrome (meconium		**Toxic/Metabolic Disorders**	
ileus equivalent)	4	Adrenal hyperplasia	1, 2, 3
Inspissated milk syndrome and lactobezoar	1, 2	Phenylketonuria	1, 2
Duplications	1, 2, 3, 4	Other aminoacidopathies and organic acidurias	1, 2
Intussusception	3, 4	Galactosemia	1, 2
Aganglionic megacolon (Hirschsprung's disease)	1, 2, (3)	Hypercalcemia	2, 3, 4
Peptic ulcer	1, 2, 3	Uremia	1, 2, 3, 4
Trichobezoar	4	Neonatal cold injury	1
		Drugs, e.g., digoxin, cytotoxic agents,	
Food Intolerances		anticonvulsants	1, 2, 3, 4
Celiac disease	3	Vitamin A excess	3
Cow's milk protein intolerance	2, 3	Diabetes mellitus (ketoacidosis)	(3), 4
Other food intolerances	3	Poisons—many	3, 4
		Hepatic Disorders	
		Hepatitis	1, 2, 3
		Cardiac failure	1, 2, 3
		Reye syndrome	(3), 4

Key: 1 = first week; 2 = 1 week to 1 month; 3 = 1 month to 1 year; 4 = over 1 year.

opsies should be taken because visual appearances are often misleading. Endoscopy, with or without biopsy, may also confirm or rule out peptic ulcer, duodenitis, and gastritis in older children. If gastroesophageal reflux is observed or suspected, its degree is best determined by *esophageal pH monitoring* using a small glass electrode situated at the tip of a fine catheter. Good correlation exists between the presence of esophagitis shown on biopsy and prolonged exposure to gastric acid indicated by pH recording. *Gastroesophageal scintigraphy* is an even more sensitive method of demonstrating gastroesophageal reflux, but it may be too sensitive for routine use. It is also much less satisfactory than contrast radiology for demonstrating anatomic lesions. Its principal indication may be the investigation of recurrent unexplained lower respiratory infection in cases of suspected reflux and aspiration.

Formal *psychiatric investigation* is indicated if behavioral abnormalities are present. These include a history or findings suggestive of anorexia or bulimia nervosa, cyclic vomiting, narcotic drug ingestion, self-poisoning (or possible poisoning by others[50]), and trichotillomania.

METABOLIC CAUSES OF VOMITING

A number of inborn errors of metabolism may present in the newborn period with vomiting as a prominent symptom. Diagnosis is nearly always made on the basis of laboratory investigations, associated symptoms and physical signs being nonspecific. These other features include lethargy, reluctance to feed, failure to thrive, seizures, disturbances of tone (flaccidity or spasticity), and coma. Nonspecific metabolic abnormalities that may be found include hyperammonemia, metabolic acidosis, hypoglycemia, and ketonuria. Table 2 lists some of the more important disorders.

PSYCHOGENIC VOMITING

"My bowels cannot hide her woes
But like a drunkard I must vomit them."
William Shakespeare, Titus Andronicus, 1584

Vomiting is a well-recognized response to acute psychological distress in both children and adults. During stress and

TABLE 2
Inborn Metabolic Disorders Causing Vomiting
in Early Infancy

Urea Cycle Defects
    Carbamyl phosphate synthetase deficiency
    Ornithine transcarbamylase (OTC) deficiency
    Citrullinemia (argininosuccinate synthetase deficiency)
    Argininosuccinic aciduria (argininosuccinase deficiency)
    Hyperargininemia (arginase deficiency)

Congenital lysine intolerance

Familial (lysinuric) protein intolerance
Propionic acidemia (ketotic hyperglycinaemia)
Methylmalonic acidemia
Isovaleric acidemia
Maple syrup urine disease

Phenylketonuria
Hereditary tyrosinemia
Hypervalinemia
Galactosemia
Hyperglycinemia (nonketotic)

Congenital adrenal hyperplasia
    21-hydroxylase deficiency

Leigh's disease (subacute necrotizing encephalomyelopathy)

Idiopathic hypercalcemia

Renal tubular acidosis

From Stanbury et al.[51]

anxiety, adrenaline levels in the cerebrospinal fluid rise and may stimulate the chemoreceptor trigger zone (area postrema). Direct intraventricular injection of adrenaline evokes vomiting in cats,[52] and other endogenous neurochemicals may act in the same way.

The proposition that nausea and emesis are part of a protective reflex[24] greatly helps to explain some disorders of childhood characterized by persistent vomiting. According to this hypothesis, the vomiting constitutes a learned behavioral response to an unpleasant or potentially toxic substance. Carnivorous animals very quickly learn that certain types of potential prey are poisonous, and it is interesting to note that vomiting is a much more highly developed reflex in carnivores than in herbivores. Induction of vomiting in man by apomorphine administered with the stimulus that the subject wishes to avoid is an established method of aversion therapy. In the same way much infant vomiting could be a learned behavioral response to a particular food with unpleasant associations, and may for example follow a GI infection or a contaminated feed that induced vomiting. The usual food given at this time would be a cow's milk formula. A good clinical response to withdrawal of the offending food (milk) would then be expected and would not constitute confirmation of cow's milk "allergy" or intolerance. The absence of objective laboratory evidence of hypersensitivity, or of atopic features, in many vomiting infants labeled "allergic" is then readily understood.

Other clinical disorders that some authors believe to be psychogenic include the uncommon condition of cyclic vomiting. This was first described more than 100 years ago by Samuel Gee, who noted the varying intervals of apparently normal health between episodes of vomiting which continue for periods of a few hours to a few days. Affected children may become severely dehydrated and often require intravenous fluids until the attacks end, usually as abruptly as they began. Radiologic and other investigations, by definition, reveal no apparent cause for the episodes, and the prognosis is uncertain. Pediatricians tend to consider it a disorder of childhood, but several studies have shown that it continues into adult life.[53,55] In one series of 16 patients, all were found to have significant psychological problems. The authors considered the main abnormality to be a prolonged symbiotic relationship between the child and the parents and failure of the child to become independent.[54] It is important to avoid surgery, which not only fails to find a cause for the vomiting attacks but raises the question of possible adhesions being responsible for subsequent episodes. Some authors have reported avoidance conditioning with electric shock treatment, which has a certain logic if the vomiting itself is considered an aversion response to threatening situations,[70,71] but seems rather drastic. Resistance to psychotherapy on the part of patients and parents is frequent.[54] In another series of 44 patients, 36 percent had associated headache, and a family history of migraine was obtained in 25 percent.[56] These features are quite compatible with a psychogenic process, stress being a well-known trigger factor provoking attacks of migraine. The diagnosis of cyclic vomiting cannot be made during the first episode, and is important to rule out organic causes, including the possibility of intracranial neoplasms, when the child first presents.

The observation that infantile hypertrophic pyloric stenosis occurs more often in firstborns than would be expected by chance led to the suggestion that maternal anxiety might be a contributory cause.[57,58] Support for this suggestion comes from the finding of an excess of adverse, stressful life events during the last trimester of pregnancies producing a baby with pyloric stenosis.[59] The physiologic pathway for such a reaction remains speculative but would presumably be humoral.

Self-induced vomiting frequently occurs in anorexia nervosa, and rumination in infants is also induced by the child, with or without the use of his fingers. Mild degrees of rumination are generally regarded as a self-gratification activity. It is particularly likely to occur when the mother-infant relationship is disturbed. A particularly severe case leading to gross emaciation was an 8-month-old child of a schizophrenic mother. Extensive investigations revealed no physical cause for his vomiting, and gastrostomy feeding resulted in regurgitation. After 1 month in hospital it was realized that the baby was regurgitating voluntarily, and successful treatment was thereafter carried out by nursing staff who cuddled him, smiled, talked, and played with him.[60]

COMPLICATIONS OF VOMITING

Apart from the features of the underlying cause, vomiting itself may give rise to complications.

Mallory-Weiss Syndrome

Forcible thrusting of the gastric fundus through the hiatus during retching and vomiting sometimes produces small longitudinal tears in the mucosa. This may be suspected clinically when after several cycles of retching or vomiting the patient starts to bring up blood. The lesions can be visualized endoscopically. The bleeding is rarely serious, and the lesions usually heal without further complications.

Aspiration of Gastric Contents

Bronchial aspiration of vomitus may cause acute asphyxia. Much more commonly, repeated small episodes of aspiration give rise to recurrent respiratory infections. This may occur as a consequence of gastroesophageal reflux even without frank vomiting.[61]

Failure to Thrive

Frequent vomiting in infancy, if of adequate degree, causes failure to gain weight and malnutrition. This is not common with simple regurgitation and should stimulate efforts to find a more satisfactory diagnosis.

Dehydration and Electrolyte Disturbances

The metabolic consequences of vomiting are best exemplified in the case of infants with pyloric stenosis. Loss of hydrogen ions and chloride leads to metabolic alkalosis and hypokalemia. If unrecognized, in extreme cases it can lead to cardiac arrest. The virtual elimination of mortality from pyloric stenosis has followed recognition of the need to restore fluid and electrolyte balance before surgery.

TREATMENT OF NAUSEA AND VOMITING

Oral antiemetic drugs are clearly unlikely to be useful in the management of children with acute nausea and vomiting, unless they can be rapidly absorbed from the mouth or stomach. They are more useful when vomiting can be anticipated, as in the treatment of children with malignant disease by cytotoxic drugs or radiotherapy, or in troublesome vomiting during acute hepatitis.

Metoclopramide is a widely used and effective antiemetic agent that blocks dopamine receptors in the chemoreceptor trigger zone, thereby influencing the central control of nausea and vomiting. It commonly causes dystonic and dyskinetic reactions with oculogyric crises, particularly in children and adolescents.[62] The difference between effective and toxic doses is insufficient to justify its continued use in patients under 20 years of age.

Domperidone is a much safer drug that also blocks dopamine receptors, both in the area postrema and in the gut.[63] It may be given by mouth or rectal suppository. Bioavailability is low, because of extensive first-pass metabolism in the gut wall and liver, and it enters the brain much less readily than metoclopramide.

In comparative clinical studies, oral domperidone (up to 1 mg per kilogram body weight) was more effective than metoclopramide (0.5 mg per kilogram body weight) in preventing nausea and vomiting in children receiving cyclic cytotoxic chemotherapy.[64] The recommended dose range for children is 0.2 to 0.4 mg per kilogram by mouth at 4- to 8-hour intervals, or one to four suppositories per day according to body weight (about 4 mg per kilogram).

Cisapride is a new prokinetic drug that enhances physiologic release of acetylcholine selectively at the level of the postganglionic nerves of the myenteric plexus. It does not have dopamine-blocking properties but enhances gastroduodenal peristalsis and inhibits gastroesophageal reflux. Reported use is rapidly increasing in children, in whom it has been shown to be effective in preventing reflux and in improving clearance of refluxed material from the esophagus.[65,66,72]

Bethanechol is a stable choline ester with a selective action on muscarinic receptors. It is related to methacholine but has a longer duration of action. It has been used in the treatment of gastroesophageal reflux in children,[67,68] in whom it was shown to be significantly better than placebo in reducing the number of vomiting episodes. The pediatric dose is 0.6 mg per kilogram daily in three divided doses by mouth, or 0.15 to 0.2 mg per kilogram daily subcutaneously. No major side effects have been reported in children, but headache, abdominal pain, and hypertension have been described in adults.

A recent interesting development has been the use of selective *5-HT-3 receptor antagonists*.[69] Receptors for 5-HT are located on vagal afferent neurons and this, together with the observation that specific receptor antagonists blocked radiation-associated vomiting and also vomiting induced by the cytotoxic drug cisplatin, provides support for the hypothesis that these agents activate vagal afferents by the release of local 5-HT. Further studies of this class of drugs in animals and adults will be needed before their possible toxic effects and application to pediatrics are known.

REFERENCES

1. Borison HL, Wang SC. Physiology and pharmacology of vomiting. Pharmacol Rev 1953; 5:193–230.
2. You CH, Chey WY. Study of electromechanical activity of the stomach in humans and dogs with particular attention to tachygastria. Gastroenterology 1984; 86:1460–1468.
3. Stern RM, Koch KL, Stewart WR, Lindblad IM. Spectral analysis of tachygastria recorded during motion sickness. Gastroenterology 1987; 92:92–97.
4. Geldof H, van der Schee EJ, van Blankenstein M, Grashuis JL. Electrogastrographic study of gastric myoelectrical activity in patients with unexplained nausea and vomiting. Gut 1986; 27:799–808.
5. Barclay AE. The digestive tract. 2nd ed. London: Cambridge University Press, 1936.
6. Lumsden K, Holden WS. The act of vomiting in man. Gut 1969; 10:173–179.
7. Azpiroz F, Malagelada JR. Pressure activity patterns in the canine proximal stomach: response to distension. Am J Physiol 1984; 247:G265–272.
8. Schindler R. Gastroscopy. Chicago: University of Chicago Press, 1937.
9. Tan LK, Miller AD. Innervation of perioesophageal region of cat's diaphragm: implications for studies of control of vomiting. Neurosci Lett 1986; 68:339–344.
10. Johnson HD, Lewis JN. The cardia in swallowing, eructation and vomiting. Lancet 1966; ii:1268–1273.
11. McCarthy LE, Borison HL, Spiegel PK, Friedlander RN. Vomiting: radiographic and oscillographic correlates in the decerebrate cat. Gastroenterology 1974; 67:1126–1130.

12. Roviralta E. Les images radiologiques de la stenose hypertrophique du pylore. Arch Franc Malad Appar Digest 1950; 39:1103–1110.
13. Carré IJ. Thesis for degree of MD, University of Cambridge, 1959.
14. Dodge JA. Infantile pyloric stenosis: a multifactorial condition. In: Bergsma D, ed. Birth defects: original article series 1972; Vol VIII: 15–21. Baltimore: Williams & Wilkins.
15. Castell DO, Harris LD. Hormonal control of gastroesophageal sphincter strength. New Engl J Med 1970; 282:886–889.
16. Dodge JA. Production of duodenal ulcers and hypertrophic pyloric stenosis by administration of pentagastrin to pregnant and newborn dogs. Nature 1970; 225:284–285.
17. Dodge JA, Karim AA. Induction of pyloric hypertrophy by pentagastrin: an animal model for infantile hypertrophic pyloric stenosis. Gut 1976; 17:280–284.
18. Moroz SP, Beiko P. Relationship between low esophageal sphincter pressure and serum gastrin concentration in the newborn infant. J Pediat 1981; 99:725–728.
19. Dent J, Dodds WJ, Sekiguchi T, Hogan WJ, Arndorfer RC. Interdigestive phasic contractions of the human lower esophageal sphincter. Gastroenterology 1983; 84:453–460.
20. Rode H, Gywes S, Davies MRQ. The phreno-pyloric syndrome in symptomatic gastroesophageal reflux. J Pediatr Surg 1982; 17:280–284.
21. McLellan DL, Park DM. Failure to vomit in hereditary ataxia. Report of a family. Neurology 1973; 23:725–728.
22. Miller AD, Wilson VJ. 'Vomiting centre' reanalyzed: an electrical stimulation study. Brain Res 1983; 270:154–158.
23. Brizzee KR, Mehler WR. The central nervous connections involved in the vomiting reflex. In: Davis CJ, Lake-Bakaar GV, Grahame-Smith DG, eds. Nausea and vomiting: mechanisms and treatment. Berlin: Springer-Verlag, 1986:31.
24. Davis CJ, Harding RK, Leslie RA, Andrews PLR. The organisation of vomiting as a protective reflex: a commentary on the first day's discussion. In: Davis CJ, Lake-Bakaar GV, Grahame-Smith DG, eds. Nausea and vomiting: mechanisms and treatment. Berlin: Springer-Verlag, 1986.
25. Andrews PLR, Hawthorn J. The neurophysiology of vomiting. Clin Gastroenterol 1988; 2:141–168.
26. Glenn JF, Erickson RP. Gastric modulation of gustatory afferent activity. Physiol Behav 1976; 16:561–568.
27. Darling D, Fisher JH, Gellis SS. Hiatal hernia and gastroesophageal reflux in infants and children: analysis of the incidence in North American children. Pediatrics 1974; 54:450–455.
28. Grundy D, Scratcherd T. Sensory afferents from the gastrointestinal tract. In: Wood JD, ed. Motility and circulation of the gastrointestinal system. Handbook of Physiology. Bethesda: American Physiological Society, 1980.
29. Andrews PLR, Wood KL. Vagally mediated gastric motor and emetic reflexes evoked by stimulation of the antral mucosa in anaesthetized ferrets. J Physiol 1988; 395:1–16.
30. Leslie RA. Neuroactive substances in the dorsal vagal complex of the medulla oblongata. Neurochem Int 1985; 7:191–211.
31. Carpenter DO, Briggs DB, Strominger N. Responses of neurons of canine area postrema to neurotransmitters and peptides. Cell Mol Neurobiol 1983; 43:2952–2954.
32. Stewart JJ, Burks TF, Weistbrodt NW. Intestinal myoelectric activity after activation of central emetic mechanisms. Am J Physiol 1977; 233:E131–137.
33. Harding RK, McDonald TJ, Hugenholtz H, Kucharczyk J. Characteristics of a new emesis producing intestinal factor. Physiologist 1984; 27:279.
34. Spitz L. Vomiting after pyloromyotomy for infantile hypertrophic pyloric stenosis. Arch Dis Child 1979; 54:886–889.
35. Botha GSM. The gastro-esophageal region in infants. Arch Dis Child 1958; 33:78–94.
36. Gryboski JD. Gastrointestinal function in the infant and young child. Clin Gastroenterol 1977; 6:253–265.
37. Carré IJ. Clinical significance of gastro-oesophageal reflux. Arch Dis Child, 1984; 59:911–912.
38. Friedland GW, Dodds WJ, Sunshine P, Zboralske FF. The apparent disparity in incidence of hiatal herniae in infants and children in Britain and the United States. Am J Radiol 1974; 2:205–214.
39. Toccalino H, Licastro R, Guastavino E, Oritiz J, Carpaneto E, Schiavi J, Ciocca M, Cervetto J, Garcia H. Vomiting and regurgitation. Clin Gastroenterol 1977; 6:267–282.
40. Moroz SP, Espinoza J, Cuming WA, Diamant NE. Lower esophageal sphincter function in children with and without gastroesophageal reflux. Gastroenterology 1976; 71:236–241.
41. Boix-Ochoa J, Canals J. Maturation of the lower esophagus. J Pediatr Surg 1976; 11:749–756.
42. Vandenplas Y, Sacre-Smits L. Continuous 24-hour esophageal pH monitoring in 285 asymptomatic infants 0-15 months old. J Pediatr Gastroenterol Nutr 1987; 6:220–224.
43. Weihrauch TR. Gastro-esophageal reflux—pathogenesis and clinical implications. Eur J Pediatr 1985; 144:215–218.
44. Holloway RH, Hongo M, Berger K. Gastric distension: a mechanism for postprandial gastroesophageal reflux. Gastroenterology 1985; 89:779–784.
45. Hillemeier AC, Lange R, McCallum R, Seashore J, Gryboski J. Delayed gastric emptying in infants with gastroesophageal reflux. J Pediatr 1981; 98:190–193.
46. Di Lorenzo C, Piepsz A, Ham H, Cadranel S. Gastric emptying with gastro-oesophageal reflux. Arch Dis Child 1987; 62:449–453.
47. Jackson PT, Glasgow JFT, Thomas PS, Carré IJ. Children with gastroesophageal reflux with or without partial thoracic stomach (hiatal hernia) have normal gastric emptying time. J Pediatr Gastroenterol Nutr 1989; 8:37–40.
48. Shrand H. Vomiting in utero with intestinal atresia. Pediatrics 1972; 49:767–768.
49. Jackson RH. Genetic studies in peptic ulcer in childhood. Acta Paediatr Scand 1971; 61:493–494.
50. Colletti RB, Wasserman RC. Recurrent infantile vomiting due to intentional ipecacc poisoning. J Pediatr Gastroenterol Nutr 1989; 8:394–396.
51. Stanbury JB, Wyngaarden JB, Fredrickson DS, Goldstein JL, Brown MS. The metabolic basis of inherited disease. 5th ed. New York: McGraw-Hill, 1983.
52. Beleslin DB, Strbac M. Noradrenaline induced emesis. Alpha-2-adrenoreceptor mediation in the area postrema. Neuropharmacology 1987; 26:1157–1165.
53. Hammond J. The late sequelae of recurrent vomiting of childhood. Dev Med Child Neurol 1974; 16:15–22.
54. Reinhart JB, Evans SL, McFadden DL. Cyclic vomiting in children: seen through the psychiatrist's eye. Pediatrics 1977; 59:371–377.
55. Hill OW. Psychogenic vomiting. Gut 1968; 9:348–352.
56. Hoyt CS, Stickler GB. A study of 44 children with the syndrome of recurrent (cyclic) vomiting. Pediatrics 1960; 25:775–780.
57. McGregor RR. Some interesting cases of hypertrophic pyloric stenosis. Can Med Assoc J 1931; 24:269–271.
58. Spock B. Etiological factors in hypertrophic pyloric stenosis and infantile colic. J Psychosom Med 1944; 6:162–165.
59. Revill SI, Dodge JA. Psychological determinants of infantile pyloric stenosis. Arch Dis Child 1978; 53:66–68.
60. Menking M, Wagnitz JG, Burton JJ, Coddington RD, Sotos JF. Rumination—a near fatal psychiatric disease of infancy. N Engl J Med 1969; 280:802.
61. McFadyen UM, Hendry GMA, Simpson H. Gastro-esophageal reflux in near-miss sudden infant death syndrome or suspected recurrent aspiration. Arch Dis Child 1983; 58:87–91.
62. Bateman DN, Rawlins MD, Simpson JM. Extrapyramidal reactions with metoclopramide. 1985; 291:930–932.
63. Brogden RN, Carmine AA, Heal RC, Speight TM, Avery GS. Domperidone. A review of its pharmacological activity, pharmacokinetics and therapeutic efficacy in the symptomatic treatment of chronic dyspepsia and as an antiemetic. Drugs 1982; 24:360–400.
64. Swann IL, Thompson EN, Qureshi K. Domperidone or metoclopromide in preventing chemotherapeutically induced nausea and vomiting. Br Med J 1979; 2:1118.
65. Saye Z, Forget P, Geubelle F. Effect of cisapride on gastroesophageal reflux in children with chronic bronchopulmonary disease. Pediatr Pulmonol 1987; 3:8–12.
66. Cucchiara S, Staiano A, Capozzi C, Di Lorenzo C, Boccieri A, Auricchio S. Cisapride for gastro-esophageal reflux and peptic oesophagitis. Arch Dis Child 1987; 62:454–457.
67. Euler AR. Use of bethanechol for the treatment of gastroesophageal reflux. J Pediatr 1980; 96:321–324.
68. Strickland AD, Chang JHT. Results of treatment of gastroesophageal reflux with bethanechol. J Pediatr 1983; 103:311.
69. Miner GWD, Sanger GJ. Inhibition of cis-platin-induced vomiting by

selective 5-hydroxytryptamine M-receptor antagonism. Br J Pharmacol 1986; 88:497–499.

70. Wright L, Thalassinos P. Success with electroshock in habitual vomiting: report of two cases in young children. Clin Pediatr 1973; 12:594–597.

71. Lang PJ, Melamet BG. Avoidance condition therapy of an infant with chronic ruminative vomiting. J Abnorm Psychol 1969; 74:1–8.

72. Cucchiara S, Gobio-Casali L, Balli F, Magazzu G, Staiano A, Astolfi R, Amarri S, Conti-Nibali S, Guandalini S. Cimetidine treatment of reflux esophagitis in children: an Italian multicentre study. J Pediatr Gastroenterol Nutr 1989; 8:150–156.

CHAPTER 4

Acute Abdominal Pain

Arthur J. Ross, III, M.D.

The evaluation of acute abdominal pain in the child is never easy. The patient and his family are usually both frightened by and anxious about the child's discomfort, and often the clinician is forced to make assessments and decisions under less than optimal circumstances. Obviously, the most important specific issue to be resolved by the assessment of an abdominal emergency is whether or not the child requires an operative procedure. Although the answer to this issue may be obvious, most frequently a serious, thoughtful, and thorough approach to the child is required before the true acuteness of the abdominal emergency is appreciated and the significance of the problem fully understood. Specific disease entities are discussed elsewhere in this text. This chapter outlines an approach to the child who has presented with acute abdominal pain.

PATHOPHYSIOLOGY

An understanding of acute abdominal pain in the pediatric patient requires an understanding of the general pathophysiology of most abdominal emergencies.[1-7] These are inflammation, mechanical obstruction, and hemorrhage. Inflammation is generally the result of an infectious process, although it may also be an autoimmune or physiologic reaction in the child who has undergone chemotherapy or radiation therapy. Inflammatory responses usually begin as either mucositis or serositis, and inflammation alone may lead to obstruction and distention. Intestinal obstruction may occur on either a congenital or an acquired basis and may also lead to distention. The causes of newborn obstruction differ from those that present later in life. Beyond the neonatal period, an incarcerated hernia is a common source of obstruction in a previously unoperated child. In children who have undergone prior operative procedures, adhesive bands represent the most common cause of obstruction. The presence of hemorrhage may herald either prior inflammation or obstruction but occasionally presents as a singular finding. Although both dramatic and emergent, hemorrhage is not usually painful if it is the sole abnormality.

The most common cause of acute abdominal pain is distention of a hollow viscus, which can result from inflammation, obstruction, or both. Distention, especially acute, of a hollow viscus is the only way that the viscus itself may be responsible for pain. To understand the pain of distention, one must appreciate the difference between visceral and somatic pain, as this distinction is critical in understanding the pathophysiology of the acute abdomen. The visceral peritoneum is innervated by the autonomic nervous system. Stretching of the fibers in the bowel wall, usually due to acute gaseous distention, is the only "pain" stimulus that is generated from the bowel, and it is generally appreciated in the midepigastrium as a nonspecific, vague, poorly localizing discomfort. Inflammation of the visceral peritoneum is perceived as a similar sensation. On the other hand, innervation of the parietal peritoneum and abdominal musculature is via the same specific cerebrospinal somatic pathways that innervate dermatomes, so that the same specific localization of cutaneous pain can occur with the stimulation of the parietal peritoneum and the abdominal musculature. Thus, specific pain and/or spasm of muscles such as the rectus, lateral abdominal, and psoas can help one to better appreciate and delineate the specific underlying pathology. Localization of the problem is often possible by appreciating specific areas of inflammation of the parietal peritoneum. This is often demonstrable as acute, reproducible pain in one specific area. An example is lateral rectal wall tenderness with a localized pelvic process. In contrast, diffuse irritation of parietal peritoneal surfaces may be manifested as less well localized but specific discomfort with motion or stretching of the parietal peritoneal surface. This generalized peritoneal irritation is also known as diffuse peritonitis.

One must also understand the distribution of segmental nerves so that radiating or "referred" pain can be appreciated. Perhaps the best example of this is the referred pain from irritation or inflammation of the diaphragm to the upper back and lower neck regions.

MEDICAL HISTORY

As the abdominal cavity is not readily visualized with the naked eye, it becomes incumbent upon the physician assessing the child with an acute abdomen to use all of his powers of history taking and physical diagnosis; repeated examinations and observation are often needed to arrive at an accurate diagnosis. In general, these principles, along with the careful use of selective diagnostic studies and laboratory tests, allow the child who requires acute surgical intervention to be differentiated from one who will benefit most from conservative medical management.

One of the most important aids to the physician in the diagnosis of the acute abdomen is to proceed in an atmosphere that gains the child's trust and helps him to relax as much as possible. Much can be gleaned from the history itself, and it is best obtained prior to any attempt to examine the child.

The ideal situation allows the examiner to sit and chat with the child and his family. The child may act as he pleases, and the examiner has the opportunity to observe the child during this period of time.

Pain is the single most significant indicator of an acute abdominal process, and its quality and characteristics are of the utmost importance. Therefore, careful attention should be paid to the historical presence and progression of these features. The initial assessment of the patient's pain is also greatly enhanced by a clear understanding of the child's past history, especially with regard to prior operative procedures. The child's age, as well as the most exact possible time and mode of onset of his pain, is important to understand. The acuteness of onset of the abdominal pain may give the examiner several clues as to its etiology; in particular, an inflammatory process first involving visceral peritoneum usually has a vague onset. The pain and its presentation, as well as its relationship to nausea, vomiting, diarrhea, and constipation, are all important, as is the timing of the onset of these symptoms relative to the presence of constitutional problems such as fever and chills. The history of blood in the vomitus or stool should be sought; as should the onset of distention and/or the cessation or passage of flatus.

In the child who vomits, the relationship of the pain to the vomiting—i.e., whether it began before or after the vomiting—is an important feature. For example, with gastroenteritis one usually has nausea and vomiting before pain, whereas the opposite is true with appendicitis. The relationship of pain to vomiting is important because the etiologies of vomiting are rather specific. When it occurs as a primary event preceding any pain or discomfort, it is likely caused by the effect of an absorbed toxin upon the medullary center, as in an acute gastroenteritis. On the other hand, when it follows pain, it may be due to either acute obstruction of a viscus or severe irritation of either peritoneal or mesenteric nerves, such as an inflammatory process like appendicitis. Also, the nature of the vomitus (bilious versus nonbilious) is a critical distinction. Bilious vomiting should be considered to be indicative of bowel obstruction until proven otherwise.

Changes in the characteristics of the pain from the time of onset to the time of presentation are important. This is most vividly demonstrated in appendicitis, which often presents as visceral, vague pain when the visceral peritoneum overlying the appendix becomes inflamed. As the inflammation progresses to involve somatic innervated surfaces such as parietal peritoneum, the pain localizes. Radiation of the pain as well as the nature of the pain (e.g., colicky) also needs to be understood. Colic results from the intermittent distention of a hollow viscus; radiation requires the physician to consider the somatic pathways of pain distribution to determine the pathophysiology of the child's discomfort. It is surprising how often and how well children are able to participate in this discussion; with their parents' added observations, one can often sort out many features regarding the characteristics of their pain.

PHYSICAL EXAMINATION

While the history is being taken, the examiner should observe the child closely to determine the acuteness and nature of the discomfort. It is also helpful, before beginning the physical examination, to have the child perform simple tasks that may indicate the degree of irritation of the peritoneum. If the child is able to hop up and down on one foot and jump onto and off of the examining table, it is unlikely that significant peritoneal irritation is present. With regard to the physical examination itself, one must keep in mind that no child readily submits to physical examination and successful evaluation of the uncomfortable child may require full use of one's bedside and diagnostic skills. Because children are often frightened, hurt, and incredibly frustrated by pain in their abdomen, the time spent interrelating with the child before beginning the examination in order to win his trust and confidence enhances the examiner's ability to make the necessary assessments. One should perform as much of the examination as possible without causing the child discomfort before examining the areas that may cause distress. Diversionary tactics are often helpful; allowing the child, especially the older child, to participate in the examination is also beneficial. Once the child is undressed and on the examining table, the clinician's observation continues to be a critical component in assessing the child's discomfort and the presence of peritoneal irritation. Is the child lying motionless on the bed, or is he or she willing to move about? Does the child wince with cough, movement, or motion of the bed? Does the child's abdomen appear scaphoid or distended? Is there evidence of cutaneous lesions or abnormalities that may contribute to his or her discomfort? Much may also be gained by auscultation. One of the simplest and most critical judgments to be made early in the evaluation is whether ileus or obstruction exists; differentiation between these two entities is possible in even the sickest and most compromised of children by a careful assessment of the presence or absence of bowel sounds. Gentle palpation during auscultation has much to offer in the evaluation of the child with acute abdominal pain. Whereas the concept of palpation may frighten a child, palpation may be done with the stethoscope during auscultation without the child's perceiving it, and much information can be gleaned from this maneuver. Although deeper palpation to determine the presence or absence of masses and tenderness is an important component of any abdominal examination, much information can be gleaned without resorting to deep palpation. Spasm, guarding, and tenderness can be assessed without an aggressive examination. Testing for rebound tenderness (pushing down on the abdomen and then letting go quickly to see if pain is elicited) is to be condemned. Acute distention of the bowel creates abdominal pain, and performing the maneuver necessary for rebound tenderness produces sudden acute abdominal distention. The purpose of the test is to see if peritoneal irritation exists and specifically to determine whether spasm and guarding are present or stretching the parietal peritoneum and involuntarily musculature elicits pain, but these features can easily be assessed without performing the rebound maneuver. Indeed, if one causes the child sudden, unexpected pain by performing a rebound maneuver, all of the trust that one has gained will be lost; moreover, future examinations will be compromised, as the child will now guard voluntarily to prevent himself from being hurt again. The reproducibility of the pain is important and may require diversionary tactics in children of any age. It is also important to recall that an entire physical examination must be performed. Pneumonia may well masquerade as an acute abdominal complaint. Furthermore, one must not underestimate the value of the rectal examination: It is not only an examination for perianal and anorectal disease but also an additional means of evaluating the peritoneal cavity in the child. The presence or absence of masses and peritoneal irritation is often best assessed with this exam. In a child with an "acute" abdomen, the correct assessment is a potentially life-saving decision, so there is absolutely no contraindication to a gentle rectal examination done by an experienced examiner.

Having established the presence or absence of bowel sounds, localizing tenderness, peritoneal irritation, and masses or dilated loops of bowel, one often is able to correlate the physical findings with the laboratory and diagnostic modalities available to arrive at the correct plan for management.

LABORATORY

One must use laboratory and diagnostic tests selectively to produce the most information with the least expense and discomfort to the patient.

Most children with acute abdominal pain should have a complete blood count performed. In addition to the white blood cell count, the absolute numbers of granulocytes and any relative shift in the differential count are of significance. The presence of a lymphocytosis rather than a leukocytosis is reassuring. A thrombocytopenia may be reflective of severe sepsis and is also an important feature. Although the hemoglobin is a reliable indicator of ongoing blood loss in a chronic problem, it may well be grossly misleading in assessing acute, sudden changes in red cell volume due to gastrointestinal (GI) hemorrhage. Electrolyte determinations are also important, as many abdominal processes cause severe metabolic deficits due to fluid shifts long before they become clinically apparent. Assessment of the nasogastric aspirate for blood and of stool for blood and specific pathogens may be of great value.

Although radiologic examinations have become increasingly sophisticated, routine plain abdominal films showing both the flat and erect or decubitus views remain the most useful radiologic study in initially assessing the child with an acute abdomen. Ultrasound examinations, computed tomography, and MR scans, as well as contrast studies, radionuclide exams, and angiography, all need to be available to the child's physician/caretaker as part of their diagnostic armamentarium.

Abdominal paracentesis and diagnostic lavage are useful in situations in which it is otherwise impossible to assess the child for extraluminal bleeding or a GI perforation. One must remember that following a "tap," the presence of free abdominal air may be iatrogenic and misleading. The value of paracentesis with Gram's stain, culture, and microscopic analysis of the peritoneum cannot be understated in a patient in whom significant uncertainty exists regarding the presence of a perforative process.

SUMMARY

A multitude of specific disease entities that can produce or mimic the acute abdomen will be described in this text. Without question, any condition is more easily defined if the clinician approaches the child with the utmost patience and gentleness. Time spent in obtaining a good history and in gaining the child's trust permits the examiner to perform a more thorough and reliable physical examination. The result should be greater diagnostic accuracy and a better ability to direct the management of the child with acute abdominal pain.

REFERENCES

1. Botsford TW, Wilson RE. The acute abdomen. 2nd ed. Philadelphia: WB Saunders, 1977.
2. Brewer RJ, Golden GT, Hitch DC, et al. Abdominal pain: an analysis of 1,000 consecutive cases in a university hospital emergency room. Am J Surg 1976; 131:219.
3. Cheung LY, Ballinger WF. Manifestations and diagnosis of gastrointestinal diseases. In: Hardy JD, ed. Textbook of surgery. 2nd ed. Philadelphia: JB Lippincott, 1988:460.
4. Diethelm AG. The acute abdomen. In: Sabiston DC, ed. Textbook of surgery. 13th ed. Philadelphia: WB Saunders, 1986:790.
5. Menacker GJ. The physiology and mechanism of acute abdominal pain. Surg Clin North Am 1962; 42:241.
6. Silen W. Cope's early diagnosis of the acute abdomen. 16th ed. Oxford: Oxford University Press, 1983.
7. Way LW. Abdominal pain and the acute abdomen. In: Sleisenger MH, Fordtran JS, eds. Gastrointestinal disease: pathophysiology, diagnosis and management. 3rd ed. Philadelphia: WB Saunders, 1983, 207.

CHAPTER 5

Chronic Abdominal Pain

John T. Boyle, M.D.

Chronic abdominal pain is one of the most commonly encountered symptoms in childhood and adolescence. There is general agreement that abdominal pain becomes chronic when episodic attacks occur over a period of 3 months.[1] Chronic abdominal pain that affects normal activity or usual levels of performance has been reported to occur in 10 to 15 percent of school-age children between the ages of 5 and 14 years.[2-5] Recent evidence suggests that at least as many children experience chronic abdominal pain but maintain normal activity and rarely come to the attention of the physician.[5] In excess of 90 percent of children with chronic abdominal pain are believed to have a "functional gastrointestinal (GI) disorder."[1,6-10] The modifier "functional" is used if no specific structural, infectious, inflammatory, or biochemical cause for the abdominal pain can be determined. This does not imply that the pathophysiology of the disorder has been clearly identified or that we know exactly how to treat the symptom complex. Current speculation is that functional abdominal pain represents a disturbance of GI motility provoked by physical and psychological stress.

The most widely used diagnostic term for functional chronic abdominal pain is recurrent abdominal pain (RAP).[2-10] I believe that a heterogeneous group of patients is included under this broad descriptive term. When it is evaluated critically, there are three clinical presentations of RAP in children and adolescents: primary periumbilical paroxysmal pain, primary "peptic symptoms," and lower abdominal pain associated with altered bowel pattern. The first presentation is the most common and in this chapter is designated functional abdominal pain. Patients with peptic symptoms complain of recurrent upper abdominal pain that may or may not be related to meals, nausea, postprandial epigastric fullness and distention, belching, hiccups, and early satiety. This group can be considered to be afflicted with "nonulcer dyspepsia." Patients with a temporal association between lower abdominal pain and an altered bowel pattern are more characteristic of irritable bowel syndrome in adults. The purpose of this chapter is to discuss the pathophysiology of RAP and the clinical presentations, differential diagnosis, and management of each of the three variants.

PATHOPHYSIOLOGY

There is general agreement that recurrent abdominal pain is genuine and not simply social modeling or imitation of parental pain or a means to avoid an unwanted experience (e.g., school phobia or malingering). The etiology and pathogenesis

of the pain are unknown. There appears to be a genetic vulnerability because of the high frequency of pain complaints in family members.[1] Recent studies suggest that patients with functional abdominal pain who make their way to a subspecialty setting commonly exhibit "internalizing" behavior characterized by anxiety, mild depression, withdrawal, and low self-esteem.[11,12] Such a behavioral profile may be primary and part of the genetic vulnerability of such patients. Alternatively, it has been postulated that such internalizing behavior is fostered within a family structure characterized by maternal depression, enmeshment, overprotectiveness, rigidity, and lack of conflict resolution.[13] A third possibility is that the internalizing behavior is a common psychological adaptation to both organic and nonorganic chronic conditions. Whether primary or secondary, both the behavior pattern of the child and the family structure may influence how the disorder is experienced and acted upon.

Despite the lack of direct evidence, the best conceptual model for the pathogenesis of functional abdominal pain depicts a sequence of a heterogeneous group of physical and psychosocial stressful stimuli that provoke an alteration in intensity or imbalance in intestinal motor activity in susceptible patients. The consequence is the abdominal pain. Examples of physical stress include viral infections, developmental lactose intolerance, and chronic stool retention. Examples of psychosocial stress include anxiety, school problems, and preoccupation with illness. Attempts to describe pain relief after withdrawal of a single provocative stimulus have been controversial. This is illustrated by examining the role of lactose intolerance as a cause of recurrent abdominal pain. Barr et al have reported lactose malabsorption diagnosed by breath hydrogen testing in 40 percent of a group of school children with recurrent abdominal pain.[14] They observed that such children lack an awareness of intolerance to lactose because there was no temporal relationship between lactose ingestion and abdominal discomfort. They reported a qualitative improvement in pain symptoms in 70 percent of intolerant children treated with a lactose-free diet and thus concluded that lactose malabsorption was the cause of pain in a subgroup of patients who fit the criteria for chronic abdominal pain. However, a subsequent study claimed a similar prevalence of lactose intolerance in a group of patients with functional abdominal pain and a separate group of age-matched patients with diarrhea but without pain.[15] This result suggests that lactose intolerance is not directly the cause of the pain, but the initiating factor of a sequence in which pain is the consequence of altered intestinal function provoked by lactose malabsorption in susceptible patients. That lactose is but one provocative stimulus in patients with recurrent abdominal pain is supported by observations that a lactose-free diet does not induce complete resolution of the pain or alter the natural history of the condition.[14-16]

Three studies have described altered intestinal motor activity in heterogeneous populations of patients with recurrent abdominal pain. Dimson reported delayed intestinal transit of carmine red dye in patients with functional abdominal pain triggered by emotional factors.[17] No statistical analysis of the data was performed, however. The data suggested that delayed transit is more likely in patients with tenderness over the left colon on physical examination and in patients with associated constipation. In an earlier study, Kopel et al were more specific in addressing the question of an altered intraluminal manometric GI response to a provocative stimulus.[18] They described increased amplitude and duration of rectosigmoid pressure waves in response to the parasympathetic agonist prostigmine methyl sulfate in 78 percent of patients with recurrent abdominal pain versus 33 percent of controls. Although available methodologic technology at the time of Kopel's study limited quantitative analysis of the data, the study strongly implied that patients with recurrent abdominal pain responded with increased intensity of muscle contraction compared with control patients following a provocative stimulus. These observations must be counterbalanced by the lack of direct evidence linking the symptom of abdominal pain to the altered intestinal function that they described. In a recent study Pineiro-Carrero et al described a temporal relationship between altered gastroduodenal motility and the presence of abdominal pain.[19] Specific motility patterns associated with pain included high-amplitude duodenal contractions and activity of the migrating motor complex (MMC). The major weakness of the findings, however, was lack of an aged-matched control population. Also, there was no direct evidence linking environmental stress to the specific patterns of gut motility. The three studies do point out that functional GI disorders may be associated with both upper and lower manometric abnormalities and altered intestinal transit. The predominance of one or more of these variables may explain the variation in clinical presentation that characterizes recurrent abdominal pain.

One speculation is that alteration of intestinal motility in patients with recurrent abdominal pain results from dysfunction of the autonomic nervous system.[18] The autonomic nervous system functions as an important participant in homeostasis of the intestine by modulating the sensory and motor responses to various internal and external stimuli. Vagotomy often leads to the development of a characteristic group of symptoms, including abdominal pain, nausea, and bloating, which arise as a result of impaired gastric function and are presumably signaled via splanchnic afferents.[20] Perhaps recurrent abdominal pain represents an imbalance of splanchnic afferent activity in the bowel. Alternatively, autonomic dysfunction may be more generalized in these patients. Many of the associated symptoms in patients with functional abdominal pain, including headache, pallor, dizziness, and nausea, are also "autonomic" symptoms. Rubin et al have described an abnormal pupillary response to cold stress characterized by enhanced pupillary dilatation and delay in the recovery phase in patients with nonorganic abdominal pain compared with a control group.[21] However, this observation could not be duplicated by Apley et al.[22] Furthermore

Feuerstein et al were not able to demonstrate a differential perception of distress measured by heart rate, peripheral vasomotor tone, or facial expression following a cold stress between controls and patients with nonorganic abdominal pain.[23] The above studies utilized a physical stimulus outside the GI tract, which may explain the variable results.

In the next few years, we are going to see a growing controversy regarding the role of microscopic inflammation in the pathogenesis of chronic abdominal pain, particularly in the variants similar to adult nonulcer dyspepsia and irritable bowel syndrome. The concept of microscopic esophagitis has already altered the diagnostic evaluation and management of gastroesophageal reflux in children.[24] The new frontier will be histologic colitis, gastritis, and duodenitis.[25-28] The rapid growth of pediatric endoscopic technology, the growing number of pediatric gastroenterologists, the standard practice of routine biopsy during pediatric endoscopy despite macroscopic normality, and the growing tendency of pathologists to describe nonspecific mild inflammatory changes in small punch biopsy specimens all have contributed to the growth of "microscopic inflammation." The role of mild to moderate nonspecific inflammation in the pathogenesis of nonulcer dyspepsia and irritable bowel in adults is controversial.[28] It has been speculated that such low-grade inflammation may be the cause or the effect of altered intestinal motility. The significance of such mild inflammatory changes is even questioned, since it is common in biopsies of asymptomatic control adult patients. Unfortunately, given the invasiveness of endoscopy, pediatric gastroenterologists are not going to have access to pediatric control data. In the context of what has happened in gastroesophageal reflux, it will be very interesting to see how histologic colitis, gastritis, and duodenitis affect our concept of recurrent abdominal pain.

The morbidity associated with recurrent abdominal pain is not physical but results from interference in normal school attendance and performance, peer relationships, and participation in organizations, sports, and personal and family activities. Liebman found that only one of 10 children with functional abdominal pain attended school regularly and that absenteeism was greater than one day in 10 in 28 percent of patients.[9] A common misconception is that pain is the direct cause of the morbidity. In fact, the environmental consequences of the pain probably contribute significantly to the morbidity. Fordyce et al have observed that while pain does not originate from its consequences, much pain behavior is accounted for and modified by its consequences.[29] As described below, the usual parental, school, and medical management of recurrent abdominal pain is focused on symptom relief, which reinforces the pain behavior with attention, rest, and medication. This approach fails to reinforce nonpain responses such as normal activity.

FUNCTIONAL ABDOMINAL PAIN

Clinical Presentation

The characteristics of the abdominal pain in this group are listed in Table 1. In the individual patient, pain episodes tend to cluster, alternating with pain-free periods of variable length. Most episodes begin gradually and last less than 1 hour in

TABLE 1
Characteristic Pain Pattern in Functional
Abdominal Pain

Paroxysmal (variable in severity)

Clustering of pain episodes lasting several weeks to months during
which time pain occurs daily to several times per week

Gradual beginning

Periumbilical or midepigastric location

Inability to describe the nature of the pain (stabbing, burning, dull)

Inability to ascribe temporal relationship of pain to meals, exercise,
stress (often occurs at same time of day)

Interruption of normal activity

---

50 percent and less than 3 hours in another 40 percent of
children.[1,10] Continuous pain has been described in less than
10 percent of patients.[1,10] In 90 percent of patients the pain
is periumbilical or midepigastric in location.[1,6,10] The child
usually gives a vague description of the pain, although typically it is constant rather than colicky. Radiation of the pain
to the back, chest, or hips is rare. A temporal relationship
to meals, activity, and bowel habits is unusual. Rarely do children give a history that particular foods cause the symptoms.
The pain rarely awakens the child from sleep, but it is not
uncommon for pain in the evening to affect the ability to fall
asleep. Parents describe the patient as miserable and listless
during most episodes of pain. During severe attacks, the child
may exhibit a variety of motor behaviors including doubling
over, grimacing, crying, and clenching and pushing on the
abdomen.

Commonly associated symptoms inlcude headache, pallor,
nausea, dizziness, and fatigability, at least one of which is
observed in 50 to 70 percent of cases.[1,9] Vomiting, regurgitation, gaseous distention, diarrhea, and constipation are uncommon in my experience. Many patients report fever, which,
on questioning, turns out to mean more than 99 °F but less
than 100 °F. Weight loss, constitutional symptoms of chronic
organic illness (e.g., fever, joint pains, rash, growth failure),
rectal bleeding, and sleepiness after attacks are not symptoms
of functional abdominal pain.

In addition to the clinical features of the pain and associated symptoms, there is a constellation of historical features
that facilitate recognition of functional abdominal pain:

1. Relatively high incidences of concurrent stressful life
   events are often reported, including death or separation
   of a significant family member, physical illness or
   chronic handicap in parents or siblings, school problems,
   poverty or financial problems, and recent geographical
   moves. The parents and child rarely relate the pain symptoms directly to environmental stress.
2. Family history is likely to be positve for irritable bowel
   syndrome, peptic ulcer, previous appendectomy, and
   migraine headaches.[1] Symptoms of irritable bowl syndrome are more common in the mother than in the father.
3. The pain behavior evokes a characteristic reinforcement
   response from parents, school, and primary physician.[30]

The pain behavior is often reinforced by rest periods,
social attention, and medication. The characteristic
parental response following a report of pain includes
requesting that the child lie down on the couch or bed;
providing TV, toys, books, drinks, or food to distract the
child; and administering some type of symptomatic therapy, either tactile (massaging abdomen or heating pad)
or medication (Tylenol, Donnatal, Bentyl, etc.).
Although the pain usually lasts less than 1 hour, the child
is kept home all day from school. Usually the child
resumes normal home routine after the pain subsides.
Schools reinforce the pain consequence behavior by send-
ing the child home when he or she complains of pain
while at school. The family physician or pediatrician may
reinforce the pain consequence behavior by prescribing
a steady stream of medication on an as-needed basis.

Diagnostic Approach

At the time of referral to the gastroenterologist, about 50
percent of patients will have been symptomatic for less than
1 year, and the remaining 50 percent report pain for 1 to 5
years. The specialist is often at a disadvantage by being the
second or third physician to evaluate the child. Primary care
physicians often have difficulty making a positive diagnosis
of a functional GI disorder. Instead, they attempt a stepwise
series of diagnostic studies to make a negative diagnosis of
organic pain. Rather than being reassured by a negative diagnosis, parents tend to become more frustrated and anxious,
particularly if the only alternative diagnosis is perceived by
them to be an emotional or behavioral disorder. Parental
uncertainty only increases the stressful environment that provokes or reinforces the pain behavior, which in turn usually
results in further diagnostic tests or hospitalization.

I strongly believe functional abdominal pain can and should
be a positive diagnosis. Rather than having a specific diagnostic marker, the diagnosis is established by a constellation
of criteria based on a careful history, physical examination,
and minimum laboratory investigation (Table 2). Management
can be instituted if these criteria are met without further work-
up, provided that routine follow-up is assured.

TABLE 2
Diagnostic Criteria for Functional Abdominal
Pain

Documentation of chronicity

Compatible age range, age of onset

Characteristic features of abdominal pain

Evidence of physical or psychological stressful stimuli

Environmental reinforcement of pain behavior

Normal physical examination (including rectal examination and stool
guaiac)

Normal laboratory evaluation (complete blood count, erythrocyte
sedimentation rate, urinalysis, urine culture, stool ova and parasites,
lactose breath test)

TABLE 3
"Red Flags" in Evaluation of Chronic
Abdominal Pain

Well-localized pain away from the umbilicus

Altered bowel pattern (diarrhea, constipation) associated with the
　abdominal pain

Vomiting

Recurrent isolated episodes of pain that come on suddenly and last
　several minutes to a few days

Pain awakening patient from sleep

Radiation of pain to back, shoulder, scapula, lower extremities

Involuntary weight loss or growth deceleration

Rectal bleeding, constitutional symptoms (including temperature above
　100° F, arthralgias, rash)

Intermittent fecal incontinence

Consistent sleepiness following pain attacks

Positive family history of peptic ulcer, inflammatory bowel disease

---

The age distribution is between 4 and 14 years, with the mean age of onset variably reported between 5 and 8 years of age. Apley observed that males and females are equally affected in early childhood until the age of 9, at which point the incidence decreases in males.[1] The incidence in females continues to increase until age 11 to 12 years, such that between 9 and 12 years the female:male ratio approaches 1.5:1. Onset of symptom after 14 is rare, at which time more traditional symptoms of irritable bowel syndrome are usually observed. Onset of chronic pain in a child less than 4 years old requires a more in-depth organic work-up, particularly for structural abnormalities. Age of onset greater than 12 years requires a more detailed evaluation of emotional disturbances (conversion reaction), systemic inflammatory conditions, and gynecologic disorders. Table 1 lists the characteristics of the

TABLE 4
Stressful Stimuli in Patients with Functional
Abdominal Pain

1. **Physical Stress**
　a. Recent physical illness
　b. Lactose intolerance
　c. Other carbohydrate intolerance (e.g., sorbitol, sucrose, fructose,
　　　dietary starch including wheat, corn, oats, potatoes)
　d. Aerophagia
　e. Recent intake of medication (either prescription or non-
　　　prescription)
　f. Simple constipation

2. **Psychosocial Stress**
　a. Death of a significant family member
　b. Separation from a significant family member (divorce, sibling
　　　going to college)
　c. Physical illness or chronic handicap in parents or sibling
　　　(including positive family history of inflammatory bowel
　　　disease, peptic ulcer)
　d. School problems
　e. Altered peer relationships
　f. Family poverty or financial problems
　g. Recent geographic move

TABLE 5
Signs of Environmental Reinforcement of
Pain Behavior

Specific attention at time of pain

Rest period during pain

Medication at time of pain

Absence from school on days of pain

Normal home activity during pain-free periods (especially on days of
　school absence)

---

pain pattern. Consistent deviation from this pattern or the "red flags" listed in Table 3 suggest the need for further organic evaluation.

Sex, intelligence, and personality traits do not distinguish patients with functional pain from those with organic pain. The majority of patients are of average intelligence. The generalization that patients with functional abdominal pain are superintellects, perfectionists, overachievers, bad mixers, or constant worriers is without foundation.

Table 4 lists potential stressful stimuli, both physical and psychological, that may be present in patients with functional abdominal pain. Although the child is often unable to confirm a temporal association between stress and the presence of abdominal pain, one or more of these historical signs of stress can be identified in most patients. Likewise, another confirming signal is the environmental response that follows most pain episodes, the characteristics of which have been discussed and are listed in Table 5.

The physical examination of these patients is often described as nonspecific. Although many children claim to have pain at the time of examination, their behavior, affect, and activity are seldom consistent with the degree of expressed discomfort. The physician may elicit tenderness during palpation, without rebound, which is usually not localized to a particular quadrant of the abdomen. Documentation of specific parts of the physical examination are critical, however, including normal growth parameters and absence of (a) linea alba hernia, (b) hepatomegaly, (c) splenomegaly, (d) costovertebral angle tenderness, (e) right lower quadrant mass or fullness, (f) perianal fistula, fissure, or ucleration, (g) perianal fecal staining, (h) patulous anal tone, (i) capacious rectum with stool palpable to the anal verge, (j) guaiac-positive stool, and (k) joint swelling. The basic laboratory evaluation listed in Table 2 is targeted at screening for occult systemic inflammatory conditions, urinary tract infection, parasitic infection, and lactose intolerance and should be standard procedure in all patients with chronic abdominal pain.

Differential Diagnosis

There are over 100 organic disorders that may present with chronic abdominal pain as the primary symptom.[6] The organic disorders listed below represent those that may on rare occasions have to be differentiated from functional abdominal pain. The brief descriptions provided demonstrate how symptom criteria of each organic disease allow the gastroenterologist to distinguish these disorders from functional abdominal pain.

Primary Peptic Ulcer. Abdominal pain has been reported to be the sole presenting symptom in 55 percent of a small population of patients between 10 and 17 years of age diagnosed with primary peptic ulcer.[31] Unfortunately, pain location and character were not described, nor was the relationship of the pain to meals. Silverman and Roy have reported that the pain-food-relief cycle is not characteristic of primary peptic ulcer disease in children and adolescents.[32] They suggest that peptic ulcer should be considered in the following circumstances: (1) chronic abdominal pain if it is present at night or in the early morning hours, (2) recurrent vomiting if related to eating, (3) anemia if occult blood is present in the stools, and (4) a positive family history of duodenal ulcer. Tomomasa et al have described similar variables that are highly discriminate of peptic ulcer, including (1) epigastric location of abdominal pain, (2) relationship of pain to eating (before or after meal), (3) vomiting, (4) evidence of GI blood loss, and (5) positive family history within a second-degree relative.[33] It is very rare for an ulcer to be missed if the gastroenterologist pays attention to "red flags" in the history.

Inflammatory Bowel Disease. The pattern of intestinal signs and symptoms of inflammatory bowel disease depends upon the site of involvement. Colitis is associated with either diarrhea or evidence of GI blood loss. This is true not only for ulcerative colitis but also for the "microscopic colitis" syndromes described to date.[25-27] Abdominal pain associated with colitis is usually lower abdominal, maximal prior to and during defecation, and relieved by the passage of stool or flatus. In small bowel Crohn's disease, symptoms tend to be obstructive in nature, with pain associated with meals. Crohn's disease should be suspected when pressure tenderness is localized to the right lower quadrant, especially if associated with fullness, or mass effect, elevated erythrocyte sedimentation rate, or extraintestinal symptoms such as fever, rash, or joint pains.

Biliary Colic. The pain is acute in onset, frequently follows a meal, and is usually localized to the epigastrium or right upper quadrant. In children, however, the pain may occur in the periumbilical area. Characteristically the pain rises to a plateau of intensity over 5 to 20 minutes and resolves gradually over 1 to 4 hours. Referred pain is common, particularly to the back near the tip of the right scapula. Associated symptoms include nausea, vomiting, and occasionally scleral icterus. Laboratory tests are nonspecific. Patients should have ultrasonography of the gallbladder to document the presence of gallstones.

Ureteropelvic Junction (UPJ) Obstruction. UPJ obstruction has been described in children with distinct episodes of periumbilical, crampy pain occurring as frequently as two times per week. In a series of three cases reported by Byrne et al, vomiting was asociated with the pain in all patients.[34] CBC, urinalysis, BUN, and creatinine were normal in all patients. Abdominal ultrasonography established the correct diagnosis in the two patients in whom it was performed.

Chronic Fibrosing Pancreatitis[35] and Hereditary Pancreatitis.[36] Pancreatitis should be considered in patients with distinct episodes of sharp recurrent abdominal pain that are localized to the epigastrium or periumbilical area. The pain is usually associated with nausea and vomiting and lasts 1 to 3 days. Hereditary pancreatitis is inherited as an autosomal dominant trait that demonstrates complete penetrance but variable expression. Because serum amylase may rapidly return to normal within the first 24 to 48 hours, abdominal ultrasonography is indicated to demonstrate an edematous pancreas or pseudocyst in such patients.

Partial Small Bowel Obstruction. Potential etiologies of recurrent small bowel obstruction include malrotation with volvulus, intussusception caused by Meckel's diverticulum, and adhesions. Patients present with the acute onset of crampy, paroxysmal periumbilical pain, vomiting, abdominal distention, and failure to pass flatus. Abdominal radiography at the time of pain reveals abnormally large quantities of gas in the bowel and air-fluid levels on upright films, Meckel's diverticulum should not be included in the differential diagnosis of chronic abdominal pain unless there are signs of obstruction or GI bleeding.[37,38]

Appendiceal Colic. Schisgall has described recurrent abdominal pain caused by inspissated casts of fecal material within the appendix.[39] Diagnostic criteria include (1) recurrent crampy right lower quadrant or periumbilical pain, (2) right lower quadrant pressure tenderness demonstrated on several examinations, and (3) one of three radiographic findings demonstrated on upper GI small bowel follow-through, including (a) filling defects in the appendix, (b) focal globular or diffuse distention of the appendix, and (c) retained barium in the appendix 72 hours or more after contrast study. Schisgall has reported 96 percent resolution of abdominal pain following appendectomy in 10 children between the ages of 4 and 16 years who fulfilled the above criteria. Despite skepticism regarding the numbers of patients, I have anecdotal experience of one patient who met the above criteria for 3 months of observation and who had complete resolution of symptoms following appendectomy.

Cystic Teratoma of the Ovary. Cystic teratoma has been described in prepubertal patients presenting with right or left lower quadrant pain. Ahmed described ten such patients, nine of whom had either ascites or a palpable abdominal mass.[40] Pelvic ultrasonography should be considered in girls with well-defined pain above the iliac fossa in either quadrant.

Musculoskeletal Pain. Muscle pain is usually well-localized and sharp and may be triggered by exercise or change in body position. It is usually located near the insertion of the rectus muscle or oblique muscles into the costal margins or iliac crest. Slipping rib syndrome is a sprain disorder frequently confused with intra-abdominal conditions.[41] The symptoms are sharp or dull pain in one of the upper abdominal quadrants "under the ribs," frequently accompanied by a sensation of "something rubbing" in the anterior costal area. Diagnosis is made by a positive hooking maneuver in which the physician elicits pain by hooking his curved finger under the inferior rib margins on the affected side and pulling anteriorly. The condition frequently requires surgical resection of the affected cartilages. Another localized musculofascial problem exacerbated by exercise is a linea alba hernia, which is midline and may be either infra- or supraumbilical.[42] The anatomic defect is detected in the midline while the child performs sit-up exercises.

Giardia lamblia, Dientamoeba fragilis,* and *Blastocystis hominis. Parasitic infection with these agents should be considered as primary etiology for chronic abdominal pain in the presence of anorexia, nausea, epigastric fullness, and watery diarrhea. In the face of negative stool examination for ova and parasites performed in the basic laboratory evaluation, further work-up requires obtaining duodenal fluid by intubation or string test.[42] A chronic carrier state may be a provocative stimulus of altered bowel function in patients with functional abdominal pain.

Carbohydrate Intolerance. Carbohydrate intolerance should be considered as the primary etiology for chronic abdominal pain in the presence of diarrhea, bloating, and increased flatulence. Dietary lactose and sorbitol are the principal offending sugars in such patients.[44,45] More commonly, intolerance of dietary lactose, fructose, starches, and sorbitol acts as one of several provocative stimuli to induce altered intestinal function in patients with functional abdominal pain.

Abdominal Epilepsy. This is a controversial disorder characterized by the temporal association of paroxysmal abdominal pain and a variety of central nervous system symptoms including headache, dizziness, syncope, confusion, memory loss, feeling of exhaustion, and transient blindness.[46,47] Associated GI symptoms may include nausea, bloating, and watery diarrhea. The disease is suspected by sleep EEG abnormalities (bursts of sharp waves or spikes) emanating from the temporal lobe and confirmed by resolution of symptoms after treatment with anticonvulsive therapy.

Acute Intermittent Porphyria (AIP). Porphyria is often considered in the differential diagnosis of chronic abdominal pain but should rarely be confused with functional abdominal pain. AIP is an autosomal dominant disorder associated with a deficiency of the enzyme porphobilinogen deaminase.[48] Abdominal pain in this condition is usually severe and associated with nausea and vomiting and neurologic symptoms including muscle weakness, confusion, hallucinations, and seizures. Hospitalization is often required for acute attacks. The disorder usually becomes manifested after puberty. Abdominal pain is often precipitated by low intake of carbohydrate or specific drugs such as barbiturates or sulfonamides. Premenstrual attacks are not uncommon, often resolving quickly following onset of menses.

Conversion Reaction. Psychic pain generated by environmental stress or critical life setbacks and expressed through the use of bodily sensations is by definition a conversion reaction.[49] In conversion reaction, abdominal pain is an unconscious expression of psychological conflict. Abdominal pain was the presenting symptom in 26 percent of a series of 105 cases of conversion reaction reported by Maloney.[49] Several factors should suggest a conversion reaction, including (a) age at onset after 12 (88 percent of patients), (b) precipitating unresolved grief reaction or family stress (identified in 97 percent of patients), (c) an hysterical personality (dramatic, exhibitionist, labile, excitable, egocentric, seductive), and (d) a parent who is clinically depressed (85 percent of families). Prompt resolution of symptoms usually follows psychotherapy.

Treatment

The objective of treatment of functional abdominal pain is to restore "normality" of patient functioning. It need not be defined as total freedom from pain symptoms. Treatment must be individualized if it is to have more than a transient effect on this condition.

Management begins with a positive diagnosis using the terminology of *functional abdominal pain. Recurrent abdominal pain* is too vague a term and not clinically useful. It is unreasonable to expect a parent whose child has chronic abdominal pain to accept a diagnosis that merely reiterates the symptom. It is mandatory to explain the nature of the symptoms and something of the presumed pathophysiology. I explain that the pain is real and is caused by an increased intensity of intestinal motor function in response to a wide variety of stressful stimuli. I emphasize that in many instances the child many experience normal amounts of stress, but the reaction of the intestines to stress results in abnormal function. I emphasize that the specific cause of the pain response is unknown but that there is a potential genetic vulnerability in those families with a strong history of pain. I explain that the condition is chronic and that pain periods may be interspersed with partial or complete remissions. It is important to reassure the parents and child that no serious organic disease exists. I review radiographic studies that the patient may have had before referral, naming disorders that are ruled out. I discuss symptom criteria and physical findings that are absent in the clinical presentation which preclude further in-depth evaluation. I specifically discuss such disorders as peptic ulcer, inflammatory bowel disease, and cancer. Reassurance is then made operational by a system of regular return visits to the primary pediatrician to monitor symptoms and physical examination.

The rational therapy of functional abdominal pain is directed toward environmental modification. The first goal is to identify, clarify, and reverse stresses that may provoke pain (see Table 4). Equally important is to reverse environmental reinforcement of the pain behavior (see Table 5). Parents and school must be engaged to support the child rather than the pain.[50] Life style must be normalized regardless of the presence of pain. Regular school attendance is essential. In many cases it is helpful for the physician to communicate directly with school officials to explain the nature of the problem. School officials must be encouraged to be responsive to the pain behavior but not to let it disrupt attendance, class activity, or performance expectations. At home, parents should foster more independent dealing with the pain on the part of the child, and less social attention should be directed toward the symptoms.

In lactose-intolerant individuals, a strict diet eliminating all food sources of lactose is instituted for 2 weeks as a therapeutic trial. Milk intake may continue during this time by pretreatment of milk with a lactase enzyme replacement such as Lact-aid (10 drops per quart, effectively removing 92 percent of the lactose). Depending on the symptom response, foods containing minimal amounts of lactose may be reintroduced, allowing the child to determine his or her own threshold of tolerance to pain. It is important to remember that the quantity of lactose consumed before a lactose breath test (1 g per kilogram to maximum of 50 g) may exceed the normal daily lactose intake of a child (50 g lactose is roughly equivalent to a quart of milk). If a child dislikes milk or drinks small quantities per day, it is not necessary to hydrolyze all of the lactose. The usual recommended dosage of Lact-aid (5 drops per quart, which removes 70 percent of the lactose) or commercially available lactose-free milk is recommended in such patients. Recent evidence suggests that yogurt is well-tolerated in lactose-intolerant patients because bacterial cultures in yogurt utilize lactose as a substrate and enzymatically break it down.[51] This is true only for homemade yogurts and specific brands without added milk solids.

Because other dietary carbohydrates may be malabsorbed and act as provocative stimuli in functional abdominal pain, a 3- to 7-day food record often uncovers excessive intakes of carbonated beverages (fructose), dietary starches (corn, potatoes, wheat, oats), or sorbitol-containing products (vehicle for oral medication, sugar substitute in gum and candy, ingredient in toothpaste, and a plasticizer in gelatin capsules). A similar 2-week diagnostic and therapeutic trial, as described above for lactose, eliminating the potential offending sugar may be tried.

A controversial issue in the management of functional abdominal pain is the use of a high-fiber diet or bulk-producing agents. Such therapy is a mainstay of adult IBS, in which constipation is a major feature. Only one study in children has suggested that increased fiber may be beneficial in terms of pain frequency or severity. In a double crossover study, Feldman et al observed a significant decrease in pain attacks in patients whose diet was supplemented with 10 g of corn fiber per day, compared with placebo.[52] The number of patients in this study was small, and the inclusion criteria did not satisfy Apley's definition of chronicity. Nevertheless, I usually recommend a high-fiber diet in patients with functional abdominal pain, although I do not specify quantity. I do stress that excessive fiber in the diet may result in increased gas and distention (as described above) and actually provoke pain. The use of bulk-producing agents is probably not indicated in functional abdominal pain unless there is associated constipation.

There are no data that support the use of drug therapy (anticholinergics, antispasmodics, anticonvulsants, etc.) in patients with functional abdominal pain. However, it is rare for the gastroenterologist to see such patients who have not been treated with Donnatal or Bentyl, as needed. Such therapy is probably one of the major reinforcers of pain behavior in these patients. Nevertheless, many gastroenterologists quote anecdotal evidence of clinical improvement when antispasmodics are given on a regular schedule for a finite period of time following diagnosis of functional abdominal pain. Efficacy is difficult to evaluate in the context of simultaneous environmental modification in such patients. These types of drugs in the low doses given have a relatively good safety record. I have used such medication for finite periods in rare patients whom I feel need a "face-saving device" to ease their return to a normal life style.

Hospitalization is rarely indicated for patients with functional abdominal pain. Stone and Barbero demonstrated that 50 percent of patients experience relief of symptoms during hospitalization.[10] However, no data have been presented that the natural history of the pain is affected. Hospitalization does not enhance the fundamental goals of environmental modification. More commonly it reinforces pain behavior.

Consultation with a child psychiatrist or psychologist is indicated if the gastroenterologist is concerned about (1) conversion reaction, (2) extreme internalizing behavior in the child (anxiety, depression, low self-esteem), (3) modeling or imitation of family pain behavior, (4) maladaptive family coping mechanisms, or (5) failure of the initial attempts at environmental modification to result in return to a normal life style. Following referral, the gastroenterologist must communicate with the psychiatrist or psychologist and continue to see the patient to assure parental compliance. If environmental modification is not possible or not successful, a behavioral approach is a practical alternative. I have become increasingly impressed by the beneficial effects of teaching the child relaxation techniques on the frequency and severity of pain episodes.

Prognosis

There are no prospective studies of the outcome of functional abdominal pain. Reassuringly, retrospective studies suggest that organic disease is rarely masked in the context of a functional disorder.[6,7,49,50] Once functional abdominal pain is diagnosed, subsequent follow-up rarely identifies an occult organic disorder. Interestingly, pain resolves completely in 30 to 50 percent of patients by 2 to 6 weeks after diagnosis.[6,7,53,54] This high incidence of early resolution suggests that in most instances child and parent accept reassurance that the pain is not organic and that environmental modification is effective treatment. Nevertheless, more long-term studies suggest 30 to 50 percent of children with functional abdominal pain in childhood experience pain as adults, although in 70 percent of such individuals the pain does not limit normal activity. Both Christensen and Mortensen[53] and Apley and Hale[54] report that the clinical symptoms in adults are more consistent with irritable bowel syndrome. Thirty percent of patients with functional abdominal pain develop other chronic complaints as adults, including headaches, backaches, and menstrual irregularities.[54] Based on a small number of patients, Apley and Hale have described several factors that influence prognosis for a lasting resolution of pain symptoms during childhood (Table 6).[54]

SPECIFIC VARIANTS OF FUNCTIONAL ABDOMINAL PAIN

Nonulcer Dyspepsia

Unlike functional abdominal pain, nonulcer dyspepsia is a diagnosis that has received little attention in the pediatric literature. Heretofore, this group of patients has been included

TABLE 6
Factors That Affect Long-term Resolution of Functional Abdominal Pain

Factor	Prognosis Better	Prognosis Worse
Family	Normal	"Painful family"
Sex	Female	Male
Age of onset	Over 6 years	Under 6 years
Period before treatment	Under 6 months	Over 6 months

From Apley and Hale.[54]

under the RAP designation. They should be considered separately, however, because of differences in clinical presentation, diagnostic evaluation, and management. This subset of patients complains of chronic (greater than 3 months) epigastric or midepigastric abdominal pain, which may or may not be associated with eating. Associated symptoms include nausea, bloating, regurgitation, heartburn, belching, hiccups, and "gastric rumblings." I am impressed that patients characteristically answer "yes" to inquiries of each of these symptoms. Vomiting, evidence of GI blood loss, weight loss, and systemic symptoms are rare. The "peptic symptoms" often alternate with more classic symptoms of irritable bowel syndrome discussed below. Physical examination is normal. One is struck by how well the patient appears. The disorder in my experience occurs in the same age distribution as functional abdominal pain. Most commonly, the age of onset is after 10 years. The same pain consequences as observed in functional abdominal pain tend to occur. Indeed, pain reinforcement is often greater because the symptoms more clearly suggest an organic problem.

Nonulcer dyspepsia is probably not a homogeneous entity. Genetic, environmental, and psychological factors have been suggested to play a role in the pathogenesis of nonulcer dyspepsia in adults.[28,55] Alterations in gastric acid secretion and gastroduodenal and small bowel motility have been described.[56] Thirty to 50 percent of adult patients have mild chronic histologic gastritis and/or duodenitis, usually associated with macroscopically normal mucosa at endoscopy.[28] Such nonspecific findings have been described in asymptomatic controls.[57,58] and have also been observed in 62 percent of patients with irritable bowel syndrome.[59] Evidence is mounting that *Campylobacter pylori* colonizes the gastric antrum in one-third to one-half of adults with nonulcer dyspepsia.[28,60] Whether *C. pylori* causes or is only coincidentally associated with dyspepsia is currently unknown.[61] *C. pylori*–associated gastritis should be regarded as a separate entity at this time.

The principal differential diagnoses to be considered in nonulcer dyspepsia include peptic ulcer, gastroesophageal reflux (reflux esophagitis), *C. pylori*–associated gastritis, and drug-associated gastritis. Primary gastroesophageal reflux should be considered in a patient with a clinical history of chronic regurgitation since early childhood, dysphagia, GI blood loss, or pulmonary complaints such as chronic cough, bronchitis, and asthma. Less common causes of "peptic symptoms" include marked aerophagy, eosinophilic gastroenteritis, parasitic infestation, lactose intolerance, biliary tract disease, chronic pancreatitis, inflammatory bowel disease, and angioneurotic edema.

Laboratory evaluation should include complete blood count, white blood count, differential, erythrocyte sedimentation rate, SMA 20, amylase, lipase, and stool ova and parasites. If vomiting or GI blood loss is present, the first study should be an air-contrast upper GI series with small bowel follow-through. Such an evaluation, in addition to evaluation for ulcer, also rules out gross esophagitis, gastric outlet disorder, malrotation, and inflammatory bowel disease of the duodenum and distal small bowel. In the vast majority of patients who do not vomit, upper endoscopy is the procedure of choice. Peptic ulceration and macroscopic esophagitis (erosion, esophageal ulcer) are ruled out by endoscopy. Bi-

opsies of the duodenum, gastric antrum, and esophagus should be obtained for histologic review. Separate antral biopsies should be evaluated for urease production and cultured for *C. pylori*.[63,64] Primary gastroesophageal reflux is usually ruled out by finding histologic changes of mild gastritis and/or duodenitis in antral and duodenal biopsies. In the absence of documentation of *C. pylori*, the finding of mild nonspecific upper GI inflammation should not deter a positive diagnosis of nonulcer dyspepsia.

Management begins with a clear positive diagnosis using the terminology *nonulcer dyspepsia*. Clinical improvement is often observed by the simple act of applying a name to the disorder. As with functional abdominal pain, it is mandatory to explain the natue of the symptoms and discuss speculations on pathophysiology. Therapy is directed toward environmental modification. Parents are advised to avoid exposing their children to cigarette smoke, caffeine, nonsteroidal anti-inflammatory medications, and specific foods that exacerbate symptoms. Attempts should be made to identify, clarify, and reverse stresses that may provoke symptoms (see Table 4). Equally important is to reverse reinforcement of the pain behavior (see Table 5). If environmental modification is not possible or not successful, teaching the child relaxation techniques may be helpful.[65]

Because of uncertainty of pathogenesis, I currently treat all patients with evidence of histologic inflammation with short-term therapy (6 weeks) with an H_2 receptor blocker (cimetidine 7.5 mg per kilogram orally three times a day or ranitidine 2 mg per kilogram orally twice a day). I have been unimpressed with the results of this therapy to date. Antacids are not recommended primarily because of compliance problems in this age group, especially when there is no clearcut therapeutic response. Anticholinergics (propantheline bromide) may occasionally temporize postprandial symptoms if given before a meal.

Prognosis of nonulcer dyspepsia is unknown. Until better understanding of this condition is achieved, close follow-up is required because of the potential of complications, including peptic ulcer and reflux esophagitis.

Irritable Bowel Syndrome

Onset of chronic abdominal pain in adolescence is more commonly associated with altered bowel habits. The clinical presentation of alternating diarrhea and constipation, flatulence, and lower abdominal pain is characteristic of irritable bowel syndrome (IBS) in adults.[66,67] Because of age, however, such patients are usually referred for diagnostic evaluation of inflammatory bowel disease. Further confusing the presentation is the frequent co-existence of features of functional dyspepsia.

Typical symptoms in the context of a normal physical examination should suggest the diagnosis of IBS to the experienced gastroenterologist. It is essential that IBS be included in the initial differential diagnosis explained to the patient and parent. The principal differential diagoses to be considered include inflammatory bowel disease, lactose intolerance, parasitic infestation, and laxative abuse. Stepwise diagnostic evaluation should include complete blood count, erythrocyte sedimentation rate, urinalysis, urine culture, analysis of the stool for blood and parasites, lactose breath H_2 test, and pelvic examination in girls. Total colonscopy is recommended for all patients with guaiac-positive stool, weight loss, or significant diarrhea. Patients with IBS may exhibit microscopic inflammation of the colon, despite normal macroscopic endoscopic appearance.[59] Based on current reports in the literature, these patients should not be treated for chronic inflammatory bowel disease in the absence of small bowel radiographic changes, systemic symptoms, growth retardation, or elevated erythrocyte sedimentation rate.

Therapy of IBS begins with a positive diagnosis. As in other variants of functional abdominal pain, environmental modification is an important focus of management. High-fiber diet and psyllium preparations are logical agents for the treatment of irritable bowel syndrome, particularly when there is alternating constipation and diarrhea. A low-fat diet may also be helpful. The patient whose life style is disrupted by diarrhea may benefit from taking loperamide prior to anticipated stressful events. Antispasmodics (dicyclomine 10 to 20 mg) may occasionally help individual patients. Anticholinergics may also occasionally temporize postprandial abdominal pain and diarrhea. Management of excessive gas is difficult. Patients are advised to eat slowly and to avoid chewing gum, carbonated beverages, artificial sweeteners containing sorbitol, legumes, and foods of the cabbage family. Simethicone or activated charcoal may help individual patients.

SUMMARY

One can appreciate the evolution of a biopsychosocial model of functional abdominal pain in children and adolescents which provides a framework for diagnosis and management and a blueprint of future research. Diagnostic criteria can be established for three variants of functional pain which occur in the pediatric patient. A management approach can be defined which attempts modifications of the contingencies operating with a child's environment to maintain the pain behavior. Prospective studies are needed to determine the long-term outcome of such an approach. Basic studies are needed to better define how stressful stimuli affect intestinal function and why in some patients altered intestinal motor activity is perceived as pain.

REFERENCES

1. Apley J. The child with abdominal pains. London: Blackwell Scientific Publications, 1975.
2. Apley J, Naish N. Recurrent abdominal pains: a field survey of 1000 school children. Arch Dis Child 1958; 33:165–170.
3. Oster J. Recurrent abdominal pain, headache, and limb pains in children and adolescents. Pediatrics 1972; 50:429–436.
4. Pringle MLK, Butler NR, Davie R. 11,000 seven year olds. London: Longmans, 1966.
5. Faull C, Nicol AR. Abdominal pain in six-year olds: an epidemiological study in a new town. J Child Psychol Psychiatry 1986; 27:251–260.
6. Barr RG. Recurrent abdominal pain. In: Levine MD, Carey WP, Crocker AC, Gross RT, eds. Developmental-behavioral pediatrics. Philadelphia: WB Saunders, 1983.
7. Stickler GB, Murphy DB. Recurrent abdominal pain. Am J Dis Child 1979; 133:486–489.
8. Galler JR, Neustein S, Walker WA. Clinical aspects of recurrent abdominal pain in children. Adv Pediatr 1980; 27:31–53.
9. Liebman WM. Recurrent abdominal pain in children: a retrospective survey of 119 patients. Clin Pediatr 1978; 17:149–153.
10. Stone RJ, Barbero GJ. Recurrent abdominal pain in childhood. Pediatrics 1970; 45:732–738.
11. Raymor D, Weininger O, Hamilton JR. Psychological problems in children with abdominal pain. Lancet 1984; i:439–440.
12. Wood B. A biopsychosocial model for the treatment of pediatric gastrointestinal disease. In: Walker W, Durie PR, Hamilton JR, Walker-Smith JA, Watkins JB, eds. Pediatric gastrointestinal disease: pathophysiology, diagnosis, management. Philadelphia: BC Decker, 1989.
13. Minuchin S. Rosman BL, Baker L. Psychosomatic families: anorexia nervosa in context. Cambridge, MA: Harvard University Press, 1978.
14. Barr RG, Levine MD, Watkins J. Recurrent abdominal pain in children due to lactose intolerance. A prospective study. N Engl J Med 1979; 300:1449–1452.
15. Lebenthal E, Rossi TM, Nord KS, Branski D. Recurrent abdominal pain and lactose absorption in children. Pediatrics 1981; 67:828–832.
16. Wald A, Chandra R, Fisher SE, Gartner JC, Zitelli B. Lactose malabsorption in recurrent abdominal pain in childhood. J Pediatr 1982; 100:65–68.
17. Dimson SB. Transit time related to clinical findings in children with recurrent abdominal pain. Pediatrics 1972; 47:666–674.
18. Kopel FB, Kim IC, Barbero GJ. Comparison of rectosigmoid motility in normal children, children with RAP, and children with ulcerative colitis. Pediatrics 1967; 39:539–544.
19. Pineiro-Carrero VM, Andres JM, Davis RH, Mathias JR. Abnormal gastroduodenal motility in children and adolescents with recurrent functional abdominal pain. J Pediatr 1988; 113:820–825.
20. Andrews PLR. Vagal afferent innervation of the gastrointestinal tract. Prog Brain Res 1986; 67:65–86.
21. Rubin LS, Barbero GJ, Sibinga MS. Pupillary reactivity in children with recurrent abdominal pain. Psychosom Med 1967; 29:111–120.
22. Apley J, Haslam DR, Tulloch G. Pupillary reaction in children with recurrent pain. Arch Dis Child 1971; 46:337–340.
23. Feuerstein M, Barr RG, Francoeur TE, Houle M, Rafman S. Potential biobehavioral mechanisms of recurrent abdominal pain in children. Pain 1982; 13:287–298.
24. Boyle JT. Gastroesophageal reflux in the pediatric patient. Gastroenterol Clin North Am 1989; 18:315–337.
25. Bo-Linn GW, Vendrell DD, Lee E, Fordtran JS. An evaluation of the significance of microscopic colitis in patients with chronic diarrhea. J Clin Invest 1985; 75:1559–1569.
26. Elliot PR, Williams CB, Lennard-Jones JE, Dawson AM, Bartram CL, Thomas BM, Swarbrick ET, Morson BC. Colonscopic diagnosis of minimal change colitis in patients with normal sigmoidoscopy and normal air-contrast barium enema. Lancet 1982; i:650–651.
27. Heyman MB, Prman JA,. Ferrell LD, Thaler MM. Chronic nonspecific inflammatory bowel disease of the cecum and proximal colon in children with grossly normal appearing colonic mucosa; diagnosis by colonoscopic biopsies. Pediatrics 1987; 80:255–261.
28. Talley NJ, Phillips SF. Non-ulcer dyspepsia: potential causes and pathophysiology. Ann Intern Med 1988; 108:865–879.
29. Fordyce WE, Fowler RS, Lehmann JR, Delateur BJ. Some implications of learning in problems of chronic pain. J Chron Dis 1968; 2:179–190.
30. Miller AJ, Kratochwill TR. Reduction of frequent stomachache complaints by time out. Behav Ther 1979; 10:211–218.
31. Drumm B, Rhoads JM, Stringer DA, Sherman PM, Ellis LE, Durie PR. Peptic ulcer disease in children: etiology, clinical findings, and clinical course. Pediatrics 1988; 82:410–414.
32. Silverman A, Roy CC. Peptic disease. In: Pediatric clinical gastroenterology. 3rd ed. St. Louis: CV Mosby, 1983.
33. Tomomasa T, Hsu JY, Shigeta M, et al. Statistical analyses of symptoms and signs in pediatric patients with peptic ulcer. J Pediatr Gastroenterol Nutr 1986; 5:711–715.
34. Byrne WJ, Arnold WC, Stannard MW, Redman JF. Ureteropelvic junction obstruction presenting with recurrent abdominal pain: diagnosis by ultrasound. Pediatrics 1985; 76:934–937.
35. Williams TE, Sherman NJ, Clatworthy HW. Chronic fibrosing pancreatitis in childhood: a cause of recurrent abdominal pain. Pediatrics 1967; 40:1019.
36. Rothstein FC, Gauderer MWL. Hereditary pancreatitis and recurrent abdominal pain of childhood. J Pediatr Surg 1985; 20:535–537.
37. Soltero MJ, Bill AH. The natural history of Meckel's diverticulum and its relation to incidental removal. Am J Surg 1976; 132:168.

38. Nielsen OV, Christiansen J. Chronic abdominal pain and Meckel's diverticulum. Acta Chir Scand 1973; 139:739–741.
39. Schisgall RM. Appendiceal colic in childhood. The role of inspissated casts of stool within the appendix. Ann Surg 1980; 192:687–693.
40. Ahmed S. Ovarian cysts in childhood. Aust NZ J Surg 1975; 45:398–404.
41. Porter GE. Slipping rib syndrome: an infrequently recognized entity in children: A report of three cases and review of the literature. Pediatrics 1985; 76:810–813.
42. Bugensten RH, Phibbs CM. Abdominal pain in children caused by linea alba hernias. Pediatrics 1975; 56:1073–1074.
43. Rosenthal P, Liebman WM. Comparative study of stool examinations, duodenal aspiration, and pediatric Entero-Test for giardiasis in children. J Pediatr 1980; 96:278–279.
44. Committee on Nutrition, American Academy of Pediatrics. The practical significance of lactose intolerance in children. Pediatrics 1978; 62:240–245.
45. Hyams JS. Chronic abdominal pain caused by sorbitol malabsorption. J Pediatr 1982; 100:772–773.
46. Babb RR, Eckman PB. Abdominal epilepsy. JAMA 1972; 222:65–66.
47. Zarline EJ. Abdominal epilepsy: an unusual cause of recurrent abdominal pain. Am J Gastroenterol 1984; 79:687–688.
48. Stein JA, Tschudy DP. Acute intermittent porphyria: a clinical and biochemical study of 46 patients. Medicine 1970; 49:1–16.
49. Maloney MJ. Diagnosing hysterical conversion reactions in children. J Pediatr 1980; 97:1016–1020.
50. Berger HG, Honig PJ, Liebman R. Recurrent abdominal pain. Gaining control of the symptom. Am J Dis Child 1977; 131:1340–1344.
51. Kolars JC, Levitt MD, Mostafa A, Savaiano DA. Yogurt: an autodigesting source of lactose. N Engl J Med 1984; 310:1–3.
52. Feldman W, McGrath P, Hodgson C, Ritter H, Shipman RT. The use of dietary fiber in the management of simple, childhood, idiopathic, recurrent abdominal pain. Am J Dis Child 1985; 130:1216–1218.
53. Christensen MF, Mortensen O. Long-term prognosis in children with recurrent abdominal pain. Arch Dis Child 1975; 50:110–114.
54. Apley J, Hale B. Children with recurrent abdominal pain: How do they grow up? Br Med J 1973; 3:7–9.
55. Talley NJ, McNeil D, Hayden A, Colreauy C, Piper DW. Prognosis of chronic unexplained dyspepsia. Gastroenterology 1987; 92:1060–1066.
56. Malagelada JR, Stanghellini V. Manometric evaluations of functional upper gut symptoms. Gastroenterology 1985; 88:1223–1231.
57. Kruening J, Bossman FT, Kuiper G, Wal AM, Lindeman J. Gastric and duodenal mucosa in "healthy" individuals. An endoscopic and histopathological study of 50 volunteers. J Clin Pathol 1978; 31:69–77.
58. Myren J, Sereck-Hanssen A. Gastroscopic observations related to bioptical histology in healthy medical students. Scand J Gastroenterol 1975; 37:353–355.
59. Fielding JF, Doyle GO. The prevalence and significance of gastritis in patients with lower intestinal irritable bowel (irritable colon) syndrome. J Clin Gastroenterol 1982; 4:507–510.
60. Dooley CP, Cohen H. The clinical significance of *Campylobacter pylori*. Ann Intern Med 1988; 108:70–79.
61. Bartlett JG. Campylobacter pylori: fact or fancy? Gastroenterology 1988; 94:229–232.
62. Czinn SJ, Carr H. Rapid diagnosis of *Campylobacter pyloridis* associated gastritis. J Pediatr 1987; 110:569–570.
63. Drumm B, O'Brien A, Cutz E, Sherman P. *Campylobacter pyloridis*-associated primary gastritis in children. Pediatrics 1987; 80:192–195.
64. Kilbridge PM, Dahms BB, Czinn SJ. *Campylobacter pylori* associated gastritis and peptic ulcer disease in children. Am J Dis Child 1988; 142:1149–1152.
65. Olness K. Hypnotherapy: a cyberphysiologic strategy in pain management. Pediatr Clin North Am 1989, in press.
66. Kruis W, Thieme CH, Weinzier LM, Schussler P, Holl J, Paulis W. A diagnostic score for irritable bowel syndrome. Gastroenterology 1984; 87:1–7.
67. Schuster MM. Irritable bowel syndrome. In: Sleisenger MH, Fordtran JS, eds. Pathophysiology, diagnosis, management. 4th ed. Philadelphia: WB Saunders, 1989.

6

CHAPTER

Colic and Gas

Ronald G. Barr, M.A., M.D.C.M., FRCPC

The term *colic* and the entities to which it refers are ill-defined and poorly understood in children compared with the complaint in adults. Colic is thought of as a *symptom*, a synonym for abdominal pain that is acute and unexpected, but in children it refers also to a *syndrome* characterized by a self-limited cluster of behaviors in the first 3 months of life, presumed to be secondary to underlying gastrointestinal (GI) disturbances. Also, older infants and children are described sometimes as "colicky," implying a *predisposition* to irritability and GI upset. It is telling that neither the presumption that its source is gastrointestinal nor that it is a painful condition has been demonstrated. Our understanding of its etiology, its pathophysiology, and its treatment is far from complete.

Frequently gas is associated with colic. It is so deeply embedded in the lay description of colic that the syndrome is often referred to as "colic and gas," or just "wind."[1-3] After crying, gas is the second most common defining symptom (Table 1). Observations of abdominal distention and acute relief when gas is released per rectum lend credence to its role, but it is unclear whether the role of this ubiquitous gas in the syndrome is primary or secondary.

Systematic descriptions of "colic" have provided some understanding of the nature of the complaint, identified certain behavioral characteristics that putative mechanisms should explain, delimited the role of familiar hypotheses, and suggested rational approaches to management. Interest in possible GI determinants of colic continues to command attention because of a perceived relationship between diet and symptoms, but evidence supporting such relationships remains tentative at best.

DEFINITIONS

Colic refers to a behavioral *syndrome* occurring during the first 3 months of life; in about 30 percent of cases, symptoms persist into the fourth and fifth months.[1,4] It has been proposed that some underlying mechanisms leading to colic in babies are associated with such problems as difficult temperament, sleep disturbance, diarrhea, child abuse, and recurrent abdominal pain later in life, but these associations have not been proven.[5-8] It is unclear whether infants with colic are actually "normal."[9] In clinical practice, colic usually implies normality (nondisease), a conclusion supported by prevailing opinion and most clinical series.[4,5,10,11] For most infants, the characteristic behaviors of "colic" most likely represent normal, albeit dysfunctional, functioning, but in

a few cases, colic may be the manifestation of an organic disease. The extent to which the clinical syndrome of colic "matches" similar behaviors in normal infants remains completely unknown.

It is proposed that the definition of colic be restricted to a behavioral *syndrome* brought as a concern to the physician, leaving open the question of its normality, putative etiologies, or prognosis. Such a definitional strategy takes the reported behavior as the starting point, refrains from making assumptions about what is not known (e.g., whether its source is gastrointestinal and/or pain), and permits an evaluation of various predisposing factors, such as characteristics of the child, the child's environment, and parental perceptions.

Clinicians differ on what they consider to be constituent behaviors of the syndrome (Table 1). Almost all accept some level of crying (or fussing) behavior, and most qualify the crying as being more typical in the evening, reaching a peak sometime in the second month, and resolving if left untreated by 3 to 4 months of age. The most frequently applied diagnostic criterion is Wessel's "rule of threes," that is, crying more than 3 hours per day for more than 3 days per week for more than 3 weeks.[4] Other criteria include characteristic motor behaviors (legs over the abdomen, clenched fists), atypical facial expression (pain facies), GI symptoms (abdominal distention, gas, regurgitation), and lack of responsivity to soothing stimulation.

Whether these criteria define a distinct entity or simply the extreme end of the spectrum of crying of normal infants remains unresolved. The *pattern* of crying with evening clustering peaking at 2 months is identical to that seen in infants without colic.[12,13] Severity of crying has not been demonstrated to correlate consistently with other possible determinants of the syndrome.[5,10,11] Furthermore, the associated motor, facial, gastrointestinal, and lack of responsiveness criteria could be sequelae of prolonged active crying bouts rather than specific signs of a distinct condition. The possibility that there may be qualitative differences between the cries of normal infants and those with colic, although often suggested, has not been assessed objectively.

When colic is described as a *symptom* in infants having an identifiable organic disease, usually it refers to unexplained, unremitting crying for a short period and is often not limited to the age group typical of the colic syndrome. Whether any organic disease conditions present with the crying pattern seen in colic *syndrome* remains undetermined. In older infants and verbal children, the complaint is less likely to denote crying and more likely to refer to abdominal pain.

TABLE 1
Definitions That "Recognize" These Features as Relevant to Identification of "Colic"
(n = 50 Articles)*

Features of "Colic"	Articles Including This Feature (%)	Features of "Colic"	Articles Including This Feature (%)
General Characteristics		**Motor Characterisitics**	
Paroxysmal (in nature)	42	Taut legs, knees up	28
Unresponsive to intervention	24	Clenched fists	10
Otherwise well infant (unexplained cry)	30	Increased activity	4
No definition given	8	**Gastrointestinal Characteristics**	
Cry Characteristics		Gas-related	30
Presence of cry/fuss	82	Distended abdomen	10
Duration of cry/fuss		Other GI symptoms	
≥90 minutes	6	Vomiting, regurgitation	6
≥3 hours/day	14	Diarrhea	6
≥3 days/week	8	**Interpretation of Origin**	
≥3 weeks	6	Pain experience	26
Nonspecific duration	4	GI origin	12
Frequency of cry/fuss		**Other Characteristics**	
Frequency bouts	8	Altered sleep/feed pattern	14
≥1 episode/day	6	Distress to parents	6
Varying	2		
Daily pattern of cry/fuss			
Late afternoon/evening	28		
Postprandial	12		
Same time each day	2		
Age of onset of "colic"			
≤3 weeks	20		
Age of cessation of "colic"			
≤3 months	38		
>3 months	10		
Prolonged bouts of crying	20		
Quality of cry (screaming)	18		

* Definitions from 50 articles culled from three review articles on infant colic. (Table prepared by S. McMullan.)

PATHOGENESIS

Despite definitional uncertainties, the behavioral features of colic suggest potential underlying mechanisms; such mechanisms should explain *both* the early increase in crying *and* its subsequent decline, the most reliable feature of the crying of both colicky and noncolicky infants.[4,10–13] Similarly, crying during the day is not random, but tends to cluster in the evening hours ("evening colic"). Finally, there is increasing evidence in normal infants that the malleable component of early crying is duration (or bout length) and not frequency,[13,14] but a colic "episode" is difficult to terminate after it starts. This observation suggests that mechanisms underlying colic may relate to intrinsic or extrinsic proximal factors, which tend not so much to initiate crying as to maintain the crying state once it has begun.

The Concept of State

Infant behavior is not organized as a continuum of arousal, but rather as a set of discontinuous and distinct modes of activity representing central nervous system conditions. Three of the important features of behavioral states are that (1) they are self-organizing in the sense that a state is maintained until that pattern of necessary and/or sufficient events occurs which results in a "shift" to another state, (2) they are relatively stable over time (minutes rather than seconds), and (3) the same input stimulus experienced in different states results in nonlinear, state-specific output responses. In Wolff's classification, crying is defined in terms of persistent cry vocalizations (from whimpering to loud screaming), diffuse motor activity or rigid extended trunk posture, resistance of limbs to passive movement, and facial cry grimace sometimes accompanied by flushing.[15] In support of the concept of a cry state, Wolff notes that it is a specific property of the behavior of human infants not seen in other animal young that crying and the accompanying rhythmic limb movements frequently continue after removal of an offending stimulus.[15] Fussing is conceptualized as a state of transition, characterized by intermittent vocalizations and less intense and nonrhythmic motor activity.[15] One of the waking states, waking activity, is characterized by bursts of generalized motor activity and open eyes. Occasional moaning, grunting, or whimpering can occur, but it is always unsustained. In principle, then, a soothing stimulus applied to an infant who has just begun to cry (in whom a crying "state" has not been organized) is more likely to be successful in aborting the transition from awake activity to crying than when it is applied to the infant after the crying has become sustained. Similarly, the soothing stimulus is less likely to be successful if it occurs with another stimulus (e.g., a pain stimulus) sufficient to establish transition to and/or maintenance of a crying state.

The features of vocalization, motor behavior, facial expression, and vascular reactivity that characterize crying as a self-organizing state closely parallel the clusters of behavior which are "recognized" as typical of colic. Therefore, what is being described as colic probably is not a disease entity, but rather a "discontinuous" concatenation of behaviors. This concept helps to explain how the crying of colic may be distinct from common fussing and intermittent crying while being a manifestation of normal behavior. It helps to explain why a soothing maneuver successful for the unsustained whimpering of fussiness might fail if initiated during the crying state. More generally, the problem of colic may be the problem of understanding the conditions that provoke or terminate the crying *state*, not just crying vocalizations.

Central Nervous System Maturation and Self-Regulation

Probably the rapid growth and differentiation of the central nervous system during early postnatal life is an important determinant of the behavioral states manifest as colic syndrome. Infant states undergo significant change during the second to fourth month of life, including periodic organization of sleep and waking[15,16] and emergence of the waking state of "alert activity."[15] The overall amount of wakefulness continuously increases during this period, but its quality changes rapidly at 6 to 8 weeks. Alert activity is characterized principally by goal-directed activity (e.g., visual pursuit, smiling, vocalizing with social pattern) without reciprocal inhibition of continuous limb movements.[15] The organizational shift reflected in this emerging maturation of the central nervous system is probably prerequisite to the infant's attainment of state control and ability to maintain a stable waking state less affected by extrinsic or intrinsic perturbations. The decline in crying following the early peak at 2 months probably represents only one manifestation of central nervous system organization of state control in the infant.

The development of cognitive, affective, and motor function makes maintenance of a stable state of noncrying wakefulness less dependent on environmental factors. For example, the infant becomes more responsive to psychologically significant environmental stimuli during the first 3 months, including the human voice (compared with nonhuman sounds) and human figures (compared with visual distraction in general).[15] The onset of the "social" smile at about 6 weeks serves to prolong infant interaction with caregivers and stabilize alert waking states. Similarly, the increase in thumb-sucking provided by hand control permits the infant to achieve a quiet awake state through co-ordinated rhythmic motor activity.[12] In general, the infant's increasing competence pro-

vides more options than are available earlier for self-regulation of state in the second and third months. Most etiologic hypotheses fail to account for the "spontaneous remission" of colicky behavior despite persistence of etiologic factors. The infant's maturing ability to regulate state may explain this remission in part. This increasing competence could modify the crying response in the face of persistent stimuli that otherwise predispose to transition to and/or maintenance of a crying state.

Feeding and Colic

The dietary causes most commonly implicated in colic relate to the constituents of the feeding, particularly its protein content. Dietary cow's milk proteins are presumed to act as antigenic stimuli for a GI hypersensitivity reaction. If this were an important consideration, change or modification of the ingested protein to a less antigenic form should reduce the colicky behavior. In breast versus formula comparisons, two contradictory predictions are possible depending on which mechanism is operative. On the one hand, formula-fed infants should develop colic because of the presence of potentially antigenic protein. On the other hand, breast feeding may produce an "insufficient milk syndrome" due to increased hunger and crying. In controlled studies, neither prediction has been confirmed. The prevalence, pattern, and amount of crying associated with colic have been similar in breast and formula feeders in referred and nonreferred infants.[2,10,11,17,18] In theory, this lack of difference could have occurred because both hypotheses are true, with the opposing effects acting to diminish group differences. Also, the most likely protein antigen in cow's milk, beta-lactoglobulin, is found in human milk,[19] a finding that could diminish group differences in colic incidence. Furthermore, variables such as socioeconomic status, infant care, and attitudinal differences probably co-vary with choice of feeding, making it difficult to identify independent effects attributable to diet. Nevertheless, the clinical impression of crying differences in breast- and formula-fed infants is not substantiated when such potential confounders are controlled.[18]

Cow's milk protein intolerance could be implicated by immunologic or local toxic mchanisms. True cow's milk hypersensitivity occurs in recognized clincial syndromes,[20,21] but there are inadequate data relating it to colic. Classic GI hypersensitivity manifestations of vomiting and diarrhea are not part of colic syndrome, and colic is often not seen in other protein intolerance syndromes.[20] The incidence of family atopic history and other atopic manifestations is not increased in colic patients.[10,11,22] The quantity of ingested antigen, the relative permeability of the small intestine to dietary protein, and reduced secretory IgA typical of the infant may predispose patients to dietary antigen sensitization, but the confusing spectrum of clinical presentations of hypersensitivity reactions,[23] the number of potential protein antigens in cow's milk (about 20), the possible role of digestive products, and the variety of possible humoral or cellular mechanisms both local and systemic make demonstration of a specific immunologic relationship to colic difficult.[21] Evidence of increased plasma cell content in the lamina propria of small intestinal mucosa in response to milk challenge has been reported in infants with colic and with other milk protein intolerance syndromes consistent with an IgE-mediated hypersensitivity reaction.[24] Both immunologic and toxic mechanisms imply tissue damage in the intestine, but indirect evidence of intestinal damage as indexed by fecal alpha[1]-antitrypsin and hemoglobin concentrations is lacking in colic.[25]

Diet trials have been conducted in infants with colic to provide indirect evidence implicating protein intolerance. Evans et al did not demonstrate symptomatic improvement in breast-fed infants despite a measureable reducton in the presence of cow's milk antigen on control days.[22] However, Jakobsson and colleagues did find symptomatic improvement in select subgroups of infants with colic symptoms in response to elimination of cow's milk from the diet of the infant or mother in formula- and breast-fed infants, respectively.[26,27] In three breast-fed infants, symptomatic improvement occurred in association with reduction in detectable beta-lactoglobulin in the breast milk.[19] At best, current evidence supports the possibility of protein intolerance in a small proportion of infants with colic symptoms.

Despite the emphasis on dietary content, other elements of feeding practices may also be determinants of crying behavior. In particular, feeding *style* represented by frequency (or interfeed interval) is closely related to infant state. Under conditions in which usual feeding patterns are suspended, an endogenous 4-hour sleep-wake cycle, presumably under control of GI physiologic rhythms, becomes manifest and can be manipulated by changes in the feeding schedule.[28,29] The sleep-wake cycles of breast-fed infants of La Leche League mothers, whose interfeed intervals are shorter than those of "standard care" mothers, do not develop the typical "settling through the night" at 4 months.[30] If colic is conceptualized as transition to and maintenance of the crying state, such gastrointestinal-state interdependence might be expected to be reflected in early crying behavior. Indeed, less frequent and fewer prolonged crying bouts are observed in infants whose mothers have an a priori commitment to frequent feeding, suggesting that feeding style is a proximal cause of less crying.[31] If so, the practice of scheduled and widely spaced feedings may exacerbate the tendency to prolong the wakeful crying state.

Intestinal Gas

Intestinal gas may be derived from air swallowing, diffusion from the blood, and intraluminal production.[32] Air swallowing is the main source of gastric gas, which is predominantly nitrogen and oxygen. Intraluminal production of carbon dioxide derives from the interaction of hydrogen ion and bicarbonate in the small intestine and as a direct or indirect product of bacterial fermentation in the colon. Hydrogen and methane, the other major GI gases, are produced by bacterial metabolism in the colon in adults and probably in infants.[32,33] Passive diffusion of gas between blood and lumen is dependent on relative partial pressures of the gases in the two compartments, with the probable result that carbon dioxide enters the stomach, nitrogen the small intestine and colon, and oxygen the colon. Gas is removed from the intestine through eructation, lumen-to-blood diffusion with

subsequent expiration through the lungs, flatus, and bacterial catabolism in the colon.[32]

Factors affecting accumulation and distribution of gas in the intestine may be implicated in the mechanisms of colic. Obligate air swallowing with sucking is thought to be exacerbated by poor feeding technique or inappropriately sized holes in artificial nipples. Crying itself may result in additional gastric gas, which remains after the crying episode itself has ended.[34] Lying supine may inhibit gas escape if the posteriorly placed gastroesophageal junction is covered by gastric liquid. Gastric accumulation itself may be irrelevant, symptoms depending on passage of gas through the pylorus,[35] but this is unknown.

Colonic gas produced in the gut may be the major contributor to abdominal gas. Colonic bacteria utilize as substrate exogenous carbohydrate, protein, and endogenous glycoproteins, but exogenous carbohydrate (usually lactose) results in relatively more gas per gram of substrate.[36] Extrapolating from in vitro estimates of small intestinal lactase activity, Auricchio et al predicted that the newborn small intestine, despite a maximum level of lactase activity at birth, might not be able to hydrolyze the quantity of lactose presented to it.[37] Incomplete lactose digestion unassociated with clinical disease has been confirmed in vivo by breath hydrogen testing in response to typical feeding conditions in normal infants[33,38]; in fact, some proportion of all carbohydrates in formulae are incompletely absorbed.[39] There is significant interindividual variability, but the "functional" lactose insufficiency persists into the third month of life in most infants.[33] Colonic gas is influenced by a variety of factors affecting substrate levels and relative composition of bacterial flora and their function; these include feeding patterns, colonic acidity, and antibiotics. Intermittent incomplete absorption of lactose after the first 2 months of life implies a developmental increase in small intestinal capacity to handle carbohydrate loads, change in nonsubstrate factors related to gas production, or both.

In principle, a primary role for colonic gas secondary to incomplete carbohydrate absorption in colic is attractive because it is consistent with the clinical pattern observed in patients. Colic could be related to a large individual variability in colonic gas production; both breast- and formula-fed infants are equally likely to be affected, and increased absorption occurs at approximately the same ages as the "spontaneous" reduction in crying. Evening crying could be related to accumulation of partial, incompletely absorbed carbohydrate from the more frequent daytime feeds. The hypothesis is consistent with persistent postfeed crying (Table 1), since colonic gas would still be present even with adequate burping. However, mechanisms by which gas might be implicated in producing distress and crying have not been elucidated. The usual presumptions are that increased gas volume or localized accumulations of gas occur, but there is little radiologic evidence to indicate increased intestinal gas volume in colic.[10,34,40] Another theoretical possibility is that distressing sensations may be related to intestinal gas volume *change*, producing reactive gut contractions rather than a steady state of distention. Alternatively, pain may be related to motility patterns that permit retrograde gas passage from the colon rather than volume differences.[41] Unfortunately, to date, attempts to modify crying behavior by interventions designed to reduce intestinal gas volume using lactase pretreatment of formulae or surface-active agents (Simethicone) have been unsuccessful.[42,43]

Motility

Theoretically, alterations in intestinal motor activity could predispose to colic as a direct source of abdominal distress or indirectly by affecting the distribution, accumulation/ elimination, or transit of stimulus substances in the intestinal contents, including gas. Jorup[40] reported colonic hyperperistalsis, increased rectal pressure, and responsiveness to anticholinergics in "dyspeptic" infants in whom frequent stools were a prominent symptom. The motility changes were limited to the colon, stimulated by sucking, equally likely with breast or cow's milk, and noticeable for individual differences in pressure fluctuations. Although the finding of loose stools was somewhat atypical, Jorup believes that the majority of cases of colic can be accounted for by this mechanism. In favor of motility disturbances as determinants of colic is the clinical usefulness of dicyclomine hydrochloride, the only medication supported by proper clinical trials, to date.[44,45] Dicyclomine is thought to decrease GI spasm by a direct relaxant action on smooth muscle. As with any therapy, its success suggests but does not establish cause.

Prostaglandins and Gut Hormones

Because prostaglandins affect smooth muscle contraction and GI motility, are present in high concentrations in breast milk, and can induce colic and diarrhea symptoms as a side effect of intravenous administration in newborns, they are candidates as proximal mediators of colic symptoms.[46–48] There is preliminary evidence that maternal ingestion of prostaglandin synthetase inhibitors (aspirin) reduces colic symptoms in breast-fed infants.[49] Which of the prostaglandins is involved and whether the effect is local or systemic are uncertain. Most clinical syndromes in which prostaglandins are implicated involve stimulation of an intestinal secretory process with secondary motility changes; since diarrhea is not part of the colic syndrome, a role for prostaglandins would have to be explained in terms of their impact at physiologic dose levels.

A case can be made for the role of several classes of the gut hormones in colic, but direct evidence is sparse. Basal motilin levels are raised in colic infants independent of feeding type, vasoactive intestinal peptide (VIP) and gastrin levels are not, and all three are raised in other symptomatic GI syndromes, suggesting a degree of specificity for the role of motilin.[50] A subgroup of formula-fed colic infants had high VIP levels, probably related to feeding type rather than colic. The specific role of motilin is unknown, but because it stimulates gastric emtying, small intestinal peristalsis, and shorter transit time, it could contribute to passage of stimuli to the colon.

If motility changes contribute significantly to colic symptoms, endogenous opiates that have strong biologic effects on motility and secretion are likely to be implicated. These effects are not likely to be understood in isolation from cholecystokinin (CCK), which under many conditions acts to oppose the effects of the opiates. Both opiates and CCK have been implicated in the regulation of pain perception and feeding behavior (satiety).[51] The demonstration in animal models that their roles in endogenous control of pain and satiety become important only during the nursing-suckling period[52,53] could be of particular interest in understanding the decline in crying and colic behavior after 3 months of age.

Infant Care-Giving Style

Because the early crying peak is present despite varying styles of care-giving, and colic tends to be unresponsive to maternal interventions, the concept that GI factors rather than care-giving style are important in colic syndrome is supported. However, systematic observation does confirm the common wisdom that care-taking practices such as carrying and rocking are effective soothing behaviors in already crying infants; they shift arousal to states of increased visual and auditory alertness and produce soothing effects that persist.[13,15] Psychologically significant interventions, e.g., human voice and figures versus nonhuman sounds and visual distraction, become increasingly important as effective soothing agents during the early months.[15] Use of a pacifier to induce an organized rhythmic motor pattern will attenuate the crying state in response to pain[54] and probably reduce spontaneous fussing.[15] However, crying due to hunger is arrested only by gastric filling, not by sucking and swallowing.[15] In general, behaviors and environmental stimuli that involve postural change, repetitiveness, constancy and/or rhythmicity, and close proximity between mother and infant tend to maintain a noncrying state.

The effect of systematically changing infant care-giving was demonstrated by a randomized controlled trial in which parents increased carrying of their normal infants. Approximately 2 hours per day of increased carrying reduced daily cry/fuss behavior at 6 weeks by 43 percent and evening crying by 54 percent and eliminated the 6-week peak.[13] Whether such a change would have therapeutic or preventive value in relation to colic has not been demonstrated. However, a regimen of behavioral counseling aimed at increasing parental responsiveness significantly reduced crying time by 70 percent to the level seen in noncolic controls.[55] The magnitude of these effects is of the same order as that seen with medication, suggesting multiple paths for modulating the behavioral syndrome. As with medication, its effectiveness suggests, but does not demonstrate, possible etiologies.

Biobehavioral Interactions

Gastrointestinal and behavioral factors may be complementary systems modulating crying behavior. In a cross-species comparison, Blurton Jones reported that species in whom the protein and fat content of breast milk is low also demonstrate low sucking rates, frequent feeding at short intervals, and continuous proximity ("carrying species"), whereas species with high protein and fat content in breast milk exhibit the opposite behaviors ("caching species").[56] Extrapolating from human breast milk composition, infant sucking rates are, and caretaking "should" be, characteristic of carrying species. The small, frequent feeds might, for example, reduce "hunger" cries, result in less fermentable substrate delivered to the colon, and increase rhythmic sucking behavior. Indeed, care-taking in the !Kung hunter-gatherers is characterized by close mother-infant contact, constant carrying, upright posture, immediate responsivity, and frequent feeding (approximately four times per hour),[57] all features that might be expected to reduce crying behavior. Preliminary data suggest that crying and fretting in !Kung infants do show a peak in the early months and are characterized by frequent but short episodes.[14] With data from Western societies, these findings support the concept that there is an early, maturationally based predisposition to cry but that prolonged crying bouts are amenable to change by biologic and behavioral factors associated with infant care-giving style.

POPULAR MISCONCEPTIONS

Assumptions concerning colic derived from cultural and medical lore may achieve the status of facts on which treatment is based. There is accumulating evidence sufficient to reclassify a number of assumptions more appropriately as "misconceptions" than facts:

1. Neither crying and fussing nor colic has been shown to be more common in breast- or bottle-fed infants.
2. With the exception of dicyclomine hydrochloride, evidence for the effectiveness of medications is missing. The most common in current use are combinations that include alcohol, phenobarbital, and/or anticholinergics.[58,59] "Gripe water," whose active ingredients are sodium bicarbonate and alcohol, may "work" by producing an increase of gastric gas through contact with gastric acid and thus stimulating burping,[3] but its effectiveness remains untested.
3. By including "sham" diaper changes, Wolff showed that wet diapers were not a sufficient cause of infant crying.[15]
4. The advice not to respond to a crying infant because it would be "spoiled" is based usually on an operant conditioning learning paradigm. To leave the infant is difficult and ineffective,[55] and evidence to support negative consequences of "responding" is absent. Immediate responsivity and picking up activate multisensory channels demonstrably effective in soothing crying infants.
5. There is no systematic evidence that changing from breast to formula feeding reduces colic or that, with the possible exception of a small subgroup of infants, changes to special formulae are effective. There has yet to be a diet trial that appropriately controls for the "spontaneous decline" in crying which is part of the natural history of colic. The belief in the practice is out of proportion to the evidence supporting it.
6. There is no systematic evidence for, and much against, the proposition that maternal personality or anxiety causes colic. Whether prepartum maternal anxiety may contribute to postpartum infant colic has not been satisfactorily examined.

MANAGEMENT PRINCIPLES

In the absence of adequate studies, approaches to management must remain tentative. Consistent findings are the typical pattern of a crying peak in the second month and clustering in the evening, the absence of a difference between breast- and formula-fed infants, and the distress and anxiety produced in the parents. Medication and care-taking changes are the most effective measures, formula changes the least. If the conceptualization of colic as a self-organizing, prolonged crying "state" persisting after the original stimulus has resolved is correct, then recommendations likely to diminish transition to or maintenance of the crying state are in order. On these bases, rational approaches to management include the following:

1. Information for the parent(s) aimed at reducing anxiety attributable to not knowing basic facts about early crying and colic *syndrome*. Primary among these are the fact that crying increases into the second month and the absence of disease underlying the syndrome.
2. A history and physical examination aimed at detecting other symptoms and signs of underlying pathology that might produce colic *symptoms*.
3. Recommendations aimed at focusing parental anxiety and providing clinically helpful information— specifically, keeping a diary of crying and infant weight gain. Presence of the diurnal crying pattern and weight gain makes disease less likely.
4. Changes in infant care-taking styles which encourage in the infant a state of alert wakefulness rather than crying. These approaches include increased carrying and rocking, immediate responsivity to infant signals, decreased interfeed intervals, and use of a pacifier. The effectiveness of these practices probably varies as a function of the "dose," the effective dose often being greater than that which is typical of Western care-taking.[9,13,31]
5. Changes in the environment which predispose to a noncrying state by capitalizing on the responsiveness of infants to constant, rhythmic stimulation. Techniques include background music and rides in the car or stroller, as well as a variety of technical substitutes available commercially.
6. Because of reports of associated respiratory distress and apnea, dicyclomine is not generally recommended for colic. Currently there is no rationale for the use of other medications.
7. For refractory cases, a trial feeding change may be indicated in subgroups of infants with colic. It is most likely to be helpful in infants with manifestations other than crying, such as visible GI peristalsis within minutes following cow's milk protein (immediate hypersensitivity reaction), weight loss, persistent regurgitation, or diarrhea. Removal of cow's milk from the mother's diet may be tried for a breast-fed baby, but there is no evidence that a "switch" to formula is ever indicated. Changing formula for its placebo effect is not indicated and increases maternal perception of infant vulnerability.[17]

Despite lack of evidence for a primary etiologic role, the complaint of colic will continue to be understood as gastrointestinal in origin until the relevant mechanisms are better understood. The dilemma of responding to the distress of the infants and parents in the absence of demonstrable pathogenesis remains problematic.

REFERENCES

1. Illingworth RS. Crying in infants and children. Br Med J 1955; 1:75–78.
2. Stahlberg M-R. Infantile colic: occurrence and risk factors. Eur J Pediatr 1984; 143:108–111.
3. Levin S. Gripe water. South Afr Med J 1968; 42:753–757.
4. Wessel MA, Cobb JC, Jackson EB, Harris GS, Detwiler AC. Paroxysmal fussing in infancy, sometimes called "colic." Pediatrics 1954; 14:421–434.
5. Carey WB. "Colic"—primary excessive crying as an infant-environment interaction. Pediatr Clin North Am 1984; 31:993–1005.
6. Adams LM, Davidson M. Present concepts of infant colic. Pediatr Ann 1987; 16:817–820.
7. Weissbluth M. Sleep and the colicky infant. In: Guilleminault C, ed. Sleep and its disorders in children. New York: Raven, 1987; 129.
8. Frodi AM. Contribution of infant characteristics to child abuse. Am J Ment Defic 1981; 85:341–349.
9. Barr RG. Recasting a clinical enigma: The problem of early infant crying (and colic). In: Zelazo PH, Barr RG, eds. Challenges to developmental paradigms. New York: Erlbaum, in press.
10. Illingworth RS. Three months colic. Arch Dis Child 1954; 29:165–174.
11. Paradise JL. Maternal and other factors in the etiology of infantile colic. JAMA 1966; 197:123–131.
12. Brazelton TB. Crying in infancy. Pediatrics 1962; 29:579–588.
13. Hunziker UA, Barr RG. Increased carrying reduces infant crying: a randomized controlled trial. Pediatrics 1986; 77:641–648.
14. Barr RG, Konner M, Bakeman R, Adamson L. Crying in !Kung infants: A test of the cultural specificity hypothesis. Pediatr Res 1987; 21:178A.
15. Wolff PH. The development of behavioral states and the expression of emotions in early infancy: new proposals for investigation. Chicago: University of Chicago Press, 1987.
16. Weissbluth M. Sleep and the colicky infant. In: Guilleminault C, ed. Sleep and its disorders in children. New York: Raven, 1987: 129.
17. Forsyth BWC, McCarthy PL, Leventhal JM. Problems of early infancy, formula changes, and mothers' beliefs about their infants. J Pediatr 1985; 106:1012–1017.
18. Barr RG, Kramer M, Pless IB, Boisjoly C, Leduc D. Feeding and temperament as determinants of early infant cry/fuss behaviour. Pediatrics 1989.
19. Jakobsson I, Lindberg T, Benediktsson B, Hansson B-G. Dietary bovine beta-lactoglobulin is transferred to human milk. Acta Paediatr Scand 1985; 74:342–345.
20. Lake AM, Whitington PF, Hamilton SR. Dietary protein-induced colitis in breast-fed infants. J Pediatr 1982; 101:906–910.
21. Eastham EJ, Walker WA. Adverse effects of milk formula ingestion on the gastrointestinal tract: an update. Gastroenterology 1979; 76:365–374.
22. Evans RW, Fergusson DM, Allardyce RA, Taylor B. Maternal diet and infantile colic in breast-fed infants. Lancet 1981; i:1340–1342.
23. Hill DJ, Firer MA, Shelton MJ, Hosking CS. Manifestations of milk allergy in infancy: clinical and immunologic findings. J Pediatr 1986; 109:270–276.
24. Harris MJ, Petts V, Penny R. Cow's milk allergy as a cause of infantile colic: immunofluorescent studies on jejunal mucosa. Aust Paediatr J 1977; 13:276–281.
25. Thomas DW, McGilligan K, Eisenberg LD, Lieberman HM, Rissman EM. Infantile colic and type of milk feeding. Am J Dis Child 1987; 141:451–453.
26. Lothe L, Lindberg T, Jakobsson I. Cow's milk formula as a cause of infantile colic: a double-blind study. Pediatrics 1981; 70:7–10.
27. Jakobsson I, Lindberg T. Cow's milk proteins cause infantile colic in breast-fed infants: a double-blind crossover study. Pediatrics 1983; 71:268–271.
28. Mills JN. Development of circadian rhythms in infancy. In: Davis JA, Dobbing J, eds. Scientific foundations of paediatrics. London: Heinemann, 1974: 758.
29. Salzarulo P, Fagioli I, Salomon F, Ricour C, Rimbault G, Ambrosi S, Cicchi O, Duhamel JF, Rigoard MT. Sleep patterns in infants under continuous feeding from birth. Electroencephalogr Clin Neurophysiol 1980; 49:330–336.
30. Elias MF, Nicolson NA, Bora C, Johnston J. Sleep/wake patterns of breast-fed infants in the first 2 years of life. Pediatrics 1986; 77:322–329.
31. Barr RG, Elias MF. Nursing interval and maternal responsivity: effect on early infant crying. Pediatrics 1988; 81:529–536.
32. Levitt MD, Bond JH. Intestinal gas. In: Sleisenger MH, Fordtran JS, eds. Gastrointestinal disease: pathophysiology, diagnosis, and treatment. 3rd ed. Philadelphia: WB Saunders, 1983: 221.
33. Barr RG, Hanley J, Patterson DK, Wooldridge JA. Breath hydrogen excretion of normal newborn infants in response to usual feeding patterns: evidence for "functional lactase insufficiency" beyond the first month of life. J Pediatr 1984; 104:527–533.
34. Harley LM. Fussing and crying in young infants: clinical considerations and practical management. Clin Pediatr 1985; 8:139–141.
35. Snow W. The postural treatment of infant colic. AJR 1937; 38:799–780.
36. Perman JA, Modler S. Glycoproteins as substrates for production of hydrogen and methane by colonic bacterial flora. Gastroenterology 1982; 83:388–393.
37. Auricchio S, Rubino A, Murset G. Intestinal glycosidase activities in the human embryo, fetus, and newborn. Pediatrics 1965; 35:944–954.
38. Lifshitz CH, O'Brian Smith E, Garza C. Delayed complete functional lactase sufficiency in breast-fed infants. J Pediatr Gastroenterol Nutr 1983; 2:478–482.
39. Schulman RJ, Wong WW, Irving CS, Nichols BL, Klein PD. Utilization of dietary cereal by young infants. J Pediatr 1983; 103:23–28.
40. Jorup S. Colonic hyperperistalsis in neurolabile infants: studies in so-called dyspepsia in breast-fed infants. Acta Paediatr Scand 1952; Suppl 85.
41. Lasser RN, Bond JH, Levitt MD. The role of intestinal gas in functional abdominal pain. N Engl J Med 1975; 293:524–526.
42. Danielsson B, Hwang CP. Treatment of infantile colic with surface active substance (Simethicone). Acta Pediatr Scand 1985; 74:446–450.
43. Stahlberg M-R, Savilahti E. Infantile colic and feeding. Arch Dis Child 1986; 61:1232–1233.
44. Weissbluth M, Christoffel KK, Davis AT. Treatment of infantile colic with dicyclomine hydrochloride. J Pediatr 1984; 104:951–955.
45. Illingworth RS. Evening colic in infants: a double-blind trial of dicyclomine hydrochloride. Lancet 1959; ii:1119–1120.
46. Lucas A, Mitchell MD. Prostaglandins in human milk. Arch Dis Child 1980; 55:950–952.
47. Dodge JA, Hamdi IA, Burns GM, Yamashiro Y. Toddler diarrhea and prostaglandins. Arch Dis Child 1981; 56:705–707.
48. Sankaran K, Conly J, Boyle CAJ, Tyrrell M. Intestinal colic and diarrhea as side effects of intravenous alprostadil administration. Am J Dis Child 1981; 135:664–665.
49. Butler D. Infantile colic and aspirin. Med J Aust 1987; 146:179.
50. Lothe L, Ivarsson SA, Lindberg T. Motilin, vasoactive intestinal peptide and gastrin in infantile colic. Acta Paediatr Scand 1987; 76:316–320.
51. Stacher G. Effects of cholecystokinin and caerulein on human eating behavior and pain sensation: a review. Psychoneuroendocrinology 1986; 11:39–48.
52. Blass EM, Beardsley W, Hall WG. Age-dependent inhibition of suckling by cholecystokinin. Am J Physiol 1979; 236:567–570.
53. Faris PL, Komisaruk BR, Watkins LR, Mayer DJ. Evidence for the neuropeptide cholecystokinin as an antagonist of opiate analgesia. Science 1983; 219:310–312.
54. Field T, Goldson E. Pacifying effects of nonnutritive sucking on term and preterm neonates during heelstick procedures. Pediatrics 1984; 74:1012–1015.
55. Taubman B. Clinical trial of the treatment of colic by modification of parent-infant interaction. Pediatrics 1984; 74:998–1003.
56. Blurton Jones N. Comparative aspects of mother-infant contact. In: Blurton Jones N, ed. Ethological studies of child behaviour. Cambridge: Cambridge University Press, 1972: 305.
57. Konner M, Worthman C. Nursing frequency, gonadal function, and birth spacing among !Kung hunter-gatherers. Science 1980; 207:788–791.
58. O'Donovan JC, Bradstock AS. The failure of conventional drug therapy in the management of infantile colic. Am J Dis Child 1979; 133:999–1001.
59. Robinson LA, Brown AL. Colic: pharmaceutic and medical intervention. Pediatr Nursing 1979; Nov/Dec:61–64.

CHAPTER 7

Diarrhea

Jon Marc Rhoads, M.D.
Don W. Powell, M.D.

"Infantile age... is very sensitive, more sensitive than advanced age.... There is fever, also diarrhoea and pain. When the catarrh begins in the stomach, there is vomiting. When catarrh descends to, or begins in the rectum, there is tenesmus.... The % of water in the evacuations is very large....The babies are pale, and draw up their lower extremities. The odorless condition of the evacuations changes very soon, for it becomes fecal, afterwards acid, and in protracted cases,...it is cadaveric."
A. Jacobi, Acute intestinal catarrh, 1887[1]

Each year, approximately 5 million infants and children in Latin America, Asia, and Africa die of diarrheal dehydration.[2] In comparing poor with rich countries, as infant mortality rises, deaths attributed to diarrhea rise in direct proportion. In fact, in the absence of diarrheal disease, infant mortality in developing countries would probably not exceed mortality in developed nations.[3] Although some of these deaths undoubtedly occur in chronically debilitated or malnourished children, the larger proportion are preventable deaths in otherwise healthy hosts. A recent 10 year survey demonstrated that about 500 American children, almost all of them from families of low income, die of diarrheal disease each year.[4]

To consider the magnitude of the problem, one must recognize that the average child living in a developing country develops enteritis four times a year.[5] In North America, the annual rate is about 0.9 episode per child—unless the child attends a daycare center, a risk factor increasing the diarrhea attack rate to 4.5 episodes per year in some centers.[6] In the United States, diarrhea accounts for 14 hospital admissions each year per 1,000 children under 1 year old, at an average cost $1,000 to $3,000 per child.[7]

DEFINITION

Diarrhea, derived from a Greek word meaning "to flow through," is a disease characterized by deranged intestinal water and electrolyte transport. Abnormalities of muscle function, manifesting as alterations in the frequency of bowel movements, may accompany diarrhea, but healthy infants also show tremendous variation in motility pattern. For instance, stool frequency among healthy breast-fed infants ranges from once every 2 to 3 weeks to about 12 times per day. The normal formula-fed infant shows less variation, typically passing one to seven stools per day.[8] After 4 years of age, it is rare for normal infants to pass more than three stools per day.[8] Stool texture and color are also unreliable indicators of diarrhea. When toddlers ingest iron or banana fibers, their stools may assume a black color; when they consume vegetables, particularly corn and peas, virtually unaltered fiber matter may pass per rectum. Stool volume is the best predictor of whether intestinal fluid and electrolyte transport is normal in infants and children. Since stool is 60 to 95 percent water, fecal excretion is conveniently expressed by weight. Normal infants excrete 5 to 10 g per kilogram per day[9] and healthy adults, 100 to 200 g per day. A typical 15-kg 3-year-old may pass as much stool as his parents! Stool output in a healthy individual may double or triple when dietary fiber is increased, but in general a stool weight greater than 10 g per kilogram per 24 hours in infants or greater than 200 g per day in children defines diarrhea. For clinical purposes, the physician may have to rely on the assessment of the parents, that is, what they consider to be abnormal frequency or consistency.

Diarrhea commences when the normal intestinal fluid and electolyte transport is disturbed. The most common causes of diarrhea in children are intestinal colonization or invasion by microorganisms or viruses, the establishment of inflammatory processes, and drugs. The change in stool volume in infectious diarrhea is usually not subtle. Stool losses in rotavirus and enterotoxigenic *Escherichia coli* diarrheas are increased 20-fold above normal and approximate the infant's maintenance fluid requirements.[10]

NORMAL INTESTINAL FUNCTION

Fluid and Electrolyte Transport

Permeability Gradient of the Intestine. Both the apical and basolateral membranes of the intestinal epthelial cell have similar electrolyte and fluid permeabilities, regardless of the enterocyte's location along the gastrointestinal (GI) tract. However, these membrane permeabilities are modified somewhat by the active electrolyte transport mechanisms and/or conductance channels that reside in the various membranes.[11] In general, it is the permeability of the paracellular pathway (the tight junction and intercellular space) that governs the permeability characteristics of the intestinal tract. This paracellular pathway appears to be under cellular control and can vary in its permeabilty (see below).

There is a gradient of permeability along the GI tract: The duodenum is the most "leaky" segment of the intestine, whereas the rectum has the lowest permeability. The duodenal permeability allows for the rapid osmotic flow of fluid into the upper GI tract, rendering the intestinal contents essentially isotonic. In contrast, the tightness of the colonic epithelium allows the distal part of the intestinal tract to efficiently extract sodium (Na) and fluid from the luminal contents without reverse flux into the lumen. Therefore, water and electolytes are conserved and the luminal contents converted into a semisolid form that is more easily processed and eliminated by the mechanical (muscular) elements of the colon and rectum.[12]

Segmental Fluid and Electrolyte Flows. The primary function of the small bowel is to absorb nutrients, electrolytes, and water against steep gradients. The infant gut, comparatively deficient in key transport functions necessary for maximal solute and water absorption,[13-15] is challenged by the necessity to absorb, proportionally, more nutrients and fluid than the adult bowel. Quantitative regional perfusion studies of small and large intestine, which have yielded so much information on absorption in adults,[16] have not been performed in children. However, data compiled from separate pediatric studies of salivary,[17] gastric,[18] pancreaticobiliary,[19] ileostomy,[20] and stool[9,21] output allow several conclusions (Table 1). First, compared with the adult bowel, the child's small intestine is presented with more than twice the quantity of water and electrolyte (per kilogram of body weight), owing primarily to greater dietary intake and salivary output. Second, electrolyte compositions of fluids in the various parts of the small bowel and colon in infants and adults are virtually identical. Third, compared with adults, children absorb the same percentage of delivered electrolyte and water (more than 98 percent of all water and ions entering the intestinal tract) (Table 2). However, pediatric ileostomy and

stool output studies[9,20,21] indicate that the healthy child's colon is challenged by the task of absorbing two to three times as much fluid as its adult counterpart (60 versus 25 ml per kilogram per 24 hours). In the pediatric ileostomate who has lost significant Na- and water-retaining capacity of the colon, chronic volume depletion leads to increased aldosterone secretion. Mineralocorticoid excess results in expression of an ileal amiloride-inhibitable Na channel, which is normally present only in the distal colon.[22] The result is a dramatic increase in the absolute amount and percent of Na and water absorption by the small intestine.[23] Table 2 shows that an infant with a newly created ileostomy absorbs 80 percent of the estimated small bowel fluid load, whereas a child with an "established" ileostomy absorbs more than 90 percent of the same volume. In fact, output in the ileostomate is 25 ml per kilogram per day; a volume less than 50 percent of that produced from a new ileostomy.

Segmental Intestinal Function. The various regions of the intestine function as highly specialized transport organs working in series. As mentioned, the duodenum serves as a permeable mixing segment and regulator of pH and osmotic pressure. In the normal human jejunum, active chloride secretion has been observed under resting conditions. Active transport of amino acids and sugars, coupled to Na and accompanied by water absorption, is the chief function of the jejunum.[24] Dipeptides and tripeptides formed from the hydrolysis of proteins by the intraluminal pancreatic enzymes and brush border proteases are absorbed by the jejunal enterocytes, either intact or after hydrolysis to constituent amino acids.[25] Whereas amino acid transport is driven by the

TABLE 1
Volume and Ionic Composition of Fluid in the Human Intestine: Comparison of Infants with Adults

	Water Flow (ml/kg/24 hr)	Ion Concentration (mEq/L)			Ion Flow (mEq/kg/24 hr)		
		Na	K	Cl	Na	K	Cl
Entering Duodenum							
Infant							
Dietary	100	30	20	30			
Saliva	70	3	25	20			
Gastric juice*	70	50	7.5	140			
Pancreaticobiliary*	45	100	3	30			
Total	285				11	5	16
Adult							
Dietary	35	75	25	100			
Saliva	30	3	30	20			
Gastric juice	30	50	7.5	140			
Pancreaticobiliary	45	100	3	30			
Total	120				9	2	17
Entering Cecum							
Infant	60†	100‡	26†	—	2.5‡	0.7‡	—
Adult	25	125	9	60	3.0	0.2	1.5
Stool							
Infant	5–10	22	54	21	0.2	0.4	0.1
Adult	1–3	32	75	16	0.1	0.2	0.1

Data from references 9, 16–21, and 23.
* Gastric and pancreaticobiliary electrolyte concentrations based on adult data.[16]
† Volume of output from a ''new'' ileostomy.[20] Volume from an established pediatric ileostomy is 25 ml/kg/24 hr.[23]
‡ Pediatric ileostomy electrolyte concentrations obtained from reference 23.

TABLE 2
Estimated Efficiency of Water Absorption in
Small Intestine and Colon: Comparison of
Children with Adults

	Percentage Absorption of Delivered Fluid		
	In Small Bowel	In Colon	Whole Gut
Infant	—	88*	98
New ileostomy	79	—	—
Established ileostomy	91[†]	—	—
Adult[‡]	80	92	98

* Estimated from difference in normal output per rectum[9] and output from "new" ileostomy.[20]
† From Schwartz et al.[23]
‡ From in vivo perfusion studies.[16]

Na gradient, several dipeptides are transported across the brush border coupled to the hydrogen ion. In summary, in the proximal small bowel, there is net absorption of Na, potassium (K), Cl (chloride), bicarbonate (HCO_3), sugars, amino acids, vitamins, and trace elements.

By the time the luminal contents reach the ileum, concentrations of amino acid and glucose are low. Most of the remaining organic solutes are absorbed by high-affinity, low-capacity transport systems. NaCl is absorbed either by a coupled process or by pH-coupled Na/H and Cl/HCO_3 ex-

changes (see below). Bile acids are transported by Na-coupled carriers located specifically in the ileum.[26] Cobalamin (vitamin B_{12}) enters by an ileal receptor-mediated process that may involve endocytosis.[27]

The colon is a scavenger of Na, Cl, and water. Whereas the jejunum does not absorb Na when the luminal concentration is less than 130 mEq per liter, the colon is able to extract Na when the luminal concentration is as low as 30 mEq per liter. Although malabsorbed sugars and amino acids are not actively transported in adult mammalian colon, Na-coupled absorption of these nutrients occurs in the colon of some species briefly after birth.[28] The bulk of the carbohydrate that is not absorbed is metabolized by colonic microorganisms to short-chain fatty acids (SCFA), which are actively absorbed by highly efficient mechanisms.[29] In various disease states, the colon may be called upon to increase its salvage of fluid and electrolytes and can compensate for a 50 percent reduction in small bowel absorption. In adults, three times the normal water load may be handled before colonic absorption mechanisms are overwhelmed.[30] The precise transport capacity of the infant colon is not known, although in infants with small bowel resection, the value of retaining as much colon as possible in continuity with the small intestine is recognized.

Figure 1 shows the ionic composition of fluid at various locations in the adult GI tract. Proximal intestinal electrolytes are similar in composition to plasma. In the ileum, Cl

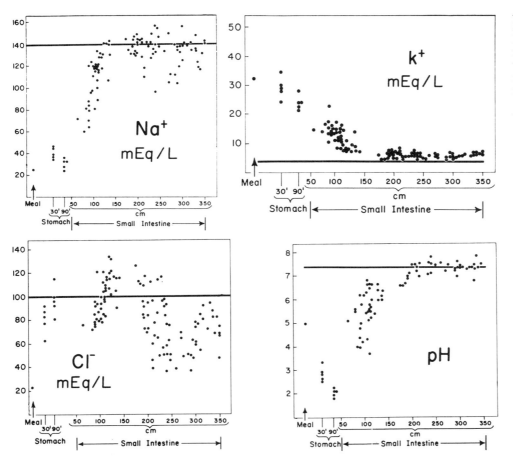

FIGURE 1 Concentrations of Na^+, K^+, and Cl^- and intraluminal pH in the adult gastrointestinal tract following a steak meal. The heavy horizontal line in each box indicates the normal plasma value. (From Fordtran and Locklear.[31])

normally decreases in the lumen from 90 to 60 mEq per liter and HCO_3 increases from 40 to 70 mEq per liter. As stool passes through the colon, Na and Cl are actively absorbed and HCO_3 and K are secreted. Measurement of electrolytes in stool water indicates a K concentration in excess of that of Na (Fig. 2).[32] In the absence of secretory diarrhea a large "anion gap" is present, reflecting the major contribution of volatile (short-chain) fatty acids (mainly acetate, propionate, and butyrate) to the anionic composition of normal stools.[32]

Cellular Mechanisms of Fluid and Electrolyte Transport

General Principles. There are several general principles germane to intestinal solute and water absorption and secretion.[12] The first important principle is that the sodium pump (Na,K-ATPase) on the basolateral membrane of the enterocyte, by creating low intracellular Na content and thus a Na concentration gradient across the cell membrane, is the prime moving force for both intestinal absorption and secretion. The second general principle is that active transport of Na is linked to fluid absorption, whereas active transport of Cl is associated with fluid secretion. The third principle follows from the second: There is no active transport of water. Its movement is always secondary to the active transport of solute from one side of the epithelium to the other.

Na,K-ATPase (the Na Gradient). The fundamental driving force for both Na and fluid absorption and Cl and fluid secretion is the low intracellular Na content of the enterocyte, which is created by the exchange of three Na molecules for two K molecules by Na,K-ATPase.[33] Essentially all cells in the mammalian body contain a Na,K-ATPase, which transduces the energy of ATP to transport. In the so-called symmetric cell, such as the red blood cell, the Na,K-ATPase is present at all cell borders. The epithelial cell is altered so that over 95 percent of the Na,K-ATPase resides on the basolateral membrane below the tight junction, vectorially directing Na out of the cell toward the blood. In the fasting state, the metabolic fuels used for synthesizing ATP are glutamine, ketone bodies such as acetoacetate and beta-hydroxybutyrate, SCFA, and to a lesser extent glucose. Glutamine is the crucial metabolic fuel after feeding, accounting for more than 75 percent of all postprandial oxidative metabolism. There are a sufficient number of Na,K "pump" sites on the intestinal epithelial cell (1.5×10^5 pump sites per rat enterocyte with a turnover rate of 8×10^3 per minute) to theoretically quickly deplete the intracellular Na concentration (maintained at about 20 mM) in a very short time (1 to 2 minutes).[33] Obviously, there must be Na entry mechanisms that prevent this from happening.

Na and Fluid Absorption. Na transport is a two-step process: entry across the apical (brush border) membrane and exit at the basolateral membrane. The rate-limiting step for Na (and water) absorption is the movement of Na from lumen to cell as a result of the low intracellular Na content. There are at least four, and perhaps five, important mechanisms for Na entry, and these operate at various capacities during the interdigestive and postprandial states.[12,34] In the fasting animal, Na entry into the cell takes place by diffusion across the membrane, by movement through Na-specific

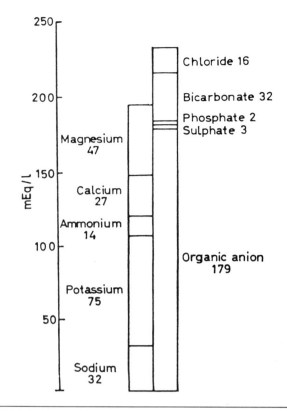

FIGURE 2 Mean electrolyte concentrations in adult stool water. Note the low sodium and high potassium concentrations and the high concentration of organic anions (SCFA). (From Wrong, et al[32]; ©1965 by The Biochemical Society, London.)

conductance channels, and by protein carriers that couple the movement of Na to that of the Cl ion (Fig. 3). It was once thought that diffusion was the most important mechanism for Na movement across the small intestinal brush border. More recent work suggests that Na enters across specific Na-conductance channels, which are recognized by their sensitivity to agents such as phenamil, an analogue of the diuretic amiloride.[35] Amiloride-sensitive Na-conductance channels are the most important Na entry mechanism in the mammalian colon, particularly in the distal colon. These channels are under the important regulatory control of glucocorticoids and mineralocorticoids.[12,36]

The NaCl-coupled entry mechanism in the small intestine and ascending colon is particularly interesting because it is regulated by changes in intracellular content of ionized Ca^{2+} and cyclic nucleotides (see below). This key transport mechanism is modified in several diarrheal states.[37] Currently, there is controversy as to whether this coupled NaCl carrier represents a transport protein that directly couples the movement of Na to Cl, or a combination of a Na/H and Cl/HCO_3 exchanges[38] (Fig. 4). A dual exchange mechanism is tantamount to a coupled NaCl entry mechanism because the luminal movements of HCO_3 and H titrate each other to form H_2O and CO_2.[39] The importance of coupled Na/H and Cl/HCO_3 exchanges in the human small intestine is support-

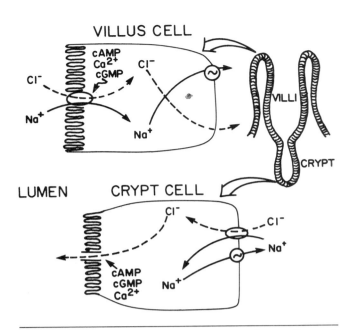

FIGURE 3 NaCl absorptive mechanisms in the small intestinal villous cell and Cl⁻ secretory processes in the crypt cell. (Modified from Field, et al[37]; ©1979 by the American Gastroenterological Association.)

ed by findings in children with congenital chloride diarrhea. In vivo perfusion studies in afflicted children have shown that this is a disorder of ileal Cl/HCO₃ exchange. It is characterized clinically by dehydration, systemic alkalosis, and a stool electrolyte pattern showing Cl concentrations in excess of those of (Na + K).[40]

In the postprandial state, it is the coupling of the transport of monosaccharides and amino acids to the Na ion that drives Na and fluid absorption in the small bowel. The monosaccharide carrier, which recognizes all sugars with a D-glucose pyranose ring-chair conformation, co-transports two Na molecules with each monosaccharide. In adults, increasing jejunal glucose or galactose concentrations up to 50 mM stimulate Na and water transport by a factor of four- and six-fold, respectively. The enhancement of Na absorption caused by glucose results in a potential difference (lumen-to-serosa), which stimulates Cl absorption in vivo. The coupling of glucose to Na transport is the basic premise behind the use of oral replacement solutions (ORS) for the treatment of infants with dehydration. Although they were first used in India and Bangladesh to treat the severe dehydration caused by cholera, similar solutions are now widely used in developing and developed nations for treatment for both bacterial and viral diarrhea. They restore fluid and electrolyte balance in 85 to 90 percent of infants, avoiding the need for intravenous fluid therapy.

Because there are at least five different types of Na-coupled intestinal amino acid carriers (neutral, aromatic, imino, dibasic, and acidic), amino acid–Na co-transport quantitatively accounts for much more sodium absorption in the postprandial state than does monosaccharide-Na co-transport.[34] Amino acid–linked mechanisms may account for as much as 50 percent of the Na transport after meals,

whereas the coupling of glucose to Na may account for only 10 percent. Investigators are now exploring the simultaneous use of amino acids with glucose and the use of solutions containing cooked rice or dried seeds (dal moong), hoping to create an improved ORS that would even more efficiently replenish fluid and electrolyte losses in diarrheal states.

The importance of glucose-Na co-transport in maintaining normal intestinal fluid balance is underscored by a disease called glucose-galactose malabsorption.[41] The hallmark of this disease is severe diarrhea due to reduced Na-coupled hexose transport in the small bowel. In vitro, the intestine and kidneys of these individuals, while demonstrating reduced glucose uptake, are capable of normal transport of amino acid driven by Na, and the specific activity of mucosal Na, K-ATPase in these patients is normal. Thus, this disease is due to a specific hexose-transport defect, rather than to abnormalities in brush border permeability or in the lumen-to-cell Na electrochemical gradient.

All transepithelial movement of water is brought about by osmotic gradients created by the transport of solute.[42] In the case of intestinal water absorption, it is the active transport of Na that creates the lumen-to-blood flow of water. The Na,K-ATPase translocates Na into the intercellular space, a relatively confined compartment where, along with simultaneously transported Cl, glucose, or amino acid, it increases the osmotic pressure of this compartment. Although the increase in osmotic pressure is only a few milliosmoles, it is sufficient to effect the net bulk transfer of water from the lumen into the space. Some fluid and solute may regurgitate back across the tight junction into the lumen. However, because the resistance to fluid flow is less at the basal (or serosal) end of the intercellular space than it is at the tight junctional end, the net direction of fluid and solute movement is across the basement membrane, into the interstitium, and from there into the lymphatics and capillaries.

Although the transcellular transport mechanisms described earlier account for a considerable proportion of Na and water absorption in the intestine, as much as 40 percent of solute and fluid absorption by the jejunum may take place by pas-

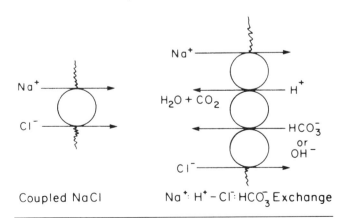

FIGURE 4 Proposed models for NaCl absorption in the small intestine. *Left*, NaCl process in the brush border membrane that involves direct coupling between Na⁺ and Cl⁻. *Right*, Na⁺ and Cl⁻ entry, which occurs via dual exchange mechanisms for Na/H and Cl/HCO₃. (From Turnberg et al.[38])

sive, paracellular mechanisms.[43] Under this scheme, when organic solutes such as glucose or amino acid are present in the lumen in high concentrations (i.e., 100 to 200 mM), the concentration gradients between lumen and blood result in diffusion across the tight junction. Recent studies suggest that the coupled, transcellular movement of Na with glucose or amino acid triggers a contraction of the perijunctional actin-mysosin complex, which further opens this paracellular route.[44] Thus, active transport of solute from lumen to intercellular space creates an osmotically driven flow of water and at the same time opens the tight junctions to allow the bulk movement of luminal contents, including its dissolved nutrients and electrolytes, from lumen to blood.

In the healthy adult, as much as 50 g of carbohydrate each 24 hours escape absorption in the small intestine. These sugars are then metabolized by colonic bacteria into SCFAs. The SCFAs are the predominant anion in stool fluid, ranging in concentration from 50 to 250 mM.[12,45] The predominant anion in adult stool is acetate (50 to 70 mol percent) followed by proprionate and butyrate, with lesser quantities of lactate, fumarate, succinate, and valerate. SCFAs play a key role in maintaining normal absorption by stimulating Na (and fluid) absorption in the colon (Fig. 5). SCFAs appears to be absorbed in the protonated form and then dissociate in the cell cytoplasm into H and anion, supplying H for the Na/H exchange and anion for a Cl/SCFA exchange mechanism.[46] The net result is the coupled absorption of Na and Cl. This mechanism may explain why children develop diarrhea when they take oral antibiotics, as these drugs reduce the population of normal colonic flora that produce SCFAs.

Cl and Fluid Secretion. Just as Na absorption is the primary moving force for the lumen-to-blood movement of water, the active secretion of Cl is the primary driving force for intestinal fluid secretion.[37] As is the case for Na absorption, the low intracellular Na concentration created by the basolateral Na,K-ATPase is the primary driving force for intestinal secretion (see Fig. 3). The Na gradient promotes the uphill entry of Cl across the basolateral membrane by way of a NaCl or a Na/K/2Cl transport process. The Na ion is recycled back across the basolateral membrane by the Na,K-ATPase. Chloride is then accumulated in the cell at concentrations above its electrochemical equilibrium. Increases in intracellular cyclic AMP, cyclic GMP, or free ionized Ca^{2+} initiate phosphorylation of specific membrane proteins by protein kinases, and these proteins open Cl conductance channels in the apical membrane of the crypt cells. The Cl ion is "poised" to egress down its electrochemical gradient from the enterocyte into the lumen of the intestine, once the channels are opened. It is possible that Cl channels might also exist on villous cells of the small intestine and the surface epithelium of the colon; however, evidence indicates that it is the crypt cells that are mainly responsible for secretion. The lumen-negative potential difference generated by Cl secretion is the driving force for Na secretion. The fluid movement from blood to lumen that accompanies active Cl secretion must occur in response to an osmotic gradient created by the Cl transport. The site of this osmotic pressure excess is not apparent, although it has been postulated that it is the relatively unstirred region in the lumen of the crypts.

Recent evidence suggests that cystic fibrosis (CF), a disorder characterized by pancreatic insufficiency, malabsorp-

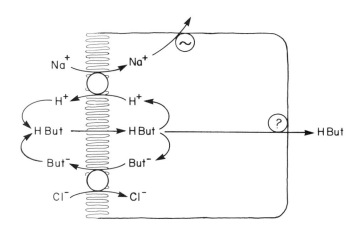

FIGURE 5 Proposed model for the stimulation of colonic Na absorption by SCFAs. The protonated form of butyrate (H But) enters the cell by nonionic diffusion and there is metabolized to H^+ and butyrate (But^-), which exchange for Na^+ and Cl^-, respectively. (From Binder and Mehta.[46])

tion, and recurrent chest infections, results from a defect in regulation of epithelial Cl secretion. Recently, Berschneider et al[47] demonstrated failure of the CF intestine (ileum and colon) to secrete Cl in vitro in response to cyclic AMP–mediated stimuli (theophylline and prostaglandin E_2) or to increases in intracellular Ca (Ca ionophore or bethanechol). Thus, the diarrhea of CF is paradoxical: It occurs in an intestine that cannot secrete Cl and water! Therefore, it must be entirely osmotic or malabsorptive in etiology.

HCO_3 Transport. The exact mechanisms responsible for HCO_3 transport in the intestine are not clear.[12,36,45,48] Duodenal and pancreatic HCO_3 secretion buffers gastric acid, which is emptied into the proximal small intestine. The mechanism of HCO_3 absorption in the jejunum, which serves to recapture the previously secreted HCO_3, is uncertain. H secretion into the lumen in stomach and duodenum titrates luminal HCO_3, and the CO_2 thus formed diffuses into the blood, where it is rehydrated to HCO_3. Thus, jejunal HCO_3 "absorption" is in part the result of H ion secretion (Na/H exchange) into the gut lumen. Similarly, the mechanisms responsible for HCO_3 secretion in the terminal ileum and colon (where it titrates SCFAs and maintains intraluminal pH at levels conducive to bacterial growth) are not clear. There may be prostaglandin-stimulated, cyclic AMP–mediated active HCO_3 secretion in both duodenum and colon. Certainly part of ileal and colonic HCO_3 secretion is the result of Cl/HCO_3 exchange.

K Transport. In the more permeable small intestine, K moves out of or into the bowel lumen across leaky intercellular junctions in response to the prevailing concentration gradients.[49] In the colon, there are active absorptive and secretory mechanisms for K (Fig. 6).[50] Absorption (perhaps occurring mainly in surface cells) is the result of an energy-dependent K/H exchange at the apical membrane, with egress of K through conductance channels in the basolateral membrane. K secretion (perhaps occurring in crypt cells) is by a mechanism similar to that for Cl secretion: K enters across the basolateral membrane via a Na/K/2Cl carrier, with K

Mucosa   Serosa

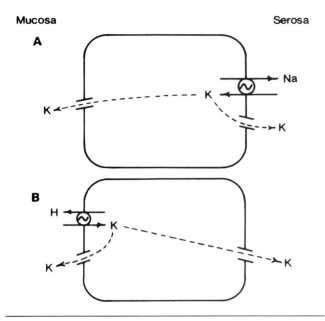

FIGURE 6 Models for transcellular K transport by the colonocyte. *A,* K secretion in which the Na,K-ATPase creates an electrochemical gradient for subsequent K diffusion across the two cell membranes. The direction of net transport in this model is governed by the relative K conductances at the two cell borders; secretion results when the mucosal membrane is more permeable to potassium than the serosal membrane. *B,* K absorption in which a K,H-ATPase mediates entry across the apical membrane to achieve intracellular concentrations above electrochemical equilibrium. The basolateral conductances of potassium are greater than the apical conductance, so K absorption occurs. (From Smith and McCabe.[50])

egress across the apical membrane through cyclic AMP– or Ca^{2+}-regulated conductance channels. K transport is markedly disturbed in several diarrheal states, including viral diarrhea. It is possible that active K transport mechanisms could be present in the small intestinal enterocyte as well as the colonocyte.

Regulation of Water and Electrolyte Transport

The regulation of Na and water absoption and of electrogenic Cl and water secretion is under the control of three separate regulatory systems:[36,48,51-53] (1) the enteric nervous system (ENS), (2) the endocrine system, and (3) the immune system. Bacterial enterotoxins constitute a fourth, or external, regulatory system, if pathophysiology is also to be considered. Mediators released by these four systems alter transport by changing the intracellular concentrations of one or more intracellular messengers: cyclic AMP, cyclic GMP, or ionized Ca^{2+}. These intracellular messengers are increased through stimulation of receptor-activated enzymes—adenylate cyclase, guanylate cyclase, or phospholipase C—often with participation of important guanine nucleotide membrane regulatory proteins, the so-called G-proteins. Once the intracellular levels of the messengers are increased, they regu-

late the electrolyte carriers or channels through activation of protein kinases, which directly phosphorylate membrane transport proteins or phosphorylate some regulatory protein that governs these carriers or channels.

Intracellular Messengers. The concentration of cyclic AMP in the intestinal epithelial cell may be increased by neurotransmitters, hormones, bacterial enterotoxins, and both endogenous and exogenous laxative compounds (Tables 3 and 4).[54] The catalytic subunit of adenylate cyclase is coupled to membrane receptors through stimulatory (G_S) and inhibitory (G_I) proteins that regulate the cyclase activity. Neurotransmitters such as vasoactive intestinal peptide (VIP), paracrine agents such as prostaglandins, or bacterial enterotoxins such as cholera toxin, heat-labile *E. coli* toxin, and *Campylobacter jejuni* toxin activate the G_S proteins with resulting stimulation of the catalytic subunit. Similarly, alpha$_2$-adrenergic agents inhibit the cyclase by receptor-mediated activation of the G_I proteins.

An example of cyclic GMP-stimulated control of intestinal transport is the effect of the heat-stable enterotoxins of *E. coli*.[55,56] These toxins, which bind receptors different from those for cholera toxin, activate a brush border–located (particulate) guanylate cyclase through mechanisms that do not involve ADP ribosylation. Once elevated, intracellular cyclic GMP activates protein kinases (perhaps the same ones activated by cyclic AMP), and these inhibit neutral NaCl entry and stimulate Cl exit in a manner similar to that of cyclic AMP. Although atrial natriuretic factor activates guanylate cyclase in intestinal cells,[57] its role in the regulation of mammalian intestinal electrolyte and its mechanism of effect (if any) remain to be clarified.

Several hormones, the most important being acetylcholine (ACh) and serotonin (5-HT), and, less clearly, some bacterial enterotoxins (such as *Bordetella pertussis* toxin) and laxatives (such as the anthraquinones) increase the intracellular concentrations of ionized Ca^{2+}.[48] Increased intracellular Ca^{2+} decreases neutral NaCl absorption and/or promotes electrogenic Cl secretion, perhaps through calmodulin-regulated protein kinases. ACh stimulates receptor-mediated activation of phospholipase C with subsequent phosphoinositol (PI) metabolism (Fig. 7), which releases diacylglycerol (DAG) and inositol 1,4,5-trisphosphate (IP$_3$).[58] DAG activates protein kinase C and IP$_3$ releases Ca^{2+} from intracellular stores and

TABLE 3
Bacterial Enterotoxins That Affect Intestinal Electrolyte Transport Through Stimulation of Adenylate or Guanylate Cyclase

Adenylate cyclase–cyclic AMP
  Cholera toxin
  Heat-labile *Escherichia coli* enterotoxin
  Salmonella enterotoxin
  Campylobacter jejuni enterotoxin
  Pseudomonas aeruginosa enterotoxin
  Shigella enterotoxin

Guanylate cyclase–cyclic GMP
  Heat-stable *Escherichia coli* enterotoxin
  Yersinia enterocolitica enterotoxin
  Klebsiella pneumoniae enterotoxin

Modified from Donowitz and Welsh.[48]

TABLE 4
Mechanism of Action of Endogenous and Exogenous ''Laxatives'' on
Intestinal Electrolyte Transport

	Decrease Na,K-ATPase	Increase Adenylate Cyclase–Cyclic AMP	Increase Permeability	Histologic Damage
Triarylmethane derivatives				
Phenolphthalein	+/−	−	NS	+/−
Bisacodyl	+	+	NS	+
Oxyphenisatin	+	−	+	NS
Anionic surfactants				
Bile salts (e.g., deoxycholate)	+	+/−	+	+
Ricinoleic acid (e.g., castor oil)	+	+/−	+	+
C-18 fatty acids	−	NS	NS	+
Dioctyl sodium sulfosuccinate	+	+/−	+	+/−
Anthraquinones	NS	−	+	+/−
Magnesium	NS	−	NS	−

NS = not studied; +/− = contradictory data reported.
Modified from Donowitz and Welsh[48] and Nell and Tummel.[54]

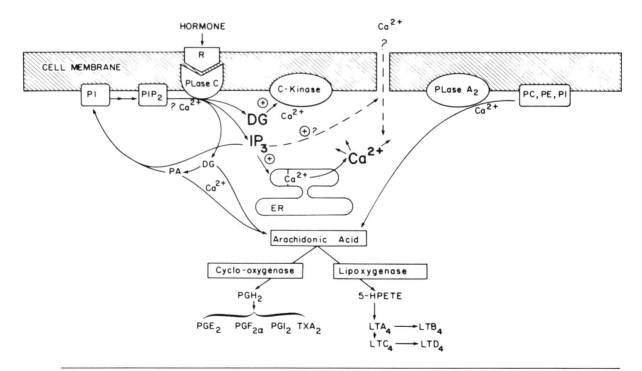

FIGURE 7 Control of intracellular Ca^{2+} by phosphoinositol hydrolysis. Phosphatidylinositol 4,5-bisphosphate (PIP_2) hydrolysis yields diacylglycerol (DG), phosphatidic acid (PA), inositol 1,4,5-trisphosphate (IP_3), and arachidonic acid metabolites of the cyclo-oxygenase and lipoxygenase pathways. PIP_2 is synthesized from phosphatidylinositol (PI) and hydrolysed by receptor-activated (Ca^{2+}-dependent) phospholipase C (PLase C). The products of hydrolysis are DG, which activates protein kinase C (C-kinase) in a Ca^{2+}-dependent fashion, and IP_3, which releases Ca^{2+} from endoplasmic reticulum (ER). Arachidonic acid, formed by specific lipase hydrolysis of DG and PA or by phospholipase A_2 (PLase A_2) hydrolysis of phosphatidylcholine (PC), phosphatidylethanolamine (PE), or PI, is converted to prostaglandins (PGs) or to hydroperoxyeicosatetraenoic acid (5-HPETE) and the leukotrienes (LTs). (From Powell, et al.[55])

may indirectly gate Ca^{2+} across the external cell membrane. Free arachidonic acid is also liberated, and prostaglandins and leukotrienes may be formed during the activation of the PI metabolism. Some believe that these lipids may also play a role as intracellular messengers, although evidence for that is still scant at the present time.

Regulatory Systems. The ENS is a separate component of the autonomic nervous system, along with the sympathetic and parasympathetic systems.[51] Some authorities divide the ENS into three parts: extrinsic nerves, mucosal endocrine cells, and the enteric neural plexuses.

The extrinsic autonomic nervous supply is made up of the cranial (vagal) and sacral parasympathetic nerves together with the sympathetic nerves ramifying from the various prevertebral ganglia. ACh and norepinephrine (NE) are the principal neurotransmitters in these nerves; however, substance P, enkephalins, VIP, gastrin/cholecystokinin (CCK), and somatostatin (SOM) are also found in these extrinsic nerves.

The endocrine-paracrine system is made up of several different mucosal endocrine cells that reside in the epithelium, sandwiched between columnar epithelial cells.[51] They discharge their hormones in response either to luminal stimuli or, since they are often innervated, to neurotransmitters. Gastrin cells in the antrum of the stomach and CCK cells in the duodenum are classic examples of such endocrine cells. In the intestine, 5-HT, SOM, and various cells containing other peptides such as bombesin, substance P, neurotensin, and motilin are also present and may affect adjacent epithelial cell function.

The most important segment of the ENS is the intrinsic neural network: the myenteric (Auerbach's) plexus and the submucosal (Meissner's) plexus.[51] The myenteric plexus is located between the longitudinal and circular layers of the muscularis propria and presumably is primarily concerned with gut motility. The submucosal plexus, located between the circular muscle layer and the muscularis mucosae, has extensive axonal ramification into the lamina propria with terminal endings on both crypt and villous cells. Presumably, it is primarily concerned with regulation of water electrolyte transport. Although over 20 neurotransmitters and hormones have been localized to either neurons or endocrine cells of the ENS, the majority of these neurotransmitters and hormones serve to regulate other nerves rather than to affect the epithelial cells directly. To date, enterocyte receptors have been documented only for the neurotransmitters/hormones ACh, VIP, and secretin, which stimulate intestinal secretion, and for NE and perhaps SOM, which promote fluid and electrolyte absorption. There is indirect evidence suggesting enterocyte receptors for substance P, gastrin-releasing peptide/bombesin, and neuropeptide Y. Thus, neurotransmitters might promote intestinal secretion or absorption both by activating neurons in the plexus and by activating receptors on the enterocyte.

The most important elements of the endocrine system affecting intestinal electrolyte transport are the adrenal glucocorticoids and mineralocorticoids.[36,45] Both adrenal hormones stimulate Na and water absorption by increasing the number of amiloride-blockable Na channels in the surface epithelium of the colon and, in some species, in the villous cells of the terminal ileum. Adrenal corticoids also increase basolateral Na,K-ATPase activity in colon and in ileum. Available evidence suggests that the primary physiologic hormone is aldosterone rather than glucocorticoid, although this issue remains controversial.

The immune system has been recently recognized to be an important regulator of water and electrolyte transport.[52,53,59] The primary effector cells in this system are phagocytes (macrophages, eosinophils, and neutrophils) and the mucosal mast cell. Phagocytes release reactive oxygen species (such as superoxide anion and hydrogen peroxide) and various soluble mediators of inflammation, such as the prostaglandins (PGs), leukotrienes (LTs), and platelet activating factor (PAF). LTs, H_2O_2, and PAF are capable of releasing more PGs from other gut immune cells and mesenchymal cells (fibroblasts, muscle cells, and endothelium), thus augmenting the signal. The prostaglandins themselves may stimulate the epithelium directly, including Cl secretion, and may activate secretory nerves in the ENS. PAF, PGs, and LTs are also important products of mast cell degranulation. However, mast cells also release other intestinal secretagogues, including 5-HT, adenosine, and histamine, which stimulate Cl secretion and inhibit NaCl absorption. Inflammatory mediators may activate nerves in the ENS, and immune cells actually have receptors for neurotransmitters released by the ENS. Thus, there is a complex interaction between the immune system and the neuroendocrine system in regulating water and electrolyte transport by the intestine.

The intestinal epithelial cell is unique in that it has receptors for regulation of ion transport on the apical as well as on the basolateral membrane.[48] The apical receptors are for bacterial enterotoxins. The mechanism of enterotoxin-mediated Cl secretion is described below under "Enterotoxigenic *E. coli* Enteritis."

INTESTINAL FUNCTION IN DISEASE

General Mechanisms of Diarrhea

In general terms, diarrhea results when the volume presented to the colon is greater than its absorptive capacity. This can occur with small bowel disease, because of either decreased absorption or increased secretion or both. Likewise, if the small intestinal function is normal, diarrhea may result if the colon is incapable of absorbing its normal volume of absorbate or if the colon is actually secreting in response to some stimulus. For example, we estimate a 10-kg child's small intestine normally absorbs approximately 2,250 ml (2,850 ml is converted to 600 ml) per 24 hours (see Table 1). This child's colon, in health, is capable of processing up to 600 ml. If small intestinal absorption were reduced by 50 percent, more than 1,725 ml would be presented to the colon ($2,850 - 0.5 \times 2,250$ ml). The adult colon can increase basal absorption by a factor of two to three, an indication that the adult enjoys considerable compensatory capacity. The reserve capacity of the human infant's colon has not been determined, but since it is already absorbing 2.5 times the relative volume of its adult counterpart, probably it is absorbing at rates near its capacity. Therefore, the infant may have little reserve to handle any increase in flow resulting from small intestinal dysfunction. There is evidence from studies in newborn animals (piglets) that the immature colon has a reduced reserve capacity.[60] Any bacterial enterotoxin or drug that would actually stimulate the small intestine to secrete could overwhelm the colon, resulting in severe diarrhea. Finally, in the child with colitis, a 50 percent reduction in the volume absorbed by the colon of a 10-kg infant, in the face of normal small intestine transport, would result in 300 ml of stool output per 24 hours, or more than three times the normal stool output.

There are two ways to categorize diarrheal diseases:[61] by etiology and by mechanism. Mechanisms include either decreased absorption (malabsorption) or active secretion (secretory diarrhea). Below we attempt to categorize, by mechanism, the major causes of diarrhea in children and infants. However, it is clear from the study of animal models that such a classification is often too simple: Many diarrheas are both malabsorptive and secretory. To illustrate this important point, we will describe what bas been learned about the pathophysiology from animal models of three important causes of diarrhea: enterotoxigenic *E. coli* diarrhea, viral diarrhea, and intestinal anaphylaxis.

Malabsorption

Selective Malabsorption. Malabsorption may be generalized, as the case in celiac sprue, or it may be selective, as is the case with magnesium hydroxide ingestion, congenital sucrase-isomaltase deficiency, or adult-onset lactase deficiency.[62] In each of these conditions, nonabsorbed solutes make up an important part of the osmolality of the intestinal luminal fluid, because of either insufficient absorptive surface with abnormal absorptive function (in severe mucosal disease) or absence of normal digestion or transport of a specific solute. For example, the ingestion of magnesium hydroxide (e.g., Milk of Magnesia) places large amounts of nonabsorbable magnesium (Mg) in the lumen of the proximal small intestine. Similarly, a deficiency of lactase, either congenital or acquired, leaves lactose present in high concentrations in proximal intestinal luminal fluid.[63] Water flows into the permeable jejunum in response to the osmotic pressure difference between blood and lumen, and Na moves into the lumen down its concentration difference. The end result is a large volume of intraluminal isotonic fluid with a normal Na concentration. Some Na and fluid are absorbed, but most of the water is held within the lumen because of the osmotic pressure generated by the nonabsorbable solute (Mg, glucose, sucrose, or lactose) (Fig. 8). The volume of ileal effluent exceeds the absorptive capacity of the colon and diarrhea results. Marginal malabsorption of the carbohydrates of fruit juices, most of which are hypertonic and some which contain sorbitol, has similar effects. Excess juice intake may play a role in the common entity called chronic nonspecific diarrhea of infancy, or "toddler's diarrhea."[64] Ingestion of large quantities of chewing gum, candy, dried fruits, or other food sweetened with sorbitol may also induce diarrhea by the same mechanism.

Generalized Malabsorption. In generalized conditions such as the short bowel syndrome or celiac disease, proteins, peptides, starches, and even individual amino acids and monosaccharides may contribute to osmotic movement of fluid into

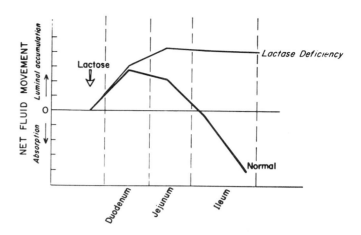

FIGURE 8 Net fluid movement in the intestine of normal and lactase-deficient subjects. This figure demonstrates the failure to reabsorb fluid from the jejunum and ileum when lactose cannot be hydrolyzed to glucose and galactose, monosaccharides that can be transported by the small intestinal epithelium. This presents a large volume of lactose-rich fluid to the colon, where bacterial fermentation creates short-chain fatty acids, which lower the pH and produce gas (CO_2 and H_2). (From Bayless TM, et al,[56] and from data in Christopher and Bayless.[63])

the bowel lumen. Damage to the cells that normally absorb Na and water may result from viral enteritis or bacterial enterocolitis (*Salmonella, Shigella,* or *Campylobacter*) (Table 5). These absorptive cells are damaged in idiopathic inflammatory bowel disease also and when certain drugs or toxins are present (Table 5). The characteristic feature of diseases that cause small intestinal malabsorption is partial or total villous atrophy. Furthermore, certain microorganisms (fecal organisms colonizing the small bowel in the bacterial overgrowth syndrome, giardiasis, and enteroadherent *E. coli*) may cause malabsorption of nutrients by altering brush border membrane structure without extensive anatomic derangement of the mucosa. Lastly, maldigestion of complete proteins, carbohydrates, and triglycerides, resulting from pancreatic exocrine insufficiency, may lead to significant malabsorption, thus causing an "osmotic diarrhea."[65] Steatorrhea differs from protein and carbohydrate malabsorption in that intraluminal long-chain fatty acids not only cause an osmotic diarrhea but also promote colonic Cl secretion (see Table 4).

Secretory Diarrheas

Crypt Hyperplasia. If the intestinal crypts are indeed the primary anatomic site of intestinal secretion, then any disease that results in crypt hyperplasia could, theoretically, cause net intestinal secretion and diarrhea. Most of these diseases (Table 5) also induce villous atrophy, so it is inappropriate to assign the responsibility for increased luminal fluidity to either crypt hypersecretion or decreased villous absorption alone.

Luminal Secretagogues. As mentioned, there are two types of luminal substances that stimulate intestinal secretion:[48] (1) bacterial enterotoxins (see Table 3) and (2) certain

TABLE 5
Causes of Small Bowel Villous Damage and
Crypt Hyperplasia

Infectious Agents
  Rotavirus
  Norwalk agent
  Other viruses: adenovirus, mini-reovirus, calicivirus, astrovirus*
  Giardia lamblia†
  Cryptosporidium
  Enteroadherent Escherichia coli
  Yersinia‡
  Campylobacter jejuni‡
  Strongyloides
Food Intolerance
  Celiac disease
  Cow's milk or soy milk protein intolerance
Drugs
  Chemotherapeutic agents (e.g., cytosine arabinoside, methotrexate)
  Ipecac
  Neomycin
  Para-amino salicylic acid
Crohn's Disease‡
Irradiation
Autoimmune Enteropathy
Small Bowel Ischemia
Eosinophilic Gastroenteropathy

* Biopsy data not yet available, but clinical features suggest a rotavirus-like enteritis.
† Villous damage often occurs in the presence of other potentially causative factors, such as tropical sprue, small bowel bacterial overgrowth, and malnutrition.
‡ Ulceration and inflammation of ileal mucosa have been reported.

secretory chemicals (e.g., laxatives, dihydroxy bile salts, or long-chain fatty acids) (see Table 4). The mechanisms of enterotoxin-stimulated intestinal secretion are described below. The mechanisms of action of exogenous and endogenous laxatives are less clear. These drugs have variable effects on Na,K-ATPase activity; some increase the intracellular concentration of cyclic AMP, presumably initiating secretion; many increase intestinal permeability; and most cause some degree of histologic damage. Certainly, for most of these drugs, intestinal secretion is the end result. Thus, malabsorptive diseases that increase colonic concentrations of bile salts or fat, e.g., ileal resection and Crohn's disease, may represent secretory disorders as well.

Blood-Borne Secretagogues. In children in developing countries, secretory diarrhea is most often due to enterotoxigenic E. coli or cholera. In developed countries, secretory diarrhea is rare. When recognized, it is usually due to drugs or tumors such as ganglioneuromas or neuroblastomas that secrete hormones, primarily VIP.[66] In adults, severe secretory diarrheas result from non–beta cell islet neoplasms of the pancreas that secrete VIP, pancreatic polypeptide, and other secretory hormones (watery diarrhea hypokalemia achlorhydria [WDHA] syndrome).[67] The diarrhea that results from these tumors represents the purest form of secretory diarrhea.

Animal Models

Enterotoxigenic E. coli (ETEC) Enteritis. E. coli cause diarrhea in humans by several mechanisms[68]: (1) invading the colonic mucosa and inciting an inflammatory colitis

(enteroinvasive E. coli), (2) adhering to small intestinal enterocytes and interfering with absorption (enteroadherent E. coli), (3) damaging colonic enterocytes without inducing significant inflammation (enterohemorrhagic E. coli), or (4) producing toxins (enterotoxigenic E. coli). By far the most common of these is the leading cause of diarrhea in older children in developing countries—enterotoxigenic E. coli. These organisms are well known to travelers who develop "Montezuma's revenge." E. coli may produce one or both of two enterotoxins: heat-labile toxin (LT) or heat-stable toxin (ST). Forms of E. coli that produce LT are the cause of traveler's diarrhea in adults, whereas ST producers are a more frequent cause of watery diarrhea in young children who live in developing countries. These infections are diagnosed by bioassays such as the infant suckling mouse assay and adrenal cell assay, and also by enzyme-linked immunosorbent assay (ELISA).

ETEC are spread by the fecal-oral route.[69] In the intestinal lumen, the virulent strains adhere to cells via pili, or plasmid-mediated structural proteins on their external surface. After attachment, they grow to high concentrations (10^6 to 10^9 per milliliter) in the small bowel lumen. The LT produced, strikingly similar to cholera toxin, is composed of multiple binding (B) subunits and a single active (A) subunit. The A subunit binds the GM_1 ganglioside receptor rapidly and irreversibly and activates adenylate cyclase, thereby increasing intracellular cyclic AMP. A lag period of 18 to 24 hours after exposure is required before Cl secretion becomes evident.

ST binds to an unidentified receptor and almost instantaneously induces secretion by activating guanylate cyclase and increasing intracellular cyclic nucleotide. In both ST- and LT-induced diarrhea, elevation of intracellular cyclic nucleotide causes phosphorylation of key brush border membrane proteins, opening the apical chloride channel and also inhibiting NaCl absorption.[70] Studies of in vitro rabbit ileal transport have shown that ST, at concentrations as low as 1 ng per milliliter on the luminal side, abolishes NaCl absorption.[71,72] ST is as effective at inhibiting NaCl absorption as theophylline, a phosphodiesterase inhibitor that increases cell cyclic AMP. However, compared to theophylline, ST is a less potent stimulator of Cl secretion. Crypt cells contain far less guanylate cyclase activity than villous cells,[73] whereas adenylate cyclase activity is evenly distributed along the crypt-villous axis. This is a possible explanation for why E. coli LT-induced diarrhea is more severe than E. coli ST-associated diarrhea.

Clearly, a major component of the alteration in water and electrolyte transport induced by bacterial enterotoxins is due to direct effects of toxin on membrane receptors. However, recent work by Lundgren and colleagues demonstrated that endocrine cells in the mucosa also respond to these toxins with release of peptides or amines (e.g., 5-HT).[74,75] The hormones released activate afferent nerves, which synapse with the submucosal plexus and, through a reflex arc, further promote intestinal secretion. As much as 50 percent of the change in intestinal electrolyte transport brought about by bacterial enterotoxins may come about through this complex involvement of the enteric nervous system. Thus, as is the case with the immune system, the enteric nervous system also plays an important role in the response to bacterial enterotoxins.

Viral Enteritis. World-wide, viral enteritis is the leading cause of diarrhea in infants and toddlers less than 2 years old. Although at least seven or eight viruses have been implicated as potential human pathogens, one particular virus, rotavirus, leads to about 22,000 pediatric hospitalizations per year in the United States.[76] Clinical studies in infants infected with rotavirus or Norwalk virus have shown jejunal villi are damaged and large amounts of carbohydrates and organic acids are detected in their stools.[77] The study of animal models, including piglet rotavirus, piglet coronavirus (transmissible gastroenteritis [TGE]), murine rotavirus (EDIM agent), and calf rotavirus (Nebraska calf diarrhea virus enteritis), has clarified several of the puzzling features about this disease. We will focus on swine enteritis, which uniformly causes villous damage and severe diarrhea and in which the intestinal transport abnormalities have been defined.

The first event after virus reaches the intestine is viral attachment and entry of viral genome into the enterocyte cytoplasm. The site of injury is the jejunoileum, whereas stomach, duodenum, and colon appear to be spared. Thus the term *viral gastroenteritis* is a misnomer. Rotavirus appears to directly invade the cell across the brush border, whereas TGE virus enters by pinocytosis. Host susceptibility is determined by the animal's age: newborn animals less than 1 week old uniformly develop diarrhea and severe small intestinal morphologic damage, whereas adult pigs are resistant.[78,79] Although development of immunity may play a role, the lining enterocytes also demonstrate a progressively increasing resistance to viral invasion and/or cell destruction shortly after birth.[79] As viral replication proceeds, the microvilli on the epithelial cells become disorganized, the terminal web begins to disintegrate, and the villous cells are sloughed. Maximal injury and stooling do not appear until about 2 days after exposure to virus,[80] at a time when most of the virus has been shed from the mucosa.

At the height of diarrhea the small intestinal epithelium is characterized by blunted villi, deepened crypts, and increased inflammation in the lamina propria.[81,82] The crypt-type cells, which dominate the cell population, have altered transport and enzymatic function[82] (Table 6).[77-90] In viral enteritis, neither resting Cl secretion nor mucosal cyclic AMP content is increased; instead, glucose-Na co-transport is consistently diminished or absent. The abnormality has been demonstrated in perfused jejunal loops in vivo[81] and in vitro in jejunum[80,83] and ileum.[82] Studies of purified jejunal brush border membrane vesicles[84] demonstrated the absence of high-affinity Na-coupled D-glucose uptake in virus-damaged tissue. Therefore, glucose malabsorption and reduced glucose-facilitated Na absorption in piglet enteritis are defects of brush border membrane transport, not simply an indirect reflection of reduced mucosal absorptive surface. In piglet enteritis, in vitro studies have also demonstrated that jejunal Na-coupled neutral amino acid (L-alanine) transport[85,91] and electroneutral NaCl absorption[86] are markedly reduced.

These animal studies, combined with clinical investigations in babies,[92] suggest that diarrheal purging in viral enteritis is due primarily to lack of efficient salt and solute absorption. Crypt-cell Cl secretion is not balanced by NaCl absorption in the villi. Acidic stools are due to carbohydrate malabsorption followed by bacterial degradation to organic acids in the colon. Systemic acidosis may result from colon-

TABLE 6
Comparison Between Characteristics of Intestinal Mucosa in Viral Enteritis and Isolated Intestinal Crypt Cells

Mucosal and Transport Abnormalities in Viral Enteritis

Diminished villus height and reduced sucrase, lactase, and alkaline phosphatase activities in brush border[77-82]
Reduced Na,K-ATPase activity[81,84,85]
Impaired small intestinal and colonic Na, Cl, and water absorption[60,81]
Decreased D-glucose–facilitated Na absorption[80,82-85]
Decreased L-alanine–stimulated Na absorption[85]
Impaired NaCl transport[85]

Characteristics of Intestinal Crypt Cells

Diminished dissaccharidase activities[87,88]
Reduced Na,K-ATPase activity[89]
Reduced glucose-stimulated Na absorption and absence of apical membrane depolarization after D-glucose[89,90]
Decreased L-alanine uptake compared with villous cells[91]

ic titration of fecal SCFA by secreted HCO_3.[12] In summary, viral diarrhea, like other diarrheal conditions, is both a malabsorptive and a secretory state.

Intestinal Anaphylaxis. Inflammation in the bowel, whether the result of intestinal infection, inflammatory bowel disease, or food allergy, causes decreased absorption. Often bleeding and exudation of a protein-rich fluid can be demonstrated as well. Severe abnormalities of the surface epithelium may be demonstrated microscopically, and these may correlate with demonstrable decreases in intestinal Na and fluid absorption. Disruption of the underlying capillaries may account for hemorrhage and protein exudation. Much of this damage may be due to the explosive release of reactive oxygen metabolites, proteases, lipases, and other enzymes from mast cells and phagocytes.[93] Emerging knowledge of phagocyte and mast cell-mediated intestinal secretion and study of experimental models of gut anaphylaxis make it clear, however, that there is also a secretory component to the diarrhea of inflammation.[52,53,59]

Models of immediate hypersensitivity (anaphylaxis) can be created by injecting animals with egg albumin, feeding them cow's milk, or infecting them with nematodes such as *Nippostrongylus* or *Trichinella*.[94-97] When the animals are challenged subsequently in vivo with specific antigen or nematode (intraluminally, parenterally, or when intestinal lamina propria is re-exposed to antigen in vitro), profound changes in water and electrolyte transport are observed. At a stage occurring prior to the epithelial damage, inhibition of neutral NaCl absorption and stimulation of electrogenic Cl secretion can be demonstrated. These effects of the antigen can be inhibited by antagonists of histamine (H_1-receptor blockers) or serotonin and by inhibitors of prostaglandin synthesis, indicating that mediators are being released from degranulating mucosal mast cells. Furthermore, inhibitors of the enteric nervous system (tetrodotoxin, hexamethonium, and atropine) also reduce the secretory response, indicating that the inflammatory mediators are not only affecting the epithelium directly, but also are affecting the ENS, which stimulates the epithelium to secrete. Thus, what may be viewed as an inflammatory (and therefore malabsorptive) diarrhea clearly also possesses a secretory component. The relevance of these models to human disease (milk hypersensitivity, celiac sprue, and nematode infestation) should be obvious.

Since infiltration of the lamina propria with phagocytes accompanies other inflammatory and infectious diarrhea (viral, bacterial, or parasitic) and since mast cells, as well as phagocytes, proliferate in many parasitic and inflammatory intestinal diseases, it seems likely that the secretion of soluble mediators of inflammation such as PGs, LTs, PAF, histamine, and serotonin may play a role in these diarrheas as well.

VALUE OF STOOL ANALYSIS

An analysis of diarrheal stools can give useful clinical information concerning etiology, as long as the results are not over-interpreted. There are four aspects of stool analysis: (1) quantity and gross appearance, including changes in fecal volume with fasting; (2) chemical determinations that suggest malabsorption of nutrients: fat examination and tests for carbohydrate wastage; (3) examination for fecal leukocytes; and (4) analysis of stool electrolytes (Na and K) and osmolality.

Although purely secretory diarrheas and malabsorptive diarrheas may seem separable by virtue of difference in stool appearance (watery stools without form as opposed to greasy, bulky stools), rarely do these pure states present in the pediatric population. One distinguishing feature is that the volume of malabsorptive stool often returns to normal (less than 10 g per kilogram per 24 hours) when the patient fasts, whereas the volume of secretory diarrheas may decrease somewhat on fast but remains higher than normal. The problem in the pediatric patient is the accurate assessment of stool excretion in a functionally incontinent subject. The dry and wet weight of diapers can be useful in this regard.

Stool analysis for fat and reducing substances can be very useful, provided that certain limitations are kept in mind. Infants have a low coefficient of fat absorption, but after 1 year of age, a fat absorption of more than 93 percent of intake is considered normal. Incomplete stool collections make quantitative fat determinations difficult. Examinations of a stool smear mixed with a drop of Sudan red or black on a microscope slide will indicate whether triglyceride droplets are present. Triglyceride (neutral fat) malabsorption suggests small bowel malabsorption or pancreatic insufficiency. The finding of significant quantities of reducing susbstances (carbohydrate) in an infant's stool (more than 0.5 per 100 ml) points to a defect in small bowel absorption. However, there are problems with standard testing using the Clinitest tablet. Non-reducing sugars (such as sucrose) are not measurable unless stool carbohydrate is first hydrolyzed by boiling with acid. Also, the test underestimates total fecal carbohydrate excretion by 67 to 90 percent.[98] Clinitest examination is most useful when combined with pH testing of the stool with nitrazine paper: A fecal pH of 5.5 or less even in the absence of intact reducing sugars, suggests carbohydrate malabsorption and fermentation to SCFAs in the colon. Finally, fecal leukocytes, which can be stained with a drop of methylene blue, indicate colonic inflammation and suggest bacterial or inflammatory colitis.

Stool Na, K, and osmolality have been proposed as helpful in differentiating between malabsorptive and secretory diarrheas.[61,99] Since Na and K are the major cations in stool, the value derived from multiplying by two the stool concentrations of Na and K ($2 \times ([Na] + [K])$), to account for the accompanying anions, should nearly equal the measure osmolality (milliosmoles per kilogram of H_2O). An osmotic gap of less than 50 (stool mOsm $- 2 \times ([Na] + [K])$) was thought to be normal if stool volume was normal and to indicate a secretory diarrhea when fasting stool volumes were greater than normal. This follows because electrolytes are the osmotic solutes that account for the liquid component in normal stools and the fluidity of stool in secretory states. Conversely, in malabsorption, the increased fluidity is due to the osmotic properties of nonabsorbed, non-electrolyte solutes. In both specific and generalized malabsorption, an osmotic gap of greater than 50 is usually found.

There are two problems with the use of stool osmotic gap. First, stool osmolality increases steadily after stool excretion as a result of continued bacterial fermentation of fecal carbohydrates.[100,101] This has led to the recommendation that a plasma osmolality of 290 mOsm per kilogram H_2O should be used as the value from which to subtract $2 \times ([Na] + [K])$, and/or that an osmotic gap of 100 should be used to differentiate between malabsorptive and secretory diarrheas.[101] Second, healthy children's stools often contain some malabsorbed nutrients and thus may show a significant osmotic gap.

Table 7 shows stool volume and electrolyte composition of normal infants and those admitted with different infections to a diarrheal treatment center in Bangladesh. A good general rule is that when fecal volume is high (greater than 150 ml per kilogram per day), Na concentration is high (greater than 70 mEq per liter), and stool osmotic gap is low (less than 100 mOsm per liter), a severe secretory state such as cholera is likely. When diarrheal feces have a low Na (less than 50 mEq per liter) and an increased osmotic gap (greater than 100 mOsm per liter), a viral etiology or other cause of malabsorption is suggested;[9,92] tests for reducing substances and fat may provide further evidence for malabsorption. In enterotoxigenic E. coli diarrhea, stool analyses of electrolytes and osmolarity fall between these extremes, and therefore appear to be of limited value. The most likely explanation is that ETEC induces some villous damage and malabsorption as well as crypt cell–mediated secretion. Also, infants in developing countries infected with ETEC are often coinfected with Giardia or colonized in the proximal small bowel with colonic flora ("bacterial overgrowth"). These are conditions that can lead to both malabsorption and secretion.

SYSTEMIC IMPACT OF ACUTE DIARRHEA IN CHILDREN

Fluid and Electrolyte Imbalance. The age at which humans are most susceptible to virtually all enteric pathogens, with the exception of cholera, is 6 to 24 months. It is children of this same age group who suffer most frequently from diarrheal dehydration. This dangerous complication is observed

TABLE 7
Comparison of Volume and Electrolyte Composition of Diarrhea Caused by
Different Agents in Children[10]

	Peak Stool Volume	Electrolytes (mMol/L)				Osmotic Gap (mOsm/L)
	(ml/kg/day)	Na$^+$	K$^+$	Cl$^-$	HCO$_3^-$	$(290 - 2[(Na)+(K)])$
Cholera	180	80	30	86	32	70
Enterotoxigenic *Escherichia coli*	160	53	37	24	18	110
Rotavirus	130–160	37	38	22	6	140
Normal stools*	5–10	22	54	21	ND	140

ND = not determined in children. For adult data, see Figure 2.
*From Anderson [9] and Silverman and Roy.[21]
Modified from Molla et al.[10]

in up to 10 percent of rotavirus-infected infants[76] and a smaller percentage of those suffering from ETEC or bacterial colitis. Increased susceptibility to infection in this age group coincides with the normal nadir in maternally-acquired serum IgG at 6 months. Increased severity in this age group also reflects the inability of the newborn's kidney to adequately retain salt and water (Table 8). The infant's intake is dictated entirely by his parents and physician. After infection, exclusive adminstration of hyperosmolar sugar-containing solutions, such as fruit juices (700 to 900 mOm per liter), may further increase intestinal fluid losses. Evaporative losses and water loss due to fever are increased in the infant host who has an increased body surface area-to-volume ratio. Finally, both small bowel transport and colonic absorption are deficient in neonatal mammals, and probably including humans. Decreased colonization of the colon by beneficial SCFA-producing flora during the first weeks of life, and shifts in flora concomitant with antibiotic treatment later in infancy, may impair the colonic "salvage" of malabsorbed carbohydrate, Na, and water.[60] As discussed, the common feature of all diarrheal diseases is presentation to the infant colon of a volume greater than it can handle.

In North America, where cholera and ETEC are rare, infants normally experience mild diarrhea, but each year hundreds of North American infants die of acute diarrhea, usually children from poor families who become infected during the winter months.[4] Postmortem findings in one report from Canada of a winter rotavirus outbreak indicated that vir-

TABLE 8
Factors Contributing to Increased Morbidity and Mortality in Infants with Diarrhea

Increased fluid and electrolyte requirements

Inadequate caloric reserves

Renal immaturity—impaired ability to conserve sodium and water

Incompletely developed absorption in the small intestine

(?) lack of colonic reserve

Lack of immunity to enteric infection

tually all infants who died showed evidence of electrolyte imbalance, aspiration, or seizures.[102] In some cases of severe diarrhea, hyperglycemia and glycosuria may cause the dehydration to worsen and may contribute further to the metabolic acidosis.[103]

Chronic Diarrhea. By definition, acute diarrhea resolves within 2 weeks of onset. ETEC infection usually lasts 2 to 3 days, *C. jejuni* enterocolitis 4 to 5 days, and rotavirus enteritis 4 to 5 days. When the illness extends beyond 2 weeks, particularly in the very young infant (less than 3 months old), diarrhea assumes a more ominous course; in severe cases many months of parenteral nutrition may be necessary for survival.[104] In the majority no cause for the diarrhea can be found. In some infants, chronic diarrhea is the result of infection by organisms such as *Cryptosporidium*[105] or enteroadherent *E. coli*,[106] which do not respond to antibiotics. Other infants are infected simultaneously by several pathogens.[107] Fortunately, some children with food allergies or gluten intolerance will respond to restriction of milk protein or gluten from the diet. Rarely, autoimmune disease causes chronic enteropathy; afflicted patients have high titers of anti-enterocyte antibodies and may respond to immunosuppressive therapy.[108] Certainly, most infants with "chronic protracted diarrhea of infancy" respond to no specific therapy. Massive fluid losses persist for months and then suddenly resolve.

Malnutrition. Intestinal infections during infancy are less prevalent than upper respiratory illnesses but are much more closely linked to subsequent malnutrition.[109] Shigellosis is particularly likely to lead to malnutrition. Patients with diarrhea are more likely to become malnourished than those with other infections because they develop anorexia and vomiting, because they malabsorb nutrients, and because increased calories are required for intestinal secretion and repair. Normal infant growth and development, the major "tasks" of the first year of life, depend on normal appetite and normal nutrient absorption. Even a mild injury to the intestine, if persistent, can lead to malnutrition. For example, after acute enteritis, the infant's nutrition may be threatened by prolonged steatorrhea, whether due to bile salt malabsorption[110] or to a persistent reduction in mucosal absorptive surface. Bile salt deconjugation in the proximal intestine, resulting from bacterial overgrowth or chronic giardiasis, can also lead to chronic malabsorption of fat.

The impoverished child repeatedly assailed by enteric infection or the child in a developed country with inflammatory bowel disease may have blunted growth, so that height and weight are proportionately decreased, compared with normal children (marasmus). Micronutrient deficiencies (Table 9) are also common, both in developed and in developing countries. The specific deficiencies are influenced by dietary omissions and by the site of the intestinal lesion. For example, in celiac disease, gluten-induced injury to the duodenum, the primary site of iron absorption, is the likely cause of iron-deficiency anemia. Chronic damage to the proximal and mid-jejunum may lead to folate deficiency. Resection of ileum in the child with Crohn's disease can lead to vitamin B_{12}-deficiency anemia and/or steatorrhea due to bile salt depletion. In chronic malabsorptive diarrheas, fat-soluble vitamin deficiencies and depletion of divalent cations (Zn and Mg) are common. Vitamin A deficiency, particularly frequent in India and Southeast Asia, leads to xerophthalmia, night blindness, and delayed repair of epithelial surfaces. Deficiency of both iron and zinc may cause intestinal epithelial abnormalities.

The vicious circle of diarrhea-malnutrition-diarrhea is a menace to children in both developing and industrialized nations. Future research in diarrheal disease will be needed to identify pathogens currently not recognized and to design treatments that will facilitate repair of the severely damaged gut.

TABLE 9
Micronutrient Deficiencies Seen in Children with Chronic Diarrhea

Deficiency	Signs/Symptoms
Trace Metals	
Iron	Anemia
	Glossitis
Zinc	Anorexia
	Poor growth
	Ageusia
	Rash
Copper	Anemia
	Depigmented hair
	Osteopenia
	Neutropenia
Magnesium	Tremors
	Anorexia
	Abnormal reflexes
Calcium	Rickets
Vitamins	
Vitamin K	Coagulopathy
Vitamin A	Night blindness
	Xerophthalmia
	Urinary infection
Vitamin E	Hemolysis
	Neuropathy
Vitamin D	Rickets
Folic acid	Megaloblastic anemia
	Glossitis
	Irritability
	Sleeplessness
Vitamin B_{12}	Megaloblastic anemia
	Glossitis
	Peripheral neuropathy
	Loss of position and vibration sense
	Depression, psychosis

REFERENCES

1. Jacobi A. Acute intestinal catarrh. In: Intestinal diseases of infancy and childhood. Physiology, hygiene, pathology and therapeutics. Detroit: GS Davis, 1887: 190.
2. Snyder JD, Merson MH. The magnitude of the global problem of acute diarrhoeal disease: a review of active surveillance data. Bull WHO 1982; 60:605–613.
3. Kumate J, Armando I. Pediatric diarheal diseases: a global perspective. Pediatr Infect Dis 1986; 5:S21–S28.
4. Ho M-S, Glass RI, Pinsky PF, Young-Okoh N, Sappenfield W, Buehler JW, Gunter N, Anderson LJ. Diarrheal deaths in American children. Are they preventable? JAMA 1988; 260:3281–3285.
5. Persistent diarrhoea in children in developing countries. World Health Organization, Publication CCD/88.27, 1988.
6. Bartlett AV, Moore M, Gary GW, Starko KM, Erben JJ, Meredith BA. Diarrheal illness among infants and toddlers in daycare centers. II. Comparison with daycare homes and households. J Pediatr 1985; 107:503–509.
7. Recommends GRTR use of oral rehydration therapy in the U.S. Pediatr News Oct 1988; 22:1.
8. Weaver LT. Bowel habit from birth to old age. J Pediatr Gastroenterol Nutr 1988; 7:637–640.
9. Anderson DH. Celiac syndrome. I: Determination of fat in feces; reliability of two chemical methods and microscopic estimate; excretion of feces and of fecal fat in normal children. Am J Dis Child 1945; 69:141–151.
10. Molla AM, Rahman M, Sarker SA, Sack DA, Molla A. Stool electrolyte content and purging rates in diarrhea caused by rotavirus, enterotoxigenic *E. coli*, and *V. cholerae* in children. J Pediatr 1981; 98:835–838.
11. Powell DW. Barrier function of epithelia. Am J Physiol 1981; 241:G275–G288.
12. Powell DW. Ion and water transport in the intestine. In: Andreoli TE, Hoffman JF, Fanestil DD, Schultz SG, eds. Physiology of membrane disorders. New York: Plenum, 1986: 559.
13. Cooke HJ, Dawson DC. Transport characteristics of isolated newborn rabbit ileum. Am J Physiol 1978; 234:E257–E261.
14. Shepherd RW, Hamilton JR, Gall DG. The postnatal development of sodium transport in the proximal small intestine of the rabbit. Pediatr Res 1980; 14:250–253.
15. Ghishan FK, Wilson FA. Developmental maturation of D-glucose transport by rat jejunum brush-border membrane vesicles. Am J Physiol (Gastrointest Liver Physiol 11) 1985; 248:G87–G92.
16. Phillips SF. Diarrhea: a current view of the pathophysiology. Gastroenterology 1972; 63:495–518.
17. Twetman S, Linder A, Modéer T. Lysozyme and salivary immunoglobin A in caries-free and caries-susceptible pre-school children. Swed Dent J 1981; 5:9–14.
18. Gilman RH, Partanen R, Brown KH, Spira WM, Khanam S, Greenburg B, Bloom SR, Ali A. Decreased gastric acid secretion and bacterial colonization of the stomach in severely malnourished Bangladeshi children. Gastroenterology 1988; 94:1308–1314.
19. Kopelman H, Durie P, Gaskin K, Weizman Z, Forstner G. Pancreatic fluid secretion and protein hyperconcentration in cystic fibrosis. N Engl J Med 1985; 312:229–334.
20. Ho TF, Yip WCL, Tay JSH, Vellayappan K. Rice water and milk: effect on ileal fluid osmolality and volume. Lancet 1982; I:169.
21. Silverman A, Roy CC, eds. Pediatric clinical gastroenterology. 3rd ed. St. Louis: CV Mosby Co, 1983: 204.
22. Will PC, Cortright RN, Groseclose RG, Hopfer U. Amiloride-sensitive salt and fluid absorption in small intestine of sodium-depleted rats. Am J Physiol (Gastrointest Liver Physiol 11) 1985; 248:G133–G141.
23. Schwartz KB, Ternberg JL, Bell MJ, Keating JP. Sodium needs of infants and children with ileostomy. J Pediatr 1983; 102:509–513.
24. Fordtran JS. Speculations on the pathogenesis of diarrhea. Fed Proc 1967; 26:1405–1414.
25. Adibi SA, Kim YS. Peptide absorption and hydolysis. In: Johnson LR,

ed. Physiology of the gastrointestinal tract. New York: Raven Press, 1981: 1073.

26. Moyer MS, Heubi JE, Goodrich AL, Balistreri WF, Suchy FJ. Ontogeny of bile acid transport in brush border membrane vesicles from rat ileum. Gastroenterology 1986; 90:1188-1196.

27. Donaldson RM Jr. How does cobalamin (vitamin B_{12}) enter and traverse the ileal cell? Gastroenterology 1985; 88:1069-1076.

28. Potter GD, Burlingame SM. Glucose-coupled sodium absorption in the developing rat colon. Am J Physiol (Gastrointest Liver Physiol 13) 1986; 250:G221-G226.

29. Ruppin H, Bar-Meir S, Soergel KH, Wood CM, Schmitt MG Jr. Absorption of short-chain fatty acids by the colon. Gastroenterology 1980; 78:1500-1507.

30. Phillips SF, Giller J. The contribution of the colon to electrolyte and water conservation in man. J Lab Clin Med 1973; 81:733-746.

31. Fordtran J, Locklear T. Ionic constituents and osmolality of gastric and small intestinal fluids after eating. Am J Dig Dis 1966; 11:503-521.

32. Wrong O, Metcalfe-Gibson A, Morrison RBI, Ng ST, Howard AV. *In vivo* dialysis of faeces as a method of stool analysis. Clin Sci 1965; 28:357-372.

33. Harms V, Wright EM. Some characteristics of Na/K-ATPase from rat intestinal basal lateral membranes. J Membr Biol 1980; 53:119-128.

34. Gunther R, Wright E. Na$^+$, Li$^+$ and Cl$^-$ transport by brush border membranes from rabbit jejunum. J Membr Biol 1983; 74:85-94.

35. Sellin JA, Dyarzabal HA. Phenamil blocks electrogenic Na absorption in rabbit ileum. Gastroenterology 1988; 94:A419.

36. Powell DW. Intestinal water and electrolyte transport. In: Johnson LR, ed. Physiology of the gastrointestinal tract. 2nd ed. New York: Raven Press, 1987: 1267.

37. Field M. Intracellular mediators of secretion in the small intestine. In: Binder HJ, ed. Mechanisms of intestinal secretion. New York: Alan R. Liss, 1979: 83.

38. Turnberg LA, Bieberdorf FA, Morawski SG, Fordtran JS. Interrelationships of chloride, bicarbonate, sodium, and hydrogen transport in the human ileum. J Clin Invest 1970; 49:557-567.

39. Armstrong WM. Cellular mechanism of ion transport in the small intestine. In: Johnson LR, ed. Physiology of the gastrointestinal tract. 2nd ed. New York: Raven Press, 1987: 1251.

40. Bieberdorf FA, Gorden P, Fordtran JS. Pathogenesis of congenital alkalosis with diarrhea. Implications for the physiology of normal ileal electrolyte absorption and secretion. J Clin Invest 1972; 51:1958-1968.

41. Elsas LJ, Hillman RE, Patterson JH, Rosenberg LE. Renal and intestinal hexose transport in familial glucose-galactose malabsorption. J Clin Invest 1970; 49:576-585.

42. Diamond JM. Solute-linked water transport in epithelia. In: Hoffman JF, ed. Membrane transport processes. New York: Raven Press, 1978: 257.

43. Fordtran J. Stimulation of active and passive sodium absorption by sugars in the human jejunum. J Clin Invest 1975; 55:728-737.

44. Pappenheimer JR. Physiological regulation of transepithelial impedance in the intestinal mucosa of rats and hamsters. J Membrane Biol 1987; 100:137-148.

45. Binder HJ, Sandle GI. Electrolyte absorption and secretion in the mammalian colon. In: Johnson LR, ed. Physiology of the gastrointestinal tract. 2nd ed. New York: Raven Press, 1987: 1389.

46. Binder HJ, Mehta P. Short-chained fatty acids stimulate active Na and Cl absorption in vitro in the rat distal colon. Gastroenterology 1989; 96:989-996.

47. Berschneider HM, Knowles MR, Azizkhan RG, Boucher RC, Tobey NA, Orlando RC, Powell DW. Altered intestinal chloride transport in cystic fibrosis. FASEB J 1988; 2:2625-2629.

48. Donowitz M, Welsh MJ. Regulation of mammalian small intestinal electrolyte secretion. In: Johnson LR, ed. Physiology of the gastrointestinal tract. 2nd ed. New York: Raven Press, 1987: 1351.

49. Turnberg L. Potassium transport in the human small bowel. Gut 1971; 12:811-818.

50. Smith P, McCabe R. Mechanism and regulation of transcellular potassium transport by the colon. Am J Physiol (Gastrointest Liver Physiol 10) 1984; 247:G445-G456.

51. Cooke HJ. Neural and humoral regulation of small intestinal electrolyte transport. In: Johnson, LR, ed. Physiology of the gastrointestinal tract. 2nd ed. New York: Raven Press, 1987: 1307.

52. Castro GA. Immunological regulation of epithelial function. Am J Physiol (Gastrointest Liver Physiol 6) 1982; 243:G321-G329.

53. Powell DW. The immunophysiology of intestinal electrolyte transport.

In: Schultz SG, ed. Handbook of physiology: The gastrointestinal system. Vol 4. Frizzell RA, Field M, vol eds. Absorptive and secretory processes of the intestine. Bethesda: American Physiological Society (in press).

54. Nell A, Tummel W. Action mechanisms of secretagogue drugs. In: Csaky TZ, ed. Pharmacology of intestinal permeations. New York: Springer-Verlag, 1984: 461.

55. Powell DW, Berschneider HM, Lawson LD, Martens H. Regulation of water and ion movement in intestine. In: Evered D, Whalen J, eds. Microbial toxins and diarrhoeal disease. Ciba Foundation Symposium 112. London: Pitman, 1985: 14.

56. Bayless TM, Whiting DS. Pathophysiology of diarrhea. In: Binder HJ, ed. The undergraduate teaching project in gastroenterology liver disease. Timonium, MD: Milner-Fenwick, Inc, 1979.

57. O'Grady SM, Field M, Nash NT, Rao MC. Atrial natriuretic factor inhibits Na-K-Cl cotransport in teleost intestine. Am J Physiol (Cell Physiol 18) 1985; 249:C531-C534.

58. Berridge MJ. Inositol trisphosphate and diacylglycerol: two interacting second messengers. Ann Rev Biochem 1987; 56:159-193.

59. Bern MJ, Sturbaum CW, Karayalcin SS, Berschneider HM, Wachsman JT, Powell DW. Immune system control of rat and rabbit colonic electrolyte transport: role of prostaglandins and enteric nervous system. J Clin Invest 1989; 83:1810-1820.

60. Argenzio RA, Moon HW, Kemeny LJ, Whipp SC. Colonic compensation in transmissible gastroenteritis of swine. Gastroenterology 1984; 86:1501-1509.

61. Krejs GJ, Fordtran JS. Diarrhea. In: Sleisenger MH, Fordtran JS, eds. Gastrointestinal disease: pathophysiology, diagnosis, management. 3rd ed. Philadelphia: WB Saunders, 1983: 257.

62. Gray GM. Maldigestion and malabsorption: clinical manifestations and specific diagnosis. In: Sleisenger MH, Fordtran JS, eds. Gastrointestinal disease: pathophysiology, diagnosis, management. 3rd ed. Philadelphia: WB Saunders, 1983: 228.

63. Christopher NL, Bayless TM. Role of the small bowel and colon in lactose-induced diarrhea. Gastroenterology 1971; 60:845-852.

64. Hyams JS, Etienne NL, Leichtner AM, Theuer RC. Carbohydrate malabsorption following fruit juice ingestion in young children. Pediatrics 1988; 82:64-68.

65. Zentler-Munro PL. Cystic fibrosis—a gastroenterological cornucopia. Gut 1987; 28:1531-1547.

66. Scheibel E, Rechnitzer C, Fahrenkrug J, Hertz H. Vasoactive intestinal polypeptide (VIP) in children with neural crest tumours. Acta Pediatr Scand 1982; 71:721-725.

67. Krejs GJ. VIPoma syndrome. Am J Med 1987; 82:37-47.

68. Levine MM, Edelman R. Enteropathogenic *Escherichia coli* of classic serotypes associated with infant diarrhea: epidemiology and pathogenesis. Epidemiol Rev 1984; 6:31-50.

69. Sack RB. Acute diarrheal diseases in humans caused by bacteria. In: Tyrell DAJ, Kapickian AZ, eds. Virus infections of the gastrointestinal tract. New York: Marcel Dekker Inc, 1982:239.

70. Shlatz LJ, Kimberg DV, Cattieu KA. Phosphorylation of specific rat intestinal microvillus and basal-lateral membrane proteins by cyclic nucleotides. Gastroenterology 1979; 76:293-299.

71. Field M, Graf LH, Laird WJ, Smith PL. Heat-stable enterotoxin of *Escherichia coli: in vitro* effects on guanylate cyclase activity, cyclic GMP concentration, and ion transport in small intestine. Proc Natl Acad Sci USA 1978; 75:2800-2804.

72. Hughes JM, Murad F, Chang B, Guerrant RL. Role of cyclic GMP in the action of heat-stable enterotoxin of *Escherichia coli*. Nature 1978; 271:755-756.

73. Quill H, Weiser MM. Adenylate and guanylate cyclase activities and cellular differentiation in rat small intestine. Gastroenterology 1975; 69:470-478.

74. Cassuto J, Jodal M, Tuttle R, Lundgren O. On the role of intramural nerves in the pathogenesis of cholera toxin-induced intestinal secretion. Scand J Gastroenterol 1981; 16:377-384.

75. Eklund S, Jodal M, Lundgren O. The enteric nervous system participates in the secretory response to the heat stable enterotoxins of *Escherichia coli* in rats and cats. Neuroscience 1985; 14:673-681.

76. DuPont HL. Rotaviral gastroenteritis—some recent developments. J Infect Dis 1984; 149:663-666.

77. Torres-Pinedo R, Lavastida M, Rivera CL, Rodriguez H, Ortiz A. Studies on infant diarrhea. I. A comparison of the effects of milk feeding and intravenous therapy upon the composition and volume of the stool and urine. J Clin Invest 1966; 45:469-480.

78. Moon HW, Normal JO, Lambert G. Age dependent resistance to transmissible gastroenteritis of swine (TGE). I. Clinical signs and some mucosal dimensions in small intestine. Can J Comp Med 1973; 37:157–166.

79. Kirstein CG, Clarke DA, Lecce JG. Development of resistance of enterocytes to rotavirus in neonatal, agammaglobulinemic piglets. J Virol 1985; 55:567–573.

80. Kerzner B, Kelly MH, Gall DG, Butler DG, Hamilton JR. Transmissible gastroenteritis: sodium transport and the intestinal epithelium during the course of viral enteritis. Gastroenterology 1977; 72:457–461.

81. Butler DG, Gall DG, Kelly MN, Hamilton JR. Transmissible gastroenteritis. Mechanisms responsible for diarrhea in an acute viral enteritis in piglets. J Clin Invest 1974; 53:1335–1342.

82. Shepherd RW, Gall DG, Butler DG, Hamilton JR. Determinants of diarrhea in viral enteritis. The role of ion transport and epithelial changes in the ileum in transmissible gastroenteritis in piglets. Gastroenterology 1979; 76:20–24.

83. McClung HJ, Butler DG, Kerzner B, Gall DG, Hamilton JR. Transmissible gastroenteritis: mucosal ion transport in acute viral enteritis. Gastroenterology 1976; 70:1091–1095.

84. Keljo DJ, MacLeod RJ, Perdue MH, Butler DG, Hamilton JR. D-Glucose transport in piglet jejunal brush-border membranes: insights from a disease model. Am J Physiol (Gastrointest Liver Physiol 12) 1985; 249:G751–G760.

85. Rhoads JM, MacLeod RJ, Hamilton JR. Alanine enhances jejunal sodium absorption in the presence of glucose: studies in piglet viral diarrhea. Pediatr Res 1986; 20:879–883.

86. MacLeod RJ, Hamilton R. Absence of a cAMP-mediated antiabsorptive effect in an undifferentiated jejunal epithelium. Am J Physiol (Gastrointest Liver Physiol 15) 1987; 252:G776–G782.

87. Riby JE, Kretchmer N. Effect of dietary sucrose on synthesis and degradation of intestinal sucrose. Am J Physiol (Gastrointest Liver Physiol 9) 1984; 246:G757–G763.

88. Boyle JT, Kelly K, Krulich L, Koldovsky O. Site of thyroxine-evoked decreased of jejunal lactase in the rat. Am J Physiol (Gastrointest Liver Physiol 6) 1982; 243:G359–G364.

89. Gall DG, Chapman D, Kelly M, Hamilton JR. Na^+ transport in jejunal crypt cells. Gastroenterology 1977; 72:452–456.

90. Stewart CP, Turnberg LA. Glucose depolarizes villous but not crypt cell apical membrane potential difference: a micropuncture study of crypt-villus heterogeneity in the rat. Biochim Biophys Acta 1987; 902:293–300.

91. Smith MW. Expression of digestive and absorptive function in differentiating enterocytes. Ann Rev Physiol 1985; 47:247–260.

92. Sack DA, Rhoads M, Molla A, Molla AM, Wahed A. Carbohydrate malabsorption in infants with rotavirus diarrhea. Am J Clin Nutr 1982; 36:1112–1118.

93. Granger DN, Hernandez LA, Grisham MB. Reactive oxygen metabolites: mediators of cell injury in the digestive system. Viewpoints Dig Dis 1986; 18:13–16.

94. Perdue MH, Gall DG. Intestinal anaphylaxis in the rat: jejunal response to *in vitro* antigen exposure. Am J Physiol (Gastrointest Liver Physiol 13) 1986; 250:G427–G431.

95. Cuthbert AW, McLaughlan P, Coombs RRA. Immediate hypersensitivity reaction to β-lactoglobulin in the epithelium lining the colon of guinea pigs fed cows' milk. Int Arch Allergy Appl Imunol 1983; 72:34–40.

96. Baird AW, Coombs RRA, McLaughlan P, Cuthbert AW. Immediate hypersensitivity reactions to cow milk proteins in isolated epithelium from ileum of milk-drinking guinea-pigs: comparisons with colonic epithelia. Int Arch Allergy Appl Immunol 1984; 75:255–263.

97. Castro GA, Harari Y, Russell D. Mediators of anaphylaxis-induced ion transport changes in small intestine. Am J Physiol (Gastrointest Liver Physiol 16) 1987; 253:G540–G548.

98. Ameen VZ, Powell GK, Jonas LA. Quantitation of fecal carbohydrate excretion in patients with short bowel syndrome. Gastroenterology 1987; 92:493–500.

99. Read NW, Krejs GJ, Read MG, Santa Ana CA, Morawski SG, Fordtran JS. Chronic diarrhea of unknown origin. Gastroenterology 1980; 78:264–271.

100. Shiau YF, Feldman GM, Resnick MA, Coff PM. Stool electrolyte and osmolality measurements in the evaluation of diarrheal disorders. Ann Intern Med 1985; 102:773–775.

101. Ladefoged K, Schaffalitzky de Muckadell OB, Jarnum S. Faecal osmolality and electrolyte concentrations in chronic diarrhoea: do they provide diagnostic clues? Scand J Gastroenterol 1987; 22:813–820.

102. Carlson JAK, Middleton PJ, Szymanski MT, Huber H, Petric M. Fatal rotavirus gastroenteritis. Am J Dis Child 1978; 132:477–479.

103. Rabinowitz L, Joffe BI, Abkiewicz C, Shires R, Greef MC, Seftel HC. Hyperglycemia in infantile gastroenteritis. Arch Dis Child 1984; 59:771–775.

104. Lo CW, Walker WA. Chronic protracted diarrhea of infancy: a nutritional disease. Pediatrics 1983; 72:786–800.

105. Sallon S, Deckelbaum RJ, Schmid II, Harlap S, Baras M, Spira DT. *Cryptosporidium*, malnutrition, and chronic diarrhea in children. Am J Dis Child 1988; 142:312–315.

106. Rothbaum R, McAdams AJ, Giannella R, Partin JC. A clinicopathologic study of enterocyte-adherent *Escherichia coli*: a cause of protracted diarrhea in infants. Gastroenterology 1982; 83:441–454.

107. McAuliffe JF, Shields DS, Auxiliadora de Sousa M, Sakell J, Schorling J, Guerrant RL. Prolonged and recurring diarrhea in the northwest of Brazil: examination of cases from a community-based study. J Pediatr Gastroenterol Nutr 1986; 5:902–906.

108. Mirakian R, Richardson A, Milla PJ, Walker-Smith JA, Unsworth J, Savage MO, Bottazzo GF. Protracted diarrhoea of infancy: evidence in support of an autoimmune variant. Br Med J 1986; 293:113–1136.

109. Martorell R, Habicht J-P, Yarbrough C, Lechtig A, Klein RE, Western KA. Acute morbidity and physical growth in rural Guatemalan children. Am J Dis Child 1975; 129:1296–1301.

110. Jonas A, Avigad S, Diver-Haber A, Katznelson D. Distributed fat absorption following infectious gastroenteritis in children. J Pediatr 1979; 95:366–372.

CHAPTER 8

Malabsorption

Jacques Schmitz, M.D.

Malabsorption syndromes are characterized by the association of chronic diarrhea, abdominal distention, and failure to thrive.[1-3] During the period between 1955 and 1970, the widespread use of intestinal biopsy, the emergence of basic concepts such as lipolysis at an interface, micellar solubilization, Na$^+$-coupled solute transport, and brush border as a digestive-absorptive organelle permitted the breakdown of clinical malabsorption into many distinct congenital and acquired conditions affecting one or several of the different steps in hydrolysis or transport of nutrients. Thus the term *malabsorption syndrome* now designates also such different situations as those characterized by exocrine pancreatic insufficiency (for example, cystic fibrosis), intestinal villous atrophy (like celiac disease), specific hydrolysis (for example, congenital lipase or sucrase deficiencies), or transport (such as glucose-galactose malabsorption) defects. In order to understand how the clinician should interpret chronic diarrhea, the main symptom of these disease states, and how he should orient his approach to the precise defect involved, it is necessary to recall the physiology and pathophysiology of digestion and absorption.

PATHOPHYSIOLOGY OF DIGESTION AND ABSORPTION

Carbohydrates

Physiology of Digestion and Absorption

Carbohydrates in food comprise mainly starch (50 to 60 percent of total energy supplied by carbohydrates), sucrose (30 to 40 percent), and lactose (from 0 to 20 percent in adults, 40 to 50 percent in infants.)[4] Only starch molecules (amylose and amylopectin), which are glucose polymers of high molecular weight (M.W.), require preliminary intraluminal digestion by salivary and (predominantly) pancreatic amylases.[5] These structurally related endoamylases only split alpha$_{1-4}$ bonds at some distance from the ends of the glycosidic chains and from the branching (alpha$_{1-6}$) positions. They release mainly maltose, maltotriose, and residues of higher degree of polymerization (branched-alpha-limit dextrins, if the substrate is amylopectin) but no glucose. Intraluminal alpha-amylase activity is 10 times that required for digesting the amount of starch ingested daily.[6]

The final hydrolysis of di- and oligosaccharides occurs at the brush border of enterocytes where act three glycoproteins of high M.W. (greater than 200 kilodaltons [kDa]), the disaccharidases: (1) sucrase-isomaltase (S-I), which accounts for 75 to 80 percent of the hydrolysis of maltose in the intestinal mucosa, the total hydrolysis of sucrose, and the nearly total hydrolysis of isomaltose (alpha$_{1-6}$ bonds in dextrins); (2) glucoamylase, an exoamylase that is responsible for 20 to 25 percent of total mucosal maltase activity and releases glucose from glucose polymers of four or more residues; (3) lactase-phlorizin hydrolase, which accounts for over 95 percent of lactase activity in the intestinal mucosa and for the hydrolysis of glycosyl ceramides, complex glycolipids that are important constituents of milk globule membranes.[7] The ingested disaccharides, which physiologically are not absorbed as such, are thus ultimately broken down into their constituent monosaccharides: glucose, galactose, fructose.

Entry into the enterocytes through the brush border membrane occurs via carrier molecules. Entry of glucose and of galactose, occurring through the same carrier, is linked to the entry of Na$^+$ along its electrochemical gradient; the latter blocks glucose exit from the cell and eventually provides the energy necessary for its accumulation in the cell against a concentration gradient. The electrochemical Na$^+$ gradient is maintained by the Na$^+$,K$^+$-ATPase located in the basolateral membrane of the enterocyte. Thus, glucose and galactose absorptions are indirectly active.[8] Entry of fructose occurs through another specific carrier. It is not Na$^+$-dependent. Fructose is more metabolized in the enterocyte than glucose, whose exit from the cell occurs via a facilitated transport system (a carrier) similar to the one present in red blood cell membranes.[8]

Final hydrolysis and absorption of carbohydrates are closely integrated in the brush border so that when sucrose is perfused into the jejunum, no or low amounts of glucose diffuse back into the intestinal lumen. Perfusion studies in adults as in children have shown that the limiting factor in the overall process of disaccharide absorption is absorption of glucose and fructose in the case of sucrose and of maltose, but lactase activity in the case of lactose. This relationship is not modified in case of mucosal atrophy.[9]

Pathophysiology

Pancreatic amylase insufficiency occurs normally in newborns (see "Development"), whose amylase activity remains extremely low during the first weeks of life. Yet substantial amounts of starch (greater than 40 grams per sq meter per day) can be given to 1-month-old infants before the sign of carbohydrate malabsorption, fermentation, occurs.[10] Similarly, in cases of exocrine pancreatic insufficiency (cystic fibrosis or Shwachman's syndrome), symptoms related to amylase insufficiency are modest. In the stools, volatile fatty acids are notably increased, but lactic acid is low or absent and pH is above 5.5. This is probably due to the fact that starch is a poorer substrate for colonic bacteria than are oligosaccharides.[11]

Indeed, congenital or acquired defects of intestinal digestion and absorption of oligosaccharides lead to a major digestive symptom: fermentative diarrhea. It is characterized by watery stools whose volume is roughly proportional to the amount of ingested carbohydrates. Stool volume may thus be extremely variable from one day to another. Stools have an acidic smell, resembling that of rotten apples or of vinegar. They have an acidic pH (5.5 to 4.0) and usually contain unabsorbed reducing sugars or undigested disaccharides. The child often is thirsty and presents some degree of abdominal distention, the more impressive the younger he is.[1-3]

Diarrhea and abdominal distention (with gas-fluid levels on plain abdominal radiographs) are secondary to a cascade of events: Maldigested di- or trisaccharides or malabsorbed monosaccharides are small, osmotically active molecules that drive water inside the lumen of the gut in direct proportion to their amount. The increased volume of chyme leads in turn to an increased peristaltic activity and a reduced transit time, decreasing the chance of digestion and/or of absorption.[12] In the cecum, the unabsorbed small carbohydrate molecules are readily fermented by colonic bacteria. The latter produce CO_2, H_2, and mainly acetic but also butyric and propionic acids. If availability of carbohydrates further increases, lactic acid, a strong acid with a low pKa, is produced and pH decreases below 5.5 (a stool pH less than 5.5 indicates lactic acid in the stools[1,2]). This low pH disturbs Na^+ absorption by the colonic mucosa, which tends to further increase stool volume, as does the presence of the osmotically active molecules of volatile fatty acids in the lumen of the colon.

The same mechanism applies in all cases of carbohydrate malabsorption: in isolated congenital defects of intestinal hydrolysis (congenital sucrase-isomaltase, lactase, or trehalase deficiencies, or late-onset lactase deficiency) or of absorption (congenital glucose-galactose malabsorption) or as a consequence of mucosal atrophy (mainly in cow's milk protein intolerance and in celiac disease). Excluding the malabsorbed carbohydrate(s) from the diet stops diarrhea in a few hours; it is again triggered in a similar short period of time if the malabsorbed oligosaccharide is reintroduced in the diet. Dextrins or starch, however, may lead to diarrhea only after several (2 to 6) days in sucrase-isomaltase deficiency, probably because of the complementary glucoamylase activity.[13]

Proteins

Physiology

Digestion of proteins starts in the lumen of the stomach, where gastric acid denatures them and activates pepsinogens I and II into the corresponding pepsins. The latter are inactive at pH of less than 5 and have a broad specificity, splitting peptide bonds mostly involving phenylalanine, tyrosine, leucine.[14] In view of the buffering capacity of food, it is unlikely that gastric secretion plays a major role in protein digestion. In contrast, the efficiency of pancreatic proteolysis is demonstrated by the fact that as soon as 15 minutes after a test meal, about half of amino acids in the lumen are free or in the form of small peptides.[15] After activation by enterokinase, a glycoprotein of high M.W. synthesized by and anchored in the brush border membrane of enterocytes in the proximal small intestine, trypsinogen is converted into trypsin, which, in its turn, activates the other zymogens into active proteases. The endopeptidases—trypsin, chymotrypsin, and elastase—are serine proteases of similar M.W. (25 to 28 kDa) but with different and strictly defined specificities. Trypsin splits only bonds involving at the amino end basic amino acids (lysine and arginine), chymotrypsin splits those involving aromatic amino acids (phenylalanine, tyrosine, tryptophan), and elastase splits those involving uncharged small amino acids (such as alanine, glycine, and serine); these amino acids are left at the carboxy end of the newly formed peptide. They are released by exopeptidases, by carboxypeptidase A, which releases from a peptide its last amino acid when it is aromatic, neutral or acid, and by carboxypeptidase B, when the last amino acid is basic.[16]

In contrast to carbohydrates, peptides enter enterocytes either after preliminary digestion by brush border peptidases into amino acids, or as such, in the case of di- or tripeptides, which are then split inside the cell by cytoplasmic peptidases.[17,18] In man, at least eight brush border peptidases are now well defined: three aminopeptidases (oligoaminopeptidase or neutral aminopeptidase, the main brush border peptidase, acid aminopeptidase, dipeptidyl-peptidase IV), two carboxypeptidases (carboxypeptidase P and ACE, angiotensin-converting enzyme), two endopeptidases (including PABA peptidase), and gamma-glutamyl-transpeptidase. These enzymes are glycoproteins of M.W. somewhat lower than that of disaccharidases and altogether are able to hydrolyze all peptide bonds except those involving a proline at the carboxyl side.[7] The released amino acids are absorbed through at least four amino acid transport systems: one for neutral amino acids, mostly studied with alanine and having the broader specificity, one for imino acids (proline, hydroxyproline), one for dicarboxylic amino acids, and a fourth one for dibasic amino acids. Transport of all amino acids is active and, except for dibasic amino acids for which it is still debated, Na^+-dependent.[8]

Di- and tripeptides can also cross the brush border membrane as such via a (main) peptide transport system that has been shown to have a broad specificity. This carrier protein is able to transport dibasic as well as diacid peptides and di- as well as tripeptides (but no tetrapeptides).[17,18] Transport of peptide seems to be coupled to a proton rather than to a Na^+ gradient.[19] The existence of more than one system is still discussed. Once in the absorbing cell, di- and tripeptides are split into amino acids by soluble peptidases of which are known gly-leu dipeptidase, a prolidase hydrolyzing X-Pro bonds, and a tripeptidase.[18]

Small peptides are the form in which amino acids are, in general, the more readily absorbed. Even when a di- or tripeptide is susceptible to rapid hydrolysis by brush border peptidases, an important proportion of it (30 to 50 percent, depending on its concentration) is directly absorbed as such.[18] Thus, peptides represent the main physiologic route of entry of amino acids in the enterocytes.

Pathophysiology

In adults, nitrogen absorption is not affected by gastrectomy, which indicates that gastric acid and pepsins do not play a critical role in protein digestion. In contrast, selective absence of pancreatic protease activities—in congenital enterokinase deficiency, for example—leads to dramatic situations: Although stools are only moderately overabundant and foul smelling, fecal losses of nitrogen are massive with the consequence of early failure to thrive. The latter is more probable and severe, as the protein content of milk is low (as in human milk). Hypoproteinemia develops, leading to edema. Replacing the standard formula by a formula containing a protein hydrolysate is usually enough to normalize the stools, to decrease the fecal loss of nitrogen, and for the infant to start catching up its growth retardation.[20]

The consequences of pancreatic exocrine insufficiency on protein digestion are similar to those of selective pancreatic proteolytic deficiency. They are associated with significant losses of energy in the stools due to the defect in starch and, mostly, in fat digestion with a massive steatorrhea. The stools are often whitish, greasy, soft but not liquid, and extremely foul smelling. Malnutrition and growth failure follow when food intakes are not sufficient to compensate for the fecal losses.

No specific congenital defect of peptide digestion or absorption by the intestinal mucosa is known, although assays of the main peptidase activities have been systematically included in the work-up of diarrheal states in several pediatric gastroenterology teams for several years now. This is not surprising considering the fact that peptides may enter enterocytes by two routes of roughly similar physiologic importance: When one is blocked, the other one still can be used. Indeed, such defects may exist but may go undiagnosed. Similarly, specific absorption defects involving neutral (Hartnup's disease), basic (cystinuria), or imino (prolinuria) acids are well known. Yet they have not been recognized because of digestive symptoms, which do not exist in these conditions, but because of associated specific aminoaciduria, reflecting defective tubular reabsorption of the homologous amino acids by the kidney.[21] The absence of diarrhea in these diseases is clearly due to the fact that the specifically malabsorbed amino acids can cross the brush border membrane as peptides.[17] Indeed, the only known disease affecting amino acid absorption in which diarrhea is a real problem, often associated with severe malnutrition, is protein intolerance with lysinuria (or lysinuric protein intolerance). In this condition, the congenital defect does not affect the entry of arginine, lysine, and ornithine into the absorptive cell, but their exit out of the cell through the basolateral membrane. Whatever the way of entry into enterocytes, these basic amino acids cannot get out and symptoms occur.[22] Diarrhea is usually liquid, being probably mainly osmotic in its mechanism.

Nonspecific inflammatory alterations of the intestinal mucosa, such as those seen in celiac disease, do not lead to symptoms that can easily be assigned to protein or peptide maldigestion or absorption. A certain degree of creatorrhea exists in children with mucosal atrophy, yet it is usually mild and, because of the complex origin—both endogenous and exogenous—and the fate of protein in the human gut— absorbed or utilized by colonic bacteria, it is difficult to relate it directly to malabsorption. Similarly, it is difficult to decide whether the fecal losses of nitrogen observed in cases of intestinal malabsorption are the only explanation of the hypoalbuminemia that may be seen in severe celiac disease when anorexia (and consequently, decreased protein intake) and protein-losing enteropathy are also symptoms of the disease.

Fat

Physiology

Unlike carbohydrates and proteins, fats are insoluble in water; while they diffuse through the lipid phases of the brush border and basolateral membranes of enterocytes, they have to be "wrapped" in outwardly hydrophilic, inwardly lipophilic particles—bile salt micelles in the gut lumen, chylomicrons in the absorbing cell and circulation—to reach their site of metabolic utilization.[23]

Digestion of fat starts in the stomach, acted upon by a lipase that has been shown recently to originate exclusively from the gastric fundus in man,[24] whereas it is produced by the serous glands of von Ebner at the base of the tongue in the rat (hence the often-used term "lingual lipase"). In man, this lipase has an acidic optimum pH (3.5 to 5.5), it hydrolyzes medium-chain triglycerides (MCT) five to eight times more rapidly than long-chain triglycerides (LCT), it preferentially splits the outer ester bonds of triglycerides (TG), and it is not appreciably dependent on bile salts. It acts as a "starter" of pancreatic lipolysis by favoring emulsification of lipid droplets by the free fatty acids it releases. It plays a particularly important role in neonates whose pancreatic lipase activity is low.[25]

In the duodenum, pancreatic lipase acts at the oil/water interface, adsorbed to the lipid droplets. Bile salts both increase the interface by emulsifying the ingested lipid droplets, thus favouring lipase activity, and, on the contrary, by forming a film between oil and lipase, inhibit its action. Colipase restores lipase activity by anchoring lipase to the interface, thus giving it access to its substrate. In the presence of bile salts, pancreatic lipase has an optimum pH of 8. It has an absolute specificity for the outer ester bonds (positions 1 and 3) of the glyceride molecule and releases free fatty acids (FFA) and 2-monoglycerides (2 MGs).[26] Other lipolytic enzymes are secreted by the pancreas: (1) carboxylesterhydrolase, whose structure resembles that of human milk, bile-salt dependent lipase, acts on soluble substrates. In the presence of bile salts, it becomes active toward cholesterol esters and esters of vitamin A and E, whose absorption is thus dependent on normal bile salt secretion[27]; (2) phospholipase A_2 releases lysophosphoglycerides and fatty acids from phosphoglycerides, major membrane constituents.

From the onset of lipolysis, FFAs and 2 MGs are solubilized in bile salt micelles, forming bigger "mixed micelles" which, in their turn, can solubilize more hydrophobic lipids such as diglycerides, un-ionized FFA, cholesterol esters, and lipid-soluble vitamins whose absorption is therefore improved when ingested with other fats.

Primary bile acids (cholic and chenodeoxycholic acids) are synthesized in the liver from cholesterol; they are glyco and tauro conjugated, excreted, and transformed by colonic bacteria into secondary acids (deoxycholic and lithocholic acids). Because of their lower pKa, conjugated bile acids allow a much better micellar solubilization of the products of lipolysis.[28] Bile acids, whose pool amounts to 1 to 2.5 g, are efficiently reabsorbed in the distal ileum by an Na^+-dependent, carrier-mediated process that is responsible for the reabsorption (and recirculation) of 95 percent of the bile salts secreted in bile.[28]

Micelles diffuse from the gut lumen through the unstirred water layers lining the luminal surface of brush borders, where the products of lipolysis are liberated. They diffuse across the apical cell membrane. In enterocytes, FFA of 12 atoms of carbon or more bind to a small carrier protein, the fatty acid binding protein (FABP). In the smooth endoplasmic reticulum, long-chain FA are activated in acyl-CoA before entering the monoglyceride pathway responsible for at least 70 percent of postprandial TG resynthesis (while the role of glycerophosphate pathway in TG resynthesis increases between meals and during fast).[23] In the rough endoplasmic reticulum, resynthesized TG, phospholipids, and cholesterol are joined by newly synthesized apolipoproteins AI, AIV, and B48, which is supposed to be necessary for chylomicron formation in the Golgi apparatus. Chylomicron-containing Golgi vesicles are released from Golgi apparatus. After fusion of these vesicles with the basolateral membrane, chylomicrons are excreted by exocytosis into the intercellular spaces, from which they reach the lymphatics and, by the thoracic duct, the systemic circulation.[29]

Pathophysiology

Because of their hydrophobicity, digestion and absorption of dietary fats are dependent on many auxiliary molecules other than enzymes and carriers: bile salts, colipase, FABP, apolipoproteins. It is thus remarkable that, given this complexity, more than 95 percent of ingested fat should be ultimately absorbed in children over the age of 1 year.

However, these auxiliary mechanisms are also sites for potential disturbances; indeed, causes of fat malabsorption and steatorrhea are much more numerous than those of carbohydrate and protein malabsorption. Fat malabsorption may result from lipase and/or colipase deficiency(ies); abnormal bile salt synthesis, excretion, deconjugation, reabsorption; impaired TG resynthesis, chylomicron formation and/or excretion; or obstruction of intestinal lymphatics.

Isolated fat malabsorption is extremely rare. In the case of congenital lipase deficiency, for example, stools are greasy but not liquid nor even soft: nonabsorbed fat constitutes an oil phase distinct from, or surrounding, otherwise nearly normal stools. Steatorrhea is massive, with fat absorption coefficient being less than 50 percent. Such a steatorrhea is painless and may have no other consequence for the patient than greasy soiling and a strong appetite to compensate for the loss of energy in the stools.[30] Colipase deficiency leads to less severe steatorrhea, and biliary atresia, although leading to no other digestive symptom, presents usually with its own signs such as jaundice and hepatomegaly.

In most cases, fat malabsorption is part of a more general pathologic condition. It may result from exocrine pancreatic insufficiency: Severely reduced lipase and colipase secretions

result in abnormally great quantities of neutral TG reaching the colon where the bacterial flora hydrolyzes part of them, releasing FFA and glycerol. Steatorrhea is usually severe, fat absorption being reduced to 70 to 40 percent of ingested fat. Because undigested starch is not so osmotically active, stools are soft or pasty, not liquid, like mastic.

Bile salt metabolism abnormalities other than reduced or absent secretion may disturb fat absorption. Bile salts may be deconjugated by certain bacterial species in cases of bacterial overgrowth. Nonconjugated bile salts are less ionized than conjugated ones at the pH of the gut lumen; they have thus a lower ability to form micelles than the latter. Significant steatorrhea may follow. It is usually associated with other symptoms of bacterial overgrowth in a stagnant loop: increased degradation of protein and particularly of vitamin B_{12} binding proteins, fermentation of carbohydrates with production of H_2 released in breath and of volatile fatty acids resulting in diarrhea, hypoproteinemia, loss of weight, and megaloblastic anemia.[31] Bile salts also may not be absorbed because of a congenital defect or ileal disease (Crohn's disease) or because of ileal resection with two consequences: On the one hand, abnormally high amounts of nonabsorbed bile salts reach the colon where they inhibit Na^+ and water absorption; on the other hand, depletion of bile salt pool progressively leads to poor micellar solubilization and steatorrhea. In this situation, however, the direct effect of bile salts on colonic mucosa is probably more responsible for the abnormal loose or watery stools than is the increased fecal loss of fat.

Intestinal mucosal abnormalities never affect only fat absorption, even when, as in abnormal chylomicron formation and/or excretion, fat transport alone is disturbed by the disease. Most frequently fat malabsorption is secondary to nonspecific intestinal mucosal atrophy as observed in celiac disease or cow's milk protein intolerance. In these conditions, malabsorption of fat, as of other nutrients, results both from decreased absorptive surface and from disturbed enterocyte metabolism. In fact, abnormal accumulation of lipid droplets occurs in active celiac disease by mechanisms that are not completely elucidated but may involve impaired apolipoprotein synthesis. It is not clear whether lipids in the stools originate directly from ingested fat or indirectly from desquamated fat-filled enterocytes. In any case, fat lost in the stools is mainly FFA partly hydroxylated by the colonic flora, which accounts for at least 1 g daily of obligatory loss of fat in the stools.[32] Interestingly, steatorrhea is usually far less severe in intestinal mucosal disorders than in exocrine pancreatic insufficiency. This may be due to the fact that most intestinal pathologic conditions, such as celiac disease, affect only the proximal small intestine, or to the existence of "accessory" pathways of fat absorption as suggested by the paradoxic absorption of 50 to 70 percent of ingested fats in situations in which no absorption at all is expected, as in congenitally impaired formation or excretion of chylomicrons. The moderate steatorrhea observed in conditions with subtotal villous atrophy is usually not sufficient to make the stools grossly greasy; in fact, stool features in these situations result more from the degree of associated carbohydrate fermentation than from the degree of steatorrhea.

Even when chylomicron formation and/or excretion is blocked, as in abetalipoproteinemia or Anderson's disease with enterocytes filled with fat droplets, malabsorption is not restricted to fat. Balance studies in these conditions show fecal excretion of fat, nitrogen, and volatile fatty acids that is similar to that observed in celiac disease. Stools have the same aspect. Yet a fat-free diet is sufficient to normalize the fecal excretions of nitrogen and of volatile fatty acids. This indicates that nitrogen and carbohydrate malabsorption is induced by the accumulation of fat observed in enterocytes in these conditions.

Similarly, in intestinal lymphangiectasia, reflux of absorbed fat into the intestinal lumen because of blocked lymph flow is never isolated, and steatorrhoea, usually moderate, is associated with signs of enteric loss of the other constituents of intestinal lymph: albumin, immunoglobulins, and T lymphocytes. However, fats lost in the lumen are excreted in the stools, whereas proteins are easily digested and reabsorbed, and balance studies usually fail to find a significant increase in fecal nitrogen. Diarrhea is often moderate in this condition, in which low serum albumin levels and edema are major symptoms.[33]

NUTRITIONAL CONSEQUENCES OF MALABSORPTION

Malabsorption may have no or minor nutritional consequences (for example, lipase deficiency) or, at the opposite extreme, may lead to severe malnutrition and eventually death (for example, celiac disease). Furthermore, the same disease may be life threatening in infancy and well tolerated in adolescence (celiac disease or congenital sucrase-isomaltase deficiency). Finally, malnutrition may become the consequence of a stable state of malabsorption under the influence of exogenous factors (bronchopulmonary infection in cystic fibrosis, for example). Thus, a given nutritional disturbance is not strictly linked to a given malabsorption syndrome and it seems appropriate, in dealing with nutritional consequences of malabsorption, to describe first the different consequences that malabsorption syndromes may have on the nutritional status of the child and then to analyze the general mechanisms by which malnutrition occurs. Nutritional disturbances involving micronutrients will not be considered here.

States of Malnutrition

The most obvious nutritional consequences of malabsorption syndromes concern the growth of the child. Malabsorption always first reduces weight gain before it slows down growth rate. The clinical situation may deteriorate with disappearance of subcutaneous fat, muscle wasting, and the appearance of the skin as too large for the child. Growth stops. Life may be threatened. Such a severe evolution was described in toddlers with historic celiac disease. Nutritional consequences are not so dramatic in older children with celiac disease, for example: A certain equilibrium may be reached, the child having a weight roughly adapted to his height, yet growth is retarded and the child may progressively become a dwarf. In adolescents, puberty may be delayed.[34,35]

In most severe and/or rapidly evolving malabsorption syndromes, not only is growth affected, but also other general functions: Malabsorption of vitamin K, whatever its mechanism (mucosal atrophy, fat malabsorption, bacterial overgrowth), may result in decreased synthesis of blood clotting factors and disturbed hemostasis, with hematomas and easy bleeding; long-term Ca^{2+} and vitamin D malabsorption leads usually to osteoporosis, with hypocalcemia, hypocalciuria, and, in severe cases, "spontaneous" bone fractures, rarely to rickets.[34] Severe protein-losing enteropathy, often associated with malabsorption syndromes (celiac disease, bacterial overgrowth, Crohn's disease, intestinal lymphangiectasia), may be an additional factor responsible for hypoalbuminemia and edema and for hypogammaglobulinemia.[33]

Other biologic anomalies, also present in children with overt malnutrition, may be used in others to detect malnutrition when it is not clinically certain. They include hyposideremia, microcytic anemia with low reticulocyte counts secondary to iron malabsorption, low serum folate levels usually without hematologic consequences in case of mucosal atrophy,[36] low serum vitamin A levels (whose ophthalmologic consequences are nonetheless rare), and low vitamin E levels, which may lead, after years of evolution, to loss of proprioception and tendon reflexes and to ataxia, in cases of fat malabsorption; vitamin E deficiency is most severe in biliary atresia and in abetalipoproteinemia.[37]

Mechanisms of Development of Malnutrition

Our knowledge concerning the mechanisms resulting in malnutrition is limited because of the complexity of a phenomenon with intricate causes, always studied when already present, with often only crude parameters (weight and height).

Although malabsorption per se is the most obvious mechanism leading to malnutrition, it is probably less often responsible for failure to thrive than decreased food intake. This has been clearly demonstrated in the case of Crohn's disease,[38] but it may be also true for active celiac disease in which anorexia is a major symptom; more generally, decreased food intake may be a main factor of malnutrition in all situations in which fermentation is a major consequence of malabsorption (congenital disaccharidase deficiencies or disaccharidase deficiencies secondary to villous atrophy) leading to abdominal distention, discomfort, and poor appetite, whereas fecal losses of protein and energy are usually modest. At the opposite end of the spectrum, fecal losses of up to 40 percent of ingested protein and energy in cases of exocrine pancreatic insufficiency, associated with no major discomfort, do not lead to malnutrition as long as they are compensated by an increased appetite. In this situation, any factor decreasing food intake—bronchopulmonary infection in cystic fibrosis, for example—triggers malnutrition and retards growth.

Malabsorption per se—independently from anorexia—may induce malnutrition only when fecal loss cannot be compensated by increased intake; this is the case in infants with undiagnosed exocrine pancreatic insufficiency when nutrient intakes are low, particularly proteins, whose levels in commercial formulas tend to parallel those of human milk. Weight gain decreases and hypoalbuminemia and edema develop. The same symptoms occur in the short bowel syndrome when losses of nutrients in the stools are too high to be compensated by increased intakes without digestive symptoms.

Other mechanisms may induce or contribute to malnutrition: (1) chronic inflammation, which has been shown, as in Crohn's disease, to increase protein degradation and thus protein turnover, with consequent increased energy needs for rest metabolism[39]; (2) protein-losing enteropathy, which may exceed the capacity of the liver to synthesize albumin and occurs not only in intestinal lymphangiectasia, but also in celiac disease and Crohn's disease; (3) bacterial overgrowth, which results in energy losses (fermented carbohydrates, malabsorbed fat) and leads to diversion of nitrogen fluxes toward bacterial growth, with the ultimate consequences of hypoalbuminemia and loss of lean body mass.[40] In all these situations, protein malnutrition is responsible for low plasma levels of insulin-like growth factor-I (IGF-I, or somatomedin C), whereas growth hormone secretion is normal.[35,41] Thus, decreased plasma levels of IGF-I explain, at least in part, growth retardation during malnutrition, and IGF-I levels may be used as accurate markers of nutritional sufficiency.[41]

Finally, impaired absorption appears as much more harmful than impaired digestion, because in the vast majority of cases mucosal lesions affect not only absorption of major nutrients but also of vitamins (lipid-soluble vitamins [A, D, E, K] and folic acid, when intestinal lesions are proximal, as in celiac disease; vitamin B_{12} when they are distal, as in ileal Crohn's disease), of major minerals like iron and Ca^{2+}, and of trace minerals. These deficiencies hasten and aggravate malnutrition, whereas their absence, in states of impaired pancreatic digestion, contribute to the relatively satisfactory nutritional tolerance of the latter conditions.

PRACTICAL APPROACH TO MALABSORPTION

The main clinical expression of malabsorption is diarrhea. It is the direct consequence of malabsorption which, in its turn, when chronic, may result in malnutrition and failure to thrive, the usual other features of malabsorption syndromes. Since the consequences of malabsorption on growth have already been dealt with elsewhere, this part of the chapter focuses on chronic diarrhea, or more properly on "abnormal stools,"[3] as the main clue to the diagnosis and etiology of malabsorption.

Recognizing Chronic Diarrhea

Chronic diarrhea is usually defined as diarrhea lasting for more than 14 days. In toddlers who already control their stools, abnormal stools are not missed by the family, who often tends to exaggerate their importance. On the contrary, when diarrhea starts from birth or soon after, the abnormal features of the stools are less easily recognized, especially if the infant is breast-fed and is the first child in the family.

A careful clinical history remains the most important step in getting to the diagnosis of malabsorption. The fluidity, number, size, color, and smell of the stools should first be ascertained. Stools may be as liquid as water and mistaken

for urine in infants in case of congenital chloride diarrhea, for example[42]; passed noisily with flatus in cases of sugar intolerance; loose and bulky in celiac disease; or pasty and yellowish in exocrine pancreatic insufficiency. The number of stools may vary from two (bulky) to 10 or more (small and liquid). Stools may be homogeneous or, on the contrary, may contain undigested pieces of vegetables and mucus. Whether the stools are greasy or not is often difficult to ascertain; the less liquid the stools are, the easier it is. Liquid stools may be odorless, or they may have an acidic smell due to fermentation. Smell is usually offensive in celiac disease. In exocrine pancreatic insufficiency stools have a penetrating cheesy odor. Finally, the mode of evolution of diarrhea should be recorded: Stools may be abnormal every day or periodically.[3]

Recognizing the Cause of Chronic Diarrhea

First, the necessary time should be spent in trying to correlate the occurrence of diarrhea with modifications in the diet—introduction or elimination of cow's milk proteins, wheat flour, lactose, sucrose, and vegetables, for example. Associated symptoms should be systematically looked for: anorexia (intestinal malabsorption), increased appetite (exocrine pancreatic insufficiency), thirst (when diarrhea is fluid and severe as in sugar intolerance), abdominal pain, cramps, discomfort, bloating (indicative of fermentation), vomiting (protein intolerance), asthenia, weakness (celiac disease, Crohn's disease).

Equally important is to establish whether the growth of the child is normal or not by recording carefully his growth charts from birth, for height and weight. Clinical examination will appreciate the activity and psychomotor development of the child. One should look for abdominal distention, best observed in the standing position in profile, taking into account the physiologic distention in toddlers, and for finger clubbing. It is important to evaluate the state of nutrition by recording skinfold thickness, muscle tone and volume, paleness of the skin and conjunctiva, color and quality of hair, and dryness of the skin.

At the end of this clinical evaluation, the most frequent cause of chronic diarrhea in childhood—"non-specific chronic diarrhea" or "toddler's diarrhea"[43] (characterized by periods of frequent, heterogeneous [with vegetable matter] often mucus-containing, foul smelling stools, often alternating with periods of normal stools or even constipation, and a normal state of nutrition)—has been eliminated. Frequently, the clinical history, the growth charts, and the physical examination of the child lead to the diagnosis of celiac disease or cystic fibrosis; an intestinal biopsy or a sweat test rapidly confirms the diagnosis.

In many cases, however, other investigations are necessary—among those, balance studies with recording of ingested foods and collection of the stools during at least three days. Thus will be differentiated chronic diarrhea due to major pathophysiologic mechanisms: impaired intraluminal digestion, intestinal malabsorption, and fermentation. Once one of these has been established, further laboratory tests usually lead to the precise etiology of malabsorption.[1,2]

Diarrhea Due to Impaired Intraluminal Digestion (IID)

Diarrhea due to exocrine pancreatic insufficiency (EPI), the predominant cause of IID, is remarkable by the macroscopic appearance of the stools: They are more frequently loose and pasty than liquid, homogeneous, often obviously greasy with undigested triglycerides oozing like oil from the stool when it is passed in a "pot" or floating on the surface of the water in the toilet, pale (hence the mastic aspect of the stools), with an offensive cheese smell. Balance studies show that volume of the stools is rather constant from one day to another. They contain large amounts of fat, nitrogen, and volatile fatty acids; steatorrhea may amount to 10 g per day in infants or toddlers and to 30 g per day in children of 5 to 10 years of age, with a fat absorption coefficient varying from 40 to 70 percent; excretion of nitrogen is also massively increased, from 1 to 3 or 4 g per day (normal is less than 0.5 g per day); volatile fatty acids are usually above 30 mmol per day (normal is less than 10), whereas the stools contain no or small amounts of lactic acid (Table 1).[44]

Apart from acquired surgical conditions (short bowel syndrome, stagnant loop), such a massive fecal loss of the three classes of nutrients can only be explained by EPI, whose most frequent cause in children is, by far, *cystic fibrosis*. Most often, however, the sweat test has been performed before balance studies. If chloride concentration in sweat is normal, EPI is due to congenital hypoplasia of the pancreas. Hypoplasia may be associated with lipomatous infiltration. Such is the case when EPI is part of several syndromes, the most frequent of which is *Shwachman syndrome*. In this rather rare condition EPI is associated with chronic or cyclic neutropenia or other hematologic abnormalities, with metaphyseal chondrodysplasia, especially in ribs and hips, often with severe growth retardation.[45] Rarer is *Johanson-Blizzard syndrome*, in which EPI is associated with morphologic abnormalities: congenital aplasia of the alae nasi, ectoder-

mal scalp defects, and imperforate anus.[46] Pancreatic hypoplasia is linked to fibrosis in the few reported cases in which EPI is associated with refractory sideroblastic anemia and vacuolization of marrow precursors.[47] Finally, seldom in children is EPI due to *chronic pancreatitis*. It has been described in the course of cystinosis.[48] In all cases, EPI is confirmed by direct assay of pancreatic enzyme activities in the duodenal juice (Table 2).

IID rarely involves only one class of nutrient. A massive isolated steatorrhea may be due to *isolated congenital lipase or colipase deficiency*, which can be confirmed by the direct assay of lipase activity in the duodenal juice.[49,50] In this situation, normal lipase activity would orient the diagnosis toward defective micellar solubilization due to *congenital absence of bile acid synthesis,*[51] abnormal biliary excretion (*congenital biliary atresia*),[52] interrupted bile acid enterohepatic circulation because of *bacterial overgrowth,*[31] *ileal resection,*[53] *Crohn's disease* or *congenital bile acid malabsorption.*[54] Bile acid assay in blood or the duodenal juice, or, less easily, in stools, may lead to one of these diagnostic possibilities. Isolated pancreatic proteolytic insufficiency has also been described; *congenital trypsinogen deficiency* has been reported, yet it is less well established than *congenital enterokinase deficiency* suspected in a malnourished infant, failing to thrive, with abnormal stools from birth.[20] Diagnosis is suspected when exogenous enterokinase restores a previously severely reduced or absent proteolytic activity in the duodenal juice; it is confirmed by the direct measurement of enterokinase activity in the duodenal mucosa (Table 2).

Diarrhea Due to Intestinal Malabsorption

Diarrhea due to intestinal malabsorption is loose or liquid, often with an acidic smell, rarely greasy. Balance studies show that stool volume is more variable than in EPI; they demonstrate a usually mild steatorrhea (rarely above 10 g per day), fat absorption coefficient varying from 70 to 85 percent, a

TABLE 1
Results of Balance Studies in Children with Chronic Diarrhea, According to Pathophysiologic Mechanisms

Pathophysiologic Mechanism	Etiology (n)*	Stools				
		Fresh Weight (g/day)	Nitrogen (g/day)	Fat (g/day)	Volatile Fatty Acids (mmol/day)	Lactic Acid (mmol/day)
Intraluminal digestion insufficiency	Cystic fibrosis Shwachman syndrome } (9)	235 ± 36[†]	3.2 ± 0.5	24.9 ± 3.5 (42 ± 9)[‡]	42.3 ± 8.0	2.8 ± 5.1
Intestinal malabsorption	Celiac disease <3 years (28)	118 ± 75	0.88 ± 0.27	6.7 ± 2.0 (75 ± 8)	16.6 ± 11.3	4.4 ± 5.8
	>3 years (22)	161 ± 88	1.48 ± 0.39	7.3 ± 3.2 (85 ± 7)	24.9 ± 11.5	2.1 ± 2.8
	CMPI (11)	118 ± 68	0.64 ± 0.26	4.7 ± 2.4 (76 ± 8)	15.1 ± 8.0	9.2 ± 12.1
Fermentation	CSID§ (13)	413 ± 175	0.95 ± 0.79	4.6 ± 2.3 (85 ± 7)	44.6 ± 17.9	30 ± 15.3

* n = number of children studied during 6-day balances.
† Mean ± 1SD (personal data)
‡ Fat absorption coefficient
§ Congenital sucrase-isomaltase deficiency

TABLE 2
Diarrhea Due to Impaired Intraluminal Digestion

| | Diagnosis | |
Pathophysiology	Suspected	Evidence for Probable or Certain Diagnosis
Impaired digestion affecting all nutrients	Cystic fibrosis	Sweat test positive
	Pancreatic hypoplasia with lipomatosis part of	
	Shwachman syndrome	Neutropenia
		Metaphyseal chondrodysplasia
	Johanson-Blizzard syndrome	Morphologic anomalies
	fibrosis, part of Pearson syndrome	Sideroblastic anemia
	Cystinosis	Tubular acidosis
Impaired digestion affecting fat and proteins		
Fat	Isolated lipase or colipase deficiency	Direct assay in duodenal juice
	Abnormal micellar solubilization	
	Impaired bile acid synthesis	Bile acid assay in blood, duodenal juice, stools
	Bile duct atresia	Cholestasis
	Interrupted enterohepatic circulation	
	Ileal resection	Clinical history
	Crohn's disease	Clinical history
	Congenital malabsorption of bile acids	Bile acid assay in blood, duodenal juice, stools
	Blind loop syndrome	Clinical history, H_2, breath test
Proteins	Congenital trypsinogen deficiency	Direct assay in duodenal juice
	Congenital enterokinase deficiency	Assay in duodenal mucosa

modest creatorrhea (1 to 2 g per day), and an increased excretion of volatile fatty acids often associated with the abnormal presence of high amounts of lactic acid[1] (see Table 1).

Such a diarrhea indicates that an intestinal biopsy should be performed. It may disclose either specific or nonspecific inflammatory alterations of the intestinal mucosa. The latter include the various degrees of villous atrophy. A flat mucosa (total villous atrophy) in a child of more than 1 year of age is highly suggestive of *celiac disease*, which can be confirmed several years later by relapse of the intestinal lesions after challenge with gluten.[55] Partial villous atrophy in an infant of less than 6 months of age is most often secondary to *sensitization to food proteins*, most often cow's milk proteins, more seldom to soya, rice, or wheat proteins.[56] Given the lack of a reliable laboratory test to confirm such a sensitization, proof of it relies on the curative effect of an exclusion diet and eventually on relapse of symptoms after challenge with the suspected protein. Partial villous atrophy may also occur in the *postgastroenteritis syndrome*, or in *Giardia lamblia infestation*; motile trophozoites may then be seen on histologic sections in the mucous layer covering the mucosa. Finally, partial villous atrophy and chronic diarrhea may reveal a state of immunodeficiency: *hypogammaglobulinemia, combined immunodeficiency syndromes*, of which some may be linked to the *absence of expression of HLA antigens*.[57] Measurements of immunoglobulin levels and of specific antibodies, counts of Ig-containing cells in the intestinal mucosa, should be performed in these situations as studies of delayed-type hypersensitivity. Although it is probable that intestinal lesions, in these situations, are linked to *bacterial overgrowth*,[58] the latter is often difficult to demonstrate, either indirectly by H_2 breath measurements after a glucose load[59] or directly by bacterial counts in the intestinal juice. A combination of several of these factors—

food sensitization, depressed immune status, bacterial overgrowth—probably explains the partial villous atrophy often observed in children with *protracted diarrhea* (Table 3).

In other, much rarer cases, the intestinal biopsy reveals specific lesions. The mucosal architecture is normal, but enterocytes appear full of lipid droplets that reflect abnormal chylomicron assembly or excretion. Such a disorder may reveal *abetalipoproteinemia*, which will be quickly confirmed by the finding of acanthocytosis, absence of LDL and apoprotein B from the plasma, loss of tendon reflexes, and eventually retinitis[60]; the same intestinal lesions may also be the main finding in favor of *Anderson's disease* (or *chylomicron retention disease*), whose clinical features are similar to those of celiac disease.[61,62] In other cases *lymphangiectasia* distorts the shape of villi. Lymphopenia, hypoalbuminemia with eventual edema, and hypogammaglobulinemia are usually associated with a modest steatorrhea. Measurement of alpha$_1$ antiprotease clearance confirms the loss of lymph in the digestive tract.[33] Finally, the lamina propria of the intestinal mucosa may be densely infiltrated by a monomorphic lymphoplasmocytic population, composed of packed plasma cells or later of lymphoblasts, which disrupts crypts and widens and flattens villi whose epithelium is barely altered. In such cases, *alpha chain disease* should be suspected. The presence of an abnormal monoclonal IgA in plasma confirms the diagnosis (Table 3).[63]

Diarrhea Due to Fermentation

Diarrhea due to fermentation is liquid, acid (pH less than 5.5), and often passed with flatus, and its volume is variable and roughly proportional to the amount of malabsorbed carbohydrate that has been ingested. Balance studies show that there is no steatorrhea (except in cases of extremely rapid transit time) and no significant creatorrhea. Stools contain

TABLE 3
Diarrhea Due to Intestinal Malabsorption

	Diagnosis	
Pathophysiology	Suspected	Evidence for Probable or Certain Diagnosis
Intestinal biopsy: nonspecific inflammatory lesions		
Total villous atrophy (flat mucosa)	Celiac disease	Relapse at gluten challenge
Partial villous atrophy*	Sensitization to food proteins: CMP, rice, soya, wheat	Relapse at challenge
	Dermatitis herpetiformis	Dermal IgA deposit
	Giardia lamblia infestation	*Giardia* on biopsy specimen
	Immunodeficiency status, among these: absence of HLA expression	HLA typing
	Bacterial overgrowth	Bacterial counts in duodenal juice, H_2 test
	"Intractable diarrhea" syndrome (may be postgastroenteritis)	Clinical history
Intestinal biopsy: specific lesions		
Fat-filled enterocytes	Abetalipoproteinemia	Absence of plasma LDL, apo B; acanthocytosis
	Anderson's disease	Decreased levels of plasma LDL, apo B
Villi distorted by ectatic lymphatics	Lymphangiectasia	Lymphopenia, hypoalbuminemia, increased alpha$_1$ PI clearance
Dense monomorphic lymphoplasmocytic infiltrate	Alpha chain disease	Monoclonal abnormal IgA in plasma
Normal intestinal biopsy	Lysinuric protein intolerance	Dibasic aminoaciduria Severe osteoporosis

* In severe cases, villous atrophy may be subtotal.

large amounts of volatile fatty acids (acetic, butyric, and propionic acids) and lactic acid. These small, osmotically active molecules determine the volume of the stools, lactic acid being responsible for the stool pH below 5.5. Such an acidic pH is extremely evocative of fermentation due to carbohydrate intolerance and must lead to a systematic search for reducing substances in the stools[1] (see Table 1).

Although overexcretion of H_2 in breath after an oral load of a suspected sugar may orient the diagnosis, the most useful investigation is an intestinal biopsy. The intestinal mucosa appears normal on histologic sections in cases of congenital (or primary) sugar intolerance. The assay of dissacharidase activities in an homogenate of the mucosa more often detects *sucrase-isomaltase deficiency*,[64] the most frequent of these

intolerances, than *congenital lactase deficiency*,[65] which has been ascertained principally in Finland. In children or adolescents of non-Caucasian origin, *late-onset lactase deficiency*[66] is, on the contrary, frequently the cause of a mild lactose intolerance. Normal enzyme activities, as well as clinical trials with different sugars, lead to the possibility of *congenital glucose-galactose malabsorption*, which can be proven by studies in an Ussing chamber (glucose does not trigger any short-circuit current as it should) or with brush border vesicles (glucose is not taken up even in the presence of Na$^+$) (Table 4).[67]

However, much more frequently, the intestinal mucosa looks abnormal with more or less severe villous atrophy. Disaccharidase activities are, like peptidase activities, nonspe-

TABLE 4
Diarrhea Due to Fermentation

	Diagnosis	
Pathophysiology	Suspected	Conditions of Probable or Certain Diagnosis
Intestinal biopsy: normal or subnormal intestinal mucosa	CSID Congenital lactase deficiency Late-onset lactase deficiency Congenital trehalase deficiency[69] Congenital glucose-galactose malabsorption	Assay of saccharidases in mucosal homogenate: *one* activity affected

Absence of glucose-induced short-circuit current in Ussing chamber |
| Intestinal biopsy: nonspecific inflammatory lesions | All causes of villous atrophy (cf. Table 3), mainly: Celiac disease CMPI Postgastroenteritis syndrome | *All* saccharidase activities affected Cf. Table 3 Cf. Table 3 Cf. Table 3 |

TABLE 5
Chronic Diarrhea Starting in the Neonatal*Period

Condition (in Order of Decreasing Severity)	Distinctive Clinical Features	Key Laboratory Investigation	Therapeutic Decision
Congenital microvillous atrophy[70]	Intractable† watery diarrhea	Intestinal biopsy (PAS stain)	Total parenteral nutrition
Congenital glucose-galactose malabsorption	Acid diarrhea	Intestinal biopsy (Ussing chamber, brush border vesicles)	Replacement of glucose and galactose by fructose in the diet
Congenital lactase deficiency	Acid diarrhea	Intestinal biopsy (assay of activity)	Lactose-free diet
Congenital chloride diarrhea	Hydramnios, intractable watery diarrhea	Assay of electrolytes in stools	IV then oral Cl^- supplementation
Congenital defective jejunal Na^+/H^+ exchange[71]	Hydramnios, intractable watery diarrhea	Assay of electrolytes in stools	IV then oral Na^+ supplementation
Congenital bile acid malabsorption	Steatorrhea	Bile acid assay in plasma, stools	MCT, cholestyramine
Congenital enterokinase deficiency	Failure to thrive, edema	Intestinal biopsy (assay of enterokinase activity)	Protein hydrolysate

* Neonatal = within the first week of life.
† Intractable = persisting despite nothing by mouth.

cifically decreased as a consequence of mucosal damage. Sugar intolerance and fermentation are, then, secondary to villous atrophy, as in *celiac disease*.[68] In the latter condition, *secondary sugar intolerance* is probably the main factor responsible for the volume of stools (Table 4).[1,69]

Diarrhea Starting in the Neonatal Period

Chronic diarrhea starting in the hours or days following birth is usually extremely severe, leading in a few weeks to life-threatening malnutrition. The features of a malabsorption syndrome are thus gathered, although in some of the conditions characterized by such a diarrhea, malabsorption may involve only one ion. The age at which these conditions are discovered—the neonatal period, the often abundant and watery character of the stools, the severity of the dehydration and of malnutrition resulting from diarrhea, and the fact that these conditions are all familial justify their grouping independently from their pathophysiology (Table 5). Keeping in mind these conditions, in the presence of any newborn presenting with a persistent diarrhea, should improve the quality of the care offered to these neonates at risk.

REFERENCES

1. Lamy M, Frezal J, Rey J, Nezelof C, Fortier-Beaulieu M, Jos J. Les stéatorrhées par troubles de l'absorption intestinale. XIX Congrès de l'Association des Pédiatres de langue française. Paris 18-20 June 1963. Paris: Expansion Scientifique Française. 1963: vol I, p 1.
2. Weijers HA, Van de Kamer JH, Wauters EAK, Pikaar NA. Diagnosis of malabsorption. XIIIème Congrès International de Pédiatrie, Vienne, 1971, Section II, pp 13–23.
3. Anderson CM. The child with persistently abnormal stools: classification and general clinical and diagnostic approach. In: Anderson CM, Burke V, Gracey M, eds. Paediatric gastroenterology. London: Blackwell Scientific, 1987:329.
4. Gray GM. Carbohydrate digestion and absorption. Gastroenterology 1970; 58:96-107.
5. Stiefel DJ, Keller PJ. Preparation and some properties of human pancreatic amylase including a comparison with human parotid amylase. Biochim Biophys Acta 1973; 302:345-361.
6. Fogel MR, Gray GM. Starch hydrolysis in man: an intraluminal process not requiring membrane digestion. J Appl Physiol 1973; 35:263-267.
7. Semenza G. Anchoring and biosynthesis of stalked brush border membrane proteins: glycosidases and peptidases of enterocytes and renal tubuli. Ann Rev Cell Biol 1986; 2:255-313.
8. Stevens BR, Kaunitz JD, Wright EM. Intestinal transport of amino acids and sugars: advances using membrane vesicles. Ann Rev Physiol 1984; 46:417-433.
9. Gray GM, Santiago NA. Disaccharide absorption in normal and diseased human intestine. Gastroenterology 1966; 51:489-498.
10. De Vizia B, Ciccimarra F, De Cicco N, Auricchio S. Digestibility of starches in infants and children. J Pediatr 1975; 86:50-55.
11. Salyers AA, Leedle JAZ. Carbohydrate metabolism in the human colon. In: Hentges DJ, ed. Human intestinal microflora in health and disease. New York: Academic Press, 1983:129.
12. Launiala K. The mechanism of diarrhoea in congenital disaccharide malabsorption. Acta Paediatr Scand 1968; 57:425-432.
13. Rey J, Frézal J. Les anomalies des disaccharidases. Arch Fr Pédiatr 1967; 24:65-101.
14. Samloff IM. Pepsinogens I and II: purification from gastric mucosa and radioimmunoassay in serum. Gastroenterology 1982; 82:26-33.
15. Nixon SE, Mawer GE. The digestion and absorption of protein in man. The site of absorption. Br J Nutr 1970; 24:227-240.
16. Gray GM, Cooper HL. Protein digestion and absorption. Gastroenterology 1971; 61:535-544.
17. Matthews DM, Adibi SA. Peptide absorption. Gastroenterology 1976; 71:151-161.
18. Schmitz J, Triadou N. Digestion et absorption intestinales des peptides. Gastroenterol Clin Biol 1982; 6:651-661.
19. Ganapathy V, Leibach FH. Role of pH gradient and membrane potential in dipeptide transport in intestinal and renal brush-border membrane vesicles from the rabbit. J Biol Chem 1983; 258:14189-14192.
20. Tarlow MJ, Hadorn B, Arthurton MW, Lloyd JK. Intestinal enterokinase deficiency. a newly-recognized disorder of protein digestion. Arch Dis Child 1970; 45:651-655.
21. Frézal J, Rey J. Genetics of disorders of intestinal digestion and absorption. In: Harris H, Hirschorn K, eds. Advances in human genetics. Vol I. New York: Plenum Press, 1970: 275.
22. Desjeux JF, Rajantie J, Simell O, Dumontier AM, Perheentupa J. Lysine fluxes across the jejunal epithelium in lysinuric protein intolerance. J Clin Invest 1980; 65:1382-1387.
23. Carey MC, Small DM, Bliss CM. Lipid digestion and absorption. Annu Rev Physiol 1983; 45:651-677.
24. Moreau H, Laugier R, Gargouri Y, Ferrato F, Verger R. Human preduodenal lipase is entirely of gastric fundic origin. Gastroenterology 1988; 95:1221-1226.
25. Hamosh M. A review. Fat digestion in the newborn: role of lingual lipase and preduodenal digestion. Pediatr Res 1979; 13:615-622.
26. Desnuelle P. The lipase-colipase system. In: Rommel K, Goebell H, eds. Lipid absorption: biochemical and clinical aspects. Lancaster: MTP Press, 1976: 23.
27. Lombardo D, Guy O. Studies on the substrate specificity of a carboxyl ester hydrolase from human pancreatic juice. II. Action on cholesterol esters and lipid-soluble vitamin esters. Biochim Biophys Acta 1980; 611:147-155.
28. Hofmann AF. Functions of bile in the alimentary canal. In: Code CF, ed. Handbook of physiology. Section 6: Alimentary canal, Vol V. Washington, DC: American Physiological Society, 1968: 2507.

29. Bisgaier CL, Glickman RM. Intestinal synthesis, secretion and transport of lipoproteins. Annu Rev Physiol 1983; 45:625–636.
30. Rey J, Frézal J, Royer P, Lamy M. L'absence congénitale de lipase pancréatique. Arch Fr Pédiatr 1966; 23:5–14.
31. Gracey M. Intestinal absorption in the 'contaminated' small-bowel syndrome. Gut 1971; 12:403–410.
32. Cotton PB. Non-dietary lipid in the intestinal lumen. Gut 1972; 13:675–681.
33. Schmitz J. Protein-losing enteropathies. In: Milla PJ, Muller DPR, eds. Harries' paediatric gastroenterology. London: Churchill Livingstone, 1988: 260.
34. Hamilton JR, Lynch MJ, Reilly BJ. Active coeliac disease in childhood. Clinical and laboratory findings of forty-two cases. Q J Med 1969; 38:135–158.
35. Bresson JL, Prevot C, Rappaport R, Czernichow P, Schmitz J, Rey J. Activité somatomédine circulante et sécrétion d'hormone de croissance. Arch Fr Pédiatr 1979; 36(suppl):XIII–XVIII.
36. Hoffbrand AV. Folate absorption. J Clin Pathol 1971; 24 Suppl (R Coll Pathol) 5:66–76.
37. Thompson GR. Absorption of fat-soluble vitamins and sterols. J Clin Pathol 1971; 24 Suppl (R Coll Pathol) 5:85–89.
38. Kelts DG, Grand RJ, Shen G, Watkins JB, Werlin SL, Boehme C. Nutritional basis of growth failure in children and adolescents with Crohn's disease. Gastroenterology 1979; 76:720–727.
39. Powell-Tuck J, Garlick PJ, Lennard-Jones JE, Waterlow JC. Rates of whole body protein synthesis and breakdown increase with the severity of inflammatory bowel disease. Gut 1984; 25:460–464.
40. Jones EA, Smallwood RA, Craigie A, Rosenoer VM. The enterohepatic circulation of urea nitrogen. Clin Sci 1969; 37:825–836.
41. Kirschner BS, Sutton MM. Somatomedin-C levels in growth-impaired children and adolescents with chronic inflammatory bowel disease. Gastroenterology 1986; 91:830–836.
42. Holmberg C, Perheentupa J, Launiala K, Hallman N. Congenital chloride diarrhoea. Clinical analysis of 21 Finnish patients. Arch Dis Child 1977; 52:255–267.
43. Davidson M, Wasserman R. The irritable colon of childhood (chronic nonspecific diarrhea syndrome). J Pediatr 1966; 69:1027–1038.
44. Shmerling DH, Forrer JCW, Prader A. Fecal fat and nitrogen in healthy children and in children with malabsorption or maldigestion. Pediatrics 1970; 46:690–695.
45. Aggett PJ, Cavanagh NPC, Matthew DJ, Pincott JR, Sutcliffe J, Harries JT. Shwachman's syndrome. A review of 21 cases. Arch Dis Child 1980; 55:331–347.
46. Johanson A, Blizzard R. A syndrome of congenital aplasia of the alae nasi, deafness, hypothyroidism, dwarfism, absent permanent teeth, and malabsorption. J Pediatr 1971; 79:982–987.
47. Pearson HA, Lobel JS, Kocoshis SA, Naiman JL, Windmiller J, Lammi AT, Hoffman R, Marsh JC. A new syndrome of refractory sideroblastic anemia with vacuolization of marrow precursors and exocrine pancreatic dysfunction. J Pediatr 1979; 95:976–984.
48. Fivush B, Flick JA, Gahl WA. Pancreatic exocrine insufficiency in a patient with nephropathic cystinosis. J Pediatr 1988; 112:49–51.
49. Rey J, Frézal J, Royer P, Lamy M. L'absence congénitale de lipase pancréatique. Arch Fr Pédiatr 1966; 23:5–14.
50. Hildebrand H, Borgström B, Bekassy A, Erlanson-Albertsson C, Helin I. Isolated co-lipase deficiency in two brothers. Gut 1982; 23:243–246.
51. Vanderpas JB, Koopman BJ, Cadranel S, Vandenbergen C, Rickaert F, Quenon M, Wolthers BG, Brauherz G, Vertongen F, Tondeur M. Malabsorption of liposoluble vitamins in a child with bile acid deficiency. J Pediatr Gastroenterol Nutr 1987; 6:33–41.
52. Kobayashi A, Ohbe Y, Yonekubo A. Fat absorption in patients with surgically repaired biliary atresia. Helv Pediatr Acta 1983; 38:307–314.
53. Poley JR, Hofmann AF. Role of fat maldigestion in pathogenesis of steatorrhea in ileal resection. Fat digestion after two sequential test meals with and without cholestyramine. Gastroenterology 1976; 71:38–44.
54. Popovic OS, Kostic KM, Milovic VB, Milutinovic-Djuric S, Miletic VD, Sesic L, Djordjevic M, Bulajic M, Bojic P, Rubinic M, Borisavljevic N. Primary bile acid malabsorption. Histologic and immunologic study in three patients. Gastroenterology 1987; 92:1851–1858.
55. Weijers HA, Lindquist B, Anderson CM, Rey J, Shmerling KH, Visakorpi JK, Hadorn B, Gruttner R. European Society for Paediatric Gastroenterology. Round table discussion. Diagnostic criteria in coeliac disease. Acta Paediatr Scand 1970; 59:461–464.
56. Kuitunen P, Rapola J, Savilahti E, Visakorpi JK. Response of the jejunal mucosa to cow's milk in the malabsorption syndrome with cow's milk intolerance. A light- and electron-microscopic study. Acta Paediatr Scand 1973; 62:585–595.
57. Arnaud-Battandier F, Cerf-Bensussan N, Schmitz J, Griscelli C. Defective expression of HLA-DR antigens (DR-Ag): another cause of chronic diarrhea. Pediatr Res 1986; 20:694 (abstract).
58. Ament ME, Shimoda SS, Saunders DR, Rubin CE. Pathogenesis of steatorrhea in three cases of small intestinal stasis syndrome. Gastroenterology 1972; 63:728–747.
59. Davidson GP, Robb TA, Kirubakaran CP. Bacterial contamination of the small intestine as an important cause of chronic diarrhea and abdominal pain: diagnosis by breath hydrogen test. Pediatrics 1984; 74:229–235.
60. Lamy M, Frézal J, Polonovski J, Druez G, Rey J. Congenital absence of beta-lipoproteins. Pediatrics 1963; 31:277–289.
61. Bouma ME, Beucler I, Aggerbeck LP, Infante R, Schmitz J. Hypobetalipoproteinemia with accumulation of an apoprotein B-like protein in intestinal cells. Immunoenzymatic and biochemical characterization of seven cases of Anderson's disease. J Clin Invest 1986; 78:398–410.
62. Roy CC, Levy E, Green PHR, Sniderman A, Letarte J, Buts JP, Orquin J, Brochu P, Weber AM, Morin CL, Marcel Y, Deckelbaum RJ. Malabsorption, hypocholesterolemia, and fat-filled enterocytes with increased intestinal apoprotein B. Chylomicron retention disease. Gastroenterology 1987; 92:390–399.
63. Rambaud JC. Small intestinal lymphomas and alpha-chain disease. Clin Gastroenterol 1983; 12:743–766.
64. Naim HY, Roth J, Sterchi EE, Lentze M, Milla P, Schmitz J, Hauri HP. Sucrase-isomaltase deficiency in humans. Different mutations disrupt intracellular transport, processing, and function of an intestinal brush border enzyme. J Clin Invest 1988; 82:667–679.
65. Savilahti E, Launiala K, Kuitunen P. Congenital lactase deficiency. A clinical study on 16 patients. Arch Dis Child 1983; 58:246–252.
66. Simoons FJ. The geographic hypothesis and lactose malabsorption. A weighing of the evidence. Dig Dis 1978; 23:963–980.
67. Booth IW, Patel PB, Sule D, Brown GA, Buick R, Beyreiss K. Glucose-galactose malabsorption: demonstration of specific jejunal brush border membrane defect. Gut 1988; 29:1661–1665.
68. Berg NO, Dahlqvist A, Lindberg T, Norden A. Correlation between morphological alterations and enzyme activities in the mucosa of the small intestine. Scand J Gastroenterol 1973; 8:703–712.
69. Fraisse F, Schmitz J, Rey J. Valeurs normales des principaux constituants des selles de un an à la puberté. Arch Fr Pédiatr 1981; 38:667–670.
70. Bergoz R, Vallotton MC, Loizeau E. Trehalase deficiency. Prevalence and relation to single-cell protein food. Ann Nutr Metab 1982; 26:291–295.
71. Cutz E, Rhoads JM, Drumm B, Sherman PM, Durie PR, Forstner GG. Microvillus inclusion disease: an inherited defect of brush-border assembly and differentiation. N Engl J Med 1989; 320:646–651.
72. Booth IW, Murer H, Stange G, Fenton TR, Milla PJ. Defective jejunal brush-border Na^+/H^+ exchange: a cause of congenital secretory diarrhoea. Lancet 1985; i:1066–1069.

CHAPTER 9

Constipation

M. Stephen Murphy, B.Sc., M.B., B.Ch., M.R.C.P.

The patterns of motility that exist in the colon and anorectum are, in part, adapted to permit control of fecal elimination. It has been suggested that this adaptation of the distal gastrointestinal (GI) tract provides important biologic advantages to animals in the avoidance of predators that track by scent.[1] In human beings the enormous social and biologic importance of fecal continence is obvious—uncontrolled passage of feces is associated not only with grave social repercussions but also with an increased risk for the transmission of infectious pathogens. This capacity for control is not obtained, however, without cost; constipation is one of the most common ailments occurring in man, and the consequences of impaired fecal elimination may sometimes prove serious.

Concern about the child who appears to have a disorder of defecation is commonplace, as is obvious from the frequency with which professional advice is sought.[2] By far the most common parental anxieties concerning the child's "bowel habit" relate to a group of symptoms often considered to be synonymous with the term "constipation."

DEFINITION

A clear definition of constipation is not available. It is often stated that, like "cough," constipation should be considered a symptom and not a diagnosis; that is, constipation may be a manifestation of a wide variety of disorders. In practice the term commonly includes a number of symptoms and signs that suggest either undue difficulty with defecation or abnormal fecal retention. Some children may pass small, excessively firm stools at infrequent intervals and with difficulty. They may, in addition, suffer from intermittent abdominal pain, and on occasion defecation may be associated with anal discomfort and bleeding. In such cases the diagnosis may seem clear, although confusion frequently arises from failure to appreciate the wide variation in bowel habit in normal subjects. The diagnosis is further complicated by the subjective nature of the assessment. Sometimes, despite an apparently normal bowel habit, chronic fecal retention is present.[2,3] Unsuspected severe fecal impaction may first present with severe abdominal pain and vomiting, and such children may undergo unnecessary surgery for suspected small bowel obstruction.[4] Children with chronic fecal retention may, at intervals, pass stools of very large caliber.[2] A frequent and serious consequence of chronic fecal retention in childhood is its association with fecal soiling, or encopresis, which is often the presenting symptom.[2] Examination of the abdomen may, in some children, reveal the presence of severe colonic or rectal fecal loading. On rectal examination large quantities of feces may be found in a voluminous rectal ampulla.

In many studies of patients with constipation, the criteria employed for inclusion have been imprecise; they have included, in varying combinations, subjective reports of stool infrequency, abnormal stool consistency and size, and a sense of incomplete evacuation following defecation. Although encopresis is frequently associated with chronic constipation, a history of soiling cannot invariably be assumed to indicate the presence of fecal retention.[5] Parental impressions of excessive straining at stool may be misleading,[5] but such reports have often been considered diagnostically significant.[6] The presence of feces in the rectum is sometimes considered abnormal, but unless the quantity is large or the stool is unduly hard, this is not a reliable indicator of dysfunction. A plain radiograph of the abdomen may show evidence of excessive fecal retention, but interpretation of films is subjective. Measurement of intestinal transit time has been employed in an effort to provide an objective approach to the study of fecal elimination[7]; although the total gut transit time is significantly longer in chronically constipated children, it is not always abnormal.[8]

"Normal" Bowel Habit

As with constipation, efforts to provide a simple definition of normal bowel habit have been problematic. Weaver[9] has pointed out the surprising scarcity of systematically performed studies in this important area. Bowel habit may be described in terms of stool frequency, consistency, and size. In order to identify patients with constipation in terms of these criteria, it is essential to consider the information available from studies of normal populations. Unfortunately, even a thorough description of the bowel habits of a healthy population may not provide ideal data, as they are affected by various environmental influences. A wide variation in bowel habits exists within healthy adult populations,[10] and further diversity is found in different population groups[11,12] and as a consequence of dietary variation.[13,14]

Stool Frequency

Stool frequency is the most easily quantified aspect of bowel habit and so has been the best studied (Fig. 1).[9] Studies from western societies have indicated that 94 to 99 percent of adults have a bowel action between three times daily and three times weekly.[15,16] A similar frequency has been report-

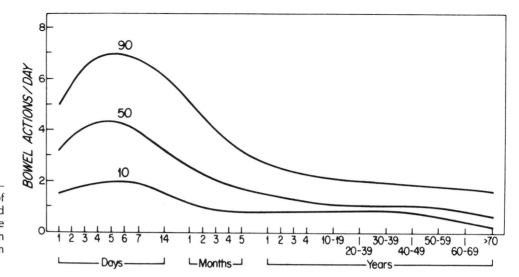

FIGURE 1 Daily frequency of defecation from birth to old age. The curves represent the range; the 10th, 50th, and 90th percentiles are shown. (From Weaver.[9])

ed in preschool children.[17] In infancy, however, the frequency is higher. Ninety-seven percent of a group of 800 infants were reported to have between one and nine bowel actions daily during the first week of life.[18] Another study reported that among 240 infants between the ages of 2 and 20 weeks, half of whom were fed breast milk and half cow's milk formula, 93 percent had between one and seven bowel actions each day (Fig. 2).[19] These results were based on prospective records kept by the infants' mothers over a 7-day period. Among breast-fed infants after the first week of life, during which there was a relatively smaller number of bowel movements, the stool frequency was significantly higher than in formula-fed infants. This difference persisted until at least 8 weeks of age. By 16 weeks, when most of the infants from both groups had been introduced to solid foods, no difference in stool frequency could be identified. Not all of the breast-fed infants followed this pattern, however; one apparently healthy infant, for example, had only 14 bowel actions in the first 16 weeks of life.

Significant variation in stool frequency exists between population groups studied. Subjects on high-fiber diets[13] and those on vegetarian diets[14] have been shown to have a larger number of bowel movements. Data obtained from subjects in western countries are also different from data from developing countries, a lower stool frequency being found.[11,12]

Stool Consistency and Size

Much less information is available on children in relation to the other important facets of normal bowel habit—stool size and consistency—owing to the difficulties entailed in obtaining precise information on these characteristics from large numbers of patients.[9] Normal values for the weight of stool output vary widely as a consequence of dietary variations, but variation occurs even within individual subjects on a fixed caloric and fiber intake.[4] This may be due to changes in colonic bacterial flora, as bacterial content accounts for almost 50 percent of stool bulk.[4] Little information is available on the weight of daily stool output during childhood, especially in those from western countries (Table 1).[11] In infants the mean daily stool volume has been reported to remain constant (approximately 5 ml per day) from the second to the twentieth weeks of life, but prior to weaning breast-fed infants produced significantly larger stools than did cow's milk formula-fed infants (Fig. 3).[19]

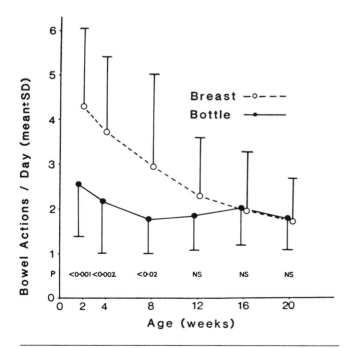

FIGURE 2 Daily frequency of bowel actions in breast-fed and cow's milk formula–fed infants from 2 to 20 weeks. (From Weaver et al.[19])

TABLE 1
Transit Time and Weight of Stools Passed by Children from Different Geographic Areas

Origin	Age (yr)	Mean (range) Time of Marker Appearance (hr)	Mean (range) Transit Time (hr)	Mean (range) Stool Weight/Day (g)
African (n = 500) traditional diet*	13–18	13 (5–28)	34 (20–48)	275 (150–350)
African (n = 500) part western diet*	13–18	29 (9–40)	45 (24–59)	165 (120–260)
African (n = 30) part western diet*	10–12	10 (8–15)§		75 (55–90)
Canadian (n = 46)†	3–13	33 (14–96)	49 (20–101)	78 (30–205)
English (n = 65) (normal)‡	3–12	26 (24–96)§		
English (n = 65) (constipated)‡	3–12	80 (48–168)§		

*Walker ARP. Unpublished data. †Habbick BF, et al. Unpublished data. ‡Dimson SB.[42]
§Carmine red marker; radiopaque markers were used for the other studies.
From Burkitt et al.[11]

ANATOMIC, PHYSIOLOGIC, AND DEVELOPMENTAL CONSIDERATIONS

Anatomy and Embryology of the Colon and Anorectum

The anatomy, embryology, and development of the GI tract, including colon and anorectum, are described in Chapter 13. Certain anatomic features are particularly germane to the bowel's capacity for controlled fecal elimination.

Although it is increasingly recognized that the colon is an organ with a variety of important functions,[20] its capacious appearance emphasizes its most obvious role as an organ for the containment of food residue prior to evacuation. In this capacity it does not merely serve as an inert container but is subject to complex intrinsic and extrinsic controls that regulate the delivery of its contents to the anorectum.

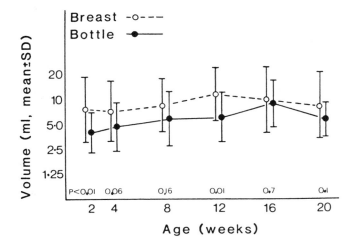

FIGURE 3 The daily stool volume passed (logarithmic scale) by breast-fed and cow's milk formula–fed infants from 2 to 20 weeks. (From Weaver et al.[19])

The extrinsic innervation of the distal gut and its sphincters has been discussed in detail by Gonella et al.[21] The extrinsic nerve supply consists of efferent sympathetic and parasympathetic nerves, together with afferent nerves. These provide connections between two centers of neural control—the central and the enteric nervous systems. The enteric nervous system receives and processes input from both extrinsic and intrinsic sources. The myenteric plexus lies between the circular and longitudinal smooth muscle layers of the intestinal wall and appears to be the component of the enteric nervous system most closely involved in the control of motility. In the colon the ganglion cells of the myenteric plexus are largely concentrated beneath the longitudinal fibers of the taenia coli.[22] The density of ganglion cells decreases distally, so that in the rectum it is only 5 percent of that in the proximal colon, and in the lower part of the anal canal ganglia are almost absent.[1]

The myenteric plexus of the distal colon contains neural fascicles, or ascending nerves, running longitudinally in the plane of the plexus, which may play a part in colocolonic or colorectal reflex pathways.[1] Okamoto and Ueda[23] first studied the embryogenesis of human intramural ganglia and demonstrated the progressive appearance of neuroblasts in an apparently craniocaudal direction between 5 and 12 weeks' gestation. Smith[24] studied their development throughout pregnancy and into the first years of life. Neuroblasts first appear in the myenteric plexus of the 12-mm embryo and become progressively more numerous up to the end of the second trimester. Their appearance then becomes more differentiated, and cells with an axon emerging from one pole can be identified. By the beginning of the third trimester, cells of the rectal myenteric plexus still appear as sheets of undifferentiated cells, and ganglia can be identified more proximally. By this time unipolar and bipolar cells are numerous, and multipolar cells are beginning to appear. In the first month of postnatal life, multipolar cells predominate and nerve fibers are identifiable. Throughout the first 2 years of life histologic evidence of incomplete neural maturation persists, ganglia in different stages of development being present; neurons with profuse dendritic processes are now numerous, however, and the appearance of the plexuses in the rectum is very similar to those in the upper intestine. Between the ages of 2 and 5 years, the appearances are almost fully mature, although occasional neurons with an immature appearance can be seen. In a recent study, the concept of a craniocaudal wave of neuronal migration from the neural crest to the gut and of progressive craniocaudal maturation of the cells of the intrinsic nervous system has been questioned.[25] Ganglion development and the appearance of neural interconnections were studied using neuron-specific enolase staining between 9 and 21 weeks of gestation; maturation was most advanced in the pylorus, less so in the colon, and least so in the ileum, evidence that the neuronal population may follow a dual gradient of maturation.

The structures of the anorectum are highly adapted to achieving continence and incorporate a variety of mechanisms that are subject to both reflex and conscious controls.[26] At the level of the third sacral vertebra the sigmoid colon becomes the rectum, and this lies in contact with the posterior pelvic wall in the concavity of the sacrum and coccyx. Toward its distal end the rectum widens to form the rectal ampulla. Just beyond the coccyx the rectum narrows and turns posteroinferiorly to form the anal canal, which passes through the pelvic diaphragm. The angle formed between the axes of the rectum and anus is considered an important factor in the maintenance of continence. The pelvic diaphragm forms the floor of the pelvis and supports the pelvic viscera. It is composed of the levator ani and coccygeal muscles and their fasciae. This diaphragm stretches like a hammock from the pubis anteriorly to the coccyx posteriorly and is attached laterally to a band of fascia along the side walls of the pelvis known as the tendinous arch. The muscles of the pelvic floor are supplied by somatic nerves from the third, fourth, and fifth sacral roots via branches of the pudendal nerves. The levator ani and coccygeal muscles support the pelvic floor during forced expiration. The puborectal muscle, which is a part of the levator ani muscle, arises from the dorsal surface of the pubis and passes posteriorly to form a sling around the rectum; contraction of this sling draws the lower rectum anteriorly, occluding its lumen.

The internal and external anal sphincter muscles lie in the posterior half of the perineum, which is a diamond-shaped space lying immediately beneath the outlet of the pelvis. The internal sphincter, which is formed from the circular fibers of the intestine, surrounds the proximal portion of the anal canal. It is supplied by fibers of the autonomic nervous system and is therefore an involuntary muscle. The external sphincter, which is composed of striated muscle, surrounds the more distal anal canal and is in contact with the lower border of the internal sphincter. It is an elliptical flat muscle composed of subcutaneous, superficial, and deep parts. The subcutaneous part surrounds the anal orifice, arising anteriorly from the perineal body, a fibromuscular structure in the midline of the perineum, and passing posteriorly to the anococcygeal ligament. The superficial part, which lies deep to the subcutaneous, surrounds the anal canal and also passes from the perineal body to the anococcygeal ligament. The deep part of the external sphincter lies adjacent to the internal sphincter, its fibers interlacing with those of the puborectal muscles. It too arises from the perineal body and forms a complete sphincter, its fibers frequently decussating in front

of and behind the anal canal and blending with the levator superiorly. The external sphincter and the puborectal muscles are supplied by somatic innervation from the fourth sacral roots via the pudendal nerves. It is a voluntary muscle that is in a state of tonic contraction, but it contracts more strongly when necessary to maintain closure of the anal canal.

Physiology of Colonic and Anorectal Motility

Colonic Motility

The motility patterns of the colon differ in character in its proximal, middle, and distal parts. Animal experiments employing direct observation of the colon and radiologic studies demonstrated more than 80 years ago that the contents of the proximal colon do not simply move progressively to the rectum, but rather are repeatedly driven back toward the cecum by waves of "antiperistalsis" originating in the transverse or ascending colon.[27,28] There is now much evidence that a similar pattern of motility occurs in human subjects, thus permitting thorough and prolonged mixing of intestinal contents in the proximal colon.[1] In studies of whole-gut transit time, it appears that the longest delay in the passage of markers occurs in the cecum and the sigmoid colon.[29] In the transverse and descending colon the most usual form of motility which has been observed is apparently random segmental contractions, leading to the formation of colonic haustrations. These contractions are not associated with any consistent direction of flow of colonic contents, but rather they displace the contents in either direction in a process known as "haustral shuttling" (Fig. 4).[30] Finally, infrequent waves of peristalsis are intermittently observed in the colon and tend to travel farther than those observed in the small intestine. These may commence in the transverse colon and travel rapidly as far as the rectum, causing rapid transfer of luminal contents; such patterns of contraction are referred to as "mass peristalsis."

It is widely known that a defecation urge frequently occurs after the ingestion of a meal, reflecting an increase in colonic contractions and the occurrence of mass peristalsis. Manometric studies have shown that motility in the postprandial period is increased throughout the colon, but the maximal augmentation is in the distal colon.[31] The evidence suggests that receptors in the duodenum are important in this response to eating, although the entry of chyme from the distal small intestine into the colon may also play a part.[1] The factors responsible for the postprandial response are unclear, but both neural pathways and humoral agents such as gastrin and cholecystokinin may be involved.

The regulation of colonic contraction and flow is complex, being potentially influenced by the intrinsic myogenic properties of the colon, the enteric nervous system, extrinsic nerve pathways that may carry neural signals to and from the central nervous system at any level, and humoral influences. Myogenic factors are important in both the initiation and the control of colonic motility.[20] The muscle of the large bowel of human subjects exhibits "slow wave" activity or an electrical oscillation similar to that which occurs in the small bowel, although in the colon it is lower in amplitude and more variable in frequency. This governs the occurrence of smooth

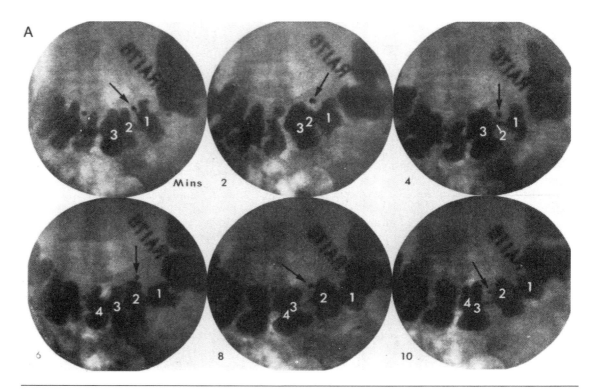

FIGURE 4 Cinefluorography frames (2-min intervals) showing movement of segmental constrictions in the human colon. The studies demonstrate changes in the position of the constrictions in relation to a diverticulum (*arrow*). *A*, Aboral movement of segmental constrictions. In the first frame the diverticulum is in continuity with colonic segment 1. At 2 minutes segment 1 has contracted, closing off the neck of the diverticulum, and the annular constriction separating segments 2 and 3 has disappeared. At 6 minutes the constriction has reformed and has moved distally, because segment 2 is now opposite the diverticulum. By 10 minutes segment 2 has reached the section of bowel just distal to the diverticulum which was originally occupied by 1.

muscle action potentials and hence of contractile activity, although the precise interactions in colonic smooth muscle are poorly understood. Neurocrine, paracrine, and endocrine influences may all interact in the control of myogenic activity and hence in the regulation of colonic motility.[20] The result is that luminal flow proceeds at a rate that permits the rescue of excess water, electrolytes, and some nutrients from the colonic contents, the preservation of the colonic bacterial flora, and the delivery of feces to the anorectum intermittently and with a consistency that aids in the control of elimination.

The Anal Sphincter Mechanism

The internal sphincter is in a state of tonic contraction, an important factor in maintaining continence. Rectal distention is associated with reflex relaxation of the internal sphincter. The location of the mechanoreceptors and the pathway of the neural connections involved in this reflex are uncertain. The intrinsic innervation of the anorectum is likely involved, since relaxation cannot usually be elicited in Hirschsprung's disease, in which the intramural plexus of the rectum is absent (Fig. 5),[32,33] and since the reflex is abolished by transection and reanastomosis of the distal rectum.[34] There is evidence, however, that extrinsic nervous pathways are also involved because the reflex may be impaired in patients with myelo-meningocele.[21] The rectoanal inhibitory reflex may be absent in premature infants, but it can usually be elicited at a postconceptual age of 39 weeks irrespective of the gestational age at birth.[35]

The external sphincter, similarly, has a degree of tonic contraction, but this is not of prime importance in maintaining closure of the anal canal. Electrophysiologic studies have shown that the external anal sphincter contracts in response to rapid rectal distention; this reflex response can first be elicited at about the age at which voluntary control of defecation is achieved.[36] Manometric studies have shown that external sphincter tone increases during rises in intra-abdominal pressure, except during defecation, when it decreases (Figs. 5 and 6).[33,37] It is thought that at rest the internal sphincter contributes most to anal sphincteric tone but that during episodes of sudden rectal distention when the internal sphincter relaxes the external sphincter becomes important in maintaining continence, thus allowing the rectum time to adapt to its contents.[38] Although moderate distention causes reflex contraction, more marked distention results in reflex sphincteric relaxation. The reflex responses of the external sphincter involve extrinsic nerve pathways, which appear to be multiple. This, together with the existence of cross-innervation to each side of the sphincter, may explain the frequent preservation of function in various neurologic disease states.[1]

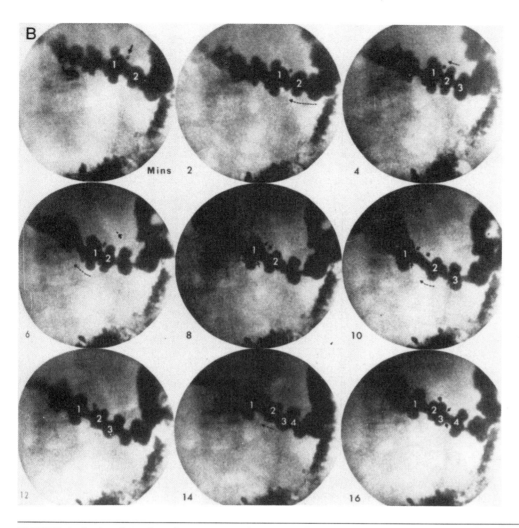

FIGURE 4 *Continued B*, Aboral movement of segmental constrictions. From 6 minutes the constriction between 1 and 2 begins to extend proximally, displacing segment 1 toward the hepatic flexure. At this time the neck of the diverticulum becomes occluded and remains so until 12 minutes. At 12 minutes the distal end of the annular constriction begins to relax, and this section of bowel is distended by segment 2. At this time, the neck of the diverticulum is again patent and is in continuity with segment 2. Segment 2 is seen advancing past the diverticulum ahead of another retropulsive wave at 16 minutes. (From Ritchie.[30])

The Integrated Processes of Defecation

At intervals, often during the postprandial period, the colon delivers stool to the rectal ampulla. The resulting distention may lead to reflex relaxation of the internal anal sphincter, and small quantities of the rectal contents then enter the anal canal. Mucosal receptors, which are probably located in and just above the anal canal,[1,38,39] detect the presence of these contents and can distinguish between solid and fluid matter; the individual is thus made aware of the "call to stool." Stimulation of these receptors may also result in reflex colonic and rectal contraction.[1] If the circumstances are inappropriate defecation is delayed, assisted by voluntary contraction of the puborectalis and external anal sphincter muscles. The rectum then undergoes a process of adaptation to accommodate its contents, and stimulation of anal canal receptors diminishes. During defecation the individual adopts a sitting or squatting position and performs a Valsalva maneuver, thus increasing intra-abdominal pressure. These voluntary acts are accompanied by contraction of the levator ani and coccygeal muscles, which oppose downward descent of the pelvic floor. Simultaneously the external sphincter relaxes, permitting the passage of feces through the anal canal. Increased intra-abdominal pressure and hip flexion both tend to straighten the anorectal angle, which may also aid the passage of feces. In the flexed position the angle formed by the puborectalis is such that its contraction cannot occlude the lumen of the distal rectum. Increased intra-abdominal pressure promotes the forward movement of feces from both the distal colon and the rectum, and defecation occurs.

Achievement of Voluntary Control

Stool frequency is maximal at about 1 week of age and gradually decreases during the first 12 months of life, so that

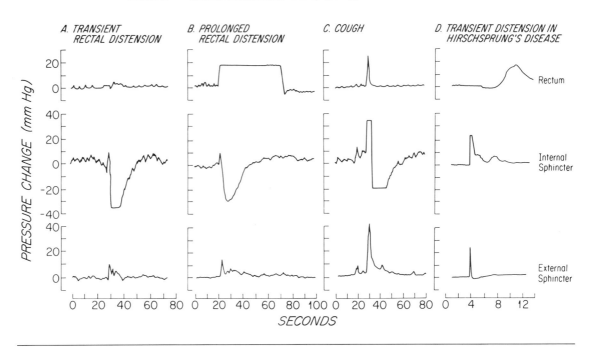

FIGURE 5 Manometric tracings showing the rectal and the internal and external anal sphincter responses. *A,* With transient rectal distention. *B,* With prolonged rectal distention. *C,* During a cough. *D,* In a subject with Hirschsprung's disease during transient distention. (Adapted from Tobin et al[33] and Schuster et al.[48])

by 1 year most infants have fewer than three stools daily (see Fig. 1).[9] During infancy and early childhood there is also a gradual tendency toward the production of stools of increased consistency.[19] These changes in bowel habit assist in the achievement of controlled defecation. In the newborn infant fecal evacuation occurs as a reflex process. Mothers recognize that defecation frequently occurs in the immediate postprandial period and so changing the diaper is usually postponed until after feeding. Subsequently, with progressive cortical maturation and its increasing participation in motor control, voluntary effort becomes increasingly important in defecation, and the possibility of voluntary control gradually emerges. Some infants may be trained very early to defecate when placed on the pot, but initially this represents a process of reflex conditioning. Understanding also develops progressively throughout infancy, and later, and in the second year of life, demands begin to be made on the child to conform socially. By 15 months of age the child may begin to indicate when he has wet or soiled his pants. Many children achieve voluntary bowel control around 18 months, but the age at which complete control is attained is very variable. Different cultures appear to accept different norms.[40] In western societies the limit has often been considered to be 2 to 3 years of age, whereas in some other cultures a much more gradual and stepwise program of training is traditional, with the child gradually being taken farther and farther from the dwelling place to attend to his bowel functions.[40]

Motility Study Techniques

A variety of new techniques and modifications of older methods have been introduced in recent years for the study of intestinal motility, and these are discussed in detail elsewhere. Some of these have been employed for the investigation of colonic and anorectal motility in human subjects. It has been stated that the ideal method for the study of intestinal motility would simultaneously provide detailed information about muscle activity and changes in intraluminal pressure and about the movement of luminal contents.[41] It would also be safe, noninvasive, and applicable to subjects as they go about their normal daily activities. The absence of such an ideal technique, together with the difficulties of selecting homogeneous patient groups for investigation, have impaired the design of satisfactory study protocols and have caused difficulty with comparison of the results of the many investigations that have been reported.

Intestinal transit of luminal contents may be examined by studying the rate at which orally administered markers pass through the GI tract; this approach provides indirect information about intestinal motility. The whole-gut transit time may be simply measured by timing the passage of solid or liquid materials; as mouth-to-cecum transit time is normally relatively brief, whole-gut transit time largely reflects the rate of passage from cecum to anus (Table 1).[8,11,42] The movement of colonic contents can be studied in more detail by using serial radiography to follow the transit of radiopaque particles, such as fragments of nasogastric tubing, as they pass along the large bowel.[8,43]

Relatively few electrophysiologic studies of the human colon have been performed. Attempts have been made to record the colonic electromyogram using mucosal electrodes; alternately, the electrical activity of the external anal sphincter has been recorded by inserting fine electrodes into the external anal sphincter[37,44] or by applying cutaneous electrodes at the anal margin.[36,45-47]

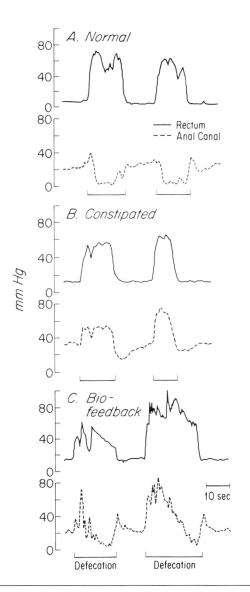

FIGURE 6 Manometric tracings from the rectum and anal canal during attempted defecation. *A*, Normal defecation. During straining the pressure rises within the rectum while it decreases in the anal canal as the sphincters relax. *B*, Paradoxical anal closure during defecation in a constipated child. The anal canal contracts, creating a pressure which may exceed that in the rectum. *C*, Pressure recording during biofeedback therapy. At the beginning of defecation the anal canal contracts, but afterwards it relaxes. This is an intermediate pattern between normal anal relaxation and paradoxical closure. (From Keren et al[55]; © by American College of Gastroenterology.)

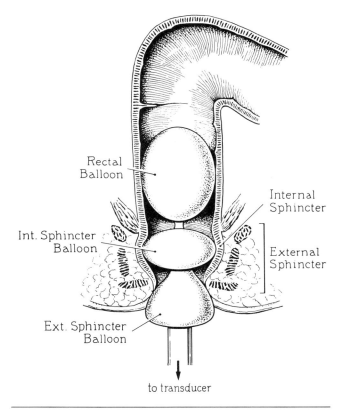

FIGURE 7 Balloon manometric assembly employed to simultaneously measure intraluminal pressure changes in the rectum and changes in internal and external anal sphincter tone. (Redrawn after Schuster et al.[48])

The technique most frequently used for the study of colonic and anorectal motility in children has been the recording of intraluminal pressure changes. This provides an indirect measure of intestinal muscular activity, so the interpretation of results may be complex. Pressure recordings have been obtained using either air-filled[32,36,45,48,49] or water-filled balloons[35,37,50,51] connected via tubing to an external sensor (Fig. 7). More recently studies have commonly employed systems in which an open-ended tube is perfused with water and pressure is transmitted by the column of liquid. Multilumen tubes with openings located at regular intervals are frequently used, thus permitting simultaneous pressure recording at various fixed levels in the digestive tract.[52–55] An alternative technique has been the use of intraluminal probes that use strain gauge pressure transducers (Fig. 8).[43,45,46,56–59] Finally, pressure-sensitive radiotelemetry capsules have occasionally been employed.[44] Manometric techniques have made it possible to study rectal intraluminal pressure and the activity of the internal and external anal sphincters simultaneously (see Figs. 5 and 7).[48,49]

Dynamic studies of anorectal motility have been performed by visualizing the rectum radiologically during the expulsion of a semisolid radiopaque contrast medium.[44] The dynamics of defecation have also been examined by studying the ability of subjects to expel balloons or other forms of simulated stool from the rectum.[47,60]

Because of the special difficulties associated with the investigation of motility in the human colon, particularly in children, studies have been largely restricted to the sigmoid colon and anorectum.

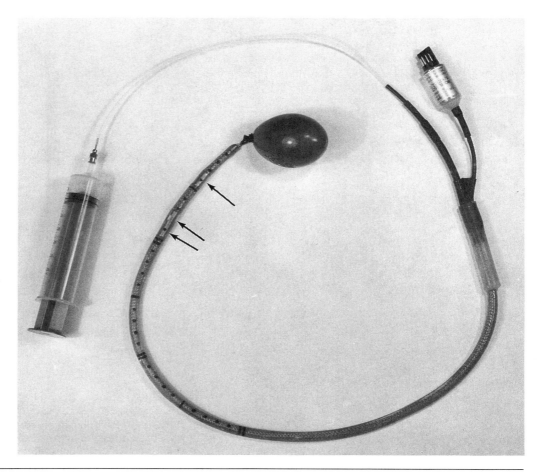

FIGURE 8 Manometric assembly with strain gauges (*arrows*) orientated at 120-degree angles around the circumference of the probe to permit measurement of pressure changes in rectum and anal canal. The rectum is distended by inflating the terminal balloon.

IDIOPATHIC CONSTIPATION

"Clinical Syndromes"

In the majority of patients with chronic constipation, no underlying cause can be clearly identified. It is possible, however, to describe a variety of "constipation syndromes," the clinical patterns of which are characteristically seen at different stages in life.

Constipation in Infancy and Childhood

Constipation is usually said to be relatively uncommon in the first months of life.[5,61] However, this view may relate to the lack of precise measures of normality, and the emergence of overt symptoms and signs at a later time may in fact follow a period of subtle dysfunction present from early infancy.

In later infancy and in the toddler period, symptoms of constipation become much more common. At this stage the frequency of defecation normally decreases. Most children experience transient periods of constipation. Occasionally a more persistent decrease in the frequency or effectiveness of defecation occurs, resulting in progressive fecal retention. In these children the rectum may eventually become voluminous and distended with large quantities of feces. In some, fecal soiling continues after the age at which continence is normally expected, and the child is found to have previously unsuspected fecal impaction and "megarectum," the rectum being dilated down to the anal canal. Less commonly, true tubular dilatation of the colon—idiopathic megacolon—is present.[62] The child usually denies awareness of the urge to defecate and often appears to be unaware of the passage of stool.[2,40] Intermittently a stool of unusually large caliber and volume may be passed with voluntary effort.[2] Soiling has been reported in 1.5 percent of 7-year-old children.[40] Although it occurs three to six times more commonly in boys,[2,40] the sex distribution for chronic constipation unassociated with soiling may be more nearly equal.[3]

Constipation in Adolescence, Adulthood, and Old Age

Although the natural history of severe chronic constipation in childhood is not well studied, it is clear that encopresis, at least, tends to resolve in or before adolescence.

Many adults with chronic or recurrent constipation suffer from "irritable bowel syndrome."[63] This disorder is characterized by the presence of abnormal bowel motility associated with the clinical features of abdominal pain and abnormal bowel habit, in the absence of detectable organic pathology. In its most common form constipation is the major complaint, although in some cases constipation alternates with diarrhea. Other features include intermittent abdominal distention, relief of abdominal pain following defecation, and a sense of incomplete evacuation. The stools are usually hard and either narrow in caliber or scybalous. Less commonly, irritable bowel syndrome is characterized by painless diarrhea. Patients with irritable bowel syndrome usually present to a physician between the ages of 20 and 50, but in many cases symptoms begin in adolescence or even in childhood.[64,65]

Irritable bowel syndrome is one of the most commonly encountered GI disorders in adult patients and consequently was first described as a disorder of adult life. It has been suggested that the common functional disorders of nonspecific diarrhea as seen in the preschool child,[66] and recurrent abdominal pain usually seen in the school-age child,[67] may be considered early forms of irritable bowel syndrome.[68] The precise relationship between these varied disorders is unclear, however, and it is noteworthy that the female predominance that is found in irritable bowel syndrome in adults is not a feature of the functional gut disorders of childhood.

Mild constipation is a common complaint in adult life, but occasionally severe chronic constipation occurs. This differs clinically from irritable bowel syndrome in that fecal retention is severe, bowel movements occur at infrequent intervals, and diarrhea is absent. The psychological overtones that are a feature of irritable bowel syndrome are typically absent, patients often presenting with symptoms they have endured for many years.[4] This condition is resistant to treatment with dietary fiber, and abdominal pain is not a prominent feature. In this type of constipation the rectum and colon are not grossly distended. The onset is often between the ages of 10 and 20 years,[69,70] and, in contrast to idiopathic constipation of childhood, there is a striking female predominance.[4]

Although idiopathic megacolon is much more common in childhood, a proportion of adults with severe chronic constipation are also found to have a grossly dilated colon. The relationship between idiopathic megacolon in childhood and that in adult life is unclear. It has been reported, however, that in young adults so affected there is often a history of fecal impaction and encopresis in childhood, and the sex distribution is equal.[71,72]

Finally, constipation in the elderly is usually associated with a marked degree of rectal fecal impaction.[73] This may be due to various factors including immobility, weakness, and psychiatric disorder. Elderly patients with impaction frequently leak feculent material.

Theories of Origin: Predisposing and Precipitating Factors

Initiating Factors—The "Vicious Circle" Concept

Traditionally it has been said that chronic constipation in childhood may initiated by environmental influences.[5] Suggested precipitating factors have included transient illness, inappropriately early or overzealous attempts at toilet training, and difficulties of access to toilet facilities.[5,74,75] Such potential precipitants may lead to increased difficulty with defecation or deliberate withholding behavior. Retained stool becomes progressively more difficult to evacuate as a result of prolonged absorption of its water content, leading to a vicious circle in which the rectum is increasingly distended by abnormally firm fecal contents.[76] If the passage of hard stools then results in injury to the sensitive anal canal, with fissure formation, anticipation of discomfort or pain may further inhibit voluntary efforts at defecation.[76] Finally, chronic rectal distention may lead to loss of rectal sensitivity and hence of the normal defecation urge.[2,3,52,62,77] Although it is likely that this hypothesis incorporates a number of important components in the pathophysiology of constipation in childhood, it remains unproven and is unsatisfactory from several points of view.

Genetic Factors

There is some evidence that children with chronic constipation may have an inherited predisposition to this disorder. One study has reported that concordance for constipation was fourfold higher in monozygotic than in dizygotic twins.[78] Most children are likely to have encountered some of the proposed precipitating factors at some time in early life, yet the majority do not develop a persistent problem with fecal retention. Although the onset of constipation is commonly reported to occur after the age of 1 year,[5] in some studies a history of constipation from the early months of life has been recorded, suggesting that voluntary repression of defecation is not a primary precipitant.[43]

Psychosocial Factors

In the past there has been a strong tendency to attribute chronic fecal retention in childhood, particularly when accompanied by encopresis, to an underlying psychological disorder.[40] Indeed, chronic constipation without an apparent organic cause is sometimes referred to as "psychogenic constipation."[75] It is noteworthy that the incidences of both constipation and encopresis do increase markedly at a time when the processes of development are allowing the toddler to gain control over defecation. The second year of life is a period of intense attachment between parent and child, and it is also a period during which the quality of their relationship undergoes great change. The child becomes aware that he can exert his own authority and can oppose his parents. The parent in turn is beginning to provide guidelines for acceptable social behavior. A key element in the parent-child interaction at this time relates to the process of toilet training, and this may assume a symbolic significance to both parent and child. To the parent, successful toilet training is a milestone in the process of normal social development. For the child, cooperation with the training process may be a rewarding experience, or the process may become a focus of the child's determination to exert his own will. Many authors have suggested that improper handling of toilet training may therefore predispose to constipation.[76,79–81]

Various studies have suggested that personality and emotional factors may play a role in the etiology of constipation. There is some evidence that subjects with positive, outgoing personality traits may have relatively higher weights of stool output, and it has been suggested therefore that personality factors may predispose individuals to dysfunction.[82] Studies of the personalities of children with chronic constipation and encopresis have varied in their findings. Bellman[40] found that children with encopresis were described as anxious, lacking in self-assurance, and less able to cope with demands than were controls. They were said to frequently exhibit excessive or poor control of aggressive reactions, to be immature in their behavior, and to have difficulties relating to their peers. Other studies have reported difficulties such as poor self-esteem, social withdrawal, and affective disorders.[83,84] Children with hyperactivity and attention deficits have been said to be over-represented among those with bowel dysfunction, and these may be especially resistant to treatment.[5] Although severe constipation may be found more frequently in association with mental retardation, the I.Q.'s of children with chronic constipation and encopresis are similar to those of normal controls.[40] It has been suggested that stressful events may provoke bowel dysfunction in some children,[5] but convincing evidence for this has not been forthcoming.[2]

Encopresis is sometimes classified as primary or secondary, depending on whether the child has always soiled or the disorder has appeared following successful toilet training. Both primary and secondary encopresis may be associated with chronic constipation and megacolon.[2] When the characteristics of children with primary and secondary encopresis have been compared, the secondary form has been reported in 60 percent; this is in marked contrast to enuresis, which is usually primary.[2] No significant differences in personality traits or behavioral characteristics have been identified between those with primary and secondary encopresis.[2,40]

There is evidence that many of the behavioral abnormalities that have been described in association with encopresis may be secondary to the disorder rather than its cause; a strong tendency toward resolution has been demonstrated when encopresis is successfully treated.[83]

Evidence of psychological dysfunction has also been reported in association with irritable bowel syndrome, although it is possible that this also arises as a consequence of illness rather than predisposing to it.[40] By comparison with irritable bowel syndrome, such characteristics are not frequently associated with chronic severe constipation in adulthood.[4] Adult patients suffering from psychotic illness, particularly schizophrenia, are prone to severe constipation with megacolon.[85]

Dietary Influences

It has been observed that, in societies in which the fiber content of the average diet is high, constipation is uncommon.[86] Although the addition of bran to the diet may be beneficial in patients with constipation of mild to moderate severity, there is no clear evidence that those who present with severe constipation have a less-than-average level of fiber intake.[73] The use of bran in the treatment of irritable bowel syndrome may have a useful role in the alleviation of consti-

pation,[63] but it may worsen other symptoms associated with this disorder.[73] The results of studies in which severely constipated women have been treated with bran have also been disappointing, with only a minority showing any improvement.[73] These observations suggest that although a low-fiber diet may contribute to the incidence of constipation in western societies, it may not provide an explanation for many of the more severe cases.

Colonic Absorption of Water

Although it has been shown that constipated children absorb more water from the colon when this is infused rectally, it appears that this can be explained on the basis of delayed transit rather than altered mucosal function.[87]

Histologic Abnormalities

It has been reported that the clinical syndrome of chronic severe constipation in adults is associated with a distinct abnormality of the colonic myenteric plexus; in a group of 12 women with this disorder who underwent subtotal colectomy, silver staining of the myenteric plexus revealed reduced numbers of argyrophilic neurons in 83 percent, reduced numbers of neuronal processes in 92 percent, and the presence of clusters of variably sized nuclei within the ganglia in all cases (Fig. 9).[88] The authors speculate that the abnormalities revealed by silver staining represent a disorder of neuronal maturation.

Motility Studies in Idiopathic Constipation

Intestinal Transit Time—Pediatric Subjects

The whole-gut transit time as judged by the passage of the markers has been reported to be significantly prolonged in children with simple constipation.[8,42] Detailed studies of intestinal transit in children have been somewhat limited because of the difficulties involved in the use of radiologic methods on young subjects.[8,43] In one study of 176 children with chronic constipation, the mean transit time in different segments was studied by administering radiopaque markers and obtaining abdominal radiographs at intervals of 12 hours.[43] Markers were found to occupy various segments of the colon and the rectum for prolonged periods in 61 percent of those with constipation. Clearance was reported to be delayed in the distal colon and/or rectum in 42 percent and in the proximal colon and distal colon and rectum in 19 percent. When constipation is due to "colonic inertia," the passage of markers is delayed, and they may remain distributed throughout the left and right colon for more than 5 days.[4] Outlet obstruction may be suggested by the persistence of markers in the rectosigmoid region.[7] Interpretation of these patterns of marker distribution is not simple, however, owing to the nondynamic nature of the study technique.

A recent study employed the breath hydrogen method to estimate orocecal transit time in children suffering from constipation.[89] It was reported that while the transit rate of the commonly used lactulose test solution was unaltered, that of a semisolid nutrient meal was significantly prolonged. This delay in transit was small, however, and would not have con-

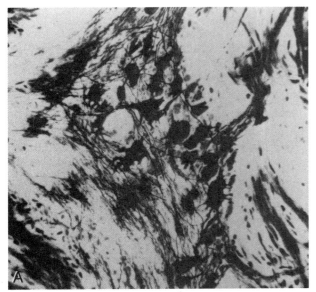

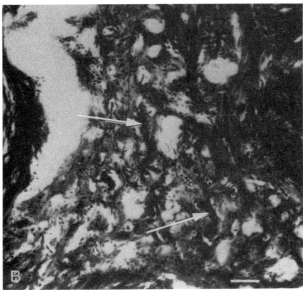

FIGURE 9 *A,* Ganglionic area from the colon of a control subject showing plentiful normal argyrophilic neurons with multiple nerve processes and nerve fibers. *B,* Ganglionic area of colon from an adult with severe idiopathic constipation showing lack of argyrophilic neurons, paucity of nerve fibers, and presence of multiple nuclei. The arrows denote muscle fibers. (Silver, both × 166; scale bar = 50 µm.) (From Krishnamurthy et al[88]; © 1985 by The American Gastroenterological Association.)

tributed much to the overall increase in whole-gut transit time commonly associated with constipation. Prolongation of orocecal transit might be explained merely as a phenomenon secondary to colonic distention,[90] or, alternately, it may reflect a generalized disturbance of intestinal motility.

Intestinal Transit Time—Adult Subjects

In adults with constipation associated with irritable bowel syndrome, both the orocecal and whole-gut transit times have been reported to be significantly prolonged when compared with normal subjects.[91] The delay in mouth-to-cecum transit is small, however, and the whole-gut transit time falls within the normal range in the majority of cases. In adults with chronic constipation associated with megacolon, whole-gut transit time is often prolonged.[71] In those with chronic severe constipation unassociated with megarectum or megacolon, small bowel transit time is prolonged,[72] and whole-gut transit time is usually greatly prolonged.[91]

Manometric and Electrophysiologic Studies— Pediatric Subjects

Studies of anorectal and distal colonic motility in children with chronic constipation have demonstrated some functional abnormality in nearly all cases (Table 2). This is so despite the fact that the precise methodologies and parameter definitions employed have differed widely, and the patient groups studied have tended to be heterogeneous in terms of age distribution, clinical manifestations, and severity. This variability in experimental design may explain many of the inconsistencies that exist between the findings in various studies. Some observations have, however, been fairly consistently reported.

Because many children with fecal retention and encopresis claim to have little awareness of the defecation urge, a large number of studies have been aimed at examining conscious rectal sensation. These experiments have been performed by inflating balloons in the rectal ampulla and noting the threshold volume at which the subject reports awareness of distention. Studies have reported on the "threshold of transient sensation," defined as the minimal distention volume required to produce a transient sense of fullness. Others have studied the "threshold of fullness," defined as the minimal volume at which a constant sensation of fullness occurs. Finally, the "critical volume," defined as the level at which lasting pain or an urge to defecate is experienced, has also been studied. The threshold of transient sensation has been reported to be increased in children with chronic constipation in several[51-54,92-94] but not all[49,77] studies. One study has reported that the incidence of encopresis among a group of 61 children with radiologically confirmed megarectum was related to the severity of the decrease in conscious sensation.[52] In one of the few reports in which the threshold of transient sensation was not altered, the threshold of fullness and the critical volume were both significantly elevated.[77] An increased critical volume in childhood constipation has also been reported by others.[50] These experiments have been dependent on the child's subjective responses, and so it is necessary to exercise some caution in their interpretation. The consistent trends do nevertheless provide quite convincing evidence of a physiologic basis for the clinical impression of diminished rectal sensitivity in these patients.

Attempts have been made to study the function of the anal sphincter mechanism using a variety of techniques. Anal tone has been studied by manometric recording of the rectoanal pressure profile.[53,54,58] This has been done by manually withdrawing a perfused catheter system while recording the changing pressure level. Meunier et al[53] calculated the maximal anal resting closure pressure by subtracting the recorded rectal pressure from the maximal anal pressure measured during the pull-through procedure; they found this to be significantly

TABLE 2
Summary of Results of Manometric and Electrophysiologic Studies Performed on Children with Chronic Idiopathic Constipation

Reference	TTS	TF	CV	RACP	MASP	RAIRT	VCR	MRC	ESRD
Porter, 1961[92]	Inc								
Callaghan and Nixon, 1964[93]	Inc								
Lawson, 1975[94]	Inc								
Clayden and Lawson, 1976[50]				Inc					
Meunier et al, 1976[52]	Inc					0			
Meunier et al, 1979[53]	Inc			Inc		0			
Molnar et al, 1983[51]	Inc								
Meunier et al, 1984[54]	Inc			Inc		0		Inc	
Loening-Baucke and Younoszai, 1984[59]	0	Inc	Inc			0	Inc		
Wald et al, 1984[49]	0					0			Inc
Loening-Baucke, 1984[58]				Dec	0	0			
Suzuki et al, 1980[97]				Inc		Inc			
Arhan et al, 1983[43]				Inc		Inc			
Loening-Baucke and Younoszai, 1982[56]				Dec		0			
Arhan et al, 1972[99]						Inc			
Schuster, 1973[101]						Inc			
Tobin and Schuster, 1974[100]						Inc			
Meunier, 1985[102]									Inc
Keren et al, 1988[55]									Inc
Loening-Baucke and Cruikshank, 1986[46]				Inc				Inc	Inc

TTS = threshold of transient sensation; TF = threshold of fullness; CV = critical volume; RACP = resting anal canal pressure; MASP = maximal anal canal squeeze pressure; RAIRT = rectoanal inhibitory response threshold; VCR = volume of constant relaxation; MRC = maximal rectal compliance; ESRD = external anal sphincter response on defecation. Inc = increased; Dec = decreased; 0 = no difference from normal response.

higher in children with constipation than in controls. Approximately half of those with constipation had a value that was above the control range. They suggested that anal hypertony might explain the outlet obstruction that had recently been described in some adult patients with chronic constipation.[7] They suggested that an elevated maximal anal resting closure pressure might provide a means of selecting patients who would benefit from anal sphincterotomy; this approach has been advocated for the treatment of both adults[7] and children with chronic constipation.[95,96] Increased anal pressure in chronic constipation has subsequently been reported in several studies using varied measurement techniques.[43,54,97] Arhan et al[43] recorded the luminal pressure in the rectal ampulla, in the upper part of the anal canal, and at the anal margin; they found the resting pressure in the rectum and upper canal to be increased in children with constipation, but there was no difference from controls at the anal margin. In one study, however, in which resting anal tone was recorded with a pressure transducer located statically in the anal canal, it was found to be significantly reduced.[56] In a subsequent report from the same group, in which resting tone was measured both by a step-wise pull-through method and also by the rapid pull-through method employed by Meunier et al[53] a significantly lower resting tone was also recorded.[58] The authors suggested that the discrepancy between their findings and those of other groups might have been due to differences in their patient population; they separately analyzed the measurements obtained from those children with chronic constipation with and without encopresis and found that only those with encopresis had a significant reduction in resting anal pressure.[58] In addition to assessing resting anal tone, Leoning-Baucke et al[58] attempted to study external anal sphincter function by measuring the maximal anal squeeze pressure. This was done by asking the subjects to squeeze maximally for a period of 1 minute while the intraluminal transducer was withdrawn step-wise through the anal canal; the pressure increase above anal resting tone produced during external anal sphincter squeeze was not significantly different in constipated children from that in controls.

In normal subjects balloon distention of the rectum leads to reflex relaxation of the internal anal sphincter (see Fig. 5). This reflex has been the subject of intensive study because it is absent in patients with rectal aganglionosis and so provides a valuable test for the identification of patients with constipation due to Hirschsprung's disease (see Fig. 5).[32,35,98-100] Studies have been performed of the "rectoanal inhibitory response threshold," the minimal distending volume required to elicit the rectoanal inhibitory reflex. Using manometric techniques, internal anal sphincter relaxation is studied while the rectum is transiently distended by balloon to known volumes. The majority of these studies have not shown a significant difference in the threshold volume between children with constipation and controls.[49,52-54,56,58,77] In most of these studies, however, individual patients have had threshold volumes greater than those of the control group,[50-54,57] and in a few studies a significantly increased threshold volume has been reported.[43,97,99-101] The "volume of constant relaxation," or threshold volume required to induce a long-lasting relaxation of the internal sphincter, has also been reported to be increased in children with chronic constipation.[77] The percentage relaxation of the internal sphincter following rectal distention to a fixed volume has been studied, and although this has been reported to be significantly reduced in constipated children,[58] this finding has not been consistently observed.[55]

Some authors have pointed out that in normal subjects the rectoanal inhibitory reflex threshold is close to the threshold for conscious rectal sensation, but in children with chronic constipation the increase in the minimal volume required to induce conscious rectal sensation in association with an unchanged threshold for reflex internal anal sphincter relaxation may be conducive to soiling.[51,52]

Meunier et al[54] examined the rectometrogram or pressure-volume relationship in the rectum and demonstrated a significant increase in the "maximal rectal compliance," defined as the ratio of the maximal tolerable rectal volume and the maximal tolerable rectal pressure in children with chronic constipation. This supports the view that the increase in volume required to produce conscious rectal sensation or to induce the rectoanal inhibitory reflex may reflect a change in the viscoelastic properties of the rectum. The authors suggested that the rectometrogram might provide a rational technique for the assessment of the degree of rectal wall dysfunction and hence of the severity of the constipation disorder.

A variety of techniques have been employed to study the dynamics of defecation in children with chronic constipation. Wald et al[49] studied expulson dynamics by recording the manometric profile when the child was requested to simulate defecation by attempting to expel the manometric apparatus. This apparatus consisted of three inflatable balloons placed in the anorectum so as to permit simultaneous recording of pressure in the rectum and at the level of the internal and external sphincters. In normal children this device recorded an increase in pressure in the rectum and at the level of the internal sphincter during attempted expulsion while the pressure at the level of the external sphincter simultaneously decreased. Thirty-six percent of the children with encopresis exhibited an inappropriate increase in pressure at the level of the external sphincter during simulated defecation, compared with 10 percent of the control children. Meunier et al[102] studied anal relaxation manometrically during Valsalva maneuvers in a group of chronically constipated children

without encopresis who had been unsuccessfully treated with lactulose. "Rectal dysynergia," defined as a failure of anal relaxation during the Valsalva maneuver, was present in 77 percent of patients and in none of the control subjects. The authors suggested that this finding could explain, at least in part, the failure of lactulose therapy in these children; they proposed that "rectal dysynergia" is an indication for biofeedback therapy. Keren et al,[55] using a multichannel catheter perfusion technique to study pressure responses in the rectum and anal canal, demonstrated an increase in anal pressure during attempted defecation in 78 percent of children with chronic constipation and encopresis (see Fig. 6). In control subjects there was a decrease in anal pressure during attempted defecation, and the paradoxical closure of the canal seen in the patient group differed from that seen during voluntary anal squeeze in that there was an associated rise in rectal pressure. Loening-Baucke and Cruikshank[46] examined the defecation dynamics of constipated encopretic children by studying their ability to expel water-filled balloons of various volumes. During the attempted expulsions they measured the pressure exerted on the balloon by recording its intraluminal pressure, and they studied changes in rectal and anal canal pressure using a motility probe; simultaneously external anal sphincter activity was assessed electrophysiologically using cutaneous electrodes placed close to the anal margin. Although constipated children exerted pressures on the water-filled rectal balloons similar to those of control children, their ability to expel them was significantly decreased. The external cutaneous electrodes detected a decrease in activity in the external sphincter during defecation in all of the control children but in only 42 percent of the constipated children, and 50 percent had an actual increase in activity. The electrical response was normal in only one of 15 constipated children who were unable to defecate balloons, compared with 11 of 19 who were successful in expelling them. They failed to identify any clinical characteristics that separated those patients able to defecate the balloons from those unable to do so. The critical volume and the volume of constant relaxation, although increased in the patients with constipation, were not significantly different between those able or unable to expel the balloons. It thus appears that the ability or inability to defecate balloons was independent of rectal sensation or rectal size. There is thus considerable evidence that some chronically constipated children may have an abnormality of defecation dynamics characterized by a failure of external anal sphincter relaxation. It appears likely that the closely related puborectalis muscle is similarly affected, and the results of an electrophysiologic study on adult women with constipation associated with failure of external anal sphincter relaxation tend to confirm this possibility.[44] It remains uncertain whether these motor abnormalities are due to deliberate or unconscious motor behavior or such children have a primary or maturational disorder of sphincter function.

In a number of studies children with constipation have been followed up manometrically over periods of months to years, and the effects of successful treatment on abnormal motility patterns have been examined. In a 3-year follow-up of 11 chronically constipated children treated with milk of magnesia and bowel training, only eight had recovered symptomatically.[77] In five of these clinically recovered patients, rectal sensory responses were persistently abnormal, despite the fact that rectal size had returned to normal. It has also been reported that among chronically constipated children, those with evidence of outlet obstruction, as judged by their inability to expel balloons placed in the rectum, were much less likely to respond satisfactorily to treatment with milk of magnesia over a 6-month period.[46] Keren et al[55] treated 12 children with constipation and encopresis associated with paradoxical external anal sphincter contraction using a biofeedback method designed to condition these patients to relax the external anal sphincter during defecation. In most cases they recorded a gradual transition to a normal manometric pattern, and in general there was an improvement in clinical symptoms which usually, but not in every case, paralleled normalization of the anal sphincter response.

In summary, children with idiopathic chronic constipation have evidence of an increased threshold of sensation for rectal distention, but the threshold for reflex inhibition of the internal sphincter appears to be well preserved in most cases. This may predispose them to fecal soiling. In some children there is evidence of anal outlet obstruction—they have difficulties with the expulsion of simulated stools from the rectum, and they fail to relax or actively contract the external anal sphincter during attempted defecation; this subgroup may be resistant to treatment with medications. It is unclear whether outlet obstruction is a primary or a secondary phenomenon in these children.

Manometric and Electrophysiologic Studies— Adult Subjects

There is evidence of an abnormality of smooth muscle function in patients with irritable bowel syndrome—a decreased colonic slow wave frequency of three cycles per minute occurring for a much larger proportion of time than in normal subjects.[4] Patients with irritable bowel syndrome associated with constipation have an increased frequency of nonpropagated contractions leading to functional partial colonic obstruction.[103] After meals many patients with irritable bowel syndrome experience abdominal pain, and studies have demonstrated a delay in the postprandial colonic motility response.[104] The threshold for pain on balloon distention of the rectum is believed to be reduced.[63] Studies have shown that normal subjects experience difficulty in expelling small, hard simulated stools when these are placed in the rectum.[60] It has been proposed that in patients with irritable bowel syndrome the hyperactive, poorly propulsive colon delivers small pellets of stool to the hypersensitive rectum, resulting in difficulty in defecation and a sense of incomplete evacuation.[73]

Motility studies in adults with chronic severe constipation have demonstrated anorectal outlet obstruction in about one-third of cases.[4,7] Inadequate relaxation of the puborectalis can also cause outlet obstruction.[105] Electrophysiologic studies have suggested that during attempted defecation patients may contract both the puborectal muscle and the external anal sphincter instead of relaxing them.[44] It is uncertain whether these anomalies are primary factors or merely secondary findings. Some patients with chronic severe constipation have "colonic inertia" associated with per-

sistence of radiopaque markers throughout the colon; this may be due to increased segmenting nonpropulsive contractions.[4]

In elderly patients with chronic constipation associated with fecal impaction, rectal sensation is usually diminished and rectal capacity is markedly increased.[73]

CONSTIPATION SECONDARY TO ORGANIC DISEASE

Although in the great majority of cases the etiology of chronic constipation remains obscure, it may arise secondary to a variety of disorders of the GI tract or in association with a wide range of systemic disorders.

Anatomic Disorders of the Colon and Anorectum

Congenital structural disorders of the distal bowel or anorectum may be found in association with constipation. Rare congenital colonic strictures or strictures acquired secondary to such disorders as necrotizing enterocolitis may lead to constipation. Constipation may also be caused by the presence of a sacrococcygeal teratoma. The majority of severe congenital anorectal anomalies declare their presence within a short period, being associated with obvious obstructive symptoms. Some less severe anomalies may, however, be overlooked and can result in a chronic disorder of fecal evacuation.

Anal stenosis may result in constipation associated with severe fecal retention, and if undiagnosed these children may be subjected to prolonged and ineffective therapy. Typically they have symptoms of constipation from an early age and pass stools of small caliber.

Anterior ectopic anus has been reported by several authors as a common cause of intractable constipation in childhood.[106-108] The onset of constipation has characteristically been in early infancy, and it has rarely been reported to commence after the first year of life. In some children overflow incontinence may occur.[107] On rectal examination the anal canal is usually of normal size, but there may be a prominent "rectal shelf" posterior to the anal orifice. Studies of the anal sphincter mechanism have been performed in these children using electromyographic and manometric techniques; these studies have suggested that the internal sphincter may frequently function normally and that the difficulties with defecation may arise directly as a consequence of the abnormal oblique direction of the anal canal.[109] In some children the anal orifice is located well forward of its normal location, but in others the anterior displacement may be subtle.[106] Reisner et al[110] studied the location of the anal orifice in normal infants and children. They calculated the distance ratios of anus-fourchette:coccyx-fourchette in the female and anus-scrotum:coccyx-scrotum in the male; anterior displacement was defined as a ratio of less than 0.34 in females and less than 0.46 in males. The existence of such displacement in a child with chronic constipation should at least raise the possibility that an anatomic basis for the condition may be present.

Constipation and Chronic Intestinal Pseudo-obstruction

Intestinal pseudo-obstruction is defined as the presence of symptoms and signs of intestinal obstruction in the absence of a mechanical obstructing lesion.[111] Chronic intestinal pseudo-obstruction syndrome is associated with disturbances of motility that may affect the digestive tract at any or all levels. Consequently, apart from the classic features of small intestinal obstruction, other dysmotility symptoms including dysphagia, gastric outlet obstruction, and constipation may predominate. A broad spectrum of disease states has been classified under the heading of chronic intestinal pseudo-obstruction and may be associated with severe chronic constipation; some of these are localized to the GI tract, whereas others are systemic disorders that result in secondary involvement of the GI tract.[111]

Familial and Nonfamilial Visceral Myopathies

Rare familial and nonfamilial visceral myopathies have been described which are characterized histologically by the presence of degenerating muscle cells and fibrosis, chiefly affecting the external layer of the muscularis propria.[111] Familial type I visceral myopathy, which has an autosomal dominant mode of transmission, may present after the first decade of life, and is characterized by a wide range of dysmotility symptoms, including constipation. It is usually associated with a good prognosis, as pseudo-obstruction is uncommon and is often amenable to surgery.

Congenital Aganglionosis—Hirschsprung's Disease

Hirschsprung's disease is characterized by a congenital absence of ganglion cells in the myenteric and submucosal plexuses. In the great majority of cases the affected segment extends proximally for a variable distance from the internal anal sphincter. The length of aganglionic bowel varies, ranging from that seen in short-segment Hirschsprung's disease, in which only the region of the anal sphincter may be affected, to that in more extensively affected cases, in which the entire colon or rarely even the small intestine is without ganglion cells.[112–114] In 80 percent of cases the affected segment extends no farther than the sigmoid colon, in 3 percent it involves the entire colon, and total intestinal aganglionosis extending from rectum to duodenum has been reported in a small number of infants.[113] Hirschsprung's disease has an incidence of one in 5,000 live births.[115] It is approximately three times more common in males, and this difference in incidence between the sexes is more pronounced in the long-segment forms of the disorder. The risk of recurrence in the siblings of an affected child is increased in cases of long-segment disease, and if the patient is female or the sibling male. The recurrence rate varies from 0.6 percent in the female sibling of a male with short-segment disease to 18 percent in the male sibling of a female with long-segment involvement.[115] While familial occurrence of Hirschsprung's disease is usually attributed to multifactorial inheritance, the evidence is that the rare disorder of total intestinal aganglionosis may be transmitted as an autosomal inheritance.[113]

Hirschsprung's disease has been said to result from a failure of neural cells to complete their normal pathway of migration from the neural crest. Recent evidence of a dual gradient of development of the enteric nervous system proceeding from each end of the gut toward its middle has, however, raised the possibility that aganglionosis may arise from a failure of differentiation or of neuronal survival in the affected regions rather that from a failure of craniocaudal cell migration.[25] The existence of rare cases of "zonal aganglionosis," in which isolated segments of colon proximal to the rectum are affected, suggests that, at least in these individuals, regression of neural elements may be important, or alternately precursor cells may indeed be multifocal in origin.[116,117] Congenital aganglionosis has been described in association with a wide range of congenital abnormalities and syndromes, including Down's syndrome, which accounts for 2 percent of cases.

Histologic examination of the affected segment of intestine, in addition to demonstrating aganglionosis, also reveals the presence of numerous abnormally thickened nerve fibers that stain positively for acetylcholinesterase, indicating that they are derived from the parasympathic nervous system (Fig. 10).[118] These are the intramural ramifications of parasympathic preganglionic lumbosacral nerves, and it is uncertain if their presence contributes to the disordered motility found in this disease.[118]

In subjects with Hirschsprung's disease, balloon distention of the rectum fails to induce the reflex relaxation of the internal anal sphincter that is found in normal subjects (see Fig. 5).[32,33,35,98,99] The aganglionic segment is tonically contracted and lacks the intrinsic inhibitory neural reflex that normally exists in the intestine. Consequently, there is a functional obstruction at the level of the aganglionic segment, and the bowel proximal to this is dilated. In the majority of cases there is, therefore, a significant delay in the first passage of meconium, and in many cases symptoms of intestinal obstruction with vomiting and abdominal distention appear after the second day of life. In others the obstruction is partial, and symptoms may be less severe, with abdominal distention and constipation predominating. Those patients with the mildest symptoms typically have short-segment aganglionosis, and the diagnosis of Hirschsprung's disease may often be delayed even into adult life.[119] The severity of symptoms is not always directly related to the length of the aganglionic segment, however, so the functional disability associated with aganglionosis in individual patients must be influenced by other less well defined factors.[120] On rectal examination patients with aganglionosis classically have an anal canal and rectal ampulla of small caliber, unlike those with idiopathic constipation, in whom the rectum is frequently voluminous. An exception to this occurs in patients with very short segment aganglionosis in whom feces may accumulate in the rectum. Soiling and the passage of stools of unusually large caliber, both of which are frequently associated with idiopathic constipation in childhood, are not features of Hirschsprung's disease, although ultra-short segment aganglionosis may again prove an exception.[121] The clinical manifestations and management of Hirschsprung's disease are discussed in detail in a later chapter.

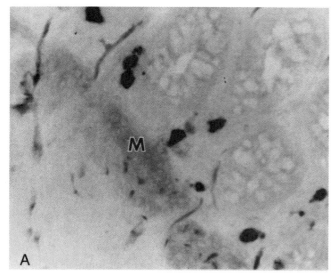

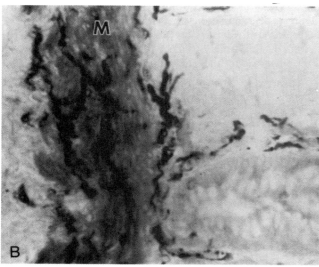

FIGURE 10 Acetlycholinesterase staining of colonic tissue for the diagnosis of Hirschsprung's disease. *A*, Normal rectal mucosa and muscularis mucosae (M) with colonic glands to the right and submucosa to the left. The muscularis mucosae is traversed by several nerve fibers. The dense staining in the lamina propria represents nonspecific cholinesterase within macrophages. *B*, In Hirschsprung's disease, thick nerve fibers staining positively for acetylcholinesterase are found within the muscularis mucosae (M). These extend into the lamina propria between colonic glands. (From Weinberg.[118])

Acquired Aganglionosis

Rare cases of acquired aganglionosis in infancy have been reported. Animal studies have shown that the intramural ganglion cells are very susceptible to anoxic injury.[122] An infant born at 30 weeks' gestation, who had been subject to moderate anoxia and acidosis and who had suspected necrotizing enterocolitis in the early days of life, developed intermittent signs of obstruction thereafter, and although a submucosal rectal biopsy obtained at 10 weeks of age was normal, full-thickness colonic biopsies and submucosal rectal biopsies at 18 weeks demonstrated aganglionosis.[123] It is of interest that a report exists of premature monozygotic twins in which the smaller twin, who had suffered respiratory complications and necrotizing enterocolitis in the early days of life, was subsequently found to have distal aganglionosis.[124] Acquired aganglionosis has also been reported in a full-term infant who had not been subject to any apparent perinatal risk factors and who had obstructive symptoms from birth; a deep rectal biopsy obtained within the first 2 weeks of life was normal, but at 4 months biopsies at the level of the sigmoid and rectum demonstrated aganglionosis.[125] It should be borne in mind, however, that on rare occasions ganglia may have a patchy distribution in the hind gut; two infants have been described with signs of subacute obstruction in whom ganglion cells were identified by suction biopsy, but in whom detailed histologic examination of resected rectal tissue revealed the presence of zones of aganglionosis alternating with normal areas.[126]

Other Disorders of Intrinsic Innervation

During the past two decades it has increasingly been recognized that other rare disorders of the enteric nervous system exist.[120,127] Intestinal neuronal dysplasia,[127] or hyperganglionosis,[120] is characterized by the presence of hyperplastic parasympathetic nerve fibers in the submucosa and circular muscles associated with increased acetylcholinesterase activity. In some cases hyperplasia of the plexuses, giant ganglia, or displaced neurons in the lamina propria may be seen. Neuronal dysplasia has been described in a localized form limited to the colon.[127] A disseminated form affecting the entire GI tract has also been reported, and this may be associated with megacystis and megaureter.[128] In a few cases the dysplastic appearance has occurred immediately proximal to an aganglionic distal segment.[128,129] Localized neuronal dysplasia may be associated with symptoms suggestive of Hirschsprung's disease. The disseminated forms have all proved fatal.

Neuronal intestinal dysplasia has been found on rare occasions in adults and children with megacolon in association with neurofibromatosis.[130] It has also been described in infancy and childhood in association with the syndrome of multiple endocrine neoplasia type 2.[131,132] This disorder is characterized by the presence of medullary thyroid carcinoma, pheochromocytoma, and swelling of the lips which reflects the diffuse alimentary tract ganglioneuromatosis.

In the transition zone between normal bowel and the aganglionic segment in Hirschsprung's disease, the number of ganglion cells is reduced, but isolated hypoganglionosis has also been described in patients with chronic constipation.[120] Precise quantitative data are not available on the distribution of ganglia in the colon and anorectum, and this causes difficulty in the identification of hypoganglionosis. In addition, the distinction between hypoganglionosis and Hirschsprung's disease may be problematic, as conventional staining may fail to identify the small numbers of ganglia present. It is said that unlike Hirschsprung's disease there is a paucity of cholinesterase-positive nerves, and this may prove helpful in making the diagnosis.[120]

Congenital Segmental Dilatation of the Colon

Segmental dilatation of the colon is a disorder that may be associated with constipation from early infancy.[133-135] Barium enema reveals the presence of focal dilatation of the colon. The dilated segment appears nonmotile, but the colon proximal and distal to it appears to function normally. No abnormality of the submucosal or myenteric ganglia has been identified, but the muscle layers of the dilated segment may be hypertrophied.

Cathartic Colon

This is a poorly defined clinical entity in which patients have had an atonic dilated colon that has been attributed to chronic use of laxatives.[136] Damage to the myenteric plexus, smooth muscle atrophy, and melanosis coli have been reported in these patients. Histologic abnormalities have been induced in mice by administering syrup of senna, but the doses employed were extremely large.[137] No prospective histologic studies have been performed, however, on patients receiving these drugs, and the effects of drug withdrawal on histologic changes have not been assessed. Similar abnormal histologic appearances have been seen in patients with chronic intestinal pseudo-obstruction with no history of laxative abuse.[138] The existence of this entity is therefore in some doubt, and its relevance in the management of childhood constipation is at present unclear.

Systemic Disorders Associated with Constipation

A wide range of systemic disorders may be associated with constipation. Hypothyroidism is commonly associated with chronic constipation in childhood and may be the presenting complaint. Severe constipation has been reported in 20 percent of patients with diabetes mellitus and clinical evidence of neuropathy, but this is rare in childhood.[139] In progressive systemic sclerosis symptoms of dysmotility, including dysphagia and constipation alternating with diarrhea, may occur, and reduced rectal compliance and absence of the rectoanal inhibitory reflex have been reported.[140,141] Other rare disorders that may result in chronic constipation in childhood include pheochromocytoma, porphyria, and various disorders associated with hypercalcemia such as hyperparathyroidism and vitamin D excess. Chronic lead poisoning may be associated with anorexia, vomiting, abdominal pain, and constipation. Finally, constipation may be associated with a wide range of frequently administered drugs.

Lesions of the Spinal Cord

Spinal cord lesions that affect the sacral reflex centers may be associated with loss of rectal tone and sensation and reduced anal closure pressure as a consequence of paralysis of the external anal sphincter. The rectoanal inhibitory reflex is usually preserved, but distention of the rectum does not initiate the normal reflex rectal contractions. Spinal cord injury may also eliminate the postprandial gastrocolic reflex.[142] These patients are therefore prone to chronic fecal retention associated with overflow incontinence.

Spinal dysraphism, or defective embryogenesis of the spinal cord and associated structures, is commonly associated with disordered defecation. Myelomeningocele, which is one of the most common serious congenital disorders seen in infants and children, occurs most frequently in the lumbosacral region, and in the majority of patients the nerve supply to the bladder and the anorectum is affected. Many such children, therefore, suffer from some degree of urinary and fecal incontinence. The loss of nerve conduction, however, may not be complete, and pseudocontinence may be possible with proper dietary and drug management.[143] Disorders of continence are most obvious in those with sacral lesions, while in children with lumbar or dorsolumbar lesions, despite complete paralysis of the lower limbs, continence may be preserved.[143] Spina bifida occulta, in which there is a failure of fusion of the vertebral arches, may also be associated with abnormal development of the underlying cord. An overlying cutaneous anomaly may provide a clue to the diagnosis. Minor occult vertebral defects in the lumbosacral region are extremely common on radiologic examination and are usually asymptomatic. In some cases, however, motor and sensory defects may affect the lower limbs and occasionally control of the bladder and anorectum. Other congenital disorders of the spine, including diastematomyelia, in which the cord is divided longitudinally; tethering of the cord by an abnormally tight filum terminale or by fibrous bands; the presence of neurenteric cysts, intradural lipomata, or dermoid cysts; and sacrococcygeal agenesis may lead to similar problems of sphincter dysfunction. It is important to be aware that progressive deterioration in function may occur in these children owing to the normal differential pattern of growth in the spinal cord and vertebral column. It is thus possible for a child with a hidden spinal dysraphic state, having achieved continence at an appropriate age, to later lose it.

Acquired disorders of the spinal cord may also lead to disorders of defecation. Spinal cord tumors are rare and occur least commonly in the lumbosacral area. Their presence is associated with regression of bladder or bowel control in one third of children, however, and this sign is often overlooked initially in children.[144] Other acquired lesions affecting the cord, including trauma, vascular insults, infection, and transverse myelitis, may all lead to similar problems.

CONCLUSION

Chronic constipation is a common and often serious disorder in childhood. Definition in terms of altered bowel habit is difficult because studies of normal populations have been limited and because the normal pattern is highly variable, especially during infancy and childhood. A precise physiologic definition has also proved elusive. These ambiguities are important, particularly in the design of studies of childhood constipation. In clinical practice, however, many children are seen who clearly suffer from undue difficulty with fecal elimination and who develop chronic fecal retention. Although a wide range of disorders, both systemic and local, may be associated with constipation, in the majority of cases the etiology is obscure and subject to much speculation. In recent years some light has been cast on the mechanisms that may underlie idiopathic constipation in childhood. Intensive study of sensory and motor function in the anorectum of these children has been undertaken. This has provided important information about the accompanying pathophysiologic phenomena, and an understanding of these abnormalities may prove of considerable importance, not alone in attempting to define the primary factors responsible for the disorder but also in assisting in the development of rational approaches to therapy.

REFERENCES

1. Christensen J. Motility of the colon. In: Johnson LR, ed. Physiology of the gastrointestinal tract. 2nd ed. New York: Raven Press, 1987: 665.
2. Levine MD. Children with encopresis: a descriptive analysis. Pediatrics 1975; 56:412–416.
3. Davidson M, Kugler MM, Bauer CH. Diagnosis and management in children with severe and protracted constipation and obstipation. J Pediatr 1963; 62:261–275.
4. Reynolds JC. Chronic severe constipation. In: Cohen S, Soloway RD, eds. Functional disorders of the gastrointestinal tract. Contemporary issues in gastroenterology. Vol. 6. New York: Churchill Livingstone, 1987: 95.
5. Rappaport LA, Levine MD. The prevention of constipation and encopresis: a developmental model and approach. Pediatr Clin North Am 1986; 33:859–869.
6. Hendren WH. Constipation caused by anterior location of the anus and its surgical correction. J Pediatr Surg 1978; 13:505–512.
7. Martelli H, Devroede G, Arhan P, Duguay C. Mechanisms of idiopathic constipation: outlet obstruction. Gastroenterology 1978; 75:623–631.
8. Corazziari E, Cucchiara S, Staiano A, Romaniello G, Tamburrini O, Torsoli A, Auricchio S. Gastrointestinal transit time, frequency of defecation, and anorectal manometry in healthy and constipated children. J Pediatr 1985; 106:379–382.
9. Weaver LT. Bowel habit from birth to old age. J Pediatr Gastroenterol Nutr 1988; 7:637–640.
10. Wyman JB, Heaton KW, Manning AP, Wicks ACB. Variations of colonic function in healthy subjects. Gut 1978; 19:146–150.
11. Burkitt D, Morley D, Walker A. Dietary fiber in under- and overnutrition in childhood. Arch Dis Child 1980; 55:803–807.
12. Walker ARP, Walker BF. Bowel behaviour in young black and white children. Arch Dis Child 1985; 60:967–970.
13. Kelsay JL, Behall KM, Prather ES. Effects of fiber from fruits and vegetables on metabolic responses of human subjects. I. Bowel transit time, number of defecations, fecal weight, urinary excretions of energy and nitrogen and apparent digestibilities of energy, nitrogen and fat. Am J Clin Nutr 1978; 31:1149–1153.
14. Davies GJ, Crowder M, Reid B, Dickerson JWT. Bowel function measurements of individuals with different eating patterns. Gut 1986; 27:164–169.
15. Connell AM, Hilton C, Irvine G, Lennard-Jones JE, Miesewicz JJ. Variation in bowel habit in two population samples. Br Med J 1965; 2:1095–1099.
16. Drossman DA, Sandler RS, McKee DC, Lovitz AJ. Bowel patterns among subjects not seeking health care. Gastroenterology 1982; 83:529–534.
17. Weaver LT, Steiner H. The bowel habit of young children. Arch Dis Child 1984; 59:649–652.
18. Nyhan WL. Stool frequency of normal infants in the first weeks of life. Pediatrics 1952; 10:414–425.
19. Weaver LT, Ewing G, Taylor LC. The bowel habit of milk-fed infants. J Pediatr Gastroenterol Nutr 1988; 7:568–571.
20. Huizinga JD. Electrophysiology of human colon motility in health and disease. Clin Gastroenterol 1986; 15:879–901.
21. Gonella J, Bouvier M, Blanquet F. Extrinsic nervous control of motility of small and large intestines and related sphincters. Physiol Rev 1987; 67:902–961.
22. Schofield GC. Anatomy of muscular and neural tissues in the alimentary canal. In: Heidel W, Code CF, eds. Handbook of physiology. Sec 6. Alimentary Canal. Vol IV. Motility. Washington, DC: American Physiological Society, 1968: 1579.
23. Okamoto E, Ueda T. Embryogenesis of intramural ganglia of the gut and its relation to Hirschsprung's disease. J Pediatr Surg 1967; 2:437–443.
24. Smith B. Pre- and postnatal development of the ganglion cells of the rectum and its surgical implications. J Pediatr Surg 1968; 3:386–391.
25. Tam PKH. An immunochemical study with neuro-specific enolase and substance P of human enteric innervation. The normal developmental pattern and abnormal deviations in Hirschsprung's disease and pyloric stenosis. J Pediatr Surg 1986; 21:227–232.
26. Clement CD, ed. Anatomy of the human body, by H. Gray. 30th ed. Philadelphia: Lea & Febiger, 1985.
27. Elliot TR, Barclay-Smith E. Antiperistalsis and other activities of the colon. J Physiol (Lond) 1904; 31:272–304.
28. Cannon WB. The movements of the intestines: Studies by means of Röntgen rays. Am J Physiol 1902; 6:251–277.
29. Hansky J, Connell AM. Measurement of gastrointestinal transit using radioactive chromium. Gut 1962; 3:187–188.
30. Ritchie JA. Movement of segmental constrictions in the human colon. Gut 1971; 12:350–355.
31. Misiewicz JJ, Connell AM, Pontes FA. Comparison of the effects of meals and prostigmine on the proximal and distal colon in patients with and without diarrhoea. Gut 1966; 7:468–473.
32. Lawson JON, Nixon HH. Anal canal pressures in the diagnosis of Hirschsprung's disease. J Pediatr Surg 1967; 2:544–552.
33. Tobon F, Reid NCRW, Talbert JL, Schuster MM. Nonsurgical test for the diagnosis of Hirschsprung's disease. N Engl J Med 1968; 278:188–194.
34. Schuster MM, Hendrix TR, Mendeloff AI. The internal anal sphincter response: manometric studies on its normal physiology, neural pathways and alteration in bowel disorders. J Clin Invest 1963; 42:196–207.
35. Ito Y, Donahoe PK, Hendren WH. Maturation of the rectoanal response in premature and perinatal infants. J Pediatr Surg 1977; 12:477–482.
36. Molander M-L, Frenckner B. Electrical activity of the external anal sphincter at different ages in childhood. Gut 1983; 24:218–221.
37. Duthie HL, Watts JM. Contribution of the external anal sphincter to the pressure zone in the anal canal. Gut 1965; 6:64–68.
38. Duthie HL, Gairns FW. Sensory nerve-endings and sensation in the anal region of man. Br J Surg 1960; 47:585–595.
39. Duthie HL, Bennet RC. The relation of sensation in the anal canal to the functional anal sphincter: a possible factor in anal continence. Gut 1963; 4:179–182.
40. Bellman M. Studies on encopresis. Acta Pediatr Scand 1966; 170(Suppl):1–138.
41. Wingate DL. Motility of the small intestine. In: Chadwick VS, Phillips SF, eds. Gastroenterology 2. Small intestine. Butterworth international medical reviews. London: Butterworth Scientific, 1982; 119.
42. Dimson SB. Carmine as an index of transit time in children with simple constipation. Arch Dis Child 1970; 45:232–235.
43. Arhan P, Devroede G, Jehannin B, Faverdin C, Revillon Y, Lefebvre D, Gignier P, Pellerin D. Idiopathic disorders of fecal continence in children. Pediatrics 1983; 71:774–779.
44. Womack NR, Williams NS, Holmfield JHM, Morrison JFB, Simpkins KC. New method for the dynamic assessment of anorectal function in constipation. Br J Surg 1985; 72:994–998.
45. Howard ER, Nixon HH. Internal anal sphincter. Observations on development and mechanism of inhibitory responses in premature infants and children with Hirschsprung's disease. Arch Dis Child 1968; 43:569–578.
46. Loening-Baucke VA, Cruikshank BM. Abnormal defecation dynamics in chronically constipated children with encopresis. J Pediatr 1986; 108:562–566.
47. Loening-Baucke V, Cruikshank B, Savage C. Defecation dynamics and behaviour profiles in encopretic children. Pediatrics 1987; 80:672–679.
48. Schuster MM, Hookman P, Hendrix TR, Mendeloff AI. Simultaneous manometric recording of internal and external anal sphincteric reflexes. Bull Johns Hopkins Hosp 1965; 116:79–88.
49. Wald A, Chandra R, Chiponis D, Gabel S. Anorectal function and continence mechanisms in childhood encopresis. J Pediatr Gastroenterol Nutr 1986; 5:346–351.
50. Clayden GS, Lawson JON. Investigation and management of longstanding chronic constipation in childhood. Arch Dis Child 1976; 51:918–923.
51. Molnar D, Taitz LS, Urwin OM, Wales JKH. Anorectal manometry results in defecation disorders. Arch Dis Child 1983; 58:257–261.

52. Meunier P, Mollard P, Marechal J-M. Physiology of megarectum: the association of megarectum with encopresis. Gut 1976; 17:224–227.

53. Meunier P, Marechal JM, de Beaujeu MJ. Rectoanal pressures and rectal sensitivity studies in chronic constipation. Gastroenterology 1979; 77:330–336.

54. Meunier P, Louis D, Jaubert M, de Beaujeu J. Physiologic investigation of primary chronic constipation in children: comparison with the barium enema study. Gastroenterology 1984; 87:1351–1357.

55. Keren S, Wagner Y, Heldenberg D, Golan M. Studies of manometric abnormalities of the rectoanal region during defecation in constipated and soiling children: modification through biofeedback therapy. Am J Gastroenterol 1988; 83:827–831.

56. Loening-Baucke VA, Younoszai MK. Abnormal anal sphincter response in chronically constipated children. J Pediatr 1982; 100:213–218.

57. Loening-Baucke VA. Ano-rectal manometry: experience with strain gauge pressure transducers for the diagnosis of Hirschsprung's disease. J Pediatr Surg 1983; 18:595–600.

58. Loening-Baucke VA. Abnormal rectoanal function in children recovered from chronic constipation and encopresis. Gastroenterology 1984; 87:1299–1304.

59. Loening-Baucke VA, Younoszai MK. Effect of treatment on rectal and sigmoid motility in chronically constipated children. Pediatrics 1984; 73:199–205.

60. Bannister JJ, Davison P, Timms JM, Gibbons C, Read NW. The effect of stool size and consistency on defecation. Gut 1987; 28:1246–1250.

61. Pettei M, Davidson M. Constipation. In: Silverberg M, Daum F, eds. Textbook of pediatric gastroenterology. 2nd ed. Chicago: Year Book Medical Publishers, 1988: 180.

62. Nixon HH. Megarectum in the older child. Proc R Soc Med 1967; 60:801–803.

63. Snape WJ. Irritable bowel syndrome. In: Cohen S, Soloway RD, eds. Functional disorders of the gastrointestinal tract. Contemporary issues in gastroenterology. Vol 6. New York: Churchill Livingstone, 1987: 95.

64. Schuster MM. Irritable bowel syndrome. In: Sleisenger MH, Fordtran JS, eds. Gastrointestinal disease. Pathophysiology, diagnosis, management. 4th ed. Philadelphia: WB Saunders, 1989: 1402.

65. Fielding JF. A year in outpatients with irritable bowel syndrome. Irish J Med Sci 1977; 146:162–166.

66. Davidson M, Wasserman R. The irritable colon of childhood (chronic, non-specific diarrhoea syndrome). J Pediatr 1966; 69:1027–1038.

67. Apley J, Naish N. Recurrent abdominal pain: a full survey of 1000 school children. Arch Dis Child 1958; 33:165–170.

68. Peteii M, Davidson M. Irritable bowel syndrome. In: Silverberg M, Daum F, eds. Textbook of pediatric gastroenterology. 2nd ed. Chicago: Year Book Medical Publishers, 1988: 189.

69. Watier A, Devroede G, Duarnceau A, Abdel-Rahman M, Duguay C, Forand M, Tetreault L, Arhan P, Lamarche J, Elhilali M. Constipation with colonic inertia. A manifestation of systemic disease? Dig Dis Sci 1983; 28:1025–1033.

70. Preston DM, Lennard-Jones JE. Severe chronic constipation in young women: idiopathic slow transit constipation. Gut 1986; 27:41–48.

71. Barnes PRH, Lennard-Jones JE. Balloon expulsion from the rectum in constipation of different types. Gut 1985; 26:1049–1052.

72. Preston JE, Lennard-Jones JE. Pelvic motility and response to intraluminal bisacodyl in slow-transit constipation. Dig Dis Sci 1985; 30:289–294.

73. Read NW, Timms JM. Defecation and the pathophysiology of constipation. Clin Gastroenterol 1986; 15:937–965.

74. Pinkerton P. Psychogenic megacolon in children: the implications of negativism. Arch Dis Child 1958; 33:371–380.

75. Silverman A, Roy CC. Pediatric clinical gastroenterology. 3rd ed. St. Louis: CV Mosby, 1983: 391.

76. Oppe TE. Megacolon and megarectum in older children. Proc R Soc Med 1967; 60:803–805.

77. Loening-Baucke VA. Sensitivity of the sigmoid colon and rectum in children treated for chronic constipation. J Pediatr Gastroenterol Nutr 1984; 3:454–459.

78. Bakwin H, Davidson M. Constipation in twins. Am J Dis Child 1971; 121:179–181.

79. Huschka M. The child's response to coercive bowel training. Psychosom Med 1942; 4:301–308.

80. Garrard SD, Richmond JB. Psychogenic megacolon manifested by fecal soiling. Pediatrics 1952; 10:474–481.

81. Prugh DG. Childhood experience and colonic disorders. Ann NY Acad Sci 1954; 58:355–376.

82. Tucker DM, Sandstead HH, Logan GM, Klevay LM, Mahalko J, Johnson LK, Inman L, Inglett GE. Dietary fiber and personality factors as determinants of stool output. Gastroenterology 1981; 81:879–883.

83. Levine MD, Mazonson P, Bakow H. Behavioural symptom substitution in children cured of encopresis. Am J Dis Child 1980; 134:663–667.

84. Landman GB, Rappaport L, Fenton T, Levine MD. Locus of control and self-esteem in children with encopresis. J Dev Behav Pediatr 1986; 7:111–113.

85. Ehrentheil OF, Wells EP. Megacolon in psychotic patients. A clinical entity. Gastroenterology 1955; 29:285–294.

86. Burkitt DP, Walker ARP, Painter NS. Effect of dietary fibre on stools and transit times and its role in the causation of disease. Lancet 1972; ii:1408–1412.

87. Devroede G, Soffie M. Colonic absorption in idiopathic constipation. Gastroenterology 1973; 64:552–561.

88. Krishnamurthy S, Schuffler MD, Rohrmann CA, Pope CE. Severe idiopathic constipation is associated with a distinctive abnormality of the colonic myenteric plexus. Gastroenterology 1985; 88:26–34.

89. Vajro P, Silano G, Longo D, Staiano A, Fontanella A. Orocaecal transit time in healthy and constipated children. Acta Paediatr Scand 1988; 77:583–586.

90. Youle MS, Read NW. Effects of painless rectal distension on gastrointestinal transit of a solid meal. Dig Dis Sci 1984; 29:902–906.

91. Cann PA, Read NW, Brown C, Hobson N, Holdsworth CD. Irritable bowel syndrome: relationship of disorders in the transit of a single solid meal to symptom pattern. Gut 1983; 24:405–411.

92. Porter NH. Megacolon: a physiological study. Proc R Soc Med 1961; 54:1043–1047.

93. Callaghan RP, Nixon HH. Megarectum: physiological observations. Arch Dis Child 1964; 39:153–157.

94. Lawson JON. The soiling child. Practitioner 1975; 214:807–808.

95. Schandling B, Desjardins JG. Anal myomectomy for constipation. J Pediatr Surg 1969; 4:115–118.

96. Bentley JFR. Constipation in infants and children. Gut 1971; 12:85–90.

97. Suzuki H, Amano S, Honzumi M, Saijo H, Sakakura K. Rectoanal pressures and rectal compliance in constipated infants and children. Z Kinderchir Grenzgeb 1980; 29:330–336.

98. Schnaufer L, Taubert JL, Haller JA, Reid NCR, Tobon F, Schuster MM. Differential sphincteric studies in the diagnosis of anorectal disorders of childhood. J Pediatr Surg 1967; 2:538–543.

99. Arhan P, Faverdin C, Thouvenot J. Anorectal motility in sick children. Scand J Gastroenterol 1972; 7:309–314.

100. Tobon F, Schuster MM. Megacolon: special diagnostic and therapeutic features. Johns Hopkins Med J 1974; 135:91–105.

101. Schuster MM. Diagnostic value of anal sphincter pressure measurements. Hosp Pract 1973; 8:115–122.

102. Meunier P. Rectoanal dysynergia in constipated children. Dig Dis Sci 1985; 30:784A.

103. Misiewicz JT. Colonic motility. Gut 1975; 16:311–314.

104. Sullivan MA, Cohen S, Snape WJ. Colonic myoelectrical activity in irritable bowel syndrome—effect of eating and anticholinergics. N Engl J Med 1978; 298:878–883.

105. Preston DM, Lennard-Jones JE, Thomas GM. Towards a radiological definition of idiopathic megacolon. Gastrointest Radiol 1984; 10:167–169.

106. Bill AH, Johnson RJ, Foster RA. Anteriorly placed rectal opening in the perineum, "ectopic anus." A report of 30 cases. Ann Surg 1958; 147:173–179.

107. Hendren WH. Constipation caused by anterior location of the anus and its surgical correction. J Pediatr Surg 1978; 13:505–512.

108. Leape LL, Ramenofsky ML. Anterior ectopic anus: a common cause of constipation in children. J Pediatr Surg 1978; 13:627–629.

109. Kerremans PH, Penninck MA, Beckers PV. Functional evaluation of ectopic anus and its surgical consequences. Am J Dis Child 1974; 128:811–814.

110. Reisner SH, Sivan Y, Nitzan M, Merlob P. Determination of anterior displacement of the anus in newborn infants and children. Pediatrics 1984; 73:216–217.

111. Anuras S. Intestinal pseudo-obstruction syndrome. In: Cohen S, Soloway RD, eds. Functional disorders of the gastrointestinal tract. Contemporary issues in gastroenterology. Vol 6. New York: Churchill Livingstone, 1987: 139.

112. Frech RS. Aganglionosis involving the entire colon and a variable length of small bowel. Radiology 1968; 90:249–257.

113. Caniano DA, Ormsbee HS, Polito W, Sun C-C, Barone FC, Hill JL. Total intestinal aganglionosis. J Pediatr Surg 1985; 20:456–460.

114. Dykes EH, Guiney EJ. Total colonic aganglionosis. J Pediatr Gastroenterol Nutr 1989; 8:129–132.

115. Passarge E. Genetics of Hirschsprung's disease. Clin Gastroenterol 1973; 2:507–513.

116. Martin LW, Buchino JJ, LeCoultre C, Ballard ET, Neblett WW. Hirschsprung's disease with skip area. (Segmental aganglionosis). J Pediatr Surg 1979; 14:686–687.

117. De Chadarévian J-P, Akel S. Double zonal aganglionosis in long segment Hirschsprung's disease with a "skip area" in transverse colon. J Pediatr Surg 1982; 17:195–197.

118. Weinberg AG. Acetylcholinesterase and Hirschsprung's disease. J Pediatr Gastroenterol Nutr 1986; 5:837–843.

119. Todd IA. Adult Hirschsprung's disease. Br J Surg 1977; 64:311–312.

120. Howard ER, Garett JR, Kidd A. Constipation and congenital disorders of the myenteric plexus. J R Soc Med 1984; 77:13–19.

121. Udassin R, Nissan S, Lernau O, Hod G. The mild form of Hirschsprung's disease (short segment). Fourteen-years experience in diagnosis and treatment. Ann Surg 1981; 194:767–770

122. Cannon WB, Burket IR. The endurance of anaemia by nerve cells in the myenteric plexus. Am J Physiol 1913; 32:347–357.

123. Touloukian RJ, Duncan R. Acquired aganglionic megacolon in a premature infant: report of a case. Pediatrics 1975; 56:459–462.

124. Moore TC, Landers DB, Lachman RS, Ament ME. Hirschsprung's disease discordant in monozygotic twins: a study of possible environmental factors in the production of colonic aganglionosis. J Pediatr Surg 1979; 14:158–161.

125. Towne BH, Stocker JT, Thompson HE, Chang JHT. Acquired aganglionosis. J Pediatr Surg 1979; 14:688–690.

126. MacMahon RA, Moore CCM, Cussen IJ. J Pediatr Surg 1981; 16:835–839.

127. Schärli AF, Meier-Ruge W. Localized and disseminated forms of neuronal intestinal dysplasia mimicking Hirschsprung's disease. J Pediatr Surg 1981; 16:164–170.

128. Berdon WE, Baker DH, Blanc WA. Megacystis-microcolon-intestinal hypoperistalsis syndrome. A new cause of intestinal obstruction in the newborn: report of radiologic findings in five newborn girls. Am J Roentgenol Rad Ther Nucl Med 1976; 126:956.

129. Puri P, Lake BD, Nixon HH, Mishalany H, Claireaux AE. Neuronal colonic dysplasia: an unusual association of Hirschsprung's disease. J Pediatr Surg 1977; 12:681–685.

130. Feinstat T, Tesluk H, Schuffler MD, Krishnamurthy S, Verlenden L, Gilles W, Frey C, Trudeau W. Megacolon and neurofibromatosis: a neuronal intestinal dysplasia. Case report and review of the literature. Gastroenterology 1984; 86:1573–1579.

131. Carney JA, Hayles AB. Alimentary tract manifestations of multiple endocrine neoplasia, type 2b. Mayo Clin Proc 1977; 52:543–548.

132. Verdy M, Weber AM, Roy CC, Morin CL, Cadotte M, Brochu P. Hirschsprung's disease in a family with multiple endocrine neoplasia type 2. J Pediatr Gastroenterol Nutr 1982; 1:603–607.

133. Swenson O, Rathauser F. Segmental dilatation of the colon: a new entity. Am J Surg 1959; 97:734–738.

134. Brawner J, Schafer AD. Segmental dilatation of the colon. J Pediatr Surg 1973; 8:957–958.

135. Helikson MA, Schapiro MB, Garfinkel DJ, Shermeta DW. Congenital segmental dilatation of the colon. J Pediatr Surg 1982; 17:201–202.

136. Anuras S, Shirazi SS. Colonic pseudoobstruction. Am J Gastroenterol 1984; 79:525–532.

137. Smith B. Effect of irritant purgative on the myenteric plexus in man and the mouse. Gut 1968; 9:139–143.

138. Schuffler MD, Jonak Z. Chronic idiopathic pseudoobstruction caused by a degenerative disorder of the myenteric plexus: the use of Smith's method to define the neuropathology. Gastroenterology 1982; 82:476–486.

139. Mayne N. Neuropathy in diabetic and non-diabetic populations. Lancet 1965; 2:1313–1316.

140. Hamel-Roy J, Devroede G, Arhan P, Tetreault JP, Duranceau A, Menard HA. Comparative esophageal and anorectal manometry in scleroderma. Gastroenterology 1985; 88:1–7.

141. Whitehead WE, Taitelbaum G, Wigley FM, Schuster MM. Rectosigmoid motility and myoelectric activity in progressive systemic sclerosis. Gastroenterology 1989; 96:428–432.

142. Aaronson MJ, Freed MM, Burakoff R. Colonic myoelectric activity in persons with spinal cord injury. Dig Dis Sci 1985; 30:295–300.

143. Eckstein HB. Myelomengocele. In: Brett EM, ed. Pediatric neurology. Edinburgh, Churchill Livingstone, 1983: 385.

144. Brett EM. Intracranial and spinal cord tumours. In: Brett EM, ed. Pediatric neurology. Edinburgh, Churchill Livingstone, 1983: 430.

CHAPTER 10

Gastrointestinal Bleeding

Ravi Berry, M.D.
Jean Perrault, M.D.

Gastrointestinal (GI) hemorrhage in infants and children ranges from a worrisome to a panic-provoking acute episode. While this clinical situation has not changed over the years, advances in endoscopy and radiology, as well as new therapeutic modalities, permit us to pinpoint the cause of bleeding more easily and to treat it effectively. GI bleeding, however, can still be a catastrophic event and requires a team approach with prompt assessment, diagnosis, and treatment.

We will define the types of GI bleeding encountered, discuss the different settings in which GI bleeding can present and the diagnostic techniques available, and offer a plan of management. A separate section discusses special forms of GI bleeding, namely in the infant and in the immunosuppressed patient, and also the challenging problem of chronic occult bleeding.

Hematemesis is the vomiting of bright red blood or of denatured blood that can look like "coffee grounds"; usually this represents a bleeding source proximal to the ligament of Treitz. Hematochezia is the passage of bright red blood per rectum, indicating a lower GI source for the bleeding. This blood may precede or follow a bowel movement or be mixed with or coat the stool, or bleeding may occur independently of a bowel movement. The cathartic action of blood can cause an upper GI bleeding source to produce bright red blood per rectum; in this instance, the bleeding is massive, not simply streaks. The distinction is important when attempting to identify a source of bleeding. Perianal lesions such as hemorrhoids or fissures commonly coat the stool with bright red blood and may be accompanied by a hard bowel movement. Blood mixed with stool indicates a bleeding source higher up, whereas blood alone following a bowel movement points to the perianal area or the rectum, i.e., hemorrhoid or polyp. Blood with mucus in the stool suggests an inflammatory or infectious condition; currant jelly-like material indicates vascular congestion and hyperemia, as seen with intussusception. Maroon-colored stools indicate a voluminous bleed anywhere proximal to the rectosigmoid area. Melena, the rectal passage of black, sticky (tarry) stools representing denatured blood, suggests upper GI tract bleeding, although the bleeding site can be found distally in the right colon. These symptoms, because of their subjective nature, are only indirect predictors of the severity of the bleeding episode.[1] Nevertheless, frank hematemesis seems not only to indicate a large bleed, but also to warn of a likely recurrence, whereas melena alone represents less voluminous bleeding.[2]

Another important distinction is the "nonbleeding, bleeding episode." Spurious GI bleeds due to various ingested substances often provoke unnecessary panic. Red food coloring as in Jell-O, Kool Aid, amoxicillin and other medicines, and certain fruits and fruit juices like tomato, cranberry, and beets may look like blood when vomited or passed per rectum by a child who often has diarrhea. Bismuth, iron supplements, spinach, and dark chocolate may impart a dark coloration to stools, often mistaken for melena. *Serratia marcescens* causes a pink discoloration in diapers if some time elapses prior to their disposal.[3]

In other instances, true blood is recovered, but it does not necessarily originate from the GI tract. Blood can be swallowed during vigorous or nocturnal epistaxis, with resultant hematemesis or melena. In the pubertal female patient with apparent hematochezia, consider the onset of menarche.

PATHOPHYSIOLOGY

Not only does the GI tract cover a wide surface area, but it also benefits from a rich vasculature, in large part to provide enzyme secretion, osmotic balance, and appropriate absorption. It becomes immediately apparent that bleeding can occur anywhere along the GI tract from such sources as a venous ooze, an arterial "pumper," or a vascular malformation.

Acute GI bleeding presents suddenly, often unheralded by any symptom, although nonspecific symptoms such as weakness, fatigue, or pain might be mentioned. Hematemesis or hematochezia is the usual manifestation.

Chronic GI bleeding, on the other hand, presents primarily as lower GI tract bleeding. The patient may have recurrent melena or hematochezia or may present with recurrent heme-positive stools with or without anemia. In some patients, the blood loss is continuous and slow, with partial compensation of increased hematopoiesis. In others, there are recurrent episodes of blood loss accompanied by an acute fall in hematocrit. The bleeding site in all these patients, however, is usually identifiable.

In contrast, patients with obscure GI bleeding may also have either a continuous slow blood loss and anemia or acute episodes of bleeding of varying severity, all without an identifiable bleeding site, despite extensive and repetitive investigations. In others, the bleeding is occult, with chronic or recurrent iron deficiency anemia and heme-positive stools but no gross evidence of GI bleeding and no other identifiable site of blood loss. These are the patients who present the greatest diagnostic challenge and therapeutic dilemma. Table 1 presents examples of clinical conditions with acute, chronic, or occult bleeding; the classification is not exclusive, since some conditions can present differently at times.

A known underlying condition cannot always account for an episode of GI hemorrhage. For example, pre-existing esophageal varices are not necessarily the cause of blood loss in many bleeding patients with portal hypertension,[4,5] but this knowledge is still valuable in quickly orienting the evaluation. Similarly, many other conditions, if known or detected, can suggest an etiology to an otherwise challenging situation. One should look in particular for congenital or hereditary lesions, drugs, underlying medical conditions, and even external signs of child abuse.

Coagulopathies

Patients with hemophilia A or B (Factor VIII or IX deficiency) have a reported incidence of GI hemorrhage varying from 10 to 25 percent[6]; peptic ulcer disease and gastritis are the most frequent diagnoses. This applies to patients with moderate or severe factor deficiency; patients with mild factor deficiency do not seem to be at increased risk for bleeding. Other bleeding diatheses, including easy bruisability in family members, should be sought.

Patients on anticoagulants can be at increased risk for bleeding, especially if the dosage pushes the coagulation factors out of therapeutic range. The long list of medications that can affect coagulation factors or potentiate the effect of coumarin derivatives includes antibiotics (chloramphenicol, metronidazole, trimethoprim and sulfamethoxazole, in particular), phenytoin, barbiturates, and salicylates.[7]

Patients with chronic liver disease not only can develop portal hypertension with esophageal, gastric, and duodenal varices, but also can have a deficiency of many coagulation factors because of poor synthetic function; moreover, because of bile acid deficiency, these patients can have malabsorption of vitamin K.

Similarly, any malabsorption syndrome can be complicated by vitamin K deficiency with the potential for a bleeding tendency[8]; spontaneous bleeding from the GI tract would be unusual, but a potential bleeding site would bleed more briskly or more readily in the case of hypoprothrombinemia.

Portal Hypertension

When the portal flow is impaired, portosystemic shunts are spontaneously created that can result in the development of large venous channels in vulnerable locations such as the esophagus, gastric fundus, duodenum, and even as remote as the rectum.

Prehepatic lesions are more common in children than in adults, with portal vein thrombosis (e.g., after umbilical vein catheterization[9]) or splenic vein thrombosis (e.g., in chronic pancreatitis[10]). Certain fibrotic lesions of the liver give a similar picture (schistosomiasis, congenital hepatic fibrosis). In all these instances, the wedged hepatic pressure is normal.

Cirrhosis, whatever its cause, can be accompanied by portal hypertension; the wedged hepatic pressure is elevated. Obstruction of the normal flow of blood beyond the liver (suprahepatic portal hypertension) is less common, but is seen with hepatic vein obstruction, severe congestive heart failure, or pericarditis. We have seen patients with portal hypertension present with occult bleeding, but usually the bleeding is brisk, presenting as melena and/or hematemesis, and most of the time it is intermittent.

Vascular Lesions

A family history of chronic occult GI bleeding, repeated blood transfusions, and/or evidence of GI hemorrhage should alert the physician to the possibility of hereditary hemorrhagic telangiectasia (Osler-Weber-Rendu disease),[11] an autosomal dominant condition. In the younger patient, the typical skin lesions are notoriously absent at a time when GI bleeding manifests itself.[12] The Klippel-Trenaunay syndrome with characteristic limb deformities is another cutaneous vascular malformation with possible GI tract involvement[13,14]; these patients may develop hemangiomas of the intestine. Turner's syndrome can be complicated by telangiectasias of the GI tract[15]; moreover, these patients have an increased incidence of inflammatory bowel disease.[16] The identification or past history of hemangiomata[17,18] or blue rubber bleb nevi[19-21] on the skin suggests similar lesions of the GI tract.

The association of hypermobile joints, hyperextensible skin, and GI bleeding favor the diagnosis of a group of inherited disorders of connective tissue, the Ehlers-Danlos syndrome, especially type IV.[22,23] Endoscopy, and more specifically therapeutic endoscopy, has to be attempted with caution because of poor healing and the possibility of perforation.[24]

TABLE 1
Clinical Conditions Presenting with Acute, Chronic, or Occult Bleeding

Acute	Chronic	Occult Bleeding
Mallory-Weiss tear	Gastritis	Esophagitis
Esophageal varices	Infectious entero-	Telangiectasia
Peptic ulcer	colitis	
Meckel's	Inflammatory bowel	Cow, soy protein
diverticulum	disease	allergy
Intussusception		
Duplication cyst	Hemangioma	Blue rubber nevus
		syndrome
Hemolytic uremic	Peutz-Jeghers	
syndrome	syndrome	
Henoch-Schönlein	Nodular lymphoid	
syndrome	hyperplasia	
Intestinal infarction		
Necrotizing		
enterocolitis		
Juvenile polyps		
Hemorrhoids		
Anal fissure		

Pseudoxanthoma elasticum is another inherited disorder of elastic tissue; vascular lesions with GI bleeding occur in 10 percent of patients, although the exact location of hemorrhage might remain unidentified.[25,26]

Mucosal Lesions

In the upper GI tract, peptic ulcer disease is a frequent offender, from severe erosions and ulcerations of the esophagus secondary to gastroesophageal reflux to ulceration of the antrum and/or duodenum from *Campylobacter pylori* infection. A positive family history is obtained in 25 to 50 percent of young patients.[27] Acetylsalicylic acid (aspirin) is certainly the most frequently implicated medication in cases of GI tract bleeding; a common scenario is an episode of bleeding developing on the heels of an acute infectious episode during which aspirin was used, sometimes only once. Bleeding may arise from local erosions or diffuse gastritis which may be enhanced because of decreased platelet adhesiveness.[28-30] Nonsteroidal anti-inflammatory drugs (NSAIDs) of other classes are also known to cause erosions of the upper GI tract.[31] Whether corticosteroids have the same propensity remains debatable.[31-32] Chronic renal failure can be accompanied by bleeding from ulcerations or erosions of the GI tract[33,34]; the lesion is identifiable by endoscopy and improves with correction of the uremic state.

Inflammatory bowel disease is another important and frequent cause of bleeding, whether from an infectious or an idiopathic (Crohn's disease or ulcerative colitis) source. The bleeding is rarely massive but is often continuous from large surface areas, causing a gradual fall in hemoglobin.

Juvenile polyps can present with painless bright red blood in and on the stool; physical examination and laboratory screening are negative. A positive family history for multiple adenomatous colonic polyps may indicate familial polyposis, an autosomal dominant condition with mild rectal bleeding in children but frequent carcinomatous changes in young adults.[35] The identification of mucosal pigmentation in a young patient with intestinal polyps suggests the diagnosis of Peutz-Jeghers syndrome[36]; these hamartomatous polyps seldom progress to carcinoma.[37]

As already demonstrated in adult patients,[38] children with severe medical conditions requiring hospitalization in an intensive care unit have a propensity for upper GI tract bleeding,[39] especially those with central nervous system lesions[40] or with burns[41]; the lesions observed are either ulcers (so-called stress ulcers) or erosions.

Finally, prior suspicion of child abuse or external signs of physical abuse in a child with GI tract bleeding raise the possibility of an intramural hematoma of the intestine.[42]

GASTROINTESTINAL BLEEDING IN THE INFANT

The parent or care-giver facing an infant with GI bleeding is panic stricken, and with good reason: The blood volume is limited, the compensatory mechanisms are as yet immature, and the diagnostic approach is somewhat limited. The clinician's concerted approach should quickly focus on the infant and provide reassurance to the parents, since most instances of bleeding are self-limited, except of course for a few surgical conditions (Meckel's diverticulum, for instance).

Pathophysiology

Most of the information known in neonates with hemorrhagic shock has been gained through animal studies. Horton and Coln conducted studies in neonatal and older puppies[43] after inducing hemorrhagic shock and compared the results with similar studies in adult dogs.[43a] Neonatal puppies responded to a similar volume bleed with a more modest drop in blood pressure than did adult dogs. There was also a smaller reduction in the extracellular fluid compartment in the puppies (−27 percent) than in the dogs (−42 percent). Yet the puppies demonstrated an inadequate sympathetic-adrenal response to hypovolemia; bradycardia persisted, increase in systemic vascular resistance was inadequate, reduction in myocardial blood flow was sustained, while the reflex compensatory response to maintain coronary blood flow was inadequate. Myocardial contractility was impaired during shock, and importantly, persisted after resuscitative measures, possibly related to accompanying acidosis. These observations suggest a more precarious condition of the bleeding infant.

Assessment and Differential Diagnosis (Table 2)

As in older children, what appears as blood may not indicate bleeding in the infant. In the newborn, swallowed maternal blood explains 30 percent of instances of GI bleeding[44] and should be ruled out by the Apt-Downey test (see "Diagnosis"). A bleeding site on the nipple of a nursing mother

TABLE 2
Causes of Gastrointestinal Bleeding in the Infant

Source	Common	Less Common
Upper tract	Nasopharyngeal bleeding	Bleeding disorders
	Swallowed maternal blood	Duplication cyst
	Esophagitis	Foreign body
	Peptic ulcer	Tube trauma
	Gastritis	Vascular malformation
Lower tract	Anal fissure	Milk allergy
	Enteric infections	Pseudomembranous colitis
	Intussusception	Duplication cyst
	Upper GI source	Meckel's diverticulum
	Necrotizing enterocolitis	Enterocolitis with Hirschsprung's disease
		Gangrenous intestine
		Vascular malformation

might lead to traces of heme in the stool of a breast-fed infant. Finally, foods, coloring agents, and even bismuth[45] always need to be considered, especially when the infant looks fine.

In an otherwise healthy newborn infant, hemophilia or inherited coagulation factor deficits are rarely accompanied by bleeding unless other conditions are superimposed. Inquiry should be made of bleeding problems in other members of the family or of a difficult course or fatal outcome of previous pregnancies. Was the mother affected by any illness, especially infectious, during pregnancy?[46] Any medication taken by the mother or the infant should be carefully detailed; warfarin sodium, promethazine, and phenytoin cross the placenta, limiting an already immature production of vitamin K-dependent factors.[47,48] It is important to verify that vitamin K was indeed administered to a newborn, as it should be done prophylactically. On examination, petechiae and edema soon after birth suggest trauma from the delivery, whereas progressive petechiae and ecchymoses indicate a platelet defect. Diffuse bleeding, in particular from previous puncture sites, raises the specter of consumption coagulopathy and fibrinolysis (disseminated intravascular coagulation), usually complicating septicemia, varied infections, giant hemangiomas, or liver failure. If there is any abnormality in the prothrombin time, activated partial thromboplastin time, platelet count, or bleeding time, more specific factor determination and function studies should be undertaken.

Peptic ulcers or hemorrhagic gastritis is rare in the infant but may be more common in the newborn, particularly after a stormy delivery or possible asphyxia. Even more unusual is the instance of an ulcer induced by the tip of a catheter. Unfortunately, in either circumstance, perforation may complicate the clinical picture. A negative flat plate radiograph of the abdomen should be followed by upper GI endoscopy with a bronchoscope or pediatric endoscope,[49] but the presence of free air in the abdomen mandates surgery.

Esophagitis or esophageal ulcer occurs later in an infant with gastroesophageal reflux (GER). In spite of the frequency of GER, erosion or ulceration is quite rare. Barium studies of the esophagus are notoriously insensitive at demonstrating inflammatory changes; scintigraphy or pH monitoring studies can only confirm the presence or absence of reflux. Esophagoscopy is the procedure of choice. In an older infant, a foreign object lodged in the esophagus is always a consideration. A Mallory-Weiss tear at the gastroesophageal junction has also been described in an infant.[50]

Necrotizing enterocolitis usually manifests early after initiation of feeding but can present as late as 1 month after the start of oral intake of food.[51] The first signs include abdominal distention, decreased activity, and poor feeding, and it may develop into sepsis and shock. Pneumatosis intestinalis on a flat plate radiograph of the abdomen is very suggestive of the diagnosis.

Cow or soy milk protein allergy, whether induced directly[52-54] or indirectly through breast milk[55] or transplacental sensitization,[56] can cause occult blood loss or even frank colitis with gross bleeding. If the stool is positive for occult blood, the formula should be changed, unless another cause for the bleeding is identified, remembering that these patients are also prone to soy protein allergy.[57] When fecal leukocytes are also seen, gentle proctoscopic examination

should be done. Repeated challenges, done under close supervision, should be conducted only if the diagnosis is in doubt. The offending protein can later be reintroduced, usually by 18 to 24 months of age.

Many infectious agents, either bacterial (e.g., *Salmonella, Shigella, Yersinia enterocolitica, Campylobacter jejuni* or *coli*) or parasitic (*Entamoeba histolytica, Dientamoeba fragilis*), have the propensity to induce a colitis that is often indistinguishable from formula protein allergy or idiopathic inflammatory bowel disease. The bleeding is usually mild, with blood mixed with mucus and stool, but the patient can appear quite toxic. Stool culture and examination for parasites are essential. *Clostridium difficile* can also present with a similar clinical and endoscopic picture of diffuse colitis, but in the newborn period the identification of the agent and/or its toxin in stool is often considered normal, since certain nurseries have reported a recovery rate varying from 10 to 50 percent in otherwise healthy babies.[58-60] Although rare, idiopathic inflammatory bowel disease has been well described in infancy; the clinical picture and endoscopic appearance are similar to those of its counterpart in older patients, but the course often progresses rapidly to require surgical intervention.[61] Another diagnostic consideration in a young patient with a picture of colitis is Hirschsprung's disease, especially if constipation preceded the bleeding episode[62]; morbidity and mortality can be high with this complication.

A history of acute abdominal pain and passage of currant-jelly stool immediately suggest intussusception. The patient is often male, 6 to 18 months of age, with intermittent vomiting, bloody mucus per rectum, and a nondistended abdomen, sometimes with a mass in the right lower quadrant. If examination of the anus and rectum is negative, a barium enema should be done. Mesenteric vascular accidents, such as venous or arterial thrombosis, are quite rare and rarely hemorrhagic; these conditions should be considered in the setting of abdominal inflammation, shock, systemic embolization, or infants of poorly controlled diabetic mothers.

In all instances of bloody stools or diapers in an otherwise healthy infant, examination of the anus and anal canal should be meticulous to rule out a simple fissure, the most common cause of hematochezia. If the perianal examination is negative, proctosigmoidoscopy in infants is applicable and often rewarding.[63]

Treatment

Treatment should be both symptomatic and directed at the primary condition. The pediatric surgeon should be consulted early, although most cases of bleeding fortunately resolve with close medical attention. The cardiac and respiratory systems need close supervision, especially in the newborn. Oro- or nasogastric aspiration should be maintained in the patient with upper GI bleeding. Intravenous lines should be kept open with appropriate solutes; peripheral alimentation may be added if the infant is kept NPO. Blood transfusions may be given intermittently, 10 ml per kilogram, to maintain the hematocrit at 35 to 40 percent.

The younger infant should be monitored carefully for evidence of hypoglycemia, hypocalcemia, or metabolic acidosis. Neonates should remain under a warmer, as indicated by the measurement of skin or core temperature.

Antacids (1 cc per kilogram) and H$_2$-blockers have been used effectively in peptic ulcer disease. Specific therapy should be instituted in all the other clinical circumstances as soon as the diagnosis is made. There is as yet no experience with therapeutic endoscopy in the infant. For the rare neonate with uncontrollable bleeding from hemorrhagic gastritis, gastric devascularization was recently advocated.[64]

GASTROINTESTINAL BLEEDING IN THE IMMUNOCOMPROMISED HOST

The body is protected by a tightly woven, integrated system of specialized cells and proteins, collectively called the immune system. Nonspecific immunity is provided by the skin and mucosal surfaces, which serve as a barrier to the free penetration of antigens or organisms. More specific immunity comes from the interrelationship of the lymphocytes (T and B cells), the phagocytic cells, the complement proteins, and the major histocompatibility system, which actively and specifically recognize and then eliminate antigenic material.[65] A defect along any of these defenses may result in disease; the defect may be genetically determined (primary immune disorders[65-67]) or may be acquired through infection (acquired immunodeficiency syndrome [AIDS]), lymphoproliferative disorders, systemic diseases, or immunosuppressive agents (chemotherapy, steroids).[65] Through its direct exposure to the environment, and because of the rapid turnover of its surface epithelium, the GI tract is a frequent target in immunologic disorders, resulting in chronic diarrhea from varied organisms,[66,68-70] malabsorption,[66] and also bleeding. We will focus on some of the conditions, usually infectious, that can present with GI bleeding (Table 3).

Primary Immunodeficiency Disorders

Any branch of the immune system may be affected by a congenital defect, singly or in combination.

Isolated T- or B-Cell Defects

Agammaglobulinemia is an X-linked disorder in which severe pyogenic infections occur owing to the absence of B cells, but there is normal T-cell function. *Campylobacter fetus* ssp *jejuni* infection has been reported, with prolonged excretion of the agent, not responding to usual therapy.[66]

Hypogammaglobulinemia, a similar but somewhat less severe condition, presents later clinically and is sometimes associated with a T-cell defect. Herpes simplex esophagitis was described in one patient,[71] while in another patient melena requiring 1,500 ml of blood transfusion developed on a background of nodular lymphoid hyperplasia, but no definite cause was identified.[71] *Salmonella, Shigella,* and *Campylobacter fetus* infections have also been identified[66,72] as were Crohn's

TABLE 3

Infectious and Inflammatory Lesions with Potential Bleeding in the Immunocompromised Host

Type of Disorder	Infection	Tumors or Inflammation
Primary Disorder		
Agammaglobulinemia	*Campylobacter*	
Hypogammaglobulinemia	Herpes simplex	Nodular lymphoid
	Cytomegalovirus	hyperplasia
	Campylobacter	Crohn's disease
	Salmonella, Shigella	Ulcerative colitis
IgA deficiency		Nodular lymphoid
		hyperplasia
		Inflammatory bowel
		disease
Severe combined	*Candida*	
immunodeficiency	*Salmonella*	
disease		
Wiskott-Aldrich syndrome		Hemorrhagic enteritis
Ataxia-telangiectasia		Adenocarcinoma
		Lymphoma
Neutrophil Defects		
Chronic granulomatous	*Salmonella*	
disease		
Cyclic neutropenia		Neutropenic colitis
Secondary Disorder		
AIDS	Herpes simplex	Kaposi's sarcoma
	Cytomegalovirus	Necrotizing jejunitis
	Salmonella	
Post-transplantation		
Kidney	Herpes simplex	Colonic bleeding
	Cytomegalovirus	
	Clostridium difficile	
Liver	Cytomegalovirus	Intestinal ischemia
		EBV-related
		lymphoma
Marrow	*Candida*	Stress ulcers
	Cytomegalovirus	Neutropenic colitis
	Herpes simplex	
	Clostridium difficile	
Chemotherapy	Herpes simplex	Mucositis
	Cytomegalovirus	Neutropenic colitis
	Candida	

disease and chronic ulcerative colitis.[66,72] Cytomegalovirus (CMV) infection, another possible complication in this disorder,[70] can be difficult to differentiate from idiopathic inflammatory bowel disease.

Secretory IgA deficiency, a common immunodeficiency disorder, is often accompanied by nodular lymphoid hyperplasia; bleeding has reportedly occurred when the colon is involved.[73] Idiopathic inflammatory bowel disease has also been reported,[66,72] but both of these associations could represent the simultaneous occurrence of two relatively common diseases.

Combined T- and B-Cell Defects

Severe combined immunodeficiency disease is secondary to a stem cell defect. Esophagitis secondary to candidiasis has been described.[66,68] If *Salmonella* infection develops, bacteremia may ensue.[71,72]

Wiskott-Aldrich syndrome presents with eczema, recurrent infections, and thrombocytopenia; the latter may predispose to severe GI bleeding.[66,71,74] One case of mucocutaneous lymph node syndrome was also reported with hemorrhagic enteritis, possibly related to focal infarctions.[71]

Ataxia-telangiectasia develops early in life with the typical features of telangiectasia, ataxia, and variable immunodeficiency, not necessarily developing simultaneously. Adenocarcinoma or lymphoma of the GI tract is a feared complication.[66]

Neutrophil Defects

Chronic granulomatous disease is an inherited disorder (X-linked or autosomal transmission) with severe infections; granulomas may be found in certain tissues. *Salmonella* enteritis, with or without bacteremia, may be identified.[71,72]

Cyclic neutropenia is characterized by alternating periods of normal, low, and even absent granulocytes. Neutropenic colitis, a severe inflammatory lesion of the cecum and ascending colon, may lead to bloody diarrhea and at times perforation.[71]

Acquired Immunodeficiency Syndrome

Few disorders have received as much attention as AIDS in recent years, and yet the syndrome pursues its relentless course. All the systems, including the GI tract, are affected by a progressive deficiency of the T helper cells secondary to human immunodeficiency virus (HIV). The distinguishing features of the tumors (Kaposi's sarcoma or lymphoma) and a variety of opportunistic infections (viral, bacterial, fungal, and protozoan) help make the diagnosis. Indeed, tumors have been reported all along the GI tract, from the mouth[75] to the anorectal area,[76] although in children tumors of the GI tract are quite rare.[77,78] On the other hand, chronic infections are frequent causes of protracted diarrhea.[69,70,77] Certain infections are more likely to be accompanied by bleeding.

Herpes simplex virus (HSV) can involve the esophagus, causing a picture very similar to that of candidiasis[69,70]; endoscopic biopsies or smears should be done in each patient to distinguish the two agents.[69,79,80] HSV and another member of the herpes virus group, CMV, both cause proctitis,[68,70,77] in some cases presenting with a picture suggestive of pseudomembranous colitis.[70] CMV has been associated with esophagitis as well, and in either instance ganciclovir has reportedly provided clinical improvement.[81] *Salmonella* infections are also common,[70,72,79,80,82] especially with unusual types,[82] and the infection is often complicated by bacteremia.[80,82] An unusual segmental necrotizing jejunitis was described in a 5½-year-old boy with colicky pain, fever, and stools positive for occult blood.[77]

Immunosuppression Following Transplantation

Availability of organs and improved surgical techniques have contributed to the success of organ transplantation, but these accomplishments would not be possible without immunosuppressive agents. The major drawback of immunosuppressives relates to the frequency of opportunistic infections, but rarely these agent may be responsible for severe GI bleeding.

After renal transplantation, esophagitis has been observed after infection with HSV[83] or CMV infection.[70,83] *Clostridium difficile*–induced pseudomembranous colitis has also been described.[84] Early colonic bleeding after renal transplantation is a rare but severe complication[85]; its cause may be multifactorial.

Many opportunistic infections may occur after liver transplantation,[86-88] but bleeding from the GI tract is infrequent. One case of intestinal ischemia did contribute to the fatal outcome in a young patient.[86] A patient presented with rectal bleeding and was found at surgery to have a perforated rectum from EBV-related lymphoma.[88] Another patient developed perforation of the Roux-en-Y limb with mucosal ulcers from CMV infection.[88]

The GI tract is more frequently involved in the graft-versus-host disease (GvHD) occurring after bone marrow transplantation. Fungal infections are common,[70,89] and in some instances *Candida* may produce severe bleeding from erosions.[89] CMV and HSV can be isolated from the esophagus[90] or from gastric and duodenal lesions,[89] whereas the toxin of *Clostridium difficile* has been isolated in cases of pseudomembranous colitis.[89] Some patients seem more prone to stress ulcers,[89] whereas others go on to develop neutropenic colitis.[70,89]

Chemotherapy

Primary malignant tumors of the GI tract in children are relatively rare,[91,92] whereas leukemic infiltrates throughout the GI tract, often with bleeding, are more frequently reported.[93-96] Even more commonly cited are lesions of the GI tract from infections,[70,72] thrombocytopenia, or even direct effects of chemotherapeutic agents, often referred to as mucositis.[67,97]

The esophagus can be the site of bacterial,[95] viral (HSV[83,95] or CMV[70]), or fungal (usually *Candida*[70,95,97]) infections. Radiation directed to the mediastinum can also damage the esophagus, which in turn can predispose it to direct chemotherapeutic (e.g., Adriamycin) toxic effects.[98] The colon is also sensitive to radiation damage, with subsequent proctocolitis, but the most feared complication is the neutropenic colitis, or typhlitis,[70,93-95,99] a severe inflammatory lesion of the right colon and cecum in particular, with bleeding and possible perforation; because the integrity of the bowel wall is altered, bacteremia often develops. In spite of the severity of the lesion, surgery is only rarely indicated.[94]

ASSESSMENT

In the acutely bleeding patient, assessment and data gathering must be co-ordinated with stabilization and initial management. A team approach, including a special care nurse, pediatrician, pediatric surgeon, and intensivist, can most effectively deliver such care by integrating early stabilization and therapeutic efforts with ongoing information gathering, patient examination, and diagnostic and therapeutic procedures. The history can be as brief or as detailed as the clinical setting dictates. It helps to characterize the bleeding episode and to define the condition of the patient when the bleeding occurred: any dizziness or fainting, the nature and probable site of bleeding (upper versus lower GI); whether it is fresh or denatured blood, whether it is blood alone or blood mixed with emesis or stool, and whether there were accompanying or preceding symptoms like emesis, diarrhea, or pain.

The initial physical examination is directed toward assessing the stability of the patient; a rapid pulse and orthostatic hypotension attest to the severity of the condition. Decompensation can set in rapidly and prove catastrophic. Once the patient has been stabilized or deemed stable, a more complete examination can follow.

Diagnosis

Even in the most favorable clinical circumstances, the GI evaluation of a child may be difficult; orifices have to be penetrated and probed, usually with uncomfortable instruments. The situation can be even more dramatic in a bleeding child who is already frightened, not only by the sight of blood, but by anxious parents and appropriately overattentive medical care workers. Moreover, the physician realizes that close attention has to be paid to vital signs throughout the investigation, and thus a sphygmomanometer is placed on one arm and an intravenous line on the other, and a nasogastric tube is often inserted, along with other monitoring devices. Psychosocial considerations are important in approaching the patient. A compassionate physician will achieve much with a friendly smile coupled with a gentle approach.

The history will help determine if it is truly blood that has been passed, but if questions remain as to the nature of the red streaks or the black discoloration, biochemical analysis can rapidly bring an answer. In gastric fluids, Gastroccult (SmithKline Diagnostics, Sunnyvale, CA 94086) provides the most reliable confirmation of blood, mainly because of its advantage over Hemoccult (SmithKline Diagnostics) in an acidic environment.[100]

The stool analysis can be performed on a specimen retrieved by rectal examination, using orthotolidine or guaiac (Table 4); the peroxidase contained in hemoglobin leads to oxidation of the reagent, resulting in a blue discoloration. With orthotolidine (Hematest, Ames Company), a fecal smear is placed on a filter paper; a Hematest tablet is placed in the specimen and a drop of water is placed on the tablet, followed 5 to 10 seconds later by a second drop of water. The water gradually permeates the paper; if a blue color appears within 2 minutes, the test is positive. The guaiac reaction has been successfully developed into a convenient kit (Hemoccult). A small stool specimen is smeared on one side of the guaiac-impregnated paper and two drops of a developing solution (hydrogen peroxide in denatured ethyl alcohol) are applied on the reverse side; again, a blue discoloration appearing within 60 seconds indicates a positive reaction.

Hemoccult II (SmithKline Diagnostics) has the added advantage of including a positive control to check the developing solution. The guaiac test is less sensitive than the orthotolidine test, but both are sufficiently sensitive to detect blood in the stool. Peroxidases are present not only in human hemoglobin, but also in animal blood and in myoglobin, so that a false-positive reaction can be obtained in a patient who recently ate red meat. Moreover, iron preparations[101] and certain plant peroxidases can also give a false-positive test, whereas large doses of ascorbic acid can inhibit the reaction.[102] In the past few years we have been using a new assay, HemoQuant (SmithKline Diagnostics) (Table 4). The chemical reaction depends on the fluorescence of porphyrin, derived from hemoglobin after removing iron.[103] Not only is it more specific, but its reaction includes the already converted porphyrin from the action of bacterial and other enzymes on heme along the GI tract. Moreover, it is also a quantitative test, not just qualitative, with a normal value of 2 mg Hb per gram of stool identified in 98 percent of normal volunteers (less than 4 mg Hb per gram of stool in patients on salicylates or a red meat diet).[104] It was hoped that this new technique would help differentiate proximal and distal GI bleeding by measuring the intestinal converted fraction and the total fecal hemoglobin separately, but the technique has not yet proved reliable.[105]

The history can also help in determining whether the site of bleeding is in the upper or lower GI tract, but more precise localization should not be expected without further evalu-

TABLE 4
Tests for Occult Blood in Stool

Test	Reagent	Result	False Positive	False Negative
Hematest (Ames Co)	Orthotolidine	Qualitative	Red meats Iron preparations Plant peroxidases	Ascorbic acid
Hemoccult (SmithKline Diagnostics)	Guaiac	Qualitative	As above, plus cimetidine	Hard stool Penicillamine Antacids Ascorbic acid
HemoQuant (SmithKline Diagnostics)	Fluorescence of porphyrin	Quantitative	Red meats	—

ation. Hematemesis localizes the bleeding above the ligament of Treitz. Streaks of blood in and/or on the stool limits the bleeding to the colon, but massive red blood in the stool can originate anywhere along the GI tract, since blood is a cathartic. Similarly, melena or maroon stool could originate in the upper GI tract or on the right side of the colon, depending on the transit time. Importantly, however, melena usually indicates a loss of blood of at least 200 ml.[106]

The approach to diagnosis depends largely on the presenting symptoms and their severity. In the following, we will describe each method of diagnosis and its application.

Evaluation for Fetal Red Cells (Apt-Downey Test)

Indication. Bleeding in a newborn. Test will determine whether red cells are fetal or maternal in origin.

The principle behind this test is that adult hemoglobin, eluted from erythrocytes, is denatured to alkaline globin hematin in an alkaline milieu with a resultant yellow-brown solution, whereas fetal hemoglobin resists the effect of alkali and imparts a pink coloration to the solution.[107]

Procedure.

1. One part bloody stool (or gastric aspirate) to five parts water in a test tube to lyse the erythrocytes.
2. Centrifuge at 2,000 rpm for 1 to 2 minutes to separate the fecal material.
3. Filter or decant the supernatant hemoglobin solution.
4. Mix 1 ml of 0.25 N (1 percent) sodium hydroxide with 5 ml of the hemoglobin solution.
5. Read the color change after 2 minutes (remains pink with fetal Hb; changes from pink to yellow-brown with adult Hb).

A control test with the newborn's blood will give an estimate of the presence of adult Hb in the infant, if any.

Note that the test should not be done with denatured blood (melena or coffee ground aspirate) because the oxyhemoglobin has already been changed to hematin and will be falsely read as representing adult Hb. A similar test can be done with an acid.[108]

Nasogastric Tube

Intubation of the upper GI tract is easily done, is accompanied by discomfort in the first 5 to 10 minutes, but is well tolerated if it needs to stay in longer. Selecting a tube with the largest bore tolerable and with a decompressing lumen (e.g., Salem sump, Sherwood Medical, St. Louis, MO 63103) is preferable. With the patient in the left lateral position (the tip of the tube often lodges in the fundus), the gastric contents are aspirated with a syringe. If the returns are clear or bilious, the bleeding is not coming from the nasopharynx, esophagus, or stomach. This does not rule out a bleeding duodenal lesion, however. A few streaks of blood recovered amid clear secretions could represent vigorous aspiration only; similarly, detection of occult blood in a grossly nonbloody gastric aspirate with Hemoccult or Hematest does not imply upper GI tract bleeding because these tests are very sensitive and a positive result could indicate very mild oozing from

the aspiration. At this point, the tube can be removed unless fresh or old blood is discovered, in which case the tube can be used to aspirate the gastric contents before endoscopy or to prevent gastric dilatation from continued bleeding. However, in a group of adult patients with negative returns, 16 percent were found to have a lesion at endoscopy.[109] If the returns are voluminous, a large bore tube (e.g., Edlich tube from Monoject, Sherwood Medical, or Mini Lavage Kit, Ethox Corporation, Buffalo, NY 14204) can be substituted in the older child to clear the stomach of clots.

A Sengstaken-Blakemore (SB) tube, or one of its modifications,[110] can be used diagnostically in a patient bleeding acutely and profusely, especially a patient known to harbor varices. The tube is available in a pediatric size or can be adapted for a young child.[111] In brief, this is a multilumen tube with (1) a gastric aspiration site, (2) a gastric balloon proximal to the aspiration site, (3) a longitudinal esophageal balloon to exert tamponade, and (4) a proximal esophageal aspiration site on the more recent variants; a separate naso- or oroesophageal tube has to be used with the original SB tube (see "Management—Therapeutic Modalities"). Once the gastric balloon is inflated and in place, a gastric aspirate that reveals fresh blood while the esophageal aspirate is dry indicates gastric or duodenal bleeding; gastric and esophageal aspirates that are dry or yield only old blood imply that the bleeding site was at the fundus, now under tamponade; if fresh blood returns from the esophageal aspirate, then the patient is bleeding from an esophageal lesion and the esophageal balloon can be inflated if varices are known. The most common error is too little tension in the gastric balloon, permitting oozing from the fundus or passage of blood from the esophagus down into the stomach, causing bloody gastric aspirates. A physician should be present at all times during the diagnostic use of this complicated tube, since even in experienced hands complications can occur frequently.[112] Upper GI endoscopy should be planned as soon as the medical condition stabilizes.

Upper GI Endoscopy

Indications. Hematemesis or aspiration of fresh or old blood from the stomach; also melena or passage of large amounts of blood per rectum. The test can rule out an actively bleeding lesion in the upper GI tract.

The introduction of fiberoptic endoscopes has radically changed the investigation of GI bleeding and more recently the approach to treatment since the addition of therapeutic modalities. Most of the endoscopes now in use have a four-way deflection tip for easier handling and a larger channel for better aspiration or for introduction of instruments (e.g., biopsy cable, foreign body retrievers). In the neonate and infant, the fiberoptic bronchoscope, with a very small external diameter but only a two-way deflection tip, is used preferentially for safety reasons, since a larger scope can lead to serious respiratory problems by compressing the trachea.

The clear advantages of fiberoptic endoscopy in upper gastrointestinal bleeding include direct visualization of lesions, many of which remain undetectable by conventional contrast radiography[113-116]; determination of the bleeding lesion when more than one lesion is identified[117]; application of therapeutic modalities such as sclerotherapy or laser therapy (see "Management"); and the immediate use of other diagnostic modalities if no lesion is found, whereas 2 or 3 days may be lost in clearing the intestinal tract of contrast material when barium is used.

In the pre-endoscopic era, 20 to 50 percent of the bleeding sites remained unidentified,[44,118] whereas most authors using fiberoptic endoscopes now report identification of more than 80 percent of the bleeding sites.[116,119,120] Even if blood and clots remain in the stomach at the time of the examination, it is important to do the endoscopy early to increase the chances of making a diagnosis[121]; the position of the patient can be changed to expose the mucosa after movement of the retained contents. When comparing the results of diagnostic studies before endoscopy was available with results gained from endoscopy (Table 5), the percentage of unknown diagnoses dropped from 50 to 20 percent, and most of these were mucosal lesions such as gastritis or esophagitis. In Table 6, data were collected from four studies in which comparisons could be made between contrast radiography and endoscopy in the diagnosis of mucosal lesions or ulcers. In the same patients, radiographs identified 18 percent of the mucosal lesions and 55 percent of the ulcers, but endoscopy diagnosed 100 percent of the mucosal lesions and 94 percent of the ulcers. In a national survey of members of the American Society of Gastrointestinal Endoscopists,[122] 269 physicians reported consecutive patients with upper GI bleeding seen during an 18-month period. They reported 2,255 patients of all ages with at least one bleeding episode, requiring blood transfusions in at least 75 percent of them. Forty-one percent of the patients were identified at endoscopy to have a mucosal lesion that probably would not have been seen by conventional radiography.

The diagnostic capabilities of the procedure are undeniable, but until recently, obtaining a more precise diagnosis did not seem to influence the requirements for blood transfusion or to decrease the mortality rate from upper GI bleeding.[123-126] These conclusions will likely be revised as therapeutic endoscopy with thermal probes or laser is gaining in popularity. Even if active bleeding had stopped at the time of endoscopy, the procedure can provide important information to determine if the lesion has the potential for rebleeding.[127]

TABLE 5
Upper GI Bleeding in Children: Diagnosis in the Pre-endoscopic and Endoscopic Era According to Age

Age (yrs)	Pre-endoscopy[118]		Endoscopy[120,121]		
	1	2–12	<2	2–7	7–18
Number of patients	90		32	26	41
Esophagitis	—	—	9	5	4
Mallory-Weiss syndrome	—	—	2	1	0
Gastritis	—	—	6	2	6
Varices	—	11	0	3	4
Gastric ulcer	8	9	2	6	5
Duodenal ulcer	10	7	6	4	13
Unknown	45 (50%)		7	5	9
Death	(70%)			(18%)	

TABLE 6
Upper GI Bleeding in Children: Comparison of Contrast Radiography (X-Ray) and Esophagogastroduodenoscopy (EGD) in Detecting Lesions

Type of Disorder	Number of Patients	Number Positive	
		X-Ray	EGD
Esophagitis, gastritis[113,114,120]*	28	5 (18%)	28 (100%)
Ulcers[27,113,114]*	38	21 (55%)	36 (94%)

* References in the text.

Upper endoscopy in children is safe in expert hands.[113,114,116,128] In the acutely bleeding patient, all resuscitative measures need to be applied before endoscopy can be undertaken. Some children can be examined endoscopically without anesthesia if they are guided appropriately by competent and friendly gastrointestinal assistants; many need sedation,[129] or even general anesthesia.[115] Complications should remain below 1 percent, whether routine or emergency upper GI endoscopy is performed, and are related to sedation (thrombophlebitis and respiratory arrest), to general anesthesia, or to the procedure itself (sore throat, aspiration pneumonia, or rare perforation).[115,116,130]

Lower Endoscopy

The examination of the lower GI tract can be as limited as anoscopy or as extensive as complete colonoscopy with distal ileoscopy.

Anoscopy. This procedure is indicated in wipe bleeding or passage of blood on or separate from stool. A special head can be fitted on the handle of a traditional otoscope, permitting easy and adequate visualization of the anal canal. A large number of bleeding lesions can be identified with this simple technique.[131]

Rigid Proctoscopy. The test is cumbersome and very uncomfortable to children and now has little indication for use, except perhaps to remove foreign objects. It has been replaced by flexible proctosigmoidoscopy.

Flexible Proctosigmoidoscopy (FPS). This procedure is indicated in patients passing blood on or mixed in the stool. The instruments have benefited from the same technology that has given us gastroscopes and colonoscopes. The instruments were designed for examination of the adult rectum and sigmoid colon but all are well suited for the child; they range in length from 30 to 65 cm.[132] Although it can induce mild mucosal changes, an enema should certainly be used when the ampulla is full with solid material, preferably 30 minutes before the procedure; enema kits in pediatric and adult sizes are readily available. Very mild sedation, such as diazepam by mouth, may be used 45 minutes before the procedure; the patient rarely reaches somnolence but feels more relaxed during the procedure. With FPS, the patient is placed in the left lateral position, and one parent can remain at the head of the table to provide comfort, if needed. In children, introduction of the full 60-cm scope can permit visualization up to the splenic flexure. All types of bleeding lesions can be easily identified by this means,[131] and biopsies are readily obtainable, if indicated. Perforation, particularly in the sigmoid colon, is a rare but feared complication.

Colonoscopy

Indications. Blood in the stool when FPS is negative; melena or severe bleeding if no evidence of upper GI tract lesions; examination of the terminal ileum if Crohn's disease is suspected.

The fiberoptic colonoscopes have a demonstrated superiority to barium examination in bleeding of the GI tract[117,133]; they are available in a wide variety of models, and in young children a fiberoptic gastroscope can be used for total colonic examination. In most instances, therapeutic modalities such as biopsy, electrocautery, and polypectomy can also be undertaken when indicated.[134] Preparation of the colon is of crucial importance to permit satisfactory visualization of the mucosa. The recent development of poorly absorbable electrolyte polyethylene glycol solutions[135] or the use in large quantities of electrolyte solutions[136] has permitted excellent evacuation of the colonic contents with few or no complications. In addition, the electrolyte polyethylene glycol preparation does not predispose to the risk of colonic explosion if electrocautery is used. Sedation is preferable to general anesthesia to limit the risk of perforation by allowing the patient to respond to increased pressure; supervision of the patient by a nurse or a trained assistant during the procedure is mandatory. Although total colonoscopy is often indicated, the procedure may be stopped once a bleeding lesion is identified. In experienced hands using the proper technique, perforation is unlikely; because the colon is thinner in young patients, precautions have to be taken during biopsies, electrocautery, or laser treatment. Sedation has to be titrated carefully to prevent respiratory depression, remembering that the effect of meperidine can be reversed by naloxone.

Intraoperative Endoscopy

The introduction of endoscopy in the operating room has expanded the application of the endoscopic techniques for both the upper and lower GI tracts.[137] In an emergency situation, when the patient is bleeding massively and needs immediate surgery, upper GI endoscopy can rule out esophageal lesions and may even direct the surgeon to a gastric or duodenal bleeding site, whereas a negative proctosigmoidoscopy can also provide valuable information.

When the diagnosis remains elusive in a young patient with evidence of continued bleeding and explorative surgery is contemplated, intraoperative endoscopy should also be considered. After proper anesthesia, the gastroscope or colonoscope is inserted into the stomach, then the abdomen is opened. The endoscope is pushed through the pylorus, at which time the surgeon can locate the tip of the instrument. The intestine is gradually telescoped over the endoscope while the endoscopist tries to identify mucosal lesions otherwise not easily reachable by conventional means.[138] Alternatively, if the colon has been adequately prepared, a gastroscope/colonoscope can be introduced into the colon and the lower small intestine can be gradually telescoped over the endoscope.

The development of a long enteroscope with easy maneuverability to permit intubation of the entire small intestine should obviate this practice. For now, only a few models are in limited use[139-141]; after the tip of the instrument is introduced into the upper small bowel, it is left in place for the contractions of the small intestine to gradually propel it to the distal ileum. At that point, it is slowly pulled back while the endoscopist surveys the mucosa for any abnormality. At present, poor control of the tip of the instrument and absence of biopsy facilities remain limiting problems.[142]

Scintigraphic Studies

Because the site of bleeding is not always apparent and bleeding is often intermittent, scintigraphic studies have now been adapted to help in the detection of aberrant gastric mucosa or in the confirmation of a bleeding site along the GI tract.

^{99m}Tc-Pertechnetate Scan (Meckel's Scan)

Indications. For identification of functional gastric mucosa in an ectopic location, i.e., Meckel's diverticulum or duplication cyst of the GI tract.

The agent used, technetium-99m pertechnetate, is injected intravenously; it is loosely bound to plasma proteins and accumulates in functional gastric mucosa, including the stomach and ectopic locations.[143,144] After the injection, the patient is placed supine under a gamma camera for anterior images of the abdomen, with a field that includes the stomach superiorly to the bladder inferiorly.[144] Images are obtained sequentially, usually every 5 minutes for 1 hour. A Meckel's diverticulum often presents as an abnormal focal collection in the mid-abdomen or right lower quadrant; a duplication cyst can be spotted anywhere in the abdominal field. Not only is the test noninvasive, but the gamma camera is also available in a portable model, making it an ideal screening test for a young patient in the intensive care unit. Since more than 90 percent of bleeding Meckel's diverticula contain gastric mucosa,[143] the scan should be very useful in that condition, but there are reports of as many as 20 percent false-positive or false-negative results (Table 7).

Conditions such as ureteral obstruction or sacral meningomyelocele can be very misleading because radionuclear

---

TABLE 7
False Results with Meckel's Scan

False-positive, nonbleeding lesion
    Ureteral obstruction
    Sacral meningomyelocele

False-positive, bleeding lesion
    Intussusception
    Hemangioma
    Arteriovenous malformation
    Inflammatory lesions (Crohn's disease)
    Peptic ulcer

False-negative
    Barium
    Bladder overdistention
    No gastric mucosa in diverticulum

activity accumulates in these areas and appears as a focal lesion on the scan, producing a false-positive result. On the other hand, other false-positive images obtained from such lesions as an arteriovenous malformation,[145] hemangioma, or inflammatory mass can be rewarding in that a potential bleeding lesion is identified, even though the final diagnosis is not an ectopic mucosa.

False-negative scans usually result from the absence of functional gastric mucosa in the diverticulum or duplication cyst, or a background that will simulate a focal image, as seen with an overdistended bladder or with retained barium.

99mTc-Labeled Red Cells (Bleeding Scan)

Indications. To better localize an intermittently bleeding site, thereby orienting the endoscopist or angiographer.

Lesions of the GI tract may bleed only intermittently, in small volumes, or at sites not easily reachable with the endoscope, thus requiring a sensitive noninvasive technique to orient the clinician in the continued evaluation of the patient.

Technetium-99m has been identified as a reliable marker. 99mTc–sulfur colloid is quite sensitive,[146,147] but its half-life is very short (2½ minutes) so that after 10 minutes only 10 percent of the radionuclide remains in circulation; moreover, it is rapidly concentrated in the reticuloendothelial system, thereby gradually obscuring the background. These factors dictate that the test be done during the stage of active bleeding.

99mTc-albumin[148] is easily and rapidly prepared, an advantage in briskly bleeding patients, but the elution of the agent is rapid, thus limiting its use in patients bleeding intermittently. 99mTc-labeled red blood cells provide an accurate and sensitive approach to both the briskly and the intermittently bleeding patient.[149-151] Over 95 percent of technetium is bound to red cells, thereby confining the label to the intravascular space; since it is not absorbed or degraded, identification of the radionuclide in the GI tract implies bleeding. In dog studies, it is possible to detect a bleeding rate of less than 0.1 ml per minute.[152] In humans, Smith et al[151] estimated that a bleeding rate greater than 0.1 ml per minute would give a positive scan, with more intense activity associated with a greater bleeding rate. These figures compare very favorably with a minimum bleeding rate of 0.5 ml per minute for positive angiography. With the bleeding scan, a sample of the patient's own red cells is labeled with 99mTc and reinjected into the blood stream,[153] and a gamma camera takes images of the abdomen every 5 minutes for the first hour, then at regular intervals until a potential site is suspected, or for as long as 24 hours if no site of bleeding has yet been identified. Once extravasation of the marker is detected on the scan, further imaging can demonstrate accumulation of the labeled red cells in the GI tract, more convincing evidence of bleeding. In controls, Winzelberg et al[149] noted progressive activity over the spleen, liver, and great vessels in all instances and over the kidneys, stomach, and bladder in 60 percent, 50 percent, and 40 percent of patients, respectively. After 24 hours, colonic activity can be detected in 50 percent of the controls who had gastric uptake initially, a possible cause of a false-positive scan. In patients with lower GI hemorrhage, these authors[149] determined that a minimum bleeding rate of 500 ml per 24 hours was necessary in order to obtain a positive scan; the greater the blood transfusion requirements, the more quickly the scan was positive. When positive, the scan should be followed by angiography or endoscopy. If the scan is negative, however, angiography should be delayed.[154] An incidental benefit of the 99mTc red blood cell study might be the demonstration of a Meckel's diverticulum with ectopic gastric mucosa, as was recently reported in a 2-year-old child,[155] or the localization of the bleeding site in hemolytic uremic syndrome[156] or intestinal hemangioma.[157] The total body radiation exposure is 0.2 rad with 99mTc-labeled red cells, less than an upper GI radiograph. However, surgery should not be planned on the basis of positive scintigraphy alone; further characterization of the site of bleeding with endoscopy or angiography should be done.

Angiography

Indications. Actively bleeding lesion or chronic or recurrent bleeding not otherwise identified by other tests.

The main requirement before considering angiography is that the estimated rate of bleeding be at least 0.5 ml per minute[158]; if a radionuclide bleeding scan is negative, angiography should be delayed.[154] In chronic GI bleeding, however, angiography has identified a potential bleeding site in approximately 50 percent of patients, adults[159,160] or children,[161] even without ongoing active bleeding.

Heavy sedation or general anesthesia is used. Through a femoral artery approach, a fine catheter is guided through selected arteries of the mesenteric system and their branches, if necessary. Once the catheter is in place, contrast medium (with iodine) is injected and filming is done in very rapid sequence. As the contrast agent is taken away, the arterial arborization and then the venous return route become visible, although with decreasing clarity due to dilution. Extravasation of the dye into the GI tract indicates a bleeding lesion, a mucosal "blush" represents a vascular lesion, and an early venous return identifies an arteriovenous malformation.[159]

Meyerovitz and Fellows[161] applied the technique to 14 acutely bleeding children (less than 17 years old) and correctly identified a site of bleeding in 10 patients but also obtained false-negative results in four patients. In nine patients who were actively bleeding, true-positive diagnoses were made in six, whereas four of five acute bleeders, not actively bleeding at the time of angiography, had true-positive findings. Once a bleeding lesion is identified, the catheter can be left in position for therapy (selective infusion of pitressin or embolization)[161] or for accurate identification of the site of bleeding during surgery, when methylene blue can be injected through the catheter.[137]

Good urine output and normal renal function are necessary to prevent renal damage from the contrast agent. Excellent compression over the site of entry of the catheter reduces the risk of hematoma.

How to Use the Diagnostic Tests

In order to provide quick and meaningful treatment, an accurate diagnosis is essential, helped by proper use of the different diagnostic modalities. Before invasive tests are employed, the presence of blood can be confirmed by the Gastroccult test in gastric secretions or by Hemoccult or HemoQuant in stool.

Upper GI Bleeding. A history of hematemesis or nasogastric aspiration of fresh or old blood is indicative of an upper GI bleeding lesion. If the bloody gastric aspirate gradually clears, upper GI endoscopy should lead to the diagnosis. Upper GI endoscopy should also be the first test used in a patient with melena, in spite of a negative gastric aspirate, to rule out a duodenal lesion.

In massive bleeding, resuscitative measures are mandatory. Continuous nasogastric suction can prevent gastric distention, and in a patient with known esophageal varices, the Sengstaken-Blakemore tube should be used preferentially, not only to achieve tamponade but also to help in localizing the site of bleeding. Once the bleeding is controlled and the patient is stabilized, upper GI endoscopy should be performed. If the bleeding persists and the condition of the patient deteriorates, endoscopy can be performed in the operating room to orient the surgeon more precisely. When the condition of the patient remains stable but there is continued active bleeding, a bleeding scan and/or angiography can be safely undertaken.

Lower GI Bleeding. Most cases of lower GI bleeding are mild to moderate, permitting a co-ordinated approach to diagnosis. The identification of leukocytes in the stools suggests an infectious or inflammatory condition and a stool specimen should be sent for identification of parasites and culture. A flexible sigmoidoscopy is then performed, and, if negative, colonoscopy can follow to visualize the whole colon and the terminal ileum.

If melena or maroon stool is the presenting symptom and upper GI endoscopy is negative, colonoscopy is the next step. If the diagnosis remains elusive, a Meckel's scan or a bleeding scan may suggest a bleeding site, to be confirmed by angiography during active bleeding.[162]

Occult Bleeding. The most frustrating condition facing the clinician is the patient with chronic iron deficiency anemia, without gross evidence of blood loss. The symptoms may be limited to pallor or fatigue, as recently described in an adolescent runner.[163]

The first step is the confirmation of blood in the stool by using the qualitative Hemoccult[102] or the quantitative HemoQuant test.[103–105] Neither test will indicate whether the bleeding is originating in the upper or lower GI tract, although with the HemoQuant test efforts are made to identify the intestinal converted fraction (heme already converted to porphyrin by the action of bacteria or other enzymes) separately from the freshly derived porphyrin.[105] It may be necessary to check stool samples at different intervals to confirm bleeding. Contrast (barium) radiography of the GI tract will follow; if a suspicious lesion is identified, confirmation can be obtained by gastroscopy or colonoscopy. If radiography is negative, it should be followed by gastroscopy and colonoscopy; in a few selected instances, enteroscopy should be considered.[140,141] In the few cases in which all these tests are unrevealing, angiography can be used to advantage, even if bleeding is not severe or active. In 11 children with chronic GI bleeding,[161] six (55 percent) had true-positive angiograms; this experience parallels a previous study by Sheedy et al in adult patients.[159] In both studies, vascular malformations were common.

When the diagnosis remains enigmatic in spite of all the above efforts, sugical exploration, including perioperative endoscopy, may be indicated if the occult bleeding is persistent.

MANAGEMENT

The approach to management of GI bleeding implies a knowledge of the different degrees of severity of presentation, conveniently divided into four classes by the American Trauma Association (Table 8).[164] The major concern is for the child who has bled significantly, presenting in shock or impending shock secondary to hypovolemia and a decrease in the overall oxygen-carrying capacity of the blood. This is manifested by hypotension with reduced arterial systolic, diastolic, and mean blood pressures. Tachycardia is observed initially with pallor, a weak pulse, and often a mildly cyanotic tinge to the skin. Extremities may be cool as a result of poor peripheral perfusion. Oliguria, when present, results from renal hypoperfusion due to a shift of blood volume from the peripheral and splanchnic beds to the central circulation. In a late stage, mental confusion may develop secondary to central nervous system hypoperfusion. Many of these known compensatory mechanisms have been observed and reproduced in animal experiments with interesting findings. An excellent review of the pathophysiology of shock in the pediatric patient is concisely presented by Wetzel in the *Textbook of Pediatric Intensive Care*[164a]; some highlights are included in the following discussion.

Pathophysiology of Acute Bleeding

After hemorrhaging down to 50 percent of normal mean arterial pressure, animals demonstrate a rise in blood pressure back toward baseline. This lasts 30 to 60 minutes, and in some animals the baseline blood pressure may be restored after several hours. In most others, unless resuscitation measures are instituted, the initial transient rise is followed by a progressive and ultimately irreversible fall in blood pressure resulting in death.

TABLE 8
Classification of Shock (in Adult Patients) According to the Subcommittee on Advanced Trauma Life Support of the American College of Surgeons[164]

Class 1	Blood volume loss ≤15%
	Normal blood pressure
	Pulse increased 10–20%
	Capillary refill unchanged
Class 2	Blood volume loss 20–25%
	Tachycardia >150 beats/min
	Tachypnea 35–40/min
	Prolonged capillary refill
	Decreased systolic and pulse pressure
	Orthostatic hypotension
	Urine output >1 ml/kg/hr
Class 3	Blood volume loss 30–35%
	Signs as in Class 2
	Urine output <1 ml/kg/hr
	Lethargy
Class 4	Blood volume loss 40–50%
	Pulses nonpalpable
	Obtunded patient

In another experiment,[164a] animals were allowed to exsanguinate into a constant-pressure reservoir until the blood pressure dropped to between 30 and 40 percent of control and then was allowed to remain constant. For the first or second hour the animals continued to lose blood, indicating vasoconstriction as the initial response to hypovolemia. Thereafter, the flow was reversed, going from the constant-pressure reservoir to the animal, implying vasodilatation. If at this point the low blood pressure persists for several hours, there is an accelerated fall in arterial pressure, leading to death despite massive transfusions. This inexorable deterioration in hemodynamic function represents irreversible shock.

From clinical experience in humans, it has been learned that hypotension and hypovolemia incite several compensatory responses. Right-heart filling pressures are initially maintained through increased systemic vascular resistance; blood flow is diverted from the peripheral and splanchnic beds to the central circulation to maintain adequate oxygenation of the central nervous system and the myocardium. When cerebral perfusion pressure falls below 40 mm Hg, cerebral blood flow also falls, causing a massive sympathetic discharge. Vagal activity increases, with a resultant bradycardia and worsening of the hypotension, especially in infants whose cardiac output depends more on heart rate than on stroke volume. Hypovolemia results in a reduced venous return and a reduced preload to the heart. Cardiac output falls, but blood pressure is initially maintained. Release of ADH and activation of the renin-angiotensin system cause salt and water retention from the kidney to help restore the intravascular volume. This is perhaps the most potent humoral response to hypovolemia. Another response to hypovolemia is an "autotransfusion" from the extracellular and intracellular compartments to the intravascular compartment, mostly at the microcirculatory level along Starling forces.[164a] The volumes involved can reach up to 15 cc per kilogram per hour in adults following an acute intravascular volume depletion. This, however, slows down considerably as the hematocrit and the colloid oncotic pressure in the intravascular compartment drop.

If the blood loss continues or even if it stops but 30 to 35 percent of the blood volume has been lost and the hypovolemia remains uncorrected, irreversible shock can result, with hypotension, anuria, and respiratory and cardiac failure.

Hypotension is a late manifestation of hypovolemia in children. Initially there is a minor fall in systolic blood pressure due to a fall in stroke volume, but an increase in peripheral vascular tone causes an increase in diastolic blood pressure with only a minor fall in pulse pressure. As the compensatory mechanism fails, diastolic blood pressure falls with a rapid fall in mean arterial pressure and a major hemodynamic compromise.

Previously healthy children without pre-existing cardiovascular disease compensate well initially following acute blood loss. They may appear alert with a stable blood pressure, mild tachycardia, and good color soon after hemorrhage, and it is at this stage that they can most effectively be treated for hypovolemia. Owing to the very real possibility of rapid deterioration, a high index of suspicion is required, with compulsive and repetitive monitoring, best provided in the intensive care (ICU) setting. Expectant treatment to prevent circulatory collapse should be promptly initiated with continuous monitoring. This is especially important in younger infants and neonates, in whom clinical assessment is fallible and hemodynamic reserves and compensatory mechanisms are inadequate.

Stabilization

Initial assessment should be directed toward the single vital question: Is shock imminent or present? One approach is to meet with the patient and parents in the emergency room (or at the bedside if the patient is already hospitalized) and as the parents are giving the details of the bleeding episode, the physician and nurse are obtaining the vital signs and ensuring good venous access. Blood can be drawn at that time for emergency studies and blood typing and crossmatching. Fluids and/or colloids can then be started; diagnostic procedures follow appropriate resuscitation. Table 8 lists the classification of shock according to approximate loss of blood and accompanying systemic symptoms and signs in adult patients according to the Subcommittee on Advanced Trauma Life Support of the American College of Surgeons.[164] Mildly ill patients (class 1 or less, no anemia, associated minor systemic signs and symptoms, obvious and minor source of bleeding, no ongoing blood loss) can be discharged to outpatient follow-up but must be followed until complete resolution of symptoms. Moderately ill patients (class 2, associated systemic signs and symptoms, ongoing blood loss, all newborns with GI bleeding regardless of associated findings) should be admitted to the hospital for further evaluation and close observation. Severely ill patients (class 3 or 4, toxic or obtunded, other systemic signs and symptoms, ongoing blood loss) should be admitted to the ICU after initial stabilization. An initial hematocrit of less than 20 percent, a hemoglobin less than 7 gm per deciliter, or a transfusion requirement equal to or exceeding total calculated blood volume prior to surgical intervention and without a recognized active bleeding site are all indications of poor outcome.[120] Presence of an associated coagulation disorder or other systemic disease is also indicative of a poor prognosis.[120]

Initial stabilization is directed toward preventing or treating hypovolemia and restoring the hematocrit to acceptable levels in order to maintain adequate tissue oxygenation. The importance of IV access cannot be overemphasized,[120] especially in the apparently stable patient in whom shock is often delayed; if shock should develop, this usually simple procedure becomes technically difficult precisely at a time when rapid access is critical. It is imperative, therefore, that a large-bore peripheral IV line (and at least two in class 2 to 4 patients), or preferably a central line, be placed and secured.[165] The aim of initial bolus fluid administration is to improve tissue perfusion. To this end an initial fluid bolus of 10 to 20 cc per kilogram is given over 10 minutes, and further boluses are later titrated to maintain adequate blood pressure and tissue perfusion. The choice of fluid for IV bolus is best based on convenience and accessibility; the choice between colloid and crystalloid remains controversial.[166-168] If more than 50 to 70 cc per kilogram is required over 4 to 6 hours, invasive monitoring should be considered to facilitate fluid management.[164a]

In the patient with 20 to 25 percent blood loss (class 2) oxygen is administered via a face mask or nasal cannula to maintain an intra-arterial oxygen saturation of 95 percent or more. Considering the metabolic derangements secondary to hypovolemia, acute hypocalcemia, possible hypothermia, or hypoxia, the initial evaluation should include a complete blood count (hemoglobin, hematocrit, red blood cell count, white blood cell count, differential, and platelets), serum calcium, serum electrolytes, anion gap and pH, arterial blood gases, prothrombin time and partial thromboplastin time, and, if indicated clinically, serum fibrinogen degradation products and fibrinogen.

While hypovolemia is being corrected, restoration of proper hematocrit should be attempted. If blood transfusion is needed urgently (class 2 patients with hemorrhage, class 3 and 4 patients), group O blood can be used until type-specific blood is available (Table 9). Packed red cells with low anti-A, anti-B titers are preferred over whole group O blood to further reduce the risk of hemolysis, since switching to type-specific blood after beginning the transfusion with group O whole blood has been reported to lead to hemolysis due to passively transfused anti-A and anti-B antibodies.[169] Blood for typing and crossmatching must be drawn before any transfusion to eliminate subsequent difficulties. In some emergency situations in which the patient's blood type is known, type-specific unmatched blood has been used without major complications,[170] provided that a sample of blood from that patient has been typed by that hospital within 48 hours. Errors have been made because the parent or the patient gave the wrong information or the patient was carrying false documents. An immediate spin (saline) crossmatch detects clinically important ABO system antibodies and takes only 15 minutes, while a more complete crossmatching takes 45 to 90 minutes.[171]

Stored red blood cells have more than 70 percent survival at 24 hours following transfusion,[172] implying that approximately 30 percent are excessively fragile and are lysed in the reticuloendothelial system, releasing hemoglobin and potassium. Stored red blood cells also have reduced 2,3-DPG and therefore an enhanced affinity for oxygen. Oxygen delivery to tissue already compromised by a low hematocrit is thus further impaired.[174] A rewarming pump should be used as soon as it is available to avoid hypothermia and a resultant increase in energy expenditure, increased potassium release from tissues, increased oxygen affinity of hemoglobin, and increased ventricular irritability. Whole blood may also introduce microaggregates into the recipient circulation, possibly causing pulmonary problems.[175-177] "Washing" takes 24 to 48 hours and is not feasible in emergency situations[175]; moreover, the unit of blood is outdated in 24 hours. Some authors have therefore suggested using ultrafresh whole blood drawn less than 4 hours prior to use.[177] Availability is currently a problem and the need unproven.

Other blood products such as packed red blood cells, platelets, fresh frozen plasma, and cryoprecipitate are available for use in specific clinical situations.

Continuous monitoring should be initiated in patients with class 2 or higher blood loss. While re-emphasizing the unquestioned importance of repetitive physical examination to check capillary refill, color, distal extremity warmth, pulse rate, respiratory rate, blood pressure, mental status, and overall appearance, it remains that by definition this is an intermittent assessment, however frequently it is done. The nature of the derangement in GI hemorrhage is dynamic, with moment-to-moment alterations causing significant changes that can be missed if not continuously monitored. At the very least, this would consist of an ICU monitor displaying constant ECG, heart rate, and respiratory rate; a urinary catheter can be used to monitor urinary output. Blood pressure is an extremely important parameter to assess status and therapeutic response, and many instruments are available.[178-182] The major problem with noninvasive monitoring lines is the lack of complete correlation with intra-arterial values and the unmonitored time lapse between measurements. Direct arterial measurements are usually 5 to 20 mm Hg higher than indirect measurements (if it is the other way around, the cause is usually a technical problem or faulty calibration). In hypothermia or hypotension, the indirect measurements may falsely read 20 to 30 mm Hg lower.[178]

Direct continuous monitoring using intra-arterial lines is preferred in the patient requiring intensive care.[183] Electronic monitors automatically read and display the highest pressure

TABLE 9
Blood Transfusions in the Acutely Bleeding Patient

Type	Availability	Comments
Group O	Immediate	Draw blood for typing and crossmatching before transfusion Give packed red cells with low anti-A, anti-B titers
Specific (e.g., A, AB), unmatched	Immediate	Provided that blood type had been determined by that hospital within 48 hours
Immediate spin (saline) crossmatch	15 min	Detects most clinically important ABO system antibodies
Complete crossmatch	45–90 min	Safest blood transfusion (other than autologous)

every 3 to 7 seconds, but disparities of more than 30 mm Hg can occur in catheter manometry systems, especially in the presence of tachycardia. The increased heart rate causes the harmonic components of the pressure wave to approach the resonance frequency of the system, causing "systolic overshoot." These problems can be minimized by careful technique to ensure a bubble-free and clot-free tubing using the stiffest and shortest possible length of arterial line. An ideal cannulation site, therefore, would be a large vessel, which would more accurately reflect the true systemic blood pressure. It should have sufficient collateral flow to distal tissues in the event of thrombotic blockage, and when the upper extremity is selected, it should be the nondominant side.

In severe shock requiring prolonged administration of IV fluids, a central venous pressure (CVP) line has been traditionally held to be helpful in fluid management.[184] In acute hemorrhagic shock, the central filling pressure does not accurately reflect intravascular volume. After pure hemorrhagic shock, CVP is low (0 to 1 mm Hg) despite adequate intravascular filling, and attempts to restore CVP to the upper range of normal (5 to 10 mm Hg) could be deleterious, with possible volume overload and tissue edema.[164a] In pure hypovolemic shock, careful clinical evaluation of capillary refill, urine output, blood pressure, and respiratory pattern may serve just as well. If myocardial and renal functions are compromised, then a CVP line can be helpful in regulating IV fluid administration.

In severe shock with myocardial compromise, a Swan-Ganz catheter can be very helpful to monitor CVP as well as cardiac output, pulmonary arterial pressure, and capillary wedge pressure.[185,186] Measurement of the ventricular output and the filling pressures of each ventricle delineates their functional characteristics, and measurements of cardiac output in children by this method have been shown to be reliable over a wide range of values.[185–187] Using this information, fluid administration can be titrated to meet tissue metabolic demands while maintaining a pulmonary capillary wedge pressure within normal limits to prevent extrusion of fluid into the pulmonary interstitial space. Use of catecholamine pressors for preload augmentation can be an adjunct to correction of hypovolemia and of the underlying etiology for the shock state.[188,189]

Therapeutic Modalities

Whatever the cause of bleeding, the specific goal is to provide therapy, either symptomatic or directly aimed at the bleeding site. It is traditional in the presence of blood from nasogastric aspirates to use iced saline lavage in an effort to stop the bleeding. Not only is its efficacy unproven, but it has been demonstrated to have deleterious effects. Since the goal of gastric lavage is more commonly the evacuation of blood and blood clots to permit better visibility during endoscopy, tap water at room temperature would meet the goal equally well.[190] In a study in dogs, iced gastric saline lavage recovered only 14 percent of the blood while 32 percent of the saline was not recovered.[190] Nicoloff et al[191] demonstrated in humans that a large amount of the lavage fluid is passed into the intestine. If the goal is to reduce or stop the hemorrhage, then iced saline might in fact do more harm than good. Waterman and Walker[192] demonstrated that with cooling, bleeding time increases to three times control, clotting time increases by 60 percent, and the prothrombin time is prolonged to more than twice control. Cold therefore appears to alter the clotting mechanism. Moreover, Menguy and Masters[193] demonstrated in rabbits that during hypovolemic shock the gastric mucosa was more susceptible to stress ulceration, with reduced gastric blood flow as the probable etiology. In addition, cooling causes reduced tissue oxygenation due to a shift of the hemoglobin-oxygen dissociation curve to the left.

Iced saline lavage therefore has been demonstrated to be harmful for gastric hemostasis and mucosal integrity and no more effective than tap water at room temperature for removing clots. In addition, it imposes on the pediatric patient a further risk of hypothermia, with resultant cardiac conduction and metabolic derangements. It is only logical, then, that it be abandoned in favor of saline or tap water at room temperature for the express purpose of diagnosis and clot removal. When large clots are present, a large-bore tube should be passed orally with the patient in the left lateral decubitus position. Pharyngeal anesthesia and intravenous sedations may be safely administered, especially with an agitated and combative individual. Oral suction should be readily available at the patient's bedside to remove any regurgitated material.

With the advent of therapeutic endoscopy, lavage with epinephrine or metaproterenol has been used in an attempt to provide a better field of vision by decreasing the bleeding transiently; the results are equivocal.

Intravascular infusion of vasoactive agents has been popularized following the successful use of selective arteriography in localizing the site of bleeding. Vasopressin has been the agent of choice, but with time it has become evident that intra-arterial injection is not without complications[194] and intravenous infusion is just as effective.[195,196] Vasopressin, 0.2 to 0.4 unit per 1.73 sq m per minute administered by continuous IV infusion, has been especially useful in prehepatic portal hypertension, Mallory-Weiss tear, and stress-induced gastritis. It reduces cardiac output and arterial blood flow through the splanchnic bed with a resultant fall in portal vein pressure. Arrhythmias, hypertension, oliguria, and seizures due to water retention from antidiuretic hormone effect have accompanied its use, so the patient should be carefully monitored. Analogues of vasopressin have also been used.[197,198]

Somatostatin has recently been advocated for upper GI hemorrhage owing to its action in reducing gastric blood flow and inhibiting gastric acid and gastrin production,[199] although one study did not confirm any benefit over placebo in upper GI hemorrhage.[200] Somatostatin has been found to be as effective as vasopressin with fewer complications in cirrhotic patients with variceal hemorrhage.[201]

Balloon Tamponade

Since the initial report by Sengstaken and Blakemore in 1950,[202] the Sengstaken-Blakemore tube and its modifications[203] have been a mainstay in initial therapy of persistent variceal hemorrhage. It has also been used for

Mallory-Weiss tears with persistent bleeding. In its original form, it consists of a triple-lumen tube to which are attached an esophageal and a gastric balloon, with the third lumen serving to aspirate intragastric contents. The esophageal and gastric balloons can be independently inflated to varying volumes. The tube comes in adult and pediatric sizes and if a pediatric size is not available, an adult size can be modified for adequate, although careful, pediatric use using heat-labile tubing to alter the size of the esophageal balloon.[111] Each balloon should be inflated and tested prior to use. It is passed through the nose or mouth into the stomach with the patient sitting; the intragastric contents are aspirated and the gastric balloon is inflated with the appropriate amount of air (range: 120 to 240 cc). The tube is gradually withdrawn until the gastroesophageal junction offers resistance and the position is maintained with traction by taping it to the nose or to the mouthpiece of a football helmet. At this point, a flat plate radiograph of the upper abdomen ensures that the gastric balloon is in proper position (the diaphragmatic leaflet and the balloon seem to juxtapose). If the esophageal balloon need not be inflated, a nasoesophageal tube should be positioned in the lower esophagus to provide appropriate drainage of blood that might accumulate. To inflate the esophageal balloon, a manometry system is used to accurately monitor the pressure used for tamponade (approximately 30 to 40 mm Hg). In this instance, the nasoesophageal draining tube is pulled out just above the esophageal balloon and kept on suction. Even in competent hands, serious complications have been reported in up to 20 percent of patients.[203,204] These are usually associated with malpositioning, resulting in upper airway obstruction from migration of the esophageal balloon into the hypopharynx due to traction on the tube, especially with an underinflated gastric balloon. Excessive pressures carry the risk of esophageal ulcer and perforation. The esophageal balloon should be decompressed in 12 to 24 hours. If fresh bleeding recurs, the esophageal balloon is reinflated and rechecked in 6 hours. Up to 24 hours of continuous use may be safe, but the incidence of mucosal damage increases with duration of use. The patient should be adequately sedated during this time for both comfort and compliance. Cough, if persistent, should be suppressed to prevent repetitive and sudden increases in intra-abdominal pressure. If bleeding stops, the esophageal balloon can be deflated, followed by deflation of the gastric balloon in 12 to 24 hours. The completely deflated tube is left in place overnight as a precaution in case rebleeding occurs.

The Linton-Nachlas tube can be used for adequate tamponade of gastric varices.[205] It has a gastric balloon capacity of 600 cc for use in adults, and inflation volume can be varied according to age.[206] Traction is maintained after inflation, using the same vigilance as with the SB tube. Similar balloon devices have been designed for tamponade of bleeding duodenal ulcers, a recent report described a flexible but noncollapsible, balloon fitted over the distal 7 cm of an end-viewing endoscope with an attached thin tube for inflation of the balloon.[207] This balloon is inflated to systolic pressure after placement under direct vision and the endoscope removed. This was left overnight in two adult patients, with complete hemostasis in both. One patient had minor rebleeding that resolved spontaneously.

If bleeding persists from esophageal varices despite SB tamponade, direct obliteration of the varices can be done using a sclerosing solution.

Sclerotherapy

This was first described in 1939 by Crafoord and Frenckner using a rigid endoscope,[208] but it is more commonly done now with a flexible endoscope to inject the sclerosing solution either directly into the varix or alongside it.[209-213] Remaining varices should be sclerosed at weekly[212-213] or monthly[209] intervals until total obliteration is achieved. Follow-up at 6 months is recommended for inspection and reinjection. Various complications are encountered with this procedure, even in experienced hands, with a complication rate of 5.8 percent in the Van Stiegmann and Stellin study[212] (esophageal perforation 0.7 percent, esophageal mucosal sloughing 0.7 percent, esophageal stricture 2.2 percent, left pleural effusion 1.5 percent) and 4.2 percent in the study of Howard et al[210] (esophageal ulceration 2.4 percent, esophageal stricture 1.7 percent). Other reported complications range from disturbances of esophageal motility to a single case report of thoracic spinal cord paralysis in a 4-year-old girl[214]; development of gastric or rectal varices after sclerosis of esophageal varices has been reported.[211,213] Rebleeding is a constant concern until sclerotherapy completely obliterates the varices. This technique does not preclude a surgical procedure in the future.

Obliteration of bleeding lesions (e.g., vascular malformations and bleeding peptic ulcers) with sclerosing solutions has also been reported.[216,217] Much more experience with this procedure is needed before recommending its routine use in children, but it appears safe and effective in adults.

Thermal Coagulation

Thermal coagulation should be considered in the presence of a visible vessel, especially with active bleeding such as spurting or streaming. A visible vessel may be found in any ulcer crater or may be exposed in a Mallory-Weiss tear. It may appear as a frankly protruding artery, an elevated red dot (sentinel clot), or densely adherent to a clot sitting within the crater.[218] The risk of rebleeding from an inactive visible vessel approaches 60 percent.[219]

Heater Probe. This involves the use of a probe consisting of a Teflon-coated hollow aluminum cylinder with an inner electronic heating coil. It has the advantage of providing tamponade as well as heat for coagulation. Water may be simultaneously injected to clear the field. Power is computer controlled for a precise regulation of the probe temperature.[220] The probe must be pushed directly and firmly into the bleeding point to effectively tamponade it. Coagulation is produced after three to four pulses. If the bleeding does not stop, the probe is repositioned and the process is repeated.[221] Its relative ease of operation, its portability, and its low complication rate[222] make it a valuable technique.

Electrocoagulation

Electrocoagulation utilizes electrical current passing through the target tissue to produce coagulation. The monopolar probe was the first device to be used. The electrical current takes a deep path, resulting in a fairly deep zone of tissue coagulation. Pooled secretions and debris may unfortunately dissipate any coagulation energy. Tissue often adheres to the probe, also reducing its efficacy. It has been largely abandoned because of these problems and because it demonstrated no added efficacy over other available probes. The BICAP (bipolar circumactive probe, ACMI, Stamford, CT) completes an electrical circuit between two electrodes 1 to 2 mm apart which are in contact with the bleeding site.[221,223] The multipolar probe has six electrode plates designed to minimize the depth of thermal penetration, thereby reducing the risk of perforation.[221] The paths taken by the electrical current through the tissue are shallow, and the power generator has limited voltage to prevent sparking. Tissue heating is self-limited; as the heated tissue dries out, electrical resistance increases and current flow drops. Initial experience with adults looks very promising.[221,223]

Each of these probes uses pressure application as well as heat, all the while controlling the depth of coagulation by the pressure applied and the amount of energy delivered. They stop bleeding effectively,[224] produce limited tissue injury, and are cheap and portable.[225] These approaches have been effective in bleeding lesions of both the upper and lower GI tract.[226,227]

Laser Photocoagulation

Laser photocoagulation requires no contact with the bleeding site. This is especially advantageous during active bleeding and in fragile lesions such as vascular malformations. The laser energy is transmitted via the endoscope using a flexible quartz fiber. The monochromatic light energy is transmitted to the tissue at low power, which creates heat and causes coagulation of its proteins.[223,228] Two devices are available. The Argon laser is absorbed by hemoglobin and produces a superficial coagulation; therefore, its use in bleeding lesions is limited.[223] The Nd:YAG (neodymium:yttrium-aluminum-garnet) laser penetrates the tissue to a greater depth (3 to 4 mm) and is not absorbed by hemoglobin; therefore, the presence of blood does not interfere with its use.[223,226] Laser effectively delivers endoscopic thermal therapy but is expensive, is not readily portable, and requires considerable expertise to obtain consistent results. There is the potential risk of causing a full-thickness injury to the gut wall resulting in perforation, especially in the cecum. Considering the relative lack of experience in children and in the thinner gut wall, its use remains a concern.[229] Studies comparing these modalities with each other and the depth of injury to the gut wall in the pediatric population need to be critically evaluated.

From what is currently known from the adult literature, it is reasonable to assume the following for children with GI bleeding:

1. The use of these endoscopic techniques should be restricted to the acutely bleeding patient or the patient with a high risk of rebleeding.[218,219]
2. Local injection of epinephrine 1:10,000 seems to offer some control of the hemorrhage[224,225] and improves the results with polar probes or laser therapy.[224]

3. The heater probe is one of the simplest techniques to use, combining tamponade and heat, but hemostasis takes longer to achieve. Accurate positioning of the probe is crucial to successful hemostasis.
4. The bi- or multipolar probes also use tamponade and are reasonable alternatives.
5. Laser needs more expertise for its use, is not portable, is quite expensive, and therefore is currently used more commonly for polypectomy or obliteration of vascular lesions of the upper and lower GI tract in children.[230]

After therapeutic endoscopy, the patient is kept NPO until stable and then gradually advanced to a soft, bland diet. H_2-blocker and cytoprotective agents are continued for at least 6 weeks, with further prophylactic use in those who have bled severely.

Surgery

The assistance of the pediatric surgeon should be sought from the early moments of the evaluation. Even though a bleeding child rarely requires surgery, the assistance of the surgeon is invaluable. A few conditions do require surgery (e.g., Meckel's diverticulum, duplication cyst), but surgery should also be considered for the severely bleeding child with continued blood transfusion requirements or for the child with undiagnosed persistent or recurrent bleeding.

REFERENCES

1. Oshita Y, Okazaki Y, Takemoto T, et al. What are the signs of recent hemorrhage and what do they mean? Criteria for massive bleeding. Endoscopy 1986; 18:11–14.
2. Northfield TC, Smith T. Haematemesis as an index of blood loss. Lancet 1971; i:990–991.
3. Green M. Rectal bleeding. In: Pediatric diagnosis: interpretation of symptoms and signs in different age periods. 3rd ed. Philadelphia: WB Saunders, 1980: 345.
4. Sutton FM. Upper gastrointestinal bleeding in patients with esophageal varices: what is the most common source? Am J Med 187; 83:273–275.
5. Hillemeier C, Gryboski JD. Gastrointestinal bleeding in the pediatric patient. Yale J Biol Med 1984; 57:135–147.
6. Mittal R, Spero JA, Lewis JH, et al. Patterns of gastrointestinal hemorrhage in hemophilia. Gastroenterology 1985; 88:515–522.
7. O'Reilly RA. Anticoagulant, antithrombotic and thrombolytic drugs. In: Gilman AG, Goodman LS, Rall TW, Murad F, eds. The pharmacological basis of therapeutics. 7th ed. New York: Macmillan, 1985: 1344.
8. Berezin S, Newman L, Russe J. Hemorrhage and shock due to intestinal malabsorption. Pediatr Emerg Care 1986; 2:91–92.
9. Alvarez F, Bernard O, Brunelle F, et al. Portal obstruction in children. I. clinical investigation and hemorrhage risk. J Pediatr 1983; 103:696–702.
10. Grendell JH, Cello JP. Chronic pancreatitis. In: Sleisenger MH, Fordtran JS, eds. Gastrointestinal disease: pathophysiology, diagnosis, management. 3rd ed. Philadelphia: WB Saunders, 1983: 1502.
11. Vase P, Grove O. Gastrointestinal lesions in hereditary hemorrhagic telangiectasia. Gastroenterology 1986; 91:1079–1083.
12. Mestre JR, Andres JM. Hereditary hemorrhagic telangiectasia causing hematemesis in an infant. J Pediatr 1982; 101:577–579.
13. Servelle M, Bastin R, Loygue J, et al. Hematuria and rectal bleeding in children with Klippel and Trenaunay syndrome. Ann Surg 1976; 183:418–428.
14. Schmitt B, Posselt HG, Waag KL, et al. Severe hemorrhage from intestinal hemangiomatosis in Klippel-Trenaunay syndrome: pitfalls in

diagnosis and management. J Pediatr Gastroenterol Nutr 1986; 5:155–158.

15. Grumbach MM, Conte FA. Disorders of sexual differentiation. In: Wilson JD, Foster DW, eds. Textbook of endocrinology. 7th ed. Philadelphia: WB Saunders, 1985: 341.

16. Price WH. A high incidence of chronic inflammatory bowel disease in patients with Turner's syndrome. J Med Genet 1979; 16:263–266.

17. Abrahamson J, Shandling B. Intestinal hemangiomata in childhood and a syndrome for diagnosis: a collective review. J Pediatr Surg 1973; 8:487–495.

18. Boley SJ, Brandt LJ, Mitsudo SM. Vascular lesions of the colon. Adv Intern Med 1984; 29:301–326.

19. Fretzin DF, Potter B. Blue rubber bleb nevus. Arch Intern Med 1965; 116:924–929.

20. McCauley RGK, Leonidas JC, Bartoshesky LE. Blue rubber blev nevus syndrome. Radiology 1979; 133:375–377.

21. Wong SH, Lau WY. Blue rubber-bleb nevus syndrome. Dis Colon Rectum 1982; 25:371–374.

22. Beighton PH, Murdoch JL, Votteler T. Gastrointestinal complications of the Ehlers-Danlos syndrome. Gut 1969; 10:1004–1008.

23. Pinnell SR, Murad S. Disorders of collagen. In: Stanbury JB, Wyngaarden JB, Fredrickson DS, Goldstein JL, Brown MS, eds. The metabolic basis of inherited disease. 5th ed. New York: McGraw-Hill, 1983: 1434.

24. Sykes EM. Colon perforation in Ehlers-Danlos syndrome. Report of two cases and review of the literature. Am J Surg 1984; 147:410–413.

25. Morgan AA. Recurrent gastrointestinal hemorrhage: an unusual cause. Am J Gastroenterol 1982; 77:925–928.

26. Case records of the Massachusetts General Hospital. Scully R, Mark EJ, McNeely BU, eds. N Engl J Med 1983; 308:579–585.

27. Nord KS, Rossi TM, Lebenthal E. Peptic ulcer in children. The predominance of gastric ulcers. Am J Gastroenterol 1981; 75:153–157.

28. Fromm D. Salicylate and gastric mucosal damage. Pediatrics 1978; 62:938–942.

29. Graham DY, Smith JL. Aspirin and the stomach. Ann Intern Med 1986; 104:390–398.

30. Levy M, Miller DR, Kaufman DW, et al. Major upper gastrointestinal tract bleeding. Relation to the use of aspirin and other nonnarcotic analgesics. Arch Intern Med 1988; 148:281–285.

31. Domschke S, Domschke W. Gastroduodenal damage due to drugs, alcohol and smoking. Clin Gastroenterol 1984; 13:405–436.

32. Conn HO, Butzer BL. Nonassociation of adrenocorticoid therapy and peptic ulcer. N Engl J Med 1976; 294:473–479.

33. Dewayne Andrews M, Papper S. The kidneys and the urinary tract. In: Berk JE, Haubrich WS, Kalser MH, Schaffner F, eds. Bockus gastroenterology. 4th ed. Philadelphia: WB Saunders, 1985; 4613.

34. Zuckerman GR, Cornette GL, Clouse RE, et al. Upper gastrointestinal bleeding in patients with chronic renal failure. Ann Intern Med 1985; 102:588–592.

35. Silverman A, Roy CC, eds. Tumors of the peritoneum, gastrointestinal tract, liver and pancreas. In: Pediatric clinical gastroenterology. 3rd ed. St. Louis: CV Mosby, 1983: 462.

36. Ibid., p 458.

37. Dozois RR, Judd ES, Dahlin DC, et al. The Peutz-Jeghers syndrome: is there a predisposition to the development of intestinal malignancy? Arch Surg 1969; 98:509–517.

38. Schuster DP, Rowley H, Feinstein S, et al. Prospective evaluation of the risk of upper gastrointestinal bleeding after admission to a medical intensive care unit. Am J Med 1984; 76:623–630.

39. Lacroix J, Infante-Rivard C, Gauthier M, et al. Upper gastrointestinal tract bleeding acquired in a pediatric intensive care unit: prophylaxis trial with cimetidine. J Pediatr 1986; 108:1015–1018.

40. Ross AJ, Siegel KR, Bell W, et al. Massive gastrointestinal hemorrhage in children with posterior fossa tumors. J Pediatr Surg 1987; 22:633–636.

41. Abramson DJ. Curling's ulcer in childhood: review of the literature and report of five cases. Surgery 1964; 55:321–336.

42. Kleinman PK, Brill PW, Winchester P. Resolving duodenal-jejunal hematoma in abused children. Radiology 1986; 160:747–750.

43. Horton JW, Coln D. Cardiovascular function and fluid compartments in newborn canine hemorrhagic shock. Am J Physiol 1985; 248:R724–R731.

43a. Horton JW, Longhurst JC, Coln CD, et al. Cardiovascular and hemodynamic effects of hemorrhagic shock in spleen intact and splenectomized dogs. J Clin Physiol 1984; 4:533–548.

44. Sherman NJ, Clatworthy HW. Gastrointestinal bleeding in neonates: a study of 94 cases. Surgery 1967; 62:614–619.

45. Stillman AE. Black heme-positive stools without gastrointestinal hemorrhage. J Pediatr 1982; 100:414–415.

46. Glader BE. Bleeding disorders in the newborn infant. In: Avery ME, Taeusch HW, eds. Schaffer's Diseases of the newborn. 5th ed. Philadelphia: WB Saunders, 1984: 560.

47. Keith DA, Gallop PM. Phenytoin therapy and hemorrhagic disease. J Pediatr 1980; 97:501.

48. Gryboski J, Walker WA, eds. Gastrointestinal problems in the infant. 2nd ed. Philadelphia: WB Saunders, 1983: 85.

49. Liebman WM, Thaler MM, Bujanover Y. Endoscopic evaluation of upper gastrointestinal bleeding in the newborn. Am J Gastroenterol 1978; 69:607–608.

50. Powell TW, Herbst CA, Ulshen M. Mallory-Weiss syndrome in a 10-month-old infant requiring surgery. J Pediatr Surg 1984; 19:596–597.

51. Kliegman RM, Fanaroff AA. Necrotizing enterocolitis. N Engl J Med 1984; 310:1093–1103.

52. Wilson JF, Heiner DC, Lahey ME. Milk-induced gastrointestinal bleeding in infants with hypochromic microcytic anemia. JAMA 1964; 189:568–572.

53. Powell GK. Milk- and soy-induced enterocolitis of infancy. J Pediatr 1978; 93:553–560.

54. Coello-Ramirez P, Larrosa-Haro A. Gastrointestinal occult hemorrhage and gastroduodenitis in cow's milk protein intolerance. J Pediatr Gastroenterol Nutr 1984; 3:215–218.

55. Lake AM, Whitington PF, Hamilton SR. Dietary protein-induced colitis in breast fed infants. J Pediatr 1982; 101:906–910.

56. Sherman MP, Cox KL. Neonatal eosinophilic colitis. J Pediatr 1982; 100:587–589.

57. Halpin TC, Byrne WJ, Ament ME. Colitis, persistent diarrhea and soy protein intolerance. J Pediatr 1977; 91:404–407.

58. Donta ST, Myers MG. Clostridium difficile toxin in asymptomatic neonates. J Pediatr 1982; 100:431–434.

59. Sheretz RJ, Sarubbi FA. The prevalence of Clostridium difficile and toxin in a nursery population: a comparison between patients and necrotizing enterocolitis and an asymptomatic group. J Pediatr 1982; 100:435–439.

60. Welch DF, Marks MI. Is Clostridium difficile pathogenic in infants? J Pediatr 1982; 100:393–395.

61. Ein SH, Lynch MJ, Stephens CA. Ulcerative colitis in children under one year: a twenty-year review. J Pediatr Surg 1971; 6:264–271.

62. Thomas DFM, Fernie DS, Bayston R, et al. Enterocolitis in Hirschsprung's disease: a controlled study of the etiologic role of Clostridium difficile. J Pediatr Surg 1986; 21:22–25.

63. Dupont C, Badoual J, Le Luyer B, et al. Rectosigmoidoscopic findings during isolated rectal bleeding in the neonate. J Pediatr Gastroenterol Nutr 1987; 6:257–264.

64. Udassin R, Nissan S, Lernau OZ. Gastric devascularization—an emergency treatment for hemorrhagic gastritis in the neonate. J Pediatr Surg 1983; 18:579–580.

65. Graziano FM, Bell CL. The normal immune response and what can go wrong. A classification of immunologic disorders. Med Clin North Am 1985; 69:439–452.

66. Ament ME. Immunodeficiency syndromes and the gut. Scand J Gastroenterol (Suppl) 1985; 114:127–135.

67. Feigin RD, Shearer WT. Opportunistic infection in children. II. In the compromised host. J Pediatr 1975; 87:677–694.

68. Lauzon D, Delage G, Brochu P, et al. Pathogens in children with severe combined immune deficiency disease or AIDS. Can Med Assoc J 1986; 135:33–38.

69. Weller IVD. AIDS and the gut. Scand J Gastroenterol (Suppl) 1985; 114:77–89.

70. Bodey GP, Fainstein V. Infections of the gastrointestinal tract in the immunocompromised patient. Annu Rev Med 1986; 37:271–281.

71. Mulholland MW, Delaney JP, Foker JE, et al. Gastrointestinal complications of congenital immunodeficiency states. Ann Surg 1983; 198:673–680.

72. Arbo A, Santos JI. Diarrheal diseases in the immunocompromised host. Pediatr Infect Dis J 1987; 6:894–906.

73. Kaplan B, Benson J, Rothstein F, et al. Lymphonodular hyperplasia

of the colon as a pathologic finding in children with lower gastrointestinal bleeding. J Pediatr Gastroenterol Nutr 1984; 3:704–708.

74. Perry GS, III, Spector BD, Schuman LM, et al. The Wiskott-Aldrich syndrome in the United States and Canada (1892–1979). J Pediatr 1980; 97:72–78.

75. Keeney K, Abaza NA, Tidwel O, et al. Oral Kaposi's sarcoma in acquired immune deficiency syndrome. J Oral Maxillofac Surg 1987; 45:815–821.

76. Ioachim HL, Weinstein MA, Robbins RD, et al. Primary anorectal lymphoma. A new manifestation of the acquired immune deficiency syndrome (AIDS). Cancer 1987; 60:1449–1453.

77. McLoughlin LC, Nord KS, Joshi VV, et al. Severe gastrointestinal involvement in children with the acquired immunodeficiency syndrome. J Pediatr Gastroenterol Nutr 1987; 6:517–524.

78. Scott GB, Buck BE, Leterman JG, et al. Acquired immunodeficiency syndrome in infants. N Engl J Med 1984; 310:76–81.

79. Bernstein LJ, Krieger BZ, Novick B, et al. Bacterial infection in the acquired immunodeficiency syndrome of children. Pediatr Infect Dis 1985; 4:472–475.

80. Oleske J, Minnefor A, Cooper R Jr, et al. Immune deficiency syndrome in children. JAMA 1983; 249:2345–2349.

81. Chachoua A, Dieterich D, Krasinski K, et al. 9-(1,3-dihydroxy-2-propoxymethyl) quanine (Ganciclovir) in the treatment of cytomegalovirus gastrointestinal disease with the acquired immunodeficiency syndrome. Ann Intern Med 1987; 107:133–137.

82. Celum CL, Chaisson RE, Rutherford GW, et al. Incidence of salmonellosis in patients with AIDS. J Infect Dis 1987; 156:998–1002.

83. Agha FP, Lee HH, Nostrant TT. Herpetic esophagitis: a diagnostic challenge in immunocompromised patients. Am J Gastroenterol 1986; 81:246–253.

84. So SKS, Najarian JS, Nevins TE, et al. Low-dose cyclosporine therapy combined with standard immunosuppression in pediatric renal transplantation. J Pediatr 1987; 111:1017–1021.

85. Siegal B, Horowitz A. Early colonic bleeding and kidney transplantation. Transplant Proc 1988; 20:446–448.

86. Kahn D, Esquivel CO, Madrigal-Torres M, et al. An analysis of the causes of death after pediatric liver transplantation. Transplant Proc 1988; 20:613–615.

87. Esquivel CO, Koneru B, Karrer F, et al. Liver transplantation before 1 year of age. J Pediatr 1987; 110:545–548.

88. Breinig MK, Zitelli B, Starzl TE, et al. Epstein-Barr virus, cytomegalovirus and other viral infections in children after liver transplantation. J Infect Dis 1987; 156:273–279.

89. McDonald GB, Shulman HM, Sullivan KM, et al. Intestinal and hepatic complications of human bone marrow transplantation. Part II. Gastroenterology 1986; 90:770–784.

90. Engelhard D, Marks MI, Good RA. Infections in bone marrow transplant recipients. J Pediatr 1986; 108:335–346.

91. Odone V, Chang L, Caces J, et al. The natural history of colorectal carcinoma in adolescents. Cancer 1982; 49:1716–1720.

92. Rose RH, Axelrod DM, Aldea PA, et al. Colorectal carcinoma in the young. Clin Pediatr 1988; 27:105–108.

93. Moss TJ, Adler R. Necrotizing enterocolitis in older infants, children and adolescents. J Pediatr 1982; 100:764–766.

94. Sherman NJ, Woolley MM. The ileocecal syndrome in acute childhood leukemia. Arch Surg 1973; 107:39–42.

95. Moir DH, Bale PM. Necropsy findings in childhood leukaemia, emphasizing neutropenic enterocolitis and cerebral calcification. Pathology 1976; 8:247–258.

96. Sallan SE, Weinstein HJ. Childhood acute leukemia. In: Nathan DG, Oski FA, eds. Hematology of infancy and childhood. 3rd ed. Philadelphia: WB Saunders, 187: 1028.

97. Mitchell EP, Schein PS. Gastrointestinal toxicity of chemotherapeutic agents. Semin Oncol 1982; 9:52–64.

98. Newburger PE, Cassady JR, Jaffe N. Esophagitis due to Adriamycin and radiation therapy for childhood malignancy. Cancer 1978; 42:417–423.

99. Shamberger RC, Weinstein HJ, Delorey MJ, et al. The medical and surgical management of typhlitis in children with acute nonlymphocytic (myelogenous) leukemia. Cancer 1986; 57:603–609.

100. Rosenthal P, Thompson J, Singh M. Detection of occult blood in gastric juice. J Clin Gastroenterol 1984; 6:119–121.

101. Lifton LJ, Kreiser J. False-positive stool occult blood tests caused by iron preparations: a controlled study and review of the literature. Gastroenterology 1982; 83:860–863.

102. Ahlquist DA, Beart RW. Use of fecal occult blood tests in the detection of colorectal neoplasia. Probl Gen Surg 1985; 2:200–210.

103. Schwartz S, Dahl J, Ellefson M, et al. The "HemoQuant" test: a specific and quantitative determination of heme (hemoglobin) in feces and other materials. Clin Chem 1983; 29:2061–2067.

104. Ahlquist DA, McGill DB, Schwartz S, et al. Fecal blood levels in health and disease. A study using HemoQuant. N Engl J Med 1985; 312:1422–1428.

105. Goldschmiedt M, Ahlquist DA, Wieand HS, et al. Measurement of degraded fecal hemoglobin-heme to estimate gastrointestinal site of occult bleeding. Appraisal of its clinical utility. Dig Dis Sci 1988; 33:605–608.

106. Schaffner J. Acute gastrointestinal bleeding. Med Clin North Am 1986; 70:1055–1066.

107. Apt L, Downey WS. "Melena" neonatorum: the swallowed blood syndrome, a simple test for the differentiation of adult and fetal hemoglobin in bloody stools. J Pediatr 1955; 47:6–12.

108. Parikh N, Sebring ES, Polesky HF. Evaluation of bloody gastric fluid from newborn infants. J Pediatr 1979; 94:967–969.

109. Gilbert DA, Silverstein FE, Tedesco FJ, et al. The National ASGE survey on upper gastrointestinal bleeding. III. Endoscopy in upper gastrointestinal bleeding. Gastrointest Endosc 1981; 27:94–102.

110. Teres J, Cecilia A, Bordas JM, et al. Esophageal tamponade for bleeding varices. Gastroenterology 1978; 75:566–569.

111. Kline J. Modification of the adult Blakemore tube for use in children with bleeding esophageal varices. J Pediatr Gastroenterol Nutr 1986; 5:153–154.

112. Chojkier M, Conn HO. Esophageal tamponade in the treatment of bleeding varices. Dig Dis Sci 1980; 25:267–272.

113. Tedesco FJ, Goldstein PD, Gleason WA, et al. Upper gastrointestinal endoscopy in the pediatric patient. Gastroenterology 1976; 70:492–494.

114. Graham DY, Klish WJ, Ferry GD, et al. Value of fiberoptic gastrointestinal endoscopy in infants and children. South Med J 1978; 71:558–560.

115. Gryboski JD. The value of upper gastrointestinal endoscopy in children. Dig Dis Sci 1981 (July suppl), 26:17S–21S.

116. Ament ME, Berquist WE, Vargas J, et al. Pediatr Clin North Am 1988; 35:141–155.

117. Cadranel S, Rodesch P, Peters JP, et al. Fiberendoscopy of the gastrointestinal tract in children. Am J Dis Child 1977; 131:41–45.

118. Spencer R. Gastrointestinal hemorrhage in infancy and childhood: 476 cases. Surgery 1964; 55:718–734.

119. Hyams JS, Leichtner AM, Schwartz AN. Recent advances in diagnosis and treatment of gastrointestinal hemorrhage in infants and children. J Pediatr 1985; 106:1–9.

120. Cox K, Ament ME. Upper gastrointestinal bleeding in children and adolescents. Pediatrics 1979; 63:408–413.

121. Hartemann E, Rigal D, Sassolas F, et al. Hemorragies digestives hautes de l'enfant: interet de la fibroscopie d'urgence. Pediatrie 1979; 34:649–658.

122. Silverstein FE, Gilbert DA, Tedesco FJ, et al. The National ASGE survey on upper gastrointestinal bleeding. I. Study design and baseline data. Gastrointest Endosc 1981; 27:73–79.

123. Peterson WL, Barnett CC, Smith HJ, et al. Routine early endoscopy in upper gastrointestinal tract bleeding. A randomized controlled trial. N Engl J Med 1981; 304:925–929.

124. Conn HO. To scope or not to scope. N Engl J Med 1981; 304:967–969.

125. Dronfield MW, Langman MJS, Atkinson M, et al. Outcome of endoscopy and barium radiography for acute upper gastrointestinal bleeding: controlled trial in 1037 patients. Br Med J 1982; 284:545–548.

126. Erickson RA, Glick ME. Why have controlled trials failed to demonstrate a benefit of esophagogastroduodenoscopy in acute upper gastrointestinal bleeding? A probability model analysis. Dig Dis Sci 1986; 31:760–768.

127. Swain CP, Storey DW, Bown SG, et al. Nature of the bleeding vessel in recurrently bleeding gastric ulcers. Gastroenterology 1986; 90:595–608.

128. Prolla JC, Diehl AS, Bemvenuti GA, et al. Upper gastrointestinal fiberoptic endoscopy in pediatric patients. Gastrointest Endosc 1983; 29:279–281.

129. Figueroa-Colon R, Grunow JE. Randomized study of premedication

for esophagogastroduodenoscopy in children and adolescents. J Pediatr Gastroenterol Nutr 188; 7:359–366.

130. Katon RM. Complications of upper gastrointestinal endoscopy in the gastrointestinal bleeder. Dig Dis Sci 1981 (July suppl); 26:47S–54S.

131. Cucchiara S, Guandalini S, Staiano A, et al. Sigmoidoscopy, colonoscopy and radiology in the evaluation of children with rectal bleeding. J Pediatr Gastroenterol Nutr 1983; 2:667–671.

132. Haubrich WS. Proctosigmoidoscopy. In: Berk JE, Haubrich WS, Kalser MH, Schaffner F, eds. Bockus Gastroenterology. 4th ed. Philadelphia: WB Saunders, 1985: 581.

133. Maxfield RG, Maxfield CM. Colonoscopy as a primary diagnostic procedure in chronic gastrointestinal tract bleeding. Arch Surg 1986; 121:401–403.

134. Williams CB, Laage NJ, Campbell CA, et al. Total colonoscopy in children. Arch Dis Child 1982; 57:49–53.

135. Caos A, Benner KG, Manier J, et al. Colonoscopy after Golytely preparation in acute rectal bleeding. J Clin Gastroenterol 1986; 8:46–49.

136. Lee JMH, Tam PKH, Saing H. Whole-gut irrigation in infants and young children. Dis Colon Rectum 1986; 29:252–254.

137. Lau WY, Fan ST, Wong SH, et al. Preoperative and intraoperative localisation of gastrointestinal bleeding of obscure origin. Gut 1987; 28:869–877.

138. Stevenson RJ. Gastrointestinal bleeding in children. Surg Clin North Am 1985; 65:1455–1480.

139. Tada M, Misaki F, Kawai K. Pediatric enteroscopy with a sonde-type small intestinal fiberscope (SSIF-type VI). Gastrointest Endosc 1983; 29:44–47.

140. Tada M, Shimizu S, Kawai K. A new transnasal sonde type fiberscope (SSIF type VII) as a pan-enteroscope. Endoscopy 1986; 18:121–124.

141. Lewis BS, Waye JD. Chronic gastrointestinal bleeding of obscure origin: role of small bowel enteroscopy. Gastroenterology 1988; 94:1117–1120.

142. Ament M. A large investment for small intestinal endoscopy. Gastrointest Endosc 1983; 29;59–60.

143. Majd M. Radionuclide imaging in pediatrics. Pediatr Clin North Am 1985; 32:1573–1579.

144. Driscoll DM. The role of radionuclide imaging in the diagnosis of gastrointestinal bleeding in children. Radiography 1986; 52:237–239.

145. Wesselhoeft CW, DeLuca FG, Luke M. Positive ^{99m}Tc-pertechnetate scan in a child with intestinal arteriovenous malformation. J Pediatr Surg 1986; 21:71–72.

146. Alavi A, Ring EJ. Localization of gastrointestinal bleeding: superiority of ^{99m}Tc sulfur colloid compared with angiography. AJR 1981; 137:741–748.

147. Alavi A. Detection of gastrointestinal bleeding with ^{99m}Tc-sulfur colloid. Semin Nucl Med 1982; 12:126–138.

148. Miskowiak J, Nielsen SL, Munck O, et al. Acute gastrointestinal bleeding detected with abdominal scintigraphy using technetium-99m-labeled albumin. Scand J Gastroenterol 1979; 14:389–394.

149. Winzelberg GG, Froelich JW, McKusick KA, et al. Radionuclide localization of lower gastrointestinal hemorrhage. Radiology 1981; 139:465–469.

150. Siddiqui AR, Schauwecker DS, Wellman HN, et al. Comparison of technetium-99m sulfur colloid and in vitro labeled technetium-99m RBCs in the detection of gastrointestinal bleeding. Clin Nucl Med 1985; 10:546–549.

151. Smith R, Copely DJ, Bolen FH. ^{99m}Tc RBC scintigraphy: correlation of gastrointestinal bleeding rates with scintigraphic findings. AJR 1987; 148:869–874.

152. Datz FL, Thorne DA, Remley K, et al. Determination of bleeding rates necessary for imaging acute gastrointestinal bleeding with Tc-99m labeled red blood cells. (Abstract) J Nucl Med 1986; 27:956.

153. Landry A Jr, Hartshorne MF, Bunker SR. Optimal technetium-^{99m} RBC labeling for gastrointestinal hemorrhage study. Clin Nucl Med 1985; 10:491–493.

154. Hattner R, Engelstad BL. An advance in identification and localization of gastrointestinal hemorrhage. Gastroenterology 1982; 83:484–492.

155. Zwas ST, Czerniak A, Wolfstein I. Unusual scintigraphic presentation of a shifting Meckel's diverticulum. Clin Nucl Med 1985; 10:252–255.

156. Riff EJ, Hayden PW, Stevenson JK. The detection of acute gastrointestinal bleeding using in vivo technetium^{99m} pertechnetate–labeled erythrocytes. J Pediatr 1980; 97:956–958.

157. Maeda M, Yamashiro Y. Diagnostic red blood cell scintigraphy in GI

158. Afshani E, Berger PE. Gastrointestinal tract angiography in infants and children. J Pediatr Gastroenterol Nutr 1986; 5:173–186.

159. Sheedy PF, Fulton RE, Atwell DT. Angiographic evaluation of patients with chronic gastrointestinal bleeding. AJR 1975; 123:338–347.

160. Thompson JN, Salem RR, Hemingway AP, et al. Specialist investigation of obscure gastrointestinal bleeding. Gut 1987; 28:47–51.

161. Meyerovitz MF, Fellows KE. Angiography in gastrointestinal bleeding in children. AJR 1984; 143:837–840.

162. Spechler SJ, Schimmel EM. Gastrointestinal tract bleeding of unknown origin. Arch Intern Med 1982; 142:236–240.

163. Schoch DR, Sullivan AL, Grand RJ, et al. Gastrointestinal bleeding in an adolescent runner. J Pediatr 1987; 111:302–304.

164. Subcommittee on Advanced Trauma Life Support of the American College of Surgeons Committee on Trauma. Collicott PE, Chairman. Advanced trauma life support course for physicians. American College of Surgeons, 1984: 185.

164a. Wetzel RC. Shock. In: Rogers MC, ed. Textbook of pediatric intensive care. Baltimore: Williams & Wilkins, 1987: 483.

165. Pryor RW, Bricker JT, Stein F, et al. An improved technique for femoral venosection in children. Pediatr Emerg Care 1986; 2:104–105.

166. Shoemaker WC, Schluchter M, Hopkins JA, et al. Comparison of the relative effectiveness of colloids and crystalloids in emergency resuscitation. Am J Surg 1981; 142:73–84.

167. Brinkmeyer S, Safer P, Motoyama E, et al. Superiority of colloid over electrolyte solution for fluid resuscitation (severe normovolemic hemodilution). Crit Care Med 1981; 9:369–370.

168. Shoemaker WC. Evaluation of colloids, crystalloids, whole blood and red cell therapy in the critically ill patient. Clin Lab Med 1982; 2:35–61.

169. Camp FR, Jr, Shields CE. Military blood banking—identification of the group O universal donor for transfusion of A, B and AB recipients—an enigma of two decades. Milit Med (June) 1967; 426–429.

170. Gervin AS, Fischer RP. Resuscitation of trauma patients with type-specific uncrossmatched blood. J Trauma 1984; 24:327–331.

171. Mintz PD, Henry JB, Boral LI. The type and antibody screen. Clin Lab Med 1982; 2:169–179.

172. Shulman IA, Nelson JM, Saxena S, et al. Experience with the routine use of an abbreviated crossmatch. Am J Clin Pathol 1984; 82:178–181.

173. Moore GL, Peck CC, Sohmer PR, et al. Some properties of blood stored in anticoagulant CPDA-1 solution. A brief summary. Transfusion 1981; 21:135–137.

174. Sohmer PR, Moore GL, Beutler E, et al. In vivo viability of red blood cells in CPDA-2. Transfusion 1982; 22:479–484.

175. Reynolds LO, Simon TL. Size distribution measurements of microaggregates in stored blood. Transfusion 1980; 20:669–677.

176. Sohmer PR, Scott RL. Massive transfusion. Clin Lab Med 1982; 2:21–33.

177. Pepe PE, Potkin RT, Reus DH, et al. Clinical predictors of the adult respiratory distress syndrome. Am J Surg 1982; 144:124–130.

178. Tabata BK, Kirsch JR, Rogers MC. Diagnostic tests and technology for pediatric intensive care. In: Rogers MC, ed. Textbook of pediatric intensive care. Baltimore: Williams & Wilkins, 1987: 1401.

179. Geddes LA, Spencer WA, Hoff HE. Graphic recording of the Korotkoff sounds. Am Heart J 1959; 57:361–370.

180. Friesen RH, Lichtor JL. Indirect measurement of blood pressure in neonates and infants utilizing an automatic noninvasive oscillometric monitor. Anesth Analg 1981; 60:742–745.

181. Hutton P, Dye J, Prys-Roberts C. An assessment of the Dinamap 845. Anaesthesia 1984; 39:261–267.

182. Sy WP. Ulnar nerve palsy possibly related to use of automatically cycled blood pressure cuff. Anesth Analg 1981; 60:687–688.

183. Kaye W. Invasive monitoring techniques: arterial cannulation, bedside pulmonary artery catheterization and arterial puncture. Heart Lung 1983; 12:395–426.

184. Packman MI, Rackow EC. Optimum left heart filling pressure during fluid resuscitation of patients with hypovolemic and septic shock. Crit Care Med 1983; 11:165–169.

185. Stanger P, Heymann MA, Hoffman JIE, et al. Use of the Swan-Ganz catheter in cardiac catheterization of infants and children. Am Heart J 1972; 83:749–754.

186. Todres ID, Crone RK, Rogers MC, et al. Swan-Ganz catheterization in the critically ill newborn. Crit Care Med 1979; 7:330–334.

187. Wyse SD, Pfitzner J, Rees A, et al. Measurement of cardiac output by thermal dilution in infants and children. Thorax 1975; 30:262–265.

188. Driscoll DJ, Gillette PC, McNamara DG. The use of dompanine in children. J Pediatr 1978; 92:309–314.

189. Perkin RM, Levin DL, Webb R, et al. Dobutamine: a hemodynamic evaluation in children with shock. J Pediatr 1982; 100:977–983.

190. Andrus CH, Ponsky JL. The effects of irrigant temperature in upper gastrointestinal hemorrhage: a requiem for iced saline lavage.

191. Nicoloff DM, Griffen WO Jr, Salmon PA, et al. Local gastric hypothermia in the management of massive gastrointestinal hemorrhage. Surg Gynecol Obstet 1962; 114:495–503.

192. Waterman NG, Walker JL. The effect of gastric cooling on hemostasis. Surg Gynecol Obstet 1973; 137:80–82.

193. Menguy R, Masters YF. Influence of cold on stress ulceration and on gastric mucosal blood flow and energy metabolism. Ann Surg 1981; 194:29–34.

194. Resnick RH. Intraarterial vasopressin: a continuing challenge. Gastroenterology 1975; 68:411–412.

195. Chojkier M, Groszmann RJ, Atterbury CE, et al. A controlled comparison of continuous intra-arterial and intravenous infusions of vasopressin in hemorrhage from esophageal varices. Gastroenterology 1979; 77:540–546.

196. Johnson WC, Widrich WC, Ansell JE, et al. Control of bleeding varices by vasopressin: a prospective randomized study. Ann Surg 1977; 186:369–376.

197. Freeman JG, Cobden I, Lishman AH, et al. Controlled trial of terlipressin ("Glypressin") versus vasopressin in the early treatment of oesophageal varices. Lancet 1982; ii:66–68.

198. Vosmik J, Jedlicka K, Mulder JL, et al. Action of the triglycyl hormonogen of vasopressin (Glypressin) in patients with liver cirrhosis and bleeding esophageal varices. Gastroenterology 1977; 72:605–609.

199. Reichlin S. Somatostatin (second of two parts). N Engl J Med 1983; 309:1556–1463.

200. Basso N, Bagarani M, Bracci F, et al. Raniditine and somatostatin. Their effects on bleeding from the upper gastrointestinal tract. Arch Surg 1986; 121:833–835.

201. Kravetz D, Bosch J, Teres J, et al. Comparison of intravenous somatostatin and vasopressin infusions in treatment of acute variceal hemorrhage. Hepatology 1984; 4:442–446.

202. Sengstaken RW, Blakemore AH. Balloon tamponage for the control of hemorrhage from esophageal varices. Ann Surg 1950; 131:781–789.

203. Pitcher JL. Safety and effectiveness of the modified Sengstaken-Blakemore tube: a prospective study. Gastroenterology 1971; 61:291–298.

204. Conn HO, Simpson JA. Excessive mortality associated with balloon tamponade of bleeding varices. JAMA 1967; 202:135–139.

205. Nachlas MM. A new triple-lumen tube for the diagnosis and treatment of gastrointestinal hemorrhage. N Engl J Med 1955; 252:720–721.

206. Portal hypertension. In: Silverman A, Roy CC, eds. Pediatric clinical gastroenterology. 3rd ed. St. Louis: CV Mosby, 1983: 757.

207. Taylor TV, Blower AL, Holt S. A new device for isolated duodenal tamponade in the management of bleeding duodenal ulcer (DU). (Abstract) Am J Gastroenterol 1987; 82:951.

208. Crafoord C, Frenckner P. New surgical treatment of varicose veins of the oesophagus. Acta Otolaryngol 1939; 27:422–429.

209. Lilly JR, Stellin G. Variceal hemorrhage in biliary atresia. J Pediatr Surg 1984; 19:476–479.

210. Howard ER, Stamatakis JD, Mowat AP. Management of esophageal varices in children by injection sclerotherapy. J Pediatr Surg 1984; 19:2–5.

211. Vane DW, Boles ET Jr, Clatworthy HW Jr. Esophageal sclerotherapy: an effective modality in children. J Pediatr Surg 1985; 20:703–707.

212. Van Stiegmann G, Stellin GP. Emergent and therapeutic upper gastrointestinal endoscopy in children. World J Surg 1985; 9:294–299.

213. Donovan TJ, Ward M, Shepherd RW. Evaluation of endoscopic sclerotherapy of esophageal varices in children. J Pediatr Gastroenterol Nutr 1986; 5:696–700.

214. Seidman E, Weber AM, Morin CL, et al. Spinal cord paralysis following sclerotherapy for esophageal varices. Hepatology 1984; 4:950–954.

215. Azmy AAF. Bleeding rectal varices following injection sclerotherapy of oesophageal varices in a child. Z Kinderchir 1987; 42:252.

216. Panes J, Viver J, Forne M, et al. Controlled trial of endoscopic sclerosis in bleeding peptic ulcers. Lancet 1987; ii:1292–1294.

217. Schuman BM. Endoscopic injection therapy for nonvariceal upper gastrointestinal hemorrhage: is it too good to be true? Gastrointest Endosc 1987; 33:121–122.

218. Johnston JH. The sentinel clot/visible vessel revisited. Gastrointest Endosc 1986; 32:238–239.

219. Swain CP, Storey DW, Brown SG, et al. Nature of the bleeding vessel in recurrently bleeding gastric ulcers. Gastroenterology 1986; 90:595–608.

220. Protell RL, Rubin CE, Auth DC, et al. The heater probe: a new endoscopic method for stopping massive gastrointestinal bleeding. Gastroenterology 1978; 74:257–262.

221. Laine L. Multipolar electrocoagulation in the treatment of active upper gastrointestinal tract hemorrhage. N Engl J Med 1987; 316:1613–1617.

222. Johnston JH, Sones JQ, Long BW, et al. Comparison of heater probe and YAG laser in endoscopic treatment of major bleeding from peptic ulcers. Gastrointest Endosc 1985; 31:175–180.

223. Silverstein FE, Gilbert DA, Auth DC. Endoscopic hemostasis using laser photocoagulation and electrocoagulation. Dig Dis Sci 1981 (July suppl); 26:31s–40s.

224. Rutgeerts P, Vantrappen G, Van Hootegem P, et al. Neodymium-YAG laser photocoagulation versus multipolar electrocoagulation for the treatment of severely bleeding ulcers: a randomized comparison. Gastrointest Endosc 1987; 33:199–202.

225. Johnston JH. Endoscopic hemostasis for bleeding peptic ulcer. Gastrointest Endosc 1987; 33:260–262.

226. Johnston JH. Endoscopic thermal treatment of upper gastrointestinal bleeding. Endos Rev, July/August 1985; 12–26.

227. Goff JS. Bipolar electrocoagulation versus Nd-YAG laser photocoagulation for upper gastrointestinal bleeding lesions. Dig Dis Sci 1986; 31:906–910.

228. Johnston JH, Jensen DM, Auth D. Experimental comparison of endoscopic yttrium-aluminum-garnet laser, electrosurgery and heater probe for canine gut arterial coagulation. Gastroenterology 1987; 92:1101–1108.

229. Tedesco FJ. Endoscopic therapy for vascular lesions: new challenges. J Pediatr Gastroenterol Nutr 1988; 7:321–322.

230. Gostout C, Ahlquist D, Perrault J, et al. Unpublished observations.

CHAPTER 11

Abdominal Masses

Lesli A. Taylor, M.D.
Arthur J. Ross, III, M.D.

Abdominal masses in children can be caused by a wide variety of entities. These may be divided most easily into the broad categories of organomegaly and normal anatomic variants; benign and malignant neoplasms; inflammatory processes; cystic collections; congenital anomalies; and the sequelae of trauma. All abdominal masses in children except organomegaly and normal anatomic variants should have surgical evaluation. A study of 653 cases of abdominal masses in 1959 found that organomegaly comprised 57 percent of abdominal masses in children. Of the remaining 43 percent, half involved the urinary tract. Of the renal masses, 50 percent were benign and 50 percent were malignant. In this study, 90 percent of the masses requiring surgical evaluation were retroperitoneal and 10 percent were intraperitoneal. Of the retroperitoneal masses, 66 percent were of renal origin. The remaining 33 percent were nonrenal and were likely to be malignant.[1] Current studies show that hydronephrosis and multicystic kidney are the two most common palpable abdominal masses in children, followed by neuroblastoma and Wilms' tumor.[2] As new imaging modalities such as computed tomography (CT) and magnetic resonance imaging (MRI) gain widespread use, the detection of abdominal masses in children, and perhaps their etiologic distribution, will change. Re-evaluation of the incidence of different entities will be needed.

The current widespread use of prenatal ultrasonography has increased the incidence of masses discovered in the fetus and neonate and thus, theoretically, has decreased those that will be detected clinically at a later age.[3-5] Despite the growing use of ultrasonography, a thorough abdominal examination and, if indicated, a rectal examination, should be part of every neonatal and well-baby visit. One should remember that while most neonatal masses are found in the first few days of life, a congenital mass may present at birth or at any other age.

Quite often, the detection of abdominal masses occurs by incidental palpation of an asymptomatic mass during a well-child examination. Masses are also discovered during evaluation of associated symptoms or abdominal distention, by incidental radiologic discovery, or because of follow-up of abnormal blood values. Abdominal masses are occasionally found when minor trauma brings the child to medical attention.

When a child is found to have an abdominal mass, a careful history should always be taken, as concurrent symptoms such as pain, tenderness, jaundice, weight loss, fever, intestinal obstruction, melena, urinary tract infection, dysuria, hematuria, and hypertension and the duration of these symptoms can provide valuable diagnostic clues. The possibility

of trauma should always be ascertained. The sex of the child may be an important determinant of the likelihood of a particular entity. For example, choledochal cysts and sacrococcygeal teratomas are much more common in girls, whereas bilateral hydronephrosis due to posterior urethral valves is found exclusively in males.[6-8] Similarly, the age of the child can give important diagnostic information. Benign renal abnormalities are the most common masses found in the first 2 days of life, whereas the incidence of Wilms' tumor peaks at age 2 to 3 years and that of neuroblastoma at 2 years.[6,9]

The abdomen of a normal neonate, infant, or toddler should be completely soft and nontender. A smooth liver edge may be the only palpable finding. Occasionally, normal kidneys are palpable in neonates. In a thin older child, the right kidney may be palpable if it assumes an anterior position.[10,11] A normal spleen tip may present as a palpable abdominal mass.[12] Any suggestion of firmness, resistance to palpation, or mass effect should be investigated further. As a child grows, the abdominal wall musculature gives greater resistance on examination, but the abdomen should still be soft to deep palpation.

For children presenting with an abdominal mass, a complete abdominal examination should always include a rectal examination and, in older females, bimanual pelvic examination. In younger females, the rectal examination can be used to give important information on the pelvic organs. These examinations should not be traumatic for the child. Indications for pelvic examination under anesthesia in the younger female include vaginal discharge or bleeding and inability to obtain the co-operation necessary to do a full examination, which is commonly the case.

The quadrant of origin of the mass provides important diagnostic information. Some authors have found it useful to think of four anatomic regions, these being the liver, the anterior abdomen, the pelvis, and the retroperitoneum. The majority of masses in neonates are retroperitoneal.[13] The estimated size of the mass can also contribute to the differential diagnosis. A very large mass may present as increased abdominal girth, with snugness of the child's waistband as the presenting complaint. Wilms' tumors frequently present when they have attained a great size, usually more than 12 cm. The tumor may be large enough to comprise 15 percent of the child's weight.[14] Determination of fixation or mobility of the mass also aids in diagnosis (Fig. 1). Children presenting with an acute abdomen should be thoroughly evaluated for a mass, which most likely represents an inflammatory process.

Diagnoses that can be eliminated early by simple maneuvers include gastric dilatation, urinary retention, and fecal impaction.[10] Passage of a nasogastric tube or Foley cathether

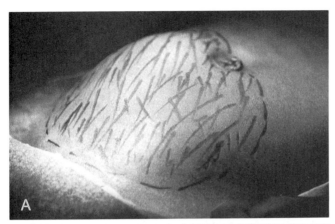

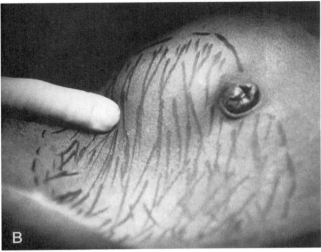

FIGURE 1 The mobility of abdominal masses is variable. Demonstrated here is a 6-year-old black female with a huge right pelvic mass (A). Its mobility is demonstrated by its ability to be displaced up beneath the right costal margin (B). At operation, an ovarian fibroma was found.

or administration of an enema may quickly provide the answer. If a mass is clearly palpable and persistent after exclusion of these functional causes, radiologic evaluation should be undertaken. Multiple imaging modalities are available and include standard radiography, ultrasonography, CT, MRI, intravenous pyelography, contrast gastrointestinal (GI) radiography, and radionuclide scintigraphy. Each modality has advantages and limitations, and these will be discussed further. Currently, masses as small as 1 cm can be reliably detected by a skillful radiologist.

ABDOMINAL WALL

In assessing an abdominal mass, it is important to distinguish whether it is intra-abdominal or part of the anterior abdominal wall. Common entities that can present as anterior abdominal wall masses or protrusions are umbilical hernia, umbilical granuloma, inguinal hernia, epiplocele, and diastasis recti. These are easily differentiated. An umbilical her-

nia protrudes at the ring of the umbilicus and should be reducible with gentle pressure. These usually close spontaneously by the age of 5 years. An umbilical granuloma is a small mound of tissue at the umbilicus that may represent a simple remnant of the cord or an abnormal persistence of the urachus or omphalomesenteric duct. Inguinal hernias protrude in the medial groin. These are usually distinguishable from inguinal adenopathy and retractile testes. A more difficult differentiation is between an inguinal hernia and a hydrocele. An isolated scrotal swelling is likely to be a hydrocele, whereas a groin swelling could be either. An epiplocele is herniation of omentum through the linea alba in the epigastric area, whereas diastasis recti is a midline protrusion of an attenuated linea alba which is demonstrated when the patient tries to sit from a supine position.

Omphalocele and gastroschisis are obvious abdominal wall abnormalities that present at birth: Omphalocele occurs when the abdominal contents herniate through the umbilical ring, often into an intact sac, whereas gastroschisis is present when the herniation is lateral to the ring. This herniation is usually to the right of the umbilicus, and there is never a peritoneal sac.

Other conditions that may present in the anterior abdominal wall include rectus hematoma from trauma and interfascial abscess from prior surgery. These are easily diagnosed with ultrasonography. Rare abdominal wall tumors include fibroma, fibrosarcoma, lipoma, and rhabdomyoma. These usually present as firm masses. Their atypical location and character alert the examiner.

ANTERIOR ABDOMEN

The anterior abdomen contains the biliary tract, the liver, the spleen, the small intestine, and the large intestine and appendix, as well as the stomach, mesentery, and omentum. All of these organs can develop masses palpable on examination.

Biliary Tract

A common mass of the biliary tract is an enlarged gallbladder. There are many processes that can cause this. These include total parenteral nutrition, fasting, beta-streptococcal infection, Kawasaki disease, acute hepatitis, and calculous and acalculous cholecystitis.[15] Calculous cholecystitis, which presents with a tender, palpable gallbladder when acute, may be idiopathic or associated with hematologic disease. Common duct obstruction by a stone may cause a distended gallbladder; this is rarely seen before adolescence. A very rare cause of common duct obstruction is biliary rhabdomyosarcoma.

A less common but important biliary mass is choledochal cyst. This is a congenital lesion that can present at any time during life but usually does so in the first decade. Five types have been delineated (Fig. 2). These include type I, a fusiform dilatation of the extrahepatic ducts which constitutes 90 percent of all such cysts, and type II, a diverticulum of the common bile duct. Type III is a duodenal choledochocele. Type IV is multiple intrahepatic and extrahepatic cystic dila-

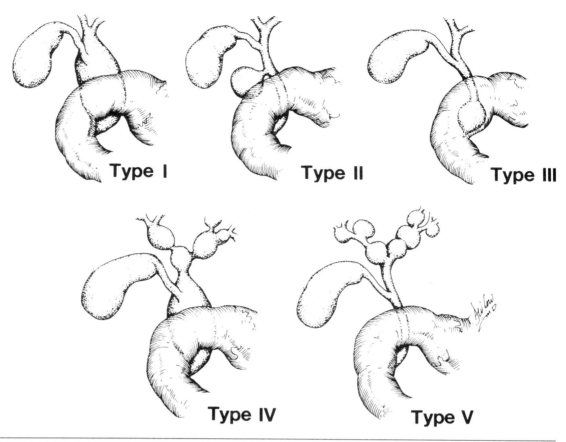

FIGURE 2 Choledochal cysts, types I to V.

tations of the bile ducts, whereas type V is a single intra-hepatic cyst. Infants present with an abdominal mass, jaundice, and failure to thrive. Older children present with a right upper quadrant mass and tenderness and jaundice. Females outnumber males 4 to 1 in incidence. Evaluation includes liver function tests and ultrasonography or radionuclide scintigraphy.[16]

Liver

Hepatomegaly is the most common cause of a liver "mass." It may be due to hepatitis, cirrhosis, glycogen storage disease, or fatty infiltration from hyperalimentation. Unique causes of neonatal hepatomegaly include excessive extrameduallary hematopoiesis, congestive heart failure, and subcapsular hematoma from birth trauma. An unusual cause of hepatomegaly is compensatory hypertrophy of one lobe of the liver after radiation atrophy of another lobe.[17]

The liver may also be enlarged by infectious processes such as liver abscesses or cystic infections such as echinococcal cyst and amebic cyst.[18] Liver abscesses are rare in children. They may be single or mutiple. The bacteriology includes *Staphylococcus aureus*, *Streptococcus fecalis*, and *Escherichia coli*. A subcapsular hematoma from blunt trauma may also produce a mass. CT scan gives excellent definition.

Liver tumors are the other main entity causing liver enlargement in children. These may be benign, malignant, or metastatic. Primary liver tumors are the third most common solid abdominal neoplasm in childhood and thereby make up 15 percent of abdominal masses in children.[19]

Benign liver tumors make up one-third of such tumors. These include hemangioendotheliomas, which present with hepatomegaly, heart failure, and cutaneous hemangiomas. Benign liver hemangiomas are usually small and asymptomatic. These are usually not palpable. The remaining liver tumors are palpable and include mesenchymal hamartoma, focal nodular hyperplasia, adenoma, and congenital cyst. Mesenchymal hamartoma usually presents as a very large liver mass in children under 2 years (Fig. 3). There is a male predominance. It is a benign tumor arising from mesenchymal rest cells of the portal tract. Treatment is excision.[20] Although focal nodular hyperplasia and adenoma are more common in adults and in relation to oral contraceptive use, they can present in childhood. Symptoms are similar to those in adults. Hepatic cyst is a rare congenital lesion that is thought to be derived from the biliary tract. It can present at any age and can be found in any lobe of the liver.[21] Malignant neoplasms comprise two-thirds of all liver tumors and usually present as a painless mass.[22] Hepatoblastoma is the most common liver tumor in children under 5 years of age. It usually presents as a single mass in the right lobe of the

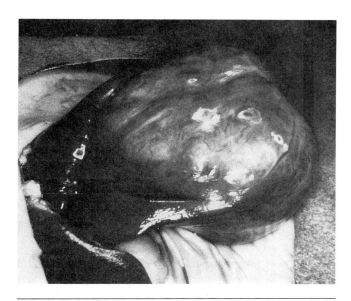

FIGURE 3 This nontender, somewhat mobile, large, left upper quadrant mass encountered in an otherwise healthy 1-year-old white male was found to be a mesenchymal hamartoma. The mass was resected completely.

liver. Hepatocellular carcinoma presents in older children, usually between the ages of 12 and 15 years.[23]

Metastatic tumors cause a large, firm liver, with diffuse mottling visible on ultrasonography.[13] Leukemia, lymphoma, and Wilms' tumor are common metastatic lesions. Stage IV neuroblastoma is a unique entity characterized by the occurrence of liver metastases in children under 6 months with the tumor. Characteristic subcutaneous lesions may be present. Spontaneous regression is likely.

Current imaging modalities are unable to distinguish benign from malignant hepatic masses, and aspiration or biopsy may still be needed for definitive diagnosis. MRI promises to be the most specific diagnostic study.[19]

Spleen

As with hepatomegaly, splenomegaly is the most common reason for diagnosis of a splenic "mass." Causes of hypersplenism include hereditary spherocytosis and other blood dyscrasias and infectious mononucleosis. Hemangiomas can also involve the spleen and may be a cavernous hemangioendothelioma.

A variety of cysts can cause mass effect in the spleen, including simple cysts, epidermoid cysts, parasitic cysts, and traumatic pseudocysts[24] (Fig. 4). Unusual causes of splenic enlargement include lymphangioma and hamartoma. As previously mentioned, an abnormally mobile spleen may present as an abdominal mass in any quadrant.[12]

Stomach

Gastric masses are uncommon in children. Gastric dilatation can give the appearance of an abdominal mass and is easily diagnosed and treated by passage of a nasogastric tube.

When gastric dilatation is found, causes of gastric outlet obstruction or ileus should be ruled out. A common abdominal mass in the neonate is the pyloric olive of pyloric stenosis.[25] Other benign causes of gastric masses include bezoar and gastric duplications. Gastric duplications present as a mid-epigastric mass. Rarely, older children can present with a phlegmon from a penetrating gastric ulcer.

Gastric tumors make up a very small component of gastric masses. Benign gastric tumors include carcinoid, hemangiopericytoma, lipoma, neurofibroma, eosinophilic granuloma, leiomyoma, and teratoma. Inflammatory polyps and adenomatous polyps may also cause a mass effect. Malignant gastric tumors constitute less than 1 percent of pediatric malignancies but may present as gastric masses. These include carcinoma, leiomyosarcoma, rhabdomyosarcoma, fibrosarcoma, and lymphoma.

Small Intestine

Several conditions of the small intestine may present as an abdominal mass. Intestinal duplications are the most common mass of the GI tract of the neonate, although they can present at any age. Of these, ileal duplications are most common[26] (Table 1 and Fig. 5).

Idiopathic ileocolic intussusception of the small bowel creates a palpable mass (Fig. 6). Associated symptoms of lethargy, crampy abdominal pain, and currant jelly stools suggest the diagnosis. Barium enema confirms and possibly reduces an ileocolic intussusception. Small bowel intussusception may occur in the postoperative period in children and create a mass but usually presents as a small bowel obstruction. Malrotation with midgut volvulus is another condition of the small bowel which could create an abdominal mass. All children who present with bilious vomiting should be evaluated for this.[27] Perforation of the small bowel from Crohn's disease or an ulcerated Meckel's diverticulum may cause a palpable phlegmon that can be diagnosed by CT scan. Occasionally, a Meckel's diverticulum is large enough to be palpable itself.

A duodenal hematoma from blunt abdominal trauma may rarely be palpable. Barium swallow shows a "coiled spring sign." Dilated loops of obstructed bowel cause abdominal distention and if asymmetric may be mistaken for an abdominal mass. In the neonatal period, intestinal atresia and meconium ileus may cause intestinal obstruction, whereas in the older child, ileocolic intussusception or postoperative adhesive bands are more likely to be the cause.

Primary tumors of the small bowel are rare and include lymphoma, especially Burkitt's, leiomyosarcoma, angiosarcoma, rhabdomyosarcoma, and carcinoid.

Colon and Appendix

A common cause of mass effect of the colon is fecal impaction (Fig. 7). This may be due to functional or organic causes. Table 2 outlines the various entities that can precipitate fecal impaction. Another benign cause of colonic mass is colon duplication, which may be cystic or tubular.[28] Tumors of the large intestine are rare in children but include

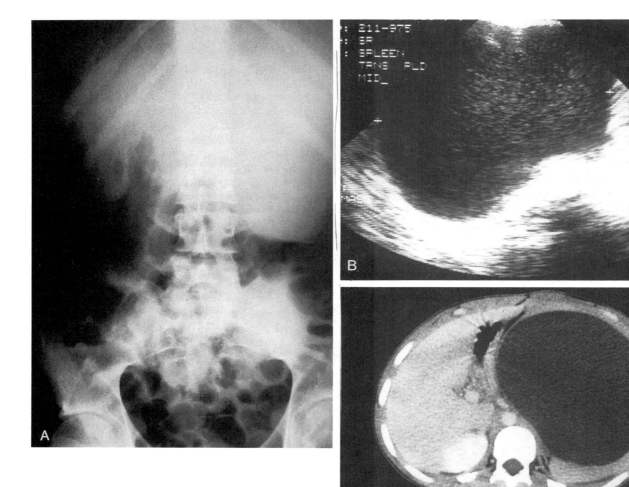

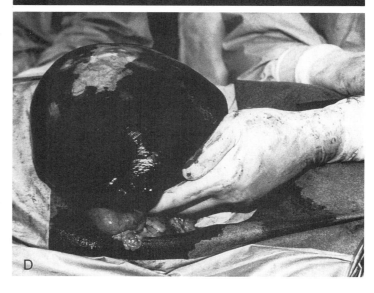

FIGURE 4 A 16-year-old white male developed symptoms of early satiety. Left upper quadrant fullness was appreciated. A survey film of the abdomen suggested a left upper quadrant mass (*A*); ultrasonography (*B*) and CT scan (*C*) demonstrated that this was a large splenic cyst. Interestingly, there was a remote history of abdominal trauma. The huge splenic cyst is seen at laparotomy (*D*). A splenorrhaphy was performed to resect the cyst yet preserve a critical mass of splenic tissue.

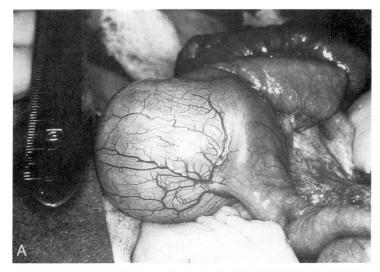

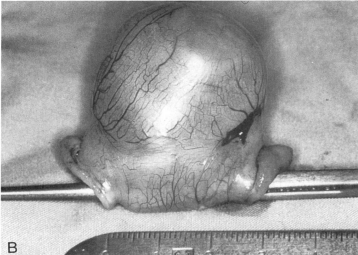

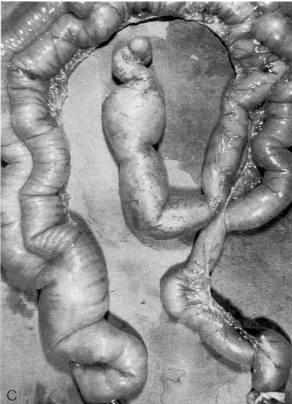

FIGURE 5 The most common site of intestinal duplications is within the ileum. They may or may not be palpable. Intestinal duplications may be cystic or tubular. *A* and *B* depict a cystic ileal duplication that was palpable as a mobile abdominal mass in a 5-month-old female. *C* depicts a long tubular ileal duplication, which presented as an abdominal mass in a 12-year-old male.

TABLE 1
Location and Type of 101 Duplications in 96 Patients

Location	Total
Esophagus	21
Thoracoabdominal	3
Gastroduodenal	10
Jejunal	12
Ileal	35
Colonic	20
TOTAL	101

Adapted from Holcomb et al.[26]

carcinoma secondary to longstanding ulcerative colitis or familial polyposis, and lymphoma.

One of the most common causes of an abdominal mass, particularly in older children, is an appendiceal abscess.[29] The mass effect is created by the omentum or the actual abscess with necrotic appendix. A rare cause of appendiceal mass is carcinoid.

Mesentery and Omentum

Both the mesentery and the omentum can be involved in conditions that cause a palpable abdominal mass.[30,31] Mesenteric masses include lymphangioma and mesenteric

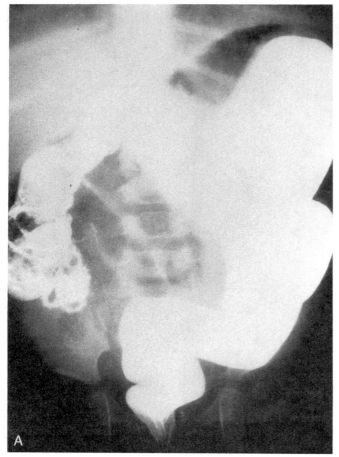

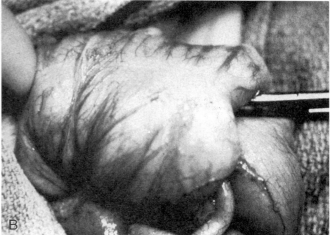

FIGURE 6 Idiopathic ileocolic intussusception is a common finding in toddlers. This 14-month-old male had intermittent colicky abdominal pain and a right lower quadrant mass. Barium enema confirmed the presence of an intussusception but was unable to reduce it (*A*); an operative reduction was performed (*B*).

cysts (Fig. 8). Such cysts present in older children with a pulling sensation, abdominal distention, and possibly intestinal obstruction. Thirty to 40 percent are asymptomatic. They are caused by obstructed lymphatics. Hematoma from blunt abdominal trauma may create a palpable mesenteric mass. A very rare cause of benign mesenteric mass is Castleman's disease, or giant lymphoid hyperplasia. This is also known as "pseudotumor of the mesentery."[32,33]

The omentum can also be involved with lymphangioma or cysts. Omental cysts differ from mesenteric cysts in that 90 percent are asymptomatic, and they are more likely to be found in younger children. They are also caused by obstructed lymphatics and are soft, mobile, and compressible. When large and thin-walled, they may have the appearance of ascites.[34] The treatment is complete resection.

RETROPERITONEUM

Structures of the retroperitoneum which may give rise to a mass are the urinary tract, including kidneys, ureters, and bladder; the adrenal glands; and the pancreas. Lymphoma and lymphangioma may also present in the retroperitoneum.

Urinary Tract

Anatomic variants of the kidney that produce a mass include duplicate kidney, horseshoe kidney, renal ectopia, fused kidney, and a hypertrophied single kidney. The most common cause of an enlarged kidney giving a mass effect is hydronephrosis, a kidney with a dilated collecting system. Hydronephrosis is most commonly caused by ureteropelvic junction obstruction, which may be due to idiopathic stenosis, extrinsic pressure by crossing vessels, an aperistaltic ureteral segment, ureterocele, or a horseshoe or ectopic kidney.[3] Nonobstructive causes of hydronephrosis include vesicoureteral reflux, primary megacalyces, prune belly syndrome, and dilatation from sepsis.[13] Hydronephrosis is bilateral in one-third of cases.

The next most common cause of a renal mass is multicystic kidney diseas. It is the most common cause of unilateral abdominal mass in the neonate.[4] Eighty percent of cases are detected before the age of 2 years.[3] It is a benign condition that presents as a large, smooth, asymptomatic flank mass. It may be bilateral in 15 percent of cases and therefore incompatible with life. It is an autosomal recessive condition. In the most common form, the ureter and pelvis are atretic. Normal renal parenchyma is replaced by cysts, and

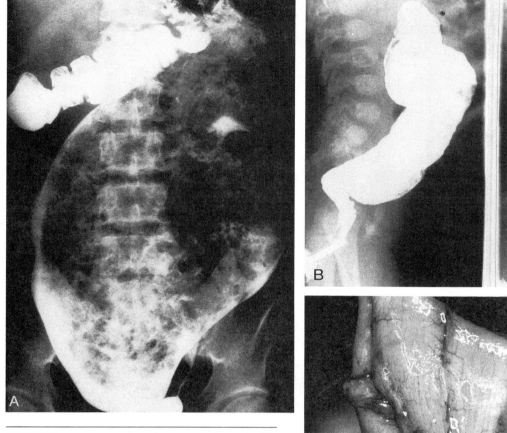

FIGURE 7 Feces are often the cause of a palpable abdominal mass. *A* demonstrates a fecal impaction due to severe constipation in a 6-year-old with profound mental retardation. An 18-month-old male presented with a palpable left lower quadrant mass and history of constipation. Shown in *B* is a typical transition zone due to congenital aganglionosis (Hirschsprung's disease). At operation, the impressive change in caliber at this transition zone is easily seen. *C*, A colostomy was performed on the child, who later underwent definitive treatment via a Duhamel pull-through procedure.

TABLE 2
Causes of Constipation

Functional	Organic
Psychogenic	Distal obstruction
Mental retardation	Tumor
Pain avoidance, e.g., anal fissure	Aganglionosis
Hypothyroidism	acquired
	congenital (Hirschsprung's)

the kidney is nonfunctioning. Multicystic kidney must be differentiated from other causes of nonfunctioning kidney, such as hydronephrosis. Ultrasonography is the radiologic modality of choice.[6]

A benign cause of massive nephromegaly is polycystic kidney, which may be inherited as autosomal recessive or autosomal dominant. The recessive form is associated with variable involvement of the kidney and liver. The kidneys are enlarged with multiple small cysts. The liver has bile duct hyperplasia, portal fibrosis, and hepatomegaly. There may be splenomegaly. The dominant form of polycystic kidney

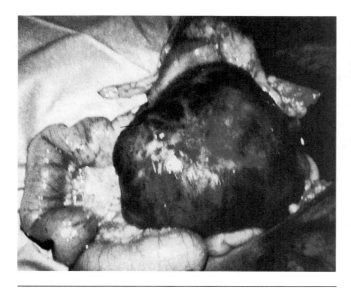

FIGURE 8 This 16-year-old black female presented with chronic abdominal pain, and examination revealed a vague mid-abdominal mass. At exploration, a large abdominal mesenteric lymphangioma was found.

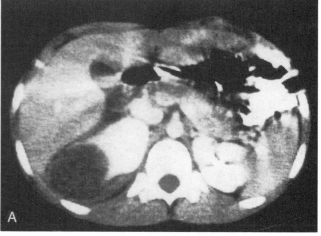

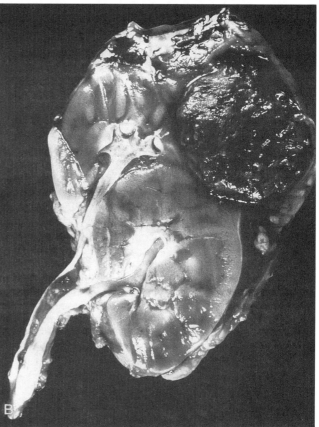

FIGURE 9 Following an episode of mild, blunt abdominal trauma, hematuria was detected in a healthy 5-year-old white male. Examination was significant for a slightly mobile, nontender right upper quadrant mass. A CT scan demonstrated the mass to be emanating from the upper pole of the right kidney (*A*). This was a Wilms' tumor (*B*).

disease is the most common genetic renal disease; it involves the kidney primarily. It usually presents in the third and fourth decade but may present in infancy or childhood with bilateral nephromegaly. Both recessive and dominant forms can be diagnosed prenatally by ultrasonography.[35,36]

Simple renal cysts are a rare cause of a renal mass in children and are believed to be retention cysts caused by obstruction of renal tubules due to local ischemia.[37] These usually present as an asymptomatic flank mass. Other benign renal masses include benign mesenchymal tumors such as hamartoma, teratoma, leiomyoma, and hemangioma. Renal abscess should also be considered as a benign cause of a renal mass.

Neoplastic renal masses include Wilms' tumor, mesoblastic nephroma, and the congenital premalignant condition nephroblastomatosis. Wilms' tumor is the most common renal neoplasm occurring in childhood (Fig. 9). It comprises 12 percent of all childhood cancers. It is frequently diagnosed during a well-child examination or when a minor complaint brings the child to medical attention. Occasionally, the appearance of hematuria after minor trauma leads to the discovery of a Wilms' tumor. Eighty percent are diagnosed by age 6 years, with most presenting at age 2 to 3 years. Approximately 5 percent of cases are bilateral; two-thirds of bilateral Wilms' tumors present synchronously. In contrast, mesoblastic nephroma is a benign condition that, although rare, is the most common renal neoplasm of the neonate.[38] It presents in infants less than 3 months of age.[13,39] Nephroblastomatosis, which is persistence of metanephric blastema, may cause enlarged kidneys. CT is the study of choice for diagnosis.[40] Renal cell carcinoma, metastatic lymphoma, angiolipoma of tuberous sclerosis, multiocular cystic nephroma, and rhabdomyosarcoma are rare causes of renal masses.

Renal vein thrombosis is an important benign vascular cause of renal enlargement, which can present as a palpable mass in the neonatal period. The thrombosis is caused by hemoconcentration from dehydration, low perfusion, and polycythemia. Symptoms include a flank mass (the kidney swollen by blood and edema), hematuria, and thrombocytopenia. Predisposing factors include perinatal asphyxia, sepsis, necrotizing enterocolitis, hyperosmolar feeds, cyanotic congenital heart disease, maternal diabetes, diuretic use, and steroid use. There may be associated ipsilateral adrenal hemorrhage.[6] Ultrasonography is diagnostic; therapy is supportive and directed toward the underlying cause.

A full bladder can easily be mistaken for an abdominal mass, particularly in neonates, in whom it is an intra-abdominal rather than a pelvic organ. Causes of bladder distention include pharmacologic blockade of the detrusor muscle, neurologic impairment, and, in boys, posterior urethral valves. Foley catheterization is a simple and quick diagnostic and therapeutic maneuver. A remnant of the urachus, a urachal cyst, may present as a palpable mass on the lower midline abdominal wall.

Adrenal Gland

Although it is the smallest retroperitoneal organ, the adrenal gland can be enlarged enough by several conditions to be palpable. Adrenal hemorrhage, usually found in a neonate stressed by systemic disease or birth trauma, can produce a mass effect. There may be associated anemia or jaundice. Adrenal hemorrhage must be differentiated from neuroblastoma by ultrasonography. An adrenal hemorrhage lique-

fies and contracts in several weeks and may appear calcified on radiography.[6,41] The treatment is expectant.

The adrenal medulla and the sympathetic chain of the retroperitoneum give rise to neuroblastoma, the most common extracranial malignancy of childhood (Fig. 10). It is the most common tumor of infancy and the most common malignancy of the newborn. The peak incidence is at 2 years of age. Seventy-five percent are retroperitoneal. Most abdominal neuroblastomas present as a palpable mass. Fifty percent have calcifications visible on plain film. Sonography is the screening study of choice, but CT scan provides excellent anatomic detail.

Other tumors of the adrenal medulla of childhood are ganglioneuroma and, rarely, pheochromocytoma.[9] Ganglioneuroma is a benign, mature lesion of neural crest tissue. Its presentation is similar to that of neuroblastoma, and these two entities must be differentiated by histology. Pheochromocytomas are a rare lesion in children and usually present with hypertension rather than a palpable mass.

Adrenal hyperplasia may cause adrenal enlargement but usually causes a microscopic focal nodule. The adrenal cortex may give rise to adrenocortical carcinoma or adenoma. These comprise less than 1 percent of all neoplasms in the pediatric age group. The clinical presentation may be due to endocrine imbalance or may be nonspecific. A mass is usually not palpable, although tumors large enough to be palpable have been reported.

Pancreas

The pancreas is also a retroperitoneal organ that can give rise to palpable masses. Post-traumatic pancreatic pseudocyst, phlegmon, and abscess are common benign causes of pan-

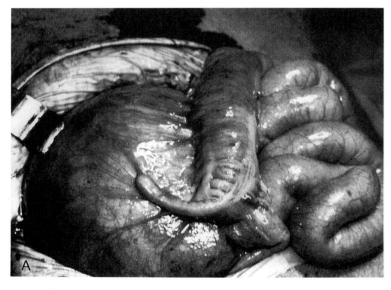
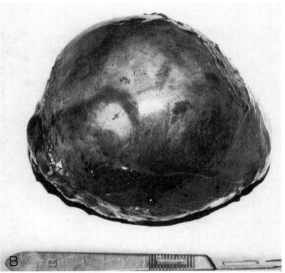

FIGURE 10 A 17-month-old white male had 3 weeks of fever and diminishing activity. The ill-appearing child had a large, fixed abdominal mass found on examination. A large right retroperitoneal neuroblastoma was found at exploration (A). The tumor was resected completely (B).

creatic mass.[42] Rare malignant causes of a mass include islet cell tumor, pancreaticoblastoma, sarcoma, and lymphoma.

PELVIC MASSES

Pelvic organs that can form masses include the ovaries, uterus, vagina, and fallopian tubes. Elements of the sacrum can also cause pelvic masses. A small percentage of neuroblastomas and rhabdomyosarcomas present in the pelvis.

Ovary

Ovarian masses present most commonly in adolescence but are not uncommon in younger girls, in whom their presence may be heralded by precocious puberty. An ovarian mass may present anywhere in the abdomen. It is usually asymptomatic but may present with dull, poorly localized pain or difficulty with urination or defecation. Fifty to 80 percent of ovarian masses are palpable and mobile on abdominal and rectal examination.

Benign cysts of the ovary include hemorrhagic cysts and follicular cysts. These are uncommon in the neonate and child compared to the adolescent, yet of ovarian tumors in the neonate, follicular cysts are the most common cause and are due to maternal placental human chorionic gonadotropin.

Primary neoplasms of the ovary include germ cell tumors, of which benign teratomas comprise 70 percent (Fig. 11). Mature cystic teratomas are known as dermoids of the ovary. Other germ cell tumors include dysgerminoma, embryonal carcinoma, and entodermal sinus tumor. Stromal neoplasms, which make up 10 percent of pediatric ovarian tumors, include the granulosa-theca cell tumor, which may cause feminizing precocious puberty; androblastoma, which

may cause virilization; and gynandroblastoma.[43] Epithelial tumors include serous cystadenoma and mucinous cystadenoma.

Ovarian torsion due to a cyst or neoplasm presents with acute pain, nausea, and vomiting. A boggy, fixed mass is palpable. In utero ovarian torsion may be detected antenatally with ultrasonography or may present as a nontender, mobile mass in the newborn female[5,44] (Fig. 12).

Uterus

Uterine enlargement in the neonate, which may be palpable as a mass, may be a normal uterus stimulated by maternal hormones in utero. Hydrometrocolpos, a uterus and/or vagina distended with secretions or blood, may also present in the neonatal period or at any age and is due to imperforate hymen (Fig. 13), cervical or vaginal atresia, cloacal anomalies, or reproductive tract duplications. There may be associated imperforate anus.[45]

In the adolescent, uterine enlargement may be due to pregnancy or to uterine stimulation by the hormones of an ovarian tumor. Phlegmons due to pelvic inflammatory disease or tubo-ovarian abscess also present in the adolescent. Ectopic pregnancy is an important differential diagnosis.

Rhabdomyosarcomas may arise in the trigone of the bladder, the prostate, seminal vesicles, spermatic cord, vagina, or uterus. Presenting symptoms include lower abdominal mass and urinary obstruction. CT scan is the imaging modality of choice.[10,43] Pelvic neuroblastomas represent approximately 4 percent of all neuroblastomas. They may present as a palpable abdominal mass. Rectal and pelvic examinations are essential in diagnosis.

Sacrococcygeal teratoma is the most common tumor recognized at birth. Eighty percent are benign. It usually

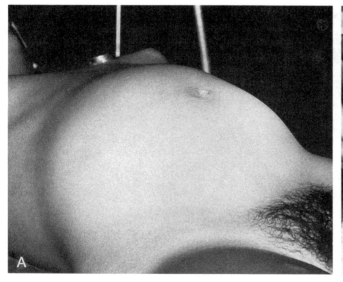
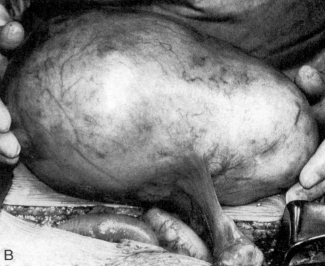

FIGURE 11 This 14-year-old white female was found to have a large, asymptomatic abdominal mass (A). Upon exploration, a huge ovarian teratoma as found (B).

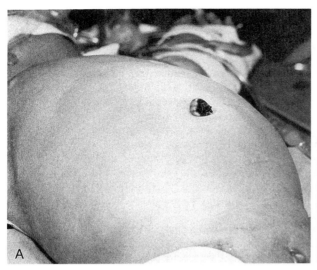
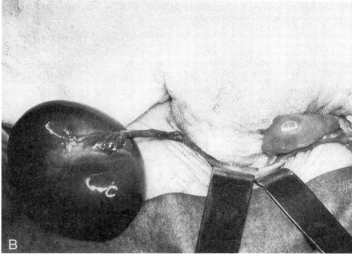

FIGURE 12 This 1-week-old white female was found on newborn evaluation to be distended and to have a mobile pelvic mass (A). The child was explored and found to have sustained an intrauterine torsion of her right fallopian tube and ovary (B).

presents as a mass of the buttocks or lower spine but may be completely intrapelvic. A rectal examination is essential for diagnosis.[46] Other presacral conditions include anterior meningomyelocele and teratoma.[2]

RADIOLOGIC ASSESSMENT

Radiologic findings that are useful in diagnosis of abdominal masses include the presence of calcifications, the consistency of the mass—e.g., cystic, solid, or mixed, and the organ or site of origin. In general, cystic masses are more likely to be benign and solid masses are more likely to be malignant. Whether the mass is discrete or poorly defined can also be diagnostic. Masses that tend to be discrete include hydronephrosis, cystic lesions, benign tumors, and Wilms' tumor. Ill-defined masses may be advanced neuroblastoma or an inflammatory process.[47] Associated skeletal anomalies can provide diagnostic information. The presence of teeth or formed bony structures in an abdominal mass indicates a dermoid or teratoma. Radiologic evaluation also provides important information for the staging of tumors by delineating

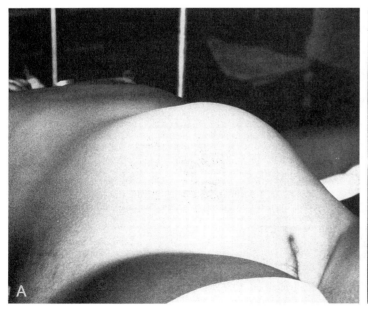
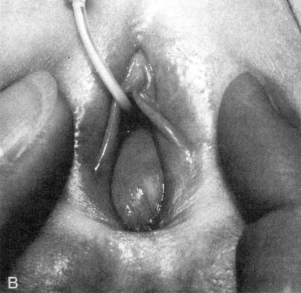

FIGURE 13 This 11-year-old white female had a sizable pelvic mass diagnosed following a 3- to 4-month history of vague abdominal pain (A). Evaluation revealed an imperforate hymen (B), and hydrometrocolpos was diagnosed.

metastases or tumor extension, parameters that are very important in planning the surgical approach.

Plain radiographs are usually obtained; masses may be suspected by displacement of bowel loops or by calcifications. Bowel obstruction as a cause of abdominal distention and mass effect should be ruled out. In the past, because the majority of abdominal masses in children are renal and adrenal in origin, the intravenous pyelogram, augmented by inferior venacavogram and total body opacification, was performed as the initial study. With the advent of ultrasonography, CT scan, and MRI, this is no longer true.[2] The intravenous pyelogram gives limited information compared with these other studies, especially when renal function is impaired, as in neonates in whom glomerular filtration rate and concentrating ability are decreased in the first week of life. It also involves radiation exposure. The intravenous pyelogram is useful in demonstrating tumor extension in the inferior vena cava in the case of renal tumors, but ultrasonography can also demonstrate this.

Ultrasonography has currently assumed the role of primary screening modality. It offers many advantages over other studies. Neither contrast nor ionizing radiation is required. It is inexpensive and portable. Although it is usually noninvasive, percutaneous needle aspiration can be done with ultrasound guidance. It is highly accurate in diagnosis and does not depend on organ function. It efficiently differentiates cystic and solid masses. The paucity of fat in children enhances the diagnostic ability of ultrasonography.[2] The only drawbacks are that it gives poor anatomic detail and is limited by the presence of intestinal gas or obesity. It is also very much operator dependent.

CT scan gives the best anatomic detail of all current modalities in common use, and it can determine the tissue density of the lesion as well as the presence of calcium and fat. The disadvantages of CT scan in children are that children have less fat and this limits organ differentiation, especially in the retroperitoneum.[2] Ionizing radiation and contrast enhancement are required, and children usually require sedation to avoid motion artifact. Longitudinal structures such as the inferior vena cava are difficult to visualize.

Radionuclide scintigraphy can demonstrate organomegaly and biliary tract abnormalities, but because of the need to use a radioactive tracer, it is not the modality of first choice. Specific indications for nuclear scans include the gallium scan or indium scan for abscesses and Meckel's scan for Meckel's diverticulitis. Similarly, because it is invasive, angiography is rarely used in pediatric cases. However, it may give important information about the vascular supply of a mass, which is useful in distinguishing benign and malignant tumors and in diagnosing hemangiomas.

The imaging capabilities of magnetic resonance are still being defined. The major limitations include the fact that respiration and bowel peristalsis cause motion artifact. Calcifications are not well seen. However, MRI does not use ionizing radiation, and metal clips do not cause streak artifacts. At present it is an expensive modality. Although MRI can accurately image the fetus and uterus, it probably will not replace ultrasonography.[48,49] With regard to imaging of specific organs, the liver and spleen are easily identified and have sharp margins. MRI is sensitive but not specific for liver disorders. For example, it cannot differentiate primary liver malignancy from metastases, but this is under active research at this time. Tumor extent can be defined. Liver cysts, abscesses, and hepatitis are well defined, whereas other infiltrates of the liver are not. The gallbladder is easily seen, as are choledochal cysts. Gallstones are not well seen.

With MRI, it is difficult to distinguish the pancreas from adjacent bowel loops, as the ideal enteral contrast agent is still being sought. Pancreatic pseudocysts are well defined, as are splenic abscesses and cysts. Lymphomas of the distal small bowel can be diagnosed. Abdominal abscesses can be defined if they are near a solid organ, such as the liver, but not if they are near bowel. The kidneys and renal cysts are usually well seen, as they are highlighted by perinephric fat. Hydronephrosis is easily diagnosed by the presence of urine, which appears dark.[50]

Vascular structures such as the portal vein, renal vein, and inferior vena cava are imaged better with MRI than with CT scan. Intravenous contrast is not required. Encasement or displacement of the vessels by Wilms' tumor or neuroblastoma is easily seen.[51]

SUMMARY

In summary, abdominal masses in children represent a wide variety of benign and malignant processes. The age and sex of the child as well as associated symptoms and physical findings provide important diagnostic leads. These clues, along with judicious use of the newer imaging modalities, readily reveal a diagnosis in most cases.

REFERENCES

1. Melicow MM, Uson AC. Palpable abdominal masses in infants and children: a report based on a review of 653 cases. J Urol 1959; 81:705–710.
2. Kirks DR, Merten DF, Grossman H, et al. Diagnostic imaging of pediatric abdominal masses: an overview. Radiol Clin North Am 1981; 19:527–545.
3. Donaldson JS, Shkolnik A. Pediatric renal masses. Semin Roentgenol 1988; 23:194–204.
4. Ault BH, Burton E, Stapleton FB. Cystic kidneys in infants: a brighter outlook. Contemp Pediatr 1988; (Oct):122–136.
5. Gaudin J, Le Treguilly C, Parent P, et al. Neonatal ovarian cysts. Twelve cysts with antenatal diagnosis. Pediatr Surg Int 1988; 3:158–164.
6. Wolfson BJ, Gainey MA, Faerber EN, et al. Renal masses in children. Urol Clin North Am 1985; 12:755–769.
7. Noseworthy J, Lack EE, Kozakewich HP, et al. Sacrococcygeal germ cell tumors in childhood: an updated experience with 118 patients. J Pediatr Surg 1981; 16:358–364.
8. Kim SH. Choledochal cyst: a survey by the Surgical Section of the American Academy of Pediatrics. J Pediatr Surg 1981; 16:402–407.
9. Daneman A. Adrenal neoplasms in children. Semin Roentgenol 1988; 23:205–215.
10. Teele RL, Henschke CI. Ultrasonography in the evaluation of 482 children with an abdominal mass. Clin Diagn Ultrasound 1984; 14:141–165.
11. Wilson DA. Ultrasound screening for abdominal masses in the neonatal period. Am J Dis Child 1982; 136:147–151.
12. Thompson JS, Ross RJ, Pizzaro ST. The wandering spleen in infancy and childhood. Clin Pediatr 1980; 19:221–224.
13. Teele RL, Share JC. The abdominal mass in the neonate. Semin Roentgenol 1988; 23:175–184.
14. Hays D. General principles of surgery. In: Pizzo P, Poplack P, eds. Principles and practice of pediatric oncology. Philadelphia: J B Lippincott, 1989: 207.
15. Barth RA, Brasch RC, Filly RA. Abdominal pseudotumor in childhood:

distended gallbladder with parenteral hyperalimentation. AJR 1981; 136:341–343.

16. O'Neill JA, Templeton JM Jr, Schnaufer LS, Bishop HC, Ziegler MM, Ross AJ III. Recent experience with choledochal cyst. Ann Surg 1987; 205:533–540.

17. Leonidas JC, Carter BL, Leape LL, et al. Computed tomography in diagnosis of abdominal masses in infancy and childhood. Arch Dis Child 1978; 53:120–125.

18. Moore S, Millar AJW, Cywes S. Liver abscess in childhood. A 13-year review. Pediatr Surg Int 1988; 3:27–32.

19. Boechat MI, Kangarloo H, Gilsanz V. Hepatic masses in children. Semin Roentgenol 1988; 23:185–193.

20. Alkalay AL, Puri AR, Pomerance JJ, el al. Mesenchymal hamartoma of the liver responsive to cyclophosphamide therapy: therapeutic approach. J Pediatr Surg 1985; 20:125–128.

21. Yandza T, Valayer J. Benign tumors of the liver in children: analysis of a series of 20 cases. J Pediatr Surg 1986; 21:419–423.

22. Dachman AH, Pakter RL, Ros PR, et al. Hepatoblastoma: radiologic-pathologic correlation in 50 cases. Radiology 1987; 164:15–19.

23. Davidson PM, Waters KD, Brown TCK, et al. Liver tumors in children. Pediatr Surg Int 1988; 3:377–381.

24. Robbins FG, Yellin AE, Lingua RW, et al. Splenic epidermoid cysts. Ann Surg 1978; 187:231–235.

25. Bishop HC. Diagnosis of pyloric stenosis by palpation. Clin Pediatr 1973; 12:226–227.

26. Holcomb GW III, Gheissari A, O'Neill JA Jr, et al. Surgical management of alimentary tract duplications. Ann Surg 1989; 209:167–174.

27. Mahaffey SM, Ryckman FC, Martin LW. Clinical aspects of abdominal masses in children. Semin Roentgenol 1988; 23:161–174.

28. Ravitch MM. Duplications of the gastrointestinal tract. In: Welch KJ, Randolph JG, Ravitch MM, O'Neill JA, Rowe MI, eds. Pediatric surgery. 4th ed. Chicago: Year Book, 1986: 911.

29. Puri P, Boyd E, Guiney EJ, et al. Appendix mass in the very young child. J Pediatr Surg 1981; 16:55–57.

30. Takiff H, Calabria R, Yin L, et al. Mesenteric cysts and intra-abdominal cystic lymphangiomas. Arch Surg 1985; 120:1266–1269.

31. Colodny AH. Mesenteric and omental cysts. In Welch KJ, Randolph JG, Ravitch MM, O'Neill JA, Rowe MI, eds. Pediatric surgery. 4th ed. Chicago, Year Book, 1986: 921.

32. Powell RW, Lightsey Al, Thomas WJ, et al. Castleman's disease in children. J Pediatr Surg 1986; 23:678–682.

33. Bove KE. Pathology of selected abdominal masses in children. Sem Roentgenol 1988; 23:147–160.

34. Bodai BI, Jung W, Marr C, et al. Omental cyst: case report and review of the literature. Contemp Surg 1983; 22:83–86.

35. Taitz LS, Brown CB, Blank CE, et al. Screening for polycystic kidney disease: importance of clinical presentation in the newborn. Arch Dis Child 1987; 62:45–49.

36. Cole BR, Conley SB, Stapleton FB. Polycystic kidney disease in the first year of life. J Pediatr 1987; 111:693–699.

37. Siegel MJ, McAlister WH. Simple cysts of the kidney in children. J Urol 1980; 123:75–78.

38. Hrabovsky EE, Othersen HB Jr, deLorimier A, et al. Wilms' tumor in the neonate: a report from the national Wilms' tumor study. J Pediatr Surg 1986; 21:385–387.

39. Gerber A, Gold JH, Bustamante S, et al. Congenital mesoblastic nephroma. J Pediatr Surg 1981; 16:758–759.

40. Fernbach SK, Feinstein KA, Donaldson JS, et al. Nephroblastomatosis: comparision of CT with US and urography. Radiology 1988; 166:153–156.

41. Butler H, Bick R, Morrison S. Unsuspected adrenal masses in the neonate: adrenal cortical carcinoma and neuroblastoma. A report of two cases. Pediatr Radiol 1988; 18:237–239.

42. Dahman B, Stephens CA. Pseudocysts of the pancreas after blunt abdominal trauma in children. J Pediatr Surg 1981; 16:17–21.

43. Sty JR, Wells RG. Other abdominal and pelvic masses in children. Semin Roentgenol 1988; 23:216–231.

44. Hartman GE, Shochat SJ. Abdominal mass lesions in the newborn: diagnosis and treatment. Clin Perinatol 1989; 16:123–135.

45. Hahn-Pedersen J, Kvist N, Nielsen OH. Hydrometrocolpos: Current views on pathogenesis and management. J Urol 1984; 132:537–540.

46. Stevenson RJ. Abdominal masses. Surg Clin North Am 1985; 65:1481–1504.

47. Swischuk LE. Abdominal masses and fluid. In: Holder TM, Ashcraft KW, eds. Pediatric surgery. Philadelphia: WB Saunders, 1980: 909.

48. Cohen MD. Gastrointestinal tract. In: Cohen MD, ed. Pediatric magnetic resonance imaging. Philadelphia: WB Saunders, 1986: 52.

49. Cohen MD. Reticuloendothelial and endocrine systems. In: Cohen MD, ed. Pediatric magnetic resonance imaging. Philadelphia: WB Saunders, 1986: 102.

50. Cohen MD. Genitourinary system. In: Cohen MD, ed. Pediatric magnetic resonance imaging. Philadelphia: WB Saunders, 1986: 62.

51. Cohen MD, Weetman R, Provisor A, et al. Magnetic resonance imaging of neuroblastoma with a 0.15-T magnet. AJR 1984; 143:1241–1248.

CHAPTER 12

Hepatic Failure

William R. Treem, M.D.

Hepatic failure is a clinical syndrome that reflects the consequences of severe hepatocyte dysfunction. In some cases, the insult to the liver is acute, resulting in fulminant injury to hepatocytes and rapid development of the clinical manifestations of hepatic failure. In others, it is the end-stage of chronic injury that has accumulated, causing a serious compromise of liver function. Regardless of the antecedent causes or duration of liver disease, hepatic failure is clinically characterized by hepatic encephalopathy, a complex coagulopathy, derangements of intrahepatic metabolic pathways, and the complications of renal dysfunction, cerebral edema, susceptibility to infection, and hemodynamic disturbances, all potentially related to impairment of hepatic synthesis or degradation of important chemical mediators of these processes. This chapter reviews the pathophysiology of hepatic failure. The various etiologies are only briefly discussed, since they are more fully covered in other chapters. Supportive modalities of therapy and newer experimental measures are discussed in light of knowledge of the pathophysiologic derangements. Methods of diagnosis and prognostic considerations are reviewed with emphasis on the appropriate selection of patients who are candidates for orthotopic liver transplantation. The reader is referred to several excellent reviews of hepatic failure for further information.[1-5]

DEFINITIONS

Traditionally, the definition of fulminant hepatic failure (FHF) has been based on the development of hepatic encephalopathy within 8 weeks of the first symptoms of illness without any previous history of underlying liver disease.[6] However, there is no general agreement on the time interval between the onset of jaundice and the development of encephalopathy. Some investigators allow only a 2-week interval to qualify the disorder as fulminant or acute liver failure.[7] Other terms such as *subfulminant, subacute,* and *late onset* hepatic failure have been substituted for cases demonstrating periods of greater than 2 weeks and less than 6 months prior to the onset of encephalopathy.[8,9] The distinction between these two groups seems arbitrary but is becoming more important in light of the availability of liver transplantation. Certain causes of acute hepatic failure are predominantly associated with a more truncated, and others with a more protracted, course. Recognition of the clinical course and prognostic indicators associated with each etiology may allow more timely inter-

vention by means of transplantation or medical therapies with a reasonable chance of promoting hepatic regeneration and recovery.

PRINCIPAL CAUSES OF HEPATIC FAILURE IN CHILDREN

Table 1 summarizes causes of hepatic failure in infancy and childhood, categorized by the age at which the liver fails and by the natural history of the disease process. The list is not exhaustive and is meant to offer a framework for differential diagnosis based on the age at presentation, the presence or absence of previous liver disease, and the evolution of clinical signs.

In adults, viral hepatitis and drug-induced hepatic toxicity are the two most common causes of FHF.[8,10-12] In the United States, hepatitis B virus (HBV) is the most common etiologic agent in many series.[11,13,14] The importance of the hepatitis delta virus (HDV) in the United States has recently been recognized. A report from Los Angeles showed that 34 percent of patients with HBV-associated fulminant hepatitis were also infected with HDV.[15]

FHF was reported in 31 children by a group of investigators from King's College Hospital in London.[16] Patients with Reye's syndrome and Wilson's disease were excluded from consideration. Acute viral hepatitis (HBsAg-negative) made up 26 of 31 cases. Three cases were due to acetaminophen overdose, one to ingestion of the mushroom *Amanita phalloides*, and one to halothane anesthesia. In Chile, a series of 28 children with fulminant hepatitis revealed 20 with hepatitis A virus (HAV), four with HBV, and four with presumed non-A non-B (NANB) hepatitis.[17] In developed countries, where the overall incidence of HAV infection in children is low, the importance of that virus as a cause of fulminant hepatic failure is minimal.

Another way to assess the relative frequencies of various etiologies of hepatic failure in children is to review mortality resulting from liver disease. Between 1976 and 1983, 81 children died of hepatic failure at a children's hospital.[18] These included 20 with biliary atresia; 22 with metabolic disorders (tyrosinemia, cystic fibrosis, alpha$_1$-antitrypsin [alpha$_1$-AT] deficiency, Wilson's disease, Zellweger's syndrome); 7 with Reye's syndrome; 15 with infections (HBV, adenovirus, cytomegalovirus, NANB hepatitis); 12 with cholestatic syndromes (Alagille's syndrome and other familial

TABLE 1
Etiology of Hepatic Failure in Infancy and Childhood

Timing of Hepatic Failure	Infancy (0–6 months)	Late Infancy (6–36 months)	Childhood
Fulminant	Congenital viral infections: Echovirus Herpesvirus Cytomegalovirus Hepatitis B Galactosemia	Hepatitis A ⟶ Hepatitis B ⟶ Delta hepatitis ⟶ Epstein-Barr virus ⟶ Drugs, toxins ⟶	Reye's syndrome
Late onset	Tyrosinemia Zellweger's syndrome Neonatal iron storage Wolman's disease	Hereditary fructose intolerance Non-A non-B hepatitis ⟶	Wilson's disease
Chronic liver disease	Hemangiomatosis	Biliary atresia Alpha₁-antitrypsin ⟶ deficiency Alagille's syndrome Nonsyndromic paucity of intrahepatic bile ducts Total parenteral nutrition Niemann-Pick disease Indian childhood cirrhosis	Wilson's disease Cystic fibrosis Byler's syndrome Sclerosing cholangitis Chronic active hepatitis Glycogen storage disease (type IV)

syndromes, and total parenteral nutrition–associated liver disease); 5 with miscellaneous causes including Budd-Chiari syndrome, autoimmune chronic active hepatitis, and primary hepatic tumors. Reye's syndrome would be less likely to account for deaths in more recent series because the incidence has fallen dramatically since 1980.[19]

A third method of estimating the contributions of various etiologies to the spectrum of hepatic failure in children is reviewing the selection of candidates for liver transplantation. In most pediatric liver transplant centers, patients with biliary atresia account for one-half to two-thirds of the total number of patients who undergo transplantation.[20,26] Inborn errors of metabolism including most prominently alpha₁-AT deficiency and smaller numbers of patients with Wilson's disease, tyrosinemia, glycogen storage disease, and Crigler-Najjar syndrome make up the second largest group, accounting for approximately 20 percent of the patients. Idiopathic cirrhosis secondary to presumed NANB hepatitis or autoimmune chronic active hepatitis is responsible for 10 to 15 percent. The balance of pediatric patients transplanted includes those with familial cholestatic syndromes, sclerosing cholangitis, primary nonmetastatic or nonmalignant liver tumors, and FHF. Seven pediatric patients who underwent transplantation at Pittsburgh Children's Hospital with FHF included five with NANB hepatitis, one with Wilson's disease, and one with valproate toxicity.[27]

Infectious Causes of Hepatic Failure

Acute Hepatitis B

In adults, acute hepatitis B either alone or together with HDV, is the most prevalent cause of fulminant viral hepatitis in Greece, France, and the United States.[8] In children, it is

a rare cause except in endemic areas such as Taiwan, where the carrier rate of HBV is 15 to 20 percent in pregnant women.[28] FHF due to HBV has been reported both in infants in the United States passed vertically from infected mothers and in older children secondary to blood transfusions.[29,30] The frequency of post-transfusion fulminant HBV infection has markedly decreased since the exclusion of HBsAg-positive blood donors from the blood supply.

Most infants infected from HBsAg-positive mothers have subclinical or mild icteric disease followed by chronic persistent hepatitis and the development of the carrier state.[31-34] Factors that promote vertical transmission include maternal infection during pregnancy, high maternal HBsAg titer, and maternal HBeAg positivity.[31,33,35] Eighty-five percent of infants born to HBeAg-positive, HBsAg-positive carrier mothers become chronic HBsAg carriers.[36,37] However, in studies from Taiwan and Japan, the occurrence of HBV-associated FHF in infants younger than 6 months was correlated with the presence of anti-HBe antibody and the absence of HBeAg in their mothers.[28,38] Fulminant hepatitis B in infants reported in the United States has also been associated with anti-HBe–positive, HBeAg-negative mothers.[29,30] Children infected at birth by HBsAg-positive, anti-HBe-positive mothers are also prone to develop acute icteric resolving hepatitis rather than subclinical infection.[39] Thus, although HBeAg is a practical marker of infectivity and confers a greater likelihood of the offspring becoming infected and developing the carrier state, the absence of HBeAg and the presence of anti-HBe antibody in a carrier mother seem to increase the risk of fulminant hepatitis B in the infant. Of five children with fulminant hepatitis B with a history of blood transfusions 2 to 5 months before the onset of fulminant hepatitis, three had received blood from anti-HBe–positive, HBV DNA–negative, HBsAg-positive carrier donors.[28] It appears that a relatively low dose of HBV infection passed from mother to infant or blood donor to recipient may cause a fulminant reaction leading to massive hepatic necrosis.[40]

Whether this overwhelming reaction is immune-mediated is unknown. Suggestions that the host immune system is playing a pivotal role come from several clinical observations. FHF due to massive liver necrosis has been reported in asymptomatic HBV chronic carriers being treated for malignancy after withdrawal of immunosuppressive drugs.[41] Several children who developed post-transfusion fulminant hepatitis B had leukemia in remission and a recent reduction in their chemotherapy, allowing recovery of a more normal immune response.[29] In a series of 65 patients with fulminant hepatitis B investigated soon after the onset of encephalopathy, serum HBV DNA was present in only 10 percent.[42] This finding indicates that viral multiplication has been interrupted early in most of these patients and suggests that host immunologic mechanisms are likely to be involved in the clearance of HBV, causing extensive necrosis of hepatocytes.

Delta Agent Infection (Hepatitis D)

The two mechanisms of delta agent (HDV) infection are co-infection with HBV in the normal person and superinfection of HBsAg-positive carriers. Whereas co-infection usually induces an acute hepatitis without long-term sequelae,[43-45] superinfection has a propensity to progress to chronic liver disease.[46,47]

Fulminant hepatitis has been reported both in patients who have simultaneous acute co-infection with HBV and HDV and in patients who have chronic hepatitis B and superimposed acute infection with HDV. In two studies of patients with HBsAg-positive fulminant hepatitis, the prevalence of delta markers was determined.[48,49] Using IgM antibody to hepatitis B core antigen as a marker of acute HBV infection, these studies showed that the prevalence of acute co-infection with HDV in patients with fulminant hepatitis B was approximately 30 percent. In contrast, a study of serologic markers in 118 patients with nonfulminant acute hepatitis B revealed only a 4.2 percent incidence of simultaneous HDV infection.[49] This finding has been interpreted as evidence that the risk of fulminant hepatitis is higher in patients with combined acute infection with HBV and HDV than in those with acute HBV infection alone.

The relative importance of acute co-infection versus superinfection of chronic hepatitis B carriers in the pathogenesis of fulminant HDV hepatitis varies according to the epidemiologic characteristics of the population studied. In tropical countries, where the rate of HBsAg carriers is very high, the majority of cases of fulminant hepatitis associated with HDV are mediated by superinfection. In contrast, the cases in more developed countries occur predominantly in drug addicts who acquire the HDV infection simultaneously with hepatitis B.[50,51] Of the patients with fulminant hepatitis and serologic markers of both hepatitis B and hepatitis D studied in Europe and the United States, a minority (23 to 47 percent) were examples of acute superinfection with the HDV in chronic carriers of hepatitis B.[48,49] However, superimposed HDV infection on the chronic carrier state of hepatitis B may carry greater risk of fulminant hepatic failure than simultaneous acute infection with the two agents. Ex-

perimental studies performed with chimpanzees have shown that more severe liver necrosis occurs when acute HDV infection is superimposed on pre-existing HBV infection than occurs with simultaneous acute infection with both the HDV and HBV.[52] Several studies have suggested but not completely documented that the mortality rate of fulminant hepatitis due to superinfection with HDV may be higher than that due to simultaneous acute co-infection in humans (Fig. 1).[48,53] In patients surviving fulminant hepatitis due to superinfection with HDV, chronic active hepatitis is a frequent development.[54-56]

A retrospective study from Europe including Italy, an endemic area, has reported that the prevalence of HDV infection in children with chronic HBsAg-positive hepatitis is approximately 12.5 percent.[57] Children with HDV antigen in the liver confirmed by direct immunofluorescent staining progress to cirrhosis more often than do HBsAg-positive, HDV antigen–negative children.[57] This progression is generally associated with serologic markers of low hepatitis B replication such as serum anti-HBe antibodies and lack of HBV DNA. However, superinfection with HDV is not the only cause of progressive liver disease in children who are HBsAg carriers. Thirty-seven HBsAg-positive pediatric patients in this study (41.5 percent) had severe progressive liver disease, including chronic active hepatitis and cirrhosis without HDV infection. An additional recent retrospective study from Taiwan (an area of high prevalence for HBV carriers but low prevalence of delta hepatitis superinfection) showed that only one of 68 children with chronic active HBV liver disease had anti-delta antibodies.[58]

HDV superinfection has also been implicated as the etiologic agent in epidemics of fulminant hepatitis in northern South America, with children under the age of 15 years most commonly affected.[59] These are endemic areas for HBV with a carrier rate of 15 to 20 percent and exposure to HBV infection documented in 90 percent of persons by age 5 years.

Non-A Non-B Hepatitis

In European patients with fulminant hepatitis the prevalence of cases attributed to sporadic NANB hepatitis was 24 percent in Athens,[12] 23 percent in France,[8] 27 percent in Denmark,[60] and 44 percent in England.[61] In a recent series from England, 43 of 47 patients with hepatic encephalopathy occurring more than 8 but less than 24 weeks after the onset of illness were thought to have NANB hepatitis, and the mortality rate was 81 percent.[9] The high mortality rate and prolonged period between the onset of jaundice and encephalopathy have been corroborated in other series of sporadic NANB-induced hepatic failure.[62] However, the absence until recently of a reliable diagnostic marker raises questions about the association between NANB hepatitis and fulminant hepatitis. Few cases called fulminant NANB hepatitis have had a history of preceding blood transfusions, administration of blood products, or intravenous drug addiction.[8] Among more than 1,000 pooled patients with post-transfusion NANB acute hepatitis in two studies, no cases of FHF were observed.[63,64]

In Western countries, children at special risk of NANB hepatitis are hemophiliacs or others who require frequent transfusions of blood products, as well as chronic dialysis

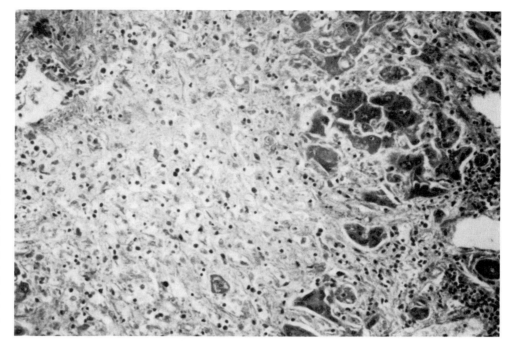

FIGURE 1 Submassive hepatic necrosis secondary to acute delta hepatitis infection superimposed on persistent hepatitis B infection. There is a rim of preserved periportal hepatocytes. The portal tracts are expanded owing to proliferation of bile ductules and a moderate lymphocyte infiltrate. The rest of the parenchyma is necrotic (Masson trichrome).

patients.[65] Most cases occur 5 to 12 weeks after a transfusion and tend to have mild anicteric disease with low levels of aminotransferases (200 to 600 IU per liter) that follow a fluctuating pattern. Although the acute disease is often mild, chronic alanine aminotransferase (ALT) elevations more than 6 months after the onset of symptoms occur in approximately 50 percent of patients, and 15 to 25 percent demonstrate histologic cirrhosis when followed for longer periods of time.[66,68] A series of 157 liver biopsy or autopsy specimens from hemophiliacs reviewed by a distinguished panel of hepatopathologists found 7 percent with severe chronic active hepatitis and 15 percent with cirrhosis thought to be attributable mainly to NANB hepatitis virus.[69] In another study, 26 percent of patients with hemophilia who had biopsies on one or more occasions had cirrhosis, and in 10 patients who had biopsies serially over an 8-year period cirrhosis developed in five. Based on this and other biopsy data, approximately 5 percent of patients with chronic NANB hepatitis may be expected to die of hepatic failure, particularly those whose transfusion requirement begins at a young age.

Herpes Simplex Virus and Epstein-Barr Virus

Severe hepatitis in the context of disseminated fatal herpes simplex virus infection (HSV) has been reported rarely in infants, older children, and adults. Neonatal infection is usually severe, generalized, and characteristically associated with retrograde spread of HSV-2 genital infection in the mother.[71,72] Infants are particularly at risk if the maternal infection is primary and not recurrent and active infection is present at the time of delivery. A clinical presentation of FHF on the fourth to seventh day of life may herald disseminated HSV infection. The liver grossly shows miliary nodules of necrosis, and microscopically there are extensive areas of bland necrosis with surrounding hemorrhage but with

minimal inflammatory reaction. Intranucleur inclusions typically can be seen (Fig. 2).

In older children and adults, fatal cases of disseminated HSV with hepatic necrosis have been reported in renal transplant patients treated with immunosuppresive drugs,[73,74] in children with kwashiorkor,[75] and in patients with primary or secondary immunodeficiency.[76,77] There have also been three reports of apparently immunocompetent children (ages 11 months, 22 months, and 13 years) whose deaths were attributed to fatal HSV hepatitis.[78] Early diagnosis requires a high index of suspicion. A characteristic clinical syndrome is fever, leukopenia, thrombocytopenia, high aminotransferase values, and normal to minimally elevated serum bilirubin levels. Typical mucocutaneous lesions may or may not be present. In immunocompromised patients, HSV infection should be considered in the differential diagnosis of FHF. With the introduction of relatively safe and effective antiviral therapy, a liver biopsy should be performed early, since characteristic histology, intranucleur inclusions, and immunoperoxidase staining can all facilitate early diagnosis and the institution of treatment.[79]

Rare fatal cases of Epstein-Barr virus (EBV)–associated fulminant hepatitis have been reported in children.[80–82] In most of these cases sensitive serologic or immunoperoxidase tissue-staining methods were not employed to exclude other hepatotropic viruses, and therefore the association is suspect. This conclusion is reinforced by the absence of serologic demonstration of acute EBV infection in any patient with FHF reported in several recent large series. Male children with an X-linked recessive lymphoproliferative syndrome can develop massive hepatic necrosis during EBV infection,[83] suggesting that immunodeficiency states are a prerequisite for the development of fulminant hepatitis with EBV. However, recently, two children with no evidence of immunodeficiency were reported to have acute EBV infection associated with

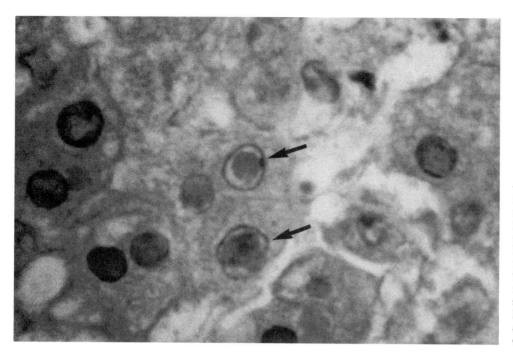

FIGURE 2 Intranuclear inclusions are found in hepatocytes just beyond the edges of areas of coagulative necrosis in this biopsy of a patient with fulminant herpes simplex hepatitis. Occasional liver cells have red Cowdry-type A viral inclusions (*arrows*). Many others have homogeneous "ground-glass" nuclei (hematoxylin and eosin).

FHF. In a 14-year-old girl, the diagnosis was serologically confirmed by an EBV VCA-IgM titer of 1:640, but a postmortem examination was not performed.[84] The second patient was a 9-year-old boy who died with a mononucleosis syndrome and FHF.[82] Epstein-Barr virus VCA-IgM was positive at a titer of 1:65, and all other hepatotropic viruses were excluded by appropriate negative serologic tests. Techniques of southern blot hybridization and in situ DNA hybrid probes were used to demonstrate the presence of highly concentrated EBV-specific DNA in liver tissue, but damaged cell structures caused by tissue necrosis prevented allocation of the EBV DNA to a certain cell type.

Echovirus

Fatal echovirus infection (types 6, 11, 14, and 19) causing massive hepatic necrosis has been documented mimicking neonatal HSV infection.[85-88] Accompanying clinical findings in these cases include focal encephalitis as well as renal and adrenal necrosis but no evidence of herpes-like intranuclear inclusions in the liver tissue.

Drug-Induced Fulminant Hepatic Failure

Table 2 lists drugs associated with hepatic failure due to massive or centrilobular hepatic necrosis, periportal necrosis, or steatosis. In children, the drugs most commonly implicated are acetaminophen; anticonvulsants including phenytoin and valproate; the anesthetic halothane; and the antituberculous drug isoniazid. Hepatocellular necrosis may occur as the result of a reactive metabolite of the drug interfering directly with a vital function within the cell or by covalent binding to intracellular targets.[89-92] An example of this process is seen with acetaminophen hepatotoxicity.[93] Toxins such as carbon tetrachloride can also damage the cell or in-

tracellular organelle membrane by other biochemical effects such as lipid peroxidation.[94] Hepatocellular damage may also elicit an immune response with features of generalized hypersensitivity such as fever, arthralgia, rash, eosinophilia, and generalized lymphadenopathy. Examples of drugs causing this syndrome are phenytoin, sulfamethoxazole, and sulfasalazine.[95-97] In other instances, the pathologic process is a combination of direct cell damage by the drug and a subsequent abnormal host immunologic response to an antigen exposed by that damage. The presence of IgG antibodies to halothane-altered hepatocyte membranes suggests that this mechanism may contribute to some cases of halothane-induced hepatotoxicity.[98-100]

Factors that influence drug metabolism in an individual affect the balance between the production of toxic metabolites via oxidation-reduction reactions (cytochrome P-450 enzymes) and detoxification of these metabolites via conjugation reactions (glucuronidation, sulfation, and glutathione conjugation).[89] Such factors include (1) genetic polymorphism affecting cytochrome hydroxylator or acetylator status,[101-103] (2) induction of enzyme systems by environmental exposure to drugs such as phenobarbital or ethanol, (3) nutritional status such as starvation or vitamin E deficiency,[104] (4) availability of co-factors such as glutathione, nicotinamide-adenine dinucleotide phosphate, or uridine diphosphoglucuronic acid,[105] and (5) hepatic zonal differences in the relative abundance of various drug metabolizing enzymes.[106] Morphologic features suggestive of drug-induced liver injury include discrete (zonal) necrosis, steatosis, bile duct damage, eosinophilia, granulomas, and unusually severe necrosis given the patient's condition and biochemical changes.[107,108]

In general, the necrosis produced by intrinsic hepatotoxins is zonal, whereas that produced by drugs causing hypersensitivity reactions is diffuse and confluent. Predominance of injury in acinar zone 3 (centrilobular) is characteristic of hepatic necrosis caused by agents converted to toxic metabo-

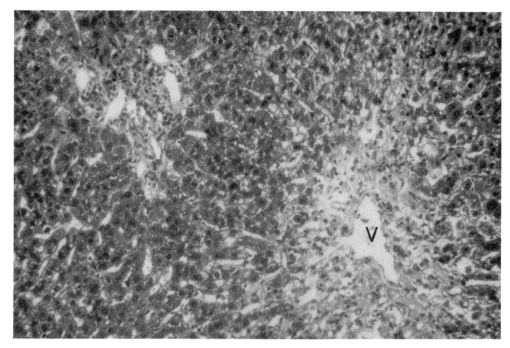

FIGURE 3 Typical zone 3 or centrilobular hepatic necrosis in a child with acetaminophen toxicity. There is necrosis of hepatocytes around the terminal hepatic venule (V) and a slight increase in fibrous tissue. The architecture in the rest of the lobule is preserved, and there is little inflammatory response (Masson trichrome).

lites by the cytochrome P-450 mixed function oxidase system, which is known to be concentrated in that zone.[109] Examples of drugs causing zone 3 necrosis are acetaminophen, carbon tetrachloride, and halothane (Figs. 3 and 4).[110] Examples of drugs causing zone 1 (periportal) necrosis are iron sulfate, phosphorus, and cocaine.[111]

The relationship between a drug and FHF may be clear or ambiguous. If the agent is hepatotoxic in a dose-related fashion (e.g., acetaminophen), levels can often be measured and the diagnosis is rarely in doubt. If the patient is taking a drug with common known hepatotoxic effects such as isoniazid or valproate, liver enzymes are serially measured and, if hepatoxicity occurs, there is a high index of suspicion. In the case of drugs known to cause hypersensitivity reactions, other simultaneous extrahepatic manifestations such as rash, peripheral eosinophilia, and arthralgias may signal drug-

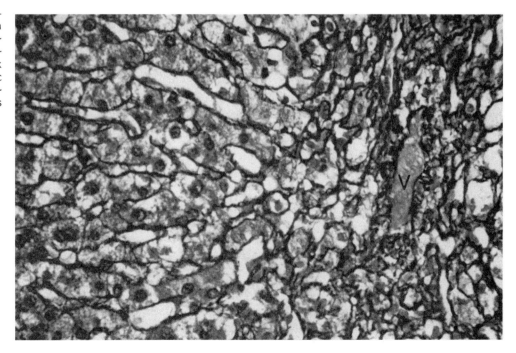

FIGURE 4 Acetaminophen toxicity. This special stain displays the disruption and collapse of the reticulin framework around the terminal hepatic venule (V) secondary to necrosis of pericentral hepatocytes (reticulin).

TABLE 2
Drugs Associated with Fulminant Hepatic Failure in Childhood:
Predominant Histologic Pattern

Massive Necrosis	Centrilobular Necrosis	Periportal Necrosis	Steatosis
Allopurinol	Acetaminophen	Iron sulfate	Valproate
Amitriptyline	Allopurinol	Phosphorus	Tetracycline
Carbamazepine	Diazepam	Cocaine	Amiodarone
Chlordiazepoxide	Enflurane		
Halothane	Halothane		
Hydralazine	Imipramine		
Indomethacin	Indomethacin		
Isoniazid	Isoniazid		
Ketoconazole	6-Mercaptopurine		
Methyldopa	Methoxyflurane		
Nitrofurantoin	Methyldopa		
Phenobarbital	Quinidine		
Phenytoin	Rifampin		
Propylthiouracil	Sulfasalazine		
Sulfamethoxazole	Valproate		
Valproate			

induced hepatotoxicity. Biopsy of the liver, if feasible, can be helpful, since it may show a pattern consistent with drug-induced hepatic failure.

Table 2 lists drugs associated with hepatic failure by histologic groupings: diffuse or massive hepatic necrosis, zone 3 or centrilobular necrosis, zone 1 or periportal necrosis, and diffuse steatosis. In the case of valproate, a commonly used anticonvulsant in pediatric patients, microvesicular steatosis is an important finding in patients with fulminant hepatic failure.[112–114]

"Ischemic" Hepatitis

FHF with jaundice, hepatic encephalopathy, and coagulopathy can accompany acute or chronic cardiac disease in children and even dominate the clinical presentation.[115–120] In 65 infants, children, and young adults with cardiovascular abnormalities evaluated by Mace and colleagues, those with low cardiac output (even without overt hypoxemia and hypotension) had the greatest derangement of bilirubin, aspartate aminotransferase, and prothrombin time.[121] A combination of chronic venous congestion and hypoxemia without low output was also associated with a high degree of abnormality on the above tests, although not to the extent of low cardiac output states. Since the liver receives a fixed 20 percent of cardiac output,[122] it compensates for a decrease in blood flow by increased oxygen extraction so that hepatic oxygen consumption is maintained at normal levels. If the hepatic blood flow drops below a critical level or the demands for oxygen increase such as with exercise or fever, this compensating mechanism becomes inadequate. In this setting, the hepatocytes around the central vein, which normally receive blood that has a lower oxygen content than the periportal hepatocytes, suffer irreversible hypoxic damage. This is manifested by the characteristic gross and microscopic histologic pattern of centrilobular hepatocyte necrosis with sparing of periportal hepatocytes seen in patients with low cardiac output during an episode of acute circulatory failure (Fig. 5). As the process becomes more chronic, there are increasing

sinusoidal engorgement, hepatocellular compression, atrophy, and collapse of the pericentral stroma, with subsequent deposition of bland fibrous tissue in the pericentral zones and central vein sclerosis[115,123] (Fig. 6).

CHRONIC LIVER DISEASE ASSOCIATED WITH HEPATIC FAILURE

Biliary Atresia

Prolonged bile flow restoration using a Roux-en-Y portoenterostomy (Kasai procedure) can be expected in 50 to 90 percent of patients with biliary atresia.[124–127] The prognosis after the Kasai procedure is related to the restoration of bile flow, which is most dependent upon early intervention. The anatomy and patency of the interlobular bile ducts at the time of surgery correlate with successful drainage in some studies[128] but not in others.[129] Data from Japan show successful bile drainage in more than 80 percent of patients undergoing the operation before 60 days of age, but in only 50 percent of those between 71 and 90 days of age when surgery was performed.[124] In a large English series of 149 cases, 71 percent of those operated on by 56 days of age were jaundice free, but the incidence fell to 25 to 35 percent in those operated on when older.[125] Even with the initial restoration of bile flow after the Kasai procedure, the long-term prognosis is a function of the pace of progressive obliteration of intrahepatic bile ducts as a result of the original insult and recurrent episodes of bacterial cholangitis. Approximately 40 percent of children with extrahepatic biliary atresia are immediate candidates for orthotopic liver transplantation, because postoperatively complete restoration of bile flow is not obtained and jaundice does not disappear.[130] Eighty percent of these children die of complications of cirrhosis before 3 years of age if transplantation is not performed.[124] Even if bile flow is restored and serum bilirubin transiently returns to normal, a significant number of patients have per-

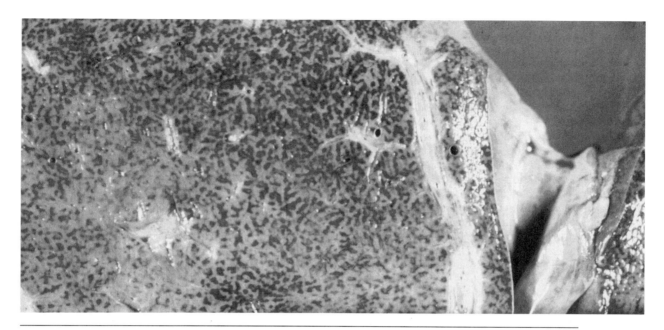

FIGURE 5 Cut surface of the liver from a child with an acute-onset cardiomyopathy and cardiogenic shock. The cut surface shows parenchymal congestion and a typical "nutmeg" pattern. The dark areas correspond to hemorrhage, sinusoidal congestion, and necrosis around the central veins and the light areas to spared periportal regions. (From Treem and Boyle.[115])

sistent cholestasis, recurrent jaundice, and progressive biliary cirrhosis. Hepatic failure may occur in these patients between 2 and 10 years after the original portoenterostomy.

FHF may develop suddenly in patients after portoenterostomy. Gartner and colleagues described four patients aged 7 to 13 months who died suddenly in FHF after episodes of presumed hypovolemia from bleeding, diuretic use, or sepsis.[131] All had undergone portoenterostomy and two of the four were stable outpatients, but only one appeared to have

adequate restoration of bile flow. At autopsy, a common feature was almost total infarction of hepatocytes with patent hepatic arteries and portal veins.

Alpha₁-Antitrypsin Deficiency

In patients with alpha₁-AT deficiency (PiZ phenotype), a significant proportion of those who present with neonatal cholestasis are at risk for the development of cirrhosis and

FIGURE 6 Autopsy section from a child with cardiogenic shock superimposed on chronic congestive heart failure. There is striking central vein dilatation, pericentral hemorrhage and necrosis, and collapse of hepatocytes. A rim of periportal hepatocytes is spared. Cholestasis is present, but there is no evidence of an inflammatory infiltrate in the portal tracts (hematoxylin and eosin). (From Treem and Boyle.[115])

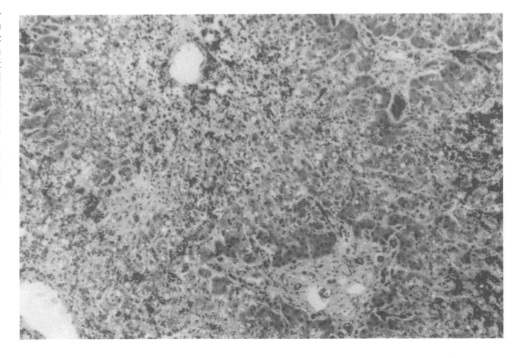

liver failure.[132] Alagille and colleagues reported that of 45 PiZ infants who presented with neonatal cholestasis, 25 patients later developed cirrhosis.[133,134] Portal hypertension was present in 19 of 25 children with cirrhosis, and eight children died in the first decade of life. In a group of 17 PiZ infants with neonatal hepatitis studied by Lutz and Cox, six developed cirrhosis and died between 6 and 12 years of age of liver failure or complications of cirrhosis.[135] Ghishan and Greene followed 15 patients with PiZ phenotype who presented with neonatal cholestatic jaundice. Three underwent liver transplantation because of decompensated cirrhosis at 3, 3½, and 7 years of age. Two additional patients died at 4 months and 3 years from complications of cirrhosis. Of the remaining 10 patients, three had histologic evidence of cirrhosis, and the remaining seven patients continued to have an enlarged liver and spleen with abnormal liver enzymes, but no follow-up biopsies were performed.[136] The only prospective study shows that 11 percent of all PiZ infants develop cirrhosis after 8 years.[137] Some investigators believe that the presence of cirrhosis associated with alpha$_1$-AT deficiency ensures that the patient will die of progressive liver failure at some time during childhood or adolescence.[130]

Wilson's Disease

The diagnosis of Wilson's disease is frequently delayed in children until jaundice, coagulopathy, and ascites signal terminal decompensated cirrhosis. Wilson's disease may also first present with FHF and encephalopathy in children without previous evidence of chronic liver or neurologic disease.[138-141] In these cases, morphologic study shows massive hepatic necrosis, nodular regeneration, and increased fat. Many clinical features of idiopathic FHF are similar to those found in patients with Wilson's disease, including elevated 24-hour urinary copper and decreased serum ceruloplasmin levels. Features that distinguish Wilson's disease from idiopathic FHF include high copper levels in serum and liver, less pronounced elevations of transaminase levels, higher concentrations of total bilirubin, and lower hemoglobin levels.[138,142] The latter two parameters may reflect significant intravascular hemolysis, which has been reported to accompany FHF in children with Wilson's disease. Serum copper is the most useful premortem biochemical test; it is high in Wilson's disease presenting with FHF and normal or low in patients with idiopathic FHF.

Patients with Wilson's disease who present with FHF are immediate candidates for liver transplantation, since none will respond to chelation therapy with D-penicillamine.[142] Based on the degree of abnormality of ALT, bilirubin, and prothrombin time, one group of investigators has developed a prognostic index that correctly predicts the response to treatment in subsequent cases.[143] A bilirubin greater than 10 mg per deciliter, an ALT greater than 200 IU per liter, and a prothrombin time greater than 12 seconds prolonged above control are predictive of a poor response to therapy and require referral for transplantation. The presence of cirrhosis confirmed histologically is also a poor prognostic sign.[149] A 5-year survival of less than 50 percent despite adequate chelation therapy was recorded in two series of patients with Wilson's disease who presented with decompensated cirrhosis.[144,145] Failure of a 2- to 3-month course of chelation therapy in patients with Wilson's disease and decompensated cirrhosis is considered an indication for liver transplantation.[142]

Autoimmune Chronic Active Hepatitis

Hepatic failure in children with autoimmune chronic active hepatitis (CAH) is uncommon. In recent reported series, few children died, but the majority had proven or suspected cirrhosis.[146-148] Identification of new autoimmune markers has allowed the subdivision of autoimmune CAH into groups that appear to be associated with a different prognosis, particularly in children. The presence of antiliver-antikidney microsomal antibodies (anti-LKM1) and absence of antimitochondrial antibodies, and only rare presence of antiactin (anti–smooth muscle) or antinuclear antibodies, appear to be associated with a higher incidence of cirrhosis and hepatic failure in children.[149] Patients with anti-LKM1 antibodies appear to have a more aggressive course, with a fulminant onset of hepatitis observed in six patients in the largest series.[150] Of 65 patients in this series, approximately half the patients who had anti-LKM1 antibodies presented with an acute hepatitis picture, and there was rapid progression to cirrhosis in 82 percent within 6 months to 3 years. The overall actuarial survival rate for all patients treated with corticosteroid therapy and followed up to 14 years was 51 percent. All but two of the survivors had residual inactive cirrhosis. Hepatic encephalopathy has appeared in 11 of the survivors, all of whom have a small atrophic liver.

Anti-LKM1 antibody–positive CAH has occurred at all ages but is most common between 2 and 14 years of age. In a series of 20 pediatric patients with anti-LKM1–positive CAH, six patients were younger than 3 years of age.[149] All but one of the 20 children reported had cirrhosis and one presented in FHF. Four children died in spite of immunosuppressive therapy, three as a direct result of hepatic failure.

HEPATIC ENCEPHALOPATHY

The hallmark of hepatic failure is encephalopathy. During the last 30 years, there have been great efforts to identify the encephalopathic agent or agents responsible for hepatic encephalopathy and devise a unifying theory. This section describes the typical clinical manifestations of hepatic failure and encephalopathy and explores proposed pathophysiologic mechanisms to explain them.

Clinical Manifestations of Hepatic Failure and Encephalopathy

The clinical appearance of hepatic encephalopathy is variable, depending on the extent and rapidity of hepatic damage, the degree of portal-systemic shunting, and the contributions of precipitating factors. FHF secondary to hepatitis A infection may progress to coma and unresponsiveness over days from the onset of jaundice, whereas a child with Wilson's disease may have intermittent mild alterations in mental status, waxing and waning, which become progressively more severe over months. A child with cirrhosis and alpha$_1$-AT deficiency may be well compensated until major gastrointestinal (GI) hemorrhage or infection precipitates the onset of hepatic encephalopathy. Table 3 lists clinical clues signifying an atypical course of viral hepatitis, suggesting that the patient is at risk of FHF.

Patients with hepatic encephalopathy are traditionally divided into stages or grades that correlate with clinical severity and prognosis. Table 4 summarizes some of the mental status changes, neurologic findings, and other physical signs seen in stages I to V of hepatic encephalopathy. Passage through these stages may be rapid, as in Reye's syndrome, so that the early phases are missed. In more gradual processes, the early subtle stages may be mistaken for behavioral or psychiatric disturbances and may be first noticed by teachers. Deterioration of school performance in the classroom may be the earliest sign. A child with the acute onset of combative or irrational behavior should always be screened for evidence of hepatic encephalopathy.

Asterixis is described as a flapping tremor of the fingers and wrist elicited by attempted dorsiflexion of the wrist with the arm extended and forearm fixed. It is absent at rest and maximum with sustained posture. During coma, the tremor disappears. Asterixis is not specific for hepatic encephalopathy.[151] It can also be present in uremia, respiratory failure, or severe congestive heart failure. Fetor hepaticus is a peculiar odor described as mildly sweet-smelling and fruity, fecal, or musty. It is specific for hepatic failure and is presumably of intestinal origin, since it becomes less intense with treatment designed to alter intestinal flora. Fetor hepaticus is thought to be due to mercaptans, such as methanethiol or its derivatives dimethyl disulfide, or dimethyl sulfide. These metabolites have been found in the blood, breath, and urine of patients with hepatic failure.[152,153] Direct measurements have established that mercaptans are normally present in breath

TABLE 3
Atypical Course of Viral Hepatitis Indicating Potential Fulminant Hepatic Failure

Persistent or deepening jaundice (bilirubin greater than 20 mg per deciliter)

Persistent anorexia and/or vomiting

Relapse of initial symptoms, fever after jaundice appears

Mental status changes

Hyperventilation and respiratory alkalosis

Shrinking liver size and falling aminotransferases in the face of an increasing bilirubin

Development of ascites

Hypoglycemia, persistent large dextrose requirement

Low BUN, albumin, cholesterol

Leukocytosis and thrombocytopenia

Vitamin K–resistant prolongation of prothrombin time

TABLE 4
Clinical Staging of Hepatic Encephalopathy

Category of Physical Signs	Stage I	Stage II	Stage III	Stage IV	Stage V
Mental Status	Alert, oriented, slow mentation	Lethargic, confused, agitated	Stupor, arousal to voice	Unarousable	Unarousable
Behavior	Restless, irritable, short attention span, disordered sleep	Combative, sullen, euphoric	Sleeps most of time, marked confusion	None	None
Spontaneous motor activity	Inco-ordination, tremor, poor handwriting	Yawning, sucking, grimacing, intention tremor present, blinking	Decreased, marked intention tremor	Absent	None
Asterixis	Absent	Present	Present (if co-operates)	Absent	Absent
Muscle tone	Normal	Increased	Increased	Increased	Flaccid
Reflexes	Normal	Hyper-reflexic	Hyper-reflexic extensor plantars	Hyper-reflexic extensor plantars	Absent
Respirations	Regular or hyperventilation	Hyperventilation	Hyperventilation	Irregular	Apnea
Verbal response	Normal	Confused, dysarthric	Incoherent	None	None
Motor response	Obeys commands	Purposeful movements, may not respond to commands	Localized appropriately to pain	Abnormal flexor, abnormal extensor	None
Pupils	Brisk	Brisk	Brisk	Sluggish	Fixed
Eye opening	Spontaneous	Verbal stimuli	Verbal stimuli	Noxious stimuli	None
Oculocephalic Oculovestibular	Normal	Normal	Normal	Partial dysconjugate	Absent

and that they increase fourfold in hepatic failure.[154] Mercaptans are metabolic products of the action of gut flora on methionine and are present in larger amounts because of liver damage and inhibition of the normal hepatic demethylating reactions.

The stage of hepatic encephalopathy is an important prognostic variable, especially in cases of FHF. One-third to two-thirds of patients survive stage II or III hepatic encephalopathy, but mortality of patients who reach stage IV is more than 80 percent. The advent of orthotopic liver transplantation appears to be modifying these statistics.

Pathogenesis of Hepatic Encephalopathy

Recent reviews of the pathophysiology of hepatic encephalopathy have concentrated on four major hypotheses. (1) The *ammonia hypothesis* suggests that ammonia accumulation in the brain is primarily responsible. (2) The *synergistic neurotoxins hypothesis* states that encephalopathy and coma are the result of synergistic effects of accumulating toxins, with coma-producing potential augmented by other endogenous metabolic abnormalities. (3) The *false neurotransmitter hypothesis* suggests that an excessive production of brain inhibitory neurotransmitter (serotonin) and false neurotransmitter (octopamine) and a deficient synthesis of excitatory neurotransmitters (norepinephrine and dopamine) are responsible for encephalopathy and coma. (4) The *GABA-ergic inhibitory neurotransmitter hypothesis* divides brain amino acids into excitatory and inhibitory neurotransmitters and concentrates on gamma-aminobutyric acid (GABA) and glycine as the main inhibitory neurotransmitters. In this hypothesis, hepatic encephalopathy is the result of increased GABA-ergic and glycinergic neurotransmission.

No single hypothesis is completely satisfactory to explain the pathophysiology of hepatic encephalopathy, which may be multifactorial and involve aspects of all of these theories. However, all explanations depend to a certain extent on several accompanying abnormalities almost universally present in hepatic failure.

Portal-Systemic Shunting

As liver destruction proceeds, more blood flow from the intestine is shunted around the liver completely or through the liver, bypassing viable hepatocytes. Thus, the liver is unable to completely remove potentially toxic metabolites normally formed by intestinal bacterial degradation of proteins, amino acids, and blood. In acute forms of hepatic failure, the shunts exist within the liver past damaged or necrotic hepatocytes, but in more chronic forms portal vein–to–hepatic vein shunts around cirrhotic nodules or even prehepatic portal-systemic shunts through large spontaneous venous collaterals can develop (Fig. 7). Although hepatic encephalopathy is rare in children with prehepatic portal-systemic shunting owing to cavernous transformation of the portal vein, it has been reported after surgical shunting procedures in spite of seemingly normal hepatocyte function.[155] This finding is analogous to the animal model of hepatic encephalopathy by surgical creation of a portacaval anastomosis (Eck fistula) and

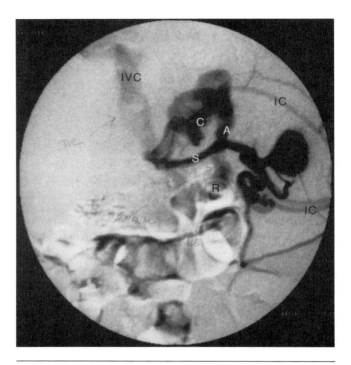

FIGURE 7 Negative-contrast percutaneous ultrasound-guided splenoportography in an infant with biliary atresia showing the spontaneous development of a splenorenal shunt via the splenic vein (S), coronary vein (C), adrenal vein (A), left renal vein (R), and inferior vena cava (IVC). Note the absence of an identifiable portal vein and also the large intercostal veins (IC) fed from large collaterals emanating from the splenic hilum.

subsequent feeding of a high-protein diet in an animal with a previously normal liver.

Blood-Brain Barrier Permeability

Alterations in the function of the blood-brain barrier (BBB) are also likely to contribute to the genesis and maintenance of hepatic encephalopathy. The BBB plays an essential role in excluding toxic substances delivered via the systemic circulation from entry into the brain. Unlike capillary systems elsewhere in the body, the endothelial cells of the cerebral capillaries are uniquely impermeable, without fenestrations, and with few pinocytotic vesicles. Furthermore, the BBB is strengthened by the endothelial basement membrane and by astrocyte processes that completely envelop the capillaries. Animal models of acute hepatic failure have been used to demonstrate increased permeability to normally excluded substances during induction of hepatic encephalopathy, including trypan blue, insulin, D-sucrose, L-glucose, and horseradish peroxidase.[156,157] In normal rats, infusion of ammonia, methyloctanoate, mercaptans, and phenolic acids has been shown to increase the permeability of the BBB.[158] Thus, accumulating toxins in hepatic encephalopathy may mediate their own increased entry into the target organ. Electron microscopic studies of the BBB in animal models of acute hepatic failure have thus far failed to demonstrate consistent recognizable alterations in intercellular tight junctions.[159]

Contributing Metabolic Alterations

Concomitant alterations in metabolism accompanying hepatic failure probably play an auxiliary role in the progression and outcome of hepatic encephalopathy. Hypoglycemia develops rapidly in the hepatectomized animal. It is also a common clinical occurrence in FHF in children and in syndromes that more specifically cause mitochondrial dysfunction interfering with gluconeogenesis, such as Reye's syndrome and genetic or acquired disorders of fatty acid oxidation.[160] Even in patients with viral hepatitis without massive or subacute necrosis, clinically inapparent fasting hypoglycemia was found in one-half of the subjects appropriately studied.[161] Hepatic glycogen stores are depleted and gluconeogenesis is impaired when hepatic necrosis is massive. Insulin metabolism is slowed, leading to elevated circulating levels. Since glucose is an important fuel for cerebral function, decreased availability could contribute to decreased brain energy metabolism. However, both in experimental animals with cirrhosis and in cirrhotic patients with coma of less than 24 hours duration, brain glucose utilization is normal.[162,163]

Decreased synthesis of proteins by the failing liver may also contribute to the development of hepatic encephalopathy. Decreased plasma albumin concentration limits albumin binding of exogenous and endogenous substances, which in the free form penetrate the BBB. Examples of such potential contributing toxins include highly bound sedative-hypnotic drugs (e.g., benzodiazepines) and free fatty acids.

Hypoxemia is common in cirrhotic patients and has been related to intrapulmonary shunting through microscopic arteriovenous fistulas.[164-166] In addition, in patients with FHF, there is a low pulmonary vascular resistance, peripheral pulmonary vasodilatation, and defective hypoxic pulmonary vasoconstriction leading to a ventilation-perfusion mismatch.[167,168] Finally, when hepatic encephalopathy develops, red cell 2,3-diphosphoglycerate increases, shifting the oxyhemoglobin dissociation curve to the right and further decreasing oxygen delivery to the tissues.[169] In animals, hypoxia and hypoxemia have been shown to increase the acute encephalopathy caused by ammonia.[170]

Acid-base abnormalities are frequently present prior to the development of hepatic encephalopathy. The respiratory center is stimulated in the presence of hepatic failure and respiratory alkalosis can develop, leading to a reduction in cerebral blood flow. Serum potassium tends to fall related to urinary losses from hyperaldosteronism, renal tubular disease, diuretic therapy, poor intake, vomiting, and high glucose infusions. This precipitates a metabolic alkalosis, potentiating the change in pH. Theoretically, in the presence of alkalosis, impermeable NH_4^+ becomes NH_3, which should favor the movement of ammonia into cells, potentiating absorption of ammonia in the gut and accumulation in the brain.

Toxic Metabolites in Hepatic Encephalopathy

There is no general agreement on which neuroactive metabolites are of importance in the pathogenesis of hepatic encephalopathy. However, several generalizations and conditions are broadly accepted in testing the various hypotheses:

(1) The metabolite is a toxic nitrogenous substance partially produced by the metabolism of enteric bacteria and normally extracted from the portal circulation by viable hepatocytes. This concept is supported by two clinical observations: First, hepatic encephalopathy is precipitated or exacerbated by the ingestion of protein or delivery of protein in the form of blood to the gut; and second, hepatic encephalopathy can be prevented or ameliorated by administering oral broad-spectrum antibiotics. (2) The metabolite must gain access to the brain by crossing the BBB and demonstrate increased permeability and abnormal accumulation in the brain in the presence of hepatic failure. (3) The metabolite should be capable of direct toxicity to neurons or modulation of neuronal function by altering the metabolism of neurotransmitters and/or the functional status of neurotransmitter receptors. The lack of structural neuropathologic changes in the brains of patients with chronic hepatocellular failure and the potential for rapid reversibility of the encephalopathy are evidence that a change in brain function and metabolism is responsible. (4) The metabolite should be capable of producing coma and a clinical picture similar to hepatic encephalopathy when infused in large amounts in normal experimental animals or in smaller amounts in animal models of cirrhosis. (5) Intervention leading to correction of the abnormal plasma or brain levels of the metabolite or intervention blocking its mode of action on the target organ, the brain, should lead to a reversal of the clinical state of hepatic encephalopathy.

Ammonia Hypothesis. Ammonia is increased in blood, and ammonia and glutamine are increased in muscle, brain, and cerebrospinal fluid (CSF) in patients with cirrhosis, hepatic encephalopathy, and FHF, as well as in animals with portacaval anastomosis.[1,2] Hyperammonemia also occurs in encephalopathies associated with Reye's syndrome[171,172] and congenital metabolic liver disease such as urea cycle defects,[173] organic acidemias, and defects in fatty acid oxidation.[160,174] Hyperammonemia and coma are also associated with valproic acid therapy in certain patients.[175]

Ammonia is generated in the bowel after ingestion of dietary protein by the action of bacterial urease and endogenous gut amino acid oxidases on nitrogenous substances, including urea and amino acids such as glutamine.[176] It appears from studies of germ-free animals and studies with isolated bowel segments that only one-half of the ammonia coming from the bowel is the result of colonic bacterial action, with the remainder arising from metabolic utilization of glutamine by the small intestine.[177] Even during fasting, endogenous glutamine and urea act as substrates for ammonia production in the gut.[178] However, under fasting conditions, ammonia coming from the kidney, muscle, and brain takes on more significance.[179] Ammonia release from the kidney is greater than normal in patients with hepatic encephalopathy and is increased further by alkalinization of urine and hypokalemia. Absorbed ammonia is carried from the gut to the liver by the portal venous system, where it is rapidly converted to glutamine via transamination of alpha-ketoglutarate to glutamate. The liver converts ammonia to urea more slowly via the enzymes of the urea cycle (Fig. 8). The capacities of the two ammonia-removal systems are approximately equal. When there is excess ammonia, the availability of ornithine becomes rate-limiting for the urea cycle. Supplemental ornithine (or arginine) enhances the conver-

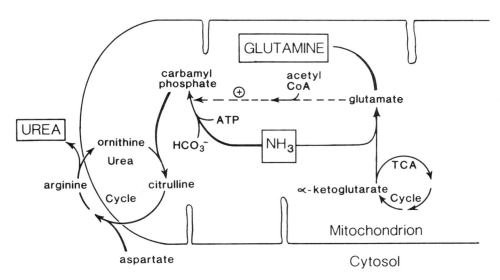

FIGURE 8 Pathways of ammonia metabolism in the liver. Ammonia is generated mainly in the intestine by metabolism of arterial glutamine and by gut bacterial metabolism of urea and dietary protein. Kidney and skeletal muscle (especially during exercise) are other sources. The liver metabolizes ammonia rapidly via conversion to glutamate and then glutamine. More slowly ammonia enters the urea cycle via the synthesis of carbamyl phosphate from bicarbonate and ammonia. This reaction requires the presence of *N*-acetylglutamate from acetyl-CoA and glutamate. Ornithine is regenerated at each turn of the cycle as arginine is hydrolyzed in the cytosol, forming urea and ornithine.

sion of ammonia to citrulline and urea by increasing carbamyl transferase activity.[180] If the urea cycle is lost, as it is in a hepatectomized dog, glutamine synthesis can expand to compensate partially for the increased ammonia load, but whether or not intrahepatic glutamine synthesis can compensate to some extent in patients with hepatic failure has not been shown. The liver also produces some ammonia when amino acids are excessive. After a meal, amino acids not utilized immediately for protein synthesis are deaminated and ammonia is produced. High blood levels of ammonia have been shown to stimulate glucagon secretion in patients with cirrhosis and portal-systemic shunts.[181] Increased glucagon secretion leads to increased deamination of amino acids for increased hepatic gluconeogenesis, which further augments ammonia production.

The liver ordinarily removes 80 percent of the portal vein ammonia in a single pass. Extensive portal-systemic shunting and disruption of the intracellular urea cycle allow large quantities of ammonia to bypass the liver and concentrate in the brain. Under normal resting conditions there is a small uptake of ammonia by peripheral tissues, but in the face of rising blood ammonia levels generated by exercise, the extraction of ammonia by the muscles of the extremities may exceed 50 percent of the arterial level.[182] This potential detoxification mechanism may be impaired in a patient with decreased skeletal muscle mass secondary to chronic liver disease, or in an infant in whom the proportion of skeletal muscle to body weight is only one-half that of the adult.

The brain, unlike the liver, has no functional urea cycle, and ammonia is primarily detoxified by conversion to glutamine and further to alpha-ketoglutaramate by brain astrocytes (Fig. 9). When blood ammonia levels are increased, brain and muscle uptake is also increased proportionally.[183] However, in general, the correlation between blood ammonia and the degree of hepatic encephalopathy is poor. Correlation between CSF glutamine and alpha-ketoglutaramate

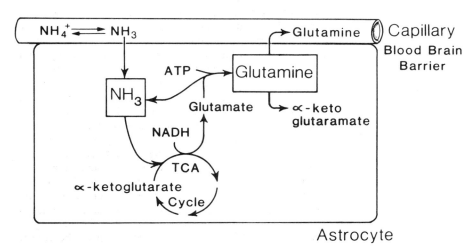

FIGURE 9 Brain metabolism of ammonia. The brain astrocyte "detoxifies" ammonia chiefly by glutamine formation in two major steps. The first is a reductive amination of alpha-ketoglutarate derived from the tricarboxylic (TCA) cycle requiring NADH and generating glutamate. The second reaction requires ATP and results in glutamine formation. Thus, an increased ammonia load could (1) deplete alpha-ketoglutarate, impairing oxidative metabolism; (2) reduce the availability of NADH for the electron transport chain, reducing energy production and oxygen consumption; and (3) consume ATP, leading to reduced stores of high-energy phosphates for other key reactions.

(presumably reflecting the brain concentrations of accumulating ammonia) and the clinical severity of encephalopathy has been much closer.[184-186]

When cirrhotic patients are fed ammonium salts, protein, amino acids, or urea, a neurologic syndrome resembling hepatic encephalopathy is induced. Therapeutic maneuvers aimed at reducing the intestinal absorption of ammonia tend to be associated with an amelioration of encephalopathy in cirrhotic patients. Other clinical evidence used to support the ammonia hypothesis includes the observation that milk and vegetable proteins, which generate less ammonia than do meat and animal proteins, are tolerated better by cirrhotics with significant portal-systemic shunting.[187-189] The congenital hyperammonemic syndromes are also thought to provide support for the role of ammonia, since these infants present with coma, similar to adult cirrhotics with hepatic encephalopathy. In animal models of portacaval shunting and a chronic low-grade state of ammonia excess, the infusion of a small, ordinarily nontoxic ammonia load results in neurologic effects similar to those documented in hepatic encephalopathy.[190] In these animals, type II astrocytes are increased, brain alpha-ketoglutarate levels are reduced, cerebral blood flow and oxygen consumption are reduced, and the concentrations of glutamate and aspartate (potential excitatory neurotransmitters) are reduced. The electroencephalogram (EEG) develops high-voltage slow waves.[191,192]

In spite of this compelling evidence, there are strong criticisms of the ammonia hypothesis. Most have centered on the issue of whether ammonia-induced encephalopathy actually resembles hepatic encephalopathy. Evidence that there is a difference is based on animal and human studies. A rabbit model of galactosamine-induced FHF combined with careful quantitative and qualitative measurements of visual evoked potentials (VEPs) has been used and compared with the VEPs produced in rabbits with acute hyperammonemic encephalopathy, postictal coma, and toxin-induced coma resulting from the administration of a combination of subcoma doses of three neurotoxins: ammonia, dimethylsulfide, and octanoic acid. In the absence of seizures, patterns of VEPs showed marked dissimilarities between any stage of galactosamine-induced hepatic failure and hyperammonemic encephalopathy or that caused by "synergistic" neurotoxins. In contrast, if seizures occurred, the pattern of VEPs in early postictal coma resembled that of late-stage hepatic encephalopathy due to galactosamine-induced FHF.[193] Other studies have supported the concept that increasing ammonia intoxication causes a preconvulsive state, progresses to seizures, and finally results in a postictal encephalopathic state that resembles hepatic encephalopathy but is caused by the seizures rather than the ammonia itself.[194,195] Hyperammonemia has failed to produce EEG changes characteristic of hepatic encephalopathy in animal models and in patients with liver disease given ammonium salts.[196,197] Ammonia reduces inhibitory neurotransmission by decreasing chloride conductance across the cell membrane of postsynaptic neurons.[198] It thus promotes neural excitation and seizures, a state distinctly different from that of neural inhibition and lack of seizures in hepatic encephalopathy. Further differences relate to studies of brain neurotransmitters. In rabbit brain, hyperammonemia leads to an increase in glutamate receptors, but in the rabbit galactosamine-induced FHF model a decreased

number of glutamate receptors are found.[199] Other neuroactive nitrogenous substances besides ammonia may be increased by the ingestion of protein or blood in patients with cirrhosis and decreased by antibiotic inhibition of gut bacteria. Finally, the correlation between arterial blood ammonia and the stage of hepatic encephalopathy is poor, and the clinical findings may develop even before the blood ammonia level is elevated.

Synergistic Neurotoxins Hypothesis. In an effort to overcome these arguments against ammonia as the sole neurotoxin, Zieve and co-workers proposed that a combination of neurotoxic metabolites (each at brain levels insufficient to cause encephalopathy if acting alone) act synergistically on the brain to produce hepatic encephalopathy.[1] Candidates include ammonia, mercaptans, fatty acids, and phenols. All accumulate in plasma and brain during hepatic failure, and all have been shown to cause reversible coma in animals when given alone in large doses.[200-204]

Mercaptans are thioalcohols largely generated in the GI tract by the action of bacteria on methionine. They are normally efficiently removed by the liver. Blood methanethiol levels are 2.5 times normal in adults with hepatic encephalopathy.[153] In one study of patients with alcoholic liver disease, blood methanethiol levels correlated well with the stage of encephalopathy.[205] However, other studies using a different assay have failed to show any difference in methanethiol metabolites in the blood of patients versus controls.[206] In vitro studies have shown that low concentrations of methanethiol can inhibit brain microsomal Na^+,K^+-ATPase activity.[207] Like fatty acids, mercaptans depress enzymes of the urea cycle, interfering with the disposition of ammonia.

Short- and medium-chain fatty acids also accumulate in the peripheral blood of adult patients with hepatic failure. In Reye's syndrome, plasma short- and medium-chain fatty acids may be markedly elevated.[208-210] Recently, elevated levels of long-chain dicarboxylic acids (indicative of inefficient or overwhelmed intramitochondrial beta-oxidation of fatty acids) have been found to correlate well with the stage of encephalopathy in patients with Reye's syndrome.[211] Infusions of octanoate, a medium-chain fatty acid, into rats and rabbits have produced reversible coma, central hyperventilation, elevated blood ammonia levels, and inhibition of Na^+,K^+-ATPase activity in brain microsomes.[212,213] Fatty acids may also augment disturbances in other metabolic pathways. In high concentrations, they depress enzymes involved in the formation of both urea and glutamine, thus inhibiting the disposition of ammonia. They also displace tryptophan and possibly drugs from albumin binding and augment brain uptake of these potential neurotoxic substances.[214]

Phenols derived from both tyrosine and tyramine have been implicated as potential synergistic toxins because of the findings of elevated levels in the plasma and CSF in patients with hepatic encephalopathy.[215] The increase correlates well with the stage of encephalopathy. Phenols were also found to be synergistic coma-producing agents in rats treated with subcoma doses of ammonia, mercaptans, and octanoate.[203]

Much smaller doses and lower blood levels of ammonia, mercaptans, fatty acids, and phenols are needed to produce coma in normal rats when these neurotoxins are used in combination rather than in infusions of each alone. Even less is required if the animal has pre-existing liver damage or in the presence of hypoglycemia and hypoxemia, two common metabolic complications accompanying severe liver disease.[170,216] Normal rats become comatose when they are given a combination of doses of the above neurotoxins, which produce blood-brain levels of ammonia and methanethiol in the range of those observed in rats with ischemia-induced hepatic coma.[217]

Again, the major objection to this hypothesis is that the encephalopathy induced by synergistic neurotoxins may be mediated by a mechanism different from that mediating hepatic encephalopathy. Studies in rats treated with synergistic neurotoxins have shown that recorded VEPs are similar to those in a rat model of FHF.[218] However, this work was not duplicated in a rabbit model.[193] Since both ammonia and mercaptans are epileptogenic, the question of a confounding postictal state has again been raised.

False Neurotransmitter Hypothesis. This hypothesis states that the accumulation of inhibitory (serotonin) and false neurotransmitters (octopamine) and the depletion of excitatory neurotransmitters (dopamine, norepinephrine) in the brain are responsible for the syndrome of hepatic encephalopathy, particularly in patients with chronic liver failure.[219] Figure 10 illustrates how proposed plasma amino

acid imbalances may contribute to altered brain neurotransmitters. Liver metabolic failure and portal-systemic shunting give rise to elevated plasma levels of aromatic amino acids (AAA), tryptophan, biogenic amines, and octopamine, a gut bacterial metabolite of tyrosine. Ordinarily, these are efficiently metabolized by the liver. Branched-chain amino acids (BCAA) (valine, leucine, isoleucine) predominantly bypass the liver and are taken up by skeletal muscle. Elevated insulin levels secondary to decreased liver degradation of the hormone enhance BCAA uptake and further exacerbate the abnormal elevated ratio, AAA:BCAA. According to this hypothesis, the amino acid imbalance permits increased entry of AAA and tryptophan into the brain by decreased competition with BCAA for the same carrier transport system at the BBB.[220] Free tryptophan is then converted to the inhibitory neurotransmitter serotonin. Phenylalanine, by competing for tyrosine oxidase, results in decreased conversion of tyrosine to the true excitatory neurotransmitters, dopamine and norepinephrine. Octopamine, a weak neurotransmitter, replaces the true neurotransmitters at nerve endings. Unmetabolized tyrosine may undergo decarboxylation to tyramine and then conversion to octopamine in the brain. Brain ammonia accumulation could potentiate the amino acid imbalance by facilitating the entry of AAA into the brain. Gluta-

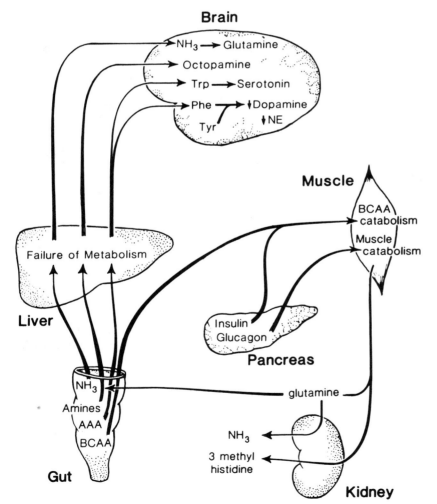

FIGURE 10 Organ interactions illustrating the pathogenesis of amino acid imbalances which may precipitate hepatic encephalopathy. Failure of liver metabolism and portal-systemic shunting allows increased passage of aromatic amino acids (AAA) and biogenic amines to the brain. Insulin excess leads to increased removal of branched-chain amino acids (BCAA) by muscle, resulting in a high AAA:BCAA ratio. Decreased competition by BCAA with tryptophan and phenylalanine for transport across the blood-brain barrier allows increased entry of neutral amino acids into the brain, which act as precursors for inhibitory and false neurotransmitters and inhibitors of the synthesis of excitatory neurotransmitters. (Adapted from Munro HN. Metabolic integration of organs in health and disease. J Parenter Enteral Nutr 1982; 6:271–279.)

mine, formed in a high concentration from brain ammonia detoxification, may exchange with blood AAA via a shared membrane carrier, enhancing AAA influx and glutamine efflux.[221]

Evidence to support this hypothesis includes elevated plasma and brain levels of tyrosine, phenylalanine, tyramine, and octopamine in patients with acute liver failure as well as elevated cerebrospinal fluid 5-hydroxyindoleacetic acid, and decreased brain levels of norepinephrine and dopamine.[219,222] In cirrhotic patients levels of octopamine are increased, and when patients with cirrhosis bleed into the GI tract, the serum octopamine concentration correlates with the serum levels of its precursors tyrosine and phenylalanine and with the stage of encephalopathy.[223,224] Animal experiments in rats and dogs with acute hepatic necrosis or portacaval shunts have shown an increased uptake of AAA by the brain, moderately increased brain serotonin and octopamine, as well as decreased norepinephrine.[225-227] Brain concentrations of tryptophan and tyrosine are greatly elevated.[214]

In spite of the demonstration of increased entry and elevated levels of AAA and false neurotransmitters in the brain of patients and animals with hepatic encephalopathy, the levels achieved have not been shown to induce coma.[1] When octopamine was administered by intraventricular injection to increase the concentration in the brains of rats 200,000-fold, a depletion of brain levels of norepinephrine and dopamine occurred, but there was no disturbance of consciousness.[228] Ingestion of large amounts of tryptophan may cause headache, dizziness, nystagmus, drowsiness, and disturbances in gait in normal subjects and cirrhotics, but hepatic encephalopathy does not occur.[229,230] In the only published study of human autopsy material to date, octopamine was decreased in brains of patients dying of hepatic failure, whereas dopamine levels were increased.[231] In controlled trials, neither L-dopa nor bromocriptine, which might be expected to restore brain dopamine levels, has been shown to be effective in ameliorating encephalopathy in cirrhotic patients.[232] Finally, the contribution of brain ammonia to increased transport of AAA across the BBB in exchange for glutamine has been challenged on kinetic grounds, since the affinity of the carrier system for glutamine is very low compared with that for AAA.[3]

GABA-ergic Inhibitory Neurotransmitter Hypothesis. It is evident from the above discussion that the main experimental strategy used in constructing the previous hypotheses is measurement of neuroactive substances in the plasma, CSF, and brain and an attempt to demonstrate their coma-producing properties in experimental animal preparations. When a positive correlation is found between the increased level of a substance and the stage of encephalopathy it can be a cause of the encephalopathy, caused by it, or merely an epiphenomenon of hepatic failure but unrelated to the encephalopathy. Recently, a different strategy was devised by Jones, Schafer, and colleagues.[5] They asked which of the established mechanisms that mediate neuronal activity in the brain could contribute to the pathogenesis of hepatic encephalopathy. Reasoning that encephalopathy is characterized by profound neural inhibition and knowing that GABA is considered the principal inhibitory neurotransmitter of the mammalian brain, they considered whether GABA and its receptors might be implicated in the pathogenesis. There was ample previous evidence to suspect that GABA might be in-

volved.[233] Twenty-five to 45 percent of all nerve endings in the brain are GABA-ergic. GABA is a potent inhibitor of single neurons. In addition, instillation of small amounts of GABA into the brain of rabbits can cause coma associated with EEG changes similar to those in rabbits and humans in deep hepatic coma.[234-236]

Most GABA in the brain is stored in cytoplasmic storage vesicles in postsynaptic neurons. When it is released, GABA enters the synaptic cleft and binds to specific receptors on the postsynaptic neuronal membrane. The binding results in increased chloride conductance, membrane hyperpolarization, and generation of an inhibitory postsynaptic potential. This same chloride ionophore can be modulated as a consequence of binding by a barbiturate or a benzodiazepine. The chloride ionophore itself is a transmembrane complex of proteins that contains binding sites for multiple ligands on its external surface. GABA is the signal that opens the chloride channel, but in the presence of GABA other ligands modulate its effects[237] (Fig. 11). Thus GABA, barbiturates, and benzodiazepines act as synergistic ligands whose sedative-hypnotic effects are mediated via the GABA receptor. Barbiturates are thought to increase the average time that chloride channels are open, and benzodiazepines to increase the frequency of chloride channel opening.[238]

GABA satisfies other requirements for an important mediator of hepatic encephalopathy. Application of a competitive radioreceptor assay using binding of ^{3}H-GABA with synaptic membranes has shown twice the GABA-like activity in the portal venous plasma versus the aortic plasma of normal rabbits.[239] *Escherichia coli* and *Bacteroides fragilis* isolated from human feces produce such activity. These findings suggest that gut bacteria are a source of GABA outside the nervous system and would therefore help explain the amelioration of encephalopathy by therapies designed to reduce the interaction between nitrogenous substances and enteric bacterial flora. Serum GABA-like activity increases 10-fold in a rabbit model of FHF prior to the onset of overt encephalopathy.[240] GABA-like activity also accumulates in the plasma of patients with acute and chronic liver failure. In cirrhotics, hemorrhage into the GI tract is consistently followed by increased serum GABA-like activity.[241] The liver appears to play a key role in the removal of gut-derived GABA-like activity from the circulation. The liver of rabbits contains most of the total body activity of GABA transaminase, the enzyme responsible for the catabolism of GABA. Hepatic uptake of intravenous ^{3}H-GABA is greatly reduced in rabbits with acute liver failure.[240]

In order to study whether GABA crosses the BBB in increased quantities during encephalopathy, an isomer of GABA, alpha-amino isobutyric acid (AIB) has been used. Unlike GABA, it is not rapidly metabolized and is rapidly taken up and trapped in brain cells at the point where it crosses the BBB. In addition, its transport does not rely on a specific amino acid carrier but rather is a function of membrane lipid solubility. Thus, an increase in the blood-to-brain transfer of AIB implies a nonspecific increase in permeability of the BBB. In normal animals, transfer of ^{14}C-AIB measured with quantitive autoradiography is minimal. After the onset of acute liver failure in a rabbit model but before overt manifestations of encephalopathy, there is a striking increase in the transfer of ^{14}C-AIB to certain areas of grey matter in

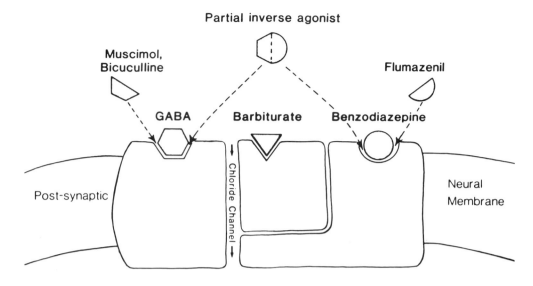

FIGURE 11 Schematic representation of the GABA transmembrane protein complex containing binding sites for multiple ligands on its outer membrane surface. GABA binding is mandatory in order to open the chloride channel, but in the presence of GABA, barbiturates and benzodiazepines can act as synergistic ligands potentiating the inhibitory post-synaptic potential that is generated and the sedative-hypnotic state. Also shown are the GABA antagonists, which act at the GABA site, inhibit GABA binding and chloride conductance, and are proconvulsant (muscimol, bicuculline). Flumazenil, a benzodiazepine antagonist, competes with an agonist at the binding site but does not promote chloride conductance or decrease GABA's effect on the chloride ionophore. Only if an exogenous ligand such as diazepam or the putative endogenous benzodiazepine is present will flumazenil have a clinical effect. Partial inverse agonists are unique ligands because they not only compete with any benzodiazepine agonist present but also decrease GABA's effect on chloride conductance. (Adapted from Schafer and Jones.[198])

the brain.[242] This increase is likely nonspecific, since hepatectomy in rabbits causes increased blood-to-brain transfer of L-glucose, D-sucrose, insulin, and trypan blue dye.[157]

All of the above evidence points to a potential role for GABA in the pathogenesis of hepatic encephalopathy. In order to measure the effects of GABA on the brain more specifically than can be done via EEG changes and to allow more quantitative comparisons with other putative neurotoxins, investigators have turned to the study of visual evoked potentials. VEPs reflect the summation of excitatory and inhibitory postsynaptic potentials in the area of the brain being monitored. Changes in behavior induced by certain pharmacologically active substances are associated with distinctive patterns of the VEP.[243] In a rabbit model of hepatic encephalopathy due to galactosamine-induced FHF, the pattern of VEPs differed fundamentally from that in ether-induced coma but was identical to that in comas induced by three drugs that activate the GABA receptor: pentobarbital, diazepam, and muscimol, a potent GABA agonist.[244] In the absence of seizures, the pattern of VEPs in rabbits given subcoma doses of three putative neurotoxins—ammonia, dimethyldisulfide, and octanoic acid—was also markedly different.[193] Only when seizures occurred did the VEPs of the animals given synergistic neurotoxins resemble those seen in late-stage hepatic encephalopathy due to galactosamine-induced FHF.

In the rat, however, the VEPs produced by a combination of ammonia, dimethyldisulfide, and octanoate were similar to the VEPs of rats in galactosamine-induced hepatic failure without any documentation of seizure activity.[218]

Recently, the use of VEPs and somatosensory evoked potentials have been applied to the study of human patients with liver failure and varying degrees of hepatic encephalopathy.[245-247] Even in patients with subclinical grade I hepatic encephalopathy, the VEP was abnormal in two-thirds of the patients, versus 0 to 8 percent of controls.[248] However, similar abnormalities in VEPs have been recorded in patients with hypothyroidism, uremia, and hypothermia. A recent study found VEPs poorly correlated with mental status changes in patients with alcohol-induced advanced chronic liver disease.[249]

A second tool recently used to further study the GABA hypothesis is the measurement of brain neurotransmitter receptors. Because of compartmentalization of brain neurotransmitters within cellular structures, mean changes in the concentration of a neurotransmitter in the entire brain or a region of the brain may not accurately reflect actual effects of compartmentalized neurotransmitters on neuronal function. Up-and-down regulation of a membrane receptor is believed to better reflect local concentrations of the functional ligands for that receptor. Much recent research has been directed toward the study of GABA and other neurotransmitter receptors in animal models of hepatic failure and encephalopathy. This research has generally relied on the binding of labeled GABA or other neurotransmitters to postsynaptic neural membranes from the brains of experimental animals.

In the rabbit model of galactosamine-induced FHF, the number of binding sites for the inhibitory neurotransmitters GABA and glycine and for benzodiazepines on postsynaptic neurons increases substantially.[250] In contrast, the densities of receptors for the excitatory amino acid neurotransmitters glutamate and aspartate decrease.[251] The numbers of dopamine, opiate, and muscarinic acetylcholine receptors are unchanged. These findings were initially corroborated in rats with hepatic encephalopathy.[252] Binding of a labeled benzodiazepine compound (^{3}H-flunitrazepam) to rabbit postsynaptic membranes was also increased. The firing rate of brain neurons isolated from this model was more profoundly decreased by flunitrazepam than that of neurons from control animals.[253] These findings suggest an experimental basis for the clinical hypersensitivity of cirrhotics with marginal liver function to benzodiazepine drugs. No changes in brain receptors for GABA or glutamate were found in rabbits with uremic encephalopathy or in rats with hypoglycemia-induced seizures, suggesting that the changes in neurotransmitter receptors in hepatic coma are not common to all metabolic encephalopathies. Differentiation of this rabbit model from that of hyperammonemic encephalopathy is evident, since the infusion of ammonium chloride was associated with an increased density and affinity of glutamate receptors but no changes in the density or affinity of GABA receptors.[199]

The experimental findings supporting the GABA hypothesis may be summarized as follows: (1) In liver failure, GABA produced by enteric flora crosses an increasingly permeable BBB and binds to postsynaptic receptors, giving rise to marked neural inhibition. (2) Increased receptor density of GABA and glycine receptors enhances binding and the effects of the inhibitory neural transmitters. (3) Increased binding sites for benzodiazepines and barbiturates mediate increased sensitivity to these drugs.

There are limitations to the above hypothesis, and more recent data have led to questions about many of the basic assumptions. It has now been shown that the assay used to measure plasma GABA-like activity overestimated the amount of GABA in serum owing to cross-reactivity with glutamine and other amino acids.[254] Most of the research cited above has been on one model of acute hepatic failure—the rabbit galactosamine model. Other animal models have failed to confirm various aspects of this previous work. Guinea pigs with galactosamine-induced and rats with thioacetamide-induced hepatic encephalopathy have not shown increased GABA binding to neural membranes.[255,256] A dog model of chronic liver disease and hepatic encephalopathy failed to show any changes in brain GABA uptake, concentration of brain GABA, or brain glutamic acid decarboxylase, the enzyme in the brain responsible for formation of GABA from glutamate.[257] Quantitative autoradiography of brain slices has been used as an alternative to binding to isolated membranes in order to measure GABA receptor density. The advantages of this method are the use of intact brain tissue instead of disrupted membranes, a high sensitivity, and high spatial resolution.

Rats subjected to portacaval shunting and severe hyperammonemia developed coma but demonstrated no increase in binding of ^{3}H-muscimol, a GABA agonist, to any area of the brain tested by autoradiography techniques.[258]

The results of scant studies of human patients and human autopsy material do not support the GABA hypothesis. Plasma and cerebrospinal fluid GABA levels have recently been measured in cirrhotic patients with and without hepatic encephalopathy.[259] Instead of using the previously mentioned nonspecific radioreceptor method, a mass fragmentographic approach was used, and no differences were found in either evolution of the neurologic symptoms to different grades of encephalopathy. GABA content of brain tissue from cirrhotic patients dying with hepatic encephalopathy was not different from that of controls dying from other causes and free from neurologic, psychiatric, or hepatic disease.[260] A recent comparison of ^{3}H-muscimol and ^{3}H-flunitrazepam binding to membrane preparations from the cortex of nine cirrhotic patients and nine controls shows no modifications in the cirrhotics dying with hepatic encephalopathy.[261] However, a recent preliminary study using positron emission tomography has reported the determination of benzodiazepine receptor density in four living human patients with portal-systemic encephalopathy. There was a two- to threefold increase in cerebral radioactivity over controls using a ^{14}C-labeled benzodiazepine antagonist.[262]

Thus, certain aspects of the GABA hypothesis have been called into question, especially the ideas of increased plasma GABA-like activity derived from the gut and increased brain uptake of GABA. It seems that the behavioral expression of hepatic encephalopathy in animals is not dependent on an increase in the number of GABA or benzodiazepine receptors in all models tested. The data in humans in relation to brain receptor density are inconclusive. However, new lines of evidence implicating GABA-ergic transmission are being developed from studies employing GABA and benzodiazepine agonists and antagonists. Bassett and co-workers used the galactosamine-induced FHF model in rabbits to test whether blocking the postsynaptic GABA supramolecular complex ameliorated encephalopathy.[263] Bicuculline, a GABA receptor blocker; Ro15-1788 (flumazenil), a benzodiazepine receptor antagonist; and isopropyl-bicyclophosphate, a chloride channel blocker, consistently induced a transient decrease in the clinical severity and corrected the abnormal pattern of VEP associated with hepatic encephalopathy in rabbits. Similar findings have been reported in galactosamine-treated rats using two different benzodiazepine antagonists.[264] Recent case reports and small series have confirmed these animal data in humans by demonstrating the blood or CSF levels of GABA in patients with or without encephalopathy. In addition, the levels did not change with improved clinical EEG and evoked potential status after treatment with flumazenil in patients with hepatic encephalopathy associated with both FHF and cirrhosis.[265-267] In an effort to reconcile conflicting data on GABA levels in CSF or brain and GABA receptor densities with the data supporting an improvement using benzodiazepine receptor antagonists, research is now focusing on the possibility that an endogenous substance with benzodiazepine agonist properties contributes to the development of hepatic encephalopathy by potentiating GABA-ergic neurotransmission.[268]

Recent work from Mullen and colleagues has shown that CSF from rabbits and humans with hepatic encephalopathy contains a substance that binds avidly to benzodiazepine receptors. This has been shown by the ability of the CSF to displace high-affinity ligands for the benzodiazepine receptor and by using a radioimmunoassay based on polyclonal rabbit antibenzodiazepine antibodies.[269,270] Preliminary work has demonstrated similar benzodiazepine receptor activity in the plasma and urine of humans with stage III to IV hepatic coma.[271] This activity is enhanced by GABA, which is characteristic of benzodiazepine agonists. The identity of this substance(s) and the site of origin remain to be determined.

COMPLICATIONS OF HEPATIC FAILURE

Cerebral Edema

Cerebral edema is a major cause of mortality in patients with FHF. In series of adult patients, the frequency of this complication has ranged from 25 to 81 percent.[272-275] Autopsy findings showed that 7 of 13 children dying with FHF had cerebral edema.[16] Cerebral edema and brain stem herniation were found to be the direct cause of death in 36 of 96 autopsied patients with FHF and stage III or IV hepatic encephalopathy.[276] Twelve of the 36 patients showed herniation of the cerebellar tonsils, and eight, of the temporal lobes. In none of these cases was papilledema detected prior to brain death. In nine patients, liver function was improving at the time of death caused by cerebral edema. There appears to be no correlation between cerebral edema and other complicating factors such as acute hemorrhage, hypoglycemia, hypotension, or the need for mechanical ventilation. Nor has any consistent relationship between the length of time in stage IV encephalopathy and the occurrence of cerebral edema been found. Adult patients with encephalopathy and underlying chronic hepatic disease or even late-onset hepatic failure[9] have a much lower incidence of cerebral edema than do those with fulminant hepatic failure.

The brain does not show striking characteristic morphologic changes in patients dying with FHF. The principal pathologic finding is swollen astrocytes.[4] The findings are more demonstrable in patients with chronic liver disease terminating with hepatic coma.[277] Here the protoplasmic astrocytes (Alzheimer type II) are increased in number and size. These cells are more numerous in all parts of the cerebral cortex, the basal ganglion, cerebellum, and brain stem, approaching twice the number seen in patients with chronic liver disease without overt encephalopathy. Similar increases in Alzheimer type II astrocytes have been observed in chronic hyperammonemia associated with urea cycle enzyme defects.[278] Animal models of portal-systemic shunts alone showed only mild significant neuropathologic changes, including astrocytic nuclear swelling and spongiform changes. However, when rats were shunted and fed ammonium chloride, coma developed and astrocytes, oligodendrocytes, and even some neurons showed more dramatic nuclear and cytoplasmic swelling. This has led some investigators to suggest that ammonia intoxication plays a key role in these structural changes.[279]

Recent work with animal models of acute FHF has begun to yield clues to the pathogenesis of cerebral edema in hepatic encephalopathy. Surgical devascularization of the liver of pigs produced coma and increased intracranial pressure and swelling of the body and foot processes of the frontal lobe astrocytes, predominantly in the grey matter.[280] Using the rabbit galactosamine-induced FHF model, Traber and colleagues demonstrated a significant increase in brain water content in cortical and hippocampal grey matter, but not in subcortical, mesencephalic, or pontine white matter or in the cerebellum.[281] The increases in grey matter edema correlated well with clinical grading of encephalopathy and increases in monitored intracranial pressure. Neither hypotension, hypoxia, nor severe hypoglycemia was present to account for the edema. Electron microscopic evaluation of brain tissue from this model showed marked swelling of the cytoplasm and perineuronal and perivascular processes of the astrocytes in cortical grey but not white matter areas.[282] The other cellular components of the brain had normal morphology. A major advantage of this study was the premortem whole-body perfusion with chilled phosphate-buffered saline and immediate antemortem perfusion fixation with 3 percent glutaraldehyde paraformaldehyde, allowing an accurate ultrastructural view of the brain edema. Using this technique, the same ultrastructural changes were found in a rat hepatectomy model of FHF.[159]

Two main mechanisms lead to cerebral edema: (1) vasogenic edema, in which a damaged BBB leads to leakage of protein-rich edema fluid into the extracellular space, and (2) cytotoxic edema, in which the edema is intracellular and the result of cellular toxicity leading to disruption of normal mechanisms for maintenance of intracellular fluid and electrolyte homeostasis. The above-described changes in brain water content in grey matter suggest primarily a cytotoxic mechanism of cerebral edema in FHF. Although evidence of alteration in the BBB has been found in animal models of FHF (see above), the vasogenic edema that results should initially develop in white matter areas, where it should be well established before affecting the grey matter.[283] The observation of edema in the grey matter in this rabbit galactosamine FHF model suggests a predominantly cytotoxic mechanism. Another known rabbit model of cytotoxic edema secondary to treatment with 6-aminonicotinamide also results in a regional pattern of water accumulation in grey matter.[284] The amelioration of cerebral edema by hyperosmolar mannitol in patients with FHF has been interpreted as being further evidence of a cytotoxic mechanism, since the osmotic action of mannitol is thought to be dependent on an intact BBB.

A possible explanation for cytotoxic edema could be disruption of intracellular osmoregulation secondary to depressed Na^+, K^+-ATPase activity. Inhibition of ouabain-sensitive sodium transport is characteristic of the cytotoxic form of cerebral edema.[285] Many of the putative neurotoxins that accumulate during FHF, including mercaptans, phenols, and fatty acids, are known to inhibit neuronal Na^+, K^+-ATPase in animal models.[213,285-287] Sera from patients with FHF inhibits Na^+, K^+-ATPase activity in rat brain.[288] This finding, however, could not be reproduced in the rabbit model of FHF.[289]

Perturbations of the BBB probably contribute to cerebral edema in FHF, since water must cross in order to increase total grey matter water content. The rabbit model described above did not demonstrate significant permeation of the BBB by the large-molecule horseradish peroxidase, but other investigators have found increases in this and smaller molecules crossing from plasma to brain more easily in FHF.[157,158] The permeability to AIB and GABA has been noted to be increased in the rabbit model of FHF localized to grey but not white matter areas.[242] Changes in the specific permeability of electrolytes and water have not been adequately studied.

The brain cell most consistently affected by hepatic failure is the astrocyte. This glial cell performs multiple functions in the modulation of the immediate extracellular environment in which neurons function. These include fluid and electrolyte regulation and the metabolism of ammonia, GABA, and other neurotransmitters. Elevated ammonia levels are known to cause morphologic changes of cultured astrocytes similar to those seen in vivo in animal models of FHF.[290,291] Ammonia has also been found to cause changes in ion fluxes and protein synthesis in brain slices from young rats.[292,293] Further research is required to determine the effects of this and other putative neurotoxins on astrocyte function and subsequent neuronal function.

Clinical signs of increased intracranial pressure (ICP) are summarized in Table 5. Papilledema is not a reliable sign, and muscle tone and posturing may be masked by muscle-paralyzing drugs. Thus, changes in pupillary responses become an important clinical sign of increased ICP in these patients. Continuous monitoring of ICP using subdural or extradural pressure transducers has been advocated for patients in stage III or IV encephalopathy in order to permit earlier recognition of increased ICP and intervention to prevent irreversible changes.[294] Measurement of ICP and simultaneous arterial pressure allows calculation of cerebral perfusion pressure, which must be greater than 40 mm Hg if cerebral perfusion is to be adequate. Extradural monitors carry a low risk of infection, since the dura remains intact. Using these monitors, clinical signs of cerebral edema described above appeared within 5 minutes of an elevation of ICP to 30 mm Hg or greater in patients with FHF.[275] In spite of the ability to monitor ICP accurately, the use of intracranial monitors has not been associated with increased survival in head trauma patients or patients with FHF.[285,295] When no ICP monitor is in place, the patients must be assiduously monitored for clinical signs of increased ICP and treated immediately if they appear. If clinical signs are obscured by muscle-paralyzing and centrally active drugs, an ICP monitor should be placed in any patient in hepatic failure and stage III or IV encephalopathy.

Coagulopathy

The liver plays a pivotal role in hemostasis. It is the major site of synthesis of most of the coagulation factors, fibrinolytic agents, and inhibitors of coagulation. As a major reticuloendothelial organ, the liver clears many of the activated factors and their by-products from the circulation. When the liver fails, it is inevitable that there will be significant derangements in coagulation. Of 96 patients dying with FHF, major hemorrhage was the proximate cause of death in 28.[276] Bleeding originated in the GI tract in 25 of 28 patients. In 31 children with FHF, 14 had massive GI bleeding, all of

TABLE 5
Clinical Signs of Increased Intracranial Pressure

Early
Increased muscle tone, myoclonus
Hyperventilation
Unequal or dilated pupils
Sluggish pupillary response to light
Focal seizures

Late
Papilledema
Trismus
Decerebrate posturing
Fixed, dilated pupils
Loss of oculocephalic reflex
Loss of oculovestibular reflex

whom died.[16] Prothrombin time was prolonged by greater than 90 seconds in 10 fatal cases but in none of the survivors. The impact of liver failure on the blood coagulation system can be divided into consideration of effects on (1) coagulation factors, (2) inhibitors of coagulation, (3) platelets, and (4) disseminated intravascular coagulation.

Fibrinogen levels are often reduced in FHF owing to the combination of decreased synthesis and increased consumption.[296] Specific and sensitive assays have shown increased circulating fibrinogen degradation products, indicative of increased consumption and decreased clearance from the circulation by the impaired liver.[297] Dysfibrinogenemia, caused by abnormal fibrin polymerization, may develop in patients with chronic liver disease.[298] Increase in the terminal sialic acid residues of the fibrinogen chains results in abnormal fibrinogen incapable of responding to thrombin.[299] Acquired dysfibrinogenemia should be suspected in any patient with an abnormal thrombin time uncorrectable with fresh frozen plasma, a normal level of fibrinogen, and elevated fibrinogen degradation products.

The most common coagulation defects are decreased levels of Factors II, V, VII, IX, and X. In an experimental rat model of FHF, 12 hours after infusion of dimethylnitrosamine, the levels of Factors V and VII were reduced to 20 percent of control and of Factors II, IX, and X to between 25 and 63 percent of control levels.[300] Since Factor VII has the shortest half-life of the coagulation factors, it has been studied as a potential sensitive indicator of hepatic function in patients with hepatic failure.[301] Although it is the earliest detectable coagulation disturbance accompanying severe acute hepatocellular disease, the levels obtained within 36 hours of the onset of encephalopathy showed no significant predictive value of the clinical outcome.[302] Serial determinations were of more value, since levels increased rapidly in those who recovered. Other studies have found that concentrations of Factor V and antithrombin III (AT III) were useful prognostic indicators.[303,304] It is generally agreed that an increased prothrombin time unresponsive to adequate parenteral vitamin K implies poor hepatic synthetic ability and severe hepatocellular disease.

In contrast to the other coagulation factors, Factor VIII is often increased in hepatic failure.[305] Factor VIII is synthesized both in hepatocytes and in other tissues, including the spleen and lymph nodes.[306] Von Willebrand factor, which is part of the Factor VIII molecule, is synthesized by vascular endothelial cells. Elevated Factor VIII levels may represent an acute-phase reaction, since Von Willebrand factor is an acute-phase reactant. Alternative explanations include continued synthesis from extrahepatic sites such as spleen or lymph nodes and hepatic release of Factor VIII during hepatocyte necrosis.[307] Owing to its characteristically high level, the plasma level of Factor VIII may help differentiate coagulation abnormalities secondary to FHF, in which Factor VIII is often elevated or normal, from those secondary to disseminated intravascular coagulation, in which the Factor VIII level is depressed.

In patients with underlying chronic cholestatic liver disease, it is important to consider the possibility of vitamin K deficiency mediating the coagulopathy. In a post-translational step, vitamin K carboxylates glutamic acid residues of the precursors of Factors II, VII, IX, and X, enabling them to bind to phospholipids and function as coagulation proteins.[308] However, in most patients with cirrhosis and hepatic failure (even those with profound cholestasis), large doses of parenteral vitamin K have no effect on the synthesis of these proteins, since there is no increase in the low levels of factors determined either by immunoassay, which measures both noncarboxylated precursors and functional molecules, or functional activity, which measures only the carboxylated species.[309]

AT III is the most important natural inhibitor of the coagulation cascade. It is synthesized by the liver and, using heparin as a co-factor, binds to and neutralizes thrombin and other activated coagulation factors, including Factors VII, IX, X, XI, and XII. Low concentrations of AT III are seen in cirrhosis and FHF secondary to reduced synthesis of the protein or increased consumption in disseminated intravascular coagulation.[296,310] A qualitatively abnormal AT III may be synthesized in liver disease (much like fibrinogen and prothrombin), since some studies have noted a discrepancy between the immunoassay and the functional assay.[311] Low levels of AT III in FHF have the effect of increasing sensitivity to heparin and lead to difficulty in controlling anticoagulation with heparin. Reduced AT III concentrations may also contribute to continued activation of the coagulation cascade and disseminated intravascular coagulation.[305]

Both quantitative and qualitative platelet abnormalities have been described in FHF. A decreased platelet count of less than $100,000 \times 10^9$ per liter is common in FHF.[312] Mean platelet counts are lower in patients who have major GI hemorrhage than in those who do not (53,000 versus 91,000).[276] Thrombocytopenia may be caused by decreased survival due to splenic sequestration, to platelet-associated antibody in chronic active hepatitis, or to disseminated intravascular coagulation. The increased appearance of small platelets suggests a component of impaired release of younger, larger platelets from the marrow and delayed clearance of older platelets by the reticuloendothelial system.[313]

Functional platelet abnormalities in FHF include a decrease in adenosine diphosphate–induced aggregation and increased adhesion to glass bead columns.[314] These defects may be mediated by alterations in plasma and platelet lipids. In patients with FHF, the concentration of platelet arachidonic acid, the precursor of prostaglandin endoperoxides and thromboxane A_2 (TxA_2), is only 20 percent of the levels in platelets

from control subjects, and this may be a factor in poor platelet aggregation.[315] The plasma from patients in FHF has been shown to stimulate prostacyclin production from vascular endothelium to a greater extent than in control subjects.[296] This may be another reason for poor platelet aggregation in FHF.

Currently available data showing increased fibrinogen catabolism and increased circulating fibrin degradation products point to the occurrence of low-grade disseminated intravascular coagulation in patients with FHF. Continued activation of the clotting cascade may be due to the release of tissue thromboplastin from necrotic hepatocytes, reduced clearance of activated coagulation proteins, reduced synthesis of inhibitors such as AT III, and circulating endotoxin.[305] Evidence of the importance of low levels of AT III comes from animal models of acute liver failure.[316] Rats with acute liver damage induced by dimethylnitrosamine form fibrin clots in hepatic sinusoids 12 hours after injection and have markedly elevated circulating fibrin monomer complexes detected 24 hours after injection. At 12 hours one group of rats was given an infusion of AT III concentrate and showed a dose-dependent improvement of values of bilirubin, ALT, prothrombin time, platelet count, plasma fibrinogen, Factor VIII, and liver histology at 24 hours. These experiments lend credence to the idea that disseminated intravascular coagulation occurs in certain types of acute liver injury and is an aggravating factor that can be partially blocked by infusions of AT III.

Renal Dysfunction in Hepatic Failure

Oliguria is a common clinical development in both acute and chronic liver failure. Three mechanisms have been recognized as mediators of oliguria in this setting: acute tubular necrosis (ATN), prerenal azotemia associated with a decreased circulating blood volume, and "functional" renal failure, commonly called the hepatorenal syndrome. In FHF, the hepatorenal syndrome accounts for the majority of cases of renal impairment and is frequently associated with a fatal outcome. Hepatorenal syndrome is defined as an unexplained progressive renal dysfunction without obvious histologic lesions. It is characterized by avid sodium retention and negligible urinary sodium; a benign urinary sediment without protein, cells, or casts; and oliguria unresponsive to intravascular volume expansion.[317] Significant urinary findings include a urine sodium concentration less than 10 mEq per liter, a urine–to–plasma creatinine ratio of greater than 30:1, and a urine osmolality at least 100 mOsm greater than plasma osmolality. These findings allow easy differentiation from the oliguria in patients with ATN but are more difficult to separate from the findings in patients with prerenal azotemia (Table 6). Much recent work has centered on the pathogenesis of hepatorenal syndrome. Although certain mechanisms may differ in the renal impairment that develops in decompensated cirrhosis versus that seen in FHF, this discussion emphasizes pathophysiologic derangements that may be pertinent to both situations and are commonly seen in severe liver disease.

Sodium retention is the major renal excretory abnormality causing fluid retention. A large free water load can be adequately excreted by patients with cirrhosis, provided that it

TABLE 6
Differentiation of Hepatorenal Syndrome from Other Causes of Oliguria

Category of Findings	Prerenal Azotemia	Hepatorenal Syndrome	Acute Renal Failure (ATN)
Urine Na^+ concentrations (mEq/L)	<10	<10	>30
Urine/plasma creatinine	>30:1	>30:1	<20:1
Urine/plasma osmolality	>1	>1	1
Fractional excretion of Na^+	<1%	<1%	>2%
Urine sediment	Unremarkable	Unremarkable	Casts, cells, etc.
Pulmonary capillary wedge pressure	<10 mm Hg	>12 mm Hg	
Acute volume expansion	Diuresis	No diuresis	No diuresis

is given without sodium.[318] Conversely, increased dietary sodium often mediates a worsening of ascites and fluid retention, even in the face of fluid restriction.

The pathogenesis of deranged sodium homeostasis is complex and the subject of much debate. Two major theories have been advanced (Fig. 12). The "underfill" theory has stressed the concept of a diminished effective blood volume perfusing the kidneys and other volume receptors, with the resulting activation of the sympathetic nervous system and the renin angiotensin-aldosterone system, leading to alterations in intrarenal blood flow and avid sodium retention. Here, the renal retention of sodium is a secondary event resulting from redistribution of plasma volume and reduction of effective circulating volume caused by ascites formation. Ascites formation is the primary event and begins with a block in hepatic sinusoidal outflow, increased formation of lymph overwhelming the clearance capacity of the thoracic duct, and accumulation of excessive fluid in the peritoneal cavity. In contrast, the "overflow" theory proposes that avid renal sodium retention is the primary abnormality present prior to the development of ascites and is mediated by either intrahepatic baroreceptors, decreased hepatic clearance of a salt-retaining hormone, or decreased hepatic synthesis of a natriuretic hormone. In this hypothesis, plasma volume is initially overfilled in the pre-ascitic phase of cirrhosis with suppression of plasma renin and aldosterone. Only after effective plasma volume is reduced secondary to ascites formation is there progressive elevation of plasma renin, aldosterone, antidiuretic hormone, and catecholamines.

Support for the underfill theory comes mainly from clinical observations, in human patients, of transient improvement in renal sodium and water handling with rapid intravascular volume expansion using saline, mannitol, or albumin.[319,320] A series of experiments by Epstein and colleagues used the technique of head-out-of-water immersion to expand the effective circulating plasma volume in cirrhotic patients who had ascites without increasing the total plasma volume.[321] Immersion resulted in a marked natriuresis (up to 20-fold greater than baseline), exceeding the response of normal subjects.[322] These studies suggest that a diminished effective intravascular volume is a major determinant of the enhanced tubular reabsorption of sodium in patients who have established cirrhosis.

Evidence supporting the overflow theory comes from a series of experiments by Levy and co-workers using two canine models of cirrhosis produced by feeding the potent hepatotoxin dimethylnitrosamine or by chronic ligation of the bile ducts.[323] In these models, ascites develops in 8 to 12 weeks and cirrhosis is well established at that time. As dogs were followed, urinary sodium retention preceded the appearance of ascites. In order to completely separate disturbances of sodium retention from the development of portal hypertension and possible subclinical sequestration of circulating plasma volume in the mesenteric circulation, similar experiments were performed on dogs that first had undergone an end-to-side portacaval shunt.[324] The same pattern emerged, that of sodium retention prior to the development of ascites. There were no observed changes in cardiac output, peripheral vascular resistance, or renal blood flow to account for the increase in renal tubular sodium retention. Further experiments in cirrhotic dogs and humans with severe ascites treated with peritoneal venous shunts have reinforced these findings.[325,326] This treatment completely mobilized the ascites, expanded plasma volume, raised glomerular filtration rate (GFR) and renal blood flow to normal or nearly normal, increased cardiac output and blood pressure, and normalized plasma circulating levels of renin and aldosterone, thus removing any previous stimulus for sodium retention. In spite of these changes, both dogs and humans were unable to excrete a sodium load.

These two hypotheses are not necessarily mutually exclusive. Early in the course of developing cirrhosis, a primary defect in renal sodium handling may mediate expansion of plasma volume. Later, with ascites formation and a reduction in effective plasma volume, secondary sodium retention may be mediated by renin, aldosterone, and other effectors of renal sodium retention.

Many candidates for the primary effector of renal sodium retention have been proposed. Urinary sodium excretion in nonascitic cirrhotics correlates strongly with antipyrine clearance, a measure of functional hepatocellular mass, and not well with other measures of portal pressure, intrahepatic shunting, and hepatic blood flow.[327] This finding suggests that in cirrhotic patients, even before ascites develops, there is impaired hepatic metabolism of a sodium retaining hormone or decreased synthesis of a circulating natriuretic fac-

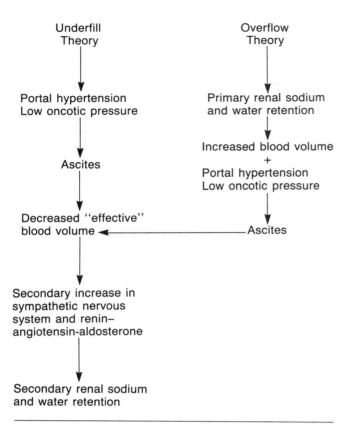

FIGURE 12 Classic theories of salt and water retention and ascites formation in advanced liver disease. The "underfill" theory stresses the importance of ascites formation and depleted "effective" plasma volume as the primary event leading to secondary renal salt and water retention. The "overflow" theory draws on experimental evidence in animal models to support the idea that sodium retention is a primary event occurring before any reduction in intravascular volume and is mediated by intrahepatic baroreceptors or the failure of normal hepatic modulation of hormones involved in renal sodium homeostasis.

tor. Currently, the role of atrial natriuretic factor (ANF) is being actively investigated. ANF is a peptide hormone stored in the myocardial cells of the human atria and released by atrial distention.[328,329] It is known that plasma ANF is stimulated in normal humans by immersion-induced central hypervolemia and that, in intact animals, synthetic ANF increases GFR and renal sodium excretion and decreases renin secretory rate, plasma renin levels, and aldosterone levels.[330] A deficiency of ANF could lead to renal arterial vasoconstriction and avid sodium retention. Supporting this hypothesis are studies showing that in contrast to normal controls, cirrhotic patients with ascites show less than one-fourth the normal increase in plasma ANF in response to increasing the effective plasma volume by head-out-of-water immersion.[331] However, cirrhotic patients with ascites treated with peritoneal-venous shunts demonstrate an intact ANF response to intravascular expansion by shunt implantation, arguing against this hormone as the causal diminished natriuretic factor.[332] Patients with the hepatorenal syndrome have also recently been shown to have an elevated plasma ANF level

equivalent to that of cirrhotic ascitic patients without functional renal failure.[333] Thus, the bulk of recent evidence suggests an intact volume-dependent release of ANF in cirrhotic patients.

A second hypothesis is that intrahepatic baroreceptors responding to increased intrasinusoidal pressure caused by inflammation and scarring in the liver modulate avid renal tubular sodium reabsorption.[334,335] The existence of such receptors has already been documented, and one group of investigators has shown that as these baroreceptors are stimulated, there is simultaneous reflex activity in the sympathetic efferents to the kidney and heart.[336] These data imply the existence of neuroanatomic pathways that may modulate renal sodium retention.

Traditionally, aldosterone has been thought of as the sodium-retaining hormone poorly metabolized by a cirrhotic liver.[337] The rate of hepatic degradation of aldosterone is related directly to hepatic blood flow, which is markedly decreased in decompensated cirrhotics with ascites. Clinical studies have shown that the aldosterone antagonist spironolactone increases sodium excretion in these patients.[338] However, the evidence for the importance of aldosterone is ambiguous. Plasma aldosterone has been found to be elevated in some patients with cirrhosis but not in others.[339] These discrepancies may be resolved by the recent categorization of cirrhotic patients as excretors and nonexcretors of a water load.[340] Those with impaired water excretion (nonexcretors) have diminished circulating blood volume and high levels of renin, catecholamines, arginine vasopressin, and aldosterone. Those who excrete a water load normally have normal levels of aldosterone and other hormones. Nonexcretors treated with head-out-of-water immersion in order to uniformly increase effective plasma volume progressively increased sodium excretion as plasma renin activity and aldosterone levels decreased.[341] In one study, only when plasma aldosterone was suppressed below a level of 50 ng per deciliter was a negative sodium balance achieved.[342] In cirrhotics with diminished effective blood volume, decreased distal tubular sodium delivery impairs the normal escape from the sodium retaining effects of aldosterone. Restoration of adequate effective blood volume effectively suppresses aldosterone and also allows increased distal tubular sodium delivery and excretion.[343]

In spite of avid sodium retention, hyponatremia is probably the single most common electrolyte defect confronting the physician caring for patients with cirrhosis. This implies that there must be a defect in water excretion as well as sodium excretion and that water retention must be disproportionately greater than sodium. Confounding variables include sources of increased sodium loss such as diuretic therapy, vomiting, diarrhea, and poor oral intake. However, even in the absence of these variables, hyponatremia with a serum sodium less than 130 mEq per liter is common. Two principal mechanisms have been proposed to explain this propensity: (1) decreased delivery of filtrate to the diluting segments of the nephron, and (2) elevated levels of the antidiuretic hormone arginine vasopressin (AVP). Elevated AVP levels have been found in studies of decompensated cirrhotic patients.[344] Demeclocycline, which inhibits the peripheral action of AVP, results in increased free water excretion and decreased urine osmolality in patients with cirrhosis and ascites.[345]

Over the last decade, interest has centered on the role of intrarenal prostaglandins in the pathogenesis of renal derangements of sodium and water-handling in patients with cirrhosis and FHF. Several observations stimulated this interest. In 1979, two groups reported that nonsteroidal antiinflammatory drugs produced acute reversible reductions of renal function in patients with chronic alcoholic liver disease.[346,347] These drugs, indomethacin and ibuprofen, are known inhibitors of arachidonic acid metabolism, inhibiting cyclo-oxygenase, which converts arachidonic acid to PGG_2. A 30 to 50 percent reduction in GFR was found in cirrhotics with ascites treated with nonsteroidal anti-inflammatory drugs, and these results were confirmed in a canine model of cirrhosis.[348] This reduction is mediated by diminished renal blood flow and increased renal vascular resistance secondary to intrarenal vasoconstriction. Studies in animals and humans have documented that endogenous intrarenal prostaglandins attenuate the vasoconstriction induced by angiotensin II, catecholamines, and renal sympathetic nerve stimulation.[349] Since these substances normally appear to serve a compensatory homeostatic role to modulate intrarenal vasoconstriction, and since inhibition of renal prostaglandin synthesis appears to produce a syndrome of functional renal impairment not unlike the hepatorenal syndrome in cirrhotics, it seems reasonable to investigate the role of prostaglandins in the control of renal function in severe hepatic disease.

Hepatorenal Syndrome

For many years, the hepatorenal syndrome (HRS) has been considered a functional renal impairment. Indirect evidence supporting this hypothesis includes the absence of consistent pathologic findings at autopsy and the preservation of tubular function in spite of severe oliguria. More direct compelling evidence comes from the successful transplantation of cadaveric kidneys from patients dying with hepatorenal syndrome into patients with normal livers.[350] Conversely, renal failure has been reversed in patients with HRS after orthotopic liver transplantation.[351] Renal angiographic studies have shown beading and tortuosity of renal interlobular and proximal arcuate arteries and an absence of vascular filling of the cortical vessels.[352] In addition, the renal arterial circulation is unstable, as indicated by minute-to-minute changes in the renal arteriogram. Postmortem angiography carried out on the kidneys of patients dying with HRS has shown complete reversal of all the above changes (Fig. 13). [133]Xe washout studies have also demonstrated a significant reduction in mean renal blood flow as well as a preferential reduction in cortical perfusion and a shift to maintaining relatively normal perfusion of the medulla.[352] This corticomedullary redistribution of renal blood flow and vasoconstriction in the renal cortex have been documented even in cirrhotic patients with normal levels of blood urea nitrogen (BUN) and creatinine and without ascites.[354]

Measurements of the urinary excretion of prostaglandins have been carried out in patients with cirrhosis and in those with HRS. Several studies have documented that renal synthesis of vasodilatory prostaglandins (PGE_2) is increased above normal in cirrhotic patients with ascites and preserved renal function but falls significantly when renal failure spontaneously develops.[347,354–356] In chronic bile duct–ligated dogs, cirrhosis is accompanied by augmented renal synthesis of PGE_2, PGF_2, and PGI_2. The synthesis of these vasodilatory prostaglandins is important in maintaining renal blood flow in this model, since administration of cyclooxygenase inhibitors reduces renal synthesis of vasodilatory prostaglandins by 75 to 90 percent and is accompanied by intense renal vasoconstriction.[357] A recent study measured renal production of the potent vasodilator prostacyclin (PGI_2) in controls, 10 patients with FHF and normal renal function, and eight with FHF and renal failure. Urinary excretion of 6-keto PGF_1, a metabolite of locally synthesized PGI_2, is highly stimulated in FHF patients without renal failure but not in patients with both FHF and renal failure. Plasma renin activity was increased in all patients, and those in renal failure had the highest levels. This local intrarenal imbalance between the intense vasoconstrictive effect of the renin angiotensin system and the potent vasodilatory effect of PGI_2 was mirrored in dramatic decreases in renal blood flow and GFR in the patients with functional renal failure.[358]

The concept of an imbalance in intrarenal vasodilatory and vasoconstrictive factors is supported by the findings of a marked decrement in urinary PGE_2 and a fivefold elevation of urinary thromboxane B_2 (TxB_2) in patients with cirrhosis and HRS compared to cirrhotic patients with ascites but without HRS, and to patients with oliguric renal failure from other causes.[359] TxB_2 is a nonenzymatic metabolite of thromboxane A_2 (TxA_2), a potent renal cortical vasoconstrictor. In contrast to patients with cirrhosis and renal failure, elevated urinary TxB_2 levels were not found in patients with FHF and renal failure.[358] This difference may be related to a more severe reduction in renal plasma flow and GFR in patients with FHF and renal failure.

Although these data offer an attractive explanation of the vascular changes involved in HRS, therapeutic trials designed to modulate either vasodilatory or vasoconstrictive prostaglandins have been inconclusive thus far. Infusions of vasodilatory PGE_1 and PGA_1 had minimal effect on renal perfusion in patients with ascites and stable renal function and in those with HRS.[360,361] A specific inhibitor of TxA_2 synthesis, dazoxiben, has been administered to eight patients with cirrhosis and HRS.[362] Although urinary excretion of TxB_2 was reduced to normal and urinary PGE_2 was unaffected, there was no consistent improvement in renal function. Recent studies using more potent experimental selective inhibitors of intrarenal TxA_2 synthesis in patients with cirrhosis and ascites have been more encouraging. OKY 046, a potent inhibitor of intrarenal TxA_2 synthesis, causes an effective decrease in plasma TxB_2 concentration and urinary TxB_2 excretion after furosemide administration without any effect on renal prostacyclin (PGE_2) production, plasma renin activity, or plasma aldosterone concentration. The potent thromboxane-synthesis inhibitor significantly increased postfurosemide natriuresis in cirrhotic patients and free water clearance in both cirrhotic patients and healthy subjects.[363] These results suggest that through a mechanism independent of other modulators of renal sodium reabsorption, intrarenal TxA_2 generation normally restricts the effects of furosemide on water and sodium diuresis. Such a reduction may be more marked in the presence of an activated intrarenal prostaglandin system found in cirrhotic patients. The use of a potent

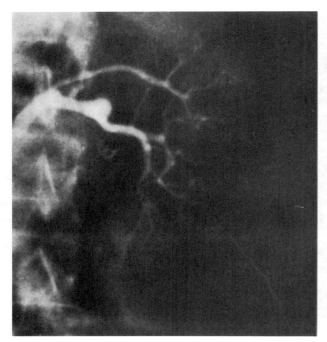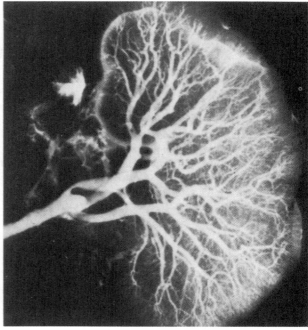

FIGURE 13 Selective renal arteriogram of a patient with cirrhosis and hepatorenal syndrome showing intense renal vasoconstriction. Only the primary and secondary branches of the main renal artery are filled (*left*). In a postmortem study of the same kidney (*right*) the entire renal arterial system was visualized and appeared normal. (From Epstein et al.[352])

inhibitor of TxA_2 may enhance sodium and water excretion and relieve the impaired responsiveness to furosemide frequently observed in cirrhotic patients with ascites.

Hemodynamic Disturbances

Both FHF and cirrhosis with chronic portal-systemic encephalopathy are characterized by a marked decrease in total peripheral resistance, lowered arterial blood pressure, and increased cardiac output. This occurs in spite of raised levels of the potent vasoconstrictors epinephrine and norepinephrine. A fall in peripheral arterial vascular resistance, including splanchnic vasodilation, has been shown to occur very early in animal models of experimental cirrhosis.[364,365] Failure of the compromised liver to metabolize a potent endogenous vasodilating substance has been proposed as the mechanism behind these hemodynamic changes.[366] Candidate compounds have included glucagon and vasoactive intestinal peptide.[367] Recently, substance P, a potent vasodilating compound originating in the intestine and inactivated by the liver, was measured in patients with hepatic encephalopathy and found to be 10 times the normal level measured both in healthy control subjects and in patients with septic shock.[368] Plasma substance P levels were also significantly higher and continued to rise in patients with hepatic failure who died, compared with those who survived. In all patients, plasma norepinephrine levels paralleled those of substance P. Substance P intravenous infusions are known to significantly lower arterial blood pressure in animals and normal

human subjects, even at concentrations less than those found in patients with hepatic failure. High plasma norepinephrine levels and their correlation with plasma substance P levels are interpreted as a reflex activation of the sympathetic nervous system in response to peripheral vasodilatation.

Another potential candidate for the arteriolar vasodilating substance is methionine enkephalin. Opiate peptides are potent vasodilators whose wide distribution of receptors includes arterial blood vessels. The source of circulating methionine enkephalin is unclear, but the peptide is known to be present in the gut. Methionine enkephalin was measured in patients with cirrhosis and ascites and the levels compared with those in patients who had cirrhosis but not ascites, and also with those in controls. The mean value of methionine enkephalin was elevated only in all patients with ascites; the range was 2.5 to 13.7 times the upper limit of normal.[369] In three patients with cirrhosis who developed ascites during the study, methionine enkephalin levels rose from normal to markedly elevated. Again, in this study, plasma norepinephrine and epinephrine rose in concert with methionine enkephalin.

In an effort to reconcile the hemodynamic changes in patients with liver failure to the hormonal and renal perturbations, a new hypothesis, the "peripheral arterial vasodilation hypothesis," has recently been developed to account for the initiation of sodium and water retention in cirrhosis.[370] This theory states that peripheral arterial vasodilation is the initiating event in cirrhotic patients that establishes the hemodynamic consequences of low arterial pressure and generates the reflex secondary increase in sympathetic tone and cardiac output (Fig. 14). In humans, it is known that the peripheral vasodilation that accompanies an arteriovenous fistula causes renal sodium retention.[371] This is mediated via a decrease in the "effective" arterial blood volume and immediate increase in circulating vasoconstrictor hormones. These compensatory hormones, including plasma norepinephrine, AVP, renin, and aldosterone, also affect renal hemodynamics, causing a fall in renal blood flow and GFR and an increase in sodium and water retention. Thus, peripheral arterial vasodilation could explain the two main objections to the classic underfill hypothesis of ascites formation[372]: (1) Renal sodium retention precedes ascites formation in animal models. (2) Plasma volume, central cardiac filling, and cardiac output are actually increased in humans with cirrhosis.[373] It also could answer the major criticism of the overflow theory—that plasma expansion by primary sodium retention should not cause a rise in compensatory vasoconstrictor substances.

Evidence that vasodilation is the primary event that may initiate raised plasma catecholamines, vasoconstrictor hormones, renal sodium retention, and ascites formation was provided in a study in which patients with refractory ascites had ascitic fluid recirculated into their vascular compartment by means of a peritoneal-venous shunt. This procedure produced a marked natriuresis and diuresis and a return of catecholamine levels to normal, but the patients remained hypotensive with a low peripheral vascular resistance.[374] Additional evidence is provided by experiments using head-out-of-water immersion in patients with cirrhosis, ascites, and impaired water excretion. Although this maneuver results in significant increases in cardiac output, intracardiac pressures, renal sodium, and water excretion and in suppression of plasma norepinephrine, AVP, renin, and aldosterone, it did not result in elevation in mean arterial pressure, since systemic vascular resistance declined further below its low baseline value. It was not until these same patients were treated with combined norepinephrine infusion and head-out-of-water immersion that mean arterial pressure normalized, urinary sodium excretion dramatically improved, and plasma aldosterone fell to its lowest levels.[342]

In this hypothesis, ascites forms when the resulting plasma volume expansion is still inadequate to completely refill the enlarged arterial vascular compartment. In cirrhosis, the major documented site of peripheral arteriolar vasodilation is the splanchnic circulation.[375] The cause of the arteriolar vasodilation of the splanchnic bed seems to be related to increases in portal pressure.[376] Thus, in spite of increased central filling and cardiac output, failure to fill regional vascular beds may activate arterial baroreceptors and perpetuate the maintenance of high levels of vasoconstrictor hormones. Further avid renal salt and water retention and increased plasma volume expansion may be modified by hypoalbuminemia and decreased colloid oncotic pressure and by increased portal pressure leading to ascites formation.

The extent of the activation of this integrative system of hemodynamic compromise and hormonal and renal compensation has been shown to correlate with the severity of the disease and the prognosis. Patients with cirrhosis who excrete less than 20 percent of an acute water load had a greater reduction in effective arterial blood volume and renal perfusion, as defined by significantly lower clearance of inulin and para-aminohippurate and significantly higher plas-

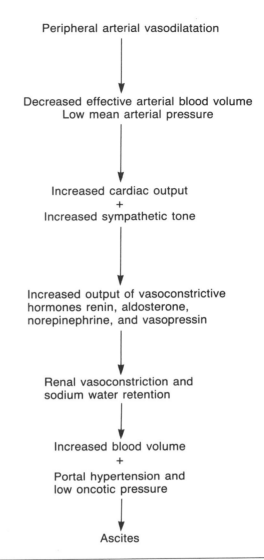

FIGURE 14 The peripheral arterial vasodilation hypothesis seeks to reconcile evidence that sodium retention occurs early in patients with cirrhosis, even before there is intravascular hypovolemia, with evidence showing that there is early stimulation of plasma hormones including renin, norepinephrine, vasopressin, and aldosterone which normally accompany intravascular hypovolemia. The primary event is arteriolar vasodilation, which stimulates compensatory vasoconstricting hormones, which in turn leads to early renal sodium and water retention and plasma volume expansion before ascites formation. (Adapted from Schrier et al.[372])

ma levels of AVP, renin, aldosterone, and norepinephrine, than those who excreted between 20 and 80 percent of an acute waterload. Six of seven patients in this former group died within 5 months. Presumably, these are patients with extreme underfilling of the peripheral arterial circulation. Patients with the hepatorenal syndrome generally have the highest observed plasma concentrations of the major vasoconstrictors seen in patients with liver disease.[355] In addition to extreme intrarenal vasoconstriction, a failure of renal vasodilatory prostaglandin synthesis and excretion may play a key role in the genesis of the hepatorenal syndrome.[377]

Infections in Fulminant Hepatic Failure

The predisposition of patients with serious liver disease to bacteremia and fungemia is well documented.[378,379] The incidence of bacteremia is five- to sevenfold higher in patients with chronic liver disease than in other hospitalized patients.[378] Infection is a major cause of morbidity and mortality in adults and children with FHF.[16,276] Deficiencies in host defenses attributed to patients with advanced liver disease and cirrhosis include (1) impaired removal of bacteria in the blood,[380] (2) impaired hepatic reticuloendothelial system phagocytosis,[381] and (3) defective serum bactericidal and opsonic activity.[382,383]

Since complement is required for leukocyte chemotaxis, phagocytosis, and intracellular killing of bacteria, studies have been performed to evaluate complement activity in patients with FHF. Opsonization of heat-killed baker's yeast, which is dependent on the integrity of the alternative pathway of complement, and C3 and C4 complement concentrations was compared in sera from 69 children with liver disease and 39 controls.[384] In all 10 children with FHF, these parameters were significantly reduced. Functional activity of complement was also measured using radial hemolytic diffusion assays and found to be reduced to less than 45 percent of control levels. These deficiencies in yeast opsonization and complement in children with FHF were of a similar order to those seen in primary complement deficiency. In children surviving FHF, these abnormalities return to normal.

Eight episodes of bacteremia and fungemia developed in seven of 15 children with FHF and grade III to IV encephalopathy.[385] The occurrence of renal failure, GI hemorrhage, and other complications was similar in the children who developed infection and those who did not. All children had normal immunoglobulin levels and none was neutropenic. Opsonization of yeast and functional activity of C4 were significantly lower in those children who developed infection than in those who did not. In five patients who developed infection and had a fatal outcome, serial studies showed a continuing reduction in opsonization and complement activity despite clearance of encephalopathy. The infusion of fresh frozen plasma has been shown to increase yeast opsonization and complement activity in children with chronic diarrhea.[386] This may be useful prophylactic therapy to prevent serious bacterial and fungal infections in children with FHF but has yet to be systematically evaluated.

Gram-positive bacteremia predominates in studies of children and adults with FHF and adults with cirrhosis.[385,387] The most common gram-positive isolates are *Streptococcus pneumoniae*, *Staphylococcus aureus*, and group A beta-hemolytic streptococci. Of the gram-negative isolates, *E. coli* is the most commonly found. The most frequent sources of infection are (1) soft-tissue infections, including cellulitis, wound infections, or phlebitis associated with intravenous catheters and arteriovenous shunts, (2) pneumonia, (3) spontaneous bacterial peritonitis in those patients with ascites, and (4) urinary tract infection, especially in those who have undergone urinary catherization. In approximately 20 percent of patients, no clinically apparent focus of infection can be found.[379]

MANAGEMENT OF HEPATIC FAILURE

The management of patients with hepatic failure requires meticulous attention to detail and co-ordination of multiple medications and regimens to combat this multisystem disorder. It is clear that most patients with FHF die because of the complications enumerated above: cerebral edema and brain herniation, renal failure, GI hemorrhage and shock, or overwhelming sepsis. Thus, prevention of these complications and prompt intervention when they do occur are the cornerstones of therapy. Recent advances in the treatment of these complications are outlined in this section. The advent of orthotopic liver transplantation as an accepted modality of therapy in patients with end-stage liver disease and its application to patients with FHF has spurred great interest in more effective management in order to allow preparation for a transplant. Finally, a clearer understanding of the pathophysiology of hepatic encephalopathy has led to experimental protocols testing new drugs and regimens designed to alter circulating toxic metabolites and their effects on the target organ, the brain.

Supportive Therapy

Table 7 outlines many of the accepted conservative methods of managing the multisystem complications of FHF. Conditions such as hypokalemia, hypoglycemia, GI hemorrhage, hypovolemia; sedatives such as benzodiazepines and barbiturates; an inappropriately high protein intake, constipation, and infection are known aggravating or precipitating factors of hepatic encephalopathy. They must be searched for and promptly corrected and treated. In spite of a desire to control agitation or combative behavior, the physician must resist the temptation to give sedatives or tranquilizers. Potassium loss due to vomiting and diarrhea or excessive diuretic therapy can precipitate metabolic alkalosis, alkalinization of the urine, and increased renal vein ammonia levels. Potassium replacement may require large amounts of potassium (0.5 mEq per kilogram per hour). Up to 3 mEq per kilogram per day of potassium can be provided as the phosphate salt in order to avoid hypophosphatemia. Hypoglycemia is a frequent metabolic complication of FHF in young children and often requires continuous glucose infusion with a hypertonic dextrose solution via a central venous catheter. It is safest to routinely start with at least a 10 percent dextrose solution, even if the serum glucose level is within normal limits, until glucose homeostasis is assured.

Reduction of the nitrogenous load to the gut and alteration of the colonic milieu to retard ammonia production have been mainstays of therapy for patients with hepatic encephalopathy. Blood in the intestinal tract is a highly ammoniagenic material, and GI bleeding is a common coma-precipitating event in patients with chronic liver disease. Meat protein is more likely than dairy protein or vegetable protein to trigger encephalopathy.[388] Azotemia is another precipitating cause of encephalopathy and contributes to the ammonia load via the enterohepatic circulation of urea and degradation of urea by bacterial ureases to ammonia and CO_2 in the gut. Con-

TABLE 7
General Supportive Measures Used in the Treatment of
Fulminant Hepatic Failure

Complication	Treatment
Electrolyte imbalance	
Hyponatremia	No NaCl unless obvious loss Restrict fluids and NaCl Aldosterone antagonist
Hypokalemia	IV KCl or KPO_4 Stop K^+-losing diuretics
Hyperkalemia, azotemia	Peritoneal dialysis or hemodialysis
Metabolic disorder	
Hypoglycemia	10% IV dextrose solution and monitor
Acidosis	Ensure adequate intravascular volume (Swan-Ganz catheter, central venous cathether) IV albumin slowly to expand volume Dialysis if no response to volume expansion
Alkalosis (hypokalemia)	IV KCl
Hypoxemia, pulmonary edema	100% O_2 Ventilation, positive end-expiratory pressure
Coagulopathy	Platelets if <50,000 Fresh frozen plasma only for active bleeding H_2 receptor antagonist (keep gastric pH >5.0) Vitamin K (0.2 mg/kg up to 10 mg) IM or IV daily × 3 days
Encephalopathy	Avoid sedatives, barbiturates Withdraw dietary protein Intubate to protect airway for stage III, IV coma Nasogastric tube Cleansing enemas Lactulose via nasogastric tube (30 cc q6h; 2-4 loose stools/day) 50% branched-chain amino acid solution IV ? Reversal with benzodiazepine antagonist
Raised intracranial pressure (ICP)	Fluid restriction (60-80 cc/kg/day) Hyperventilation ($PaCO_2$ 25-30 mm Hg) Head of bed elevated Avoid frequent movement or head flexion Darkened room, decreased noise CT scans ICP pressure monitor (extradural bolt) Mannitol (0.25-0.5 g/kg) for ICP >30 mm Hg for >5 minutes
Fever	Antipyretics, cooling blanket Cultures of blood, urine, ascites, fluids, etc. Chest radiograph Broad-spectrum antibiotics

stipation may exaggerate these phenomena and, in susceptible patients, may itself induce hepatic encephalopathy.[389]

After identifying and treating the source of a nitrogen load to the gut, the next important step is to eliminate the offending material from the GI tract. This may be accomplished by gastric emptying of blood or protein via a nasogastric tube and by use of cleansing enemas. Alkaline enemas such as soapsuds enema create a pH gradient that favors passage of ammonia from the intestinal lumen into the plasma. Dilute acetic acid enemas or lactulose enemas, which are acidic, trap ammonia and amines in the lumen and promote catharsis and excretion of these substances (Fig. 15).

The activity of gut bacteria, which are thought to be pivotal in the production of putative neurotoxins, can be suppressed with nonabsorbable antibiotics such as neomycin. Although it is traditional to use nonabsorbable antibiotics, any broad-spectrum antibiotic that is excreted in the bile such as ampicillin can be effective when administered by oral or parenteral routes. Owing to absorption of small amounts, prolonged use of oral neomycin has been associated with ototoxicity, renal tubular toxicity, and steatorrhea.[390,391]

Lactulose and Lactitol

In contrast, the use of lactulose, a synthetic disaccharide (beta-galactosidofructose), is not associated with any of these side effects. It is contraindicated only in patients with galactosemia due to small amounts of contaminating galactose. Lactulose is neither absorbed nor metabolized in the upper GI tract and is degraded by bacteria in the lower tract, causing acidification of the lumen. In controlled trials, lactulose was shown to be effective in ameliorating chronic hepatic encephalopathy in adults in approximately 80 percent of cases.[392,393] In a large controlled trial, lactulose was shown to be as effective as neomycin plus sorbitol in improving the clinical grade of encephalopathy, the degree of asterixis, and the EEG abnormalities and in reducing the arterial plasma ammonia concentration.[393] Failure of lactulose to acidify stool adequately may be attributable to antibiotic-induced suppression of lactulose-degrading bacteria or administration of inadequate amounts of lactulose. Because of dependence on gut bacteria for the salutary action of lactulose, the simultaneous administration of neomycin can interfere with its efficacy. However, studies of concurrent administration of the two drugs have shown additive or synergistic effects, as long as stool pH falls below 6. For this reason, stool pH monitoring should be employed whenever lactulose or a combination of lactulose and antibiotics is used. Lactulose can be administered orally, intragastrically, or as an enema (20 percent solution). The initial oral or intragastric dose is 15 to 30 ml every 4 hours until loose stools are produced. Then the dose is titrated to produce two to four loose stools daily.

Recently, lactitol (beta-galactosidosorbitol) has been introduced as a potential alternative to lactulose. It has the advantage of tablet or powder preparation (as opposed to liquid lactulose) and a less objectionable taste when added to beverages or taken alone. Side effects of nausea and abdominal distention commonly seen with lactulose have been minimal with lactitol.[394] In a recent randomized double-blind trial of lactitol versus lactulose given for 5 days in 24 cirrhotic patients experiencing episodes of acute hepatic encephalopathy, there was no significant difference in the effectiveness of the two drugs as judged by clinical status, EEG, and psychometric performance. However, patients given lactitol responded significantly more quickly than those given lactulose.[395] Other recent studies have demonstrated the effectiveness and patient compliance of long-term lactitol treatment in patients with chronic portal-systemic encephalopathy.[394] Lactitol has also been safely and effectively administered as an acidifying enema to patients with acute hepatic encephalopathy.[396]

Keto Acids and Branched-Chain Amino Acids

A number of specific measures to incorporate intestinal ammonia into other compounds have been tried with mixed success. Chief among these is the administration of alpha-keto analogues of amino acids which are converted to amino acids

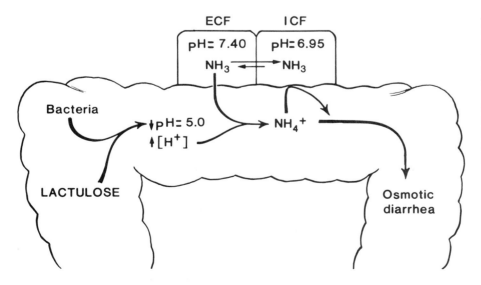

FIGURE 15 Lactulose metabolized by gut bacteria creates an acid milieu in the colon which favors the conversion of NH_3 to NH_4^+. The ammonium ion is trapped by the pH gradient and is excreted in the stool. Lactulose promotes excretion by causing an osmotic diarrhea. The lowered colonic pH also inhibits coliform growth and decreases ammonia production. (Adapted from Conn and Lieberthal.[2])

by transamination reactions within the intestinal mucosa, thus reducing the intestinal ammonia pool. In addition, ketoacids supply the carbon skeleton of the amino acid and the substrate for protein synthesis without supplying any additional nitrogen. Initial work has shown that ketoacids are converted to amino acids, are efficiently incorporated into protein, and maintain nitrogen balance in cirrhotic patients.[397,398] Ornithine salts of branched-chain ketoacids combine the provision of a substrate to prime the urea cycle (ornithine) with the keto acid analogue of BCAA. Trials in patients with hepatic encephalopathy have shown a reduction in plasma ammonia and provision of enough acceptable protein to reverse negative nitrogen balance.[399]

Malnutrition is a major problem in patients with chronic parenchymal liver disease. Previous studies have demonstrated clinical, biochemical, hematologic, and immunologic evidence of protein-calorie malnutrition in patients with alcoholic and nonalcoholic liver disease.[400,401] There is suggestive evidence of a link between malnutrition, sepsis, and mortality in patients who have end-stage liver disease and in those awaiting and undergoing liver transplantation.[402] Because it is known that patients who have cirrhosis with or without encephalopathy are catabolic and have increased rates of protein breakdown, efforts have turned to providing an adequate formulation of protein to reverse negative nitrogen balance without precipitating hepatic encephalopathy. This is of particular importance in children, in whom growth and protein synthesis are central to normal development. These efforts have been guided by research mentioned above into the false neurotransmitter hypothesis of hepatic encephalopathy.

In chronic hepatic encephalopathy, there is a two- to fourfold rise in the plasma concentration of AAA and a decrease in the plasma concentrations of the BCAAs valine, leucine, and isoleucine.[403] Concentrations of AAA are also raised in FHF, but concentrations of BCAA are normal.[404] This pattern is thought to arise largely from massive necrosis of liver cells with release of AAA into the circulation. In chronic liver disease, a combination of enhanced catabolism of peripheral muscle and impaired hepatocellular function contributes to the alteration in AAA and BCAA concentrations. Raised plasma glucagon concentrations stimulate muscle catabolism with release of amino acids for gluconeogenesis. The compromised liver does not take up the AAA, and increased portal-systemic shunting leads to increased circulating levels of AAA. In contrast, BCAA uptake by peripheral muscle and fat is enhanced by hyperinsulinemia and circulating levels decline.[405]

Although these abnormalities in plasma amino acids have been found in most studies of cirrhotic patients with and without encephalopathy, there has been no consistent correlation between amino acid levels and the degree of encephalopathy. The one exception may be plasma and CSF free tryptophan and the ratio of free tryptophan to BCAA.[406] In spite of this lack of correlation, the possibility that excessive AAAs are contributing to the development of hepatic encephalopathy by increased entry into the brain and subsequent metabolism to inhibitory and false neurotransmitters has led to clinical trials of protein formulations rich in BCAA. BCAA would be expected to be beneficial via two major mechanisms: (1) by competing with AAA for transport across the BBB and (2) by decreasing or reversing peripheral muscle catabolism and liberation of AAA from muscle.

Fischer and colleagues were the first to propose that the primary treatment of hepatic encephalopathy might be augmented by normalizing circulating amino acid profiles. Support for this hypothesis comes from studies in normal dogs of intracarotid artery infusion of a solution containing phenylalanine and free tryptophan. This is followed within 6 hours by a reversible coma accompanied by a significant rise in CSF concentrations of phenylalanine, tryptophan, tyrosine, octopamine, and phenylethanolamine. These effects can be totally prevented by the simultaneous infusion of leucine, isoleucine, and valine.[407] Initially, in uncontrolled studies, patients with hepatic encephalopathy were treated with amino acid solutions with decreased amounts of phenylalanine, tryosine, methionine, tryptophan, and glycine and increased BCAA and arginine. Investigators reported improvement in the neuropsychiatric state and reversal of negative nitrogen balance during treatment.[408] Since that time, there have been controlled trials in patients with chronic portal-systemic and acute hepatic encephalopathy. In a large 4-week double-blind controlled trial, the BCAA-supplemented diet was as effective at inducing positive nitrogen balance as an equivalent amount of whole protein but had the distinct advantage of inducing encephalopathy far less often.[409] Two smaller crossover trials of BCAA supplements failed to show any beneficial effect on the mental status of the patients.[410,411]

In patients with acute hepatic encephalopathy, BCAAs have been administered parenterally in three randomized controlled trials.[412-414] These studies are difficult to compare, since in two of them BCAAs represented the sole source of nitrogen and in the third BCAAs were part of a more comprehensive enriched amino acid solution (FO80). These considerations are of importance, since it has recently been shown that in stable cirrhotic patients without encephalopathy who receive 100 percent of their protein as BCAA without essential amino acids, any increase in protein synthesis is matched by a significant increase in protein catabolism and lack of improvement in overall protein balance.[415] Lack of tyrosine or cysteine in parenteral amino acid formulations has been shown to prevent achievement of positive nitrogen balance in some patients with cirrhosis.[416] The presence of tryptophan, phenylalanine, and methionine in some formulations may be detrimental, whereas the presence of arginine (7.5 percent of total amino acids in FO80) may be helpful, since there is evidence that treatment with arginine counteracts hyperammonemia and stimulates ureagenesis in patients with hereditary defects in the urea cycle.[417]

A comparison of the effect of BCAA plus glucose versus lactulose plus glucose as the primary therapy for grade III to IV hepatic encephalopathy showed no statistical difference in mortality or recovery from encephalopathy. BCAA therapy was just as effective as lactulose in reversing hepatic coma.[412] A second trial comparing intravenous glucose, fat, and BCAA with intravenous glucose and fat alone failed to show any benefit of BCAA with respect to either encephalopathy or mortality.[413] A double-blind randomized controlled trial using BCAA-enriched total amino acid mixture versus glucose plus neomycin has shown improved nitrogen balance and more rapid diminution of encephalopathy on the first and second days of treatment in the group given BCAA. In addition, most importantly, mortality was significantly decreased in patients treated with the BCAA-enriched formulation.

However, patients whose encephalopathy was precipitated by gastrointestinal hemorrhage were excluded from this analysis.[414]

Despite these inconclusive data on the efficacy of BCAA formulations as primary therapy for hepatic encephalopathy, a growing body of evidence suggests that BCAA may be important as nutritional therapy in conjunction with primary therapy for hepatic encephalopathy. The relationship between malnutrition and hepatic encephalopathy has recently been studied in dogs with Eck fistulas, in whom maintenance of nutrition and prevention of weight loss were shown to prevent the development of hepatic encephalopathy.[418] In human patients with cirrhosis, alterations in plasma BCAA concentrations may be dependent on the nutritional status, with decreased plasma levels occurring only in malnourished patients.[419] Previous studies showed that infusion of BCAA reduced skeletal muscle protein catabolism as measured by urinary excretion of 3-methylhistidine in cirrhotics with reduced basal levels of alanine and BCAA and elevated basal levels of AAA and free tryptophan. In addition, plasma alanine levels were restored to normal, suggesting that the rapid uptake of BCAA by muscle stimulated de novo synthesis of alanine.[420] Body protein metabolism in patients with cirrhosis was assessed using labeled (^{14}C) leucine as a tracer, and protein balance was found to be improved in patients receiving solutions containing 35 and 53 percent of total amino acids as BCAA.[415]

Benzodiazepine Antagonists

Treatment with lactulose or BCAA emphasizes manipulation of peripherally produced toxins implicated in the pathogenesis of hepatic encephalopathy. A different strategy is to administer drugs designed to work at the level of the target organ—the brain. In initial uncontrolled series, L-dopa and bromocriptine, which might be expected to restore brain dopamine levels, were reported to induce an amelioration of encephalopathy in cirrhotic patients. However, in controlled trials of L-dopa and bromocriptine, no sustained benefit was achieved.[421,422]

More recently, experimental drugs designed to reduce GABA-ergic transmission in the brain have been introduced and tested. Thus far, only case reports or small series have appeared.[265–267] The most commonly used agent is a benzodiazepine antagonist, flumazenil (Ro 15-1788), which blocks the benzodiazepine receptor but does not alter chloride conductance at the postsynaptic membrane. Flumazenil has been reported to induce clinical and electrophysiologic remissions of hepatic encephalopathy in patients with FHF and chronic portal-systemic encephalopathy. A recent report describes the successful long-term treatment of chronic intractable encephalopathy with flumazenil.[423] This patient had been previously unresponsive to protein restriction and lactulose. With the use of flumazenil, the patient was able to tolerate an unrestricted protein diet. Stopping the drug immediately precipitated abnormalities in VEPs and, soon after, attacks of hepatic encephalopathy. Restarting the medication again reversed these abnormalities. Two recent trials of intravenous flumazenil in 31 patients with hepatic encephalopathy have been carried out.[267,424] Approximately two-thirds of the patients experienced improvement in their level of consciousness. The most impressive response was seen in those patients with grade IV encephalopathy. The arousal effect occurred from 1 to 60 minutes after intravenous administration but was usually short-lived, lasting approximately 1 to 4 hours. Nonresponse to flumazenil correlated well with clinical evidence of brain edema and eventual in-hospital death.

These data suggest that arousal with intravenous flumazenil can be used as a prognostic factor in predicting short-term survival in severe hepatic encephalopathy and allowing identification of individuals whose neurologic deterioration is not due to some structural abnormality of the central nervous system such as cerebral edema, hypoxia, or hemorrhage. Other drugs are currently being tested in animal models. These ligands are known as partial inverse benzodiazepine agonists because not only do they compete with any benzodiazepine agonist present, but they also decrease the ability of GABA to promote chloride conductance. One of these drugs has the property of reversing the sedative-hypnotic effects of alcohol in the rat,[425] and another has shown a more complete reversal of hepatic encephalopathy in a rat model of FHF.[426]

Treatment of Cerebral Edema

Advances have also been made in treating complications other than hepatic encephalopathy. Controlled trials failed to show benefit from dexamethasone used prophylactically to prevent cerebral edema.[427] However, a controlled trial of the use of intracranial monitoring and intravenous mannitol for intracranial pressure (ICP) elevations of greater than 30 mm Hg for more than 5 minutes showed reductions of ICP in 80 percent of the cases and improved survival in patients with FHF.[294] Mannitol consistently reversed or arrested ICP rises when the pressure was less than 60 mm Hg. It was not effective in patients with renal failure. In these patients, mannitol should be used only when hemodialysis (or hemofiltration) is in progress, since mannitol infusion may cause hyperosmolarity and fluid overload. Mannitol must be infused rapidly in order to be maximally effective, and urine output should be monitored hourly. Plasma osmolarity should be less than 320 mOsm in order to continue treating with mannitol. Experimental studies in rats have shown that 20 percent mannitol solutions readily crystallize at room temperature and that infusion of unfiltered mannitol may cause edema and microinfarcts in the brain.[285] Therefore, mannitol should be infused through a system that incorporates a blood filter. Although there are no clinical trials of nonosmotic diuretics for the treatment of cerebral edema, combinations of albumin and loop diuretics have been shown to be as effective as mannitol in lowering ICP in experimental head injury.[428] Since hypoalbuminemia and reduced oncotic pressure are common in patients with hepatic failure, combination therapy with albumin, furosemide, and mannitol, given if ICP is greater than 30 mm Hg and there is clinical evidence of cerebral edema, appears to be a rational approach.

Other therapeutic interventions are designed to reduce cerebral blood flow and cerebral oxygen utilization and metabolism. Short-term hyperventilation via intubation and mechanical ventilation has become an accepted modality of treatment for increased ICP and is designed to maintain arterial PCO_2 between 25 and 30 mm Hg. However, a recent controlled clinical trial of elective mechanical hyperventilation in patients with FHF and ICP monitoring failed to show any reduction in mean ICP or mannitol requirements in the prophylactically ventilated group versus the control group in whom mechanical ventilation was instituted only when hypercapnia or hypoxia was present.[275]

Short-acting high-dose barbiturates have been used to control increased ICP in Reye's syndrome.[429] Their use in FHF has been limited by development of hypotension. Short-acting anesthetic agents have been tried as alternative cerebral protective agents in FHF and have proven effective when given as an intravenous bolus without marked hemodynamic disturbance.[285] Controlled trials of these agents have not been carried out.

Treatment of Bleeding and Coagulopathy

GI bleeding is a major complication and cause of death in hepatic failure. A controlled trial of intravenous cimetidine sufficient to maintain gastric pH greater than 5.0 has been shown to reduce the incidence and severity of GI bleeding and the transfusion requirement in patients with FHF.[430] In view of cimetidine's potential for causing encephalopathy in certain patients, other H_2 blockers such as ranitidine may be safer and equally efficacious agents. Prophylactic administration of fresh frozen plasma in patients without bleeding did not reduce morbidity or mortality in patients with FHF.[431] In FHF, the combination of a complex coagulopathy and thrombocytopenia greatly increases the likelihood of bleeding. In one study, the mean platelet count in those having major episodes of bleeding was $53,000 \times 10^9$ per liter compared with $91,000 \times 10^9$ per liter in the nonbleeding patients.[296] Therefore, the platelet count should be maintained greater than $50,000 \times 10^9$ per liter, especially if any invasive procedure is planned.

Two recent therapeutic developments are the use of desmopressin [D-amino-8-D-arginine vasopressin (DDAVP)] and treatment of disseminated intravascular coagulation with AT III. DDAVP increases plasma levels of Factor VIII and VIIIc (von Willebrand factor) and has proven to be a useful therapeutic agent in mild hemophilia.[432] Infusion of DDAVP in eight patients with cirrhosis increased plasma values of Factors VII, VIII, IX, and XII.[433] Recent studies have shown a shortening of bleeding and partial thromboplastin times in cirrhotics but no change in prothrombin time.[434,435] No controlled trials with assessment of bleeding episodes have been conducted in patients with cirrhosis and coagulopathy or in patients with hepatic failure. AT III concentrates have been given to patients with disseminated intravascular coagulation and FHF. In several of these small studies, including one in children, there seemed to be an association of decreased mortality with treatment.[436,437] In a recent study, 26 patients with FHF were all treated with 3,000 U daily of AT III. Maintenance of AT III levels at greater than 80 percent of control levels was associated with improved survival and no changes in platelet count. Decreases in AT III levels were accompanied by lengthening of the prothrombin time, lowering of the platelet count, and an increased bleeding tendency.[438] AT III concentrates carry the risk of transmission of hepatitis and acquired immunodeficiency syndrome. No large controlled clinical trials have yet been carried out.

Treatment of Hepatorenal Syndrome

There is no proven modality of therapy capable of reversing hepatorenal syndrome in patients with hepatic failure. Patients with oliguria secondary to intravascular volume contraction have urinary sodium concentration, urinary-to-plasma creatinine ratio, and urinary osmolality indistinguishable from those with hepatorenal syndrome. Thus, every effort should be made to ensure that intravascular volume is replete before making the diagnosis. This requires infusion of saline or albumin or both with simultaneous measurement of central venous pressure or pulmonary capillary wedge pressure and careful hourly monitoring of urine output. If other causes of renal failure are excluded and a diagnosis of hepatorenal syndrome is entertained, the mainstay of therapy is careful restriction of sodium and fluid intake and consideration of hemodialysis. A number of specific measures aimed at increasing renal blood flow such as colloid-induced volume expansion, transient ascites reinfusion, water immersion, or repeated paracentesis have resulted in only transient improvement in renal hemodynamics and function without significant improvement in outcome. Most published reports of the use of dialysis or hemofiltration in patients with hyperkalemia or fluid overload in the setting of hepatorenal syndrome have not reported any improvement in the overall high mortality rate. However, these reports concern patients with chronic end-stage liver disease.[439] In patients with FHF, dialysis is indicated, since the renal failure may reverse in conjunction with resolution of the acute hepatic insult or with successful liver transplantation.

Recent studies have reported the successful use of the peritoneal-jugular shunt (LeVeen shunt) in managing ascites and the hepatorenal syndrome.[440-442] Some of them suffer from inadequate discrimination between patients with hepatorenal syndrome and those with prerenal azotemia and oliguria.[443] Nevertheless, scattered reports satisfy accepted criteria for the diagnosis and document marked improvement in renal function and urine output.[444-446] No controlled prospective study has been done, but such a study appears to be warranted based on the uncontrolled observations. Major complications of peritoneal-jugular shunts include disseminated intravascular coagulation, bleeding, shunt occlusion, superior vena cava syndrome, sepsis, ascitic fluid leaks, and small bowel obstruction, which occur in approximately one-third of patients.[443,447-449] Experience with LeVeen shunts in children is quite limited.[450,451] Most patients have had refractory chylous ascites but normal liver function.[452,453] Thus, extrapolation of successful experiences in this group of patients may not be valid.

Greater understanding of the pathophysiology of sodium and water retention in advanced liver disease has led to a more rational pharmacologic approach to the problem. Specific inhibitors of renal TxA_2 are being tested and appear to enhance the effects of furosemide-induced sodium and water diuresis in cirrhotic patients with ascites.[363] ANF is a potent natriuretic agent that also causes vasodilation and counteracts the renin-angiotensin system in humans. Recent studies on small numbers of cirrhotic patients with ascites showed that intravenous ANF bolus therapy can induce a short-term natriuresis and diuresis.[454] This effect is attenuated by a fall in mean arterial pressure but can be restored in a rat model of portal hypertension and ascites by the addition of phenylalanine-isoleucine-ornithine vasopressin, a vasopressin receptor agonist with pressor effects but without antidiuretic effects.[455] Further testing of these new agents holds promise.

Prevention of Hepatorenal Syndrome

It has long been observed that the majority of patients who develop hepatorenal syndrome have tense ascites and often develop oliguria and functional renal failure while in the hospital undergoing vigorous attempts to mobilize the ascitic fluid with sodium and fluid restriction and the use of diuretics. A new loop diuretic, muzolimine, has been developed, which appears to be as effective as furosemide in the treatment of cirrhotic patients with ascites but is longer acting, induces less urinary potassium and chloride excretion, has a more gradual diuretic action, and, unlike furosemide, does not induce any reactive rise in plasma renin activity.[456] These properties may be beneficial, reducing the likelihood of acute intravascular volume depletion, hypokalemia, hypochloremia, metabolic alkalosis, and rebound activation of the renin-angiotensin system, with concomitant reduction in GFR and azotemia which may follow overvigorous diuresis with furosemide.

Recent studies have documented the efficacy and safety of large-volume paracentesis (approximately 5 liters over a 20- to 40-minute period) in the treatment of cirrhotic patients with tense ascites, both with and without edema.[457-459] Previously, large-volume paracentesis had been avoided because of fear of precipitating fluid shifts out of the intravascular space, leading to intravascular volume depletion, oliguria, azotemia, hyponatremia, and encephalopathy. In the recent studies, no patient developed hypotension or renal insufficiency following paracentesis. Measurements of plasma volume using ^{125}I-labeled human serum albumin showed no significant changes 24 and 48 hours after paracentesis even when no albumin was infused during or after the paracentesis.[458] A controlled study comparing large-volume paracentesis plus albumin infusion with standard diuretic therapy in cirrhotics with tense ascites was recently reported.[457] Paracentesis eliminated ascites in 96 percent of patients, whereas diuretics were similarly effective in only 72 percent. The length of hospital stay after paracentesis was also much shorter. Plasma volume and plasma renin activity were unchanged in 24 patients following paracentesis, and there was a lower incidence of hyponatremia, encephalopathy, and renal impairment in the paracentesis group. When patients were randomized to large-volume paracentesis with or without albumin infusion, those who did not receive albumin had a pronounced increase in plasma renin and aldosterone levels and a higher frequency of hyponatremia and decreased creatinine clearance.[459,460] These studies confirm the safety of large-volume paracentesis plus intravenous albumin as an alternative to chronic diuretic therapy with its attendant risks.

Artificial Liver Support

The goal of the previously described treatments is to support the patient temporarily in order to allow the injured host liver to regenerate. Support includes removing potential toxic substances normally cleared from the circulation by the liver and adding back important substances synthesized by the liver for the maintenance of homeostatic mechanisms. To these ends much effort has been directed toward the development of artificial liver support systems. These have included charcoal hemoperfusion, resin hemoperfusion, hemodialysis and hemofiltration, plasmapheresis and plasma filtration, and artificial cells. Although some of these techniques have been used in humans with FHF and have resulted in transient improvement in levels of consciousness and even in a longer duration of survival, no consistent improvement in survival rates has been demonstrated. Failure of these support systems to affect survival rates may be primarily related to two problems: (1) failure of timely liver regeneration from the initial insult sufficient to sustain hepatic function without artificial systems, and (2) limited blood flow through any of the extracorporeal systems. The amount of blood flow through a hemoperfusion column during the usual 4- to 8-hour procedure per day is approximately 2 to 4 percent of the total daily liver blood flow. In addition, the clearance of most putative toxins is inferior to that of the normal liver.

Charcoal hemoperfusion was first attempted in 1972 by Chang and co-workers using a charcoal column with an ultrathin cellulose-nitrate membrane coated onto the surface of each charcoal granule to allow removal of toxic substances but prevent embolization of charcoal particles and detrimental interactions with platelets and white cells. The system was shown to be effective in removing mercaptans, free fatty acids, GABA, phenols, AAA, and so-called middle molecules but did not remove ammonia, which is heavily ionized at physiologic pH.[461,462]

Many modifications of the original system have been made over the last 15 years. Polyhydroxylethyl methacrylate (polyhema) encapsulation of charcoal granules led to a significant reduction in platelet loss and was used in the initial large clinical trials of charcoal hemoperfusion at King's College Hospital in London.[463,464] An exterior coating of human serum albumin over the encapsulated charcoal potentiated the removal of loosely protein-bound drugs as albumin on the particle surface competed for toxins bound to carrier proteins in perfused blood. In an effort to facilitate removal of lipophilic substances, particularly those bound to plasma proteins, resins coated with albumin (Amberlite XAD-7) have been used in the hemoperfusion circuit. Bilirubin, bile acids, ammonia, and middle molecules have all been removed with this system.

One of the major advances in artificial liver support has been the use of PGI_2 infusions to prevent the formation of platelet aggregates and release of activated factors thought to be responsible for hypotension and hemodynamic instability in patients treated with charcoal hemoperfusion.[465] Platelet factor beta–thromboglobulin and platelet factor 4 were both found to be significantly increased in the plasma of patients in grade III or IV encephalopathy, indicating that even before hemoperfusion circulating platelets are preactivated.[297] PGI_2 continuous infusion during a 4-hour period of charcoal hemoperfusion was associated with maintenance of the preperfusion platelet count versus a 14 percent reduction in control patients not given PGI_2. Beta-thromboglobulin levels did not rise when PGI_2 was given, and hypotension did not develop.[466]

Two other artificial support systems have been used clinically in patients with FHF. Polyacrylonitrile-membrane hemodialysis differs from standard dialysis in that the membrane is permeable to compounds with molecular weights of 1,500 to 5,000 (middle molecules), a similar range to those substances absorbed during charcoal hemoperfusion. There have been reports of significant improvement in consciousness levels of patients with FHF and grade IV hepatic encephalopathy but no significant effect on long-term survival.[274] Plasmapheresis and plasma exchange allow removal of toxic substances from the plasma and replacement with normal donor fresh frozen plasma containing clotting factors and other substances. Improvements in coma score and coagulopathy have been documented in patients with FHF, but there has been no change in overall survival.[465,467] These donor blood products carry the risk of NANB hepatitis and also may not contain substances involved in stimulation of hepatic regeneration which are removed by the plasmapheresis.

Until recently charcoal hemoperfusion has been enthusiastically supported by several groups of investigators, and studies have been published in which the survival rates of patients with FHF treated with charcoal hemoperfusion have compared favorably with the overall survival figures for such patients treated conservatively at the time. In a series of 76 patients with FHF reported from England, increased survival (65 percent versus 20 percent) and decreased frequency of cerebral edema (49 percent versus 78 percent) were found when hemoperfusion was begun when the patients were experiencing grade III encephalopathy rather than awaiting the development of grade IV encephalopathy before intervening.[468] Survival rates were 41 percent in Japan for patients treated with hemoperfusion between 1974 and 1981[469] and 38 percent in England compared to 15 to 20 survival in large numbers of collected patients treated conservatively.

In spite of these data, no carefully controlled randomized prospective clinical trials had been carried out until recently. O'Grady and colleagues published a large series in which 62 patients with FHF of varying etiologies and established grade IV encephalopathy were randomized to have 10 hours of charcoal hemoperfusion daily versus standard intensive supportive care.[10] Overall survival rates for the two groups were the same (39 percent versus 34 percent). What is striking is that the overall survival for control patients receiving conventional supportive therapy exceeded the "improved" survival rates of patients from the same institution who were treated previously with charcoal hemoperfusion.[470] These data suggest that it is advances in the care of the complications of FHF which have improved survival, not the use of charcoal hemoperfusion.

The chief use of artificial support systems may be in buying time for either hepatocellular regeneration to take place or a suitable donor liver to be procured for liver transplantation. Charcoal hemoperfusion has been shown to prolong survival in a dog model of ischemic liver injury from a mean of 10.8 hours to between 2 and 7 days.[471] A second study

demonstrated a marked prolongation in survival of dogs transplanted with liver allografts subjected to ischemic injury prior to transplantation. When treated with three periods of hemoperfusion on days 0, 1, and 2 after transplant, survival in transplanted dogs was increased from a mean of 18 hours to a mean of 27 days.[472]

Orthotopic Liver Transplantation

Orthotopic liver transplantation (OLTx) holds the greatest potential for altering the natural history of fulminant hepatic failure. Table 8 shows preliminary results of five small series of OLTx in patients presenting with grade III or IV encephalopathy and FHP.[10,473–476] Although the numbers are small, the short-term survival rate compares very favorably with most larger series of conservatively treated patients. This is particularly evident in comparison with survival rates for patients whose FHF is caused by NANB hepatitis, drug-induced hepatic necrosis, Budd-Chiari malformation, and Wilson's disease, in which reversible liver damage and spontaneous recovery are less likely. OLTx has been successfully performed in small numbers of children with FHF secondary to fulminant hepatitis (presumed NANB hepatitis), Wilson's disease, hereditary tyrosinemia, and valproate toxicity.[21,23,141,467,477] In the Pittsburgh series, 29 adult patients met the criteria for FHF or subacute hepatic failure and grade III or IV encephalopathy when admitted.[473] Of those, 3 recovered without a transplant, 13 died awaiting transplant, and 13 received a transplant, 7 of whom survived. Thus, 13 of 16 (81 percent) died without a transplant versus only 6 of 13 (45 percent) with a transplant. It appears that liver transplantation improves survival in this particularly ill subset of patients. One-year survival rates for OLTx are approximately 70 to 75 percent for all candidates, a figure only slightly better than the 44 to 70 percent obtained in cases of FHF (Table 8).

Application of OLTx to pediatric patients with FHF is restricted by the availability of donor organs and the small size of the recipients. Recent developments enhance prospects for overcoming this difficulty in the future. Volume-reduced livers have been successfully used for both heterotopic and orthotopic liver transplantation.[478,479] The possibility of providing more than one small critically ill child with a volume-reduced

TABLE 8
Orthotopic Liver Transplantation in Fulminant Hepatic Failure

Series	Number of Patients	Patients Survived (No.)	(%)	Reference
France	17	12	(70)	474
Pittsburgh	13	7	(54)	473
UCLA	6	4	(66)	475
England	19	11	(58)	10
West Germany	16	7	(44)	476
TOTAL	71	41	(58)	

liver from one donor and even possibly of avoiding the removal of the native liver should lessen the likelihood that these patients will die awaiting transplantation.

Liver Regeneration

A major determinant of survival in FHF is the capacity of the liver to regenerate after the primary insult. Although still in its infancy, research directed toward elucidating important hepatic growth factors or stimulating substances has begun in an effort to find a successful method of treatment for FHF. Initial reports suggest a role for insulin and glucagon in liver regeneration.[480] Encouraging data in a mouse model of fulminant hepatitis indicate that simultaneous treatment with insulin and glucagon enhances survival rates.[481] However, such treatments have shown inconsistent effects in humans.

Recent research has attempted to isolate other hepatotropic or inhibitor factors by using animal models of partial hepatectomy or chemically induced hepatic failure. Diversion of portal blood supply and ablation of the pancreas and duodenum drained by the portal vein causes a delay and reduced liver regeneration after partial hepatectomy.[482] Insulin, glucagon, and regulatory peptides such as epidermal growth factor (EGF) are all carried in portal blood and all appear to be involved in stimulating liver regeneration.[483]

EGF is localized in Brunner's glands and is secreted in an exocrine fashion into duodenal contents. It stimulates the growth of many cells, including liver parenchymal cells both in vivo and in vitro.[484] A recent study of the role of EGF suggested that endogenous EGF participates in the stimulation of liver regeneration after partial hepatectomy in rats.[485] Exogenous instillation of EGF in the duodenum resulted in increased portal vein concentrations and duodenectomy decreased liver regeneration after partial hepatectomy. Oral or subcutaneous administration of EGF alone had no effect on liver regeneration but when administered with insulin and glucagon, hepatic DNA synthesis was significantly increased compared to both controls and animals given only insulin and glucagon without EGF. Administration of EGF antiserum significantly reduced hepatocyte DNA synthesis and liver regeneration. These results suggest that hepatotropic hormones and regulatory peptides co-operate with each other in enhancing hepatic regeneration and that EGF may be an important mediator of this process.

Other hepatic regenerative factors have been derived from the liver itself. LaPlante-O'Neill and colleagues showed that cell-free supernatant from hepatocyte cultures improved the survival of rats with chemically induced acute liver failure.[486] Protein fractions have been partially purified and characterized from regenerating liver cytosol which are able to stimulate hepatocyte DNA synthesis and cellular proliferation in vitro and in vivo when injected into partially hepatectomized rats.[487,488] A recent report describes the intraperitoneal injection of "hepatic stimulatory substance" and subfractions of 300,000 and 50,000 daltons prepared from regenerating rat liver into rats treated 48 hours earlier with lethal doses of D-galactosamine. Hepatic stimulatory substance (M.W. 300,000) improved survival over the saline-treated control group. The preparation studied was completely free of recognizable hormones including insulin, glucagon, and EGF.[491]

A major area of investigation in the field of liver regeneration is hepatocyte transplantation.[490] In most animal experiments, freshly isolated hepatocytes have been transplanted. Advances in tissue culture techniques have allowed isolation of hepatocytes by in situ collagenase perfusion and preservation of metabolically functioning hepatocytes for up to 3 weeks. Other technical problems have included difficulty in assuring hepatocyte attachment, proliferation, and survival in the host despite a number of different approaches. Demetriou and co-workers have recently reported a technique of intraperitoneal transplantation of hepatocytes attached to collagen-coated microcarriers into rats undergoing a 90 percent partial hepatectomy.[491] When hepatocyte transplantation was done 3 days prior to hepatectomy, there was a marked improvement in long-term survival compared to rats given injections of microcarriers, hepatocytes, or medium alone, all of whom died within 5 days of hepatectomy. Transplantation simultaneous with hepatectomy did not improve survival, suggesting that the establishment of an adequate blood supply to the transplanted cells was critical prior to hepatectomy. In addition, animals transplanted with microcarrier-attached hepatocytes exhibited a lesser degree of hypoglycemia following 90 percent partial hepatectomy, suggesting enhanced gluconeogenesis and metabolic activity. It is not clear whether this effect is a result of the metabolic function of the transplanted hepatocytes or stimulation of regeneration of the host liver by growth factors derived from the transplant. However, the number of hepatocytes transplanted only increased the remaining hepatic mass from 10 to 12 percent in 90 percent hepatectomized rats, suggesting that the modest initial increase in viable hepatocyte mass is not the only important factor in the observed increased survival.

ASSESSMENT AND PROGNOSIS IN HEPATIC FAILURE

With the advent of liver transplantation as an effective modality of therapy for fulminant hepatic failure, the importance of an early reliable prognostic evaluation of patients has become critical. Transplantation in the presence of grade IV encephalopathy, functional renal failure, spontaneous bacterial peritonitis and sepsis, or massive GI bleeding carries a poor prognosis. Thus, transplantation should be considered before these complications arise when a decision is made that the prognosis for recovery of hepatic function is poor. Table 9 suggests various etiologic, clinical, laboratory, and pathologic factors that have been associated with a poor prognosis and may point to the need for immediate transplantation. In many of these variables, the certainty of the assessment of prognosis increases with the time of observation, and several studies have shown that serial determinations give more information than single ones.[492]

The etiology of FHF figures prominently in the prognosis. For example, metabolic disease presenting with FHF such alpha₁-AT deficiency, Wilson's disease, or tyrosinemia, in which the liver is persistently exposed to a toxic insult, is generally considered irreversible liver injury requiring transplantation. Conversely, in an acute self-limited insult such

TABLE 9
Suggested Criteria for Immediate Liver
Transplantation in Patients with Fulminant
Hepatic Failure

Nonreversible disease (Wilson's, NANB hepatitis, halothane,
   idiosyncratic drug reaction, biliary atresia, metabolic liver disease)

Stage IV coma

Factor VII persistently less than 10 percent of control

Factor V persistently less than 20 percent of control

Prothrombin time greater than 50 seconds

Duration of jaundice before encephalopathy exceeds 7 days (subacute)

Metabolic acidosis, hypoglycemia

ICP responsive to mannitol

Patent portal venous system by Doppler flow study

as hepatitis A or acetaminophen overdose, the exposure to liver injury is limited and there is potentially reversible liver disease. Figure 16 shows survival data for five different subsets of patients presenting to the King's College Hospital Liver Failure Unit in London. Survival data range from 66.7 percent for those with hepatitis A to 20 percent for patients with NANB hepatitis and only 12.5 percent for those with halothane hepatitis or idiosyncratic drug reactions.[10]

Generally, laboratory data that reflect either hepatic protein synthesis or regenerative capacity are the best predictors of survival. Coagulation factors have emerged as good indicators in several studies. In a series of 31 children with FHF, the prothrombin time was prolonged by more than 90 seconds and unresponsive to parenteral vitamin K in 10 fatal cases but in none of the survivors.[16] Factor VII, with the shortest half-life of all the factors (3 to 5 hours), has been evaluated as a predictor of survival, since levels rapidly reflect hepatic synthetic dysfunction. In one study, survival was 100

percent in patients with a Factor VII level greater than 9 percent.[301] In another study, Factor VII levels did not distinguish five survivors from seven nonsurvivors on admission, but serial Factor VII levels showing a rapid elevation always predicted survival. Multivariate analysis of prognostic factors in fulminant hepatitis B revealed two indicators of imminent death: rapid deterioration of the neurologic status to grade III to IV encephalopathy and a Factor V level below 20 percent of normal. The presence of these two features was associated with a mortality rate of 95 percent. Additionally, patients who were HBsAg-positive had a worse prognosis than those who were HBsAg-negative.[493] Alpha-fetoprotein has been suggested as a marker of hepatic regeneration. Its presence has been associated with survival in 59 to 80 percent of patients with FHF, whereas, in its absence, only 9 to 24 percent survived.[494,495]

"Quantitative" liver function tests such as galactose elimination, aminopyrine metabolism, indocyanine green clearance, and bile acid conjugation have been applied to patients with FHF in order to assess prognosis. Galactose clearance measures the functional metabolic capacity of the liver determined by hepatocyte function and liver blood flow. Using a large intravenous bolus, elimination over the initial 60 minutes is zero order, and the galactose-specific metabolic system is saturated. Under these conditions, galactose elimination capacity over time is more a measure of viable hepatocyte function and less of liver blood flow.[496] In 13 patients with FHF and a galactose elimination capacity of less than 9.5 μmol per minute per kilogram, there were no survivors. Using a discrimination limit of 15 μmol per minute per kilogram, the survival of 15 patients above the limit was 57 percent and in 47 patients below the limit 19 percent.[492,497] The rate of appearance of $^{13}CO_2$ or $^{14}CO_2$ after administration of similarly labeled aminopyrine correlates with the functioning mass of the hepatic microsomal mixed function oxidase enzyme system. In a study of patients with alcoholic hepatitis, an appearance of greater than 1 percent of the administered ^{14}C-aminopyrine in breath as $^{14}CO_2$ correlated

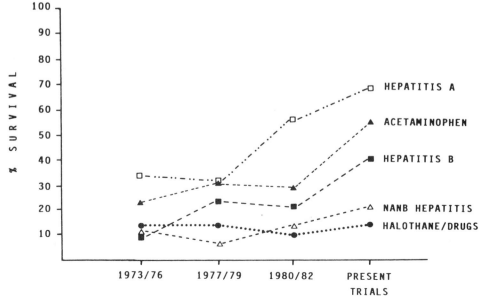

FIGURE 16 Serial survival rates in the main etiologic subgroups in the King's College Hospital Liver Failure unit, London, England. There has been steady improvement in survival rates for fulminant hepatitis due to hepatitis A, hepatitis B, and acetaminophin toxicity. However, no improved survival rates have been documented for patients with halothane toxicity or non-A, non-B, hepatitis–related hepatic failure. (From O'Grady et al.[10])

TABLE 10
Scoring System for Prediction of Mortality
from Chronic Liver Disease in Children

Weighting Factor	Variable
+15	If cholestrol ≤ 100 mg/dl
+15	If positive history of ascites
+13	If bilirubin (indirect) ≥ 6 mg/dl
+11	If bilirubin (indirect) = 3–6 mg/dl
+10	If PTT prolonged ≥ 20 seconds

Total Score	Patient Group	Risk of Dying Within 6 Months of Evaluation
0–27	Low risk	<25%
18–39	Moderate risk	25–75%
≥ 40	High risk	$\geq 75\%$

From Malatack et al.[504]

with short-term survival of 3 weeks in 31 of 32 patients, whereas 6 of 7 patients died with an aminopyrine breath test of less than 1 percent.[498] Plasma levels of bile acids are greatly increased in FHF, with no significant difference between survivors and nonsurvivors. However, a quantitative assessment of glycine conjugation of unconjugated cholic acid has correlated well with survival. Using a 60 percent conjugation limit, survival above this level was 88 percent in one study and only 17 percent below this level.[499]

Two metabolic complications of hepatic failure have been associated with an ominous prognosis. Ongoing hypoglycemia and a large requirement for intravenous dextrose (1 g per kilogram per hour) has been noted in a large percentage of nonsurvivors.[500] The presence of hypoglycemia in hepatic failure secondary to inborn errors of metabolism such as galactosemia, hereditary fructose intolerance, or Reye's syndrome does not carry the same prognostic value, since these defects involve direct inhibition of gluconeogenic pathways. Lactic acidosis with a median mixed venous lactate of 7.2 mmol per liter has been observed in 17 of 32 patients admitted in grade III or IV encephalopathy and FHF in one study.[501] Of these 17 patients, 16 subsequently died. Twelve of the remaining 15 who were also admitted with equivalent grades of encephalopathy survived, and in this group the median mixed venous lactate was 3.0 mmol per liter.

An attempt to correlate histologic findings with prognosis in FHF has been made by assessing the volume of viable hepatocytes as a fraction of the total volume of the biopsy. Normally hepatocytes make up 85 ± 5 percent of a needle biopsy specimen. A critical volume of 40 percent intact hepatocytes has been suggested, below which the prognosis is poor.[502] In a large study of causes of death in FHF, the hepatocyte volume fraction was less than 12 percent in all but one of the 17 patients who died of progressive hepatic failure without evidence of cerebral edema, bleeding, or infection. In contrast, the fraction was greater than 28 percent in all patients with FHF who died of an infectious complication.[276] In practice, since most patients with FHF have contraindications to percutaneous needle biopsy of the liver, this method has limited application.

Study of prognostic factors predictive of the imminent need for liver transplantation has also been applied to adults and children with chronic liver disease. Previously published guidelines by hepatologists with vast experience caring for adults with chronic liver disease include (1) rapidly deepening jaundice and a total bilirubin of 10 to 15 mg per deciliter or more, (2) a prothrombin time that is uncorrectable with vitamin K and greater than the control by more than 5 seconds, (3) a serum albumin of 2.5 g per deciliter or less, (4) diuretic-resistant ascites, (5) hepatic encephalopathy in spite of a protein-restricted diet and lactulose therapy, and (6) recurrent bleeding from esophageal varices poorly controlled with sclerotherapy.[503]

Recently, an effort was made by Malatack and colleagues to identify by multivariate analysis variables most predictive of risk of death in pediatric patients with chronic liver disease awaiting liver transplantation.[504] The four strongest prognostic indicators were a cholesterol level less than 100 mg per deciliter, a PTT greater than 20 seconds over control, a positive history of ascites, and an indirect bilirubin greater than 6 mg per deciliter. Using a weighted score based on these indicators, predictions could be made which correlated well with actual data obtained from patients dying awaiting transplantation. Table 10 shows the weighted scoring system used, allowing selection of patients with a 75 percent chance of dying within 6 months of the evaluation. Other variables such as a serum sodium less than 132 mEq per liter, an albumin less than 3.0 gm per deciliter, fasting ammonia level greater than 100 μmol per liter, and a positive history of variceal bleeding correlated well but did not improve on the overall predictive value of the top four variables. These investigators suggested that frequent evaluation of these variables would aid in the appropriate selection for transplantation of the sickest children among the available candidates with chronic liver disease even before obvious severe decompensation into hepatic encephalopathy and failure.

REFERENCES

1. Zieve L. The mechanism of hepatic coma. Hepatology 1981; 1:360–365.
2. Conn HO, Lieberthal MM. The hepatic coma syndromes and lactulose. Baltimore: Williams & Wilkins, 1978.
3. Hoyumpa AM, Schenker S. Perspectives in hepatic encephalopathy. J Lab Clin Med 1982; 100:477–487.
4. Fraser CL, Arieff AI. Hepatic encephalopathy. N Engl J Med 1985; 313:864–873
5. Jones EA, Schafer DF, Ferenci P, Pappas SC. The neurobiology of hepatic encephalopathy. Hepatology 1984; 4:1235–1242.
6. Trey C, Davidson C. The management of fulminant hepatic failure. Prog Liver Dis 1970; 3:282–298.
7. Rueff B, Benhamou JP. Acute hepatic necrosis and fulminant hepatic failure. Gut 1973; 14:805–815.
8. Bernuau J, Rueff B, Benhamou JP. Fulminant and subfulminant liver failure: definitions and causes. Semin Liver Dis 1986; 6:97–106.
9. Gimson AES, Ede RJ, Portmann B, Williams R. Late onset hepatic failure. Hepatology 1986; 6:288–294.
10. O'Grady JG, Gimson AES, O'Brien CJ, Pucknell A, Hughes RD, Williams R. Controlled trials of charcoal hemoperfusion and prognostic factors in fulminant hepatic failure. Gastroenterology 1988; 94:1186–1192.
11. Acute Hepatic Failure Study Group. Etiology and prognosis in fulminant hepatitis. (Abstract) Gastroenterology 1979; 77:A33.
12. Papaevangelou G, Tassopoulos N, Roumeliotou-Karayannis A, Richardson C. Etiology of fulminant viral hepatitis in Greece. Hepatology 1984; 4:369–372.

13. Berk PD, Popper H. Fulminant hepatic failure. Am J Gastroenterol 1978; 69:349–400.

14. Trey C, Lipworth L, Davidson CS. Parameters influencing survival in the first 318 patients reported to the fulminant hepatic failure surveillance study. (Abstract) Gastroenterology 1970; 58:306A.

15. Govindarajan S, Chin KP, Redeker AG, Peters RL. Fulminant B viral hepatitis: role of delta agent. Gastroenterology 1984; 86:1417–1420.

16. Psacharopoulos HT, Mowat AP, Davies M, Portmann B, Silk DBA, Williams R. Fulminant hepatic failure in childhood: an analysis of 31 cases. Arch Dis Child 1980; 55:252–258.

17. Zacarias J, Brinck P, Cordero J, Velasco M. Etiologies of fulminant hepatitis in pediatric patients in Santiago, Chile. Pediatr Infect Dis J 1987; 6:686–687.

18. Lloyd-Still JD. Mortality from liver disease in children: implications for hepatic transplantation programs. Am J Dis Chid 1985; 139:381–384.

19. Center for Infectious Disease, CDC. Reye syndrome. United States, 1985. MMWR CDC Surveill Summ 1986; 35:66–68.

20. Zitelli BJ, Malatack JJ, Gartner JC, Urback AH, Williams L, Miller JW, Kirkpatrick B. Evaluation of the pediatric patient for liver transplantation. Pediatrics 1986; 78:559–565.

21. Starzl TE, Esquival C, Gordon R, Todo S. Pediatric liver transplantation. Transplant Proc 1987; 19:3230–3235.

22. Stock PG, Ascher NL, Najarian JS. Pediatric liver transplantation using combination immunosuppressive therapy. Transplant Proc 1987; 19:3303–3308.

23. Andrews W, Fyock B, Gray S, Coln D, Hendricke W, Siegel J, Belknap B, Hogge A, Benser M, Kennard B, Stewart S, Albertson N. Pediatric liver transplantation: the Dallas experience. Transplant Proc 1987; 19:3267–3276.

24. Pett S, Pelham A, Tizard J, Barnes N, Mieli-Vergani G, Mowat AP, Williams R, Rolles K, Calne R. Pediatric liver transplantation: Cambridge/King's series, December 1983 to August 1986. Transplant Proc 1987; 19:3256–3260.

25. Hiatt JR, Ament ME, Berquist WJ, Brems JF, Brill JE, Colonna JO, El Khoury G, Quinones WJ, Ramming KP, Vargas JH, Busuttil RW. Pediatric liver transplantation at UCLA. Transplant Proc 1987; 19:3282–3288.

26. Vacanti JP, Lillehei CW, Jenkins RL, Donohoe PK, Cosimi AB, Kleinman R, Grand RJ, Cho SI. Liver transplantation in children: the Boston Center experience in the first 30 months. Transplant Proc 1987; 29:3261–3266.

27. Van Thiel DH. Liver transplantation. Pediatr Ann 1985; 14:474–480.

28. Chang MH, Lee CY, Chenn DS, Husu HC, Lai MY. Fulminant hepatitis in children in Taiwan: the important role of hepatitis B virus. J Pediatr 1987; 111:34–38.

29. Delaplane D, Yogeu R, Crussi F, Shulman ST. Fatal hepatitis B in early infancy: the importance of identifying HBsAg-positive pregnant women and providing immunoprophylaxis to their newborns. Pediatrics 1983; 72:176–180.

30. Sinatra FR, Shah P, Weissman JY, Thomas DW, Merritt RJ, Tong MJ. Perinatal transmitted acute icteric hepatitis B in infants born to hepatitis B surface antigen-positive and antihepatitis B e-positive carrier mothers. Pediatrics 1982; 70:557–559.

31. Stevens CE, Beasley RP, Tsui J, Lee WC. Vertical transmission of hepatitis B antigen in Taiwan. N Engl J Med 1975; 292:771–774.

32. Okada K, Yamada T, Miyakawa Y, Mayumi M. Hepatitis B surface antigen in the serum of infants after delivery from asymptomatic carrier mothers. J Pediatr 1975; 87:360–363.

33. Okada K, Kamiyama I, Inomata M, Mitsunobu I, Miyakawa Y, Mayumi M. e antigen in the serum of asymptomatic carrier mothers as indicators of positive and negative trnsmission of hepatitis B virus to their infants. N Engl J Med 1975; 294:746–749.

34. Dupuy JM, Kostewicz E, Alagille D. Hepatitis B in children: analysis of 80 cases of acute and chronic hepatitis B. J Pediatr 1978; 92:17–20.

35. Schweitzer IL, Wing A, McPeak C, Spears RL. Hepatitis and hepatitis-associated antigen in 56 mother-infant pairs. JAMA 1972; 220:1902–1905.

36. Lee CY, Au C, Shu CT. Hepatitis B virus as the most important cause of acute or fulminant hepatitis in Taiwan. Proceedings of the 18th International Congress of Pediatrics, Honolulu, July 7–12, 1986 (Abstract 600).

37. Beasley RP, Trepo C, Stevens CE, Szmuness W. The e antigen and vertical transmission of hepatitis B surface antigen. Am J Epidemiol 1977; 105:94–98.

38. Shiraki K, Yoshihara N, Sakurai M, Eto T, Kawana T. Acute hepatitis B in infants born to carrier mothers with the antibody to hepatitis B e antigen. J Pediatr 1980; 97:768–770.

39. Bortolotti F, Cadrobbi P, Bertaggia A, Rude L, Alberti A, Realdi G. A 7 year study of acute hepatitis B. Arch Dis Child 1983; 58:993–996.

40. Okuda K. Is fulminant B hepatitis more common among infants born to e antigen-negative carrier mothers? Hepatology 1987; 5:974–976.

41. Galbraith RM, Eddleston ALWF, Williams R, Zuckerman AJ, Bagshawe KD. Fulminant hepatic failure in leukemia and choriocarcinoma related to withdrawal of cytotoxic drug therapy. Lancet 1975; 2:528–530.

42. Brechot C, Bernuau J, Theirs V, Dubois F, Goudeau A, Rueff B, Tiollais P, Benhamou JP. Multiplication of hepatitis B virus in fulminant hepatitis B. Br Med J 1984; 288:270–271.

43. Caredda F, Rossi E, d'Arminio Monforte A, Zampini L, Tiziana R, Meroni B, Moroni M. Hepatitis B virus associated co-infection and super-infection with delta agent: indistinguishable disease with different outcome. J Infect Dis 1985; 151:925–928.

44. DeCock KM, Govindarajan S, Chin KP, Redeker AG. Delta hepatitis in the Los Angeles area: a report of 126 cases. Ann Intern Med 1986; 105:108–114.

45. Buti M, Esteban R, Jardi R, Estaban JI, Guardia J. Clinical and serological outcome of acute delta infection. Hepatology 1987; 5:59–64.

46. Rizzetto M, Verme G, Gerin JL, Purcell RH. Hepatitis delta virus disease. Prog Liver Dis 1986; 8:417–431.

47. Lee SD, Wang JY, Wu JC, Tsai YT, Lo RJ, Lai KH, Tsay SH, Govindarajan S. Hepatitis D virus (delta agent) superinfection in an endemic area of hepatitis B infection: immunopathologic and serologic findings. Scand J Infect Dis 1987; 29:173–177.

48. Smedile A, Farci P, Verme G, Caredda F, Cargnel A, Caporaso N, Dentico P, Trepo C, Opolon P, Gimson A, Vergani D, Williams R, Rizzetto M. Influence of delta infection on severity of hepatitis B. Lancet 1982; 2:945–947.

49. Govindarajan S, Chin KP, Redeker AG, Peters RL. Fulminant B viral hepatitis: role of delta agent. Gastroenterology 1984; 86:1417–1420.

50. Bensabeth G, Hadler SC, Pereira Soares MC, Fields H, Dias LB, Popper H, Maynard JE. Hepatitis delta virus infection and Labrea hepatitis. Prevalence and role in fulminant hepatitis in the Amazon basin. JAMA 1987; 258:478–483.

51. Saracco G, Macagno S, Rosina F, Rizzetto M. Serologic markers with fulminant hepatitis in HBsAg-positive persons; a world wide epidemiological and clinical survey. Ann Intern Med 1988; 108:380–383.

52. Rizzetto M, Canese MG, Gerin JL, London WT, Sly DL, Purcell RH. Transmission of the hepatitis B virus-associated delta antigen to chimpanzees. J Infect Dis 1980; 141:590–602.

53. Purcell RH, Rizzetto M, Gerin JL. Hepatitis delta virus infection of the liver. Semin Liver Dis 1984; 4:340–346.

54. Colombo M, Cambieri R, Rumi MG, Rhonchi G, Del Ninno E, De Franchis R. Long-term delta superinfection in hepatitis surface antigen carriers and its relationship to the course of chronic hepatitis. Gastroenterology 1983; 85:235–239.

55. Govindarajan S, DeCock KM, Redeker AG. Natural course of delta superinfection in chronic hepatitis B virus infected patients—histopathologic study with multiple liver biopsies. Hepatology 1986; 6:640–644.

56. Bonino F, Negro F, Baldi M. The natural history of chronic delta hepatitis. Prog Clin Biol Res 1987; 234:145–152.

57. Maggiore G, Hadchouel M, Sessa F, Vinci M, Craxi A, Marzani MD, DeGiacomo C, Alagille D. A retrospective study of the rule of delta agent infection in children with HBsAg-positive chronic hepatitis. Hepatology 1985; 5:7–9.

58. Hsu HY, Chang MH, Chen DS, Lee CY. Hepatitis D virus infection in children with acute or chronic hepatitis B virus infection in Taiwan. J Pediatr 1988; 112:888–892.

59. Buitrago B, Hadler SC, Popper H, Thung SN, Gerber MA, Purcell RH, Maynard JE. Epidemiologic aspects of Santa Marta hepatitis over a 40 year period. Hepatology 1986; 6:1292–1296.

60. Mathiesen LR, Skinej P, Nielsen JO, Purcell RH, Wong D, Ranek L. Hepatitis A, B, and non-A non-B in fulminant hepatitis. Gut 1980; 21:72–77.

61. Gimson AES, White YS, Eddleston ALWF, Williams R. Clinical and prognostic differences in fulminant hepatitis type A, B, and non-A non-B. Gut 1983; 24:1194–1198.

62. Bernau J, Margulies A, Dubois F. Asian-African non-A non-B fulminant viral hepatitis in France. (Abstract) J Hepatol (suppl) 1985; S21.

63. Dienstag JL. Non-A non-B hepatitis I. Recognition, epidemiology, and clinical features. Gastroenterology 1983; 85:439–462.

64. Feinman SV, Berris B, Bojarski S. Post-transfusion hepatitis in Toronto, Canada. Gastroenterology 1988; 95:464–469.

65. McGrath KM, Lilleyman JS, Triger DR, Underwood JCE. Liver disease complicating severe hemophilia in childhood. Arch Dis Child 1980; 55:537–540.

66. Koretz RL, Stone O, Mousa M, Gitnick GL. Non-A non-B post-transfusion hepatitis—a decade later. Gastroenterology 1985; 88:1251–1254.

67. Realdi G, Alberti A, Rugge M, Rigoli AM, Tremolada F, Schivazappa L, Ruol A. Long-term follow-up of acute and chronic non-A non-B post-transfusion hepatitis: evidence of progression to liver cirrhosis. Gut 1982; 23:270–275.

68. Seeff LB, Dienstag JL. Transfusion-associated non-A non-B hepatitis. Gastroenterology 1988; 95:530–533.

69. Aledort LM, Levine PH, Hilgartner M, Blatt P, Spero JA, Goldberg JD, Bianchi L, Desmet V, Scheuer P, Popper H, Berk PD. A study of liver biopsies and liver disease among hemophiliacs. Blood 1985; 66:367–373.

70. Hay CRM, Preston FE, Triger DR, Underwood JCE. Progressive liver disease in hemophilia: an understated problem? Lancet 1985; i:1495–1498.

71. Stagno S, Whitley RJ. Herpes virus infections of pregnancy: Part I. Cytomegalovirus and Epstein-Barr virus infections; Part II. Herpes simplex virus and varicella-zoster virus infections. N Engl J Med 1985; 313:1270–1274, 1327–1330.

72. Nahmias AJ, Josey WE, Naib ZM. Neonatal herpes simplex infection: role of genital infection in the mother as the source of virus in the newborn. JAMA 1967; 199:164–168.

73. Taylor RJ, Saul SH, Dowling JN, Hakala TR, Peel RL, Monto H. Primary disseminated herpes simplex infection with fulminant hepatitis following renal transplantation. Arch Intern Med 1981; 141:1519–1521.

74. Holdsworth SR, Atkings RC, Scott DF, Hayes K. Systemic herpes simplex infection with fulminant hepatitis post-transplantation. Aust NZ J Med 1976; 6:588–590.

75. Becker W, Naude WT, Kipps A. Virus studies in disseminated herpes simplex infections: association with malnutrition in children. S Afr Med J 1963; 37:74–76.

76. Sutton AL, Smithwick EM, Seligman SJ, Kim DS. Fetal disseminated herpes virus hominis type 2 infection in an adult with associated thymic dysplasia. Am J Med 1974; 56:545–553.

77. Orenstein JM, Castodot MJ, Wilens SL. Fatal herpes hepatitis associated with pemphigus vulgaris and steroids in an adult. Human Pathol 1974; 5:489–493.

78. Moedy JCA, Lerman SJ, White RJ. Fatal disseminated herpes simplex virus infection in a healthy child. Am J Dis Child 1981; 135:45–47.

79. Raga J, Chrystal V. Coovadia HM. Usefulness of clinical features and liver biopsy in diagnosis of disseminated herpes simplex infection. Arch Dis Child 1984; 59:820–824.

80. Harries JT, Ferguson AW. Fatal infectious mononucleosis with liver failure in two sisters. Arch Dis Child 1968; 43:480–485.

81. Chang MY, Campbell WG. Fatal infectious mononucleosis: association with liver necrosis and herpes-like virus particles. Arch Pathol 1975; 99:185–191.

82. Deutsch J, Wolf H, Becker H, Fuchs B, Goriup U, Grubbauer HM, Muntean W, Popow-Kraupp Th, Stunzer D. Demonstration of Epstein-Barr virus DNA in a previously healthy boy with fulminant hepatic failure. Eur J Pediatr 1986; 145:94–98.

83. Purtilo DT, Paquin L, Deflorio D, Virzi F, Sakhuja R. Immunodiagnosis and immunopathogenesis of the X-linked recessive lymphoproliferative syndrome. Semin Hematol 1979; 16:309–343.

84. Hart GH, Thompson WR, Schneider J, Davis NJ. Fulminant hepatic failure and fatal encephalopathy associated with Epstein-Barr virus infection. Med J Aust 1984; 141:112–113.

85. Modlin JF. Fatal echovirus eleven disease in premature neonates. Pediatrics 1980; 66:775–780.

86. Philip AGS, Larson EJ. Overwhelming neonatal infection with ECHO 19 virus. J Pediatr 1973; 82:391.

87. Hughes JR, Wilfert CM, Moore MT, Benirschke K, deHoyos-Guevara E. Echovirus 14 infection associated with fatal neonatal hepatic necrosis. Am J Dis Child 1972; 123:61–67.

88. Krous HF, Dietzman D, Ray CG. Fatal infections with echovirus types 6 and 11 in early infancy. Am J Dis Child 1973; 126:842–846.

89. Kaplowitz N, Aw TY, Simon FR, Stolz A. Drug-induced hepatotoxicity. Ann Intern Med 1986; 104:826–839.

90. Black M. Acetaminophen hepatotoxicity. Gastroenterology 1980; 78:382–392.

91. Davis M. Protective agents for acetaminophen overdose. Semin Liver Dis 1986; 6:138–147.

92. Mitchell JR, Jollow DJ, Potter WZ, Gillette JR, Brodie BB. Acetaminophen-induced hepatic necrosis: IC protective role of glutathione. J Pharmacol Exp Ther 1973; 187:211–213.

93. Porubek DJ, Rundgren M, Harvison PJ, Nelson SD, Moldeus P. Investigation of mechanisms of acetaminophen toxicity in isolated rat hepatocytes with the acetaminophen analogues 3,5-dimethyl-acetaminophen and 2,6 dimethylacetaminophen. Mol Pharmacol 1987; 31:647–653.

94. Smith MT, Thor H, Orrenius S. The role of lipid peroxidation in the toxicity of foreign compounds to liver cells. Biochem Pharmacol 1983; 32:763–764.

95. Lee TJ, Carney CN, Lapis JL, Higgin T, Fallon HJ. Diphenylhydantoin-induced hepatic necrosis. Gastroenterology 1976; 70:422–424.

96. Ransohoff DF, Jacobs G. Terminal hepatic failure following a small dose of sulfamethoxazole-trimethoprim. Gastroenterology 1981; 80:816–819.

97. Sotolongo RP, Neefe LI, Rudzki C, Ishak KG. Hypersensitivity reaction to sulfasalazine with severe hepatotoxicity. Gastroenterology 1978; 75:95–99.

98. Kenna JG, Neuberger J, Mieli-Vergani G, Mowat AP, Williams R. Halothane hepatitis in children. Br Med J 1987; 294:1209–1211.

99. Satoh H, Fukuda Y, Anderson DK, Ferrans VJ, Gillette JR, Pohl LR. Immunologic studies on the mechanism of halothane-induced hepatotoxicity: immunohistochemical evidence of trifluoroacetylated hepatocytes. J Pharmacol Exp Ther 1985; 233:857–862.

100. Kenna JG, Satoh H, Christ DD, Pohl LR. Metabolic basis for a drug hypersensitivity: antibodies in sera from patients with halothane hepatitis recognize liver neoantigens that contain the trifluoroacetyl group derived from halothane. J Pharmacol Exp Ther 1988; 245:1103–1109.

101. Kupfer A, Preisig R. Inherited defects of hepatic drug metabolism. Semin Liver Dis 1983; 3:341–354.

102. Meyer UT, Meyer UA. Genetic polymorphism of human cytochrome P450 s-mephenytoin-4-hydroxylase studies with human autoantibodies suggest a functionally altered P450 isozyme as cause of the genetic deficiency. Biochemistry 1987; 26:8466–8474.

103. Evans DAP. Survey of the human acetylator polymorphism in spontaneous disorders. J Med Genet 1984; 21:243–253.

104. Pascoe GA, Fariss MW, Olafsdottir K, Reed DJ. A role of vitamin E in protection against cell injury: maintenance of intracellular glutathione precursors and biosynthesis. Eur J Biochem 1987; 166:241–247.

105. Ketterer B. Detoxification reactions of glutathione and glutathione transferases. Xenobiotica 1986; 16:957–973.

106. Ishak KG. The liver. In: Riddel RH, ed. Pathology of drug induced and toxic diseases. New York: Churchill Livingstone, 1980; 457.

107. Zimmerman HJ, Ishak KG. Hepatic injury due to drugs and toxins. In: MacSween RNM, Antony PP, Scheuer PJ, eds. Pathology of the liver. 2nd ed. London: Churchill Livingstone, 1987; 503.

108. Bianchi L, DeGroute J, Desmet VJ, Scheuer PJ. Guidelines for diagnosis of therapeutic drug-induced liver injury in liver biopsies: review by an international group. Lancet 1974; i:854–857.

109. Mitchell JR, Jollow DJ, Potter WZ, Gillette JR, Brodie BB. Acetaminophen induced hepatonecrosis. I. Role of drug metabolism. J Pharmacol Exp Ther 1973; 187:185–194.

110. Benjamin SB, Goodman ZD, Ishak KG, Zimmerman HJ, Irey NS. The morphologic spectrum of halothane-induced hepatic injury: analysis of 77 cases. Hepatology 1985; 6:1163–1171.

111. Witzleben CL, Chaffey N. Acute ferrous sulfate poisoning. Arch Pathol 1966; 82:454.

112. Zimmerman HJ, Ishak KG. Valproate-induced hepatic injury: analysis of 23 fatal cases. Hepatology 1982; 2:591–597.

113. Powell-Jackson PR, Tredger JM, Williams R. Hepatotoxicity to sodium valproate: a review. Gut 1984; 25:673–681.

114. Suchy FJ, Balistreri WF, Buchino JJ, Sondheimer JM, Bates SR, Kearns GL, Stull JD, Bove KE. Acute hepatic failure associated with the use of sodium valproate. N Engl J Med 1979; 300:962–966.

115. Treem WR, Boyle JT. Severe cardiomyopathy simulating hepatitis in adolescence. Clin Pediatr 1986; 25:260–265.

116. Cohen JA, Kaplan MM. Left-sided heart failure presenting as hepatitis. Gastroenterology 1978; 74:583–587.

117. Kisloff B, Schaffer G. Fulminant hepatic failure secondary to congestive heart failure. Dig Dis Sci 1976; 21:895–900.

118. Nouel O, Henrion J, Bernuau J, Dogott C, Rueff B, Benhamou JP. Fulminant hepatic failure due to transient circulatory failure in patients with chronic heart disease. Dig Dis Sci 1980; 25:49–52.

119. Bagens HS, Henreksen J, Matzen P, Poulsen H. The shock liver. Acta Med Scand 1978; 204:417–421.

120. Moussavian SN, Dincsoy HP, Goodman S, Helm RA, Bozian RC. Severe hyperbilirubinemia and coma in chronic congestive heart failure. Dig Dis Sci 1982; 27:175–180.

121. Mace S, Borkat G, Leibman J. Hepatic dysfunction and cardiovascular abnormalities, occurrence in infants, children, and young adults. Am J Dis Child 1985; 139:60–65.

122. Myers JD, Hickman JB. Estimation of hepatic blood flow and splanchnic oxygen consumption in heart failure. J Clin Invest 1948; 27:620–627.

123. Dunn GD, Hayes P, Breen KJ, Schenker S. The liver in congestive heart failure. Am J Med Sci 1973; 265:174–189.

124. Ohi R, Hanamatsu M, Mochizuki I, Chiba T, Kasai M. Progress in the treatment of biliary atresia. World J Surg 1985; 9:285–293.

125. Howard ER, Mowat AP. Hepatobiliary disorders in infancy: hepatitis; extrahepatic biliary atresia; intrahepatic biliary hypoplasia. In: Thomas HC, McSween RN, eds. Recent advances in hepatology. London: Churchill Livingstone, 1983; 153.

126. Kasai M. Treatment of biliary atresia with special reference to hepatic portoenterostomy and its modification. Prog Pediatr Surg 1974; 6:6–24.

127. Smith EI, Carson JA, Tunnell WP, Hitch DC, Pysher TJ. Improved results with hepatic portoenterostomy: a reassessment of its value in the treatment of biliary atresia. Ann Surg 1982; 195:746–755.

128. Chandra RS, Altman RP. Ductal remnants in extrahepatic biliary atresia: a histological study with clinical correlation. J Pediatr 1978; 93:196–200.

129. Lawrence D, Howard ER, Tzannatos C, Mowat AP. Hepatic portoenterostomy for biliary atresia: a comparative study of histology and prognosis after surgery. Arch Dis Child 1981; 56:460–463.

130. Alagille D. Liver transplantation in children—indications in cholestatic states. Transplant Proc 1987; 19:3242–3248.

131. Gartner JG, Jaffe R, Malatack JJ, Zitelli BJ, Urbach AH. Hepatic infarction and acute liver failure in children with extrahepatic biliary atresia and cirrhosis. J Pediatr Surg 1987; 22:360–362.

132. Psacharopoulos HT, Mowat AP, Cook PJL, Carlile PA, Portmann B, Rodeck CH. Outcome of liver disease associated with alpha-1-antitrypsin deficiency (PiZ). Arch Dis Child 1983; 58:882–887.

133. Odievre M, Martin JP, Hadchouel M, Alagille D. Alpha-1-antitrypsin deficiency and liver disease in children: phenotypes, manifestations, and prognosis. Pediatrics 1976; 57:226–231.

134. Alagille D. Alpha-1-antitrypsin deficiency. Hepatology 1984; 4:115–145.

135. Lutz E, Cox DW. Alpha-1-antitrypsin deficiency: the spectrum of pathology and pathophysiology. In: Rosenberg HS, Bolande RP, eds. Perspectives in pediatric pathology. Vol 5. New York: Masson, 1979; 1.

136. Ghishan FK, Greene HL. Liver disease in children with P₁ZZ alpha-1-antitrypsin deficiency. Hepatology 1988; 8:307–310.

137. Sveger T. Prospective study of children with alpha-1-antitrypsin deficiency: eight year follow-up. J Pediatr 1984; 104:91–94.

138. McCullough AJ, Fleming CR, Thistle JL, Baldus WP, Ludwig J, McCall JT, Dickson ER. Diagnosis of Wilson's disease presenting as fulminant hepatic failure. Gastroenterology 1983; 84:161–167.

139. Kraut JR, Yogev R. Fatal fulminant hepatitis with hemolysis in Wilson's disease. Clin Pediatr 1984; 23:637–640.

140. Doering EJ, Savage RA, Dittmer TE. Hemolysis, coagulation defects, and fulminant hepatic failure as a presentation of Wilson's disease. Am J Dis Child 1979; 133:440–441.

141. Sokol RJ, Francis PD, Gold SH, Ford DM, Lum GM, Ambruso DR. Orthotopic liver transplantation for acute fulminant Wilson's disease. J Pediatr 1985; 107:549–552.

142. Sternlieb I. Wilson's disease: indications for liver transplant. Hepatology 1984; 4:155–175.

143. Mowat AP. Liver disorders in children: the indications for liver replacement in parenchymal and metabolic disease. Transplant Proc 1987; 19:3236–3241.

144. Keating JJ, Johnson RD, Johnson PJ, Williams R. Clinical course of cirrhosis in young adults and therapeutic potential of liver transplantation. Gut 1985; 26:1359–1363.

145. Scott J, Gollan JL, Samourian S, Sherlock S. Wilson's disease presenting as chronic active hepatitis. Gastroenterology 1978; 74:645–651.

146. Arasu TS, Wyllie R, Hatch TF, Fitzgerald JF. Management of chronic aggressive hepatitis in children and adolescents. J Pediatr 1979; 95:514–522.

147. Maggiore G, Bernard O, Hadchouel M, Hadchouel P, Odievre M, Alagille D. Treatment of chronic active hepatitis in childhood. J Pediatr 1984; 104:839–844.

148. Vegnente A, Larcher VF, Mowat AP, Portmann B, Williams R. Duration of chronic active hepatitis and development of cirrhosis. Arch Dis Child 1984; 59:330–335.

149. Maggiore G, Bernard O, Homberg JC, Hadchouel M, Alvarez F, Hadchouel P, Odievre M, Alagille D. Liver disease associated with anti-liver-kidney microsome antibody in children. J Pediatr 1986; 108:399–404.

150. Holmberg JC, Abuaf N, Bernard O, Islam S, Alvarez F, Khalil SH, Poupon R, Darnis F, Levy VG, Grippon P, Opolon P, Bernuau J, Benhamou JP, Alagille D. Chronic active hepatitis associated with anti-liver/kidney microsome antibody type I: a second type of "autoimmune" hepatitis. Hepatology 1987; 7:1333–1339.

151. Conn HO. Asterixis in non-hepatic disorders. Am J Med 1960; 29:647–661.

152. Challenger F, Walshe JM. Methyl mercaptan in relation to foetor hepaticus. Biochem J 1955; 59:372.

153. McClain CJ, Zieve L, Doizaki WM, Gilberstadt S, Onstad GR. Blood methanethiol in alcoholic liver disease with and without hepatic encephalopathy. Gut 1980; 21:318–323.

154. Chen S, Zieve L, Mahadevan V. Mercaptans and dimethyl sulfide in the breath of patients with cirrhosis of the liver. J Lab Clin Med 1970; 75:628–635.

155. Hassall E, Benson L, Hart M, Krieger DE. Hepatic encephalopathy after portacaval shunt in a non-cirrhotic child. J Pediatr 1984; 105:439–441.

156. Livingstone AS, Potvin M, Goresky CA, Finlayson MD, Hinchey EJ. Changes in the blood-brain barrier in hepatic coma after hepatectomy in the rat. Gastroenterology 1977; 73:697–704.

157. Zaki AEO, Ede RJ, Davis M, Williams R. Experimental studies of blood-brain barrier permeability in acute hepatic failure. Hepatology 1984; 4:359–363.

158. Zaki AEO, Wardle EN, Canalese J, Ede RJ, Williams R. Potential toxins of acute liver failure and their effects on blood-brain barrier permeability. Experientia 1983; 39:988–991.

159. Potvin M, Finlayson MH, Morrison HF, Hinchey FJ, Lough JO, Goresky CA. Cerebral abnormalities in hepatectomized rats with acute hepatic coma. Lab Invest 1984; 50:560–564.

160. Treem WR, Witzleben CA, Piccoli DA, Stanley CA, Hale DE, Coates PM, Watkins JB. Medium-chain and long-chain acyl-CoA dehydrogenase deficiency: clinical, pathologic, and ultrastructural differentiation from Reye's syndrome. Hepatology 1986; 6:1270–1278.

161. Felig P, Brown WV, Levine RA, Klatskin G. Glucose homeostasis in viral hepatitis. N Engl J Med 1970; 283:1436–1440.

162. Maiolo AT, Bianchi-Porro G, Galle C. Brain energy metabolism in hepatic coma. Exp Biol Med 1971; 4:52–70.

163. Zieve L, Nicoloff D, Doizaki W. Effect of total hepatectomy on selected cerebral substrates and enzymes of the glycolytic pathway and Krebs cycle. Surgery 1975; 78:414–423.

164. Kravath RE, Scarpelli EM, Bernstein J. Hepatogenic cyanosis: arteriovenous shunts in chronic active hepatitis. J Pediatr 1971; 78:238–245.

165. Hutchison DCS, Sapru RP, Sumerling MD, Donaldson GWK, Richmond J. Cirrhosis, cyanosis, and polycythemia: multiple pulmonary arteriovenous anastomoses. Am J Med 1968; 45:139–151.

166. Berthelot P, Walker JG, Sherlock S, Reid L. Arterial changes in the lungs in cirrhosis of the liver-lung spider nevi. N Engl J Med 1966; 274:291–298.

167. Daoud FS, Reeves JT, Schaefer JW. Failure of hypoxic pulmonary vasoconstriction in patients with liver cirrhosis. J Clin Invest 1972; 51:1076–1080.

168. Williams A, Trewby P, Williams R, Reid L. Structural alterations to

the pulmonary circulation in fulminant hepatic failure. Thorax 1979; 34:447–453.

169. Farber MO, Carlone S, Serra P, Capocaccia L, Rossi-Fanelli F, Antonini E, Manfredi F. The oxygen affinity of hemoglobin in hepatic encephalopathy. J Lab Clin Med 1981; 98:135–144.

170. Warren KS, Schenker S. Hypoxia and ammonia toxicity. Am J Physiol 1960; 199:1105–1108.

171. Heubi JE, Partin JC, Partin JS, Schubert W. Reye's syndrome: current concepts. Hepatology 1987; 7:155–164.

172. Snodgrass PJ, Delong GR. Urea-cycle enzyme deficiencies and an increased nitrogen load producing hyperammonemia in Reye's syndrome. N Engl J Med 1976; 294:855–860.

173. Flannery DB, Hsia YE, Wolf B. Current status of hyperammonemia syndromes. Hepatology 1982; 2:495–506.

174. Treem WR, Stanley CA, Finegold DN, Hale DE, Coates PM. Primary carnitine deficiency due to a failure of carnitine transport in kidney, muscle, and fibroblasts. N Engl J Med 1988; 319:1331–1336.

175. Ohtani Y, Endo F, Matsuda I. Carnitine deficiency and hyperammonemia associated with valproic acid therapy. J Pediatr 1982; 101:782–785.

176. Weber FL, Veach GI. The importance of the small intestine in gut ammonium production in the fasting dog. Gastroenterology 1979; 77:235–240.

177. Nance FC, Kaufman HJ, Kline DG. Role of urea in the hyperammonemia of germ-free Eck fistula dogs. Gastroenterology 1974; 66:108–112.

178. Onstad GR, Zieve L. What determines blood ammonia. Gastroenterology 1979; 77:803–805.

179. Dawson AM. Regulation of blood ammonia. Gut 1978; 19:504–509.

180. Goodman MW, Zieve L, Konstantinides FN, Cerra FB. Mechanism of arginine protection against ammonia intoxication in the rat. Am J Physiol 1984; 247:G290–G295.

181. Sherwin R, Joshi P, Hendler R, Felig P, Conn HO. Hyperglucagonemia in Laennec's cirrhosis. The role of portal-systemic shunting. N Engl J Med 1974; 290:239–242.

182. Bessman SP, Bradley JE. Uptake of ammonia by muscle. Its implications in ammoniagenic coma. N Engl J Med 1955; 253:1143–1147.

183. Lockwood AH, McDonald JM, Reiman RE, Gelbard AS, Laughlin JS, Duffy TE, Plum F. The dynamics of ammonia metabolism in man. Effects of liver disease and hyperammonemia. J Clin Invest 1979; 63:449–460.

184. Plum F, Hindfelt B. The neurological complications of liver disease. In: Vinken PH, Bruyn GW, eds. Handbook of clinical neurology. Vol 27. Metabolic and deficiency diseases of the nervous system, part I. New York: American Elsevier, 1976: 349.

185. Hourani BT, Hamlin EM, Reynolds TB. Cerebrospinal fluid glutamine as a measure of hepatic encephalopathy. Arch Intern Med 1971; 127:1033–1036.

186. Gilon E, Szeinberg A, Tauman G, Bodongi E. Glutamine estimation in cerebrospinal fluid in cases of liver cirrhosis and hepatic coma. J Lab Clin Med 1959; 53:714–719.

187. Uribe M, Marquez MA, Ramos GG, Ramos-Uribe MH, Vargas F, Villalobos A, Ramos C. Treatment of chronic portal systemic encephalopathy with vegetable and animal protein diets: a controlled crossover study. Dig Dis Sci 1982; 27:1109–1116.

188. DeBruijn KM, Blendis LM, Zilm DH, Carlen PL, Anderson GH. Effect of dietary protein manipulations in subclinical portal systemic encephalopathy. Gut 1983; 24:53–60.

189. Weber FL, Minco D, Fresard K, Banwell JG. Effects of vegetable diets on nitrogen metabolism in cirrhotic subjects. Gastroenterology 1985; 89:538–544.

190. Raabe W, Onstad G. Portacaval shunting changes neuronal tolerance to ammonia. (Abstract) Ann Neurol 1980; 8:106.

191. Hindfelt B, Plum F, Duffy TE. Effect of acute ammonia intoxication on cerebral metabolism in rats with portacaval shunts. J Clin Invest 1977; 59:386–396.

192. Gjedde A, Lockwood AH, Duffy TE, Plum F. Cerebral blood flow and metabolism in chronically hyperammonemic rats. Effect of an acute ammonia challenge. Ann Neurol 1978; 3:325–330.

193. Pappas SC, Ferenci P, Schafer DF, Jones EA. Visual evoked potentials in a rabbit model of hepatic encephalopathy. Gastroenterology 1984; 86:546–561.

194. Torda C. Ammonium ion content and electrical activity of the brain during the pre-convulsive and convulsive phases induced by various convulsants. J Pharmacol Exp Ther 1953; 107:193–203.

195. Kuamme E. Ammonia metabolism in the CNS. Prog Neurobiol 1983; 20:109–132.

196. Cole M, Rutherford RB, Smith FO. Experimental ammonia encephalopathy in the primate. Arch Neurol 1972; 26:130–136.

197. Cohn R, Castell DO. The effect of acute hyperammonemia on the encephalogram. J Lab Clin Med 1966; 68:195–205.

198. Schafer DF, Jones EA. Hepatic encephalopathy and the gamma-aminobutyric-acid neurotransmitter system. Lancet 1982; i:18–20.

199. Ferenci P, Pappas SC, Munson PJ, Plum F, Duffy TE. Changes in glutamate receptors on synaptic membranes associated with hepatic encephalopathy or hyperammonemia in the rabbit. Hepatology 1984; 4:25–29.

200. Zieve L, Doizaki WM, Zieve FJ. Synergism between mercaptans and ammonia or fatty acids in the pathogenesis of hepatic coma. J Lab Clin Med 1974; 83:16–28.

201. Zieve L. Coma production with NH_4^+: synergistic factors. (Abstract) Gastroenterology 1980; 78:1327A.

202. Teychenne PF, Walters I, Claveria LE, Calne DB, Price J, MacGillivray BB, Gompertz D. The encephalopathic action of five-carbon atom fatty acids in the rabbit. Clin Sci Molec Med 1976; 50:463–472.

203. Windus-Podehl G, Lyftogt C, Zieve L, Brunner G. Encephalopathic effect of phenol in rats. J Lab Clin Med 1983; 101:586–592.

204. Derr RF, Zieve L. Effect of fatty acids on the disposition of ammonia. J Pharmacol Exp Ther 1976; 197:675–680.

205. Doizaki WM, Zieve L. An improved method for measuring blood mercaptans. J Lab Clin Med 1977; 90:849–855.

206. Blom HJ, Yap SH, Tangerman A. The role of methanethiol in the pathogenesis of hepatic encephalopathy. (Abstract) Gastroenterology 1988; 94:A526.

207. Foster D, Ahrnad K, Zieve L. Action of methanethiol on $Na^+K^+ATPase$: implications for hepatic coma. Ann NY Acad Sci 1974; 242:573–576.

208. Ogburn PL, Sharp H, Lloyd-Still JD, Johnson SB, Holman RT. Abnormal polyunsaturated fatty acid pattern of serum lipids in Reye's syndrome. Proc Natl Acad Sci USA 1982; 79:908–911.

209. Mamunes P, DeVries GH, Miller CP, David RB. Fatty acid quantitation in Reye's syndrome. In: Pollack JD, ed. Reye's syndrome. New York: Grune & Stratton, 1975: 245.

210. McArthur B, Sarnaik AP, Mitchell RA. Short-chain fatty acids and encephalopathy of Reye's syndrome. Neurology 1984; 34:831–834.

211. Tonsgard JH. Serum dicarboxylic acids in patients with Reye's syndrome. J Pediatr 1986; 109:440–445.

212. Trauner DA, Adams H. Intracranial pressure elevations during octanoate infusion in rabbits: an experimental model of Reye's syndrome. Pediatr Res 1981; 15:1098–1099.

213. Dahl DR. Short-chain fatty acid inhibition of rat brain Na-K adenosine triphosphate. J Neurochem 1968; 15:815–820.

214. Curzon G, Kantamaneni BD, Winch J, Rojas-Bueno A, Murray-Lyon M, Williams R. Plasma and brain tryptophan changes in experimental acute hepatic failure. J Neurochem 1973; 21:137–145.

215. Zieve L, Brunner G. Encephalopathy due to mercaptans and phenols. In: McCandless DW, ed. Cerebral energy metabolism and metabolic encephalopathy. New York: Plenum Press, 1985: 179.

216. Zieve L, Lyftogt C, Draves K. Toxicity of a fatty acid and ammonia: interactions with hypoglycemia and Kreb's cycle inhibition. J Lab Clin Med 1983; 101:930–939.

217. Zieve L, Doizaki W, Lyftogt C. Brain methanethiol and ammonia concentrations in experimental hepatic coma and coma induced by injections of various combinations of these substances. J Lab Clin Med 1984; 104:655–664.

218. Zeneroli ML, Ventura E, Baraldi M. Visual evoked potentials in encephalopathy induced by galactosamine, ammonia, dimethyl disulfide, and octanoic acid. Hepatology 1982; 2:532–538.

219. Fischer JE, Baldessarini RJ. False neurotransmitters and hepatic failure. Lancet 1971; ii:75–80.

220. Fischer JE, Baldessarini RJ. Neurotransmitter metabolism in hepatic encephalopathy. N Engl J Med 1975; 293:1152–1153.

221. James JH, Ziparo V, Jeppsson A, Fischer JE. Hyperammonemia, plasma amino acid imbalance, and blood-brain amino acid transport: a unified theory of portal-systemic encephalopathy. Lancet 1979; ii:772–775.

222. Borg J, Warter JM, Schlienger JL, Imler M, Marescaux C, Mack G. Neurotransmitter modifications in human cerebrospinal fluid and serum during hepatic encephalopathy. J Neurol Sci 1982; 57:343–356.

223. Cangiano C, Rossi Fanelli F, Bozzi A, Calcatterra V, Cascino A, Capocaccia L. Plasma phenylethanolamine in hepatic encephalopathy. Eur J Clin Invest 1978; 8:183–184.

224. Capocaccia L, Cangiono C, Attili AF, Angelico M, Cascino A, Rossi Fanelli F. Octopamine and ammonia plasma levels in hepatic encephalopathy. Clin Chim Acta 1977; 75:99–105.

225. Cummings MG, James JH, Soeters PB, Keane JM, Foster J, Fischer JE. Regional brain study of indoleamine metabolism in the rat in acute hepatic failure. J Neurochem 1976; 27:741–746.

226. James JH, Escourrou J, Fischer JE. Blood-brain neutral amino acid transport activity is increased after portacaval anastomosis. Science 1978; 200:1395–1397.

227. Smith AR, Rossi-Fanelli F, Ziparo V, James JH, Perelle BA, Fischer JE. Alterations in plasma and CSF amino acids, amines, and metabolites in hepatic coma. Ann Surg 1978; 187:343–350.

228. Zieve L, Olsen RL. Can hepatic coma be caused by a reduction of brain noradrenaline or dopamine? Gut 1977; 18:688–691.

229. Smith B, Prockop DJ. Central nervous system effects of ingestion of L-tryptophan by normal subjects. N Engl J Med 1962; 267:1338–1341.

230. Hirayama C. Tryptophan metabolism in liver disease. Clin Chim Acta 1971; 32:191–197.

231. Cuilleret G, Pomier-Layrargues G, Pons F, Cadilhac J, Michel H. Changes in brain catecholamine levels in human cirrhotic hepatic encephalopathy. Gut 1980; 21:565–569.

232. Fischer JE, Funovics JM, Falcao H, Wesdorp RIC. L-Dopa in hepatic coma. Ann Surg 1976; 183:386–391.

233. Mandel P, Defendis FV. GABA-biochemistry and CNS functions. New York: Plenum Press, 1979.

234. Smialowski A. The effect of intrahippocampal administration of gamma-amino butyric acid (GABA). In: Fonnum E, ed. Amino acids as chemical transmitters. New York: Plenum Press, 1978: 1977.

235. Blitzer BL, Waggoner JG, Jones EA, Gralnick HR, Towne D, Butler J, Weise V, Kopin IJ, Walters I, Teychenne PF, Goodman DG, Berk PD. A model of fulminant hepatic failure in the rabbit. Gastroenerology 1978; 74:664–671.

236. Trewby PN, Casemore C, Williams R. Continuous bipolar recording of the EEG in patients with fulminant hepatic failure. Electroenceph Clin Neurophysiol 1978; 45:107–110.

237. Olsen RW. Drug interactions at the GABA receptor–ionophere complex. Ann Rev Pharmacol Toxicol 1982; 22:245–277.

238. Study RE, Barker JL. Diazepam and phenobarbital: fluctuation analysis reveals different mechanisms for potentiation of gamma-aminobutyric acid responses in cultured central neurons. Proc Natl Acad Sci USA 1981; 78:7180–7184.

239. Schafer DF, Fowler JM, Jones EA. Colonic bacteria: a source of gamma-aminobutyric acid in blood. Proc Soc Exp Biol Med 1981; 167:301–303.

240. Ferenci P, Covell D, Schafer DF, Waggoner JG, Schrager R, Jones EA. Metabolism of the inhibitory neurotransmitter gamma-aminobutyric acid in a rabbit model of fulminant hepatic failure. Hepatology 1983; 3:507–512.

241. Ferenci P, Schafer DF, Kleinberger G, Hoofnagle JH, Jones EA. Serum levels of gamma-aminobutyric acid-like activity in acute and chronic hepatocellular disease. Lancet 1983; ii:811–814.

242. Horowitz ME, Schafer DF, Molnar P, Jones EA, Blasberg RG, Patlak CS, Waggoner J, Fenstermacher JD. Increased blood-brain transfer in a rabbit model of acute liver failure. Gastroenterology 1983; 84:1003–1011.

243. Bigler ED. Neurophysiology, neuropharmacology, and behavioral relationships of the visual system evoked after discharges: a review. Biobehav Rev 1977; 1:95–112.

244. Schafer DF, Pappas SC, Brody LE, Jacobs R, Jones EA. Visual evoked potentials in a rabbit model of hepatic encephalopathy. I: sequential changes and comparisons with drug-induced comas. Gastroenterology 1984; 86:540–545.

245. Zeneroli ML, Pinelli G, Gollini G, Penne A, Messori E, Zani G, Ventura E. Visual evoked potential; a diagnostic tool for the assessment of hepatic encephalopathy. Gut 1984; 25:291–299.

246. Casellas P, Sagales T, Calzeda MD, Accarino A, Vargas V, Guarner L. Visual evoked potentials in hepatic encephalopathy. Lancet 1985; i:394–395.

247. Yange SS, Chu NS, Liaw YF. Somatosensory evoked potentials in hepatic encephalopathy. Gastroenterology 1985; 89:625–630.

248. Matos L, Paiva T, Cravo M, Fred A, Camilo ME, Pinto Correia J. Mapping of EEG and evoked potentials in subclinical hepatic encephalopathy. (Abstract) Gastroenterology 1988; 94:A569.

249. Sanford NL, Saul RE. Assessment of hepatic encephalopathy with visual evoked potentials compared with conventional methods. Hepatology 1988; 8:1094–1098.

250. Schafer DF, Fowler JM, Munson PJ, Thakur AK, Waggoner JG, Jones EA. Gamma-aminobutyric acid and benzodiazepine receptors in an animal model of fulminant hepatic failure. J Lab Clin Med 1983; 102:870–880.

251. Ferenci P, Pappas SC, Munson PJ, Henson K, Jones EA. Changes in the status of neurotransmitter receptors in a rabbit model of hepatic encephalopathy. Hepatology 1984; 4:186–191.

252. Baraldi M, Zeneroli ML. Experimental hepatic encephalopathy: changes in the binding of gamma-aminobutyric acid. Science 1982; 216:427–429.

253. Basile AE, Gammal SH, Mullen KD, Skolnick P, Jones EA. Hepatic encephalopathy: enhanced sensitivity of isolated CNS neurons to a benzodiazepine. (Abstract) Hepatology 1987; 7:1032.

254. Maddison JE, Dodd PR, Morrison M, Johnston GAR, Farrell GC. Plasma GABA, GABA-like activity and the brain GABA-benzodiazepine receptor complex in rats with chronic encephalopathy. Hepatology 1987; 7:621–628.

255. Maddison JE, Dodd PR, Johnston GAR, Farrell GC. Brain gamma-aminobutyric acid receptor binding is normal in rats with thioacetamide-induced hepatic encephalopathy despite elevated plasma gamma-aminobutyric acid-like activity. Gastroenterology 1987; 93:1062–1068.

256. Nakatsukasa H, Gordon VP, Martin P, Pappas SC. Brain gamma aminobutyric acid (GABA) binding is unaltered in two guinea pig models of fulminant hepatic failure: further evidence conflicting with the GABA hypothesis. (Abstract) Hepatology 1987; 7:1033A.

257. Roy S, Pomier-Layrargues G, Butterworth RF, Huet PM. Hepatic encephalopathy in cirrhotic and portacaval shunted dogs: lack of changes in brain GABA uptake, brain GABA levels, brain glutamic acid decarboxylase activity, and brain postsynaptic GABA receptors. Hepatology 1988; 8:845–849.

258. Rossle M, Decker J, Gerok W. Quantitative autoradiography of GABA-receptors in portasystemic and hyperammonemic encephalopathy in the rat. (Abstract) Gastroenterology 1988; 94:A586.

259. Moroni F, Riggio O, Carla V, Festuccia V, Ghinelli F, Marino IR, Merli M, Natali L, Pedretti G, Fiaccadori F, Capocaccia L. Hepatic encephalopathy: lack of changes of gamma-aminobutyric acid content in plasma and cerebrospinal fluid. Hepatology 1987; 7:816–820.

260. Lavoie J, Giguere JF, Pomier-Layrargues G, Butterworth RF. Amino acid changes in autopsied brain tissue from cirrhotic patients with hepatic encephalopathy. J Neurochem 1987; 49:692–697.

261. Butterworth RF, Lavoie J, Giguere JF, Pomier-Layrargues G. Affinities and densities of high-affinity (^{3}H) muscimol (GABA-A) binding sites and of central benzodiazepine receptors are unchanged in autopsied brain tissue from cirrhotic patients with hepatic encephalopathy. Hepatology 1988; 8:1084–1088.

262. Samson Y, Bernuau J, Pappata S, Chavoix C, Baron JC, Maziere MA. Cerebral uptake of benzodiazepine measured by positron emission tomography in hepatic encephalopathy. (Letter) N Engl J Med 1987; 316:414–415.

263. Bassett ML, Mullen KD, Skolnick P, Jones EA. Amelioration of hepatic encephalopathy by pharmacologic antagonism of the GABA$_A$-benzodiazepine receptor complex in a rabbit model of fulminant hepatic failure. Gastroenterology 1987; 93:1069–1077.

264. Baraldi M, Zeneroli ML, Ventura E, Penne A, Pinelli G, Ricci P, Santi M. Supersensitivity of benzodiazepine receptors in hepatic encephalopathy due to fulminant hepatic failure in the rat: reversal by a benzodiazepine antagonist. Clin Sci 1984; 67:167–175.

265. Scollo-Lavizzari G, Steinmann E. Reversal of hepatic coma by benzodiazepine antagonist (Ro15-1788). Lancet 1985; i:1324.

266. Bansky G, Meier PJ, Ziegler WT, Walser H, Schmid M, Huber M. Reversal of hepatic coma by benzodiazepine antagonist (Ro15-1788). Lancet 1985; i:1324–1325.

267. Grimm G, Ferenci P, Katzenschlager R, Madl C, Schneeweiss B, Laggner AN, Lenz K, Gangl A. Improvement of hepatic encephalopathy treated with flumazenil. Lancet 1988; ii:1392–1394.

268. Mullen KD, Martin JV, Mendelson WB, Bassett ML, Jones EA. Could an endogenous benzodiazepine ligand contribute to hepatic encephalopathy. Lancet 1988; i:457–459.

269. Mullen KD, Szauter KM, Galloway PG, Kaminsky K. CSF of patients with hepatic encephalopathy contains significant benzodiazepine (BZ) binding activity. Correlation with post-mortem cortical BZ binding studies. (Abstract) Hepatology 1987; 7:1103.

270. Olasmaa M, Guidotti A, Costa E, Rothstein JD, Goldman ME, Weber RU, Paul SM. Endogenous benzodiazepines in hepatic encephalopathy. Lancet 1989; i:491–492.

271. Mullen KD, Szauter KM, Kaminsky K, Matuszak SM. Characterization of "endogenous" benzodiazepine (BZ) activity detected in human hepatic encephalopathy. (Abstract) Hepatology 1988; 8:1352.

272. Pirola RC, Ham JM, Elmslie RG. Management of hepatic coma complicating virus hepatitis. Gut 1969; 10:898–903.

273. Ware AJ, D'Agostino A, Combes B. Cerebral edema: a major complication of massive hepatic necrosis. Gastroenterology 1971; 61:877–884.

274. Silk DBA, Hanid MA, Trewby PN, Davies M, Chase RA, Langley PG, Mellon PJ, Wheeler PG, Williams R. Treatment of fulminant hepatic failure by polyacrylonitrile membrane hemodialysis. Lancet 1977; ii:1–3.

275. Ede RJ, Gimson AES, Bihari D, Williams R. Controlled hyperventilation in the prevention of cerebral edema in fulminant hepatic failure. J Hepatol 1986; 2:43–51.

276. Gazzard BG, Portmann B, Murray-Lyon IM, Williams R. Causes of death in fulminant hepatic failure and relationship to quantitative histological assessment of parenchymal damage. QJ Med 1975; 176:615–626.

277. Adams RD, Foley JM, Merritt HH, Hare CC. The neurologic disorder associated with liver disease. In: Metabolic and Toxic Diseases of the Nervous System. Vol.32. Baltimore, Williams & Wilkins, 1953: 198.

278. Bruton CJ, Corsellis JAN, Russell A. Hereditary hyperammonemia. Brain 1970; 93:423–434.

279. Pilbeam CM, Anderson RM, Bhathal PS. The brain in experimental portal-systemic encephalopathy. II: Water and electrolyte changes. J Pathol 1983; 140:347–355.

280. Hanid MA, Mackenzie RL, Jenner RE, Chase RA, Mellon PJ, Trewby PN, Janota I, Davis M, Silk DBA, Williams R. Intracranial pressure in pigs with surgically induced acute liver failure. Gastroenterology 1979; 76:123–131.

281. Traber PG, Granger DR, Blei AT. Brain edema in rabbits with galactosamine-induced fulminant hepatitis. Gastroenterology 1986; 91:1247–1356.

282. Traber PG, DalCanto M, Granger DR, Blei AT. Electron microscopic evaluation of brain edema in rabbits with galactosamine-induced fulminant hepatic failure: ultrastructure and integrity of the blood brain barrier. Hepatology 1987; 7:1272–1277.

283. Fishman RA, Chan PH. Metabolic basis of brain edema. In: Cervos-Navarro J, Ferszt E, eds. Advances in neurology. Vol 28: Brain edema. New York: Raven Press, 1980; 207.

284. James HE, Laurin RA. Intracranial hypertension and brain edema in albino rabbits. Part I: Experimental models. Acta Neurochir 1981; 55:213–226.

285. Ede RJ, Williams R. Hepatic encephalopathy and cerebral edema. Semin Liver Dis 1986; 6:107–118.

286. Quarforth G, Ahmed K, Foster D, Zieve L. Action of methanethiol on membrane Na^+, K^+ ATP-ase of rat brain. Biochem Pharmacol 1976; 25:1039–1044.

287. Seda HWM, Gove CD, Hughes RD, Williams R. Inhibition of partially purified rat brain Na^+, K^+-dependent ATP-ase by bile acids, phenolic acids, and endotoxin. Clin Sci 1984; 66:415–420.

288. Seda HWM, Hughes RD, Gove CD, Williams R. Inhibition of rat brain Na^+, K^+ ATP-ase activity by serum from patients with fulminant hepatic failure. Hepatology 1984; 4:74–79.

289. Pappas SC, Ferenci P, Jones EA. Evidence against the hypothesis that cerebral edema in fulminant hepatic failure is due to decreased neural Na^+, K^+ ATPase activity. (Abstract) Hepatology 1983; 8:848.

290. Gregorios JB, Mozes LW, Norenberg L-OB, Norenberg MD. Morphologic effects of ammonia on primary astrocyte cultures. I Light microscopic studies. J Neuropathol Exp Neurol 1985; 44:397–403.

291. Gregorios JB, Mozes LW, Norenberg MD. Morphologic effects of ammonia on primary astrocyte cultures. II Electron microscopic studies. J Neuropathol Exp Neurol 1985; 44:404–414.

292. Benjamin AM, Okamoto K, Quastel JH. Effects of ammonia ions on spontaneous action potentials and on contents of sodium, potassium, ammonium, and chloride ions in brains in vitro. J Neurochem 1978; 30:131–143.

293. Nohott K, Poetter U, Neuhoff V. Ammonia inhibits protein synthesis in slices from young rat brain. J Neurochem 1984; 42:644–646.

294. Hanid MA, Davies M, Mellon PJ, Silk DBA, Strunin L, McCabe JJ, Williams R. Clinical monitoring of intracranial pressure in fulminant hepatic failure. Gut 1980; 21:866–869.

295. Bowers SA, Marshall LF. Outcome in 200 consecutive cases of severe head injury managed without intracranial pressure monitoring. Neurosurgery 1980; 6:237–242.

296. O'Grady JG, Langley PG, Isola LM, Aledort LM, Williams R. Coagulopathy of fulminant hepatic failure. Semin Liver Dis 1986; 6:159–163.

297. Hughes RD, Lane DA, Ireland H, Langley PG, Gimson AES, Williams R. Fibrinogen derivatives and platelets activation products in acute and chronic liver disease. Clin Sci 1985; 68:701–707.

298. Green FB, Thomson JM, Dymock IW, Poller L. Abnormal fibrin polymerization in liver disease. Br J Haematol 1976; 34:427–437.

299. Martines J, Palascak JE, Kwasniak D. Abnormal sialic acid content of the dysfibrinogenaemia associated with liver disease. J Clin Invest 1978; 61:3535–3547.

300. Cornillon B, Paul J, Belleville J, Aurousseau AM, Clendinnen G, Eloy R. Experimental DMNA induced hepatic necrosis: early course of hemostatic disorders in the rat. Comp Biochem Physiol 1985; 80C:277–284.

301. Dymock IW, Tucker JS, Woolf IL, Poller L, Thomson JM. Coagulation studies as a prognostic index in acute liver failure. Br J Haematol 1975; 29:385–395.

302. Gazzard BG, Henderson JM, Williams R. Factor VII levels as a guide to prognosis in fulminant hepatic failure. Gut 1976; 17:489–491.

303. Ekindjian OG, Devanley M, Duchassaing D, Leluan G, Kammerer J, Fouet P, Auget JL, Maccario J. Multivariate analysis of clinical and biological data in cirrhotic patients: application of prognosis. Eur J Clin Invest 1981; 11:213–240.

304. Nanji AA, Blank DW. Clinical status as reflected in biochemical tests on patients with chronic alcoholic liver disease. Clin Chem 1983; 29:992–993.

305. Kelly DA, Summerfield JA. Hemostasis in liver disease. Semin Liver Dis 1987; 7:182–189.

306. Wion KL, Kelly DA, Summerfield, Tuddenham EGD, Lawn RM. Distribution of factor VIII MRNA and antigen in human liver and other tissues. Nature 1985; 317:726–729.

307. Langley PG, Hughes RD, Williams R. Increased factor VIII complex in fulminant hepatic failure. Thromb Haemost 1985; 54:693–696.

308. Friedman PA. Vitamin K. In: Arias I, Popper H, Schaffner D, Shafritz DA, eds. The liver: biology and pathobiology. New York: Raven Press, 1982; 359.

309. Feldshon SD, Earnest DL, Corrigan JJ. Impaired coagulant factor synthesis is more important that impaired carboxylation in the coagulopathy of liver disease. Hepatology 1983; 3:858–863.

310. Sette H, Hughes RD, Langley PC, Gimson AES, Williams R. Heparin response and clearance in acute and chronic liver disease. Thromb Haemost 1985; 54:591–594.

311. Duchert F. Behavior of antithrombin III in liver disease. Scand J Gastroenterol 1973; 8(suppl 19):109–112.

312. Gazzard BG, Rahe MO, Flute PT, Williams R. Bleeding in relation to the coagulation defect of fulminant hepatic failure. In: Williams R, Murray-Lyon IM, eds. Artificial liver support. London: Pitman Medical Publishing, 1975; 143.

313. Weston MJ, Langley PG, Rubin MH, Hanid MA, Mellon P, Williams R. Platelet function in fulminant hepatic failure and effect of charcoal hemoperfusion. Gut 1977; 18:897–902.

314. Rubin MH, Weston MJ, Bullock G, Roberts J, Langley PG, White YS, Williams R. Abnormal platelet function and ultrastructure in fulminant hepatic failure. QJ Med 1977; 46:339–352.

315. Owen JS, Hutton RA, Day RC, Bruckdorfer KR, McIntyre N. Platelet lipid composition and platelet aggregation in human liver disease. J Lipid Res 1981; 22:423–430.

316. Fujiwara K, Ogata I, Ohta Y, Hirata K, Oka Y, Yamada S, Sato Y, Masaki N, Oka H. Intravascular coagulation in acute liver failure in rats and its treatment with antithrombin III. Gut 1988; 29:1103–1108.

317. Papper S. Renal failure in cirrhosis (the hepatorenal syndrome). In: Epstein M, ed. The kidney in liver disease. 2nd ed. New York: Elsevier Science, 1983; 87.

318. Papper S, Saxon L. The diuretic response to administered water in patients with liver disease: II. Laennec's cirrhosis of the liver. Arch Intern Med 1959; 103:750–757.

319. Tristani FE, Cohn JN. Systemic and renal hemodynamics in oliguric hepatic failure: effect of volume expansion. J Clin Invest 1967; 46:1894–1906.

320. Vlahcevic ZR, Aham NF, Jick H, Moore EW, Chalmers TC. Renal effects of acute expansion of plasma volume in cirrhosis. N Engl J Med 1965; 272:387–391.

321. Epstein M, Pins DS, Arrington R, Denunzio AG, Engstrom R. Comparison of water immersion and saline infusion as a means of inducing volume expansion in man. J Appl Physiol 1975; 39:66–70.

322. Epstein M, Pins DS, Schneider N, Levinson R. Determinants of deranged sodium and water homeostasis in decompensated cirrhosis. J Lab Clin Med 1976; 87:822–839.

323. Levy M. Sodium retention and ascites formation in dogs with experimental portal cirrhosis. Am J Physiol 1977; 233(F):572–585.

324. Levy M, Wexler MJ. Renal sodium retention and ascites formation in dogs with experimental cirrhosis but without portal hypertension or increased splanchnic vascular capacity. J Lab Clin Med 1978; 91:520–536.

325. Levy M, Wexler MJ, McCaffrey C. Sodium retention in dogs with experimental cirrhosis following removal of ascites by continuous peritoneovenous shunting. J Lab Clin Med 1979; 94:933–946.

326. Greig PD, Blendis LM, Langer B, Taylor BR, Colapinto RF. Renal and hemodynamic effects of peritoneovenous shunt. II. Long-term effects. Gastroenterology 1981; 80:119–125.

327. Wood LJ, Massie D, McLean A, Dudley FJ. Renal sodium retention in cirrhosis: tubular site and relation to hepatic dysfunction. Hepatology 1988; 8:831–836.

328. Ballerman BJ, Brenner BM. Biologically active atrial peptides. J Clin Invest 1985; 76:2041–2048.

329. Cody RJ, Atlas SA, Laragh JA, Kubo SH, Covit AB, Ryman KS, Shaknovich A, Pandolfino K, Clark M, Camargo MJF, Scarborough RM, Lewicki JA. Atrial natriuretic factor in normal subjects and patients with heart failure. J Clin Invest 1986; 78:1362–1374.

330. Maack T, Marion DN, Camargo MJF, Kleinert HD, Vaughan ED, Atlas SA. Effects of auriculin (atrial natriuretic factor) on blood pressure, renal function, and the renin aldosterone system in dogs. Am J Med 1984; 77:1069–1975.

331. Gerbes AL, Arendt RM, Riedel A, Ritter D, Liebermeister R, Jungst D, Sauerbruch T, Zohringer J, Paumgarther G. Role of the atrial natriuretic factor (ANF) in volume regulation of healthy and cirrhotic subjects: effects of water immersion. (Abstract) Gastroenterology 1986; 90:1727.

332. Klepetko W, Muller C, Hartter E, Miholics J, Schwarz C, Woloszczuk W, Moeschl P. Plasma atrial natriuretic factor in cirrhotic patients with ascites: effect of peritoneovenous shunt implantation. Gastroenterology 1988; 95:764–770.

333. Morgan TR, Imada T, Hollister AS, Inagami T. Plasma human atrial natriuretic factor in cirrhosis and ascites with and without functional renal failure. Gastroenterology 1988; 95:1641–1647.

334. Levy M. Pathophysiology of ascites formation. In: Epstein M, ed. The kidney in liver disease. 2nd ed. New York: Elsevier Biomedical, 1983; 245.

335. Levy M, Wexler MJ. Sodium excretion in dogs with low-grade caval construction: role of hepatic nerves. Am J Physiol 1987; 253:F672–F678.

336. Kostreva D, Cataner A, Kanipane JP. Reflex effects of hepatic baroreceptors on renal and cardiac sympathetic nerve activity. Am J Physiol 1980; 238:(R)390–394.

337. Rosoff L Jr, Zia P, Reynolds T, Horton R. Studies of renin and aldosterone in cirrhotic patients with ascites. Gastroenterology 1975; 69:698–705.

338. Eggert RC. Spironolactone diuresis in patients with cirrhosis and ascites. Br Med J 1970; 4:401–403.

339. Epstein M. Aldosterone in liver disease. In: Epstein M, ed. Kidney in liver disease. 2nd ed. New York: Elsevier Biomedical, 1983: 377.

340. Bichet DG, Van Putten V, Schrier RW. Potential role of sympathetic activity in the sodium and water excretion in cirrhotic patients. N Engl J Med 1982; 307:1552–1557.

341. Bichet DG, Groves BM, Schrier RW. Mechanism of improvement of water and sodium excretion by immersion in decompensated cirrhotic patients. Kidney Int 1983; 307:1552–1557.

342. Nicholls KM, Shapiro MD, Kluge R, Chung HM, Bichet DG, Schrier RW. Sodium excretion in advanced cirrhosis: effect of expansion of central blood volume and suppression of plasma aldosterone. Hepatology 1986; 6:235–238.

343. Better OS, Schrier RW. Disturbed volume homeostasis in patients with cirrhosis of the liver. Kidney Int 1983; 23:303–311.

344. Bichet DG, Szatolowicz V, Chaimovitz C, Schrier RW. Role of vasopressin in abnormal water excretion in cirrhotic patients. Ann Intern Med 1982; 96:413–417.

345. DeTroyer A, Pilloy W, Broeckaert I, Demanet JC. Demeclocycline treatment of water retention in cirrhosis. Ann Intern Med 1976; 85:336–337.

346. Boyer TD, Zia P, Reynolds TB. Effects of indomethacin and prostaglandin A on renal function and plasma renin activity in alcoholic liver disease. Gastroenterology 1979; 77:215–222.

347. Zipser RD, Hoefs JC, Speckart PF, Zia PK, Horton R. Prostaglandins: modulators of renal function and pressor resistance in chronic liver disease. J Clin Endocrinol Metab 1979; 48:895–900.

348. Levy M, Wexler MJ, Fechner C. Renal perfusion in dogs with experimental hepatic cirrhosis: role of prostaglandins. Am J Physiol 1983; 245:F521–F529.

349. Dunn MJ. Renal prostaglandins. In: Dunn MJ, ed. Renal endocrinology. Baltimore: Williams & Wilkins, 1983: 1.

350. Koppel MH, Coburn JW, Mims MM, Goldstein H, Boyle JO, Rubin ME. Transplantation of cadaveric kidneys from patients with hepatorenal syndrome. Evidence for the functional nature of renal failure in advanced liver disease. N Engl J Med 1969; 280:1367–1371.

351. Iwatsuki S, Popovtzer MM, Corman JL, Ishikawa M, Putnam CW, Katz FH, Starzl TE. Recovery from "hepatorenal syndrome" after orthotopic liver transplantation. N Engl J Med 1973; 289:1155–1159.

352. Epstein M, Berk DP, Hollenberg NK, Adams DF, Chalmers TC, Abrams HC, Merrill JP. Renal failure in the patient with cirrhosis. The role of active vasoconstriction. Am J Med 1970; 49:175–185.

353. Kew MC, Brunt PW, Varma RR, Hourigan KJ, Williams HS, Sherlock S. Renal and intrarenal blood flow in cirrhosis of the liver. Lancet 1971; ii:504–509.

354. Arroyo V, Gines P, Rimola A, Gaya J. Renal function abnormalities, prostaglandins, and the effects of nonsteroidal anti-inflammatory drugs in cirrhosis with ascites. Am J Med 1986; 81(suppl 2B):104–122.

355. Arroyo V, Planas R, Gaya J, Deulofeu R, Rimola A, Perez-Ayuso RM, Rivera F, Rodes J. Sympathetic nervous activity, renin-angiotension system and renal excretion of PGE$_2$ in cirrhosis. Relationship to functional renal failure and sodium and water excretion. Eur J Clin Invest 1983; 13:271–278.

356. Guarnar C, Colina I, Guarner F, Corzo J, Prieto J, Vilardell F. Renal prostaglandins in cirrhosis of the liver. Clin Sci 1986; 70:477–484.

357. Zambraski EJ, Dunn MJ. Importance of renal prostaglandins in control of renal function after chronic ligation of the common bile duct in dogs. J Lab Clin Med 1984; 103:549–559.

358. Guarner F, Hughes RD, Gimson AES, Williams R. Renal function in fulminant hepatic failure: haemodynamics and renal prostaglandins. Gut 1987; 28:1643–1647.

359. Zipser RD, Radvan GH, Kronborg IJ, Duke R, Little TE. Urinary thromboxane B$_2$ and prostaglandin E$_2$ in the hepatorenal syndrome: evidence for increased vasoconstrictor and decreased vasodilator factors. Gastroenterology 1983; 84:697–703.

360. Zusmara RM, Axelrod L, Tolkoff-Rubin N. The treatment of the hepatorenal syndrome with intra-arterial administration of prostaglandin E. Prostaglandin 1977; 13:819–830.

361. Arieff AI, Chidsey CC. Renal function in cirrhosis and the effect of prostaglandin A. Am J Med 1974; 56:695–703.

362. Zipser RD, Kronborg I, Rector W, Reynolds T, Daskalopoulos G. Therapeutic trial of thromboxane synthesis inhibition in the hepatorenal syndrome. Gastroenterology 1984; 87:1228–1232.

363. Pinzani M, Laffi G, Meacci E, LaVilla G, Cominelli F, Gentilini P. Intrarenal thromboxane A$_2$ generation reduces the furosemide-induced sodium and water diuresis in cirrhosis with ascites. Gastroenterology 1988; 95:1081–1087.

364. Levy M, Allotey JB, Temporal relationships between urinary salt retention and altered systemic hemodynamics in dogs with experimental cirrhosis. J Lab Clin Med 1978; 92:560–569.

365. Fernandez Munoz D, Caramelo C, Santos JC, Blanchart A, Hernando L, Lopez-Novoa JM. Systemic and splanchnic hemodynamic disturbances in conscious rats with experimental liver cirrhosis without ascites. Am J Physiol 1985; 249:G316–G320.

366. Murray IF, Dawson AM, Sherlock S. Circulatory changes in liver disease. Am J Med 1958; 24:358–367.

367. Sullivan SN, Chase RA, Christofides A, Bloom SR, Williams R. The gut hormone profile of fulminant hepatic failure. Am J Gastroenterol 1981; 76:338–341.

368. Hortnagl H, Singer EA, Lenz K, Kleinberger G, Lochs H. Substance P is markedly increased in plasma of patients with hepatic coma. Lancet 1984; i:480–483.

369. Thornton JR, Dean H, Losowsky MS. Is ascites caused by impaired hepatic inactivation of blood borne endogenous opioid peptides. Gut 1988; 29:1167–1172.

370. Arroyo V, Bernardi M, Epstein M, Henrikson JH, Schrier KW, Rodes J. Pathophysiology of ascites and functional renal failure in cirrhosis. J Hepatol 1988; 6:239–257.

371. Schrier RW. Pathogenesis of sodium and water retention in high output and low-output cardiac failure, nephrotic syndrome, cirrhosis, and pregnancy. N Engl J Med 1988; 319:1127–1134.

372. Schrier RW, Arroyo V, Bernardi M, Epstein M, Henriksen JH, Rodes J. Peripheral arterial vasodilation hypothesis: a proposal for the initiation of renal sodium and water retention in cirrhosis. Hepatology 1988; 6:1151–1157.

373. Rector WG, Hossack KF. Pathogenesis of sodium retention complicating cirrhosis: is there room for diminished "effective" arterial blood volume. Gastroenterology 1988; 95:1658–1663.

374. Blendis LM, Sole MJ, Campbell P, Lossing AG, Greig PD, Taylor BR, Langer B. The effect of peritoneovenous shunting on catecholamine metabolism in patients with hepatic ascites. Hepatology 1987; 7:143–148.

375. Vorobioff J, Bredfeldt JE, Groszmann RJ. Increased blood flow through the portal system in cirrhotic rats. Gastroenterology 1984; 87:1120–1126.

376. Blanchet L, Lebrec D. Changes in splanchnic blood flow in portal hypertensive rats. Eur J Clin Invest 1982; 12:327–330.

377. Laffi G, LaVilla G, Pinzani M, Ciabattani G, Patrignani P, Mannelli M, Cominelli F, Gentilini P. Altered renal and platelet arachidonic acid metabolism in cirrhosis. Gastroenterology 1986; 90:274–282.

378. Graudal N, Milman N, Kirkegaard E, Korner B, Thomsen AC. Bacteremia in cirrhosis of the liver. Liver 1986; 6:297–301.

379. Wyke RJ, Canalese JC, Gimson AES, Williams R. Bacteremia in patients with fulminant hepatic failure. Liver 1982; 2:45–52.

380. Ruttenberg AM, Sonnenblick E, Koven I, Schweinburg F, Fine J. Comparative response of normal and cirrhotic rats to intravenously injected bacteria. Proc Soc Exp Biol Med 1959; 101:279–281.

381. Rimola A, Soto R, Bory F, Arroyo V, Piera C, Rodes J. Reticuloendothelial system phagocytic activity in cirrhosis and its relation to bacterial infections and prognosis. Hepatology 1984; 4:53–58.

382. Fieror J, Finley F. Deficient serum bactericidal activity against *Escherichia coli* in patients with cirrhosis of the liver. J Clin Invest 1979; 63:912–921.

383. Wyke RJ, Rajkovic IA, Williams R. Impaired opsonisation by serum from patients with chronic liver disease. Clin Exp Immunol 1983; 51:91–98.

384. Larcher VF, Wyke RJ, Vergani D, Mowat AP, Williams R. Yeast opsonisation and complement in children with liver disease. Analysis of 69 cases. Pediatr Res 1983; 17:296–300.

385. Larcher VF, Wyke RJ, Mowat AP, Williams R. Bacterial and fungal infection in children with fulminant hepatic failure: possible role of opsonisation and complement deficiency. Gut 1982; 23:1037–1043.

386. Candy DCA, Larcher VF, Tripp JH, Harries JT, Harvey BAM, Soothill JF. Defective yeast opsonisation in children with chronic diarrhea. Arch Dis Child 1980; 55:189–193.

387. Barnes PF, Arevalo C, Chan LS, Wong SF, Reynolds TB. A prospective evaluation of bacteremic patients with chronic liver disease. Hepatology 1988; 8:1099–1103.

388. Uribe M, Marquez MA, Famos GG, Ramos-Uribe MH, Vargas F, Villalobos A, Ramos C. Treatment of chronic portal systemic encephalopathy with vegetable and animal protein diets: a controlled crossover study. Dig Dis Sci 1982; 27:1109–1116.

389. Lerman BB, Levin ML, Patterson R. Hepatic encephalopathy precipitated by fecal impaction. Arch Intern Med 1979; 139:707–708.

390. Berk DP, Chalmers T. Deafness complicating antibiotic therapy of hepatic encephalopathy. Ann Intern Med 1970; 73:393–396.

391. Cabrera J, Arroyo V, Ballesta AM, Rimola A, Gual J, Elena M, Rodes J. Aminoglycoside nephrotoxicity in cirrhosis: value of urinary B$_2$-microglobulin to discriminate functional renal failure from acute tubular damage. Gastroenterology 1982; 82:97–105.

392. Elkington SG, Floch MH, Conn HO. Lactulose in the treatment of chronic portal-systemic encephalopathy. A double-blind clinical trial. N Engl J Med 1969; 281:408–412.

393. Conn HO, Leevy CM, Vlahcevic ZR, Rodgers JB, Maddrey WC, Seeff L, Levy LL. Comparison of lactulose and neomycin in the treatment

394. Uribe M, Toledo H, Perez F, Vargas F, Gil S, Garcia-Ramos G, Ravelli GP, Guevara L. Lactitol, a second-generation disaccharide for treatment of chronic portal-systemic encephalopathy. Dig Dis Sci 1987; 32:1345–1353.

395. Morgan MY, Hawley KE. Lactitol vs. lactulose in the treatment of acute hepatic encephalopathy in cirrhotic patients: a double-blind randomized trial. Hepatology 1987; 7:1278–1284.

396. Uribe M, Campollo O, Vargas F, Ravelli GP, Mundo F, Zapata L, Gil S, Garcia-Ramos G. Acidifying enemas (lactitol and lactose) vs. nonacidifying enemas (tap water) to treat acute portal-systemic encephalopathy: a double-blind, randomized clinical trial. Hepatology 1987; 7:639–643.

397. Maddrey WC, Weber FL, Coulter AW, Chura CM, Chapanis NP, Walser M. Effects of ketoanalogues of essential amino acids in portal-systemic encephalopathy. Gastroenterology 1976; 71:190–195.

398. Munoz S, Walser M. Utilization of alpha-ketoisocaproate for synthesis of hepatic export proteins and peripheral proteins in normal and cirrhotic subjects. Gastroenterology 1986; 90:1834–1843.

399. Herlong HF, Maddrey WC, Walser M. The use of ornithine salts of branched-chain ketoacids in portal systemic encephalopathy. Ann Intern Med 1980; 93:545–550.

400. O'Keefe SJD, El-Zayadi A, Carraher T, Davis M, Williams R. Malnutrition and immune competence in patients with liver disease. Lancet 1980; ii:615–617.

401. Mendenhall CL, Tosch T, Wiesner RE, Garcia Pont P, Goldberg SJ, Kiernan T, Seeff LB, Sorrell M, Taburro C, Zetterman R, Chedid A, Chen T, Rabin L. VA cooperative study on alcoholic hepatitis II: Prognostic significance of protein-calorie malnutrition. Am J Clin Nutr 1986; 43:213–218.

402. Shaw BW, Wood RP, Gordon RD, Iwatsuki S, Gillquist WP, Starzl T. Influence of selected variables and operative blood loss on six-month survival following liver transplantation. Semin Liver Dis 1985; 5:385–393.

403. Rosen HM, Yoshimura M, Hodgman JM, Fisher JE. Plasma amino acid patterns in hepatic encephalopathy of differing etiology. Gastroenterology 1977; 72:483–487.

404. Chase RA, Davis M, Trewby PN, Silk DBA, Williams R. Plasma amino acid profiles in patients with fulminant hepatic failure treated by repeated polyacrylonitrate membrane haemodialysis. Gastroenterology 1978; 75:1033–1040.

405. Munro HN, Fernstrom JD, Wurtman RJ. Insulin, plasma amino acid imbalance and hepatic coma. Lancet 1975; i:722–724.

406. Cascino A, Cangiano C, Calcaterra V, Rossi-Fanelli F, Capocaccia L. Plasma amino acids imbalance in patients with liver disease. Dig Dis Sci 1978; 23:591–598.

407. Rossi-Fanelli F, Freund H, Krause R, Smith AR, James JA, Castorina-Ziparos, Fischer JE. Induction of coma in normal dogs by the infusion of aromatic amino acids and its prevention by the addition of branched chain amino acids. Gastroenterology 1982; 83:664–671.

408. Fischer JE, Rosen HM, Ebeid AM, James JH, Keane JM, Soeters PB. The effect of normalization of plasma amino acids on hepatic encephalopathy in man. Surgery 1976; 80:77–91.

409. Horst D, Grace ND, Conn HO, Schiff E, Schenker S, Viteri A, Law D, Atterbury CE. Comparison of dietary protein with an oral, branched chain-enriched amino acid supplement in chronic portal systemic encephalopathy. A randomized controlled trial. Hepatology 1984; 4:279–287.

410. Eriksson LS, Person A, Wahren J. Branched-chain amino acids in the treatment of chronic hepatic encephalopathy. Gut 1983; 23:801–806.

411. McGhee A, Henderson JM, Millikan WJ, Bleier JC, Vogel R, Kassouny M, Rudman D. Comparison of the effects of hepatic acid and a casein modular diet on encephalopathy, plasma, amino acids, and nitrogen balance in cirrhotic patients. Ann Surg 1983; 197:288–293.

412. Rossi-Fanelli F, Riggio D, Cangiano C, Cascino A, DeConcilis D, Merli M, Stortoni M, Giunchi G, Capocaccia L. Branched-chain amino acids vs. lactulose in the treatment of hepatic coma: a controlled study. Dig Dis Sci 1982; 27:929–935.

413. Wahren J, Denis J, Desurmont P, Eriksson LS, Escoffier JM, Gauthier AP, Hagenfeldt L, Michel H, Opolon P, Paris JC, Veyrac M. Is intravenous administration of branched-chain amino acids effective in the treatment of hepatic encephalopathy? A multicenter study. Hepatology 1983; 3:475–480.

414. Cerra FB, Cheung NK, Fischer JE, Kaplowitz N, Schiff ER, Dien-

stag JL, Bower RH, Mabry CD, Leevy CM, Kieman T. Disease-specific amino acid infusion (F080) in hepatic encephalopathy: a prospective, randomized, double-blind controlled trial. J Parent Enteral Nutr 1985; 9:288–295.

415. Wright PD, Holdsworth JD, Dionigi P, Clague MB, James DFW. Effect of branched-chain amino acid infusions on body protein metabolism in cirrhosis of liver. Gut 1986; 27:96–102.

416. Rudman D, Kufner M, Ansley J. Hypotyrosinemia, hypocystinemia, and failure to retain nitrogen during total parenteral nutrition of cirrhotic patients. Gastroenterology 1981; 81:1025–1035.

417. Walser M. Urea cycle disorders and other hereditary hyperammonemic syndromes. In: Stanbury JB, Wyngaarden JB, Fredrickson PS, Goldstein JL, Brown MS, eds. The metabolic basis of inherited disease. New York: McGraw-Hill, 1983; 402.

418. Thompson JS, Schafer DF, Haun J, Schafer GJ. Adequate diet prevents hepatic coma in dogs with Eck fistulas. Surg Gynecol Obstet 1986; 162:126–130.

419. Merli M, Riggio O, Iapichino S, Miazzo P, Capocaccia L. Amino acid imbalance and malnutrition in liver cirrhosis. Clin Nutr 1985; 4:249–253.

420. Marchesini G, Zoli M, Dondi C. Anticatabolic effect of branched-chain amino acid-enriched solutions in patients with liver cirrhosis. Hepatology 1982; 2:420–425.

421. Michel H, Cauvet G, Granier PM, Bali JP, Andre R, Cuilleret G. Treatment of cirrhotic hepatic encephalopathy by L-dopa: a double-blind study of 58 patients. (Abstract) Digestion 1977; 15:232.

422. Uribe M, Farca A, Marquez MA, Garcia-Ramos G, Guevara L. Treatment of chronic portal systemic encephalopathy with bromocriptine. Gastroenterology 1979; 76:1347–1351.

423. Ferenci P, Grimm G, Gangl A. Successful longtime treatment of chronic hepatic encephalopathy (HE) with a benzodiazepine antagonist. (Abstract) Hepatology 1987; 7:1064.

424. Bansky G, Meier PJ, Riederer E. Effect of a benzodiazepine antagonist in hepatic encephalopathy in man. (Abstract) Hepatology 1987; 7:1103.

425. Suzdak PD, Glowa JR, Crawley JN, Schwartz RD, Skolnick P, Paul SM. A selective imidazobenzodiazepine antagonist of ethanol in the rat. Science 1986; 234:1243–1247.

426. Gammal SH, Geller D, Skolnick P, Paul SM, Lisker-Meliman M, Jones EA. Unequivocal amelioration of hepatic encephalopathy by benzodiazepine antagonists in a rat model of fulminant hepatic failure. J Hepatol 1987; 4:S17.

427. Canalese J, Gimson AES, Davis C, Mellon PJ, Davis M, Williams R. Controlled trial of dexamethasone and mannitol for the cerebral edema of fulminant hepatic failure. Gut 1982; 23:625–629.

428. Albright AL, Latchaw RE, Robinson AG. Intracranial and systemic effects of osmotic and oncotic therapy in experimental cerebral edema. J Neurosurg 1984; 60:481–489.

429. Marshall LF, Shapiro HM, Rauscher A, Kaufman NM. Phenobarbital therapy for intracranial hypertension in metabolic coma. Reye's syndrome. Crit Care Med 1978; 6:1–5.

430. Macdougall BRD, Williams R. H₂ receptor antagonist in the prevention of acute upper gastrointestinal hemorrhage in fulminant hepatic failure. Gastroenterology 1978; 74:464–465.

431. Gazzard BG, Henderson JM, Williams R. Early changes in coagulation following a paracetamol overdose and a controlled trial of fresh frozen plasma therapy. Gut 1975; 16:617–620.

432. Manuccio PM, Canciani MT, Rota L, Donavan BS. Response of factor VIII von Willebrand's factor to DDAVP in healthy subjects and patients with haemophilia A and von Willebrand's disease. Br J Haematol 1981; 47:282–293.

433. Agnelli G, DeCunto M, Berritini M, Nenci GG. Desmopressin improvement of abnormal coagulation in chronic liver disease. Lancet 1983; i:645.

434. Mannucci PM, Vicente V, Vianello L, Cattaneo M, Alberca I, Coccato MP, Faioni E, Mari D. Controlled trial of desmopressin in liver cirrhosis and other conditions associated with a prolonged bleeding time. Blood 1985; 67:1148–1153.

435. Burroughs AK, Matthews K, Qadiri M, Thomas N, Kernoff P, Tuddenham E, McIntyre N. Desmopressin and bleeding time in patients with cirrhosis. Br Med J 1985; 1377–1381.

436. Braude P, Arias J, Hughes RD, Canalese J, Gimson AES, Williams R, Scully MF, Kakkar VV. Antithrombin III infusion during fulminant hepatic failure. (Abstract) Thromb Haemost 1981; 46:369.

437. Burghard R, Leititis JU, Rossi R, Egbring R, Brandis M. Treatment

438. of severe coagulation disturbances as a condition of improved prognosis in fulminant liver failure. Arch Dis Child 1985; 60:167–170.

438. Fujiwara K, Okita K, Akamatsu K, Abe H, Tameda Y, Sakai T, Inoue N, Kanai K, Aoki N, Oka H. Treatment with antithrombin III concentrate in fulminant hepatic failure. (Abstract) Hepatology 1987; 7:1067.

439. Perez GO, Oster JR. A critical review of the role of dialysis in the treatment of liver disease. In: Epstein M, ed. The kidney in liver disease, New York: Elsevier, 1978: 325.

440. LeVeen H, Christoudias G, Moon IP, Luft R, Falk G, Grosberg S. Peritoneovenous shunting for ascites. Ann Surg 1974; 180:580–591.

441. Grosberg SJ, Wapnick S. A retrospective comparison of functional renal failure in cirrhosis treated by conventional therapy or the peritoneovenous shunt (LeVeen). Am J Med Sci 1978; 276:281–291.

442. Kinney MJ, Schneider A, Wapnick S, Grosberg S, LeVeen H. The "hepatorenal" syndrome and refractory ascites: successful therapy with LeVeen-type peritoneal-venous shunt and valve. Nephron 1979; 23:228–232.

443. Epstein M. Peritoneovenous shunt in the management of ascites and the hepatorenal syndrome. Gastroenterology 1982; 82:790–799.

444. Pladson TR, Parrish RM. Hepatorenal syndrome: recovery after peritoneovenous shunt. Arch Intern Med 1977; 137:1248–1249.

445. Schwartz ML, Vogel SB. Treatment of hepatorenal syndrome. Am J Surg 1980; 139:370–373.

446. Schroeder ET, Anderson GH Jr, Smulyan H. Effects of a portacaval or peritoneovenous shunt on renin in the hepatorenal syndrome. Kidney Int 1979; 15:54–61.

447. Leveen HH, Wapnick S, Grosberj S, Kinney MJ. Further experience with peritoneo-venous shunt for ascites. Ann Surg 1976; 184:574–581.

448. Greig PD, Langer B, Blendis LM, Taylor BR, Glynn MFX. Complications after peritoneovenous shunting for ascites. Am J Surg 1980; 139:125–131.

449. Harmon DC, Demirjian Z, Ellman L, Fischer JE. Disseminated intravascular coagulation with the peritoneo-venous shunt. Ann Intern Med 1979; 90:774–776.

450. Altman RP, Cavett CM. The retroperitoneal approach for peritoneovenous shunting in infants and small children. J Pediatr Surg 1981; 16:965–966.

451. Gillam GL, Stokes KB, McLennan J, Smith AL. Fulminant hepatic failure with intractable ascites due to an echovirus eleven infection successfully managed with a peritoneo-venous (LeVeen) shunt. J Pediatr Gastroenterol Nutr 1986; 5:476–480.

452. Guttman FM, Montapet P, Bloss RS. Experience with peritoneo-venous shunting for congenital chylous ascites in infants and children. J Pediatr Surg 1982; 17:368–372.

453. Man DWK, Spitz L. The management of chylous ascites in children. J Pediatr Surg 1985; 20:72–75.

454. Campbell PJ, Leung WM, Logan AG, Debowski TE, Skorecki KL, Blendis LM. Effect of alpha-H atrionatriuretic peptide infusion in sodium retaining cirrhotic patients. (Abstract) Hepatology 1987; 7:1029.

455. Ganger DR, Gottstein J, Blei AT. Hemodynamic and renal effects of atrial natriuretic peptide in portal hypertensive rats. Potentiation by vasopressin. (Abstract) Hepatology 1987; 7:1029.

456. Bernardi M, DePalma R, Trevisani F, Santini C, Patrone D, Motta R, Servadei D, Gasbarrini G. Effects of a new loop diuretic (muzolimine) in cirrhosis with ascites: comparison with furosemide. Hepatology 1986; 6:400–405.

457. Gines P, Arroyo V, Quintero E, Planas R, Bory F, Cabrera J, Rimola A, Viver J, Camps J, Jimenez W, Mastai R, Gaya J, Rodes J. Comparison of paracentesis and diuretics in the treatment of cirrhotics with tense ascites. Gastroenterology 1987; 93:234–241.

458. Pinto PC, Amerian J, Reynolds TB. Large volume paracentesis in nonedematous patients with tense ascites: its effect on intravascular volume. Hepatology 1988; 8:207–210.

459. Gines P, Tito L, Arroyo V, Planas R, Panes J, Viver J, Torres M, Humbert P, Rimola PO, Llach J, Badalamenti S, Jimenez W, Gaya J, Rodes J. Randomized comparative study of therapeutic paracentesis with and without intravenous albumin in cirrhosis. Gastroenterology 1988; 94:1493–1502.

460. Simon DM, McCain JR, Bonkovsky HL, Wells JO, Hartle DK, Galambos JT. Effects of therapeutic paracentesis on systemic and hepatic hemodynamics and on renal hormonal function. Hepatology 1987; 7:423–429.

461. Chang TMS. Haemoperfusions over microencapsulated adsorbent in a patient with hepatic coma. Lancet 1972; ii:1371–1372.

462. Chang TMS. Experimental artificial liver support with emphasis on fulminant hepatic failure: concepts and review. Semin Liver Dis 1986; 6:148–158.

463. Gazzard BG, Weston MJ, Murray-Lyon IM, Flax H, Record CO, Portmann B, Langley PG, Dunlop EH, Mellon PJ, Ward MB, Williams R. Charcoal haemoperfusion in the treatment of fulminant hepatic failure. Lancet 1974; i:1301–1307.

464. Williams R. Trials and tribulations with artificial liver support. Gut 1978; 19:578–583.

465. Hughes RD, Williams R. Clinical experience with charcoal and resin hemoperfusion. Semin Liver Dis 1986; 6:164–173.

466. Gimson AES, Langley PG, Hughes RD, Canelese J, Mellon PJ, Williams R, Woods HF, Weston MJ. Prostacyclin to prevent platelet activation during charcoal haemoperfusion in fulminant hepatic failure. Lancet 1980; i:173–175.

467. Winikoff S, Glassman MS, Spivak G. Plasmapheresis in a patient with hepatic failure awaiting liver transplantation. J Pediatr 1985; 107:547–549.

468. Gimson AES, Braude S, Mellon PJ, Canalese J, Williams R. Earlier charcoal haemoperfusion in fulminant hepatic failure. Lancet 1982; ii:681–683.

469. Takahashi Y. Acute hepatic failure-in special relation to treatment. Jpn J Med 1983; 22:140–145.

470. Berk PD, Goldberg JD. Charcoal hemoperfusion. Plus ca change, plus c'est la meme chose. Gastroenterology 1988; 94:1228–1230.

471. Toledo-Pereyra LH. Role of activated carbon hemoperfusion in the recovery of livers exposed to ischemic damage. Arch Surg 1985; 120:462–465.

472. Toledo-Pereyra LH. Utilization of activated carbon hemoperfusion to assist recovery of ischemically damaged liver allografts. Artif Organs 1985; 9:243–249.

473. Peleman RR, Gavaler JS, Van Thiel DH, Esquival C, Gordon R, Iwatsaki S, Starzl TE. Orthotopic liver transplantation for acute and subacute hepatic failure in adults. Hepatology 1987; 7:484–489.

474. Bismuth H, Didier S, Gugenheim J, Castaing D, Bernuau J, Rueff B, Benhamou JP. Emergency liver transplantation for fulminant hepatitis. Ann Intern Med 1987; 107:337–341.

475. Brems JJ, Hiatt JR, Ramming KP. Fulminant hepatic failure: the role of liver transplantation as primary therapy. Am J Surg 1987; 154:137–140.

476. Ringe B, Pichmayr R, Lauchart W, Muller R. Indications and results of liver transplantation in acute hepatic failure. Transplant Proc 1986; 18:86–88.

477. Shaw BW, Wood RP, Kaufman SS, Williams L, Antonson DL, Vanderhoof J. Liver transplantation therapy for children: Part I. J Pediatr Gastroenterol Nutr 1988; 7:157–166.

478. Terpstra OT, Schalm SW, Weimar W, Willemse PJA, Baumgartner D, Groenland THN, Tenkate FWJ, Porte RJ, DeRaye S, Reuvers CB, Stribbe J, Terpstra JL. Auxiliary partial liver transplantation for end-stage chronic liver disease. N Engl J Med 1988; 319:1507–1511.

479. deHemptinne B, deVille DeGoyet J, Kestens PJ, Otte JB. Volume reduction of the liver graft before orthotopic transplantation: report of a clinical experience in 11 cases. Transplant Proc 1987; 19:3317–3322.

480. Starzl TE, Francavilla A, Porter KA, Benichou J, Jones AF. The effect of splanchnic viscera removal upon canine liver regeneration. Surg Gynecol Obstet 1973; 147:193–207.

481. Farivar M, Wands JR, Isselbacher KJ, Buchera NLR. Effect of pancreatic hormones on fulminant murine hepatitis. N Engl J Med 1976; 295:1517–1520.

482. Bucher NLF, Swaffield MN. Regeneration of liver in rats in the absence of portal splanchnic organs and a portal blood supply. Cancer Res 1973; 33:3189–3194.

483. Leffert HL, Koch KS, Moran T, Rubalcava B. Hormonal control of rat liver regeneration. Gastroenterology 1979; 76:1470–1482.

484. Gregory H. In vivo aspects of urogastrone-epidermal growth factor. J Cell Sci (suppl) 1985; 3:11–17.

485. Olsen PS, Boesby S, Kirkegaard P, Therkelsen K, Almdal T, Poulsen SS, Nexo E. Influence of epidermal growth factor on liver regeneration after partial hepatectomy in rats. Hepatology 1988; 8:992–996.

486. LaPlante-O'Neill P, Baumgartner D, Lewis WI, Zweber BA, Sutherland DER. Free supernatant from hepatocyte cultures improves survival of rats with chemically induced acute liver failure. J Surg Res 1982; 32:347–359.

487. LaBrecque Dr, Pesch LA. Preparation and partial characterization of hepatic regenerative stimulator substance (SS) from rat liver. J Physiol 1975; 248:273–284.

488. Starzl TE, Terblanch J, Porter KA, Jones AF, Usui S, Mazzoni G. Growth stimulating factor in regenerating canine liver. Lancet 1979; i:127–130.

489. Francavilla A, DiLeo A, Polimeno L, Gavaler J, Pelicci R, Todo S, Kam I, Prelich J, Makowka L, Starzl TE. The effect of hepatic stimulatory substance, isolated from regenerating hepatic cytosol, and 50,000 and 300,000 subfractions in enhancing survival in experimental acute hepatic failure in rats treated with D-galactosamine. Hepatology 1986; 6:1346–1351.

490. Bumgardner GL, Fasola C, Sutherland DER. Prospects for hepatocyte transplantation. Hepatology 1988; 8:1158–1161.

491. Demetriou AA, Reisner A, Sanchez J, Levenson SM, Moscioni AD, Chowdhury JR. Transplantation of micro carrier-attached hepatocytes into 90% partially hepatectomized rats. Hepatology 1988; 8:1006–1009.

492. Tygstrup N, Ranek L. Assessment of prognosis in fulminant hepatic failure. Semin Liver Dis 1986; 6:129–137.

493. Bernuau J, Goudeau A, Poynard T, Dubois F, Lesage G, Yvonnet B, Degott C, Bezeaud A, Rueff B, Benhamou JP. Multivariate analysis of prognostic factors in fulminant hepatitis B. Hepatology 1986; 6:648–651.

494. Karvountzis GG, Redeker AG. Relation of alpha-fetoprotein in acute hepatitis to severity and prognosis. Ann Intern Med 1974; 80:156–160.

495. Murray-Lyon IM, Orr AH, Gazzard B, Kohn J, Williams R. Prognostic value of serum alpha-fetoprotein in fulminant hepatic failure including patients treated by charcoal hemoperfusion. Gut 1976; 17:576–580.

496. Henderson JM, Kutner MH, Bain RP. First-order clearance of plasma galactose: the effect of liver disease. Gastroenterology 1982; 83:1090–1095.

497. Ranek L, Buch Andreason P, Tygstrup N. Galactose elimination capacity as a prognostic index in patients with fulminant liver failure. Gut 1976; 17:959–964.

498. Schneider JF, Baker AL, Haines NW. Aminopyrine N-demethylation: a prognostic test of liver function in patients with alcoholic liver disease. Gastroenterology 1980; 79:1145–1150.

499. Bremmelgard A, Ranek L, Bahnsen M, Buch Andreason P, Christensen E. Cholic acid conjugation test and quantitative liver function in acute liver failure. Scand J Gastroenterol 1983; 18:797–802.

500. Davis MA, Peters RL, Redeker AG, Reynolds TB. Appraisal of the mortality in acute fulminant viral hepatitis. N Engl J Med 1968; 278:1248–1253.

501. Bihari D, Gimson A, Lindridge J, Williams R. Lactic acidosis in fulminant hepatic failure—some aspects of pathogenesis and prognosis. J Hepatol 1985; 1:405–416.

502. Scotto J, Opolon P, Eteve J, et al. Liver biopsy and prognosis in acute liver failure. Gut 1973; 14:927–933.

503. Maddrey WC, Friedman LS, Munoz SJ, Hahn EG. Selection of the patient for liver transplantation and timing of surgery. In: Maddrey WC, ed. Transplantation of the liver. New York: Elsevier, 1988: 23.

504. Malatack JJ, Schaid DJ, Urbach AH, Gartner JC, Zitelli BJ, Rockette H, Fischer J, Starzl TE, Iwatsuki S, Shaw BW. Choosing a pediatric recipient for orthotopic liver transplantation. J Pediatr 1987; 111:479.

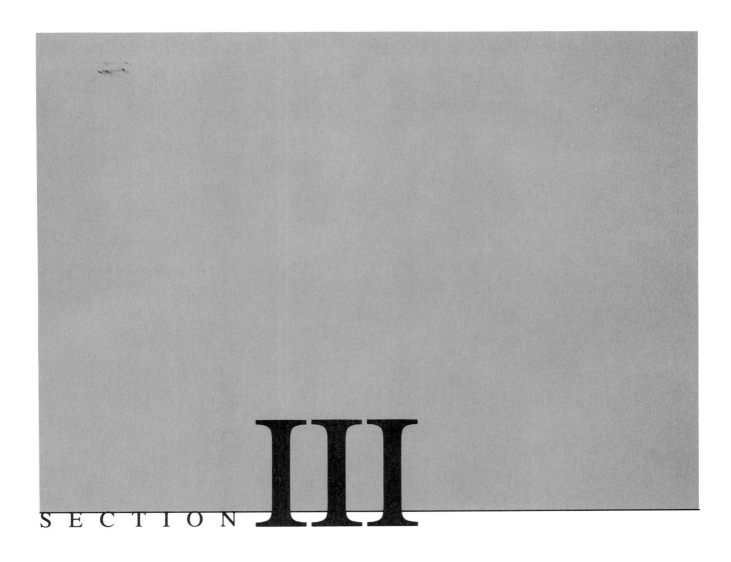

SECTION III

Development of Gastrointestinal Tract and Accessory Organs

CHAPTER 13

Anatomy and Embryology

Lawrence T. Weaver, M.A., M.D., M.R.C.P., D.C.H.

The newborn infant is a free-living organism contained within a continuous epithelium. That of endodermal origin gives rise to the lining of the gastrointestinal (GI) tract, and in terms of its surface area it represents the major interface between the organism and the environment. The human gut develops largely in utero and results in an alimentary system ready to meet the demands of extrauterine nutrition at birth.

The human GI tract has digestive, absorptive, secretory, and barrier functions, and it is also an endocrine organ and a part of the immunologic system. Its basic structure is common to all mammalian species and was achieved first by primitive chordates more than 400 million years ago. As a tube extending from mouth to anus it may be divided into three parts, each with a separate blood supply: the foregut (buccal cavity, pharynx, esophagus, stomach, and proximal duodenum) is supplied by the celiac axis; the midgut (distal duodenum, jejunum, ileum, cecum, appendix, and proximal colon) is supplied by the superior mesenteric artery; and the hindgut (distal colon and rectum) is supplied by the inferior mesenteric artery. The salivary glands, liver, gallbladder, and pancreas are outgrowths of the foregut and midgut.

In this chapter the embryology, development, and morphology of the GI tract are outlined. The topographic anatomy of the gut is not described in detail here; it may be found in a textbook of human anatomy,[1] and anatomy pertaining to particular developmental defects is discussed in the chapters on congenital anomalies. The anatomy and embryology of the liver and biliary system are covered in Chapter 22. This chapter concentrates on the functional morphology of the human gut during intrauterine and extrauterine life.

The gut of the newborn infant is adapted for the utilization of a peculiar diet—colostrum and milk. The factors regulating GI development and those involved in the transition from intrauterine to extrauterine nutrition will be discussed.

EMBRYOLOGY AND DEVELOPMENT

Stages of Gut Development

The development of the GI tract may be divided into six stages according to the major anatomic and functional events that take place between conception and maturity.

The first phase of organogenesis, soon after formation of the embryonic disc, is followed by a "chemo-architectural" phase of epithelium formation, during which the basic structure of the gut is formed. During the third phase, that of differentiation, the appearance of distinct epithelial and mesothelial cell types occurs. This is followed by a phase of maturation, during which the gut prepares for its extrauterine tasks. Birth heralds a neonatal phase of GI adaptation to the demands of enteral nutrition. Development is concluded by a weaning phase of transition from milk to solid diet. The early phases in the development of the human GI tract are summarized in Tables 1 and 2.

The Gut as a Tube

The human gut is formed from the endodermal layer of the embryo by the incorporation of the dorsal part of the yolk sac during infolding of the embryonic disc (Fig. 1). This is supported by somatic and splanchnic mesoderm. Identifiable by the fourth week after conception as a tube 4 mm long extending from mouth to cloaca, it elongates 1,000-fold by

TABLE 1
Stages in the Morphologic Development
of Human Gastrointestinal Tract in Weeks
After Conception

Weeks	Stage
2–3	Infolding of endodermal layer of embryo occurs to form primitive gut in continuity with yolk sac.
3.5	Foregut and hindgut are distinct. Liver bud is present.
4	Intestine is tubular with short esophagus, fusiform gastric and cecal swellings. Pancreatic buds are present.
5	Intestine lengthens into loop. Dorsal and ventral pancreatic buds fuse.
6	Stomach rotates. Duodenum and splenic flexure of colon become fixed. Midgut rotation begins.
7	Vacuolation of esophagus occurs. Stomach assumes final position.
	Pancreas is formed.
	Midgut herniates into umbilical cord, lengthens, and rotates.
8	Restoration of patency of small intestine occurs, with appearance of muscle layers.
9	Small intestinal villi appear with columnar epithelium.
10	Midgut returns to coelomic cavity. Crypts and gastric pits appear.
11	Villi are present throughout the intestine.
12	Colonic haustra and circular folds appear.
13	Cecum dilates and begins descent to right iliac fossa.
14	Pylorus and fundus of stomach are defined.
15	Brunner's glands present in duodenum.
18	Muscularis mucosae is clearly seen in small intestine. Peyer's patches are first seen.
20	Mature anatomic position of gut is achieved and mesenteric attachments are complete.

TABLE 2
Cellular Differentiation of Human
Gastrointestinal Tract in Weeks
After Conception

Weeks	Stage
5	Multilayered epithelium is present throughout gut.
7	Epithelium is stratified. Duodenum is temporarily occluded.
8	Villous ridges are present. Epithelium becomes columnar and enterocytes have short, irregular microvilli and terminal web. Neuroblasts are present. Circular muscle layer of small and large intestine appears.
9	Pancreatic cells bud. Goblet cells and subepithelial lymphocytes are seen. Auerbach's plexus is identifiable.
10	Esophageal epithelium ciliated. Gastric pits and small intestinal crypts are present. Enterocytes have developed microvilli and glycocalyx. Goblet and enteroendocrine cells are present. Apical tubular system is present in small intestine. Muscularis mucosae of stomach appears.
11	Entire small intestine is lined by simple columnar epithelium. Intraepithelial lymphocytes are seen.
12	Chief, parietal, and gastric neck cells are present in stomach. Pancreatic acini and islets appear. Longitudinal muscle is present in small intestine.
13	Meissner's plexus is present in small intestine.
14	Brunner's glands and M cells are present.
15	Paneth cells are clearly seen.
16	Lymphopoiesis is observed.
22	Apical tubular system disappears.
24	Zymogen cells are present in pancreas. Ganglion cells are present in rectum.
25	Stratified squamous epithelium is present in esophagus.
28	Esophageal glands are seen.

full term, generating a gut of total length between three and seven times the crown-to-heel length, and a small intestine six times the length of the large.[2,3]

At birth gastric volume is about 30 ml. The esophagus is about 10 cm long, with a diameter of 0.5 cm at full term, after which it grows by approximately 0.65 cm per year to

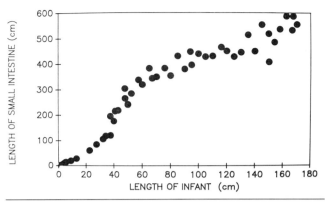

FIGURE 2 Small intestinal length from conception to maturity. (Data from several sources.[2–6,27])

an adult length of about 25 cm. The third trimester is the period of maximal rate of growth, when the gut doubles in length, the small intestine increasing 2.4-fold and the large bowel 2.1-fold.[4] The small intestine is approximately 250 to 300 cm at term. To its length at birth is added another 2 to 3 meters during growth to adulthood (Fig. 2).[5,6] The large intestine is 30 to 40 cm at birth, growing to 1.5 to 2 meters in adult life. The thickness of both the mucosa and entire GI wall increases during postnatal life.

The epithelial surface area of the mature GI tract is increased some 300 times by gastric rugae; the small intestinal valvulae connivantes; villi and crypts that project into the lumen and penetrate the lamina propria; large intestinal plicae semilunares; and microvilli that coat the luminal surfaces of the epithelial cells (Fig. 3). Between the tenth and fourteenth weeks the villi acquire a typical finger shape, with a proximodistal gradient of morphogenesis[7]; from 26 to 34 weeks both finger- and tongue-shaped villi may be identified; and thereafter a mixture of finger-, tongue-, and leaf-shaped villi are found.[8]

Amniotic Fluid

During intrauterine life the fetus is suspended in amniotic fluid. This is thought to be initially a dialysate of fetal and maternal plasma. Continuity of the gut lumen with the amniotic cavity is achieved when the buccopharyngeal membrane ruptures during the third week and the cloacal membrane during the seventh, establishing free circulation of amniotic fluid through the gastrointestinal tract. The vitello-intestinal duct closes by the fifth week.[9]

During the second half of pregnancy fetal urine is the main contributor to the volume of amniotic fluid, which is removed largely by fetal swallowing. Fluid volume rises steadily during gestation to about 700 ml at term.[10] Fetal swallowing, intestinal motility, and defecation are detectable in the second trimester, and by term the fetus ingests approximately 300 ml of amniotic fluid per day.[11] The fetal GI tract is therefore exposed to the constant passage of amniotic fluid throughout the greater part of its intrauterine development. The part played by amniotic fluid in intrauterine development is discussed at the end of this chapter.

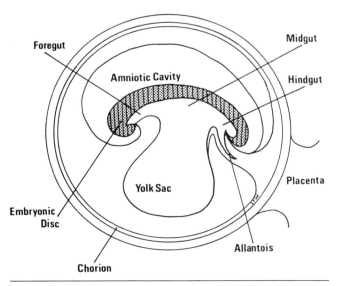

FIGURE 1 Diagram of median section of 3-week embryo showing primitive gut.

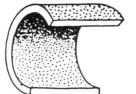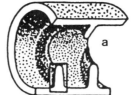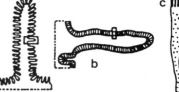

FIGURE 3 Diagram of the gut as a tube showing contributions to surface area of the small intestine by valvulae connivantes (*a*), villi (*b*), and microvilli (*c*).

Esophagus

The esophagus develops from the embryonic foregut by an anterior narrowing of the pharynx where the tracheal bud arises. It may be distinguished from the developing stomach by 4 weeks, after which it elongates rapidly, primarily by cranial extension of its proximal end.[9]

At 5 weeks the esophageal epithelium is bilayered. The lumen of the esophagus becomes vacuolated at 7 weeks, when longitudinal channels develop and its diameter increases. It is ciliated at 10 weeks, but a stratified squamous epithelium does not appear until the twenty-fifth week. Esophageal glands make their appearance at 28 weeks. Occasional neuroblasts are seen along the inner surface of the circular muscle at 5 weeks, but longitudinal muscle is not visible until 8 weeks. Myenteric plexuses demonstrate anticholinesterase reactivity by 10 weeks, and ganglion cells are differentiated by 13 weeks. By this time the muscularis mucosae is well formed. The upper third of the esophagus is supported by striated muscle, the middle third by mixed, and the lower third by smooth muscle at birth.[12]

Stomach

The stomach is identifiable by 4 weeks as a fusiform dilatation of the gut tube near the cranial pole of the embryo, between the lung buds and the pancreatic and hepatic buds. It descends to its infradiaphragmatic position by 7 weeks and broadens ventrodorsally (Figs. 4 and 5). Growth is maximal on the dorsal aspect, creating the greater curvature. At 6 weeks a 90-degree clockwise rotation places the greater curve to the left and the lesser curve to the right, with the left vagus nerve supplying the anterior wall and the right vagus nerve the posterior wall. The stomach attains its final anatomic position by 7 weeks, with the greater curve facing inferiorly and to the left and the lesser curve superiorly and to the right. The pylorus leads to the duodenum, which by this time is fixed to the posterior wall.[9]

Smooth muscle development follows a craniocaudal sequence. The circular muscles appear first during the ninth week and the longitudinal muscles soon thereafter. By the third month the pylorus is identified by its thicker musculature and pyloric glands. The muscularis mucosae differentiates first in the cardia at 10 weeks and extends to the body by the seventeenth week and to the pylorus by the eighteenth week.[12]

Parietal and enteroendocrine cells are identifiable at 10 weeks by their histochemical succinic dehydrogenase and argyrophil staining. At 12 weeks chief cells are identifiable by their abundant RNA and zymogen granules. Mucous neck cells, which appear first at this time, produce mucus by the sixteenth week. By the end of the first trimester the gastric epithelium has differentiated into pits and glands whose cells produce pepsin, hydrochloric acid, gastrin, intrinsic factor, and renin. Enzyme activity is maximal in the fundus.

Pancreas

Two diverticula of the foregut are identifiable by the fourth week of gestation. A larger dorsal bud appears first and grows rapidly toward the dorsal mesentery. A smaller ventral bud develops distally, near the insertion of the common bile duct into the duodenum. Owing to rapid growth of the foregut, the ventral bud and common bile duct rotate posterior to the duodenum and then fuse with the dorsal bud (Fig. 4). The dorsal bud forms most of the body of the pancreas, while the uncinate process and inferior part of the head of the pancreas are derived from the ventral bud. At approximately 6 weeks the ducts of each bud fuse: the main pancreatic duct (of Wirsung) is formed from the ducts of the ventral bud and the distal part of the dorsal bud, while the upper portion of

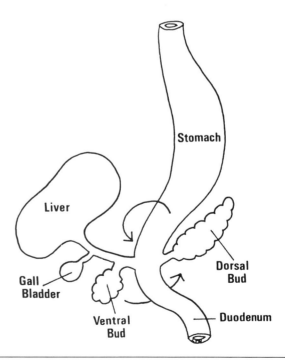

FIGURE 4 Diagram showing development of the pancreas. The dorsal and ventral buds are shown just before rotation and fusion at 5 weeks.

the head is drained by the remaining part of the dorsal duct or accessory pancreatic duct (of Santorini). By the seventh week the final form of the pancreas has been achieved.[9]

At about this time the pancreas consists of tubules with blunt ends. Pancreatic acini arise from these blind ends during the twelfth week of gestation. The acini are initially solid, but each eventually develops a lumen lined with an epithelium of cells containing zymogen granules by 20 weeks. Clumps of cells around the blunt ends are identifiable by 13 weeks as argyrophilic precursors of alpha cells. These predominate over beta and delta cells until late gestation, when the beta cells predominate.[12]

Small Intestine

Embryology and Development

The small intestine is derived from the fetal midgut and may be divided into (1) a cranial limb extending from the opening of the biliary tree to the point where it communicates with the yolk sac via the vitelline duct and (2) a caudal limb extending to the mid-transverse colon. As early as the fourth week of gestation the duodenum is recognizable by its association with the stomach, pancreas, and liver, and the cecum as a bulge in the proximal portion of the caudal limb (Fig. 5A).[9]

By the sixth week fixation of the duodenum and splenic flexure of the colon to the posterior abdominal wall by mesenteric bands has occurred. This is followed by rapid lengthening of the midgut, accompanied by considerable increase in the size of the liver, which occupies the greater part of the abdominal cavity at this time. Accommodation for the developing gut is found within the umbilical cord (extraembryonic coelom), where it undergoes a 270-degree counterclockwise rotation around an axis formed by the superior mesenteric artery. Continuity with the yolk sac via the vitellointestinal duct is lost (Fig. 5B). The vitelline vessels contribute to the portal and hepatic veins after the disappearance of the yolk sac.[9]

The jejunum returns to the abdominal cavity first, filling the left side, followed by the ileum and cecum, which settle in the right side, by the twelfth week. Thereafter the cecum dilates and descends into the right iliac fossa, and the small intestine fills the abdomen, suspended from its mesentery with roots running from the ligament of Treitz to the ileocecal junction. The final anatomic position of the GI tract is achieved by the twentieth week.[1,9]

Histiogenesis and Cytodifferentiation

Differentiation of the endoderm and its neighboring mesoderm into the epithelial, submucosal, muscular, and serosal layers of the gastrointestinal tract proceeds in a proximodistal direction.

Mucosa. The gut is lined initially by a stratified epithelium about four cells deep. Between the eighth and tenth weeks of gestation this is replaced by a columnar epithelium, first in the duodenum and then in the jejunum and ileum.

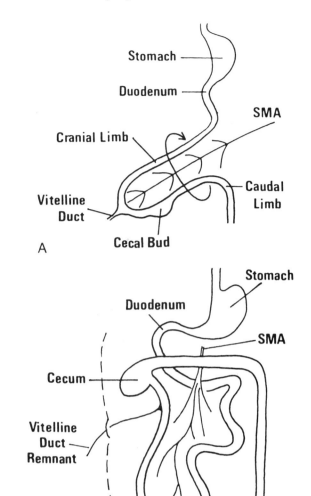

FIGURE 5 Diagram of rotation and elongation of midgut during intrauterine development. *A*, Intestinal loop before counterclockwise rotation around superior mesenteric artery (SMA) at 6 to 7 weeks. *B*, Arrangement of gut within the abdomen by 12 weeks, prior to descent of cecum to right iliac fossa.

The patency of the duodenum, occluded by rapid proliferation of stratified epithelial cells, is restored by the formation of coalescing vacuoles. This occurs pari passu with the first appearance of villi and crypts[7] (Fig. 6). Villus formation commences at 9 weeks of gestation, proceeding distally so that by 11 weeks the entire intestine is lined by short villi with a simple columnar epithelium (Fig. 7). Development of crypts also proceeds in a craniocaudal direction. These appear first at 10 to 11 weeks gestation as epithelial outgrowths into the mesenchyme between newly formed villi[13] (Fig. 8).

The simple columnar epithelial cells lining the newly formed villi of the 10- to 12-week fetus have short regular microvilli, a partially developed glycocalyx, large supranuclear and infranuclear glycogen deposits, and moderately

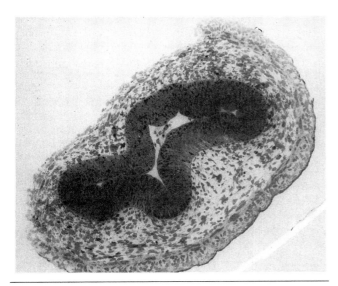

FIGURE 6 Proximal small intestine of 9-week fetus lined by stratified epithelium of undifferentiated enterocytes (1 μm epoxy section, Richardson's stain, ×200). (Reproduced with permission of Pamela C. Colony, formerly P.C. Moxey.)

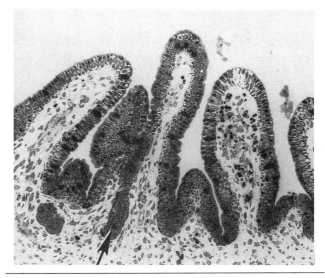

FIGURE 8 Proximal intestine of 11- to 12-week fetus showing developing crypts (*arrow*) that extend from the base of the villi into the lamina propria (1 μm epoxy section, Richardson's stain, ×150). (Reproduced with permission of Pamela C. Colony, formerly P.C. Moxey.)

well-developed Golgi complexes and mitochondria (Fig. 9). A terminal web is seen by 8 weeks, but the core filaments are less dense than in mature enterocytes. Desmosomes are present, but the zonulae occludens and adherens of the mature junctional complex are not visible until the eleventh week. Mitotic figures are frequently seen.[12] By the time the cecum has become fixed in the right lower quadrant the villi and crypts are well developed and the muscularis mucosae is present (Fig. 10).

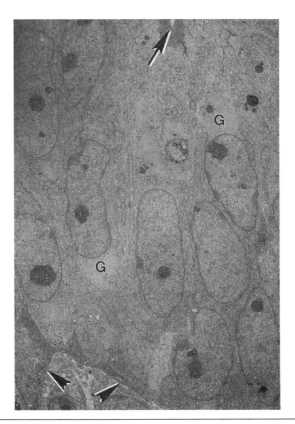

FIGURE 9 Electron micrograph of the proximal intestine of a 9- to 10-week fetus showing undifferentiated epithelial cells characteristic of this age. The large nucleus has one or more prominent nucleoli, and the cytoplasm is characterized by abundant free ribosomes, small mitochondria, and glycogen (G) deposits. The lumen is indicated by the arrow and the basal lamina by the arrowheads (×3,000). (Reproduced with permission of Pamela C. Colony, formerly P.C. Moxey.)

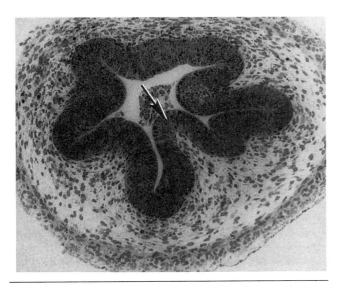

FIGURE 7 Proximal intestine of 9- to 10-week fetus showing the presumptive formation of a villus (*arrow*). Note the darkly staining glycogen deposits within the epithelial cells (1 μm epoxy section, Richardson's stain, ×200). (Reproduced with permission of Pamela C. Colony, formerly P.C. Moxey.)

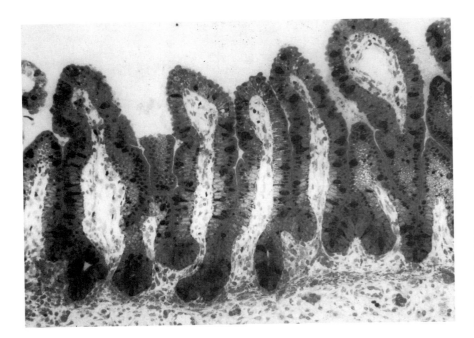

FIGURE 10 Villi and crypts of 22-week fetus. Both villi and crypts are well developed. Note the presence of the muscularis mucosae (1 μm epoxy section, Richardson's stain, ×270). (Reproduced with permission of Pamela C. Colony, formerly P.C. Moxey.)

Electron-dense lysosomal elements, vesicles, and corpuscles are visible in the apical cytoplasm of enterocytes from the tenth week. These appear to contain material ingested from the lumen by pinocytosis[14–16] and represent components of an apical tubular system (ATS) and meconium corpuscle system (MCS). The ATS is characterized by apical invaginations and tubules that resemble those of the ileum of newborn rats. The MCS is also present in the apical cytoplasm of villus enterocytes and consists of vesicles and vacuoles containing lysosomal enzymes. These systems undergo considerable differentiation during the second trimester, reaching maximal development, especially in the distal small intestine, around the twentieth week (Fig. 11). They are still present at term in some primates,[17] and it has been suggested that they are homologous with those involved in macromolecular uptake in some suckling rodents.[18]

Further differentiation of the epithelium occurs with the appearance of enteroendocrine and goblet cells at 9 to 10 weeks.[19] The former have large nuclei and abundant free ribosomes, little formed endoplasmic reticulum, many small mitochondria, and secretory granules. They are probably the precursors of the wide range of endocrine cells found in the mature GI epithelium. Their endodermal or neuroectodermal origin is unresolved. Both immature goblet cells, with small secretory granules and short strands of dilated rough endoplasmic reticulum, and mature goblet cells, with large secretory granules and well-developed Golgi complexes and abundant rough endoplasmic reticulum, are identifiable.[13]

Undifferentiated crypt cells are visible, with the formation of crypts in both the proximal and distal intestine. They are morphologically immature, with large elongate basal nuclei, abundant free ribosomes, moderately well-developed Golgi complexes, and little formed endoplasmic reticulum. Glycogen deposits, an abundance of lysosomes, and reduced size and number of secretory granules further distinguish them from mature crypt cells. Paneth cells appear first in the early part of the second trimester. They contain long strands of rough endoplasmic reticulum, well-developed Golgi complexes, and secretory granules of variable number.[13]

In the proximal intestine the crypt bases are continuous, with glandular extensions into the lamina propria resembling Brunner's glands. They are first seen at 14 to 15 weeks' gestation and are lined with simple columnar cells resembling adult secretory cells. Tuft (caveolated) cells are noted first at 16 weeks' gestation by the presence within the supranuclear region of bundles of dense filaments extending from the microvillous cores, filamentous cytoplasm, and apical multivesicular bodies. Their function is unknown.[13]

Interspersed with the columnar enterocytes, M cells are first noted in the ileum, restricted to the dome epithelium overlying aggregations of lymphocytes. The cytoplasm of these cells is attenuated to form a thin "membrane" between intestinal lumen and underlying lymphoid cells. The apical plasma membrane consists of irregular microfolds overlying a cytoplasm abundant with vesicles that appear to be involved in the uptake and transcellular transport of luminal macromolecules.[20] The appearance of M cells is coincident with the initial formation of Peyer's patches: Although lymphocytes appear in the lamina propria late in the first trimester, aggregates are not seen until 16 to 18 weeks.

Subepithelium. The lamina propria and outer layers of the GI tract are of mesenchymal origin. Interaction between mesenchymal and epithelial cells may be central to the control of proliferation and differentiation of the mucosa both pre- and postnatally.[21] In the previllous stage the mesenchyme is dense and exhibits intense metachromasia. Lymphocytes are detectable in the subepithelium from 8 weeks and within the epithelium at 11 weeks.[22] These lymphocytes are capable of a proliferative response to mitogens by 12 weeks. Lymphopoiesis is detected by 15 weeks and Peyer's patches soon after. Although plasma cells have not been observed, IgA has been detected in fetal intestine by 11 weeks.[23] The development of immune function is described in Chapter 20.

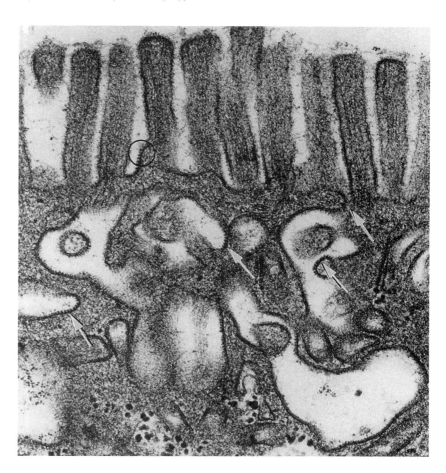

FIGURE 11 Photomicrograph of the apex of an enterocyte from a 17- to 18-week fetus showing the specialized apical tubular system (ATS). Note the ordered array of particles on the inner membrane of some elements of the ATS (*arrows*) and on the apical plasma membrane at the base of a microvillus (ringed). (From Moxey and Trier.[16] Reproduced with permission of P.C. Colony [formerly P.C. Moxey] and J.S. Trier and Alan R. Liss Inc.)

The muscularis mucosae develops from aggregates of mesenchymal cells near the bases of crypts between 17 and 20 weeks (see Fig. 10).[13] The development of the muscular coat is noted first at 6 weeks, followed by the appearance of a circular muscle layer in the proximal small intestine. By the eighth week this layer extends along the whole small intestine, and the longitudinal muscle layer is noted for the first time.[12]

Neuroblasts are visible in the midgut by 7 weeks. The autonomic plexuses of Auerbach and Meissner appear at 9 and 13 weeks, respectively, soon after which peristalsis may be detected. The vascular supply to the midgut is identifiable as thin-walled vessels within the subepithelial tissues by 9 weeks. These project into the developing villi and anastomose with vessels continuous with the superior mesenteric artery and vein and portal lymphatics.[9,12]

Large Intestine

The large intestine is derived from the distal portion of the midgut and the hindgut. The cecum is identified as a bulge in the proximal portion of the caudal limb of the midgut by the end of the fourth week (see Fig. 5A). During rotation and return of the midgut to the abdominal cavity between the sixth and twelfth weeks, the cecum and appendix come to lie in the right lower quadrant and the remaining hindgut in the left side (see Fig. 5B). As the liver decreases in size, the ascending colon and hepatic flexures become distinct from the transverse colon. The dorsal peritoneum of the ascending and descending colon fuses with the posterior abdominal wall, leaving these two parts of the large intestine in a retroperitoneal location. The dorsal mesentery of the transverse and sigmoid colon persists. The rectum is derived from the cloaca and assumes continuity with the digestive tube by the eighth week.[9]

Haustra and taeniae appear between the second and third months and extend from the cecum to the rectum. The circular muscular coat of the large intestine is identifiable by 8 weeks, and the longitudinal layer by 10 weeks. Meissner's and Auerbach's plexuses are detected at the eighth and twelfth weeks; neuroblasts migrate caudally during the fifth to twelfth weeks, and the normal distribution of ganglion cells is achieved by the sixth month of gestation. The muscularis mucosae develops craniocaudally between the fourteenth and twentieth weeks.[12]

The first appearance of longitudinal folding on the luminal surface of the hindgut during the eighth week corresponds to the development of a poorly differentiated epithelium. Between the ninth and eleventh weeks the longitudinal folds develop in size in the midcolon, and the mucosal epithelial cells display sparse microvilli. Primitive villi appear first in the distal hindgut and then aborally. Enteroendocrine cells are present in the colonic epithelium from 10 weeks, and goblet cells appear first at 12 weeks. Between 14 and 16 weeks true villi are seen throughout the colon, lined with colonocytes bearing differentiated apical microvilli. Villi persist until the end of the second trimester.[12]

ANATOMY

The Gut After Birth

The GI tract may be divided into four major organs: the esophagus, stomach, and small and large intestines. Nutrient digestion and absorption, the primary functions of the gut, are aided by secretions of the pancreas and liver. The entire GI tract is lined by a highly differentiated, plastic tissue whose constituent cells are endowed with specialized morphologic characteristics facilitating their diverse functions. This epithelium is capable of rapid proliferation and renewal throughout life to meet the changing demands of enteral nutrition.

Those changes in GI structure which occur between conception and birth were outlined under "Embryology and Development." The perinatal and weaning periods are times of further change in GI mucosal function, but by birth the basic anatomy of the human gut has been achieved. There do not appear to be further significant morphologic changes comparable to those that occur in other mammals at weaning.[24] In this section the anatomy of the "mature" GI tract and pancreas are outlined, emphasizing its functional aspects.

Esophagus

The esophagus extends from the pharynx to the stomach and carries ingested food and secretions from the mouth through the thorax, via the posterior mediastinum, to the major organs of digestion and absorption. In the healthy subject it plays no significant part in nutrient absorption.

The esophagus of the full-term infant measures from 7 to 14 cm from upper to lower esophageal sphincter, with a diameter of 5 to 6 mm. It is about 25 cm long in the adult. The esophagus is fixed superiorly where the cricopharyngeus muscle joins the cricoid bone. Inferiorly, it is fixed by the phrenoesophageal ligament at the diaphragmatic hiatus, which is the only part of the esophagus to have a serosal covering.[1]

The esophageal musculature is composed of an external longitudinal and an internal circular layer. The muscle fibers are striated in the upper third, mixed in the middle third, and smooth in the lower third of the esophagus. The upper esophageal sphincter, composed of fibers of the cricopharyngeal muscle and inferior pharyngeal constrictors, extends from 0.5 to 1.5 cm below the pharyngoesophageal junction. The lower esophageal sphincter is made up of longitudinal and circular muscles continuous with those of the body of the esophagus. It is identifiable as a ring of contracted muscle of about 2 cm in length at the esophagogastric junction, and like the upper esophageal sphincter is defined functionally rather than anatomically. Both sphincters are innervated by fibers from the vagus nerve and sympathetic ganglia.

The arterial supply to the esophagus is derived from branches of the thoracic aorta, the bronchial arteries, and the left gastric artery. Its venous drainage is by three systems: superiorly to the vena cava, centrally to the azygos vein, and inferiorly into the portal system via the gastric veins. The lymphatic drainage of the upper esophagus is to the deep cervical nodes, that of the thoracic part to the posterior mediastinal nodes, and that of the abdominal part to the left gastric lymph nodes.

The esophageal mucosa is disposed in longitudinal folds that disappear when the esophagus is distended. It is lined by a stratified squamous epithelium that extends distally to just above the gastroesophageal junction, where it changes abruptly to the simple columnar epithelium of the stomach (Z-line). Papillae project into the epithelium from the lamina propria. The muscularis mucosae divides the mucosa from the muscle layers beneath. Mucous glands, present throughout the submucosa, open into the esophageal lumen via long ducts that pierce the muscularis mucosae.[1]

Stomach

Gross Morphology

The stomach, the most dilated part of the alimentary canal, lies in the epigastric, umbilical, and left hypochondrial regions of the abdomen. It occupies a recess bounded by the upper abdominal viscera, completed in front and on the left side by the anterior abdominal wall and the diaphragm. The stomach receives ingested food, partially digests it, and prepares it for controlled delivery to the duodenum. It has a capacity of about 30 ml at birth, increasing to 1,500 ml in the adult.[1] The stomach may be divided into four anatomic regions: The cardia is that part where the esophagus communicates with the stomach. The fundus lies to the left and above the level of the cardiac orifice. The body of the stomach is the major portion and lies between the greater and lesser curves. It is continuous with the antrum, which leads via the pyloric canal to the duodenum. The gastrophrenic ligament attaches the cardia to the diaphragm, and at the pylorus the stomach is fixed by the hepatoduodenal ligament.

The stomach is completely invested in an outer serosal coat, forming the peritoneum continuous with the lesser and greater omenta. The muscular layer is divided into inner oblique, middle circular, and outer longitudinal layers. The oblique muscle, continuous with the circular muscle of the esophagus, extends over both anterior and posterior walls but is deficient along the lesser curve. The circular layer merges proximally with that of the esophagus and distally with that of the duodenum.

The stomach derives its blood supply from the celiac axis. The left gastric artery anastomoses with the right gastric artery, a branch of the hepatic artery, to supply the lesser curve and related parts of the anterior and posterior gastric surfaces. The greater curve is supplied by the right and left gastroepiploic arteries, derived from the gastroduodenal and splenic arteries, respectively. The latter also gives rise to the short gastric arteries that supply the fundus. A dense capillary network in the mucosa between and around the gastric glands is most highly developed in the acid-secreting regions.

Venous drainage is to the portal system. The right and left gastroepiploic veins drain the greater curve tributaries via the superior mesenteric and splenic veins, respectively. The lesser curve is drained by the left gastric and coronary vein into the inferior mesenteric vein and by the right gastric vein. There are anastomoses between the portal and systemic venous systems in the distal esophagus and gastric fundus.

The lymphatic drainage of the stomach follows three routes: superiorly along the lesser curve to the celiac glands and thoracic duct, inferiorly along the greater curve to subpyloric and deep celiac glands, and from the fundus along the course of the short gastric arteries to the hilum of the spleen.

The innervation of the stomach is wholly autonomic. Parasympathetic fibers from the vagus reach the stomach following a paraesophageal course in the right and left vagus nerves. They form Auerbach's plexus within the muscle layer, from which parasympathetic postganglionic cholinergic fibers arise. The sympathetic supply originates from the sixth to the tenth thoracic spinal nerves, which unite to form the splanchnic nerves of the celiac plexus, from which adrenergic postganglionic fibers accompany the arterial supply to the stomach.[1]

Gastric Mucosa

The gastric epithelium is composed of tall columnar mucous cells forming a barrier one cell thick which secretes mucus. It lines the numerous gastric pits (crypts or foveolae) that open onto the mucosal surface and communicate with the gastric glands beneath. The glands contain chief, parietal, endocrine, and mucous neck cells (Fig. 12).

The morphology of the gastric glands varies with different regions of the stomach. Cardiac glands are coiled and contain many mucus-secreting cells. Glands of the fundus and body of the stomach occupy about 60 percent of the mucosal surface. They are simple or branched tubular glands that contain mucous cells, chief (peptic) cells, and parietal (oxyntic) cells. The latter are most numerous and are found in the neck of the gland. The chief cells line the deeper region of the glands (Fig. 12). Pyloric glands are deep and rich in mucus-secreting cells as well as endocrine cells.

Surface mucous cells resemble intestinal goblet cells, with numerous mucous granules in their apical cytoplasm. They have rudimentary microvilli and basal nuclei. Mucous neck cells, found in the neck and isthmus of glands, differ from the surface cells by their larger cytoplasmic granules. Parietal cells are large oval or pyramidal cells with their base lying on the basement membrane bulging into the lamina propria. They secrete hydrochloric acid and intrinsic factor. Their cytoplasm is replete with tubulovesicular membranes and intracellular canaliculi that communicate with the luminal surface among long and numerous microvilli. These have little glycocalyx.[25]

Chief cells are typical protein-secreting exocrine cells with a cytology similar to that of pancreatic acinar cells. They synthesize, store, and secrete pepsinogen. Found mainly at the bases of the glands of the fundus and body of the stomach, they contain large secretory granules lying apical to a central nucleus surrounded by mitochondria and glandular endoplasmic reticulum. The enteroendocrine cells of the stomach, the source of several polypeptide hormones including gastrin, are found mainly in the pyloric glands. Intraepithelial lymphocytes between gastric mucosal cells are less numerous than in the intestine.

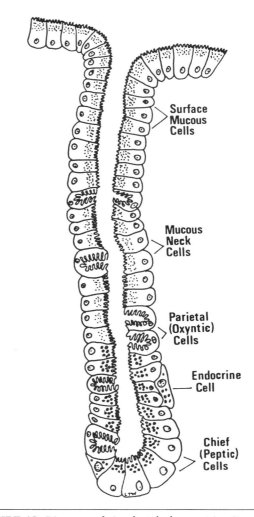

FIGURE 12 Diagram of simple tubular gastric pit and gland from the body of the stomach. (Adapted from Ito.[25])

Pancreas

Gross Morphology

The pancreas is the site of synthesis, storage, and secretion of digestive proteins and bicarbonate which facilitate nutrient digestion in the small intestine. It is also an endocrine organ that produces insulin and other hormones. It lies in the epigastrium, retroperitoneally behind the stomach and extending transversely across the posterior abdominal wall from the duodenum to the spleen. It weighs between 80 and 100 g in the adult. Its head lies within the duodenal curve, and from its lower and left part the uncinate process projects upward behind the superior mesenteric vessels. The body of the pancreas lies obliquely, extending to the left hypochondrion, where it terminates in the tail. This lies over the upper pole of the left kidney in contact with the inferior part of the gastric surface of the spleen.

The major duct (of Wirsung) traverses the pancreas from left to right. It receives ductules from the lobules of the pancreas, which join it obliquely in a herring-bone pattern. At the neck of the pancreas the duct lies in close relation to the bile duct, with which it passes into the wall of the descending part of the duodenum to unite in the formation of the ampulla of Vater. The constricted distal end of the ampulla forms the major duodenal papilla. Frequently an accessory duct (of Santorini) drains the lower half of the head of the pancreas, opening into the duodenum about 2 cm above the ampulla of Vater (see "Embryology and Development").

The blood supply of the head of the pancreas is derived from both the celiac and superior mesenteric arteries, and that of the body and tail from the splenic artery. Venous drainage is via the superior mesenteric and splenic veins. The lymph capillaries begin around the acini and follow the course of the blood vessels. Most lymph vessels end in the pancreaticosplenic lymph nodes. The pancreas is innervated by the vagus and splanchnic nerves, via the splenic plexus.[1]

Histology

The pancreas is a mixed exocrine-endocrine gland. It is made up of lobules invested by connective tissue. Each lobule is composed of many acini, each of which is made up of six to eight acinar cells, which constitute approximately 90 percent of the mass of the pancreas. Each acinus is drained by a small ductule that, connecting with those of other acini, forms an intralobular duct. The lobular ducts drain into the pancreatic ducts.

The exocrine pancreas may be divided into two general functional parts: acinar cells and duct cells. The ultrastructural appearance of the former reveals them to be specialized for pancreatic enzyme secretion. They are polar cells with a centrally located nucleus and apical zymogen granules about 1 μm in diameter. There is an elaborate network of rough endoplasmic reticulum and a Golgi complex close to the nucleus. Apical microtubules and microfilaments are probably involved in the transport and discharge of zymogen granules. Adjacent cells are attached to each other by a junctional complex. Centroacinar cells are found at the point of the final subdivision of the ductules. Smaller than acinar cells, they have sparse cytoplasm and are devoid of zymogen granules. Both acinar and centroacinar cells have short microvillous processes on their ductular surfaces.[26]

Duct cells are smaller than acinar cells and have poorly developed endoplasmic reticula and Golgi complexes, no zymogen granules, and few mitrochondria. They have large nuclei with indentations, and with increasing duct size these cells become more columnar. The structure and function of the exocrine pancreas are fully described in a later chapter.

The endocrine cells of the pancreas constitute a small but important part of the organ. They are concentrated in islets consisting of three main types of cells: 75 percent B cells which produce insulin, 20 percent A cells which produce glucagon, and 5 percent D cells which produce somatostatin, gastrin, and pancreatic polypeptide.

Small Intestine

Gross Anatomy

The small intestine is the major site of nutrient digestion and absorption. It extends from the pylorus to the cecum and is approximately 275 cm long in the neonate, growing to 5

to 6 meters in the adult (see Fig. 2).[27] The small intestine is mobile within the abdomen except for the second and third parts of the duodenum, which are retroperitoneal. The duodenum follows a C-shaped course from the pylorus, around the head of the pancreas, to the ligament of Treitz. The duodenum is approximately 25 cm long in the adult and is the site of entry of the pancreatic and biliary duct systems. The ampulla of Vater opens into the major duodenal papilla in the descending duodenum some 8 to 10 cm distal to the pylorus. The accessory duct, when present, opens 2 cm proximal to it (see "Pancreas").[1]

The jejunum lies in the upper abdomen, while the ileum generally occupies the lower abdomen and pelvis. Both are suspended by mesentery through which pass the vessels and nerves supplying them. The cecum is fixed to the posterior abdominal wall in the right iliac fossa. Abnormalities of this arrangement are discussed in later chapters.

The duodenum derives its arterial supply from the right gastric, supraduodenal, right gastroepiploic, and superior and inferior pancreaticoduodenal arteries. Its venous drainage is into the splenic, superior mesenteric, and portal veins. The jejunum and ileum are supplied by branches of the superior mesenteric artery that run between the serous and muscle coats. These divide into smaller branches that unite with adjacent branches to form arcades, themselves giving rise to secondary arcades terminating in the arterioles of the submucous tissue. The veins have a course and arrangement similar to that of the arteries. The duodenal lymphatics drain to the hepatic and preaortic lymph nodes. The superior and inferior mesenteric lymph nodes, lying on the front of the abdominal aorta close to the origins of the arteries of the same names, are the terminal groups for the GI tract from duodenal jejunal flexure to rectum. The small intestine is innervated by the vagus and splanchnic nerves through the celiac ganglia and the plexus around the superior mesenteric artery.[1]

The surface area of the duodenum and jejunum is greater than that of the ileum; there is a fourfold difference, with a reduction in the mid–small intestine.[27] In the upper small intestine the thickness of the wall of the gut and its luminal diameter are greatest. The diameter of the jejunum is about 4 cm in the adult. The valvulae connivantes or plicae circulares, folds of submucosa covered by mucosa, more abundant and well developed in this region, diminish in number and size distally (see Fig. 3). Peyer's patches (elliptical lymphoid follicles of 1 to 3 cm) are present along the antimesenteric border of the distal ileum. These are particularly prominent during infancy.[27]

The wall of the small intestine consists of four layers. The outermost, the serosa, an extension of the peritoneum, is made up of a single layer of flattened mesothelial cells lying over loose connective tissue. The muscularis comprises an outer longitudinal and an inner circular layer of smooth muscle, between which lies the myenteric plexus. Motility of the intestine is afforded by intercellular communication via specialized gap junctions between adjacent smooth muscle cells. The submucosa consists largely of dense connective tissue sparsely infiltrated by leukocytes. It also contains venous and lymphatic plexuses, which drain the capillaries of the lamina propria of the mucosa, as well as an extensive network of arterioles, ganglion cells, and nerve fibers forming the autonomic submucosal plexus which communicate with those of the muscularis. Branched acinar (Brunner's) glands are found in the submucosa of the duodenum. These glands, which contain mucous and serous secretory cells, penetrate the lamina propria of the proximal duodenal mucosa.[1,27]

Mucosal Morphology

The innermost (luminal) layer, or mucosa, of the small intestine may be divided into three further layers: the epithelium, the lamina propria, and the muscularis mucosae. The small intestinal epithelium consists of a single layer of closely packed columnar cells, or enterocytes, standing upon a basement membrane that separates it from the lamina propria. The lamina propria is a continuous layer of connective tissue dividing the epithelium from the muscularis mucosae. The epithelial surface is increased some 300 times by the valvulae connivantes, villi, and crypts, which project into the lumen and penetrate the lamina propria (Fig. 13), and microvilli that coat the luminal surfaces of the enterocytes (see Fig. 3).

The villi have different shapes and densities in different regions of the small intestine. In general, they are shorter, wider, and fewer in the duodenum; become finger-shaped and taller (up to 1.5 mm) in the jejunum, and become smaller and more pointed in the ileum. The greatest density (up to 40 per square centimeter) is found in the jejunum. The core of the villus is an extension of the lamina propria containing vascular elements.[27]

Between the villi lie the crypts (of Lieberkuhn) of about one-third the depth and three times the number of the villi (Fig. 13). These are the sites of enterocyte proliferation and renewal of the epithelium. Undifferentiated cells divide, and, as replication proceeds, new cells migrate up the wall of the crypts to the base of the villi, where they differentiate into mature cells. Differentiation continues as the cells migrate, until the upper third of the villus is reached, where absorptive capacity is at its peak. Adjacent enterocytes remain closely apposed to each other, except at the tip, where they degenerate and are extruded into the lumen. This journey from crypt base to villus tip takes 5 to 6 days in the duodenum of the adult[28] but may be slower in the newborn. Within the epithelium of the crypts, which is composed mainly of undifferentiated enterocytes in mitosis, are also found goblet cells, Paneth cells, and enteroendocrine (argentaffin) cells (Fig. 14).

As well as intraepithelial lymphocytes throughout the mucosa, the lamina propria of the distal small intestine contains collections of lymphoid nodules, which massed together form Peyer's patches. These may bulge onto the surface of the mucosa and extend through the muscularis mucosae into the submucosa, and contain plasma cells, M cells, and lymphocytes engaged in antigen handling and immunoglobulin synthesis.[20]

Within the lamina propria of the villi are found lymphocytes, plasma cells, mast cells, eosinophils, and macrophages supported by fibroblasts and noncellular elements including collagen and reticulum. A branch of the submucosal arterial plexus ascends each villus and splays at the top to give rise to a subepithelial capillary plexus. This drains into venules that descend the villus to join the submucosal venous plexus composed of branches of the portal venous system (Fig. 14). Capillary venules are closely applied to the epithelial basement membrane, which, composed of a meshwork of glycoprotein fibrils, is 30 to 50 nm thick. Their walls con-

FIGURE 13 Light micrograph of mucosa of mature proximal jejunum showing tall villi lined with enterocytes. (Approximately ×200.) (Reproduced with permission of J.S. Trier.)

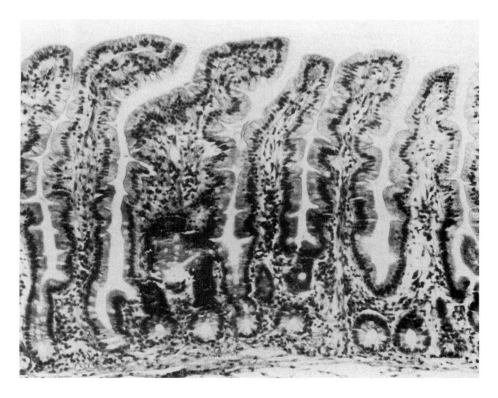

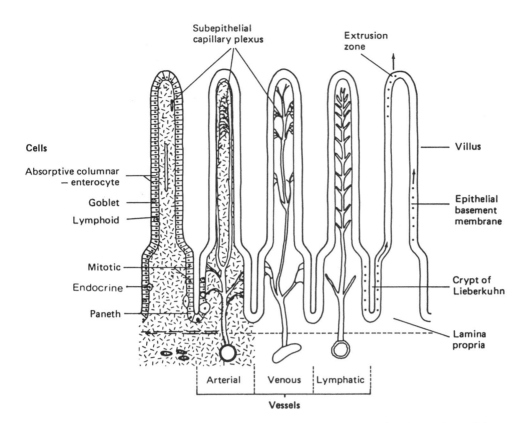

FIGURE 14 Diagram of small intestinal villi and crypts showing their vascular elements and epithelial cells.

sist of a basement membrane and endothelial cells with fenestrations 20 to 45 nm in diameter.[29] Lymphatics also drain the villus, joining to form a central lacteal in continuity with the lymphatic system of the submucosa, which drains centrally, via the thoracic duct, to the venous circulation (Fig. 14). The central lacteals have thicker walls of endothelial cells with no fenestra, but abundant vesicles and wide junctional zones.

The muscularis mucosae is a continuous thin sheet of smooth muscle three to ten cells deep lying between the mucosa and submucosa. It may play a part in mucosal motility, but its exact function is unknown.

Epithelial Cytology

The cytodifferentiation of the small intestinal epithelium is outlined in "Embryology and Development." In man it is largely completed by birth, in contrast to altricial mammals, in which considerable further morphologic and functional development of the mucosa occurs between birth and weaning.[18,24]

Enterocyte. The mature villous absorptive cell (Fig. 15) is polar and bounded by a trilaminar lipoidal plasma membrane about 7.5 nm thick. This membrane is thrown up on the apical surface into cylindric microvilli 1.0 μm long by 0.1 μm in diameter, numbering about 1,000 to 2,000 per cell, which further add to the surface area of the epithelium (Fig. 16). The microvillous membrane is 10 to 11 nm thick and rich in protein and glycoprotein, with a protein:lipid ratio of 1.7:1. The membrane lipids are largely cholesterol and glycolipids, which, together with the membrane proteins, contribute to the composition of the brush border hydrolases, receptors for certain macromolecules, and pathways for active and mediated transport of nutrients and ions.[30]

On the surface of the plasma membrane of the microvilli lies the glycocalyx (fuzzy coat), about 0.5 μm thick and composed of fine irregular filaments of glycoprotein.[31] Newly synthesized proteins are thought to be processed in the Golgi complex, from which glycoproteins are transported by vesicles or microtubules to the microvilli for insertion into the membrane or extrusion into the glycocalyx.

The microvilli are stiffened by longitudinal bundles of 20 to 30 parallel microfilaments, each 6 to 11 nm in diameter, which insert into a dense plaque at the tip (Fig. 17). These filaments are composed of actin and intermesh with a network of apical cytoplasmic microfilaments and microtubules 0.3 to 0.5 μm thick running parallel with the apical surface of the enterocyte and continuous with the junctional complexes, called the terminal web. The terminal web and microvillous skeleton act to anchor the brush border, to stabilize the microvilli and the apex of the cell, and to compartmentalize its interior. Microtubules and membrane-bound vesicles observed in this web may represent micropinocytes facilitating movement of nutrients and other substances within the enterocyte. The ultrastructure of this region of the absorptive cell is described in detail in the section "Embryology and Development." It may play an important part in intrauterine development.[18]

Adjacent enterocytes are attached to each other at the junctional complex, situated at the apical surface of the intercellular walls (Figs. 16 and 17). This complex is composed of a tight junction (zonula occludens) about 16 nm in thickness and 100 to 300 nm in depth, the fusion of the outer laminae of adjacent cell membranes forming a continuous ring around the neck of each enterocyte. Freeze-fracture studies have revealed a meshwork of interconnecting strands between tight junctions.[30] The intermediate junction (zonula adherens), ly-

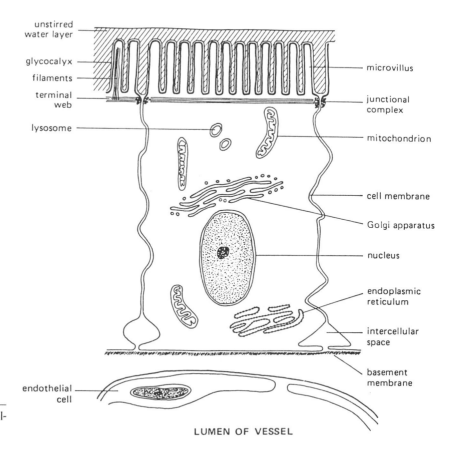

FIGURE 15 Diagram showing the morphology of a mature enterocyte.

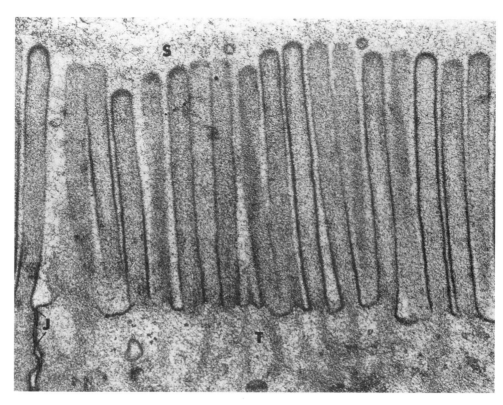

FIGURE 16 Photomicrograph of the apex of an enterocyte showing microvilli projecting at the luminal surface (S). The junctional complex (J) between two cells and the terminal web (T) are seen. (Approximately ×47,000.) (Reproduced with permission of J.S. Trier.)

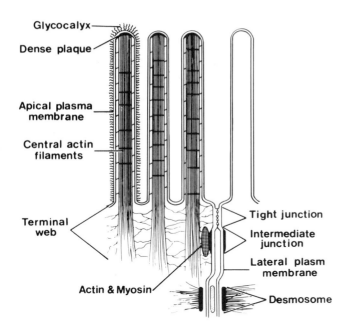

FIGURE 17 Diagram showing microvilli, the apical membrane of an enterocyte, and the junctional complex between adjacent cells. (From Madara and Trier[30] with permission of J.L. Madara and J.S. Trier and Raven Press.)

ing inferior, contains a gap of about 20 nm, filled with amorphous ground substance. The desmosome (macula adherens) lies 0.2 μm lower, enclosing a space of about 25 nm wide which contains a dense central disc of organized tissue. Within the cytoplasm adjacent to the desmosome, a series of fibrils extends into the inner laminae of the lateral membranes, maintaining cell-to-cell adhesion. There are differences in the structure of the tight junctions of different epithelial cells: those between villous enterocytes show uniformity, whereas those of crypt cells show variability in depth and strand number. There are also differences between those of the jejunum and ileum, and it is clear that tight junctions play a major role in the regulation of epithelial permeability through their control of paracellular water and solute flow.[30]

The basolateral membrane invests that part of the enterocyte beneath the junctional complexes. During net water secretion the lateral membranes of adjacent cells are closely opposed (15 to 30 nm apart). Foldlike cytoplasmic processes amplify their surfaces, projecting into and indenting the cytoplasm of neighboring cells (Fig. 18). During net water absorption the intercellular space may be widened to 2 to 3 μm, particularly between cells in the upper part of the villi. The basolateral membrane is rich in Na/K-ATPase and adenyl cyclase. Its basal part is closely applied to the basal lamina or basement membrane.

The oval nucleus of villous enterocytes is found in the basal third of the cell, contains one or more nucleoli, and is enclosed by an envelope of two closely apposed membranes that fuse at the periphery of nuclear pores. The cytoplasmic surface of the outer membrane is studded with ribosomes, which may be in continuity with the rough endoplasmic reticulum (RER). The cytoplasm beneath the terminal web contains both

RER and smooth endoplasmic reticulum (SER). Clumps of free ribosomes (polysomes) are also scattered throughout the cytoplasm. The Golgi complexes are located in the cytoplasm close to the upper pole of the nucleus, and mitochondria are found in abundance in metabolically active enterocytes. The latter appear as filamentous, rod-shaped, or spherical when sectioned (Fig. 18). Lysosomes, bounded by a membrane and containing acid phosphatase, are also found beneath the terminal web. Together with multivesicular bodies 0.25 to 1 μm in diameter, they are thought to be involved in intercellular transport and digestion of macromolecules (see "Embryology and Development"). Peroxisomes are smaller enzyme-containing cellular organelles found in the cytoplasm, whose function is unclear.

Goblet Cells. These are polarized mucus-secreting cells whose apical two-thirds are distended by many clear mucin granules. The apical microvilli are sparse and irregular, and the bulk of the cytoplasmic organelles lies lateral to the mucous granules and above the basal nucleus. There is maturation of goblet cells during migration from crypts to villi. Mucus, secreted by the goblet cells, lies as a continuous layer upon the glycocalyx, forming a physicochemical barrier (see Fig. 15). It is composed of mucoproteins and found in the greatest amount in the stomach and duodenum.[32] The glycocalyx and mucus form a barrier to large particles such as bacteria, desquamated cells, and food particles and protect the epithelium from acid and pepsin digestion. Superficial to the mucus lies the unstirred water layer, a film of fluid forming a hydrophilic barrier merging with the bulk fluid phase of the lumen.

Crypt Cells. Undifferentiated crypt cells are the most abundant cell type in the crypts of Lieberkuhn. They are the precursors of villous absorptive cells, Paneth cells, enteroendocrine cells, goblet cells, and possibly M cells. They proliferate actively and are frequently seen in mitosis. Daughter cells migrate up the wall of the crypt, where they differentiate into mature cell types as they reach the villus (see Fig. 14). The immature crypt cell has shorter and less abundant microvilli and less glycocalyx on its apical surface than the mature villous enterocyte. There is no hydrolase activity associated with the microvillous membrane, but undifferentiated crypt cells synthesize and express secretory component on the basolateral membrane, where this molecule acts as a receptor for IgA synthesized by lamina propria plasma cells (see Chapter 20).

Paneth Cells. These cells lie at the bases of the crypts. They have prominent eosinophilic cytoplasmic granules and intense basophilia of the remaining cytoplasm. They appear to derive from undifferentiated crypt cells but are not seen in mitosis. Paneth cells are pyramidal in shape, with their nuclei located in the wider basal half of the cell. They have rudimentary microvilli and a poorly developed junctional complex. Lysosomes and zymogen granules are present in the cytoplasm, although the secretory function of Paneth cells is unknown.[30]

Enteroendocrine Cells. A large group of specialized neurosecretory cells, the enteroendocrine cells, resides in the mucosa of the GI tract, lining the gastric glands, intestinal villi, and crypts. These polar cells have tufts of microvilli on their apical surface. Secretory granules, located in the subnuclear region, release their contents at the basolateral sur-

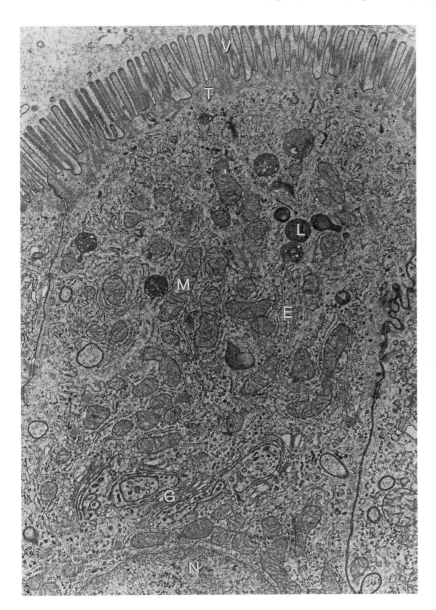

FIGURE 18 Electron micrograph of a mature jejunal enterocyte showing microvilli (V), terminal web (T), mitochondrion (M), lysosome (L), endoplasmic reticulum (E), Golgi complex (G), and basal nucleus (N). (Approximately ×6,000.) (Reproduced with permission of J.S. Trier.)

face. Junctional complexes adhere enteroendocrine cells to their neighbors. Enteroendocrine cells secrete a range of neuropeptides, including gastrin, secretin, motilin, neurotensin, glucagon, enteroglucagon, vasoactive intestinal peptide (VIP), gastric inhibitory polypeptide (GIP), neurotensin, cholecystokinin, and somatostatin.

M Cells. Specialized epithelial cells are found overlying lymphoid follicles. The apical surface of M cells has an irregularity, formed by microfolds and small microvilli, beneath which a thin sheet of cytoplasm separates the gut lumen from lymphoid cells. The Golgi complexes and mitochondria are not distinctive and lysosomes are sparse. The terminal web is incomplete, and endocytotic vesicles are abundant in the apical cytoplasm.[20] These features facilitate the transfer of intraluminal antigens across the M cell, from which they may be processed by lymphoid cells of the Peyer's patches. The part played by M cells in the immunology of the GI tract is discussed more fully in later chapters.

Large Intestine

Gross Morphology

The large intestine is the site of water and electrolyte absorption and the formation of feces. It also contains a large population of microorganisms which contributes to the metabolism of undigested dietary components. It extends from the ileocecal valve to the anus and has a length of approximately 40 cm in the newborn, growing to approximately 150 cm in the adult.[5] Its diameter decreases from cecum to rectum, where it widens before narrowing again at the anus.[1]

Cecum. The cecum is in continuity with the ileum via the ileocecal valve. Composed of an upper and lower lip, this valve, located at the posterior medial aspect of the cecum, forms a slitlike sphincter serving to regulate the passage of ileal contents into the colon and to prevent reflux of cecal contents into the small intestine. Splanchnic and vagal stimulation and cecal distention increase ileocecal valve tone, whereas distention of the terminal ileum causes its relaxation, facilitating caudal movement of luminal contents.[1]

The cecum comes to occupy the right iliac fossa after embryonic rotation between the sixth and twelfth gestational weeks (see Fig. 5 and "Embryology and Development"). Incomplete rotation may find the cecum in the right upper quadrant of the abdomen: Such malrotation predisposes the gut to intestinal volvulus. The cecum is usually invested by the posterior parietal peritoneum, and relatively immobile because it possesses no mesentery.

Appendix. The mouth of the appendix is at the apex of the cecum below the ileocecal valve where the taeniae coli converge. Its body may be attached to the posterior parietal wall by the mesoappendix or to the colon. It is variable in length, from 2 to 20 cm, and in position, located most frequently below the cecum, behind the cecum, projecting inferiorly and to the right, over the pelvic brim, or anterior or posterior to the ileum.[1]

Colon. The ascending colon extends from the cecum superiorly toward the lower pole of the right kidney where, beneath the right lobe of the liver, it turns medially at the hepatic flexure. It is usually fixed to the posterior peritoneum. The transverse colon lies between the hepatic and splenic flexures, is mobile, and lies anteriorly suspended by the transverse mesocolon. This originates from the posterior peritoneum, its upper part continuous with the lesser sac and its lower part forming a part of the greater omentum. The splenic flexure marks the junction between the transverse and descending colon. It is attached to the diaphragm by the phrenicocolic ligament, where it is in continuity with the descending colon which lies between the psoas and quadratus lumborum muscles to join the sigmoid colon at the pelvic brim. The descending colon has no mesentery. The sigmoid colon, suspended by mesentery, follows a sigmoid-shaped course from the pelvic brim to the rectum where it lies beneath the peritoneum.

Rectum and Anus. The rectum follows the curve of the sacrum, in apposition anteriorly with the uterus in the female and the bladder in the male. It becomes capacious and fusiform and has three folds, or valves of Houston, extending into its lumen before narrowing to the longitudinal columns of Morgani which end at the anal papillae. The anal canal is 2 cm long in the newborn and the rectosigmoid junction 9 cm from the anal verge. By 10 years the latter distance has lengthened to 15 cm. The anal canal passes through the internal and external sphincters, ending at the mucocutaneous junction. The internal sphincter is formed of the distal portion of the circular smooth muscle of the rectum, extending to within 1 cm of the anal orifice. The external sphincter circumscribes the canal and is separated from the internal sphincter by a thin layer of elastic fibers and the longitudinal muscle coat of the rectum. Superiorly its fibers blend with those of the levator ani muscle, and it is attached posteriorly to the coccyx and anteriorly to the perineal body.

The blood supply to the proximal large intestine, including the appendix, cecum, and ascending to mid-transverse colon (midgut derivatives), is from the colic branches of the superior mesenteric artery. The distal large intestine, extending from mid-transverse colon and including the descending and sigmoid colon, rectum, and upper half of the anal canal (hindgut), receives its blood supply largely from the inferior mesenteric artery and its branches. The arteries of the rectum and anus are the superior, middle, and inferior rectal arteries and the median sacral artery. The veins of the large intestine are the superior and inferior mesenteric veins. Those of the rectum and anal canal are the superior, middle, and inferior rectal veins.

The lymphatic vessels of the cecum and appendix are numerous because of the large amount of lymphoid tissue in this region of the GI tract. They drain into the ileocolic chain. The vessels of the ascending and transverse colon end in the superior mesenteric lymph nodes. Those of the descending and sigmoid colon end in the preaortic lymph nodes around the origin of the inferior mesenteric artery. The lymphatic drainage of the rectum is superior to the nodes of the sigmoid mesocolon. From the anal canal above the mucocutaneous junction lymph drains to the internal iliac nodes, and from below the mucocutaneous junction to the superficial inguinal lymph nodes.

The large intestine is served by both the sympathetic and parasympathetic autonomic nervous systems. The cecum, appendix, ascending colon, and right two-thirds of the transverse colon have their sympathetic supply from the celiac and superior mesenteric ganglia and their parasympathetic supply from the vagus nerve. The left third of the transverse colon, descending and sigmoid colon, rectum, and upper anal canal derive their sympathetic supply from the lumbar part of the trunk and the superior hypogastric plexus. The parasympathetic supply of the hindgut is from the pelvic splanchnic nerves.[1]

Cytology of Wall

The serosa of the colon is covered by appendices epiploicae, fatty structures attached to the peritoneum. It covers only that part of the large intestine which lies within the peritoneal cavity, excluding the rectum. The transverse and sigmoid portions of the colon are suspended by mesentery, while the cecum, ascending and descending colon, and rectum are fixed.

The wall of the colon contains an outer longitudinal and an inner circular layer of smooth muscle. The former takes the form of three longitudinal bands, the taeniae coli, which extend from the tip of the cecum to the rectum, converging on the base of the appendix. The taeniae coli are 0.5 to 1 cm in width in the adult. They are shorter in length than the colon, causing its saccular division into haustra separated by folds.[1]

The ganglion cells of the myenteric plexus of Auerbach are found between the circular and longitudinal muscle layers. From within the former, unmyelinated postganglionic fibers communicate with the submucosal plexus of Meissner. The submucosa also contains blood and lymphatic vessels, dense connective tissue infiltrated by fibroblasts, lymphocytes, plasma cells, macrophages, and eosinophils.

The mucosa of the large intestine is increased in surface area by irregular plicae semilunares and by tubular crypts (of Lieberkuhn) of up to 0.7 mm in depth, which extend into the lamina propria to the muscularis mucosae, a layer of smooth muscle cells 8 to 12 cells thick. There are no villi in the large intestine. Both the mucosal surface and the crypts are lined with a continuous sheet of columnar epithelial cells (colonocytes) and goblet cells separated from the mesen-

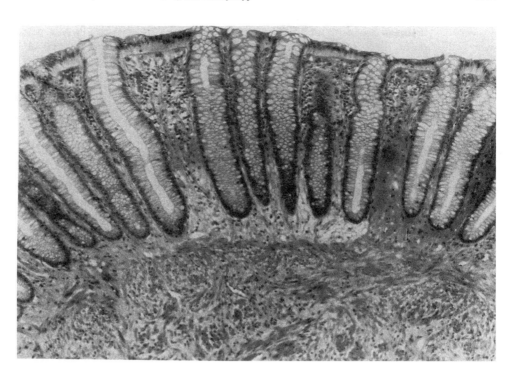

FIGURE 19 Light micrograph of mucosa of the rectum showing cylindric crypts lined by colonocytes and goblet cells. (Approximately ×200.) (Reproduced with permission of J.S. Trier.)

chymal tissue of the lamina propria by a basal lamina in apposition with the basal plasma membrane of the colonocytes (Fig. 19).

The coloncytes have fewer and shorter microvilli than their small intestinal counterparts. These are coated with a fibrillar glycocalyx and within their apical cytoplasm are many glycoprotein-containing vesicles 0.1 to 1 μm in diameter. Intraepithelial lymphocytes are found throughout the epithelium, in greater numbers in the crypts than on the surface. The epithelium of the lower part of the crypts contains proliferating undifferentiated columnar cells, mucus-secreting goblet cells, and several types of enteroendocrine cell. The upper part of the crypts contains differentiating columnar cells, goblet cells, and a few endocrine cells. The morphology of the goblet cells and enteroendocrine cells of the large intestine resembles that of comparable cells of the small intestine.

ADAPTATION TO ENTERAL NUTRITION

Challenge of Birth

Birth represents a challenge to the nutrition of the newborn infant. Delivered from the secure environment of the uterus where the fetus enjoys a continuous and regulated supply of nutrients via the mother's placenta, the neonate must adapt rapidly from parenteral to enteral nutrition. This major event demands a concerted response by the GI tract comprising coordinated sucking and swallowing; efficient gastric emptying and intestinal motility; regulated salivary, gastric, pancreatic, and hepatobiliary secretion; enterocyte function capable of synthesizing and delivering appropriate brush bord-

er enzymes and providing effective absorption, secretion, and mucosal protection; economical utilization of the products of digestion and absorption; and excretion of the waste products of digestion and metabolism.

Although the gut allows free passage of amniotic fluid in utero, it has to cope soon after birth with intermittent large volumes of milk. An adult ingesting a comparable feed volume per body weight would require 15 to 20 liters of milk.[33] Successful adaptation to extrauterine nutrition requires the hitherto untested gut to meet these demands rapidly and efficiently. The human GI tract develops under the influence of endogenous and exogenous factors. The genetic endowment of the organism, regulated by an intrinsic "biologic clock," controls this sequential development,[34] which is modulated by exogenous factors in the form of luminal influences (amniotic fluid, colostrum, and milk) and systemic influences (maternal, fetal, and neonatal neuroendocrine milieu).

The postnatal development of the function of the GI tract and its accessory organs is discussed in the succeeding chapters. In this section will be outlined the changes in GI mucosal morphology and function that occur perinatally. Two factors are of particular importance to the process of perinatal adaptation to enteral nutrition. The first is the relative maturity or gestational age of the neonate, and the second is the composition of feeds received at birth. Biologically the newborn remains an extragestate fetus until weaning, when he or she achieves nutritional independence. Until that time the growing infant relies upon a diet of closely regulated composition for which the function of the GI tract is well adapted. Weaning, the process of nutritional transition from milk to a solid diet, is a further period of GI adaptation, which will not be discussed here.

Influence of Gestational Age at Birth on Adaptation

The GI tract appears morphologically prepared for oral feeding by the end of the second trimester (Tables 1 and 2). However, many of the physiologic processes required for efficient enteral nutrition are not fully developed until 33 to 34 weeks' gestation. At birth the capacity of the gut to respond to the demands of enteral feeding depends upon the stage of development achieved, governed by endogenous factors, and the luminal and systemic environment to which it is exposed (colostrum and milk, GI secretions, and neuroendocrine influences). By full term, luminal, mucosal, and extra-GI processes co-operate to ensure an integrated response to oral feeding.

Motility. At full term a co-ordinated pattern of sucking, swallowing, esophageal peristalsis, and gastric emptying is achieved within a few days of birth. Prolonged bursts of nutritive sucking transfer milk across the pharynx, whence it is propelled through the esophagus by a peristaltic wave to the stomach, from which controlled gastric motility discharges it to the duodenum. A co-ordinated pattern of sucking and swallowing is absent in newborn infants of less than 34 weeks' gestation,[35] and over 75 percent of healthy preterm infants require gavage feeding until this gestation[36] irrespective of their weight.[37] The rate and pattern of gastric emptying in the newborn may be affected by the composition and osmolality of feeds[38,39] and posture.[40] The half-life of a feed in the stomach ranges between 30 and 90 minutes, and its emptying pattern follows a monoexponential curve.[41] Rate of gastric emptying may also be slowed in prematurity and dysmaturity.[42]

Coincident with the development of the ability to suck and swallow appears the small intestinal co-ordinated migrating motor complex of the mature newborn. Infants of less than 30 weeks' gestation exhibit disorganized random peristaltic contractions, and those of 30 to 33 weeks have short bursts of motor activity (fetal complexes). Thereafter, co-ordinated migrating motor complexes are present.[43] These may be responsible for the movement of contrast material down the intestine of infants in utero observed as early as 30 weeks' gestation.[44] There is a direct relation between increasing gestation and increasing gastroduodenal pressures, propagation, and slow wave frequency.[45] Such patterns are uninfluenced by feeding, although it is not yet known whether the onset of oral nutrition initiates such motor activity.

Gastric Digestive Function. The full-term infant is capable of secreting hydrochloric acid at birth; basal output increases over the first few hours of postnatal life.[46] The majority of preterm infants of birth weight 1 to 2.2 kg are also capable of gastric acid secretion at birth.[47] However, in both the full-term and preterm neonate this initial surge in hydrochloric acid is followed by a hyposecretory phase before a steady rise to adult levels.[48] The pattern of intrinsic factor secretion parallels that of gastric acid. Peptic activity, detected first at 16 weeks' gestation, is around 2 percent of that of adults at birth,[49] rising steadily thereafter.

Pancreatic Exocrine Function. This is relatively deficient at birth, and mature levels of pancreatic enzymes are not achieved until late infancy. Concentrations of pancreatic amylase, lipase, trypsin, and chymotrypsin are detected first in midgestation at levels of about 10 percent of adult values.[50,51] Infants of 32 to 34 weeks' gestation at birth secrete lipase and alpha-amylase, but not trypsin, at levels appreciably lower than those of mature infants,[52] but within a week pancreatic exocrine activity appears to overtake that of term neonates.[52,53] The neonatal pancreas does not appear to be responsive to the secretagogues pancreozymin and secretin.[53] In spite of apparent neonatal exocrine insufficiency, milk digestion is adequate at birth, even in the preterm infant. This is probably in part due to the contribution of enzymes in breast milk and alternate pathways of digestion in the small intestine.

Small Intestinal Function. Glucose and amino acids are transported across the gut wall of the upper small intestine as early as 10 weeks after conception, and with increasing gestation there is both a rise in active transfer capacity and a proximodistal gradient of development.[54-56] Active D-glucose absorption, as measured by changes in transmural potential difference across the jejunum, is significantly lower in infants of less than 37 weeks' gestation than in those born at term, and approximately two-thirds that of adults.[57] A postnatal surge in D-glucose and D-xylose absorption occurs between the first and third weeks[57,58] in infants of 30 to 32 weeks' gestation, and preterm infants display significantly lower values than those born at term. For both sugars, light-for-gestation infants show poorer absorption than their appropriately grown counterparts. Passive intestinal permeability to small nonmetabolizable solutes is elevated in the newborn,[59] particularly the preterm.[60,61] The initiation of enteral feeding is followed by a reduction in permeability during the first week of postnatal life in both the preterm and full-term neonate.[59-61]

Intestinal mucosal disaccharidases are first detectable coincident with the appearance of villous ridges around 8 weeks of gestation.[7] Intestinal lactase activity of the human fetus of 26 to 34 weeks' gestation is only 30 percent that of the full-term baby, but from 35 weeks onward there is a rapid rise to mature levels.[62,63] Lactase activity develops rapidly after premature delivery, independently of milk feeds.[64] Measurement of disaccharide activities in the jejunal fluid of enterally fed preterm infants of less than 32 weeks' gestation at birth has demonstrated a rapid postnatal rise in lactase activity at the end of the first week.[65] This has been confirmed by the measurement of the changing ratio of lactose and the nonmetabolizable disaccharide lactulose in the urine of the newborn: The rate of rise in lactase activity is proportional to the gestational age of the neonate at birth.[66] Sucrase and maltase activities reach mature levels earlier in gestation, even though these enzymes are not required in significant concentrations until weaning.[63] There is an aboral gradient in the mucosal activities of these disaccharidases at birth, in contrast with the highest levels of glucoamylase in the ileum. The latter enzyme may contribute to the terminal digestion of certain glucose polymers.[67]

Peptidase activity is found in both the proximal and distal fetal small intestine as early as 11 weeks, but there is no significant increase in activity between this time and 23 weeks' gestation.[68,69] Enterokinase appears late in gestation, and its activity increases during postnatal life.[63] Little is known about the perinatal transfer of dietary peptides. The uptake of intact protein by the human neonatal GI tract has been recently reviewed[18] and is summarized below.

Amniotic fluid contains very little lipid, and the functional demands for fat absorption in utero are unknown. Nevertheless, the epithelium of the 10-week fetus appears capable of taking up lipid by pinocytosis in vitro.[70] Biliary lipid secretion occurs as early as 22 weeks, and the fetal gallbladder contains cholesterol, lecithin, and bile salts. There are four major lipases active in the neonatal GI tract: lingual lipase, gastric lipase, bile salt–stimulated lipase of colostrum and milk, and pancreatic lipase.[71,72] Lingual lipase activity develops late in fetal life; there is an 80 percent increase between 25 and 34 weeks of gestation, by which time the preterm infant has sufficient intragastric activity to hydrolyze a significant proportion of milk fat.[73] Human milk contains lipases whose contribution to neonatal fat digestion is discussed below. Pancreatic lipase activity is low at birth (see above). Intraluminal bile salt concentration and bile acid size are low at birth in the preterm as opposed to the full-term infant.[74] This apparent immaturity of the capacity to digest fats at birth may be compensated for by breast milk enzymes.

Mucosal Protection. Mucosal protection is afforded by luminal, epithelial, and systemic mechanisms. Gastric acid is present within hours of birth (see above). The microvillous membrane of the neonatal epithelium appears to be immature in its barrier properties. Circulating antibodies to food proteins may be found in both the full-term and preterm neonate,[75] although their biologic significance remains unclear.[18] The uptake of macromolecules by the newborn gut may represent a persistence of the intrauterine absorptive processes present between about 12 and 22 weeks' gestation, described in "Embryology and Development." During this period the human gut mucosa appears capable of taking up intact protein and lipid.[13–16,70] Amniotic fluid contains a range of physiologically active macromolecules. Receptors for epidermal growth factor, present in amniotic fluid,[76] have been identified on fetal enterocytes as early as 12 weeks' gestation,[77] and this growth factor may play a part in intrauterine GI development.[78] However, there is no evidence that there exists in the human neonate a period of enhanced macromolecular uptake comparable to that operating in the GI mucosa of the suckling young of certain altricial mammals and essential for their neonatal adaptation.[18] The role of M cells in antigen recognition and processing in the newborn is discussed in a later chapter.

The human infant derives its circulating immunoglobulins prenatally via the placenta. Secretory IgA, with its capacity to agglutinate intraluminal antigens, is the first line of immunologic defense at the mucosal surface.[79] Its high titers in human colostrum help to protect the mucosal surfaces of the breast-fed newborn, while circulating immunoglobulins (IgG and IgM) represent a further line of defense to deal with absorbed antigens. Secretory IgA has been detected in the gut wall and contents of fetuses of 11 to 32 weeks' gestation, but not in meconium.[23] It is detectable in the saliva of full-term infants by the end of the first week of life[80] and reaches adult levels by 4 weeks. Exposure to food and microbial antigens probably induces IgA production from plasma cells in the lamina propria, where the immunoglobulin can be identified by immunofluorescence soon after birth.[81] The time of appearance of IgA is similar in preterm infants as light as 1.5 kg and full-term infants.[82]

The ability to mount a systemic immune response to ingested food antigens is not acquired until about 35 weeks' gestation. Serum antibodies to bovine serum albumin are not detectable in the circulation of infants of less than 34 weeks' gestation,[83] and such preterm infants, despite the earlier appearance of organized lymphoid tissue and immunologic evidence of albumin uptake, lack the capacity to make specific antibodies to this milk protein. The development of the protective and immune functions of the gut is discussed in a later chapter.

Large Intestinal Function. During fetal life the villi present in the colon exhibit brush-border enzymes that reach peak activity around 28 weeks.[84] It is possible that this hydrolytic activity may represent another alternate pathway of digestion available to the preterm infant.[85] After birth the large bowel becomes rapidly colonized with bacteria that contribute to the metabolism of undigested carbohydrate to short-chain fatty acids, which may be absorbed in the colon.

The major function of the colon—salt and water conservation—is immature at birth. During the first week of postnatal life the newborn may pass up to nine semiliquid stools per day.[86] Within 2 weeks this has dropped to three or four per day.[87] In infants born prematurely, stool frequency and volume appear to be directly proportional to feed frequency and volume, suggesting poorly developed colonic function in the preterm neonate (Weaver and Lucas, unpublished work).

Regulation of Responses. The adaptation of the neonate to extrauterine nutrition is in part mediated by GI hormones, which may have both regulatory and trophic functions on the developing GI tract and may be involved in intermediary metabolism.[88] In contrast to full-term infants, the first feed of human milk taken by the newborn of less than 34 weeks' gestation is not followed by a rise in blood glucose, plasma insulin, growth hormone, glucagon, enteroglucagon, gastrin, motilin, or neurotensin concentrations. However, within 3 days of birth a response comparable to that of mature infants is detectable.[89] These postnatal surges in glucose, its metabolites, and gut and other hormones, which follow the onset of oral feeding and are absent in the exclusively parenterally fed,[90] may mediate changes in GI structure and function outlined above. Motilin is thought to stimulate intestinal motility and gastric emptying in adults,[91] and its release in utero may account for the premature passage of meconium observed in the distressed fetus nearing term, but not in the very preterm fetus.[92]

Influence of Colostrum and Breast Milk on Adaptation

At birth the human neonate exchanges nutritional dependence upon two fluids of closely regulated composition (maternal blood and amniotic fluid) for a third (maternal breast milk). While varying greatly in their constituents from blood and amniotic fluid, human colostrum and milk contain all the nutrients required for the healthy growth and development of the newborn infant. In addition, human milk contains factors that may assist in digestion, the development of mucosal function and protection, and systemic metabolism.

Throughout the suckling period there exists an intimate interrelation between mammary function and GI mucosal function. During lactation the composition of colostrum and milk changes to meet the changing demands of the growing infant, and such changes are reflected by the changing pattern of GI function and metabolism during early life. This interrelation has been best studied in the young of other mammals. Altricial species, which bear relatively helpless and immature progeny (e.g., rat and mouse), are nourished on a milk high in protein, which, as well as being a nutrient source, contains active hormones, enzymes, and trophic and protective factors. Precocial species, whose young are relatively independent and mature at birth (e.g., guinea pig, foal), are reared on a milk high in energy (lactose and fat), which is relatively deficient in non-nutritive proteins. Such mammals may be weaned soon after birth.[93]

Although dependent upon a diet of milk until weaning, the human newborn is relatively mature at birth. The major phases of GI development are completed in utero, and by full term the human gut is fully prepared for enteral nutrition (see "Embryology and Development"). Moreover, it appears that while the nutrient composition of milk is critical, its source and non-nutrient composition are not: Human infants may be successfully reared not only on the modified milks of other mammals, but also on synthetic formulae devoid of animal proteins and fats. However, human colostrum and milk have macroconstituents and properties that may play an active part in perinatal adaptation to enteral nutrition and to the changes in GI function which follow birth.

Gastric emptying is delayed in the preterm infant fed cow's milk formula.[42] Intestinal transit time is longer,[94] and frequency of defecation is lower in the artificially fed newborn.[86] At 2 weeks of age breast-fed infants produce almost twice as many stools as those fed cow's milk formula.[87] The stools of the breast-fed infant are larger and softer and of lower pH and contain higher counts of bifidobacteria and fewer anaerobes than those of formula-fed infants.[95] The abundance of a range of unabsorbable oligosaccharides in breast milk may contribute to the greater volume and high numbers of saccharolytic bacteria in the stools of the naturally fed.

Such different patterns of GI motility may be related to the different patterns of gut hormone response elicited in breast-fed and cow's milk formula–fed neonates. Full-term breast-fed infants display significantly lower circulating concentration of motilin and neurotensin following milk feeds during the neonatal period. Significant differences in the serum profiles of polypeptides that are known to have trophic actions on the gut, including gastrin and enteroglucagon, and of peptides that are known to regulate intermediary metabolism, including insulin and pancreatic polypeptide (PP), have also been observed between the naturally fed and formula-fed full-term newborn.[96] Further evidence that these gut hormone responses are initiated by feeding and play a part in perinatal GI adaptation derives from the finding that minimal enteral feeding is also capable of stimulating their release.[97]

The newborn infant has an immediate requirement for carbohydrate and fat, not only for fuel and insulation but also for thermogenesis and neural tissue synthesis. Stores laid down during the last trimester of pregnancy meet these demands in the full-term infant, but the preterm infant with insufficient reserves may be vulnerable. As well as satisfying these nutritional demands, breast milk contains enzymes that assist intraluminal nutrient digestion and compensate for the relative deficiency of those secreted by the salivary, gastric, and pancreatic glands. These enzymes are present in colostrum and milk throughout lactation, and include amylase, bile salt–stimulated lipase, and esterase. All are stable within a wide pH range and make a significant contribution to intraluminal carbohydrate and fat digestion in the newborn,[71,72] even when bile salts are relatively deficient.[74] The latter enzymes are also found in preterm milk as early as 25 weeks' gestation. Fat absorption is more efficient in the breast-fed than in the cow's milk formula–fed newborn infant.[98]

Human milk contains both nutrient and non-nutrient proteins. The former consist largely of alpha-lactalbumin and casein. Cow's milk casein is less well digested than that of human milk. Immunoglobulin A is found in high concentrations in colostrum and through the enteromammary circulation may afford the newborn specific protection against exposure to microorganisms derived from the maternal GI tract.[99] Lactoferrin, lysozyme, complement, interferon, and protease inhibitors are other milk proteins that may confer protection against microbial infection. Milk also contains viable white cells, including polymorphonuclear leukocytes, macrophages, and both T and B lymphocytes, which may contribute to induction of IgA activity.[101,102]

There is a range of other physiologically active macromolecules in human milk, which, secreted against a concentration gradient, may play a role in perinatal adaptation (Table 3).[102] These include hormones, trophic factors, prostaglandins, and other anti-inflammatory agents. Of these, hydrocortisone and epidermal growth factor present in human amniotic fluid[76] and milk[103] have been shown to modulate mucosal differentiation in the human fetal small intestine.[78,104]

TABLE 3

Macromolecules in Human Colostrum and Milk, Which May Play a Part in Neonatal Adaptation to Enteral Nutrition and Extrauterine Life

Digestive Enzymes
    Amylase, bile salt–stimulated lipase, and esterase

Hormones
    Thyroxine (T_3, T_4), thyroid-stimulating hormone (TSH), thyrotrophin-releasing hormone (TRH), corticosteroids, adrenocorticotropic hormone (ACTH), insulin, luteinizing hormone–releasing factor (LHRF), gonadotropin-releasing hormone (GnRH), somatostatin, oxytocin, prolactin, erythropoietin, calcitonin

Growth Factors
    Epidermal growth factor (EGF), nerve growth factor (NGF), somatomedin-C, transforming growth factor (TGF)

Anti-inflammatory Agents
    Prostaglandin E and F, alpha₁-antitrypsin, and chymotrypsin

Anti-infective Factors
    Secretory IgA, lactoferrin, lysozyme, complement, interferon

REFERENCES

1. Williams PL, Warwick R, eds. Gray's anatomy. 36th ed. London: Churchill Livingstone, 1984: 1302.
2. Reiquam CW, Allen RP, Akers DR, Denver MD. Normal and abnormal small bowel lengths. Am J Dis Child 1965; 109:447–451.
3. Scammon RE, Kittelson JA. The growth of the gastrointestinal tract of the human fetus. Proc Soc Exp Biol Med 1926; 24:303–307.
4. Touloukian RJ, Walker-Smith GJ. Normal intestinal length in preterm infants. J Pediatr Surg 1983; 18:720–723.
5. Underhill BML. Intestinal length in man. Br Med J 1955; ii:1243–1246.
6. Siebert JR. Small intestine length in infants and children. Am J Dis Child 1980; 134:593–595.
7. Lacroix B, Kedinger M, Simon-Assmann P, Haffen K. Early organogenesis of human small intestine: scanning electron microscopy and brush border enzymology. Gut 1984; 25:925–930.
8. Ferguson A, Maxwell JD, Carr KE. Progressive changes in the small-intestinal villous pattern with increasing length of gestation. J Pathol 1969; 99:87–91.
9. Moore KL. The developing human. London: WB Saunders, 1982: 227.
10. Lind T. Amniotic fluid. In: Geigy scientific tables. 8th ed. Basel: Geigy, 1981: 197.
11. Gitlin D, Kumate J, Morales C, Noriega L, Arevalo N. The turnover of amniotic fluid protein in the human conceptus. Am J Obstet Gynecol 1972; 113:632–645.
12. Grand RJ, Watkins JB, Torti FM. Development of the human gastrointestinal tract. Gastroenterology 1976; 70:790–810.
13. Colony PC. Successive phases of human fetal intestinal development. In: Kretchmer N, Minkowski A, eds. Nutritional adaptation of the gastrointestinal tract of the newborn. New York: Raven Press, 1983: 3.
14. Bierring F, Andersen H, Egeberg J, Bro-Rasmussen F. On the nature of the meconium corpuscles in human foetal intestinal epithelium. 1. Electron microscopic studies. Acta Pathol Microbiol Scand 1964; 61:365–376.
15. Andersen H, Bierring F, Matthiessen M, Egeberg J, Bro-Rasmussen F. On the nature of the meconium corpuscles in human foetal intestinal epithelium. 2. A cytochemical study. Acta Pathol Microbiol Scand 1964; 61:377–393.
16. Moxey PC, Trier JS. Development of villus absorptive cells in the human fetal small intestine: a morphological and morphometric study. Anat Rec 1979; 195:463–482.
17. Reubner BH, Kamayama R, Bronsen RT, Blumenthal S. Meconium corpuscles in intestinal epithelium of foetal and newborn primates. Arch Pathol 1974; 98:396–399.
18. Weaver LT, Walker WA. Uptake of macromolecules. In: Lebenthal E, ed. Human gastrointestinal development. New York: Raven Press, 1989: 731.
19. Bryant MG, Buchan AMJ, Gregor M, Ghatei MA, Polak JM, Bloom SR. Development of intestinal regulatory peptides in the human fetus. Gastroenterology 1982; 83:47–54.
20. Owen WL, Jones AL. Epithelial cell specialisation within human Peyer's patches: an ultrastructural study of intestinal lymphoid follicles. Gastroenterology 1974; 66:189–203.
21. Haffen K, Kedinger M, Simon-Assmann P. Mesenchyme-dependent differentiation of epithelial progenitor cells in the gut. J Pediatr Gastroenterol Nutr 1987; 6:14–23.
22. Orlic D, Lev R. An electron microscopic study of intraepithelial lymphocytes in human fetal small intestine. Lab Invest 1977; 37:554–561.
23. Petit JE, Galinka A, Solomon JC. Immunoglobulins in the intestinal contents of the human fetus with special reference to IgA. Eur J Immunol 1973; 3:373–375.
24. Henning SJ. Functional development of the gastrointestinal tract. In: Johnson LR, ed. Physiology of the gastrointestinal tract. 2nd ed. New York: Raven Press, 1987: 285.
25. Ito S. Functional gastric morphology. In: Johnson LR, ed. Physiology of the gastrointestinal tract. 2nd ed. New York: Raven Press, 1987: 817.
26. Gorelick FS, Jamieson JD. Structure-function relationship of the pancreas. In: Johnson LR, ed. Physiology of the gastrointestinal tract. 2nd ed. New York: Raven Press, 1987: 1089.
27. Walker-Smith JA. Diseases of the small intestine in childhood. 3rd ed. London: Butterworths, 1988: 380.
28. MacDonald WC, Trier JS, Everett NB. Cell proliferation and migration in the stomach, duodenum, and rectum of man: radioautographic studies. Gastroenterology 1964; 46:405–417.
29. Clementi F, Palade GE. Intestinal capillaries. I. Permeability to peroxidase and ferritin. J Cell Biol 1969; 41:33–58.
30. Madara JL, Trier JS. Functional morphology of the mucosa of the small intestine. In: Johnson LR, ed. Physiology of the gastrointestinal tract. 2nd ed. New York: Raven Press, 1987: 1209.
31. Ito S. Structure and function of the glycocalyx. FASEB J 1969; 28:12–25.
32. Allen A, Cunliffe WJ, Pearson JP, Sellers LA, Ward R. Studies on gastrointestinal mucus. Scand J Gastroenterol 1984; 19:101–114.
33. Aynsley-Green A. The control of the adaptation to postnatal nutrition. Monogr Paediatr 16. 1982; 16:59–87.
34. Lebenthal E, Lee PC. Interactions of determinants in the ontogeny of the gastrointestinal tract: a unified concept. Pediatr Res 1983; 17:19–24.
35. Gryboski JD. The swallowing mechanism of the neonate. 1. Esophageal and gastric motility. Pediatrics 1965; 35:445–452.
36. Herbst JJ. Development of sucking and swallowing. In: Lebenthal E, ed. Textbook of gastroenterology and nutrition in infancy. New York: Raven Press, 1981: 97.
37. Hey E. Special care nurseries: admitting to a policy. Br Med J 1983; 287:1524–1527.
38. Husband J, Husband P. Gastric emptying of water and glucose solutions in the newborn. Lancet 1969; ii:409–411.
39. Costalos C, Russell G, Rahim QAL, Blumenthal I, Hanlin S, Ross I. Gastric emptying of caloreen meals in the newborn. Arch Dis Child 1980; 55:883–885.
40. Yu VYH. Effect of body position on gastric emptying in the neonate. Arch Dis Child 1975; 50:500–504.
41. Cavell B. Gastric emptying in infants. Lancet 1969; ii:904–905.
42. Cavell B. Gastric emptying in preterm infants. Acta Paediatr Scand 1979; 68:725–730.
43. Wozniak E, Fenton TR, Milla PJ. Enteral feeds and intestinal motor activity in the preterm infant. Pediatr Res 1984; 18:1051.
44. McLain CR. Amniography studies of the gastrointestinal motility of the human fetus. Am J Obstet Gynecol 1963; 86:1079–1087.
45. Bisset WM, Watt JB, Rivers RPA, Milla PJ. Ontogeny of fasting small intestinal motor activity in the human infant. Gut 1988; 29:483–488.
46. Miller RA. Observations on the gastric acidity during the first month of life. Arch Dis Child 1941; 16:22–30.
47. Ames MD. Gastric acidity in the first ten days of life in the prematurely born baby. Am J Dis Child 1960; 100:252–256.
48. Deren JS. Development of structure and function in the fetal and newborn stomach. Am J Clin Nutr 1971; 24:144–159.
49. Agunod M, Yamaguchi N, Lopez R, Lubby AL, Glass GBJ. Correlative study of hydrochloric acid, pepsin and intrinsic factor secretion in newborns and infants. Am J Dig Dis 1969; 14:400–414.
50. Lieberman J. Proteolytic enzyme activity in fetal pancreas and meconium. Gastroenterology 1966; 50:183–190.
51. Track NS, Creutzfeldt C, Bockermann M. Enzymatic, functional and ultrastructural development of the exocrine pancreas. Comp Biochem Physiol 1975; 51A:95–100.
52. Zoppi G, Andreotti G, Pajno-Ferrara F, Njai DM, Gaburro D. Exocrine pancreas function in premature and full term neonates. Pediatr Res 1972; 6:880–886.
53. Lebenthal E, Lee PC. Development of functional response in human exocrine pancreas. Pediatrics 1980; 66:556–560.
54. Koldovsky O, Heringova A, Jirsova V, Jirasek JE, Uher J. Transport of glucose against a concentration gradient in everted sacs of jejunum and ileum of human fetuses. Gastroenterology 1965; 48:185–187.
55. Jirsova V, Koldovsky O, Heringova A, Hoskova J, Jirasek J, Uher J. The development of the functions of the small intestine of the human fetus. Biol Neonate 1966; 9:44–49.
56. Levin RJ, Koldovsky O, Hoskova J, Jirsova V, Uher J. Electrical measurement of intestinal glucose absorption in man. Lancet 1968; ii:624–627.
57. McNeish AS, Ducker DA, Warren IF, Davies DP, Harran MJ, Hughes CA. The influence of gestational age and size on the absorption of D-xylose and D-glucose from the small intestine of the human neonate. In: Elliott KM, Whelan J, eds. CIBA Foundation Symposium 70. Development of mammalian absorptive processes. Amsterdam: Excerpta Medica, 1979: 267.

58. Ducker DA, Hughes CA, Warren I, McNeish AS. Neonatal gut function, measured by the one hour blood D(+) xylose test: influence of gestational age and size. Gut 1980; 21:133–136.

59. Weaver LT, Laker MF, Nelson R, Lucas A. Milk feeding and changes in intestinal permeability and morphology in the newborn. J Pediatr Gastroenterol Nutr 1987; 6:351–358.

60. Weaver LT, Laker MF, Nelson R. Intestinal permeability in the newborn. Arch Dis Child 1984; 59:236–241.

61. Beach RC, Menzies IS, Clayden GS, Scopes JW. Gastrointestinal permeability changes in the preterm neonate. Arch Dis Child 1982; 57:141–145.

62. Dahlqvist A, Lindberg T. Development of the intestinal disaccharidase and alkaline phosphatase activities in the human foetus. Clin Sci Mol Med 1966; 30:577–528.

63. Antonowicz I, Lebenthal E. Developmental pattern of small intestinal enterokinase and disaccharidase activities in the human fetus. Gastroenterology 1977; 72:1299–1303.

64. Auricchio S, Rubino A, Murset G. Intestinal glycosidase activities in the human embryo, fetus, and newborn. Pediatrics 1965; 35:944–954.

65. Mayne AJ, Brown GA, Sule D, McNeish AS. Postnatal development of disaccharidase activities in jejunal fluid in preterm neonates. Gut 1986; 27:1357–1361.

66. Weaver LT, Laker MR, Nelson R. Neonatal intestinal lactase activity. Arch Dis Child 1986; 61:896–899.

67. Lebenthal E, Lee PC. Alternate pathways of digestion and absorption in early infancy. J Pediatr Gastroenterol Nutr 1984; 3:1–3.

68. Lindberg T. Intestinal dipeptidases: characterization, development and distribution of intestinal dipeptidases of the human foetus. Clin Sci 1966; 30:505–515.

69. Auricchio S, Stellato A, De Vizia D. Development of brush border peptidases in human and rat small intestine during fetal and neonatal life. Pediatr Res 1981; 15:991–995.

70. Kelley RJ. An ultrastructural and cytochemical study of developing small intestine in man. J Embryol Exp Morphol 1973; 29:411–430.

71. Hamosh M, Scanlon JW, Ganot D, Likel M, Scanlon KB, Hamosh P. Fat digestion in the newborn: characterization of lipase in gastric aspirates of premature and term infants. J Clin Invest 1981; 67:838–846.

72. Hamosh M. Lingual and breast milk lipases. Adv Pediatr 1982; 29:33–67.

73. Harries JT. Fat absorption in the newborn. Acta Paediatr Scand 1982; 299(Suppl):17–23.

74. Watkins JB, Szczepanik P, Gould JP, Klein P, Lester R. Bile salt metabolism in the human premature infant. Gastroenterology 1975; 69:706–713.

75. Roberton DM, Paganelli R, Dinwiddie R, Levinsky RJ. Milk antigen absorption in the preterm and term neonate. Arch Dis Child 1982; 57:369–372.

76. Weaver LT, Freiberg E, Israel EJ, Walker WA. Epidermal growth factor in human amniotic fluid. Gastroenterology 1988;1436.

77. Pothier P, Menard D. Presence and characteristics of epidermal growth factor receptors in human fetal small intestine and colon. FEBS Lett 1988; 228:113–117.

78. Weaver LT, Walker WA. Epidermal growth factor and the developing human gut. Gastroenterology 1988; 94:845–847.

79. McNabb PC, Tomasi TB. Host defence mechanisms at mucosal surfaces. Annu Rev Microbiol 1981; 85:477–496.

80. Selner JC, Merrill DA, Claman HN. Salivary immunoglobulin and albumin: development during the newborn period. J Pediatr 1968; 72:685–689.

81. Bridges RA, Condie RM, Zak SJ, Good R. The morphologic basis of antibody formation development during the neonatal period. J Lab Clin Med 1959; 53:331–357.

82. Rothberg RM. Immunoglobulin and specific antibody synthesis during the first weeks of life of premature infants. J Pediatr 1969; 75:391–399.

83. Rieger CHL, Rothberg RM. Development of the capacity to produce specific antibody to an ingested food antigen in the preterm infant. J Pediatr 1975; 87:515–518.

84. Lacroix B, Kedinger M, Simon-Assmann P, Rousset M, Zweibaum A, Haffen K. Development pattern of brush border enzymes in the human fetal colon: correlation with some morphogenic events. Early Hum Dev 1984; 9:95–103.

85. Potter GD, Lester R. The developing colon and nutrition. J Pediatr Gastroenterol Nutr 1984; 3:485–487.

86. Nyhan WL. Stool frequency of normal infants in the first week of life. Pediatrics 1952; 10:414–425.

87. Weaver LT, Ewing G, Taylor LC. The bowel habit of milk-fed infants. J Pediatr Gastroenterol Nutr 1988; 7:568–571.

88. Aynsley-Green A. Metabolic and endocrine interrelations in the human fetus and neonate. Am J Clin Nutr 1985; 41:339–417.

89. Lucas A, Bloom SR, Aynsley-Green A. Metabolic and endocrine events at the time of the first feed of human milk in preterm and term infants. Arch Dis Child 1978; 53:731–736.

90. Lucas A, Bloom SR, Aynsley-Green A. Metabolic and endocrine consequences of depriving preterm infants of enteral nutrition. Acta Paediatr Scand 1983; 72:245–249.

91. Ruppin H, Sturm G, Westhoff D, Domschke S, Domschke W, Winsch E, Demling L. Effect of B NLe motilin on small intestinal transit time in healthy subjects. Scand J Gastroenterol 1976; (Suppl 39)11:85–88.

92. Lucas A, Christofides ND, Adrian TE, Bloom SR, Aynsley-Green A. Fetal distress, meconium and motilin. Lancet 1979; ii:968.

93. Weaver LT. Milk and the neonatal gut: comparative lessons to be learnt. Equine Vet J 1986; 18:427–429.

94. Lesné E, Binet L, Paulin A. La traversée digestive chez le nourisson variations biologiques et pathologiques. Arch Méd Enfants 1920; 23:449–456.

95. Bullen CL, Tearle PV. Bifidobacteria in the intestinal tract of infants: an in-vitro study. J Med Microbiol 1976; 9:335–344.

96. Lucas A, Blackburn AM, Aynsley-Green A, Sarson DL, Adrian TE, Bloom SR. Breast vs bottle: endocrine responses are different with formula feeding. Lancet 1980; i:1267–1269.

97. Lucas A, Bloom SR, Aynsley-Green A. Gut hormones and 'minimal enteral feeding.' Acta Paediatr Scand 1986; 75:719–723.

98. Koldovsky O. Digestion and absorption of carbohydrates, protein, and fats in infants and children. In: Walker WA, Watkins JB, eds. Nutrition in pediatrics. Basic science and clinical application. Boston: Little, Brown & Co, 1985: 253.

99. Kleinman RE, Walker WA. The enteromammary immune system. Dig Dis Sci 1979; 24:876–882.

100. Welsh JK, May JT. Anti-infective properties of breast milk. J Pediatr 1979; 94:1–9.

101. Juto P. Human milk stimulates B cell function. Arch Dis Child 1985; 60:610–613.

102. Koldovsky O, Thornburg W. Hormones in milk. J Pediatr Gastroenterol Nutr 1987; 6:172–196.

103. Read LC, Upton FM, Francis GL, Wallace JC, Dahlenberg GW, Ballard FJ. Changes in the growth promoting activity of human milk during lactation. Pediatr Res 1984; 18:133–138.

104. Menard D, Arsenault P, Pothier P. Biologic effects of epidermal growth factor in human fetal jejunum. Gastroenterology 1988; 94:656–663.

Feeding, Tasting, and Sucking

Peter J. Milla, M.Sc., M.B.B.S., F.R.C.P.

An essential feature of childhood is growth, and for this to be optimal an adequate supply of energy is required. In this chapter the mechanisms involved in the delivery of food to the gastrointestinal (GI) tract for the eventual production of such energy are examined, and an account of our state of knowledge regarding their development is given.

DEFINITIONS

Feeding concerns the overall process whereby the infant or child ingests food. It is a very complex process in which a number of different factors interact; these are shown in Figure 1. This chapter is concerned largely with the development of structure and function of the oropharynx, which finally allows a child to eat in such a way as to be able to satisfy his nutritional needs. Psychological factors determine whether the child eats in a socially approved manner, which is in general a particular pattern of learned behavior acquired primarily from parental and sibling example. Consideration of these elements of feeding are beyond the scope of this chapter.

Taste is the sensation associated with the detection of sweet, sour, salty, and bitter chemicals in food eaten. The sensation appears to be associated with specialized receptor cells found in the lingual epithelium of the tongue whose output is transferred to higher centers via different nerve fibers in the seventh and ninth cranial nerves to the thalamus via the tractus solitarius and eventually higher cerebral centers. Little is known about the selectivity in taste processing by higher centers or the development of these processes in infants.

Sucking is due to muscular movements involving lips, mouth, and tongue and may or may not involve the presence of food or a teat in the mouth. Observational studies have described two patterns of sucking in the preterm infant: nonnutritive and nutritive sucking. Non-nutritive sucking develops first and is not associated with any purposeful ingestion of feeds, whereas nutritive sucking, which develops later at around 34 weeks of gestation, results in the ingestion of feeds and is associated with the development of co-ordinated peristalsis further down the gut and the control of respiratory movements.

Swallowing is a complex process whereby a bolus of food or mouthful of fluid is transferred from the mouth to the stomach. Solids require active peristalsis of the pharynx and esophagus, whereas in the upright position liquids require only relaxation of the upper esophogeal sphincter and gravity in order to reach the stomach. A considerable body of information has now accumulated regarding sucking and swallowing in the infant and the factors that may affect it.

EMBRYOLOGY

A detailed account of morphogenesis and differentiation is given elsewhere in this book. The area of the gut we are largely concerned with in this chapter is, in brief, developed mostly from ectoderm and mesoderm, but the epithelium of the tongue is derived from endoderm. The mouth is formed partly from the stomodeum or primitive mouth and partly from the floor of the cephalic portion of the foregut. The epithelium of the lips, the gums, and the enamel of the teeth are ectodermal and are derived from the walls of the stomodeum. The tongue is formed from the tuberculum imper in the endodermal floor of the pharynx and the lingual swellings of the first branchial or mandibular arch. The pharynx develops from the cephalic end of the foregut, the branchial arches, and pharyngeal pouches. The endodermal aspect of the mandibular arch forms the lateral wall of the nasopharynx. The second arch forms the palatoglossal arch, the third arch the lateral glossoepiglottic fold, and the fourth arch the epiglottis.

The muscle mass of the mandibular arch forms the tensor palati and the muscles of mastication. The muscle mass of the second or hyoid arch largely forms the muscles of facial expression. The muscles of the pharynx, soft palate, and larynx are formed from the remaining branchial arches. The portion of the foregut that succeeds the pharynx remains tubular and is elongated to form the esophagus.

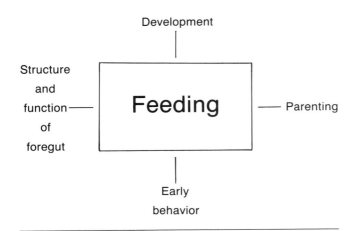

FIGURE 1 The factors that affect feeding.

217

SUCKING AND SWALLOWING

Sucking and swallowing are mechanisms that are established prenatally but are not fully developed until after birth. The fully developed mechanism has been extensively reviewed[1,2] and is considered only in outline below.

Intrauterine Swallowing

For many years it has been recognized that the fetus is able to swallow from as early as 11 to 12 weeks' gestation. Using ^{51}Cr-tagged red blood cells given by amniocentesis into the amniotic fluid, the volume of fluid swallowed increases from an initial 2 to 7 ml per day to 13 to 16 ml per day at 20 weeks' gestation and up to 450 ml per day at term.[3] Why the fetus swallows amniotic fluid is not clear, but it may serve a variety of purposes. It probably allows the fetal gut, which has well-developed absorptive mechanisms by 12 to 14 weeks' gestation, to regulate amniotic fluid volume. The importance of this function is underlined by the fact that polyhydramnios is frequently associated with esophageal, duodenal, and small bowel atresias. There are perhaps trophic factors in the amniotic fluid that are important in the development of internal structure and function; this may be particularly true for the enteric endocrine cells.

The Ontogeny of Sucking and Swallowing

Although it is well-recognized that swallowing occurs in utero and is described above, the earliest signs of sucking do not occur until between 18 and 24 weeks of gestation.[4] The early sucking movements of very premature infants do not result in effective ingestion of milk feeds and have been termed *non-nutritive sucking* to differentiate them from the much more effective nutritive sucking mechanism that develops at about 34 to 35 weeks of gestation.[5,6]

Sucking in the infant, both nutritive and non-nutritive, is a reflex behavior and, not surprisingly, most studies have shown that its development is related to gestational age.

However, a number of other factors have also been shown to affect sucking, and these include maternal sedation,[6] the presence of a nipple and the flow rate of milk,[7] the length of the feeding experience,[6,8] the taste of the fluid,[9] and even visual stimuli.[10] It is, however, gestational age and neurologic development of both the central and enteric nervous systems that are the strongest determinants of the type and efficiency of sucking. In this context it is of interest that several studies have noticed that effective nutritive sucking does not develop until 34 to 35 weeks' gestation. A study of the ontogeny of small intestinal motor activity[11] showed clearly that the onset of such sucking behavior parallels the acquisition of mature patterns (cyclic fasting migratory motor complexes and continuous postprandial pattern) of gastric antral and small intestinal motor activity, as shown in Figure 2. This pattern of development represents an exception to the usual craniocaudal gradient but ensures that the ability to transport food along the gut is developed appropriately with the acquisition of the ability to ingest large amounts of food.

Sucking and Swallowing After Birth

The Mechanisms of Sucking and Swallowing

Although sucking and swallowing movements are established before birth, as discussed above, they do not develop fully until a variable period of time after birth. It is also clear from the above discussion that ability to feed is related both to gestational age and to length of feeding experience.[6] The details of the feeding mechanism in normal infants,[12] in full-term neonates,[13] and in preterm infants[14,15] have been described in detail. Sucking movements precede swallowing, which in turn inhibits respiration and is closely co-ordinated with relaxation of the lower esophageal sphincter and receptive relaxation of the fundus of the stomach. In older infants the first stage of swallowing is voluntary in character but at term or before term is an involuntary reflex.

A bolus of fluid is delivered to the mouth by the forces of nipple compression by the mandible and intraoral suction. It is carried back to the pharynx by tongue action against the

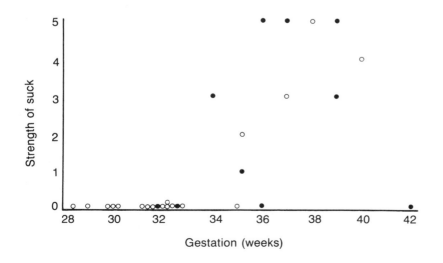

FIGURE 2 Gestational age and the acquisition of nutritive sucking. Open circles = born before 29 weeks' gestation. Closed circles = born after 29 weeks' gestation. (Courtesy of Dr. W.M. Bisset.)

palate. The movement commences at the tip of the tongue and spreads rapidly backward, thus passing the bolus to the posterior part of the mouth. The posterior part of the tongue then moves upward and backward, protruding into the oropharynx and propelling the bolus into the pharynx. A series of co-ordinated contractions of muscles associated with the pharynx, soft palate, and larynx then pushes the bolus toward the esophagus without entering the nasopharynx or larynx. The nasopharynx is closed by elevation of the soft palate and contraction of the superior constrictors of the pharynx. At the same time the larynx is drawn upward behind the hyoid and the aryepiglottic folds close, thus preventing fluid from entering the larynx. The bolus of fluid moves onward, partly under the influence of gravity and partly by successive contraction of the superior and middle constrictors. This process is aided by the posterior pharyngeal wall being converted into an inclined plane directed downward and backward by the action of the palatopharyngei; the bolus descends on its undersurface. The aryepiglottic folds also act as lateral channels, leading the bolus toward the esophagus. The last stage of swallowing is effected by the inferior constrictor, which allows food to pass into the esophagus. This muscle consists of two parts—the thyropharyngeal muscle above, which is propulsive, and the cricopharyngeal below, which is sphincteric in function and is otherwise known as the superior esophageal sphincter.

Non-nutritive Sucking

Non-nutritive sucking is characterized by a rapid rate of sucking, usually exceeding two sucks per second, which is approximately twice as fast as later nutritive sucking.[16] In its most immature form, non-nutritive sucking consists of mouthing movements only, and this may be seen as early as 18 to 24 weeks' gestation.[4] In a longitudinal study of preterm infants from 32 weeks' gestation to term, Gryboski[14] found that the initial response to a nipple was mouthing followed after a variable period of time by short bursts of sucks initially not associated with swallowing and often preceded and followed by considerable mouthing. The period of time before sucking occurred was longer in the most premature infants (3 to 10 days) than in full-term infants, in whom sucking occurred on the first day. The initial rate of sucking was slowest in the most premature (approximately one suck per second), rising to two sucks per second as the infants grew older and achieved longer bursts of sucking with intermittent swallowing. By the time infants were at 35 to 36 weeks' postconceptional age they sucked in bursts of up to 30 consecutive sucks and could swallow frequently during sucking. Gryboski termed this latter pattern "mature suck-swallow," characterized by bursts of over 30 sucks and a rate of two sucks per second, with swallows occurring frequently during sucking bursts. The first pattern seen after initial mouthing—"the immature suck-swallow"—consisted of short sucking bursts at one to one and one-half sucks per second at pressures of −5 to −15 mm Hg alternating with positive pressures of 5 to 20 mm Hg and preceded or followed by swallows, but in the older preterm infant swallows always followed each burst. Pharyngeal pressure peaks occurring with swallows measure 10 to 20 mm Hg.

The superior esophageal sphincter is located 6.5 to 8 cm from the lips and is 0.5 to 1 cm in length. It is an area of increased pressure some 2 to 4 mm Hg higher than the resting esophageal pressure. With swallows the sphincter relaxes; the pressure falls some 3 to 7 mm Hg and lasts 0.5 to 1 second and is followed by a return to resting pressure, then by a positive pressure wave of 2 to 6 mm Hg. The acquisition of the mature suck-swallow pattern is associated with pressure increases of −10 to 20 mm Hg and +15 to 30 mm Hg. Pharyngeal contractions are likewise more powerful, increasing to 15 to 30 mm Hg. The superior esophageal sphincter function seems much the same as in younger preterm infants. In all infants respiration was inhibited by swallows and prior to 33 weeks' postconceptional age, when infants had the early suck-swallow pattern, esophageal peristalsis was not recorded, but simultaneous contractions indicative of tertiary contractions were. At about 35 weeks after conception and by the time the infants had a mature suck-swallow, propagative esophageal contractions were recorded, although these were often biphasic, ill-formed, and of low amplitude (6 to 16 mm Hg). The tone of the lower esophageal sphincter was similarly low (0 to 5 mm Hg) but relaxed with swallowing. These patterns are very reminiscent of those seen in older infants with severe gastroesophageal reflux (GER) and esophagitis. Some have speculated in children with esophagitis that there is an inherent developmental delay of the esophageal myenteric plexus.[17] Clearly, in the premature infant there are developmental processes affecting both the myenteric plexus and esophageal muscle. Studies in the small intestine and experimental animal have suggested that the reflex patterns that develop around 35 weeks after conception are associated with the acquisition of particular neuronal networks.[11]

Previous studies have shown that non-nutritive sucking enhances the rate of weight gain in preterm infants.[18] A recent study of polypeptide hormone release and gastric emptying has shown that preterm infants who were tube fed and sucked a pacifier emptied their stomachs more quickly.[19] In addition, these infants were found to secrete more gastrin (a hormone known to be important in postprandial GI motor activity) and less somatostatin (a hormone associated with fasting motor activity). The authors speculated that the effects on the pattern of polypeptide hormone secretion were vagally mediated and that they may also have influenced gastric emptying. Thus, encouraging non-nutritive sucking may enhance postprandial motor activity and allow earlier feeding to be tolerated.

Nutritive Sucking

Nutritive sucking develops somewhat later than early non-nutritive sucking and seems to be related to the acquisition of the mature non-nutritive suck-swallow pattern and the development of organized patterns of motor activity in the esophagus,[20] antrum, and small intestine.[11] In the normal full-term infant, a clear pattern of sucking and swallowing develops within a few days of birth. The pattern consists of prolonged bursts of rhythmic sucking of 10 to 30 sucks, with pressures of −10 to −25 mm Hg and swallowing one to four times during each burst. During swallowing, pharyngeal con-

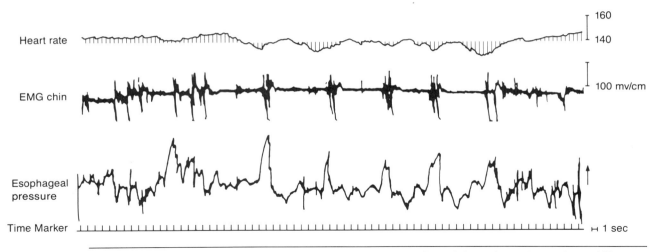

FIGURE 3 Inefficient sucking pattern in premature infants. (Adapted from data of Daniels et al.[15])

tractions transport nutrients across the pharynx when the superior esophageal sphincter relaxes, and food is admitted to the esophagus and is propelled into the stomach, relaxation of the lower esophageal sphincter being co-ordinated with the esophageal peristaltic sequences.

In premature infants two patterns of nutritive sucking have been described which broadly correlate with Gryboski's mature and immature patterns. Daniels et al[15] studied nutritive sucking in 18 preterm infants from 29 to 33 weeks' gestation at birth. Unfortunately, no details of the infants postconceptional age at the time of study are given. They observed two patterns of sucking—an inefficient pattern shown in Figure 3 and an efficient pattern in Figure 4. The sucking rate was the same in both patterns and was about one suck per second, which is comparable to that in other studies of nutritive sucking in preterm[21] and full-term infants.[16,22] Thus, unlike non-nutritive sucking, no correlation with gestational age was apparent. Daniels et al[15] also state that the sucking rate did not significantly correlate with feeding experience or with differences in feeding efficiency. Infants who needed to suck longer per milliliter of milk intake had lower suck burst-to-pause time ratio owing to shorter sucking bursts with

longer pauses. The inefficient pattern, as seen in Figure 3, was characterized by short sucking bursts and by a small volume of milk intake during each sucking movement. The efficient pattern shown in Figure 4 consists of long sucking bursts and a large amount of milk intake during each sucking movement. This pattern seems highly similar to the mature suck-swallow pattern described with non-nutritive sucking.

Whether the infants were drinking efficiently or inefficiently, they could suck, swallow, and breathe simultaneously. Respiratory arrests that have been previously described[14] were not seen, but a decrease in respiratory rate during sucking was observed.[15]

Nutritive sucking can also be modulated by a number of different inputs to the tractus solitarius of the brain from the facial, glossopharyngeal, and vagal nerves. These inputs can be stimulated by the presence of a nipple[7] and by taste and nutrient content. For example, there is more sucking activity with milk than with either dextrose or water.[23] Taste also seems to affect sucking activity. Sucking increased with increasing concentrations of glucose, fructose, sucrose, or lactose in various test feeds. Interestingly, the test feeds that

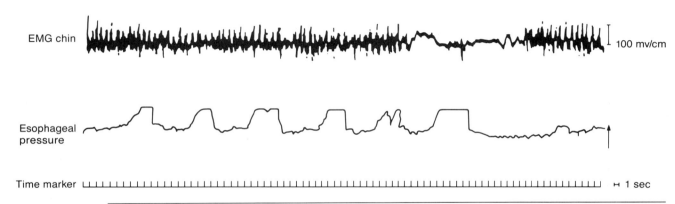

FIGURE 4 Efficient sucking pattern in premature infants. (Adapted from data of Daniels et al.[15])

provoked most sucking were those judged sweetest by the investigators.[9] In a study of sucking mechanisms, others showed that when infants sucked sucrose solutions, sucking bursts were stronger and more prolonged with less resting time between bursts than with water.[24] As infants grow older (3 to 5 months of age) different inputs such as visual stimuli can affect sucking.[10]

LATER DEVELOPMENT OF SUCKING AND CHEWING

Oral-pharyngeal motor development follows a sequential pattern summarized in Table 1. Initially two reflexes are important: rooting, which is an orientating response to assist the baby in locating food, and a suck-swallow reflex, which is described in detail above. The initial rooting reflex consists of turning the head from side to side, alternately toward and away from the stimulus, and this occurs for the first 2 to 3 weeks of life. From 3 weeks until rooting disappears at about 3 months, the infant deliberately turns the head to the stimulus, grasps the nipple, and sucks.

Similarly, the suck-swallow reflex of the term infant displays two stages in addition to those previously described for the preterm infant.[25] The initial stage in nutritive sucking,

sometimes known as suckling, is different from that of mature sucking seen at around 4 to 6 months of age. Initially the lips are loosely approximated around the nipple, allowing some loss of liquid, and the tongue moves in and out in a licking motion. In later mature sucking the teat is firmly grasped with lips and jaw closed and the tongue moves rhythmically up and down, creating a negative pressure in the mouth.

There are also changes in the pattern of swallowing. When the neonate swallows, the infant's mouth opens preceding a swallow, and the tongue protrudes and then retracts as the swallow proceeds and the mouth closes. Between 6 and 12 weeks of age, tongue protrusion diminishes and is followed by the tongue elevating and moving backward to actively help form a bolus.[26]

Biting and Chewing

In preparation for the later ingestion of solid food, a number of further developmental steps occur that are designed to break food down into small lumps to form a bolus.

Bite Reflex. In response to pressure on the anterior and lower aspects of the upper and lower gums, the infant exhibits a rhythmic vertical bite-and-release movement. This is seen shortly after birth and persists until about 5 months of age, when it is integrated into chewing.[25]

Chewing. From about 5 months onward, early chewing or munching occurs in which the jaw moves up and down with no tongue lateralization. At 6 to 7 months, isolated movements of tongue, lips, and jaw combine for chewing, and then the tongue develops lateral movements to carry food from side to side. These movements progress, and around the age of 1 year the jaw is able to make rotary movements and rotary chewing begins. This is followed by development of control of lip closure and cheek action to keep food over the molars for grinding. So by 24 months of age a mature rotary chewing action has developed, which requires the smoothly co-ordinated function of tongue, lips, jaws, and cheeks.

Spoon Feeding and Drinking from a Cup

Spoon feeding of solids initially pureed is possible when lip control progresses from undifferentiated mass movement patterns seen in the primitive reflexes to isolated control of one lip from the other. Such discrete movements allow a child to grasp a nipple firmly when lateral lip closure is incorporated and later, about 7 months of age, to clear food from a spoon with the upper lip and remove food from the lip by brushing one lip over the other. These movements are necessary for later self-feeding.

Drinking from a cup is not possible until the 6-month stage of development is reached and requires the development of tongue tip elevation during swallowing, lip control, and the maturation of jaw stabilization so that the baby can stabilize the jaw on the cup rim by muscular control rather than biting. Control of this process is not complete until 2 to 3 years of age.

TABLE 1
Development of Oral-Pharyngeal Motor Activity

Age	Food	Oral Skill
0–12 weeks	Milk	Preterm nutritive sucking Suckling Bite reflex Losing liquid from corner of mouth
12–20 weeks	May begin cereals and pureed foods	Mature sucking/swallowing Bite reflex Decrease in loss of liquid from mouth Increasing strength of suck
20–28 weeks	Strained foods Teething biscuits	Bite/suck reflexes go Smacking lips Moving lips in eating
28–32 weeks	Strained and mashed foods	Clearing spoon with lips Moving tongue laterally Early chewing
8–10 months	Mashed and mineral foods Finger foods	Biting on objects Munching Closing mouth on rims
10–12 months	Mashed-chopped fine foods	Playing with tongue Moving tongue from side to side Licking food off of lip Rotary chewing movements
12–15 months	Chopped fine foods	Spitting food Decrease in drooling
15–24 months	Ordinary food Some meat chopped fine	Mature rotary chewing movements

FEEDING PROBLEMS

It is easy to see that the above complex developmental process is open to perturbation at many different stages and that this will result in difficulty in feeding. Thus, anatomic abnormalities of the mouth, such as cleft palate, Pierre-Robin syndrome, neurologic disorders, and muscle disease, may all influence the process.

In infants with neurologic disorders, the pattern of development may be extremely slow, analogous to the delays in motor development seen elsewhere, or it may be arrested at a particular stage as, for example, in the persistence of primitive reflexes. The use of primitive oral functions will hinder progress to more textured foods, and such progress can be made only at the speed with which oral motor development takes place.

Other functional disorders may also result in feeding problems. The most common of these appears to be GER. Mahoney et al[17] showed that in those with more severe forms of GER feeding problems may occur. The feeding problem usually takes the form of inability to progress from very smooth purees to more lumpy and textured foods. Persistence in feeding lumpy foods may result in a degree of oral sensitivity to them, as described below. The mechanism of the lack of progression to lumpy foods is not known but may be due to a delay in the development of appropriate oral motor function or to difficulty in co-ordinating active pharyngeal contraction with the upper esophageal sphincter and esophageal peristalsis.

Babies who are exclusively tube fed may exaggerate oral tactile sensitivity. Mueller[27] and others[28] have suggested that lack of oral experience at a critical period of 6 to 12 months of age results in difficulty in eating solid food. However, the hypersensitivity that is associated with the lack of oral experience results in uncontrolled over-reaction to the nipple, spoon, or cup, with resulting choking, gagging, tongue-thrusting, and refusal of solids. Such difficulties can be overcome by a period of densitization and probably are not a result of loss of a critical period of development.

TASTE

The sensation of taste is initiated by small populations of specialized receptor cells found in the lingual epithelium of the tongue. The taste receptor cells are neuroepithelial cells located in the taste buds of the tongue. Each taste bud in the adult contains some 60 to 100 receptor cells with a tiny portion of its membrane exposed in a taste pore on the mucosal surface of the tongue. The afferent sensory fibers are in the base of each taste bud and travel in the facial, glossopharyngeal, or vagus nerves to primary gustatory nuclei in the brain (Fig. 5). Taste transduction has recently been the subject of an excellent review to which interested readers are referred.[29]

Classically it was suggested that taste sensation is initiated by sapid chemicals of food that interact with specific receptors on the apical microvillous membrane of the receptor cells. Binding of the chemicals results in depolarization of the receptor and a membrane conductance change. Depolarization of the receptor cell causes transmitter release and excitation of

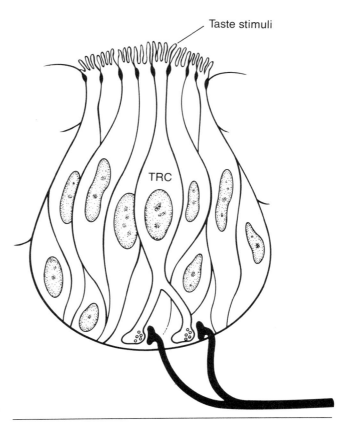

FIGURE 5 Taste receptor cells (TRC) and their innervation.

the sensory nerve fiber.[30] Recent advances in taste cell isolation have allowed the use of modern electrophysiologic methods in isolated cells. As a result, it now appears that specific membrane receptors are not required for all taste stimuli and that membrane conductance changes in response to taste stimulation are controlled by voltage-dependent selective ion channels similar to those in neurons and other epithelial cells.

Specific Taste Transduction

Sour taste is produced by acids, the degree of sourness depending on proton concentration. A very recent study shows that voltage-dependent K^+ channels are restricted to the apical membrane, whereas Na^+ and Ca^{2+} channels are present in both apical and basolateral membranes. Acid blocks K^+ channels but not Na^+ or Ca^{2+} channels; thus, the cells depolarize and the taste is transduced.[31]

Salt taste transduction also does not require specific receptors. Increasing evidence from a variety of studies shows that amiloride-sensitive voltage-independent Na^+ channels mediate Na^+ salt taste.[32] This channel appears to be identical to the passive amiloride-sensitive apical Na^+ channel found in other transporting epithelia. This mechanism is known to be present in the human.[33]

Unlike the mechanisms for salt and acid taste, sweetness appears to involve specific membrane receptors. There are probably two mechanisms: One involves receptor-mediated stimulation of adenylate cyclase and cyclic adenosine monophosphate–induced phosphorylation of basolateral K^+ channels, with consequent attenuation of the channel[34]; there is some evidence that there is another sweetness mechanism that involves an amiloride-sensitive Na^+ channel.[33]

Preliminary results of studies involving bitter and amino acid taste transduction have recently appeared and suggest that bitter taste involves receptor-mediated release of intracellular Ca^{2+}.[35] Amino acids appear to involve direct ligand gating.[36]

Thus, in some cases (acid and Na^+ salt) taste cells have utilized common membrane properties of epithelial cells and neurons in unique ways to achieve stimulus transduction, whereas special receptors are required in other cases (sweet and bitter taste).

Appreciation of Taste

How does the tongue tell the brain about taste? The diversity of mechanisms described above are unusual in sensory systems. Both vision and hearing utilize only single mechanisms that respond to homogeneous stimuli. Thus the diversity of taste mechanisms may reflect the molecular diversity of sapid chemicals. In addition, afferent nerves fibers tend to synapse with similar taste cells and respond better to a single taste modality. Different primary tastes may therefore be localized in separate receptor cells that are specialized to detect one or a few tastes. Little is known, however, about selectivity in taste cells or the processing of taste in higher centers.

Ontogeny of Taste

Only a very limited amount of information is available regarding the ontogeny of the above taste transduction mechanisms or the processing of taste sensation in higher centers. Such data that are available rely on very indirect observations, some of which have been considered regarding the modulation of sucking. It is clear that sweetness is appreciated in the early neonatal period in full-term infants.[9,24] Similarly, salty tastes have been shown to affect the amount of feeds consumed, suggesting that this taste modality is also present early on. However, there is no information regarding acid taste, although clinical experience suggests that bitter and amino acid tastes develop some time after birth. Much work remains to be done to provide clear information regarding taste that may be useful in the formulation of therapeutic feeds.

REFERENCES

1. Miller AJ. Deglutition. Physiol Rev 1982; 62:129–184.
2. Miller AJ. Neurophysiological basis of swallowing. Dysphagia 1986; 1:91–100.
3. Pritchard JA. Fetal swallowing and amniotic fluid volume. Obstet Gynecol 1966; 28:606–610.
4. Golubera EL, Shuleikina KV, Vaenshsteinii V. Development of reflex and spontaneous activity of the human fetus in the process of embryogenesis. Obstet Gynecol (USSR) 1959; 3:59–62.
5. Herbst JJ. Development of suck and swallow. J Pediatr Gastroentorol Nutr 1983; 2:S131–S135.
6. Casaer P, Daniels H, Devlieger H, DeCock P, Eggermont E. Feeding behaviour in preterm neonates. Early Human Dev 1982; 7:331–346.
7. Peiper A. Cerebral functioning in infancy and childhood. New York: Consultants Bureau, 1963.
8. Crump EP, Gore PM, Morton C. The sucking behaviour in premature infants. Hum Biol 1958; 30:334–340.
9. Maller O, Turner RE. Taste in acceptance of sugars in human infants. J Comp Physiol 1973; 84:496–501.
10. Milewski AK, Sigueland ER. Discrimination of color and pattern novelty in one month old infants. J Exp Child Psychol 1975; 19:122–136.
11. Bisset WM, Watt JB, Rivers RPA, Milla PJ. The ontogeny of small intestinal fasting motor activity in the human infant. Gut 1988; 29:483–488.
12. Logan WJ, Bosma JF. Oral and pharyngeal dysphagia in infancy. Pediatr Clin North Am 1967; 14:47–54.
13. Gryboski JD. The swallowing mechanism of the neonate: I. Esophageal and gastric motility. Pediatrics 1965; 35:445–452.
14. Gryboski JD. Suck and swallow in the premature infant. Pediatrics 1969; 43:96–101.
15. Daniels H, Casaer P, Devlieger H, Eggermont E. Mechanisms of feeding efficiency in preterm infants. J Pediatr Gastroenterol Nutr 1986; 5:593–596.
16. Wolff PH. The serial organisation of sucking in the young infant. Pediatrics 1968; 42:943–956.
17. Mahoney MJ, Spitz L, Milla PJ. Motor disorders of the oesophagus in gastro-oesophageal reflux. Arch Dis Child 1988; 63:1333–1338.
18. Measel CP, Anderson GC. Non-nutritive sucking during tube feeding: effect on clinical course in premature infants. J Obstet Gynecol Neonatal 1979; 8:265–272.
19. Widstrom AM, Marchini G, Matthiesen AS, Werner S, Winberg J, Uvnas-moberg K. Non-nutritive sucking in tube fed preterm infants: effects on gastric motility and gastric contents of somatostatin. J Pediatr Gastroenterol Nutr 1988; 8:517–523.
20. Gryboski JD. Suck and swallow. In: Schaeffer AJ, Markowitz M, eds. Gastrointestinal problems in the infant. Philadelphia: WB Saunders, 1975.
21. Cortial C, Lezine I. Comparative study of nutritive sucking in the newborn (premature and full term). Early Child Dev Care 1974; 3:211–228.
22. Colley JRT, Creamer B. Sucking and swallowing in infants. Br Med J 1958; 2:422–423.
23. Dubignon J, Campbell D. Sucking in the newborn in three conditions: non-nutritive, nutritive, and a feed. J Exp Child Psychol 1969; 6:335–350.
24. Ashmead DH, Reilly BM, Lipsitt LP. Neonates heart-rate, sucking rhythm, and sucking amplitude as a function of sweet taste. J Exp Child Psychol 1980; 29:264–281.
25. Morris SE. Assessment of children with oral motor dysfunction. In: Wilson JM, ed. Oral motor function and dysfunction in children. Chapel Hill: University of North Carolina, 1978.
26. Ingram TTS. Clinical significance of the infantile feeding reflexes. Dev Med Clin Neurol 1962; 4:159–169.
27. Mueller HA. Facilitating feeding and pre-speech. In: Pearson PH, Williams CE, eds. Physical therapy services in the developmental disabilities. Springfield, IL: Charles C Thomas, 1972.
28. Illingworth RS, Lister J. The critical or sensitive period, with special reference to feeding problems in infants and children. J Pediatr 1964; 65:839–848.
29. Kinnamon SC. Taste transduction: a diversity of mechanisms. Trends Neuro Sci 1988; 11:491–496.
30. Beidler LM. The chemical senses. Ann Rev Psychol 1961; 12:363–388.
31. McBride D, Roper S. Voltage dependent K^+ channels are restricted to the apical membrane of taste receptor cells. Biophys J 1988; 51:11a.
32. Heck GL, Mierson S, DeSimone JA. Salt taste transduction occurs through an anicloride-sensitive sodium transport pathway. Science 1984; 223:403–405.
33. Schiffman SS, Lockhead E, Maes FW. Anicloride reduces the taste intensity of Na^+ and Li^+ salts and sweeteners. Proc Natl Acad Sci USA 1983; 80:6136–6140.
34. Tonosaki K, Funakoshi M. Cyclic nucleotides may mediate taste transduction. Nature 1988; 331:354–356.
35. Akabas MH, Dodd J, Al Awqati Q. Calcium medicates bitter taste transduction. (Abstract) Soc Neuro-Sci 1987; 13:361.
36. Tester JH, Branel JG. Reconstituted L-arginine sensitive channels from catfish taste epithelia. (Abstract) Soc Neuro-Sci 1987; 13:361.

CHAPTER 15

Esophageal Motility

Samuel Nurko, M.D.

The primary function of the esophagus is to propel the fluid or food it receives from the mouth to the stomach and to prevent the retrograde flow of gastric contents between swallows. The last decade has witnessed major advances in the understanding of normal esophageal development, its physiology, and the pathophysiology of the motor disorders of the esophagus. This chapter reviews normal esophageal function and development; a later chapter provides a detailed description of the pathophysiology, diagnostic criteria, and the approach to motility disorders of the esophagus in children.

NORMAL ESOPHAGEAL FUNCTION AND DEVELOPMENT

The esophagus is a hollow organ of three major components: the upper esophageal sphincter (UES), the esophageal body, and the lower esophageal sphincter (LES).[1]

The esophagus extends from the pharynx into the stomach. In the newborn infant it measures from 7.5 to 13 cm in length[2] and for infants and children tables are available to determine approximate esophageal length on the basis of age,[3-5] or it can be estimated by the use of regression equations employing height.[5] In the adult its length varies from 27 to 45 cm in cadavers,[5] and when measured endoscopically or manometrically it ususally measures 40 cm.[6] The esophagus is closed at its rostral end by the UES and at its caudal end by the LES. From a physiologic point of view, the esophagus has four parts: two sphincters (UES and LES), and a body with two components—an upper third consisting of striated muscle and a lower third composed of smooth muscle,[7] with the middle being a combination of both.

As mentioned above, the esophagus has two main functions. The first to propel to the stomach the fluid or food it receives from the mouth during the act of swallowing, and the second is to prevent the retrograde flow of gastric contents. The first requires an organized sequence of aborally progressive peristaltic contractions and sphincter relaxations, and the second depends on its anatomic integrity and adequate function of the sphincters and smooth muscle.

The act of swallowing has been divided in three phases: the *oral phase*, which is voluntary and transfers food from the mouth into the pharynx; the *pharyngeal phase*, which cannot be stopped once it begins and which transfers food from the pharynx into the esophagus; and the *esophageal phase*, which transports food from the esophagus into the stomach. In this chapter we focus mainly on the esophageal phase.

THE UPPER ESOPHAGEAL SPHINCTER

The major functions of the UES appear to be prevention of esophageal distention during respiration and protection against lung aspiration from gastroesophageal reflux (GER).[8,9] The UES is located at a position that varies directly with the height of the patient.[10] It is located in infants somewhere between 7 and 9 cm from the nares,[11] and in adults it is usually between C5 and C7.[9]

The UES muscle is 1 cm in width, although when the UES is defined manometrically, the area of high intraluminal pressure ranges in the adult from 2 to 4 cm,[7-9] a fact that has raised questions regarding its anatomic correlate, although recently it has been suggested that the cricopharyngeus and the caudal portion of the inferior pharyngeal constrictor are its main muscular elements.[8,12] Some authors, however, believe that the circular muscle fibers of the proximal esophagus make up the remainder of the UES.[13] It is interesting to note that cricopharyngeal myotomy in humans reduces but does not abolish the high pressure zone.[14]

The UES is maintained closed between swallows by tonic stimulation of the somatic nerves, thus preventing esophageal contents from refluxing into the pharynx and lungs and preventing esophageal distention during respiration.[15] This tonic stimulation of the UES is characterized by continuous electrical spike potentials.[12] During swallowing this tonic stimulation ceases, and the UES relaxes for a short time during swallowing. It also relaxes during vomiting, belching, retching, and gagging.[16] UES relaxation is thought to result from a programmed inhibitory stimulation that travels from the swallowing center in the brain stem via the vagus nerve.[7]

During swallowing the muscles of the pharynx contract in an orderly fashion and push the bolus into the esophagus[13] through an open UES. The co-ordination of events is such that UES pressure falls at the time a swallow is initiated, and this relaxation remains until the bolus has reached the pharynx.[17] As can been seen in Figure 1, the pharyngeal contraction appears as a propagated wave that occurs in the middle of the UES relaxation period.

The manometric study of the UES has been difficult.[18] Using perfused manometric techniques there has been a lack of reproducibility of recorded pressures and a marked variability.[15] The pressures recorded depend on the directional orientation of the recording orifices, and it has been difficult to record accurately the rapid pressure changes and movement that occur in this region.[18] It is known that the UES makes an oral excursion with swallowing,[19] and it has even

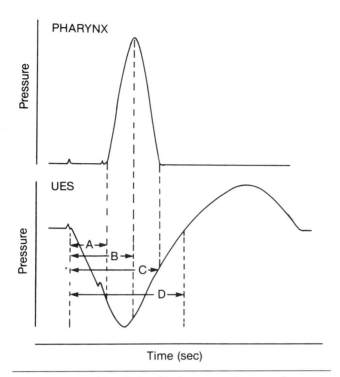

FIGURE 1 Graphic relationship between pharyngeal contraction and UES relaxation. Pressure and time units specified as A (0.58 ± 0.05 sec), B (0.98 ± 0.06 sec), and C (1.26 ± 0.07 sec) define the position of the pharyngeal pressure wave within the period of UES relaxation (D, 1.58 ± 0.07 sec). (From Green and Castell[17]; © 1987 by Elsevier Science Publishing Co., Inc.)

been suggested that the manometric recording of UES relaxation may be artifactual,[20] particularly with the high compliance perfused systems. With the advent of low-compliance, continuously perfused catheters that can record rapid pressure changes greater than 400 mm Hg per second[21] or distal transducer manometry catheters, accurate measurement of the UES has become more feasible.[22] Manometrically the UES has been shown to have radial asymmetry, with the posterior pressures being significantly higher than the anterior.[15] It has been estimated that the normal UES pressure in the adult varies from 60 to 142 mm Hg, with a mean of 101 mm Hg in the posterior quadrant.[9,17,23] It has also been shown that the peak posterior pressure does not occur at the same level in the manometric pull-through; peak posterior pressures occurred 0.55 cm more distally than anterior peak pressures.[9] Figure 1 also shows the temporal relationship between the pharyngeal contraction and UES relaxation, as measured by Knuff et al.[23] In adults it has been suggested that during deglution peak pharyngeal pressure may normally occur within 0.1 to 0.2 sec after the nadir of UES relaxation[23] and that the pharynx is capable of injecting fluid into the esophagus at a velocity of 70 cm per second.[24] As can be seen from Figure 1, total UES relaxation is always longer than pharyngeal contraction, and peak pharyngeal contraction was simultaneous with the nadir in UES.[10]

The UES exists in the newborn period [11,25] and seems to have an intact function at that age. It has also been shown to be present as early as 32 weeks of gestation.[26] In the original studies of Gryboski[11] using nonperfused systems, it was found about 7 to 9 cm from the lips of normal newborns and was 0.5 to 1 cm in length; the UES relaxation was measured to occur 0.1 sec after the pharyngeal contraction, and the UES pressure was described as being 1 to 7 mm Hg higher than that of the esophageal body. Moroz et al[27] found the UES pressures to be slightly lower in children less than 1 year than in older children. Recently, Sondheimer, using new low-compliance perfused catheters, found in a study of 11 normal infants that the mean UES pressure was 28.9 ± 10 cm H_2O (range from 18.0 to 44.0), and the pharyngeal peristaltic waves had an amplitude of 79.7 ± 19.9 cm H_2O, a velocity of 8.5 ± 3.6 cm per second, and a duration of 0.59 ± 0.18 sec.[10] It has also been shown that the UES in normal infants and children relaxes to cervical esophageal baseline pressures and that UES relaxation is completely co-ordinated with pharyngeal contraction.[10,22]

UES relaxation is thought to result from a programmed inhibitory stimulation from the swallowing center in the brain stem. These signals travel via the vagus nerve, and although sensory receptors in the smooth muscle portion of the esophageal body allow for local modulation of the UES pressure, it is clear that this modulation also relies on the central nervous system,[7] as shown by the fact that the increase in UES pressure associated with esophageal distention is lost with transection of the vagosympathetic trunk in the laboratory.[7]

UES pressures have been shown to increase in response to intraesophageal fluid infused distal to the UES, to intraluminal fluid boluses, or to intraesophageal balloon distention.[9,15] It was originally suggested in adults that UES resting tone is increased by the presence of acid in the esophagus,[15] an observation that was later replicated in normal infants and infants with GER.[10] It was observed that normal infants less than 10 weeks of age did not show this response, a finding that was attributed to the length of the esophagus and the distance from the UES to the site of acid administration.[10] This apparent reflex increase in UES has been replicated in dogs, and it has been eliminated after cryovagotomy.[28] In these three cases the UES was measured using continuously perfused catheters, and the observation was made with the artificial intraesophageal instillation of 0.1 N HCl acid; it was concluded that the UES response was greater the closer or the faster the instillation of acid occurred. This observation has been challenged recently in a study of eight normal volunteers in which the UES was continuously recorded with a sleeve device, together with simultaneous intraesophageal pH measurements.[8] The authors found that the UES pressure during episodes of acid exposure during spontaneous GER was almost identical to UES pressure during intervals without any acid exposure. They found, however, that UES pressure decreases significantly during sleep, from a mean of 40 ± 17 mm Hg during periods of wakefulness to 20 ± 17 mm Hg in stage 1 sleep, and to 8 ± 3 mm Hg during deep sleep. Both findings, namely that the UES tone is virtually absent during sleep, and that there does not seem to be a reflex increase of the UES pressure during spontaneous GER, may have implications concerning the pathophysiology of regurgitation and aspiration. Clearly more studies, particularly in children, need to be performed to address these questions. It has also been shown that UES pressure is not affected postprandially,[8] unlike LES pressure, which tends to decrease.[29] UES pressure was also observed to increase transiently with each inspiration during episodes of restfulness and sleep, a response consistent with the hypothesis that one function of the upper esophageal sphincter is to exclude air from the esophagus during inspiration.[8]

There has also been controversy about the role of the UES in the pathogenesis of GER-associated respiratory problems.[8,10,27,30] In a prospective study in which normal infants were compared with infants with GER, it was shown that there was no difference between the two groups in any of the UES parameters studied (pressure, amplitude, duration and velocity of pharyngeal contractions, UES pharyngeal co-ordination, and UES response to exogenous acid adminstration).[10]

ESOPHAGEAL BODY

After the food bolus has passed through the UES, it starts its journey into the stomach via the esophageal body. This structure starts at the lower portion of the UES and ends at the LES. Its length is variable, ranging between 18 and 24 cm in the adult, although at birth it measures approximately 10 cm.[1,26] In its proximal portion it consists of striated muscle in both the inner and the outer muscular layer, and in the lower third it has smooth muscle. The middle third is said to be a transition zone. However, recently in a series of autopsies of 11 adults it was found that on the average the distal 62 percent of the circular muscle and 54 percent of the lon-

gitudinal muscle were smooth muscle. The transition zone occupied 34.5 percent of the inner circular muscle and 41.1 percent of the longitudinal muscle, and only 4.2 percent of the inner circular muscle and 5.7 percent of the longitudinal muscle were exclusively striated muscle.[1] No similar information is available in infants and children. In the animal kingdom there is great interspecies variability in the distribution of the different types of muscle in the esophagus. Opossums, primates, and cats are more similar to the human; but dogs, rabbits, sheep, guinea pigs, rats, horses and giraffes have exclusively striated muscle, whereas amphibians, birds, and reptiles have exclusively smooth muscle.[31] One should therefore be cautious when interspecies extrapolation of physiologic data is done.

The resting pressure in the esophageal body varies with respiration from −5 to −15 mm Hg with inspiration and from −2 to +5 with expiration[31]; the intragastric pressure is slightly positive, usually +5 mm Hg.[1,7,31] After swallowing, an orderly and progressive series of peristaltic contractions begins in the pharynx and advances aborally (Fig. 2). Different types of esophageal contractions can occur: *Primary peristalsis* is the term given to the responses initiated by swallowing and is associated with a pharyngeal contraction and UES relaxation. *Secondary peristalsis* refers to the progressive esophageal contractions originating by an intraesophageal distention, either in the form of a bolus or distention with a balloon; this is not accompanied by pharyngeal contraction and UES relaxation, and it is important in clearing remaining food in the esophagus, as well as any gastric contents that might reflux into the esophagus. *Tertiary*

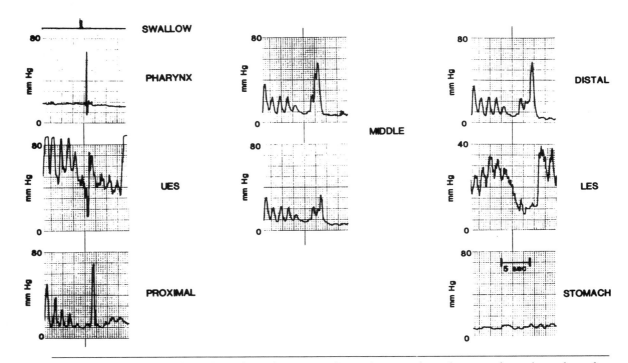

FIGURE 2 Normal esophageal motility. This tracing shows the recording of a normal esophageal motility in a 10-year-old child. Note the UES and LES relaxation and the propagation of normal peristalsis advancing from the pharynx to the esophageal body (proximal, middle, and distal esophagus), and then reaching the stomach.

peristalsis refers to simultaneous contractions in the body of the esophagus; they are nonperistaltic and do not appear to be physiologic.[1,31]

In primary peristalsis the esophageal contraction occurs in the most cephalad portion of the esophagus, shortly after the UES relaxation is terminated. This is followed by a series of aborally propagated contractions. Peristalsis passes through the esophagus in approximately 7 sec, with the average speed of peristalsis being 4 cm per second.[1,31,32] The amplitude, duration, and propagation velocity of peristalsis in the esophagus remain constant within the same individual. However, the characteristics of the contraction vary according to the age of the patient and the esophageal segment being studied.

During the esophageal phase of swallowing there is a closely co-ordinated process between the upper esophageal sphincter (UES), the esophageal body, and the lower esophageal sphincter (LES). Swallowing has been described in the 12-week-old fetus,[31] and near birth the fetus is capable of swallowing approximately 600 ml of amniotic fluid per day.[31] Sucking occurs only in short bursts of three to five in premature and newborn infants, and a swallow wave occurs inconsistently either before or after each burst.[26] The esophagus appears capable of well-developed peristalsis in the premature infant,[11,33] although in newborns less than 12 hours of age and in infants of 1,500 g the swallowing and sucking show poorly co-ordinated responses to deglutition, with rapid biphasic and often nonpropagative repetitive esophageal waves (tertiary waves).[11,33,34] In the first 12 hours of life the esophageal peristalsis is progressive and more rapid in the upper (8 to 20 cm per second) than in the lower esophagus (4 to 12 cm per second).[11]

In the 3-day-old newborn, swallowing co-ordination is beginning to take place.[11,33] As infants grow older, sucking increases to bursts of 10 to 30, peristalsis become more co-ordinated, the peristaltic rate slows, and the simultaneous contractions decrease in frequency,[11,33] the latter occurring in less than 10 percent of children over 2 years of age.[26,33] The speed of peristalsis in the lower esophageal body after deglutition is 0.8 to 2 cm per second during the first week of life[34]; in the older child and adult peristaltic speed is approximately 3 cm per second in the upper esophagus, in the lower third it accelerates to 5 cm per second, and close to the LES it slows down to 2.5 cm per second.[32] The duration of the contraction is 2 to 4 sec, and it increases down the esophagus.[31,32] The peristaltic amplitude, when studied by an intraesophageal transducer system, has been shown to be 53.4 ± 9.0 mm Hg in the upper esophagus 35.0±6.4 mm Hg in the middle segments, and 69.5± 12.1 mm Hg in the lower esophagus.[32] As can be noted, there is a low-pressure zone that has been identified in the middle esophagus. This usually occurs 4 to 6 cm below the UES, extends 2 to 3 cm in length, and in many normal individuals the peristaltic amplitude of this area can be less than 20 mm Hg.[1] This area seems to represent the region where the esophageal striated and smooth muscle intermix.[1]

The amplitude and propagation of peristalsis are influenced by several factors. Bolus size has been shown to alter to some degree the esophageal responses. A dry swallow does not give reproducible reponses; boluses with greater than 2 cm³ give reproducible results.[35,36] Esophageal peristalsis associated with a fluid bolus results in a decreased velocity and an increased amplitude as compared with a dry swallow.[31,35,36] It has been shown that 15-cm³ boluses give the same response as 5-cm³ boluses.[37] Temperature changes of the bolus can either inhibit (cold) or augment (warm) the peristalsic contraction,[1,31] and increases in intra-abdominal pressure slow the speed of the peristalsis.

The human esophagus also displays a phenomenon called *deglutitive inhibition*. This term describes the finding that when a person takes frequent rapid swallows the esophageal body activity is inhibited, with peristalsis being suspended until after the last swallow, at which time a normal peristaltic wave progresses along the esophageal body.[31] This phenomenon occurs normally while drinking fluids, and it is important in allowing only a single peristaltic wave to progress along the esophagus in response to multiple swallows. Two main explanations have been suggested for this phenomenon. One suggests that when repeated rapid swallows are voluntarily taken, deglutitive inhibition occurs because there is an inhibitory neural discharge that arises from the central swallowing center which inhibits the activity of the esophageal striated muscle, immediately arresting the contraction[1,31]; this information has been strong evidence supporting the concept that a wave of inhibition invariably precedes a peristaltic wave following deglutition and that because there is no basal activity present in the esophagus, this phenomenon becomes manifest only when two or more swallows are taken within a few seconds of each other.[1,31] The second explanation suggests that there may also be a refractory period in the esophageal muscle that prevents rapid peristalsis.[1,31,37-39] In a recent study in normal human volunteers, three main interactive phenomena between closely related swallows were identified: deglutitive inhibition, whereby the second swallow inhibits the first swallow wave, disruption by the first swallow of the normal progression of the second swallow wave, and reduction in the amplitude of the second swallow by the first swallow.[40] These suggest that the interactions are predominantly neurogenic and they have a significant neural component.

The neuromuscular mechanisms responsible for regulating peristaltic activity in the esophagus are located within the brain (central) as well as within the wall of the esophagus itself (peripheral).

Central Mechanisms

The primary peristalsis is initiated by activation of the "swallowing center" in the brain stem. As mentioned above, this activation results in the stimulation of brain stem vagal efferents whose axons project either to the striated muscle or to the smooth muscle of the esophagus. There are important differences between the function and innervation of both types of esophageal muscle:

Striated Muscle. This esophageal portion has no ability to produce a contraction and is dependent on the excitatory nerve activity that comes through lower motor neurons, in this case from the dorsal aspect of the rostral part of the nucleus ambiguus of the vagus nerve in the medulla oblongata.[1,31,41,42] During primary peristalsis these motor neurons are activated sequentially by the "swallowing center" in such a way as to sequentially activate motor neurons destined for progressively more caudal levels of esophageal striated muscle.[31,43] The contraction of the striated muscle starts with the onset of the nerve stimulation, is sustained during the period of the stimulation, and ceases when the stimulation is stopped. In animals with striated muscle predominating in the esophagus, bilateral vagotomy at the cervical level results in abolition of peristalsis.[31,44] Secondary peristalsis in the striated muscle segment of the dog and sheep is entirely dependent on central vagal pathways.[31,45] In humans, esophageal balloon distention has been shown to induce UES relaxation followed by peristalsis that passes through the striated muscle segment and into the smooth muscle.[46]

Smooth Muscle. On the other hand, even though the smooth portion of the esophageal body is also innervated through the vagus nerve, the nucleus involved is the dorsal motor nucleus (also located in the medulla oblongata). The vagal fibers do not directly innervate the smooth muscle, but instead synapse with intrinsic neurons located in both the submucosal (Meissner's) and myenteric (Auerbach's) plexus. These intrinsic nerves then send nerves that directly innervate the smooth muscle; in contrast to the striated muscle, the smooth muscle portion possesses an intramural neuromuscular mechanism that can produce peristalsis independently from the central nervous system.[1,13,31] It is clear, however, that swallow-induced primary peristalsis in the smooth muscle portion of the esophagus is also dependent upon activation of the swallowing center. This becomes evident after bilateral cervical vagotomy or vagal cooling abolishes primary peristalsis in the esophagus.[31,47,48] During primary peristalsis the preganglionic neurons located in the dorsal motor nucleus are activated by the "swallowing center," and these fibers then activate the postganglionic intramural neurons of the esophagus.[1,7,31] In contrast to the vagal fibers innervating the striated muscle, the ones innervating the smooth muscle do not appear to follow sequential activation, and it is now believed that activation of the vagal nuclei in the dorsal motor nucleus in the swallowing center may be simultaneous rather than sequential and that the peristaltic contractions in the smooth muscle of the esophagus are due to "peripheral mechanisms."[7,31] It is likely that in addition to initiating primary peristalsis, vagal efferent fibers also modulate speed, amplitude, and duration of the peristaltic wave,[47,49] even though intrinsic neural mechanisms are predominant in the generation of the wave. Secondary peristalsis produced by balloon distention in the smooth muscle segment, in contrast to the secondary peristalsis produced in the striated muscle, is not affected by bilateral vagotomy,[31,45] or vagal cooling,[31] providing further evidence for peripheral control of the esophageal smooth muscle.

Peripheral Mechanisms

Peripheral control of the smooth muscle portion of the esophagus is further suggested by the temporal dissociation between the nerve stimulation and the fact that the circular muscle reponse occurs after a latency period.[7,32,50,51] Moreover, the latency of contractions is not the same throughout the length of the esophagus; it increases aborally and manifests as peristalsis.[50,51] This latency gradient after vagal stimulation is not secondary to nerve delays along the nerve, as the speed of propagation of impulses is very fast (5 to 6 meters per second[49]). It has been shown that each esophageal contraction in response to vagal stimulation is preceded by a period of inhibition; interestingly the duration of this initial inhibition increases distally along the esophagus and corresponds to the latency of esophageal contraction to vagal stimulation.[52] The latency gradient along the esophagus noted after vagal stimulation is also observed in circular smooth muscle preparations of different levels of the esophagus, with the smooth muscle strips of the proximal esophagus having a shorter latency response than the ones from the distal portions.[32]

The circular smooth muscle has two types of contraction responses to vagal, balloon, or electrical stimulation.[7] These are termed "off" and "on" contractions.[7,31,53] When the muscle is stimulated electrically the contractions initially occur during the onset of the stimulus (on response) and after the stimulation ends following a variable delay (off response). The on response is cholinergic and the off response is nerve-mediated, but is nonadrenergic noncholinergic in nature.[1,7,31,53] The off response is strong and progressively more delayed in more distal muscle strips.[7] It has been suggested that the off responses are responsible for peristalsis as seen with swallowing,[31,53] and it is now believed that there is a gradient of cholinergic and noncholinergic neurons involved in the peristalsis along the esophagus. Cholinergic nerves predominate proximally, whereas noncholinergic predominate distally; thus, physiologic peristalsis involves both cholinergic and noncholinergic contractions.[53] These cholinergic influences on peristalsis appear to be mediated by M_2 muscarinic receptors,[54] and the neurotransmitter involved in the nonadrenergic noncholinergic response is unknown. It is then apparent that the latency of contraction and the latency gradient are of fundamental importance in the generation of the peristaltic sequence of contraction,[31] and primary peristalsis is the likely result of the interaction between peripheral and central mechanisms.[7]

To produce co-ordinated peristalsis there has to be a smooth transition in the peristaltic wave as it goes from the striated to the smooth muscle, and it is likely that vagal efferent fibers are involved in this transition.[31] Interaction between the circular and the longitudinal layer is also important for the production of co-ordinated peristalsis.[31] The longitudinal muscle contracts during peristalsis, shortening the esophageal body.[55] Contraction is faster in onset and velocity and is more prolonged than that observed in circular smooth muscle,[7,55] and there is a peripherally mediated, aborally increasing gradient in the duration of the longitudinal muscle contraction so that contraction of the distal esophageal longitudinal muscle lasts for a much longer time than the contraction of the circular muscle.[55] It may serve to help slide the esophagus over the bolus and provide rigidity during peristalsis, and the esophageal shortening that occurs will increase the density of circular muscle fibers so that more force can be generated by circular muscle contractions.[7,55]

LOWER ESOPHAGEAL SPHINCTER

The LES is a well-localized area that exists between the esophageal body and the stomach, and it has two main functions: (1) It prevents the reflux of gastric contents into the lower esophagus, and (2) it relaxes during swallowing to allow the passage of ingested material into the stomach.[9] It is found only manometrically as a zone of high pressure (see Fig. 2), although it has never been shown anatomically.[9,31] The thickened muscle seen at autopsy in the LES is related to muscle contraction and disappears as the sphincter segment is distended to a size comparable to the rest of the esophagus.[31] Ultrastructural studies of the sphincter muscle in the opossum suggest that muscle cells from the LES are of larger diameter and form fewer gap junctions than do those of the esophageal body,[57] and it has been suggested that the number of mitochondria and the mass of smooth endoplasmic reticulum are greater in the LES than in the esophageal body.[58]

Manometrically, using perfused catheters, it averages 1 cm (0.75 to 2 cm) in children less than 3 months, 1.6 cm (0.75 to 3 cm) in those older than 1 year, and 2 to 4 cm in the adult.[9,31,56] The LES is kept closed at rest, creating a zone of high pressure, and in the adult there is some radial asymmetry,[31] with the left side having a higher pressure.[39] It is probable that this is related to some mechanical factors (like the diaphragm), although it persists even in patients with hiatal hernia.[31] This asymmetry is less marked than in the UES, and it has not been studied in children.

The basal pressure of the LES is not constant, with pressure fluctuations in phase with the respiratory cycle.[39,59] Because of the location of the LES, it is subject in its proximal location to thoracic influences and distally to abdominal influences so that during inspiration there is a decrease in the LES pressure proximally and an increase distally.[59] The point at which the respiratory pressure transition occurs is called the point of respiratory reversal, or pressure inversion point, and it is thought to be related to the crura of the diaphragm or the attachment of the phrenoesophageal membrane.[31]

Because of the above-mentioned factors, together with variations in recording techniques, it is difficult to validate a single value for LES pressure.[31] Several techniques have been suggested to obtain a single reliable value for LES pressure. The rapid pull-through (RPT) is one that has been proposed. It consists in a rapid withdrawal of the manometric apparatus from the stomach across the LES during suspended respiration.[31,60,61] It has the disadvantage that it measures the LES at one point in time; esophageal peristalsis can change the measurements, and there is significant variability when repeated measurements are made in the same subjects.[60,61] Most importantly for pediatric gastroenterologists, this technique requires a great deal of patient co-operation, so it cannot be used in young patients. The other technique is called station or slow pull-through (SPT), and it is performed by withdrawing the catheter 0.5 cm at a time, allowing pressure to be recorded for a time with the catheter in one position. With this technique it is possible to observe LES relaxation (Fig. 2), although the sphincter pressure demonstrates respiration-related fluctuations, and scoring the pressure using the peak pressure is the easiest and has the lowest interobserver variability.[60] In a recent prospective study of 95 healthy adult volunteers (age range 22 to 79; mean 43 ± 2.5) using the best manometric techniques available today, the mean LES pressure was found in adults to be 29.0 ± 12.1 mm Hg by RPT and 24.4 ± 10.1 mm Hg by SPT.[62] Most authors using low-compliance, continuously perfused catheters consider a normal resting pressure of the LES in the adult to vary between 10 and 35 mm Hg above the intragastric pressure.[9,31,62]

The normal values available for children have been the subject of confusion, and it was initially suggested that the LES undergoes maturation after birth, thereby explaining the high incidence of gastroesophageal reflux observed in infants. These initial studies in the sixties using nonperfused systems [11,33,34,63] showed that the LES pressures in the newborn were low and matured in the first weeks of life, as can be seen in Table 1. Initial studies by Gryboski et al[11,33] suggested that the LES measured 0.5 to 1 cm in length and that the pressure was low, 6 mm Hg. Strawczynski et al,[63] also using nonperfused systems, studied normal infants as young as 1 week and found that the pressure in the younger children is very low (1.6 ± 1.3 mm Hg; 0.5 to 1 cm in length) but approximates adult levels between 3 and 6 weeks (5.7 ± 3.0 mm Hg; 3 to 5 cm in length). In 1976 Boix-Ochoa et al again suggested that the LES of newborn infants is lower.[64] They studied normal babies from 33 to 40 weeks using perfused systems. They found that the LES pressure at birth was low, that it correlated with age after birth and not with gestational age, and that it matured to levels that are sufficient to present an effective antireflux barrier in the first 5 to 7 weeks after birth[64] (as defined by LES pressure higher than abdominal pressure). They report mean LES values in the pars abdominals that go from 4.66 ± 1.73 mm Hg at 34 weeks to 5.48 ± 2.41 mm Hg at 40 weeks. Dividing the patients by weight, they report a pressure of 4.51 ± 1.95 mm Hg for infants less than 2,000 g and 5.95 ± 2.77 mm Hg for infants more than 3,500 g. After 5 to 7 weeks the exact values are not reported but can be inferred from the figure to be 11 (2,000 g infants) to 15 mm Hg (3,500 g). This suggestion of lower LES pressure at birth with subsequent maturation in the first weeks was reinforced by studies in the developing opossum, beagle, and cat, in which it was shown that the LES undergoes a maturational process after birth.[65-67]

This concept, however, has been challenged by several recent studies, which have shown that the LES is well developed during the first hours of life in healthy newborns. (Table 1).[27,68-70] Espinoza and Heitmann in 1971,[68] using continuously perfused chatheters, reported that 60 to 65 healthy infants between 7 days and 11 months of age had an LES mean pressure of 21.5 mm Hg (range 5 to 50). The mean pressure for infants less than 6 months was 23.9 ± 2.2 mm Hg. Moroz et al [27] studied LES pressures in 62 "normal" children with an age range of 2 weeks to 12 years. They found a mean LES pressure of 46.3 ± 7.7 mm Hg in infants 2 to 6 weeks of age, 43.3 ± 2.4 mm Hg in children less and 1 year, 30.6 ± 2.3 mm Hg in children older than 1 year, and 29.1 ± 2.4 mm Hg in those older than 3 years, suggesting that the LES pressure tends to fall with increasing age. The length of the sphincter gradually increased from 1.0 cm (0.75 to 2 cm) in children

TABLE 1
Normal Lower Esophageal Sphincter Pressure in Infants and Children

Author	Year	Age Studied	No. of Patients	LES Pressure (mm Hg)	LES Length (cm)	Comments
Gryboski[33]	1963	<7 days	20	1.6 ± 2.6	0.5–1.0	Nonperfused system
		7 days–1 year	15	4.0 ± 0.9	0.5–1.0	
Strawczynski[63]	1964	1 week	40	1.6 ± 1.3	0.5–1.0	Nonperfused system
		2 weeks	15	1.5 ± 2.2	0.5–2.0	
		1 month	15	5.6 ± 3.1	0.5–2.0	
		Adults	15	5.7 ± 3.0	3.0–5.0	Note low values in the adult
Gryboski[11]	1965	Prematures				a. Nonperfused system
		3–7 days	15	2.4 ± 1.4		b. Birth weight of the prematures 2,000 to 2,400 g
		Full term				c. The full-term infants were studied longitudinally.
		<12 hours	30	2.5 ± 1.6		
		60 hours	30	2.7 ± 1.6		
Espinoza[68]	1971	<6 months	45	23.9 ± 2.2		a. Perfused system
		>6 months	25	14.1 ± 1.7		b. 5 children less than 6 months had no detectable LES pressure.
Boix-Ochoa[64]	1976	Prematures				a. Perfused system
		34 weeks	53	4.6 ± 1.7		b. Found correlation between LES pressure and postnatal age, and no correlation with post-conceptual age
		34–36 weeks	29	5.1 ± 2.9		
		36–38 weeks	62	4.7 ± 2.1		
		Full term				
		38–40 weeks	58	6.2 ± 2.6		
		40 weeks	80	5.4 ± 2.4		
		5–7 weeks postnatal	—	11.0 – 15.0		
Moroz[27]	1976	2–6 weeks	62	46.3 ± 7.7	0.75–2	Perfused system
		<1 year		43.3 ± 2.4		
		>1 year		30.6 ± 2.3	0.75–3	
		>3 years		29.1 ± 2.4		
Vanderhoof[69]	1978	24–72 hours	10	39.0 ± 3.2		a. Perfused system
						b. Found no difference after sedation with chloral hydrate
Moroz[70]	1981	1 day (8 hours)	22	41.9 ± 10.9		a. Perfused system
		2 days	14	39.1 ± 11.5		b. Infants in the second group were originally studied at 8 hours.
Newell[71]	1988	Prematures	25		0.65	a. Perfused system
		27–28 weeks		5.0 ± 0.7		b. Correlation between postconceptual age and sphincter pressure
		29–30 weeks		8.9 ± 0.7		c. Longitudinal study
		31–32 weeks		12.1 ± 1.2		
		33–34 weeks		13.7 ± 0.7		
		35–36 weeks		16.6 ± 1.2		
		Full term		22.9 ± 1.7	1.00	

less than 3 months to 1.62 cm (0.75 to 3 cm) in children older than 1 year. Vanderhoof et al[69] in 1978 studied 10 healthy infants 24 to 72 hours of age and found a mean LES pressure of 39 ± 3.2 mm Hg in nonsedated infants as compared with 42 ± 2.5 mm Hg in infants sedated with chloral hydrate, thus providing evidence that the LES pressures of the newborn are in the normal adult range and probably higher and also that sedation with chloral hydrate does not alter LES pressures.

In 1981, Moroz et al[70] studied 22 healthy unsedated full-term newborns. The mean age at examination was 8.25 hours, and 18 infants had a repeat study at 4 days. They found a mean LES pressure of 41.9 ± 10.9 mm Hg on day 1 and 39.1 ± 11.5 mm Hg on day 4, confirming the fact that the full-term newborn has a well-developed LES pressure even in the first few hours of life, and they suggested that the pressure may be even higher than the one observed in the adult. As can be appreciated in Table 1, great variability in the meas-

ured LES pressure exists. This can be accounted for by different methodologies. Clearly the use of nonperfused systems[11,33,63] is now regarded as inaccurate, and even if perfused low-compliance catheters are used there can be variables that have to be controlled. It has been shown recently in developing kittens that the relative amount of stretch the catheter provides to the LES area affects the measurement of the LES pressure.[25,66] The results obtained by Boix-Ochoa et al[64] differ markedly from the rest of the literature when perfused catheters are employed, and their methodology has been questioned, particularly because in their paper no mention is made of the perfusion rate or the system response to pressure change.[71]

It is now accepted that the normal values for LES pressure in children and full-term infants are similar to the adult values, although some authors even suggest they are higher at birth and decrease to normal adult values sometime between 6 months and 1 year.[26,69–71] There is also overall agreement in the idea that the length of the sphincter increases with age.[11,27,33,34,63,64,68-70] In one study[27] the length of the sphincter gradually increased from 1.0 cm (0.75 to 2 cm) in children less than 3 months to 1.62 cm (0.75 to 3 cm) in children older than 1 year.

The problem of the LES function in the premature infant seems to be different. Newell et al,[71] in 1988, used a newly devised high-sensitivity, low-compliance, continuously perfused system to study the LES in infants less than 1,000 g. They studied 25 infants with a mean weight of 1,460 g (range 690 to 3,300 g) and a mean gestation age of 31.2 weeks (range 27 to 41 weeks). They found that even in the most premature infants the sphincter could be defined and that there was a strong correlation between postconceptual age and sphincter pressure, and, in contrast to the studies by Boix-Ochoa et al[64] they found that the pressure is not correlated with postnatal age. They noted that the pressures of the sphincter were low at 27 weeks (5 ± 0.7 mm Hg) and increased with conceptual age to the point where they were 22.9 ± 1.7 mm Hg at 37 weeks. This trend was confirmed in the longitudinal study of seven of the infants. Of interest is the fact that even though the more premature babies had a low sphincter pressure, it was always higher than the fundal pressure (effective sphincter pressure, ESP). The ESP varied from 3.9 ± 0.5 mm Hg at 27 weeks, to 18.1 ± 1.0 mm Hg at 37 weeks, also showing a strong correlation with postconceptual age. In Figure 3 we can observe the longitudinal increase in the ESP from 27 weeks to term. This ESP represents the pressure gradient responsible for the prevention of gastroesophageal reflux, and it seems that even in the smallest premature infants the ESP is providing a definite, albeit small pressure gradient between the esophagus and the stomach. The length of the sphincter also varied from a mean of 6.5 ± 0.96 mm Hg in the youngest infants to 10 ± 1.1 mm Hg at term. Sphincter pressure was unaffected by weight for gestational age and by illness or use of xanthines. They concluded that the LES pressure in the premature infant is lower, correlating with gestational age and reaching normal when full-term age is achieved.[71]

The LES pressure is controlled by the following factors: smooth muscle, nerves, and hormones.[9,31] There has been controversy regarding the mechanisms by which the LES maintains a tonic closure. It is now believed that this is due primarily to intrinsic smooth muscle activity,[9] although the cellular mechanisms responsible for the intrinsic tone of the muscle are not fully understood.[9] It has been shown in the opossum that even though the LES shows continuous spike activity, a major portion of the maintained sphincter tone in vivo persists in the absence of any spike activity.[72] Using direct intracellular recordings, it has been shown that the LES muscle is in a relatively depolarized condition in the resting state (−40 mv as compared with −50 mv in the esophageal body).[73] Studies in animals in which all the neutral input to the sphincter was destroyed by the administration of the neurotoxin tetrodotoxin showed that the resting LES pressure was maintained,[74] further suggesting that the tone of the LES is intrinsic in nature.

The role played by the autonomic innervation of the esophagus in maintaining the resting pressure has been the subject of some controversy. Even though alpha-adrenergic neurotransmitters increase LES pressure, alpha-blockade decreases it, beta stimulation lowers it, and beta blockers increase it,[9] there does not seem to be a tonic adrenergic activity that maintains LES pressure.[9,31,75] Even though there have been studies that show that alpha-blockade reduces LES pressure[75] and that propranolol in humans increases resting LES pressures,[76] these effects are short-lived and sphincter pressure soon returns to normal levels, even when the presence of the antagonist can still be demonstrated.

The cholinergic innervation comes through the vagus, which activates postganglionic neurons. The vagus is now considered to produce LES relaxation after stimulation.[9,31,77] It is also known that the M_2 subtype of muscarinic receptors mediates smooth-muscle contraction of the LES,[78] but there is still controversy in the literature regarding the influence of cholinergic innervation in the generation of the basal sphincter tone. In humans high abdominal truncal vagotomy does not influence resting LES pressure,[79] and the influence of anticholinergic administration on this basal pressure is controversial. Some studies suggest that they lower the pressure significantly,[9] whereas most find minor decreases in LES pressure that are not statistically significant.[31,80] Moroz et al,[27] administered bethanecol (0.1 mg per kilogram) subcutaneously in nine control children and showed that the LES pressure increased significantly over the basal levels, with a mean increase of 32.4 ± 6.1 mm Hg (to a mean value of 63.2 ± 4.9 mm Hg). The maximum response was achieved within 10 min (range 5 to 20 min), and it lasted a mean of 34 min (range 22 to 60 min).

There has been a great deal of interest in the possibility that circulating hormones maintain basal LES pressure. Gas-

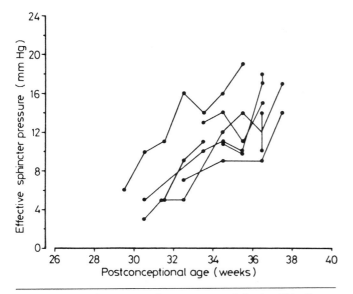

FIGURE 3 LES pressure in premature infants. This figure represents the relationship between effective sphincter pressure (defined as the difference between the LES and the gastric fundal pressure) and postconceptual age. Each line represents sequential measurements made on the same infant. Note that there is a rise in effective sphincter pressure from 27 weeks postconceptual age to term. (From Newell et al.[71])

trin was originally suggested because it was observed that it produced LES contraction and that gastrin antiserum caused an 80 percent reduction in basal sphincter pressure.[81] Recently, however, multiple studies have been reported which refute a physiologic role for gastrin.[70,82] No studies of the hormonal sensitivity of the LES in the developing human fetus or newborn are available. It was originally suggested that in the opossum the postnatal maturation of the LES was related to an increase in the responsiveness of the LES to exogenously administered gastrin in in vivo or in vitro muscle strips.[65] More recently in beagles it was found that the age-dependent maturation of the LES in the first weeks occurs at a time of tissue resistance to gastrin or pentagastrin, suggesting that the observed increase is independent of gastrin concentration.[67] In humans there has also been some speculation regarding gastrin and LES function and maturity in the newborn, particularly because of the higher serum gastrin levels usually observed in this age group.[70] One prospective study of 22 healthy neonates concluded that the LES pressure was already well developed in the neonate and that although neonatal gastrin concentrations were higher than in the adult, there was no correlation with LES pressure.[70]

It is also clear that the basal sphincter pressure can be modified by extrinsic nerves, neuropeptides, hormones, and exogenously ingested substances (Table 2).[9] Gastric acidification[83] and a protein meal[84] have been shown to increase LES pressure, whereas a fatty meal lowers LES pressure.[85] Smoking,[86] chocolate,[87] and coffee[88] lower LES pressure. Those effects may be due to the local effects of different neuropeptides such as pancreatic polypeptide, which has been shown in the dog to correlate with the increased LES pressure seen after a protein meal,[89] or neurotensin, which may mediate LES relaxation secondary to a fatty meal.[90] The effect of chocolate may be mediated by xanthines,[91] which are used clinically very often in the nursery and in children with asthma.

TABLE 2
Effects of Pharmacologic and Other Agents
on LES

Increases LES	Decreases LES
Alpha-adrenergic agonists	Beta-adrenergic agonists
Cholinergic agonists	Alpha-adrenergic antagonists
Beta-adrenergic antagonists	Anticholinergics
Metoclopramide	Dopamine
Domperidone	Calcium-channel blockers
Cisapride	Caffeine
Protein meals	Theophylline
Gastrin	Cholecystokinin
Substance P	Vasoactive intestinal peptide
Motilin	Gastric inhibitory peptide
Raised intra-abdominal pressure	Smoking
	Pregnancy
	Fat
	Chocolate
	Ethanol
	Peppermint

* Adapted from Castell DO. Anatomy and physiology of the esophagus and its sphincters. In: Castell DO, Richter JE, Dalton CB, eds. Esophageal motility testing. New York: Elsevier Biomedical, 1987:24.

At the time of swallowing the LES relaxes in response as soon as the first neural impulses originate from the swallowing center and stays relaxed until the peristaltic wave reaches it[31] (see Fig. 2). The LES relaxation usually occurs within 2 sec after the initiation of swallowing, lasts for a total of 8 to 10 sec,[92] and can be followed by an aftercontraction that is in continuity with the peristaltic contraction in the esophageal body. The pressure measured in the sphincter falls to intragastric pressure during LES relaxation.[92] LES relaxation is due to activation of preganglionic vagal fibers that synapse and activate postganglionic intramural neurons through the stimulation of both nicotinic and muscarinic receptors.[93] The activation of the postganglionic neuron releases a noncholinergic nonadrenergic neurotransmitter that produces LES relaxation. Although the nature of this neurotransmitter is still unknown, vasoactive intestinal peptide has been one of the main candidates,[93] and it is clear that this relaxation may be mediated by multiple neurotransmitters.

LES relaxation can also occur after secondary peristalsis, vomiting, belching, and rumination,[31] and it has also been shown to occur spontaneously, transiently, and inappropriately[29] when it can produce gastroesophageal reflux and actually lead to reflux esophagitis.[94]

Because of the difficulty of performing esophageal motility studies in the infant and child, it is usually necessary to sedate them. It has therefore been necessary to find a drug that does not alter the esophageal physiology. Sedation with morphine sulfate, pethidine hydrochloride, and diazepam has been shown in adults to decrease LES pressure.[95] Vanderhoof et al[69] showed that in neonates chloral hydrate does not alter LES pressure, and most studies are now performed after the administration of chloral hydrate (50 mg per kilogram).

DIAGNOSIS OF ESOPHAGEAL MOTOR DISORDERS

Since the major esophageal functions are to transport food from the mouth to the stomach and to prevent reflux of gastric contents, the main manifestations of disease in this organ are either feeding difficulties or regurgitation.

Swallowing disorders are not infrequent in infants and children.[96] They may present as isolated feeding disorders but are commonly seen in infants with multiple problems, especially neurologic, myopathic, or anatomic problems.

The feeding difficulties can manifest as dysphagia, which reflects interference with bolus transit. Dysphagia is the cardinal symptom of esophageal disease, and it refers to the subjective sensation of food being obstructed as it passes from the mouth to the stomach. Dysphagia can be divided in two main groups: that produced by abnormalities affecting the neuromuscular mechanism of the pharynx and upper esophageal sphincter (oropharyngeal dysphagia) and that produced by disorders affecting the esophagus itself (esophageal dysphagia).[22,96] To the patient it may signify problems swallowing, if the disease occurs in the pharyngoesophageal section, or problems with "food getting stuck" in the retrosternal region when the problem is in the distal esophagus. Oropharyngeal dysphagia refers to difficulty in either the initiation of swallowing or the transfer of food from the mouth into the upper esophagus, and it may represent disorders of the oral, pharyngeal, or cricopharyngeal phases of swallowing. If there are abnormalities in the oral phase, the child presents with poor sucking. Problems with the pharyngeal phase usually present as coughing, gagging, nasopharyngeal regurgitation, and pulmonary aspiration.

Esophageal dysphagia usually occurs after the solids and liquids leave the mouth without difficulty. The dysphagia is insidious in onset and not abrupt, and its severity may be variable over time. There may or may not be an association with particular foods ingested, particularly with very cold liquids, and it tends to occur for both solids and liquids. Patients with mechanical obstruction, on the other hand, usually initially experience dysphagia for solids only.

Odynophagia refers to pain when swallowing. It is usually sharp and is not present between swallows. This symptom is usually related to severe esophageal inflammation.

Regurgitation of food back into the mouth is also a common symptom of esophageal motor problems. It is crucial to differentiate whether the regurgitated material is from esophageal contents, indicating an obstruction proximal to the LES (for example, achalasia), or from gastric contents, indicating probably an inappropriate function of the LES barrier (for example, GER). Heartburn can occur frequently in cases of reflux, and in infants it can manifest only as irritability. Aspiration of food into the tracheobronchial tree may be a manifestation of esophageal problems. This may result from "overflow" of obstructed food (as in achalasia), direct aspiration (swallowing problems), or regurgitation of food from the stomach (GER). The aspiration does not have to be massive, and it can just manifest as chronic cough or wheezing, although at times it can present as recurrent aspiration pneumonia.

Chest pain is a common presenting problem in the adult, but in children it is rare. This pain is usually described as substernal or retrosternal and may be referred cephalad and it can at times be provoked by food ingestion. The pain can sometimes mimic pain of cardiac origin, and in adults it has sometimes been impossible to differentiate esophageal from cardiac pain without the use of invasive studies.

Younger children may manifest the problem by refusing to eat, and weight loss and failure to thrive can be common presentations of esophageal motor disorders in infants and children. The nutritional impact of esophageal motor disorders can be of great magnitude, and nutritional rehabilitation has to be a priority in the treatment plan of these children.

Once the diagnosis of an esophageal motor disorder is suspected, there are several techniques that can be used to evaluate the patient:

Radiologic Tests. The barium swallow is readily available and usually useful in providing information about the transit of barium from the mouth to the stomach. It also provides a good view of the anatomic configuration of the patient. To better evaluate the cervical events of a swallow, cinefluoroscopy has been developed, and it permits a more accurate examination because of the rapidity with which the radiographs can be taken.[97] There are some disadvantages to radiography. It is a subjective test to evaluate transit, and because of radiation exposure the number of swallows is usually very limited. It is also not very sensitive to motility alterations that do not produce problems with esophageal transit, and it does not allow quantification of sphincteric function.

Radionuclide Tests. Esophageal scintiscanning provides objective information regarding the rate of emptying of the esophageal body. The test is usually performed with the administration of an oral bolus marked with ^{99}Tc and a gamma camera that measures the amount of radioactivity in the esophageal body and stomach. The rate of emptying of the radionuclide has allowed the differentiation of various broad categories of motor problems, like aperistalsis from poorly co-ordinated contractions.[98] As compared with radiographic studies, radionuclide tests have less radiation, permit a longer examination, and are more sensitive.[98] They do not, however, provide any information about the swallowing mechanism, more subtle motor abnormalities, or quantitative sphincter function. Because of their lack of radiation and noninvasive nature, radionuclide tests are now also frequently used in the follow-up evaluation of patients with esophageal motor disorder, particularly after specific treatments have been undertaken, like dilatations or drugs for achalasia.[98]

Manometric Evaluation. This continues at present to be the best way to define and diagnose esophageal motor disorders. The technique uses an assembly of pressure-sensing catheters to record intraluminal pressures at various sites along the esophagus. The catheter assembly usually consists of a number of individual tubes having recording orifices at different sites along the length of the assembly. There are two main types of assemblies. The most commonly used type consists of continuously perfused, low-compliance catheters, but recently assemblies with nonperfused intraluminal pressure transducers have been introduced. During the study the catheter assembly is introduced into the patient's esophagus and stomach, and the whole esophagus is examined. When the patient swallows, the function of the sphincters can be examined as well as the nature and characteristics of the peristalsis. This technique provides a way to quantitate the events that occur in the esophagus and to measure subtle alterations that are otherwise inaccessible with other modalities. Furthermore, esophageal motor disorders have been classified based on manometric findings.[99-101] It is the best way to study sphincter function. It has the main disadvantage that it involves intubation of the GI tract, which can be a problem in children. Premedication is usually not required in the adult but is very necessary in young children. Chloral hydrate at a dose of 50 mg per kilogram is the drug usually used, as it has been shown not to interefere with esophageal motility.[69] The lack of co-operation of children, particularly when they are required not to swallow, can sometimes interfere with the study and make the evaluation more difficult. The opposite problem also exists, as it is sometimes difficult to obtain a swallow, particularly a wet one. Manometry also has some limitations in the study of the pharyngeal region, which is better studied by cinefluoroscopy. In spite of some of its disadvantages, esophageal manometry continues to be the best and most objective tool available today for the study of esophageal motor disorders, and it has been our experience that it can be performed safely and successfully in children.

SUMMARY

This chapter has presented a review of the pathophysiology of esophageal dysfunction and the diagnostic approaches to defining this dysfunction as the basis of more detailed discussion of esophageal motility disorders in Chapter 25, Part 4.

REFERENCES

1. Meyer GW, Castell DO. Anatomy and physiology of the esophageal body. In: Castell DO, Johnson LE, eds. Esophageal function in health and disease. 1st ed. New York: Elsevier Biomedical, 1983: 1.
2. Henderson SG. The gastrointestinal tract in the healthy newborn infant. Am J Radiol 1942; 48:302–308.
3. Jackson C, Jackson CL. Notes on the anatomy and physiology of the esophagus. In: Bronchoesophagology. Philadelphia: WB Saunders, 1950: 229.
4. Holinger PH. The esophagus. In: Vaughan VC, McKay RJ, eds. Nelson's textbook of pediatrics. 10th ed. Philadelphia: WB Saunders, 1975: 803.
5. Strobel CT, Byrne WJ, Ament ME, Euler AR. Correlation of esophageal lengths in children with height. Application to the Tuttle test without prior esophageal manometry. J Pediatr 1979; 94:81.
6. Kallor GJ, Deshpande AH, Collins JL. Observations on esophageal length. Thorax 1976; 31:284–290.
7. Weinstock LB, Clouse RE. Esophageal physiology: normal and abnormal motor function. Am J Gastroenterol 1987; 82:399–405.
8. Kahrilas PJ, Dodds WJ, Haeberle DB, Hogan WJ, Arndorfer RC. Effect of sleep, spontaneous gastroesophageal reflux, and a meal on upper esophageal sphincter pressure in normal human volunteers. Gastroenterology 1987; 92:466–471.
9. Gerhardt DC, Castell DO. Anatomy and physiology of the esophageal sphincters. In: Castell DO, Johnson LE, eds. Esophageal function in health and disease. 1st ed. New York: Elsevier Biomedical, 1983: 17.
10. Sondeheimer JM. Upper esophageal sphincter and pharyngoesophageal motor function in infants with and without gastroesophageal reflux. Gastroenterology 1983; 85:301–305.
11. Gryboski JD. The swallowing mechanism of the neonate. I. Esophageal and gastric motility. Pediatrics 1965; 35:445–452.
12. Asoh R, Goyal RK. Manometry and electromyography of the upper esophageal sphincter in the opossum. Gastroenterology 1978; 74:514–520.
13. Ellis FH. Upper esophageal sphincter in health and disease. Surg Clin North Am 1971; 51:553–565.
14. Hurwitz AL, Duranceau A. Upper esophageal sphincter dysfunction. Pathogenesis and treatment. Am J Dig Dis 1978; 23:275–281.
15. Gerhardt DC, Shuck TJ, Bordeaux RA, Winship DH. Human upper esophageal sphincter. Response to volume, osmotic and acid stimuli. Gastroenterology 1978; 75:268–274.
16. Ingelfinger FJ. Esophageal motility. Physiol Rev 1958; 38:533–584.
17. Green RE, Castell DO. The upper esophageal sphincter. In: Castell DO, Richter JE, Dalton CB, eds. Esophageal motility testing. Elsevier: New York, 1987: 183.
18. Dodds WJ, Stewart ET, Hogan WJ, Steff JJ, Arndorfer RC. Effect of esophageal movement on intraluminal esophageal pressure recording. Gastroenterology 1974; 67:592–600.
19. Sokol EM, Heitman P, Wolf BS, Cohen BR. Simultaneous cineradiographic and manometric study of the pharynx, hypopharynx and cervical esophagus. Gastroenterology 1966; 51:960–974.
20. Dodds WJ, Steff JJ, Hogan WJ. Factors determining pressure measurements accuracy by intraluminal esophageal manometry. Gastroenterology 1974; 67:592–600.
21. Arndorfer RC, Steff JJ, Dodds WJ, Linehan JH, Horan WJ. Improved infusion system for intraluminal esophageal manometry. Gastroenterology 1977; 73:23–37.
22. Staiano A, Cucchiara S, Vizia B, Andreotti M, Auricchio S. Disorders of upper esophageal sphincter motility in children. J Pediatr Gastroenterol Nutr 1987; 6:892–898.
23. Knuff TE, Benjamin SB, Castell DO. Pharyngoesophageal (Zenkers') diverticulum: a reappraisal. Gastroenterology 1982; 82:734–736.
24. Fisher MA, Hendrix TR, Hunt JN, Murrills AJ. Relation between volume swallowed and velocity of the bolus ejected from the pharynx into the esophagus. Gastroenterology 1978; 74:1328–1333.
25. Hillemeier C. Esophageal manometrics in children. (Editorial) J Pediatr Gastroenterol Nutr 1986; 5:840–842.
26. Diamant NE. Development of esophageal function. Am Rev Respir Dis 1985; 131(Suppl):S29–S32.
27. Moroz S, Espinoza J, Cumming W, Diamant N. Lower esophageal sphincter function in children with and without gastroesophageal reflux. Gastroenterology 1976; 71:236–241.
28. Freiman JM, El-Sharkawy TW, Diamant NE. Effect of bilateral vagosympathetic nerve blockade on response of the dog upper esophageal sphincter to intraesophageal distention and acid. Gastroenterology 1981; 81:78–84.
29. Dent J, Dodds WJ, Friedman RH, Sekiguchi T, Hogan WJ, Arndorfer RC, Petrie DJ. Mechanism of gastroesophageal reflux in recumbent asymptomatic human subjects. J Clin Invest 1980; 65:256–267.
30. Allen CJ, Newhouse MT. Gastroesophageal reflux and chronic respiratory disease. Am Rev Respir Dis 1984; 129:645–647.
31. Goyal RK, Cobb BW. Motility of the pharynx, esophagus and esophageal sphincters. In: Johnson LR, ed. Physiology of the gastrointestinal tract. New York: Raven Press, 1981: 359.
32. Humphries TJ, Castell DO. Pressure profile of esophageal peristalsis in normal humans as measured by direct intraesophageal transducers. Am J Dig Dis 1977; 22:641–645.
33. Gryboski JD, Thayer WR, Spiro HM. Esophageal motility in infants and children. Pediatrics 1963; 31:382–395.
34. Grand RJ, Watkins JB, Torti FM. Development of the human gastrointestinal tract. Gastroenterology 1976; 70:790–810.
35. Dodds WJ, Steff JJ, Hogan WJ, Hoke SE, Stewart ET, Arndorfer AC. A comparison between primary esophageal peristalsis following wet and dry swallows. J Appl Physiol 1973; 35:851–857.
36. Hollis JB, Castell DO. Effect of dry swallows and wet swallows of different volumes on esophageal peristalsis. J Appl Physiol 1975; 38:1161–1164.
37. Meyer GW, Gerhardt DC, Castell DO. Human esophageal response to rapid swallowing: muscle refractory period or neural inhibition. Am J Physiol 1981; 241:G129–G136.
38. Dodds WJ, Hogan ET, Stewart JJ, Arndorfer RC. Effects of increased intra-abdominal pressure on esophageal peristalsis. J Appl Physiol 1974; 37:378–383.
39. Welch RW, Gray JE. Influence of respiration on recordings of lower esophageal sphincter pressure in humans. Gastroenterology 1982; 83:590–594.
40. Vanek AW, Diamant NE. Responses of the human esophagus to paired swallows. Gastroenterology 1987; 92:643–650.
41. Holstage G, Gravelan G, Bijker-Biedmond C, Schuddeboom I. Location of motoneurons innervating soft palate, pharynx, and upper esophagus. Anatomical evidence for a possible swallowing center in the pontine reticular formation. Brain Behav Evol 1983; 23:47–62.
42. Fryscak T, Zenker W, Kantner D. Afferent and efferent innervation of the rat esophagus; a tracing study with horseradish peroxidase and nuclear yellow. Anat Embryol 1984; 170:63–70.
43. Roman C. Nervous control of peristalsis in the esophagus. J Physiol (Paris) 1966; 58:79–108.
44. Carveth SW, Schlegaal JF, Code CF. Esophageal motility after vagotomy, phrenicotomy, myotomy and myomectomy in dogs. Surg Gynecol Obstet 1962; 114:31–42.
45. Dodds WJ, Christensen J, Dent JD, Wood JD, Arndorfer RC. Esophageal contractions induced by vagal stimulation in the opossum. Am J Physiol 1978; 4:E392–E401.
46. Siegel CI, Hendrix TR. Evidence for the central mediation of secondary peristalsis in the esophagus. Bull Johns Hopkins Hosp 1961; 108:297–307.
47. Patterson WG, Rattan S, Goyal RK. Experimental induction of isolated lower esophageal sphincter relaxation in anesthetised opossums. J Clin Invest 1986; 77:1187–1193.
48. Reynolds RP, El-Sharkawy TY, Diamant NE. Esophageal peristalsis in the cat: the role of central innervation assessed by transient vagal blockade. Can J Physiol Pharmacol 1984; 63:122–130.
49. Gidda JS, Goyal RK. Swallow-evoked action potentials in vagal preganglionic efferents. J Neurphysiol 1984; 52:1169–1180.
50. Dodds WJ, Christensen J, Dent JD, Wood JD, Arndorfer RC. Esophageal contractions induced by vagal stimulation in the opossum. Am J Physiol 1978; 4:E392–E410.
51. Dodds WJ, Christensen J, Dent JD, Wood JD, Arndorfer RC. Pharmacologic investigation of primary peristalsis in smooth muscle portion of opossum esophagus. Am J Physiol 1979; 6:E561–E566.
52. Gidda JS, Goyal RK. Regional gradient of initial inhibition and refrac-

toriness in esophageal smooth muscle. Gastroenterology 1985; 89:843–851.

53. Crist J, Gidda JS, Goyal RK. Intramural mechanism of esophageal peristalsis: roles of cholinergic and noncholinergic nerves. Proc Natl Acad Sci USA 1984; 81:3595–3599.

54. Blackwell JN, Dalton CB, Castell DO. Oral pirenzipine does not affect esophageal pressure in man. Dig Dis Sci 1986; 31:230–235.

55. Sugarbaker DJ, Rattan S, Goyal RK. Swallowing induces sequential activation of esophageal longitudinal smooth muscle. Am J Physiol 1984; 247:G515–G519.

56. Gastroesophageal reflux. In: Silverman A, Roy CC, eds. Pediatric clinical gastroenterology. 3rd ed. St Louis: CV Mosby, 1983: 149.

57. Daniel EE, Posey-Daniel V. Neuromuscular structures in opossum esophagus: role of interstitial cells of Cajal. Am J Physiol 1984; 246:G305–315.

58. Christensen J, Roberts RL. Differences between esophageal body and lower esophageal sphincter in mitochondria of smooth muscle in opossum. Gastroenterology 1983; 85:650–656.

59. DeMeester TR, Lafontaine E, Joelsson BE, Skinner DB, Ryan JW, O'Sullivan GC, Brunsden BS, Johnson LF. Relationship of a hiatal hernia to the function of the body of the esophagus and gastroesophageal junction. J Thorac Cardiovasc Surg 1981: 82:547–558.

60. Welch RW, Drake ST. Normal lower esophageal sphincter pressure: a comparison of rapid vs slow pull-through technique. Gastroenterology 1980; 78:1446–1451.

61. Dodds WJ, Hogan WJ. Measurement of LES pressure. (Editorial) Gastroenterology 1980; 79:588–591.

62. Richter JE, Wu WC, Johns DN, Blackwell JN, Nelson JL, Castell JA, Castell DO. Esophageal manometry in 95 healthy adult volunteers: variability of pressures with age and frequency of "abnormal contractions." Dig Dis Sci 1987; 32:583–592.

63. Strawzynski H, Beck IT, McKenna RD, Nickerson GH. The behavior of lower esophageal sphincter in infants and its relationship to gastroesophageal function. J Pediatr 1964; 64:17–23.

64. Boix-Ochoa J, Lafuente JM, Gil-vernet JM. Maturation of the lower esophagus. J Pediatr Surg 1976; 11:749–756.

65. Cohen S. Developmental characteristics of lower esophageal sphincter function: a possible mechanism for infantile chalasia. Gastroenterology 1974; 67:252–258.

66. Hillemeier C, Gryboski J, McCallum R, Biancani P. Developmental characteristics of the lower esophageal sphincter in the kitten. Gastroenterology 1985; 89:760–766.

67. Spedale SB, Weisbrodt NW, Morriss FH. Ontogenic studies of gastrointestinal function. II. Lower esophageal sphincter maturation in neonatal beagle puppies. Pediatr Res 1982; 16:851–855.

68. Espinoza J, Heitmann P. The gastroesophageal sphincter in the first year of life. (Abstract) Gastroenterology 1971; 60:775.

69. Vanderhoof JA, Rappaport PJ, Paxson CL. Manometric diagnosis of lower esophageal sphincter incompetence in infants: use of a small, single lumen perfused catheter. Pediatrics 1978; 62:805–808.

70. Moroz SP, Beiko P. Relationship between lower esophageal sphincter pressure and serum gastrin concentration in the newborn infant. J Pediatr 1981; 99:725–728.

71. Newell SJ, Sarkar PK, Durbin GM, Booth JW, McNeish AS. Maturation of the lower oesophageal sphincter in the preterm baby. Gut 1988; 29:167–172.

72. Asoh R, Goyal RK. Electrical activity of the opossum lower esophageal sphincter in vivo: its role in the basal sphincter pressure. Gastroenterology 1978; 74:835–840.

73. Zelcer E, Weisbrodt NW. Electrical and mechanical activity in the lower esophageal sphincter of the cat. Am J Physiol 1984; 246:G243–247.

74. Goyal RK, Rattan S. Genesis of basal sphincter pressure: effect of tetrodotoxin on the lower esophageal sphincter of the opossum in vivo. Gastroenterology 1976; 71:62–67.

75. Behar JM, Kerstein M, Biancani P. Neural control of the lower esophageal sphincter in the cat: studies on the excitatory pathways the lower esophageal sphincter. Gastroenterolgoy 1982; 82:680–688.

76. Thorpe JA. Effect of propranolol on the lower esophageal sphincter in man. Curr Med Res Opin 1980; 7:91–95.

77. Kravitz JJ, Snape WJ, Cohen S. Effect of thoracic vagotomy and vagal stimulation on esophageal function. Am J Physiol 1978; 234:E359–E364.

78. Gilbert R, Rattan S, Goyal RK. Pharmacological identification, activation and antagonism of two muscarinic receptor subtypes in the lower esophageal sphincter. J Pharmacol Exp Ther 1984; 230:284–291.

79. Temple JG, Godall RJ, Hay DJ, Miller D. Effect of highly selective vagotomy upon the lower esophageal sphincter. Gut 1981; 22:368–370.

80. Blackwell JN, Dalton CB, Castell DO. Oral pirenzipine does not affect esophageal pressures in man. Dig Dis Sci 1986; 31:230–235.

81. Lipshutz WH, Hughes W, Cohen S. The genesis of lower esophageal sphincter pressure: its identification through the use of gastrin antiserum. J Clin Invest 1972; 51:522–529.

82. Csendes A, Oster M, Brandsborg O, Moller J, Bransborg M, Amdrup E. Gastroesophageal sphincter pressure and serum gastrin: reaction to food stimulation in normal subjects and in patients with gastric or duodenal ulcer. Scand J Gastroenterol 1978; 13:363–368.

83. Kaye MD. On the relationship between gastric pH and pressure in the normal human lower esophageal sphincter. Gut 1979; 29:69–63.

84. Nebel OT, Castell DO. Lower esophageal sphincter pressure changes after food ingestion. Gastroenterology 1972; 63:778–783.

85. Nebel OT, Castell DO. Inhibition of lower esophageal sphincter by fat—a mechanism for fatty food intolerance. Gut 1973; 14:270–274.

86. Dennish G, Castell DO. Effect of smoking on lower esophageal sphincter pressure. N Engl J Med 1971; 284:1136–1137.

87. Wright LE, Castell DO. The adverse effect of chocolate on lower esophageal sphincter pressure. Am J Dig Dis 1975; 20:703–707.

88. Cohen S, Booth GH. Gastric acid secretion and lower esophageal sphincter pressure in response to coffee and caffeine. N Engl J Med 1975; 293:897–899.

89. Maher JW, Olinde AJ, McGuigan JE. Suppression of postprandial lower esophageal sphincter pressure and pancreatic polypetide by duodenal exclusion. J Surg Res 1984; 37:467–471.

90. Thor K, Rokaeus A. Studies on the mechanism by which (GLn^4)-neurotensin reduces lower esophageal sphincter pressure in man. Acta Physiol Scand 1983; 118:373–377.

91. Johannesson N, Andersoon KE, Joelsson B, Persson AG. Relaxation of the lower esophageal sphincter and stimulation of gastric secretion and diuresis by antiasthmatic xanthines: role of adenosine antagonism. Am Rev Respir Dis 1985; 131:26–31.

92. Katz PO, Richter JE, Cowan R, Castell DO. Apparent complete lower esophageal sphincter relaxation in achalasia. Gastroenterology 1986; 90:978–983.

93. Goyal RK, Rattan S, Said S. VIP as a possible neurotransmitter of non-cholinergic, non-adrenergic inhibitory neurons. Nature 1980; 288:378–380.

94. Dodds WJ, Dent J, Hogan WJ, Helm JF, Hauser R, Patel GK, Egide MS. Mechanisms of gastroesophageal reflux in patients with reflux esophagitis. N Engl J Med 1982; 307:1547–1552.

95. Hall AW, Moosa AR, Clark J. the effects of premedication drugs on lower esophageal high pressure zone and reflux status of Rhesus monkeys and man. Gut 1975; 16:347–352.

96. Dinari G, Danzinger Y, Mimouni M, Rosenbach Y, Zahavi I, Grunebaum M. Cricopharyngeal dysfunction in childhood: treatment by dilatations. J Pediatr Gastroenterol Nutr 1987; 6:212–216.

97. Hurwitz AL, Nelson JA, Haddad JK. Oropharyngeal dysphagia: manometric and cine-esophagographic findings. Am J Dig Dis 1975; 20:313–324.

98. Russell CO, Hill LD, Holmes ER, Hull DA, Gannon R, Pope CE. Radionuclide transit: a sensitive screening test for esophageal dysfunction. Gastroenterology 1981; 80:887–892.

99. Vantrappen G, Janssens H, Hellemans J, Coremans G. Achalasia, diffuse esophageal spasm, and related motility disorders. Gastroenterology 1979; 76:450–457.

100. McCallum RW. The management of esophageal motility disorders. Hosp Practice 1988; 131–142.

101. Benjamin SB, Richter JE, Cordova CM, Knuff TE, Castell DO. Prospective manometric evaluation with pharmacological provocation of patients with suspected esophageal motility dysfunction. Gastroenterology 1984; 84:893–901.

16

CHAPTER

Endocrine Function of the Gut in Early Life

Albert Aynsley-Green, M.A., D.Phil., M.B., B.S., F.R.C.P.(Lon.), F.R.C.P.(Edin.)

HISTORICAL BACKGROUND

The modern science of endocrinology can be said to have commenced on January 16, 1902, in the Department of Physiology at University College in London, England. William Maddock Bayliss and Ernest Henry Starling were investigating the manner by which the pancreas was excited to activity. In 1927, Sir Charles Martin, in his obituary on Ernest Starling,[1] described the scene on that day in 1902:

I happened to be present at their discovery. In an anaesthetised dog a loop of jejenum was tied at both ends and the nerves supplying it dissected out and divided so that it was connected with the rest of the body only by its blood vessels. On the introduction of some weak HCl into the duodenum, secretion from the pancreas occurred and continued for some minutes. After this had subsided a few cubic centimetres of acid were introduced into the denervated loop of duodenum. To our surprise a similarly marked secretion was produced. I remember Starling saying "then it must be a chemical reflex." Rapidly cutting off a further piece of jejunum he rubbed its mucous membrane with sand and weak HCl, filtered and injected it into the jugular vein of the animal. After a few moments the pancreas responded by a much greater secretion than had occurred before. It was a great afternoon.

The experimenters suggested that an internal secretion was made in the duodenum and that this chemical messenger circulated in the blood stream to affect the activity of the pancreas. This postulated substance was called "secretin." In his Croonian lectures at the Royal College of Physicians, London, in June of 1905, Starling proposed that these chemical messengers should be called "hormones" (from δρμαω, meaning "I excite" or "arouse").

Although the new science of endocrinology had begun with the recognition that the gut was an endocrine organ, further progress in the field of gut endocrinology during the next 60 years was overshadowed by the spectacular advances in the endocrinology of the discrete glands such as the pancreas, pituitary, adrenal, and thyroid. It is easy to understand why progress in those areas of the subject was much faster than in gastrointestinal (GI) endocrinology. Thus, it was easy to remove the discrete glands and to define the physiologic consequences of hormone deficiencies; it was also relatively easy to extract from the isolated glands the active proteins and to confirm their physiologic effects by their reintroduction into animals from whom the glands had been removed. However,

the gut is a discrete endocrine organ; in other words, the cells secreting the active peptides lie indirectly throughout the mucosa and cannot be extirpated. Furthermore, the cells are widely scattered through a great bulk of tissue, and different endocrine cell systems may overlap. Moreover, tissue extracts inevitably contain several different hormonal substances submerged in a substantial bulk of interfering protein and peptide material. Although gastrin had been discovered by John Sidney Edkins in 1905, and cholecystokinin, the gallbladder-emptying factor, was discovered in 1928 by Ivy and Oldberg, little further progress was possible until the development of substantially improved chemical purification techniques. The recent introduction and availability of such techniques as ion exchange chromatography, gel chromatography, affinity chromatography, and isoelectric focusing have now enabled chemists to extract specific hormonal peptides with comparative ease.

Following the identification and isolation of a new active peptide, the next stage in its investigation is to develop an assay system capable of detecting it in low concentrations and in complex situations, for example in plasma. Its exact localization in the tissues of the body and its dynamic response to stimuli can then be investigated. The ability of the immune system of higher vertebrates to produce protein antibodies that combine with substantial avidity and high specificity to any peptide appropriately administered has enabled an explosion of knowledge during the last 15 years in the field of GI endocrinology. Thus, not only are there now highly sensitive and specific radioimmunoassays for the measurement of peptides in body fluids, but specific immunocytochemical techniques have allowed the precise anatomic localization of single cells producing a given hormone from within a mass of tissue containing many other different types of cells and endocrine products.

It is important to emphasize at this point that it is now clear that peptide-secreting cells in the GI tract may exert their effects by one of three mechanisms, working as endocrine, paracrine, or neurocrine substances. As has been indicated previously, endocrine cells exert their effects by the release of their products into the blood stream, and they are then carried through the circulation to affect target tissues distally. Paracrine substances act locally, exerting their effects on cells adjacent to those producing the peptide; neurocrine agents, on the other hand, are released from nerve endings. It will be obvious immediately that it has proved to be exceedingly difficult to define precisely the regulation of, the secretion of, and the interaction and mechanism of action of these three types of cell in the gut mucosa, particularly since a peptide may have more than one mode of action, acting, for example, as both an endocrine and a paracrine substance. Nonetheless, a substantial body of evidence has accumulated to indicate the principal actions of the peptides.

It is beyond the scope of this chapter to consider in substantial detail the analytic techniques that are currently in use and the physiology of the peptides, but the interested reader is referred to Jerzy Glass[2] and to Bloom and Polak[3] for further background information.

OVERVIEW OF THE ROLE OF HORMONES AND OF REGULATORY PEPTIDES FROM THE GASTROINTESTINAL TRACT

The efficient utilization of food in the human adult subject depends upon the integration of the functions of several physiologic systems. Food is introduced into the oral cavity, is chewed and swallowed, and enters the stomach. Thereafter, the foodstuff has to be propelled through the gut, and this requires the co-ordination of gut motor activities to ensure the orderly transit of the foodstuff through the different regions of the alimentary tract. The gut motor system is so carefully organized that there are few outward manifestations of the process that ensures that the appropriate length of time is spent in each of the anatomic sections of the GI tract. The importance of the co-ordination of the motor activity is further emphasized by the disastrous consequences of abnormal motility, which manifests itself either as vomiting or diarrhea, or, occasionally, through abnormal symptoms such as gut colic. The passage of food through the intestinal tract leads to local trauma, and this necessitates a continuous process of regeneration of the gut mucosa. Failure to maintain the integrity of the mucosa threatens the existence of the organism.

Digestive secretions have to be introduced into the gut lumen at the appropriate times, and co-ordinated with this is a redistribution of blood flow to carry the products of digestion and absorption through the visceral and then the systemic circulations. The influx of nutrients leads to changes in metabolic hormone secretion to ensure postprandial metabolic homeostasis, and this in turn has to be integrated with other adaptive metabolic changes as the individual enters into the interprandial starvation period. All of these facets of the utilization of food are also accomplished with little external evidence of the magnitude of the problems that have to be overcome to ensure normal digestion, absorption, and metabolic homeostasis.

It is important to note at this point that normal gut mucosal structure and function in the adult depend upon the presence of food in the gut lumen; in animals and adult man, gut hypoplasia rapidly occurs when enteral feeding is discontinued and is replaced by intravenous nutrition (see below).

It follows from this brief introduction that the integration and co-ordination of these facets of physiology must require a highly complex and efficient regulatory system; it is equally obvious that many factors are likely to be involved, since the dependence upon one single factor could have life-threatening consequences if that factor were to be deranged. Nonetheless, the available evidence to date suggests that the secretion of hormones and of regulatory peptides from the gut and from the classic endocrine organs has a key role to play in this process.

Table 1 outlines the human hormones and GI regulatory peptides, their main anatomic source, their mode of action, and their possible physiologic actions.

Figure 1 schematically represents the distribution in the human adult of the cells secreting specific GI hormones.

The following sections summarize briefly the chemistry, localization, physiology, and pathophysiology of the more important hormones and regulatory peptides in the human adult. Armed with this information, one can examine in perspective the importance of these substances in early life.

Gastrin

Edkins in 1905 gave the name gastrin to the active ingredient of extracts of the anterior region of the stomach which stimulated gastric acid secretion when injected into the blood stream of cats. Although the existence of gastrin remained controversial for many years (because it was suggested that the actions of the extracts were due to the effects of their histamine content), it was finally isolated and purified, and in 1964 Gregory and colleagues were able to publish the full structure and report the synthesis of active gastrin.[4]

Gastrin was initially thought to be a 17-amino acid linear peptide, but in 1970 Yalow and Berson[5] showed that the major circulating form of gastrin is a much larger molecule, "big gastrin," which was subsequently shown to consist of 34 amino acids. Big gastrin (G-34) is composed of "little gastrin" (G-17) with an additional extension of 17 amino acids at its N-terminus. Further work with gel chromatography has resulted in the discovery of small amounts of other gastrin-like immunoreactivity in tissue extracts and within the circulation.[6] These include "big big gastrin" and "mini gastrin." It has also been shown that the smallest fragment that exerts the diverse actions of gastrin is the C-terminal tetrapeptide amide.[7] The same C-terminal tetrapeptide is also found in the structurally related hormonal peptide cholecystokinin (CCK).

The major source of gastrin is the pyloric antrum; considerable quantities are present in the duodenum, but it is virtually absent from the jejunum. Gastrin-like peptides have also been observed in the central nervous system, where they are thought to act as neurotransmitter substances[8] (see below).

Gastrin affects most major GI functions, including secretion, absorption, and motility. Its main physiologic role appears to be the stimulation of gastric acid secretion; it also stimulates water and electrolyte secretion from the stomach, upper small intestine, and pancreas but inhibits the absorption of water and electrolytes from the lower small intestine.[9]

Gastrin inhibits the contraction of the sphincter of Oddi and causes contraction of the lower esophageal sphincter and gastric smooth muscle.[10] It increases gastric mucosal blood flow, releases histamine, and stimulates amino acid uptake into protein and the gastric mucosa.[11,12] Gastrin also stimulates the growth of the gastric mucosa and, when present in

TABLE 1
Human Gastrointestinal Regulatory Peptides: Main Anatomic Source,
Mode of Action, and Possible Main Physiologic Action

Regulatory Peptide	Main Source(s)	Mode of Action	Main Action
Gastrin	Antrum	Hormone	Stimulates gastric acid secretion
Cholecystokinin	Upper small intestine and CNS	Hormone/ neurotransmitter	Gallbladder contraction and pancreatic enzyme secretion
Secretin	Upper small intestine	Hormone	Pancreatic bicarbonate secretion
Pancreatic glucagon	Pancreas	Hormone	Stimulates hepatic glucose output
Enteroglucagon	Ileum and colon	Hormone	Gut mucosal growth, gut motility
Pancreatic polypeptide	Pancreas	Hormone	Inhibits pancreatic enzyme secretion and gallbladder contraction
Gastric inhibitory polypeptide	Upper small intestine	Hormone	Enhancement of insulin secretion
Motilin	Upper small intestine	Hormone	Stimulates gastrointestinal motility
Vasoactive intestinal polypeptide	All tissues	Neurotransmitter	Neurotransmitter (secretomotor, vasodilator, and smooth muscle relaxation)
Bombesin	Gut, CNS, and lung	Neurotransmitter/ paracrine	Stimulates gut hormone release
Somatostatin	Gut and CNS	Paracrine/ neurotransmitter	Inhibits hormone release and hormone target tissues
Neurotensin	Ileum and CNS	Hormone/ neurotransmitter	Inhibits gastric emptying and acid secretion
Substance P	Gut, CNS, and skin	Neurotransmitter	Sensory neurotransmitter (especially pain)
Leu-enkephalin and met-enkephalin	Gut and CNS	Neurotransmitter	Opiate-like (endorphin system)
Peptide HI	Gut and CNS	Unknown	Unknown
Peptide YY	Gut and CNS	Hormone	Inhibits gastric acid secretion and gut motility

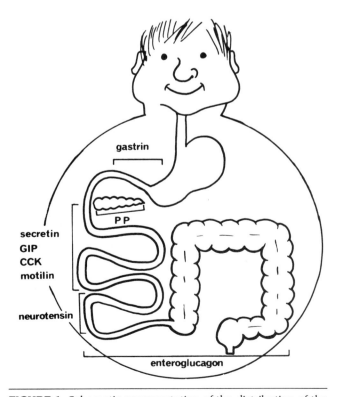

FIGURE 1 Schematic representation of the distribution of the cells secreting specific GI hormones in the human adult.

excessive concentrations in the circulation, results in gastric mucosal hypertrophy.[13]

Abnormally high plasma gastrin concentrations are found in hypochlorhydric patients with pernicious anemia[14] and also in some patients who have excessive acid secretion due to gastrin-producing pancreatic tumors.[15] Although the latter syndrome (Zollinger-Ellison) is rare, it can be suspected on the basis of excessive acid secretion with hypergastrinemia. There is considerable controversy as to whether gastrin has any role to play in the etiology of duodenal ulceration.

Cholecystokinin

CCK was discovered in 1928 when Ivy and Oldberg observed that gallbladder contraction is caused by fat entering the duodenum and also by an extract of duodenum injected intravenously. In 1964, Jorpes et al[16] isolated the CCK molecule and showed it to be a basic 33-amino acid straight-chain peptide, CCK-33. A 39-amino acid peptide was also found to be present,[17] although the C-terminal octapeptide of cholecystokinin, CCK-8, exhibited the full biologic activity of the larger molecule.[18]

It was suggested in 1975[19] that a gastrin-like peptide was present in the central nervous system, but it is now established that much of this material is CCK, which cross-reacts with antigastrin antibodies because of the common C-terminal sequence.[20] The octapeptide form of the peptide exists naturally and is the most abundant form of CCK in both brain and gut, suggesting that the larger molecular weight forms are earlier stages in the intracellular enzymic processing from a common precursor molecule.

Serious difficulties have faced all groups that have attempted to develop a specific radioimmunoassay for CCK because of its cross-reactivity with gastrin.

The classic assumption that CCK is responsible for the postprandial release of pancreatic enzymes and bile is almost certainly too simplistic.[21] Such a phenomenon also depends upon vagal innervation and possibly upon other hormones as well. As a brain peptide, it fulfills most of the requirements for a neurotransmitter, being in particular a potent activator of postsynaptic membranes.[22] However, it must be concluded that the precise physiologic roles of the various forms of CCK have yet to be elucidated with certainty.

Secretin

As reported earlier in this chapter, secretin was the first hormone to be described in 1902 by Bayliss and Starling, who demonstrated that acidification of denervated small intestine causes the prompt secretion of alkaline pancreatic juice. Sixty years elapsed before Jorpes and Mutt purified secretin,[23] and after its amino acid sequence had been established it was found to be composed of 27 amino acids, 14 of which occupy the same position as in glucagon.[24] Moreover, considerable similarities were subsequently found to gastric inhibitory polypeptide (GIP) and vasoactive intestinal polypeptide (VIP), and together these four polypeptides are considered to be one hormonal family that may have evolved from a single precursor hormone.

Secretin has been localized to the S cell, which occurs in highest concentrations in the duodenum, although significant amounts are also present in the jejunum. It appears that there is only one well-defined mechanism for the release of secretin into plasma, and this is the acidification of the upper small intestine when endogenous acid is delivered from the stomach to the duodenum. No release of secretin occurs with the ingestion of protein, fat, or carbohydrate. The main physiologic effect of secretin is to stimulate the secretion of bicarbonate from the pancreas. It must be emphasized, however, that the magnitude of the change in circulating secretion levels after the ingestion of food is very small indeed when compared with some other gut hormones,[25] and, moreover, the pattern of secretin change varies considerably among individuals.

It has been demonstrated that patients with active celiac disease fail to increase the release of secretin after intraduodenal acid perfusion, but this returns to normal after treatment with a gluten-free diet.[26]

Elevated plasma levels of secretin have been reported in patients with chronic renal failure,[27] in whom the elevation in the levels may be due to a slower rate of degradation of the hormone than in normal patients.

Pancreatic Glucagon

The explosion of interest that followed the demonstration by Banting and Best that insulin is made in the endocrine pancreas led Murlin in 1923 to show that certain pancreatic extracts give an unexpected hyperglycemic response in animals. This hyperglycemia factor was named glucagon.

Unger and co-workers were the first to describe in 1959 a specific radioimmunoassay for this hormone,[28] and in 1967 Wunsch reported the first successful complete chemical synthesis of glucagon. The amino acid sequence has been shown to consist of a 29-amino acid straight-chain polypeptide with a molecular weight of 3,485. Its sequence appears to be identical in most mammals, and it is secreted by the alpha cells of the islets of Langerhans. Although identical cells may be present in the GI tract of some other mammals, there is no hard evidence to suggest that extrapancreatic true glucagon is to be found in man. However, some antibodies to glucagon (N-terminal specific) cross-react with a material from the intestine called glucagon-like immunoreactivity, or enteroglucagon (see below).

Pancreatic glucagon is released into the portal circulation, where its primary role is to stimulate glycogenolysis and gluconeogenesis in the liver, thereby converting the liver from an organ of glucose storage to an organ of glucose production. The opposing and counterbalancing actions of glucagon and insulin on the liver make possible large changes in glucose flux rates without important changes in glucose concentrations. In the absence of stress or diabetes, hyperglycemia is the single most potent inhibitor of glucagon release, whereas hypoglycemia stimulates glucagon release, although the greatest elevations are seen after amino acid administration. Glucagon plays a vital role in elevating blood glucose concentrations at times of stress. In these circumstances, pancreatic glucagon is elevated despite the presence of hyperglycemia.

In 1974, several patients were reported, all of whom suffered a peculiar skin rash, necrolytic migratory erythema.[29] All the cases were associated with pancreatic tumors characterized by islet alpha cells containing glucagon. The subjects had very high glucagon levels in plasma, and in one case when the tumor was resected the hyperglucagonemia and rash disappeared. The glucagonoma syndrome is also associated with impaired glucose tolerance, anemia, and glossitis. As in the case of secretin, hyperglucagonemia is also seen in patients suffering from renal failure, in which there is an inability of the kidney to clear biologically active glucagon fragments. Hyperglucagonemia is associated with hepatic failure, and established diabetics may also have slightly raised fasting glucagon concentrations, which are inappropriate for the level of blood glucose concentrations.

Enteroglucagon

Shortly after the development of radioimmunoassays for glucagon at the beginning of the 1960s, it became apparent that the antibody cross-reacts with a glucagon-like substance that is present in the gut as well as in the pancreas. To differentiate between the two types of glucagon immunoreactivity, several alternative and competing terms were invented for the intestinal material, the most common being glucagon-like immunoreactivity, gut glucagon, or enteroglucagon. Antibody specificities with synthetic glucagon fragments revealed that those antibodies reacting with enteroglucagon are directed toward the N-terminal and central regions of the glucagon molecule, whereas the antibodies more specific to pancreatic glucagon are directed toward the C-terminal region.[30]

Early studies suggested that enteroglucagon exists in the intestine in several molecular forms, these being reflected in the circulating concentrations. More recently, the most abundant form of enteroglucagon in the pig has been isolated; since it was initially thought to be composed of 100 amino acids, the term *glicentin* was introduced.[31] Subsequently it was found to have only 69 amino acids, but the name has been retained.[32] This peptide contains the entire sequence of pancreatic glucagon, and the C-terminal region appears to be almost identical to that of the peptide initially extracted from the pancreas as "pro-glucagon."[33] High concentrations of enteroglucagon are found throughout the GI tract of man and mammals, being maximal in the ileum. Moreover, there appears to be only one specific type of intestinal enteroglucagon-secreting cell.

In view of the substantial difficulties that have been encountered in purifying enteroglucagon, there is little information on its pharmacology. However, after the oral ingestion of glucose, peripheral blood concentrations of enteroglucagon rise, and in man it is also released after oral administration of long-chain triglycerides or of carbohydrates and after the ingestion of a normal mixed meal. Intrajejunal and intracolonic infusions of glucose and fatty acids directly stimulate the secretion of enteroglucagon.

A case of a renal endocrine tumor producing enteroglucagon has been described, the patient being found to have marked intestinal villous hypertrophy and greatly increased intestinal transit time.[34] Resection of the tumor led to resolution of these findings. It is important to emphasize that whenever an excess of enteroglucagon has been found it has invariably been associated with mucosal hypertrophy or regeneration. Thus, high concentrations of enteroglucagon have been found in patients with active celiac disease,[35] tropical sprue,[36] cystic fibrosis,[37] acute bowel infection, and dumping syndrome[38] and also following small intestinal resection or bypass surgery.[39] These observations suggest that enteroglucagon may have a physiologic role as a trophic stimulus to gut regeneration whenever there is a loss of effective small intestinal mucosal absorptive surface.

Enteroglucagon is also elevated following gastric surgery,[40] suggesting that under these circumstances it might be released in an attempt to achieve an inhibitory effect on gastric motility and acid secretion.

Pancreatic Polypeptide

Pancreatic polypeptide (PP) was discovered as a major contaminant during the isolation of human proinsulin from pancreatic tissue.[41] It is a unique hormone in the sense that it was purified before the assessment of its biologic activity, whereas most hormones are purified only after a biologic effect has been described.

The amino acid sequence shows the peptide to have 36 amino acids in the straight chain, and it is localized in the pancreas to endocrine cells distinct from the alpha, beta, and D cells. These cells are found between the acini and the lining of the ducts of the exocrine parenchyma as well as in the periphery of the islets of Langerhans, especially in the head of the pancreas.[42] PP circulates in plasma and is released from the pancreas in response to the ingestion of food, particularly fat and protein.[43] Moreover, after infusion its in-

hibitory effects on the secretion of trypsin from the exocrine pancreas and on gallbladder contractility in man occur at plasma levels similar to those seen after a normal mixed meal.[44]

Basal and postprandial concentrations of the hormone appear to rise with increasing age.[43] Protein- and fat-containing foods cause a prompt increase in the circulating concentrations, the elevation in plasma levels being maintained for several hours so that in the usual course of adult feeding the PP levels remain high throughout the day, with only a relatively small peak following each meal.[45,46] Since little or no change in fasting levels is observed during intravenous nutrient infusions, it is suggested that the normal release of this peptide is dependent on an indirect enteropancreatic axis. The mechanism for the release of PP by food is complex, involving the vagus as well as humoral factors. Thus vagal stimulation, for example during insulin-induced hypoglycemia, is a particularly potent signal for PP production. PP has no known metabolic effects in man.

PP secretion in adults is abnormal in two particular pathologic situations, namely, pancreatic exocrine insufficiency and pancreatic endocrine tumors. Thus, patients with chronic pancreatitis and steatorrhea have low PP levels in the fasting state, with an obtundation after food.[47,48] PP concentrations may be quite normal, however, in patients with chronic pancreatitis who have no steatorrhea.

PP cells are often found in pancreatic endocrine tumors, particularly VIPomas, which produce the watery diarrhea syndrome, and in glucagonomas.[49] Plasma PP can be used as a marker for pancreatic endocrine tumors in adults.

Gastric Inhibitory Polypeptide

In 1970 a peptide was isolated which is capable of inhibiting gastric acid secretion from the upper small intestine of the pig.[50] This substance was named gastric inhibitory polypeptide (GIP) by Brown and Pederson. It was later shown to release insulin potently in the presence of hyperglycemia, and an alternative name is often applied to it, namely, glucose-dependent insulinotrophic polypeptide (thus maintaining the acronym GIP).

GIP is a straight-chain polypeptide consisting of 42 amino acids with a molecular weight of 4,977. Its structure contains several sequence homologies to pancreatic glucagon, vasoactive intestinal polypeptide, and secretin. It has been suggested that GIP is derived from mucosal endocrine cells, the K cell. These cells are numerous in the duodenum and jejunum and are also found throughout the remainder of the upper small gut.[51]

The ingestion of a mixed meal results in a three- to four-fold rise in plasma GIP concentrations, with a peak between 45 and 60 minutes after the meal; the major dietary components producing this release are glucose and fat.[52] GIP has several pharmacologic actions, namely, inhibition of gastric acid secretion, of pepsin secretion, and of gastric motor activity and stimulation of jejunal water and electrolyte flow and of glucagon and insulin release.

The secretion of GIP has been implicated as the fat-induced inhibitor of gastric acid secretion which occurs in most mammals, but in man the acid-inhibitory properties of GIP are of doubtful physiologic significance. Thus, infusion studies have shown that a fourfold increase over the peak postprandial GIP concentration is required to inhibit significantly acid secretion.[53] More attention has been focused on its role as a component of the enteroinsular axis.[54,55] Thus, infusion of GIP during intravenous glucose administration in man significantly augments the insulin release seen with glucose alone, and this effect can also be mimicked by giving oral fat to release endogenous GIP. The insulinotropic effect of GIP seems to be dependent upon the presence of hyperglycemia, and it seems entirely possible that a hyperglycemic threshold exists for GIP-induced insulin release, thereby preventing inappropriate GIP-induced release of insulin when glucose concentrations are low.[55]

Substantial interest has focused on GIP as a potential factor in the etiology of duodenal ulcer disease and of diabetes mellitus. However, studies of GIP secretion in patients with duodenal ulceration with respect to GIP have been contradictory and inconsistent.[56] Thus, paradoxically, higher postprandial GIP concentrations have been found in duodenal ulcer patients when a lack of an acid-inhibitory factor might have been expected. Similar controversy concerns the role of GIP as a causal factor in diabetes mellitus.

On much firmer ground are the reduced postprandial GIP concentrations that have been noted in patients with upper small intestinal disease, for example, adult patients with celiac disease and tropical malabsorption.[56] Moreover, reduced GIP and insulin release are also seen after jejunoileal bypass surgery for obesity. In these circumstances decreased GIP release is reflected in decreased insulin secretion.[56] As yet, no disease can be attributed to the hyper- or hyposecretion of this peptide.

Motilin

Brown et al in 1966[57] suggested the existence of motilin following their observation in dogs that there was increased gut motor activity in denervated transplanted pouches of the body of the stomach following duodenal alkalinization. Motilin is a basic polypeptide of 22 amino acids, and synthesis of the peptide has been achieved.[58] It is localized in endocrine cells, which also sometimes contain 5-hydroxytryptamine in the duodenum and jejunum.[58] Small amounts may be present in the gastric antrum.

When natural porcine motilin is infused in man,[59] there is a significant acceleration of the gastric emptying rate of solids and liquids. Gastric distention appears to be a potent stimulus of motilin secretion, and it in turn may be a physiologic agent for the control of gastric emptying. Moreover, it has been known for some time that stimulation of the stomach by distention stimulates colonic activity, as is demonstrated by recording increased electrical and mechanical activity.[60] Infusions of motilin to achieve concentrations similar to those seen postprandially were able to produce such changes in the colon.[60]

Aynsley-Green and Bloom have concluded in a comprehensive review of GI diseases that motilin is considerably elevated in all groups of patients with diarrhea.[61] However, the cause of the elevation of motilin under individual disease circumstances and its precise role in the motor abnormalities producing diarrhea have yet to be conclusively estab-

lished. No tumor producing motilin has yet been described, but patients with other endocrine tumors may have significantly elevated mean plasma motilin concentrations.

Vasoactive Intestinal Polypeptide

This substance was isolated in 1970 by Said and Mutt,[62] who noted that the infusion of this polypeptide substance extracted from porcine small intestine caused in dogs a gradual but prolonged systemic vasodilatation. On the basis of this action, the name *vasoactive intestinal polypeptide* was suggested. It has been shown subsequently that VIP occurs in high concentrations throughout the gut and also in the brain.[63] In both circumstances, VIP is present predominantly in nerves rather than in cells; therefore, its probable physiologic role is more likely that of a neurotransmitter than of a paracrine or an endocrine agent.

VIP is a basic straight-chain polypeptide consisting of 28 amino acids, with a molecular weight of 3,326. Its amino acid sequence shares numerous homologies with those of GIP, secretin, and PP. There is increasing evidence of multiple molecular forms of VIP, large molecular forms being found particularly in plasma and tumor extracts of patients with VIPomas.

Intravenous infusions of VIP cause net fluid secretion into the bowel lumen throughout the small and large bowel; there is also a fall in basal and stimulated gastric acid output, stimulation of pancreatic bicarbonate secretion, stimulation of glycogenolysis and of insulin secretion, a rise in plasma total and ionized calcium concentration, a relaxation of intestinal smooth muscle and of blood vessels, and an increase in small intestinal cyclic AMP concentrations.[64]

High concentrations of VIP have been demonstrated in the plasma of patients with diarrhea associated with pancreatic endocrine tumors (the Verner-Morrison syndrome).[65] The VIPoma syndrome may be associated with a non–insulin-secreting pancreatic islet cell adenoma or a ganglioneuroblastoma in children.[61,66] High VIP concentrations have been found in patients with severe liver failure[67] and also in the gut tissues of patients with Crohn's disease.[68] On the other hand, low concentrations of VIP have been found in patients with Chagas' disease[69] and in the aganglionic segments of colon in patients with Hirschsprung's disease.[70] These observations have led to the suggestion that estimation of tissue VIP concentrations may be helpful in rectal biopsies for diagnosis of Crohn's, Chagas', or Hirschsprung's disease.

Bombesin

Bombesin was first isolated from the skin of the frog *Bombina bombina* and is a potent stimulant to the secretion of gastrin and other gut hormones in man.[71] Bombesin has several powerful actions on the GI, vascular, and nervous systems in humans and experimental animals, as summarized in Table 2. The peptide is distributed widely in the neurons of the central and peripheral nervous systems of all mammalian species that have been examined to date.[72] It is also detectable by radioimmunoassay in human neonatal lung. Although the peptide has now been successfully purified and is known to have powerful pharmacologic effects, its precise physiologic role has yet to be established.

TABLE 2
Some Pharmacologic Actions of Bombesin

Endocrine system	Release of gastrin, glucagon, insulin, pancreatic polypeptide, motilin, neurotensin, enteroglucagon, cholecystokinin, insulin, growth hormone, prolactin, TSH, TRH, catecholamines, and calcitonin. Decreased secretion of parathyroid hormone.
Central nervous system	Intracisternal injection causes hypothermia, analgesia, diminished appetite, and inhibition of gastric acid secretion.
Lungs	Bronchoconstriction.
Kidneys	Vasoconstriction with secondary hypertension and inhibition of diuresis.
Exocrine pancreas	Adenylate cyclase activation, calcium efflux, and pancreatic enzyme secretion.
Gastrointestinal tract	Gastric acid and pancreatic enzyme secretion, lower esophageal sphincter constriction, interdigestive myoelectric activity, and gallbladder contraction.

Somatostatin

In 1973 Brazeau et al[73] discovered an ovine hypothalamic peptide that potently inhibits growth hormone release from the anterior pituitary. The peptide is also known by its acronym SRIF, representing somatotropin release–inhibiting factor. Somatostatin has been found in neurons throughout the brain and spinal cord and in the D cells of the GI tract. A particularly relevant observation is that in the fetus and neonate of man it is the second most abundant hormone after insulin in the pancreas, but a rapid reversal occurs in maturity and this peptide then takes fourth place, after insulin, pancreatic polypeptide, and glucagon in the adult pancreas.

Infusions of the synthetic peptide into man have demonstrated that pharmacologically it possesses powerful inhibitory effects on a number of diverse physiologic systems, as listed in Table 3. Somatostatin also appears to have the unique

TABLE 3
Some Inhibitory Actions of Pharmacologic
Doses of Somatostatin

Endogenous Hormone Release	Gastrointestinal Secretion
Growth hormone	Gastric acid
Thyroid-stimulating hormone and TSH-stimulated T₃ and T₄	Pepsin
Gastrin	Pancreatic exocrine
Glucagon (pancreatic and enteric)	Choleresis
Gastric inhibitory peptide	Small intestinal secretions
Insulin	
Motilin	
Neurotensin	
Pancreatic polypeptide	
Secretin	
Calcitonin	
Renin	

property of acting as an endocrine or paracrine substance and as a neurotransmitter. However, it has become accepted that the main peripheral action of somatostatin is that of a paracrine agent, being released locally to act as a modulator of neighboring cells.

A number of patients with somatostatinomas[74,75] have been described; the somatostatinomas are usually pancreatic endocrine tumors, although medullary carcinoma of the thyroid and oat cell carcinoma of the bronchus may also be associated with its release.[76] In such patients, common symptoms and physical signs result from steatorrhea, diabetes mellitus, and gallstones, and these problems correlate well with the known inhibitory effects that are observed with pharmacologic administration of the peptide. Rectal biopsies of patients with chronic Chagas' disease exhibit a reduced somatostatin content.[77] The devastating consequences of abnormal paracrine interrelationships between somatostatin- and insulin-secreting cells in the pancreas are vividly exemplified in the syndrome of nesidioblastosis of the pancreas in infancy.[78]

It is fair to conclude that the physiology and pathophysiology of somatostatin are still incompletely understood. It is likely that the study of tissue concentrations and, more importantly, the pattern of local release may offer a fruitful area of further research.

Neurotensin

Neurotensin was discovered during the isolation of substance P from the bovine hypothalamus when it was noticed that certain chromatographic fractions of the tissue extract caused marked vasodilatation in the exposed skin of anesthetized rats. This effect was also accompanied by transient hypotension, and Carraway and Leeman, on isolating the active constituent, named it neurotensin because of its presence in neural tissue and its ability to affect blood pressure.[79] Subsequently the peptide was also isolated from bovine and human small intestine and has been shown to be identical to the peptide originating from bovine hypothalamus.

It contains 13 amino acids and has a molecular weight of 1,674. In the calf central nervous system there is a distinct regional variation, with the hypothalamus and basal ganglia having the greatest concentrations.[80] In the rat, on the other hand, more than 10 times as much neurotensin is present in extracts of small intestine as in the brain, the highest concentrations being in the jejunoileal region.[81] In man, cells containing neurotensin are found most abundantly in the ileum.

The exact physiologic role of neurotensin has yet to be defined with precision. However, neurotensin may well have its most important role as a neurotransmitter or a neuromodulator in the central nervous system. It is released into the circulation by the ingestion of food,[82] excessive release being found in association with the dumping syndrome[83] or after jejunoileal bypass for morbid obesity.[84] Neurotensin is also released in man by the injection of intravenous bombesin[85] and is inhibited by somatostatin.[86]

Infusions of small doses of neurotensin in man have no discernible cardiovascular effects, and when it is infused against a background of mild hyperglycemia, plasma concentrations of insulin and glucagon are unaffected.[86,87] However, a large release of insulin is produced by neurotensin in mildly hyperglycemic calves, clearly demonstrating species- and age-specific differences in response to the peptide.[88] Infusions to induce physiologic concentrations in man show the substance to have a significant inhibitory effect on the motor and secretory aspects of gastric function,[89] as well as stimulating water and bicarbonate secretion from the pancreas.[90]

The increase of plasma neurotensin levels in response to a standardized meal is greatly in excess in patients who have undergone jejunoileal bypass.[84] These observations suggest that circulating neurotensin may be involved in secondary, compensatory mechanisms such as the slowing of gastric emptying and of intestinal transit.

Substance P

This substance is one of a group of peptides found in both the brain[91] and GI tract.[92] It was first described in 1931[93] and is believed to be confined to nerve cells within both the central and peripheral nervous systems. Within the CNS it acts as a neurotransmitter or a neuromodulator. Its presence within the autonomic innervation of a number of organs such as the pancreas and urogenital tract, as well as in the intrinsic innervation of the GI tract, suggests that it may play an important role in the nervous control of physiologic processes.

Substance P is a potent vasodilator and is strongly spasmogenic, having a direct effect on smooth muscle.[94] Pharmacologic studies in vivo and in vitro have demonstrated that it has an influence on both pancreatic endocrine and exocrine function by decreasing basal insulin concentration, raising glucagon secretion, and increasing bicarbonate and amylase output from the pancreas. There is an inhibition of biliary flow, but it directly stimulates salivation in a number of species, whereas in all regions of the GI tract it contracts smooth muscle. It has been found to be a potent natriuretic and diuretic substance. Within the central nervous system there is evidence that substance P interacts with enkephalins in pain perception[94]; moreover, changes in its concentration occur in a number of neurologic disorders, such as Huntington's chorea, in which abnormally low levels of substance P occur in the substantia nigra.[95] In the GI tract, local reduction in the substance P levels occur in Hirschsprung's and Chagas' diseases, both of which are associated with megacolon and aganglionosis.[69] High levels of the substance have been found in some carcinoid tumors, suggesting that the peptide may play a role in the pathogenesis of some of the features of this syndrome.

Conspectus

The above paragraphs have briefly outlined the relevance of gut hormones and regulatory peptides in GI physiology in the adult. Although much has yet to be learned of the interregulation and interaction of the peptidergic systems, it is evident that they have a key role to play in the efficient utilization of enteral food. More extensive reviews of the functions of individual peptides can be found in references 2, 3, 96, and 97.

If these factors are important for the adult, then it follows that they may have an even more important role in early life, particularly in the newborn infant at a time when the gut has to adapt to postnatal enteral feeding.

ADAPTATION TO POSTNATAL NUTRITION

The cutting of the umbilical cord at birth is an event of immense psychological and physiologic importance. The survival and growth of the newborn infant in the hostile extrauterine environment depend crucially upon successful adaptive changes occurring in a number of the body's physiologic systems. Events occurring in the cardiovascular and respiratory systems are evident immediately after birth, but other adaptive changes at least as complex in nature and as important in terms of survival occur during the process of adaptation to extrauterine metabolism and nutrition.

Before birth the fetus is fed largely by transplacental transfer of nutrients into the umbilical vein, the enteral assimilation of amniotic fluid being of considerably less importance in terms of nutritive value. Maternal metabolism clearly has an important regulatory influence on fetal metabolism by controlling the delivery of substrates across the placenta, and the delivery of substrates to the fetus is probably the most important factor controlling prenatal growth. After birth, the infant has to be metabolically independent and needs, moreover, to adapt to a totally new form of nutrition—the intermittent delivery of enteral milk into the gut. During the postnatal period major changes occur in GI structure, motility, and digestive and absorptive function, together with critically important adjustments in intermediary metabolism. A number of publications have appeared documenting evidence for these changes in both experimental animals and man.[98-102] Some of these postnatal adaptive changes are urgent, such as the need to maintain glucose homeostasis following the sudden cessation of the maternal supply, whereas others occur more gradually over a period of hours or days as the enteral feeding is introduced.

It has been suggested that the adaptation to postnatal nutrition depends critically upon the secretion of regulatory peptides released from the specialized cells in the gut, together with those products of the more classic endocrine organs of the pancreas, thyroid, pituitary, and adrenal glands.[103]

Significance of Postnatal Adaptation to Feeding

During fetal life an orderly sequence of developmental changes occurs in the gut in terms of structure and function which prepares it for postnatal nutrition. Structural development precedes that of function,[98-100] which is limited before 26 weeks of gestation in the human fetus.[100,104,105] Lebenthal[100] has emphasized the importance of the "biologic time clock" in the regulation of these changes, but it is evident that this natural rate of development can be influenced profoundly by environmental triggers, as suggested by the fact that prematurely born infants may adapt to enteral feeding as much as 12 weeks "too soon" in biologic terms.

Enteral feeding itself may be such a key environmental trigger, and this contention is supported by animal studies. Thus, in piglets and rats[101,106-108] oral feeding after birth results in marked structural changes and in the growth of the digestive tract; these changes are not seen in animals deprived of enteral feeding. Moreover, oral feeding enhances gut enzyme activity[105] and initiates important changes in intermediary metabolism, such as the increased responsiveness to glucose by pancreatic insulin-secreting cells which is seen in enterally fed newborn piglets.[107,108]

The fetus swallows amniotic fluid containing a significant protein content which can be digested and absorbed,[99] but when milk feeds commence after birth the gut is exposed for the first time to a diet containing high concentrations of fat and lactose as well as protein. Moreover, microorganisms enter the gut lumen for the first time. These intraluminal factors have a significant effect on the development of gut function.[109] For example, lactase activity and pancreatic lipase and trypsinogen activities are induced by feeding and occur much earlier than normal in infants born prematurely.

Intraluminal secretions themselves may have an essential role to play in gut development, evidence for this being the bile activation of enteropeptidase[104] and the increased turnover of brush border proteins by pancreatic proteases.[110] Finally, it has been shown that milk itself contains high concentrations of hormones and growth factors (Table 4). Thus, concentrations of calcitonin, epidermal growth factor, prostaglandins E and F, neurotensin, and melatonin, together with classic pituitary, thyroid, and adrenal hormones, are all detectable in milk. These ingested hormones could exert their effects "topically" on the gut or may even be absorbed intact to affect the body systemically.[111-113]

However, we have suggested previously in a number of publications that a major contribution to the regulation of postnatal gut development may be through the endogenous secretion of regulatory peptides in response to food in the gut. Our working hypothesis[103] suggested that enteral feeding triggers the secretion of gut regulatory peptides, and, through the endocrine, paracrine, and neurocrine effects that have been reviewed above, a cascade of developmental changes is stimulated which affect gut growth, gut motility, development of intestinal secretions and transport mechanisms, initiation of the enteroinsular axis, modulation of pancreatic endocrine function, and hence development of hepatic metabolism. The validation of this hypothesis requires a number of conditions to be met: (1) the gut endocrine cell lines for these peptides should be present in the fetus; (2) postnatally, gut hormones should be released by enteral feeding and not released in neonates deprived of nutrition by this route; (3) gut peptide receptors should be responsive in the neonatal period; (4) there should be a temporal relationship between postnatal gut hormone secretion and the adaptive changes proposed to be influenced by them, and (5) there should be direct experimental evidence that either inhibition of endogenous hormone release or exogenous hormone administration inhibits or induces, respectively, their proposed actions. The evidence to prove this hypothesis conclusively

is as yet incomplete. Nevertheless, the body of data considered in the following sections is strongly supportive of the basic postulate.

Prenatal Metabolic and Endocrine Milieu of the Human Fetus

The study of fetal endocrinology and metabolism in experimental animals has advanced rapidly following the development of new biochemical and physiologic techniques. Of particular relevance is the development of the chronically catheterized fetal lamb preparation, which allows frequent sampling of fetal blood vessels without manipulation and stress. However, the applicability of most of the data derived from animals to man still awaits confirmation because, as yet, it has not been possible to sample both fetal umbilical vessels simultaneously, let alone measure blood flow under unstressed conditions. Most of the information available on circulating concentrations of fetal fuels and hormones in man is based on measurements in blood samples drawn at delivery or during hysterotomy under circumstances that cannot be regarded as physiologic. Nonetheless, a number of publications have appeared using these data; a good review is to be found in reference 115. Studies have also been performed more recently in which blood samples have been drawn from fetal unbilical vessels by the process of fetoscopy in order to define the metabolic milieu of the human fetus between 16 and 20 weeks of gestation.[116,117]

Regulatory peptides, together with their corresponding cell lines, have been identified in the human fetal gut from 6 to 16 weeks after conception.[118,119] For most of the peptides examined to date, the gut tissue concentrations rise to values found in the last 10 weeks of gestation, which are at least as high as those seen in adults.[119] As the gut is relatively large in the perinatal period, this may indicate a correspondingly larger gut endocrine cell mass for some lines in this period of development. Moreover, there is a changing spectrum of molecular forms during fetal life, and, indeed, certain peptides appear and disappear from different regions of the gut during development.[119] These observations suggest that cells secreting regulatory peptides, through changes in anatomic localization and in the products and potency of their secretions, may have a key role as local inducing agents regulating the growth and functional development of the fetal intestine.

Substantial concentrations of regulatory peptides can be measured in blood drawn by fetoscopy from the umbilical blood vessels and in amniotic fluid in the human fetus between 16 and 20 weeks of gestation. Figures 2 and 3 show the concentration of enteroglucagon, gastrin, gastric inhibitory polypeptide, pancreatic polypeptide, and motilin in the maternal and fetal circulation, together with values from the assay of amniotic fluid.

In contrast to the absence of significant differences between the maternal and fetal concentrations of insulin and glucagon (despite high levels of insulinogenic and glucagonogenic amino acids in the fetal circulation),[117] there are substantially elevated concentrations of enteroglucagon in the fetal circulation. On the other hand, gastrin concentrations are much higher in the maternal circulation than in the fetal circula-

TABLE 4
Hormones Reported in Breast Milk

Steroids	Prolactin
Thyroxine	Erythropoietin
Gonadotropins	Melatonin
LHRH	Epidermal growth factor
TRH	Prostaglandins
TSH	Calcitonin
ACTH	

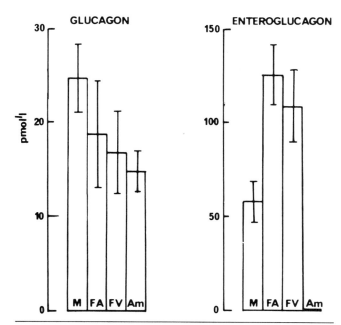

FIGURE 2 Maternal (M), fetal (FV = fetal vein, FA = fetal artery), and amniotic fluid (Am) concentrations in the human fetus at 16 to 20 weeks of gestation. (From Aynsley-Green et al.[158])

It is known that the fetus swallows and can utilize the constituents of amniotic fluid[99] and, moreover, that amniotic fluid is in continuous circulation with the fetal lung. Could these peptides have an important role to play as local inducing agents in the development of the fetal lung as well as the alimentary tract? Whatever the final answers to these questions are, the observations listed above suggest that the study of the ontogeny and the control of the fetal secretion of hormones and regulatory peptides may well throw further light on the orderly sequence of development of the lung and gut and may provide further insight into pathologic development. As mentioned previously, nesidioblastosis of the pancreas is an excellent example of a serious disorder of pancreatic endocrine cell development in which a "maturation arrest" appears to have occurred.[120]

Endocrine Milieu at Birth

GI peptides are found in significant concentrations in venous cord blood at birth in infants delivered by the normal vaginal route at full term (Table 5). It is interesting that most of the measured hormone concentrations at birth are similar to those seen in healthy fasting adults, but it is particularly noteworthy that the concentrations of gastrin and VIP are significantly higher than fasting adult values. Hypergastrinemia at birth has been reported by others[121,122] who have suggested that gastrin might be released by vagal stimuli at delivery; this accords with other data which show that plasma gastrin concentrations fall sharply toward adult fasting levels in the early hours postnatally prior to the commencement of enteral feeding.[123,124]

The observations implying that gut peptide–releasing mechanisms may operate at birth are further supported by observations that full-term infants born following fetal distress show a selective venous cord plasma elevation of motilin, VIP, pancreatic polypeptide, pancreatic glucagon, neurotensin, and enteroglucagon[125,126] (Table 5). The rise in plasma motilin in fetal distress is especially marked, and it has been suggested that this might account for the passage of meconium, an event pathognomonic of this condition. The

tion, as are the concentrations of pancreatic polypeptide. Fetal concentrations of GIP, on the other hand, are higher than those in the maternal circulation, the highest levels of this peptide being found in amniotic fluid.

Several questions follow from these observations. First, why are some hormones present in lower concentrations in the fetus than in the mother, whereas others are present in higher concentrations? What is the significance of the high concentration of GIP and the very low concentration of enteroglucagon in amniotic fluid? From where do amniotic concentrations arise? Are the molecular forms of the hormone similar in mother, amniotic fluid, and fetus?

FIGURE 3 Maternal (M), fetal (FV = fetal vein, FA = fetal artery), and amniotic fluid (Am) concentrations (m ± SEM) of gastrin, GIP, and PP. (From Aynsley-Green et al.[158])

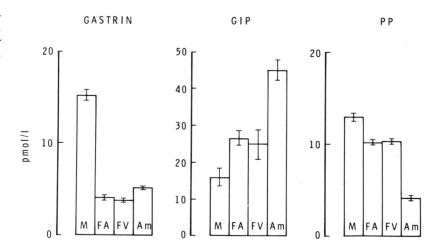

TABLE 5
Enteroinsular Hormone Concentrations in Venous
Cord Plasma from Normal Deliveries Compared with
Those from Infants Showing Fetal Distress

Hormone	Normal Deliveries (n = 20)	Fetal Distress (n = 8)	p*
Motilin	34 ± 4†	127 ± 24	<0.001
Gastric inhibitory peptide	10 ± 2	28 ± 6	<0.01
Pancreatic polypeptide	13 ± 3	44 ± 10	<0.01
Pancreatic glucagon	4 ± 2	14 ± 4	<0.05
Neurotensin	33 ± 3	48 ± 4	<0.01
Enteroglucagon	77 ± 5	107 ± 10	<0.05
Gastrin	42 ± 5	39 ± 3	NS
Secretin	6 ± 1	5 ± 1	NS

* Mann-Whitney rank sum test. NS = not significant.
† Mean ± SE. Concentrations in picomoles per liter.

elevation of plasma glucagon occurring in infants suffering fetal distress accounts for the rapid mobilization of glycogen which occurs under hypoxic conditions, with the consequent induction of hypoglycemia after the asphyxia has been resolved. The significance of the changes in plasma VIP, PP, and neurotensin is uncertain at the present time, but the former peptide may affect redistribution of visceral blood flow in the distressed fetus.

It is also worth emphasizing that the metabolic milieu at delivery is profoundly influenced by the administration of glucose to mothers during labor. Thus, a retrospective analysis of plasma insulin concentrations in the cord blood of infants born after normal delivery noted[127] that mothers given "routine" dextrose infusions during labor produced neonates with hyperinsulinism in cord blood. That the magnitude of the hyperinsulinism is related to the amount of glucose given to mothers during delivery demonstrates that transplacental passage of glucose is a potent stimulus to insulin at this time. Others[128] have confirmed this finding and have demonstrated that high cord plasma insulin concentrations may be accompanied by rebound hypoglycemia during the first hours after delivery.

Cord concentrations of regulatory peptides in preterm infants can be seen in Figure 4, and in comparing these values with those in Table 5, which outlines the concentrations in normal infants at term, it can be seen that plasma GIP, gastrin, and enteroglucagon concentrations are similar in both groups of infants, whereas there are some differences in the cord levels of PP, motilin, and neurotensin.

Metabolic and Endocrine Milieu in Relation to Postnatal Feeding

After preparation of the fetal gut for postnatal feeding, an important event that occurs immediately after birth is the first feed of milk. This is an event of considerable physiologic significance, since it is the first time that the alimentary tract has been challenged by an exogenous foodstuff. Rodgers et al[122] showed that gastrin and enteroglucagon increase in the plasma of human neonates during the first 4 days, Lichtenberger and Johnson[106] confirming that the early postnatal

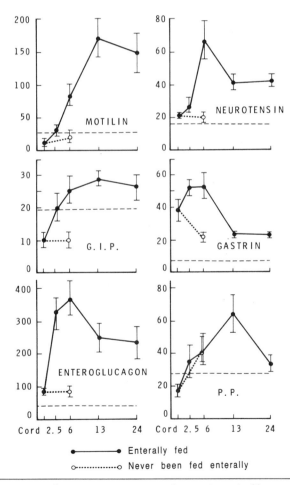

FIGURE 4 Plasma concentrations of gastrointestinal hormones in preterm infants during the first 24 days after birth: in preprandial blood samples drawn from infants fed from birth with regular boluses of human milk and from a similar group of infants who had never received any enteral feeding. The dashed line represents the mean fasting concentration in adults.

elevation in gastrin in rats is due to enteral feeding. Von Berger and colleagues demonstrated that gastrin rises in the plasma after the first feed in the human neonate.[129] In a rather more extensive study it has been demonstrated that the first feed of human milk given to full-term infants causes a significant increase in blood glucose concentrations, together with increases in insulin, growth hormone, gastrin, and enteroglucagon but not in GIP or pancreatic glucagon.[130] The lack of GIP response accords with the findings of King and colleagues,[131] who failed to identify an active enteroinsular axis in the immediate postpartum period. This, together with the absent feed response for pancreatic glucagon, supports the view that the glucagon surge after birth[102] is of importance in the initiation of glycogenolysis and gluconeogenesis independently of enteral feeding. It seems to be particularly appropriate for the newborn infant to achieve rapid regulation of blood glucose immediately after birth independently of the precise timing of the initiation of enteral feeding and to ensure that insulin dominance does not occur at a time of glucose instability.

The consequences of abnormal pancreatic endocrine development at this time of life are vividly revealed in infants born with nesidioblastosis of the pancreas. It has been demonstrated that normal pancreatic islet cell hormone control is of major importance in preventing hypoglycemia and its consequent risk of neonatal death or brain damage.[120] The investigation and management of this most difficult neonatal problem are beyond the scope of this review, but the interested reader is referred to reference 120 for further information. What is clear from these experiments of nature, however, is that the endocrine pancreas has a crucial role to play in the stabilization of blood glucose levels during the first hours after birth and in the maintenance of normoglycemia until enteral feeding is established. Moreover, normal function is entirely dependent upon the normal aggregation of discrete endocrine cells into functional units—the islets of Langerhans.

It is concluded from these studies that the infant born at term is prepared for enteral feeding and that within hours of birth demonstrable postprandial changes occur in intermediary metabolism together with changes in the secretion of hormones from the gut, pancreas, and pituitary gland. However, in contrast to these impressive changes in the infant born at term, when the same study was repeated in infants born prematurely, it was found that no change occurred after the first feed in the concentration of any metabolite or hormone that was measured.[132] This implies that developmental changes occur during the last few weeks of gestation which prepare the infant born at term to respond immediately.

A series of papers has now been published documenting the development of postnatal hormone concentrations in preterm infants, and some of the more important conclusions from these studies are summarized in the following paragraphs.

It should be obvious to the informed reader that a number of different feeding practices are used routinely in newborn nurseries. Prematurely born infants may receive milk directly into the stomach or into the small bowel, the milk may be given continuously or intermittently, and the composition of the milk may vary widely from "drip" breast milk to expressed breast milk to a variety of specially designed formulae for the low-birth-weight infant. There is evidence that the

mode of delivery and the composition of the feed have important influences on the development of the metabolic and endocrine milieu of the newborn infant.

Indeed, the effects of different feed composition can be documented in the infant born at term as early as the very first feed after birth. Thus, the gut appears to have the ability to increase enteroglucagon concentrations in response to milk but not to dextrose.[133] With particular reference to the prematurely born infant, it has been shown that infants who are given milk feeds by regular boluses directly into the stomach experience multiple gut hormonal surges during the first postnatal days.[124] Thus, although no demonstrable change occurred after the first feed, within 2½ days of birth, preprandial hormone concentrations have increased markedly in six of the peptides measured (Fig. 4), and by the sixth day there had been a highly significant three- to fourfold rise above the levels at birth in, for example, the basal plasma concentrations of neurotensin and enteroglucagon. By 13 days of age, the basal plasma motilin concentration had risen 13-fold and PP threefold. Plasma concentrations of all of these substances rose significantly above adult values—in the case of enteroglucagon by a factor of 10.

In addition to the rise in basal hormone concentrations, during the postnatal period in preterm infants, there are progressive changes in the effect of a feed on postprandial plasma concentrations of motilin, neurotensin, GIP, enteroglucagon, gastrin, secretin, glucose, growth hormone, and insulin. In the early neonatal days the responses to a feed are small or absent, whereas by 24 days the responses are marked[123,134-139] (Figs. 5 to 7).

More limited data from the term breast-fed infant show that significant postnatal hormonal surges do occur in preprandial blood samples but are smaller than those seen in pre-

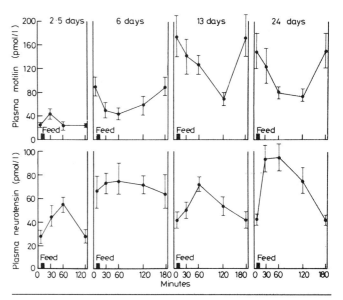

FIGURE 5 The development of postprandial feed-induced cycles of changes in plasma concentrations of motilin and neurotensin in preterm infants receiving regular boluses of milk from birth. (From Lucas et al.[124])

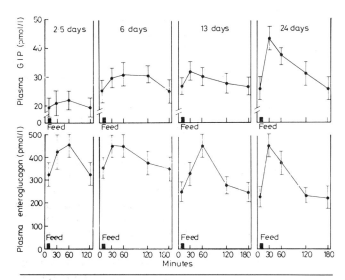

FIGURE 6 The development of postprandial feed-induced cycles of changes in plasma concentrations of enteroglucagon and GIP in preterm infants receiving regular boluses of milk from birth. (From Lucas et al.[124])

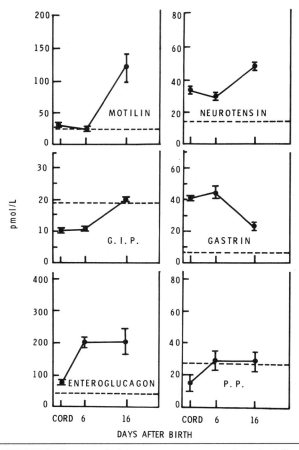

FIGURE 8 Preprandial hormone concentrations in full-term infants during the first 6 days after birth (infants receiving formula from birth). The dashed line represents the mean fasting concentration in adults.

term infants[103] (Fig. 8). There are several explanations for this difference (which is rather contrary to expectation) between premature and term infants. It may, for example, be explained by the fact that lactation takes some days to become established for breast-fed infants and that enteral feed volumes are lower on a body weight per kilogram basis in term infants than in preterm neonates. The precise mechanism for the unexpectedly high concentrations of peptides in preterm infants still requires explanation, including the need to examine the possibility that the preterm infant may have a decreased ability to degrade and eliminate these peptides.

That it is enteral feeding which has triggered the postnatal hormonal surges is confirmed in Figure 4, which also shows basal (preprandial) concentrations of six substances in preterm infants who had received regular boluses of milk into the stomach compared with another group of infants who had received no enteral feeds. With the exception of the change

in PP, none of the other five hormones increased in concentration after birth, suggesting that food introduced into the gut in the form of milk is indeed a powerful stimulus to the secretion of gut hormones and that these changes do not occur in infants who have never been fed.[140]

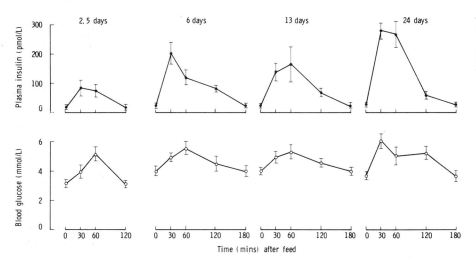

FIGURE 7 Plasma insulin and blood glucose concentrations after feeding in preterm infants (n = 8 to 12 infants for each time period; mean ± SEM).

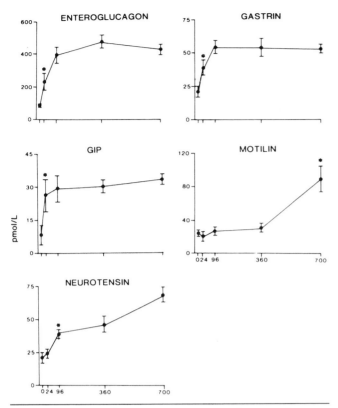

FIGURE 9 Mean plasma concentrations of enteroglucagon, gastrin, GIP, motilin, and neurotensin (pmol per liter ± SEM) according to the total (ml) cumulative enteral feed volume (human milk) since birth in preterm infants. (From Lucas et al.[141])

More recently, the amount of milk that must be given to induce gut hormone secretion has been studied.[141] Figure 9 shows the relationship between hormone concentrations and the volume of milk consumed since birth. Figure 10 shows hormone levels in three groups of preterm infants—those receiving only intravenous fluids, those healthy infants receiving total enteral feeds from birth, and those with respiratory disease who had received only half of the volume of milk given to healthy infants. From Figure 9 it is evident that a highly significant increase in enteroglucagon concentrations occurs after a total cumulative volume of milk as low as 24 ml has been given, whereas rather larger volumes are needed for the induction of motilin surges. However, initial deprivation of enteral feeding is followed rapidly by hormonal surges close to those of healthy infants.

These data can be used to question current policy of routinely feeding small premature infants entirely by the intravenous route. These infants are deprived not only of enteral milk, but also of the amniotic fluid they would be swallowing in utero. Experimental deprivation of enteral feeding is known to result in delay in gut development. Thus, in animal studies,[142,143] total parenteral nutrition results in rapid changes in the gut within a few days, including marked mucosal hypotrophy, decrease in brush border enzyme activities, and reduction in absorptive surface as evidenced by diminished xylose absorption; indeed, xylose absorption is reduced also in human neonates fed parenterally.

In neonatal clinical practice, enteral feeds are usually tolerated in premature and full-term infants within a few days after reintroduction of food after short periods of total parenteral nutrition. However, in certain circumstances, for instance in extreme prematurity and, in particular, following surgery for congenital abnormalities in the gut, it may be necessary to employ parenteral nutrition for prolonged periods from birth. The above data suggest that the use of milk should be considered not only as a nutrient but also as a pharmacologic agent to maintain the stimulus to gut development. It needs to be proved conclusively that this practice of "minimal enteral feeding" has a beneficial effect on gut development and tolerance to enteral feeding in seriously ill neonatal patients, although recent evidence is highly supportive[144] of this concept.

A further interesting issue concerns the effects of continuous intragastric infusions of milk compared with regular intermittent bolus administration of the same total daily food

FIGURE 10 Mean plasma concentrations of enteroglucagon, gastrin, GIP, motilin, and neurotensin (pmol per liter ± SEM) at birth (venous cord blood) and at 6 days: in infants who had received no enteral feeds since birth (unfed), in well enterally fed infants, and in those with respiratory disease (RDS) on restricted enteral intake. (Redrawn from Lucas et al.[141])

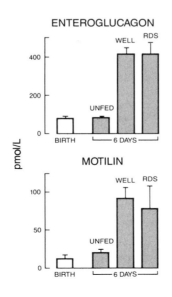
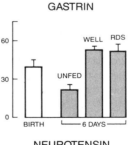
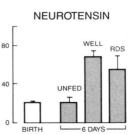
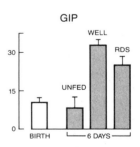

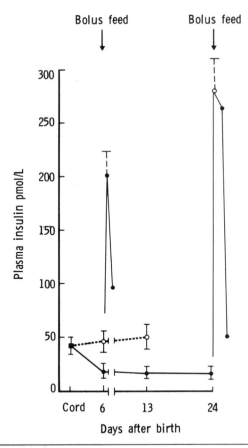

FIGURE 11 Plasma insulin concentrations in preterm infants receiving a continuous infusion of human milk from birth (*dotted line*) and in preprandial blood samples drawn from similar preterm infants receiving regular boluses of milk from birth. Superimposed are shown the magnitude of the insulin pulse after a bolus feed on day 6 and day 24. (From Aynsley-Green et al.[145])

volume. A study has been performed to examine the endocrine milieu induced by these practices, and it is evident that the continuously fed infant, although demonstrating an increase in basal concentrations of several peptides, does not experience the regular cyclic responses of hormones, particularly the anabolic hormones insulin and growth hormone, which are seen in babies given regular boluses of milk (Fig. 11).[145] Although it could be argued that feed-induced surges of anabolic hormones in relation to bolus feeding may stimulate faster growth (and this has yet to be proved), it could be postulated equally well that postprandial hormone changes after bolus feeding can be deleterious by inducing changes in blood pressure and cerebral blood flow which might predispose to further problems, such as intraventricular hemorrhage.[145,146] Some preliminary data have been published suggesting that the bolus-fed infant may grow rather faster than the continuously fed infant, but again this needs to be proved conclusively.[145]

The composition of the milk given to premature infants also appears to have effects on the milieu during the first 3 to 4 weeks after birth. Infants fed on a proprietary formula for premature babies have higher plasma GIP concentrations around the second week after birth, whereas pancreatic polypeptide concentrations are higher in human milk–fed infants around 3 weeks after birth.[147] The mechanism and significance of these differences are unclear, but it does suggest that not only the method of feeding but also the composition of the feed may influence the development of postnatal hormone concentrations for some of the peptides.

The concept of differences induced by feed composition are more vividly exemplified in the context of the full-term infant in the first week after birth. Impressive differences between the breast-fed and formula-fed infant are evident on the sixth postnatal day. Thus, there is a greater insulin response to the feed at this age in formula-fed infants than in the breast-fed infants, and this appears to be related to difference in GIP secretions.[148,149] There are also differences in the response of the motor hormones of the gut, motilin and neurotensin, together with a tendency to a greater growth hormone secretion. The functional and long-term consequences of these differences remain to be clarified. One obvious area of immediate relevance concerns the stool frequency of normal term neonates. It has been known for a long time that the breast-fed infant has his bowels open less frequently than the formula-fed infant, this difference having been attributed to differences in the residue of the two milks. However, the observation of differences in motor hormone secretion suggests that they may be more relevant in this context, and this could be relevant to the later development of "infant colic."

It has been shown that differences in the endocrine responses to a mild feed are still present at 9 months of age in infants who have been exclusively breast fed until that age when compared to others who have been formula fed from birth and weaned early.[150] It is also fascinating to deliberate upon whether or not these endocrine differences could have an effect on the programming of the central nervous system in relation to satiety and food intake in later life. It should be remembered that the premature infant, born at a time when it should be receiving only amniotic fluid into its gut, is given routinely in most newborn nurseries volumes of milk on the order of 150 to 200 ml per kilogram per 24 hours. These volumes of milk, if given to an adult, would amount to approximately 20 liters per day! It would be an extremely interesting study to determine whether or not the food intake, feeding pattern, and satiety of infants in the first 1 to 5 years after birth differ with the mode of neonatal nutrition.

Finally, it should be emphasized that other hormones may have important effects on postnatal adaptation. These include cortisol secretion, prolactin, and thyroxine release.[151] The latter may be particularly important in view of the suggestion that it is relevant in the induction of hepatic receptors for the metabolic hormones. Of particular interest, however, is the demonstration that a feed-related (and possibly sleep-related) rhythm in plasma cortisol concentrations is evident within a few days of birth.[151] Other "new" hormones are being discovered which will extend still further the repertoire of regulatory peptides. One such example, peptide tyrosine, tyrosine, or PYY, which has powerful effects on inhibiting gastric acid secretion and gut motility, has also been shown to increase dramatically after birth in response to feeding.[152]

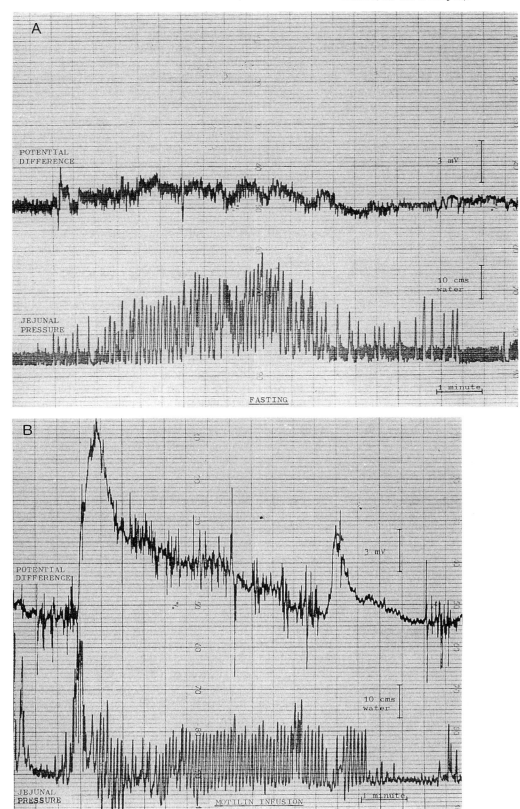

FIGURE 12 *A*, Transmural potential difference and jejunal pressure changes in a preterm infant with pseudo-obstructive ileus before receiving motilin. *B*, Transmural potential difference and jejunal pressure changes in a preterm infant with pseudo-obstructive ileus during an infusion of motilin. (*A* and *B* courtesy of Dr. P. Milla.)

Physiologic Significance of the Metabolic and Endocrine Milieu of the Fetus and Neonate

The factors regulating the ontogeny of the intestinal tract have been well reviewed.[99,100,105] Many factors are known to be involved in this process, including the genetic endowment and the existence of a biologic clock regulating developmental chronology, as well as other endogenous mechanisms and environmental influences. The expression of the genetic endowment at various stages of fetal GI development is accomplished by way of regulatory mechanisms; although most of those postulated mechanisms have been studied in experimental animals, the above additional evidence suggests that parallelism exists for the human fetus and that regulatory peptides and hormones in general may be of fundamental importance.

The interaction of environmental influences on the ontogeny of the gut appears to be well exemplified by the adaptation, up to 3 months "too soon," of the premature infant to postnatal feeding. One unexplained point relates to why preterm infants, and to a lesser extent infants at term, have concentrations of peptides that are considerably greater than those seen in the adult. These elevated concentrations could relate to deficient plasma clearance mechanisms in the immature infant, or, alternately, could result from the relatively large endocrine cell mass of the developing gut. Whatever the mechanism, it is possible that high concentrations of hormones and regulatory peptides are needed in both preterm and term neonates to induce receptor activity and hence the functional effects in target tissues. This raises a whole new issue of further work to be performed. The data reported above represent "phenomenology," and there is an urgent need to relate these observations to the actual functional development of gut activity. There is already some evidence demonstrating effects of regulatory peptides on the growth and development of intestinal cells cultured in vitro.[153-154]

Of greater practical significance are the implications of these data for the feeding practices currently employed in newborn nurseries. It is evident that differences in practice, which may seem at first glance to be innocuous, may indeed have fundamental effects on the metabolic and endocrine milieu and may even have unexpected long-term effects on nutritional management of different groups of newborn infants and on the investigation and treatment of disorders interfering with normal adaptation to postnatal nutrition.

Although the concept that regulatory peptides can be used therapeutically in pediatric practice is not well developed, there are two pieces of evidence to suggest that this is a reasonable suggestion that warrants further exploration. First, somatostatin has been used in adult patients suffering from GI hemorrhage due to peptic ulceration, in cases of hormone overproduction associated with malignant tumors, and in acute pancreatitis.[155] These problems are obviously very uncommon in children. However, in pediatric practice, somatostatin has been used to control the severe hyperinsulinism resulting from islet cell dysregulation syndromes, including nesidioblastosis and benign insulinomas in childhood,[156] although the effects of this powerful inhibitory peptide on the neonatal adaptive processes in the gut have not been studied. Second, and of possibly greater academic interest, is the observation that an infusion of exogenous motilin normalized the generation of action potentials and migrating myoelectric complexes in an infant with pseudo-obstructive ileus (Fig. 12). This interesting observation raises a fascinating possibility that some gut motility disorders in early infancy not only may be due to endocrine dysfunction but also may be helped by hormone administration.

It has been demonstrated that diarrheal states in adults and children are associated with deranged secretion of gut peptides.[61] More recently it has been shown that dramatic changes in enteroglucagon secretion occur in babies experiencing acute infectious diarrhea,[157] in turn raising another possibility that this hormone might be used as a marker to monitor gut recovery. Perhaps enteroglucagon itself (or a related peptide) might in due course be given to speed up the process of gut growth, regeneration, and repair.

SUMMARY AND CONCLUSIONS

During the last 20 years there has been an explosion of interest in and knowledge of hormones and regulatory peptides manufactured by specialized cells in the gut. Evidence has been presented to suggest that these substances have a central role to play in the effective utilization of food in the human adult. There is also rather more limited evidence to suggest that the peptides may have an essential role to play in the differentiation and functional development of the fetal gut. Knowledge of the role of these substances at this critical stage of gut development may prove to be important in understanding the control of normal gut development and in understanding the pathogenesis of abnormal gut function in the neonatal period.

It is during this period of life that gut regulatory peptides may have their most important influence, in determining the successful adaptation to postnatal enteral feeding. Although the circulating concentrations of substances may be influenced profoundly by the milieu of the infant at the moment of birth, there is good evidence that the initiation of enteral feeding is an important environmental trigger that provokes massive surges in the concentrations of these peptides in the first postnatal days.

The interrelationships and magnitude of the changes are further influenced by prematurity, by the mode of administration of feeds, and by the composition of the feed. Deprivation of enteral feeding prevents the appearance of postnatal hormonal surges; in view of the fact that subnutritional volumes of milk are capable of inducing these surges, there is an important concept to investigate further, namely, that of minimal enteral feeding in seriously ill premature and full-term neonates.

The imposition of feeding regimens that are based more on empiricism than on science may have very important and even long-term effects on the human organism.

Disease processes after birth are associated with abnormal circulating concentrations of gut peptides, raising the possibility that dietary regimens designed to manipulate hormone concentrations, or the administration of hormones themselves, may have therapeutic importance.

It is evident that much more study is required to define the ontogeny, regulation of secretion, interaction, and mechanism of effect of these fascinating substances.

REFERENCES

1. Martin CJ. Obituary, Ernest Henry Starling. Br Med J 1927; 1:900–905.
2. Jerzy Glass GB, ed. Gastrointestinal hormones. New York: Raven Press, 1980.
3. Bloom SR, Polak JM, ed. Gut hormones. Edinburgh: Churchill Livingstone, 1981.
4. Anderson JD, Barton MA, Gregory RA, Hardy PM, Kenner GQ, Macleod JK, Preston J, Sheppard RC, Morley JS. The antral hormone gastrin II. Synthesis of gastrin. Nature 1964; 204:933–934.
5. Yalow RS, Berson SA. Size and charge distinctions between endogenous human plasma gastrin in peripheral blood and heptadecapeptide gastrins. Gastroenterology 1970; 58:609–615.
6. Walsh JH, Grossman MI. Gastrin. N Engl J Med 1975; 292:1324–1332.
7. Grossman MI. Gastrin and its activities. Nature 1970; 228:1147–1150.
8. Rehfeld JF, Fottermann NR. Immunochemical evidence of cholecystokinin tetrapeptides in hog brain. J Neurochem 1979; 32:1339–1341.
9. Gingel JC, Davies MW, Shields R. Effect of a synthetic gastrin-like pentapeptide upon the intestinal transport of sodium, potassium and water. Gut 1968; 9:111–116.
10. Lin TM, Spry GF. Effect of pentagastrin, cholecystokinin, caerulein and glucagon on the choledochal resistance and bile flow of the conscious dog. Gastroenterology 1969; 56:1178.
11. Castell DO, Harris LD. Hormonal control of gastroesophageal sphincter strength. N Engl J Med 1970; 282:886–890.
12. Caren JF, Aures D, Johnson LR. Effect of secretin and cholecystokinin on histidine decarboxylase activity in the rat stomach. Proc Soc Exp Biol Med 1969; 131:1194–1197.
13. Crean GP, Marshall MW, Rumsey RDE. Parietal cell hyperplasia induced by the administration of pentagastrin to rats. Gastroenterology 1969; 57:147–155.
14. Ganguli PC, Cullen DR, Irvine WJ. Radioimmunoassay of plasma gastrin in pernicious anaemia, achlorhydria with gut pernicious anaemia, hypochlorhydria and controls. Lancet 1971; i:155–158.
15. Zollinger RM, Ellison EH. Primary peptide ulceration of the jejunum associated with islet cell tumour of the pancreas. Ann Surg 1955; 142:709–728.
16. Jorpes JE, Mutt V, Toczko K. Further purification of cholecystokinin and pancreozymin. Acta Clin Scand 1964; 18:2408–2410.
17. Mutt V. Further investigations on intestinal hormonal polypeptides. Clin Endocrinol 1976; 5(Suppl):183–187.
18. Jorpes JE, Mutt V. Secretin cholecystokinin (CCK). In: Jorpes JE, Mutt V, eds. Secretin cholecystokinin, pancreozymin and gastrin. Berlin: Springer-Verlag, 1976: 1.
19. Vanderhaegen JJ, Signeau JC, Gepts W. New peptide in the vertebrate CNS reacting with antigastrin antibodies. Nature 1975; 257:604–605.
20. Rehfeld JF. Immunochemical studies on cholecystokinin II. Distribution and molecular heterogeneity in the central nervous system and small intestine of man and hog. J Biol Chem 1978; 253:4022–4030.
21. Mellanby J. The mechanism of pancreatic digestion—the function of secretin. J Physiol 1925; 60:85–91.
22. Rehfeld JE, Goltermann N, Larsson L-I, Emson PM, Lee CM. Gastrin and cholecystokinin in central and peripheral neurons. Fed Proc 1979; 38:2325–2329.
23. Jorpes JE, Mutt V. On the biological activity and amino acid composition of secretin. Acta Chem Scand 1961; 15:1790–1791.
24. Mutt V, Jorpes JE. Secretin: isolation and determination of structure. Proceedings, International Symposium on the Chemistry of Natural Products, Stockholm 1966, 26 June: Section 2C-3.
25. Greenberg GR, McCloy RF, Baron JH, Bryant MG, Bloom SR. Gastric acid regulates plasma secretin in man. Eur J Clin Invest 1982.
26. Besterman HS, Bloom SR, Sarson DL, Blackburn AM, Johnstone D, Patel HR, Stewaret JS, Modigliani R, Guerin S, Mallinson CN. Gut hormone profile in coeliac disease. Lancet 1968; i:785–788.
27. Chey WY, Rhodes RA, Tai HH. Roles of secretin in man. In: Bloom SR, ed. Gut hormones. Edinburgh: Churchill Livingstone, 1978: 193.
28. Unger RH, Eisentraut AM, McCall MS, Keller S, Lanz HD, Madison LL. Glucagon antibodies and their use for immunoassay of glucagon. Proc Soc Exp Biol Med 1959; 102:621–623.
29. Mallinson CN, Blood SR, Warin AP, Salmon PR, Cox B. A glucagonoma syndrome. Lancet 1974; ii:1–5.
30. Assam R, Slusher N. Structure/function and structure/immunoreactivity relationships of the glucagon molecule and related synthetic peptides. Diabetes 1972; 21:843–855.
31. Sundy ES, Jacobson H, Moody AJ. Purification and characterisation of a protein from porcine gut with glucagon-like immunoreactivity. Sequence analysis of porcine gut GLI-I. Biochim Biophys Acta 1977; 493:452–459.
32. Thim L, Moody AJ. The primary structure of porcine glicentin (proglucagon). Regul Pept 1981; 2:139–150.
33. Moody AJ, Holst JJ, Thim L, Jenson SL. Relationship of glicentin to proglucagon and glucagon in porcine pancreas. Nature 1981; 289:514–516.
34. Bloom SR. An enteroglucagon tumour. Gut 1972; 13:520–523.
35. Bloom SR, Polak JM. Hormone profiles. In: Bloom SR, Polak JM, eds. Gut hormones. Edinburgh: Churchill Livingston, 1981: 550.
36. Besterman HS, Cook GC, Sarson DL, Christofides ND, Bryant MG, Gregor M, Blood SR. Gut hormones in tropical malabsorption. Br Med J 1979; i:1252–1255.
37. Adrian TE, McKiernan J, Johnstone DJ, Hiller EJ, Vyas H, Sarson DL, Bloom SR. Hormonal abnormalities of the pancreas and gut in cystic fibrosis. Gastroenterology 1980; 79:460–465.
38. Besterman HS, Sarson DL, Rambaud JC, Stewart JS, Guerin S, Bloom SR. Gut hormone responses in the irritable bowel syndrome. Digestion 1981; 21:219–224.
39. Bloom SR. Hormonal changes after jejuno-ileal bypass and their physiological significance. In: Maxwell JD, Gazet JC, Pilkington TR, eds. Surgical management of obesity. London: Academic Press, 1980: 115.
40. Sagor GR, Ghatei MA, McGregor GP, Mitchenere P, Kirk RM, Bloom SR. The influence of intact pylorus on postprandial enteroglucagon and neurotensin release after upper gastric surgery. Br J Surg 1981; 68:190–192.
41. Lin TM, Chance RE. Bovine pancreatic polypeptide (BPP) and avian pancreatic polypeptide (APP). Gastroenterology 1974; 67:737–738.
42. Heitz Ph, Polak JM, Bloom SR. Identification of the D_1 cell as the source of human pancreatic polypeptide. Gut 1976; 17:755–758.
43. Floyd JC, Fajans SS, Pek S. Regulation in healthy subjects of the secretion of human pancreatic polypeptide, a newly recognised pancreatic islet polypeptide. Trans Assoc Am Phys 1976; 89:146–158.
44. Greenberg GR, McCloy RF, Adrian TE, Chadwick VS, Baron JH, Bloom SR. Inhibition of pancreatic and gall bladder functions by pancreatic polypeptide in man. Lancet 1978; ii:1280–1283.
45. Floyd JC, Fajans SS, Ped S, Chance RE. A newly-recognised pancreatic polypeptide: plasma levels in health and disease. Recent Prog Horm Res 1977; 33:519–570.
46. Marco J, Hedo J, Villanueva M. Control of pancreatic polypeptide secretion of glucose in man. J Clin Endocrinol Metab 1978; 46:140–145.
47. Sive A, Vinik AI, Van Tonder S, Lond A. Impaired pancreatic polypeptide secretion in chronic pancreatitis. J Clin Endocrinol Metab 1978; 47:556–559.
48. Adrian TE, Besterman HS, Mallinson CN, Carolotis C, Bloom SR. Impaired pancreatic polypeptide release in patients with chronic pancreatitis with steatorrhoea. Gut 1979; 20:98–101.
49. Polak JM, Bloom SR, Adrian TE, Heitz Ph. Pancreatic polypeptide in insulinomas, gastrinomas, VIPomas and glucagonomas. Lancet 1976; i:326–330.
50. Brown JC, Pederson RA. A multiparameter study on the action of preparations containing cholecystokinin-pancreozymin. Scand J Gastroenterol 1970; 5:537–541.
51. Bryant MG, Bloom SR. Distribution of the gut hormones in the primate intestinal tract. Gut 1979; 20:653–659.
52. Gleator IGM, Gourlay RH. Release of immunoreactive gastric inhibitory polypeptide (IRGIP) by oral ingestion of food substance. Am Surg 1975; 130:128–135.
53. Soon-Shiong P, Debas HT, Brown JC. The evaluation of gastric inhibitory polypeptic (GIP) as the enterogastrone. J Surg Res 1979; 26:1681–1686.
54. Dupre J, Ross SA, Watson D, Brown JC. Stimulation of insulin secretion by gastric inhibitory polypeptide in man. J Clin Endocrinol Metab 1973; 37:826–828.
55. Anderson DK, Elahi D, Bron JC, Tobin JD, Andres R. Oral glucose augmentation of insulin release. J Clin Invest 1978; 62:152–161.
56. Sarson DL. Gastric inhibitory polypeptide. J Clin Pathol 1980; 33(suppl 8 Assoc Clin Pathol):31–37.
57. Brown JC, Johnson LP, Magee DF. Effect of duodenal alkalinisation on gastric motility. Gastroenterology 1966; 50:333–339.
58. Shimizu F, Imagawa K, Mihara S, Yanaihara N. Synthesis of porcine motilin by fragment condensation using three protected peptide fragments. Bull Chem Sci Jpn 1976; 49:3594–3596.

59. Christofides ND, Long RG, Fitzpatrick M., McGregor GP, Bloom SR. Effect of motilin on the gastric emptying of glucose and fat in humans. Gastroenterology 1981; 80:456–560.

60. Rennie JA, Christofides ND, Bloom SR, Johnson AG. Stimulation of human colonic activity by motilin. Gut 1979; 20:A912.

61. Aynsley-Green A, Bloom SR. The role of hormones in the pathophysiology of acute and chronic diarrhoea. In: Lebenthal E, ed. Chronic diarrhoea in children. New York: Raven Press, 1984: 289.

62. Said SI, Mutt V. Polypeptide with broad biological activity: isolation from small intestine. Science 1970; 169:1217–1218.

63. Bryant MG, Polak JM, Modlin I, Bloom SR, Alburquerque RH, Pearse AGE. Possible dual role for vasoactive intestinal peptide as gastrointestinal hormone and neurotransmitter substance. Lancet 1976; i:991–993.

64. Said SI. VIP overview. In: Bloom SR, Polak JM, eds. Gut hormones. London: Churchill Livingstone, 1981: 379.

65. Bloom SR, Polak JK, Pearse AGE. Vasoactive intestinal polypeptide and watery diarrhoea syndrome. Lancet 1973; ii:14–15.

66. Long RG, Bryant MG, Mitchell SJ, Adrian TE, Polak JM, Bloom SR. Clinicopathological study of pancreatic and ganglioneuroblastoma tumours secreting vasoactive intestinal polypeptide (VIPomas). Br Med J 1981; 282:1767–1771.

67. Said SI, Faloona GR, Deon H, Unger RH, Siegel SR. Vasoactive intestinal polypeptide: elevated levels in patients with hepatic cirrhosis. Clin Res 1974; 22:367A.

68. Bishop AE, Polak JM, Bryant MR, Bloom SR. VIP nerves in Crohn's disease. Gut 1978; 19:A990.

69. Long RG, Bishop AE, Barnes AJ, Albuquerque RH, O'Shaughnessy DJ, McGregor GP, Bannister R, Polak M, Bloom SR. Neural and hormonal peptides in rectal biopsy specimens from patients with Chagas' disease and chronic autonomic failure. Lancet 1980; i:559–562.

70. Freund HR, Humphrey CS, Fletcher JE. Reduced tissue content of vasoactive intestinal peptide in aganglionic colon of Hirchsprung's disease. Gastroenterology 1979; 76:1135.

71. McDonald TJ, Jornvall H, Nilsson G, Vagne M, Ghatei M, Blood SR, Mutt V. Characterisation of gastrin releasing peptide from porcine nonantral gastric tissue. Biochem Biophys Res Comm 1979; 90:227–233.

72. Polak JM, Ghatei MA, Wharton J, Bishop AE, Bloom SR, Solcia E, Brown MR, Pearse AGE. Bombesin-like immunoreactivity in the gastrointestinal tract, lung and central nervous system. Scand J Gastroenterol 1978; 13(Suppl): 149.

73. Brazeau P, Vale W, Burgus R, Ling N, Butcher M, Rivier J, Gueillemin R. Hypothalamic polypeptide that inhibits the secretion of immunoreactive pituitary growth hormone. Science 1973; 179:77–79.

74. Ganda OP, Weir GC, Soeldner JS, Legg MA, Chick WL, Patel YC, Ebeid AM, Gabbay KH, Reichlin S. "Somatostatinoma"—a somatostatin-containing tumor of the endocrine pancreas. N Engl J Med 1977; 296:963–967.

75. Penman E, Lowry PJ, Wass JAH, Marks V, Dawson AM, Besser GM, Rees LH. Molecular forms of somatostatin in normal subjects and in patients with pancreatic somatostatinoma. Clin Endocrinol 1980; 12:611–620.

76. Penman E, Wass JAH, Besser GM, Rees LH. Somatostatin secretion by lung and thymic tumors. Clin Endocrinol 1980; 13:613–620.

77. Long RG, Bishop AE, Barnes AJ, Alburquerque RH, O'Shaughnessy DJ, McGregor GP, Bannister R, Polak JM, Bloom SR. Neural and hormonal peptides in rectal biopsy specimens from patients with Chagas' disease and chronic autonomic failure. Lancet 1980; i:559–562.

78. Bishop AE, Garin Chesa P, Polak JM, Timson CM, Bryant MG, Bloom SR. Decrease of pancreatic somatostatin in neonatal "nesidioblastosis." Diabetes 1981; 30:122–126.

79. Carraway R, Leeman SE. The isolation of a new hypotensive peptide, neurotensin from bovine hypothalami. J Biol Chem 1973; J Biol Chem 1973; 248:6854–6861.

80. Uhl GR, Synder SH. Regional and subcellular distributions of brain neurotensin. Life Sci 1976; 19:1827–1832.

81. Carraway R, Leeman SE. Characterisation of radioimmunoassayable neurotensin in rat; its differential distribution in the CNS, small intestine and stomach. J Biol Chem 1976; 251:7045–7052.

82. Blackburn AM, Bloom SR. A radioimmunoassay for neurotensin in human plasma. J Endocrinol 1979; 83:175–181.

83. Blackburn AM, Christofides ND, Ghatei MA, Sarson DL, Ebeid FH, Ralphs DNL, Bloom SR. Elevation of plasma neurotensin in the dumping syndrome. Clin Sci 1980; 59:237–243.

84. Besterman HS, Sarson DL, Blackburn AM, Cleary J, Pilkington TRE, Gazet JC, Bloom SR. The gut hormone profile in morbid obesity and following jejuno-ileal bypass. Scand J Gastroenterol 1978; 3(Suppl): 49, 15.

85. Lezoche E, Ghatei MA, Carlei F, Blackburn AM, Basso N, Adrian TE, Speranzo V, Bloom SR. Gut hormone responses to bombesin in man. Gastroenterology 1979; 76:1185.

86. Adrian TE, Barnes AJ, Long RG, O'Shaughnessy D, Brown MR, Rivier J, Vale W, Blackburn AM, Bloom SR. Effect of somatostatin analogues on secretion of growth hormone, pancreatic and gastrointestinal hormones in man. J Clin Endocrinol Metab 1981; 53:675–681.

87. Blackburn AM, Fletcher DR, Adrian TE, Bloom SR. Neurotensin infusion in man: pharmokinetics and effect on gastrointestinal and pituitary hormones. J Clin Endocrinol Metab 1980; 51:1257–1261.

88. Blackburn AM, Bloom SR, Edwards AV. Pancreatic endocrine response to exogenous neurotensin in the conscious calf. J Physiol 1981; 314:11–21.

89. Blackburn AM, Fletcher DR, Bloom SR, Christofides ND, Long RG, Fitzpatrick ML, Baron JH. Effect of neurotensin on gastric function. Lancet 1980; i:987–989.

90. Fletcher DR, Blackburn AM, Adrian TE, Chadwick VS, Bloom SR. Effect of neurotensin on pancreatic function in man. Life Sci 1981; 29:2157–2161.

91. Chang MM, Llman SE. Isolation of a sialogogic peptide from bovine hypothalamic tissue and its characterisation as substance P. J Biol Chem 1970; 245:4784–4790.

92. Studer RD, Trazeciak H, Lergier W. Substance P from horse intestine: its isolation, structure and synthesis. In: von Euler US, Prnow B, eds. Substance P. New York: Raven Press, 1977: 15.

93. Euler US von, Goddum JH. An unidentified depressor substance in certain tissue extracts. J Physiol Lond 1931; 72:74–87.

94. Skrabanck P, Powell D. Substance P. In: Annual research reviews, Vols 1 and 2. Toronto: Eden Press, 1978 and 1980.

95. Pearse AGE. Peptides in brain and intestine. Nature 1976; 262:92–94.

96. Creutzfeldt W, ed. Gastrointestinal hormones. London: WB Saunders, 1980.

97. Polak JM, Bloom SR, Wright WA, Butler AG, eds. Gut hormones in disease. Scand J Gastroenterol 1982; 18(Suppl 82):1–234.

98. Elliott K, Whelan J, eds. Development of mammalian absorptive processes. Amsterdam: Excerpta Medica, 1979.

99. Grand RJ, Watkins JB, Torti FM. Development of the human gastrointestinal tract: a review. Gastroenterology 1976; 70:790–810.

100. Lebenthal E. Gastrointestinal ontogeny and its impact on infant feeding. Monogr Paediatr 1982; 16:17–38.

101. Widdowson EM, Colombo VE, Artavanis CA. Changes in the organs of pigs in response to feeding for the first 24 hours after birth. II. The digestive tract. Biol Neonate 1976; 28:272–281.

102. Sperling M. Integration of fuel homeostasis by insulin and glucagon in the newborn. Monogr Paediatr 1982; 16:39–58.

103. Lucas A, Aynsley-Green A, Bloom SR. Gut hormones and the first meals. Clin Sci 1981; 60:349–353.

104. Milla PJ. Development of intestinal structure and function. In: Tanner MS, Stocks RJ, eds. Neonatal gastroenterology. Newcastle-upon-Tyne: Intercept, 1984; 1.

105. Lebenthal E, Lee PC. Development of functional response in human exocrine pancreas. Pediatrics 1980; 60:556–560.

106. Lichtenberger L, Johnson LR. Gastrin in the ontogenic development of the small intestine. Am J Physiol 1974; 227:390–395.

107. Gentz J, Persson B, Kellum M, Bengtsson G, Thorell J. Effect of feeding on intravenous glucose tolerance and insulin response in piglets during the first few days of life. Life Sci 1971; 10:137–144.

108. Asplund K. Effects of postnatal feeding on the functional maturation of pancreatic islet B-cells of neonatal rats. Diabetologia 1972; 8:143–149.

109. Green GM, Nasset ES. Importance of bile in regulation of intraluminal proteolytic enzyme activities in the rat. Gastroenterology 1980; 79:695–702.

110. Alpers DH, Tedesco FJ. The possible role of pancreatic proteases in the turnover of intestinal brush border proteins. Biochim Biophys Acta 1975; 401:28–40.

111. Starkey RH, Orth DN. Radioimmunoassay of human epidermal growth factor (urogastrone). J Clin Endocrinol Metab 1977; 45:1144–1153.

112. Lucas A, Mitchell MD. Prostaglandins in human milk. Arch Dis Child 1980; 55:950–952.

113. Sack J. Human milk, its biological and social value. In: Frier S, Eidelman AI, eds. Amsterdam: Excerpta Medica, 1980: 56.

114. Werner S, Widstrom AM, Wahlberg V, Enroth P, Winberg J. Early Hum Dev 1982; 6:77.

115. Girard J. Paediatric nutrition. In: Arneil GC, Metcalfe J, eds. Sevenoaks: Butterworth, 1985: 3.

116. Aynsley-Green A, Soltesz G, Jenkins PA, Mackenzie IZ. The metabolic and endocrine milieu of the human fetus at 18–21 weeks of gestation. II. Blood glucose, lactate, pyruvate and ketone body concentrations. Biol Neonate 1985; 19:91–93.

117. Soltesz G, Harris D, Mackenzie IZ, Aynsley-Green A. The metabolic and endocrine milieu of the human fetus and mother at 18–21 weeks gestation. I. Plasma amino acid concentrations. Pediatr Res 1985; 19:91–93.

118. Larson L-I. Gastrointestinal cells producing endocrine, neurocrine and paracrine messengers. Clin Gastroenterol 1980; 9:485–516.

119. Bloom SR. Development of regulatory peptides in the human fetal intestine. In: Bloom SR, Polak JM, eds. Gut hormones. Edinburgh: Churchill Livingstone, 1981: 119.

120. Soltesz G, Aynsley-Green A. Hyperinsulinism in infancy and childhood. Adv Intern Med Pediatr 1984; 51:151–202.

121. Euler AR, Bryne WJ, Meis PJ, Leaks RD, Ament ME. Basal and pentagastrin stimulated acid secretion in newborn human infants. Pediatr Res 1979; 13:36–37.

122. Rodgers RM, Dix PM, Talbert JL, MacGuigan JE. Fasting and postprandial serum gastrin in normal human neonates. J Pediatr Surg 1978; 13:13–16.

123. Lucas A, Adrian TE, Bloom SR, Aynsley-Green A. Plasma motilin, gastrin and enteroglucagon and feeding in the human newborn. Arch Dis Child 1980; 55:673–677.

124. Lucas A, Bloom SR, Aynsley-Green A. Development of gut hormone responses to feeding in neonates. Arch Dis Child 1980; 55:678–682.

125. Lucas A, Bloom SR, Aynsley-Green A. Gut hormones in fetal distress. Lancet 1979; ii:968.

126. Lucas A, Christofides ND, Adrian TE, Bloom SR, Aynsley-Green A. Fetal distress, meconium and motilin. Lancet 1979; i:718.

127. Lucas A, Adrian TE, Bloom SR, Aynsley-Green A. Iatrogenic hyperinsulinism at birth. Lancet 1980; i:144–145.

128. Kenepp ND, Shelley WC, Gabbe SG, Kumar S, Stanley CA, Gutsche BB. Fetal and neonatal hazards of maternal hydration with 5% dextrose before caesarian section. Lancet 1982; i:1150–1152.

129. Von Berger L, Henrichs I, Raptis S, et al. Gastrin concentrations in plasma of the neonate at birth and after the first feeding. Pediatrics 1976; 58:264–267.

130. Aynsley-Green A, Bloom SR, Williamson DH, Turner RC. Endocrine and metabolic response in the human newborn to first feed of breast milk. Arch Dis Child 1977; 52:291–295.

131. King KC, Schwartz R, Yomaguchi K, Adam PJ. lack of gastrointestinal enhancement of the insulin response to glucose in newborn infants. J Pediatr 1977; 91:783–786.

132. Lucas A, Bloom SR, Aynsley-Green A. Metabolic and endocrine events at the time of the first feed of human milk in preterm and term infants. Arch Dis Child 1978; 53:731–736.

133. Aynsley-Green A, Lucas A, Bloom SR. The effect of feeds of different composition on entero-insular hormone secretion in the first hours of life in human neonates. Acta Paediatr Scand 1979; 68:265–270.

134. Lucas A, Adrian TE, Bloom SR, Aynsley-Green A. Plasma pancreatic polypeptides in the human neonate. Acta Paediatr Scand 1980; 69:211–214.

135. Lucas A, Sarson D, Bloom SR, Aynsley-Green A. Developmental physiology of gastric inhibitory polypeptide and its role in the entero-insular axis in preterm neonates. Acta Paediatr Scand 1980; 69:321–325.

136. Lucas A, Aysley-Green A, Blackburn AM, Adrian T, Bloom SR. Plasma neurotensin in term and preterm neonates. Acta Paediatr Scand 1981; 70:201–206.

137. Lucas A, Bloom SR, Aynsley-Green A. Postnatal surges in gut hormones in term and preterm infants. Biol Neonate 1982; 41:63–67.

138. Lucas A, Bloom Sr, Aynsley-Green A. Plasma vasoactive intestinal peptide (VIP) in the neonate. Acta Paediatr Scand 1982; 71:71–74.

139. Adrian TE, Lucas A, Bloom SR, Aynsley-Green A. Growth hormone response to feeding in the term and preterm neonates. Acta Paediatr Scand 1983; 72:251–254.

140. Lucas A, Bloom SR, Aynsley-Green A. Metabolic and endocrine consequences of depriving preterm infants of enteral nutrition. Acta Paediatr Scand 1983; 72:245–249.

141. Lucas A, Bloom SR, Aynsley-Green A. Gut hormones and "minimal enteral feeding." Acta Paediatr Scand 1986; 75:719–723.

142. Hughes CA, Dowling RH. Speed of onset of adaptive mucosal hypoplasia and hypofunction in the intestine of parenterally fed rats. Clin Sci 1980; 59:317–327.

143. Hughes CA, Breuer RS, Ducker DA, Hatoff DE, Dowling RH. The effect of cholecystokinin and secretin on intestinal and pancreatic structure and function. In: Robinson JWL, Dowling RH, Riecken EL, eds. Mechanisms of intestinal adaptation. Lancaster: MTP Press, 1982: 435.

144. Dunn L, Hulman S, Weiner J, Kliegman R. Beneficial effects of early hypocaloric enteral feeding on neonatal gastrointestinal function: preliminary report of a randomized trial. J Pediatr 1988; 112:622–629.

145. Aynsley-Green A, Adrian TE, Bloom SR. Feeding and the development of enteroinsular hormone secretion in the preterm infant: effects of continuous gastric infusions of human milk compared with intermittent boluses. Acta Paediatr Scand 1982; 71:379–383.

146. Lucas A, Aynsley-Green A. Effect of sleep state and feeding on cranial blood flow of the human neonate. Arch Dis Child 1980; 55:741.

147. Calvert SA, Soltesz G, Jenkins PA, Harris D, Newman C, Adrian TE, Bloom SR, Aynsley-Green A. Feeding premature infants with human milk or preterm milk or preterm mild formula: effects of postnatal growth, intermediary metabolism and regulatory peptides. Biol Neonate 1985; 47:189–198.

148. Lucas A, Boyes S, Bloom SR, Aynsley-Green A. Metabolic and endocrine responses to a milk feed in six day old term infants: differences between breast and cow's milk formula feeding. Acta Paediatr Scand 1981; 70:201–206.

149. Lucas A, Adrian TE, Sarson DL, Blackburn AM, Aynsley-Green A, Bloom SR. Breast vs bottle: endocrine responses are different with formula feeding. Lancet 1980; i:1267–1269.

150. Salmenpera L, Perheentupa J, Siimes MA, Adrian TE, Bloom SR, Aynsley-Green A. Effects of feeding regimen on blood glucose levels and plasma concentrations of pancreatic hormones and gut regulatory peptides at 9 months of age: comparison between infants fed with milk formula and infants exclusively breast-fed from birth. J Pediatr Gastroenterol Nutr 1988; 7:651–656.

151. Aynsley-Green A. The adaptation of the human neonate to extrauterine nutrition: a pre-requisite for postnatal growth. In: Cockburn F, ed. Fetal and neonatal growth. London: John Wiley & Sons Ltd, 1988: 153.

152. Adrian TE, Smith HA, Calvert SA, Aynsley-Green A, Bloom SR. Elevated plasma peptide YY in human neonates and infants. Pediatr Res 1986; 20:1225–1227.

153. Johnson SR, Guthrie PD. Stimulation of DNA synthesis by big and little gastrin (G34 and G17). Gastroenterology 1976; 71:599–602.

154. Strange EF, Schneider A, Seiffer E, Ditshuneit H. Effect of pentagastrin secretion and cholecystokinin on growth and differentiation in organ cultured rabbit small intestine. Horm Metabol Res 1986; 18:303–307.

155. Arnold R, Lankisch PG. Somatostatin and the gastrointestinal tract. In: Creutzfeld W, ed. Gastrointestinal hormones. London: WB Saunders, 1980: 733.

156. Aynsley-Green A, Barnes ND, Adrian TE, Kingston I, Boyes S, Bloom SR. Effect of somatostatin infusion on intermediary metabolism and entero-insular hormone release in infants with hyperinsulinaemic hypoglycaemia. Acta Paediatr Scand 1981; 70:889–895.

157. Lawson G, Aynsley-Green A, Bloom SR. Plasma gut hormone profiles in acute infectious diarrhoea in infancy. J Pediatr; in press.

158. Aynsley-Green A, Mackenzie IZ, Jenkins PA, Soltesz G, Bloom SR. The metabolic and endocrine milieu of the human fetus at 16–20 weeks gestation. In: Jones CT, Nathaniels PW, eds. The physiological development of the fetus and newborn. London: Academic Press, 1985: 771–775.

CHAPTER 17

Gastric Function*

Barry K. Wershil, M.D.

The stomach is a deceptively complex organ that serves in the digestive process. It acts as a reservoir for food and continues the digestive process that has been initiated in the oral cavity. The stomach mixes ingested food with acid and digestive enzymes and then empties its contents in a coordinated manner for further digestion and absorption in the small intestine.

The stomach relies on three basic physiologic processes to accomplish its function: (1) secretory activity, (2) endocrine function, and (3) motility. Accordingly, the gross and fine structures of the stomach are organized in a way that facilitates these processes.

The developmental aspects of gastric function are discussed in this chapter. Developmental anatomy and histology are emphasized with the intent that a study of the morphology of a cell during a period of functional development may give important insight into correlations between cell morphology and function.[1,2] Developmental physiology is discussed as well, as it is now clear that the physiologic controls in infants are organized differently than in adults and change with various stages of development.[3]

Our understanding of these developmental aspects of gastric function is oversimplified and incomplete at the present time, particularly in relation to the development of human gastric function. Experimental data from animal studies have been helpful in shedding light on the development of gastric function and are discussed; however, this information may not directly relate to human development. Significant differences in gastric development are seen among various species,[1] and these differences should be kept in mind.

NORMAL ANATOMY AND HISTOLOGY OF THE STOMACH

The stomach can be divided into three regions for descriptive purposes: cardia, fundus, and antrum.† The cardia, which is poorly defined, lies just distal to the esophagogastric junction. The antrum comprises the distal third of the stomach, just proximal to the pyloric sphincter. The remainder of the stomach is the fundus. The boundary between the fundus and antrum is poorly defined and varies with age.[4,5]

Histologically, the stomach can be divided into zones roughly corresponding to these anatomic regions.[4] The entire surface of the glandular stomach is lined by a simple columnar epithelium made up of surface mucous cells containing a neutral mucin that stains with periodic acid–Schiff (PAS) stain. The epithelium forms glandular invaginations that become gastric pits and glands. These gastric glands are coiled and show regional specialization.[4,5] The glands in the cardia and antrum of the stomach are predominantly mucus-secreting glands. On the other hand, while the fundic mucosa also contains mucus-secreting neck cells, these fundic glands are the major site of acid secretion (parietal cells) and pepsin production (chief cells). The fundic glands are also known as oxyntic glands (see Fig. 12, Chapter 13).

The stomach also contains a wide variety of hormone-producing cells. These are generally scattered throughout the stomach, and although they make up only a small portion of the glands, they produce a wide variety of important hormones and biogenic amines. There are at least eight different enteroendocrine cell types in the mammalian stomach,[6,7] and probably more that have not yet been discovered. These cells are typically identified by their granular morphology and ultrastructural characteristics. These cells are also classified by their peptide or amine content. A variety of immunocytochemical techniques have been extremely useful in the study of the cellular localization of particular polypeptide hormones.[8] However, there are some technical difficulties with these methods that should be taken into consideration. In particular, immunocytochemical methods depend on the preservation of antigenic determinants on the peptide molecule which may be limited by current fixation techniques.[8] In addition, the localization of a polypeptide to a particular cell does not prove that the cell is actually synthesizing that peptide. In some cases, hormonal content remains in question, and some cells may contain more than one peptide or amine.[10] These questions will be answered as better techniques for cell purification and in vitro cell growth are developed and as molecular probes become available for in situ localization of messenger RNA.

Gastric hormones have been found throughout the stomach in various cells or nervous tissue. Gastrin, somatostatin, and motilin[10-12] are found in endocrine cells of the stomach. Gastrin is produced and stored in G cells found predominantly in the antrum,[13] whereas somatostatin is localized in D cells in both the antrum and fundus.[14] Gastrin is known to be a potent stimulator of acid secretion,[15] whereas somatostatin has been shown to inhibit acid secretion.[14,16]

The opposing physiologic actions of these two hormones may have an anatomic correlate. In the antrum, D cells are close but not adjacent to G cells and other cell types. The D cell has been shown to have slender processes that arise

---

*Supported in part by USPHS Grants K-11-DK01543 and P01-DK33506.
†Some authors include a fourth area referred to as the body: however this is structurally and functionally similar to the fundus and the two are considered a single region in this review.

from the base of the cell and reach out to contact other cell types. In the antrum the process can contact a G cell, and in the fundus it may contact a parietal cell or another cell type, such as an enterochromaffin cell.[14,17] This suggests a pathway by which the peptide somatostatin may be directly delivered to effector cells.

The precise location of certain peptides has not been determined. For example, it is not entirely clear if vasoactive intestinal polypeptide (VIP) is contained within gastric mucosa cells or is found exclusively in the autonomic innervation of the gut.[18-20] Likewise, the cell type containing motilin has not been identified with certainty.

In the fundic mucosa are found cells that contain vasoactive amines. Enterochromaffin cells (EC cells) can be identified by their argentaffin reaction and have been shown to contain serotonin.[21] EC cells are relatively sparse in man. Another amine-containing cell is the enterochromaffin-like cell (ECL cell). In some species, this cell type has been shown to contain histamine,[22] but this has not been clearly demonstrated in man.

Finally, there are a variety of enteroendocrine cells in the gastric mucosa whose content and function have not been identified.[5,22-24]

The stomach receives parasympathetic innervation from the dorsal motor nucleus of the vagus and sympathetic fibers from T6 to T10. Numerous peptidergic neurons are found throughout multiple layers of the stomach. VIP-immunoreactive fibers are found in close association with blood vessels, smooth muscle, and epithelial cells.[25] Intense VIP-immunostaining nerve bundles have been identified in a tight association with oxyntic glands in the stomach.[26] The physiologic significance of this association is not known.

Substance P immunoreactivity has been demonstrated in the gastric mucosa of man. Likewise, met-enkephalin and bombesin-like immunoreactivity has also been seen in the stomach.[26] Other neuropeptides such as calcitonin gene-related peptide, neuropeptide Y, and galanin immunoreactive nerves have been found in the stomach of certain species but have not been well documented in man.[27]

The function of these various peptides and hormones is discussed elsewhere[28] but in many cases remains speculative. It is of interest that in several species, many gut endocrine cells are seen in increased numbers during fetal development and then decrease in adult animals.[29-31] This suggests that fetal endocrine cells may exert functions different from their adult counterparts. Since many gut hormones also have trophic actions, it has been hypothesized that fetal endocrine cells exert functions important for growth and perhaps differentiation of the gut.[31]

Ontogeny

The stomach is identifiable approximately 4 weeks after fertilization as it arises from the foregut caudal to the primitive lung. Initially, the stomach is lined by a simple columnar epithelium that is soon replaced by an undifferentiated stratified or pseudostratified epithelium.[1,32] Primitive gastric pits form at 6 to 9 weeks,[33,34] and gland-like structures can be seen by 11 to 13 weeks. The expansion of gastric glands has been studied in detail in the hamster[35] and occurs by the process of dichotomous branching, or fission (Fig. 1). Epithelial cell number increases at the neck of the gastric gland. As the cell number increases, some cells fuse together to form a bridge across the neck, resulting in the formation of two lumens. The smaller lumen then grows to form a new pit and begins to expand downward toward the muscularis propria.[32] In humans, gastric glands become extensively branched and convoluted in the fifth to sixth month of gestation.[34]

An undifferentiated cell type can be seen at the base of the gastric pit and in the upper gland. Intermediate forms in the same area have suggested that these undifferentiated cells can transform into surface pit cells, mucous neck cells, and parietal cells.[36,37] Matsuyama and Suzuki[38] have demonstrated that when glandular segments of the stomach from neonatal mice are grafted into the subcutaneous tissues of littermates, immature mucous cells can give rise to mature mucous, parietal, argyrophil, and chief cells. This concept of undifferentiated cells giving rise to many, if not all, of the differentiated cell lines in the stomach has been termed the "unitarian hypothesis." This hypothesis is strongly supported by experimental evidence in the small intestine and, to a lesser extent, the large intestine as well.[32]

Parietal cells and mucous neck cells appear at about 10 to 11 weeks, whereas immature zymogen cells are seen at 12 weeks. Although the origin of these cell types is probably the same, experimental evidence suggests that parietal cell renewal is derived from precursor cells, whereas zymogen and endocrine cell populations are slowly self-renewing.[32]

Endocrine cells appear between 8 and 9 weeks, and development is seen through about 22 weeks of gestation.[34] The exact origin of gastrointestinal (GI) cells is not known. There are currently two major theories as to their origin.[39] The endodermal theory states that all intestinal cells are produced by stem cells found at the base of the crypts.[40] The second theory suggests a neuroectodermal origin for endocrine cells based on morphologic and cytochemical similarities between neural and endocrine cells.[41,42] Grafting experiments performed in embryos refute the concept of a neural crest origin for gut endocrine cells.[43] At present, the endodermal theory is better supported.[9,32,43,44]

The ontogeny of most neurotransmitters in the human stomach is unknown; however, the development of vasoactive intestinal polypeptide has been examined in human fetal stomach.[45] VIP can be detected in the fetal stomach by radioimmunoassay at 8 to 10 weeks' gestation. Immunoreactive VIP can be seen in nerve fibers in the muscle coat at 15 weeks. The distribution of VIP in the stomach at 15 to 21 weeks is similar to that seen in adults with VIP seen in both antrum and fundus.[46]

At birth, all the cell types of the stomach are clearly discernible, but the neonatal stomach is much thinner than that of an adult.[1,33] The stomach increases in thickness in both its glandular and muscular portions during the postnatal period. Enteral nutrition may be another important factor in the postnatal development of the stomach; however, all of the endogenous and exogenous trophic factors and their precise interactions with the GI tract have not been fully defined. Such factors such as gastrin, VIP, thyroxine, cortisol, and epidermal growth factor may be responsible for gastric growth and maturation.[47-49]

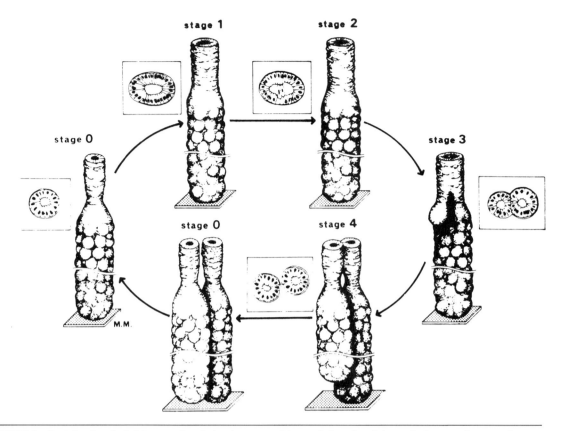

FIGURE 1 Gastric gland division cycle of the hamster. Most of the glandular tubules are in a stationary state (stage 0). Hyperplasia of the tubular portion occurs, to double its column count at stage 1. In stage 2 a thickened generative cell tubule is divided into two smaller ones by a partition formed by the newly proliferated cells. At stage 3 a bud of the new gastric gland appears below the level of the constriction. This new gland grows toward the muscularis mucosae. At stage 4 the new pit separates from its "parent" glandular tubule by penetration of connective tissue and a blood vessel of the venular plexus between two tubules. This stage 4 marks the end of the gland division cycle, and a complete pair of pits and glands is formed. Each illustration of the cross-section reveals the cell arrangement of the tubule at the level of the constriction. (From Wright and Allison.[32])

DEVELOPMENT OF SECRETORY FUNCTION OF THE STOMACH

Hydrochloride Acid Secretion

Acid secretion by the human stomach can be demonstrated a short time after birth and "matures" over the first several months of life, but the precise developmental sequence and the regulating influences affecting acid secretion are not entirely clear. Reported studies vary in such parameters as age of subjects, fasting period before gastric collections, methods of acid titration, and the agents used to stimulate acid secretion. These methodologic differences create some confusion in our understanding of the development of acid secretion.

It is now clear that acid secretion begins shortly after birth.[50-53] Ebers[51] demonstrated that initial removal of the gastric contents allowed determination of an acid pH in the stomach when sampled at 1 to 2 hours after birth. It was presumed that amniotic fluid, which has an alkaline pH, would affect the pH of gastric aspirates. Avery et al[50] demonstrat-ed a gastric pH of less than 4 immediately after birth if the stomach was first lavaged with normal saline (Fig. 2).

There is considerable controversy in the literature as to the amount of acid produced by infants during the first months of life. Gastric acidity has been reported to be constant over the first 10 days of life regardless of gestational age,[54] whereas others have reported a decline[55,56] or rise[1] in acid concentration. Interpretation of these studies is difficult because there was no consideration of factors known to correlate with acid production, such as body weight.[57,58] Several studies agree that the highest acid concentration occurs within 10 days[1,54-56] and the lowest between the tenth[55] and thirtieth[1] days of life (Fig. 3). Gastric acid production approaches adult levels by 3 months of age.[59,60]

Recent studies have examined basal acid output (BAO) and maximal acid output (MAO) in order to determine more precisely the development of gastric acid secretory function (Tables 1 and 2). Euler et al[61] examined BAO in 32 healthy, full-term newborns by continuous aspirations of gastric contents during the first 8 hours of life. They reported that the BAO, on a milliequivalent per kilogram basis, was extreme-

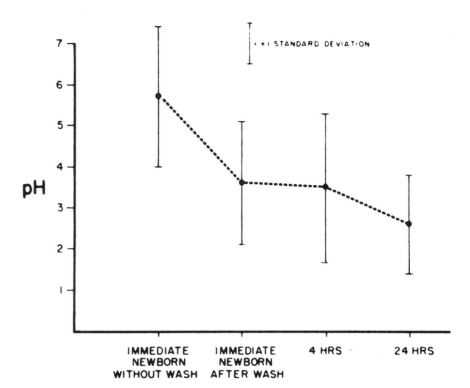

FIGURE 2 The effect of gastric washing on gastric pH in newborn and gastric pH over time. (From Avery et al[50]; reproduced by permission of Pediatrics.)

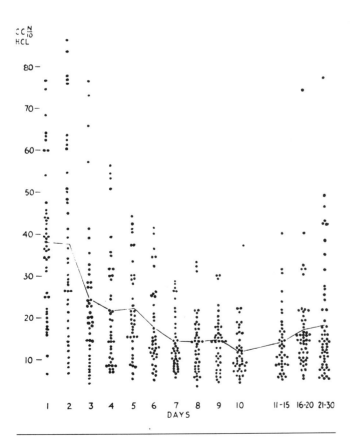

FIGURE 3 Total acidity of gastric contents in the first month of life, expressed in cubic centimeters of N/10 HCl per 100 cc of stomach contents. (From Miller.[55])

ly low during the first 5 hours of life and approached controls by 6 to 8 hours. When pentagastrin was administered to stimulate acid production, no effect was seen during the first 2 days of life.[62] The authors suggested that either acid secretion in newborns is maximal under basal conditions or newborn parietal cells are unresponsive to pentagastrin in the first 2 days of life.[62]

Hyman et al[63] examined the basal and stimulated acid production in 34 healthy, preterm infants (gestational age < 37 weeks) at 1 week of age. They found that the mean BAO of the preterm infant was lower than values reported for term infants. This finding has been supported in a subsequent study of preterm infants.[64] Hyman et al also reported that the BAO determined at 1 week of age increased over the next 4 weeks and then leveled off (Fig. 4). This increase in BAO was dependent on postnatal but not postconceptional age, suggesting that extrauterine environmental factors may influence the changes in BAO that were seen. Although no data were presented, the authors suggested that enteral feedings may be one such extrauterine factor, as it has been shown that enteral feeding does influence gastric secretory function.[65]

A response to pentagastrin was also seen in 1-week-old premature infants[63] (Fig. 4), suggesting the presence of gastrin receptors on parietal cells at 1 week of age. This response also increased over the next 4 weeks and was in part dependent on both postnatal and postconceptional age. The authors point out that although the preterm infants did respond to pentagastrin at 1 week of age, the magnitude of the response was less than that normally seen in older children.[66,67]

Studies have suggested that there may be differential development of the parietal cells' ability to respond to various secretagogues. For example, as mentioned above, no response

TABLE 1
Development of Acid Secretion

| Age | Basal HCl Secretion | | | |
	Volume ml/hr	mEq/L	mEq/hr	mEq/kg/hr
1 hr	2.7	10.9	0.029	0.0115
2 hr	3.1	17.1	0.053	0.0170
6 hr	2.9	30.4	0.088	0.0290
7 hr	3.2	28.2	0.090	0.0310
8 hr	3.5	27.0	0.094	0.0310
1 day	7.0	—	0.378 ± 0.060	0.110 ± 0.016
2 day	6.9	—	0.388 ± 0.053	0.114 ± 0.014
28 day	3.0	26.4	0.08	0.02
12 wk	3.4	34.8	0.47	0.1
1–4 yr	—	—	—	0.094
5–14 yr	—	—	—	0.067
12.1 yr	—	—	1.3 ± 0.4	0.035 ± 0.010

Modified from Christie,[60] Euler,[61] and Grand.[59]

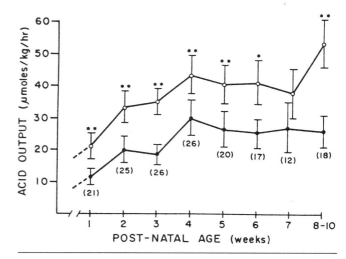

FIGURE 4 Basal acid output (*closed circles*) and pentagastrin-stimulated acid output (*open circles*) in preterm infants (<37 weeks' gestation) studied at 1 week post conception. Number of infants studied in parentheses. Asterisks denote significant differences. (From Hyman et al.[63])

to pentagastrin was seen in the first 2 days of life. Agunod et al[68] studied acid secretion stimulated by betazole, a histamine analogue. A response could be seen in the first 24 hours of life from a basal rate of 3.3 mEq per liter to 8.1 mEq per liter. This is a smaller response than seen at 3 months of age, when acid concentration reaches 34.8 mEq per liter.[68] Histamine is no longer used to test stimulated gastric acid production, but it is an important physiologic stimulus of acid secretion. In addition, histamine can potentiate the effects of both cholinergic stimulants and gastrin.[69] As such, it will be important to understand the regulation of the response to histamine and how it compares to other stimuli of acid secretion.

In most species, including man, the morphologic components necessary for acid secretion are complete shortly before birth.[1,70] The question is then why acid secretion is depressed at birth. Lichtenberger suggested that the underdeveloped secretory rate at birth may be caused by a decrease in the number of mature parietal cells, a decrease in parietal cell sensitivity to physiologic stimuli, or a combination of these factors.[71] The MAO has been shown to be proportional to parietal cell mass,[72] and the parietal cell density in the stomach has been reported to be increased in the neonatal compared to the adult stomach.[73] However, in this study, the parietal cell mass per kilogram of body weight was not de-

termined, which is the critical factor at this age.[59] Further histologic studies will be necessary to determine the precise density of parietal cells in the newborn.

The responsiveness of parietal cells to various secretory stimuli has been extensively investigated in animal models. In the rat, basal acid secretion is minimal until approximately 15 to 20 days after birth[74,75] but is still only about 25 percent of adult basal secretion levels. This significantly increases during the third week of life,[75,76] which is the time of weaning. An adult BAO level is reached by day 40 of life.[70]

In the rat, there is a parallel between the development of basal acid secretion and the development of the response to stimuli.[70,77,78] The responsiveness of the parietal cell develops in an orderly fashion,[76] but the control of this development is poorly understood. For example, 5-day-old rat pups are insensitive to gastrin.[79] The ability to respond to gastrin occurs at approximately day 20. This lack of responsiveness to gastrin in young rats has been shown to be due to a lack of the gastrin receptor on parietal cells[75] and can be influenced by corticosteroid administration[80]; however, the precise controlling influence(s) have yet to be defined.

This inability of rat pups to secrete basal acid or respond to stimuli of acid secretion correlates with the capacity of their gut to passively absorb maternally derived antibodies. It has been suggested that impaired acid secretion prevents protein precipitation and inactivation.[1] This is supported by the observation that at the time of weaning, antibody absorption stops and significant acid production begins.

TABLE 2
Development of Acid Secretion to Secretagogues

| Mean Age | Secretagogue | Stimulated HCl Secretion | |
		mEq/hr	mEq/kg/hr
1 day	P (2 μg/kg)	0.413 ± 0.053	0.122 ± 0.015
1 day	B (1 mg/kg)	0.03	0.01
2 days	P (2 μg/kg)	0.452 ± 0.065	0.133 ± 0.018
3–8 days	B (1 mg/kg)	0.06	0.02
10–11 days	B (1 mg/kg)	0.12	0.04
11.7 mo	P (6 μg/kg)	—	0.221
4.6 yr	P (6 μg/kg)	—	0.34 ± 0.06
10 yr	P (6 μg/kg)	—	0.343

Modified from Christie,[60] Euler,[62] Agunod,[68] and Lari.[67]
P = pentagastrin, B = betazole.

Gastrin

Numerous investigators have reported that neonatal levels of gastrin are significantly elevated.[60,81,82] Euler et al[82] measured gastrin levels in umbilical cord blood and found a mean level of 135 pg per milliliter. This is in contrast to normal adult levels of 49 pg per milliliter. The newborn's gastrin level is elevated compared to the mother's as well.[83-85] There is some conflict in the evidence; however, the vast majority of studies support the concept that this gastrin is of fetal origin.[71] This neonatal hypergastrinemia is persistent for variable periods of time, but several reports suggest that gastrin levels are elevated for days after birth.[82,83]

The cause of neonatal hypergastrinemia is probably multifactorial (Fig. 5). Gastric acid is a potent inhibitor of gastrin release. Elevated luminal pH has been shown to be associated with increased circulating gastrin levels.[70,75] Swallowed amniotic fluid as well as the low BAO seen during the first 8 hours of life may act in concert to promote elevated gastrin levels. Likewise, dietary factors may also influence circulating gastrin levels. The high protein and calcium content of a milk diet can stimulate gastrin release.[71]

The local regulation of gastrin release may be another important factor that contributes to the elevated gastrin levels seen in the newborn. At present, this factor is poorly understood, and further investigations into the development of gastrin synthesis and processing in the stomach will be necessary to understand the regulation of neonatal gastrin levels.

The physiologic significance of this neonatal hypergastrinemia is not known. It has been suggested that the elevated gastrin levels in neonates contribute to both the maturation of GI function and accelerated mucosal growth seen in the newborn period.[83]

Pepsin

Pepsin is an important proteolytic enzyme found in normal gastric secretions. It is packaged and stored in an inactive zymogen form, i.e., pepsinogen. The developmental aspects of pepsin have been studied in detail. Pepsinogen has been identified by immunoelectrophoresis in human stomach at the eighth week of gestation.[86] There are a variety of forms of pepsinogen differing in specificity and origin,[87] and these molecular forms exhibit differential development.[88] The predominant pepsinogen in fetal stomach is pepsinogen IV (Pg IV), which is localized to the superficial epithelium.[86] The role of Pg IV and the control of its expression in humans are not known. Animal studies have shown that exogenously administered steroid hormones can affect the development of gastric peptic activity.[89] Peptic activity has been identified in the fetal stomach at 16 weeks' gestation and increases throughout gestation.[90] The state of maturity of the neonate correlates with the activity of pepsins at birth.[91] Premature infants weighing 1,000 g have approximately half the peptic activity of term infants.[88] However, while peptic activity can be demonstrated early in gestation, histochemical demonstration of pepsin in the gastric mucosa is not found until 3 to 4 months' gestation[86] or until the weight of the newborn is greater than 2,300 g.[92]

The development of techniques to culture chief cells in vitro has allowed pepsinogen synthesis and chief cell secretory function to be studied in detail[93]; however, the developmental aspects of chief cell function in this system have not been examined.

Intrinsic Factor

Intrinsic factor is another secreted product of the gastric mucosa; however, we know relatively little about its developmental biology in man. Parietal cells have been shown to be the source of intrinsic factor in humans.[94] Intrinsic factor has been identified in the human fetus by radioimmunoassay at 11 weeks' gestation.[95] Rodbro et al[85] studied histamine-stimulated secretion of intrinsic factor in infants 9 to 30 months old. They found a more mature pattern of intrinsic factor secretion compared with acid secretion, implying a dissociation of acid and intrinsic factor secretion by parietal cells.

Several studies have suggested that parietal cells of newborns have a greater capacity to produce intrinsic factor than acid.[1,64,68] Marino et al[64] studied basal intrinsic factor production in term and premature infants. They found that parietal cell production of intrinsic factor was similar in both groups and occurred independent of enteral feeding. Acid secretion was found to be significantly less in the premature group than in term infants; however, the premature infants were not receiving enteral feedings, which probably affected acid production.

Agunod et al[68] (Fig. 6) examined histamine-stimulated intrinsic factor secretion and noted an increase over the first

---

FIGURE 5 Schematic representation of factors that might contribute to neonatal hypergastrinemia. (From Lichtenberger.[71])

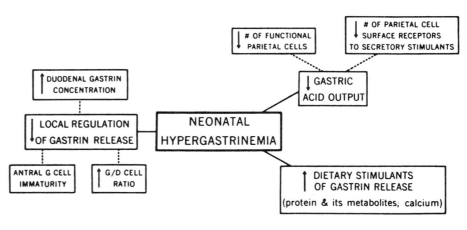

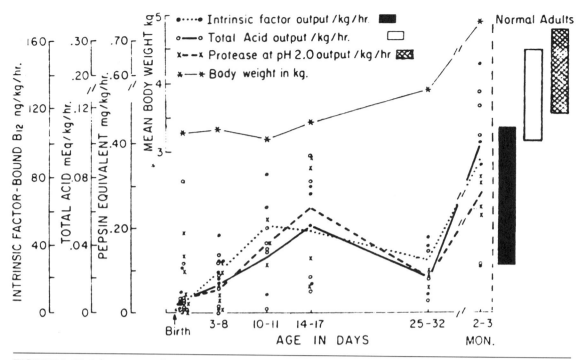

FIGURE 6 Weight-corrected gastric secretion of acid, pepsin, and intrinsic factor in newborns and infants. (From Agunod et al.[68])

2 weeks of life to approximately half the levels seen in normal adults and to adult levels by 3 months.

Intrinsic factor in rats, unlike humans, has been shown to be a product of chief cells.[94,96] Recently, a cDNA clone encoding rat intrinsic factor has been isolated,[97] which has begun to allow the analysis of the regulation of intrinsic factor production. Dieckgraefe et al[96] have shown that mRNA concentration increases with postnatal age, peaking at about day 30. More interestingly, cortisol administration increased intrinsic factor mRNA, whereas adrenalectomy led to a decrease in this message.[96] Other hormones such as pentagastrin and thyroid hormones had no effect.

Ontogeny and Developmental Physiology of Gastric Motility

The motility and emptying of the stomach involve a number of complex interactions between myenteric, neurologic, and hormonal factors.[98,99] These factors act in a co-ordinated manner to facilitate gastric digestion as well as digestion that will follow later in the small intestinal tract. Normal gastric motility is discussed in detail elsewhere (Chapter 15); this section discusses developmental aspects of gastric motility.

The stomach is initially made up of homogeneous mesenchymal cells that will differentiate to form the various muscle layers. The circular muscle develops in a craniocaudal manner so that the pyloric musculature develops later. Circular muscle development is followed by the longitudinal muscle and then the muscularis mucosae.[100,101]

Myoblasts are present in the circular muscles by 8 to 9 weeks of gestation.[98,100] By 3½ months of gestation the circular muscle in the fundus has formed bundles but remains incomplete in the antrum and pyorus until approximately 4 to 5 months. The outer longitudinal muscle does not develop in a craniocaudal fashion but rather appears over the entire stomach by 11 to 12 weeks.[100] The musculature of the stomach is complete by 7 months of gestation, although it is considerably thinner than the adult muscle wall. The innervation of the stomach by the vagus nerve occurs at approximately 4½ weeks.[101,103] Innervation of the entire stomach by vagal and sympathetic fibers is complete by approximately 9 weeks gestation[94] and mature by 7 months.

The normal physiology of gastric motility has been well described in adults.[104] Briefly, under normal circumstances, the proximal stomach relaxes in response to swallowing in order to accommodate ingested food. Contractions slowly move the ingested contents toward the distal stomach. Liquids tend to pass quickly into the duodenum. Solids, on the other hand, are retained in the distal stomach, where controlled antral contractions act to grind solids down in size as well as to mix in digestive enzymes.

A variety of contractile patterns have been identified in the stomach. Fasting gastric emptying is maintained by a cyclic pattern of activity which occurs during fasting (interdigestive rhythm) and migrates caudally. This motility pattern is intrinsically set. Another motility pattern occurs after eating and involves antrum contractions and the process of gastric emptying. Postprandial gastric emptying is modulated by a variety of factors.[105] At the present time, very little is known about the development of motility in humans and has been better characterized in a variety of animal models.[106]

Initially after birth, contractions in the stomach are not rhythmic or progressive in intensity but tend to be continuations of esophageal peristaltic waves as measured by pressure changes.[107] This pattern continues for at least the first 4 days of life.[103] Barium studies of gastric emptying in infants have shown that in 2- to 4-day-old infants the stomach empties by a combination of increased tone, antral contraction, and hydrostatic pressure.[108] Tomomasa et al[109] studied GI motility in 20 infants. They noted the dominant pattern of contraction after feeding was a high-amplitude, repetitive, but nonmigrating rhythmic contraction. Some differences from the adult pattern were noted in the fasting (interdigestive) and postprandial (nonmigrating) gastric motility pattern of infants. However, the precise patterns are not clear, since both preterm and term infants were studied and no distinction was made by gestational age.

Hancock et al[110] did measure gastric pressure tracings in premature infants from 27 to 35 weeks' gestation. They were able to identify well-defined gastric contractions in these neonates when measured more than 4 days after delivery. Bisset et al[111] found that gastric antral pressure increases from 28 weeks' gestation to term (Fig. 7).

Many questions pertaining to the development of gastric motility remain to be examined, particularly the potential influencing factors. Small bowel contractions have been shown to increase in frequency, number, and amplitude from 29 to 32 weeks' gestation.[112] In addition, if beta-methasone was administered to the mother, small bowel contraction increased at an earlier age than in controls.[112]

At present, it is believed that the ontogeny of the fasting small intestinal motor activity is a species-specific pattern of development with a clear pattern of maturation with increasing gestational age, which is similar to that seen in animal studies.[106] It will require further human studies to document a similar phenomenon with regard to gastric motility.

FUTURE DIRECTIONS

At present, there are enormous gaps in our understanding of the development of human gastric secretory and endocrine function as well as the development of gastric motility. Further clinical studies are needed to define the normal physiologic parameters at various gestational ages and the modulating influences.

Throughout this chapter, areas where further basic research is needed have been pointed out. As mentioned, new and better techniques in cell isolation and culture are needed so that long-term cultures of gastric cellular elements can be maintained and cloned cell lines developed. In addition, the application of molecular biologic techniques will greatly improve our ability to answer questions concerning development and regulation of gastric secretory function.

Another area of gastric function deserving attention is alkaline production by the stomach. The stomach has been shown to produce a significant amount of bicarbonate under a variety of circumstances[113] and may represent an important cytoprotective mechanism. Virtually nothing is known about bicarbonate secretion in neonates or the development of this secretory capacity.

An exciting area of research involves the examination of the inductive interactions between epithelium and mesenchyme.[114] For example, Fukamachi et al[115] have shown that transplants of glandular stomach in contact with homotypic mesenchyme give rise to typical glandular development; however, if heterotypic intestinal mesenchyme is used, the glandular stomach epithelium develops into an atypical intestinal crypt-villi structure. It is hoped that further research into this area will elucidate the riddle of normal organogenesis and also give important clues into the processes of intestinal metaplasia, cancer, normal healing processes, and ulcer pathogenesis.

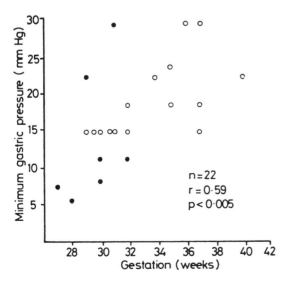

FIGURE 7 Changes in gastric antral pressure with increasing gestational age in "well" (*open circles*) and "ill" (*closed circles*) infants. (From Tomomasa.[109])

REFERENCES

1. Deren JS. Development of structure and function in the fetal and newborn stomach. Am J Clin Nutr 1971; 24:144–159.
2. Rohrer GV. Human gastric mucosa: correlation of structure and function. Am J Clin Nutr 1971; 24:137–143.
3. Hofer MA. Symposium: recent approaches in developmental physiology. Proc Soc Exp Biol Med 1984; 175:117.
4. Owen DA. Normal histology of the stomach. Am J Surg Pathol 1986; 101:48–61.
5. Owen DA. Gastritis and duodentitis. In: Appelman HD, ed. Contemporary issues in surgical pathology. Pathology of the esophagus, stomach, and duodenum. Vol 4. New York: Churchill Livingstone, 1984: 37.
6. Ito S. Functional gastric morphology. In: Johnson LR, ed. Physiology of the gastrointestinal tract. 2nd ed. Vol 1. New York: Raven Press, 1981: 817.
7. Solcia E, Capella C, Vassallo G, Butta R. Endocrine cells in the gastric mucosa. Int Rev Cytol 1975; 42:223–286.
8. Pearse AGE, Polak JM, Bloom SR. The newer gut hormones: cellular sources, physiology, and clinical aspects. Gastroenterology 1977; 72:746–761.

9. Solcia E, Capella C, Buffa R, Usellini L, Fiocca R, Sessa F. Endocrine cells of the digestive system. In: Johnson LR, ed. Physiology of the gastrointestinal tract. New York: Raven Press, 1981: 39.
10. Polak JM, Bloom SR. Regulatory peptides of the gut: the essential mechanism of gut control. In: Wright R. Recent advances in gastrointestinal pathology. Philadelphia: WB Saunders, 1980: 23.
11. Thompson JC, Marx M. Gastrointestinal hormones. Curr Probl Surg 1984; 21:1–80.
12. Chey WY, Lee KY. Motilin. Clin Gastroenterol 1980; 9:645–656.
13. McGuigan JE, Greider MH, Grawe L. Staining characteristics of the gastrin cell. Gastroenterology 1972; 62:959–969.
14. McIntosh CHS. Gastrointestinal somatostatin: distribution, secretion, and physiological significance. Life Sci 1985; 37:2043–2058.
15. Walsh JH, Grossman MI. Gastrin. N Engl J Med 1975; 292:1324–1332.
16. Creutzfeldt W, Arnold R. Somatostatin and the stomach: exocrine and endocrine aspects. Metabolism 1978; 27:1309–1315.
17. Larson L-I, Goltermann N, De Magistris L, Rehfeld JF, Schwartz TW. Somatostatin cell processes as pathways for paracrine secretion. Science 1979; 205:1393–1395.
18. Polak JM, Pearse AGE, Garaud J-C, Bloom SR. Cellular localization of a vasoactive intestinal peptide in the mammalian and avian gastrointestinal tract. Gut 1974; 15:720–724.
19. Buffa R, Capella C, Solcia E, Frigerio B, Daid SI. Vasoactive intestinal peptide (VIP) cells in the pancreas and astro-intestinal mucosa. An immunohistochemical and ultrastructural study. Histochemistry 1977; 50:217–227.
20. Larsson L-I, Fahrenkrug J, Schaffalitzky DeMuckadell O, Sundler F, Hakanson R, Rehfeld JF. Localization of vasoactive intestinal polypeptide (VIP) to central and peripheral neurons. Proc Natl Acad Sci USA 1976; 73:3197–3200.
21. Solcia E, Capella C, Buffa R, Frigerio B. Histochemical and ultrastructural studies on argentaffin and argyrophil cells of the gut. In: Couplan RE, Fujita T, ed. Chromaffin, enterochromaffin and related cells. Amsterdam: Elsevier, 1976: 223.
22. Vassallo G, Capella C, Solcia E. Endocrine cells of the human gastric mucosa. Z Zellforschung 1971; 118:49–67.
23. Capella C, Hage E, Solcia E, Usellini L. Ultrastructural similarity of endocrine-like cells of the human lung and some related cells of the gut. Cell Tissue Res 1978; 186:25–37.
24. Solcia E, Cappella C, Buffa R, Fiocca R, Frigerio B, Usellini L. Identification, ultrastructure and classification of gut endocrine cells and related growths. Invest Cell Pathol 1980; 3:37–49.
25. Fahrenkrug J. Vasoactive intestinal polypeptide. Clin Gastroenterol 1985; 9:633–643.
26. Ferri G-L, Botti P, Biliotti G, Rebecchi L, Bloom SR, Tonelli L, Labo G, Polak JM. VIP-, substance P-, and met-enkephalin-immunoreactive innervation of the human gastroduodenal mucosa and Brunner's glands. Gut 1984; 25:948–952.
27. Su HC, Bishop AE, Power RF, Hamada Y, Polak JM. Dual intrinsic and extrinsic origins of CGRP- and NPY- immunoreactive nerves of rat gut and pancreas. J Neurosci 1987; 7:2674–2687.
28. Nicholl CG, Polak JM, Bloom SR. The hormonal regulation of food intake, digestion, and absorption. Ann Rev Nutr 1985; 5:213–239.
29. Larsson L-I, Jorgensen LM. Ultrastructural and cytochemical studies on the cytodifferentiation of duodenal endocrine cells. Cell Tissue Res 1978; 194:79–102.
30. Larsson L-I, Rehfeld JF, Sundler F, Hakanson R. Pancreatic gastrin in foetal and neonatal rats. Nature (London) 1976; 262:609–610.
31. Larsson L-I. Peptide secretory pathways in GI tract: cytochemical contributions to regulatory physiology of the gut. Am J Physiol 1980; 239:G237–G246.
32. Wright N, Alison M. Morphological aspects of cell renewal systems. In: Wright N, Alison M, eds. The biology of epithelial cell populations. Vol 2. Oxford: Clarendon Press, 1984: 539.
33. Salenius P. On the ontogenesis of the human gastric epithelial cells. Acta Anat (Basel) 1962; 50:1–76.
34. Delemos C. The ultrastructure of endocrine cells in the corpus of the stomach of human fetuses. Am J Anat 1977; 148:359–384.
35. Hattori T, Fujita S. Fractographic study on the growth and multiplication of the gastric gland of the hamster. Cell Tissue Res 1974; 153:145–149.
36. Corpron RE. The ultrastructure of the gastric mucosa in normal and hypophysectomized rats. Am J Anat 1966; 118:53–90.
37. Rubin W, Ross LL, Sleisenger MH, Jeffries GH. The normal human gastric epithelia. A fine structural study. Lab Invest 1968; 19:598–626.
38. Matsuyama M, Susuki H. Differentiation of immature mucus cells into parietal, argyrophil and chief cells in stomach grafts. Science 1970; 169:385–387.
39. Buchan AMJ, Polak JM. The classification of human gastroenteropancreatic endocrine cells. Invest Cell Pathol 1980; 3:51–71.
40. Cheng H. Origin, differentiation, and renewal of the four major epithelial cell types in the mouse small intestine. III Enteroendocrine cells. Am J Anat 1974; 141:461–480.
41. Pearse AGE. Peptides in brain and intestine. Nature (London) 1976; 262:92–94.
42. Pearse AGE, Polak JM. The diffuse neuroendocrine system and the APUD concept. In: Bloom SR, ed. Gut hormones. Edinburgh: Churchill-Livingstone, 1978: 33.
43. Le Douarin NM. The embryological origin of the endocrine cell associated with the digestive tract: experimental analysis based on the use of a stable cell marking technique. In: Bloom SR, ed. Gut hormones. Edinburgh: Churchill-Livingstone, 1978: 558.
44. Andrew A. Further evidence that enterochromaffin cells are not derived from the neural crest. J Embryol Exp Morphol 1974; 31:589–598.
45. Chavyvialle JA, Paulin C, Descos F, Dubois PM. Ontogeny of vasoactive intestinal peptide in the human fetal digestive tract. Regul Pept 1983; 5:245–256.
46. Fahrenkrug J. Vasoactive intestinal polypeptide: measurement, distribution, and putative neurotransmitter function. Digestion 1979; 19:149–169.
47. Aynsley-Green A. Hormones and postnatal adaptation to enteral nutrition. J Pediatr Gastroenterol Nutr 1983; 2:418–427.
48. O'Loughlin EV, Chung M, Hollenberg M, Hayden J, Zahavi I, Gall DG: Effect of epidermal growth factor on ontogeny of the gastrointestinal tract. Am J Physiol 1985; 249:G674–G678.
49. Woll PJ, Rozegent E. Neuropeptides as growth regulators. Br Med Bull 1989; 45:492–505.
50. Avery GB, Randolph JG, Weaver T. Gastric acidity in the first day of life. Pediatrics 1966; 37:1005–1007.
51. Ebers DW, Smith DI, Gibbs GE. Gastric acidity on the first day of life. Pediatrics 1956; 18:800–802.
52. Griswold C, Sholh AT. Gastric digestion in newborn infants. Am J Dis Child 1925; 30:541–549.
53. Hess AF. The gastric secretion of infants at birth. Am J Dis Child 1913; 6:264–276.
54. Ames MD. Gastric acidity in the first ten days of life in the prematurely born baby. Am J Dis Child 1960; 100:123–126.
55. Miller RA. Observations on the gastric acidity during the first month of life. Arch Dis Child 1941; 16:22–30.
56. Ahn CI, Kim YJ. Acidity and volume of gastric contents in the first week of life. J Korean Med Assoc 1963; 6:948–950.
57. Baron JH. The clinical use of gastric function tests. Scand J Gastroenterol 1970; 6(Suppl):9–46.
58. Ghai OP, Meharban S, Walia BN, et al. The assessment of gastric acid secretory response with "maximal" augmented histamine stimulation in children with peptic ulcer disease. Arch Dis Child 1965; 40:77–79.
59. Grand RJ, Watkins JB, Torti FM. Development of the human gastrointestinal tract. Gastroenterology 1976; 70:790–810.
60. Christie DL. Development of gastric function during the first month of life. In: Lebenthal E, ed. Textbook of gastroenterology and nutrition in infancy. New York: Raven Press, 1981, 109.
61. Euler AR, Byrne WJ, Cousins LM, Ament ME, Leake RD, Walsh JH. Increased serum gastrin concentrations and gastric acid hyposecretion in the immediate newborn period. Gastroenterology 1977; 72:1271–1273.
62. Euler AR, Byrne WJ, Meis PJ, Leake RD, Ament ME. Basal and pentagastrin-stimulated acid secretion in newborn human infants. Pediatr Res 1979; 13:36–37.
63. Hyman PE, Clarke DP, Everett SL, Sonne B, Stewart D, Harada T, Walsh JH, Taylor IL. Gastric acid secretory function in preterm infants. J Pediatr 1985; 106:467–471.
64. Marino LR, Bacon BR, Kine JD, Halpin TC. Parietal cell function of full-term and premature infants: unstimulated gastric acid and intrinsic factor secretion. J Pediatr Gastroenterol Nutr 1984; 3:23–27.
65. Hyman PE, Feldman DJ, Ament ME, Byrne WJ, Euler AR. Effect of enteral feeding on the maintenance of gastric acid secretory function. Gastroenterology 1983; 84:341–345.

66. Euler AR, Byrne WJ, Campbell MF. Basal and pentagastrin-stimulated gastric acid secretory rates in normal children and in those with peptic ulcer disease. J Pediatr 1983; 103:766–768.

67. Lari J, Lister J, Duthie HL. Response to gastrin pentapeptide in children. J Pediatr Surg 1968; 3:682–690.

68. Agunod M, Yamaguchi N, Lopez R, Luhby A, Glass GBJ. Correlative study of hydrochloride acid, pepsin, and intrinsic factor secretion in newborns and infants. Am J Dig Dis 1969; 14:400–414.

69. Soll AH. The interaction of histamine with gastrin and carbamylcholine on oxygen uptake by isolated mammalian parietal cells. J Clin Invest 1978; 61:381–389.

70. Johnson LR. Functional development of the stomach. Ann Rev Physiol 1985; 47:199–215.

71. Lichtenberger L. A search for the origin of neonatal hypergastrinemia. J Pediatr Gastroenterol Nutr 1984; 3:161–166.

72. Card WI, Marks IN. The relationship between the acid output of the stomach following "maximal" histamine stimulation and the parietal cell mass. Clin Sci 1960; 19:147–163.

73. Polacek MA, Ellison EH. Gastric acid secretion and parietal cell mass in the stomach of a newborn infant. Am J Surg 1966; 111:777–781.

74. Garzon B, Ducroc R, Geloso J-P. Ontogenesis of gastric acid secretion in fetal rat. Pediatr Res 1981; 15:921–925.

75. Takeuchi K, Peitsch W, Johnson LR. Mucosal gastrin receptor V. Development in newborn rats. Am J Physiol 1981; 240:G163–G169.

76. Ackerman SH. Ontogeny of gastric acid secretion in the rat: evidence for multiple response systems. Science 1982; 217:75–77.

77. Garzon B, Ducroc R, Geloso J-P. Ontogenesis of gastric response to agonists and antagonists of acid secretion in fetal rat. J Devel Physiol 1982; 4:195–205.

78. Ikezaki M, Johnson LR. Development of sensitivity to different secretagogues in the rat stomach. Am J Physiol 1983; 244:G165–G170.

79. Garzon B, Ducroc R, Onoflo J-P, Desjeux J-F, Geloso J-P. Biphasic development of pentagastrin sensitivity in rat stomach. Am J Physiol 1982; 242:G111–G115.

80. Peitsch W, Takeuchi K, Johnson LR. Mucosal gastrin receptor. VI. Induction by corticosterone in newborn rats. Am J Physiol 1981; 240:G442–G449.

81. Roger IM, Davidson DC, Lawrence J, et al. Neonatal secretion of gastrin and glucagon. Arch Dis Child 1974; 49:796–800.

82. Euler AR, Ament ME, Walsh JH. Human newborn hypergastrinemia: An investigation of prenatal and perinatal factors and their effects on gastrin. Pediatr Res 1978; 12:652–654.

83. Lucas A, Aynsley-Green A, Bloom SR. Gut hormones and the first meals. Clin Sci 1981; 60:349–353.

84. Bell AW, Cranwell PD, Hansky J. Does gastrin cross the placenta? Proc Nutr Soc Aust 1980; 5:212–215.

85. Rodbro P, Krasilnikoff PA, Christiansen PM. Parietal cell secretory function in early childhood. Scand J Gastroenterol 1967; 2:209–213.

86. Hirsch-Marie H, Loisillier F, Touboul JP, Burtin P. Immunochemical study and cellular localization of human pepsinogens during ontogenesis and in gastric cancers. Lab Invest 1976; 34:623–632.

87. Kushner I, Rapp W, Burtin P. Electrophoretic and immunochemical demonstration of the existence of four human pepsinogens. J Clin Invest 1964; 43:1983–1993.

88. Adamson I, Esangbedo A, Okolo AA, Omene JA. Pepsin and its multiple forms in early life. Biol Neonate 1988; 53:267–273.

89. Furihata C, Kagachi T, Sugimura T. Premature induction of pepsinogen in developing rat gastric mucosa by hormones. Biochem Biophys Res Commun 1972; 47:705–711.

90. Keene MFL, Hewer EE. Digestive enzymes of the human foetus. Lancet 1929; i:767–769.

91. Malpress FH. Renin and the gastric secretion of normal infants. Nature (London) 1967; 215:855–857.

92. Werner B. Pepsin and pancreas proteinase in premature as compared with full term infants. Ann Paediatr 1948; 170:8–14.

93. Defize J, Meuwissen SGM. Pepsinogens: an update of biochemical, physiological, and clinical aspects. J Pediatr Gastroenterol Nutr 1987; 6:493–508.

94. Schepp W, Miederer SE, Ruoff HJ. Intrinsic factor secretion from isolated gastric mucosal cells of rat and man—two different patterns of secretagogue control. Agents Actions 1984; 14:522–528.

95. Schwartz M, Weber J. Gastric intrinsic factor in the human foetus. Scand J Gastroenterol 1971; 6 (Suppl):57–59.

96. Dieckgraefe BK, Seetharam B, Alper DH. Developmental regulation of rat intrinsic factor mRNA. Am J Physiol 1988; 254:G913–G919.

97. Dieckgraefe BK, Seetharam B, Banaszak L, Leykam JF, Alpers DH. Isolation and structural characterization of a cDNA clone encoding rat gastric intrinsic factor. Proc Natl Acad Sci USA 1988; 85:46–50.

98. Siegel M, Lebenthal E. Development of gastrointestinal motility and gastric emptying during the fetal and newborn periods. In: Lebenthal E, ed. Textbook of gastroenterology and nutrition in infancy. New York: Raven Press, 1982: 121.

99. Kelly KA. Motility of the stomach and gastroduodenal junction. In: Johnson LR, ed. Physiology of the gastrointestinal tract. New York: Raven Press, 1981: 393.

100. Bremner CG. Studies on the pyloric muscle. S Afr J Surg 1968; 6:79–85.

101. Jit J. The development of the muscular coats of the human oesophagus, stomach, and small intestine. J Anat Soc India 1956; 5:1–13.

102. Indir J. The development of the nerve supply of the human esophagus and stomach. J Anat Soc India 1955; 4:55–68.

103. MeGeady TA, Sack WO. The development of vagal innervation of the bovine stomach. Am J Anat 1967; 121:121–130.

104. Heading RC. Gastric motility. Front Gastrointest Res 1980; 6:35–56.

105. Lebenthal E, Siegel M. Understanding gastric emptying: implications for feeding the healthy and compromised infant. J Pediatr Gastroenterol Nutr 1985; 4:1–3.

106. Ruckebush Y. Development of digestive motor patterns during perinatal life: mechanisms and significance. J Pediatr Gastroenterol Nutr 1986; 5:523–536.

107. Gryboski JD. The swallowing mechanism of the neonate. I. Esophageal and gastric motility. Pediatrics 1965; 62:445–452.

108. Tornwall L, Lind J, Peltonen T, Wegelius C. The gastrointestinal tract of the newborn. Anal Paediatr Fenn 1958; 4:209–214.

109. Tomomasa T, Itoh Z, Koizumi T, Kuroume T. Nonmigrating rhythmic activity in the stomach and duodenum of neonates. Biol Neonate 1985; 48:1–9.

110. Hancock PJ, Bancalari E. Gastric motility in premature infants fed two different formulas. J Pediatr Gastroenterol Nutr 1984; 3:696–699.

111. Bisset WM, Watt JB, River RPA, Milla PJ. Ontogeny of fasting small intestinal motor activity in the human infant. Gut 1988; 29:483–488.

112. Morriss FH Jr, Moore M, Weisbradt NW, West MS. Ontogenic development of gastrointestinal motility. IV. Duodenal contractions in preterm infants. Pediatrics 1986; 78:1106–1113.

113. Rees WDW, Gibbons LC, Warhurst G, Turnberg LA. Studies of bicarbonate secretion by the normal human stomach in vivo: effect of aspirin, sodium taurocholate, and prostaglandin E_2. In: Allen A, et al, eds. Mechanisms of mucosal protection in the upper gastrointestinal tract. New York: Raven Press, 1984: 119.

114. Sakagami Y, Inaguma Y, Sakakura T, Nishizuka Y. Intestine-like remodeling of adult mouse glandular stomach by implanting of fetal intestinal mesenchyme. Cancer Res 1984; 44:5845–5849.

115. Fukamachi J, Miauno T, Takayama S. Epithelial-mesenchymal interactions in differentiation of stomach epithelium in fetal mice. Anat Embryol 1979; 157:151–160.

CHAPTER 18

Digestive and Absorptive Function

Jacques Schmitz, M.D.

In most mammalian species, intestinal functions develop in two main stages. The first one occurs in utero and enables the newborn to digest and absorb its mother's milk; the second one, at the time of weaning, may be considered a "redifferentiation" that adapts these functions to the more diverse food of the adult animal.[1] In man, as probably in primates,[2] this redifferentiation does not exist; the intestine of the newborn is immediately able to digest and absorb not only his mother's milk but also most of his mother's food.

The bases of our knowledge concerning intestinal development in man were established between 1955 and 1970, when the concept of the brush border as an organelle of digestion and absorption emerged. This knowledge was remarkably reviewed by Grand and co-workers in 1976.[3] However, since then major advances have been made regarding, for example, the development of colonic structure and functions, and some insights are being gained regarding the mechanisms at work in intestinal differentiation in man. Nevertheless, our knowledge remains somehow patchy and data are still lacking in certain areas of great physiologic interest, such as amino acid and peptide absorption and fat absorption. In these cases, available information from animal studies will be given when relevant.

SMALL BOWEL

Development of Structures

Formation of the Intestinal Tract

The primitive gut is formed during the fourth week of intrauterine life by invagination of the dorsal part of the yolk sac. The epithelium of the gut and associated glands develop from endoderm, while the connective tissue and muscular elements derive from mesoderm. The primitive tub can be divided into three segments, each one having a separate blood supply: the foregut— esophagus, stomach, duodenum—and its derivatives (liver, gallbladder, pancreas); the midgut— small intestine and two-thirds of the colon; and the hindgut, which extends to the upper part of the anal canal, are supplied respectively by the celiac trunk and the superior and inferior mesenteric arteries. At the end of the third week and during the seventh week of gestation, respectively, the buccopharyngeal and cloacal dermal-endodermal membranes rupture. A continuity between the amniotic cavity and the intestinal tract is thus established. It is essential for the circulation of amniotic fluid during intrauterine life.[4,5]

From the fifth week of gestation up to term, the intestine lengthens one thousand–fold.[5] This dramatic increase in length, together with the rapid development of the liver, results in a temporary herniation of the primitive intestinal loops into the umbilical cord which starts the sixth week of gestation. The proximal limb of the primitive loop develops more rapidly and forms the jejunal and ileal loops, as far as Meckel's diverticulum, while the distal limb forms the terminal ileum, cecum, and right half of the colon. From the tenth to the twelfth week the intestine re-enters the abdominal cavity from its cranial end and carries on its 270-degree counterclockwise rotation.[4] At 11 to 13 weeks of gestation, the small intestine measures between 25 and 40 cm, at the twentieth week approximately 1 m, 1.70 m between the twenty-seventh and the thirty-fifth weeks, and from 2 to 2.5 m at term, while the colon lengthens from 25 to 50 cm during the same period of time.[6] The length of the small intestine increases little after the age of 4 years, when it measures 4 m at autopsy.[7]

Morphogenesis of Villi and Crypts

It is during the period of herniation that the villi begin to differentiate. Villus formation starts in the duodenum at about the eighth week, and, proceeding distally, reaches the jejunum at 9 to 10 weeks and the ileum at 11 to 12 weeks of gestation. By the fourteenth week, scanning electron microscopy shows that the villi have acquired their typical finger-shaped appearance in the proximal intestine.[8,9] The epithelium is multilayered up to the tenth week. At 8 weeks, it is made of two to four layers of undifferentiated columnar cells, with short irregular cytoplasmic projections bordering the lumen, small intracytoplasmic deposits of glycogen; and frequent mitotic figures suggesting a high proliferative capacity,[10] which is confirmed by the scatter of ^{3}H-thymidine uptake in nuclei throughout the stratified epithelium.[11] Indeed, the rapidly proliferating epithelium soon completely fills the duodenal lumen, which is again patent by the ninth to tenth week. Despite similar proliferative activity, total occlusion of the gut lumen does not occur distal to the duodenum.[5,8]

Crypt development also proceeds distally. The first crypts appear in the proximal intestine at 10 to 11 weeks of gestation as downward buddings of the epithelium into the mesenchyme, between the new villi. They are present in the ileum and the colon 1 to 2 weeks later. Circular folds appear at this time in the midintestine and extend to the entire small intestine by 32 weeks of gestation.[5] This early appearance of villi and crypts in humans contrasts markedly with intestinal development in other species such as the rat, in which villi appear late in gestation and crypts well after birth.[8,12]

As villi form, the epithelium becomes columnar, and by 12 weeks villi are lined by a single layer of epithelial cells. In the proximal intestine, between the sixth and ninth weeks of gestation, vacuoles develop within the stratified epithelium. They resemble "secondary lumina" in that the epithelial cells that limit these vacuoles have their luminal plasma membrane forming well-defined microvilli and are joined by continuous tight junctional strands.[10] The precise role of these "secondary lumina" in the transition from stratified to single-layered epithelium is not yet totally clear in humans. In the rat they expand and contribute to the formation of short

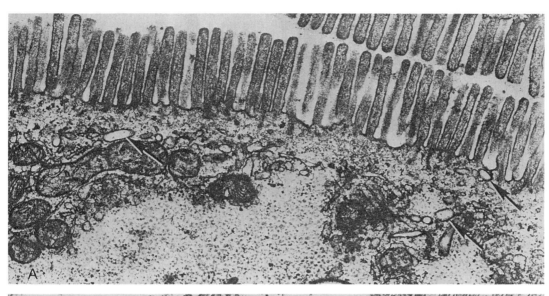

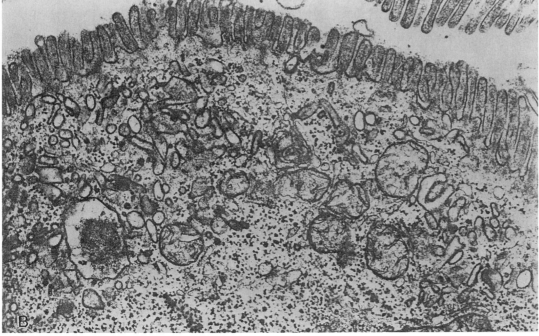

FIGURE 1 Apical cytoplasm of an enterocyte from the proximal (A) and distal (B) intestine of a 15-week fetus (×19,800). Well-developed microvilli are already present in the proximal intestine, while they are shorter and less regularly arranged in the distal intestine. In contrast, the apical tubular system is much more developed in the distal than in the proximal intestine (arrows). (With permission of P. Moxey and the Wistar Institute Press.)

villi, which are lined by a simple columnar epithelium.[12] It is suggested that in the human fetal intestine these vacuoles are part of the same process.[8]

Cellular Differentiation

Overlapping with the formation of the crypt-villus axis, distinct cell types differentiate.

Crypt Cells. Undifferentiated crypt cells appear as crypts form in both the proximal and distal intestines. They have large basal nuclei, abundant free ribosomes, little formed endoplasmic reticulum (ER), and, in contrast to undifferentiated crypt cells in adults, prominent glycogen deposits and nearly no lysosomes.[10]

Paneth cells appear in crypts during the twelfth to fourteenth weeks of gestation. They rapidly acquire long strands of rough ER (RER) and well-developed Golgi complexes. Secretory granules with electron-dense cores are highly heterogeneous in both size and number. As the fetus develops, the secretory granules become more homogeneous, as in adults, and restricted to the apical cytoplasm.[10]

Glandular extensions leading to acini deep in the lamina propria and resembling Brunner's glands are seen in the proximal intestine at 14 to 15 weeks of gestation. The columnar cells forming the glandular acini have a less well-organized RER and smaller secretory granules than corresponding cells in adults.[10]

Epithelial Absorptive Cells. Epithelial absorptive cells represent by far the most important class of cells in the epithelium, and their ultrastructure has been extensively studied.[13-15] From 6 to 8 weeks of gestation, immature cells lining the lumen present occasional cytoplasmic projections but no true microvilli.[13,14] However, by the eighth to tenth postfertilization week, absorptive cells show at their apical pole numerous, well-ordered microvilli that average 1.0 μm in length and 0.2 μm in width, their mature dimensions, and their central core is made of filaments variable in number but of consistent diameter (3.5 to 5 nm).[13] Simultaneously, brush border cytoskeleton proteins, calmodulin-binding proteins (110 kDa protein, caldesmon, fodrin), at first (eighth week) uniformly present throughout the epithelium, become localized to the apical part of the epithelial cells (twelfth week).[16] At 8 weeks, desmosomes are already present, but junctional complexes are absent. They appear by the tenth week, and the cell membranes beneath the developing terminal web are interdigitated.[15] At the same time, glycogen accumulates in large supranuclear and infranuclear vacuoles. Irregular, electron-dense lysosomal elements, also termed "meconium corpuscles," appear around the twelfth week of gestation in the supranuclear cytoplasma.[14,15] By the fourteenth week of gestation, proximal and distal enterocytes are morphologically similar, with a well-organized terminal web and a brush border that shows its typical appearance by both transmission and scanning electron microscopy.[9,15] At that time an apical tubular system, whose membranes are similar in width and density to the apical plasma membrane, and "meconium corpuscles" are prominent features of the absorptive cell[15] (Fig. 1). Between 15 and 17 weeks, both cell substructures show a marked development in the distal but not the proximal intestine, followed by a progressive decrease from the eighteenth to the twenty-second week of gestation,

after which they may be undetectable.[15,17] Both systems are supposed to be involved in the uptake of luminal macromolecules[17,18] (see below). Finally, during the fourth month of gestation, a reduction in glycogen content and a further development of the smooth ER occur. Thus the absorptive cell is morphologically not different from the adult one during at least the last trimester of gestation. This is at variance with what is seen in other laboratory animals and particularly in the rat, in which a mature brush border is not seen before birth.[12]

Endocrine Cells. Several ultrastructural[14,19] as well as immunohistochemical[20-23] studies have shown endocrine cells to be present in the fetal intestine by the tenth to twelfth week of gestation. Primitive and precursor endocrine cells, characterized by their pale cytoplasm, the presence of free ribosomes, and little formed ER, but with secretory granules denser and smaller in the primitive than in the precursor cells, already appear in the stratified epithelium of the proximal intestine at 9 to 10 weeks of gestation.[19] During the two following weeks appear "transitional" cells characterized by the simultaneous presence of secretory granules of the precursor type (large—1 μm in diameter—and pale) and of the type of one of the four specific adult endocrine cells (EC, S, I, G). These "transitional" cells are rarely seen after the sixteenth to eighteenth week of gestation. Finally, mature appearing S cells (secreting secretin) with granules of 100 to 200 nm diameter, EC cells (secreting motilin, serotonin, substance P) with dense granules of 250 to 380 nm diameter, I cells (secreting cholecystokinin) with granules of 220 to 280 nm diameter, and G cells (secreting gastrin) with granules of variable densities and of 250 to 480 nm diameter, are present in the proximal intestine between the ninth and twelfth weeks of gestation and approximately 1 week later in the distal intestine.[19] S, EC, and I cells are found only in crypts. Cells secreting somatostatin (D cells) and GIP (D_1 cells) appear during the same period. Enteroglucagon-secreting cells (L cells), unlike the other fetal endocrine cells, appear in the distal small intestine before (tenth to eleventh week) appearing in its proximal part (thirteenth week of gestation).[19] It is likely that "primitive," "precursor," and "transitional" cells represent immature precursors of adult endocrine cells. The fact that G,[20,21] D,[23] I,[20] and L[22] cells have also been characterized immunologically indicates that these fetal cells synthesize and store adult-like, probably active, peptides that may play a role during development.[19] Indeed, gastrin, secretin, motilin, GIP, VIP, enteroglucagon, and somatostatin are found in fetal intestinal tissue extracts as soon as the eighth week of gestation, their concentrations increasing steadily until term, when they are close to adult levels.[22] Furthermore, functional and specific receptors for VIP can be detected in isolated epithelial cells of fetuses aged 18 to 23 weeks (no data available earlier).[24]

Other Specialized Cells. Goblet cells differentiate as early as endocrine cells, being recognizable within the stratified epithelium of 9- to 10-week-old fetuses. Immature cells have a moderately developed RER and small, dense secretory granules. Mature fetal cells show the characteristic well-developed Golgi complex, abundant RER, and large secretory granules packed in the supranuclear region. Some of these cells, however, have their secretory granules in the infranuclear region, oriented toward the basal lamina.[10,25]

Tuft or caveolated cells, characterized by bundles of dense filaments extending from the microvillous cores deep into the supranuclear region and by apical multivesicular bodies, are first noted at 16 weeks of gestation in the villi. Their role is still unknown.[10]

M cells, known to be involved in the transfer of macromolecules from the lumen to the cells of the underlying lymphoid follicles, are first noted at 17 to 18 weeks of gestation in the distal epithelium overlying aggregated lymphocytes. Characteristic microfolds are already present along their luminal plasma membrane, and membrane-bound vesicles are abundant in their apical cytoplasm.[10] Since individual lymphocytes appear in the lamina propria late in the first trimester, and aggregates not until the sixteenth to twentieth week, it has been suggested that there is a temporal relationship between the differentiation of M cells and formation of lymphoid follicles. That this phenomenon might be linked to some kind of interaction between epithelial and lymphoid cells is supported by the frequently observed direct contracts between these two populations of cells in the fetal intestine.[8]

Biochemical Maturation of the Small Intestinal Surface

Although the small intestinal surface appears morphologically mature well before birth in humans, recent biochemical studies of one of its main components, the brush border membrane, have revealed that the membrane exhibits subtle differences in the fetus compared to the adult. This has been particularly well demonstrated for a group of its integral proteins, the hydrolytic enzymes.[26] Thus, although sucrase activity is similar in 16- to 24-week-old fetuses and in adults, sucrase-isomaltase exists in these fetuses only as an uncleaved high molecular weight precursor[27] of slightly lower molecular weight than the adult precursor.[28] Furthermore, sucrase-isomaltase and dipeptidylpeptidase IV (DPPIV) and oligoaminopeptidase isolated from meconium or from brush borders of 4-month-old fetuses have a faster anodal electrophoretic mobility and show a weaker affinity for *Helix pomatia* lectin, than do adult enzymes.[26,29]

These differences are probably related to differences in glycosylation, as suggested by studies of the interactions of these enzymes with lectins.[30] Such modifications of glycosylation during postnatal development have been described in rabbits[31] and rats,[32,33] in which they are probably linked to developmental changes in glycosyl-transferase activities.[34] Increased sensitivity and response to *Escherichia coli* heat-stable enterotoxin in young rats,[35] increased cholera toxin binding to rabbit and rat newborn brush border membranes[36,37] compared with that in adult animals, as well as the appearance of receptor activity for enteropathogenic *E. coli* RDEC-I in rabbit,[38] might be linked to these modifications of glycosylation. Such age-related differences in sensitivity to *E. coli* heat-stable enterotoxin have also been demonstrated in children, in whom the number of receptors for and the degree of stimulation of guanylate cyclase by the toxin rapidly decrease with age.[39]

In the rat, the mucus, another important component of the intestinal surface, also undergoes developmental changes: the molar ratio of carbohydrate to protein is lower in newborn that in adult animals, primarily owing to a decreased fucose and N-acetyl galactosamine content; these changes are also related to incomplete glycosylation.[40] Such changes might be physiologically relevant in view of the function of the mucus in maintaining the intestinal surface acid microclimate, whose role in the absorption of folates and peptides is probably critical.[41]

Experiments in laboratory animals suggest that not only brush border membrane proteins and mucus but also the lipid phase of the membrane undergoes biochemical changes during development. Such changes include higher lipid-to-protein and lower cholesterol-to-phospholipid ratios,[42] leading to an increased membrane fluidity in newborn compared to adult animals, as shown by electron spin resonance[43] or fluorescence polarization spectrometry.[44,45] Also, Ca^{2+} ion exerts a greater ordering effect in microvillous membranes from immature than from mature rats and binds to two classes of binding sites in newborn rat membranes instead of one class in adult membranes.[43] Such developmental differences may directly influence the maturation of enterocyte transport functions[46] as well as of antigen uptake.[18]

Although similar data are still lacking, such changes in composition of the intestinal surface most probably also occur in humans, in whom their importance remains to be established.

Development of Digestion and Absorption of Carbohydrates

Carbohydrates in food must be reduced to monosaccharides before they can be absorbed. Three enzymes only— lactase, sucrase-isomaltase, and glucoamylase—are necessary to digest lactose, sucrose, and maltodextrins. Even fewer transport systems are involved in absorbing the released monosaccharides. The development of most of these proteins is well known.

Oligosaccharidases

Lactase. Lactase activity is extremely low during the first months of gestation. It is barely assayable in homogenates of whole intestinal mucosa or even of lower half of fetuses until the third month of gestation; it remains low until the sixth month and increases steadily during the last trimester of intrauterine life to reach maximum values around birth.[47] Activities fitting in this pattern were found by others who measured lactase activity in a narrower range of gestational age (tenth to twentieth week), during which it was low and stable.[48-51] However, when more accurate methods of dating the fetuses[52] and assaying disaccharidase activities (in isolated brush border membranes) are used, lactase activity is detected in the proximal part of the intestine as soon as the eighth and ninth weeks of gestation, as sucrase activity, when microvillus-like formations appear.[9] During the following weeks, lactase activity remains low until the twelfth week and starts rising during the fourteenth week of gestation; it is then 25 percent of adult activity.[9] It remains at that level during the second trimester and rises significantly again during the third trimester of gestation, reaching the highest activity at birth.[51,53] The proximodistal gradient of activity exists as soon as the eleventh week (Fig. 2).[9]

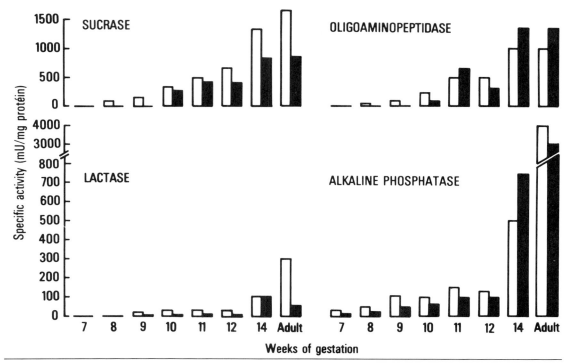

FIGURE 2 Development of brush border membrane hydrolase activities in isolated brush border membranes from jejunum (*empty columns*) and ileum (*black columns*) of human fetuses. (From Lacroix et al.[9])

After birth, lactase activity drops slightly in Caucasians to reach adult values after the first years of life.[54] In most non-Caucasians, however, lactase activity decreases slowly, during the following 2 to 20 years, and reaches low adult levels, which are usually one-tenth of values at birth.[55] This pattern of variation of lactase activity from intrauterine life to adulthood is similar to the one observed in most mammalian species,[56] including primates.[2,57]

Sucrase-isomaltase. Sucrase activity is first measurable in the proximal half of the intestine at 8 weeks of gestation when microvilli appear. It rises steadily until the fourteenth week, reaching activities two-thirds of values at birth. It continues to rise more slowly during the second and third trimesters of gestation; at birth it is not different from activity during adulthood.[9,47-51] As for lactase, the proximodistal gradient of activity is clearly noticeable as early as the tenth week of gestation, activity in the ileum appearing later (ninth week) in agreement with morphologic data and being always lower than in the jejunum.[9,53,58] Although of identical specific activity, the molecular form of sucrase isomaltase is different in fetuses than in adults, being differently glycosylated (see above). Isomaltase activity follows the same pattern of development as sucrase activity,[47,49] which is consistent with the fact that sucrase and isomaltase activities are born by the same proenzyme[59] (Fig. 2).

This pattern of development is strikingly different from the one observed in experimental animals, in which sucrase activity, undetectable at birth, begins to rise at weaning when lactase activity begins to fall.[56] In nonhuman primates, however, sucrase activity is already high at birth, as in humans.[57] Despite these differences, in rabbits as in humans, sucrase-isomaltase activity development closely parallels that

of sucrase-isomaltase mRNA, which suggests that, in the human embryo also, the biosynthesis of sucrase-isomaltase is controlled at the level of transcription.[60]

Glucoamylase. Glucoamylase activity has rarely been measured in fetuses. Early studies have reported the development of thermoresistant maltase activities, which most probably correspond to glucoamylase.[61] Thermoresistant maltase activities seem to develop late during gestation. Undetectable until the twenty-third week[49] or not measured before 6 months of gestation,[47] the level of maltase II activity is similar to adult levels as soon as it is measured, after 6 months, whereas maltase I activity is still very low at birth.[47] Recently, glucoamylase activity, assayed with soluble starch as substrate, was measured in isolated epithelial cells of fetuses from 13 to 20 weeks of gestation. Activity is low (one-fourth to one-fifth of sucrase activity) but does not vary during this period of time[62]; yet it is already significant in preterm newborns.[53] Since maltase activity is mainly (up to 75 percent) born by sucrase-isomaltase, its pattern of development follows closely the one of sucrase isomaltase and it is not possible to deduce from both patterns the development of glucoamylase.

Trehalase. Trehalase activity is found in fetal intestinal mucosa at 3 months of intrauterine life. It then rises steadily and by 23 weeks of gestation has reached values comparable to those in adult mucosa.[47,49,62]

Transport Systems

As with lactase and sucrase activities, transepithelial glucose transport develops in parallel with the brush border. Using everted gut sacs obtained from fetuses aged 11 to 19 weeks, it has been shown that glucose is already transported against a concentration gradient in the jejunum at 11 weeks, although at a low rate (S/M=1.25); it then increases markedly, being fourfold higher by 16 weeks of gestation.[63,64] Glucose transport appears and rises later in the ileum,[63] reaching at 21 weeks of gestation a level similar to the level in the jejunum at 16 weeks.[65] Similar results have been obtained by recording from the fourteenth to the twenty-first week of gestation increasing potential differences evoked by glucose; this indicates that, as soon as it appears, glucose transport is coupled to Na^+ transport (Fig. 3).[65] The increase in glucose transport capacity during gestation corresponds to an increase of the number of transport sites, the affinity of the carrier for its substrate being constant during the period of gestation considered (10 to 24 weeks).[66] At 21 weeks, maximum potential differences are three-fifths[65] and at birth two-thirds[67] of published adult values. It is worthwhile noting that lactose does not generate any potential difference in a jejunum from a 14.5-week fetus, whereas sucrose at the same concentration (3.5 mM) generates a potential difference, although of lower magnitude than glucose (7 mM).[65] This finding is consistent with the low lactase and nearly mature sucrase activities recorded at that age.

In vivo perfusion studies have shown that glucose transport rate continues to increase in the first year(s) after birth, maximal glucose absorption rates in the infant proximal intestine being one-fourth to one-fifth of adult rates, whereas apparent Km (half saturation constant) increases also from 5.8 mM in infants to 20 mM in adults.[68] Whether these differences in glucose absorption rates between infants and adults are artifactual (in relation to the unstirred water layer?) or reflect true differences (or both) is still unknown.

As galactose is transported across the intestinal mucosa through the same carrier protein as glucose, it is supposed that development of galactose absorption during gestation follows the same pattern as the one of glucose absorption. However, no experimental data are available to confirm this supposition. This is particularly unfortunate, since data have recently accumulated pointing to the possibility that in humans[69] glucose and galactose may, in fact, use two transport systems with overlapping specificities. Few in vivo studies have been concerned with intestinal absorption of galactose in infants. The maximum capacity and apparent Km for galactose absorption are similar to those for glucose[70] and several-fold lower in infants than in adults.[71]

No data are available in humans concerning the development of fructose absorption during gestation. We know only that D-fructose (7 mM) does not elicit any potential difference in the jejunal mucosa from a 13-week-old fetus.[65] In animals it has been shown that the third-trimester fetal lamb is able to absorb fructose, although less efficiently than glucose.[72]

Development of Digestion and Absorption of Peptides

In contrast to carbohydrates, peptides may be absorbed either as such, before being hydrolyzed in the intestinal absorptive cells by cytoplasmic peptidases into amino acids, or as amino acids, after preliminary hydrolysis by brush border peptidases. Intestinal digestion and absorption of peptides thus involve many more proteins and are much more complex processes than intestinal digestion and absorption of carbohydrates. Their development in humans is also less well known.

Enterokinase

Enterokinase activity, which triggers the activation of trypsinogen into trypsin and therefore plays a key role in protein digestion initiation, but has no digestive function in itself, is first detected in duodenal mucosa of 24- to 26-week-old fetuses. Between the twenty-sixth week of gestation and term, it increases three to four times, being at birth 25 percent of the activity of infants less than 1 year of age and 17 percent of that of children between 1 and 4 years of age.[51] Activity is always the highest in duodenum and the lowest in ileum, in contrast to disaccharidase activities, which are highest in jejunum. This proximodistal gradient is clearly noticeable only after the thirtieth week of gestation. The simultaneous appearance of tryptic activity in meconium and of enterokinase activity in the intestinal mucosa suggests that enterokinase is the factor limiting detection of tryptic activity in the fetal small intestinal lumen (Fig. 4).[51]

Brush Border Peptidases

Few studies are concerned with the development of human brush border peptidases.[9,73,74] Oligoaminopeptidase (OAP), aminopeptidase A (APA), dipeptidylpeptidase IV (DPPIV), carboxypeptidase (CP), and gamma-glutamyl-transpeptidase (gamma-GTP) activities are already present in the intestinal mucosa of 8-week-old fetuses. OAP activity is the only one to increase significantly from the eighth to the twenty-second

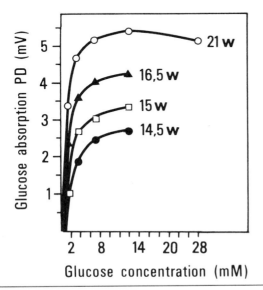

FIGURE 3 Development of glucose absorption in everted sacs of jejunum of human fetuses. Glucose absorption was estimated by the potential difference induced by glucose across the intestinal wall. (From Levin et al.[65])

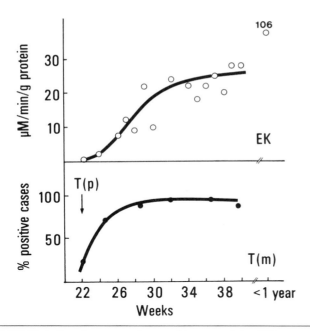

FIGURE 4 Development of enterokinase activity (EK, upper part of the figure) in the duodenal mucosa of human fetuses compared to the appearance of spontaneous trypsin activity (lower part of the figure) in meconium (Tm). The arrow T(p) indicates the appearance of trypsin activity in homogenates of pancreas after addition of EK. (From Antonowicz and Lebenthal,[51] and Lieberman J. Proteolytic enzyme activity in fetal pancreas and meconium. Gastroenterology 1966; 50:183–190; © 1966 by The American Gastroenterological Association.)

week of gestation; it is twice as high in fetuses older than 13 weeks than in fetuses younger than 13 weeks,[9,74] the increase being greater in the distal than in the proximal small intestine after the twelfth week of gestation[9,73,74] (see Fig. 2). Activities of DPP IV, CP, and OAP in fetuses of more than 13 weeks of age are similar to activities in children 7 months to 11 years old and in adults; gamma GTP activity is three times higher, whereas APA activity is four times lower in fetuses than in children (for the latter) and in adults (for both).[74] As for disaccharidases, molecular forms of these enzymes in fetuses are different from those in adults, probably because of differences in glycosylation (see above).[29,75]

Transport of Amino Acids and Peptides

Like glucose, alanine elicits an immediate increase in the potential difference recorded across the wall of everted gut sacs of fetuses 12 to 15 weeks of age,[65] which indicates that, as soon as it appears and similar to glucose transport, alanine transfer across the intestinal mucosa is coupled to Na^+ transfer. Evoked potentials increase from the fifteenth to the twenty-fourth week of gestation. As in the case of glucose, this increase is due to an increase in the number of transport sites, the affinity of the carrier for alanine remaining constant during this period (Km = 10 mM).[66] In fetuses of the same age, glycine, L-forms of neutral amino acids such as serine, valine, methionine, and phenylalanine, and acid amino

acids like aspartic acid also generate electrical potential differences of significant magnitudes, whereas basic amino acids do not.[66]

Data on development of peptide transport in humans are rare. In fetuses of 15 to 24 weeks of gestation, glycyl-glycine and glycyl-glycyl-glycine generate high transmucosal potentials.[66] In guinea pigs, glycyl-glycine and glycyl L-leucine uptakes are significantly greater in sucklings than in weanlings and greater in the latter than in adult animals. These differences are more prominent in jejunum than in ileum and are related to differences in maximum influxes, not in affinities of the carriers for peptides.[76] Similarly, in rabbits, uptake of glycyl-L-proline, a dipeptide not hydrolyzed by brush border peptidases, increases during the last days of gestation, reaches a maximum at birth, and thereafter decreases sharply during the first 10 days of life and more slowly later on.[77] The late maturation of guinea pig functions and the "redifferentiation" of rabbit intestinal mucosa at weaning make it difficult to extend these findings to humans.

Soluble Peptidases

Once absorbed, dipeptides or tripeptides are reduced to amino acids by several poorly known cytoplasmic peptidases that have been studied in humans only in homogenates of intestinal mucosa. Peptidase activities against L-alanyl-L-glutamine, L-alanyl-L-proline, glycyl-glycine, glycyl-L-leucine, and glycyl-L-valine are already present in human intestinal mucosa of 11-week-old fetuses; they do not vary until 23 weeks of age. No gradient of activity along the intestine appears during this period.[78] Similarly, dipeptidase activities toward glutaminyl-L-proline and glycyl-L-proline, probably born by separate enzymes, are present in intestinal mucosa of 15-week-old fetuses and do not vary later on until birth; these activities are always twice as high in the proximal as in the distal third of intestine.[79]

Development of Digestion and Absorption of Fat

Although fat digestion is an exclusively intraluminal process, it is dependent upon an adequate bile salt enterohepatic circulation and hence on efficient bile salt absorption.

Active Absorption of Bile Salts

Active transfer of bile salts is not found in fetal or neonatal ileal mucosa but is fully developed at the age of 8 months. It is not known exactly when it appears, since no data are available between birth and that age.[80] Immaturity of bile salt absorption in the neonate is confirmed by the fact that cholate turnover is higher before the age of 10 months than in older children.[81]

Lipid Absorption

Lipid absorption in human fetuses is poorly documented. Morphologic studies have shown that 10-week-old fetuses absorb corn oil, probably not simply by pinocytosis.[13]

However, our knowledge concerning the development of the various stages of fat absorption by the intestinal mucosa, i.e., diffusion of free fatty acids and monoglycerides through the lipid structures of the brush border and basolateral plasma membranes, their binding to FABP, the resynthesis of triglycerides in the endoplasmic reticulum, and the formation of chylomicrons after local synthesis of apolipoprotein B_{48}, is drawn nearly exclusively from animal studies.

In the rat, FABP is present at adult levels from the sixth day of gestation, and in the rat and the guinea pig the enzymes of triglyceride resynthesis (acyl-CoA synthetase, acyl-CoA-mono- and di-acyl transferases) are well developed before birth.[82-84] The early appearance of chylomicrons in circulation after ingestion of long-chain triglycerides in infants[3] suggests a similar prenatal development of these enzymes in humans and the synthesis of apo B before birth. In fact, apo B synthesis already occurs in intestines of 6-week-old fetuses.[85] However, in contrast to the situation in adult intestine, where the apo B_{48} form of the apolipoprotein B is synthesized, only the apo B_{100} form is synthesized in fetal intestine, at least until the twentieth week of gestation.[85,86]

Development of Alkaline Phosphatase and of Lysosomal Enzymes

Alkaline Phosphatase

Although alkaline phosphatase (AP) has been extensively studied, its function remains largely unknown. In the intestine, it is predominantly a brush border enzyme whose activity is histoenzymatically detected at the luminal surface of epithelial cells in fetuses of 7 weeks of gestational age, when villi begin to appear.[25,87] The surface epithelial staining is then irregular, with a beady appearance. During the following weeks it becomes thicker and more evenly distributed.[25] In homogenates of intestinal mucosa, AP activity is already high in 11-week-old fetuses (see Fig. 2). It increases fourfold during gestation.[49] At 23 weeks, however, it is still at least five times lower than in children[88] and adults.[48] At that age it is higher in jejunum than in ileum.[49] Before 1 year of age AP activity is higher (+50 percent) but also more dispersed than in older children and in adults.[88] This pattern of development is different from the one in mouse and rat duodenum, in which AP appears just before birth, remains low during the suckling period, and rises sharply at weaning.[1,89] In humans as in rodents,[89] the fetal molecular form of the enzyme is different from the adult form; it has a higher sialic acid content[90,91] but also a different polypeptide structure coded by a different gene.[92]

Lysosomal Enzymes

Acid phosphatase appears histoenzymatically confined to supranuclear particles in intestinal mucosa of 8- to 12-week-old fetuses. As the fetus matures, the number and prominence of these particles increase. In ileum from fetuses of 14 weeks and more, meconium particles also react for the enzyme.[87] In fetuses of 10 to 24 weeks of gestational age, the specific activities of acid phosphatase as well as of alpha-glucosidase, beta-glucosidase, beta-galactosidase, beta-glucuronidase, N-acetyl-beta-glucosaminidase, and arylsulfatase are comparable to those of older infants, even at the earlier time studied.[93] Beta-fucosidase activity is present in intestinal mucosa of 17-week and 18-week-old fetuses.[94] In fetuses aged 17 to 24 weeks, alpha-glucosidase activity is higher in the proximal jejunum than in ileum, whereas beta-galactosidase, beta-glucosidase, beta-glucuronidase, N-acetyl-beta-glucosaminidase, and phosphatase activities are highest in the mid–small intestine and arylsulfatase activity remains constant along the small intestine.[93]

Permeability to Macromolecules

In ruminants (cows, horses, sheep) and in pigs, which receive passive immunity (immunoglobulins) from colostrum and milk during a few days of enhanced intestinal permeability to all macromolecules, feeding induces a rapid maturation of gut morphology, which results in functional gut closure to proteins; in rodents (rats, mice), which have a specific permeability to immunoglobulins while suckling, it is thought that maternal milk induces maturation of the antigen-excluding function of the gut, absorption of immunoglobulins stopping just before weaning.[18] In fact, transepithelial transport of a nonspecific protein like horseradish peroxidase via small cytoplasmic vesicles already occurs in the still stratified small intestinal epithelium of fetal rats at 16 and 17 days of gestation. Later, during the days preceding birth, it occurs via the tubulovesicular system, which is present in the apical cytoplasm of the enterocytes,[95,96] is used by immunoglobulins during the suckling period, and is no longer seen after weaning, once closure has occurred.[97]

In contrast to ruminants and rodents, the human infant receives its passive immunity by transplacental transfer during the third trimester of intrauterine life. Thus he is not dependent on intestinal absorption of macromolecules to acquire immunoglobulins. Furthermore, maturation of the intestinal epithelial cells occurs much earlier in humans. Indeed, particles of colloidal thorium are taken up by pinocytosis and transported in vesicles to intercellular spaces already in the intestinal mucosa of 10-week-old human fetuses.[13] Also, ferritin is taken up in apical vesicles from the twelfth week of gestation by the fetal intestinal mucosa and is found in the apical tubular system from the fifteenth to the twenty-second week of gestation, when it is well developed, before its involution.[15] However, it is never found in the intercellular spaces, which does not exclude the transport of more physiologically relevant molecules (immunoglobulins, hormones) as some evidence seems to indicate.[98]

Despite early morphologic closure, shown by the disappearance during the third trimester of gestation, of the apicotubular system, enhanced permeability to macromolecules around birth seems to exist in humans, at least in premature newborns. Thus beta-lactoglobulin concentrations in plasma of preterm babies (less than 33 weeks) are 10 to 100 times higher than in plasma of term babies, whereas in term babies they are identical to concentrations in adults receiving proportionate amounts of cow's milk.[99] Human alpha-lactalbumin concentrations are also higher in preterm than in term neonates receiving human milk; however, in term neonates, they are also six times more elevated in the first days of life than 2 to 6 months later, which seems to indicate that, in contrast to what is found with beta-lactoglobulin, an enhanced permeability to macromolecules exists during the first months of life even in term babies.[100] The observed difference between beta-lactoglobulin and human alpha-lactalbumin with regard to their handling by the human intestinal mucosa remains unclear. It could relate, as has been proposed during intrauterine life, to the physiologic relevance of these proteins. The facts that IgG levels on day 5 are higher in colostrum-fed than in colostrum-deprived term newborns[101] and that colostral polio IgA antibody may be found in sera from newborns[102] are not in contradiction to this hypothesis.

A state of increased intestinal permeability during the immediate neonatal period is also demonstrated for smaller carbohydrate molecules like lactulose, mannitol, and rhamnose. Thus lactulose-to-rhamnose[103] or lactulose-to-mannitol[104] ratios are higher in preterm babies born before the thirty-fourth to thirty-sixth week of gestation than in term babies, and in both groups they are higher on day 1 than on day 4. That a "mature" ratio is achieved in 4 days in preterm as in term babies indicates a vigorous adaptation to oral feeds, which might be aimed at achieving mature functions as soon as possible.[104] Such maturation seems to be somewhat quicker with breast milk than with infant formulae.[105] However, the relationship of this increased permeability to small saccharidic molecules with the permeability to macromolecules like proteins remains unknown in humans.[106]

Meconium and Amniotic Fluid as Indicators of Intestinal Development

Meconium

Meconium, the material that collects in the intestine during fetal life, originates from secretions and desquamated cells of the fetal digestive tract as well as, to a lesser degree, from swallowed amniotic fluid. It is first found in the terminal ileum at the beginning of the second trimester of fetal life (thirteenth to seventeenth week).[87] It then accumulates and starts filling the colon, in which it is abundant around the twenty-first week of gestation.[78]

Its water content varies from 70 to 80 percent and 80 percent of its dry weight is made up of mucopolysaccharides.[107] It contains small quantities of serum proteins and many enzymes. Among them, those originating from the digestive tract have been particularly studied. Lactase and trehalase activities are low, yet they are higher in ileal than in colonic meconium and higher in fetal than in newborn meconium where they may be undetectable.[49,107] Sucrase-isomaltase and maltase activities, on the contrary, are higher in large than in small intestinal and in fetal than in newborn meconium; they are extremely variable also from one subject to another.[49,94,107] In general, activities in the meconium are higher than in the intestinal wall.[49] Meconium from preterm and from term newborns contains also high levels of OAP activity. DPP IV, APA, CP, gamma-GTP activities are higher in preterm than in term meconium samples.[29] Finally, alkaline phosphatase activity is 10 times higher in large than in small intestinal meconium,[49] and it increases with fetal age,

being higher in newborns than in fetuses.[107] It is less variable than disaccharidase activities, probably because of a greater resistance to the proteolytic activities present in meconium. The molecular forms of some of the enzymes present in meconium (sucrase-isomaltase, OAP, DPP IV, alkaline phosphatase) are different from the adult forms of the homologous enzymes (see above).

In contrast to disaccharidase activities, soluble dipeptidase activities against L-alanyl-L-glutamine, L-alanyl-L-proline, glycyl-glycine, glycyl-L-valine, and glycyl-L-leucine are rather low in fetal meconium compared to the intestinal mucosa and even lower in meconium from newborns.[78] Lysosomal enzyme activities (alpha-glucosidase, beta-D-fucosidase activities) are also found in meconium samples from 17- and 18-week-old fetuses.[94]

Trypsin activity can be measured in meconium at the end of the second trimester of gestation and in meconium from prematures less than 34 weeks of gestational age. Chymotrypsin activity is more variable and is still detectable in meconium from newborns. These activities do not account for the total proteolytic activity at pH 8 present in meconium, which probably results from a complex mixture of enzymes.[107]

Amniotic Fluid

At the start of fetal development, amniotic fluid is an extension of the extracellular compartment of the fetus. During the second half of pregnancy fetal urine becomes the chief source of amniotic fluid and its ingestion the most important route for its elimination. The volume of amniotic fluid increases from 20 to 30 ml at 10 weeks to 200 to 300 ml at 20 weeks and amounts to 800 to 1000 ml from the thirtieth week to term. The fetus, which starts to swallow from the sixteenth to seventeenth week of intrauterine life, ingests an average 450 ml of amniotic fluid per day at term.[108] Any congenital esophageal or proximal intestinal obstruction is thus usually accompanied by hydramnios.

The analysis of fetal enzymatic activities in the amniotic fluid has been suggested as a method for dating pregnancy. It is with this aim in view that digestive enzymes have been investigated. In fact, pepsinogens are present in the amniotic fluid from the fifteenth week of gestation.[3] Similarly alpha-amylase is present in the fluid from the twelfth week of intrauterine life. At that time, it is chiefly or exclusively salivary in origin,[109] the pancreatic isoenzyme being not found up to term.[110]

Brush border membrane and lysosomal enzyme activities have also been demonstrated in amniotic fluid. From the tenth week of gestation, sucrase-isomaltase activities are present in the fluid; they increase up to the eighteenth week, then decrease rapidly and are very low from the twenty-second week (Fig. 5).[94,111] The same pattern applies to the intestinal isoenzyme of alkaline phosphatase and to gamma-glutamyl-transpeptidase.[112] In contrast, glucoamylase activity is not found in the amniotic fluid of fetuses aged 16 to 24 weeks,[113] and lactase activity remains very low or is not detected throughout gestation.[94,111] Lysosomal enzyme activities (beta-D-fucosidase, alpha-D-glucosidase, N-acetyl-beta-glucosaminidase) are also present in amniotic fluid as early as the fourteenth week of gestation.[94] The first two activities tend

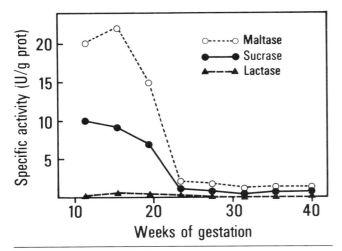

FIGURE 5 Variation of disaccharidase activities in amniotic fluid according to the duration of pregnancy. (From Potier et al.[111])

to increase or remain high until the eighteenth week, after which they decrease steadily and are low after the twenty-second week. In contrast, N-acetyl-beta-glucosaminidase activity remains roughly constant until the twenty-fourth week of gestation, which might suggest a different source(s) for this enzyme than for the other two.[94]

The fall in amniotic fluid brush border enzyme activities between the eighteenth and twenty-first weeks is contemporary with the accumulation of meconium in the terminal ileum and colon and with the functional closure of the anal sphincter. It is thus probably due to the reduced excretion of desquamated intestinal cells into the amniotic fluid. The similar pattern of decrease of several lysosomal enzymatic activities corroborates such an assumption. The fall of brush border enzyme activities occurs significantly earlier in the amniotic fluid of fetuses with cystic fibrosis. The assay of these activities in amniotic fluid of fetuses aged 16 to 18 weeks can thus be used to make the prenatal diagnosis of this condition.[114]

DEVELOPMENT OF THE COLON

Interest in the morphologic and functional development of the human colon during gestation is recent.[115] Data are still not numerous despite the possibility that the colon might subserve a nutritional role during fetal life.[116]

Morphogenesis

Like the small intestine, the colon is first a simple tube with a slit-like lumen until the eighth to ninth week of gestation, when large longitudinal folds appear which are prominent in the midcolon at 11 weeks of gestation. These previllous ridges then fold longitudinally, forming a zig-zag pattern.[117] This pattern is transient and by the thirteenth week gives way to primary villi, which split longitudinally into smaller secondary villi. Simultaneously the epithelium at the base of the

primary villi proliferates rapidly, forming knob-like projections that are the developing crypts.[117] The first outgrowth of villi occurs in the distal colon when longitudinal folds are still present in the proximal colon, the maturation process extending in a distoproximal direction, in contrast to what occurs in the small intestine.[115] Between 14 and 16 weeks of gestation villi are present in the whole colon. They are still well developed at 22 to 25 weeks of gestation; afterwards they regress and have completely disappeared at term; at which time the mucosa has its typical flat appearance with scattered crypt mouths.

Until the tenth week of gestation the lumen is lined by a pseudostratified columnar epithelium three to four layers thick. As "secondary" lumina appear and ridges become villi, the epithelium becomes monostratified. At 11 to 12 weeks, the epithelial cells display sparse microvilli and contain large supranuclear glycogen-rich areas within the cytoplasm. At 16 weeks the brush border is well developed. By 12 weeks goblet cells are present along the crests of the folds.[117] They also extend distoproximally along the colon and become prominent by the thirteenth week along the sides of the villi.[115] As in the small intestine, endocrine cells are present in the fetal colonic mucosa extremely early, as soon as the fifth to sixth week of gestation.[118] Enterochromaffin cells (secreting motilin, serotonin) and cells secreting somatostatin, glucagon-like polypeptide, and pancreatic polypeptide are found in relatively large numbers along the entire length of the colon from the ninth to the twenty-fourth week of gestation. Substance P–containing cells first appear during the fourteenth to seventeenth weeks.[119]

Development of Colonic Functions

Digestive Functions

Although always much lower (up to 10 times in brush border preparations)[115] than in the small intestine, sucrase-isomaltase activities are present in the colonic mucosa from the eleventh week of gestation, being nearly unmeasurable before.[49,115] This rise in activity corresponds to the development of villi and the appearance of microvilli in the epithelial cells. Activities increase until the twentieth week, remain high until 28 weeks, and then begin to decrease[28,53,115] to extremely low or undetectable levels at birth (Fig. 6).[47] This pattern closely parallels the development and regression of colonic villi. Interestingly, the molecular forms of fetal colonic and small intestinal sucrase-isomaltase are identical[28] and also identical to the molecular form of the enzyme expressed in human colon cancer cell lines.[120] Although lower than in the small intestine, glucoamylase activity is present in the colonic mucosa from the thirteenth week of gestation. It seems not to vary greatly until the eighteenth week.[62] It is still present in preterm colonic mucosa.[53] Lactase activity is extremely low in homogenates of whole mucosa or of isolated epithelial colonic cells[49,62] and undetectable in brush border preparations during the entire intrauterine life.[53,115] It is not expressed by human colon cancer cell lines.[120]

Brush border peptidase activities (OAP, APA, DPP IV, gamma-GT activities) are present in the fetal colonic mucosa.[62,74] OAP, like sucrase-isomaltase, rises from the eleventh

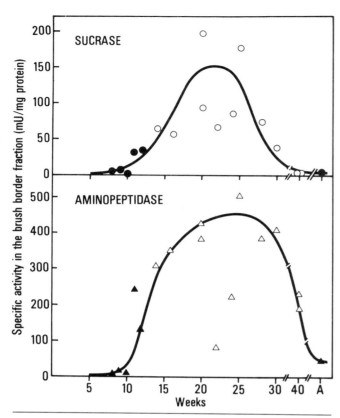

FIGURE 6 Development of brush border enzymes in the human fetal colon. (From Lacroix et al.[115])

week, reaches its highest values between 20 and 28 weeks of gestation, and then decreases.[115] However, in contrast to sucrase-isomaltase activities, OAP activity remains rather high until term and persists in the adult colonic mucosa at lower levels.[53,115] Soluble peptidase activities against five dipeptides (L-alanyl-L-glutamine, L-alanyl-L-proline, glycyl-glycine, glycyl-L-valine, glycyl-L-leucine) are also found in fetal colonic mucosa at the same level as in the small intestinal fetal mucosa. They do not vary with fetal age.[78]

Finally, alkaline phosphatase activity is very low in homogenates of colonic mucosa or of isolated epithelial colonic cells of fetuses less than 22 weeks of gestational age.[49,62,107] Yet in contrast to OAP and sucrase-isomaltase activities, alkaline phosphatase activity is already present in sizeable amounts in brush border preparations from the eighth week of gestation. It then follows the pattern of development of OAP, rising until the twentieth week, decreasing after the twenty-eighth week of gestation, and remaining higher at term than in adult colonic mucosa.[115]

Absorptive Functions

Nothing is known about the absorptive capacity of the human fetal colon for macronutrients. We know only that the anion-exchange mechanism whereby chloride is absorbed and bicarbonate secreted is poorly developed in preterm neonates.[121] In the rat, fetal colon taken on the twentieth day of a 22-day gestation is able to absorb both glucose and ala-

nine, and absorption of both solutes is Na^+-dependent. This absorptive function persists during the first days of extrauterine life.[116,122]

Thus, in humans as in rats, the colon develops during intrauterine life, first as the small intestine, although somewhat later, and it has anatomic and functional features similar to those of the small intestine from the twentieth to the twenty-eighth week of gestation in humans and a few days before and after birth in the rat; then, in a second stage, during the last 2 to 3 months of gestation in humans, these features progressively disappear, leaving the newborn colonic mucosa similar to the adult one, essentially without any digestive and absorptive capacity except for water and electrolytes.[53,121] The reason for this pattern of development and for this later "regression," which seems to be suspended in certain human colon cancer cell lines, is not known. There is a possibility that the colon plays a nutritional role during gestation. It may have the same function in (very) preterm newborns.[116]

FACTORS THAT REGULATE INTESTINAL DEVELOPMENT

Development may be viewed as the orderly expression of genes elicited or repressed by specific exogenous regulatory factors. After the pioneering experiences of Moog which demonstrated the role of glucocorticoid hormones in the development of mouse and chick small intestine and opened the vast field of the hormonal control of intestinal development,[1] the role of epitheliomesenchymal interactions for ontogenesis was recently stressed in a series of elegant experiments using xenoplastic tissue recombinants.[123,124] It appears clear now that hormones act as "triggers," affecting the timing and rate of differentiation but not altering the sequence of events that normally occurs according to an "intrinsic program" in which tissue interactions play a central role. Our knowledge concerning the respective importance of these factors has been gained nearly exclusively in laboratory animals. It is worth summarizing it to introduce the few data recently obtained in the human fetus.

Animal Studies

In animals, in vivo studies indicate a considerable diversity among species concerning the hormonal requirements for intestinal development. For example, in the chick embryo, thyroid hormones are implicated in the differentiation of the intestinal epithelium, whereas in rodents, glucocorticoid hormones are the main factor responsible for the intestinal changes that occur at weaning and, in particular, for sucrase appearance; however, thyroxine, insulin, and EGF have also been shown to be involved in postnatal maturation processes in the latter species.[1,124] More precisely, it has been shown in organ culture of fetal rat intestine that glucocorticoids are not involved in the onset of lactase activity but elicit its enhancement in the perinatal period and that they can precociously induce sucrase activity as soon as 19 days of gestation. In both cases they act at the transcriptional level, increasing the amount of newly synthesized mRNA.[125,126] In the same experiments, thyroid hormones were found to decrease significantly dexamethasone-stimulated lactase rise before birth. They are likely to be involved also in the postnatal decrease of lactase activity.[124]

Nutritional substrates are also implicated in the small intestinal functional differentiation in rodents. In vivo and organ culture experiments have shown that mono- and disaccharides synergize the effects of glucocorticoids on sucrase and maltase activities.[127,128]

Studies in Humans

Development of human gut is characterized by a high degree of differentiation at birth, which is related to the long duration of gestation. During intrauterine life, it can be summarized into three successive periods: (1) a period when the brush border becomes organized and many enzymes appear, around the eighth week of gestation; (2) a second period when most of these enzymic activities show a clear increase around the fourteenth week of gestation; and (3) a third period when lactase, glucoamylase, and enterokinase, which have been low or absent, rise again or appear.[124]

The first period is extremely early and difficult to study. It can only be speculated that the organization of the brush border and the first expression of enzymes are an intrinsic property of the intestinal endoderm, dependent, as in rodents, upon tissue interactions. Although no direct evidence is available, the fact that human fetal mesenchymal cells are able to trigger the developmental capacities of rat and chicken intestinal endoderm, thus exerting a "permissive influence," and in particular are able to induce the precocious induction of sucrase activity in rat gut endoderm, supports this assumption.[129]

Only within the last few years, when organ culture of human fetal intestine has been established,[130] has the second period become open to study of the role of hormones on fetal gut development. The first finding is that the explantation of human fetal gut for 3 to 5 days in serum-free medium elicits a spontaneous increase of brush border enzyme activities[130,131] which is of much greater amplitude than what is observed in similar conditions in the fetal rat or the chick embryo. This increase suggests that an inhibitor normally present during intrauterine life is absent from the culture medium.[131] This inhibitor is not present in organic extracts of amniotic fluid, since, added to the culture medium of 11- to 13-week-old fetuses, these extracts have no effect on several enzyme activities. It is worth noting that they do not exert any stimulatory effect either, inasmuch as the rise of enzyme activities during the second period of development is roughly coincident with the stage when the fetus begins to swallow amniotic fluid.[131]

Glucocorticoid hormones added to the culture medium of intestines from 8- to 14-week-old fetuses are ineffective in modifying epithelial morphology[132] and levels of sucrase, trehalase, glucoamylase, and amino-oligopeptidase activities. In contrast, they induce a significant increase of lactase activity and, in the oldest fetuses (12 to 14 weeks), of alkaline phosphatase activity.[131,132] Glucocorticoid hormones thus appear less active than in laboratory animals. Similarly, insulin added to the culture medium has no effect on enzyme activities.[131] In contrast, in the presence of epidermal growth factor (EGF), DNA synthesis and labeling index decrease and the normal rise of brush border enzyme activities is inhibited, except in the case of lactase, the activity of which is significantly increased over the level reached without EGF. This effect was not found in organ culture of fetal mouse intestine, in which DNA synthesis is not affected and lactase activity does not rise when EGF is present in the culture medium.[133]

Clearly, the humoral factors that regulate intestinal development in rodents and chickens are different from and/or do not exert a role of equal magnitude to those in humans. Whether this is due to a real lack of genetic susceptibility or to an inadequate timing of the experiments performed during a phase of low sensitivity is not known.[124] These uncertainties underline the difficulties in extrapolating to humans results obtained in laboratory animals.

REFERENCES

1. Moog F. Endocrine influences on the functional differentiation of the small intestine. J Anim Sci 1979; 49:239–249.
2. Welsh JD, Russell LC, Walker AW Jr. Changes in intestinal lactase and alkaline phosphatase activity levels with age in the baboon (Papio papio). Gastroenterology 1974; 66:993–997.
3. Grand RJ, Watkins JB, Torti FM. Development of the human gastrointestinal tract. A review. Gastroenterology 1976; 70:790–810.
4. Moore KL. The digestive system. In: The developing human—clinically oriented embryology, Philadelphia: WB Saunders, 1973:175.
5. Arey LB. The digestive tube and associated glands. In: Developmental anatomy. Philadelphia: WB Saunders, 1974:241.
6. Touloukian RJ, Walker-Smith GJ. Normal intestinal length in preterm infants. J Pediatr Surg 1983; 18:720–723.
7. Siebert JR. Small-intestine length in infants and children. Am J Dis Child 1980; 134:593–595.
8. Colony PC. Successive phases of human fetal intestinal development. In: Kretchmer N, Minkowski A, eds. Nutritional adaptation of the gastrointestinal tract of the newborn. New York: Nestlé, Vevey/Raven Press, 1983:3.
9. Lacroix B, Kedinger M, Simon-Assmann P, Haffen K. Early organogenesis of human small intestine: scanning electron microscopy and brush border enzymology. Gut 1984; 25:925–930.
10. Moxey PC, Trier JS. Specialized cell types in the human fetal small intestine. Anat Rec 1978; 191:269–286.
11. Arsenault P, Menard D. Cell proliferation in developing human jejunum. Biol Neonate 1987; 51:297–304.
12. Mathan M, Moxey PC, Trier JS. Morphogenesis of fetal rat duodenal villi. Am J Anat 1976; 146:73–92.
13. Kelley RO. An ultrastructural and cytochemical study of developing small intestine in man. J Embryol Exp Morphol 1973; 29:411–430.
14. Varkonyi T, Gergely G, Varro V. The ultrastructure of the small intestinal mucosa in the developing human fetus. Scand J Gastroenterol 1974; 9:495–500.
15. Moxey PC, Trier JS. Development of villus absorptive cells in the human fetal small intestine: a morphological and morphometric study. Anat Rec 1979; 195:463–482.
16. Rochette-Egly C, Lacroix B, Kedinger M, Haffen K. Calmodulin and calmodulin binding proteins during differentiation of human intestinal brush borders. Differentiation 1987; 35:219–227.
17. Verma KBL. Development of mucosa of the human ileum. J Anat 1979; 128:513–521.
18. Walker WA, Isselbacher KJ. Uptake and transport of macromolecules by the intestine. Possible role in clinical disorders. Gastroenterology 1974; 67:531–550.
19. Moxey PC, Trier JS. Endocrine cells in the human fetal small intestine. Cell Tissue Res 1977; 183:33–50.
20. Dubois PM, Paulin C, Chayvialle JA. Identification of gastrin-secreting cells and cholecystokinin-secreting cells in the gastrointestinal tract of the human fetus and adult man. Cell Tissue Res 1976; 175:351–356.

21. Larsson LI, Rehfeld JF, Goltermann N. Gastrin in the human fetus. Distribution and molecular forms of gastrin in the antro-pyloric gland area, duodenum and pancreas. Scand J Gastroenterol 1977; 12:869–872.

22. Bryant MG, Buchan AMJ, Gregor M, Ghatei MA, Polak JM, Bloom SR. Development of intestinal regulatory peptides in the human fetus. Gastroenterology 1982; 83:47–54.

23. Dubois PM, Paulin C, Dubois MP. Gastrointestinal somatostatin cells in the human fetus. Cell Tissue Res 1976; 166:179–184.

24. Gespach C, Chastre E, Emami S, Mulliez N. Vasoactive intestinal peptide receptor activity in human fetal enterocytes. FEBS Lett 1985; 180:196–202.

25. Lev R, Siegel HI, Bartman J. Histochemical studies of developing human fetal small intestine. Histochemie 1972; 29:103–119.

26. Auricchio S. Fetal forms of enzymes of intestinal brush border. In: Kretchmer N, Minkowski A, eds. Nutritional adaptation of the gastrointestinal tract of the newborn. New York: Nestlé, Vevey/Raven Press, 1983:53.

27. Skovbjerg H. High molecular weight pro-sucrase-isomaltase in human fetal intestine. Pediatr Res 1982; 16:948–949.

28. Triadou N, Zweibaum A. Maturation of sucrase-isomaltase complex in human fetal small and large intestine during gestation. Pediatr Res 1985; 19:136–138.

29. Auricchio S, Caporale C, Santamaria F, Skovbjerg H. Fetal forms of oligoaminopeptidase, dipeptidylaminopeptidase IV, and sucrase in human intestine and meconium. J Pediatr Gastroenterol Nutr 1984; 3:28–36.

30. Triadou N, Audran E. Interaction of the brush-border hydrolases of the human small intestine with lectins. Digestion 1983; 27:1–7.

31. Olson AD, Pysher TJ, Larrosa-Haro A, Mahmood A, Torres-Pinedo R. Differential toxicity of RCA$_{II}$ (Ricin) on rabbit intestinal epithelium in relation to postnatal maturation. Pediatr Res 1985; 19:868–872.

32. Mahmood A, Torres-Pinedo R. Postnatal changes in lectin binding to microvillus membranes from rat intestine. Biochem Biophys Res Comm 1983; 113:400–406.

33. Pang KY, Bresson JL, Walker WA. Development of gastrointestinal surface. VIII. Lectin identification of carbohydrate differences. Am J Physiol 1987; 252:G685–691.

34. Biol MC, Martin A, Richard M, Louisot P. Developmental changes in intestinal glycosyl-transferase activities. Pediatr Res 1987; 22:250–256.

35. Cohen MB, Moyer MS, Luttrell M, Gianella RA. The immature rat small intestine exhibits an increased sensitivity and response to Escherichia coli heat-stable enterotoxin. Pediatr Res 1986; 20:555–560.

36. Bresson JL, Pang KY, Walker WA. Microvillus membrane differentiation: quantitative difference in cholera toxin binding to the intestinal surface of newborn and adult rabbits. Pediatr Res 1984; 18:984–987.

37. Lencer WI, Chu SHW, Walker WA. Differential binding kinetics of cholera toxin to intestinal microvillus membrane during development. Infect Immun 1987; 55:3126–3130.

38. Cheney CP, Boedeker EC. Rabbit mucosal receptors for an enteropathogenic Escherichia coli strain: appearance of bacterial receptor activity at weaning. Gastroenterology 1984; 87:821–826.

39. Cohen MB, Guarino A, Shukla R, Giannella RA. Age-related differences in receptors for Escherichia coli heat-stable enterotoxin in the small and large intestine of children. Gastroenterology 1988; 94:367–373.

40. Shub MD, Pang KY, Swann DA, Walker WA. Age-related changes in chemical composition and physical properties of mucus glycoproteins from rat small intestine. Biochem J 1983; 215:405–411.

41. Said HM, Smith R, Redha R. Studies on the intestinal surface acid microclimate: developmental aspects. Pediatr Res 1987; 22:497–499.

42. Chu SHW, Walker WA. Development of the gastrointestinal mucosal barrier: changes in phospholipid head groups and fatty acid composition of intestinal microvillus membranes from newborn and adult rats. Pediatr Res 1988; 23:439–442.

43. Pang KY, Bresson JL, Walker WA. Development of the gastrointestinal mucosal barrier. V. Comparative effect of calcium binding on microvillus membrane structure in newborn and adult rats. Pediatr Res 1983; 17:856–861.

44. Schwarz SM, Ling S, Hostetler B, Draper JP, Watkins JB. Lipid composition and membrane fluidity in the small intestine of the developing rabbit. Gastroenterology 1984; 86:1544–1551.

45. Brasitus TA, Yeh KY, Holt PR, Schachter D. Lipid fluidity and composition of intestinal microvillus membranes isolated from rats of different ages. Biochim Biophys Acta 1984; 778:341–348.

46. Hayashi K, Kawasaki T. The characteristic changes of amino acid transport during development in brush border membrane vesicles of the guinea pig ileum. Biochim Biophys Acta 1982; 691:83–90.

47. Auricchio S, Rubino A, Murset G. Intestinal glycosidase activities in the human embryo, fetus, and newborn. Pediatrics 1965; 35:944–954.

48. Dahlqvist A, Lindberg T. Fetal development of the small-intestinal disaccharidase and alkaline phosphatase activities in the human. Biol Neonate 1965/66; 9:24–32.

49. Dahlqvist A, Lindberg T. Development of the intestinal disaccharidase and alkaline phosphatase activities in the human fetus. Clin Sci 1966; 30:517–528.

50. Sheehy TW, Anderson PR. Fetal disaccharidases. Am J Dis Child 1971; 121:464–468.

51. Antonowicz I, Lebenthal E. Developmental pattern of small intestinal enterokinase and disaccharidase activities in the human fetus. Gastroenterology 1977; 72:1299–1303.

52. Lacroix B, Wolff-Quenot MJ, Haffen K. Early human hand morphology: an estimation of fetal age. Early Hum Dev 1984; 9:127–136.

53. Raul F, Lacroix B, Aprahamian M. Longitudinal distribution of brush border hydrolases and morphological maturation in the intestine of the preterm infant. Early Hum Dev 1986; 13:225–234.

54. Welsh JD, Poley JR, Bhatia M, Stevenson DE. Intestinal disaccharidase activities in relation to age, race, and mucosal damage. Gastroenterology 1978; 75:847–855.

55. Simoons FJ. Primary adult lactose intolerance and the milking habit: a problem in biological and cultural interrelations. I. Review of the medical research. Am J Dig Dis 1969; 14:819–836.

56. Henning SJ, Kretchmer N. Development of intestinal function in mammals. Enzyme 1973; 15:3–23.

57. Bataille J, Pletincx M, Schmitz J. Postnatal development of sucrase and lactase in the non human primate papio. Pediatr Res 1981; 15:1194. (Abstract)

58. Jirsova V, Koldovsky O, Heringova A, Uher J, Jodl J. Development of invertase activity in the intestines of human fetuses, appearance of jejunoileal differences. Biol Neonate 1968; 13:143–146.

59. Hunziker W, Spiess M, Semenza G, Lodish HF. The sucrase-isomaltase complex: primary structure, membrane-orientation, and evolution of a stalked, intrinsic brush border protein. Cell 1986; 46:227–234.

60. Sebastio G, Hunziker W, O'Neill B, Malo C, Menard D, Auricchio S, Semenza G. The biosynthesis of intestinal sucrase-isomaltase in human embryo is most likely controlled at the level of transcription. Biochem Biophys Res Comm 1987; 149:830–839.

61. Semenza G. Intestinal oligo- and disaccharidases. In: Randle PJ, Steiner DF, Whelan WJ, eds. Carbohydrate metabolism and its disorders. Vol 3. London: Academic Press, 1981:425–479.

62. Menard D, Pothier P. Differential distribution of digestive enzymes in isolated epithelial cells from developing human fetal small intestine and colon. J Pediatr Gastroenterol Nutr 1987; 6:509–516.

63. Koldovsky O, Heringova A, Jirsova V, Jirasek JE, Uher J. Transport of glucose against a concentration gradient in everted sacs of jejunum and ileum of human fetuses. Gastroenterology 1965; 48:185–187.

64. Jirsova V, Koldovsky O, Heringova A, Hoskova J, Jirasek J, Uher J. The development of the functions of the small intestine of the human fetus. Biol Neonate 1965/66; 9:44–49.

65. Levin RJ, Koldovsky O, Hoskova J, Jirsova V, Uher J. Electrical activity across human foetal small intestine associated with absorption processes. Gut 1968; 9:206–213.

66. Sagawa N, Nishimura T, Ogawa M, Inouye A. Electrogenic absorption of sugars and amino acids in the small intestine of the human fetus. Membrane Biochem 1979; 2:393–404.

67. McNeish AS, Ducker DA, Warren IF, Davies DP, Harran MJ, Hughes CA. The influence of gestational age and size on the absorption of D-xylose and D-glucose from the small intestine of the human neonate. In: Development of mammalian absorptive processes. Ciba Foundation Symposium 70. Amsterdam: Excerpta Medica, 1979:267.

68. Younoszai MK. Jejunal absorption of hexose in infants and adults. J Pediatr 1974; 85:446–448.

69. Evans L, Grasset E, Heyman M, Dumontier AM, Beau JP, Desjeux JF. Congenital selective malabsorption of glucose and galactose. J Pediatr Gastroenterol Nutr 1985; 4:878–886.

70. Lugo-De-Rivera C, Rodriguez H, Torres-Pinedo R. Studies on the mechanism of sugar malabsorption in infantile infectious diarrhea. Am J Clin Nutr 1972; 25:1248–1253.

71. Holdsworth CD, Dawson AM. The absorption of monosaccharides in man. Clin Sci 1964; 27:371–379.

72. Char VC, Rudolph AM. Digestion and absorption of carbohydrates by the fetal lamb in utero. Pediatr Res 1979; 13:1018–1023.

73. Heringova A, Koldovsky O, Jirsova V, Uher J, Noack R, Friedrich M, Schenk G. Proteolytic and peptidase activities of the small intestine of human fetuses. Gastroenterology 1966; 51:1023–1027.

74. Auricchio S, Stellato A, De Vizia B. Development of brush border peptidases in human and rat small intestine during fetal and neonatal life. Pediatr Res 1981; 15:991–995.

75. Caporale C, Fontana P, Fontanella A, Murolo E, Santamaria F, Auricchio S. Isolation and characterization of two particle-bound oligoaminopeptidases from human meconium that are different from oligoaminopeptidase of adult small intestine. J Pediatr Gastroenterol Nutr 1985; 4:908–916.

76. Himukai M, Konno T, Hoshi T. Age-dependent change in intestinal absorption of dipeptides and their constituent amino acids in the guinea pig. Pediatr Res 1980; 14:1272–1275.

77. Guandalini S, Rubino A. Development of dipeptide transport in the intestinal mucosa of rabbits. Pediatr Res 1982; 16:99–103.

78. Lindberg T. Intestinal dipeptidases: characterization, development and distribution of intestinal dipeptidases of the human foetus. Clin Sci 1966; 30:505–515.

79. Rubino A, Pierro M, La Torretta G, Vetrella M, Di Martino D, Auricchio S. Studies on intestinal hydrolysis of peptides. II. Dipeptidase activity toward L-glutaminyl-L-proline and glycyl-L-proline in the small intestine of the human fetus. Pediatr Res 1969; 3:313–319.

80. De Belle RC, Vaupshas V, Vitullo BB, Haber LR, Shaffer E, Mackie GG, Owen H, Little JM, Lester R. Intestinal absorption of bile salts: immature development in the neonate. J Pediatr 1979; 94:472–476.

81. Heubi JE, Balistreri WF, Suchy FJ. Bile salt metabolism in the first year of life. J Lab Clin Med 1982; 100:127–136.

82. Short VJ, Dils R, Brindley DN. Enzymes of glycerolipid synthesis in small-intestinal mucosa of foetal and neonatal guinea pigs. Biochem J 1975; 152:675–679.

83. Holtzapple PG, Smith G, Koldovsky O. Uptake, activation, and esterification of fatty acids in the small intestine of the suckling rat. Pediatr Res 1975; 9:786–791.

84. Shiau YF, Umstetter C, Kendall K, Koldovsky O. Development of fatty acid esterification mechanisms in rat small intestine. Am J Physiol 1979; 237:E399–E403.

85. Hopkins B, Brice AL, Schofield PN, Baralle FE, Graham CF. Identity of cells containing apolipoprotein B messenger RNA, in 6-week to 12-week postfertilization human embryos. Development 1987; 100:83–93.

86. Glickman RM, Rogers M, Glickman JN. Apolipoprotein B synthesis by human liver and intestine in vitro. Proc Natl Acad Sci USA 1986; 83:296–300.

87. Jirasek JE, Uher J, Koldovsky O. A histochemical analysis of the development of the small intestine of human fetuses. Acta Histochem 1965; 22:33–39.

88. Welsh JD, Stevenson DE, Poley JR, Walker AW Jr. Intestinal alkaline phosphatase activity in relation to age in humans. J Pediatr Gastroenterol Nutr 1985; 4:954–959.

89. Tojyo Y. Developmental changeover in rat duodenal alkaline phosphatase. Comp Biochem Physiol 1984; 77B:437–441.

90. Miki K, Suzuki H, Iino S, Oda T, Hirano K, Sugiura M. Human fetal intestinal alkaline phosphatase. Clin Chim Acta 1977; 79:21–30.

91. Mulivor RA, Hannig VL, Harris H. Developmental change in human intestinal alkaline phosphatase. Proc Natl Acad Sci USA 1978; 75:3909–3912.

92. Mueller HD, Leung RA, Stinson RA. Different genes code for alkaline phosphatases from human fetal and adult intestine. Biochem Biophys Res Com 1985; 126:427–433.

93. Antonowicz I, Chang SK, Grand RJ. Development and distribution of lysosomal enzymes and disaccharidases in human fetal intestine. Gastroenterology 1974; 67:51–58.

94. Antonowicz I, Milunsky A, Lebenthal E, Shwachman H. Disaccharidase and lysosomal enzyme activities in amniotic fluid, intestinal mucosa and meconium. Biol Neonate 1977; 32:280–289.

95. Colony PC, Neutra MR. Macromolecular transport in the fetal rat intestine. Gastroenterology 1985; 89:294–306.

96. Orlic D, Lev R. Fetal rat intestinal absorption of horseradish peroxidase from swallowed amniotic fluid. J Cell Biol 1973; 56:106–119.

97. Rodewald R. Intestinal transport of antibodies in the newborn rat. J Cell Biol 1973; 58:189–211.

98. Gitlin D, Kumate J, Morales C, Noriega L, Arevalo N. The turnover of amniotic fluid protein in the human conceptus. Am J Obstet Gynecol 1972; 113:632–645.

99. Roberton DM, Paganelli R, Dinwiddie R, Levinsky RJ. Milk antigen absorption in the preterm and term neonate. Arch Dis Child 1982; 57:369–372.

100. Jakobsson I, Lindberg T, Lothe L, Axelsson I, Benediktsson B. Human α-lactalbumin as a marker of macromolecular absorption. Gut 1986; 27:1029–1034.

101. Iyengar L, Selvaraj RJ. Intestinal absorption of immunoglobulins by newborn infants. Arch Dis Child 1972; 47:411–414.

102. Ogra SS, Weintraub D, Ogra PL. Immunologic aspects of human colostrum and milk. III. Fate and absorption of cellular and soluble components in the gastrointestinal tract of the newborn. J Immunol 1977; 119:245–248.

103. Beach RC, Menzies IS, Clayden GS, Scopes JW. Gastrointestinal permeability changes in the preterm neonate. Arch Dis Child 1982; 57:141–145.

104. Weaver LT, Laker MF, Nelson R. Intestinal permeability in the newborn. Arch Dis Child 1984; 59:236–241.

105. Weaver LT, Laker MF, Nelson R, Lucas A. Milk feeding and changes in intestinal permeability and morphology in the newborn. J Pediatr Gastroenterol Nutr 1987; 6:351–358.

106. Weaver LT, Coombs RRA. Does "sugar" permeability reflect macromolecular absorption? A comparison of the gastro-intestinal uptake of lactulose and beta-lactoglobulin in the neonatal guinea pig. Int Arch Allergy Appl Immunol 1988; 85:133–135.

107. Eggermont E. Enzymic activities in meconium from human foetuses and newborns. Biol Neonate 1966; 10:266–280.

108. Wallenburg HCS. The amniotic fluid. Water and electrolyte homeostasis. J Perinat Med 1977; 5:191–205.

109. Wolf RO, Taussig LM. Human amniotic fluid isoamylases. Obstet Gynecol 1973; 41:337–342.

110. Laxova R. Antenal development of amylase isoenzymes. J Med Genet 1972; 9:321–332.

111. Potier M, Melancon SB, Dallaire L. Developmental patterns of intestinal disaccharidases in human amniotic fluid. Am J Obstet Gynecol 1978; 131:73–76.

112. Palekar AG, Maddaiah VI, Collipp PJ, Macri JN. γ-Glutamyl transpeptidase of human amniotic fluid. Am J Obstet Gynecol 1981; 141:788–791.

113. Claass AHW, Van Diggelen OP, Hauri HP, Sterchi EE, Sips HJ. Characteristics of maltase activity in amniotic fluid. Clin Chim Acta 1985; 145:275–281.

114. Boue A, Brock DJH. Prenatal diagnosis of cystic fibrosis. Lancet 1985; 2:47–48.

115. Lacroix B, Kedinger M, Simon-Assmann P, Rousset M, Zweibaum A, Haffen K. Developmental pattern of brush border enzymes in the human fetal colon. Correlation with some morphogenetic events. Early Hum Dev 1984; 9:95–103.

116. Potter GD, Lester R. Nutrient absorption in the developing colon. In: Lebenthal E, ed. Chronic diarrhea in children. New York: Nestlé, Vevey/Raven Press, 1984:193.

117. Bell L, Williams L. A scanning and transmission electron microscopical study of the morphogenesis of human colonic villi. Anat Embryol 1982; 165:437–455.

118. Cristina ML, Lehy T, Peranzi G. Etude ultrastrusturale des cellules endocrines dans le colon humain foetal. Ontogenèse et distribution. Gastroenterol Clin Biol 1978; 2:1011–1023.

119. Lehy T, Cristina ML. Ontogeny and distribution of certain endocrine cells in the human fetal large intestine. Histochemical and immunocytochemical studies. Cell Tissue Res 1979; 203:415–426.

120. Zweibaum A, Hauri HP, Sterchi E, Chantret I, Haffen K, Bamat J, Sordat B. Immunohistological evidence, obtained with monoclonal antibodies, of small intestinal brush border hydrolases in human colon cancers and foetal colons. Int J Cancer 1984; 34:591–598.

121. Jenkins HR, Milla PJ. The development of colonic transport mechanisms in early life: evidence for reduced anion exchange. Early Hum Dev 1988; 16:213–218.

122. Potter GD, Schmidt KL, Lester R. Glucose absorption by in vitro perfused colon of the fetal rat. Am J Physiol 1983; 245:G424–G430.

123. Haffen K, Kedinger M, Simon-Assmann P. Mesenchyme-dependent differentiation of epithelial progenitor cells in the gut. J Pediatr Gastroenterol Nutr 1987; 6:14–23.

124. Kedinger M, Haffen K, Simon-Assmann P. Control mechanisms in the ontogenesis of villus cells. In: Desnuelle P, Sjostrom H, Noren O, eds. Molecular and cellular basis of digestion. Amsterdam: Elsevier, 1986:323.

125. Simon-Assmann PM, Kedinger M, Grenier JF, Haffen K. Control of brush border enzyme by dexamethasone in the fetal rat intestine cultured in vitro. J Pediatr Gastroenterol Nutr 1982; 1:257-265.

126. Simon-Assmann P, Kedinger M, Grenier JF, Haffen K. Organ culture of fetal rat intestine. Effects on brush border enzyme activities of the combined administration of dexamethasone and cycloheximide or actinomycin D. Enzyme 1984; 31:65-72.

127. Lebenthal E, Sunshine P, Kretchmer N. Effect of carbohydrate and corticosteroids on activity of α-glucosidases in intestine of the infant rat. J Clin Invest 1972; 51:1244-1250.

128. Raul F, Kedinger M, Simon PM, Grenier JF, Haffen K. Comparative in vivo and in vitro effect of mono- and disaccharides on intestinal brush border enzyme activities in suckling rats. Biol Neonate 1981; 39:200-207.

129. Lacroix B, Kedinger M, Simon-Assmann PM, Haffen K. Effects of human fetal gastroenteric mesenchymal cells on some developmental aspects of animal gut endoderm. Differentiation 1984; 28:129-235.

130. Menard D, Arsenault P. Explant culture of human fetal small intestine. Gastroenterology 1985; 88:691-700.

131. Simon-Assmann P, Lacroix B, Kedinger M, Haffen K. Maturation of brush border hydrolases in human fetal intestine maintained in organ culture. Early Hum Dev 1986; 13:65-74.

132. Arsenault P, Menard D. Influence of hydrocortisone on human fetal small intestine in organ culture. J Pediatr Gastroenterol Nutr 1985; 4:893-901.

133. Menard D, Arsenault P, Pothier P. Biologic effects of epidermal growth factor in human fetal jejunum. Gastroenterology 1988; 94:656-663.

CHAPTER 19

Flora of the Gut and Protective Function*

Edgar C. Boedeker, M.D.
John S. Latimer, M.D.

The gastrointestinal (GI) tract of the normal infant is colonized during the first weeks of life with a complex, predominantly anaerobic flora. Over 400 different species have been cultured. Although variations in final flora composition occur among individuals, the variations are limited to minor species, and each individual tends to retain a flora of stable composition. The stages of development of the flora are influenced to some degree by substrate availability from the diet and in particular by breast-feeding. However, once the composition of the mature flora is established, it remains remarkably resistant to day-to-day dietary changes.

The development of the normal bacterial population of the intestine is closely inter-related with normal host development. Of particular relevance is the relation of the intestinal flora to the development of normal host systems, both immune and nonimmune, for exclusion of foreign microorganisms, toxins, and antigens. The flora stimulates the normal maturation and development of host mucosal defense mechanisms and is in turn limited by these mechanisms as well as by self-limiting elements of the mature flora.

In this chapter, we first review the characteristics of the normal stable flora, and the host and bacterial mechanisms that are currently known to influence its composition. We then review the stages of colonization of the newborn gut and the dietary and developmental factors that are known to modulate this process. Finally, we discuss abnormalities of bowel function and disease states that can be related to an immature or abnormal flora.

IMPORTANCE OF COLONIZATION IN HOST DEFENSE

Immune System Development. The normal gut is in a state of "physiologic inflammation" induced by the intestinal flora. This is best shown by comparison of mucosal immunocyte populations of normal hosts to those of germ-free animals. The presence of bacteria in the GI tract induces the activation, proliferation, and full development of the mucosal immune system,[1,2] which is characterized by the population of the lamina propria with committed antigen-specific, antibody-producing B cells, T helper and suppressor cells, mast cells, and accessory cells, including macrophages. These cells arise

from precursor cells in the Peyer's patches and other organized intestinal lymphoid tissue following bacterial antigen stimulation. These precursors circulate and mature systemically before they "home" to densely populate the lamina propria and other mucosal sites.[2] IgA antibody produced by lamina propria B cells is taken up and secreted at the mucosal surface by epithelial cells[3] to provide a protective barrier to foreign antigen uptake.

Epithelial Barrier Function. The presence of organisms in the gut induces major changes in host mucosal morphology, as shown by comparison of the intestinal tracts of germ-free and conventional animals. Germ-free animals have a sparsely populated lamina propria, longer intestinal villi, and shorter crypts.[4] These morphologic differences have functional correlates in terms of increased hydrolytic (digestive) enzyme activity, slower epithelial turnover, and altered mucosal permeability. The flora and their products may have direct effects on epithelial cell function. It has recently been shown that luminally provided products of bacterial fermentation (principally short-chain fatty acids [SCFAs]) are critical for the maintenance of normal epithelial integrity in the colon.[5] Such products are not available in the absence of flora. The flora (and in particular the anaerobic flora) may also exert degradative effects on the host glycoproteins and glycolipids that characterize the epithelial cell surface, primarily through alterations in glycoconjugates expressed on receptors and enzymes. The ability of organisms to degrade and utilize available host-specific substrates, such as the ability to degrade blood group substances, in turn gives them a selective advantage in colonizing a particular host.[6] Many of the morphologic changes associated with acquisition of the flora may be related to the expansion of the mucosal immune system with an increased mass of lamina propria immunocytes. The immunologic regulation of epithelial cell function[7] through local production of cytokines and eicosanoids, and the converse regulation of lamina propria and intraepithelial lymphocytes by epithelial cells functioning as antigen presenting cells (through their expression of HLA class I and class II molecules),[8] are areas of expanding research interest.

Colonization Resistance. An established flora in the intestinal tract has the ability to exclude subsequently introduced nonindigenous organisms and prevent them from colonizing. This property of the established flora has been termed "colonization resistance,"[9,10] and it is of particular importance in preventing colonization of the intestinal tract by pathogens. Recently the enteric flora, primarily its anaerobes, has also been implicated in limiting bacterial

* The views expressed herein are those of the author and not necessarily those of the United States Army, the United States Air Force, the Uniformed Services University of the Health Sciences, or the Department of Defense.

translocation[11-13] (as opposed to luminal or mucosal surface colonization), which is defined as the passage of viable bacteria from the lumen, through the mucosa, into the lamina propria and to mesenteric lymph nodes. Insights into the mechanisms of these protective functions of the flora have been derived both from animal studies and from studies in in vitro model systems such as continuous-flow cultures. Treatment of animals with antibiotics at doses sufficient to alter their normal anaerobic flora renders them susceptible to subsequent colonization by enteropathogens such as *Shigella* species.[14] Moreover, organisms such as *Escherichia coli*, which can readily colonize the intestine of germ-free animals if introduced as monocontaminants, are effectively excluded if introduced after the animals have been "conventionalized" by the introduction of a normal flora. In vitro studies in continuous-flow systems, which serve as models of the GI environment, suggest that this protective function resides in colonic populations of strict anaerobes and/or facultative anaerobes. Mechanisms whereby an established flora could inhibit an invading strain include the production of volatile fatty acids (VFAs), antibiotics such as colicins (bacteriocins), and other inhibitory metabolic products to which the invader is susceptible; successful competition with the intruder for nutrients in a reducing environment; and competition for attachment sites.

GASTROINTESTINAL FACTORS AFFECTING COLONIZATION

Limiting Factors. Host factors limiting bacterial proliferation operate at each level of the GI tract. *E. coli* can divide every 20 minutes; thus it could reach extraordinary mass if it could proliferate unchecked. Instead, it remains a relatively minor component of the GI flora, in part because of colonization resistance[9,15] of the competing flora, but also because of host factors that limit its survival.

Host factors limiting the proliferation of the enteric flora include (1) salivary factors including immunoglobulins; (2) gastric factors, primarily acid and pepsin secretion; (3) biliary and pancreatic factors, including proteolytic enzymes and bile salts; (4) mucin, either functioning as a barrier or promoting clearance; (5) intestinal motility; (6) immune function, which is initially provided passively but develops rapidly.

Host factors promoting the proliferation of the enteric flora

include (1) mucin, as a site for colonization and a nutrient source of endogenous substrate; (2) epithelial cell receptors; (3) dietary factors, providing exogenous substrate for bacterial growth. Substrate availability in the distal bowel is determined by the development of proximal digestive and absorptive function. Immature proximal absorptive function provides increased substrate for distal bacterial growth and fermentation in the colon.

NORMAL FLORA

Nature of Normal Flora

The normal intestinal flora is an ecosystem maintained in a dynamic steady state in the environment of the intestinal tract of the mature host. The mature conventional flora may be viewed as an "ecologic climax stage," sometimes termed "C flora."[16] This flora maintains a gradient of concentration from relatively sterile proximal regions to feces with concentrations of 10^{11-12} organisms per gram. In the distal intestine, beyond the ileocecal valve, anaerobes predominate over aerobes.

Determination of the genera and species of the flora of the GI tract or in feces by culture techniques and biochemical testing is time-consuming and difficult; nevertheless, the work of numerous investigators has yielded a fairly complete and consistent picture of the fecal flora.[17-19] The normal fecal flora consists of 90 percent obligate anaerobes. A typical analysis[17] yields the following distribution of genera and species: 25 percent *Bacteroides* (five species), 25 percent *Eubacterium* (four species), 8 percent *Fusobacterium* (one species), 9 percent *Peptostreptococcus* (one species), 12 percent *Bifidobacterium* (four species) (Table 1). The fecal flora is essentially similar to that in colon, with the exception that special populations may exist at the mucosal surface.[20]

Because of the difficulty of the determinations, exhaustive studies have not been performed on the composition of the flora from all regions of the GI tract or under all different conditions of diet, age, and development. In the end, such studies may not be definitive, since the more than 400 species that have been assigned on the basis of biochemical tests do not necessarily fully reflect the variable, but important metabolic activities of individual strains. Two newer techniques should increase the ease of analysis of the fecal flora

TABLE 1
Distribution of Major Genera of the Normal Flora

Site	Stomach	Upper Small Intestine	Distal Small Intestine	Colon/Feces
Total anaerobes	0	$0-10^3$	10^{5-7}	10^{10-12}
Bacteroides	0	$0-10^2$	10^{3-7}	10^{9-12}
Eubacterium	0	0–rare	0–rare	10^{9-12}
Bifidobacterium	0	$0-10^3$	10^{3-5}	10^{8-12}
Clostridium	0	0–rare	10^{2-4}	10^{6-9}
Total aerobes*	10^3	10^{3-4}	10^{3-7}	10^{7-11}
Enterobacter	$0-10^2$	$0-10^3$	10^{2-7}	10^{5-10}
Lactobacillus	$0-10^3$	$0-10^4$	10^{2-5}	10^{6-10}
Staphylococcus	$0-10^2$	$0-10^3$	10^{2-5}	10^{3-7}
Streptococcus	$0-10^3$	$0-10^4$	10^{2-4}	10^{5-9}

* Includes facultative anaerobes.

as well as provide new data on their function. These include the measurement of specific metabolic products in feces or culture media with gas chromatography and mass spectroscopy as well as the use of newly produced DNA probes on a quantitative basis.[17]

Studies of "conventionalization" of germ-free animals may be relevant to the initial colonization of the newborn and its development of a stable ecosystem. As flora are acquired, either by the newborn or by germ-free animals, they pass through stages of ecologic succession termed S flora.[16] Freter[21-24] has developed a mathematic model for the factors involved in successful competition and colonization, using data from such systems as gnotobiotic animals and continuous-flow cultures. The models explain colonization in terms of substrate availability and numbers of bacterial adhesion sites, with an advantage accruing to the organisms that occupy the sites first or can compete for substrate. The model predicts that a metabolically less efficient strain can compete if it has specific adhesion sites available or if it can compete successfully for nonspecific attachment sites, thereby permitting growth to exceed excretion. This model supports the important concept that growth of a successful colonizer takes place at a wall, where attachment sites are likely to be provided and unique substrates may be available.

E. coli (as well as *Clostridium difficile* and other potential invaders) are difficult to implant into the intestinal tract or into continuous-flow cultures of mature mouse cecal flora unless they are the first organisms introduced into the culture (or into germ-free animals).[22] However, in either setting, once an *E. coli* strain becomes established, it can persist following addition of the conventional flora. Factors are present in cultures of the conventional flora that inhibit *E. coli*, but the effects of these factors on *E. coli* growth can be overcome by adding glucose. This suggests that competition for rate-limiting substrate is an important factor in limiting growth. To determine the importance of substrates actually available in colon, Wilson and Freter[25] examined interactions between the entire cecal flora of masters and introduced pathogens (including *C. difficile* and *E. coli*) in in vitro culture systems. Factors accounting for the suppressive effect of the normal flora could be found in the culture supernatants if the growth medium was provided by sterile fecal pellets from germ-free mice, but no suppressive factors were found if conventional media, rather than fecal pellets, were used as a nutrient source. These results indicate that the mature conventional flora produces factors in culture which suppress the growth of invaders but that the production of these factors depends on the presence of host-derived components (provided by mucins and shed cells) that are also present in fecal pellets.

To determine which species were responsible for the production of suppressive factors, Wilson at al[16] obtained 100 isolates of anaerobic flora from adult conventional mouse feces. They found that many combinations of flora from different stages of ecologic succession inhibited colonization by *E. coli* (and by *C. difficile*), but no combination was as effective as the total natural flora. Thus the production of suppressive factors seems to involve co-operative interactions between different species present in the normal flora. A complex picture emerges in which strains compete for attachment sites with different affinities and for available substrate, some

strains utilizing specific nutrients provided by the host to provide for the specific metabolic requirements of themselves and of other strains.

Since *E. coli* introduced as the sole contaminant into germ-free animals can survive after addition of the conventional flora, whereas it cannot readily be introduced into conventional animals, it seems that the physiologic state of an already adapted bacterium may also give some advantage and that phenotypic phase variation may be involved. When an *E. coli* strain is introduced, there may be a long lag phase prior to induction of necessary enzyme systems or expression of surface adhesive factors, which would lower initial rates of multiplication to rates insufficient to permit colonization in the face of a competing flora. Trans acting inhibitors might also work at this level so that SCFAs produced in fermentation may delay multiplication of nonadapted invading bacteria but not of established bacteria. Such survival advantages would depend on strain (or even phenotypic) differences, rather than on more readily observable species differences.

Factors Affecting Colonization[26,27]

Bacterial Factors

Attachment. It may be useful to distinguish between the terms *attachment* and *adherence* by defining attachment as a preliminary, relatively weak, initial association with host surfaces that results from generic physicochemical forces (including Van der Waals, hydrogen, electrostatic, and hydrophobic bonding) shared by many bacterial species. These generic forces tend to operate over long range; therefore, they may be involved in initial steps of bacteria-host interaction, which are often reversible. Shear forces present in the gut are effective in overcoming such reversible attachment at a distance; thus organisms that are simply "attached" can be washed off.

Since both microbial and host biologic surfaces are negatively charged, they tend to repulse each other. The maximum force of electrostatic repulsion (primary energy maximum) occurs at a distance of about 5 nm (50 Å). However, there is a secondary energy minimum at 10 nm (100 Å) and a primary minimum even closer at about 2 nm (20 Å) where organisms may temporarily attach.[27] Since increased ionic strength results in a decreased thickness of the diffuse layer of countercharges over bacterial and host surfaces, increased electrolyte concentrations decrease the repulsive forces and promote attachment. Nonspecific hydrophobic forces, which generate increased interfacial tension, are even stronger than electrostatic interactions and become increasingly strong as the attaching objects approach each other. These two types of attachment forces may be sufficient to give colonization advantages to a strain. Stronger and more specific adherence forces may take over at shorter ranges of a few nanometers.

Adherence. Adherence may be defined as a stronger interaction, which approaches irreversible binding in the face of ordinarily generated shear forces in the gut. Adherent organisms cannot be washed off. Nonspecific adherence requires strongly hydrophobic structures or the presence of very high ionic strength or divalent cations. Adherence may also result from the bacterial expression of specific surface structures termed *adhesins*, which provide specific molecular recognition sites for host binding sites (host receptors). Such adhesin-receptor interactions have affinities of the order of enzyme substrate interactions. They may be strengthened by co-operative interactions among multiple sites. Adhesins prominently include pili (or fimbriae), which are hairlike protein appendages composed of multiple repeating structural subunits.[28,29] Some pili have minor subunits that contain the actual binding sites, often arrayed at the pilus tip.[30] An advantage of the hairlike morphology of pili is that they can span the distance between an attached bacterial cell and the host surface while experiencing minimal repulsion from electrostatic forces because of their small radii. Electron micrographs of piliated adherent organisms picture them tethered at distances of 100 nm (1,000 Å) or greater from the mucosal surface. Adhesins may also take other forms, including finer fibrillar structures and complex, bridging polymers, which are exported by the bacterial cells.

It is important to distinguish factors involved in pathologic colonization of the small intestine and proximal sites from those involved in normal colonization of the colon and distal sites. Many of the best-described bacterial colonization factors have been defined for those pathogens that have developed specialized mechanisms for adhering to the small intestine. Recent studies have provided evidence that such adherence alone can cause diarrhea in the small intestine,[31] even in the absence of the production of enterotoxins or other bacterial virulence factors. However, the relevance of such pathogenic mechanisms, selected to colonize proximal sites in regions where peristalsis is active, to those operative in normal colonization of the colon is not clear. By these definitions it is more likely that bacteria attach in the colon but do not adhere.[17] The relative stagnation of cecal and colonic contents favors intraluminal growth of organisms that may not be avidly adherent but can successfully compete for available nutrients. During slow transit, organisms can proliferate in the lumen, perhaps adhering to particulate matter, colonizing the biofilm, or attaching to and digesting mucus (mucin layer).

Motility of Organisms. Motile organisms may achieve bacterial velocities of 100 μ per second with kinetic energy sufficient to overcome a small energy barrier (1.5 kT). Such motility may be conferred by flagellae.[32] Motile variants of some pathogens, such as cholera,[33] have been shown to have a selective advantage in colonizing the mucus and intervillous spaces.

Enzyme Systems. Specific bacterial enzyme systems, which may be inducible for nutrient utilization, can confer a selective advantage. Of particular importance are enzyme systems for carbohydrate uptake and utilization and for complete degradation of those complex carbohydrates of host and exogenous origin which are present in the colon.[6]

Inhibitors. Some strains can achieve selective colonization advantage by the production of inhibitors of competing strains. These inhibitors include the volatile SCFAs and the colicins. Since *E. coli* is not sensitive to volatile SCFAs, these probably cannot be implicated in the suppression of *E. coli* growth by the normal flora.

Maintenance of Redox Potential. Facultative anaerobes growing at the mucosal surface maintain a reducing environment, which provides growth conditions suitable for strict anaerobes but inhibits colonization by aerobes. The facultative anaerobes and the environment they provide can be eliminated with tetracycline. This maintenance of redox potential is an example of symbiotic relations between different species.

Phase Variation. This is a genetic mechanism for maintaining an advantageous bacterial phenotype. Phase variation results from the rearrangement of genetic material, without actual mutation or gene loss, into a semistable conformation favoring expression of a particular phenotypic trait. The ability to switch to and maintain a particular phenotype (or phase) favorable for survival in a particular ecologic niche by phase variation confers an obvious survival advantage. Phase variation provides for the maintenance of an advantageous phenotype selected for or induced by the availability of a particular substrate or receptor site. The mechanism is reversible, so that if ecologic conditions change, alternate phenotypes of a particular strain can emerge and survive.

Host Factors

The mucosa presents successive layers of sites for bacteria-host interaction through attachment, adherence, and colonization within the mucous layer, the glycocalyx, and the apical membrane of absorptive epithelial cells. Progression from layer to layer is not assured, since each layer may be viewed as a potential barrier or site to which the organisms may be confined prior to clearance. Mucus may be cleared, the glycocalyx degraded, and apical membranes shed. As these sites are altered during the course of intestinal development, they present opportunities for evolving interactions with the intestinal flora. In rodents weaning occurs at 3 to 6 weeks and is a landmark of host development associated with "redifferentiation" of epithelial surface components. In humans, however, many of these host developmental changes take place before birth, whereas weaning occurs later in humans than in rodents, at a variable time from 6 months to 4 years. Thus, in breast-fed infants, the gradual transition to a typical mature flora associated with weaning may be predominantly determined by diet and the environment.

The Mucous Gel Layer (Biofilm). The 40 μm (40,000 Å) mucous layer can be viewed as a biofilm, or colonized gel, organized into an even thickness by "endogenous lectins."[34] Careful morphologic studies of the stabilized gel, combined with quantitative culture of successively removed layers, indicate that most organisms live in the biofilm, whereas only a few colonize the microvillar surface. Costerton's work emphasizes the analogies between organisms in the mucous layer and marine organisms colonizing submerged surfaces. In both systems, there are marked phenotypic differences between free-living species in the bulk fluid (lumen) and those same species adapted to growth at surfaces where they often express capsules, or slime layers.

Organisms can thrive in the mucous layer because of their ability to degrade mucins. Hoskins[35] has provided strong evidence for the role of degradation of gut mucins in the population ecology of the human enteric flora, particularly the anaerobic populations. Fermentable carbohydrate is the likely limiting nutrient in colonic microbial ecosystems, since nitrogen is available from diffused urea or shed cells. The enteric flora possesses glycosidases, not present in host tissue, which degrade mucin glycoproteins. The bacterial glycosidases are substrate-specific exoglycosidases that degrade specific carbohydrates from the nonreducing end. Endogenous substrate can be degraded by the sequential action of alpha- and beta-glycosidases. Estimates of the populations (performed by the most probable number method of serial dilutions of cultures) expressing these activities is 10^7 to 10^8 per gram, i.e., a rather small percentage of the total anaerobes.[36] Genetic and developmental traits of the host can determine the population densities of subpopulations of the bacterial flora. This is true for blood group antigens, since the bacterial glycosidases have blood group specificity. It may also be true for different carbohydrate specificities that successively appear and develop with growth and development. Mucin composition changes with age, but a specific relationship to age-related changes in flora composition has only been suggested.

The mucous gel serves a site for bacterial proliferation, but it also functions as a barrier to adherence of pathogens to epithelial cells. This has been demonstrated in cell culture for *Campylobacter jejuni*,[32] where the barrier effect is enhanced by the presence of antibody in the mucous layer. Binding to receptors in mucus[37] may be viewed either as protective against mucosal colonization or as a mechanism for growth and luminal colonization. This concept has been developed by the Forstners.[38] It is difficult to predict which side of the equation (growth vs clearance) will predominate for a given bacterial species.

Glycocalyx and Microvillous Membrane. Studies in rodents indicate that the microvillous surface undergoes marked redifferentiation at weaning associated with a change in the presence of binding sites for several commensals and pathogens. This has been best demonstrated for the small bowel attachment of pathogens. These changes at weaning, however, may be correlated with changes in the normal flora.[39]

Dietary (Exogenous) and Endogenous Substrates. In general, the colonic flora is stable to dietary changes,[40,41] at least in terms of the percentages of major subgroups and species. The biomass, i.e., the total number of organisms, can vary with diet. One-third of the colon contents is bacteria, and the bacterial mass in the colon can double as often as once every 6 hours, depending on substrate availability. Faster growth occurs in the ascending colon, slower growth distally.

Carbohydrates. The colonic flora ferments carbohydrates to CO_2, VFAs and ammonia if amino sugars are digested. The total flora can survive on plant polysaccharides and host glycoproteins.[42] Half of the celluloses and hemicelluloses are degraded in colonic passage; resulting VFAs are absorbed by the host. Bacterial enzyme systems are specific for their complex carbohydrate substrates; these include steps for enzyme binding to bacterial outer membrane components and for carbohydrate degradation. Such specificities in ability to digest a particular carbohydrate give advantages to some strains over others. Selective pressure favors strains with high affinity for growth-limiting nutrients.[43] However, the enzyme systems are inducible by the presence of substrate, which is efficient and permits the maintenance of species through differing conditions of substrate availability. In in vitro systems, populations can be favored by adding a particular substrate (such as rhamnose); however, these populations persist after the substrate is withdrawn. Although many of these individual species cannot break down naturally occurring plant carbohydrate, they may be able to utilize oligomeric digestion products produced by other species in the ecosystem, enabling mixed cultures to utilize substrates that pure cultures cannot.

A decrease in the biomass accompanies the ingestion of an elemental diet; however, this does not appreciably affect the relative composition of the flora. A chemically defined diet that provides no fat and no fiber, so that little exogenous substrate reaches the colon, can increase enterobacteria and decrease enterococci and other lactic acid bacteria. In this situation, total fecal mass decreases, but there is no change in concentration of anaerobes.[44] A high beef diet, on the other hand, does increase total anaerobes, primarily manifest by increased numbers of *Bacteroides*. Dietary fiber (i.e., nondigestible plant carbohydrate) supplementation increases total anaerobic counts. With this supplementation, trends in change of bacterial genus are not significant; total aerobic counts are stable.[17,45] Salyers[42] has examined the breakdown of the endogenous substrate chondroitin sulfate in continuous culture with results similar to those for endogenous substrates.

Dietary Lectins. As shown by the work of Banwell et al,[46,47] the feeding of plant lectins, particularly phytohemagglutinin derived from the red kidney bean, can promote both bacterial overgrowth and mucosal alteration. Although it was initially postulated that the lectin might have provided a bridge between mucosal components and the colonizing bacterial strains, it now appears more likely that a lectin-induced alteration in the apical epithelial cell surface, including a shedding of microvilli and increased turnover of surface components such as glycosphingolipids,[48] may provide a rich source of specific endogenous carbohydrate substrate for bacterial overgrowth. Lectins have been used extensively as probes for epithelial cell surface development and differentiation; thus, it is likely that specific cell surface receptors must be present for lectin-induced injury to occur. In addition, lectins are known to induce mucus release from goblet cells, thus providing an additional potential source of endogenous substrate for bacterial overgrowth.

Iron. When free iron is low, only bacteria that secrete iron-chelating agents (enterochelins) can successfully compete for available iron stores and proliferate. *Bacteroides* are inhibited by low iron conditions.[49] Clostridia and Enterobacteriaceae may not be as fastidious in their requirements, but they are inhibited by low iron during the first week of life. Breast milk is relatively low in iron, as is cow's milk. Supplementation of cow's milk with iron promotes the development of a complex flora with Enterobacteriaceae as well as *Bacteroides* and *Clostridium* species (note the predominance of bifidobacteria seen with breast-fed infants).[49]

Host Immune Mechanisms. The gut-associated lymphoid tissue (GALT) makes up 25 percent of GI mucosal mass, which can be divided into three anatomically and functionally separate areas: (1) the organized lymphoid tissue, (2) the lymphoid tissue of the lamina propria, and (3) the intraepithelial lymphocytes.[50] The organized lymphoid tissue of the gut is localized to the Peyer's patches of the small intestine, which serve as the site of initial antigen sampling and of antigen stimulation of precursor cells that migrate and mature to populate the lamina propria with immunocompetent cells. Since the population of the lamina propria is the result of trafficking of cells stimulated by contact with antigen, the development and expansion of this population of mononuclear cells are directly related to exposure to the flora as a major source of antigenic stimulation. Migrating cells also return to the Peyer's patches, to which they are targeted by recognition sites on high endothelial venules. This stimulation and migration result in increase in size of the Peyer's patch, which parallels the acquisition of the flora. The intraepithelial lymphocytes[51] are a population of predominantly suppressor/cytotoxic T cells that are located in a position uniquely suited for interactions with host epithelial cells and luminal organisms. They may also contain mast cell progenitors.

Role of Antibodies. Luminal antibodies, particularly of the IgA class, can inhibit colonization (by adherent pathogens), probably by bacterial agglutination or binding to adhesins.[52] They also are believed to block uptake of toxic macromolecules and absorption of luminal antigens. The presence of antibody can also induce genetic alterations in bacteria, in particular by inducing loss of plasmids responsible for virulence by exerting selective pressure against the organisms expressing virulence factors.[53] In this way, luminal antibody could, in theory, exert a selective pressure upon the normal flora.

Dimeric IgA antibodies are secreted by lamina propria B cells, then taken up by the epithelial cells upon interaction with secretory component in the basolateral membrane, translocated, and released by exocytosis into the lumen. This process is under some degree of neural and endocrine control.[54] IgA translocation is under autonomic control. It is stimulated by cholinergic agonists and by cholecystokinin, although this stimulation may be independent of the secretory component–mediated mechanisms. The peptide neuroendocrine hormones[55] somatostatin and vasoactive intestinal peptide both inhibit IgA production, whereas substance P stimulates lymphocyte proliferation and immunoglobulin synthesis.

Antibody to different types of antigen (protein versus carbohydrate) is secreted into different parts of the mucosal immune system. Hanson's group[56] (using monocontaminated and then conventionalized germ-free mice) has recently described differential secretion of antipilus protein (type 1) IgA into milk, whereas there is a preferential secretion of anti-lipopolysaccharide (LPS) IgA into bile. The mechanisms regulating this differential secretion of antibody of differing specificities into different regions have not been described.

Before the development of the mucosal antibody response, IgA in breast milk can provide passive protection and prevent adhesion and/or disease caused by pathogenic challenge. This passive protection of breast milk antibody has been best described in studies of neonatal diarrheas of calves and swine caused by enterotoxigenic *E. coli.*[57] Other immunoprotective factors may also be present in milk.

Role of the M Cell. The follicle-associated dome epithelium overlying the Peyer's patch contains a specialized population of distinctive cells with sparse microvilli, termed *M* (for membranous) *cells.*[58] M cells are capable of taking up by pinocytosis soluble or particulate antigens, including viruses and bacteria, and transferring them, largely unaltered, to closely underlying immunocompetent T cells, B cells, and macrophages. By this means, M cells appear to be capable of regulating the initiation of the mucosal immune response.

Evidence of the selective uptake of organisms by M cells has been best described for reovirus systems in the mouse,[59,60] in which uptake is determined by the viral hemagglutinin. M cells increase in numbers over the Peyer's patch dome with age, and their ability to take up viral particles also changes with age. Differences in selective uptake of different strains of bacteria and the bacterial and host determinants of this selectivity have not been well described, although live organisms are selectively taken up more readily than killed organisms.[61] Evidence from some bacterial systems suggests that the M cells may also serve as a site of colonization (i.e., RDEC-1 microcolonies).[62]

Role of Cellular Immunity. T cells exert important influence on the development of IgA-committed B cells in the Peyer's patch and gut mucosal lymphoid follicles. Factors produced by helper T cells in the Peyer's patch in response to MHC class II restricted antigen presentation promote B-cell activation, proliferation, and isotype switch to production of antibody of the IgA class,[50] which is the principal recognized immune effector mechanism in the gut. It is not clear that T-cell cytotoxic cellular effector mechanisms are important in the control of mucosal or luminal bacterial populations, although the possibility of IgA-mediated antibody-dependent cytotoxicity for invasive organisms such as *Salmonella* has been suggested by Tagliabue et al.[63] The presence of a population of intraepithelial lymphocytes that are predominantly of the T-cytotoxic suppressor phenotype may prove to have increased importance of regulation of bacterial populations in the gut, particularly in view of the increasing recognition of antigen-processing and presenting capability of the absorptive epithelial cells. It has been known for some time that gut epithelial cells can take up luminal antigen[64]; however, the recent recognition that these cells can express MHC class II antigens[8] under conditions of inflammation suggests that epithelial cells may serve as antigen-presenting cells, thereby stimulating cytotoxic or suppressor T cells in the intraepithelial (or lamina propria) compartments. Such T cells may play a variety of roles, including cytotoxicity for microorganisms, as suppressor cells mediating tolerance to luminal antigen, and in providing help for antibody synthesis.

Importance of Colonization to Bowel Function

The growth-stimulating and nutrient-sparing effects of administration of antibiotics with animal feed have been well-documented in animal nutrition.[65] These effects have been attributed to suppressive effects on the intestinal flora and suggest that the presence of the normal flora has a negative influence on absorptive function. It is not clear whether the growth-promoting effects of antibiotics are mediated by decreasing pathogenic organisms or by promoting growth of beneficial species.

Comparisons of intestinal structure and function of animals in the germ-free state with conventional animals provide some of the best evidence of the importance of the flora to bowel function.[4] In germ-free animals the intestinal epithelial cell turnover rate is low, and crypt–to–villous tip migration time is long compared to the situation in conventionalized animals. The changes of decreased villous height, increased crypt depth, and decreased surface area of individual villi induced by the acquisition of the normal flora (and the transition from the germ-free to the conventionalized state) are in the same direction as (but less extreme than) those further changes induced by infection and inflammation. In severe inflammatory states, villous atrophy and crypt hyperplasia result from increased cell turnover and increased epithelial cell proliferation and migration rates. Goblet cell hyperplasia and mucous depletion are also observed.

In parasite-infected rats, brush border membranes undergo changes in glycoconjugates manifest as a decreased lectin-binding capacity of the membranes, associated with decreased absorptive capacity and brush border enzyme hydrolytic activity.[66] Loss of brush border membrane enzymes and glycoproteins may be the result of increased shedding into the lumen.

Evidence is accumulating that some of the functional, structural, and morphologic epithelial changes associated with infection (and possibly with acquisition of the normal flora) may be local paracrine effects mediated by the peptide regulatory factors or other inflammatory mediator products of the cells of the mucosal immune system.[7,67] This fits well with the concept of the presence of the normal flora as a state of "physiologic inflammation." The lymphokine/cytokine products from lymphocytes include the interleukins and interferons, and those from macrophages include cachectin/tumor necrosis factor (TNF) and interleukin 1. Potential mast cell products include adenosine, histamine, serotonin, and platelet-activating factor (PAF).

The effect of immune mediators on gut epithelial function is perhaps best exemplified in an infection model of *Trichinella spiralis* in the rat. When an immune host is challenged with the larvae of the parasite, there is rapid induction of intestinal secretion. In this case, release of mast cell products has been invoked to explain both the secretory and motor responses that result in rapid clearing of the parasite.[7,67]

Despite marked differences in morphology (i.e., structure) between germ-free and conventionalized hosts, there are fewer well-defined corresponding differences in absorptive function. The total increase in gut surface area seen with conventional animals may compensate for decreased height of individual villi and decreased levels of hydrolytic enzymes associated with the brush border membranes of conventional animals.

Enzymatic activity of the flora also accounts for some of the structural and functional differences between germ-free and conventional animals. In the germ-free rodent, the cecum is enlarged. This is probably the result of the water-retentive capacity of complex carbohydrates of dietary and host origin, which are neither hydrolyzed nor fermented in the germ-free animal.[68] The presence of a mature flora capable of fermentation permits colonic salvage of unabsorbed simple and complex carbohydrates via their hydrolysis and fermentation to SCFAs. In turn, the SCFAs (VFAs—acetic, propionic, and butyric) produced by bacterial fermentation are the preferred energy source of colonic epithelial cells. Their presence (particularly N-butyrate) is important to normal colonic epithelial function.[69] This has been demonstrated in vitro with isolated colon epithelial cells and, more recently, in perfusion studies of human colons[5] of patients with diversion colitis. The importance of SCFA production to colonic functional development and the occurrence of dis-

ease is also illustrated by the case of transmissible gastroenteritis of swine.[70] Young animals, which lack a colonic flora capable of carbohydrate fermentation, are susceptible to severe diarrheal disease associated with carbohydrate malabsorption. In contrast, older animals, with a mature fecal flora, are able to develop a compensatory increase in colonic absorption mediated by the production of SCFA from fermentation of nonabsorbed dietary carbohydrate.

The production of D-lactic acid by intestinal bacteria, occasionally recognized in patients following intestinal bypass surgery, leads to a syndrome resembling ethanol intoxication with impaired cerebral function when it is absorbed.[71] Intestinal bacteria hydrolyze dietary triglycerides to fatty acids. They can also synthesize branched-chain and hydroxylated lipids from acetate. Some of these bacterial products have secretory effects. Intestinal bacteria degrade protein and urea to ammonia within the gut lumen. A limited amount of protein fermentation can occur, leading to the production of the SCFAs isobutyrate, valerate, and isovalerate,[72] although these are quantitatively less important than the products of carbohydrate fermentation. Elevated blood ammonia correlates with encephalopathy in the presence of hepatic insufficiency. There is no convincing evidence, however, that this ammonia can be reutilized by the host for the synthesis of nonessential amino acids.

Bacterial hydrolytic and dehydroxylase enzymes are also of importance to normal bile salt and metabolism. Intestinal bacteria hydrolyze conjugated bile acids secreted by the liver. Bacterial 7 alpha dehydroxylase converts primary bile acids (cholic and chenodeoxycholic acid) to the corresponding secondary bile acids (deoxycholic acid and lithocholic acid). Lithocholic acid is a potentially hepatotoxic bacterial product.

COLONIZATION OF THE NEWBORN GUT

Colonization of the newborn's intestinal tract is a process that begins at birth and proceeds rapidly during the first few days of postnatal life. The fetus emerges from a sterile amniotic cavity to encounter resident microorganisms of the mother and environment. The nature of this ambient flora and the form and sequence of exposure can significantly affect the composition of early intestinal microbial colonization. The type and composition of the infant's feeding also has been shown to affect the distribution of species in the developing flora, which will, in turn, affect the development of host defense factors. These factors include nonspecific mechanisms as well as immune-specific mechanisms determining interaction between the immature host and the enteric microflora. While many external factors are associated with the ontogeny of colonization, immaturity of neonatal intestinal structure and function also seems to affect the colonization process and enhance susceptibility to pathologic processes related to the developing flora.

Associated with the rapid evolution of fecal bacterial colony counts in the first few days of life are rapid adjustments in the quantities of specific species with attendant fluctuations in the prevalence of species. A relatively steady state in quantity and types of intestinal microorganisms is reached in most healthy newborns during the first 1 to 2 weeks of postnatal life. This flora typically remains quite stable, with

TABLE 2
Changes in Some Major Genera of the
Flora with Development

	Stage of Development			
	Two Weeks of Age (Breast-fed)	Early Weaning	Late Weaning	Mature
Enterobacter	10^{5-7}	Increasing	Decreasing	10^{4-8}
Bifidobacterium	10^{8-12}	Stable	Stable	10^{8-12}
Bacteroides	$<10^6$	Increasing	Increasing	10^{10-12}
Clostridium	$<10^6$	Increasing	Decreasing	10^{6-12}

persistent differences between breast-fed and formula-fed infants, until supplementary feedings are introduced (Table 2). With the process of weaning, a gradual change in the distribution of the flora occurs with shifts toward the characteristic pattern of the adult (see Table 1).

Description of the Developing Flora

The ontogeny of the colonic flora has been largely deduced from qualitative and quantitative studies of bacterial species in sequential postnatal fecal samples. In healthy infants, these studies typically show the initial appearance of Enterobacteriaceae and streptococci.[73] These aerobic organisms are rapidly followed by the appearance of anaerobes, with lactobacilli and *Bifidobacterium* predominating but also including *Clostridium* and *Bacteroides*.[74,75] Concentrations of enterobacteria peak in the first few days at approximately 10^9 per gram of feces.[73,76] Most studies of healthy breast-fed infants show a subsequent decline of enterobacteria by the second week of life. By the end of the first week the stools of breast-fed infants typically show *Bifidobacterium* in concentrations of 10^8 to 10^{10} per gram of feces. Other anaerobic species, including *Clostridium* and *Bacteroides*, are usually present in much lower concentrations or disappear. In contrast, the stools of formula-fed infants show a slightly lower concentration of *Bifidobacterium* by the second week,[73,76] with greater concentrations of other anaerobes, including *Bacteroides* and *Clostridium*. Although some studies have failed to show a normal predominance of *Bifidobacterium* in the stools of breast-fed infants,[77] most show as much as a 1,000:1 ratio of bifidobacilli to enterobacteria by the end of the first week. The stools of the formula-fed infants usually show enterobacteria predominating at that time.

Changes occur in the intestinal flora of breast-fed infants with the process of weaning. Weaning for human breast-fed infants is often a gradual process with progressive addition of supplemental foods and declining intake of maternal milk. Few detailed studies have been conducted during this extremely variable period with regard to type and amount of feedings and relationships to fecal flora. *E. coli*, streptococci, and clostridia increase in concentration.[78] Isolation rates of *Bacteroides* and anaerobic gram-positive cocci increase. Differences between the fecal flora composition of breast-fed and formula-fed infants begin to disappear. With completion of weaning, a conversion to the typical adult flora occurs over a period of a few months. *Bacteroides* and anaerobic

gram-positive organisms continue to increase and become approximately equal in concentration to *Bifidobacterium*. Concentrations of *E. coli*, streptococci, and clostridia again decline to levels of approximately 10^6 to 10^8 per gram of feces.

In contrast to estimates of the developing colonic flora based on studies of the fecal flora, attempts to define the microflora of the small intestine of healthy infants and children have varied widely with respect to age of subjects and methodologic approach. An intrinsic difficulty with these studies is the problem of distinguishing resident small bowel flora from bacteria that are transiently passing through following oral ingestion. This problem is compounded by the wide disparity among studies as relates to geographic localization and developmental level of study populations, factors that affect the nature of contamination from ingested sources. Because of these problems, it is not possible to construct an accurate longitudinal progression of small bowel flora with respect to age, and generalizations with respect to anatomic distribution must be interpreted cautiously. The stomach is generally relatively sterile, with small numbers of bacteria characteristic of nasopharyngeal and oral flora including *Staphylococcus epidermidis*, alpha-hemolytic streptococci, lactobacilli, and anaerobic cocci. The duodenum is typically sterile but may contain gram-positive and gram-negative aerobic organisms that are simultaneously present in the oropharynx and gastric juice. The proximal jejunum in healthy infants and children is often sterile but may contain up to 10^4 organisms per milliliter of a predominantly "oral type" of flora. Some investigations have occasionally yielded Enterobacteriaceae[79] and higher overall colony counts.[80] A recent study of the jejunal flora of healthy Danish children[80] showed a greater frequency of isolation of *H. parainfluenzae* and *H. influenzae* than from studies of adults. A gradual increase in bacterial colony counts probably occurs along the small intestine with increasing prevalence of coliforms. In the distal ileum the flora begins to resemble that of the colon in composition but remains several log concentrations lower, secondary in part to the barrier effect of the ileocecal valve.

Factors Affecting the Process (Table 3)

Maternal and Environmental Exposure

The indigenous flora of the mother and the environment provide the sources of microorganisms for neonatal gut colonization. Brook et al[81] examined the bacterial flora of the maternal cervix and newborn gastric fluid. They found a very extensive and heterogeneous group of anaerobic as well as aerobic species. There was marked overall similarity of the types and prevalence of organisms from these sites but not always concordance when comparing cultures of mothers with those of their own infants. While it is generally assumed that the rectovaginal flora of the mother is an important source for colonization of the newborn gut, data concerning the importance of this vertical transmission are somewhat conflicting. This has been most frequently studied for *E. coli*. Bettelheim and co-workers,[82] utilizing several markers of serotype and biotype, found that the majority of *E. coli* species in neonatal fecal samples were identical to those culled from

TABLE 3
Factors Affecting Newborn Colonization

Immaturity
    Immune system
    Receptors
    Secretory mechanisms
    Enzymatic mechanisms
    Motility

Exposure
    Maternal flora
    Environmental flora
    Type of delivery
    Gestational age

Feeding
    Type: breast versus formula
    Route: enteric versus parenteral
    Adequacy of nutrition

---

the mothers. Gareau and colleagues,[83] however, found that only 25 percent of full-term infants exhibited the same O group E. coli serotypes as their mothers. In another study that examined sequential paired maternal and infant fecal samples for several weeks after delivery,[84] nearly half of the cases never had any dominant fecal E. coli O type in common. The study showed a pattern of transient as well as resident fecal E. coli serotypes which was similar in infants and their mothers. The importance of environmental acquisition of organisms was further suggested by a predominating E. coli strain developing in some infants before subsequent appearance in their respective mothers. Some investigations have shown that the first strains of E. coli colonizing newborn infants persist longer than those that colonize them later.[85,86] Hospital-acquired strains are particularly likely to become residential.

The distribution of organisms in the feces of infants during the first days of life can be affected by gestational age and route of delivery. Long and Swenson[87] found a significantly lower rate of colonization with anaerobic bacteria in infants delivered by cesarean section than in infants delivered by the vaginal route. Preterm infants delivered by the vaginal route had lower anaerobic isolation rates than did their term counterparts. In contrast to the typical complex flora that evolves in the first week in infants born by vaginal delivery, the intestinal flora of infants delivered by cesarean section remains considerably more simple with fewer species present. It has been shown that the environment most typically serves as the important early source of colonization for infants delivered by cesarean section.[88,89] Whereas colonization with E. coli followed by strict anaerobes is the typical sequence for vaginally delivered infants, other enterobacteriaceae like Citrobacter, Enterobacter, and Klebsiella are more likely to be found with delayed appearance of anaerobes in infants deprived of contamination associated with vaginal delivery. The decreased bacterial exposure of infants born prematurely or by cesarean section with resultant slower colonization by anaerobes may increase the risk of invasion by pathogens. These studies also suggest that for most healthy infants the initial heavy exposure to maternal flora probably serves as the major source of the rapid development of a het-

erogeneous flora. Alterations of this exposure seem to enhance the importance of the environment as a reservoir for colonization and potential disease.

Nature of Feeding

There are probably several nonspecific as well as immune-specific factors in breast milk which contribute to the differences in the fecal flora of breast-fed and formula-fed infants. In both breast-fed and formula-fed infants the stool pH declines during the first few days, coincident with the appearance of E. coli and streptococci. By the end of the second week the stool pH of breast-fed infants has stabilized at 5 to 5.5 and acetic acid, probably produced largely by the predominating bifidobacteria, is the major detectable volatile fatty acid.[90] Bullen et al[91] have demonstrated that the acetate buffer in the stools of breast-fed infants inhibits the growth of gram-negative facultative anaerobes in vitro. Formula-fed infants have a slight rise in stool pH with the appearance of the more heterogeneous prevalent anaerobic flora. The stools of these infants contain greater quantities of other volatile fatty acids such as butyric and propionic acids.[90] Early work by Gyorgy and co-workers[92-94] in search of the "bifidus factor" of human milk identified N-acetyl-D-glucosamine and other nonprotein factors as stimulatory to the growth of Lactobacillus bifidus var. pennsylvanius. These investigators also showed the importance of lactose in promoting and glucose as well as casein in inhibiting the growth of lactobacilli.

Certain nonspecific antibacterial factors in human milk, including lysozyme and lactoferrin, may influence the spectrum of colonization by suppressing the growth of coliforms. Less marked differences from breast-fed infants occur in the fecal flora of formula-fed infants if the artificial milk preparations are chemically formulated to resemble human milk. Mevissen-Verhage and colleagues[95] have observed that infants fed a cow's milk preparation with the amount of iron decreased to concentrations found in breast milk have colonization counts of bifidobacteria similar to those of breast-fed infants and lower rates of E. coli isolation than infants fed an iron-fortified formula.

In addition to nonspecific factors, breast milk may affect susceptibility to colonization or pathogenicity of microorganisms by immune-specific mechanisms. The predominant antibody type in breast milk is SIgA.[96] The antibody secreted in breast milk is probably mostly synthesized by IgA-producing cells in the mammary glands. Breast milk contains antibodies directed to a variety of antigens, including those of bacteria colonizing the maternal gut.[97] The specificity of this response is presumed secondary to homing lymphoid cells from Peyer's patches to sites of IgA production. The role of these antibodies in protection against colonization of the newborn gut is still incompletely understood. Carlsson et al[98] found a rather constant daily secretion of SIgA antibodies to a wide variety of E. coli antigens into breast milk during the first few months of lactation. IgG antibodies to these antigens were present in cord blood, usually in much higher concentrations than in maternal serum. Further studies by this same group[84] found that these colostral IgA antibodies and transplacental IgG antibodies did not prevent intestinal colonization of infants by homologous *E. coli* strains. Similarly, human milk contains secretory IgA antibodies to K antigens, but these antibodies do not correlate with the particular K strains of *E. coli* present in the mother's flora and do not prevent colonization of the infants with *E. coli* strains carrying the corresponding K antigens.[99]

It remains unclear what specific role breast milk antibodies may play in the colonization process. They may function in ways that prevent tissue invasion or small bowel colonization while not necessarily preventing colonic colonization by homologous bacterial strains. In a prospective study on the clinical effect of breast-milk IgA antibodies against cholera, Glass et al[100] found no differences in fecal shedding of cholera by breast-fed infants as related to the antibody levels in milk but did find protection against disease in those colonized who had received higher levels of IgA antibodies to both cholera toxin and lipopolysaccharide. In addition to high levels of SIgA, breast milk contains a variety of functional immunologic cells, including macrophages, granulocytes, and T as well as B lymphocytes, but understanding of their biologic role awaits further investigation.

Host Development

The human infant is particularly susceptible to a variety of disease states that can be attributed to altered host defense mechanisms associated with an immature gut. For most animal species, the process of weaning is associated with significant changes of intestinal mucosal membrane structure and function, termed redifferentiation. Although this process is less well defined for humans, it is probable that factors of postnatal immaturity of human neonatal intestinal structure, function, and responsivity affect the colonization process as well as susceptibility to pathogenicity. It is also probable that colonization affects intestinal structure and function and that the pattern of colonization influences pathogenic susceptibility. The process of bacterial colonization requires some degree of attachment. Many nonspecific as well as immune-specific mechanisms can affect this process. Immaturity of neonatal immune function as well as nonspecific host mechanisms can influence the nature of this interaction. Differences in receptors for attachment and in responsivity to this attachment by the neonatal as compared with adult gut mucous membranes may affect susceptibility to disease. Maturational changes in quantity and physicochemical properties of intestinal secretions can influence colonization and disease process. Immaturity of intestinal motility in premature infants as well as the development of disease states that can alter motility may predispose to intestinal bacterial overgrowth.

Gastric acidity is one of the first lines of defense against orally acquired bacteria. Gastric acid secretory capacity remains low in the first months of life,[101] allowing more viable passage of ingested bacteria to the lower intestinal tract. Endogenous proteases have a role in degrading antigen, as well as affecting the expression of carbohydrate receptors on the microvillous membranes.[102] Selective deficiencies of exocrine pancreatic excretion in newborns[103] may directly affect bactericidal capability as well as antigen adherence and absorption.[104] Intestinal mucus serves as a mechanical matrix as well as offering potential carbohydrate attachment

sites for bacterial antigens. Although some of the antigenic properties of mucins in human neonates appear similar to those of adults, alteration of terminal sugars of the oligosaccharide chains could affect bacterial binding properties. Shub et al[105] have shown a reduced ratio of carbohydrate to protein as well as decreased amounts of fucose and *N*-acetylgalactosamine in newborn rat mucus. Additionally, potential alterations of stimulatory mechanisms for mucus-secreting cells in the immature intestine could affect susceptibility to microbial pathogenicity. Antigen-antibody complexes at the mucosal surface have been shown to stimulate release of mucin from goblet cells.[106] The relative deficiency of secretory antibody in neonates may affect this process.

Developmental immaturity of the microvillous membranes and alterations of the response of the epithelial cell to antigen binding by bacteria and their toxins may affect pathogenicity. Thaler et al[107] found enhanced attachment of *E. coli* to intestinal epithelial cells of infant rabbits as compared to adults. These investigators also showed enhanced adherence of *Vibrio cholerae* to preweanling as compared to weanling rat enterocytes. Pang et al[108] have found that the microvillous membrane of newborn rabbits is more fluid and disorganized than that of adult animals. They have shown age-related changes in the carbohydrate portion of microvillous membranes in rat.[109] Studies by these investigators of age and regional changes of sialyltransferase and fucosyltransferase activities[110] suggest that age-dependent regional changes in glycosyltransferase regulation play a role in the expression of altered carbohydrate characteristics of microvillous membranes during postnatal development. Cohen et al[111] have shown a greater sensitivity of immature rat intestine compared with that of the adult to heat-stable enterotoxin. *E. coli*, which liberates this toxin, is a major cause of secretory diarrhea in infants.[112,113] The increased sensitivity and secretory response are correlated with an increased number of receptors for this toxin in the jejunum of the immature animal. There is a markedly greater secretory response to cholera toxin by the proximal intestine of preweanling than of postweanling rats.[114] Seo et al[115] have demonstrated that suckling rats are much more sensitive than weanling rats to adenylate cyclase activation and cAMP accumulation induced by cholera toxin. These findings may correlate with an increased secretory response in the immature proximal intestine.

Intestinal motility serves a major protective role against overgrowth of bacteria in the small intestine. Premature infants less than 30 weeks' gestation have disorganized jejunal contraction patterns.[116] The frequency of jejunal and duodenal contractions increases at about 30 weeks postconception, and migrating myoelectric (housekeeper) complexes (MMCs) are seen at approximately 34 weeks. It is likely that immaturity of intestinal motor function encourages the development of an abnormal flora and may contribute to disease states in some preterm infants. The type of feeding can affect the GI motility of infants. Cavell[117] found that infants fed human milk have more rapid gastric emptying than formula-fed infants. Recently, Tomomasa et al[118] utilizing manometric techniques, demonstrated that a return to the interdigestive (fasting) state with MMCs occurred within 3 hours of a feeding much more frequently in breast-fed than in formula-fed infants. It is therefore possible that some influences of the type of feeding on intestinal flora may be related to motility. Disease states frequently have indirect effects on infant intestinal motility. Sick neonates are particularly prone to development of ileus and features of intestinal injury consistent with blind loop pathophysiology.

The development of immune mechanisms of the gut is dependent on exposure to luminal antigens, including those expressed on microbial organisms. The magnitude as well as the specificity of the response of the immature secretory and cellular immune system may be important in the protection against enteric infections. Intestinal colonization with *E. coli* induces a secretory SIgA response as well as the formation of serum antibodies. Salivary SIgA levels against *E. coli* O antigens in infants have been shown to be higher after 1 week of age in infants from Pakistan (an environment of heavy microbial exposure) than in Swedish infants. Feeding may also modulate the intestinal immune response to early colonization. Stephens et al[119] have demonstrated a greater response of serum antibodies to commensal *E. coli* O antigens in formula-fed than in breast-fed infants. These results suggest an increased exposure of the systemic immune system to these antigens in artificially fed infants.

Other Factors Affecting the Process

Malnutrition

Protein-calorie malnutrition results in many alterations of intestinal structure and function that may predispose to pathogenic alterations of intestinal microflora. Many of the abnormalities that occur in association with malnutrition are similar to and may aggravate the state of immaturity of newborn intestinal structure and function. These abnormalities include decreased production of secretory enzymes as well as immunoglobulins,[120,121] atrophy of small intestinal mucosa with alteration of microvillous structure and function,[122,123] and alterations of intestinal motility.[124] Diarrhea is a frequent part of the clinical picture of protein-calorie malnutrition. In infants with postnatal malnutrition, diarrhea may be related to the propensity to develop an abnormal flora due to alterations in structure and immunity. In infants demonstrating intrauterine malnutrition, altered capacity of host response and maturation in response to intestinal colonization may predispose to pathogenicity.

Contamination of the small bowel with an increase in total bacterial growth and a prevalence of coliforms has been documented by several studies of malnourished children with diarrhea in developing countries.[125-128] It is difficult to determine from these studies the cause and effect relationships among malnutrition, chronic diarrhea, and an altered intestinal microflora. Small intestinal bacterial overgrowth has been documented in numerous studies of acute[129-134] as well as chronic diarrhea[125-128] in infants and young children. Most of these studies show a qualitative shift in the type of flora from that of an "oral" type with predominance of streptococci, lactobacilli and *Candida* sp to that of a "fecal type" with predominance of *E. coli* and other coliforms. Abnormal small bowel colonization with normal colonic bacterial species has been reported in association with diarrhea caused by enteropathogens[135-137] as well as acute and chronic diarrhea in which no pathogen has been identified.[128,132,133,138] While it

is possible that unrecognized pathogens (viral or bacterial) initiated the mechanisms responsible for overgrowth, persistence of overgrowth in chronic cases suggests a potential role in the perpetuation of intestinal physiologic disturbances. The support for this hypothesis is enhanced by several studies showing a prompt response of chronic diarrhea to the administration of antibacterials.[132,139,140] Although the mechanisms resulting in small intestinal overgrowth of coliforms in malnourished children remain speculative, it is almost certain that a vicious circle ensues whereby the overgrowth aggravates the malnourished state, and consequences of malnutrition and intestinal dysfunction seem to perpetuate the overgrowth. The mechanism by which enteric overgrowth of the small intestine may promote malabsorption and structural abnormalities are numerous. They include abnormal interactions with the host defense mechanisms as well as the production of injurious metabolites and toxins. Malabsorption resulting from intestinal immaturity or injury may provide better nutrient support for establishment and maintenance of an abnormal small intestinal flora. A parallel in severity of disaccharide malabsorption and the degree of small bowel bacterial overgrowth in acute diarrhea of infancy has been noted.[134] Monosaccharide intolerance has been reported in association with bacterial overgrowth in animals.[141,142] In view of the observation in animals that glucose transport across the small intestinal mucosa is inhibited by free bile acids but not by conjugated bile salts,[143] some investigations have explored this relationship in clinical diarrhea of infancy. Some studies have revealed the co-existence of bacterial overgrowth of the small intestine and the presence of deconjugated bile salts or bacteria capable of deconjugation.[144,145] Others, however, have challenged the association and suggest a more multifactorial etiology of monosaccharide intolerance.[146] Abnormalities of intestinal motility secondary to immaturity, acute injury, or established blind loop pathophysiology may serve to encourage the persistence of an abnormal flora. Immaturities of the neonatal intestinal immune system, especially SIgA secretion, predispose to establishment of an abnormal small bowel flora initiated by a variety of potential risk factors. The often progressive state of malnutrition seen in association with chronic diarrhea states in infants of developing countries likely interferes with normal maturational development of pancreatic and intestinal function as well as important immune-specific defenses. Few studies, even of animals, have examined the recovery of intestinal structure and function following severe postnatal malnutrition. That nutrition may be a critical factor in breaking the vicious circle of diarrhea and malnutrition is suggested by observed declining small bowel bacterial populations in Guatemalan infants undergoing nutritional rehabilitation.[125]

Route of Nutrient Delivery

In developed countries, total parenteral nutrition (TPN) is often employed to abrogate the perils of malnutrition. Evidence is accruing, however, to suggest that intravenous delivery of an otherwise adequate diet for overall nutritional maintenance or growth may have a significant impact on the state of intestinal structure, function, and colonization. Studies employing weanling rats[147,148] and piglets[149] have demonstrated a significant decrease in the weights of the stomach, small intestine, and pancreas after short periods of TPN compared with matched controls receiving a nearly isocaloric standard enteral diet. The significance of these observations is enhanced by the apparent adequacy of the parenteral nutrition employed in these studies as reflected in similar overall weight gain[148,149] or similar final weights of other visceral organs in the parenterally fed compared with chow-fed animals.[147,149] Additional findings from these studies include parenteral nutrition–associated decreases in antral gastrin levels,[147] decreases in some intestinal brush border enzyme activities, and histologic mucosal hypoplasia affecting the villi more than the crypts and the jejunum more than the ileum.[148,149] Studies in more immature animal models including suckling rats[150] and neonatal piglets[151] have examined aspects of intestinal development in parenterally fed compared to enterally fed animals. These investigations have shown that the lack of intraluminal nutrition results in a retardation of intestinal growth[150,151] as well as altered maturation of mucosal enzymes.[151]

The relevance to humans of the observed intestinal hypoplasia or maturational delay in animals deprived of luminal nutrition must await further investigations. The probability that TPN affects the colonization process, perhaps related to alterations of intestinal structure and function, develops from several lines of evidence. In a recent study examining bacterial translocation from the gut as it relates to the type and route of feeding,[152] rats were randomized to receive TPN intravenously, TPN orally, or standard food. After 2 weeks, two-thirds of the parenterally fed group had culture-positive lymph nodes, compared to one-third of the group given the TPN solution orally and none of the group given standard oral feedings. A significant reduction in biliary SIgA levels was demonstrated in the parenterally fed group. A significant increase in cecal bacterial counts was noted in the animals fed by TPN, regardless of route. The most common translocating organism was *E. coli*.

A study of the effects of TPN in patients with Crohn's disease[153] has suggested the related development of alterations of some specific microflora-associated characteristics in the feces. The changes observed could be consistent with alterations of anaerobic colonization. In another study of patients with inflammatory bowel disease on TPN,[154] biliary concentrations of lithocholic acid were shown to be higher in patients who developed hepatic abnormalities than in those in whom hepatic function remained normal. Since the 7-alpha-dehydroxylation of chenodeoxycholic acid to form lithocholic acid is mainly performed by anaerobic gram-positive rods, possible mechanisms include an overgrowth of certain anaerobic species in some patients receiving TPN. Further support for the hypothesis that TPN may induce an overgrowth of intestinal anaerobic bacteria derives from several reports suggesting an amelioration of hepatic enzyme abnormalities in patients on TPN who received metronidazole.[155-157]

Investigations are clearly warranted to explore the effects of TPN on intestinal colonization in neonates and infants whose risk may be enhanced by pre-existing immaturities of intestinal colonization. Alterations of intestinal maturation and development of the flora could have significant implications for the development of disease states in this at-risk group.

CONSEQUENCES OF AN IMMATURE OR ABNORMAL FLORA

Understanding influences of the intestinal flora on host function has been greatly advanced by investigations comparing specific host parameters in germ-free animals compared with counterparts subjected to microbial association. Many of the important morphologic and physiologic implications from such studies have been delineated in this chapter as they relate to development of the host immune system and epithelial barrier function. Recent application of knowledge derived from studies on germ-free animals has permitted longitudinal investigations of microflora-associated changes in developing infants. Such tracking is made possible by the existence of specific markers of microbe-host interaction which have qualitative or quantitative differences between germ-free and conventional animals similar to the differences between newborn infants and adult humans. Preliminary findings from such studies in infants and children[158,159] suggest a slower development of a functionally active flora than might have been deduced from descriptive studies of fecal speciation and a considerable disparity in the time of onset and rate of development of different functions. It seems certain that such probes will enable further clarification of the complex interactions between the developing gut, the immature flora, and the diet. Immaturity of the host and of the intestinal flora predisposes to a variety of disease states, which underscores the delicate balance between these developing factors.

Disease States

Necrotizing Enterocolitis

Necrotizing enterocolitis (NEC) is a disease state that most frequently affects premature infants within the setting of a newborn intensive care unit (NICU). No unifying cause has been found or likely exists; however, many observations suggest that a pathogenic intestinal flora is important for the induction of this disease state. Because of the lack of any recognized absolute prerequisite for development of NEC, most hypotheses regarding pathogenesis have implicated some combination of predisposing factors. Santulli et al[160] postulated the requirements of an initiating injury to the intestinal mucosa, the presence of intestinal bacteria, and the supply of metabolic substrate in the form of feeding. These requirements are met by the majority of premature infants who develop NEC.

The occurrence of NEC in the minority of infants who do not meet all of these criteria has been postulated to represent extremes of at least two of the apparent predisposing factors.[161] A predominant importance of the early intestinal colonization process in the NICU has been proposed by Lawrence et al.[162] These investigators as well as others have shown a delay in the colonization process in the relatively aseptic NICU environment. They postulated that this delay in establishment of a typical flora predisposed infants to a greater likelihood of establishing an abnormal flora. Although the bacterial species that have most frequently been reported in association with NEC are common in healthy newborns, factors that interrupt the normal sequence of colonization may predispose to disease by allowing an overgrowth of potential pathogens. Such organisms as *E. coli*, *Klebsiella*, and *Clostridium* have often been implicated,[163-169] and epidemics of NEC have been linked to emergence of particular strains of these organisms in specific NICUs.[170-172] Lawrence and associates[162] postulated that enteritis in susceptible newborns may result from an excessive production of bacterial toxins similar to that seen in models of germ-free animals emerging from a germ-free environment. In addition to affecting susceptibility for development of disease, the degree of maturity of the neonatal intestinal mucosal barrier can affect the clinical outcome of NEC. Utilizing a neonatal animal model for NEC, Israel et al[173] have shown that treatment of mothers with steroids in late gestation results in a decreased rate of intestinal bacterial colonization and translocation which correlates with decreased severity of intestinal injury. The implications from these observations warrant further investigations regarding potential modification by intestinal growth factors of disease susceptibility and outcome in the clinical setting.

The influence of intestinal immaturity on the consequences of colonization by specific bacterial species is illustrated by the observations concerning *Clostridium difficile* and its toxins. Some clinical reports have suggested an association between a high rate of stool colonization with this organism and nursery epidemics of NEC.[174] Despite this, other studies have suggested nosocomial spread of *C. difficile* but have failed to show a difference in incidence or toxin titers in asymptomatic infants compared with those with NEC.[175,176] It is of interest that newborn infants can show a high rate of carriage of this pathogenic organism and its toxins without manifesting clinical disease. Speculations have included the possibilities that toxin receptors on the intestinal epithelium may not be fully developed and that the toxin may be more readily inactivated or blocked by products or metabolites of other bacteria.[177,178] Recently it has been shown that even if *C. difficile* and its toxins have no direct causal relationship with the development of NEC, the conditions that permit the nosocomial spread of *C. difficile* in NICUs may reflect the spread of other organisms that are pathogenic.[179] This observation provides an explanation for the disparity between colonization and lack of disease in newborns and suggests that if the organism and its toxins are pathogenic in some newborns, a coincidence of risk factors likely exists. Reports of NEC epidemics have also occasionally implicated pathogens that are not part of the typical early colonization process. Viruses as well as bacteria are among the group and include coronovirus,[180] coxsackievirus,[181] rotavirus,[182] and *Salmonella*.[183]

NEC is rare among infants who have never been fed as well as those who have been exclusively breast-fed. This observation reinforces the probability that substrate and its influences on the colonization process are important in the susceptibility to NEC. As noted earlier, breast milk provides passive immune factors and stimulates the growth of *Bifidobacterium*. The immune-specific as well as nonspecific factors that may be protective against the development of NEC can be destroyed by the denaturing effects of breast milk–banking processes.[184,185] Excessive formula feedings have been postulated to interfere with the proteolytic destruction of bacterial exotoxins.[168]

Whatever the varied and complex interactions between risk factors, it is quite certain that disturbances in the bacterial colonization process play a significant role in the development of NEC. The immaturity of GI structure and function, the risks of systemic insults leading to intestinal ischemia, and nosocomial factors are probably all important in pathogenesis.

Gastroenteritis

Acute diarrheal illness remains a major world-wide cause of childhood morbidity and mortality. There are approximately 750 million cases, with an estimated 5 million gastroenteritis deaths annually in children less than 5 years of age.[186] The etiologic agents responsible for gastroenteritis as well as the severity of clinical illness are influenced by many environmental and host-related factors. The importance of the indigenous intestinal microflora as a significant component of host defense against enteric pathogens is suggested by a variety of in vitro as well as epidemiologic clinical studies. Perhaps the single most important factor affecting the risk of diarrheal disease in infancy is breast-feeding. A World Health Organization review of the effect of breast-feeding on diarrheal illness[187] concluded that during the first 6 months of life the risk of developing diarrheal illness is nearly five times greater and the risk of death is 25 times greater for infants receiving no breast-milk than for those on exclusive breast-feeding. Although breast-feeding affords many important immune-specific advantages for the infant, its protective role likely includes its substantial effect on the development and maintenance of a unique intestinal microflora. The intestinal flora of infants who are partially breast-fed differs from that of those who are exclusively breast-fed as well as from those who are receiving no breast milk. The incidence of diarrheal illness is greatest for those receiving no breast milk and least for those exclusively breast-fed.[187] Similarly, the severity of diarrheal illnesses is greatest for exclusively formula-fed and least for exclusively breast-fed infants. If the protective effects of breast milk were due exclusively to immunologic and antimicrobial properties, the relative risk of disease for infants receiving no breast-feeding compared with partial breast-feeding should approximate that of infants receiving partial breast-feeding compared to exclusive breast-feeding. These relative risks are quite different. The literature does not suggest a higher morbidity for bottle-fed infants from poor families compared with wealthy families. Additionally, the protective effects of breast-feeding against diarrheal illness have been documented for infants in families of high socioeconomic status in developed countries[188,189] as well as those of indigent status in underdeveloped countries. The protective effects of breast-feeding against diarrheal illness in underdeveloped countries is related to factors other than just protection against exposure to enteric pathogens. In a prospective study of Guatemalan children,[78] breast-fed infants from rural areas with prevailing poor sanitation were found to have negligible infection rates with enteropathogenic *E. coli*. When weaning was initiated the incidence rose to 3.3 percent and peaked at 3.8 percent in the second year. Sequential studies of the fecal flora of the rural children showed a predominance of bifidobacteria during the period of exclusive breast-feeding, and increase in facultative organisms with early weaning, and a progressive increase in anaerobic gram-negative organisms with progressive supplementation. If protection by breast-feeding against diarrheal illness were due exclusively to protection against contamination of artificial foods, the relative risk of no breast-feeding compared with exclusive breast-feeding should approximate that of partial breast-feeding compared with exclusive breast-feeding. It does not. Protection by breast-feeding is likely provided by a combination of breast milk properties, protection from contamination, and the stimulation of a bifidus flora.

The pathogenic microbial organisms most frequently associated with gastroenteritis seem to vary according to the developmental level of the society. In contrast to underdeveloped countries where enteropathogenic bacteria have been associated with a significant percentage of diarrheal illnesses, viruses seem to cause the majority of cases of acute gastroenteritis in developed countries. In a study conducted on Swedish children with acute gastroenteritis,[190] viral, bacterial, and parasitic agents were found in 58 percent, 14 percent, and 1 percent of patients, respectively. Rotavirus was the major cause of gastroenteritis in the population and predominated as the etiologic agent in children admitted to the hospital as well as in those with milder disease who remained outpatients.

As is true of enteropathogenic bacteria, there is evidence that breast-feeding offers protection against illness from enteropathogenic viruses. There is interest in the potential role of the indigenous intestinal flora of breast-fed infants in promoting host resistance to viral enteric disease. In a prospective study of infants during a single rotavirus season, Duffy and associates[191] found no apparent difference in the infection rates of rotavirus enteritis in breast-fed and bottle-fed infants. They did observe, however, milder clinical manifestations of illness in the infected breast-fed infants. These investigators noted, in agreement with other studies, that exclusively breast-fed infants maintained a flora predominantly of bifidobacteria, whereas bottle-fed infants showed a greater diversity of flora. Analysis of the number of rotavirus particles in the stools of infected infants showed an inverse trend with the observed bifidobacteria levels.

Because of the many immune-specific components of breast milk that enhance resistance of the infant to enteropathogenic bacteria as well as viruses, it has been difficult to establish a clear cause and effect relationship between the associated characteristic normal flora and enhanced host resistance. However, the in vitro studies of Bullen and Willis[91] supported the earlier conclusions of Ross and Dawes[192] that the preponderance of lactobacilli and the acid pH of the large bowel of breast-fed infants were major factors in providing resistance to enteric infections. Studies on growth of a variety of strains of gram-negative aerobic bacilli in emulsions of feces from breast-fed and bottle-fed infants have shown clear differences. While bacterial strains multiply in fecal emulsions from bottle-fed infants at a rate comparable to that in control nutrient media, pronounced reduction in viability is noted in cultures using fecal emulsions from breast-fed infants. By reversing the pH values of the fecal emulsions, the growth patterns can be reversed. Although factors other than the differences in buffering capacity between breast milk and cow's milk have been advanced as relevant, it is apparent that factors in breast milk

are favorable for the growth of a lactobacillary flora and maintenance of an acid pH which suppress the growth of E. coli as well as other enterobacteria. The occurrence rates of enteropathogenic E. coli as well as salmonella diseases are significantly lower in breast-fed than in bottle-fed infants.[78,193] If a cause and effect relationship exists between the indigenous microflora and host resistance to enteropathogenic viruses, further research will be needed to explore possible mechanisms. Possibilities include effects of interactions of the native flora with the immune-specific defenses.

Sepsis

The risk of developing sepsis is higher in infancy than in childhood and is particularly significant for premature and otherwise "high-risk" newborns. The GI tract of infants serves as an important portal of entry for the systemic spread of organisms. This is especially evident in cases in which sepsis occurs in association with such disease states as NEC or transmissible gastroenteritis and blood cultures correlate with a predominance of a particular pathogen in stool. It is less evident but probably no less important when no obvious intestinal disease state exists. The GI tract of newborns is, as has been discussed, presented with a heterogeneous but variable load of maternal and environmental flora. The nature, timing, and sequence of exposure to this ambient flora is probably important not only to patterns of intestinal colonization but also to risk of systemic infection. Although immunologic factors clearly play an important role in the defense against invasion by potential pathogens, interactions between bacteria can influence this process. Studies employing gnotobiotic mice models have demonstrated the importance of bacterial interactions within the gut as well as immune factors in the susceptibility to translocation of bacteria across the intestinal mucosa. Germ-free mice inoculated intragastrically with a bacterial suspension prepared from the entire ceca of adult control-specific pathogen-free mice show a high rate of translocation of bacteria to the mesenteric lymph nodes.[194] Viable bacteria are not detected in the mesenteric lymph nodes of control-specific pathogen-free mice intragastrically inoculated with the same suspension. Of interest, certain bacteria, including Lactobacillus acidophilus and E. coli, preferentially translocate in the gnotobiotes despite the prevalence of anaerobes in both the inoculum and the resultant intestinal flora of the inoculated animals. Additional studies with this model[12] have shown that certain indigenous bacteria translocate to the mesenteric lymph nodes more readily if gnotobiotic mice are inoculated with a single bacterial strain rather than whole cecal flora. Germ-free animals, when provided a gastric inoculum of E. coli alone, have a much higher incidence of recovery of the organism from mesenteric lymph nodes than do germ-free animals inoculated with E. coli associated with the cecal contents of pathogen-free animals. It has also been shown that the GI population by E. coli persisted at much higher levels in the monoassociated animals compared to the gnotobiotes associated with both E. coli and a cecal flora. Such studies have provided insights into the probable importance of bacterial antagonism of GI population levels of certain indigenous bacteria by other species of the normal flora. Such antagonism also appears to be an important defense against translocation of indigenous bacteria across the intestinal mucosa. The germ-free model is in some important respects similar to the human newborn. To the extent that the animal studies are relevant to humans, factors that interrupt the normal sequence toward development of a healthy heterogeneous flora may predispose to intestinal or systemic disease states.

Chronic Intestinal Disease States

The idea that the early intestinal colonization process may affect the potential for development of chronic disease states is an intriguing possibility. Using animal models, numerous investigators have shown a difference in the immune response to intestinal antigens depending on the age of exposure. Whereas the normal adult response to intestinal exposure of foreign antigens is the development of immune tolerance, neonatal animals are likely to manifest hypersensitivity.[195] The mechanism leading to immune tolerance includes the stimulation of T suppressor cells by absorbed antigen, with consequent blocking of a systemic response. The primary response seen with exposure in the neonatal period seems related to a net gain in T help, which prevents the induction of hyporesponsiveness. Although immaturity of the neonatal immune system may predispose to this altered response, other GI immaturities could be important. Permeability of the neonatal gut mucosa to macromolecules is increased.[64,196] Immaturity of digestive factors, including quantity and types of luminal proteases, may alter the nature of antigen exposure from food as well as bacterial proteins and toxins. Digestion of certain proteins such as ovalbumin in the adult GI tract produces both tolerogenic and immunogenic fragments.[197] Consequently, incomplete proteolysis of proteins with greater capacity of absorption in neonates may be important for the development of hypersensitivity states. The relevance of priming of the immune system by exposure to antigens has certainly received considerable attention in the context of the pathogenesis of food allergies. Shorter and colleagues[198] proposed that such mechanisms may be relevant to the development of chronic inflammatory bowel diseases. They speculated that hypersensitivity to normal intestinal bacterial antigens may occur in infancy owing to immaturity of the mucosal barrier. The primed GALT can later be exposed to cross-reacting antigens as a result of an intercurrent disease disrupting the intestinal mucosa. This exposure could then lead to the formation of humoral antibodies with cross-reactivity to antigens present on both bacteria and colonic epithelial cells. Other chronic intestinal disease states such as celiac disease may share a similar mechanism of predisposition. Kagnoff[199] has noted that patients with HLA genotypes frequently associated with celiac disease have an increased likelihood of early GALT priming to certain adenoenteric viruses. One strain of such a virus shares a homologous peptide sequence with gliadin peptides associated with mucosal injury in celiac disease.

Although the pathogenesis of many chronic intestinal disease states awaits further research, it remains probable that for many a combination of predisposing factors is necessary. Just as they affect the development of such overt neonatal intestinal disease states as necrotizing enterocolitis, it is likely that factors related to early neonatal intestinal colonization in association with intestinal immaturity can participate in susceptibility to later pathologic host responses.

SUMMARY

The mature intestinal microflora constitutes a stable ecosystem with important effects on bowel function and host protection. Factors that maintain the equilibrium of this system include complex regulatory interactions of microorganisms with each other and with the host. The immature gut manifests underdevelopment of virtually all recognized host factors that either encourage or limit enteric microbial proliferation. This state imparts a unique vulnerability to the newborn upon exposure to ambient flora. For most newborns, initial exposure to organisms colonizing the mother provides a safe transition from the "germ-free" disease-susceptible state to a rapidly established "conventional" host-protective state. The colonization process results in maturational changes of those host factors that regulate the process. Breast-feeding provides additional protection by modulating the developing microflora while the infant's own regulatory mechanisms are developing. Newborns deprived of normal maternal exposure and nurturance are more susceptible to the acquisition of an abnormal and even hostile flora that may adversely affect host development at a most critical stage and impart susceptibility to a variety of disease states. A greater understanding of the long-term influences of the early colonization process on host function may eventually enable us to elucidate the pathogenesis of many chronic disease states.

REFERENCES

1. Simon GL, Gorbach SL. Intestinal flora and gastrointestinal function. In: Johnson LR, ed. Physiology of the gastrointestinal tract. 2nd ed. New York: Raven Press, 1987:1729.
2. Craig SW, Cebra JJ. Peyer's patches: an enriched source of precursors for IgA-producing precursors in the rabbit. J Exp Med 1971; 134:188–195.
3. Solari R, Kraehenbuhl JP. The biosynthesis of secretory component and its role in the transepithelial transport of IgA dimer. Immunol Today 1985; 6:17–20.
4. Abrams GD, Bauer H, Sprinz H. Influence of the normal flora on mucosal morphology and cellular renewal in the ileum. A comparison of germ free and conventional mice. Lab Invest 1962; 12:355–364.
5. Harig JM, Soergel MS, Komorowski RA, Wood CM. Treatment of diversion colitis with short-chain fatty acid irrigation. N Engl J Med 1989; 320:23–28.
6. Hoskins LC. Human enteric population ecology and degradation of gut mucins. Dig Dis Sci 1981; 26:769–772.
7. Castro GA. Immunological regulation of epithelial function. Am J Physiol 1982; 243:G321–G329.
8. Mayer L, Shlien R. Evidence for function of Ia molecules on gut epithelial cells in man. J Exp Med 1987; 166:1471–1483.
9. van der Waaij D, Berghouis de Vries JM, Lekkerherk van deer Wees JEC. Colonization resistance of the digestive tract in conventional and antibiotic treated mice. J Hyg (Lond) 1971; 69:405–411.
10. Hentges DJ. Role of the intestinal microflora in host defense against infection. In: Hentges DJ, ed. Human intestinal microflora in health and disease. New York: Academic Press, 1983:311.
11. Berg RD, Garlington AW. Translocation of certain indigenous bacteria from the gastrointestinal tract to mesenteric lymph nodes and other organs in a gnotobiotic mouse model. Infect Immun 1979; 23:403–404.
12. Berg RD, Owens WE. Inhibition of viable *Escherichia coli* from the gastrointestinal tract of mice by bacterial antagonism. Infect Immun 1979; 25:820–827.
13. Wells CL, Maddaus MA, Jechorek RP, Simmons RL. Role of intestinal anaerobic bacteria in colonization resistance. Eur J Clin Microbiol Infect Dis 1988; 7:107–113.
14. Freter R. Experimental enteric *Shigella* and *Vibrio* infection in mice and guinea pigs. J Exp Med 1956; 104:411–418.

15. Gorbach SL, Barza M, Giuliano M, Jacobus NV. Colonization resistance of the human intestinal microflora: testing the hypothesis in normal volunteers. Eur J Clin Microbiol Infect Dis 1988; 7:98–102.

16. Wilson KH, Patel M, Permoad P, Moore L. Ecologic succession—use in development of synthetic microfloras. Microecol Ther 1986; 16:181–189.

17. Salyers AA, Kuritza AP, McCarthy RE. Influence of dietary fiber on the intestinal environment. Proc Soc Exp Biol Med 1985; 180:415–421.

18. Moore WEC, Holdeman LV. The normal flora of 8 Japanese-Hawaiians. Appl Microbiol 1978; 7:961–979.

19. Bingen E, Lambert-Exchovsky N. Technical aspects of the quantitative and differential analysis of the microbial intestinal ecosystem. Antibiotic therapy and intestinal microbial ecosystem in the neonate. Dev Pharmacol Ther 1984; 7(suppl 1):134–137.

20. Tannock GW. Demonstration of mucosa-associated microbial populations in the colons of mice. Appl Environ Microbiol 1987; 53:1965–1968.

21. Freter R, Stauffer E, Cleven DD, Holdeman LV, Moore WEC. Continuous flow cultures as in vitro models of the ecology of large intestinal flora. Infect Immun 1983; 39:666–675.

22. Freter R, Brickner H, Botney M, Cleven D, Aranki A. Mechanisms that control bacterial populations in continuous flow culture models of mouse large intestinal flora. Infect Immun 1983; 39:676–685.

23. Freter R, Brickner H, Fekete J, Vickerman MM, Carey KE. Survival and implantation of Escherichia coli in the intestinal tract. Infect Immun 1983; 39:686–703.

24. McKay IC, Speekenbrink A. Implications of Freter's model of bacterial colonization. Infect Immun 1984; 44:199–203.

25. Wilson KH, Freter R. Interaction of Clostridium difficile and Escherichia coli with microfloras in continuous flow cultures and gnotobiotic mice. Infect Immun 1986; 54:354–358.

26. Ofek I, Beachey EH. General concepts and principles of bacterial adherence in animals and man. In: Beachey EG, ed. Bacterial adherence. London: Chapman and Hall, 1980:1.

27. Gristina AG, Taylor PT, Myrvik Q. The race for the surface: microbes, tissue cells and biomaterials. In: Switalski L, Hook M, Beachey E, eds. Molecular mechanisms of microbial adhesion. New York: Springer Verlag, 1989:177.

28. Klemm P. Fimbrial adhesions of Escherichia coli. Rev Infect Dis 1985; 7:321–340.

29. Rose AH, Tempest DW. The physiology and biochemistry of pili. Adv Microb Physiol 1988; 29:53–114.

30. Hanson MS, Brinton CC. Identification and characterization of Escherichia coli type-1 pius tip adhesion protein. Nature 1988; 332:265–268.

31. Wahnke C, Nellans HS, Guerrant RL. Small bowel colonization alone is a cause of diarrhea. Infect Immun 1987; 55:1924–1926.

32. McSweegan E, Burr DH, Walker R. Intestinal mucus gel and secretory antibody are barriers to Campylobacter jejuni adherence to int 407 cells. Infect Immun 1987; 55:131–135.

33. Freter R, Jones GW. Adhesive properties of Vibrio cholerae: nature of the interaction with intact mucosal surfaces. Infect Immun 1976; 14:246–256.

34. Costerton JW. The microbial colonization of the gut—a balance between host factors and ecological relationships. Microecol Ther 1986; 16:191–193.

35. Hoskins LC, Boulding ET. Degradation of blood group antigens in human colon ecosystems II, a gene interaction in man that affects fecal population density of certain enteric bacteria. J Clin Invest 1976; 57:74–78.

36. Miller RS, Hoskins LC. Mucin degradation in human colon ecosystems. Fecal population densities of mucin-degrading bacteria estimated by a "most probable number" method. Gastroenterology 1981; 81:758–765.

37. Cohen PA, Waldowski JC, Laux D. Adhesion of a human fecal Escherichia coli strain to a 50.5 kD receptor present in mouse colonic mucus. Microecol Ther 1986; 16:231–243.

38. Forstner G, Sherman P, Forstner J. Mucus: function and structure. In: Boedeker EC, ed. Attachment of organisms to the gut mucosa, Vol II. Boca Raton, FL: CRC Press, 1985:13.

39. Schiffrin EJ, Israel EJ, Carter EA, Benjamin J, Walker WA. Influence of prenatal mucosal barrier maturation on bacterial colonization in the newborn. Gastroenterology 1989; 96:A448.

40. Bjornside GH. Stability of the human fecal flora. Am J Clin Nutr 1983; 31:S1–9.

41. Hentges DJ. Does diet influence human fecal microflora composition? Nutr Rev 1980; 38:39–336.

42. Salyers AA, Vercellotti JR, West SEH, Wilkins D. Fermentation of mucins and polysaccharides by anaerobic bacteria from the human colon. Appl Environ Microbiol 1977; 33:319–332.

43. Mason TG, Richardson G. Observations on the in vivo and in vitro competition between strains of E. coli isolated from the human gut. J Appl Bacteriol 1982; 53:19–27.

44. Crowther S, Drasar BS, Goddard P, Hill MJ, Johnson K. The effect of a chemically defined diet on the faecal flora and faecal steroid concentration. Gut 1983; 14:790–793.

45. Fuchs H-M, Dorfaman S, Floch MH. The effect of dietary fiber supplementation in man. II. Alteration in fecal physiology and bacterial flora. Am J Clin Nutr 1976; 29:1443–1447.

46. Banwell JG, Bolut FM, Meyers J, Weber FL. Phytohemagglutinin derived from the red kidney bean (phaseolus vulgaris): a cause for intestinal malabsorption associated with bacterial overgrowth in the rat. Gastroenterology 1984; 84:500–515.

47. Ceri H, Falkenberg-Anderson K, Fang R, Costerton JW, Howard R, Banwell JG. Bacteria-lectin interactions in phytohemagglutinin-induced bacterial overgrowth of the small intestine. Can J Microbiol 1988; 34:1003–1008.

48. Larson G, Watsfeld P, Falk P, Leffler H, Koprowski H. Fecal excretion of intestinal glycosphingolipids by newborns and young children. FEBS Lett 1987; 214:41–44.

49. Mevissen-Verhage EA, Marcelis JH, de Vos MN, Harmsen-van Amerongen WCM, Verhoef J. Bifidobacterium, Bacteroides, and Clostridium spp. in fecal samples from breast-fed and bottle-fed infants with and without iron supplement. J Clin Microbiol 1987; 25:285–289.

50. Kawanishi H. Recent progress in immune responses in the gut. Dig Dis 1989; 7:113–124.

51. Cerf-Bensussan N, Guy-Grand D, Griscelli C. Intraepithelial lymphocytes of human gut: isolation, characterization and study of natural killer activity. Gut 1985; 26:81–88.

52. Fubara ES, Freter R. Protection against enteric bacterial infection by secretory IgA antibodies. J Immunol 1973; 111:395–403.

53. Linggood MA, Porter P. Antibody-induced elimination of the plasmid controlled K88 adhesion factor from a porcine enteropathogen. Immunology 1978; 35:125–127.

54. Freier S, Lebenthal E. Neuroendocrine-immune interactions in the gut. J Pediatr Gastroenterol Nutr 1989; 9:4–12.

55. Stanisz AM, Befus D, Bienenstock J. Differential effect of vasoactive intestinal peptide, substance P and somatostatin on immunoglobulin synthesis and proliferation by lymphocytes from Peyer's patches, mesenteric lymph nodes and spleen. J Immunol 1986; 136:152–156.

56. Nilsson K, Dahlgren UI, Hanson LA. Different origins of IgA antibodies with various antigen specificities appearing in rat bile. Scand J Immunol 1988; 28:547–551.

57. Rutter M, Jones GW, Brown GTH, Burrows MR, Luther PD. Antibacterial activity in colostrum and milk associated with protection of piglets against enteric disease caused by K88 positive Escherichia coli. Infect Immun 1976; 13:667–676.

58. Sneller MC, Strober W. M cells and host defense. J Infect Dis 1986; 154:737–741.

59. Wolf JL, Rubin DH, Finberg R, Kauffman RS, Sharpe AH, Trier JS, Fields BN. Intestinal M cells: a pathway for entry of reovirus into the host. Science 1981; 212:471–472.

60. Wolf JL, Kauffman RS, Finberg R, Dambrauskas R, Fields BN, Trier JS. Determinants of reovirus interaction with intestinal M cells and absorptive cells of murine intestine. Gastroenterology 1983; 85:291–300.

61. Owen RL, Pierce NF, Apple RT, Cray WC. M cell transport of Vibrio cholerae from the intestinal lumen into Peyer's patches: a mechanism for antigen sampling and for microbial transepithelial migration. J Infect Dis 1986; 153:1108–1118.

62. Inman LR, Cantey JR. Specific adherence of Escherichia coli (Strain RDEC-1) to membranous (M) cells of the Peyer's patch in Escherichia coli diarrhea in the rabbit. J Clin Invest 1983; 71:1–8.

63. Tagliabue A, Nencioni L, Villa L, Kerren DF, Lowell GF, Borashi D. Antibody dependent, cell-mediated antibacterial activity of intestinal lymphocytes with secretory IgA. Nature 1983; 306:185–186.

64. Walker WA, Isselbacher KJ. Uptake and transport of macromolecules by the intestine: possible role in clinical disorders. Gastroenterology 1974; 67:531–550.

65. Stokstad ELR. Antibiotics in animal nutrition. Physiol Rev 1954; 34:515–548.
66. Castro GA, Harari Y. Intestinal epithelial membrane change in rats immune to *Trichinella spiralis*. Mol Biochem Parasitol 1982; 6:191–202.
67. Russell DA, Castro GA. Physiology of the gastrointestinal tract in the parasitized host. In: Johnson LR. Physiology of the gastrointestinal tract. 2nd ed. New York: Raven Press 1987:1749.
68. Loesche WJ. Effect of bacterial contamination on cecal size and cecal contents of gnotobiotic rodents. J Bacteriol 1969; 99:520–526.
69. Roediger WEW. Role of anaerobic bacteria in the metabolic welfare of the colonic mucosa in man. Gut 1980; 212:793–798.
70. Argenzio RA, Moon HW, Kenny LJ, Whipp SC. Colonic compensation in transmissible gastroenteritis of swine. Gastroenterology 1984; 86:1501–1509.
71. Perlmutter DH, Boyle JT, Campos JM, Egler JM, Watkins JB. D-lactic acidosis in children: an unusual metabolic complication of small bowel resection. J Pediatr 1983; 102:234–238.
72. Rasmussen HS, Holtug K, Morensen PB. Degradation of amino acids to short chain fatty acids in humans. An in vitro study. Scand J Gastroenterol 1988; 23:178–182.
73. Grutte FK, Horn R, Haenel H. Ernahrung und biochemisch-mikrookologische vorgange im enddarm von saulingen. Z Kinderchir 1965; 93:28–39.
74. Cooperstock MS, Zedd AJ. Intestinal flora of infants. In: Hentges D, ed. Human intestinal microflora in health and disease. New York: Academic Press, 1983:79.
75. Hoogkamp-Korstanje JAA, Lindner JGEM, Marcelis JH. Den Daas-Slagt H, DeVos NM. Composition and ecology of the human intestinal flora. Antonie Van Leeuwenhoek 1979: 45:35–40.
76. Willis AT, Bullen CL, Williams K, Fagg CG, Bourne A, Vignon M. Breast milk substitute: a bacteriologic study. Br Med J 1973; 4:67–72.
77. Simhon A, Douglas JR, Drasar BS, Soothill JF. Effect of feeding on infant's fecal flora. Arch Dis Child 1982; 57:54–58.
78. Mata LV, Urrutia JJ. Intestinal colonization of breast- fed children in a rural area of low socio-economic level. Ann NY Acad Sci 1971; 176:93–109.
79. Albert MJ, Phat P, Rajan D. Jejunal microbial flora of southern Indian infants in health and with acute gastroenteritis. J Med Microbiol 1978; 11:433–440.
80. Justesen T, Nielsen DH, Hjelt K, Krasilnikoff PA. Normal cultivable microflora in upper jejunal fluid in children without gastrointestinal disorders. J Pediatr Gastroenterol Nutr 1984; 3:683–686.
81. Brook I, Barrett CT, Brinkman CR III, Martin WD, Finegold SM. Aerobic and anaerobic flora of the maternal cervix and newborn gastric fluid and conjunctiva: a prospective study. Pediatrics 1979; 63:451–455.
82. Bettelheim KA, Teoh-Chan CH, Chandler ME, O'Farrell SM, Rahamin L, Shaur EJ, Shooter RA. Further studies of *Escherichia coli* in babies after normal deliveries. J Hyg Camb 1974; 73:277–285.
83. Gareau FE, Mackel DC, Boring JR III, Payne FJ, Hammett FL. The acquisition of fecal flora by infants from their mothers during birth. J Pediatr 1959; 54:313–318.
84. Gothefors L, Carlsson B, Ahlstedt S, Hanson LA, Winberg J. Influence of maternal gut flora and colostrum and cord serum antibodies on presence of *Escherichia coli* in faeces of the newborn infant. Acta Paediatr Scand 1976; 65:225–232.
85. Gage P, Gunther CB, Spaulding EH. Persistence of *E. coli* serotypes in the stools of infants. Bact Proc 1961; 61:117.
86. Kuhn I, Tullus K, Mollby R. Colonization and persistence of *Escherichia coli* phenotypes in the intestines of children aged 0 to 18 months. Infection 1986; 14:7–12.
87. Long SS, Swenson RM. Development of anaerobic fecal flora in healthy newborn infants. J Pediatr 1977; 91:298–301.
88. Rotimi VO, Duerden B. The development of the bacterial flora in normal neonates. J Med Microbiol 1981; 14:51–62.
89. Neut C, Bezirtzoglou E, Romand C, Beerens H, Delcrois M, Noel AM. Bacterial colonization of the large intestine in newborns delivered by cesarean section. Zentralbl Bakteriol Hyg 1987; A266:330–337.
90. Bullen CL, Tearle PV, Stewart MG. The effect of "humanized" milks and supplemented breast feeding on the faecal flora of infants. J Med Microbiol 1977; 10:403–413.
91. Bullen CL, Willis AT. Resistance of the breast-fed infant to gastroenteritis. Br Med J 1971; 3:338–343.
92. Gyorgy P, Kuhn R, Rose CS. Bifidus factor: II. Its occurrence in milk from different species and in other natural products. Arch Biochem Biophys 1954; 48:202–208.
93. Gyorgy P. A hitherto unrecognized biochemical difference between human milk and cows milk. Pediatrics 1953; 11:98–107.
94. Gauhe A, Gyorgy P, Hoover RE, Kuhn R, Rose CS, Ruelius HW, Zilliken F. Bifidus factor IV. Preparation obtained from human milk. Arch Biochem Biophys 1954; 48:214–224.
95. Mevissen-Verhage EAE, Marcelis JH, Harmsen-van Amerongen WCM, deVos NM, Berkel J, Verhoef J. Effect of iron on neonatal gut flora during the first week of life. Eur J Clin Microbiol 1985; 4:14–18.
96. McClelland DBL, McGrath J, Samson RR. Antimicrobial factors in human milk. Acta Paediatr Scand (Suppl) 1978; 271:1–20.
97. Goldblum RM, Ahlstedt S, Carlsson B. Antibody-forming cells in human colostrum after oral immunization. Nature 1975; 257:797–798.
98. Carlsson B, Gothefors L, Ahlstedt S, Hanson LA, Winberg J. Studies of *Escherichia coli* O antigen specific antibodies in human milk, maternal serum and cord blood. Acta Paediatr Scand 1976; 65:216–224.
99. Carlsson B, Kaijser B, Ahlstedt S, Gothefors L, Hanson LA. Antibodies against *Escherichia coli* capsular (K) antigens in human milk and serum. Acta Paediatr Scand 1982; 71:313–318.
100. Glass RI, Svennerholm A, Stoll BJ, Khan MR, Hussain KM, Huq MI, Holmgren J. Protection against cholera in breast- fed children by antibodies in breast milk. N Engl J Med 1983; 308:1389–1392.
101. Hyman PE, Clarke DD, Everett SL, Sonne B, Stewart D, Harada T, Walsh JH, Taylor IL. Gastric acid secretory function in preterm infants. J Pediatr 1985; 106:467–471.
102. Alpers DH, Tedesco FJ. The possible role of pancreatic proteases in the turnover of intestinal brush border proteins. Biochim Biophys Acta 1975; 401:28–40.
103. Lebenthal E, Lee PC. Development of functional response in human exocrine pancreas. Pediatrics 1980; 66:556–560.
104. Udall JN, Bloch KJ, Vachino G, Feldman P, Walker WA. Development of the gastrointestinal mucosal barrier IV. The effect of inhibition of proteolysis on the uptake of macromolecules by the intestine of the newborn rabbit before and after weaning. Biol Neonate 1984; 45:289–295.
105. Shub MD, Pang KY, Wan DA, Walker WA. Age-related changes in chemical composition and physical properties of mucus glycoproteins from rat small intestine. Biochem J 1982; 215:405–411.
106. Walker WA, Wu M, Bloch K. Stimulation by immune complexes of mucus release from goblet cells of the rat small intestine. Science 1977; 197:370–372.
107. Thaler MM, Hirschberger M, Mirelman D. Adherence of *E. coli* to immature intestine is mediated by mucosal receptors of mannose-specific bacterial toxins. Clin Res 1977; 25:469A.
108. Pang KY, Bresson JL, Walker WA. Development of the gastrointestinal mucosal barrier. III. Evidence for structural differences in microvillus membranes from newborn and adult rabbits. Biochem Biophys Acta 1983; 727:201–208.
109. Pang KY, Bresson JL, Walker WA. Development of gastrointestinal surface VIII. Lectin identification of carbohydrate differences. Am J Physiol 1987; 252:G685–G691.
110. Chu SH, Walker WA. Developmental changes in the activities of sialyl- and fucosyl-transferases in rat small intestine. Biochim Biophys Acta 1986; 883:496–500.
111. Cohen MB, Moyer MS, Luttrell M, Giannella RA. The immature rat small intestine exhibits an increased sensitivity and response to *Escherichia coli* heat stable enterotoxin. Pediatr Res 1986; 20:555–560.
112. Guerrant RL, Moore RA, Kirshen PM, Sande MA. Role of toxigenic and invasive bacteria in acute diarrhea of childhood. N Engl J Med 1975; 293:567–573.
113. Levine MM, Caplan ES, Waterman D, Cash RA, Hornick RB, Snyder MJ. Diarrhea caused by *Escherichia coli* that produce only heat-stable enterotoxin. Infect Immun 1977; 17:78–82.
114. Chu SH, Ely IG, Walker WA. Age and cortisone alter host responsiveness to cholera toxin in the developing gut. Am J Phys 1989; 256:G220–G225.
115. Seo JK, Chu SW, Walker WA. Development of intestinal host defense: an increased sensitivity in the adenylate cyclase response to cholera toxin in suckling rats. Pediatr Res 1989 25:225–227.
116. Morriss FV, Moore M, Weisbrodt NW, West MS. Ontogenic development of gastrointestinal motility, IV. Duodenal contractions in preterm infants. Pediatrics 1986; 78:1106–1113.

117. Cavell B. Gastric emptying in infants fed human milk or infant formula. Acta Paediatr Scand 1981; 70:639–641.
118. Tomomasa T, Hyman PE, Itoh K, Hsu JY, Koizumi T, Itoh Z, Kuroume T. Gastroduodenal motility in neonates: response to human milk compared with cow's milk formula. Pediatrics 1987; 80:434–438.
119. Stephens S. Development of secretory immunity in breast fed and bottle fed infants. Arch Dis Child 1986; 61:263–269.
120. Barbezat GO, Hansen JDL. The exocrine pancreas and protein-calorie malnutrition. Pediatrics 1968; 42:77–92.
121. Gomez F, Galvan RR, Cravioto J, Frenk S. Studies on the undernourished child: XI. Enzymatic activity of the duodenal contents in children affected with third degree malnutrition. Pediatrics 1954; 413:548–552.
122. Brunser O, Caslillo C, Araya M. Fine structure of the small intestinal mucosa in infantile marasmic malnutrition. Gastroenterology 1976; 70:495–507.
123. Stanfield JP, Hutt MSR, Tunnicliffe R. Intestinal biopsy in kwashiorkor. Lancet 1965; ii:519–523.
124. James WPT. Sugar absorption and intestinal motility in children when malnourished and after treatment. Clin Sci 1970; 39:305–318.
125. Mata LJ, Kimenez F, Cordon MSM, Rosales R, Prera B, Schneider RE, Viteri F. Gastrointestinal flora of children with protein-calorie malnutrition. Am J Clin Nutr 1972; 25:1118–1126.
126. Heyworth B, Brown J. Jejunal microflora in malnourished Gambian children. Arch Dis Child 1974; 50:27–33.
127. Gracey M, Suharjono, Sunoto, Stone DE. Microbial contamination of the gut: another feature of malnutrition. Am J Clin Nutr 1973; 26:1170–1174.
128. Gracey M, Stone DE. Small-intestinal microflora in Australian aboriginal children with chronic diarrhea. Aust NZ J Med 1972; 3:215–219.
129. Fagundes Neto F, Toccalino H, Dujoveney F. Stool bacterial aerobic overgrowth in the small intestine of children with acute diarrhea. Acta Paediatr Scand 1976; 65:609–615.
130. Bishop RF, Barnes GL, Townley RRW. Microbial flora of the stomach and small intestine in infantile gastroenteritis. Acta Paediatr Scand 1974; 63:418–422.
131. Stintzing G, Mollby R. Colonization of the upper jejunum by enteropathogenic and enterotoxigenic Escherichia coli in paediatric diarrhoea. Acta Paediatr Scand 1982; 71:459–465.
132. Househam KC, Mann MD, Mitchell J, Bowie MD. Duodenal microflora in infants with acute diarrheal disease. J Peadiatr Gastroenterol Nutr 1986; 5:721–725.
133. Hill ID, Mann MD, Moore L, Bowie MD. Duodenal microflora in infants with acute and persistent diarrhea. Arch Dis Child 1983; 58:330–343.
134. Coello-Ramirez P, Lifshitz F. Enteric microflora and carbohydrate intolerance in infants with diarrhea. Pediatrics 1972; 49:233–242.
135. Black RE, Brown KH, Becker S. Effect of diarrhea associated with specific enteropathogens on the growth of children in rural Bangladesh. Pediatrics 1984; 73:799–805.
136. Smalley JR, Klish WJ, Brown MR, Campbell MA. Chronic diarrhea associated with Campylobacter. Clin Pediatr 1982; 21:220.
137. Pignata C, Guandalini S, Guarino B, Devizia B, Capano G, DeRitis G. Chronic diarrhea and failure to thrive in an infant with Campylobacter jejuni. J Pediatr Gastroenterol Nutr 1984; 3:812–814.
138. Challacombe DN, Richardson JM, Rowe B, Anderson CM. Bacterial microflora of the upper gastrointestinal tract in infants with protracted diarrhoea. Arch Dis Child 1974; 49:270–277.
139. Bowie MD, Mann MD, Hill ID. Commentaries: the bowel cocktail. Pediatrics 1981; 67:920–921.
140. Hill ID, Mann MD, Househam KC, Bowie MD. Use of oral gentamicin, metronidazole and cholestyramine in the treatment of severe persistent diarrhea in infants. Pediatrics 1986; 77:477–481.
141. Gracey M, Burke V, Thomas JA, Stone DE. Effect of microorganisms isolated from the upper gut of malnourished children on intestinal sugar absorption in vivo. Am J Clin Nutr 1975; 28:841–845.
142. Lifshitz F, Wapnir RA, Wehman HJ, Hawkins RL, Diaz- Bensussen S. Enteric microflora effects on intestinal transport of carbohydrates. Fed Proc 1974; 33:673.
143. Dawson AM, Isselbacher KJ. Studies on lipid metabolism in the small intestine with observations on the role of bile salts. J Clin Invest 1960; 39:730–740.
144. Hill MJ, Draser BS. Degradation of bile salts by human intestinal bacteria. Gut 1968; 9:22–27.
145. Gracey M, Burke V, Anderson CM. Association of monosaccharide

146. Kilby AM, Dolby JM, Honour P, Walker-Smith JA. Duodenal bacterial flora in early stages of transient monosaccharide intolerance in infants. Arch Dis Child 1977; 52:228–234.
147. Johnson LR, Copeland EM, Dudrick SJ, Lichtenberger LM, Castro GA. Structural and hormonal alterations in the gastrointestinal tract of parenterally fed rats. Gastroenterology 1975; 68:1177–1183.
148. Hughes CA, Dowling RH. Speed of onset of adaptive mucosal hypoplasia and hypofunction in the intestine of parenterally fed rats. Clin Sci 1980; 59:317–327.
149. Goldstein RM, Hebiguchi T, Luk GD, Taqi F, Guitarte TR, Franklin FA Jr, Niemiec PW, Dudgeon DL. The effects of total parenteral nutrition on gastrointestinal growth and development. J Pediatr Surg 1985; 20:785–791.
150. Castillo RO, Pittler A, Costa F. Intestinal maturation in the rat: the role of enteral nutrients. J Parenter Enter Nutr 1988; 12:490–495.
151. Morgan W III, Yardley J, Luk G, Niemiec P, Dudgeon D. Total parenteral nutrition and intestinal development: a neonatal model. J Pediatr Surg 1987; 22:541–545.
152. Alverdy JC, Aoys E, Muss GS. Total parenteral nutrition promotes bacterial translocation from the gut. Surgery 1988; 104:185–190.
153. Leijonmarck CE, Bergstrand LO, Carlstedt-Duke B, Gustafsson A, Midtvedt AC, Norin KE, Saxerholt H, Midtvedt T. Total parenteral nutrition and the function of the intestinal microflora in Crohn's disease. Scand J Gastroenterol 1988; 23:59–64.
154. Fouin-Fortunet H, Le Quernec L, Erlinger S. Hepatic alterations during total parenteral nutrition in patients with inflammatory bowel disease: a possible consequence of lithocholate toxicity. Gastroenterology 1982; 82:932–937.
155. Capron JP, Gineston L, Herve MA, Braillon A. Metronidazole in prevention of cholelithiasis associated with total parenteral nutrition. Lancet 1983; i:446–447.
156. Elleby H, Solhaug H. Metronidazole, cholestasis and total parenteral nutrition. Lancet 1983; i:1161.
157. Lambert R, Thomas SM. Metronidazole prevention of serum liver enzyme abnormalities during total parenteral nutrition. J Parenter Enter Nutr 1985; 9:501–503.
158. Norin KE, Gustafsson BE, Lindblad BS, Midtvedt T. The establishment of some microflora-associated biochemical characteristics in feces from children during the first year of life. Acta Paediatr Scand 1985; 74:207–212.
159. Midtvedt AC, Carlstedt-Duke B, Norin KE, Saxerholt H, Midtvedt T. Development of five metabolic activities associated with the intestinal microflora of healthy infants. J Pediatr Gastroenterol Nutr 1988; 7:559–567.
160. Santulli TV, Schullinger JN, Heird WC, Gongaware RG, Wigger J, Barlow B, Blanc WA, Berdon WE. Acute necrotizing enterocolitis in infancy: a review of 64 cases. Pediatrics 1975; 55:376–387.
161. Kosloske AM. Pathogenesis and prevention of necrotizing enterocolitis: a hypothesis based on personal observation and a review of the literature. Pediatrics 1984; 74:1086–1092.
162. Lawrence G, Bates J, Gaul A. Pathogenesis of neonatal necrotizing enterocolitis. Lancet 1982; i:137–139.
163. Bell MJ, Feigin RD, Ternberg JL, Brotherton T. Evaluation of gastrointestinal microflora in necrotizing enterocolitis. J Pediatr 1978; 92:589–592.
164. Speer ME, Taber LH, Yow MD, Rudolph AJ, Urteaga J, Waller S. Fulminant neonatal sepsis and necrotizing enterocolitis associated with a "nonenteropathogenic" strain of Escherichia coli. J Pediatr 1976; 89:91–95.
165. Guinan M, Schaberg D, Bruhn FW, Richardson CJ, Fox WW. Epidemic occurrence of neonatal necrotizing enterocolitis. Am J Dis Child 1979; 133:594–597.
166. Howard FM, Flynn DM, Bradley JM, Noone P, Szawatkowski M. Outbreak of necrotizing enterocolitis caused by Clostridium butyricum. Lancet 1977; 2:1099–1102.
167. Kliegman RM, Fanaroff AA, Izant R, Speck WT. Clostridia as pathogens in neonatal necrotizing enterocolitis. J Pediatr 1979; 95:287–289.
168. Kosloske AM, Ulrich JA, Hoffman H. Fulminant necrotizing enterocolitis associated with clostridia. Lancet 1978; ii:1014–1016.
169. Strum R, Staneck JL, Stauffer LR, Neblett WW II. Neonatal necrotizing enterocolitis associated with penicillin-resistant, toxigenic Clostridium butyricum. Pediatrics 1980; 66:928–931.
170. Powell J, Bureau MA, Pare C, Gaildry ML, Cabana D, Pitriquin H.

Necrotizing enterocolitis: epidemic following an outbreak of *Enterobacter Cloacae* type 3305573 in a neonatal intensive care unit. Am J Dis Child 1980; 134:1152–1154.

171. Stanley MD, Null DM Jr, de Lemos RA. Relationship between intestinal colonization with specific bacteria and the development of necrotizing enterocolitis. Pediatr Res 1977; 11:543.

172. Bell MJ, Shackelford P, Feigin RD. Epidemiologic and bacteriologic evaluation of neonatal necrotizing enterocolitis. J Pediatr Surg 1977; 14:1–4.

173. Israel EJ, Schiffrin EJ, Carter EA, Freiberg E, Walker WA. Corticosteroids as prophylaxis against necrotizing enterocolitis. Pediatr Res 1989; 25:219a.

174. Cashore WJ, Peter G, Lauermann M, Stonestreet BS, Oh W. Clostridia colonization and clostridial toxin in neonatal necrotizing enterocolitis. J Pediatr 1981; 98:308–311.

175. Sherertz RJ, Sarubbi FA. The prevalence of *Clostridium difficile* and toxin in a nursery population: a comparison between patients with necrotizing enterocolitis and an asymptomatic group. J Pediatr 1982; 100:435–439.

176. Donta ST, Myers MG. *Clostridium difficile* toxin in asymptomatic neonates. J Pediatr 1982; 100:431–434.

177. Rolfe RD, Helebian S, Finegold SM. Bacterial interference between *Clostridium difficile* and normal fecal flora. J Infec Dis 1981; 143:470–475.

178. Ryan RW, Kwasnik I, Tilton RC. Rapid detection of *Clostridium difficile* toxin in human feces. J Clin Microbiol 1980; 12:776–779.

179. Burdon DW, Thompson H, Candy DCA, Kearns M, Lees D, Stephen J. Enterotoxin(s) of clostridium difficile. Lancet 1981; ii:258–259.

180. Chany C, Moscovici O, Lebon P, Rousset S. Association of coronavirus infection with neonatal necrotizing enterocolitis. Pediatrics 1982; 69:209–214.

181. Johnson FE, Crnic DM, Simmons MA. Association of fatal coxsackie B2 viral infection and necrotizing enterocolitis. Arch Dis Child 1977; 52:802–804.

182. Rotbart HA, Leven MJ, Yolken RH, Manchester DK, Jantzen J. An outbreak of rotavirus-associated neonatal necrotizing enterocolitis. J Pediatr 1983; 103:454–459.

183. Stein H. Necrotizing enterocolitis in black neonates. S Afr Med J 1977; 51:199–200.

184. Kliegman RM, Pittard WB, Fanaroff AA. Necrotizing enterocolitis in neonates fed human milk. J Pediatr 1979; 95:450–453.

185. Barrie H. Human milk banks. Lancet 1982; i:284.

186. Cohen JP, Giannella RA. Bacterial diarrheal disease: host and bacterial factors involved in intestinal infection. Viewp Dig Dis 1987; 19:1–4.

187. Feacham RG, Koblisnky MA. Interventions for the control of diarrheal diseases among young children: promotion of breastfeeding. Bull WHO 1984; 62:271–286.

188. Ironside AG, Tuxford AF, Heyworth B. A survey of infantile gastroenteritis. Br Med J 1970; 3:20–24.

189. Larsen SA, Homer DR. Relation of breast versus bottle feeding to hospitalization for gastroenteritis in a middle-class U.S. population. J Pediatr 1978; 92:417–418.

190. Uhnoo I, Wadell G, Svensson L, Olding-Stenkvist E, Ekwall E, Molby R. Aetiology and epidemiology of acute gastro-enteritis in Swedish children. J Infect 1986; 13:73–89.

191. Duffy LC, Riepenhoff-Talty M, Byers TE, La Scolea LJ, Zeilezny MA, Dryja DM, Ogra PL. Modulation of rotavirus enteritis during breastfeeding. Arch Dis Child 1986; 140:1164–1168.

192. Ross CAC, Dawes EA. Resistance of the breast-fed infant to gastroenteritis. Lancet 1954; i:994–998.

193. France GL, Marmer DJ, Steele RW. Breast-feeding and *Salmonella* infection. Am J Dis Child 1980; 134:147–152.

194. Berg RD, Garlington AW. Translocation of certain indigenous bacteria from the gastrointestinal tract to the mesenteric lymph nodes and other organs in a gnotobiotic mouse model. Infect Immun 1979; 23:403–411.

195. Strobel S, Ferguson A. Immune responses to fed protein antigens in mice. III. Systemic tolerance or priming is related to age at which antigen is first encountered. Pediatr Res 1984; 18:588–594.

196. Robertson DM, Paganelli R, Dinwiddie R, Levinsky RJ. Milk antigen absorption in the preterm and term neonate. Arch Dis Child 1982; 57:369–372.

197. Dosa S, Pesce AJ, Ford DJ, Muckerheide A, Michael JG. Immunological properties of peptic fragments of bovine serum albumin. Immunology 1979; 38:509–517.

198. Shorter RG, Huizenga KA, Spencer RJ. A working hypothesis for the etiology and pathogenesis of nonspecific inflammatory bowel disease. Am J Dig Dis 1972; 17:1024–1032.

199. Kagnoff MF. Celiac disease: genetic, immunological and environmental factors in disease pathogenesis. Scand J Gastroenterol 1985; 114:45–54.

CHAPTER 20

Development of Immune Function

John N. Udall Jr., M.D., Ph.D.
Ronald R. Watson, Ph.D.

The intestine is a complex organ with diversified functions that include digestion, absorption, and excretion. It also functions to protect the host from a large number of chemicals, potential antigens, and pathogens. The protective function of the gastrointestinal (GI) tract can be divided into nonimmunologic and immunologic host defense mechanisms, neither of which is fully developed in infancy. Nonimmunologic mechanisms of host defense include gastric acidity, intestinal lysozyme, lactoferrin, proteolytic enzymes, bile acids, and peristalsis. These mechanisms are enhanced by specific humoral and cellular immunologic defenses.

Immunoglobulins constitute the humoral arm of immunity and are present in saliva, intestinal fluid, and bile. They complex with noxious substances, pathogenic organisms, or potential allergens, impeding their absorption from the intestine. Immunoglobulins in the intestine are produced in large part by plasma cells (B lymphocytes) present in the lamina propria. The cellular arm of the immune system is mediated via T lymphocytes, which are particularly effective in protecting the host against fungi, parasites, intracellular viral infections, neoplastic cells, and foreign tissue. The humoral and cellular components of immunity provide overlapping protection and are to some extent interdependent. In addition to B and T lymphocytes, macrophages, mast cells, mucous cells, and other nonlymphoid cells are important to immunologic surveillance of the GI tract (Table 1).

This chapter discusses the development of GI immune function. The development of nonimmunologic mechanisms of intestinal host defense has been reviewed elsewhere.[1,2]

TABLE 1
Cells Potentially Important For
Normal Immunologic Surveillance of the
Gastrointestinal Tract

Humoral immune system
  B lymphocytes
  Plasma cells

Cellular immune system
  Helper T lymphocytes
  Suppressor T lymphocytes
  Killer T lymphocytes

Accessory cells
  Macrophages
  Mast cells
  Mucous cells
  Hepatic cells

IMMATURITY OF IMMUNE FUNCTION

There are several lines of evidence to suggest that immune function of the intestine is immature early in life. Studies of the intestinal uptake of macromolecules suggest that increased amounts of undigested molecules are taken up intact by the newborn compared with the adult.[1-3] This may be a mechanism by which some animals acquire passive immunity, since immunoglobulins present in maternal milk are transported across the intestine of the suckling young of certain species. In addition, there also appears to be increased transport of nonimmunoglobulin macromolecules in most, if not all, newborn animals.[1,2]

We have attempted to systematically quantitate macromolecular absorption in developing animals using electroimmunodiffusion of blood samples obtained from animals following a feeding of bovine serum albumin.[4,5] Blood obtained from newborn rabbits 4 hours after the gavage of a physiologic amount of bovine serum albumin (BSA) contained approximately $5\mu g$ of immunoreactive BSA (iBSA) per milliliter of plasma (Table 2). Weaned animals given the same amount of BSA per unit of body weight did not have detectable plasma iBSA after the feed. Even when blood was obtained from older animals over 24 hours following the BSA feed we were unable to detect iBSA in the plasma of the mature animals using electroimmunodiffusion. However, with a more sensitive radioimmunoassay, nanogram quantities of BSA were detected in the plasma of older animals. The vascular clearance of radiolabeled BSA was also assessed. Newborn animals had an increased clearance of plasma BSA compared with adult animals.[4] We concluded that the increased levels of plasma iBSA in newborn animals following BSA feeding did not represent a decrease in the clearance of the intravascular protein but instead indicated an increased absorption of intact BSA.

There is also evidence that the intestine of human infants is more permeable to the uptake of macromolecules than the intestine of adults. Infants and children have increased amounts of anti-milk antibodies in their serum compared with adults, perhaps secondary to an increased transport of intact protein across the intestine and subsequent stimulation of systemic immunity.[6]

We have attempted to obtain direct evidence of intestinal permeability in humans during development. The intestinal uptake and excretion of lactose in newborns and adults were compared.[7] Normal newborns and adults were given lactose as a standard formula or a 20 percent solution, respectively. Newborns and adults ingested the same amount of lactose

TABLE 2
Plasma Immunoreactive Bovine Serum Albumin (iBSA)
in Rabbits Four Hours After Feeding Bovine Serum
Albumin (BSA)

Age	Dose of BSA (mg per 100 g Bodyweight)	ND/NT	iBSA (μg per ml Plasma)
1 day (suckling)	200	8/9	5.5 ± 1.5*
1 week (suckling)	100	14/15	6.1 ± 0.8
2 weeks (suckling)	200	5/5	3.8 ± 0.5
4 weeks (weaning)	200	0/10	ND
52 weeks (weaned)	100	0/2	ND

* $\bar{x}$ ± SEM.
ND/NT = number of animals with detectable iBSA per number of animals tested.
ND = not detectable.
From Udall et al.[5]

per kilogram of body weight. Baseline and three hourly breath samples were obtained for determination of breath hydrogen concentration to eliminate lactose malabsorption as a variable. No newborn or adult had lactose malabsorption, defined as a breath hydrogen concentration after lactose ingestion of greater than 20 ppm above the baseline breath hydrogen. Urine was collected over a 3-hour interval following lactose ingestion, and lactose, galactose, and creatinine urine concentrations were determined. (It is important to note that absorbed lactose is not hydrolyzed but is excreted unchanged in the urine.) We found a dramatic increase in the urinary excretion of lactose in newborns compared with adults when both groups ingested similar amounts of lactose (Table 3). A smaller subset of adults was given lactose as standard infant formula in a dose similar to the amount the infants ingested. Lactose excretion in the urine of adults remained low compared with that in infants. Therefore, we conclude that the intestinal uptake of intact lactose is increased in the newborn.[7] The observation that the young transport increased amounts of macromolecules across the intestinal epithelium compared with adults may be related to immaturity of both immunologic and nonimmunologic host defense factors.[1,2]

The increased macromolecular uptake across the intestine early in life is associated with a high incidence of cow's milk protein intolerance in infants. This has been reported to be 0.3 to 7.5 percent in different series.[6] Cow's milk sensitivity is largely a disease of infancy and is uncommonly diagnosed beyond age 3 years. Although this sensitivity may be secondary to the increased permeability of the intestine of newborns, it may also be due in part to the fact that infants are exposed to increased amounts of cow's milk protein, or infants may have altered immune function compared with adults, accounting for an increased reactivity to exogenous proteins. It is possible that all these factors may be operating to put the infant at risk for the development of allergies.

Additional evidence for immaturity of intestinal immune function early in life relates to the observation made by a number of investigators that the level of secretory IgA (SIgA) lining the intestine has not reached adult levels in this age group (Fig. 1 and 2). Burgio et al measured SIgA in the saliva of healthy human subjects from 2 months to 27 years of age.[8] They suggested that there is a physiologic deficiency of SIgA and secretory antibodies in infancy and childhood. Their findings are supported by the findings of Perkkio and Savilahti.[9] These investigators noted a deficiency of immunoglobulin-containing cells in the gut of newborn humans up to 12 days of age. They suggested that a reduction in immunoglobulin-producing cells and SIgA in the intestine of infants may account for the increased incidence of infection at mucosal surfaces early in life and may also be a factor in the development of atopic diseases.[9]

Additional studies have shown that the ability of the GI immune system of premature newborns must be compromised, as judged by a humoral response to the feeding of an exogenous protein. This was shown by Reiger and Rothberg, who fed BSA to human newborns at different gestational ages and followed the development of serum anti-BSA antibodies.[10] Four of five infants 35 weeks' gestation or older developed antibody to BSA, whereas none of eight infants younger than 35 weeks' gestation produced anti-BSA. However, factors other than gestational age appear to be important for a normal humoral immune response following protein ingestion. Newborn and germ-free animals exposed to a paucity of intestinal antigens have a striking absence of antibody-producing cells in the intestine and little humoral response.[11–14] Age plus antigenic exposure appears important in contributing to the normal development of intestinal immune function. Additional factors may also be necessary to

TABLE 3
Urinary Lactose Excretion ($\bar{x}$ 2 SEM) of Infants
and Adults Following the Ingestion of Lactose

Group	Lactose Intake (mg/kg)	Urine Volume (ml/kg)	Urine Lactose (mg/ml/kg)	Urine Lactose/ Creatinine (mg/mg)
Newborn (N = 10)	0.71 ± 0.11	5.8 ± 0.8	5.4 ± 1.26	2.37 ± 0.39
Adult (N = 18)	0.72 ± 0.05	4.7 ± 0.8	0.3 ± 0.06	0.12 ± 0.02
P value	N/S	N/S	<0.001	<0.001

N/S = not significant.
From Bezerra et al[7]; with permission of John Wiley & Sons, Inc, © 1988.

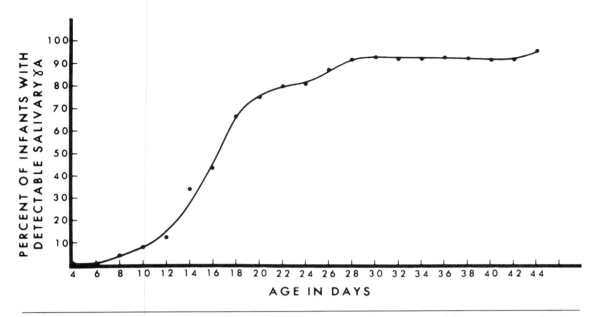

FIGURE 1 Cumulative percentage of infants with detectable salivary IgA at different ages. Each point represents a minimum of 18 and a maximum of 30 infants studied. (From Selner et al.[88])

complete the process of immune maturation, such as T lymphocytes, macrophages, and possibly soluble adjuvants in breast milk.[15-17] These factors may be important in antigen presentation and helping plasma cells (B lymphocytes) to produce antibodies to T-dependent antigens.

As noted above, the immaturity of intestinal immune function may increase the risk of GI infection in infants and children. It was noted as early as 1900 that infants had an increased death rate from enteric infections compared with older children.[18] In 1900 the death rate in New York City from dysentery, diarrhea, and enteritis in the first year of life was 5,603 per 100,000 infants per year, compared with preschool children of 1 to 4 years, who had a death rate from enteric infections of 399 per 100,000 children per year.[18] More recently, the increased susceptibility of infants to infectious enteritis has been suggested by data from the Centers for Disease Control. In 1981, salmonellosis in children under 4 years in the United States accounted for 35 percent of the reported cases of salmonellosis in all age groups.[19] However, it is important to point out that the reporting system may have inherent bias. Many factors, including intensity of surveillance, severity of illness, access to medical care, and association with a recovered outbreak affect whether an infection is reported.[20]

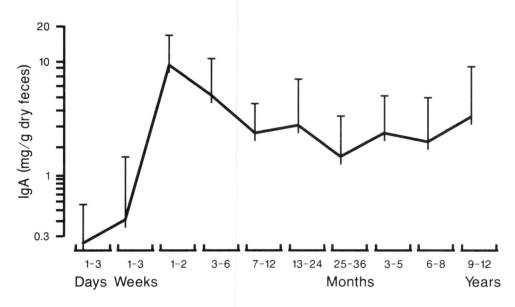

FIGURE 2 The mean concentrations of IgA in extracts of single small samples of feces from infants and children of various age groups. The material collected at 1 to 3 days of age was meconium. The upper standard deviations are indicated by vertical lines. The number of individuals in each age group varied from 9 to 22. (From Bradtzaeg et al[64]; © CRC Press, Inc.)

ABSORPTION OF MATERNAL ANTIBODIES

Maternal antibodies, especially IgG, help protect the newborn during the susceptible neonatal period from pathogenic organisms and potential allergies. These antibodies are transported from mother to developing animal in utero in humans and rabbits.[21] In other mammalian species maternal IgG is acquired not in utero, but postnatally from breast milk. Newborn sheep, cows, and horses transport IgG intact from the intestinal lumen into the blood.[21] Although the absorption and transport of maternal IgG from breast milk are not thought to occur in humans, several studies oppose this view. Iyengar and Selvaraj measured serum immunoglobulin levels from birth to 5 days of age.[22] Levels of serum IgA, IgM, and IgG on the fifth day of life were significantly higher in human colostrum-fed newborns compared with infants who were fed a cow's milk–based formula.[22] Vukavic has also attempted to determine if newborn infants absorb IgA from maternal milk.[23] On the third day of life, she detected IgA in the serum of all infants who were breast-fed. On the other hand, infants fed pasteurized human breast milk, which is devoid of immunoreactive IgA, had no detectable IgA in their blood.[23] Finally, Ogra and colleagues administered human colostrum, rich in IgA antibody against poliovirus, in a single feed to newborns whose umbilical cord blood was negative for anti-polio antibody.[24] The anti-polio antibody was detected in the blood of three of seven infants fed the colostrum, further suggesting that transport of intact immunoglobulin across the human intestine occurs in human infants.[24]

GASTROINTESTINAL-ASSOCIATED LYMPHOID TISSUE

Gastrointestinal-associated lymphoid tissue (GALT) is the basis of immune host defense of the intestinal tract. GALT includes lymphocytes scattered throughout the lamina propria of the intestine between the epithelial cells and organized into aggregates such as are found in Peyer's patches, the tonsils, and the appendix. It is generally considered that the aggregated lymphoid structures are the principal sites in the mucosa where interaction of antigen from the gut lumen and circulating lymphocytes takes place. On the other hand, the scattered lymphocytes in the lamina propria and epithelium are the effector cells that mediate immune responses.[25]

Peyer's patches, located in the ileum, are made up of clusters of lymphoid follicles having well-defined structures.[26] They consist of four compartments: (1) Lymphoid *follicles* are localized below the muscularis mucosa and show all the signs of active lymphocytopoiesis. (2) Small mature lymphocytes surround the follicles, forming the *corona*. These are mainly B lymphocytes. (3) The *intrafollicular area* can be recognized by the presence of specialized venules with a high cobblestone type epithelium. The interfollicular area contains mainly T lymphocytes and also has been called the traffic area, because of the constant influx of lymphocytes from the blood, enabling an exchange of immunologic information. (4) The follicles cause the epithelium to bulge into the lumen like the dome of a church, and this protuberance is called the *dome area*.[26]

Peyer's patches are well developed early in fetal life.[26] However, it is a few weeks after birth before activated lymphoid follicles appear in the intestine. Antigenic stimulation is necessary to activate the lymphoid follicles. The size and number of human Peyer's patches increase up to puberty. After puberty there is a rapid falling off in number of Peyer's patches, although patches remain in older mammals (Fig. 3).

Overlying Peyer's patches are specialized cells that appear to sample antigen, viral particles, and bacteria present in the intestinal tract. These microfold-cells (M cells), as they are called, have a paucity of microvilli, a poorly developed glycocalyx, and an absence of lysosomal organelles (Fig. 4). Horseradish peroxidase has been used by Owen and Jones to study macromolecular uptake by M cells.[27,28] The marker is taken up into the specialized cells, rapidly released into the interstitial space, and processed by lymphoid cells circulating through Peyer's patches. This mechanism of macromolecular transport appears to represent an important specialized access route for ingested antigens to reach lymphoid tissues and thereby stimulate the local and distant immune systems.

Intact macromolecules as well as viral and bacterial particles are processed by M cells. Wolf and colleagues inoculated reovirus into the intestinal lumen of mice; then, using electron microscopy, they noted that viruses were adherent to the surface of the intestinal M cells but not to other epitheli-

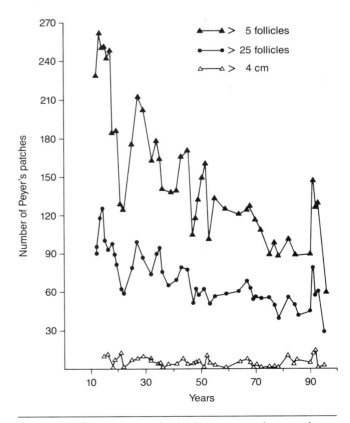

FIGURE 3 The number and size of Peyer's patches are shown for different age groups. The graph was drawn according to data from Cornes.[89] (From Pabst.[26])

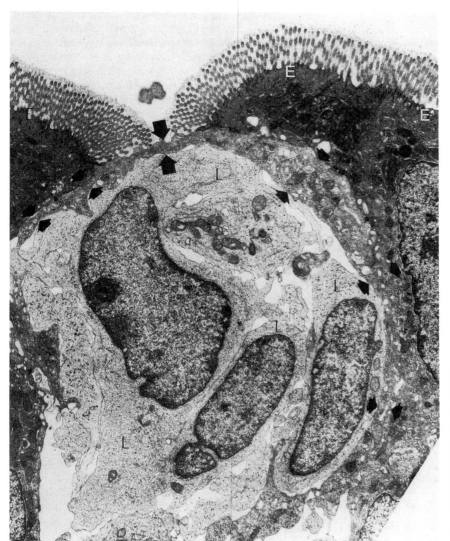

FIGURE 4 Transmission electron micrograph from the noncolumnar region of the Peyer's patch epithelium, showing a cross-sectional view of the apex of an M cell, associated microvillus-covered epithelial cells (E), and at least three lymphoid cells (L). Note attenuated cytoplasm of the M cells (*between arrows*) that bridges the surface between microvillus-covered cells, forms a tight junction with them, and produces a barrier between the lymphoid cells and the intestinal lumen. (From Owen and Jones[27]; © by Williams & Wilkins, 1974.)

al cells.[29] At 1 hour, virus particles were observed in M cell cytoplasm and were also associated with mononuclear cells in the adjacent intercellular space. Inman and Cantey demonstrated that RDEC-1 *Escherichia coli*, an organism that causes diarrhea in rabbits, attaches to M cells but not other epithelial cells in the small intestine of these animals.[30] The organism is not engulfed by M cells as are the reoviruses. However, the bacteria do interact with the M cells to stimulate a polymorphonuclear response. This response culminates in polymorphonuclear cells being extruded into the intestinal lumen to phagocytose and destroy the bacteria. The studies of Owen and Jones,[27,28] Wolf et al,[29] and Inman and Cantey[30] indicate that M cells may be important in processing or destroying antigens and pathogens not eliminated in the proximal small intestine. There is no information concerning the adequacy of M cell function during the entire lifespan of an animal.

B LYMPHOCYTES AND IMMUNOGLOBULINS

The most studied aspect of immunologic host defense of the intestine is the synthesis and release of a special form of the immunoglobulin A (IgA), secretory IgA (SIgA), which is the predominant immunoglobulin of the GI tract (Fig. 5). There are two subclasses of this immunoglobulin in humans: IgA1 and IgA2. These subclasses differ in the amino acid structure of the hinge region of IgA. The IgA1 molecule has an amino acid sequence in the hinge region which is susceptible to degradation by proteases produced by various species of *Neisseria*, *Haemophilus*, and *Streptococcus*. The IgA1 subclass is the predominant form in both monomeric and dimeric IgA present in serum and on mucosal surfaces, respectively.

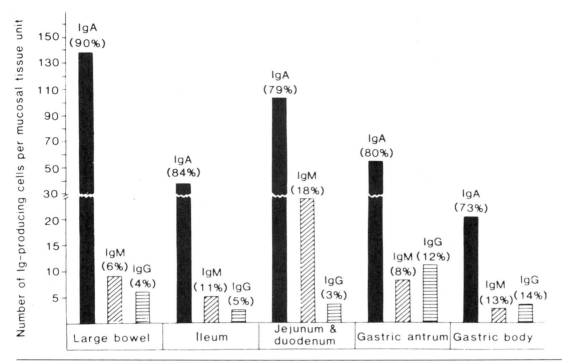

FIGURE 5 Number of IgA-, IgM-, and IgG-producing cells in various segments of normal human GI mucosa. The counts are based on a "tissue unit," which consists of a 6 μm-thick, 500 μm-wide mucosal block extending from the muscularis mucosae to the lumen. The percentage of isotype distribution of the immunocytes is indicated above the columns. (From Bradtzaeg et al[64]; © CRC Press, Inc.)

The IgA2 molecule has an amino acid sequence that is resistant to these proteases.

Immunoglobulin A is produced by plasma cells that have differentiated from B lymphocytes. The plasma cells, located in the lamina propria, synthesize dimeric IgA (two IgA molecules connected by a joint, or J-piece). The columnar epithelial cells of the small intestine express an epithelial glycoprotein on the basolateral surface, i.e., a secretory component that acts as a receptor for the dimeric IgA.[26] The secretory component has been localized by immunohistochemistry and immunoelectron microscopy to the basolateral membrane of intestinal epithelial cells; it has also been identified on the basolateral membrane of epithelial cells lining exocrine glands, ductal epithelial cells in salivary, bile pancreatic, and lacrimal ducts and on hepatocyte membranes of certain species, where it allows for the transport of IgA and immune complexes involving IgA through liver cells in bile.[26,31] Secretory IgA is then excreted onto the mucosal surface of the intestine. This immunoglobulin binds antigen, thereby preventing its attachment to the epithelial surface.[32-34] It has also been suggested that SIgA may prevent bacterial adhesion to the intestinal epithelial surface, thereby suppressing the growth of certain bacterial pathogens.[35-37] Secretory IgA may also be important in enhancing resistance against viral enteritis. The quest for other potential actions of SIgA, such as opsonization and complement fixation, has been largely unsuccessful.[38]

As noted above, intestinal IgA levels are decreased early in life. This physiologic deficiency is partially compensated

for in breast-fed infants, since IgA is present in significant amounts in human breast milk.

Recently, Pappo and Owen have examined the location of secretory component overlying Peyer's patches.[39] Using monoclonal antibodies to secretory component, these investigators showed intense staining of the epithelial cells from interdome regions between Peyer's patches, suggesting the presence of secretory piece associated with epithelial cells. However, no secretory component was identified on M cells overlying lymphoid follicles. As cells emerged from the crypt, there was a sharp demarcation of secretory component–positive cells. Those destined to populate the dome epithelium overlying Peyer's patches were secretory component–negative, whereas those destined to populate the villi were secretory component–positive. These findings demonstrate a unique difference in the expression of the receptor for IgA between follicle-associated and non-follicle-associated epithelium. This observation may explain in part the increased uptake of macromolecules across the epithelium overlying Peyer's patches.[40]

Intestinal B-Cell Traffic

Plasma cells that produce SIgA in the small intestine have been shown to be derived from precursor cells initially stimulated in the distal ileum. The antigens absorbed via M cells participate in the activation of uncommitted lymphocytes, which are modified on contact, released, and then pass through mesenteric nodes into the thoracic duct lymph. These cells can ultimately be identified as specific IgA antibody–producing plasma cells in the lamina propria (Fig. 6).

Pierce and Gowans have studied this migration in rats using cholera toxin.[41] They identified antitoxin-containing cells in thoracic duct lymph following the intraduodenal presentation of toxin. The cells eventually appeared in the lamina propria, particularly at sites where the antigen was first presented. Their studies and those of others demonstrate that cells stimulated by antigen to differentiate into IgA producers appear to "home back" to the site where the antigen was originally present. This traffic pattern of migrating cells from the gut back to the intestinal mucosal surface also occurs between the gut and the mucosa of the bronchus, mammary gland, salivary glands, and female genital tract. Since numerous mucosal surfaces have been shown to be involved in this "homing" phenomenon, Bienenstock and Befus have coined the term "mucosa-associated lymphoid tissue."[42]

The homing phenomenon is not completely understood, and the hypothesis that factors other than antigen may be important to homing is substantiated by recent experiments.

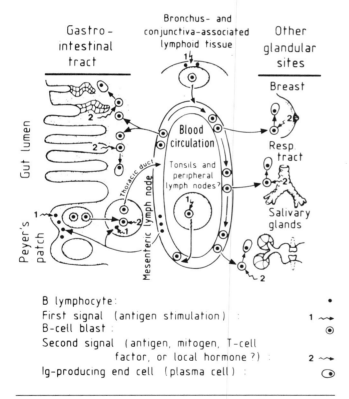

B lymphocyte:
First signal (antigen stimulation) :   1 ⤳
B-cell blast :   ◉
Second signal (antigen, mitogen, T-cell
                factor, or local hormone ?) :   2 ⤳
Ig-producing end cell (plasma cell) :   ◎

FIGURE 6 Schematic representation of B-cell traffic in the secretory immune system. B lymphocytes receive antigen-induced stimulatory "first signals" in Peyer's patches, tonsils, and peripheral lymph nodes. Most stimulated B cells migrate from Peyer's patches through lymph and peripleural blood to various secretory tissues, including the gut lamina propria, salivary glands, respiratory tract, and breast tissue of lactating women. Differentiation into plasma cells at secretory sites is induced by "second signals" that are largely antigen dependent, at least in the gut. (From Bradtzaeg et al[64]; © CRC Press, Inc.)

Mesenteric lymphocytes obtained from mice injected intravenously home to antigen-free intestine located under the kidney capsule of adult animals.[43] Other studies have demonstrated that cells committed to IgA synthesis may persist only at sites where there are sufficient IgA helper T cells.[42,44] T-lymphocyte helper and suppressor activity for IgA synthesis varies for different tissues. Peyer's patches, although having a high level of nonspecific suppressor activity, have increased amounts of specific IgA T-lymphocyte helper activity compared to the spleen and peripheral lymph nodes.[44] Therefore, it is possible that antigenic stimulation in Peyer's patches could induce a strong IgA response and, at the same time, suppress IgG and IgM responses. An additional explanation for why specific lymphocytes home to the intestinal tract could relate to surface receptors on lymphocytes which interact with a specific component in the GI tract.[42] Alternatively, random seeding of cells to the intestine followed by selective proliferation of lymphocytes in areas especially rich in secretory component may be contributing to this homing phenomenon. There are obviously a number of additional factors that may affect the localization of IgA lymphoblasts in the gut, including blood flow, endothelium of postcapillary venules, and receptors for T-lymphocyte products.[45,46]

T LYMPHOCYTES

Intraepithelial lymphocytes have ultrastructural characteristics of other lymphocytes, but some features distinguish them from the classic blood-borne lymphocytes. Intraepithelial lymphocytes may be confused with "immature mast cells." In humans, intraepithelial lymphocytes appear as early as the twentieth gestational week and increase in numbers of up to 6 to 40 per 100 epithelial cells in the normal adult human small intestine.[47] In mice there is a steady increase of these cells after birth from 0.3 to 0.5 per 100 epithelial cells at 2 days of age to around 11 per 100 epithelial cells in adult mice. The exact number of intraepithelial T lymphocytes can vary depending on infections occurring in the animals and on the strain of mice used.[48]

It is of note that the intraepithelial lymphocyte population of both rodents and humans consists almost exclusively of T cells, whereas only 30 to 40 percent of the lamina propria lymphocytes are T cells. The majority of T cells in the intraepithelial lymphocyte pool are of the suppressor/cytotoxic phenotype (T8+ in man, Lyt 2+ in mouse, and 0X8+ in rat), but in the lamina propria more of the T cells carry the helper/inducer marker (T4+ in man, Lyt 1+ in mouse, and W3/25+ in rat).[49] Cell surface marker studies emphasize the fact that intraepithelial and lamina propria populations must be investigated separately in order to elucidate the role of each in GI immune responses.

There is recent evidence which suggests that intraepithelial T lymphocytes migrate to mucosal surfaces in a manner similar to that of B lymphocytes. Cahill has shown that when ^{51}Cr-labeled small T lymphocytes from intestinal lymph are infused intravenously, their relative recovery in intestinal lymph is about twice the recovery of these cells from systemic nodal lymph.[50] In contrast, small T lymphocytes obtained from lymph nodes labeled with ^{51}Cr and injected intravenously were found preferentially in lymph nodal fluid and not intestinal lymph.[50,51]

Once T lymphocytes arrive in the intestine they are dispersed throughout the organ. Intraepithelial lymphocytes cannot remain between the same epithelial cells for long or they would be shed into the intestinal lumen with the epithelial cells when they reach the top of the villi.[51] There is little evidence that many lymphocytes enter the lumen this way.[51] The intraepithelial lymphocytes may move between the epithelial cells and then back into the lamina propria.

Antigen may modify the traffic of lymphocytes into the epithelium in the same way that it influences B-lymphocyte traffic in the lamina propria.[52] However, in studies of the intestine of developing lambs it has been noted that some epithelial lymphocytes are present in the intestine before birth.[53] With increasing age, the number of these lymphocytes increased markedly (Fig. 7). Although it is known that there are subsets of helper and suppressor T lymphocytes within the intestine which may enhance or suppress specific antibody productions, information concerning intestinal T-lymphocyte function is incomplete.

NATURAL KILLER CELLS

The importance of natural killer (NK) lymphocytes in the intestine has been reviewed elsewhere.[54–54b] NK cells represent a population of rapidly acting effector lymphocytes that function in the absence of specific immunization and without clear antigenic specificity. Located in the superficial layer of the intestinal mucosa, these cells are effective against target cells infected by intracellular parasites and are thus particularly suited to mount a rapid defense of a mucosal surface. Evi-

dence indicates that the intestinal epithelium is rich in cells with a considerable potential for NK cell activity.

Thus, the intestinal immune system has evolved in such a way that its nonspecific cytotoxic effector lymphocytes are concentrated in the most superficial layer of the mucosa, where antigenic contact is most frequent and rapid elimination of infected and tumor cells is most required.[54]

TOLERANCE

Antigens ingested by the host may stimulate the local immune system, resulting in SIgA production by B lymphocytes that have homed to the lamina propria. Antigens may also penetrate the intestinal mucosal barrier and stimulate the systemic immune system, resulting in the synthesis of specific circulating IgG antibodies. In addition, macromolecules acting as antigens may induce a state of unresponsiveness or tolerance. Immunologic tolerance may be defined as a refractory state that is antigen-directed. Its development requires previous contact with a specific antigen.[55]

Both B and T lymphocytes may be involved in the development of tolerance. In addition, tolerance may develop by different mechanisms. It has become obvious that there are diverse tolerant states, all having unresponsiveness as the end result, albeit by different mechanisms. Whether an immune response or tolerance develops following an antigen challenge depends on age and on the quality and quantity of the antigen, as well as on a number of other unappreciated factors. Additional studies are necessary to better define the different mechanisms of tolerance and to determine if tolerance can be used advantageously to protect individuals predisposed to allergic or other immune-mediated disorders.

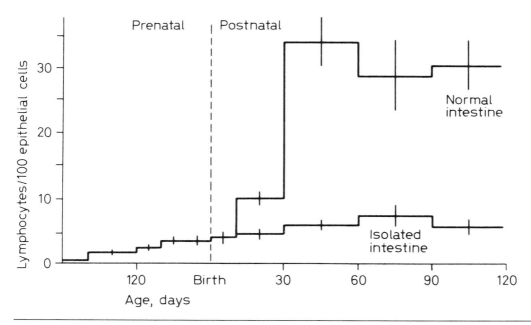

FIGURE 7 Intestinal epithelial lymphocytes in developing lambs. Data obtained from normal antigen-exposed ileal segments and surgically isolated ileal segments not exposed to antigens. The results of each group are expressed as the mean ± standard error of the mean. (From Reynolds.[53])

ACCESSORY CELLS

Macrophages

Although macrophages of the lung, peritoneal cavity, spleen, and liver have been studied in great detail,[56,57] few studies have dealt directly with the origin, distribution, and activity of intestinal macrophages. We are, however, accumulating more information concerning intestinal macrophages, as noted in a recent review.[58] These cells are found associated with GALT, surrounding the crypts of Lieberkuhn, and in the villous core. They are similar to macrophages in other parts of the body but they lack several characteristics, including a specific nuclear and lysosomal morphologic appearance characteristic of extraintestinal macrophages. They also lack membrane receptors for complement and the Fc portion of the IgG molecule.[56-58]

Macrophages carry out diverse functions in the intestinal tract, including phagocytosis, secretion, and participation in certain humoral and cellular immune responses. However, additional studies are necessary to better delineate the importance of these functions.

Mast Cells

Recent evidence indicates that mast cells, a type of lymphoid cell present in the intestine, may also be involved in immune function.[54a,59] There are at least two kinds of mast cells present in the intestinal tract.[59] One type appears to be the typical connective tissue mast cell and is confined to the submucosa. A second type is an atypical appearing mast cell that is present in the epithelium. Both cell types proliferate rapidly during certain parasite infections, have IgE receptors on their surface, and degranulate in response to antigen.[60-64] The mast cell can concentrate IgE on its surface by means of Fc receptors. There are 100,000 to 500,000 Fc receptors per mast cell, and these receptors can bind IgE. Bound IgE antibodies on the mast cell provide it with specificity for antigen-dependent degranulation and subsequent release of mediators like histamine, which cause atopic allergy (type 1 hypersensitivity).

IgE-positive cells are present in increased quantities in allergic proctitis and infantile allergic colitis.[65,66] One cannot readily distinguish between IgE-positive mast cells and IgE-producing B cells. IgE-bearing cells not only have a key role in intestinal allergy, but they may also enhance immune elimination and thus contribute significantly to mucosal defense against parasitic helminths.[65,66]

Mucous Cells

Secretory immunoglobulin has a mucinlike glycoprotein sequence at the hinge region between its Fc and Fab subunits.[67,68] It has been suggested that this hinge region of the SIgA molecule sits at the interface between mucin and overlying fluid, with its mucinlike portion in the mucin phase and the rest of the molecule in the overlying aqueous phase, like a detergent or a phospholipid at the interface between a lipid and an aqueous phase.[69] The SIgA may then form a monolayer on the surface of the mucin, where it is needed in defense against antigens and pathogens.

Mucin not only may function to anchor SIgA but also may act in many other ways to augment intestinal immune function (Table 4). These functions have recently been reviewed and are supported by some experimental observations. Nimmerfall and Rosenthaler have noted that diffusion of a substance through mucin is dependent upon the hydrated radius of the molecule and the ability of the substance to form hydrogen bonds.[70] In addition, they have found the intestinal absorption of molecules in the rat correlates inversely with molecular weight. Hence, high molecular weight molecules are retarded in their passage through the mucin layer and therefore are not absorbed as extensively as smaller molecules. In addition to possibly retarding the penetration of macromolecules and potential antigens, mucins may also act as a physical barrier to enterotoxins.

The interaction of noxious substances with the intestinal surface, i.e., cholera toxin binding to a microvillous receptor or bacterial adherence to the epithelial membrane, is necessary before pathologic reactions can occur (penetration, secretory diarrhea, and bacterial proliferation). Any physical barrier that interferes with intestinal attachment represents an important protective process within the GI tract. Some evidence exists that glycoproteins present in mucin may specifically bind with enterotoxins and thereby inhibit their interactions with the microvillous receptor. Walker and

TABLE 4
Summary of Protective Functions of the
Mucin Gel Layer of the Intestinal Tract

I. Protection
  A. Physical barrier
    1. Unstirred layer
       To maintain a pH gradient in the stomach and duodenum.
    2. Gel-permeation or molecular sieve properties
       Molecules larger than about 17,000 tend to be excluded from the gel.
    3. Phase-partition properties
       Non–mucin-type molecules tend to be excluded from the gel phase.
  B. Biologic barrier
    1. Nonspecific trapping
       Particles trapped by general "stickiness."
    2. Specific trapping
       Mucin oligosaccharides mirror the epithelial cell surface and therefore offer spurious attachment sites to lectins, toxins, and pathogens.
    3. Lysozyme
       A small bacteriolytic enzyme that can enter the gel and is retained, thereby interacting with mucin.
    4. Lactoferrin
       Maintains an iron-free environment at the mucosal surface for bacteriostasis and to prevent catalytic production of hydroxyl radicals.
    5. Secretory IgA
       SIgA1 with its mucinlike hinge associates with gel, whereas SIgA2 is excluded.
II. Mucin release and clearance
    Triggered by irritants, toxins, lectins, immune complexes, proteolytic enzymes, etc. Net flow from epithelium to lumen is therefore increased.

From Clamp.[87]

co-workers have demonstrated that formation of immune complexes, particularly IgA-specific immune complexes, may contribute to the release of goblet cell mucus onto the intestinal surface, thus preventing the interaction of immune complexes with the intestinal microvillous surface.[71] Mucin glycoproteins may also coat the external surface of bacteria and thus interfere with their attachment to, and proliferation on, the intestinal surface.[71] Shigella,[72] Staphylococcus,[73] Klebsiella,[74] and antibody-antigen complexes[71] all stimulate mucin release and/or synthesis, and the mucin then forms a protective coat for the intestinal epithelium. Furthermore, peristaltic movement of mucus along the intestinal surface may act to wash immune complexes formed in the lumen free of, or dislodge particulate antigens from, the epithelium and thereby prevent their attachment at that site.

Hepatic Cells

The liver receives absorbed molecules from the GI tract. Approximately 15 percent of the total liver mass is composed of reticuloendothelial cells or Kupffer cells,[75] which have an enormous capacity to phagocytize noxious substances that enter the portal circulation. However, the route of intestinal absorption may be critical. Haptens or small molecules are absorbed intact into the portal circulation and gain access initially to Kupffer cells, whereas larger molecules such as bovine serum albumin may be absorbed more extensively via the lymphatics and reach other organs to stimulate an immune response.[76] If absorption occurs through the portal vein, the normal liver seems to trap particulate antigen but not soluble antigen unless it is complexed with homologous antibody. Although the liver may be considered a "second line of defense" against invasion of biologically active substances, it may also play a central role in the development of tolerance.[77] In addition to the Kupffer cell function, recent studies in animals and man have demonstrated that hepatocytes are involved in the intestinal immune system. These cells have been shown to clear the circulation of SIgA. Secretory IgA is transported from the blood into bile free or complexed to various substances.[79-80] The hepatic transport of SIgA from serum to bile may not only be a means of eliminating antigen from the circulation, but may also serve to bolster intestinal host defenses by recirculating IgA to the intestinal lumen. The human serum IgA level is increased in association with several liver diseases, such as the liver disease associated with alcohol abuse. In addition, overactivity of mucosal immunocyte populations is likely to be reflected by a raised serum level of polymeric IgA. However, there is probably a complex network of homeostatic mechanisms normally keeping mucosal immune responses compatible with the local glandular capacity for the removal of dimeric IgA by secretory component–mediated external translocation. Gamma-interferon may also enhance secretory component expression and is important in this context.

NUTRITION AND MUCOSAL IMMUNE DEFENSES

The nutrient requirements of infants are dramatically increased compared with those of adults, and nutrient deficiencies may therefore occur quite readily. It is important to point out that these nutritional deficiencies impair secretory and cellular responsiveness, thus reducing antimicrobial protection.[81,82] This may be very important to mucosal immunity, sensitization to new antigens, and allergy development in children.

Protein-calorie malnutrition is prevalent not only in "underdeveloped" countries but also in hospitalized patients in "developed" countries. This occurs especially in hospitalized children and adults with cancer or chronic diseases. Individuals suffering from malnutrition are at risk for the consequences of impaired intestinal immune function, i.e., increased GI infections and infestations and increased macromolecular uptake.[81,82]

THE CENTRAL NERVOUS SYSTEM AND MUCOSAL IMMUNE DEFENSE

Investigators have recently suggested that the central nervous system may affect immune function.[83] Russell et al note that there have been many anecdotal reports of associative learning with allergic reactions as early as the nineteenth century. It was noted then that asthmatic patients who had allergic reactions to roses experienced an attack when exposed to an artificial rose.[84] Russell and his colleagues recently tested the possibility that histamine release could be a learned response. In a classical conditioning experiment in which an immunologic challenge was paired with the presentation of an odor, guinea pigs showed a plasma histamine increase when the odor was presented alone. This suggested that the immune response may be enhanced through activity of the central nervous system.[84]

MacQueen et al have also investigated the interaction of the central nervous and immune systems.[85] They injected rats with egg albumin and found that this stimulated mucosal mast cells to secrete mediators. This injection was paired with an audiovisual cue. After re-exposure to the audiovisual cue, the mediator (rat mast cell protease II) was measured with a sensitive and specific assay. Animals re-exposed to only the audiovisual cue released a quantity of protease similar to that of animals re-exposed to both the audiovisual cue and the antigen. These groups released significantly more protease than animals that had received the cue and antigen in a noncontingent manner. Like Russell et al, the results of MacQueen and coworkers support a role for the central nervous system as a functional effector of immune response.

Finally, Olness and her co-investigators have recently shown that hypnotized children can be influenced through suggestion to secrete greater quantities of salivary IgA than controls.[86]

These studies taken together provide strong evidence that the central nervous system and immune function are linked. The central nervous system may influence the immune system through the stress of emotion or malnutrition. Corticosteroid levels can increase, decreasing the size of the thymus and altering its function. This gland and its hormones may then play a key role in the development of functional T cells and hence helper T cells for SIgA production. Additional studies are necessary to better determine how the central nervous system interacts with intestinal immunity during development.

The importance of intestinal immune function as a host defense mechanism is just beginning to be appreciated. At the present time it is apparent that when functioning normally, the immune system of the intestine acts to protect the host from a diversity of foreign substances and agents. However, inadequate or abnormal function may be associated with a variety of GI and/or systemic disease processes.

REFERENCES

1. Udall JN, Walker WA. The physiologic and pathologic basis for the transport of macromolecules across the intestinal tract. J Pediatr Gastroenterol Nutr 1982; 1:295–301.
2. Udall JN, Walker WA. Mucosal defense mechanisms. In: Marsh MN, ed. Immunopathology of the small intestine. London: John Wiley and Sons, 1987: 3.
3. Gardner MLG. Gastrointestinal absorption of intact proteins. Annu Rev Nutr 1988; 8:329–350.
4. Udall JN, Pang K, Fritze L, Kleinman R, Walker WA. Development of gastrointestinal mucosal barrier. I. The effect of age on intestinal permeability to macromolecules. Pediatr Res 1981; 15:241–244.
5. Udall JN, Bloch KJ, Walker WA. Transport of proteases across neonatal intestine and development of liver disease in infants with alpha₁-antitrypsin deficiency. Lancet 1982; i:1441–1443.
6. Lee EJ, Heiner DC. Allergy to cow milk—1985. Pediatr Rev 1986; 7(7):195–203.
7. Bezerra J, Thompson S, Dos Santos B, Koldovsky O, Udall J. Urinary lactose excretion of infants and adults following ingestion of disaccharide. J Am Coll Nutr 1988; 7:417.
8. Burgio GR, Lanzavecchia A, Plebani A, Jayakar S, Ugazio AG. Ontogeny of secretory immunity: Levels of secretory IgA and natural antibodies in saliva. Pediatr Res 1980; 14:1111–1114.
9. Perkkio M, Savilahti E. Time of appearance of immunoglobulin-containing cells in the mucosa of the neonatal intestine. Pediatr Res 1980; 14:953–955.
10. Rieger CHL, Rothberg RM. Development of the capacity to produce specific antibody to an ingested food antigen in the premature infant. J Pediatr 1975; 87:515–518.
11. Abrams GD. Effects of the normal flora on the host defenses against microbial invasion. Adv Exp Med Biol 1969; 3:197–206.
12. Crabbe PA, Nash DR, Bazin H, Eyssen H, Heremans JF. Immunohistochemical observations on lymphoid tissues from conventional and germ-free mice. Lab Invest 1970; 22:448–457.
13. Ferguson A, Parrott DMV. The effect of antigen deprivation on thymus-dependent and thymus-independent lymphocytes in the small intestine of the mouse. Clin Exp Immunol 1972; 12:477–488.
14. Pollard M, Sharon N. Responses of the Peyer's patches in germ-free mice to antigenic stimulation. Infect Immun 1970; 2:96–100.
15. Ogra PL. Ontogeny of the local immune system. Pediatrics (Host Defense Supplement) 1979; 64:765–774.
16. Pittard WB III, Bill K. Immunoregulation by breast milk cells. Cell Immunol 1979; 42:437–441.
17. Pittard WB III, Bill K. Differentiation of cord blood lymphocytes into IgA-producing cells in response to breast milk stimulatory factor. Clin Immunol Immunopathol 1979; 13:430–434.
18. Gordon JE, Chitkara IO, Wyon JB. Weanling Diarrhea. Am J Med Sci 1963; 245:345–377.
19. MMWR 1982; 30:79.
20. MMWR 1987; 37:25–31.
21. Kraehenbuhl JP, Campiche MA. Early stages of intestinal absorption of specific antibodies in the newborn. An ultrastructural, cytochemical and immunological study in the pig, rat, and rabbit. J Cell Biol 1969; 42:345–365.
22. Iyengar L, Selvaraj RJ. Intestinal absorption of immunoglobulins by newborn infants. Arch Dis Child 1972; 47:411–414.
23. Vukavic T. Intestinal absorption of IgA in the newborn. J Pediatr Gastroenterol Nutr 1983; 2:248–251.
24. Ogra SS, Weintraub D, Ogra PL. Immunologic aspects of human colostrum and milk. III. Fate and absorption of cellular and soluble components in the gastrointestinal tract of the newborn. J Immunol 1977; 119:245–248.
25. Udall J. Immunologic aspects of gut function. In: Walker WA, Watkins JB, eds. Nutrition in pediatrics; basic science and clinical aspects. Boston: Little, Brown, 1985: 301.
26. Pabst R. Review article: the anatomical basis for the immune function of the gut. Anat Embryol 1987; 176:135–144.
27. Owen RL, Jones AL. Epithelial cell specialization within human Peyer's patches: an ultrastructural study of intestinal lymphoid follicles. Gastroenterology 1974; 66:189–203.
28. Owen RL. Sequential uptake of horseradish peroxidase by lymphoid follicle epithelium of Peyer's patches in the normal unobstructed mouse intestine: an ultrastructural study. Gastroenterology 1977; 72:440–451.
29. Wolf JL, Rubin DH, Finberg RS, Kauffman RS, Sharpe AH, Trier JS, Fields BN. Intestinal M cells: a pathway for entry of reovirus into the host. Science 1981; 212:471–472.
30. Inman LR, Cantey JR. Specific adherence of Escherichia coli (strain RDEC-1) to membranous (M) cells of the Peyer's patch in Escherichia coli diarrhea in the rabbit. J Clin Invest 1983; 71:1–8.
31. Crago SS, Tomasi TB. Mucosal antibodies. In: Brostoff SJ, Challacombe SJ, eds. Food allergy and intolerance. London: Bailliere Tindall, 1987: 167.
32. Heremans JF. Immunoglobulin A. In: Sela M, ed. The antigens, Vol II. New York: Academic Press, 1974: 365.
33. Walker WA, Isselbacher KJ. Intestinal antibodies. N Engl J Med 1977; 297:767–773.
34. Walker WA. Antigen handling by the gut. Arch Dis Child 1978; 53:527–531.
35. Williams RC, Gibbons RJ. Inhibition of bacterial adherence by secretory immunoglobulin A: a mechanism of antigen disposal. Science 1972; 177:697–699.
36. Wright R. Normal immune responses in the gut and immunodeficiency disorders. In: Tuck J, ed. Immunology of gastrointestinal and liver disease. London: Edward Arnold, 1977: 1.
37. Rogers HJ, Synge C. Bacteriostatic effect of human milk on Escherichia coli: the role of IgA. Immunology 1978; 34:19–28.
38. Ottaway CA, Rose ML, Parrott DM. The gut as an immunological system. In: Crane RK, ed. Gastrointestinal physiology III, international review of physiology, Vol 19. Baltimore: University Park Press, 1979: 323.
39. Pappo J, Owen RL. Absence of secretory component expression by epithelial cells overlying rabbit gut-associated lymphoid tissue. Gastroenterology 1988; 95:1173–1177.
40. Wolf JL. Why antigens are attracted to the dome epithelium: Another clue. Gastroenterology 1988; 95:1419–1421.
41. Pierce NF, Gowans JL. Cellular kinetics of the intestinal immune response to cholera toxoid in rats. J Exp Med 1975; 142:1550–1563.
42. Bienenstock J, Befus AD. Review: mucosal immunology. Immunology 1980; 41:249–270.
43. Parrott DMV, Ferguson A. Selective migration of lymphocytes within the mouse small intestine. Immunology 1974; 26:571–588.
44. Elson CO, Heck JA, Strober W. T-cell regulation of murine IgA synthesis. J Exp Med 1979; 149:632–643.
45. Bienenstock J. Review and discussion of homing of lymphoid cells to mucosa membranes: the selection localization of cells in mucosal tissues. In: Strober W, Hanson LA, Sell KW, eds. Recent advances in mucosal immunity. New York: Raven Press, 1982: 35.
46. Ottaway CA. Lymphoid cell migration to the intestine in health and disease. In: Losowsky MS, Heatley RV, eds. Gut defenses in clinical practice. Edinburgh: Churchill Livingstone, 1986: 48–66.
47. Ferguson A. Intra-epithelial lymphocytes of the small intestine. Gut 1977; 18:921–937.
48. Guy-Grand D, Griscelli C, Vassalli P. The mouse gut T lymphocyte, a novel type of T cell. Nature, origin and traffic in mice in normal and graft-versus-host conditions. J Exp Med 1978; 148:1661–1677.
49. Strobel S, Shields JG. The mucosal T-cell. In: Brostoff J, Challacombe SJ, eds. Food allergy and tolerance. London: Bailliere Tindall, 1987: 103.
50. Cahill RNP, Poskitt DC, Frost H, Trnka Z. Two distinct pools of recirculating T lymphocytes: migratory characteristics of nodal and intestinal T lymphocytes. J Exp Med 1977; 145:420–428.
51. Chin W, Hay JB. A comparison of lymphocyte migration through intestinal lymph nodes, subcutaneous lymph nodes, and chronic inflammatory sites of sheep. Gastroenterology 1980; 79:1231–1242.
52. Guy-Grand D, Griscelli C, Vassalli P. The gut-associated lymphoid system: nature and properties of the large dividing cells. Eur J Immunol 1974; 4:435–443.
53. Reynolds J. Gut-associated lymphoid tissues in lamb before and after birth. Monogr Allergy 1980; 16:187–202.

54. Mowat A. Natural killer cells and intestinal immunity. In: Brostoff J, Challacombe SJ, eds. Food allergy and intolerance. London: Bailliere Tindall, 1987: 156.

54a. Elson CO, Kagnoff MF, Fiocchi C, Befus AD, Targan S. Intestinal immunity and inflammation: recent progress. 1986:91:746–768.

54b. Gibson PR. Intestinal cytotoxic cells. Gastroenterology 1987; 93:437–438.

55. Weigle WO. Immunological tolerance. In: Samter M, ed. Immunological diseases. Boston: Little, Brown, 1978: 389.

56. Carr I. The fixed macrophage. In: The macrophage. A review of ultrastructure and function. London: Academic Press, 1973: 20.

57. Carr I, Wright J. The reticuloendothelial and mononuclear phagocyte systems and the macrophage. Can Med Assoc J 1978; 118:882–885.

58. Bockman DE. Gut-associated macrophages. In: Brostoff J, Challacombe SJ, eds. Food allergy and intolerance. London: Bailliere Tindall, 1987: 67.

59. Kaliner MA. Is a mast cell a mast cell? J Allergy Clin Immunol 1980; 66:1–4.

60. Miller HRP, Jarrett WFH. Immune reactions in mucous membranes I. Intestinal mast cell response during helminth expulsion in the rat. Immunology 1971; 20:277–288.

61. Enerback L, Lundin PM. Ultrastructure of mucosal mast cells in normal and compound 48/80-treated rats. Cell Tissue Res 1974; 150:95–105.

62. Enerback L. Mast cells in rat gastrointestinal mucosa II. Dye-binding and metachromatic properties. Acta Pathol Microbiol Immunol Scand 1966; 66:303–312.

63. Mayrhofer G, Bazin H, Gowans JL. Nature of cells binding anti-IgE in rats immunized with *Nippostrongylus brasiliensis*: IgE synthesis in regional nodes and concentration in mucosal mast cells. Eur J Immunol 1976; 6:537–545.

64. Bradtzaeg P, Baklien K, Bjerke K, Rognum TO, Scott H, Valnes K. Nature and properties of the human gastrointestinal immune system. In: Miller K, Nicklin S, eds. Immunology of the gastrointestinal tract, Vol I. Boca Raton, FL: CRC Press, 1987: 1.

65. Rosekrans PCM, Meijer CJLM, Van Der Wal AM, Lindeman J. Allergic proctitis, a clinical and immunopathological entity. Gut 1980; 21:1017–1023.

66. Jenkins HR, Pincott JR, Soothill JF, Milla PJ, Harries JT. Food allergy: the major cause of infantile colitis. Arch Dis Child 1984; 59:326–329.

67. Schrager J. The chemical composition and function of gastrointestinal mucus. Gut 1970; 11:450–456.

68. Yu-Sheng VL, Low TLK, Infante A, Putnam FW. Complete covalent structure of a human IgA1 immunoglobulin. Science 1976; 193:1017–1020.

69. Edwards PAW. Is mucus a selective barrier to macromolecules? Br Med Bull 1978; 34:55–56.

70. Nimmerfall F, Rosenthaler J. Significance of the goblet cell mucin layer, the outermost luminal barrier to passage through the gut wall. Biochem Biophys Res Commun 1980; 94:960–966.

71. Walker WA, Wu M, Bloch KJ. Stimulation by immune complexes of mucus release from goblet cells of the rat small intestine. Science 1977; 197:370–372.

72. Keusch GT, Grady GF, Takeuchi A, Sprinz H. The pathogenesis of Shigella diarrhea. II. Enterotoxin-induced acute enteritis in the rabbit ileum. J Infect Dis 1972; 126:92–95.

73. Sheahan DG, Jervis HR, Takeuchi A, Sprinz H. The effect of staphylococcal enterotoxin on the epithelial mucosubstances of the small intestine of Rhesus monkeys. Am J Pathol 1970; 60:1–18.

74. Klipstein FA, Schenk EA. Enterotoxigenic intestinal bacteria in tropical sprue II. Effect of the bacteria and their enterotoxins on intestinal structure. Gastroenterology 1975; 68:642–655.

75. Gates GA, Henley KS, Pollard HM, Schmidt E, Schmidt FW. The cell population of human liver. J Lab Clin Med 1961; 57:182–184.

76. Wright R. Normal immune responses in the gut and immunodeficiency disorders. In: Tuck J, ed. Immunology of gastrointestinal and liver disease. London: Edward Arnold, 1977: 1.

77. Rogoff TM, Lipsky PE. Role of the Kupffer cells in local and systemic immune responses. Gastroenterology 1981; 80:854–860.

78. Nagura H, Smith PD, Nakane PK, Brown WR. IgA in human bile and liver. J Immunol 1981; 126:587–595.

79. Peppard J, Orlans E, Payne AWR, Andrew E. The elimination of circulating complexes containing polymeric IgA by excretion in the bile. Immunology 1981; 42:83–89.

80. Socken DJ, Simms ES, Nagy BR, Fisher MM, Underdown BJ. Secretory component-dependent hepatic transport of IgA antibody antigen complexes. J Immunol 1981; 127:316–319.

81. Watson RR, McMurray DN, Martin P, Reyes MA. Effect of age, malnutrition and renutrition on free secretory component and IgA in secretions. J Clin Nutr 1985; 42:281–288.

82. Watson RR. Mucosal immune defenses. II. Effects of low and high nutrient intakes. Immunol Allergy Pract 1985; 7:270–278.

83. Borbjerg D, Cohen N, Ader R. The central nervous system and learning: a strategy for immune regulation. Immunol Today 1982; 3:287–291.

84. Russell M, Dark KA, Cummins RW, Ellman G, Callaway E, Peeke HVS. Learned histamine release. Science 1984; 225:733–734.

85. MacQueen G, Marshall J, Perdue M, Siegel S, Bienenstock J. Pavlovian conditioning of rat mucosal mast cells to secrete rat mast cell protease II. Science 1989; 243:83–85.

86. Olness K, Culbert T, Uden D. Self-regulation of salivary immunoglobulin A by children. Pediatrics 1989; 83:66–71.

87. Clamp JR. The properties of the mucus gel layer in the gastrointestinal tract. In: Brostoff J, Challacombe SJ, eds. Food allergy and intolerance. London: Bailliere Tindall, 1987: 190.

88. Selner JC, Merrill DAK, Claman HN. Salivary immunoglobulin and albumin: development during the newborn period. Pediatr 1968; 72:685–689.

89. Cornes JS. Number, size and distribution of Peyer's patches in the human small intestine. Gut 1965; 6:225–233.

CHAPTER 21

Transport of Water and Ions

Jehan-François Desjeux, M.D.

The intestinal epithelium controls the exchange of water and solutes between the environment and the body. Two important characteristics of this exchange are the following: (1) Water-soluble solutes, including lipids dissolved in water, are dragged by the movement of water and absorbed across the intestinal epithelium. (2) Water movement across epithela follows the movement of electrolytes. In that respect the Na^+,K^+-ATPase plays a crucial role in the circulation of water in the body.

The intestinal epithelium early in life is characterized by high permeability, poor selectivity, and high transepithelial fluxes of water and solutes.

RELEVANCE OF ANIMAL MODELS

Water and Electrolyte Transport in the Developing Rat

Our current understanding of the maturation of mammalian water and electrolyte transport is based on experiments performed in animals. Descriptive experiments were performed in the rat,[1-4] an animal in which between birth and weaning (3 weeks) the intestinal development pattern approximates preterm development in humans.

Intestinal transport of water and electrolytes was compared first in suckling, weanling, and adolescent rats. In the absence of glucose, there was minimal net secretion of *water* in intestinal segments of the 2-week-old rats but net absorption in 3- and 8-week-old rats, with rates of *water* and *sodium* (Na^+) transport lower in ileal than in jejunal segments. In jejunum, the rate of *chloride* (Cl^-) absorption was much greater in the 2- and 3-week-old than in the 8-week-old rats. In the ileal segment, the rate of chloride absorption was similar at all three age periods. *Bicarbonate*, (HCO_3^-) usually absorbed from both the jejunal and ileal segments of the 2- and 3-week-old rats, was secreted in the ileal segment of the 8-week-old rats. Glucose significantly enhanced absorption of water and sodium; the magnitude of this effect was greater in 2-week-old rats than in 8-week-old rats.

In the jejunum at all three levels of intraluminal osmolality, the rate of water secretion in response to intraluminal hyperosmolality was greater in the 2-week-old than in the 7-week-old rats. This age-related difference was not as striking in ileum as in jejunum. Further studies in which rats were perfused with HCO_3^- and made hypertonic (500 mOsm per kilogram) with mannitol demonstrated decreased HCO_3^- absorption in the jejunum of the 8-week-old rats and HCO_3^- secretion in the 2-week-old rats. In the ileum large amounts

of HCO_3^- were secreted at both age periods. In addition, the 2-week-old rats showed relatively severe metabolic acidosis, whereas the 8-week-old rats appeared to be in a normal state of acid-base balance.

Postnatal development of colonic water and electrolyte transport in the rat follows a pattern similar to that described above for the small bowel: high water and electrolyte transport in the first 2 weeks of life.[5]

Taken together, these results indicate that in the suckling rat, the intestinal epithelium is the site of intense exchange between lumen and blood across a barrier nonselective toward hypertonicity and HCO_3^-, the jejunum being relatively more immature than the ileum. Immaturity does not mean inefficiency, as the intestinal barrier is probably adapted to the suckling situation, but a minor imbalance between intestinal lumen and blood may lead to severe dehydration and acidosis. The development of the intestine is probably characterized by the appearance of specific transport mechanisms for absorption and secretion of specific solutes, together with an effective barrier function between lumen and blood.[6]

General Principles in Water and Electrolyte Transport

Most current concepts of intestinal transport are derived from animal studies performed in the late 1960s under the influence of the laws of irreversible thermodynamics.[7]

The mechanism of water absorption by the intestine of adult animals was particularly puzzling because it takes place in the absence of or against an osmotic gradient between lumen and blood. Initially these observations were interpreted as an indication that water movement was directly ("water pump") or indirectly coupled to an energetic process.

The relationship between water movement and osmotic gradient and the movement of electrolytes and metabolism were studied in the rat colon and the small intestine of a variety of animals.[8] For example, water is absorbed in isolated rat jejunal loops filled with Ringer's solution. Glucose stimulates the absorption of water, whereas cholera toxin evokes secretion, inhibited by glucose. A plot of water versus Na^+ absorption and secretion indicates a perfect linear relationship, the slope of which is an index of the osmolality of the fluid transported across the intestinal epithelium. The osmolality of the fluid transported increases with the tightness of the epithelium from 325 mOsm per kilogram in the leaky jejunum to 515 mOsm per kilogram in the tighter colon. In the absence of Na^+ movement there is no water movement. This observation indicates that water movement is passive and

FIGURE 1 Water movement in immature and mature intestinal epithelium; Na$^+$,K$^+$-ATPase located in basolateral membrane (bl) allows Na$^+$ to be pumped out of the cell, creating water movement in the lateral space (Ls). In immature intestine, water can move back to the lumen across the loose tight junction (Tj). Osmotic pressure difference between lumen and blood is main force that controls direction of water movement. In mature intestine, the tight junction is more selective to ions, so osmotic pressure can develop in the lateral space; resulting fluid accumulation is the source of hydrostatic pressure that drives water to the blood. In addition, the brush border membrane (bbm) may develop specific transport systems and a change in hydraulic conductivity.[6]

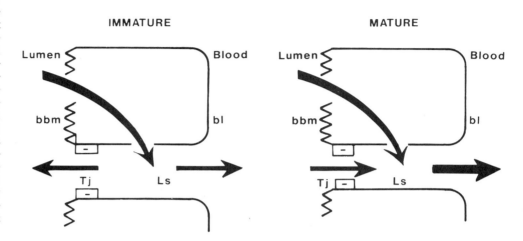

follows the movement of the actively transported electrolytes.[8-10] The mechanism of the coupling between water and Na$^+$ fluxes implies (1) a source of energy, which is the Na$^+$,K$^+$-ATPase pumping Na$^+$ from the cell to the lateral space across the basolateral membrane; (2) an asymmetric electrolyte permeability of epithelial membranes, essentially the tight junction and the loose basement membrane; and (3) a space containing a fluid rendered hypertonic ($\simeq 310$ mOsm per kilogram) by the Na$^+$ pumping where hydrostatic pressure can develop, represented by the lateral space between the epithelial cells.[11]

The results observed in the developing rat are best explained by the development of membrane selectivity, the tight junction, and also the luminal membrane, which is permeable to water (Fig. 1).

The mechanism of Na$^+$ absorption was elucidated using a method developed by Ussing. In 1964, Schultz and Zalusky[12] mounted a rabbit ileum in an Ussing chamber in order to evaluate epithelial function under steady-state conditions in the absence of pressure, temperature, and concentration gradients across the epithelium. Net transport of an uncharged solute across the isolated epithelium under these conditions is interpreted as active transport. For electrolytes that are electrically charged solutes, transepithelial electrical potential (PD), albeit small (2 to 5 mV serosa positive) is a direct force that causes cation (Na$^+$ or K$^+$) secretion and anion (Cl$^-$ or HCO$_3^-$) absorption. In the Ussing chamber it is possible to clamp the PD to zero and to record this short-circuiting current (Isc). Representing the sum of all the ionic net fluxes transported by the epithelium in the absence of transepithelial electrochemical gradient, the steady-state Isc expressed in microamperes per square centimeter or in microequivalents per hour per square centimeter is an index of active electrolyte transport. The transepithelial conductance (G) is the slope of the linear relationship between Isc

and PD. It is expressed in millisiemens per square centimeter and is an estimate of the leakiness of the epithelium for the electrolytes.

Schultz and Zalusky found that active Na$^+$ absorption by rabbit ileum is the result of a spatial discrimination between diffusion and active transport; i.e., the Na$^+$ enters the cell through the luminal membrane by diffusion, following its

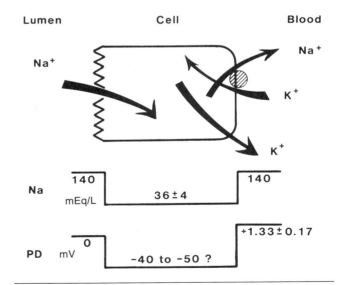

FIGURE 2 Schematic view of enterocyte Na$^+$ absorption. Energy provided by hydrolysis of ATP to ADP (Na$^+$,K$^+$-ATPase) expels 3 Na$^+$, while permitting 2 K$^+$ into the cell. An electrochemical gradient is maintained which allows Na$^+$ to enter and K$^+$ to leave the cell by diffusion. Ouabain inhibits Na$^+$,K$^+$-ATPase and barium blocks the K$^+$ channel.

electrochemical gradient, and it is pumped out of the cell actively by the Na$^+$,K$^+$-ATPase located at the basolateral membrane (Fig. 2).

The postnatal development of sodium transport was studied in the jejunum of the rabbit using the same methodology.[13] The transepithelial conductance and the unidirectional Na$^+$ fluxes both fell with increasing age, suggesting a decrease of the ionic paracellular permeability during rabbit small intestine development. In addition, Isc increased and there was a tendency for the net Na$^+$ absorption (J^{Na^+}) to increase, suggesting that active Na$^+$ absorption increases during small intestinal development in the rabbit. Similarly, the ileum of newborn rabbit has a high conductance and it absorbs Na$^+$ and Cl$^-$ actively.[14]

In jejunal biopsies from children as young as 2 months, studied in the Ussing chamber,[15] electrical parameters are not dependent on age (Table 1). This finding suggests that the jejunum of children does not mature significantly after the age of 2 months.

In search for *the energy required to absorb glucose*, Crane[16] postulated that glucose and Na$^+$ are co-transported, that the Na$^+$ electrochemical gradient across the luminal membrane is the driving force for glucose uptake, and that glucose at the luminal membrane stimulates Na$^+$ entry across this membrane.[17] Later experiments conducted on isolated brush border membrane vesicles where glucose uptake or overshoot is demonstrated in the presence of a Na$^+$ concentration gradient confirmed this hypothesis.[18,19]

DEVELOPMENT OF Na$^+$, Cl$^-$, AND HCO$_3^-$ TRANSPORT CELLULAR MECHANISMS

The mechanisms of ion transport by the intestinal epithelial cells have been studied extensively,[10,20,21] but little is known of the development of these transport systems.

Cellular Localization

It is generally accepted that electrolyte absorptive (from lumen to blood) and secretory systems are present in two separate epithelial cell types; absorption is predominant in villous cells and secretion in crypt cells. Thus, many transported electrolytes and also water enter an intestinal or enterosystemic cycle.[22] This spatial distribution is a complex phenomenon, since crypt cells differentiate into villous cells. The balance between absorption and secretion is dependent

TABLE 1
Electrical Parameters of the Isolated
Jejunal Epithelium of Children

ISC (μEq/hr • cm^2)	PD (mV)	G (mS/cm^2)
1.6	1.33	32.4
(0.3)	(0.17)	(4.5)

Isc = short-circuit current; PD = potential difference; G = conductance.

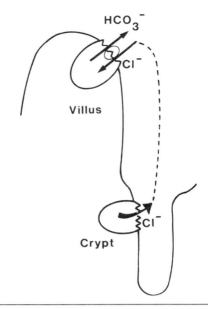

FIGURE 3 Possible interactions between crypt and villous cell transport. Here, Cl$^-$, secreted in the crypts, may be recaptured by the Cl$^-$/HCO$_3^-$ exchanger of the villous cells, producing HCO$_3^-$ secretion. This system is dynamic; the ratio of villous to crypt cell mass determines overall ionic and water transport capacities.

not only on the relative mass of villous to crypt cells but also on the rate of turnover and differentiation of the cells. It can be postulated that an increase in cell turnover and reduced differentiation will decrease absorption and increase secretion (Fig. 3).

The Source of Energy

Absorptive and secretory processes have a common source of cellular energy; Na$^+$,K$^+$-ATPase, coupled with K$^+$ permeability[23] located at the basolateral membrane, maintains a low intracellular Na$^+$ concentration, a high intracellular K$^+$ concentration, and a negative cell voltage. During development Na$^+$,K$^+$-ATPase increases threefold in isolated villous enterocytes from 3 to 5 days old to adult rabbit.[13] As the Na pump is not the limiting step in electrolyte transport under control conditions, the significance of this observation remains uncertain. In the rat colonic mucosa, Na$^+$,K$^+$-ATPase activity remains constant from day 10 to day 20, without any apparent correlation with water and Na$^+$ transport in vivo.[5]

Na$^+$ Transport Processes

Na$^+$ Absorption. This occurs by several pathways that are the limiting steps in luminal membranes of mature cells. *Several distinct solute Na$^+$ co-transport systems* (symports) are under different genetic control, one or several for glucose and galactose but not for fructose, several for groups of amino acids (neutral, basic, acidic, and imino acids), several for specific amino acids where the system for proline is the best defined,[24] and one or several systems for dipeptides or tripeptides. Thus, in mature cells Na$^+$ absorption is stimulated by food-derived solutes.

In the rabbit, the effect of glucose on Na$^+$ absorption in the jejunum but not in the ileum appears to be blunted in the suckling period.[13,14]

Everted sacs from 10-week human fetuses absorb glucose against a concentration gradient. By the age of 16 weeks, this absorption almost triples.[25] Glucose stimulates transmural PD in the fetal jejunum as early as the fifteenth week of gestation.[26] The main characteristics of a glucose-Na co-transport were present in children studied after 2 months of age.[15] All these observations suggest that the glucose-Na co-transport system is present at birth in healthy children.

Although, in the mature intestine, the solutes are mainly absorbed in the jejunum, recent evidence indicates that in the rat colon, 24 hours before birth, glucose stimulates Na$^+$ absorption; this system disappears 2 days after birth.[27] Also in human fetal colon, sucrase activity and possibly glucose transport are present transiently.

The NaCl Absorption Processes. Turnberg and Fordtran[28] during in vivo ileal perfusion in human volunteers observed that Na and Cl absorption was associated with HCO$_3$ secretion. They proposed the presence of a double exchange system: Na$^+$ absorption against H$^+$ secretion and Cl$^-$ absorption against HCO$_3^-$ secretion. The Na$^+$/H$^+$ exchanger has been identified in human jejunum and probably is present in the ileum. In contrast, the Cl$^-$/HCO$_3^-$ exchanger is present only in the ileum, together with other anion exchangers, but not in the jejunum. When coupled, these two exchangers behave like a coupled NaCl co-transporter. The coupling between these two systems is probably due to the intracellular pH.

Unidentified Na$^+$ Entry. In the small intestine, as much as 50 percent of Na absorption remains unaccounted for by the Na$^+$ entry pathways mentioned above.

Na Secretion. Na secretion, the consequence of a positive transepithelial PD, may be considered a normal phenomenon that is part of the enterosystemic cycle of water and Na$^+$, stimulated during a meal in healthy adults.[29] In infancy, this phenomenon has not been studied but probably is important, since, at that age epithelial permeability is high.

Moreover, Na secretion has been found in vitro in the form of a neutral NaCl flux in several species; its functional significance remains uncertain.[30,31]

The Amiloride-sensitive Na$^+$ Channel. In the colon, Na$^+$ enters the luminal membrane through a amiloride-sensitive Na$^+$ channel. It is inhibited by increased intracellular Na$^+$ concentration and stimulated by circulating aldosterone. In children this system is present as early as 30 to 33 weeks of gestation in the left colon, where probably it is stimulated by aldosterone.[32] This Na$^+$ channel, which exists in parallel with a Cl$^-$/HCO$_3^-$ exchanger, also may be stimulated by acetate[33,34] and short-chain fatty acids produced in the colon a few weeks after birth.[35]

Cl$^-$ Transport Processes

Chloride Absorption. Chloride is absorbed passively down its electrical gradient through the paracellular pathway. In addition, it is absorbed coupled to Na$^+$ or exchanged for HCO$_3^-$ in the ileum and the colon. In the colon, Cl$^-$/HCO$_3^-$ exchange does not appear to function before birth; it may not be fully functional until the end of the first year of life,[33] so the young infant, especially the preterm infant, may be particularly susceptible to chloride depletion.

Chloride Secretion. Chloride secretion is intimately linked with diarrhea. Entry from blood to cell across the basolateral membrane occurs through a co-transporter NaKCl$_2$, inhibited by loop diuretics and bumetanide. The driving force is the Na$^+$ electrochemical gradient produced by Na$^+$,K$^+$-ATPase and K$^+$ permeability. The Cl$^-$, thus accumulated in the cell, crosses the luminal membrane through a Cl$^-$ channel not yet identified in human intestine but well studied in tracheal epithelium. In cystic fibrosis opening of the Cl$^-$ channel is defective because its phosphorylation by the intracellular messengers is impaired.[36] In human intestinal cancer cells (CacO-2), which resemble fetal crypt cells, the Cl$^-$ channel is present in the absence of the NaKCl$_2$ co-transporter, suggesting that these two important transport systems can develop at different rates and stages.[37,38]

HCO$_3^-$ Transport Processes

HCO$_3^-$ Absorption. In the jejunum HCO$_3^-$ is absorbed against a steep electrochemical gradient by a neutral system that is Na$^+$ dependent, either a Na$^+$-HCO$_3^-$ co-transporter or a Na$^+$/H$^+$ exchanger. This exchanger has been identified in jejunal rabbit brush border membrane.[39]

HCO$_3^-$ Secretion. In the ileum, HCO$_3^-$ is secreted against an electrochemical gradient by two transport processes: (1) the well-defined Cl$^-$/HCO$_3^-$ exchanger located in the villous cell and (2) a possible Na$^+$-HCO$_3^-$ co-transporter responsible for electroneutral Na-dependent HCO$_3^-$ secretion.[40]

Intestinal transport of H$^+$ and HCO$_3^-$ is an important determinant of H$^+$ concentration in the microclimate at the surface of the luminal membrane. In the suckling and weanling rat, the pH of the surface microclimate is Na$^+$ dependent and dependent on intracellular metabolism. Also, surface mucus appears to play a role in maintaining this microclimate, most probably through retaining H$^+$ at the intestinal surface.[41] The relationship between anion transport systems and the intracellular microclimate is not yet clear.

In conclusion, the small intestine and the colon play an important role in water and electrolyte balance and the regulation of acid-base balance. Dehydration and metabolic acidosis are common consequences of intestinal insufficiency.

Regulation of Ion Transport

Multiple Levels of Regulation

Ion transport across the intestinal epithelium is regulated by extracellular and intracellular molecules. Typical extracellular molecules are glucose and amino acids that stimulate

Na entry across the luminal membrane. The main intracellular messengers are cyclic AMP, cyclic GMP, ionized calcium, the metabolites of the inositol phosphate pathways, intracellular ionic concentrations, and transmembrane electrical potential. In addition, molecules may act on the outer surface of the cells to modulate the intracellular messengers; this is the case for nutrients (fatty acids) and toxins acting from the luminal side and for hormones, circulating or produced locally and acting from the serosal side. Finally, there is a transepithelial regulation of ion transport. Very little is known about the development of these regulatory mechanisms, but there is a need for an integrated view of this regulation to understand the pathophysiology of diarrhea in children.

Intracellular Regulation

The recognition of intracellular regulation of ionic transport stems from the observation that cholera toxin, while stimulating water and electrolyte secretion, also stimulates intracellular cyclic AMP production.[42] Now the main intracellular messengers can be measured in well-characterized intestinal epithelial cells. For example, in the human colonic cell line HT 29, intracellular ionized calcium, as measured by use of the fluorescent molecule Quin-2, increased after bradykinine, adrenaline (alpha$_1$ effect), neurotensin, and carbachol.[43] In jejunal biopsies of children, adenylate cyclase and Na$^+$,K$^+$-ATPase activities have been measured.[44] By simultaneous determination of ionic transport and intracellular biochemical events, it becomes possible to investigate the regulation of ionic transport.[45]

Adenylate cyclase activity in intestinal membranes was studied in the human fetus. The basal activity tripled from the tenth to the seventeenth week of gestation, and it was stimulated by in vitro incubation with cholera toxin.[46] Probably this system is fully developed at birth. It catalyzes the synthesis of cyclic AMP from ATP. The catalytic units located in the basolateral membrane are under the control of a series of proteins called G (Gi for inhibitor and Gs for stimulator) that may be located in the luminal membrane.[47,48] Thus, pertussis toxin acts on Gi and cholera toxin on Gs. Cholera toxin acts after binding to specific gangliosides located on the outer surface of the luminal membrane, this binding being higher in the newborn period.[49]

Guanylate cyclase catalyzes the synthesis of cyclic GMP from GTP. In the small intestine guanylate cyclase exists predominantly in the particulate form and is located mainly in the brush border membrane. The enzymic activity is greatest in differentiated villous cells and least in proliferating crypt cells; in children, it is similar in small intestine and colon. In the small intestine, guanylate cyclase activity varies with age, being maximal at 1 day of age and decreasing thereafter. Activators of guanylate cyclase include unsaturated lipids, free radicals, oxidants, and *Escherichia coli* heat-stable enterotoxin (ST). Interestingly, the number of ST receptors present in infants is high, and this number rapidly decreases with increasing age. The degree of guanylate cyclase stimulation by ST is correlated with the density of ST receptors.[50,51]

Inositol phosphates modulate ion transport by diacylglycerol, which activates an 80-KD C-kinase, and inositol triphosphate (IP$_3$), which does not act directly on a kinase but enhances the release of free calcium from endoplasmic reticulum. The calcium thus liberated participates in the activation of the C-kinase, which in turn activates electrolyte secretion.[52] Development of this regulatory system is poorly understood.

Extracellular Regulation

The development of the extracellular regulation of ion transport, which has not been studied as such, must take into account the dynamic aspects of food and digestive secretions at the different periods of life. The development of the hormonal, neuronal, and immune systems probably plays an important role in determining enterocytic function. Furthermore, enterocytes lie on a matrix or basement membrane that is essential for cell differentiation. Because of these interactions, the basolateral membrane must be considered not only as a plasma membrane having the transport systems common to many nonepithelial cells (e.g., Na$^+$,K$^+$-ATPase, K$^+$ channel) but also as a membrane having a role in the development and maintenance of epithelial (asymmetric) functions.

Transepithelial regulation of ion transport occurs through the effect of substances present in the intestinal lumen activating mechanisms situated on the blood side of the epithelium. For example, ovalbumin placed in the lumen of a previously sensitized intestine stimulates Cl secretion by the epithelial cells.[53] Another example is the role of cholera toxin on water and electrolyte secretion. This toxin binds to the luminal membrane of the enterocytes, which, after stimulation of adenylate cyclase activity, produce an electrogenic Cl secretion. In addition to this direct effect on the enterocytes, cholera toxin also indirectly modulates a NaCl flux through

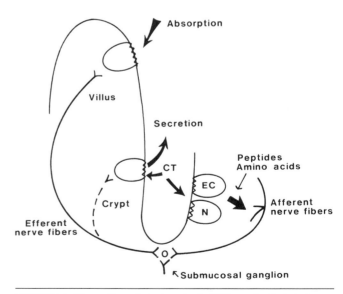

FIGURE 4 The action of cholera toxin (CT) on electrolyte transport. CT binds by its B subunits to the gangliosides of the brush border membrane; the A subunit stimulates cyclic AMP and thus electrogenic chloride secretion. This cellular effect is well documented (secretory diarrhea). In addition, it has been postulated that CT, by acting on enterochromaffin (EC) or neurotensin (N) cells, stimulates the submucosal plexus, which may control electrolyte transport, mainly the absorptive transport.

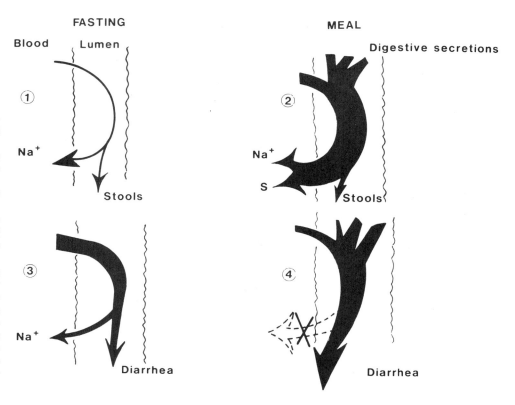

FIGURE 5 The enterosystemic water cycle. (1) During fasting, water that enters the lumen is reabsorbed following Na$^+$ absorption from lumen to blood. Therefore, very little water is lost in stools. (2) During a meal, much water enters the intestinal lumen as a consequence of digestive secretions (saliva, gastric, biliopancreatic, intestinal). Water is reabsorbed following Na$^+$ reabsorption, mainly through the solute-Na$^+$ cotransport systems; again, little water is lost in stools. In this system, diarrhea is a consequence of imbalance between absorption and secretion—due to increased secretion (3) or decreased reabsorption (4).

a complex neuronal reflex system (Fig. 4).[54,55] In addition, all luminal substances that modulate changes in transepithelial electrical potential modulate a transepithelial passive flux, which is particularly important in the immature intestine. For example, glucose that stimulates the transepithelial potential difference (the lumen being more negative) also stimulates K$^+$ secretion from blood to lumen.

In summary, the regulation of ion transport is due to a multiplicity of interactions that have been difficult to analyze in vivo. At the cellular level, these interactions are best studied in intestinal cell lines in culture. In such secreting cells the effects of calcium and cyclic AMP seem to be additive. At the mucosal level, these interactions are best studied in isolated intestine comprising mucosal and submucosal cells. For example, the phorbol esters evoke a Cl$^-$ secretion in isolated epithelium, secretion that is inhibited by indomethacin and naproxene, which inhibit the prostaglandin synthesis. In that case one postulates that phorbol ester–stimulated C-kinase stimulates the release of arachidonic acid, initiating the production of prostaglandins in the submucosal tissue. The prostaglandins thus produced stimulate the adenylate cyclase. This example indicates that ionic secretion is under the control of intracellular factors and the submucosal nervous and immune systems (Fig. 4).

Regulation of ion transport regulates the movement of water between the environment and the body and within the body. The balance between secretion and absorption is a dynamic process represented by the enterosystemic water cycle[9,22] (Fig. 5). The small intestine is the site where the quantity of water and electrolytes transported is the most important. However, from the clinical point of view, the colon is the site

of water and electrolyte salvage, which is usually important for the regulation of stool volume. The enterosystemic water cycle is best evaluated by measuring total body weight and intake and output volumes. In the immature intestine this water cycle is probably turning over rapidly, and an increase in stool output that causes dehydration may be the result of a relative increase in secretion compared with absorption or a relative decrease in absorption compared with secretion. Therefore, the treatment of secretory diarrhea could be approached by decreasing secretion and/or stimulating absorption.

REFERENCES

1. Younoszai MK, Sapario RS, Laughlin M. Maturation of jejunum and ileum in rats. Water and electrolyte transport during in vivo perfusion of hypertonic solutions. J Clin Invest 1978; 62:271–280.
2. Younoszai MK, Robillard JE. In vivo intestinal bicarbonate transport in infant rats. Pediatr Res 1980; 14:839–843.
3. Ghishan FK, Jenkins JT, Younoszai MK. Intestinal calcium loss in infant rats. Proc Soc Exp Biol Med 1979; 161:70–73.
4. Younoszai MK. Development of water and electrolyte transport in the small intestine. In: Lebenthal E, ed. Textbook of gastroenterology and nutrition in infancy. New York: Raven Press, 1981: 615.
5. Findel Y, Aperia A, Eklöf AC. Development of colonic fluid and electrolyte transport: influence of weaning pattern. J Pediatr Gastroenterol Nutr 1985; 4:457–462.
6. Wisser J, Horster M. In vitro perfused, non-isolated small intestine: ontogeny of transmural hydraulic permeability. Pflügers Arch 1978; 373:205–208.
7. Katchalsky A, Curran PF. Nonequilibrium thermodynamics in biophysics. Cambridge, MA: Harvard University Press, 1967: 248.
8. Curran PF. Twelfth Bowditch lecture: coupling between transport processes in intestine. Physiologist 1968; 2:3–23.

9. Desjeux JF, Heyman M, Ben Mansour A. Water and ion movement in intestine. In: Viral enteritis. Paris: INSERM, 1980: 39.

10. Powell DW. Intestinal water and electrolyte transport. In: Johnson LR, ed. Physiology of the gastrointestinal tract. 2nd ed. New York: Raven Press, 1987: 1267.

11. Curran PF, Macintosh J. A model system for biological water transport. Nature 1962; 193:347–348.

12. Schultz SG, Zalusky R. Ion transport in isolated rabbit ileum. I. Short-circuit current and Na fluxes. J Gen Physiol 1964; 47:1043–1059.

13. Shepherd RW, Hamilton JR, Gall DG. The postnatal development of sodium transport in the proximal small intestine of the rabbit. Pediatr Res 1980; 14:250–253.

14. Cook HJ, Dawson DC. Transport characteristics of isolated newborn rabbit ileum. Am J Physiol 1978; 234(3):E257–E261.

15. Grasset E, Heyman M, Dumontier AM, Lestradet H, Desjeux JF. Possible sodium and D-glucose cotransport in isolated jejunal epithelium of children. Pediatr Res 1979; 13:1240–1246.

16. Crane RK. Hypothesis for mechanism of intestinal active transport of sugars. Fed Proc 1962; 21:891–895.

17. Schultz SG, Curran PF. Coupled transport of sodium and organic solutes. Physiol Rev 1970; 50:637–718.

18. Hopfer U, Nelson K, Perrotto J, Isselbacher KJ. Glucose transport in isolated brush border membranes from rat small intestine. J Biol Chem 1973; 2248:25–32.

19. Hopfer U. Membrane transport mechanisms for hexoses and amino acids in the small intestine. In: Johnson LR, ed. Physiology of the gastrointestinal tract. 2nd ed. New York: Raven Press, 1987: 1499.

20. Field M. Secretion of electrolytes and water by mammalian small intestine. In: Johnson LR, ed. Physiology of the gastrointestinal tract. New York: Raven Press, 1981: 963.

21. Donowitz M, Welsh MJ. Regulation of mammalian small intestinal electrolyte secretion. In: Johnson LR, ed. Physiology of the gastrointestinal tract. 2nd ed. New York: Raven Press, 1987: 1351.

22. Desjeux JF, Tannenbaum C, Tai YH, Curran PF. Effects of sugars and amino acids on sodium movement across small intestine. Am J Dis Child 1977; 131:331–340.

23. Grasset E, Gunter-Smith P, Schultz SG. Effects of Na- coupled alanine transport on intracellular K activities and the K conductance of the basolateral membrane of necturus small intestine. J Membr Biol 1983; 71:89–94.

24. Peerce BE, Wright EM. Conformational changes in the Na/proline cotransporter of intestinal brush borders. Ann NY Acad Sci 1985; 456:118–120.

25. Jirosova V, Koldovsky O, Heringova A, Hoskova J, Jirasek JE, Uker J. The development of the functions of the small intestine of human fetus. Biol Neonate 1966; 9:44.

26. Koldovsky O, Heringova A, Jirosova V, Jirasek JE, Uker J. Transport of glucose against a concentration gradient in everted sacs of jejunum and ileum of human fetuses. Gastroenterology 1965; 48:185.

27. Potter GD, Burlingame SM. Glucose-coupled sodium absorption in the developing rat colon. Am J Physiol 1986; 250:G221–G226.

28. Turnberg L, Bieberdorf F, Morawski S, Fordtran J. Interrelationships of chloride, bicarbonate, sodium and hydrogen transport in the human ileum. J Clin Invest 1970; 49:557–567.

29. Miazza B, Palma R, Lachance JR, Chayvialle JA, Jonard PP, Modigliani R. Rejunal secretory effect of intraduodenal food in humans. Gastroenterology 1985; 88:1215–1222.

30. Powell DW, Binder HJ, Curran PF. Electrolyte secretion by the guinea pig ileum in vitro. Am J Physiol 1972; 223:531–537.

31. Desjeux JF, Tai YH, Curran PF. Characteristics of sodium flux from serosa to mucosa in rabbit ileum. J Gen Physiol 1974; 64:274–292.

32. Jenkins HR, Fenton TR, McIntosh N, Dillon MJ, Milla PJ. Development of epithelial electrolyte transport process in early childhood. Pediatr Res 1987; 22:97.

33. Jenkins HR, Milla PJ. The development of colonic transport mechanisms in early life: evidence for reduced anion exchange. In press.

34. Jenkins HR, Schnackenberg U, Milla PJ. Mechanisms of transport of sodium and chloride and the effects of short-chain fatty acids in the human infant. Pediatr Res 1987; 22:97.

35. Murray RD, Mcclung HJ, Ulysses B, Li K, Ailabouni A. Short- chain fatty acid profile in the colon of newborn piglets using fecal water analysis. Pediatr Res 1987; 22:720–724.

36. Schoumacher RA, Shoemaker RL, Halm DR, Tallant EA, Wallace RW, Frizzell RA. Phosphorylation fails to activate chloride channels from cystic fibrosis airway cells. Nature 1987; 330:752–754.

37. Grasset E, Pinto M, Dussaulx E, Zweibaum A, Desjeux JF. Epithelial properties of human colonic carcinoma cell line Caco-2: electrical parameters. Am J Physiol 1984; 247:C260–C267.

38. Grasset E, Bernabeu J, Pinto M. Epithelial properties of human colonic carcinoma cell line Caco-2: effect of secretagogues. Am J Physiol 1985; 248:C410–C418.

39. Gunther R, Wright E. Na$^+$, Li$^+$ and Cl$^-$ transport by brush border membranes from rabbit jejunum. J Membr Biol 1983; 74:85–94.

40. Smith PL, Cascairo MA, Sullivan SK. Sodium dependence of luminal alkalinisation by rabbit ileal mucosa. Am J Physiol 1985; 249:G358–G368.

41. Said HM, Smith R, Redha R. Studies on the intestinal surface acid microclimate: developmental aspects. Pediatr Res 1987; 22:497–499.

42. Schafer DE, Lust WD, Sircar B, Goldberg ND. Elevation of 3-5' cyclic monophosphate concentration in intestinal mucosa after treatment with cholera toxin. Proc Natl Acad Sci 1970; 67:851–857.

43. De Jonge HR, Vaandrager AB. Signal transduction in mammalian enterocytes: protein phosphorylation and polyinositide cycling in the brush border membrane. Gastroenterology. In press.

44. Tripp JH, Muller DPR, Harries JT. Mucosal (Na$^+$- K$^+$)-ATPase and adenylate cyclase activities in children with toddler diarrhea and the postenteritis syndrome. Pediatr Res 1980; 14:1382–1386.

45. Desjeux JF, Ben Mansour A, Nath S. Les mécanismes cellulaires de la sécrétion intestinale. In: Rambaud JC, Modigliani R, eds. l'Intestin grêle. Amsterdam: Excerpta Medica, 1988: 102.

46. Grand RJ, Torti FM, Jaksina S. Development of intestinal adenyl cyclase and its response to cholera enterotoxin. J Clin Invest 1973; 52:2053–2059.

47. Gill DM, Woolkalis M. Toxins which activate adenylate cyclase. Ciba Found Symp 1985; 112:57–73.

48. Dominguez P, Velasco G, Barros F, Lazo PS. Intestinal brush border membranes contain regulatory subunits of adenylate cyclase. Proc Natl Acad Sci USA 1987; 84:6965–6969.

49. Bresson JL, Pang KY, Walker WA. Microvillus membrane differentiation: quantitative difference in cholera toxin binding to the intestinal surface of newborn and adult rabbits. Pediatr Res 1984; 18:984–987.

50. Guarino A, Cohen M, Giannella RA. Small and large intestinal guanylate cyclase activity in children: effect of age and stimulation by *Escherichia coli* heat-stable enterotoxin. Pediatr Res 1987; 21:551–555.

51. Cohen MB, Guarino A, Shukla R, Giannella RA. Age-related differences in receptors for *Escherichia coli* heat-stable enterotoxin in the small and large intestine of children. Gastroenterology 1988; 94:367–373.

52. Weikel CS, Sando JJ, Guerrant RL. Stimulation of porcine jejunal in secretion in vivo by protein kinase-C activators. J Clin Invest 1985; 76:2430–2435.

53. Perdue MH, Gall DG. Intestinal anaphylaxis in the rat: jejunal response to in vitro antigen exposure. Am J Physiol 1986; 250:G427–G431.

54. Cassuto J, Siewert A, Jodal M, Lundgren O. The involvement of intramural nerves in cholera-toxin induced intestinal secretion. Acta Physiol Scand 1983; 117:195–202.

55. Ben Mansour A, Rautureau M, Tomé D, Bisalli A, Desjeux JF. Neurotoxins and opiates stimulate neutral NaCl absorption in control and cholera-toxin treated intestine. Gastroenterol 1987; 25: 614.

CHAPTER 22

Hepatobiliary System: Structure and Function

Eldon A. Shaffer, M.D., FRCPC, F.A.C.P.

BILE FORMATION AND GALLBLADDER FUNCTION

The liver is an exocrine organ producing a unique secretion, bile. This complex fluid consists of organic compounds, predominantly lipids, held in an aqueous electrolyte solution. These lipids interact to be solubilized and transported in bile through the biliary system into the small intestine. The solubilizing components of bile (mainly bile salts and phospholipids) aid in the excretion of endogenous lipids (e.g., cholesterol), potentially toxic metabolites (e.g., steroid hormones, bilirubin), and exogenous agents (e.g., drugs, environmental chemicals).[1,2] In the intestine, bile promotes the lipolysis and absorption of dietary fats.

For the fetus, the placenta provides the excretory and nutritional functions that must be assumed by the liver after birth. Adaptation to extrauterine life includes, therefore, the development of hepatic excretory function. The importance of neonatal physiology is highlighted by the increased susceptibility of the newborn to cholestatic agents such as parenteral hyperalimentation and endotoxin from gram-negative microorganisms. Further, impaired fat digestion due to decreased intraluminal bile acids carries an adverse nutritional impact. All these risks are compounded in the premature infant.

This section will explore hepatic secretory and biliary tract functions, emphasizing known aspects of its immaturity in early life and postnatal development. Information concerning bile formation and delivery via the biliary system is relevant to the pathogenesis of bile secretory failure (cholestasis), gallstone formation, and fat malabsorption.

Functional Anatomy of the Hepatobiliary System

The liver postnatally receives blood from two sources: 25 percent from the hepatic artery (a branch of the celiac artery that carries highly oxygenated blood) and 75 percent from the portal vein (a confluence of the superior mesenteric and splenic veins, that is loaded with nutrients). These two afferent vessels enter the liver through a fissure, the porta hepatis, and divide into branches. A hemodynamic interaction between the two vascular beds maintains a constant total blood flow: When hepatic arterial flow decreases, portal venous flow increases, and vice versa. Both streams mix in the hepatic sinusoids and leave via the terminal hepatic venules (central veins), which converge to form the right and left hepatic veins and then the inferior vena cava. Thus, the liver is strategically located between the splanchnic and systemic circulations. This site allows it to regulate and metabolize substances absorbed by the intestine or hormones produced in organs drained by the splanchnic bed, before being passed to other parts of the body by the systemic circulation or via excretion into bile.

The traditional unit of liver architecture is the *lobule.* The classic lobule is hexagonal but may be viewed as a wheel: the central vein in the middle being the axle, the sinusoids as the spokes, and the portal tracts lying on the circumference. Five to seven portal tracts (portal triads) located at the periphery contain branches of the portal vein, bile ducts, and hepatic arteries, along with nerves and lymphatics. Between the central and peripheral (or central and portal) systems lie columns of liver cells whose adjacent surfaces act as blood-filled sinusoids and bile conduits. The sinusoids are vascular channels lined by endothelial cells and macrophages termed Kupffer cells. The sinusoids run perpendicular to the central veins. They receive blood separately from the portal venous and hepatic arterial systems and drain to the central veins. In the lobule, therefore, blood flows centripetally from portal tracts to central vein.

Sinusoids are larger than capillaries. Their endothelial lining is incomplete with fenestrations and lack of a complete basal lamina (Fig. 1). Such an incomplete barrier allows plasma to freely enter the perisinusoidal space of Disse, yet restricts the entry of blood cells (Fig. 2). This sinusoidal space not only provides contact between plasma and hepatocytes but also drains interstitial fluid to the lymphatics and the portal tract. The liver cells or hepatocytes are arranged in sheets, one cell thick, lying between the sinusoids. This microcirculatory anatomy allows the liver to transport tightly protein-bound substances like bilirubin. A "limiting plate" of liver cells surrounds each portal tract.

The *hepatic acinus* is a more functional organization that divides the liver into tridimensional microcirculatory units[2] (Fig. 3). In this scheme, hepatocytes receive their blood supply from a central axis formed by the terminal portal venule and the terminal hepatic arteriole in the portal triad. Both of these small vessels enter from the portal tract, providing portal venous and hepatic arterial blood, respectively. The incoming arterial and portal branches form the center; the outgoing hepatic vein branches lie at the periphery. Sinusoids

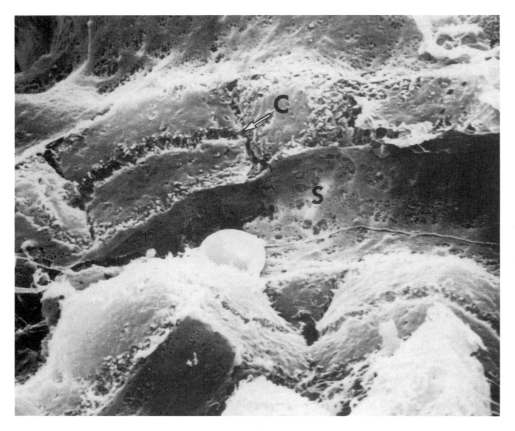

FIGURE 1 Scanning electron micrograph showing a canaliculus, the lateral groove between two adjacent hepatocytes (C, denoted by the white arrow). Tiny microvilli protrude into the canalicular lumen and are also present on the sinusoidal membrane surface of the hepatocyte. S is the adjacent wall of the sinusoid. The many small depressions in the endothelial cell lining the sinusoid are perforations or small fenestrae. (Courtesy of Dr. R.S. Hannah.)

radiate from the central axis and distribute blood centrifugally throughout the acinus, sequentially from acinar zone 1 near the portal triad through zone 2 to acinar zone 3. In zone 3, one or more terminal hepatic veins (central veins) interdigitate from adjacent acini.

Hepatocytes may be separated into these three zones depending on distance from their central vascular supply. In zone 1, periportal hepatocytes are exposed to the highest level of nutrients (from hepatic portal blood) and oxygen (from the hepatic artery). Zone 3, the centrilobular region, is situ-

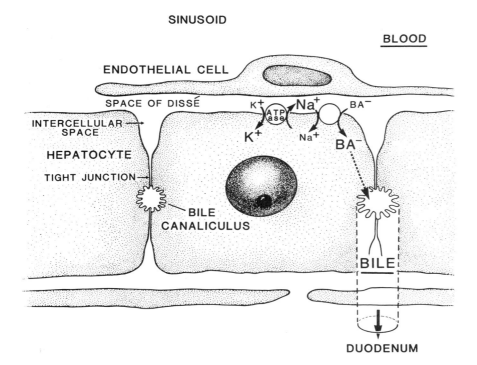

FIGURE 2 Model of hepatic bile formation and schematic representation of a liver cell plate. The liver plate is a single cell thick, separated from blood on either side by the space of Dissé. The sinusoidal endothelial cells have fenestrae and lack a basal lamina, allowing plasma but not blood cells access to the space of Dissé. The bile canaliculus is formed by the lateral groove between adjacent hepatocytes. Tight junctions separate the canaliculus from the sinusoidal and lateral surfaces of the liver cells. As with the sinusoidal surface (not shown here), the canaliculus has many microvilli enlarging its surface area. Bile acid (BA⁻) uptake from the space of Dissé is coupled to sodium (Na⁺) uptake. The inwardly directed Na⁺ gradient for this is established by the sodium pump (Na⁺,K⁺-ATPase). This electrogenic pump also creates a negative intracellular potential difference of about −35 mV, which assists the secretion of BA⁻ anions into the less negative canaliculus. (From Shaffer.[2])

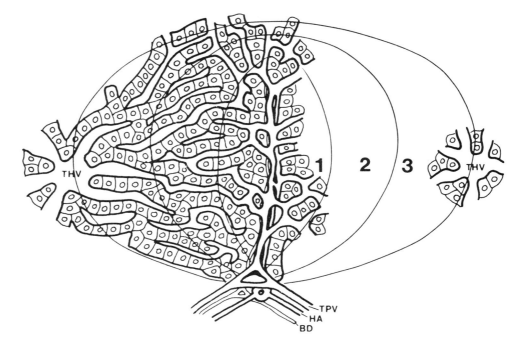

FIGURE 3 Hepatic acinus as a microcirculatory unit. The central axis consists of the blood supply to the acinar sinusoids from the terminal portal vein (TPV) and the hepatic artery (HA). Both enter from the portal tract, which also contains the bile ductule (BD). Blood first enters zone 1 and subsequently flows through zone 2 to zone 3, a peripheral area that drains radially to the terminal hepatic vein (THV).

ated in the microcirculatory periphery near the central vein, far from the supplying vessels. Zone 2 is an intermediate area between the central and peripheral regions. Oxygen, some carbohydrates, and other substances in sinusoidal blood have higher concentrations in zone 1 than in zone 3, creating an oxygen-nutrient concentration gradient between these areas.[4,5] This results in an increased vulnerability of zone 3 to toxic, anoxic, or metabolic injury.

The microcirculatory concept of the acinus and its zonal organization also has functional consequences relative to bile formation. A lobular gradient exists in the sinusoids, resulting in *functional heterogeneity*. Cells near the portal vein in zone 1 have greater access to incoming plasma solutes compared to hepatocytes further from the central supply in zone 3. For substances like bile salts, which are avidly cleared by the mature liver, hepatocytes in zone 1 readily take up large quantities, leaving a serially decreasing concentration in the sinusoid for hepatocytes in zone 3, which is perfused last. Any increase in the incoming supply of solute causes a progressive recruitment of hepatocytes in zone 2 and eventually zone 3. Recent work has suggested that the transport of bile salts is similar in cells from zone 1 and zone 3, although transit through and secretion from hepatocytes in zone 3 may be slower. Heterogeneity between periportal and centrilobular hepatocytes is also evident histologically and biochemically: Periportal hepatocytes are heavier, their bile canaliculi are larger, and they are more active in terms of gluconeogenesis and oxidative metabolism.[5] Such heterogeneity does not exist in the suckling rat liver in contrast to the adult.[6] The developing liver is deficient in its ability to take up bile salts and is unable to establish a concentration gradient from the periportal (zone 1) to the central (zone 3) areas. The entire acinus is used but still remains relatively inefficient for bile salt transport in the very young.[7,8]

Hepatocytes form their own secretory-drainage system. The contact surface of adjacent liver cells forms 1-μm grooves, the bile canaliculus. The integrity of the canalicular space is maintained by tight junctions that are stabilized by desmosomes and microfilaments. Tiny microvilli project into the canalicular lumen. These extracellular channels begin blindly and form anastomosing networks that convey bile from the centrilobular area toward the periphery of the lobule to the portal triads. Here, canalicular bile enters the small terminal bile ductules or canals of Hering (preferred term: cholangioles). These short channels pass through the limiting plate of liver cells into larger interlobular bile ducts (diameter less than 100 μm) within the portal triad. These and the progressively larger drainage system (in order: septal bile ducts, segmental bile ducts, and then the right and left hepatic ducts) are lined by cuboidal epithelium.

The liver is a transporting epithelium conveying a variety of substrates from blood to bile. This vectoral transport is made possible by the high degree of polarization of the plasma membrane of the hepatocyte. The hexagonal-shaped liver cell has three interfaces: (1) sinusoidal, bathed by plasma; (2) contiguous, cell-cell contact, and (3) bile canaliculi, limited by the tight junction (see Fig. 2). These three domains of the liver cell membrane possess important morphologic, biochemical, and enzymatic differences that are necessary for transepithelial transport. For example, sodium-potassium–activated adenosine triphosphatase (Na+, K+-ATPase) is located in the sinusoidal and intercellular membrane, with little or no activity on the canalicular membrane.[9] Further, receptors for several hormones and proteins have been identified in the plasma but not the canalicular membrane. Similarly, there are specific enzymes (e.g., alkaline phosphatase) and proteins in canalicular membrane. For the hepatocyte, the sinusoidal and intercellular membrane is the equivalent of the "basolateral" membrane of other transporting epithelial cells. The canalicular domain represents the "apical" surface. The liver cell is therefore polarized with a relatively large surface for uptake (the basolateral domain may comprise as much as 87 percent of the hepatocyte membrane surface), but a small surface for excretion into bile (13 percent of the total cell surface is the canalicular membrane). The surface area of both the sinusoidal and canalicular membranes is increased by the presence of microvilli. This relation is not different in the developing liver. The surface area of the sinusoidal space may be less in the neonatal rat liver but still represents about 10 percent of the liver volume, as in the adult rat.[10] Transport is further enhanced by a countercurrent flow between blood and bile: sinusoidal plasma flowing in a direction opposite to canalicular bile flow.

The *tight junction* is the sealing structure between the lumen of the bile canaliculus and the intercellular space (see Fig. 2). It represents the principal barrier to free movement of molecules from blood to bile. Despite the term "tight," there is a gradation of permeability among tight junctions depending upon the epithelial tissue of origin. The "relatively loose" tight junction in the liver acts as a paracellular pathway for water and electrolyte permeation from blood through the lateral intercellular space and tight junction to the bile canalicular lumen.[2,9]

Bile Composition

Bile formed by the liver is predominantly water with a 3 percent (g per deciliter) solid concentration (Table 1). When concentrated by the gallbladder, this rises to 10 g per deciliter, but the osmolarity remains 295 to 300 mOsmol per liter, like plasma. Bile salts comprise two-thirds of the organic anions. Lecithin (phosphatidyl choline—the phospholipid in bile) and cholesterol (in the free or unesterified form) are both water-insoluble lipids. They represent another 22 and 4 percent, respectively, of the organic solids in bile. Bilirubin (as the diglucuronide conjugate) is the predominant bile pigment. Little glucose is present; presumably any glucose secreted by the liver is reabsorbed in the biliary system.[11] The pro-

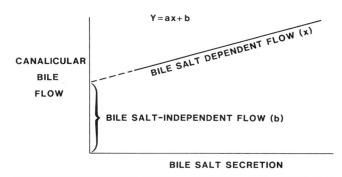

FIGURE 4 Relationship between canalicular bile flow and bile salt secretion. Canalicular flow is commonly estimated by erythritol clearance, a small inert marker. The relation between bile flow and bile salt secretion rate is linear. This bile salt–dependent flow varies directly with bile salt output. The slope of this line, given as *a* in the formula $Y = ax + b$, represents the osmotic or "choleretic activity" of the bile salt (i.e., increases in units of volume per increment in mass of bile salt secreted). Extrapolation back to a theoretical zero bile salt secretion (shown as dashed line and represented by *b* in the formula) yields an apparent output of bile in the absence of bile salt secretion, termed *bile salt–independent flow*. A third component, not shown, is *ductular flow*, which would correspondingly modify the resultant total bile output.

teins present include plasma proteins (like albumin), liver-specific proteins (e.g., secretory component, 5'-nucleotidase, and lysosomal enzymes), and polymeric IgA. Hepatic bile with a relatively high concentration of bicarbonate has a pH of 7 to 8, whereas bicarbonate absorption in the gallbladder yields a lower pH of 6 to 7. The inorganic electrolytes in hepatic bile closely reflect their plasma concentrations. The major cation is sodium.

Canalicular Bile Formation

Canalicular bile flow is believed to be induced by active secretion of solutes, followed osmotically by obligatory water flow.[12,13] Bile salts, the most abundant organic anion in the bile, are considered the major driving force for bile formation. A linear relation exists between bile flow and bile salt output in man and a variety of animals (Fig. 4). The slope of this line (the increment in bile volume accompanying each increase in bile salt secretion) indicates the choleretic potency of the bile salt: water movement occurring in response to bile salt secretion, termed *bile salt–dependent bile flow*. This fits conceptually with the transport of bile salts into the canalicular lumen, creating an osmotic gradient to which water passively flows.

The osmotic activity of bile salts depends on their presence in bile as monomers; an additional contribution comes from their counter ion, sodium (Na^+). Above a certain concentration, bile salt molecules self-aggregate, forming simple micelles. Micelle formation should decrease the number of osmotically active particles and reduce the apparent choleretic activity. For those bile salts that aggregate at high concen-

TABLE 1
Average Composition of Human Gallbladder Bile

Contents	g/dl	Gallbladder Solids (Organic) (% Total)	mM*
Bile salts	12.00	} 91	3–45
Lecithin	3.00		
Cholesterol	0.50		
Bilirubin	0.15	} 9	
Protein	0.10		
Ions			
Potassium	0.05		2.7–4.9
Calcium and magnesium	0.06		1.2–4.8 / 1.4–3.0
Chloride	0.08		88–115
Bicarbonate	0.09		27–55
Sodium			146–156
Osmolarity (mOsmol/L)			295–330

*Reported range depends on whether the bile is hepatic or from the gallbladder.

trations (a high "critical micellar concentration"), relatively more will remain in solution as osmotically active monomers. Their apparent choleretic activity will approach a theoretical maximal bile salt–dependent bile flow: e.g., for deoxycholate, 13 to 17 μl per micromole is secreted in the rat and hamster. Non–micellar-forming bile acids therefore would be quite choleretic. The osmotic behavior of individual bile acids, however, cannot fully account for differences in their choleretic activities. The effect of bile acids on bile flow is also a function of their molecular structure. Tri- and dihydroxy bile salts are choleretic, whereas monohydroxy bile salts are cholestatic. Choleretic activity further depends on the polarity of the molecule: Lipophilic bile acids are more choleretic than polar bile acids; unconjugated bile acids are more choleretic than conjugated ones. Lastly, other ion transport systems modify bile formation.[15] "Hypercholeretic" bile acids such as ursodeoxycholic acid have an apparent choleretic activity exceeding 20 μl per micromole. For them, bile flow is too great to be explained solely by the principle of their osmotic activity in bile.[14]

Extrapolation of the line relating bile flow (*y*-axis) to bile salt secretion (*x*-axis) to the ordinant arbitrarily defines a component of canalicular flow which theoretically would be present if no bile salts were secreted (Fig. 4). This *bile salt–independent flow* varies in magnitude between animals but in human adults represents about 50 percent of total canalicular bile flow.[16] The appearance of bile salt-independent bile formation is also an important landmark in the postnatal development of hepatic excretory function, becoming evident at the time of weaning.[17]

A portion of bile output relates to the addition of water and electrolytes distally in the bile duct system. This has been termed *ductular bile flow* and in certain species is increased by the hormone, secretin.

The concept directly relating bile flow to bile salt secretion may be an oversimplification.[9] Depending upon experimental conditions, the choleretic activity of a specific bile salt varies. Even a curvilinear relation between bile flow and bile salt secretion is possible at low rates of bile salt secretion. Altered permeability of the hepatobiliary epithelium, the presence of hepatic electrolyte transport systems, and the secretion of other organic anions all could modify canalicular bile flow. The permeability properties of the hepatobiliary epithelium, particularly the paracellular barriers between cells, are influenced by bile salts per se and by cholestatic agents such as estrogen.[18] Besides the sodium-coupled bile salt transport system (described later), bile salts may stimulate flow through other transport mechanisms. The osmotic effect of concentrative bile salt transport might cause electrolytes to secondarily enter bile via the paracellular route by solvent drag with water or by diffusion. This would not require specific ion transport mechanisms. The hypercholeresis induced by ursodeoxycholic acid is associated with increased bicarbonate secretion.[14] Such excessive bile flow may represent an example of electrolyte transport being induced by bile salt secretion. Ursodeoxycholic acid enhances basolateral Na^+/H^+ exchange, increasing bicarbonate (HCO_3^-) activity in the liver cell and secretion into the canaliculus.[19] Alternately, ursodeoxycholic acid could stimulate a Cl^-/HCO_3^- exchange in the canalicular membrane causing HCO_3^- secretion into bile.

A different mechanism for this hypercholeresis with active bicarbonate secretion has been postulated for unconjugated dihydroxy bile acids such as ursodeoxycholic acid. These unconjugated dihydroxy bile acids are lipophilic; when protonated, they easily pass across epithelial cells. Once secreted, they could be reabsorbed further downstream by the biliary epithelium and returned via the periductular capillary plexus to the sinusoid for reuptake and secretion by the liver cells, a "cholehepatic shunt."[20,21] Carbonic acid would provide the protons allowing the passive uptake of ursodeoxycholic acid while generating HCO_3^-. The osmotic activity is thus passed to bicarbonate while the bile acid is recycled.

Bile salt–independent flow is not due to altered biliary permeability nor to the sodium pump (Na^+,K^+-ATPase), which is located on the sinusoidal pole of the hepatocyte. Most ion transport models such as bicarbonate or chloride use the Na^+ gradient established by Na^+,K^+-ATPase.[15] None explains bile salt–independent flow. Instead, biliary permeability and electrolyte secretion into bile are more likely to modulate the effect of bile salts on bile flow, i.e., their choleretic activity. One attractive hypothesis suggests that the active secretion of one or more organic anions other than bile salts independently stimulates bile flow. Of the endogenous compounds that enter bile, glutathione and its metabolites are likely candidates.[22]

Enterohepatic Circulation of Bile Salts

The hepatic secretion of bile salts is the driving force behind bile flow and the principal determinant of biliary solute secretion. Bile salt flux through the liver depends upon their

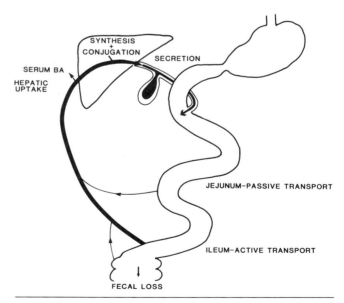

FIGURE 5 Enterohepatic circulation of bile salts in a human adult. Typical kinetic values are hepatic synthesis (0.2–0.6 g/day), hepatic secretion = pool (3 g) × cycles (5–15/day) = (15–40 g/day), fecal excretion (0.2–0.6 g/day), and portal venous return (more than 95 percent of hepatic secretion). Little escapes into the systemic circulation or is lost by fecal elimination.

cycling from the intestine, the enterohepatic circulation (Fig. 5). Hepatic clearance and intestinal transport in the adult are quite efficient.[23] Bile salts are synthesized exclusively in the liver from cholesterol. Secreted by the liver, they are then stored in the gallbladder during the interdigestive period. In the jejunum, bile salts act as detergents to promote fat absorption; their active absorption occurs later in the terminal ileum. Some passive absorption also occurs along the jejunum and in the colon. Once absorbed into the portal vein, bile acids return to the liver, where they are effectively cleared and secreted once again into the bile. The major source for hepatic secretion during the day is bile salts recirculated from the intestine, with only a small portion being derived from de novo synthesis. The latter may represent only 1.5 percent of the total 24-hour bile salt input in the presence of an intact enterohepatic circulation. Put another way, the efficiency of the enterohepatic circulation allows cycling of bile salts to exceed the bile salt synthesis rate by more than 10-fold.

Hepatic clearance and intestinal absorption are rapid and efficient in healthy adults. Although first-pass clearance of bile salts by the liver is extremely high, there is some spill into the systemic circulation. Normally only low levels of serum bile acids are detectable. The serum concentration therefore represents a balance between input from the intestine and clearance by the liver.[24]

The total mass of bile salts within the enterohepatic circulation represents the bile salt pool. The size of this pool and the rate at which it circulates produce the bile salt secretion rate. This efficient recycling system allows a small pool of bile salts (about 50 mg per kilogram of body weight in adults)

to recirculate 5 to 15 times a day: about twice with each meal but less rapidly when fasting.[25] With each circuit, some 3 to 5 percent of bile salts are lost via fecal excretion. These small losses are accurately replaced by hepatic synthesis, maintaining a stable bile salt pool. Bile salt synthesis from cholesterol accounts for about half of the cholesterol removed from the body each day; biliary cholesterol excretion represents another major route of elimination.

Bile salt synthesis is regulated by the rate at which bile salts return to the liver in a negative feedback manner.[26] The mechanism for this inhibition is the down-regulation of the activity of cholesterol 7 alpha-hydroxylase, the rate-limiting step in the bile acid biosynthetic pathway (Fig. 6).[27] A low rate of return stimulates synthesis, whereas a high rate is inhibitory. Loss of the bile salt pool, such as from biliary drainage or ileal loss, decreases the rate of bile salt return. The liver responds by augmenting synthesis. Complete interruption of the enterohepatic circulation yields a maximum stimulus, increasing synthesis 10-fold in most mammals. Under such circumstances, synthesis becomes the major source of bile salts for secretion.

Bile acid synthesis is controlled not only by the rate of bile salt return, but also by the availability of microsomal free cholesterol as substrate and by the type of bile acid fluxing through the liver. More hydrophobic bile salts (like cholic, chenodeoxycholic, and deoxycholic acids) inhibit cholesterol 7 alpha-hydroxylase to a greater extent than hydrophilic bile salts (like ursodeoxycholic acid).[27]

The enterohepatic circulation is thus powered by two active transport sites (the liver and terminal ileum), two mechan-

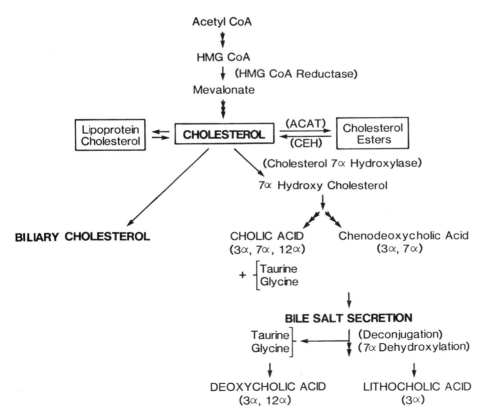

FIGURE 6 Cholesterol and bile salt biosynthetic pathways and secretion into bile. Hepatic microsomal cholesterol receives input from lipoprotein cholesterol, newly synthesized cholesterol from acetate (the rate-limiting step being HMG CoA reductase), and cholesterol stored as cholesterol ester. This pool of free cholesterol is either converted into bile acids (rate-limiting enzyme is cholesterol 7 alpha-hydroxylase) or secreted as biliary cholesterol. The primary bile acids synthesized in humans are cholic acid and chenodeoxycholic acid. Before being secreted into bile, they are conjugated with either taurine or glycine. Bacterial transformation occurs in the intestine: first deconjugation splitting off the taurine or glycine moiety, then dehydroxylation removing the 7 alpha-OH and forming secondary bile acids. Only lithocholic acid, which is water-insoluble, normally is not reabsorbed to any appreciable extent.

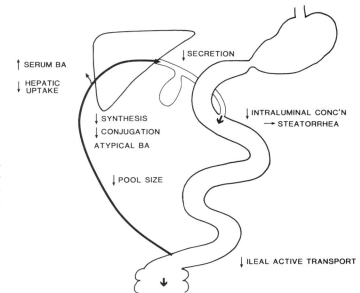

↑ SERUM BA

↓ HEPATIC
   UPTAKE

↓ SECRETION

↓ SYNTHESIS
↓ CONJUGATION
ATYPICAL BA

↓ INTRALUMINAL CONC'N
  → STEATORRHEA

↓ POOL SIZE

↓ ILEAL ACTIVE TRANSPORT

FIGURE 7 Enterohepatic circulation of bile acids in the neonate. Compared to the adult (see Fig. 5), most facets of the enterohepatic circulation are defective, allowing loss via fecal elimination and spillover into the systemic circulation. Transport in the liver and the intestine is impaired; intestinal motility is not well developed. Failure to conserve and secrete the bile acid pool results in decreased intraluminal concentrations impairing fat absorption. Atypical bile acids, perhaps a vestige of an important fetal pathway, are also present.

ical pumps (the gallbladder and small intestine), and a rapidly flowing conduit (the portal vein) (see Fig. 5). The two rate-limiting steps, however, are storage in the gallbladder and transit through the small intestine.

For the newborn and especially the fetus, the enterohepatic circulation of bile acids (Fig. 7) is immature, with defects occurring at several levels[7,8] as follows:

Hepatic Synthesis

The fetal liver is capable of synthesizing bile acid from cholesterol at a low rate,[28] which progressively increases throughout gestation.[29] Transfer across the placenta is bidirectional.[30] Near term, placental transfer from fetus to mother is an important route of elimination of the primary bile salt taurocholate. (Taurocholate is the major bile salt in most young animals and human newborns.) Bidirectional transfer of this trihydroxy bile salt and the dihydroxy bile salts allows the fetus a mechanism to excrete the primary bile salts, which it synthesizes (synthesis exceeding fetal-to-maternal transfer three- to fivefold), and to receive secondary bile acids like deoxycholate from the mother.[31]

Besides an overall reduction in bile acid synthesis, the fetus demonstrates qualitative differences in the bile acids present. The predominant ones are the *primary* bile acids, cholic acid and chenodeoxycholic acid, which are synthesized in the liver (see Fig. 6). Deoxycholic acid is also present but is derived from the mother via placental transfer, as the fetal intestine is sterile. This *secondary* bile salt usually represents a bacterial degradation product from cholic acid. Indeed, a complex array of bile acids is found in the human fetus and newborn.[32] One of these *atypical* bile acids, 3 beta-hydroxycholenoic acid, a direct hepatic metabolite of 26-hydroxycholesterol, is synthesized via a recently established pathway in the adult and perhaps a predominant one in the fetus. This bile acid, along with another monohydroxy bile acid, lithocholic acid, is cholestatic. Both have been identified in the normal fetus and in urine of infants with neonatal hepati-

tis and biliary atresia. A toxic role has been postulated but unproven. Being lipophilic or water-insoluble, these bile acids might alter the functional integrity of the canalicular membrane and induce cholestasis by reducing membrane permeability to water and ions. Fortunately, the standard di- and trihydroxy bile acids prevent or rapidly reverse lithocholate-induced cholestasis, perhaps by solubilizing the offending bile acid and removing it from the canaliculus.[33] Also, they are extensively sulfated in the liver, kidney, intestine, and placenta, increasing their water solubility and enhancing their elimination from the body.[34] Sulfation also abolishes the detergent properties of bile acids, which lessens their likelihood of depleting phospholipid from the canalicular membrane and changes a cholestatic bile acid into a choleretic one.[35] Conjugation of sulfated lithocholate with taurine also eliminates this cholestatic property. How this protective effect works is not truly known, but bile acid sulfation is another process that increases postnatally. These atypical bile acids are likely synthesized in minute amounts in the normal adult; their association with neonatal cholestasis may simply represent an unmasking of their existence rather than resurrection of an atavistic pathway.

Typical bile acids are acidic sterols containing a total of 24 carbon atoms with a 5-carbon-atom side-chain (see Fig. 9). Recently, shorter-chain bile acids have been identified in the meconium, some with only 20 carbon atoms.[32] Although the short-chain bile acids are cleared from plasma into bile quite effectively, they tend to be conjugated with glucuronide. Any influence on the bile secretory apparatus is unknown.

The patterns of hepatic bile acid conjugation with taurine and glycine have parallel ontogenic and phylogenetic development. Glycine conjugation occurs late in evolution and then only among the placental mammals.[36] It appears well after birth. In the human infant, taurine conjugation predominates in fetal bile and in the immediate postnatal period when human breast milk provides a major source of taurine. The human liver preferentially uses taurine but has a limited supply.

After birth both bile acid–conjugating enzymes increase, in parallel with the increase in bile acid synthesis. In human adults most bile salts are conjugated with glycine.

Bile Acid Pool Size

The bile acid pool is small but enlarges in the fetal rat.[37] For example, there is a 50-fold increase in the taurocholate pool size between gestational days 15 and 19. This rapid expansion coincides with the period of development of the fetal hepatic enzymes necessary for taurocholate synthesis. The onset of synthesis increases the bile acid pool. The pool continues to increase through the remainder of gestation into the neonatal period, peaking after weaning. In the newborn child (especially if premature), bile acid metabolism is immature relative to that in adults, but the pool size and synthesis rate increase as the infant becomes older [38,39]

Because of a lag between the onset of bile acid synthesis and the development of an efficient hepatic secretory process, the bile acid pool is localized in the liver of the fetal rat.[37] As the pool enlarges and presumably as the hepatic secretory apparatus develops, the distribution of bile acids shifts to the rat's intestine. After birth, the pattern approaches that in adult rats. The rat, however, lacks a gallbladder. In animals possessing a gallbladder, such as the rabbit, a large proportion of the bile acid pool may reside in the gallbladder. In the newborn rabbit, frequent suckling stimulates the gallbladder to empty and bile acids largely reside in the intestine.[40] The resultant intraduodenal concentration of bile acids, however, is low in newborns, especially premature human infants.[38]

Hepatic Uptake and Secretion

The hepatic translocation of bile salts from plasma to bile involves at least three distinct steps: (1) hepatic uptake at the sinusoidal and lateral (basolateral) membrane surface of the hepatocyte, (2) intracellular or transcellular processing, and (3) excretion across the canalicular membrane.

Hepatocellular uptake of bile salts represents the primary cellular event in bile formation. Bile salt uptake from the sinusoidal surface membrane is a carrier-mediated, active, sodium-dependent co-transport process. This is a "secondary active" transport process: The concentrative driving force is derived from an inwardly directed sodium gradient established across the sinusoidal membrane. The energy for this sodium gradient is generated by Na^+,K^+-ATPase (the primary active transport deriving its metabolic energy from ATP hydrolysis). The sodium pump drives three Na^+ ions out of the cell in exchange for entry to two K^+ ions (see Fig. 2). This process maintains both a concentrative (low intracellular Na^+) and an electrical (negative intracellular potential) gradient for sodium, providing the free energy for co-transport. Hydrophobic unconjugated di- and monohydroxy bile acids appear to enter the liver cell independent of sodium coupling. More than one uptake mechanism likely exists.

Bile acids bind to albumin and to high-density lipoproteins in plasma. Uptake would seem dependent on the free or unbound fraction present at the sinusoidal membrane, implying that albumin binding inhibits uptake. A more recent concept suggests that the rate of uptake depends on the concentration of the fraction bound to albumin; albumin would then facilitate uptake via an albumin receptor on the hepatocyte membrane.[41,42] Uptake may still depend on the unbound fraction present at the membrane, i.e., the dissociation of ligand from albumin. Bile acid–binding proteins on the plasma membrane further assist the uptake process.

Bile acid uptake and clearance by the liver are impaired in the infant.[6] Hepatic Na^+,K^+-ATPase activity matures relatively early, unlike the sodium pump in other tissues, which appears during late gestation but becomes well developed only during postnatal life.[43] Thus, the sodium pump is unlikely to be rate-limiting for the transport of bile acids across the basolateral membrane of the hepatocyte. The plasma membrane carriers for taurocholate develop later, accounting for the limited uptake and secretion by the liver in the perinatal period. The reduced uptake and secretion by the liver impair hepatic clearance and result in the newborn having increased serum bile acid levels.

In transit through the liver cell, several events transpire: conjugation with taurine or glycine, inhibition of cholesterol synthesis by depressing 7 alpha-hydroxylase activity, stimulation of lecithin synthesis, and perhaps induction of bile salt receptors and certain plasma membrane enzymes such as alkaline phosphatase and Na^+,K^+-ATPase. Transit through the cell occurs by either binding with cytosolic proteins or associating with a vesicle or organelle.[45] Canalicular secretion is the rate-limiting step in the transfer of conjugated bile salts from portal blood to bile. Conjugation is one factor influencing (and in some cases enhancing) the "maximum transport secretory rate" (SRm). Hepatic secretion reaches a maximum and then declines along with bile flow even as the exogenous bile acid infusion rate is further increased.[46] The maximum output attained is considered the SRm. The decline is likely a toxic effect of the high bile acid concentrations on the liver—a functional cholestasis. The measured SRm is often inversely proportional to the toxicity of that particular bile acid. Canalicular transport is saturable, sodium-independent, and concentrative. Translocation across the canalicular membrane is driven by the electrical gradient: The resting liver cell potential is about -35 mV, whereas that in the canaliculus may be -5 mV, allowing a potential difference of -30 mV across the membrane. This potential-dependent transport process aids the movement of the negatively charged bile acids. But such passive driving forces alone cannot fully account for the efflux of bile acids, given the adverse chemical gradient: about 0.2 to 0.3 mM intracellularly versus 1 to 2 mM in the canalicular lumen. As canalicular secretion of bile acids is both concentrative and saturable, carrier-facilitated diffusion or active transport may also be involved.

In the early newborn period, the decreased circulating bile salt pool results in a reduced bile salt secretion, which progressively increases to nearly adult levels at the time of weaning in rabbits.[17] Bile flow increases with age from the rise in bile salt secretion and the appearance of bile salt–independent flow at the time of weaning. Bile salt–independent flow is absent in the neonate. The appearance of bile salt–independent bile formation may result from either the development of an ion pump, such as the sodium pump in the rabbit, or the appearance of a secretory pathway separate from bile acids, such as from an organic solute like glutathione. Bile flow in infant rabbits, although low, appears to be maintained by increased biliary permeability. This allows a relative increase in water movement per unit of bile acid (or increased bile salt–dependent flow) to maintain flow despite a depressed bile acid secretion rate.[17]

Developmental findings are similar in puppies compared to adult dogs.[47] Here too there is an age-related increase in canalicular bile flow, gallbladder bile acid content, and ductular reabsorption. Suckling rats also exhibit altered membrane permeability, maintaining bile flow at a time of decreased bile acid secretion.[48]

Intestinal Absorption

Intestinal absorption occurs actively in the ileum[49] and passively throughout the gastrointestinal (GI) tract and perhaps even the biliary system. Ileal absorption of bile salts exhibits the characteristic features of *active transport:* (1) occurring against concentration gradients, (2) requiring cellular energy, being blocked by metabolic inhibitors and hypoxia, (3) exhibiting competition for the same transport process because individual bile salts inhibit the absorption of other bile salts, and (4) demonstrating saturation kinetics. Ionized bile salts, especially the taurine conjugates, depend on active, sodium-coupled transport in the distal ileum for their absorption. Active absorption in the ileum occurs into mature villous rather than the undifferentiated crypt cells.[50] Energy for this process comes from the sodium pump, which maintains a Na^+ electrochemical gradient for coupled Na^+–bile acid co-transport,[51] similar to hepatic uptake.

Passive transport in the jejunum and colon is characterized by (1) flux proportional to the electrochemical gradients, (2) energy not being necessary, and (3) the absence of evidence for competitive inhibition, saturation kinetics, or dependence on the presence of Na^+. Passive absorption may occur by two mechanisms: ionic diffusion and nonionic diffusion. The relative contribution of each process depends on the intraluminal pH, the dissociation constant (pKa) of the bile salt, and the permeability and partition coefficients of the ionic and nonionic species. Because nonionized forms (HA) traverse lipid plasma membranes more readily than ionized forms (Na^+A^-), absorption for practical purposes is by nonionic diffusion. In fact, nonionic diffusion is about 10-fold greater than the diffusion of ionized bile salts. At the normal pH of the upper intestine (pH 5.5 to 6.5), about half of the unconjugated bile acids (with pKa 5.5 to 6.5) are not ionized. A minor amount of glycine-conjugated bile salts (pKa 3.5 to 5.2) is protonated at this pH. No taurine-conjugated bile salts (pKa < 1.8) are protonated. To be absorbed by passive nonionic diffusion, dissociated bile acids must remain in solution. This can occur in the presence of the ionized species, which can solubilize their protonated partner as mixed micelles.

An unstirred water layer exists adjacent to the epithelial cell membrane and extends the aqueous-membrane interface in a series of water lamellae from the surface of the enterocyte: Each is progressively stirred, blending imperceptibly with the bulk water phase in the intestinal lumen. Bile salt micelles, being groupings of molecules, diffuse relatively slowly through the unstirred water layer, limiting bile salt uptake. The unstirred layer also impairs passive transport of lipophilic bile acids, whereas polar species are more limited by the mucosal membrane.[52]

A reciprocal structural-activity relationship exists between active and passive transport rates. The more polar bile salts are absorbed poorly by passive diffusion in the upper small intestine but are maximally transported across the ileum. Conversely, less polar bile acids are well absorbed in the upper intestine by passive diffusion but have lower rates of maximal transport in the ileum. The relatively hydrophobic glycine conjugates of chenodeoxycholate and deoxycholate are easily absorbed by passive nonionic diffusion in the upper small intestine. Similarly, free chenodeoxycholic and deoxycholic acids are passively taken up in the colon. In contrast, ursodeoxycholate, which precipitates at pH 8.0, and cholate, which is ionized, are less well absorbed. Even though passive permeability of the jejunum is greater than that of the ileum, sulfated and glucuronidated bile salts are poorly absorbed from the intestine by either transport mechanism.

Conceptually, then, three sites of bile salt absorption exist in adults: glycine-conjugated dihydroxy bile salts passively absorbed in the jejunum, taurine and glycine conjugated di- and trihydroxy bile salts actively taken up in the distal ileum, and free bile acids passively transported in the colon. The relative significance of these three mechanisms is not fully understood, but as much as 50 percent of bile salts in the enterohepatic circulation may be absorbed passively in the upper small intestine and colon. If the capacity of active ileal transport is exceeded, any overflow into the large bowel still allows some opportunity for recapture by passive absorption.

In early life, many aspects of intestinal structure and function are immature. The fetal gut absorbs taurocholate passively; the ileum is no more efficient than the jejunum.[53] Active ileal transport appears after birth at a species-dependent rate.[54,55] The postnatal development of the active transport system appears linked to changes in membrane lipid composition and fluidity.[56]

Fasting small intestinal motor activity also regulates the enterohepatic circulation of bile salts and hence hepatic secretion, periodically driving bile salts through the small intestine.[57] This migratory myoelectric complex (MMC) exhibits a gestational pattern of postnatal development that is species-specific. The organizational development in human infants is characterized by an increase in the amplitude and frequency of contraction of the intestinal smooth muscle associated with increased propagative activity.[58] In premature infants less than 30 weeks of gestational age, the intestinal motility pattern is disorganized. Between 31 and 34 weeks of gestation, there are repetitive bursts of activity. By term a well-defined cyclic pattern develops, which is characteristic of the fasting intestinal motility pattern in older children and adults.

Thus, multiple components of the enterohepatic circulation of bile acids appear during gestation, yet are impaired at birth in terms of decreased bile acid synthesis, pool size, and hepatic clearance. Thereafter hepatic synthesis and uptake and ileal transport mature to expand the bile acid pool even to levels exceeding those present in adults. Hepatic excretion and intestinal reabsorption may not develop in a synchronous manner.

Regulation of Developmental Changes

Although portions of the enterohepatic circulation and bile acid metabolism seem to develop at dyssynchrous times, there is a remarkable degree of coordination between the diverse array of physiologic and biochemical processes. Each event may be governed by an intrinsic timing mechanism, but a central trigger is most likely. The best candidates for ontogenic changes postpartum are weaning, thyroxine, and glucocorticoids.[59]

Weaning certainly correlates with the appearance of bile salt–independent flow in the rabbit[17] and has been associated with other digestive and metabolic events. Animal studies on the effects of weaning have been hampered by the stress of early transition to food instead of breast milk, which may not even be the cue for intestinal enzyme development. Dietary intake, however, may be a factor modulating the process. Malnutrition, in weaning rabbits at least, causes a reduction in liver growth, bile flow, and bile salt–independent flow.[60] Any beneficial effect from weight gain remains undefined.

Hormones undoubtedly mediate some developmental changes in the liver. Adrenocorticosteroids stimulate the early maturation of factors controlling the bile acid pool in the fetal rat[37] and human.[38] Epidermal growth factor (EGF), a polypeptide similar in structure and function to urogastrone, is a powerful mitogen that influences the growth and differentiation of several tissues, including the GI tract and liver.[61] EGF is produced in the salivary glands, Brunner's glands, and pancreas. Its presence in breast milk assures the suckling young of significant quantities of EGF within the lumen of the GI tract, where it can be absorbed and delivered to the liver. The liver avidly sequesters EGF from the plasma and translocates it in lysosomal vesicles into bile. EGF, administered to suckling rabbits increases the liver weight without causing fatty infiltration and increases bile salt secretion and pool size, findings that suggest that EGF may play a role in the postnatal growth and maturation of the liver.[62]

Gallbladder and Sphincter of Oddi

The gallbladder, cystic duct, and sphincter of Oddi control the flow of hepatic bile through the biliary tract and out into the duodenum.

Gallbladder Storage

During fasting, hepatic bile is partitioned between entering the gallbladder to be stored and directly exiting through the sphincter of Oddi into the duodenum. Of the 500 to 1,000 ml of bile produced each day in adult humans, more than 50 percent enters the gallbladder. Tone in the sphincter of Oddi regulates duodenal bile output: A tight sphincter and a relatively relaxed gallbladder cause more hepatic bile to enter the gallbladder. Spincter of Oddi tone may also regulate gallbladder filling, depending on the resistance at the cystic duct and intraluminal pressure in the gallbladder.[63] As the gallbladder fills, the intraluminal pressure increases and compliance decreases.[64] The gallbladder accommodates this increased distention by receptive relaxation without substantial

pressure changes. Stress relaxation is a general property of smooth muscle tissue which decreases tension with time under sustained stretch or volume distention. An additional adaptive mechanism is gallbladder absorption.

Gallbladder Absorption

The gallbladder is able to absorb 10 to 30 percent of its luminal volume each hour. This change results in a marked increase in bile salt and sodium concentrations but decreased chloride and bicarbonate concentrations. Bile salt anions remain in the lumen, obligating an equivalent number of Na^+ counterions to remain behind. As bile salt concentration increases, micelle formation reduces the osmotic activity of the luminal fluid. Hence, the effective osmolality of gallbladder bile is about half of that predicted from its molar concentrations. This allows bile to remain isotonic relative to plasma despite Na^+ plus bile salt concentrations exceeding 300 mEq per liter (Table 1).

The gallbladder chiefly absorbs NaCl and $NaHCO_3$, along with water in the isotonic proportions, leaving behind the organic solids whose absorption by passive diffusion is extremely slow. Both Na^+ and Cl^- are absorbed at a rapid but equal rate, meaning that absorption is electrically neutral: one anion with one cation.[65] The speed of transcellular sodium movement is determined by the rate of passive Na^+ entry across the luminal membrane and its active transport across the basolateral membrane—another "secondary active transport" system. The energy is derived from the sodium pump, which is located in the basolateral membrane, just like the liver cell and the enterocyte. The gallbladder is a relatively "leaky" epithelium. Such leaky epithelia tend to be characterized by NaCl co-transport and the presence of a significant intercellular or paracellular route for ion and water flow. Also, the presence of low-resistance shunt pathways inhibit their developing a significant transepithelial potential difference. The presence of bicarbonate stimulates NaCl absorption, perhaps via a Cl^-/HCO_3^- exchange mechanism at the basolateral membrane on the serosal surface. In addition, bicarbonate is absorbed from the lumen and H^+ is secreted. This may account for the acidification of gallbladder bile, whose pH is 6.5 compared to hepatic bile at pH 8.2. This also may be responsible for the diurnal variation in the pH of gallbladder bile, which tends to acidify with time. The movement of water is passive, maintaining osmotic equilibrium secondary to active solute transport. Water absorption can occur via either the transcellular or paracellular route. In the duct system, bile water is also absorbed (0.2 μl per minute per gram of liver in the dog) via a sodium-coupled transport system similar to that in the gallbladder.

Gallbladder Contraction

During fasting, the gallbladder does not remain dormant. Evacuations occur at about 90-minute intervals in higher mammals and coincide with late phase II of the intestinal migratory myoelectric complex. This periodic delivery of bile into the duodenum is coordinated with propulsive small intestinal contractions. Thus, even during fasting, enterohepatic cycling continues, both from hepatic bile which bypasses the gallbladder to enter the duodenum and from periodic gallbladder emptying timed with the migratory myoelectric complex traveling down the small intestine.[57,63]

Eating triggers contraction through cephalic and hormonal influences, causing more than 70 percent of the gallbladder contents to be discharged into the duodenum. The cephalic phase empties some 25 percent via cholinergic nerves in the vagus. The principal hormone for gallbladder contraction is cholecystokinin (CCK). CCK is released from the duodenum and jejunum by fatty acids and amino acids. It directly causes gallbladder contraction and indirectly (via inhibitory nerves) relaxes the sphincter of Oddi. Gallbladder emptying in response to eating delivers a bolus of bile salts into the upper small intestine to aid in the digestion and absorption of dietary fat.

BILIARY LIPIDS

Bile Salts—Properties

Bile salts are C22 to C28 carboxylic acids with a cyclopentanophenanthrene nucleus, most commonly as a 24-carbon-atom steroid.[66] The carboxy group on the side chain is usually conjugated with glycine or taurine, a prerequisite for secretion into bile[23,25] (see Fig. 6). Although the terms *bile salt* and *bile acid* are used interchangeably, the "salt" that is ionized is the form more commonly found in biologic fluids. Bile salts are predominantly unprotonated, more polar and more water soluble, and therefore have greater physiologic significance. Bile acids, often unconjugated, un-ionized, and sparingly soluble, are found principally in the colon and portal venous blood. The properties of these

molecules represent a balance between the hydrophobic (water-hating) steroid ring structure and the hydrophilic (water-loving) regions (the juxtaposed OH groups on the ring and the charged conjugated anion (see Fig. 9). This hydrophobic-hydrophilic balance[67] determines many characteristics: hepatic transport, choleretic effect, influence on bile salt synthesis, toxicity, intestinal absorption, and biliary cholesterol secretion. Bile salts, although amphophilic, are quite water soluble because of their hydroxyl groups and taurine (or glycine) conjugates.

Cholesterol in Bile

The hepatic metabolism of cholesterol and its subsequent secretion into bile is complex, as illustrated in Figures 6 and 8. The liver and the intestine are the key organs regulating cholesterol metabolism in the body, even though cholesterol synthesis transpires in virtually every tissue, including the skin. The intestine regulates cholesterol entry into the body. The liver is the major site of cholesterol synthesis, provides the principal route for cholesterol elimination (in bile), and also distributes cholesterol to several major pathways: conversion to bile salts and secretion into plasma as lipoproteins (see Fig. 6). Lipoproteins in turn deliver cholesterol to peripheral tissues, where cholesterol serves a necessary structural function in cell membranes. Lipoprotein-cholesterol influences the synthetic rates of cholesterol in peripheral tissues, whereas intrahepatic cholesterol regulates its own synthesis by negative feedback on the rate-limiting step in cholesterol synthesis, the enzyme beta-hydroxy-beta-methylglutaryl-CoA (HMG CoA) reductase. Indeed, cholesterol synthesis begins from two carbon acetate fragments in an activated form,

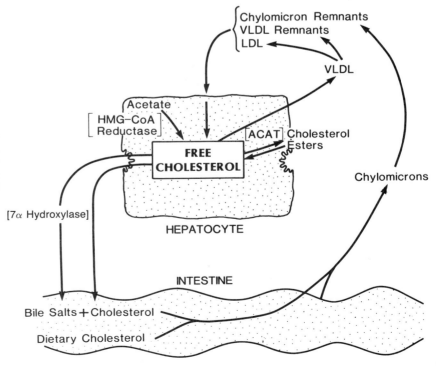

FIGURE 8 Cholesterol metabolism by the liver. Cholesterol input to the liver comes from three sources: (1) chylomicron remnants (cholesterol absorbed from the diet and from biliary cholesterol plus cholesterol synthesized by the small intestine), (2) plasma lipoproteins (containing cholesterol from peripheral tissues—VLDL, LDL, and possibly HDL), and (3) hepatic synthesis from acetate. Cholesterol may then be (1) secreted into plasma as lipoproteins (primarily as VLDL), (2) stored as cholesterol ester (esterification by ACAT), (3) converted into bile salts (bile salt synthesis), and (4) excreted into bile.

acetyl-CoA. Successive condensations of three molecules of acetyl-CoA form HMG CoA. HMG CoA is then reduced to mevalonate, the first unique step in the total sequence of cholesterogenesis (see Fig. 6). The final product, cholesterol, consists of 27 carbon atoms. The cholesterol excreted into bile is free (or unconjugated) and insoluble in water. The liver accounts for about 50 percent of endogenous cholesterol synthesis. Hepatic cholesterol synthesis is controlled by the quantity of free cholesterol available and is also regulated to a minor extent by certain bile acids[27] and other agents. In healthy adults, about 400 mg of cholesterol are synthesized in the liver each day.

Another source of cholesterol is that reabsorbed from the intestine. This consists of dietary cholesterol (approximately 200 mg per day, although dietary intake in American adults may be double this) plus a biliary contribution (750 to 1250 mg per day).[69,70] As about 50 percent is absorbed, 200 mg probably originates from a dietary source and 600 mg from the cholesterol in bile. Cholesterol either absorbed or synthesized in the intestinal mucosa is esterified by the enzyme acyl-coenzyme-A-cholesterol-acyl-transferase (ACAT). This mucosal cholesterol is incorporated into triglyceride-enriched lipoproteins, termed chylomicrons (Fig. 8). Chylomicrons enter the intestinal lymphatics to the thoracic duct and then the systemic circulation. En passant, they come in contact with lipoprotein lipase at the surface of capillary endothelial cells; here the triglyceride component undergoes hydrolysis, forming fatty acids and glycerol. A cholesterol-rich residual lipoprotein (chylomicron remnants) results, is released into the circulation, and is rapidly cleared by the liver. Thus, most of the newly absorbed cholesterol ends up being transported directly to the liver. Besides chylomicron remnants, hepatic cholesterol is derived from plasma lipoproteins containing cholesterol which originated in peripheral tissues. There is also a cyclic pathway for liver cholesterol. In it, the liver secretes cholesterol in the form of very low density lipoprotein (VLDL). VLDL is degraded into VLDL remnants; these can be either cleared by the liver or catabolized to low density lipoprotein (LDL), which returns to the liver (Fig. 8).

The pool of free hepatic cholesterol in the liver can be removed through either esterification by ACAT into cholesterol ester, synthesis into bile acids (about 500 mg per day in adults), or secretion into bile (about 1,000 mg per day). Despite considerable day-to-day fluctuations in cholesterol intake and excretion, the liver (and intestine plus other organs) maintains a stable cholesterol balance. Close regulation of cholesterol synthesis (suppressed or increased) prevents rapid sterol accumulation or loss, respectively. This reciprocal adaptive response maintains a fairly stable rate of bile salt synthesis and secretion and biliary cholesterol secretion. Biliary cholesterol is traditionally considered to be derived from a common hepatic pool consisting of a mixture of cholesterol from esterified cholesterol (the storage form of cholesterol), new hepatic synthesis, chylomicron remnants, and lipoproteins. There may also be a more direct shunting of cholesterol through the liver cell and into bile, termed "metabolic channeling." Putative candidates for this direct route include VLDL remnants, LDL, and even HDL-cholesterol. Esterified cholesterol and newly synthesized cholesterol probably contribute little to the cholesterol in bile. Dietary cholesterol has a slightly more important role in hu-

mans, as biliary cholesterol secretion increases with marked rises in dietary cholesterol. Similarly, during mobilization of peripheral cholesterol stores, as occurs in obese people undergoing rapid weight reduction and during drug therapy (e.g., clofibrate) for hyperlipidemia, biliary cholesterol increases. At best, perhaps only 20 percent of biliary cholesterol in man is derived from hepatic synthesis. This newly synthesized cholesterol may be excreted into bile without equilibrating in the liver.[71] Cholesterol secretion is relatively resistant to moderate changes in production. The majority of cholesterol exported into bile is preformed.[72,73] In fact, much of this preformed cholesterol originally was synthesized in the liver, exported to peripheral tissues, and then recycled to the liver in the form of lipoproteins.[74] The rate of biliary cholesterol secretion is thus determined primarily by the size of a metabolically active precursor pool of free cholesterol in the liver.[70,75] The source of this preformed biliary cholesterol may even reside in canalicular membranes.

Lecithin in Bile

The phospholipids in bile and plasma are synthesized only in the liver. Despite this common origin, the phospholipid secreted into bile is a lecithin whose fatty acids differ from other hepatic lecithins and from that in plasma. Bile lecithin generally contains a saturated fatty acid (palmitic acid) in position one (R in Fig. 9) and an unsaturated fatty acid (linoleic or oleic acids) in the second position (R' in Fig. 9). This unique composition of biliary phospholipids originates in a specific pool of phosphatidylcholine, located in hepatic microsomes and destined for biliary secretion.[73,76] The synthesis of lecithin and its secretion into bile, however, are linked: Both are dependent on bile salt secretion. It is even possible that biliary phospholipid vesicles are transported to the bile canalicular membrane, enter it, and form highly fluid, lipid microdomains. Subsequent solubilization of these regions by bile salts would transport these phospholipids with their distinctive composition into bile.[45] Replacement would occur via hepatic synthesis.

Once lecithin reaches the intestinal lumen, it undergoes partial hydrolysis to lysolecithin and fatty acids, which are absorbed. These products are not substantially reused as a source of bile lecithin, so there is little enterohepatic circulation of lecithin. The choline moiety may be preserved for de novo hepatic synthesis.

Physical Chemistry of Lipids in Bile

Although bile is the major route for cholesterol elimination from the body, cholesterol is virtually insoluble in aqueous solution, whereas bile is predominantly water, with solids accounting for only 5 to 10 g per deciliter (w/v). More than 90 percent of the total solids in bile consist of three organic components: bile salts, lecithin, and free cholesterol (Table 1). The conventional chemical formulae depicted in the upper portion of Figure 9 provide less information than the schematic drawings in the lower panel, which represent the physical state of the molecules at an oil-water interface. Each substance is *amphophilic* ("loving both sides"): part of the

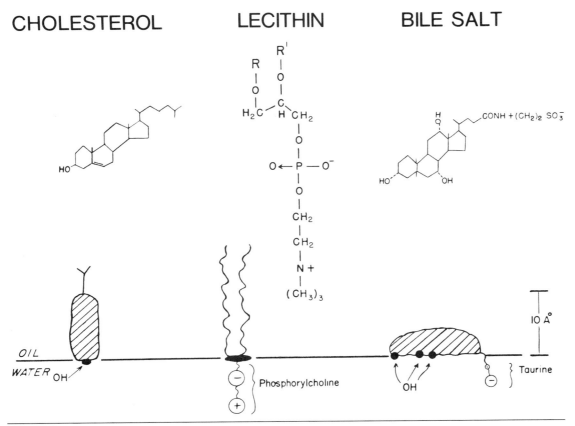

FIGURE 9 Chemical formula and physical state of cholesterol, lecithin, and bile salts at an oil-water interface. The upper part of the figure shows chemical formulae of cholesterol, lecithin, and sodium taurocholate. For lecithin, the R and R' represent long-chain fatty acids attached to the glycerol skeleton by ester linkages. The lower part is the schematic representation of molecules as space-filled models at an oil-water interface. Shaded areas represent the hydrophobic steroid nuclei of cholesterol and bile salt. Closed circles and ovals represent hydroxyl and ester groups, respectively. + and − are the positive and negative charges on the respective groups. Wavy lines are lipid-soluble hydrocarbon alkyl chains of lecithin. (From Shaffer.[68])

molecule is attracted to water and part to oil. At the oil-water interface, the water-soluble parts are oriented in the aqueous phase (downward in Fig. 9), whereas the oil-soluble parts are in the oil phase (upward in Fig. 9). Cholesterol has a single hydroxyl group, which is water soluble. The remainder of the molecule is the water-insoluble (oil-soluble) 27-carbon steroid ring. The single OH group cannot possibly pull the bulky hydrocarbon moiety deep within the water phase. Thus, cholesterol has only modest surface solubility on water and negligible solubility within water.

Lecithin (80 to 95 percent being phosphatidylcholine) contains a phosphoryl choline group—OP (O_3)-Ch_2-Ch_2N^+ $(CH_3)_3$—which is hydrophilic and seeks water. The other portion of the lecithin molecule, the two long-chain fatty acids (R and R') esterified through glycerol, is hydrophobic and seeks the oil phase. The phosphorylcholine and ester groups therefore lie below the water surface, whereas the long hydrocarbon chains point upward into the oil phase like a tuning fork. Lecithin is insoluble in water on its own and forms crystals of bimolecular leaflets. The hydrophilic end sticks into water and the hydrophobic portions adhere to one another. Water penetrates between the hydrophilic phosphoryl choline groups, causing the crystals to swell, forming "liquid

crystals." Thus, aggregates of lecithin, although insoluble in water, become extremely hydrated, forming bilayers of lipid molecules interwoven with multiple layers of water.[25] When the solute concentration is low, lecithin liquid crystals can form closed, spherical structures, termed *vesicles*. When sufficiently large, they can be seen on a polarizing microscopy as Maltese crosses. Cholesterol possesses the ability to interdigitate between the lecithin molecules, with its hydroxyl group sitting in the water layer and the remainder of the molecule buried deep within the fatty acid–hydrocarbon interior of the lecithin bilayer.

Bile salts, in contrast, are quite soluble, with their polar hydroxyl groups and taurine or glycine conjugates attracted into the water. In aqueous solution above the limited concentration (the "critical micellar concentration"), bile salts are attracted into the bulk phase of water and aggregate by association of their hydrophobic sides, forming "simple micelles."[77] Lecithin can be dissolved by these bile salt aggregates, creating "mixed micelles." These bilayer disks appear like stout drums with a water-soluble coating and a water-insoluble core. Cholesterol can then be dissolved within the hydrophobic core between the fatty acid chains of lecithin. As lecithin is hydrated with its molecules separated by water, the micelle is capable of incorporating more cholesterol than could be contained by simple bile-salt micelles alone. Thus, bile salts are biologically active detergents that co-operate with lecithin to keep cholesterol in solution. In bile, then, bile salts plus lecithin solubilize cholesterol in two forms: *unilamellar vesicles*, closed, spherical, membrane-like fragments often with relatively small amounts of bile salts, or smaller *mixed micelles*, in which the solubilizing potential of the polar lipids is relatively limited. For example, in micellar solution only about five molecules of cholesterol can be dissolved by 94 molecules of bile salts and lecithin.[78]

Biliary Lipid Secretion

The physical coupling of these biliary lipids and their secretion into bile may occur at or near the canalicular membrane, either within the membrane during translocation or adjacent to the membrane in the newly formed bile.[45] In the first instance, vesicles of bile salts, lecithin, and cholesterol would form in the hepatocyte, then fuse with the canalicular membrane and finally leave the cell via exocytosis into bile. Alternatively, bile salts may either be secreted into the bile canaliculi first and then leach cholesterol and lecithin out of the canalicular membranes, or else acquire their lipid component en route. Where biliary lipids are solubilized and in what physical form they journey across the cell and exit into the canaliculus (more likely as vesicles than micelles) is unknown.

Cholesterol and lecithin are present in bile both as vesicles and as mixed micelles with bile salts.[79] The balance between these two forms represents a shifting equilibrium with less stable vesicles becoming more stable as mixed micelles. Lipid vesicles are capable of maintaining a higher cholesterol-phospholipid ratio than micelles. Conversion to micelles can thus overwhelm the cholesterol-carrying capacity, forming bile with excess cholesterol. Variations in bile output alter the distribution of cholesterol transported by biliary micelles versus vesicles. At low bile salt secretion rates (e.g., after an overnight fast), more cholesterol is carried as vesicles.[80]

Because biliary cholesterol excretion requires solubilization by bile salts and lecithin (as micelles and/or vesicles) and as lecithin secretion is tightly controlled by bile salt secretion, biliary cholesterol and lecithin secretion rates are also coupled under physiologic conditions. Thus, cholesterol output into bile is generally coupled to the rate of bile salt secretion, while a close association exists between lecithin and bile salt secretion (Fig. 10). The relation between these three is

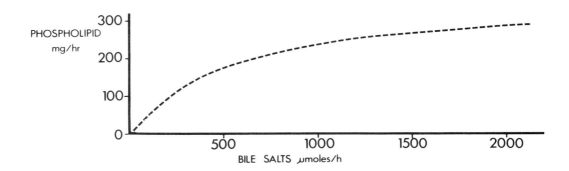

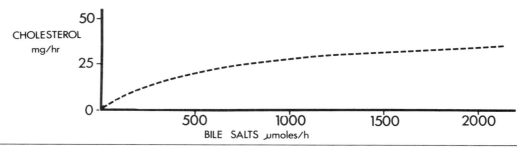

FIGURE 10 Influence of bile salt secretion on phospholipid and cholesterol secretion. Secretion of both phospholipid and cholesterol is closely related in a curvilinear manner to that of bile salts. (Human data from Shaffer and Small.[70]) The curve and asymptote for cholesterol may be slightly shifted to the left so that at low bile salt secretion, there is relatively more cholesterol secreted. Cholesterol saturation of bile tends to be higher at reduced bile salt secretion rates, as occurs with fasting.

not fixed, but is curvilinear. At low rates of bile salt secretion, there is little secretion of lecithin. Cholesterol secretion is also low, but less so than the other two, so that the amount of cholesterol in bile compared with the other two components is greater. Conversely, at high rates of bile salt secretion, the lecithin and cholesterol outputs plateau and the relative proportion of cholesterol diminishes. The rate of bile salt secretion is thus the principal determinant of biliary lipid composition, but several modifying factors exist. For example, in humans the cholesterol-lecithin ratio is higher than in animals. Biliary lipid composition also is governed by a diurnal variation that may be partially influenced by changes in the enterohepatic cycling of bile acids but also has an intrinsic, circadian rhythm of its own.

Although the rate of bile salt flux through the liver is the major determinant of the amount of cholesterol and lecithin entering bile, the species of bile salts is also important. Different bile salts with different physicochemical properties vary in their abilities to recruit cholesterol and phospholipid.[81] The hydrophilic-hydrophobic balance (the relative contributions of the water-loving and water-hating parts of an amphophile, respectively, to the overall polarity of the molecule) is a physicochemical property that determines aqueous solubility. The ability of a given bile salt to interact with and to solubilize cholesterol is directly related to the hydrophobicity of that bile salt: With increasing hydrophobicity, the phospholipid–bile salt ratio and cholesterol–bile salt ratio are both increased. The cholesterol-solubilizing capacity of bile salt micelles therefore increases as the hydrophobicity of the monomeric bile acid species increases.[67] For example, sodium glycodeoxycholate is more hydrophobic and has a greater cholesterol-solubilizing capacity than does sodium taurocholate. A more hydrophilic bile salt like ursodeoxycholate is associated with reduced biliary cholesterol secretion.

REFERENCES

1. Klaassen CD, Watkins JB. Mechanisms of bile formation, hepatic uptake and biliary excretion. Physiol Rev 1984; 36:1–67.
2. Shaffer EA. Hepatobiliary secretion. In: Davison JS, ed. Gastrointestinal secretion. London: Wright (Butterworth & Co.), 1989: 123.
3. Rappaport AM. Anatomic considerations. In: Schiff L, ed. Diseases of the liver. Philadelphia: JB Lippincott, 1985: 1.
4. Jones AL, Schmucker DL, Renston RH, Murakami T. The architecture of bile secretion: a morphological perspective of physiology. Dig Dis Sci 1980; 25:609–629.
5. Traber PG, Chianale J, Gumucio JJ. Physiologic significance and regulation of hepatocellular heterogeneity. Gastroenterology 1988; 95:1130–1143.
6. Suchy FJ, Balisteri WF, Breslin JS, Dumaswain R, Setchell KDR, Garfield SA. Absence of an acinar gradient for bile acid uptake in developing rat liver. Pediatr Res 1987; 21:417–421.
7. Balisteri WF. Immaturity of hepatic excretory function and the ontogeny of bile acid metabolism. J Pediatr Gastroenterol Nutr 1983; 2(suppl 1):S207–S214.
8. Shaffer EA. Ontogeny of hepatic bile formation and the enterohepatic circulation of bile acids. In: Davison JS, Shaffer EA, eds. Gastrointestinal and hepatic secretions: mechanism and control. Calgary: The University of Calgary Press, 1988: 56.
9. Blitzer BL, Boyer JL. Cellular mechanisms of bile formation. Gastroenterology 1982; 82:346–357.
10. Daimon T, David H, Azlinicki TV, Marx E. Correlated ultrastructural and morphometric studies on the liver during perinatal development of rats. Exp Pathol 1982; 21:237–250.
11. Guzelian P, Boyer JL. Glucose reabsorption from bile. Evidence for biliohepatic circulation. J Clin Invest 1974; 53:526–535.
12. Sperber I. Secretion of organic anions in the formation of urine and bile. Pharmacol Rev 1959; 11:109–134.
13. Scharschmidt BF, Van Dyke RW. Mechanisms of hepatic electrolyte transport. Gastroenterology 1983; 85:1199–1214.
14. Dumont M, Erlinger S, Uchman S. Hypercholeresis induced by ursodeoxycholic acid and 7-ketolithocholic acid in the rat: possible role of bicarbonate transport. Gastroenterology 1980; 79:82–89.
15. Bear CE, Shaffer EA. Hepatocellular water and electrolyte secretion. Can J Physiol Pharmacol 1988; 66:1253–1260.
16. Boyer JL, Bloomer JR. Canalicular bile secretion in man: studies utilizing the biliary clearance of ^{14}C-mannitol. J Clin Invest 1974; 54:773–781.
17. Shaffer EA, Zahavi I, Gall DG. Postnatal development of hepatic bile formation in the rabbit. Dig Dis Sci 1985; 30:558–562.
18. Forker IL. The effect of estrogen on bile formation in the rat. J Clin Invest 1969; 48:654–663.
19. Moseley RH, Ballatori N, Smith DJ, Boyer JL. Ursodeoxycholate stimulates Na$^+$-H$^+$ exchange in rat basolateral plasma membrane vesicles. J Clin Invest 1987; 80:684–690.
20. Hofmann AF, Gurantz D, Hagey LR, Schteingart C, Yoon YB, Clayton LR, Palmer KR, Neoptolemos JP, Rossi SS, Steinbach J, Clerici C. The key role of bile acid biotransformation in bile acid dependent bile flow. In: Davison JS, Shaffer EA, eds. Gastrointestinal and hepatic secretions: mechanisms and control. Calgary: The University of Calgary Press, 1988: 56.
21. Lake JR, Renner EL, Scharschmidt BF, Cragoe EJ, Hagey LR, Lambert KJ, Burantz D, Hofmann AF. Inhibition of Na$^+$/H$^+$ exchange in the rat is associated with decreased ursodeoxycholate hydrocholeresis, decreased secretion of unconjugated ursodeoxycholate, and increased ursodeoxycholate glucuronidation. Gastroenterology 1988; 95:454–463.
22. Boyer JL. Mechanisms of bile acid independent bile flow. In: Davison JS, Shaffer EA, eds. Gastrointestinal and hepatic secretions: mechanism and control. Calgary: The University of Calgary Press, 1988: 12.
23. Carey MC, Cahalane MJ. Enterohepatic circulation. In: Arias IM, Jakoby WB, Popper H, Schachter D, Shafritz DA, eds. The liver: biology and pathobiology. 2nd ed. New York: Raven Press. 1988: 573.
24. Shaffer EA, Gordon ER. Serum bile acids as related to bile acid secretion in liver disease. Dig Dis Sci 1978; 23:392–397.
25. Shaffer EA, Small DM. Gallstone disease: pathogenesis and management. Curr Probl Surg 1976; 13:1–72.
26. Eriksson S. Biliary excretion of bile acids and cholesterol in bile fistula rats. Proc Soc Exp Biol Med 1957; 94:578–582.
27. Heuman DM, Vlahcevic ZR, Bailey ML, Hylemon PB. Regulation of bile acid synthesis. II. Effect of bile acid feeding on enzymes regulating hepatic cholesterol and bile acid synthesis in the rat. Hepatology 1988; 8:892–897.
28. Smallwood RA, Jablonski P, Watts JMcK. Bile acid synthesis in the developing sheep liver. Clin Sci Mol Med 1973; 45:403–406.
29. Graham TO, Van Thiel DH, Little JM, Lester R. Synthesis of taurocholate by the rat fetal liver in organ culture: effects of cortisol in vitro. Am J Physiol 1979; 237:E177–184.
30. Jackson BT, Smallwood RA, Piasecki GJ, Brown AS, Rauschecker HFG, Lester R. Fetal bile rat metabolism. I. The metabolism of sodium cholate ^{14}C in the fetal dog. J Clin Invest 1971; 50:1286–1294.
31. Sewell RB, Hardy KJ, Smallwood RA, Hoffman NE. Fetal bile salt metabolism: placental transfer of dihydroxy bile salts in sheep. Am J Physiol 1982; 243:G172–G175.
32. Lester R, St Pyrek J, Little JM, Adcock EW. Diversity of bile acids in the fetus and newborn infant. J Pediatr Gastroenterol Nutr 1983; 2:355–364.
33. Kakis G, Yousef IM. Mechanisms of cholic acid protection in lithocholate-induced intrahepatic cholestasis in rats. Gastroenterology 1980; 78:1402–1411.
34. Watkins JB. Placental transport: bile acid conjugation and sulfation in the fetus. J Pediatr Gastroenterol Nutr 1983; 2:365–373.
35. Yousef IM, Barnwell SG, Tuchweber B, Weber A, Roy CC. Effect of complete sulfation of bile acids on bile formation in rats. Hepatology 1987; 7:535–542.
36. Haslewood GAD. The biological importance of bile salts. Amsterdam: North Holland Publishing, 1978.
37. Little JM, Richey JE, Van Thiel DH, Lester R. Taurocholate pool size and distribution in the fetal rat. J Clin Invest 1979; 63:1042–1049.

38. Watkins JB, Szcepanik P, Gould JB, Klein P, Lester R. Bile salt metabolism in the human premature infant. Gastroenterology 1975; 69:706–713.
39. Heubi JE, Balisteri WF, Suchy FJ. Bile salt metabolism in the first year of life. J Lab Clin Med 1982; 100:127–136.
40. Subbiah MTR, Marai L, Dinh DM, Penner JW. Sterol and bile acid metabolism during development. I. Studies on the gallbladder and intestinal bile acids of newborn and fetal rabbit. Steroids 1977; 29:83–92.
41. Forker EL, Luxon BA. Albumin helps mediate removal of taurocholate by rat liver. J Clin Invest 1981; 67:1517–1522.
42. Ockner R, Weisiger RA, Gollan JA. Hepatic uptake of albumin-bound substances: albumin receptor concept. Am J Physiol 1983; 245:G13–G18.
43. Suchy FJ, Bucuvalas JC, Goodrich AL, Moyer MS, Blitzer BL. Taurocholate transport and Na$^+$-K$^+$-ATPase activity in fetal and neonatal rat liver plasma membrane vesicles. Am J Physiol 1986; 251:G665–G673.
44. Balisteri WF, Heubi JE, Suchy FJ. Immaturity of the enterohepatic circulation in early life: factors predisposing to "physiologic" maldigestion and cholestasis. J Pediatr Gastroenterol Nutr 1983; 2:346–354.
45. Coleman R. Biochemistry of bile secretion. Biochem J 1987; 244:249–261.
46. Hardison WGM, Hatoff DE, Miyai D, Weiner RG. Nature of bile acid maximum secretory rate in the rat. Am J Physiol 1981; 241:G337–G343.
47. Tavoloni N, Jones MJT, Berk PD. Postnatal development of bile secretory physiology in the dog. J Pediatr Gastroenterol Nutr 1985; 4:256–267.
48. Piccoli DA, Treem WR, Vanderslice RR, Watkins JW. Mechanism for water and solute entry into bile: developmental studies using perfused rat liver. Hepatology 1985; 5:1043. (Abstract)
49. Lack L, Weiner IM. In vitro absorption of bile salts by small intestine of rats and guinea pigs. Am J Physiol 1961; 200:313–317.
50. Kapaida CR, Essandoh LK. Active absorption of vitamin B$_{12}$ and conjugated bile salts by guinea pig ileum occurs in villous and not crypt cells. Dig Dis Sci 1988; 33:1377–1382.
51. Wilson FA, Treanor LL. Studies of relationships among bile acid uptake, Na$^+$,K$^+$-ATPase, and Na$^+$ gradient in isolated cells from rat ileum. Gastroenterology 1981; 81:54–60.
52. Wilson FA. Intestinal absorption of bile acids. Am J Physiol 1981; 241:G83–G92.
53. Lester R, Smallwood RA, Little JM, Brown AS, Piasecki GJ, Jackson BT. Fetal bile salt metabolism. The intestinal absorption of bile salt. J Clin Invest 1977; 59:1009–1016.
54. de Belle RC, Vaupshas VV, Vitullo BB, Haber LR, Shaffer E, Mackie GG, Owen H, Lester R. Intestinal development of bile salts: immature development in the neonate. J Pediatr 1979; 94:472–476.
55. Heubi JE, Fondacaro JD. Postnatal development of intestinal bile salt transport in the guinea pig. Am J Physiol 1982; 243:G89–G94.
56. Heubi JE, Fellows JL. Postnatal development of intestinal bile salt transport. Relationship to membrane physicochemical changes. J Lipid Res 1985; 25:797–805.
57. Scott RB, Strasberg SM, El-Sharkawy TY, Diamant NE. Regulation of the canine fasting enterohepatic circulation by the migratory myoelectric complex. J Clin Invest 1983; 71:644–654.
58. Bisset WM, Watt JB, Rivers RPA, Milla PJ. Ontogeny of fasing small intestinal motor activity in the human infant. Gut 1988; 29:483–488.
59. Henning SJ. Postnatal development: coordination of feeding, digestion, and metabolism. Am J Physiol 1981; 241:G199–G214.
60. Opleta K, Butzner JD, Shaffer EA, Gall DG. The effect of protein-calorie malnutrition on the developing liver. Pediatr Res 1988; 23:505–508.
61. St Hilaire RJ, Jones AL. Epidermal growth factor: its biologic and metabolic effects with emphasis on the hepatocyte. Hepatology 1982; 2:601–613.
62. Opleta K, O'Laughlin EV, Shaffer EA, Hayden J, Hollenberg M, Gall DG. Effect of epidermal growth factor on growth and postnatal development of the rabbit liver. Am J Physiol 1987; 253:G622–G626.
63. Scott RB, Eidt PB, Shaffer EA. Regulation of fasting canine duodenal bile acid delivery by sphincter of Oddi and gallbladder. Am J Physiol 1985; 249:G622–G633.
64. Cole MJ, Shaffer EA, Scott RB. Gallbladder pressure, compliance, and hysteresis during cyclic volume change. Can J Physiol Pharmacol 1987; 65:2124–2130.
65. Rose RC. Absorptive function of the gallbladder. In: Johnson LR, Christensen J, Jackson MJ, Jacobson ED, Walsh JH, eds. Physiology of the gastrointestinal tract. 2nd ed. New York: Raven Press. 1987: 1455.
66. Nair PP, Kritchevsky D, eds. The bile acids. New York: Plenum Press, 1971.
67. Armstrong MJ, Carey MC. The hydrophobic-hydrophilic balance of bile salts. Inverse correlation between reverse-phase high performance liquid chromatographic mobilities and micellar cholesterol solubilizing capacities. J Lipid Res 1982; 23:70–80.
68. Shaffer EA. Gallstones: current concepts of pathogenesis and medical dissolution. Can J Surg 1980; 6:517–532.
69. Grundy SM, Metzger AL. A physiological method for estimation of hepatic secretion of biliary lipids. Gastroenterology 1972; 62:1200–1217.
70. Shaffer EA, Small DM. Biliary lipid secretion in cholesterol gallstone disease. The effect of cholecystectomy and obesity. J Clin Invest 1977; 59:828–840.
71. Robins SJ, Fasulo JM, Collins MA, Patton GM. Evidence for separate pathways of transport of newly synthesized and preformed cholesterol into bile. J Biol Chem 1985; 260:6511–6513.
72. Turley SD, Dietschy JM. Regulation of biliary cholesterol output in the rat: dissociation from the rate of hepatic cholesterol synthesis, the size of the hepatic cholesteryl ester pool, and the hepatic uptake of chylomicron cholesterol. J Lipid Res 1979; 20:923–934.
73. Robins SJ, Brunengraber H. Origin of biliary cholesterol and lecithin in the rat: contribution of new synthesis and preformed hepatic stores. J Lipid Res 1982; 23:604–608.
74. Schwartz CC, Berman M, Vlahcevic ZR, Halloran LG, Gregory DH, Swell L. Multicompoartmental analysis of cholesterol metabolism in man. Characterization of the hepatic bile acid and biliary cholesterol precursor sites. J Clin Invest 1978; 61:408–423.
75. Stone BG, Erickson SK, Craig WY, Cooper AD. Regulation of rat biliary cholesterol secretion by agents that alter intrahepatic cholesterol metabolism. Evidence for a distinct biliary precursor pool. J Clin Invest 1985; 76:1773–1781.
76. Gregory DH, Vlahcevic ZR, Schatzki P, Swell L. Mechanism of secretion of biliary lipids. I. Role of bile canalicular and microsomal membranes in the synthesis and transport of biliary lecithin and cholesterol. J Clin Invest 1975; 55:105–141.
77. Carey MC, Small DM. Micelle formation by bile salts: physical-chemical and thermodynamic considerations. Arch Intern Med 1972; 130:506–527.
78. Carey MC, Small DM. The physical chemistry of cholesterol solubility in bile. Relationship to gallstone formation and dissolution in man. J Clin Invest 1978; 61:998–1026.
79. Somjen G, Gilat T. Contribution of vesicular and micellar carriers to cholesterol transport in human bile. J Lipid Res 1985; 26:699–704.
80. Pattinson NR, Chapman BA. Distribution of biliary cholesterol between mixed micelles and nonmicelles in relation to fasting and feeding in humans. Gastroenterology 1986; 697–702.
81. Bilhartz LE, Dietschy JM. Bile salt hydrophobicity influences cholesterol recruitment from rat liver in vivo when cholesterol synthesis and lipoprotein uptake are constant. Gastroenterology 1988; 95:771–779.

CHAPTER 23

Exocrine Pancreas: Structure and Function

Steven L. Werlin, M.D.

EMBRYOLOGY AND HISTOGENESIS OF THE HUMAN PANCREAS

The dorsal and ventral anlagen of the human pancreas first become visible as evaginations of the primitive foregut the fifth week of gestation (Fig. 1).[1] The larger, dorsal anlage, which develops into the tail, body, and part of the head of the pancreas, grows directly from the duodenum. The ventral anlage develops from one or two buds from the primitive liver and eventually forms the major part of the head of the pancreas. At about 17 weeks of gestation, the dorsal and ventral anlagen fuse as the buds develop and the gut rotates. The ventral duct forms the proximal portion of the major pancreatic duct of Wirsung. The dorsal duct forms the distal portion of the duct of Wirsung and the accessory duct of Santorini. Variations in fusion account for the variety of developmental abnormalities of the pancreas. The final appearance of the pancreas and its relationship to neighboring structures is shown in Figure 2.

Histologic examination of the early pancreas reveals predominantly undifferentiated epithelial cells, which by 9 to 12 weeks form a lobular-tubular pattern; zymogen granules are absent but the Golgi apparatus is present[2-5] (Fig. 3A and B). Primitive acini containing rough endoplasmic reticulum and recognizable zymogen granules are present by 14 to 16 weeks. Golgi vesicles become prominent at this time. Activity of secretory enzymes is first detectable at this age. By 16 to 20 weeks, large numbers of zymogen granules are present (Fig. 3C). As the pancreas matures, the luminal volume decreases and acinar cell volume increases. Connective tissue continues to decrease both throughout gestation and in the postnatal period. By 20 weeks of gestation, the acinar cells contain mature-appearing zymogen granules, well-developed endoplasmic reticulum, and highly developed basolateral membranes. The pancreas from the 6-day-old rat shows a similar increase in acinar volume and small lumina. Stroma continues to decrease. Acinar cells have a mature appearance (Fig. 3D).

The mature acinar cell is pyramidal in shape with a basal nucleus. The most prominent organelles in the fasted state are the large numbers of zymogen granules, located apically. Abundant rough endoplasmic reticulum (RER), the location of protein synthesis, and Golgi apparatus, the focus of packaging proteins for export, are present. Junctional complexes join between adjacent acinar cells. The apical membrane contains abundant microvilli projecting into the lumen.

The final three-dimensional structure of the pancreas consists of a complex series of branching ducts surrounded by grape-like clusters of acinar cells (Fig. 4).

Postnatally, the volume of the exocrine pancreas continues to grow, nearly tripling in size during the first year of life (Table 1).[6] During the first 4 months the ratio of acinar cells to connective tissue increases fourfold.

Centroacinar and duct cells, which are responsible for water, electrolyte, and bicarbonate secretion, are also found by 20 weeks. The ductal system contains less than 5 percent of the volume of the exocrine pancreas. In the postnatal period, lumen volume increases along with the increase in acinar cell volume.

Islets are first identifiable at 12 to 16 weeks, at which time immunoreactive insulin is present in beta cells. Mixed cells, those with characteristics of both acinar and islet cells which are only rarely seen in the adult, may be seen. The histologic appearance of the term pancreas is similar to that of the adult.

While the signals controlling both cytodifferentiation, the process by which pancreatic cells differentiate into the various structural elements, and morphogenesis have not been well described in the human, abundant information on these processes is now being derived from studies on rodents. The control of cytodifferentiation and morphogenesis in the rodent is described below.

While duodenal and stool protease activity has been clearly demonstrated by many investigators, the time of first appearance of pancreatic enzymes in the fetal pancreas has been variably described. Unfortunately, not only is much of the currently available data derived from methods no longer considered scientifically acceptable, but they are also contradictory. The presence of trypsinogen was found as early as 22 weeks of gestation by Keene and Hewer.[7] Using modern biochemical techniques, Lieberman found proteolytic activity both in the pancreas of the 500-g fetus after activation of pancreatic homogenate with enterokinase and in the meconium from fetuses of similar age.[8] Recently, Track and colleagues have determined the levels of five pancreatic enzymes in a group of 42 fetuses of gestational age 14 to 40 weeks (Fig. 5).[3] Trypsin, chymotrypsin, phospholipase A, and lipase were all present in the 14-cm (14-week) fetus in low concentrations, and these steadily increased with gestational age. Amylase was not found in any fetus studied.

Lipase activity has been reported to be present as early as 16 weeks of gestation[9] and absent until nearly 32 weeks.[7] Madey and Dancis found trypsin activity in duodenal aspirates

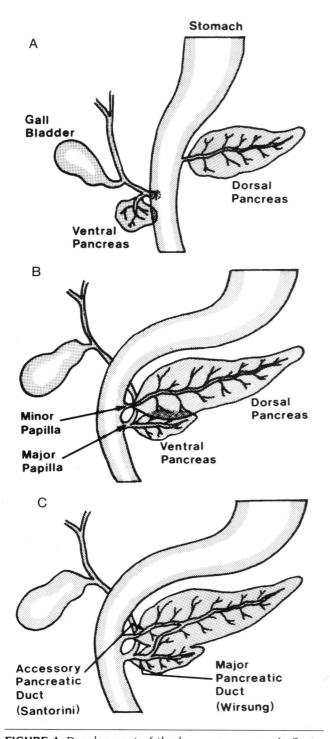

FIGURE 1 Development of the human pancreas. *A*, Gestational age 6 weeks. *B*, Gestational age 7 to 8 weeks. The ventral pancreas has rotated but has not yet fused with the dorsal pancreas. *C*, The ventral and dorsal pancreatic ductal systems have fused. (From Werlin SL. The exocrine pancreas. In: Kelley VC, ed. Practice of pediatrics, Vol V, Chap 23. Philadelphia: Harper & Row, 1987; with permission.)

from 16 premature infants weighing between 1120 and 1740 g.[10] Borgstrom and colleagues demonstrated both amylase and trypsin in the duodenal fluid of preterm infants.[11]

De Filippi and colleagues found that stool from 28 to 30 infants would hydrolyze x-ray gel on day 1 of life.[12] Jodl et al determined chymotrypsin activity in the stools collected from 42 low-birth-weight infants ranging in weight from 750 to 2570 g.[13] All 42 babies had chymotrypsin activity in concentrations that increased with gestational age. Chymotrypsin activity was low at birth, peaked at age 3 days, then declined slightly. Similarly, Mullinger and Palasi detected trypsin and chymotrypsin in stool of neonates.[14] A wide day-to-day variation of enzyme concentration is found.

The ontogeny of amniotic and pancreatic amylase has been investigated in numerous studies with contradictory results. Pancreatic amylase has been both found and not found in the fetus and in amniotic fluid by a variety of techniques. Wolf and Taussing found pancreatic isoamylase in amniotic fluid at 16 to 18 weeks of gestation.[15] De Castro et al found increasing levels of amniotic fluid amylase with increasing gestational age but did not differentiate between the pancreatic and salivary forms.[16]

Other investigators found no pancreatic amylase in amniotic fluid. For example, Laxova found only salivary amylase in 40 amniotic fluid specimens taken from fetuses of gestational age 12 to 40 weeks.[17] Track et al found no amylase in their series of 39 fetuses.[3] Using polyacrylamide gel electrophoresis, Tye et al found pancreatic amylase in only 25 percent of urine specimens collected from 36 newborn infants.[18] Auricchio et al found that amylase in pancreatic homogenates from newborn infants was 10 percent of that found in adults.[19]

Davis and colleagues, using a variety of the most up-to-date techniques, including electrophoresis and immunohistochemistry with monoclonal antibodies, have clearly and definitively shown that pancreatic amylase is present in amniotic fluid as early as 14 weeks of gestation (Fig. 6).[20] Immunologic activity is present in the pancreas at 16 weeks of gestation. Although it appears that all enzymes are present by 16 weeks of gestation, the time of rapid development of zymogen granules, the definitive ontogenic profiles of other pancreatic proteins in the human must await the application of this type of approach.

ONTOGENY OF SECRETORY FUNCTION

Because of both the technical difficulties and the ethical concerns of performing invasive procedures on well infants, few studies of pancreatic secretory function in the human infant have been published. Since direct collection of pancreatic juice is not possible in the infant and young child, pancreatic secretions must be collected in the duodenum in the fasted or basal state, after indirect stimulation with a meal or direct stimulation with secretagogues such as secretin and/or cholecystokinin (CCK). Pancreatic function may be indirectly determined by the measurement of pancreatic enzymes in stool and by fat balance studies.

In a series of studies, Zoppi and colleagues measured stimulated pancreatic secretion in normal infants and children.[21-24]

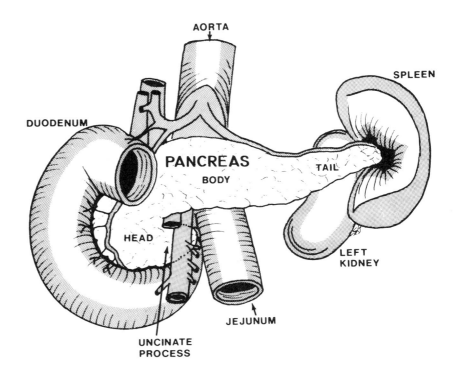

FIGURE 2 Anterior view of the pancreas: Relationship to neighboring structures. (From Werlin SL. The exocrine pancreas. In: Kelley VC, ed. Practice of pediatrics, Vol V, Chap 23. Philadelphia: Harper & Row, 1987; with permission.)

In premature infants with gestational age 32 weeks before first feeding, duodenal trypsin, lipase, and amylase were present in levels considerably lower than those found in term infants. Enzyme levels were even lower at 24 hours. The levels found at age 1 week depended on the carbohydrate of the ingested formula. Infants fed a high-starch formula had higher amylase while those fed a high-glucose formula had lower amylase but higher trypsin and lipase. Although infants fed a low-fat formula had the highest trypsin levels and no change in lipase, secretion of trypsin was lower than that found in older children and adults. The major problems with these early studies are the qualitative nature of the collections and the lack of separation between the pancreatic and salivary amylase and lipase isoenzymes. Thus the presence and changes of concentration of either or both of these enzymes may well have been due to contamination with the salivary isoenzyme.

In a small group of older children, they demonstrated that amylase continues to increase with age; the oldest child studied was 13 years old. While output of lipase, proteinases, fluid, and bicarbonate was independent of age, a good correlation was found between protein secretion and enzyme activity.

Norman et al measured pancreatic secretion in eight healthy full-term infants 3 to 15 days of age after a test meal of breast milk.[25] While the trypsin/chymotrypsin ratio was relatively constant, the levels of the individual enzymes varied considerably between infants. Salivary but not pancreatic amylase was present in low levels.

Lebenthal and Lee studied basal and stimulated pancreatic secretion in a group of well premature and full-term infants, infants 1 month of age, and toddlers 2 years of age (Fig. 7).[26] The results obtained from full-term and premature in-

fants were similar and data were pooled in the report. While total protein content was similar in the pancreatic secretions collected from the duodenum of all three groups, each of the five individual secretory proteins studied had its own developmental profile. Trypsin was low at 1 day, but at 1 month it was similar to the level seen at 2 years. Chymotrypsin remained low at 1 month. Carboxypeptidase was very low at 1 day and at 1 month when compared with the level found at 2 years. Amylase was not found until age 2 years. Similarly, lipase was almost unmeasureable at 1 day and at 1 month. Thus, the ontogeny of the various enzymes is not parallel, a finding that has also been documented in rodents. Responses to secretin and CCK were poor in the newborn and infant. Responses at 1 month were similar whether the infants were fed a cow's milk-based or a soy formula.

These data confirm previous reports concerning proteinases but are contradictory with respect to amylase and lipase. It has clearly been shown that pancreatic amylase is present early in gestation; similarly, salivary amylase is secreted in high concentration in the newborn. Serum pancreatic isoamylase and lipase are both low at birth and increase with age. These findings suggest that the newborn pancreas can synthesize but not secrete amylase. The failure to find any amylase at all may reflect the fasted state of the infants. A similar argument can be constructed to explain the extremely low levels of lipase.

Not only is enzyme secretion decreased in the infant and young child, but secretion of water and bicarbonate is blunted. An increase in ductal cell function also occurs with increasing age. Secretion of water increases 10 times by age 9 months.[24]

In spite of this pancreatic insensitivity described above, the human newborn infant and indeed the premature infant ab-

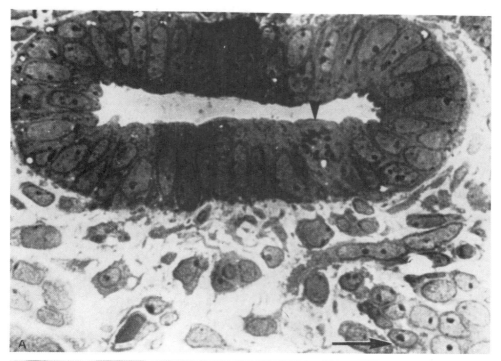

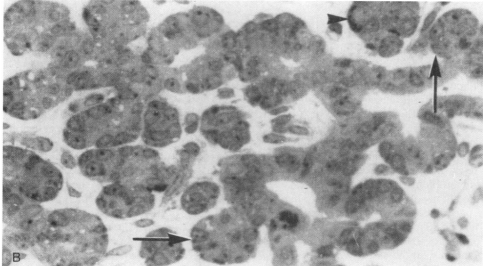

FIGURE 3 Light micrographs of developing human pancreas. *A,* Nine fetal weeks. At the top is a small duct lined by tall columnar cells containing elongated nuclei and a mitotic figure (*arrowhead*). Solid islands of similar cells are seen in the loose connective tissue (*arrow*). *B,* Twelve weeks. Pushing out from the small ducts are numerous clumps of epithelial cells (*arrows*). Some of these are endocrine cells (*arrowhead*). No zymogen granules are seen.

sorb both fat and carbohydrate with seemingly little difficulty. In elegant studies, Fomon and colleagues evaluated fat absorption in a group of infants ingesting a variety of formulas.[27] While an adult-type coefficient of fat absorption was not seen until 4 to 6 months of life, "clinically" important malabsorption is not seen unless an additional pancreatic insult, such as cystic fibrosis, is present. The lack of significant malabsorption is almost certainly due to the presence of the non-pancreatic lingual and gastric lipases.

Although the ontogeny of complex carbohydrate digestion and absorption has not yet been as carefully examined as that of fat absorption, there is some information regarding the ability of the newborn to digest starches. Husband et al showed that there is only a minimal rise in blood sugar after the in-

gestion of cooked starch.[28] Aurricchio et al showed that intestinal hydrolysis of starch is rapid in the 1-year-old child.[29] In contrast, at age 6 months, hydrolysis of amylopectin is incomplete and duodenal amylase activity is low. In spite of this lack of rise of serum glucose and the poor duodenal hydrolysis of starch, only minimal carbohydrate is found in the stool of infants fed formulas containing complex carbohydrates. This seeming paradox has been explained as being secondary to salvage of colonic carbohydrate by bacterial fermentation and absorption of short-chain organic acids.[30] It is also clear that the digestability of starches, modified starches, and complex carbohydrates varies considerably.[31] Levitt et al have shown in adults that the breath hydrogen increase after ingestion of meals containing complex carbohy-

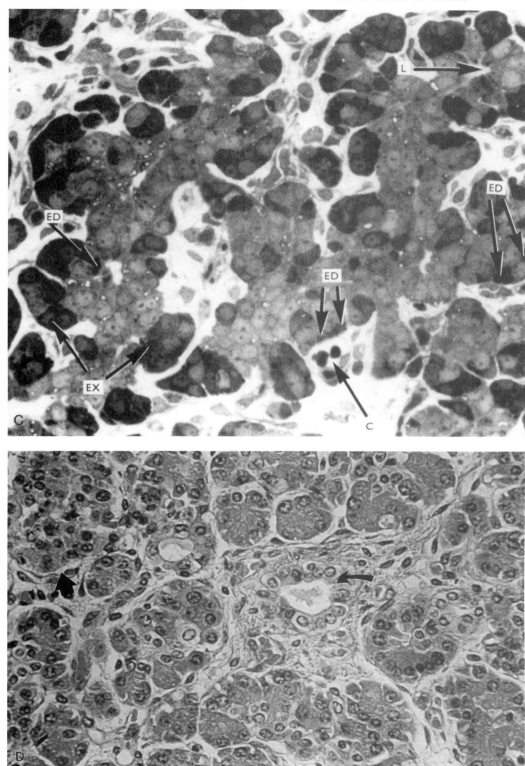

FIGURE 3 *(Continued) C*, Twenty weeks. There is extensive periductal proliferation. Note the clumps of darkly staining exocrine cells (EX) and scattered endocrine cells (ED). Numerous lightly staining duct cells and centroacinar cells are also seen. L = duct lumen; C = capillary. (A to C from Laitio, et al.[2] Reprinted with the permission of Cambridge University Press.) *D*, Six days old (postnatal). Pancreatic acini are mature appearing. Acinar cell borders are indistinct; nuclei are basal. Stromal volume is further decreased. An intralobular duct is present (*curved arrow*). An islet of Langerhans is present (*short arrow*). (Courtesy of Herbert Oechler, M.D.)

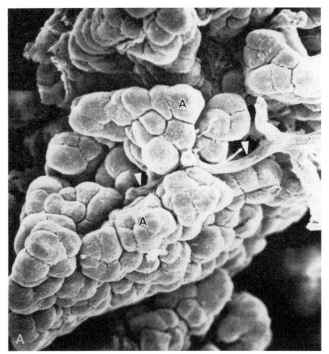

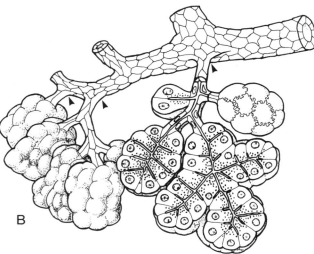

FIGURE 4 *A*, Scanning electron microscopic view of rat pancreatic lobule. Arrowheads indicate a long intercalated duct that connects with numerous acini (A). *B*, A three-dimensional schematic representation of the architecture of the exocrine pancreas. An excretory duct branches and the intercalated ducts (*arrowheads*), which are fairly constant in thickness, originate from both proximal and distal portions. Pancreatic acini are of varying sizes and shapes. Acinar lumina are narrow secretory canaliculi. (From Takahashi H. Scanning electron microscopy of rat exocrine pancreas. Arch Histol Jpn 1984; 47:387–404; with permission.)

TABLE 1
Growth of the Pancreas

Age	Pancreas Weight (g)
Neonate	5.1
1 month	5.6
3–6 months	11
6–12 months	14.5
2–4 years	19
4–6 years	22
6–12 years	29
15 years	68
Adult	85

Adapted from Schulz et al.[6]

drates varies considerably, suggesting that a large amount of fermentable material escapes small bowel absorption even in the adult.[32] Also present is glucoamylase, a brush border enzyme, which aids in the digestion of starch but also contributes intraluminal glucose, which increases the serum glucose.

It is clear that most infants, even those born prematurely, thrive on formulas that contain glucose polymers or corn syrup solids as their carbohydrate source.[33] It is this author's experience, which is supported by a small number of published case reports, that a number of infants develop watery diarrhea when fed such formulas.[34–36] This diarrhea resolves when the formula is changed to a sucrose-containing formula.

Diet modulates pancreatic enzyme secretion in the human as it does in the animal models discussed below. While these changes may occur at the level of synthesis, some changes reported to occur in animals clearly occur faster than can be explained by changes in synthesis. A high-starch diet fed to premature infants for 30 days increases amylase, whereas a high-protein diet increases stimulated secretion of lipase and trypsin.[24] In contrast, a high-fat diet had no effect on lipase secretion. Feeding a soy-based formula to premature infants

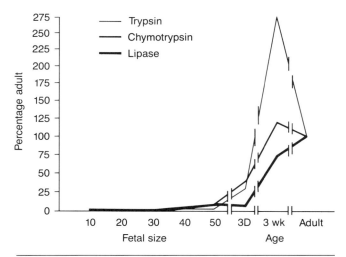

FIGURE 5 Increase in concentration of amylase, lipase, chymotrypsin, and trypsin in the human fetal (in 10-cm growth intervals) and postpartum pancreas. (Adapted from Track et al.[3])

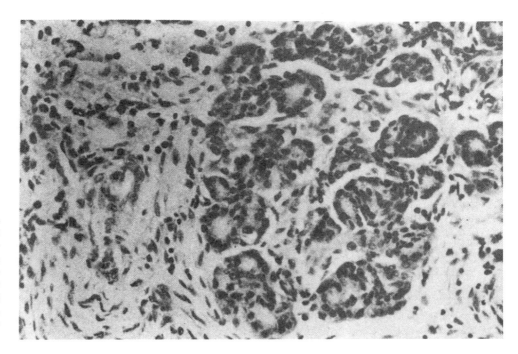

FIGURE 6 Pancreas from 24-weeks' gestation human fetus. There is faint to moderate staining of acinar cells for pancreatic amylase. The positivity of the acinar cells contrasts with the negative stroma. (From Davis et al,[20] with permission.)

increases stimulated pancreatic secretion of lipase and trypsin compared to infants fed a cow's milk-based formula.[37] Total parenteral nutrition induces reversible pancreatic atrophy in animals and pancreatic hyposecretion in humans. In spite of this potential problem, clinical experience has demonstrated that extended parenteral nutrition seems to have no long-term deleterious effects on pancreatic function in the human infant. Thus, as in the animal models described below, some changes in pancreatic enzyme secretion are programmed, whereas others are inducible by diet.

SECRETION FROM THE EXOCRINE PANCREAS

Although there is a continuous slow basal secretion of pancreatic enzymes, physiologically important secretion occurs only after stimulation by a secretagogue. While a large number of agents have been described that are effective secretagogues in the experimental animal, only acetylcholine and CCK are probably of significance in man. Acetylcholine is released locally in the pancreas after vagal stimulation. CCK is synthesized and stored in the intestinal amine precursor uptake and decarboxylation (APUD) cells and released after ingestion of a protein or fatty meal. The secretagogue then interacts with its specific receptor on the acinar cell membrane (Fig. 8). Intracellular second and third messengers include Ca^{2+}, protein kinase C, diacylglycerol, and inositol phosphates.[38-40] This complex and as yet inadequately understood process eventually leads to fusion of zymogen granules and cell membranes and exocytosis of pancreatic protein into the ductal system. While nonparallel secretion of pancreatic proteins has also been described, at the present time,

most authors feel that nonparallel secretion is probably the exception and not the norm.[41]

Fluid and electrolyte secretions from the centroacinar and ductal cells are controlled by secretin, the first hormone to be discovered (Fig. 8). Intracellular messengers in this system are cyclic AMP and protein kinase A. The concentrations of bicarbonate and chloride in pancreatic secretion are dependent on the flow rate. At low flow rates, the concentration of bicarbonate is low and that of chloride is high.[41] As the rate increases, bicarbonate secretion increases and chloride secretion decreases while sodium and potassium secretion remains constant.

The pancreas synthesizes more than 20 proteins specifically designed for export. After synthesis it must segregate those proteins designated for export from those synthesized for internal use.[38-43] Classic studies have demonstrated the synthetic pathway using the pulse chase technique. Newly synthesized proteins travel from the endoplasmic reticulum to the Golgi apparatus, where they are "packaged" to the condensing vacuoles, which are then converted into mature zymogen granules in the apical portion of the cell. There is little or no processing of individual proteins from the time they leave the rough endoplasmic reticulum until the time they leave the cell. This entire process takes less than 1 hour.[43]

HISTOGENESIS AND CYTODIFFERENTIATION OF THE RODENT PANCREAS

Since the ontogeny of the pancreas has been more extensively studied in the rat than in the human, many of our concepts concerning human pancreatic development are based

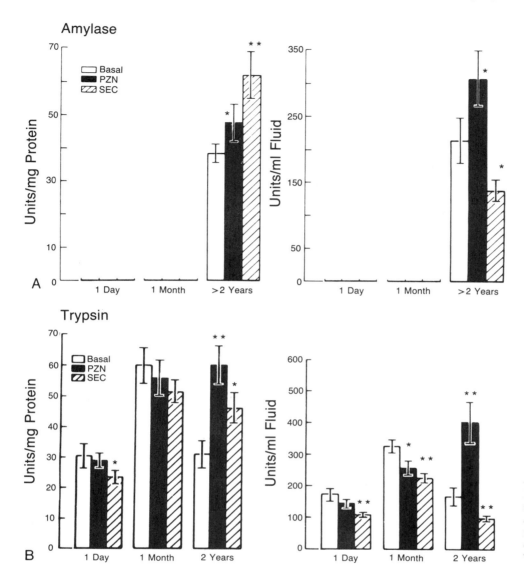

FIGURE 7 Effect of cholecystokinin and secretin on specific activities of pancreatic enzymes in duodenal fluid in infants and children. *A*, Amylase. *B*, Trypsin.

on data derived from these rodent studies. While the time span is different, the developmental stages of rat and human pancreas are believed to be similar. Pictet and Rutter have carefully documented and correlated the morphologic, histologic, ultrastructural, and biochemical development of the rat pancreas and have defined several distinct prenatal developmental periods (Table 2).[44]

The *predifferentiated* stage lasts until day 10 to 11 of gestation. During this phase pancreatic cells are indistinguishable from other embryonic gut cells and contain no pancreas-specific proteins. An as-yet-unknown *primary event* occurs that releases the apparent restriction of pancreatic gene expression and initiates the *protodifferentiated* stage of development. At this time, the two pancreatic anlagen bud from the duodenum, the dorsal pancreas appearing about 12 hours after the ventral bud. The early pancreatic epithelial cells form a single layer of primitive polarized cells facing the lumen and joined by junctional complexes. Mesodermal cells condense with the pancreatic diverticulum and initiate a phase of cellular proliferation, morphogenesis, and cytodifferenti-

ation, which results in the final tubuloacinar gland, which therefore contains both epidermal and mesenchymal components. Pancreas-specific proteins, such as amylase and lipase, are first found during this stage.

At day 16, the *secondary* transition occurs, initiating the third or *differentiated* stage of development. Recognizable acinar cells, acini, and collecting ducts are found at 16 to 17 days of gestation, the time of final fusion of the dorsal and ventral pancreatic bud. This is followed first by the appearance of endoplasmic reticulum, then by the development of zymogen granules, signifying full differentiation. By day 22 of gestation, the acinar cells are so packed with zymogen granules that other organelles are often obscured (Fig. 9*A*). Postnatally, RER increases while zymogen granules decrease both in number and in size [45,46] (Fig. 9*B*). Zymogen granule volume decreases from 45 percent of cytoplasmic volume at birth to 18 percent at age 3 weeks.

Responsiveness of the gland to secretagogues released when the newborn animal feeds depletes the acinar cell of stored secretory product. A *tertiary* event occurs after birth which

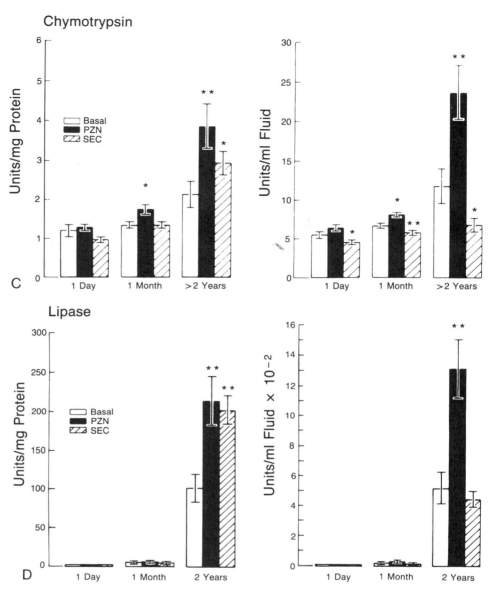

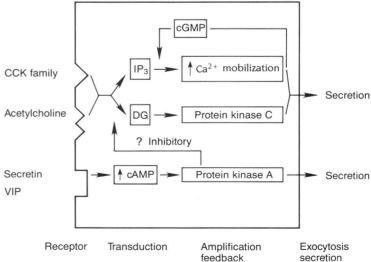

FIGURE 7 *(Continued) C,* Chymotrypsin. *D,* Lipase. (From Lebenthal and Lee.[26] Reproduced by permission of Pediatrics.)

FIGURE 8 Schematic drawing of pancreatic acinar cell demonstrating the four phases of stimulation-secretion coupling. Abbreviations: CCK = cholecystokinin; DG = 1,2-diacylglycerol; IP$_3$ = inositol 1,4,5-triphosphate; VIP = vasoactive intestinal peptide.

TABLE 2
Stages of Rat Pancreatic Development

Stage	Gestational Age	Characteristics
Predifferentiated	0–11	No pancreas-specific proteins
Protodifferentiated	12–14	Differentiated exocrine cells not present Embryonic proteins present Extensive morphogenesis Few zymogen granules Low levels of pancreas-specific proteins Onset of cytodifferentiation
Differentiated	15–21	Cell surface glycoproteins appear and mature Ductal cells appear Large number of zymogen granules synthesized Polarization Rapid increase of protein synthesis Rough endoplasmic reticulum develops Specific mRNA transcripts present Very high levels of secretory proteins
Modulated	Postnatal	Change in relative concentrations of secretory proteins Decreased numbers of zymogen granules Modified levels of secretory proteins

modifies the exocrine pancreas. Decreased numbers of zymogen granules and lower levels of secretory enzymes are then found.

In organ culture, normal morphogenesis and cytodifferentiation occur in primitive explants, demonstrating that nerves and factors from distant organs are not required for these processes. Local factors, however, are required, as a mesenchymal factor, probably basal lamina components, such as type IV collagen or laminin, is required for orderly cytodifferentiation and cell polarity but not for morphogenesis.[44,47,48] Without mesenchymal factor, which is neither tissue-nor species-specific, acinar structures do not develop. Other studies using 5-bromodeoxyuridine (BrdU), an inhibitor of acinar cell differentiation, have clearly shown that cytodifferentiation and morphogenesis are separable events.[49] In organ culture, fetal pancreas incubated in the presence of BrdU develops ductlike structures with lectin-binding characteristics similar to those of centroacinar cells. Acinar-like cells do not grow in this system, and pancreatic-specific proteins do not accumulate. Thus, extracellular factors are required for differentiation into acinar cells.

The ontogeny of cell-surface glycoproteins is critical for normal cell-cell interactions leading to normal morphogenesis.[50] Studies of the ontogeny of lectin-binding patterns have clearly demonstrated that the primitive pancreatic cells most resemble the centroacinar cells. The expression of the mature phenotype can first be detected at gestational age 15 days, the onset of the differentiated stage. Inhibition of glycoprotein synthesis in pancreatic rudiments between days 15 and 17 with tunicamycin delays histogenesis as well as the normal increase in amylase found at this age.[51] At 17 days acinar lumina are first seen coincident with differentiation of the apical and basolateral domains of the acinar cell membrane. The adult pattern is fully developed at age 19 days.

The temporal profiles of secretory proteins in the prenatal pancreas have been defined.[52-54] Until day 14 of gestation, little or no secretory product, specific mRNA for secretory proteins, or zymogen granules are found. From days 14 to 18, synthesis of embryonic proteins also found in a wide variety of other fetal tissues, but not in zymogen granules, continues. A constant low level of a few pancreas-specific secretory proteins is found. From days 18 to 21, a rapid increase in specific mRNA transcripts occurs, followed by a nonparallel increase in pancreas-specific proteins and zymogen granules.[55,56] RNA synthesis peaks at day 18, followed by a peak in protein synthesis 1 day later. During this period, while total pancreatic protein synthesis increases only 25 percent, synthesis of certain pancreas-specific proteins such as amylase and chymotrypsinogen increase by more than 100 percent. During the final days of gestation and during early neonatal life, synthesis of secretory proteins accounts for more than 90 percent of all pancreatic synthesis.

The appearance of the various secretory proteins is not parallel, suggesting independent regulation of gene expression.[53,54] Amylase and chymotrypsinogen appear synchronously at day 15. Other proteins that also appear in pairs are trypsinogen and procarboxypeptidase B and specific lipase and procarboxypeptidase A. Nonspecific lipase and ribonuclease accumulate independently. Amylase-specific mRNA increases 600-fold between gestational days 14 and 20, coincident with the above-described 1,000-fold increase in amylase specific activity. Synthesis of amylase and presumably other secretory proteins is regulated at the level of transcription or mRNA turnover.

Thus, both the timing of initiation of synthesis of individual proteins and final levels are different. While the curves for the appearance of each protein are quite similar, they are time shifted. The final adult level of each enzyme is related neither to the onset of synthesis nor to the peak fetal level. In fact, the final adult concentration of a given enzyme may be less than or greater than the peak fetal concentration. Concentrations of enzyme change considerably after birth. For example, the level of amylase specific mRNA at day 20 is less than 20 percent of that found in the adult, while the level of amylase is greater in the 20-day fetus.[52] This can be explained by the fact that the fetal pancreas synthesizes but does not secrete amylase. In contrast, the level of amylase in the mature pancreas represents the balance between synthesis and secretion. These changes seem to be related both to internal programming and to the influence of diet.

Pancreatic content of exportable proteins and zymogen granules falls dramatically after birth.[45,46] This fall is not preprogrammed but rather relates to feeding and stimulation of secretion.[57,58] Alterations in diet, time of weaning, and time of first feeding by induction of postmaturity all affect the levels of secretory proteins in predictable ways.

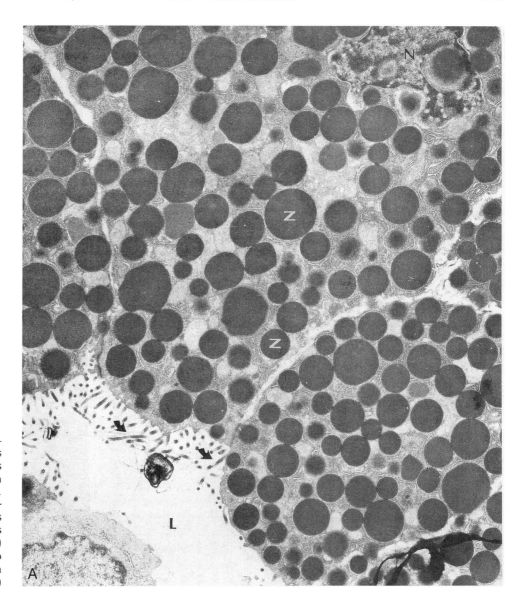

FIGURE 9 *A*, Pancreatic acinus from newborn rat. The cells contain abundant zymogen granules of variable size (Z). The nucleus (N) is located basally and shows indentations where zymogen granules press against it. Microvilli (*arrows*) from acinocytes project into the acinar lumen (L). (From Harb et al,[46] with permission.)

DEVELOPMENT OF SECRETORY FUNCTION IN THE RODENT PANCREAS

The pancreas of the newborn rat is both histologically and ultrastructurally fully developed and is packed with secretory proteins. Although it appears poised to secrete, it is functionally immature. Immaturity has been documented at a number of locations along the stimulus-secretion chain. Responsiveness to cholinergic and peptidergic (CCK) secretagogues in a manner similar to but not identical with the adult gland does not occur until age 24 to 48 hours.[59–61] The newborn pancreas, while unresponsive to cholingergic agents and to CCK, does respond with increased secretion of amylase to the calcium ionophore A23187, suggesting that the secretory mechanism distal to calcium mobilization is intact.[61,62] In contrast, Chang and Jamieson failed to find responsiveness to A23187 in fetal pancreas.[63]

Morisset and colleagues have defined the ontogeny of the muscarinic receptor.[64] Receptor density, low in the fetal and newborn periods, steadily increases with age, reaching maximum levels at age 1 month, then decreases steadily until age 1 year. They found a parallel increase in secretory response and receptor density.

The ontogeny of the CCK receptor has been similarly evaluated by Leung et al[65] and Werlin et al.[66] Binding of radiolabeled CCK, low at birth, also rises rapidly, reaching levels of the mature pancreas at age 3 weeks. In contrast, Chang and Jamieson found that the postnatal increase in secretory responsiveness is not associated with increased CCK binding.[63] They found that in both the fetal and neonatal pancreas, calcium is mobilized by CCK. These studies imply that decreased receptor density cannot explain the lack of secretory responsiveness in the immature pancreas and that the immaturity is distal to calcium mobilization.

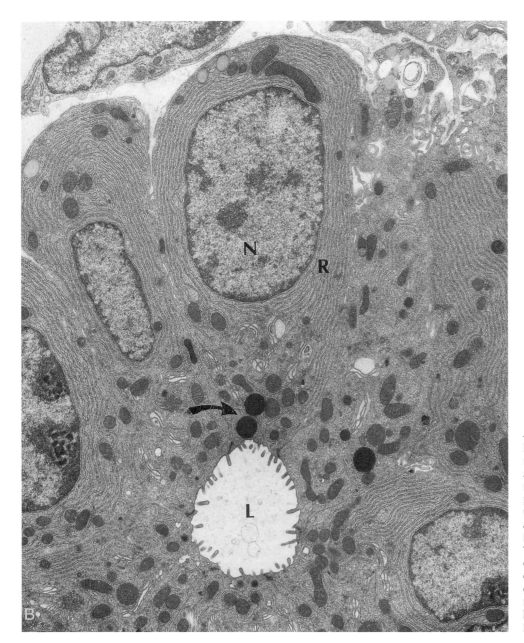

FIGURE 9 *(Continued) B,* Acinus of 24-hour-old rat. Zymogen granule content is markedly reduced when compared with *A.* Remaining granules *(arrow)* are located in the apical cytoplasm. The lumen (L) is small with short microvilli. The nucleus (N) is large with clumped and marginated heterochromatin. Abundant rough endoplasmic reticulum (R) is arranged into parallel stacked lamellae. (Courtesy of Joseph Harb, Ph.D.)

Since protein phosphorylation appears to play an important role in the pancreatic response to secretagogues, the roles of protein kinases have been examined. Calcium-calmodulin–dependent protein kinase increases in parallel with responsiveness to secretagogues from the late fetal to the newborn period.[67] Similarly, protein kinase C was found to be low in the term fetus. Levels increase in the newborn period, reaching adult values by age 2 days.[68] Newborn rat pancreas was unresponsive to 12-0-tetradecanoylphorbol 13-acetate (TPA), an activator of protein kinase C, but 2-day-old pancreas responded to TPA with increased amylase secretion. These studies of protein kinases suggest immaturity of the secretory response to regulatory peptides at a number of levels.

Thus, immaturity both of receptors to secretagogues and of protein kinases is found in the neonatal rat. At this time,

the lack of responsiveness to secretagogues in the neonatal rat cannot be attributed to any one pharmacologic deficiency and may in fact be multifactorial.

CONTROLS OF GROWTH IN THE RODENT PANCREAS

Pancreatic growth in the mature animal can be altered by a variety of agents, diets, and experimental procedures.[69] The trophic effects of CCK and CCK-like peptides have been well documented.[69] Glucocorticoids induce hypertrophy in the mature rat, with particular increases in concentrations of amylase and chymotrypsin. Hydrocortisone also potentiates the trophic effect of cerulein, a CCK analogue. While secretin has only a mild trophic effect, it potentiates the trophic effect of CCK. Although high doses of cholingeric agents induce hypertrophy in rat pancreas, the physiologic importance of this effect is uncertain. Epidermal growth factor (EGF) has also been shown to have trophic effects. Pancreatic biliary diversion, small bowel resection, and ingestion of raw soy flour all induce pancreatic growth in the mature animal. The roles of ornithine decarboxylase and polyamines remain controversial.

While there are published studies concerning the roles of many of the above agents and treatments on the immature pancreas, interpretation and comparison of these studies present numerous difficulties in data analysis, including the following: (1) The various agents tested were given in different doses, at different ages, and for different lengths of time, and (2) the animals were evaluated for effects on growth in different ways. A major overlooked fact is that the growth rate and the rates of synthesis of both DNA and protein vary considerably with developmental ages.[70]

Werlin and colleagues have shown that the concentrations of DNA and protein in immature rat pancreas do not parallel the rates of their synthesis.[70] DNA concentration increases rapidly from a low level in the first day of life, peaks between 3 and 14 days, then slowly falls to a lower adult level. In contrast, DNA synthesis decreases in the first 24 hours, peaks at 3 days at a rate of 30 times the adult rate, then falls slowly to the adult rate (Fig. 10). Similarly, protein concentration, which is nearly as high at birth as it is in the adult, plummets at day 3 before it slowly begins to rise to adult levels. Protein synthesis, in contrast, is as low at birth as it is in the adult but is three to five times higher at all intermediate ages tested (Fig. 11).

In spite of these controversies and the many gaps in our knowledge that remain, a great deal has been learned concerning the effects of many agents on the growth of the exocrine pancreas in the developing animal. CCK and CCK-like peptides have a variety of effects that seem to be age dependent. DNA synthesis is not increased before age 28 days by CCK. Hypertrophy, atrophy, hyperplasia, and no effects on growth have been described depending on age, dosage, and CCK analogue studied.[71-75]

Hydrocortisone decreases protein synthesis in the first week of life but has no effect on DNA synthesis in the immature animal.[71] Other studies have described hypertrophy and hyperplasia or hypertrophy alone,[75,76] depending on age. Cerulein and hydrocortisone potentiate each other's trophic effects. The lack of increase in DNA synthesis in the suckling animal after treatment with either CCK or hydrocortisone may be due to the fact that synthesis is already proceeding at the maximum rate possible.

A temporal relationship exists among corticosterone levels, cytoplasmic corticosteroid receptors, and increases in pancreatic secretory products in the developing pancreas.[76,77] Corticosterone levels and dexamethasone binding increase from birth, reach a peak at about 25 days, then decrease to adult levels. Increases in circulating levels of steroids precede the sharp increases in receptor density after age 15 days. These increases parallel those of both amylase and hydrolase activities, which can be induced by exogenous steroids. Early weaning, which augments corticosterone levels, causes similar changes in content of exportable proteins in the pancreas. The highest density of steroid receptors occurs at age 21 to 28 days, the period of peak responsiveness of the pancreas to hydrocortisone in DNA and protein synthesis.

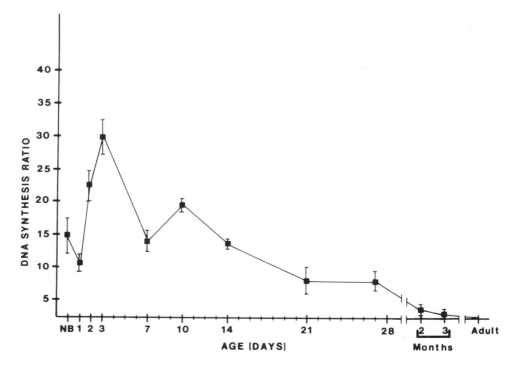

FIGURE 10 The DNA synthesis ratio in developing rat pancreas. The DNA synthesis ratio in counts per minute of ^{3}[H]-thymidine incorporated per milligram of DNA at each time point was divided by the mean adult rate to obtain the DNA synthesis ratio. (From Werlin et al,[70] with permission.)

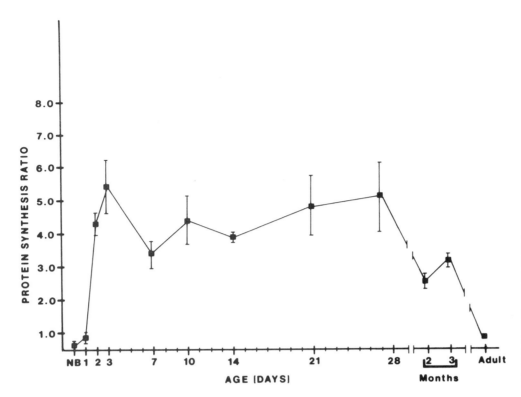

FIGURE 11 The protein synthesis ratio in developing rat pancreas. The protein synthesis ratio in counts per minute of ^{14}[C]-leucine incorporated per milligram of protein at each time point was divided by the mean adult rate to obtain the protein synthesis ratio. (From Werlin et al,[70] with permission.)

Thus, glucocorticoids clearly modulate postnatal pancreatic development.

Among the less well-studied factors, thyroxine induces precocious increases of amylase, lipase, chymotrypsin, and trypsin in neonatal rats, whereas chemical thryoidectomy retards pancreatic development.[78] Endogenous thyroxine peaks between days 10 and 16, the time when amylase levels are also increasing. Parenteral but not oral EGF increases pancreatic amylase in suckling rabbits.[79] Inhibition of ornithine decarboxylase (and thus polyamine metabolism) inhibits pancreatic development, suggesting a possible role in normal growth.[80] Secretin increases DNA, amylase, and chymotrypsin in 6-day-old rats. Bombesin induces hypertrophy and hyperplasia in newborn rats.[81] Thus, while a variety of agents have been shown to alter pancreatic development in the young rat, the physiologic role and interrelationships among them remain to be clarified.

Studies in which the diets of immature animals are altered have shown that the changes in concentrations of the various enzymes are not all preprogrammed. Changing the diet from high fat, low carbohydrate to high carbohyrate, low fat by early weaning increases chymotrypsin and lipase and decreases amylase. Delaying weaning by prolonged nursing postpones these changes in enzyme concentration.[82] Animals weaned on a high-fat diet similar to mother's milk had changes in enzyme pattern similar to those found in animals prematurely weaned. Interestingly, the changes found with early weaning are similar to those induced by glucocorticoids, and premature weaning induces an increase in corticosteroid levels in the infant rat. Changes in diet after 21 days of age induce characteristic changes in pancreatic enzyme composition; increasing the dietary intake of starch increases amylase, increasing intake of fat increases lipase, and increasing protein intake increases trypsin. Thus, glucocorticoids may modulate some effects of feeding, whereas others seem to be preprogrammed.

REFERENCES

1. Moore KL. The developing human. Philadelphia: WB Saunders, 1982.
2. Laitio M, Lev R, Orlic D. The developing human fetal pancreas: an ultrastructural and histochemical study with special reference to exocrine cells. J Anat 1974; 117:619–634.
3. Track NS, Creutzfeldt C, Bokermann M. Enzymatic, functional and ultrastructural development of the exocrine pancreas II. The human pancreas. Comp Biochem Physiol 1975; 51A:95–100.
4. Grand RJ, Watkins JB, Torti FM. Development of the human gastrointestinal tract. Gastroenterology 1976; 70:790–810.
5. Sturgess JM. Structural and developmental abnormalities of the exocrine pancreas in cystic fibrosis. J Pediatr Gastroenterol Nutr 1984; 3:S55–S66.
6. Schulz DM, Giordano DA, Schulz DH, et al. Weight of organs of fetuses and infants. Arch Pathol 1962; 74:244.
7. Keene MFL, Hewer EE. Digestive enzymes of the human fetus. Lancet 1929; i:767–769.
8. Lieberman J. Proteolytic enzyme activity in fetal pancreas and meconium, demonstration of plasminogen and trypsinogen activators in pancreatic tissue. Gastroenterology 1966; 50:183–190.
9. Tachibana T: Physiological investigation of the fetus: lipase in the pancreas. Jpn J Obstet Gynecol 1929; 11:92–99
10. Madey S, Dancis J. Proteolytic enzymes of the premature infant, with special reference to his ability to digest unsplit protein food. Pediatrics 1949; 4:177–182.
11. Borgstrom B, Lindquist B, Lundh G. Enzyme concentration and absorption of protein and glucose in duodenum of premature infants. Am J Dis Child 1960; 99:338–343.
12. De Filippi F, Giussani AA, Rivelis L. Assay of the tryptic activity of the feces of the newborn infant, at term or premature. Pediatrics 1954; 15:114–126.

13. Jodl J, Kornfalt R. Svenningsen NW. Chymotryptic activity in stool of low birth weight infants in the first week of life. Acta Pediatr Scand 1975; 64:619–623.
14. Mullinger M, Palasi M. Tryptic and chymotryptic activity of stools of newborn infants. Pediatrics 1966; 38:657–659.
15. Wolf RO, Taussig LM. Human amniotic fluid isoamylases, functional development of fetal pancreas and salivary glands. Obstet Gynceol 1973; 41:337–342.
16. De Castro AF, Usategui-Gomez M, Spellacy WN. Amniotic fluid amylase. Am J Obstet Gynecol 1973; 116:931–936.
17. Laxova R. Antenatal development of amylase isoenzymes. J Med Genet 1972; 9:321–323.
18. Tye JG, Karn RC, Merritt AD. Differential expression of salivary (Amy$_1$) and pancreatic (Amy$_2$) human amylase loci in prenatal and postnatal development. J Med Genet 1976; 13:96–102.
19. Auricchio S, Rubino A, Murset G. Intestinal glycosidase activities in the human embryo, fetus and newborn. Pediatrics 1965; 35:944–954.
20. Davis MM, Hodes MR, Munsick RA, Ulbright TM, Goldstein DJ. Pancreatic amylase expression in human pancreatic development. Hybridoma 1986; 5:137–145.
21. Hadorn B, Zoppi G. Shmerling DH, Prader A, McIntrye I, Anderson CM. Quantitative assessment of exocrine pancreatic function in infants and children. J Pediatr 1968; 73:39–50.
22. Zoppi G, Hitzig WH, Shmerling DH, Plus H, Hadorn B, Prader A. Protein content and pancreatic enzyme activities of duodenal juice in normal children and in children with exocrine pancreatic insufficiency. Helv Paediatr Acta 1968; 23:577–590.
23. Zoppi G, Shmerling DH, Gaburro D, Prader A. The electrolyte and protein contents and outputs in duodenal juice after pancreozymin and secretin stimulation in normal children and in patients with cystic fibrosis. Acta Paediatr Scand 1970; 59:692–696.
24. Zoppi G, Andreotti G, Pajno-Ferrara F, Njai DM. Guburro D. Exocrine pancreas function in premature and full term infants. Pediatr Res 1972; 6:880–886.
25. Norm A. Strandvik B, Ojamae O. Bile acids and pancreatic enzymes during absorption in the newborn. Acta Paediatr Scand 1972; 61:571–576.
26. Lebenthal E, Lee PC. Development of functional response in human exocrine pancreas. Pediatrics 1980; 66:556–560.
27. Fomon SJ, Ziegler EE, Thomas LN, Jensen RL, Filer LJ. Excretion of fat by normal full-term infants fed various milks and formulas. Am J Clin Nutr 1970; 23:1299–1313.
28. Husband J, Husband P, Mallinson CN. Gastric emptying of starch meal in the newborn. Lancet 1970; ii:290–292.
29. Auricchio S. Pietra DD. Vegnente A. Studies on intestinal digestion of starch in man. II. Intestinal hydrolysis of amylopectin in infants and children. Pediatrics 1967; 39:853–862.
30. Shulman RJ, Wong WW, Irving CS, Nichols BL, Klein PD. Utilization of dietary cereal by young infants. J. Pediatr 1983; 103:23–28.
31. De Vizia B, Ciccimarra F, De Cicco N, Auricchio S. Digestibility of starches in infants and children. J Pediatr 1975; 86:50–55.
32. Levitt MD, Hirsh P, Fetzer CA, Sheahan M, Levine AS. H$_2$ excretion after ingestion of complex carbohydrates. Gastroenterology 1987; 92:383–389.
33. Cicco R, Holzman IR, Brown DR, Becker DJ. Glucose polymer tolerance in premature infants. Pediatrics 1981; 67:498–501.
34. Lilibridge CB, Townes PL, Physiologic deficiency of pancreatic amylase in infancy: a factor in iatrogenic diarrhea. J Pediatr 1973; 82:279–282.
35. Fisher SE, Leone G, Kelly RH. Chronic protracted diarrhea: intolerance to dietary glucose polymers. Pediatrics 1981; 67:271–273.
36. Fagundes-Neto U, Viaro T. Lifshitz F. Tolerance to glucose polymers in malnourished infants with diarrhea and disaccharide intolerance. Am J Clin Nutr 1985; 41:228–234.
37. Lebenthal E, Choi TS, Lee PC. The development of pancreatic function in premature infants after milk-based and soy-based formulas. Pediatr Res 1981; 15:1240–1244.
38. Grossman A. An overview of pancreatic exocrine secretion. Comp Biochem Physiol 1984; 78B:1–13.
39. Nishizuka Y. The role of protein kinase C in cell surface signal transduction and tumor promotion. Nature 1984; 308:693–698.
40. Nishizuka Y. Studies and perspectives of protein kinase C. Science 1986; 233:305–312.
41. Scheele G. Cellular processing of proteins in the exocrine pancreas. In: Go VLW, Gardner JD, Brooks FP, Lebenthal E, DiMagno EP,

42. Scheele G, eds. The exocrine pancreas: biology, pathophysiology, and diseases. New York: Raven Press, 1986:69.
43. Bro-Rasmussen F, Killman SA, Thaysen JH. The composition of pancreatic juice as compared to sweat, parotid saliva and tears. Acta Physiol Scand 1956; 37:97–113.
44. Scheele GA. The secretory process in the pancreatic exocrine cells. Mayo Clin Proc 1979; 54:420–427.
45. Pictet R, Rutter WJ. Development of the embryonic endocrine pancreas. In: Steiner DF, Freinkel N, eds. Handbook of physiology, Sec 7, Endocrinology, Vol 1. Washington, DC: American Physiological Society, 1972:250.
46. Ermak TH, Rothman SS, Large decrease in zymogen granule size in the postnatal rat pancreas. J. Ultrastruct Res 1980; 70:242–256.
47. Harb JM, Werlin SL, Taylor TJ, Stefaniak J. Effects of cholecystokinin octapeptide and hydrocortisone on the exocrine pancreas of fed and fasted 24-hour-old-rats: an electron microscopic study. Exp Molec Pathol 1982; 37:92–100.
48. Spooner BS, Walther BT, Rutter WJ. The development of the dorsal and ventral mammalian pancreas in vivo and in vitro. J Cell Biol 1970; 47:235–246.
49. Pictet RL, Clark WR, Williams RH, Rutter WJ. An ultrastructural analysis of the developing embryonic pancreas. Dev Biol 1972; 29:436–467.
50. Maylie-Pfenninger MF, Jamieson JD. Effect of 5-bromodeoxyuridine on appearance of cell-surface saccharides in organ cultures of embryonic pancreas. Dev Biol 1981; 87:16–23.
51. Jamieson JD. Plasmalemmal glycoproteins and basal lamina: involvement in pancreatic morphogenesis. In: Hoffman J, Giebisch G, eds. Membranes in growth and development, New York: Alan R. Liss, 1982.
52. Sarras MP, Maylie-Pfenninger MF, Manzi RRM, Jamieson JD. The effect of tunicamycin on development of the mammalian embryonic pancreas. Dev Biol 1981; 87:1–15.
53. Sanders TG, Rutter WJ. The developmental regulation of amylolytic and proteolytic enzymes in the embryonic rat pancreas. J Biol Chem 1974; 249:3500–3509.
54. Kemp JD, Walther BT, Rutter WJ. Protein synthesis during the secondary developmental transition of the embryonic rat pancreas. J Biol Chem 1972; 247:3941–3952.
55. Van Nest GA, MacDonald RJ, Raman RK, Rutter WJ. Proteins synthesized and secreted during rat pancreatic development. J Cell Biol 1980; 86:784–794.
56. Harding JD, Rutter WJ. Rat pancreatic amylase mRNA. J Biol Chem 1978; 253:8736–8740.
57. Przybyla AE, MacDonald RJ, Harding JD, Pictet RL, Rutter WJ. Accumulation of the predominant pancreatic mRNAs during embryonic development. J. Biol Chem 1979; 254:2154–2159.
58. Lee PC, Kim OK, Lebenthal E. Effect of early weaning and prolonged nursing on development of rat pancreas. Pediatr Res 1982; 16:470–473.
59. Merchant Z, Jiang LX, Lebenthal E, Lee PC. Pancreatic exocrine enzymes during the neonatal period in postmature rats. Int J Pancreat 1987; 2:325–335.
60. Larose L, Morisset J. Acinar cell responsiveness to urecholine in the rat pancreas during fetal and early postnatal growth. Gastroenterology 1977; 73:530–533.
61. Doyle CM, Jamieson JD. Development of secretagogue response in rat pancreatic acinar cells. Develop Biol 1978; 65:11–27.
62. Werlin SL, Grand RJ. Development of secretory mechanisms in rat pancreas. Am J Physiol 1979; 236:E446–E450.
63. Werlin SL, Stefaniak J. Maturation of secretory function in rat pancreas. Pediatr Res 1982; 16:123–125.
64. Chang A, Jamieson JD. Stimulus-secretion coupling in the developing exocrine pancreas: secretory responsiveness to cholecystokinin. J Cell Biol 1986; 103:2353–2365.
65. Dumont Y, Larose L, Morisset J, Poirier GG. Parallel maturation of the pancreatic secretory response to cholinergic stimulation and the muscarinic receptor population. Br J Pharmacol 1981; 73:347–354.
66. Leung YK, Lee PC, Lebenthal E. Maturation of cholecystokinin receptors in pancreatic acini of rats. Am J Physiol 1986; 250:G594–G597.
67. Werlin SL, Colton DG, Harb J, Reynolds E, Hoffman RG, Williams JA. Ontogeny of secretory function and cholecystokinin binding capacity in immature rat pancreas. Life Sci 1987; 40:2237–2245.
68. Gorelick FS, Chang A, Jamieson JD. Calcium-calmodulin-stimulated protein kinase in developing pancreas. Am J Physiol 1987; 253:G469–G476.
69. Shimizu K, Lebenthal E, Lee PC. Immature stimulus-secretion coupling

in the developing exocrine pancreas and ontogenic changes of protein kinase C. Biochim Biophys Acta 1988; 968:186-191.

69. Folsch UR. Regulation of pancreatic growth. Clin Gastroenterol 1984; 13:679-699.

70. Werlin SL, Colton DG, Virojanavat S, Reynolds E. DNA and protein synthesis in developing rat pancreas. Pediatr Res 1987; 22:34-38.

71. Werlin SL, Virojanavat S, Reynolds E, Hoffman RG, Colton DG. Effects of cholecystokinin and hydrocortisone on DNA and protein synthesis in immature rat pancreas. Pancreas 1988; 3:274-278.

72. Brants F, Morisset J. Trophic effect of cholecystokinin-pancreaozymin on pancreatic acinar cells from rats of different ages (39583). Proc Soc Exp Biol Med 1976; 153:523-527.

73. Morisset J. Stimulation of pancreatic growth by secretin and caerulein in suckling rats. Biomed Res 1980; 1:405-409.

74. Morisset J, Jolicoeur L. Effect of hydrocortisone on pancreatic growth in rat. Am J Physiol 1980; 239:G95-G98.

75. Werlin SL, Stefaniak J. Effects of hydrocortisone and cholecystokinin-octapeptide on neonatal rat pancreas. J Pediatr Gastroenterol Nutr 1982; 1:591-595.

76. Grossman A, Boctor AM, Band P, Lane B. Role of steroids in secretion-modulating effect of triamcinolone and estradiol on protein synthesis and secretion from the rat exocrine pancreas. J Steroid Biochem 1983; 19:1069-1081.

77. Lu RB, Lebenthal E, Lee PC. Developmental changes of glucocorticoid receptors in the rat pancreas. J Steroid Biochem 1987; 26:213-218.

78. Lu RB, Chaichanwatankul K, Lin CH, Lebenthal E, Lee PC. Thyroxine effect on exocrine pancreatic development in rats. Am J Physiol 1988; 254:G315-G321.

79. O'Loughlin EV, Chung M, Hollenberg M, Hayden J, Zahavi I, Gall DG. Effect of epidermal growth factor on ontogeny of the gastrointestinal tract. Am J Physiol 1985; 249:G674-G678.

80. Morisset J, Grondin G. Implication of ornithine decarboxylase and polyamines in pancreatic growth of neonatal rats. Pancreas 1987; 2:303-311.

81. Lehy T, Puccio F, Chariot J, LaBeille D. Stimulating effect of bombesin on the growth of gastrointestinal tract and pancreas in suckling rats. Gastroenterology 1986; 90:1942-1949.

82. Snook JT. Effect of diet on development of exocrine pancreas of the neonatal rat. Am J Physiol 1971; 221:1388-1391.

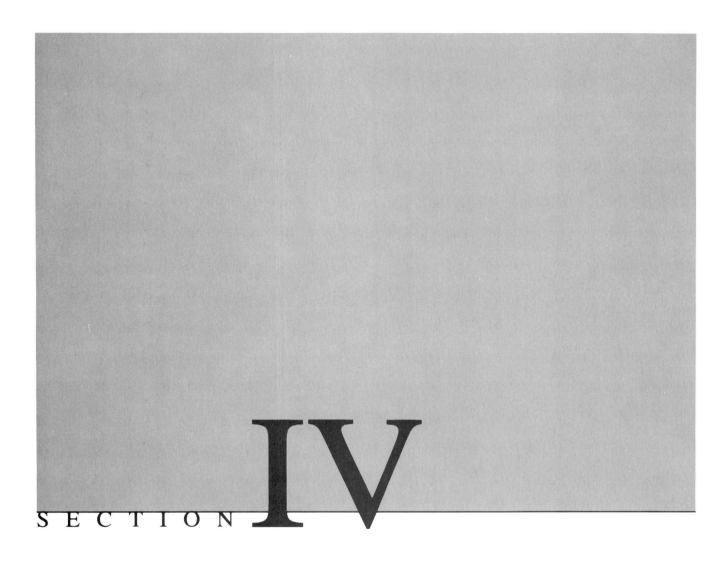

SECTION IV

Clinical Manifestations and Management

PART 1

Disorders of the Oral Cavity

David C. Rule, B.D.S., F.D.S., D.Orth., M.C.C.D.

The precise relationship between ulcerative or granulomatous lesions of the oral mucosa and similar manifestations elsewhere in the gastrointestinal (GI) tract remains in some cases obscure, whereas in others the initial recognition of such lesions may be a precise diagnostic pointer toward the general underlying disease process.

RECURRENT APHTHOUS ULCERATION

The most common form of ulceration affecting the oral mucosa is the so-called aphthous type. This condition is characterized by the presence of one or more oral ulcers, which heal within days or sometimes weeks only to reappear at regular intervals. The associated constitutional effects may vary from minor discomfort from the ulcers themselves to a severely incapacitating illness caused by persistent oral ulceration.[1] The overall prevalence of the condition has been shown to be 20 to 30 percent,[2] and it has been estimated that 30 percent of affected individuals have experienced their first attack of oral ulceration by the age of 14 years, with 10 percent having ulcers before the age of 10 years.[3] An associated family history has been demonstrated in 24 to 46 percent of cases,[2-4] with a very high incidence in patients whose parents both suffered from the condition.[5] Furthermore, in a study carried out on twins, a 90 percent concordance between identical twins was found, in contrast to a 57 percent concordance between nonidentical twins.[6]

This group of disorders may be further subdivided into three distinct subgroups,[7] largely on the basis of the clinical appearance and history of the individual lesions. All three types of recurrent aphthous ulceration (RAU) may be seen in children and are referred to as minor aphthous ulceration (MiAU), major aphthous ulceration (MjAU), and herpetiform ulceration (HU).

Minor aphthous ulcers account for 80 percent of the total and are most common in patients between 10 and 40 years of age. Ulcers of this type, referred to previously as Mikulicz's aphthae, affect characteristically the nonkeratinized oral mucosa of the lips, cheeks, vestibule, and margins of the tongue. The hard palate, gingivae, and dorsum of the tongue are typically unaffected. The appearance of a painful ulcer is frequently preceded by a prodromal phase of 1 to 3 days, during which the patient may complain of a burning or pricking sensation accompanied by a degree of paresthesia at the site of future ulceration.[8] The ulcers, which may occur alone or in groups of three or four during a single episode, usually last between 10 and 14 days, reaching a maximum size at 4 to 5 days. Healing is complete with no residual scarring, but recurrent episodes of ulceration tend to occur regularly at 1- to 4-month intervals. Individual ulcers are shallow, surrounded by an area of reddened mucosa, and vary in shape depending upon the site. Those affecting the cheeks may appear rounded, whereas a more linear presentation is common in the depths of the buccal and lingual sulci. The base is covered with a greyish yellow slough.

There are no distinguishing histopathologic features, microscopy revealing an appearance similar to that seen in cases of traumatic ulceration of the oral mucosa.[9] The epithelium shows no diagnostic features, and the underlying connective tissue is infiltrated with inflammatory cells, predominantly lymphocytes and plasma cells.

In MjAU, formerly known as periadenitis mucosa necrotica recurrens,[10] the ulcers are much larger than those seen in MiAU. They may appear singly or up to three or four at one time, are very painful, and give rise to extensive tissue destruction.

Both keratinized and nonkeratinized oral mucosa may be affected, including that of the dorsum of the tongue and oropharynx. The appearance of an individual ulcer is preceded by a submucous nodule that breaks down after several days to produce a central deep necrotic area. Healing occurs over a period of weeks, leaving an area of scarred, distorted tissue.[11] During the period when an ulcer is present, the patient may feel generally unwell, and a marked lymphadenitis may be observed.

Herpetiform ulcers occur with frequency similar to that of MjAU[3] and also involve both the keratinized and nonkeratinized oral mucosa, typically of the floor of the mouth, lateral borders, and ventral surface of the tongue.[12] Females tend to be affected more commonly than males.[7] At the outset of an episode of ulceration, numerous discrete ulcers approximately 1 to 2 mm in diameter appear. These may later coalesce to form a single, large, painful lesion with a serpiginous outline. The ulcers usually heal within 10 days without mucosal scarring, although recurrent episodes of ulceration may supervene within days. Repeated attacks of this type may give rise to severe dysphagia.

Etiology

The etiology of RAU remains unclear despite the many factors, both local and general, that have been identified with the appearance of mucosal ulceration.

Minor mucosal trauma, such as that caused during dental treatment, has long been linked with RAU, and in a recent review,[13] the authors suggest that trauma may be an initiating factor in the susceptible patient.

Although stress has been implicated in the occurrence of RAU,[14,15] there is some evidence to suggest that RAU patients are no more anxious than general medical or surgical patients.

In a small number of patients, the occurrence of oral ulceration may coincide with certain phases of the menstrual cycle and puberty. It has also been reported that RAU is not encountered during pregnancy.[16] However, a direct hormonal link with RAU is as yet unproven.

Attempts to implicate specific bacteria in the etiology of RAU have, in general, been unsuccessful. Delayed skin hypersensitivity to a vaccine prepared from an L-form of *Streptococcus sanguis* has been reported in a significant number of RAU patients,[17] but the importance of this finding has been questioned[18] because the particular organism has been found commonly in the mouths of patients who do not suffer from RAU, and furthermore it has been shown[19] to stimulate lymphocyte transformation less in RAU patients than in unaffected individuals.

It has been suggested that RAU patients have increased cell-mediated immunity and humoral immunity against streptococcal and human oral mucosal antigens. One study[20] has indicated that there is a significant increase in cell-mediated immunity during an exacerbation of RAU.

The evidence for a viral etiology in RAU is far from convincing, although a type I adenovirus has been identified by culture and immunofluorescent staining of ulcer scrapings in affected patients.[21]

Despite the accepted view that the herpes simplex virus (HSV) type I is not the primary etiologic factor responsible for RAU, the results of one study[22] have led to the suggestion that the virus may, in fact, play some part in the immunopathogenesis. Using viral DNA probes, these workers were able to demonstrate significant RNA hybridization to HSV type I DNA in mononuclear cells from patients with minor aphthous ulceration and ocular or arthritic types of Behçet's syndrome.

Although RAU is regarded as not being associated with general autoimmune disease,[18] the evidence to suggest that cellular immune responses play a major role in the pathogenesis of the condition is very strong.[23] Hemagglutinating antibodies to saline homogenates of oral fetal mucosa have also been demonstrated in a significantly greater proportion of RAU patients than in controls.[24] The antibodies identified were mainly of the IgM and to a lesser extent IgG class.

Hematologic abnormalities, including anemia, have been reported in 7 to 14 percent of patients suffering from RAU,[25] although in some cases they were secondary to GI disease. An extensive study[26] to investigate the potential role of anemia, vitamin B_{12}, folate, and iron deficiency in the occurrence of RAU failed to identify anemia, sideropenia, reduced folate, and vitamin B_{12} deficiency as primary etiologic factors. However, the depression of serum ferritin in patients with MiAU and MjAU has led to the suggestion that low body iron stores may predispose to oral ulceration.[18] Recurrent ulcers of the aphthous type are typically seen in patients suffering from either chronic or cyclic neutropenia.

A strong association between GI disease (including celiac and Crohn's disease) and RAU has frequently been suggested, although the proportion of patients with RAU who have been shown to be affected is very low in most reported studies.[2,25,27,28]

Treatment

There is no universally effective treatment for aphthous ulceration, although clearly before any therapy is started, general conditions associated with oral ulceration should be excluded. A full hematologic investigation, although of particular importance for patients developing ulcers late in life, seldom reveals any marked abnormality in child patients.

Oral hygiene may be assisted during episodes of ulceration by the use of a mouthwash containing 0.2 percent chlorhexidine gluconate. The use of topical steroid preparations, e.g., Corlan pellets (containing 2.5 mg hydrocortisone sodium succinate) and Adcortyl A in Orabase (0.1 percent triamcinolone acetonide), if applied early, may reduce the severity and duration of ulceration. Systemic corticosteroids are seldom prescribed, except in severe cases of MjAU. Systemic antibiotics may be prescribed to control secondary infection, and a mouthwash containing mysteclin (compound tablet: tetracycline hydrochloride 250 mg and nystatin 250,000 IU) is particularly useful in younger children. This should not be swallowed because there is a danger of the tetracycline component causing staining of the permanent teeth.

BEHÇET'S DISEASE

Oral ulceration has been demonstrated in 98 percent of patients with Behçet's disease. The ulcers are clinically and histologically indistinguishable from those seen in RAU, and all three types of RAU may be seen in this closely related condition.[7] It has been argued that, while oral ulceration is frequently the earliest sign in the development of the disease, progression of RAU to other signs and symptoms of Behçet's disease may be regarded as uncommon, because only 3 percent of patients with RAU were diagnosed as having Behçet's disease.[30] Alternatively, it has been suggested that the interval between a diagnosis of RAU and the development of Behçet's disease may be 1 to 24 years.[7]

The local management of oral ulceration in this condition is similar to that for RAU.

ORAL MONILIASIS

The most common monilial infections seen within the oral cavity in children are caused by *Candida albicans*, which is commensal in the mouths of over 40 percent of the general population. Candidosis may present in a variety of clinical forms but is, in each case, the response to an opportunistic organism in patients who are debilitated through acute or chronic illness, in particular those on immunosuppressive therapy or showing an impaired immune response.

The typical form of acute pseudomembranous candidosis (Fig. 1), so-called thrush, is seen in the newborn and presents clinically as soft, creamy yellow areas raised above the surrounding mucosa, which leave a red bleeding surface when wiped off. The lesions may be multiple or a confluent mass and may affect all mucosal surfaces, including the soft and hard palate, tongue, and vestibule.

The diagnosis may be confirmed by taking a smear of the material; a Gram stain of the preparation reveals the typical branching hyphae of *Candida*.

Although treatment with antifungal agents is appropriate to control the local infection, it should be emphasized that in cases in which a rapid improvement is not achieved, further more extensive investigations should be undertaken to elicit the nature of possible underlying systemic diseases. The local antifungals suitable for use in neonates and infants are suspensions of nystatin (100,000 IU per milliliter) and amphotericin (100 mg per milliliter), which should be applied three times a day.

Acute atrophic candidosis is very occasionally seen in children and is the result of candidal overgrowth in patients being treated with broad-spectrum antibiotics or with immunosuppressive drugs. The mucosa is typically sore, in-

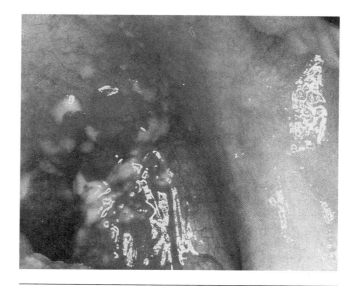

FIGURE 1 A typical appearance of acute pseudomembranous candidosis ("thrush"). The lesions are seen to involve the soft palate and anterior pillars of the fauces in a 2-year-old female patient.

flamed, and sensitive to hot and spicy foods. Nystatin pastilles (100,000 IU) or amphotericin lozenges (10 mg) may be sucked four times daily after food is taken. The treatment should be continued for 48 hours after the lesions have resolved.

Chronic atrophic candidosis (Fig. 2), which has also been termed "denture sore mouth," is characterized by a red, inflamed mucosa and is precisely limited to the area covered by a well-fitting (usually upper) denture. The condition is seen not infrequently in children who are wearing a removable orthodontic appliance, with the area of inflammation confined to the mucosa covered by the acrylic base plate. The diagnosis is confirmed by scraping the affected mucosa with

FIGURE 2 Chronic atrophic candidosis. The mucosa has a roughened appearance, which is confined to the area beneath a denture in a 4-year-old girl who had all her maxillary deciduous teeth removed with the exception of the canines.

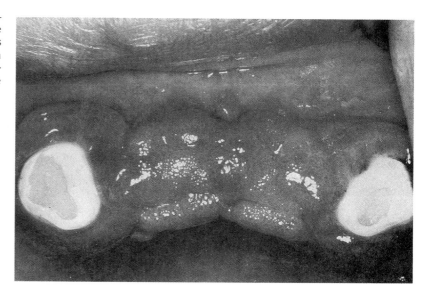

a wooden spatula and identifying candidal hyphae in the Gram stained preparation.

Local treatment for this condition is primarily the use of antifungal agents. Suspensions may be placed conveniently on the fitting surface of the intraoral appliance and lozenges or pastilles of either nystatin or amphotericin prescribed. In addition, the appliance should be immersed overnight in a weak hypochlorite solution to eliminate organisms lying within the interstices of its fitting surface.

Chronic hyperplastic candidosis in children may present as angular cheilitis, although the diagnosis should always be confirmed by swabbing the affected area and culturing for staphylococci that may have invaded the area by transference from the anterior nares. Miconazole cream (miconazole nitrate in a water-soluble base) applied three times a day to the affected area is a recommended treatment.

Chronic mucocutaneous candidosis is a very rare form occurring during the first few months of life. The lesions may extend beyond the oral cavity into the oropharynx and larynx. The underlying pathology is varied according to the particular immunodeficiency or endocrine disorder identified.[19]

TUBERCULOSIS

Oral lesions that can be identified with tuberculosis are rare and in most cases are secondary to co-existing pulmonary disease. However, isolated cases of primary oral lesions have been reported, and it has been suggested[31] that they are more common in children and adolescents (Fig. 3).

The clinical appearance of the lesions is varied, although the classic picture of a ragged, relatively painless ulcer on the dorsum of the tongue is usually associated with oral manifestations secondary to pulmonary tuberculosis. Granulomatous and diffuse inflammatory lesions of the gin-

givae have been reported, in addition to gingival ulcers, which are typical of primary lesions in childhood and adolescence.

Diagnosis is confirmed by biopsy of lesional tissue; typical epithelioid cells are seen, within which Langhans' giant cells can be identified. Caseation necrosis within the follicles is also observed. Tissue should also be sent for culture so that the *Mycobacterium tuberculosis* may be identified by appropriate staining (Ziehl-Neelsen).

Treatment with antituberculous drugs produces excellent results in cases of primary tuberculosis of the oral cavity, but success varies with the degree of pulmonary involvement when secondary oral lesions are diagnosed.

CROHN'S DISEASE

The incidence of chronic oral lesions in Crohn's disease has been reported by various sources as between 6 and 20 percent,[32] and they are said to occur more commonly in patients suffering from granulomatous colitis.[33] The oral lesions, which can precede the confirmation of bowel involvement,[34] may appear in a variety of forms, from typical aphthous ulcers to the more classic cobblestone appearance of raised mucosal nodules (Figs. 4 to 6). Diffuse gingival

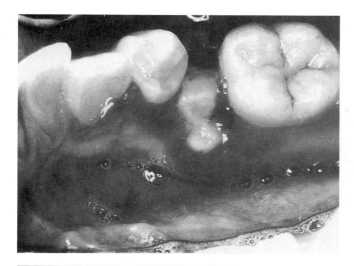

FIGURE 3 A granulomatous lesion around an erupting mandibular second premolar in a 13-year-old girl. Histologic examination of material taken at biopsy and culture of the isolated organism confirmed a diagnosis of primary tuberculosis of the oral cavity.

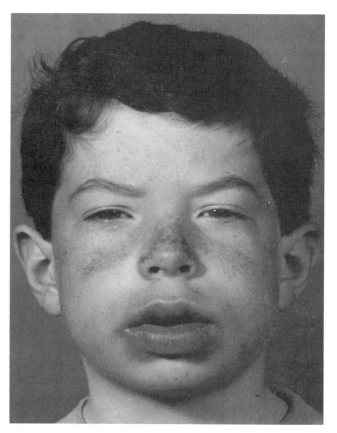

FIGURE 4 Crohn's disease. The lips and surrounding area of the face are seen to be diffusely swollen in this 12-year-old male patient.

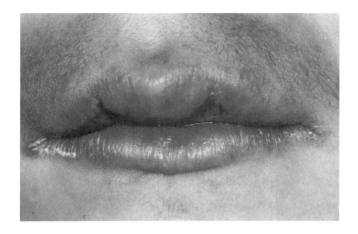

FIGURE 5 Crohn's disease. The lips in this 13-year-old male patient are swollen. They also demonstrate the characteristic fissuring and angular cheilitis seen in the condition.

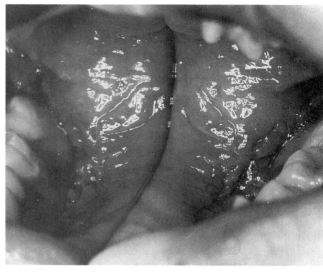

FIGURE 6 Crohn's disease. The vestibular mucosa of the patient shown in Figure 4. The "heaped-up" longitudinal furrowed appearance caused by exuberant linear granulations is evident.

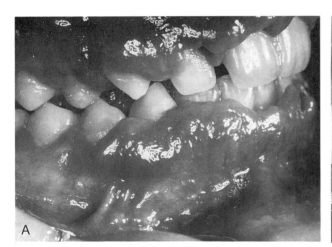

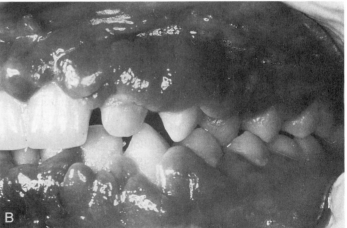

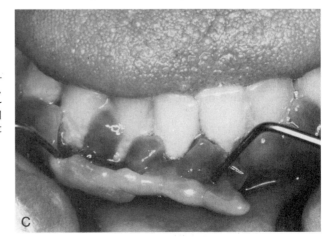

FIGURE 7 Orofacial granulomatosis. Typical gingival lesions. *A*, Right buccal view shows hyperplastic gingivae extending in the maxilla and mandible to the second premolar region. *B*, Left buccal view. *C*, View of lower buccal gingivae to demonstrate the extent of the "taglike" granulomatous lesions.

swelling may also occur, and this presentation has been reported in children especially.[35] In the buccal sulci the tissue may be heaped up in a longitudinal or furrowed "taglike" manner, and in the retromolar region linear shallow ulcers may be found that extend forward into the buccal sulci. A clearly definable clinical entity may be observed, especially in children, in whom gingival hyperplasia and retromolar/vestibular lesions are seen together with diffuse swelling of the lips, which may extend beyond the vermillion border to involve the adjacent areas of the face. In this condition, fissuring of the lips may also be present. A secondary cheilitis of inflammatory origin may supervene in the depths of the fissures owing to colonization with either *Candida* or *Staphylococcus.*

The management of the oral lesions is difficult, and local treatment is seldom any more than palliative. However, a marked improvement is usually noted when systemic treatment measures include the administration of steroids or sulfasalazine (Salazopyrin). Local treatment includes general oral hygiene measures supplemented by a mouthwash such as chlorhexidine (0.2 percent), which should be used twice daily. The use of topical steroid preparations, including Corlan, has also been found to be of benefit in some patients.

OROFACIAL GRANULOMATOSIS

The term *orofacial granulomatosis* has been used to group together disorders previously described as cheilitis granulomatosa, Melkersson-Rosenthal syndrome, sarcoidosis, and Crohn's disease.[36] It is essentially descriptive and is justified by certain similarities in the clinical presentation of the individual condition and the difficulty in distinguishing between them on the histopathologic appearance of tissue taken at biopsy. The condition is diagnosed when recurrent and persistent swelling of the lips and cheeks is associated with granulomatous lesions of the oral mucosa. It is thought to be on the increase in children and would be identified precisely with the condition described under Crohn's disease as being more common in children. The appearance can be severely disfiguring and a source of great embarrassment to affected children (Fig. 7).

Management of orofacial granulomatosis is very difficult, and treatment measures are similar to those described for Crohn's disease. Intralesional injections of triamcinolone acetonide (0.1 percent) have given only temporary relief in the treatment of lip swelling. They are also painful and therefore not well tolerated by children.

In one study, food intolerance was demonstrated in 14 of 80 patients, to agents such as cinnamaldehyde, carvone, and piperitone.[37] Elimination of carmiosine, sunset yellow, and monosodium glutamate from the diet of an 8-year-old girl has been reported to have led to a remission of the condition.[38]

REFERENCES

1. Eyre J. Recurrent aphthous ulceration. Postgrad Doctor Middle East 1984; 7:208–217.
2. Sircus W, Church R, Kelleher J. Recurrent aphthous ulceration of the mouth. Q J Med 1957; 26:235–249.
3. Cooke BED. Recurrent Mikulicz's aphthae. Dent Pract Dent Rec 1961; 12:119–124.
4. Farmer ED. Recurrent aphthous ulcers. Dent Pract Dent Rec 1958; 8:177–184.
5. Ship II. Inheritance of aphthous ulcers of the mouth. J Dent Res 1965; 44:837–844.
6. Miller MF, Garfunkel AA, Ram C, Ship II. Inheritance patterns in recurrent aphthous ulcers: twin and pedigree data. Oral Surg Oral Med Oral Pathol 1977; 43:886–891.
7. Lehner T. Recurrent oral ulcers and Behçet's syndrome: pathological immunological and clinical study. MD Thesis, University of London, 1968.
8. Soames JV, Southam JC. Oral pathology. Oxford: Oxford University Press, 1985.
9. Kramer IRH. Ulceration of the mouth in children. Aust Dent J 1967; 12:83–91.
10. Sutton RL. Periadenitis mucosa necrotica recurrens. J Cutan Dis 1911; 29:65–71.
11. Cohen L. Aetiology, pathogenesis and classification of aphthous stomatitis and Behçet's syndrome. J Oral Pathol 1978; 7:347–352.
12. Rennie JS, Reade PC, Scully C. Recurrent aphthous stomatitis. Br Dent J 1985; 159:361–367.
13. Wray D, Graykowski EA, Notkins AL. Role of mucosal injury in initiating aphthous stomatitis. Br Med J 1981; 283:1569–1570.
14. Ship II. Epidemiological aspects of recurrent aphthous ulcerations. Oral Surg Oral Med Oral Pathol 1972; 33:400–406.
15. Donatsky O. Epidemiologic study on recurrent aphthous ulceration among 512 Danish dental students. Community Dent Oral Epidemiol 1973; 1:37–40.
16. Dolby AE. Recurrent Mikulicz's aphthae. Br Dent J 1968; 124:359–360.
17. Graykowski EA, Barile EF, Lee WB Stanley HR. Recurrent aphthous stomatitis: clinical, therapeutic, histopathologic and hypersensitivity aspects. JAMA 1966; 196:637–644.
18. Scully C, Lehner T. Disorders of immunity. In: Jones JH, Mason DK. Oral manifestations of systemic disease. Philadelphia: WB Saunders, 1980:102.
19. Francis TC, Oppenheim JJ. Impaired lymphocyte stimulation by some streptococcal antigens in patients with recurrent aphthous stomatitis and rheumatic heart disease. Clin Exp Immunol 1976; 6:573–586.
20. Donatsky O. A leucocyte migration study on the cell-mediated immunity against adult human oral mucosa and streptococcal antigens in patients with recurrent aphthous stomatitis. Acta Pathol Microbiol Scand 1976; 84:227–234.
21. Sallay K, Kulesar G, Dan P, Nasz I, Geck P. Atiologic and Prophylaxe der rezidivierinden Aphthen. Dtsch Zahn Z 1975; 30:570–575.
22. Eglin RP, Lehner T, Subak-Sharpe JH. Detection of RNA complementary to herpes simplex virus in mononuclear cells from patients with Behçet's syndrome and recurrent oral ulcers. Lancet 1982; ii:1356–1361.
23. Lehner T. Progress report. Oral ulceration and Behçet's syndrome. Gut 1977; 18:491–511.
24. Lehner T. Immunologic aspects of recurrent oral ulcers. Oral Surg Oral Med Oral Pathol 1972; 33:80–85.
25. Wray D, Ferguson MM, Mason DK, Hutcheon AW, Dagg JH. Recurrent aphthae treatment with vitamin B_{12}, folic acid and iron. Br Med J 1975; 2:490–493.
26. Challacombe SJ, Barkhan P, Lehner T. Haematological features and differentiation of recurrent oral ulceration. Br J Oral Surg 1978; 15:37–48.
27. Ferguson MM, Carmichael HA, Lee FD, Russell RI, Wray D. Recurrent aphthae and coeliac disease. Int Assoc Dent Res 1977; Abstract 114.
28. Wray D, Ferguson MM, Hutcheon AW, Dagg JH. Nutritional deficiencies in recurrent aphthae. J Oral Pathol 1978; 7:418–423.
29. Oshima Y, Shimizu T, Yokohari R, Matsumoto T, Kano K, Kagami T, Nagaya H. Clinical studies on Behçet's syndrome. Ann Rheum Dis 1963; 22:36–45.
30. Williams DM, Wray D. Autoimmune mucocutaneous diseases and diseases of uncertain aetiology. In: Ivanyi L, ed. Immunological aspects of oral diseases. Lancaster: MTP Press, 1986:142.
31. Cawson RA. Tuberculosis of the mouth and throat with special reference to the incidence and management since the introduction of chemotherapy. Br J Dis Chest 1960; 54:40.
32. Basu MK. Diseases of the gastrointestinal tract. In: Jones HJ, Mason DK, eds. Oral manifestations of systemic disease. Philadelphia: WB Saunders, 1980: 229:
33. Basu MK, Asquith P, Thompson RA, Cooke WT. Oral manifestations of Crohn's disease. Gut 1975; 16:249–254.

34. Bishop RP, Brewster AC, Antonioli DA. Crohn's disease of the mouth. Gastroenterology 1972; 62:302–306.
35. Holmes A, Smith CJ. Gingival swelling as the presenting feature of Crohn's disease in children. J Paediatr Dent 1985; 1:65–69.
36. Sainsbury CPQ, Dodge JA, Walker DM. Orofacial granulomatosis in childhood. Br Dent J 1987; 163:154–157.
37. Patton DW, Ferguson MM, Forsyth A, James J. Orofacial granulomatosis: a possible allergic basis. Br J Oral Maxillofac Surg 1985; 23:235–242.
38. Sweatman MC, Tasker R, Warner JO, Ferguson MM, Mitchell DN. Orofacial granulomatosis. Response to elemental diet and provocation by food additives. Clin Allergy 1986; 16:331–338.

PART

2

Disorders of Deglutition

David N. Tuchman, M.D.

The pediatric patient with impaired or dysfunctional swallowing poses a number of unique problems for the clinician. In contrast to adults, issues such as growth and development of the swallowing apparatus, development of normal oromotor reflexes, maturation of feeding behavior, the importance of oral feeding in the development of parent-child bonding, the acquisition of adequate nutrition for somatic growth, and the effects of non-nutritive sucking on growth must be considered in the approach to this group of patients. In addition, many pediatric patients with dysfunctional swallowing lack the cognitive skills necessary to follow specific therapeutic recommendations (e.g., children with central nervous system disease), a situation that complicates patient management.

NORMAL DEGLUTITION

The function of the swallowing apparatus is to transport materials from the oral cavity to the stomach without allowing entry of substances into the airway. This is known as safe swallowing. In order to accomplish this, there must be precise co-ordination between the oral and pharyngeal phases of swallowing so that the pharyngeal swallow is initiated at the appropriate moment following onset of bolus movement. The passage of an oral bolus without aspiration is the result of a complex interaction of cranial nerves and muscles of the oral cavity, pharynx, and proximal esophagus.[1,2]

Deglutition is generally divided into three phases based on functional as well as anatomic characteristics. These divisions include the oral, pharyngeal, and esophageal phases of swallowing.[1,2] The oral stage of swallowing is voluntary and involves a preparatory phase. In the unimpaired child, the oral cavity functions as a sensory and motor organ in effecting changes in the physical properties of the food bolus in order to make it swallow-safe. The oral bolus is modified to allow passage through the pharynx without entry into the larynx or the tracheobronchial tree. Physical properties of the food bolus altered by oral activity include bolus size, shape, volume, pH, temperature, and consistency.[3]

Following oral manipulation, the food bolus moves into the pharynx, an area where the respiratory and gastrointestinal (GI) tracts interface. Passage of food through this region requires an efficient mechanism to safely direct food into the esophagus. During the pharyngeal phase, the swallow is reflexive and involves a complex sequence of co-ordinated motions. Generally the pharyngeal phase, which lasts for approximately 1 second, consists of two basic movements: elevation of the entire pharyngeal tube, including the larynx, followed by a descending peristaltic wave. In the adult, this action takes about 100 msec. Food is then injected from the pharynx into the esophagus with a large force at velocities as high as 100 cm per second.[4,5] Approximately 600 to 900 msec after the onset of the pharyngeal phase, food passes through the upper esophageal sphincter and enters the esophagus. The cricopharyngeal muscle, the main component of the upper esophageal sphincter, relaxes for approximately 500 msec during the swallow to allow passage of the bolus.[6] Normal adults complete the swallow in approximately 1,500 msec.[7] Timing data for children are not well described. Following pharyngeal transit, food enters the esophagus and via primary peristalsis is transported to the stomach.

Upper Esophageal Sphincter: Normal Function

The upper esophageal sphincter (UES), also known as the pharyngoesophageal segment, is a manometrically defined high-pressure zone located in the region distal to the hypopharynx. The UES, which is composed of striated muscle, is tonically closed at rest and opens during swallowing, vomiting, and belching.[8] The length of the high-pressure zone in adults is from 2.5 to 4.5 cm, averaging about 3 cm.[8] Although the cricopharyngeal muscle is part of the upper sphincter, its length is about 1 cm and therefore this muscle is not the only determinant of the high-pressure zone.[8–10] The relative contributions of the inferior pharyngeal constrictor muscle and the muscle fibers of the proximal esophagus to the upper sphincter remain controversial.[11,12] The pressure profile of the UES is asymmetric, with higher pressures noted in the anterior and posterior directions.[13] Orientation of the recording device must take this into account when pressures are measured in this region. Table 1 reports normal values for the pharyngoesophageal region of control infants obtained by using a low-compliance, water-perfused manom-

TABLE 1
Pharyngoesophageal Manometric
Measurements in Control Infants

Resting UES pressure (cm H$_2$O)	28.9 ± 10	(18.0–44.0)
Pharyngeal peristaltic wave		
Amplitude (cm H$_2$O)	74.7 ± 19.9	(37.0–102.0)
Velocity (cm/sec)	8.5 ± 3.6	(3.2–15.0)
Duration (sec)	0.59 ± 0.18	(0.4–0.86)

Numbers are mean ± SD; values in parentheses are ranges.
From Sondheimer.[14]

etry system in which directional orientation of the catheter is maintained.[14] Neurologic control of the sphincter has been reviewed by Palmer.[8] Although not completely understood, neurologic connections include visceral afferents that travel to the nucleus solitarius and from there to the nucleus ambiguous. Vagal efferents probably reach the muscle by the pharyngeal plexus, using the pharyngeal branch of the vagi.[8] There is probably little or no contribution by the sympathetic nervous system to cricopharyngeal control.[8,15] The response of the UES is not stereotypical but may be modified by varying bolus size, suggesting that feedback receptors, stimulated in the oral cavity and pharynx, provide afferent signals for modulating central nervous system impulses that give rise to the oral and pharyngeal phases of swallowing.[16]

Proposed functions of the UES include prevention of esophageal distention during normal breathing[8] and protection of the airway against aspiration following an episode of acid reflux.[17-19] Although the latter remains controversial, studies have demonstrated that upper esophageal sphincter pressure increases in response to intraesophageal acidification in both infants[14] and adults,[18] suggesting that the UES functions as a dynamic barrier to acid reflux and protects against aspiration. However, Sondheimer[14] found no difference in resting UES pressures between control infants and infants with gastroesophageal reflux. Interestingly, in some infants with pulmonary disease the UES failed to respond following esophageal acidification. Others have documented qualitative abnormalities of UES function in infants with reflux disease.[20]

Neurology of Deglutition

Miller[21] provides an excellent review of the neurophysiologic control of swallowing. Swallowing may be evoked by stimulating many different central pathways, including the cortex (the region of the prefrontal gyri), the subcortex, and the brain stem. The swallowing center can be activated by afferent impulses from the cerebral cortex (voluntary swallowing) and from peripheral receptors in the mouth and pharynx (reflex swallowing). The corticobulbar impulses trigger and control the initial phases of swallowing but not the later esophageal stages. The cortex is not essential for the pharyngeal and esophageal phases of swallowing to occur. In the human fetus, swallowing occurs prior to the time when the descending cortical-subcortical pathways have fully innervated

the brain stem.[22] Deglutition has been noted to occur in infants with loss of nervous tissue rostral to the midbrain.[23] Higher pathways, however, are important in allowing voluntary elicitation of deglutition and integrating facial and oral movements and other responses with swallowing.[1,21] The neurons important to the pharyngeal and esophageal phases of swallowing are located in different regions of the pons[24,25] and medulla.[1,26,27] Lesions placed in the medulla fractionate the sequence of muscle activity during pharyngeal swallowing, suggesting that interneurons located in this region are important to the pharyngeal and esophageal phases; these core interneurons are termed "central pattern generators."[22,28] The deglutition center integrates afferent impulses and coordinates the activity of the motor nuclei of the fifth, seventh, tenth, and twelfth cranial nerves. Other activities such as respiration are inhibited during swallowing.[29] Swallowing may be evoked by stimulating the oropharyngeal regions innervated by the pharyngeal branches of the glossopharyngeal nerve (ninth cranial nerve) or by the superior laryngeal and recurrent laryngeal nerves of the vagus (tenth cranial nerve). Sensory fibers from these nerves synapse in the nucleus tractus solitarius. Multiple receptive sites that elicit swallowing are present in the oral cavity and pharynx.[21] Once activated, the sequence of muscle activity during the pharyngeal phase remains the same in spite of altering the duration of this phase; this is termed a time-locked sequence.[30,31]

All phases of deglutition may be modified by sensory feedback, although each to a different degree. Oral phase activity is modulated by peripheral feedback received from the touch and pressure receptors in the oral cavity as well from the mandible and temporomandibular joints.[32] Feedback from sensory receptors modifies the duration of the pharyngeal phase, the intensity of muscle activity, and the threshold necessary to evoke a response.[6,33-37] Sensory feedback may have therapeutic implications in the clinical management of the swallowing-impaired individual. For example, maintaining jaw control during deglutition may facilitate a safe swallow by improving feedback signals from the mandible or temporomandibular joints, whereas modifying the size of an oral bolus may favorably alter motor response of the pharynx.

Prenatal Deglutition

Deglutition occurs at approximately 16 to 17 weeks of gestation, although a pharyngeal swallow has been described in a delivered fetus at a gestational age of 12.5 weeks.[38] It is estimated that the normal fetus at term swallows approximately 450 ml of amniotic fluid per day out of a total amniotic fluid volume of 850 ml. Deglutition plays an important role in maintaining normal amniotic fluid volume.[39,40]

Postnatal Development of Deglutition

Changes in Structure

Major changes in size and relative location of components of the oral and pharyngeal cavities occur during the postnatal period.[41,42] These developmental changes should be considered when interpreting pediatric imaging studies. In general, the central mobile elements of the oropharynx in the infant are large in comparison with their containing chambers. For example, the tongue is large compared with the oral cavity, and the arytenoid mass is nearly mature in size in contrast to the small-sized vestibule and ventricle of the larynx (see Fig. 2 in Kramer[42]).

In the infant, the tongue lies entirely within the oral cavity, whereas the larynx is positioned high in the neck, resulting in a small oropharynx.[43] Between 2 and 4 years of age, the tongue begins to descend so that by approximately 9 years of age its posterior third is present in the neck.[43] The larynx also moves in a caudal direction. Based on autopsy studies, the larynx descends from the level of the third to the fourth cervical body during the prenatal period, an arrangement that persists during infancy.[44] During childhood the larynx descends to a level opposite the sixth vertebra and finally moves to the level of the seventh cervical vertebra in adulthood. As maturation progresses, the face vertically elongates and the chambers of the oral cavity and oropharynx enlarge.[45]

Developmental Changes in Feeding Behavior

The development of normal feeding behavior in the infant and child has been reviewed in detail elsewhere in the text and by others.[42,45] Briefly, in the normal infant the oral phase of swallowing is characterized by a pattern known as suckle feeding. Suckle feeding is followed by the development of transitional feeding (ages 6 to 36 months) and eventually mature feeding, which is characterized by biting and chewing. Maturation of feeding behavior occurs mainly as a result of central nervous system development, with motor activity being directed by higher centers such as the thalamus and cerebral cortex.[45]

Non-nutritive Sucking

Non-nutritive sucking, defined as rhythmic movements on a nonfeeding nipple, may improve weight gain during gavage feeding in preterm infants. Bernbaum et al[46] studied the nutritional effects of non-nutritive sucking in a group of low birth weight infants receiving formula by enteral tube and found that, compared with control infants, the group receiving non-nutritive sucking gained significantly more weight. The mechanism accounting for this weight gain is not clear, although it has been hypothesized that non-nutritive sucking results in more efficient nutrient absorption or a decrease in energy requirements secondary to a lessening of infant activity or restlessness.[47,48]

Non-nutritive sucking may have effects on pulmonary function as well. In preterm infants, non-nutritive sucking is associated with an increase in transcutaneous oxygen tension and respiratory frequency.[49,50] This is in contrast to the changes in pulmonary function that occur during oral feeding (i.e., nutritive sucking). Therefore, lowered oxygen tension during oral feeding appears to be unrelated to the action of sucking per se.[50] The mechanism(s) accounting for the differing effects of nutritive versus non-nutritive sucking on pulmonary function remains unknown.

DISORDERS OF DEGLUTITION IN THE PEDIATRIC PATIENT: CLINICAL OVERVIEW

In the pediatric age group, swallowing disorders rarely present as isolated problems but more often occur in infants and children with multiple impairments. Although accurate epidemiologic data are lacking, underlying conditions that predispose to impaired swallowing in childhood include central and peripheral nervous system dysfunction, diseases of muscle, and structural anomalies of the oral cavity and pharynx. Other groups "at risk" of developing dysfunctional swallowing and its complications include premature infants with poor co-ordination of breathing and swallowing, infants with long-term deprivation of oral feeding, and infants with chronic pulmonary disease. The spectrum of pediatric swallowing disorders has been reviewed in detail by others.[42,45,51-54] Table 2 provides a broad list of disorders that result in dysphagia in pediatric patients.

Complications of Impaired Deglutition

In the severely affected child with impaired swallowing, poor oral and/or pharyngeal function may lead to decreased energy intake as a consequence of prolonged feeding time and the inability to ingest adequate volumes. As a result, protein-energy malnutrition may develop, with subsequent deleterious effects on the immune system and muscle strength. Dysfunctional swallowing may also lead to repeated episodes of aspiration and the development of chronic pulmonary disease. In the severely affected child with dysfunctional swallowing, repeated pulmonary infections become increasingly more debilitating in the face of worsening nutritional status (Fig. 1). In addition, the child with impaired swallowing has poor protection of the airway; consequently, an episode of acid reflux may result in severe pulmonary conditions such as bronchospasm, pneumonia, and apnea.[55-57]

DEGLUTITION IN THE PRETERM INFANT

An important clinical issue to consider in the preterm infant is the relationship between deglutition and breathing. Although premature infants are able to suckle feed at a gestational age of approximately 34 weeks, successful oral feeding requires co-ordination of swallowing and breathing. Poor integration of these activities may result in respiratory difficulties such as aspiration. Wilson et al[58] evaluated the co-ordination of breathing and swallowing in preterm infants and found that deglutition occurred during both inspiration and expiration and resulted in an interruption of airflow. They concluded that preterm infants are unable to breath and swallow simultaneously. Shivpuri and co-workers[59] studied the effects of oral feeding on respiratory response in preterm infants and found that during feeding by continuous sucking, tidal volume and respiratory frequency decreased, resulting in a decrease of minute ventilation and PO_2.

TABLE 2
Differential Diagnosis of Dysfunctional
Swallowing in Pediatric Patients

I. Prematurity

II. Upper airway-foodway anomalies
 A. Nasal and nasopharyngeal
  1. Choanal atresia and stenosis
  2. Nasal and sinus infections
  3. Septal deflections
  4. Tumors
 B. Oral cavity and oropharynx
  1. Defects of lips and alveolar processes
  2. Cleft lip and/or cleft palate
  3. Hypopharyngeal stenosis and webs
  4. Craniofacial syndromes, e.g., Pierre Robin, Crouzon, Treacher Collins, Goldenhar
 C. Laryngeal
  1. Laryngeal stenosis and webs
  2. Laryngeal clefts
  3. Laryngeal paralysis
  4. Laryngomalacia

III. Congenital defects of the larynx, trachea, and esophagus
 A. Laryngo-tracheo-esophageal cleft
 B. Tracheoesophageal fistula/esophageal atresia
 C. Esophageal strictures and webs
 D. Vascular anomalies
  1. Aberrant right subclavian artery (dysphagia lusorum)
  2. Double aortic arch
  3. Right aortic arch with left ligamentum

IV. Acquired anatomic defects
 A. Trauma
  1. External trauma
  2. Intubation and endoscopy

V. Neurologic defects
 A. Central nervous system disease
  1. Head trauma
  2. Hypoxic brain damage
  3. Cortical atrophy, microcephaly, anencephaly
  4. Infections, e.g., meningitis, brain abscess
  5. Myelomeningocele
 B. Peripheral nervous system disease
  1. Traumatic
  2. Congenital
 C. Neuromuscular disease
  1. Myotonic muscular dystrophy
  2. Myasthenia gravis
  3. Guillain-Barré syndrome
  4. Poliomyelitis (bulbar paralysis)
 D. Miscellaneous
  1. Achalasia
  2. Cricopharyngeal achalasia
  3. Esophageal spasm
  4. Esophagitis
  5. Dysautonomia
  6. Paralysis of esophagus (atony)
  7. Tracheoesophageal fistula/esophageal atresia–associated nerve defects
  8. Aberrant cervical thymus
  9. Conversion dysphagia

Adapted from Weiss[53] and Cohen SR. Difficulty with swallowing. In: Bluestone CD, Stool SF, eds. Pediatric otolaryngology. Philadelphia: WB Saunders, 1983.

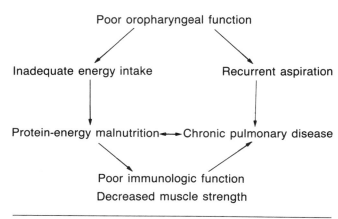

FIGURE 1 Clinical sequelae of impaired deglutition.

DEGLUTITION: CRITICAL PERIOD OF LEARNING

A critical period of development refers to a segment of time during maturation during which a specific stimulus must be applied to produce a particular action. It has been suggested that inadequate oral stimulation during a critical period may result in difficulty in re-establishing successful oral feeding at a later date. The concept of a "critical" or sensitive period as it pertains to feeding behavior has been reviewed by Illingworth and Lister,[60] and cases of infants and children developing resistance to oral feeding following long-term deprivation of oral stimulation have been reported.[61,62] Successful treatment of this problem has been accomplished by a multidisciplinary feeding team using a behavioral approach.[62]

ISOLATED CRICOPHARYNGEAL DYSFUNCTION AND CRICOPHARYNGEAL ACHALASIA

The term *cricopharyngeal achalasia* is not synonymous with cricopharyngeal dysfunction. *Achalasia* means failure to relax. This does not always accurately describe the type of cricopharyngeal dysfunction present. For example, nonrelaxation of the sphincter resulting from primary cricopharyngeal disease differs from nonopening of the sphincter secondary to weak forces of propulsion located in the proximal pharynx.[29]

Isolated cricopharyngeal dysfunction or achalasia is a rare disorder in infants and children.[63,64] Cricopharyngeal dysfunction is usually part of a more global disorder of deglutition, frequently involving the oral phase and other non–sphincter-related aspects of pharyngeal function. Most patients with cricopharyngeal achalasia present at birth with feeding difficulties, although some may present as late as 6 months. Drug-induced dysfunction of the upper esophageal sphincter has also been reported.[65]

The diagnosis of isolated cricopharyngeal dysfunction is difficult to make when based solely on radiographic studies. A horizontal bar in the proximal esophagus representing the cricopharyngeal muscle may be seen in up to 5 percent of adults undergoing radiographic examinations for all indications and may also be a normal radiologic sign in infants.[66,67] In some patients with a prominent bar seen on radiographic study, manometric studies have demonstrated normal relaxation and decreased UES pressure.[29,68] Alternatively, manometric studies may be normal in patients with clinical or radiologic evidence of cricopharyngeal dysfunction.[29,69,70] Improvement of cricopharyngeal achalasia may occur spontaneously or following dilatation.[70,71] In some cases cricopharyngeal myotomy may be required, with preoperative selection of appropriate candidates requiring motility and radiographic studies.[72] Surgery is usually contraindicated in patients with gastroesophageal reflux or those with poor pharyngeal peristalsis.

CLINICAL ASSESSMENT OF THE PEDIATRIC PATIENT WITH IMPAIRED DEGLUTITION

Successful evaluation and management of the pediatric patient with dysfunctional swallowing requires a multidisciplinary approach. It is essential that the pediatrician enlist the aid of a pediatric radiologist, speech-language pathologist, occupational therapist, and pediatric dietician with experience in the field of pediatric swallowing disorders to assist in the diagnostic evaluation and planning of therapy.

Feeding History

The diagnostic approach to the pediatric patient with dysfunctional swallowing begins with the feeding history. However, obtaining an accurate history may be difficult for a number of reasons.[73] First, pediatric patients with severe impairment of swallowing frequently include individuals with limited cognitive abilities, making direct communication with the patient impossible. As a result, the feeding history must be obtained from individuals directly involved in caring for the child, such as a parent or feeding specialist (i.e., speech-language pathologist, occupational therapist). Second, it has been our experience that severely handicapped children with dysfunctional swallowing often aspirate without coughing, a phenomenon known as "silent aspiration." A similar condition has been described in adults.[74–76] Consequently, it is difficult to accurately predict which food substances are swallowed without aspiration solely on the basis of feeding history or clinical examination.

Areas covered in the feeding history include caretakers involved in feeding the child, location or setting where feeding takes place (feeding performance may differ depending on location, e.g., school versus home), method of feeding (e.g., type of feeding utensils used), position of the head, neck, and body during feeding, volume of food offered and volume of food tolerated per swallow, consistency of food offered and tolerated per swallow, presence or absence of chewing, the amount of time required to feed, history of dysphagia or odynophagia, the presence or absence of drooling (suggestive of oral phase abnormalities), and a history of gagging, choking, or coughing associated with feeding. Determining whether these symptoms occur before, during, or after the swallow helps "localize" the affected phase.[74] Symptoms that occur prior to the swallow suggest abnormalities of oral control; those that occur during the swallow may indicate pharyngeal phase dysfunction; gagging and choking after completion of the swallow probably represent abnormalities of pharyngeal clearance secondary to pharyngeal muscle weakness and/or inco-ordination or dysfunction of the upper esophageal sphincter.

In addition to a feeding history, a complete nutritional assessment is an essential part of the evaluation of the child with dysfunctional swallowing. Clinical goals should include determining the patient's current nutritional status, estimating energy and protein requirements for establishing optimal growth, and outlining a plan for providing the route and type of feeding. Consultation with a registered pediatric dietician will aid in planning a comprehensive nutritional program.

Physical Examination

Physical examination of the child with dysfunctional swallowing should include examination of the structures of the oral cavity and oropharynx. If structural abnormalities are found and/or are suspected in the pharynx, consultation with an otolaryngologist is indicated. Presence or absence of a gag reflex should be noted, including the existence of a "hyperactive" gag reflex. Lack of a gag reflex is a contraindication to oral feeding, whereas a hyperactive gag results in significant feeding difficulties.

Observational Feeding Trial

The diagnostic yield of the observational feeding trial is greatly enhanced if it is performed in collaboration with a feeding therapist such as a speech-language pathologist or occupational therapist trained in the evaluation of swallowing disorders. Oral motor function is tested during the initial part of the feeding trial by determining the presence or absence of age-appropriate oral motor skills. The acquisition of oral feeding skills and their development have been reviewed in detail by others.[77–81] During the feeding trial, the presence of movements not observed in the normally developing infant such as jaw thrust, tongue thrust, tonic bite reflex, and jaw clenching are noted. In the impaired patient, normal reflexes or movements beyond their expected time of disappearance may persist, such as the phasic bite reflex and suckle feeding (persistent "primitive reflexes"). Normal movements seen in the older infant and retained into adulthood include jaw stabilization, chewing, and the ability to lateralize the tongue. During feeding, position of the head, neck, and body during swallowing should be noted, as well as abnormal feeding behaviors such as tongue thrust, aversion of the mouth, and symptoms of choking, gagging, or ruminating.

Diagnostic Tests of Swallowing Function

Specialized tests of deglutition allow broad categorization of swallowing abnormalities. Unfortunately, these examinations are mainly descriptive and provide the clinician with limited data regarding specific pathophysiologic mechanisms.

Videofluoroscopy

At the present time, videofluoroscopy is the procedure of choice for evaluating the patient with impaired swallowing.[74,82-84] Videofluoroscopy provides the best means of determining oral, pharyngeal, and esophageal anatomy; it provides objective evidence of oral and pharyngeal incoordination, and detects episodes of aspiration, all of which help identify children in whom oral feeding may be contraindicated. However, the clinical significance of small amounts of aspiration occurring during deglutition remains unknown. Videofluoroscopy is valuable in the management of swallowing-impaired patients by helping to determine bolus characteristics of food that make it safe to swallow (i.e., bolus size, consistency).[75] However, this procedure involves exposure to radiation and does not provide quantitative data regarding the function of oral and pharyngeal structures during deglutition.

Pharyngeal Manometry

Manometry provides quantitative data regarding pharyngeal motor function during deglutition, including amplitude of peristalsis, speed of propagation of the pharyngeal wave, response of the upper esophageal sphincter following deglutition, and co-ordination between pharyngeal peristalsis and UES relaxation.[14,20] Recording the response of the pharyngoesophageal region during deglutition is complicated by a number of factors.[85] Since motor events in the hypopharynx occur at a more rapid rate than in the esophagus, recording equipment with a rapid response time (usually greater than 300 mm Hg per second) is required.[86] Water-perfused catheters with rapid response times are acceptable, but intraluminal pressure transducers provide the most accurate readings. Second, the asymmetric pressure profile of the upper esophageal sphincter requires that close attention be given to the spatial orientation of the recording device while recording in the UES. Third, during deglutition there is significant differential axial movement of the recording catheter and oropharyngeal structures, which may result in a significant recording artifact.[85,87] A sleeve sensor has been used to monitor UES pressures over time in order to minimize the effects of catheter and sphincter movement.[37] Finally, manometry does not provide information regarding intraluminal events, such as the movement of fluid in response to recorded pressure changes. Simultaneous recording of videofluoroscopic images and manometric tracings has allowed investigators to correlate motor events with intraluminal movement of substances.[88-90]

Ultrasonography

Ultrasonography represents a new diagnostic modality for evaluation of the swallowing-impaired individual.[91] Motion of structures in the oral cavity, such as the tongue and floor of the mouth, may be imaged during feeding and deglutition by placing a transducer in the submental region and aiming the beam toward the tongue. This technique has been used to identify feeding movements of oral structures in healthy breast-fed and bottle-fed infants.[92] Disadvantages of ultrasonography include poor visualization of the oropharynx secondary to an acoustic shadow cast by bony structures in the neck and the lack of standardized measurements.

TREATMENT OF THE PEDIATRIC PATIENT WITH IMPAIRED DEGLUTITION

Treatment plans should be developed in the context of a multidisciplinary group. Specific treatment of oral and pharyngeal dysfunction in the neurologically impaired infant or child is not always possible, nor is surgical therapy frequently indicated. Different types of treatment modalities have been discussed in detail by others.[74,93-97] Therapy usually involves managing swallowing-related complications and devising compensatory strategies to minimize the morbidity and, in some cases, mortality associated with impaired oral and pharyngeal function.[98] Swallowing abnormalities arise from a diverse group of underlying disorders that alter oral and pharyngeal function in varied ways, and therefore devising effective forms of therapy in this group of patients is difficult. This heterogeneity is also reflected in the fact that patients have differing potentials for recovery. In the patient with acquired brain injury secondary to head trauma, rehabilitation with possible reacquisition of swallowing skills is a major goal, whereas compensatory and adaptive maneuvers form the basis for managing the child with severe cerebral palsy. Therapeutic regimens for the swallowing-impaired patient must take into account these and other variables and therefore require an individualized plan.

Management of dysphagia must be considered in the context of the child's level of development and cognitive abilities. Inability of the child to follow directions limits therapeutic maneuvers to "passive" procedures (e.g., bolus modification). Children with intact cognition have the potential to become actively involved with their therapy and learn specific procedures shown to be effective in promoting a safe swallow (e.g., supraglottic swallow procedure).

In general, therapeutic recommendations are based on the patient's ability to swallow safely (that is, to transfer food from the oral cavity into the esophagus without entry into the larynx or tracheal airway), the patient's nutritional status, the presence of gastroesophageal reflux, and enjoyment of feeding for parents and patient.

For a complete discussion of techniques used to facilitate oral motor function in swallowing in impaired infants and chil-

TABLE 3
Dysfunctional Swallowing: Examples of
Therapy

Modification of the oral bolus—modify volume, physical properties
  (e.g., consistency)
Appropriate position of the head, neck, and body during deglutition
Proper intraoral bolus placement
Provision of jaw control and stabilization
Modification of oral sensitivity
Extinguishing of abnormal feeding behaviors
Thermal sensitization/stimulation
Swallowing exercises
  Tongue resistance/range of motion
  Laryngeal adduction
Protective maneuvers—supraglottic swallow procedure
Cricopharyngeal myotomy
Suckle feeding—valved feeding bottle
Provide alternate means of enteral nutrition
  Nasogastric feeding
  Gastrostomy tube (surgical or endoscopic)

Adapted from Tuchman.[73]

dren who are receiving either some form of oral feeding or oral stimulation, the reader is referred to Mueller,[81] Morris,[80,99,100] and Ottenbacher.[101] Many of these techniques seek to reduce tactile hypersensitivity, stabilize body position, and optimize the motor response of the oral swallowing mechanism. Table 3 lists some therapeutic options used for the pediatric patient with dysfunctional swallowing. It should be noted that because of a paucity of well-controlled clinical trials, the use of many of these therapeutic manuevers remains empiric.

REFERENCES

1. Miller AJ. Deglutition. Physiol Rev 1982; 62:129–184.
2. Morrell RM. The neurology of swallowing. In: Groher ME, ed. Dysphagia and management. Boston: Butterworths, 1984: 3.
3. Coster ST, Schwarz WH. Rheology and the swallow-safe bolus. Dysphagia 1987; 1:113–118.
4. Buthpitiva AG, Stroud D, Russell COH. Pharyngeal pump and esophageal transit. Dig Dis Sci 1987; 32:1244–1248.
5. Fisher MA, Hendrix TR, Hunt JN, Murrills AJ. Relation between volume swallowed and velocity of the bolus ejected from the pharynx into the esophagus. Gastroenterology 1978; 74:1238–1240.
6. Shipp T, Deatsch WW, Robertson K. Pharyngo-esophageal muscle activity during swallowing in man. Laryngoscope 1970; 80:1–16.
7. Curtis DJ. Cruess DF, Dachman AH, Maso E. Timing in the normal pharyngeal swallow. Prospective selection and evaluation of 16 normal asymptomatic patients. Invest Radiol 1984; 19:523–529.
8. Palmer ED. Disorders of the cricopharyngeus muscle: a review. Gastroenterology 1976; 71:510–519.
9. Ellis FH Jr. Upper esophageal sphincter in health and disease. Surg Clin North Am 1971; 51:553–565.
10. Goyal RK. Disorders of the cricopharyngeus muscle. Otolaryngol Clin North Am 1984; 17:115–130.
11. Asoh R, Goyal RK. Manometry and electromyography of the upper esophageal sphincter in the opossum. Gastroenterology 1978; 74:514–520.
12. Welch RW, Luckmann K, Ricks PM, Drake ST, Gates GA. Manometry of the normal upper esophageal sphincter and its alteration in laryngectomy. J Clin Invest 1979; 63:1036–1041.
13. Winans CS. The pharyngoesophageal closure mechanism: a manometric study. Gastroenterology 1972; 63:768.
14. Sondheimer JM. Upper esophageal sphincter and pharyngeal motor function in infants with and without gastroesophageal reflux. Gastroenterology 1983; 85:301–305.
15. Parrish RM. Cricopharyngeus dysfunction and acute dysphagia. Can Med Assoc J 1968; 99:1167–1171.
16. Kahrilas PJ, Dodds WJ, Dent J, Logemann JA, Shaker R. Upper esophageal sphincter function during deglutition. Gastroenterology 1988; 95:52–62.
17. Hunt PS, Connell AM, Smiley TB. The cricopharyngeal sphincter in gastric reflux. Gut 1970; 11:303–306.
18. Gerhardt DC, Shuck TJ, Bordeaux RA, Winship DH. Human upper esophageal sphincter. Response to volume, osmotic, and acid stimuli. Gastroenterology 1978; 75:268–274.
19. Winship DH. Upper esophageal sphincter: does it care about reflux? Gastroenterology 1983; 85:470–472.
20. Staiano A, Cucchiara S, De Vizia B, Andreotti MR, Auricchio S. Disorders of upper esophageal motility in children. J Pediatr Gastroenterol Nutr 1987; 6:892–898.
21. Miller AJ. Neurophysiological basis of swallowing. Dysphagia 1986; 1:91–100.
22. Doty RW. Neural organization of deglutition. In: Code CF, ed. Handbook of physiology, alimentary canal. Sect 6, Vol 4. 1861–1902. Washington, DC. American Physiological Society, 1968.
23. Utter O. Ein fall von anensephalie. Acta Psychiatr Neurol 1928; 3:281–318.
24. Car A, Jean A, Roman C. A pontine primary relay for ascending projections of the superior laryngeal nerve. Exp Brain Res 1975; 22:197–210.
25. Sumi T. Reticular ascending activation of frontal cortical neurons in rabbits with special reference to the regulation of deglutition. Brain Res 1972; 46:43–54.
26. Car A, Roman C. Deglutitions et contractions oesophaglennes reflexes produit par la stimulation du bulke Rachidien. Exp Brain Res 1970; 11:75–92.
27. Miller AJ. Characteristics of the swallowing reflex induced by peripheral nerve and brain stem stimulation. Exp Neurol 1972; 34:210–220.
28. Doty RW. Influence of stimulus pattern on reflex deglutition. Am J Physiol 1951; 166:142–158.
29. Hellemans J, Agg HO. Pelemans W, Vantrappen G. Pharyngoesophageal swallowing disorders and the pharyngoesophageal sphincter. Med Clin North Am 1981; 65:1149–1171.
30. Doty RW, Bosma JF. An electromyographic analysis of reflex deglutition. J Neurophysiol 1956; 19:44–60.
31. Kawasaki M, Ogura JH, Takenouchi S. Neurophysiologic observations of normal deglutition. I. Its relationship to the respiratory cycle. Laryngoscope 1965; 74:1747–1765.
32. Dubner RB, Sessle BJ, Storey AT. The neurological basis of oral and facial function. New York: Plenum, 1978.
33. Hrychshyn AW, Basmajian JV. Electromyography of the oral stage of swallowing in man. Am J Anat 1972; 133:335–340.
34. Mansson I, Sandberg N. Effects of surface anesthesia on deglutition in man. Laryngoscope 1974; 84:427–437.
35. Mansson I, Sandberg N. Oro-pharyngeal sensitivity and elicitation of swallowing in man. Acta Otolaryngol 1975; 79:140–145.
36. Mansson I, Sandberg N. Salivary stimulus and swallowing in man. Acta Otolaryngol 1975; 79:445–450.
37. Kahrilas PJ, Dent J, Dodds WJ, Wyman JB, Hogan WJ, Arndorfer RC. A method for continuous monitoring of upper esophageal sphincter pressure. Dig Dis Sci 1987; 32:121–128.
38. Humphrey T. Reflex activity in the oral and facial arch of the human fetus. In: Bosma JF, ed. Second symposium on oral sensation and perception. Springfield: Charles C. Thomas, 1967:195.
39. Pritchard JA. Fetal swallowing and amniotic fluid volume. Obstet Gynecol 1966; 28:606–610.
40. Grand RJ, Watkins JB, Torti FM. Development of the human gastrointestinal tract: a review. Gastroenterology 1976; 70:796–810.
41. Bosma JF. Postnatal ontogeny of performances of the pharynx, larynx, and mouth. Am Rev Respir Dis 1985; 131:S10–S15.
42. Kramer SS. Special swallowing problems in children. Gastrointest Radiol 1985; 10:241–250.
43. Laitman JT, Crelin ES. Postnatal development of the basicranium and vocal tract region in man. In: Bosma JF, ed. Symposium on development of the basicranium. Washington DC: US Government Printing Office, 1976: 206.
44. Noback GJ. The developmental topography of the larynx, trachea, and lungs in the fetus, newborn, infant, and child. Am J Dis Child 1923; 26:515–533.
45. Bosma JF. Oral-pharyngeal interactions in feeding. Presented at Symposium on Dysphagia, Johns Hopkins University, February, 1986.

46. Bernbaum JC, Pereira GR, Watkins JB, Peckham GJ. Nonnutritive sucking during gavage feeding enhances growth and maturation in premature infants. Pediatrics 1983; 71:41–45.

47. Neely CA. Effects of non-nutritive sucking upon behavior arousal in the newborn. Birth Defects 1979; 15:173–200.

48. Field T, Ignatoff E, Stringer S, Brennan J, Greenberg R, Widmayer S, Anderson GC. Non-nutritive sucking during tube feedings: effects on preterm neonates in an intensive care unit. Pediatrics 1982; 70:381–384.

49. Paludetto R, Robertson SS, Hack M, Shivpuri CR, Martin RJ. Transcutaneous oxygen tension during non-nutritive sucking in preterm infants. Pediatrics 1984; 74:539–542.

50. Paludetto R, Robertson SS, Marting RJ. Interaction between non-nutritive sucking and respiration in preterm infants. Biol Neonate 1986; 49:198–203.

51. Illingworth RS. Sucking and swallowing difficulties in infancy: diagnostic problem of dysphagia. Arch Dis Child 1969; 44:655–665.

52. Fisher SE, Painter M, Milmoe G. Swallowing disorders in infancy. Pediatr Clin North Am 1981; 28:845–853.

53. Weiss MH. Dysphagia in infants and children. Otolaryngol Clin North Am 1988; 21:727–735.

54. Shapiro J, Healy GB. Dysphagia in infants. Otolaryngol Clin North Am 1988; 21:737–741.

55. Mansfield LE, Stein MR. Gastroesophageal reflux and asthma: a possible reflex mechanism. Ann Allergy 1978; 41:224–226.

56. Herbst JJ, Minton SD, Book LS. Gastroesophageal reflux causing respiratory distress and apnea in newborn infants. J Pediatr 1979; 95:763–768.

57. Boyle JT, Tuchman DN, Altschuler SM, Nixon TE, Pack AI, Cohen S. Mechanisms for the association of gastroesophageal reflux and bronchospasm. Am Rev Respir Dis 1985; 131:(Suppl):S16–S20.

58. Wilson SL, Thach BT, Brouillette RT, Abu-Osba YK. Coordination of breathing and swallowing in human infants. J Appl Physiol: Respirat Environ Exercise Physiol 1981; 50:851–858.

59. Shivpuri CR, Martin RJ, Carlo WA, Fanaroff AA. Decreased ventilation in preterm infants during oral feeding. J Pediatr 1983; 103:285–289.

60. Illingworth RS, Lister J. The critical or sensitive period, with special reference to certain feeding problems in infants and children. J Pediatr 1964; 65:839–848.

61. Geertsma MA, Hyams JS, Pelletier JM, Reiter S. Feeding resistance after parenteral hyperalimentation. Am J Dis Child 1985; 139:255–256.

62. Blackman JA, Nelson CLA. Reinstituting oral feedings in children fed by gastrostomy tube. Clin Pediatr 1985; 24:434–438.

63. Bishop HC. Cricopharyngeal achalasia in childhood. Pediatr Surg 1974; 9:775–778.

64. Reichert TJ, Bluestone CD, Stool SE, Sieber WK, Sieber AM. Congenital cricopharyngeal achalasia. Ann Otorhinolaryngol 1977; 86:603–610.

65. Wyllie E, Wyllie R, Cruse RP, Rothner AD, Erenberg G. The mechanism of nitrazepam-induced drooling and aspiration. N Engl J Med 1986; 314:35–38.

66. Seaman WB. Cineroentgenographic observation of the cricopharyngeus. AJR 1966; 96:922–911.

67. Gideon A, Nolte K. The non obstructive pharyngo-esophageal cross roll. Ann Radiol 1973; 16:129–135.

68. Hurwitz AL, Duranceau A. Upper-esophageal sphincter dysfunction. Pathogenesis and treatment. Digest Dis 1978; 23:275–281.

69. Fisher SE, Painter M, Milmoe G. Swallowing disorders in infancy. Pediatr Clin North Am 1981; 28:845–853.

70. Dinari G, Danziger Y, Mimouni M, Rosenbach Y, Zahavi I, Grunebaum M. Cricopharyngeal dysfunction in childhood: Treatment by dilatations. J Pediatr Gastroenterol Nutr 1987; 6:212–216.

71. Lernau OZ, Sherzer E, Mogle P, Nissan S. Congenital cricopharyngeal achalasia treatment by dilatations. J Pediatr Surg 1984; 19:202–203.

72. Berg HM, Jacobs JB, Persky MS, Cohen NL. Cricopharyngeal myotomy: a review of surgical results in patients with cricopharyngeal achalasia of neurogenic origin. Laryngoscope 1985; 95:1337–1340.

73. Tuchman DN. Dysfunctional swallowing in the pediatric patient: clinical considerations. Dysphagia 1988; 2:203–208.

74. Logemann JA. Evaluation and treatment of swallowing disorders. San Diego: College-Hill Press, 1983.

75. Linden P, Siebens A. Dysphagia: predicting laryngeal penetration. Arch Phys Med Rehabil 1983; 64:281–284.

76. Splaingard ML, Hutchins B, Sulton LD, Chaudhuri G. Aspiration in rehabilitation patients: videofluoroscopy vs bedside clinical assessment. Arch Phys Med Rehabil 1988; 69:637–640.

77. Bosely E. Development of sucking and swallowing. Cerebral Palsy J 1963; 24:14–16.

78. Bosma JF. Postnatal ontogeny of performances of the pharynx, larynx, and mouth. Am Rev Respir Dis 1985; 131(suppl):S10–S15.

79. Bosma JF. Development of feeding. Clin Nutr 1986; 5:210–218.

80. Morris SE. Program guidelines for children with feeding problems. Madison, WI: Childcraft Education Corp, 1977.

81. Mueller HA. Facilitating feeding and pre-speech. In: Pearson PH, Williams CE, eds. Physical therapy services in the developmental disabilities. Springfield, IL: Charles C Thomas, 1972.

82. Curtis DJ, Hudson T. Laryngotracheal aspiration. Analysis of specific neuromuscular factors. Radiology 1983; 149:517.

83. Eckberg O, Wahlgren L. Pharyngeal dysfunctions and their interrelationship in patients with dysphagia. Acta Radiol [Diagn] (Stockh) 1985; 26:659–664.

84. Jones B, Kramer SS, Donner MW. Dynamic imaging of the pharynx. Gastrointest Radiol 1985; 10:213–224.

85. Dodds WJ, Kahrilas PJ, Dent J, Hogan WJ. Considerations about pharyngeal manometry. Dysphagia 1987; 1:209–217.

86. Dodds WJ. Instrumentation and methods for intraluminal esophageal manometry. Arch Intern Med 1976; 136:515–523.

87. Isberg A, Nilsson ME, Schiratzki H. Movement of the upper esophageal sphincter and a manometric device during deglutition. A cineradiographic investigation. Acta Radiol Diagn 1985; 26:381–388.

88. Sokol EM, Heitmann P, Wolf BS, Cohen BR. Simultaneous cineradiographic and manometric study of the pharynx, hypopharynx, and cervical esophagus. Gastroenterology 1966; 51:960–974.

89. Hamilton JW, Kretzschmar CS, Robbins H, Sufit R. Evaluation of the upper esophageal sphincter using simultaneous pressure measurements with a sleeve device and videofluoroscopy. Gastroenterology 1986: 91:1054a

90. Kahrilas PJ, Dodds WJ, Dent J, Logemann JA, Shaker R. Upper esophageal sphincter function during deglutition. Gastroenterology 1988; 95:52–62.

91. Shawker TH. Sonies BC, Stone M. Sonography of speech and swallowing. In: Sanders RC, Hill M, eds. Ultrasound annual. New York: Raven Press, 1984:237.

92. Weber F, Woolridge MW, Baum JD. An ultrasonographic study of the organization of sucking and swallowing by newborn infants. Dev Med Child Neurol 1986; 28:19–24.

93. Griffin KM. Swallowing training for dysphagic patients. Arch Phys Med Rehabil 1974; 55:467–470.

94. Dobie RA. Rehabilitation of swallowing disorders. Am Fam Physician 1978; 17:84–95.

95. de Lamma Lazzara G, Lazarus C, Logemann JA. Impact of thermal stimulation on the triggering of the swallowing reflex. Dysphagia 1986; 1:73–77.

96. Logemann JA. Treatment for aspiration related to dysphagia. Dysphagia 1986; 1:34–38.

97. Groher ME. Bolus management and aspiration pneumonia in patients with pseudobulbar dysphagia. Dysphagia 1987; 1:215–216.

98. Helfrich-Miller, Rector KL, Straka JA. Dysphagia: its treatment in the profoundly retarded patient with cerebral palsy. Arch Phys Med Rehabil 1986; 67:520–525.

99. Morris SE. Prespeech and language programming for the young child with cerebral palsy. Milwaukee, WI: Curative Workshop, 1975.

100. Morris SE. Developmental implications for the management of feeding problems in neurologically impaired infants. Semin Speech Lang 1985; 6:293–314.

101. Ottenbacher K, Bundy A, Short MA. The development and treatment of oral-motor dysfunction: a review of clinical research. Phys Occup Ther Pediatr 1983; 3(2):1–13.

102. Byrne WS, Euler AR, Achcraft E. Gastroesophageal reflux in the severely retarded who vomit: criteria for and the results of surgical intervention in twenty two patients. Surgery 1982; 91:95–98.

103. Dodds WJ, Hogan WJ, Lydon SP, Stewart ET, Stef JJ, Arndorfer RC. Quantitation of pharyngeal motor function in normal human subjects. J Appl Physiol 1975; 39:692–696.

104. Sondheimer JM, Morris BA: Gastroesophageal reflux among severely retarded children. J Pediatr 1979; 94:710–714.

CHAPTER 25

The Esophagus

PART 1

Congenital Anomalies

Vanessa M. Wright, M.B., B.S., F.R.C.S., F.R.A.C.S.

Congenital anomalies of the gastrointestinal (GI) tract are those that are present at birth. Although congenital anomalies of the esophagus, namely esophageal atresia and esophageal stenosis, typically present in early infancy, later presentation is recognized.

ESOPHAGEAL ATRESIA

Incidence

An incidence of 1 per 3,000 to 3,500 live births is widely accepted, with an almost equal sex incidence.[1]

Clinical Features

The most common form of esophageal atresia has an associated distal tracheoesophageal fistula. Figure 1 illustrates the varieties of esophageal atresia and tracheoesophageal fis-tula most often encountered, with their relative incidences. The best-known classification is that of Vogt,[2] modified by Ladd[3] and Roberts et al.[4]

The first indication of the diagnosis of esophageal atresia may be maternal polyhydramnios,[5] reported to occur in 50 percent of cases. In the presence of polyhydramnios, prenatal ultrasound scanning may raise the possibility of the diagnosis of esophageal atresia if the stomach is either very small or not identified. Prematurity is common. After delivery the baby's inability to swallow saliva results in frothy saliva bubbling from mouth and nose, with episodes of coughing, choking, and cyanosis. Attempts to feed the baby exacerbate these symptoms. The presence of a distal tracheoesophageal fistula allows air to pass from trachea to GI tract; abdominal distention may be pronounced, particularly if the baby requires intermittent positive-pressure ventilation with high airway pressures. A proximal pouch tracheoesophageal fistula increases the likelihood of aspiration of saliva or feed with resultant pulmonary collapse and consolidation.

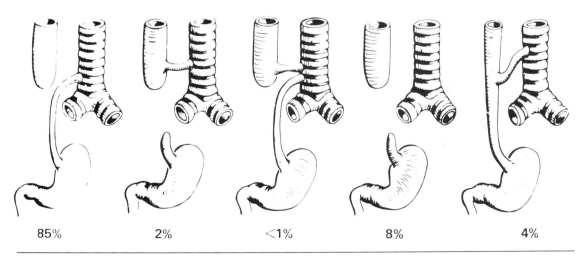

| 85% | 2% | <1% | 8% | 4% |

FIGURE 1 Types and incidence of esophageal atresia with or without fistula.

367

The incidence of associated congenital anomalies is around 50 percent.[6,7] Cardiac, anorectal, urogenital, and skeletal anomalies predominate. The term VATER is used to describe this association of anomalies when they occur together.[8]

Diagnosis

Failure to advance a size 10 or 12FG radiopaque tube beyond 9 to 11 cm when passed via nose or mouth is diagnostic. Radiographs of the chest and abdomen should be obtained with the tube in situ. These show the level of the upper pouch. In the presence of a distal tracheoesophageal fistula, air is present in the GI tract (Fig. 2). Duodenal atresia occurs in association with esophageal atresia, and the characteristic "double bubble" may be seen on the abdominal radiograph. Complete absence of air in the GI tract suggests a pure esophageal atresia (Fig. 3). The plain radiographs also demonstrate rib and vertebral anomalies and may indicate cardiac pathology. Evidence of aspiration, particularly collapse and/or consolidation of the right upper lobe, may be present. Contrast studies are rarely indicated, but early clinical or radiologic evidence of aspiration suggests the possibility of an upper pouch fistula, and a careful upper pouch study under fluoroscopic control is then indicated and should also be performed when no distal tracheoesophageal fistula is demonstrated.

Management

Following diagnosis the priorities are maintenance of the airway and prevention of aspiration pneumonia. Removal of secretions from the mouth, pharynx, and upper pouch requires frequent suction or continuous suction using a double-lumen tube.[9] Maintenance of the airway may require endotracheal intubation. The baby with respiratory distress syndrome or a severe aspiration pneumonia needs respiratory support. Reflux of gastric contents through the distal fistula into the airway is minimized by nursing the baby prone with a slight head-up tilt. Maintenance of body temperature and prevention of hypoglycemia are also important. Careful clin-

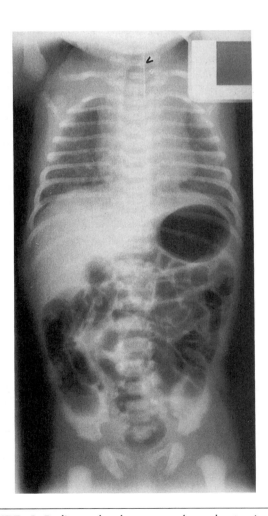

FIGURE 2 Radiograph shows esophageal atresia with tracheoesophageal fistula. Arrowhead indicates tube in upper esophagus.

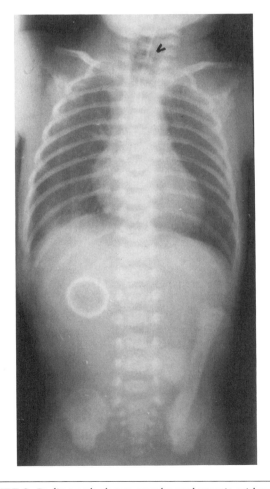

FIGURE 3 Radiograph shows esophageal atresia without fistula. Arrowhead indicates tube in upper esophagus.

ical, radiologic, ultrasound, and echocardiographic investigations confirm or identify associated anomalies. Hemoglobin should be estimated preoperatively and blood cross-matched.

With advances in neonatal intensive care, the proportion of babies with esophageal atresia and tracheoesophageal fistula treated by division of the fistula and primary anastomosis has steadily increased. This operation is performed via a right thoracotomy using an extrapleural approach. Low birth weight is not a contraindication to primary repair.[10] However, a long gap between the two ends of the esophagus, as in pure esophageal atresia, does not usually allow a primary anastomosis. When the baby requires ventilation preoperatively, escape of air via the fistula into the GI tract may produce enormous abdominal distention, embarrassing respiration. In such circumstances division of the fistula without necessarily attempting an anastomosis is advocated.[6] Formation of a gastrostomy may relieve the abdominal distention in such circumstances, but the air leak via the fistula through the gastrostomy may be such that ventilation of the lungs is impossible, necessitating urgent division of the fistula.

Should initial primary anastomosis not be possible, management may involve division of the fistula if present, formation of a feeding gastrostomy, and maintenance of a clear airway by careful aspiration of saliva from the upper pouch, a delayed esophageal anastomosis being attempted after some weeks. Some elongation of the upper pouch and hypertrophy of the lower pouch occur during the early weeks, facilitating a delayed anastomosis. Techniques such as bougienage of the upper pouch to encourage lengthening[11] and the use of an electromagnetic force to bring the upper and lower pouches closer together[12] have been advocated, but it seems likely that the normal swallowing mechanism produces upper pouch hypertrophy and that lengthening and reflux of feeds dilates and hypertrophies the lower esophagus.

To reduce tension at the anastomosis in cases in which a long gap exists between the esophageal ends and delayed esophageal anastomosis is attempted, circular myotomy of the esophagus may be performed.[13] Intra-abdominal mobilization of the stomach has also been advocated.[14]

An alternative to delayed esophageal anastomosis is to perform a cervical esophagostomy and feeding gastrostomy, with the intention of replacing the esophagus with a length of colon,[15] a tube fashioned from the stomach,[16] or complete gastric interposition.[17] These operations are usually performed between 3 and 12 months of age.

Following primary repair, ventilation may be required, but the fit, bigger baby breathes spontaneously and may simply require occasional pharyngeal suction until normal swallowing occurs. Fluid and electrolyte balance is maintained with intravenous fluids until enteral feeds are established, feeds initially being introduced via a nasogastric tube or gastrostomy. Oral feeds usually commence about the fifth postoperative day provided that an anastomotic leak is not evident either clinically or radiologically.

Immediate postoperative complications include an anastomotic leak or complete dehiscence of the anastomosis, recurrent tracheoesophageal fistula, and anastomotic stricture.

In the longer term, gastroesophageal reflux may exacerbate a tendency to stricture formation at the anastomosis. Recurrent chest infections are common and may be related to aspiration secondary to reflux or incoordinate esophageal

motility. Dysphagia for lumpy food in the first year or so is most frequently associated with incoordinate peristalsis, and in the absence of an anastomotic stricture this is also the most likely explanation for the longer-term dysphagia.[18] Tracheomalacia associated with repaired esophageal atresia presents clinically with episodes of apnea and cyanosis. If severe, a tracheopexy may be needed.[19]

The prognosis for esophageal atresia as an isolated anomaly is excellent; however, the severity of associated anomalies and the high incidence of premature low birth weight babies continue to produce an overall mortality of 10 to 15 percent.[6]

CONGENITAL ESOPHAGEAL STENOSIS AND WEBS

Incidence

This is an extremely rare condition that occurs in an estimated 1 in 25,000 to 50,000 live births. Much confusion has occurred because esophagitis secondary to gastroesophageal reflux can produce stenosis of the esophagus at a very early age. Intrinsic stenosis of the esophagus present at birth but not necessarily symptomatic can be classified in the following way:

1. Stenosis associated with ectopic tracheobronchial remnants (cartilage, glands, respiratory epithelium) in the wall of the esophagus (Fig. 4).
2. Membranous diaphragm.
3. Fibromuscular stenosis.[20]

Clinical Features

Dysphagia for liquids in the early days or weeks of life occurs when the stenosis is severe. Initial presentation commonly occurs at the time of weaning to solid food. Later presentation with dysphagia is described. Recurrent respiratory infections, dribbling of saliva, and failure to thrive all occur. Congenital esophageal stenosis has been described in association with esophageal atresia, isolated tracheoesophageal fistula, duodenal atresia, anorectal anomalies, cardiac anomalies, and Down's syndrome,[20] but the incidence of associated anomalies is much lower than the incidence of associated anomalies in esophageal atresia.

Diagnosis

The clinical picture should prompt radiologic and endoscopic investigation. Such investigation should not only define the level and extent of the stenosis but should also identify any evidence of gastroesophageal reflux, duodenal pathology, or malrotation. Stenosis associated with tracheobronchial remnants commonly occurs in the lower esophagus. Membranous webs and fibromuscular stenosis may occur in either upper or lower esophagus. Endoscopically the stenosis with tracheobronchial remnants is irregular and unyielding, the membranous web is visible as a web with regular contours, and the fibromuscular stenosis is regular, flexible, and easily dilatable.

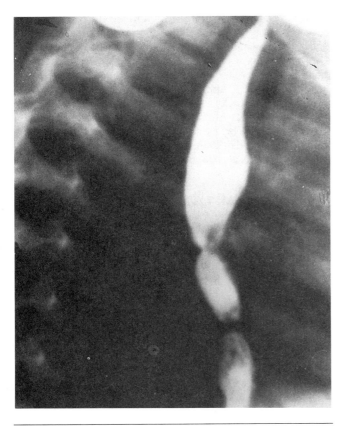

FIGURE 4 Contrast study of two webs in lower esophagus associated with tracheobronchial remnants.

Management

If a stenosis with tracheobronchial remnants seems likely, resection should be carried out either transthoracically or transabdominally. End-to-end esophageal anastomosis is usually possible, but gastroesophageal reflux must be prevented by antireflux surgery. The majority of membranous webs respond best to excision, but dilatation may be successful and the possibility of endoscopic diathermy of the web should be considered. The majority of fibromuscular stenoses respond to repeated dilatation; resection is rarely indicated.

Treatment of these congenital stenoses results in relief of symptoms and an excellent prognosis, provided that steps are taken to prevent gastroesophageal reflux, which may produce further stricturing of the esophagus.

REFERENCES

1. Cudmore RE, Rickham PP, Lister J, Irving IM, eds. Neonatal surgery. 2nd ed. London: Butterworths, 1978: 192.
2. Vogt EG. Congenital esophageal atresia. AJR 1929; 22:463–465.
3. Ladd WE. The surgical treatment of esophageal atresia and tracheo-esophageal fistulas. N Eng J Med 1944; 230:625–637.
4. Roberts KD, Carre IJ, Inglos MN. The management of congenital esophageal atresia tracheo-esophageal fistula. Thorax 1955; 10:45–52.
5. Scott JS, Wilson JK. Hydramnios as an early sign of esophageal atresia. Lancet 1957; ii:569–572.
6. Spitz L, Kiely E, Brereton RJ. Esophageal atresia. Five year experience with 148 cases. J Pediatr Surg 1987; 22:103–108.
7. Holder TM, Cloud DJ, Lewis E, Pilling GP. Esophageal atresia and tracheo-esophageal fistula. A survey of its members by the Surgical Section of the American Academy of Pediatrics. Pediatrics 1964; 34:542–549.
8. Quan L, Smith DW. The VATER association. J Pediatr 1973; 82:104–107.
9. Replogle RL. Esophageal atresia. Plastic sump catheter for drainage of the proximal pouch. Surgery 1963; 54:296–297.
10. Rickham PP. Infants with esophageal atresia weighing under three pounds. J Pediatr Surg 1981; 16:595–598.
11. Howard R, Myers NA. Esophageal atresia. A technique for elongation of the upper pouch. Surgery 1965; 58:725–727.
12. Hendren WH, Hale JR. Electromagnetic bougienage to lengthen esophageal segments in congenital esophageal atresia. N Engl J Med 1975; 293:428–432.
13. Livaditis A. Oesophageal atresia, a method of overbridging large segmental gaps. Z Kinder Chir 1973; 13:298–306.
14. Myers NA, Beasley SW, Auldist AW, Kent M, Wright V, Chetcuti P. Esophageal atresia without fistula—anastomosis or replacement. Pediatr Surg Int 1987; 2:216–222.
15. German JC, Waterston DJ. Colon interposition for the replacement of the esophagus in children. J Pediatr Surg 1976; 11:227–234.
16. Anderson KD, Randolph JG. Gastric tube interposition. A satisfactory alternative to the colon for esophageal replacement in children. Ann Thorac Surg 1978; 25:521–525.
17. Spitz L. Gastric transposition via the mediastinal route for infants with long-gap esophageal atresia. J Pediatr Surg 1984; 19:149–154.
18. Chetcuti P, Myers NA, Pheland PD, Beasley SW. Adults who survived repair of congenital oesophageal atresia and tracheo- oesophageal fistula. Br Med J 1988; 297:344–346.
19. Kiely EM, Spitz L, Brereton RJ. Management of tracheomalacia by aortopexy. Pediatr Surg Int 1987; 2:13–15.
20. Nihoul-Fekete C, DeBacker A, Lortat-Jacob S, Pellerin D. Congenital esophageal stenosis. A review of 20 cases. Pediatr Surg Int 1987; 2:86–92.
21. Nishina T, Tsuchida Y, Saito S. Congenital esophageal stenosis due to tracheobronchial remnants and its associated anomalies. J Pediatr Surg 1981; 16:190–193.

PART 2

Traumatic Injury of the Esophagus

Joyce D. Gryboski, M.D.

In children, traumatic injuries of the esophagus are most often due to caustic ingestions, direct insults from interventional procedures, foreign bodies, and blunt or penetrating injury. A precise history of ingestion or trauma is usually available, but in the young, nonverbal child and even in older children the etiology of esophageal symptoms is not always obvious, and late symptoms are often respiratory.

FOREIGN BODIES AND COINS

The type of ingested foreign bodies causing obstruction of the esophagus varies with age: In young children they are largely coins, whereas in the adult they are foods (Table 1).[1-4a] More than half of coin ingestions are by children under 2 years old and 29 percent by those under 1 year.[5] Mentally retarded or disturbed children may ingest virtually anything (Figs. 1 and 2), and toothbrush swallowing may occur in the anorectic adolescent.[6] The majority of foreign bodies (80 percent) pass spontaneously (Fig. 3). Dimes (17 mm) and pennies (18 mm) are less likely to obstruct the esophagus than are larger coins, which lodge at or just distal to the level of the cricopharyngeus. The metal of coins is usually not corrosive, but in 1982 the composition of the copper penny was changed from 95 to 2.4 percent copper and from 5 to 97.6 percent zinc, which is more corrosive.[7] Small foreign bodies that fail to pass should suggest evaluation for strictures or achalasia.

Some foreign bodies such as plastic buttons or leaves are radiolucent and not detected by radiologic means. Radiographs differentiate a coin in the esophagus from that in the trachea.[8] The anteroposterior film shows the edge of the coin if it is in the trachea and shows the flat surface if it lies in the more posterior esophagus. In lateral films, the flat surface is seen if the coin lies in the trachea, and the edge if it is in the esophagus (Fig. 4). One indication of foreign body

TABLE 1
Esophageal Foreign Bodies

Coins
Dental retainer
Pins
Plastic leaves
Toy parts
Impacted pasta
Thumbtacks
Bones
Crayons
Ballpoint pen caps
Button batteries
Meats

in a child with stridor or respiratory distress is separation of the trachea and esophagus seen on flat film. Hodge et al studied 80 children who ingested coins.[9] Radiologic examination showed the coin lodged in the esophagus in 25 (31 percent), 14 percent of whom had no symptoms. Forty-four had subdiaphragmatic coins, and 11 had no coins identified. Clinical findings that correlated with coins lodged in the esophagus were localization by the patient, choking at ingestion, drooling, vomiting, and chest pain.[10] They stressed the value of screening films, for 17 percent of asymptomatic children had an esophageal foreign body.

The sudden onset of dysphagia, stridor, wheezing, or respiratory distress should always suggest ingestion of a foreign body.[11-14] Longstanding esophageal foreign bodies can present as a neck mass or as inspiratory stridor and dysphagia.[15]

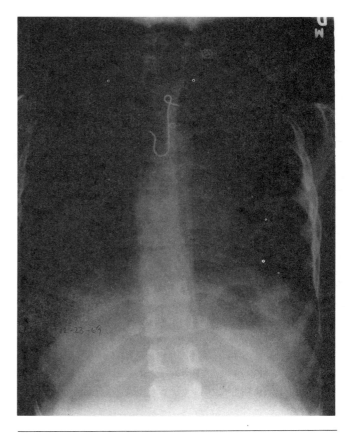

FIGURE 1 This 2½-year-old boy complained of pain in the neck shortly after he was seen playing with a Christmas ornament.

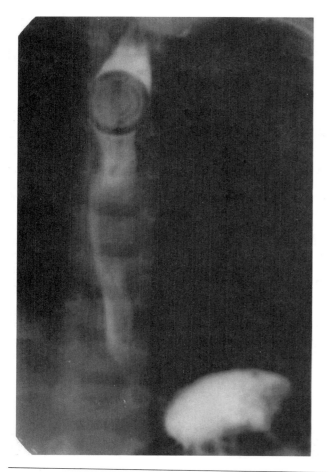

FIGURE 2 This 5-year-old boy presented with the sudden onset of crying, drooling, and inability to swallow. The parents found a box of checkers scattered on the floor. Upon endoscopic removal, the obstructing object was identified as a plastic checker.

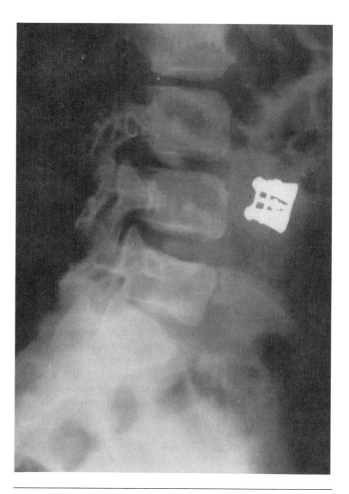

FIGURE 3 Swallowed toy binoculars 48 hours after ingestion.

Diagnosis and Treatment. The Heimlich maneuver has been reported to cause esophageal rupture.[16,17] The American Academy of Pediatrics Committee on Prevention of Accidents and Poisonings has advised against the use of the Heimlich abdominal thrust maneuver as being too forceful for infants and young children, carrying the risk of injury to abdominal organs.[18] Instead, they advise four strong back blows followed by "chest thrusts"—maneuvers that in themselves carry some risk to the child.

If the child complains after swallowing a foreign body and it cannot be visualized, study with thin barium may define the object. Whether it is identified or not, endoscopy is indicated (Fig. 5).

The most important element of treatment is maintenance of an adequate airway. In removing a foreign body from the esophagus, there is always the danger of its release from the carrier and aspiration into the respiratory tract.[19] Eighty percent of coins lodge in the upper esophagus.[20] O'Neill et al[21] and others[22,23] have used Foley balloon catheter extraction in awake patients to retrieve smooth objects. This procedure is performed under fluoroscopy with the catheter passed through the mouth and the fluoroscopy table placed in the Trendelenburg position during the period of removal. Others prefer endotracheal anesthesia and endoscopy using the polypectomy snare or grasping forceps.[19] The coin should be pulled directly out without rotating the endoscope, and if the child does not have an endotracheal tube he should be placed in the Trendelenburg position during the period of removal. As stated by Webb,[8] if the foreign body is less than 20 mm diameter it may be pushed into the stomach, from which it should pass easily. Care must be taken to examine the esophagus for the presence of a second coin whose radiologic image may have been obscured.[24]

Complications increase significantly if the foreign body remains in the esophagus for more than 24 hours.[25] Pointed and sharp objects should be removed immediately using general anesthesia and an endotracheal tube to protect the airway. Toothpicks, bones, nails, needles, razors, and even dental retainers are included in this group; those longer than 5 cm or wider than 2 cm are unlikely to pass through the pylorus.[8,26] Safety pins that are open proximally should be pushed into the stomach and removed through an overtube.

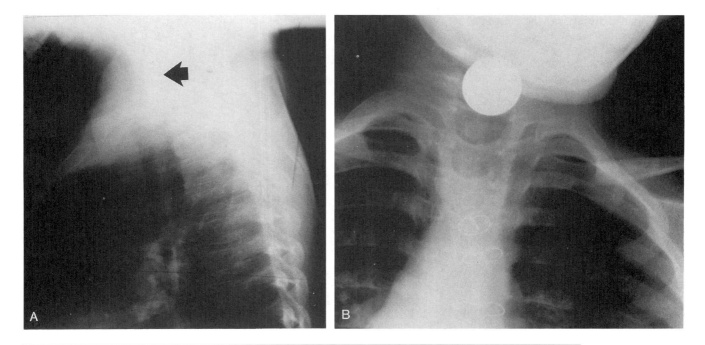

FIGURE 4 *A*, A lateral film showing the edge of an ingested coin in the esophagus. *B*, Anteroposterior film showing the flat surface of the coin in the esophagus.

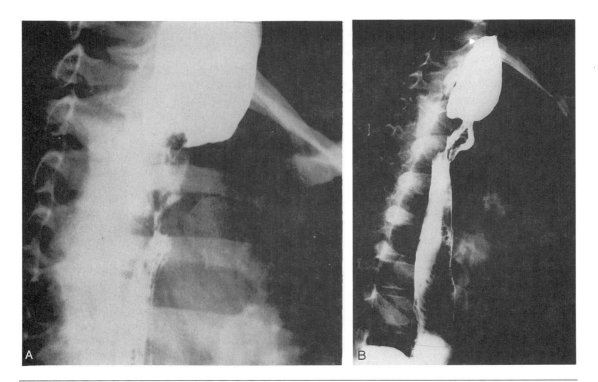

FIGURE 5 This 8-year-old male presented with dysphagia over a 6-month period, which had progressed to difficulty swallowing liquids. *A*, There is narrowing of the esophagus at the thoracic inlet. *B*, At the area of narrowing, there are two channels that distend and narrow with peristalsis, suggesting that these are not fistulous tracts. Horizontal diverticulum-like barium-filled projections suggest pseudodiverticulosis (adenosis) but were proven to indicate distended mucous glands. At surgical exploration, the filling defect was found to represent an impacted toy soldier.

Those opened distally may be pulled out by the hinge either freely or through an overtube. Razor blades are best removed through a rigid endoscope[8,27] or with an overtube (Fig. 6).

Complications. Perforation of the esophagus has been reported after coin ingestions, being either acutely symptomatic or asymptomatic.[28-30] Acquired esophageal pouch, pseudodiverticuli, aspiration pneumonia, and aortic pseudoaneurysm are less common complications.[31-33] Hemoptysis of long duration has been reported following silent chicken bone perforation of the esophagus.[34] After reviewing the literature of 321 cases of penetrating ingested foreign bodies of the upper aerodigestive tract, Remsen et al[35] reported 252 remained intraluminal and 43 were found outside the lumen. Analysis revealed that an intraluminal penetrating foreign body carried a higher mortality, although this did not correlate with the duration of foreign body retention.

DISC BATTERY INGESTION

Disc button batteries used in watches, hearing aids, cameras, toys, calculators, and even musical greeting cards are a relatively new source of caustic esophageal injury.[36-40] Because of an estimated 510 to 850 battery ingestions yearly and two reported deaths, a National Button Battery Ingestion Study was established in 1972 in the United States to review the characteristics of ingestions and provide guidelines for therapy. A review of 119 ingestions in an 11-month period determined that the majority of buttons contained silver or mercuric oxide. Less common were those of manganese dioxide, zinc, or lithium content.[41] Those most commonly ingested were the 7.9- and 11.6-mm batteries. Ingesters were primarily young, with 71.2 percent younger than 5, 16.2 percent between 6 and 12, 4.5 percent between 13 and 17, and 8.1 percent older than 17 years. Nearly half of the children found the battery loose or discarded, and surprisingly some had ingested batteries from their own hearing aids.[42] Older children and adults may test the viability of the battery by touching it to the tongue and inadvertently swallow it.

Although 89.9 percent of batteries pass spontaneously in 12 hours to 14 days, with 31 percent requiring more than 48 hours, those lodged in the esophagus (4.2 percent) require early removal.[40] Injury is attributable to one of the following: (1) electrolyte leakage from batteries, (2) alkali produced from external flow of current—it is estimated that when lodged in the esophagus, 26 to 45 percent leak sodium or potassium hydroxide, (3) mercury toxicity, (4) pressure necrosis, and (5) direct flow of 1.5 volt current.[36,43,44] Although most batteries show corrosion, they do not disassemble.

Esophageal damage occurs rapidly, and burns are noted as early as 1 hour after ingestion. Within 4 hours there may be involvement of all layers of the esophagus. In experimental studies in dogs in which batteries were placed within the esophagus, by 8 hours there was mucosal abrasion or necrosis under the muscular layer even without evidence of battery leakage.[48] Elevated urine mercury levels have been found after battery ingestion.[45]

Symptoms. Immediate symptoms are nausea, vomiting, chest pain, and abdominal pain.

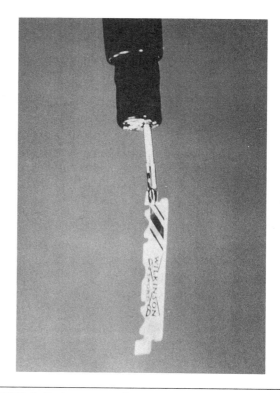

FIGURE 6 Endoscopic technique used for removal of a foreign body (razor blade) from the esophagus.

Diagnosis. The battery may be identified and radiologically distinguished from a coin. In the anterior projection it shows a double density shadow owing to its bilaminar structure. On lateral film, the edges are round and show a step-off at the junction of anode and cathode.[46]

Treatment. Ipecac is not recommended to induce vomiting, for it may lead to impaction of the disc in the respiratory tree.[42] Administration of neutralizing solutions or charcoal has not proven helpful.[47]

The treatment protocol recommended by the Button Battery Study includes an initial radiographic examination to determine the location. (1) If the battery lies lodged within the esophagus, it should be removed immediately. Endoscopic retrieval rates are 33 to 100 percent, and in children endoscopic removal is recommended rather than blind retrieval with a Fogarty catheter and balloon. (2) If the battery is beyond the esophagus, the child is discharged, and the parents are instructed to strain the stool for retrieval of the battery and to report any pain, fever, or vomiting. Metoclopramide, through stimulation of gastric emptying, is used to aid its passage from the stomach. However, if the battery measures 23 mm or more, a film should be repeated in 48 hours. If the disc remains in the stomach at that time it should be retrieved by endoscope, perhaps with a magnet attached to its end.[41]

Reported complications of esophageal lesions are tracheoesophageal fistula, perforation, stricture, and even death.[48,49]

FOREIGN BODIES IN PHARYNX AND CRICOPHARYNGEAL AREA

Foreign bodies that lodge in the pharynx or at the level of the cricopharyngeal area are often jacks (American flipping toys) or fish bones. The patient in this case is placed in the supine position and a rigid laryngoscope is used with a long surgical grasping clamp or foreign body forceps. Fish bones can often be felt with the finger and are usually on the side identified by the patient. If the foreign body cannot be retrieved, flexible endoscopy is performed. Jacks can often be grasped with a Kelly clamp (Fig. 7).[8]

FOOD AND MEAT OBSTRUCTION

Impaction of meat in the esophagus of children occurs in those with congenital anomalies, esophageal stricture, spasm, or achalasia. A review of esophageal foreign bodies identified 15 children with congenital or acquired defect[50] of the esophagus. Steak and frankfurters are frequently the offending agents and are usually lodged in the distal esophagus (Figs. 8 and 9).[51]

The approach to therapy depends upon the symptoms. If the child is comfortable and handling his secretions, one may wait several hours or overnight. Radiographic study is not necessary, for with time and relaxation many impacted meats will pass. However, the bolus should not remain for longer than 12 hours. If the patient is unable to handle secretions and is uncomfortable, the meat should be removed immediately. Endoscopy with the flexible endoscope is easier at this time with the meat intact. Later removal is more difficult as the meat fragments, and pushing it into the stomach may be easier[8] for the patient and physician. Alternative treatments should be mentioned. Enzymatic digestion with papain as in meat tenderizer is effective, but the risk of digestion of the esophageal wall itself is ever present.[52] Absolute contraindications are meat impaction for more than 36 hours, suspected perforation, and radiographic evidence of bone within the bolus. Its use can no longer be recommended. Administration of diazepam or glucagon has been successful in relieving obstruction in some adults.[20,53-56] Glucagon has been recommended for meat lodged in the distal esophagus through its action of decreasing lower esophageal sphincter pressure.[57] Contraindications are allergy to the drug, pheochromocytoma, and insulinoma. The sudden release of gas by gas-forming agents (tartaric and sodium bicarbonate) has been used by a few physicians to propel the meat into the stomach but has been associated with perforation.[58] Since few impacted foods perforate the esophagus, conservative treatment and endoscopy are usually all that are needed.

DRUG-INDUCED ESOPHAGEAL INJURY

In an extensive review of the literature describing pill-induced esophagitis, Kikendall and co-workers[59] identified 26 different pill types associated with injury (Table 2). Ten antibiotics accounted for more than half of all cases, with doxycycline being most responsible. A Swedish survey reports on incidence of 3.9 per 100,000 population per year.[60]

The majority of patients with pill-induced injury have been without esophageal disease, but transit abnormalities have been predisposing conditions in some, i.e., stricture, achalasia, esophageal compression due to valvular heart disease with left auricular enlargement, or esophageal entrapment from

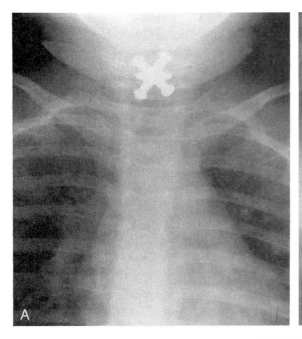
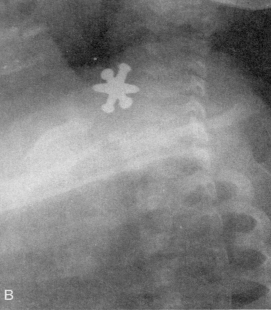

FIGURE 7 *A, B,* Ingested jack at the level of the cricopharyngeal area.

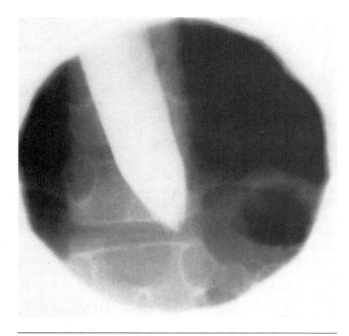

FIGURE 8 This 5-year-old mentally retarded girl had multiple congenital anomalies, including a tracheoesophageal fistula, which was repaired shortly after birth. A grape is impacted just above the narrowed end-to-end anastomosis.

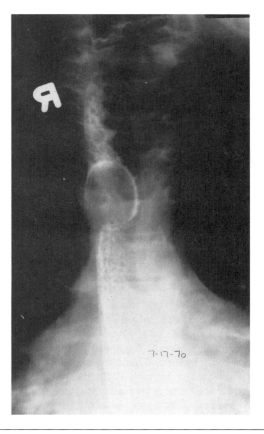

FIGURE 9 A 9-year-old boy with a 4-month history of intermittent vomiting and food, particularly meat, sticking in his chest. This follow-up contrast study, which was performed after endoscopic removal of impacted meat, shows early achalasia with smooth distal tapering of the esophagus.

adhesions after thoracic surgery. Forty percent of patients take their pills with little or no fluid, with the primary cause of injury being adherence of the drug product to the esophagus.[61] Gelatin capsules and those with cellulose fillers have the greatest tendency to adhere, with gelatin capsules remaining in the normal esophagus for longer than 10 minutes. Anhydrous pills may increase in size and adhere. Those with low adherence are film coated with aqueous dispersions or are sugar coated.[62]

The symptoms are continuous retrosternal pain and dysphagia. Less common are abdominal pain, weight loss,

TABLE 2
Medications Causing Esophageal Injury

Doxycycline
Other antibiotics: tetracycline, clindamycin, oxytetracycline, minocycline, ampicillin, erythromycin, phenoxymethyl penicillin, lincomycin, tinidazole
Emepronium bromide
Potassium chloride
Ferrous sulfate or succinate
Alprenolol chloride
Doleron
Quinidine
Aspirin
Indomethacin
Aspirin, caffeine, phenacetin
Decagesic
Phenylbutazone, prednisone
Acetaminophen and praflex compound
Estramustin phosphate
Ascorbic acid
Pantogar

hematemesis, fever, and dehydration. Direct caustic injury is suggested by the feeling that the pill has stuck in the chest (25 percent of patients) or observation of fragments of pill in the area of injury.[63,64]

The most common site of injury is at the level of the aortic arch, where the esophagus is slightly compressed and has a reduction in peristaltic amplitude owing to a transition from skeletal to smooth muscle. Lesions of the lower esophagus are less frequent and often may be erroneously attributed to gastroesophageal reflux. Doxycycline, ferrous sulfate, and slow-release emepronium bromide produce an acid pH when dissolved in water and may even injure the buccal mucosa if held in the mouth for a protracted time. Doxycycline further accumulates in the buccal layer of squamous epithelium. Stricture may be an eventual complication.

Pills should be taken with adequate water and not at bedtime when saliva is decreased and the patient is supine.[65]

BAROTRAUMA

Pressurized soft drinks or aerosols can cause significant trauma to the pharynx and esophagus owing to sudden increases in pressure. The addition of dry ice (CO_2) to screw-top plastic soft drink containers increases pressure. Children can, by clamping the screw top between their teeth and rotating the bottle, generate a violent thrust of compressed gas into the mouth, pharynx, and esophagus. Symptoms are nearly immediate: respiratory distress, neck pain, blood-stained secretions, and hemoptysis. Airway obstruction requires immediate oropharyngeal or endotracheal airway. All six of the patients reported by Conlan et al[66] had cervical and mediastinal emphysema; two had a pneumothorax. Contrast barium studies reveal pharyngeal and upper esophageal penetrating injury or pharyngeal and left lower esophageal laceration. Lacerations occur in the posterior pharynx with associated tonsillar and soft palate injury.

Treatment. Treatment is either conservative, with broad-spectrum antibiotics, and chest suction in those who develop pneumothorax, or surgical. Those who require surgery undergo cervical exploration and repair of pharyngeal or pharyngoesophageal lacerations. Feeding is through a fine-bore silicone rubber catheter or by the parenteral route, and children are encouraged to expectorate rather than to swallow oral secretions. Fortunately, airway reaction subsides within 48 hours, and the healing of the lacerations is made obvious by radiologic study within 7 to 10 days. No later complications are reported.

ELECTRICAL AND THERMAL BURNS

Electrical burns of the esophagus are extremely rare but have been reported in situations of esophageal temperature monitoring during general anesthesia and experimentally, during the use of pill electrodes for transesophageal pacing when current levels above 75 mA are applied over a period of less than 30 minutes.[67-69]

A deliberate electrical burn followed by stricture was reported in a suicide attempt involving ingestion of a severed active electrical cord.[70]

Because microwave ovens rapidly cook through to the center of heated foods, children may not appreciate that the interior of a heated delicacy is intensely hot, although the outer covering is only moderately warm. Local esophageal burns resulting from this situation are now being reported.[71,72]

CAUSTIC INJURY

Caustic ingestions number more than 5,000 per year. Those by children have decreased somewhat but remain a serious reality. Leape et al[73] estimated that approximately 5,000 cases of lye ingestion occur per year by children under 5 years old. Ingestions are largely of lye (sodium hydroxide), with injury due to liquefaction necrosis of the esophageal mucosa and its underlying tissues. Before 1967, lye was available as a drain cleaner in solid form as granules, pellets, or powder. Crystalline forms are less often associated with esophageal burns because they cause such pain in the mouth that they are quickly expelled.[74,75] If swallowed, these forms adhere to the oropharynx and esophagus, causing proximal and linear burns. Lye is now available in liquid form, and ingestion of this leads to far more serious extensive, deep circular burns.[76] Concentrations of lye in these cleaners are as follows: Liquid Plumber, 30.5 percent; Drano, 32 percent; Plunge, 25 percent; Glamorene, 25 percent; and Down the Drain, 36.5 percent, as compared with 54 to 98 percent in the granular forms.[77] Krey[78] studied the concentrations of sodium hydroxide required to cause injury in experimental animals. Normal or 3.8 percent NaOH for 10 seconds of contact necrosed mucosa, submucosa, and some fibers of the lumen muscular layer; 3N or 10.7 percent necrosed to the outer muscle layer; and 7N or 22.5 percent necrosed through the wall of the esophagus. Severe burns have followed minor exposures such as licking a bottle cap[73] or eating from an unwashed spoon used to measure liquid lye.[79] A more recent source of ingestion is a home-pregnancy test that is left to stand for color development.[80] Weaker alkalis such as ammonia and nonphosphate detergents and chlorinated alkalis as cleaning agents also cause esophageal burns, but they are of lesser severity.[81-83]

Ingestion of acids is less frequent, and esophageal damage is unusual. However, strong acids may cause coagulation necrosis of the esophagus, but their primary sites of damage are stomach and duodenum.[84] With the increasing popularity of Mexican foods esophageal burns have followed the ingestion of hot chili peppers. Preparation of such peppers requires the use of rubber gloves.

Pathology and Pathophysiology. Because of rapid liquefying necrosis, the alkalis penetrate deep into the esophageal muscle layers, often destroying the full thickness of the organ and causing edema and cell necrosis. First-degree burn is evidenced by superficial involvement of the mucosa. A second-degree burn shows transmural involvement with or without muscularis damage. There is no extension into the periesophageal or perigastric tissues. Polymorphonuclear cells infiltrate the edge of the injury, and granulation tissue forms. Vessels thrombose and bacteria invade. Within a few days the necrotic tissue sloughs and acute inflammation begins to subside. Third-degree burn represents a full-thickness injury that extends into the periesophageal or perigastric tissue and may result in mediastinitis or peritonitis. Perforation may occur within hours, or it may be delayed. The intense inflammatory reaction created can extend into the mediastinum, and bacteria can invade the mediastinum even in the absence of perforation. As healing progresses, fibrotic proliferation occurs during the second week and later collagen is deposited, leading to fibrous tissue and stricture formation.[85-88] Ulcerations may last for months. Acid burns, although they coagulate surface tissues, are more superficial and less likely to cause perforation of the esophagus, exerting their action on the stomach.

During the first 48 hours, therefore, early dysphagia is due to inflammatory edema, which may completely obstruct the esophagus. Later dysphagia is caused by stricture (Figs. 10 and 11). The esophagus is weakest at 10 to 12 days, when connective tissue begins to appear, and strictures develop between 3 and 4 weeks.

Symptoms. The child who ingests a caustic agent is usually symptomatic immediately—frightened, crying, spitting, and coughing. The bottle of ingested substance is nearby. Burns are present on the lips and in the oropharynx in most, but only one-third of these children have esophageal burns. A mild burn causes pain on swallowing for a few days. Generally, the more severe the oral burns, the more likely the

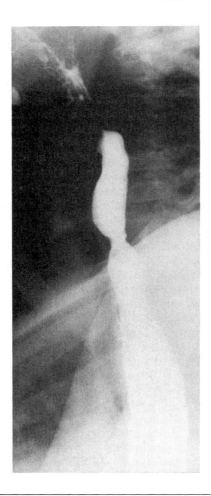

FIGURE 10 A 3-year-old who ingested liquid Drano. There is a stricture of the proximal esophagus with an ulceration above.

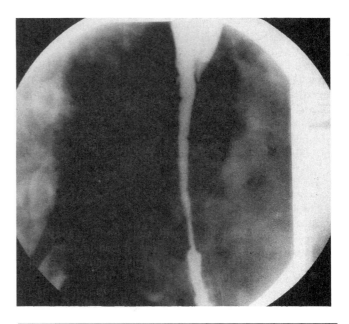

FIGURE 11 Long stricture of the esophagus following lye ingestion.

presence of esophageal lesions. However, esophageal burns may be present when no burns are seen in the oropharynx.[76]

Symptoms do not always correlate with the presence or severity of burns within the esophagus, although one study reports that if two or more symptoms of vomiting, drooling, and stridor are present, there is a 50 percent likelihood of serious esophageal injury.[89,90] As the esophagus becomes atonic in severe injury, there is drooling of mucus and saliva. Chest pain, dysphagia, difficulty in breathing, and stridor are other symptoms. Burns on the lips or in the mouth and pharynx are white, necrotic, edematous lesions. Aspiration is evident by chest examination. Respiratory symptoms may appear early or develop later, depending upon injury to the glottis and trachea. Transmural burns produce rapid symptoms, and the children are acutely ill, having fever and tachycardia.

Treatment. Vomiting should not be induced because of the risk of increasing esophageal injury and aspiration of alkali into the trachea. Shortly after ingestion there is a chemical reaction in the stomach between gastric acid and lye, which generates significant heat. A "sloshing" of this mixture occurs from stomach to esophagus, further increasing the damage.[91]

A similar creation of heat results from attempts to dilute or neutralize ingested acids, with mixtures of sulfuric acid and water attaining temperatures of 80° C. The stomach should be aspirated as completely as possible before cold water lavage is undertaken.

All children suspected of caustic ingestion should be admitted to the hospital for observation and chest film. Intravenous fluids are administered, and the child is not permitted to drink until after endoscopy. Barium studies are not performed. Early endoscopy within 12 hours should be performed under general anesthesia.[92-93] Gentle advancement of the instrument must avoid trauma and the risk of perforation. Endoscopy confirms the diagnosis and establishes the extent of burn. Early versus late endoscopy remains debatable. Those who prefer to perform endoscopy at 48 hours do so to more readily identify fibrin patches and avoid increasing arytenoid edema. Others prefer early endoscopy to identify second- or third-degree burns and the extent of injury.[94]

Endoscopic findings in superficial involvement are mucosal hyperemia and edema with occasional mucosal desquamation. Second-degree burns show sloughing of the mucosa, hemorrhagic exudates, pseudomembrane formation, ulceration, and, later, granulation tissue. Third-degree burns are full-thickness burns with mediastinal or intraperitoneal involvement and show total obliteration of the lumen from edema, charring, eschar, and full-thickness necrosis with perforation.[95]

If there is no evidence of an esophageal burn, the child is discharged to home. Those with first-degree burns are observed for 24 to 48 hours in the hospital. In some centers these patients receive no other treatment,[93,95] but in other centers they are treated with an oral broad-spectrum antibiotic and in some with steroids. Within 48 hours liquids are usually tolerated, and feedings are advanced to a soft diet. There is a general consensus that all children with second-and third-degree oropharyngeal burns and/or significant esophageal burns should be treated with broad-spectrum antibiotics and steroids (as 2 mg per kg per day of prednisone) administered daily for 3 to 4 weeks, with the steroid dose gradually tapered over that time. Steroids must be started early to counteract edema and inhibit fibrosis. Although they decrease the incidence and severity of strictures, they do not prevent all stricture formation.[77] The rationale for antibiotics is inhibition of bacterial invasion of the esophageal wall, which is believed to play a role in stricture formation. Experimentally, Butler et al[96] used beta-aminopropionitrile, which inhibits intermolecular cross-bonding in newly formed collagen. They concluded that the substance prevented stenosis as did steroids; that it prevented shortening of the esophagus that occurred in steroid-treated animals; and that animals with full-thickness injury and no stricture had thinning of the wall in the healed area.

The severity of severe second- and third-degree burns by liquid caustics has been emphasized, with high mortality rates following deep circumferential burns.[75] The stomach may be primarily affected in some cases of liquid caustic ingestion.[97] Estrera et al[95] reported that 100 percent of patients with full-thickness esophagogastric necrosis died under standard medical management. They recommend, in addition to steroids and antibiotics, early surgical intervention with laparotomy and insertion of an esophageal stent if evidence of esophagogastric necrosis is absent. If there is any question of viability, a second-look procedure is performed 36 hours later, and, if necessary, radical resection is performed and the stent is left in place for 21 days. Differentiation of transmural from extensive full-thickness necrosis is difficult by means of endoscopy alone. Children heal without stricture if the stent is left in place until the esophagus is well healed.[98] Blunt thoracic esophageal stripping through a cervicotomy and laparotomy avoids pleural exposure and respiratory complication. This may prove safer than thoracic esophagectomy in those without full-thickness burns.[99,100] DiCostanzo et al, in 1980, used normal alimentation for patients with minor burns and parenteral feedings for those with moderate to severe burns; healing occurred in 8 to 90 days, and parenteral nutrition decreased stricture formation and complications.[101]

Radiographic examination is withheld for several weeks because early radiographs can give false-negative information. Early findings are intramural retention of contrast material, gaseous dilatation of the esophagus due to air trapping, and blurred mucosal margins. Studies at 1 week show some esophageal ulcerations, with later stiffness of the esophageal wall and defective peristalsis. If no stricture is noted, the patient should be seen monthly and have radiologic studies every few months during the first year after ingestion. In acid burns, the radiologic findings are in the acute and subacute states: mucosal and submucosal edema, hemorrhage, ulcerations, sloughing of the mucosa, atony, and dilatation. In the chronic phases of both types of burns, the lesions progress to fibrosis and often to stricture.[101]

Complications. Aspiration pneumonia, mediastinitis, and sepsis are complications that develop most often during the first 48 hours after ingestion. Bleeding has occurred in some patients. Gastric burns may perforate, with patients showing abdominal pain and peritonitis. Several days may pass in a relatively asymptomatic patient before signs of perforation into the thorax, peritoneum, or mediastinum are manifest, i.e., pain, fever, and vascular collapse. Tracheoesophageal fistula is a serious complication associated more often with ingestion of liquid than of crystalline lye. Although stricture rarely develops after first- and linear second-degree burns, the complication occurs in half of second-degree burns from liquid lye and follows severe burns in more than half of untreated and in 4 to 13 percent of treated patients. Stricture may follow acid as well as caustic burns.[102] Strumboff reported his experience with 1,221 patients in 1950, listing the following complications: mediastinitis, 20 percent; esophageal perforation, 15 percent; gastric perforation, 10 percent; peritonitis, 15 percent; laryngeal edema, 16 percent; pneumonia, 14 percent; and fistula to the trachea or aorta, 20 percent.[103]

Dilations are begun cautiously when esophageal stricture is identified, using endoscopy first to determine the extent of healing.[93] Rigidity of the stricture determines whether string with metal olives and/or Maloney dilators or gastrostomy with retrograde dilation should be used. Esophageal motility is disordered from days to several years after lye ingestion, with weak to absent peristaltic contractions or repetitive ones, causing some dysphagia.[104] Other complications are shortening of the esophagus, hiatal hernia, and incompetence of the lower esophageal sphincter.

Mortality rates vary from 2.5 to 13.6 percent to 45 to 100 percent in severe liquid caustic ingestion.[77,105] Patients who have ingested caustics are at increased risk of developing esophageal squamous carcinoma—a risk that may be 1,000 times greater than in the general population. The onset of carcinoma occurs between 41 and 45 years later, with three-quarters of lesions in the midthorax at the level of the bronchial bifurcation.[106,107]

ACQUIRED ESOPHAGEAL STRICTURE

Acquired esophageal stricture is a result of peptic esophagitis, ingestion of caustics, or severe infections of the esophagus as with meningococcemia. Strictures also follow food abrasion of the esophagus in patients with epidermolysis bullosa.[108]

In peptic esophagitis, mucosal lesions tend to heal by regeneration of the mucosa while the inflammatory process continues in the deeper layers and heals by fibrosis. Although all levels of the esophagus are equally sensitive to acid-peptic digestion, the more distal esophagus is most often involved. *Barrett's esophagus* is a term used to represent replacement of areas of lower esophageal squamous epithelium by columnar epithelium containing parietal cells. Although esophagitis and stricture are often present above this epithelium, it is not subject to esophagitis. Occasionally it contains a solitary Barrett's ulcer. The diagnosis is suggested by a midesophageal stricture; endoscopy and biopsy will identify the abnormal tissue. Since Barrett's esophagus is being seen more often in infants and children with the use of endoscopy, once identified it must be treated aggressively because of a potential for the later development of carcinoma. In contrast, caustic strictures tend to be more proximal. Those associated with epidermolysis may occur in any area of the esophagus, although there is some evidence that gastroesophageal reflux may play a role in the more distal strictures in these patients.

Historically, affected children show a progression of symptoms from difficulty in swallowing solids to eventual difficulty with liquids. As the stricture becomes tighter, there may be pain referred to the neck or epigastrium as well as substernal pain. There is often choking during attempts to feed and problems in handling secretions, which lead to drooling.

Treatment. A short stricture can be successfully dilated using bougienage or balloon dilation. If dilation is unsuccessful or if the stricture is long, one must consider colon interposition procedures for relief.

ESOPHAGEAL LACERATION

Esophageal lacerations may result from endoscopic trauma or in the infant from excessively vigorous use of oropharyngeal suction or passage of a nasogastric tube. These range from small to significant tears, with treatment depending upon the degree of bleeding. Most can be managed conservatively, but long or deep tears require surgical repair.

On other occasions pharyngeal and/or esophageal lacerations have followed ingestion of hard food substances such as bay leaf or tacos.[109]

MALLORY-WEISS SYNDROME

As endoscopy is used more liberally the Mallory-Weiss syndrome in children is increasingly recognized. The syndrome represents spontaneous laceration of the esophagus after forceful or prolonged vomiting and is the most common form of esophageal trauma. Vomiting increases the intraesophageal pressure by several hundred millimeters of mercury, and the extent of tear may well depend upon whether the superior esophageal sphincter remains open or closed.[110-112]

Pathology. During vomiting, the diaphragm descends and a portion of stomach is protruded upward through the diaphragmatic hiatus. Interestingly, half of adults with Mallory-Weiss syndrome actually have hiatal hernia. The laceration is located at the esophagogastric junction and often extends into the cardia of the stomach. If through-and-through perforation occurs, it involves only the distal esophagus. The tear is either single or double and is usually superficial, extending only through the mucosa along the longitudinal axis of the esophagus. Bleeding is most serious when the gastric wall as well as the esophageal wall is torn. Fresh lesions appear as a longitudinal crack in the mucosa with little inflammatory reaction. They may be so thin as to be missed by the endoscopist, and several passages of the endoscope are often needed to identify them. After 24 hours, the tear often appears raised, with some erythema and granulation tissue.

Symptoms. The history typically involves one or more acute episodes of vomiting or of vomiting for several days, followed by the vomiting of blood. A few patients vomit alternately dark and red blood.

Diagnosis. The diagnosis is made by endoscopy and visualization of the laceration.[112-114]

Treatment. In the majority of children, bleeding stops spontaneously. The stomach should be lavaged to prevent gastric distention. If hemostasis does not occur, the tear must be sutured. Vasopressin and balloon tamponade have been recommended, but their effectiveness is unpredictable. In some instances, Gelfoam embolization of the left gastric artery has proven effective in stopping bleeding.[112] In adults, approximately 20 percent require surgical control of hemorrhage, and the mortality rate is between 7.5 and 25 percent. In children these figures are undoubtedly less, and we have seen no child who required surgery.

NEONATAL BOERHAAVE'S SYNDROME

Neonatal Boerhaave's syndrome represents true spontaneous rupture of the esophagus.[115] In older children and adults who rupture the esophagus from vomiting, coughing, or blunt chest trauma, the tear arises in the lower left lateral esophagus, an area containing the weakest musculature. In the neonate, however, spontaneous rupture is consistently on the right, suggesting a muscular defect in that region or a different etiology. Usually no cause is identified, although in one infant, the tear was above an esophageal web.[116,117]

At exploration there is a sharp right esophageal linear tear without evidence of esophagitis. Subcutaneous emphysema, mediastinitis, and right pneumothorax followed by pleural effusion are major findings.

Symptoms. The onset of symptoms in infants is sudden. As in the Mallory-Weiss syndrome, it may be preceded by one or more episodes of vomiting and then vomiting of blood. The neonate shows only the sudden onset of marked respiratory distress and has diminished or absent breath sounds in the right chest, retractions, decreased movement of the right chest, and a tympanitic percussion. There may also be subcutaneous emphysema of the neck. In older infants and children, the precipitating factor is often trauma or a paroxysm of coughing, which is followed by pain on swallowing, respiratory distress, and vomiting.

Diagnosis. The presence of a right pneumothorax may wrongly suggest a respiratory origin. This in association with subcutaneous emphysema should suggest the proper diagnosis.

An adult with spontaneous esophageal rupture presented with the only symptom of unilateral proptosis secondary to orbital emphysema.[118] Pneumomediastinum is unusual, and early chest films show only tension pneumothorax. Radiologic study of the esophagus shows extravasation along a tract extending into the pleural space. Chest drainage resembles saliva or contains milk if the pleural fluid is obtained shortly after a feeding. Later films show loculation of the fluid.

Treatment. The esophageal tear requires immediate closure with drainage of the chest and, if indicated, the mediastinum. Antibiotic therapy and gastrostomy or transpyloric feedings substantially decrease mortality, which now approximates 40 percent. Although most survivors have an uncomplicated course, esophageal stricture may be a late complication.

Pseudodiverticulum of the esophagus may follow esophageal perforation. In a review of 15 infants, the major symptoms of this complication were increased salivation and drooling, cyanosis and respiratory distress, vomiting and choking, and inability to pass a nasogastric tube.[119]

PERFORATION AND RUPTURE OF THE ESOPHAGUS

Esophageal rupture in children, as in adults, is largely secondary to direct or blunt trauma, to foreign bodies, or in the neonate to necrotizing enterocolitis[120] (Table 3). The same symptoms result from iatrogenic causes, which loom high among factors identified in esophageal perforation.[121-127] In those situations one or more hours often elapse before symptoms develop. The esophagus may be torn and even perforated by overly vigorous suctioning of the neonate,[121] by blind advancement of the fiberoptic endoscope, and by endoscopic injection sclerotherapy for esophageal varices.[122,123] Blunt trauma from motor vehicle accidents, cardiac massage, and the Heimlich maneuver have also been responsible for esophageal perforations. Tracheal injury is nearly always associated with severe blunt esophageal perforation.[124] Balloons used for tamponade of varices and for dilation of strictures as well as dilation procedures for achalasia are less usual causes of perforation.[125,126] Severe vomiting may lead to esophageal rupture,[125-127] but mediastinal emphysema from alveolar rupture in a patient with anorexia nervosa has mimicked perforation.[128] The esophageal obturator airway used in cardiopulmonary resuscitation has caused several cases of esophageal perforation through distention of the occlusive balloon at the level of the tracheal bifurcation.[129,130]

Esophageal injury must be suspected in penetrating wounds by sharp objects or in gunshot wounds whose path courses through the neck, mediastinum, or thoracic esophagus.[131,132] It is estimated that clinical evaluation will identify only 80 percent of esophageal injuries,[133] with major concern for those with no symptoms. Traumatic fracture of the cervical spine has been associated with rupture of the cervical esophagus and trachea, and meningitis as a complication has been reported.

Symptoms. Important physical findings are subcutaneous emphysema, cervical hematoma, and blood in the nasogastric tube.[134] Clinical evaluation is estimated to identify only

TABLE 3
Esophageal perforation

Iatrogenic
    Resuscitation, endotracheal intubation, nasogastric intubation,
      Heimlich maneuver, esophageal obturator airway, pneumatic
      dilation for achalasia
    Balloon dilation of stricture
    Balloon tamponade of varices
    Sclerotherapy
    Endoscopic tear
    Suction biopsy perforation
Foreign body
Shotgun injury
Blunt trauma: traumatic cervical spine fracture
Spontaneous rupture
Necrotizing enterocolitis
Compressed air or CO_2
Vomiting

---

80 percent of esophageal injuries in penetrating cervical injuries. Although thoracic injuries are more often associated with chest pain, tachycardia, respiratory distress, cyanosis, pain between the shoulder blades, and vomiting, some may have few or no symptoms, particularly the sedated or unconscious patient or the infant (Fig. 12). With mediastinal emphysema there may be a crunching sound associated with the heart beat.

Radiologic findings are cervical and/or mediastinal air widening of the mediastinum, pleural effusion, and pneumothorax.[135] Contrast examinations, best performed with metrizamide rather than barium, are not always positive (75 percent),[134] nor is endoscopy (83 percent).[135] The majority of patients suffering blunt or penetrating injuries have associated tracheal injuries.[137] Computed tomography is helpful in determining mediastinal abscess.[138]

Examination of the pleural fluid may show a mucoid appearance from extravasated saliva or even food. Amylase in the fluid represents the salivary and not the pancreatic enzyme. A low pH of pleural fluid may be due to reflux of gastric and/or bacterial or leukocytic metabolism, with experimental studies suggesting polymorphonuclear leukocyte metabolism as the major cause.[139]

Treatment. Brewer et al reviewed 90 cases of esophageal perforation in the antibiotic era and emphasized the importance of individualized treatment.[140] If the patient presents within the first 24 hours, surgical repair with two-layer closure and irrigating tube drainage is the treatment for most thoracic and abdominal perforations. An operative delay beyond 24 hours increases mortality to 33 percent.[141] If a small perforation is proven and there is no pleural involvement or constitutional symptoms, the patient may be treated medically with gastric drainage, antibiotics, and parenteral nutrition.[142-146] Mollitt et al[121] reported their experience in the treatment of nine neonates, weighing between 480 and 3,900 g, with iatrogenic perforation due to endotracheal or nasogastric intubation. Three infants with small, localized collections were treated by placement of a nasogastric tube and administration of broad-spectrum antibiotics. Two neonates with intrapleural contamination but weighing less than 1,000 g were treated with chest drainage and a nasogastric tube, and four underwent surgical repair. For large perforations with extensive contamination of the mediastinum and pleura and in gunshot wounds in which there is extensive tissue damage, esophageal exclusion through ligation of the distal esophagus, gastrostomy, and cervical esophagostomy with supportive hyperalimentation may be life saving. There is a high incidence of failure of primary repair of thoracic perforations. Lucas et al[147] used the same technique for a 16-year-old boy with delayed esophageal rupture after vehicular trauma but with staged direct closure of the esophagus buttressed by a rhomboid muscle flap. High gastric fundoplication has also been used to cover a low esophageal perforation.[148] In patients seen more than 24 hours after perforation, both the size of the perforation and the extent of mediastinal and pleural infection dictate the type of therapy.

Fulminant mediastinitis is the major threat in esophageal perforation. Although most often due to rupture in the thoracic esophagus, it may occur in rupture of the cervical esophagus if drainage is delayed and the infection spreads along periesophageal planes to the mediastinum. Peroral trans-

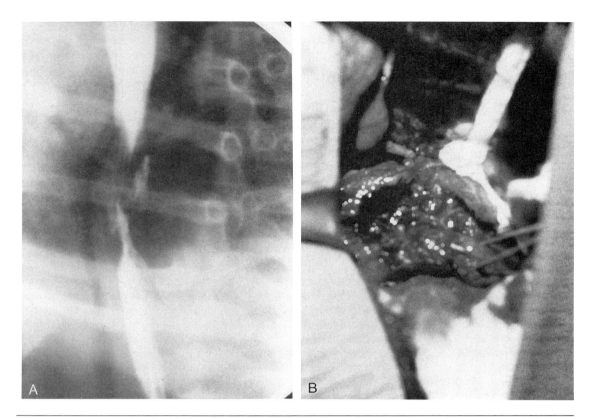

FIGURE 12 A 1-year-old with a history of stridor since birth, which had increased during the past 2 months. Physical examination was normal, but with expiration during crying, he emitted a loud sound resembling the honk of a wild goose. A lateral film of neck and chest showed separation of the esophagus and trachea. *A*, Esophagogram showed narrowing of the proximal esophagus with extravasation of contrast posteriorly. *B*, At surgery, a dark green plastic leaf was found embedded between the esophagus and trachea.

esophageal drainage of the mediastinum has been accomplished by using a nasogastric tube positioned in the upper esophagus proximal to the perforation or irrigation by mouth with drainage tubes positioned in the neck.[149]

Signs of complications and breakdown of the repair are pain, neck tenderness, dyspnea, and dysphagia with subcutaneous emphysema, crepitus, fever, and leukocytosis. Cervical osteomyelitis can follow cervical perforation. A delayed complication is tracheoesophageal fistula.[150]

Mortality rates range from 15 percent in penetrating perforation of the cervical esophagus to 45 percent in that of the thoracic esophagus, being highest in those with delayed detection. There is little difference in mortality between iatrogenic perforation and Boerhaave's syndrome as long as the diagnosis is made early and treatment is prompt.[151]

ESOPHAGEAL TRAUMA IN EPIDERMOLYSIS BULLOSA

Several clinical types of epidermolysis bullosa are associated with esophageal disease: Epidermolysis bullosa letalis is an autosomal recessive form associated with early death from fluid loss and sepsis. The autosomal dominant form displays moderate bullous skin lesions and oral, esophageal, and anal lesions without stricture formation. Acquired EB is a mild disease. In the inversus form, the skin is normal and lesions are internal. The autosomal recessive dystrophic epidermolysis bullosa (RDEB) is most frequently associated with extensive lesions of the mucous membranes of the mouth, pharynx, and esophagus.[108]

Mucosal bullae develop at any age between infancy and 30 years (Fig. 13). Some occur spontaneously along with the appearance of active skin lesions. Others are precipitated by the ingestion of coarse foods and often are associated with dysphagia. Bullae may cause a nearly complete obstruction of the esophagus, with pooling of saliva and regurgitation of food. Strictures are frequent complications, with half occurring in the proximal esophagus, one-quarter in the lower esophagus, and the remaining one-quarter randomly distributed. The primary symptom is dysphagia, which increases in severity until even liquids are not tolerated. Stricture with impaction of food is unusual, for these patients are skilled in preparing pureed diets when they are symptomatic.

Radiologic study is the safest diagnostic procedure, but since strictures may be multiple, care must be taken to provide as good filling as possible, for a tight proximal stricture often prevents good visualization of the esophagus below it. During the phase of active mucosal erosion there are detectable edema and ulcer niches (Fig. 14). Strictures vary from

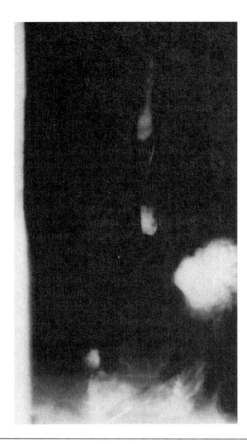

FIGURE 13 A 4-year-old child with bullous lesions of the esophagus from epidermolysis bullosa. The child was unable to swallow.

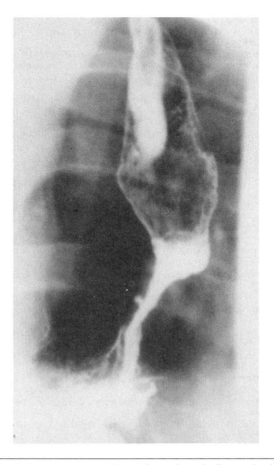

FIGURE 14 A patient with epidermolysis bullosa who has a distal esophageal stricture with ulceration.

less than 3 mm to several centimeters in length and appear either smooth or irregular.

Treatment in the acute stage is aimed at decreasing the formation of bullae, with nutrition being of primary concern. Corticosteroid treatment should be used cautiously, but high-dose steroid therapy such as prednisone, 1.5 to 2 mg per kilogram per day, or the intravenous equivalent of hydrocortisone usually decreases dysphagia in 3 to 14 days. Peripheral parenteral hyperalimentation should be used while treatment is ongoing. Steroids are tapered over 6 to 8 weeks after cessation of symptoms. Mylanta and antibiotic liquids also help to minimize symptoms.

Phenytoin (Dilantin) used in an adult dosage of 250 mg per day or in pediatric equivalents to achieve a plasma level of 10 mg per milliliter has been used successfully in young patients at the early onset of symptoms. It has been less successful when used at the time of stricture dilation.

Dilation of strictures must be done with extreme care, for perforation is an ever-present hazard. This we have seen after mercury bougienage and after balloon dilation. In those with long strictures, right colon interposition or gastric tube replacement have proven successful. There is some concern about the development of carcinoma in the bypassed esophagus.

REFERENCES

1. Healy GB. Foreign bodies of the air and food passages in children. Am J Dis Child 1987; 141:239.
2. Bloom RR, Nakano PH, Gray SW, Skandalakis JE. Foreign bodies of the gastrointestinal tract. Am Surg 1987; 52:618–621.
3. Kramer TA, Riding KH, Salkeld LJ. Tracheobronchial and esophageal foreign bodies in the pediatric population. J Otolaryngol 1986; 6:355–358.
4. Taylor RB. Esophageal foreign bodies. Emerg Med Clin North Am 1987; 5:301–311.
4a. Schunk JE, Corneli H, Bolte R. Pediatric coin ingestions. Am J Dis Child 1989; 143:546–551.
5. Jackson RM, Hawkins DB. Coins in the esophagus. What is the best management? Int J Pediatr Otorhinolaryngol 1986; 12:127–135.
6. Kirk AD, Bowers BA, Moylan JA, Meyers WC. Toothbrush swallowing. Arch Surg 1988; 123:382–384.
7. Fernbach SK, Tucker GF. Coin ingestion: unusual appearance of the penny in a child. Radiology 1986; 158:512–514.
8. Webb WA. Management of foreign bodies of the upper gastrointestinal tract. Gastroenterology 1988; 94:204–216.
9. Hodge D III, Tecklenburg F, Fleischer G. Coin ingestion: does every child need a radiograph? Ann Emerg Med 1985; 5:443–446.
10. Hess GP. An approach to throat complaints: foreign body sensation, difficulty swallowing and hoarseness. Emerg Med Clin North Am 1987; 5:313–334.
11. Beer S, Avidan G, Viure E, Starinsky R. A foreign body in the esophagus as a cause of respiratory distress. Pediatr Radiol 1982; 12:41–42.

12. Nussbaum E, Fleming DG, Wood RE, Boat TF, Doershuk CF. Stridor due to radiotransparent esophageal foreign body. Am J Dis Child 1984; 138:1081–1083.

13. Kobayashi T. Esophageal foreign bodies in children. Int J Pediatr Otorhinolaryngol 1984; 7:193–198.

14. Humphrey A, Holland WG. Unsuspected esophageal foreign bodies. J Can Assoc Radiol 1981; 32:17–20.

15. Vos GD, Heymans HS, Urbanus NA. Inspiratory stridor and dysphagia because of prolonged oesophageal foreign body. Eur J Pediatr 1987; 146:86–87.

16. Haynes DE, Haynes BE, Young YV. Esophageal rupture complicating the Heimlich maneuver. Am J Emerg Med 1984; 2:501–509.

17. Merideth MJ, Liebowitz R. Rupture of the esophagus caused by the Heimlich maneuver. Ann Emerg Med 1986; 15:106–107.

18. Day RL, Crelin ES, Dubois AB. Choking: the Heimlich abdominal thrust vs back blows. Pediatrics 1982; 70:113–119.

19. Bendig DW. Removal of blunt esophageal foreign bodies by flexible endoscopy without general anesthesia. Am J Dis Child 1986; 140:789–790.

20. Giordano S, Adams G, Boies L Jr, Meyerhoff W. Current management of esophageal foreign bodies. Arch Otolaryngol 1981; 107:249–251.

21. O'Neill JA, Holcomb GW Jr, Neblett W. Management of tracheobronchial and esophageal foreign bodies in childhood. J Pediatr Surg 1983; 18:475–479.

22. Campbell JB, Quattromain F, Foley LC. Foley catheter removal of blunt esophageal foreign bodies: experience with 100 consecutive children. Pediatr Radiol 1983: 13:116–118.

23. Ginaldi S. Removal of esophageal foreign bodies using a Foley catheter in adults. Am J Emerg Med 1985; 3:64–66.

24. Simon DJ. Coins in the esophagus: two for the price of one. Ann Emerg Med 1981; 10:489–491.

25. Chaikhouni A, Kratz JM, Crawford FA. Foreign bodies of the esophagus. Am Surg 1985; 51:173–179.

26. Hinkle FG. Ingested retainer: a case report. Am J Orthod Dentofacial Orthop 1987; 92:46–49.

27. Henderson CT, Engel J, Schlesinger P. Foreign body ingestion: review and suggested guidelines for management. Endoscopy 1987; 19:68–71.

28. Janik JS, Bailey WC, Burrington JD. Occult coin perforation of the esophagus. J Pediatr Surg 1986; 21:794–797.

29. Barber GB, Peppercorn MA, Erlich C, Thurer R. Esophageal foreign body perforation: report of an unusual case and review of the literature. Am J Gastroenterol 1984; 79:509–511.

30. Nahman BJ, Mueller CF. Asymptomatic esophageal perforation by a coin in a child. Ann Emerg Med 1984; 8:627–629.

31. Schumacher KJ, Weaver DL, Knight MR, Presberg HJ. Aortic pseudoaneurysm due to ingested foreign body. South Med J 1986; 79:246–248.

32. Ramadan MF, Rogers JH. An acquired oesophageal pouch in childhood: a problem in diagnosis. J Laryngol Otol 1981; 95:101–108.

33. Mittelman M, Perek J, Kolkov Z, Lewinski U, Djaldetti M. Fetal aspiration pneumonia caused by an esophageal foreign body. Ann Emerg Med 1985; 14:365–367.

34. So SY, Mok CK, Lam WK, Yu DY. Haemoptysis due to unsuspected foreign body penetration of the oesophagus. Aust NZ J Med 1982; 12:533–535.

35. Remsen K, Lawson W, Biller HF, Som ML. Unusual presentations of penetrating foreign bodies of the upper aerodigestive tract. Ann Otol Rhinol Laryngol 1983; 105:32–44.

36. Kost KM, Shapiro RS. Button battery ingestion: a case report and review of the literature. J Otolaryngol 1987; 16:252–257.

37. Votteler TP, Nash JC, Rudledge JC. The hazard of ingested alkaline disc batteries in children. JAMA 1983; 249:2504–2506.

38. Temple DM, McNeese MC. Hazards of battery ingestion. Pediatrics 1983; 71:100–103.

39. Katz I, Cooper MT. Danger of small children swallowing hearing aid batteries. J Otolaryngol 1978; 7:467–471.

40. Maves MD, Carithers JS, Birck HG. Esophageal burns secondary to disc battery ingestion. Ann Otol Rhinol Laryngol 1984; 93:364–369.

41. Litovitz TL. Battery ingestions: product accessability and clinical course. Pediatrics 1985; 75:469–476.

42. Litovitz TL. Button battery ingestions: a review of 56 cases. JAMA 1983; 249:2495–2500.

43. Yamashlta M, Saito S, Koyama K, Hattori H, Ogata T. Esophageal electrochemical burn by button-type alkaline batteries in dogs. Vet Hum Toxicol 1987; 29:226–230.

44. Yasui T. Hazardous effects due to alkaline button battery ingestion: an experimental study. Ann Emerg Med 1986; 15:901–906.

45. Kulig K, Rumack CM, Rumack BH, Duffy JP. Disc battery ingestion: elevated urine mercury levels and enema removal of battery fragments. JAMA 1983; 249:2502–2504.

46. Maves MD, Lloyd TV, Carithers JS. Radiographic identification of ingested disc batteries. Pediatr Radiol 1986; 16:154–156.

47. Rivera EA, Maves MD. Effects of neutralizing agents on esophageal burns caused by disc batteries. Ann Otol Rhinol Laryngol 1987; 96:362.

48. Blatnik BS, Toohill RJ, Lehman RH. Fatal complications from an alkaline battery foreign body in the esophagus. Ann Otol 1977; 86:611–615.

49. Vanasperen PP, Seeto I, Cass DT. Acquired tracheoesophageal fistula after ingestion of a mercury button battery. Med J Aust 1986; 145:412–415.

50. Buchin PJ. Foreign bodies in the esophagus. NY State J Med 1981; 81:1057–1059.

51. Vizcarrondo FJ, Brady PG, Nord H. Foreign bodies of the upper gastrointestinal tract. Gastrointest Endosc 1983; 29:208–210.

52. Holsinger JW, Fuson RI, Sealy WC. Esophageal perforation following meat impaction and papain ingestion. JAMA 1968; 204:188–189.

53. Trenker SW, Maglinte DD, Lehman GA, Chernish SM, Miller RE, Johnson CW. Esophageal food impaction: treatment with glucagon. Radiology 1983; 149:401–403.

54. Friedland GW. The treatment of acute esophageal food impaction using intravenous glucagon. Radiology 1977; 125:25–28.

55. Hogan WJ, Dodds WJ, Hoke SE, Reid DP, Kalkhoff RK, Arndorfer RD. Effect of glucagon on esophageal motor function. Gastroenterology 1975; 69:160–165.

56. Marks HW, Lousteau RJ. Glucagon and esophageal meat impaction. Arch Otolaryngol 1979; 105:367–368.

57. Jaffer SS, Makhlouf GM, Schorr BA, Zhass AM. Nature and kinetics of inhibition of lower esophageal sphincter pressure by glucagon. Gastroenterology 1974; 67:42–46.

58. Rice BT, Spiegel PK, Dombrowski PJ. Acute esophageal food impaction treated by gas forming agents. Radiology 1983; 146:299–301.

59. Kikendall JW, Friedman AC, Oyewole MA, Fleischer D, Johnson LF. Pill-induced esophageal injury: case reports and review of the medical literature. Dig Dis Sci 1983; 28:174–182.

60. Carlborg B, Kumlien A, Olsson H. Medikamentalla esofagusstrikturer. Lakartidningen 1978; 75:4609–4611.

61. Marvola M, Rajaniemi M, Martilla E, Vahervuo K, Sothmann A. Effect of dosage form and formulation factors on the adherence of drugs to the esophagus. J Pharm Sci 1983; 72:1034–1036.

62. Roach J, Martyak T, Benjamin G. Anhydrous pill ingestion: a new cause of esophageal obstruction. Ann Emerg Med 1987; 16:913–914.

63. Bonavina L, DeMeester TR, McChesney L, Schwizer W, Albertucci M, Gaily RT. Drug-induced esophageal injury. Ann Surg 1987; 206:173–183.

64. Winckler K. Tetracycline ulcers of the oesophagus— endoscopy, histology and roentgenology in 2 cases and review of the literature. Endoscopy 1981; 13:225–229.

65. Applegate GR, Malmud LS, Rock E, Reilley JR, Fisher RS. "It's a hard pill to swallow" or "Don't take it lying down." Gastroenterology 1980; 78:1132.

66. Conlan AA, Wessels A, Hammond CA, Beale PG, Katz G. Pharyngoesophageal barotrauma in children: a report of six cases. J Thorac Cardiovasc Surg 1984; 88:452–456.

67. Partar EO. Electrical surgical burn at the site of an esophageal temperature probe. Anesthesiology 1984; 61:93–95.

68. Weiss FR. Technique of avoiding esophageal burns. Anesthesiology 1985; 62:370.

69. Jenkins JM, Dick M, Collins S, O'Neill W, Campbell RM. Use of the pill electrode for transesophageal pacing. PACE 1985; 8:512–527.

70. Flisak ME, Berman S. Electrical injury in the esophagus. AJR 1988; 150:103–104.

71. Lieberman DA, Keefe EB. Esophageal burn and the microwave oven. Ann Intern Med 1982; 97:137.

72. Perlman A. Hazards of a microwave oven. N Engl J Med 1980; 302:970–971.

73. Leape L, Ashcraft KW, Scrapilli DG, Holder TM. Hazard to health— liquid lye. N Engl J Med 1971; 284:478–480.

74. Rothstein FC. Caustic injuries to the esophagus in children. Pediatr Clin North Am 1986; 33:665–674.

75. Oakes DD, Sherck JP, Mark JB. Lye ingestion: clinical patterns and

therapeutic implications. J Thorac Cardiovasc Surg 1982; 83:194–204.

76. Sellars SL, Spence RA. Chemical burns of the oesophagus. J Laryngol Otol 1987; 101:1211–1213.

77. Postlethwait RW. Chemical burns of the esophagus. Surg Clin North Am 1983; 63:915–924.

78. Krey H. On the treatment of corrosive lesions in the esophagus: an experimental study. Acta Otolaryngol 1952; 102(Suppl 1):1–12.

79. Habener SA. Letter to the editor. N Engl J Med 1971; 284:143.

80. Grenga TE. A new risk of lye ingestion by children. N Engl J Med 1983; 308:156–157.

81. Klein J, Olson KR, McKinney HE. Caustic injury from household ammonia. Am J Emerg Med 1985; 3:320–324.

82. Lee JF, Simonowitz D, Block GE. Corrosive injury of the stomach and esophagus by nonphosphate detergents. Am J Surg 1972; 126:652–657.

83. Wasserman R, Guisberg C. Caustic substance injuries. J Pediatr 1985; 107:169–174.

84. Penner GE. Acid ingestion: toxicology and treatment. Ann Emerg Med 1980; 9:374–379.

85. Goldman LP, Weigert JM. Corrosive substance ingestion: a review. Am J Gastroenterol 1984; 79:85–90.

86. Symbas PN, Vlasis SE, Hatcher CR Jr. Esophagitis secondary to ingestion of caustic material. Ann Thorac Surg 1983; 36:73–77.

87. Moore WR. Caustic ingestions: pathophysiology, diagnosis and treatment. Clin Pediatr 1986; 25:196.

88. Moazam F, Talbert JL, Miller D, Mollitt DL. Caustic ingestion and its sequelae in children. South Med J 1987; 80:187–190.

89. Crain EF, Gershel JC, Mezen AP. Caustic ingestions, symptoms as predictors of esophageal injury. Am J Dis Child 1984; 138:863–865.

90. Gandrebault P, Parent M, McGuigan MA, Chicoine L, Lovejoy FH Jr. Predictability of esophageal injury from signs and symptoms: A study of caustic ingestion in 378 children. Pediatrics 1983; 71:767–770.

91. Ray JF III, Myers WO, Lawton BR, Lee FY, Wenzel FJ, Sautter RD. The natural history of liquid lye ingestion. Arch Surg 1974; 109:436–439.

92. Sugawa C, Mullins RJ, Lucas CE, Leibold WC. The value of early endoscopy following caustic ingestion. Surg Gynecol Obstet 1981; 143:553–556.

93. Haller JA Jr, Andrews HG, White JJ, et al. Pathology and management of acute corrosive burns of the esophagus: results of treatment in 285 children. J Pediatr Surg 1971; 6:578–587.

94. Buttross S, Brouhard BH. Acute management of alkali ingestion in children: a review. Tex Med 1981; 77:57–60.

95. Estrera A, Taylor W, Mills L, Platt M. Corrosive burns of the esophagus and stomach: a recommendation of an aggressive surgical approach. Ann Thorac Surg 1986; 41:276–283.

96. Butler C, Madden JW, Davis WM, et al. Morphologic aspects of experimental esophageal lye strictures. II. Effect of steroid hormones, bougienage and induced lathyrism on acute lye burns. Surgery 1977; 81:431–437.

97. Gryboski W, Page R, Bush BF Jr. Management of total gastric necrosis following lye ingestion. Ann Surg 1965; 161:469–474.

98. Coln D, Change JH. Experience with esophageal stenting for caustic burns in children. J Pediatr Surg 1986; 21:588–591.

99. Brun JG, Celerier M, Koskas F, Dubost C. Blunt thorax oesophageal stripping: an emergency procedure for caustic ingestion. Br J Surg 1984; 71:698–700.

100. Gossot D, Sarfati E, Celerier M. Early blunt esophagectomy in severe caustic burns of the upper digestive tract. J Thorac Cardiovasc Surg 1987; 94:188–191.

101. DiCostanzo J, Noirclerc M, Jouglard J, Escoffier JM, Cavo N, Martin J, Gauthier A. New therapeutic approach to corrosive burns of the upper gastrointestinal tract. Gut 1980; 21:370–375.

102. Muhletaler CA. Gerlock AJ Jr, deSoto D, Kalter SA. Acid corrosive esophagitis: radiographic findings. AJR 1980; 134:1137–1140.

103. Strumboff AV. Chemical burns of the oral cavity and esophagus. Arch Otolaryngol 1950; 52:419–424.

104. Baldi F, Ferrarini F, Longanese A, Angeloni M, Ragazzini M, Miglioli M, Barbara L. Esophageal function before, during and after healing of erosive esophagitis. Gut 1988; 29:157–160.

105. Cardona JC, Daly JF. Current management of corrosive esophagitis—an evaluation of results in 239 cases. Ann Otol 1971; 80:521–530.

106. Appelqvist P, Salmo M. Lye corrosion carcinoma of the esophagus: a review of 63 cases. Cancer 1980; 45:2655–2658.

107. Csikos M, Horvath O, Petri A, Petri I, Imre J. Late malignant transformation of chronic corrosive oesophageal strictures. Langenbecks Arch Chir 1985; 365:131–138.

108. Gryboski JD, Touloukian R, Campanella RA. Gastrointestinal manifestations of epidermolysis bullosa in children. Arch Dermatol 1988; 124:746–752.

109. Hunter TB, Protell RL, Horsley WW. Food laceration of the esophagus: the taco tear. AJR 1983; 140:503–504.

110. Cannon RA, Lee G, Cox R. Gastrointestinal hemorrhage due to Mallory-Weiss syndrome in an infant. J Pediatr Gastroenterol Nutr 1985; 4:323–324.

111. Ross LA. Mallory-Weiss syndrome in a 10 month-old infant. Am J Dis Child 1979; 133:1069.

112. Lamiell JM, Weygandt TB. Mallory-Weiss syndrome in two children. J Pediatr 1978; 92:583–584.

113. Michel L, Serrano A, Malt R. Mallory-Weiss syndrome. Ann Surg 1980; 192:716–722.

114. Hastings PR, Peters KW, Cohn I Jr. Mallory-Weiss syndrome: review of 69 cases. Am J Surg 1981; 142:560–562.

115. Clarke TA, Coen RW, Feldman B, Papile L. Esophageal perforations in premature infants and cements on the diagnosis. Am J Dis Child 1980; 134:367–372.

116. Meyers NA. Neonatal rupture of the esophagus. Ann Clin Infant 1972; 13:213–217.

117. Harrell GS, Friedland GW, Dailey WJ, Cohn RB. Neonatal Boerhaave's syndrome. Radiology 1970; 95:665–669.

118. Schneider SM, Goodman D. Spontaneous rupture of the esophagus presenting with unilateral proptosis. Ann Emerg Med 1984; 13:374–377.

119. Urrutta J, Antonmattei S, Cordero L. Pseudodiverticulum of the esophagus in the newborn infant. Am J Dis Child 1980; 134:417–422.

120. Shepard R, Raflensperger J, Goldstein R. Pediatric esophageal perforation. J Thorac Cardiovasc Surg 1977; 74:261–268.

121. Mollitt D, Schullinger J, Santulli TV. Selective management of iatrogenic esophageal perforation in the newborn. J Pediatr Surg 1981; 16:989–996.

122. Hoffman JR, Pietrafesa CA, Orban DJ. Esophageal perforation following use of esophageal obturator airway. Am J Emerg Med 1983; 1:282–287.

123. Shemesh E, Bat L. Esophageal perforation after fiberoptic endoscopic injection sclerotherapy for esophageal varices. Arch Surg 1986; 121:243–245.

124. Stothert JC Jr, Buttorff J, Kaminski DL. Thoracic esophageal and tracheal injury following blunt trauma. J Trauma 1980; 20:992–995.

125. Turner WW Jr. Esophageal rupture: fatal complication of balloon tamponade for acute variceal hemorrhage. Tex Med 1983; 79:57–59.

126. LaBerge JM, Kerlan RK Jr, Pogany AC, Ring EJ. Esophageal rupture: complication of balloon dilatation. Radiology 1985; 157:56–58.

127. Miller RE, Tiszenkel HI. Esophageal perforation due to pneumatic dilatation for achalasia. Surg Gynecol Obstet 1988; 166:458–460.

128. Overby KJ, Litt I. Mediastinal emphysema in an adolescent with anorexia nervosa and self-induced emesis. Pediatrics 1988; 81:134–136.

129. Michael TA. The esophageal obturator airway. A critique. JAMA 1981; 246:1098–1101.

130. Smith JP, Bodai BI, Seifkin A, Palder S, Thomas V. The esophageal obturator airway. A review. JAMA 1983; 250:1081–1084.

131. Pass LJ, LeNarz LA, Schreiber JT, Estrera AS. Management of esophageal gunshot wounds. Ann Thorac Surg 1987; 44:153–156.

132. Popovsky J. Perforations of the esophagus from gunshot wounds. J Trauma 1984; 24:337–339.

133. Weigelt JA, Thall ER, Snyder WH III, Gry RE, Meier DE, Kilman WT. Diagnosis of penetrating cervical esophageal injuries. Am J Surg 1987; 154:619–622.

134. Glatterer MS Jr, Toon RS, Ellestad C, McFee AS, Rogers W, Mack JW, Trinkle JK, Grover FL. Management of blunt and penetrating external esophageal trauma. J Trauma 1985; 25:784–789.

135. Yap RG, Yap AG, Obeid FN, Horan DP. Traumatic esophageal injuries: 12 year experience at Henry Ford Hospital. J Trauma 1984; 24:623–625.

136. Kelly JP, Webb WR, Moulder PV, Moustoukas NM, Lirtzman M. Management of airway trauma. II. Combined injuries of the trachea and esophagus. Ann Thorac Surg 1987; 43:160–163.

137. Feliciano DV, Bitondo CG, Mattox KL, Romo T, Burch JM, Beall AC Jr, Jordan GL Jr. Combined tracheoesophageal injuries. Am J Surg 1985; 150:710–715.

138. Brown BM. Computed tomography of mediastinal abscess secondary to post traumatic esophageal laceration. J Comput Assist Tomogr 1984; 8:765–767.
139. Good JT Jr, Antony VB, Reller LB, Maulitz RM, Sahn SA. The pathogenesis of the low pleural fluid pH in esophageal rupture. Am Rev Respir Dis 1983; 127:702–704.
140. Brewer LA III, Carter R, Mullder GA, Stiles QR. Options in the management of perforations of the esophagus. Am J Surg 1986; 152:62–69.
141. Ajalet GH, Mulder DG. Esophageal perforation: the need for an individualized approach. Arch Surg 1984; 119:1318–1320.
142. Odell PF, LeBrun CJ. Tracheo-esophageal disruption. J Otolaryngol 1980; 9:433–437.
143. Mandal AK, Bui AD, Oparah SS. Surgical and non-surgical treatment of penetrating injuries to the cervical esophagus. Laryngoscope 1983; 93:801–804.
144. Schockley WW, Tate JL, Stucker FJ. Management of perforations of the hypopharynx and cervical esophagus. Laryngoscope 1985; 95:939–941.
145. Keszler P, Bunza E. Surgical and conservative management of esophageal perforation. Chest 1981; 80:158–162.
146. Haffner JF, Fausa O, Ryne T. Nonoperative treatment of subcervical oesophageal perforations after forced dilatation for nonmalignant disease. Acta Chir Scand 1984; 150:389–392.
147. Lucas AE, Snow N, Tobin GR, Flint LM Jr. Use of the rhomboid major muscle flap for esophageal repair. Ann Thorac Surg 1982; 33:619–623.
148. Tarkka M, Harkonen N, Lepojarvi M, Karkoli P, Pokela R. Repair of ruptured oesophagus. Acta Clin Scand 1985; 151:385–387.
149. Santos GH, Frater RW. Transesophageal irrigation for the treatment of mediastinitis produced by esophageal rupture. J Thorac Cardiovasc Surg 1986; 91:57–62.
150. Simpson ET, Lloyd DA. The management of swallowed oesophageal foreign bodies in children. S Afr Med J 1982; 62:1044.
151. Graebor GM, Niezgoda JA, Albus RA, Burton NA, Collins GJ, Lough FC, Zajtchuk R. A comparison of patients with endoscopic esophageal perforations and patients with Boerhaave's syndrome. Chest 1987; 92:995–998.

PART

3

Infections

John S. Goff, M.D.

INFECTIOUS ESOPHAGITIS

Many infectious agents have been found to cause acute and chronic esophagitis.[1] Most of these have been described in patients with some immune disorder, but clinically immunocompetent individuals have been described with fungal or viral esophagitis.[2-6] As many as one-third of leukemic patients coming to autopsy have some form of esophagitis. *Candida albicans* and herpes simplex virus are the most common pathogens, but there are reports of esophagitis due to numerous organisms including, but not limited to, varicella-zoster virus, cytomegalovirus (CMV), *Aspergillus*, gram-negative bacilli, and gram-positive cocci.[1-7] Altered local or systemic defenses are found in most patients. Gastroesophageal reflux, decreased peristalsis, mechanical obstruction, radiation therapy, ulcerations from pills sticking in the esophagus, and nasogastric tubes have all been implicated as conditions that may allow an opportunistic infection to start, because they have, in one way or another, damaged the mucosal defenses of the esophagus. Systemic defenses (immunity) are altered by malignancy, chemotherapy, prednisone, antibiotics, ethanol abuse, diabetes mellitus, and congenital or acquired immunodeficiency syndromes. Many patients have more than one of these predisposing factors.

Diagnosis

Patients with acute infectious esophagitis present with severe pain upon swallowing (odynophagia), dysphagia, atypical chest pain, or a sensation of feeling each bolus of food as it passes slowly down the esophagus. Occasionally, they complain of hoarseness. Many, but not all, who turn out to have herpes esophagitis have or give a history of recently having a fever blister or a sore in the mouth.[4] Oral candidiasis (thrush) is commonly a marker for esophageal candidal infections, especially in the immunocompromised patient, but is absent in up to 50 percent of patients.[2] Once the diagnosis is suspected clinically, one needs to confirm the presence of esophagitis and establish whether there is an infectious agent involved so that appropriate therapy can be initiated as soon as possible.

An esophagram can be a useful first step in evaluating patients with the above-mentioned complaints. It can identify any mechanical problems (obstruction, abnormal peristalsis) and may suggest that the patient has an infectious esophagitis.[8] Unfortunately, many patients have normal or nondiagnostic esophagrams because the mucosal abnormalities early in the course are subtle or because they were unable to tolerate a double-contrast study, which is mandatory in order to see fine detail in the esophageal mucosa. Endoscopy is the best way to make a definitive diagnosis.[9] Through the endoscope one can obtain brushings and biopsies for examination and culture. Brushing may actually be superior to biopsy in this setting, but it is best to do all three (brush, biopsy, and culture), since no one means of obtaining specimens has a 100 percent detection rate. Blind brushings of the esophagus can be helpful for making a diagnosis in patients who cannot undergo endoscopy for one reason or another. Serum antibody titers to the potential pathogens may prove to be useful diagnostic tools in the future, but at present candidal agents are not specific enough to reliably confirm a diagnosis of invasive *Candida albicans*, and one usually needs acute and convalescent titers to diagnose a virus as the causative agent, which would be too slow to guide initial therapy in the acute setting.[2] However, one can consider a trial of empiric treatment based on an isolated high titer for a specific pathogen, if it happens to be found early in the course.

Candida Esophagitis

Candida esophagitis is not limited to the immunocompromised population; there have been many reports of *Candida* esophagitis in patients with apparently no predisposing condition.[10,11] *Candida* is probably the most common organism implicated in infectious esophagitis. Esophagitis in patients with chronic mucocutaneous candidiasis is uncommon but has been described.

Although oral candidiasis (thrush) is present in many patients with *Candida* esophagitis, by itself it is not a very effective way to actually predict who has *Candida* in the esophagus.[2,12] In patients with acquired immunodeficiency syndrome (AIDS), the combination of thrush and esophageal symptoms may have a greater than 95 percent predictive value for a diagnosis of esophageal candidiasis.[13] Also, the development of oral or esophageal candidiasis in patients with AIDS-related complex (ARC) has a dire prognosis. These patients have a 60 percent chance of developing other severe opportunistic infections within 1 year after a diagnosis of candidiasis.[14,15] Leukemic patients with oralpharyngeal candidiasis are more likely to develop systemic candidiasis if they have mucositis and prolonged leukocyte counts less than 500.[16]

The best way to make a diagnosis of esophageal candidiasis is with endoscopy, since the gross appearance can be characteristic and one can obtain tissue specimens for histology and cytology. The mucosa can vary in appearance from moderate erythema and friability to ulcers covered with a thick white exudate to a black membrane (Fig. 1). The most classic finding is white raised lesions, usually less than 1 cm in diameter, that often extend up to the upper one-third of the esophagus. These exudative lesions are adherent and are not easily washed off the mucosal surface. The exudate may contain hyphae of the organism. Biopsies and specimens for cytology are prone to error in diagnosing true, locally invasive *Candida*, because *Candida* is frequently present in the mouth and esophagus and may be in the samples without clinical significance. Ideally, one would like to see the *Candida* associated with viable squamous cells on smears from the lesions or to find invading hyphal forms on biopsy to make a diagnosis (Fig. 2).[17] Culture is of limited value because, as mentioned above, *Candida* is frequently present in the mouth or gastrointestinal (GI) tract.

Radiographic studies of the esophagus are sometimes helpful in making a diagnosis, especially when endoscopy is contraindicated because of low platelet or low leukocyte counts. It has been shown that single-contrast studies are not sensitive enough (55 percent) to pick up some of the more subtle early findings.[18] Double-contrast studies are more sensitive (88 percent). A shaggy, irregular mucosal pattern is found in mild to moderate cases. Ulcers, abnormal motility, and nodules (cobblestone pattern) are also seen (Fig.

3).[19] *Candida* can have a very localized area of involvement and thus can be mistaken for malignancy on a barium esophagram.[20] Occasionally, the entire esophageal mucosa sloughs secondary to *Candida* infection. In this situation, the esophagram can incorrectly appear totally normal.[21]

Candida esophagitis can lead to several complications. Abnormal esophageal motility, intramural diverticula, mucosal bands, obstruction of the esophagus by a fungus ball, fistula, perforation, stricture formation, systemic candidiasis, and secondary bacterial infection with sepsis can all occur. The strictures are often painless and frequently involve the upper esophagus. Esophageal dilatation may not be adequate, and surgery has been necessary to manage this complication.[22,23]

Treatment for *Candida* esophagitis depends upon its severity and the degree of the patient's immunocompromised state. The immunocompetent patient usually responds to nystatin in methylcellulose or carboxymethylcellulose given by mouth every 2 hours for 2 to 6 weeks.[24] Nystatin is rarely helpful for the immunocompromised patient. In one study, the use of nystatin prophylaxis in leukemics undergoing chemotherapy was no better than placebo in preventing oral or systemic candidiasis from developing.[16] Alternative therapy for the immunocompetent patient and initial therapy for immunocompromised patients include clotrimazole troches four to five times per day, flucytosine 50 to 150 mg per kilogram per day orally in divided doses, miconazole 20 to 40 mg per day intravenously in divided doses, and ketoconazole 3.3 to 6.6 mg per kilogram per day orally.[2,25,26] Of these agents, ketoconazole is currently the preferred one despite the potential for developing resistant *Candida*. Amphotericin B 5 to 10 mg per day intravenously is definitive therapy for most cases of *Candida* esophagitis, but the side effects of this drug

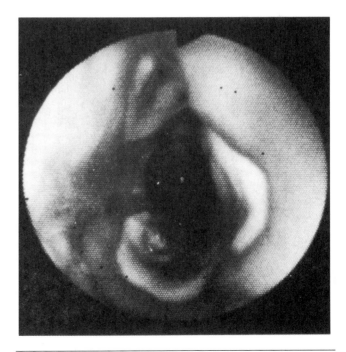

FIGURE 1 Endoscopic view of large flat ulcers with erythematous borders in the proximal esophagus secondary to *Candida* infection in an immunocompromised patient.

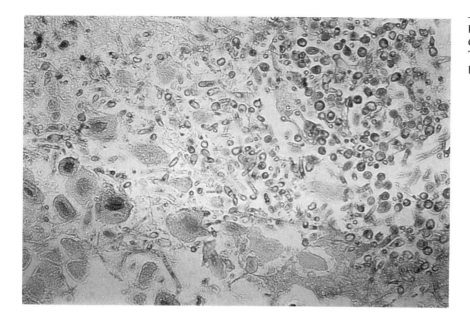

FIGURE 2 Esophageal biopsy showing *Candida* invading the squamous mucosa. There are both yeast and mycelial phases present in the specimen.

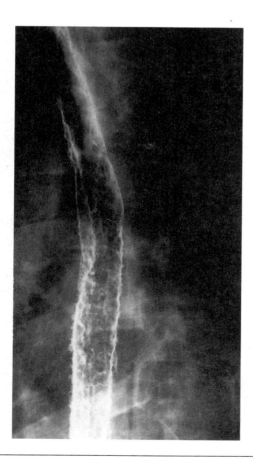

FIGURE 3 Barium swallow in a patient with severe *Candida* esophagitis showing the typical irregular mucosa with ulcers seen in profile and en face.

are sufficient to warrant using it only when other agents are not effective.[27,28] The daily dose of amphotericin B should not exceed 1.5 mg per kilogram. There is very limited experience with all of these drugs in children less than 2 to 3 years old.

Viral Esophagitis

The primary viruses that cause esophagitis are herpes simplex and CMV, with varicella-zoster being less common and other viruses even rarer.[29-31] In one autopsy series, 80 percent of patients with visceral herpes simplex had esophageal ulcers.[32] They found that many of these patients were asymptomatic premorbidly. They also found that the mucosa could appear normal in these patients even with a positive biopsy for herpes. CMV infections may be more common in patients with transplants and with AIDS. Ten percent or more of patients have CMV or herpes esophagitis following liver or kidney transplantation.[33] More than 90 percent of AIDS patients are infected with CMV and have evidence for dissemination at autopsy.[34-36] Viral esophagitis occurs in immunocompetent patients as well.[3,5,6]

Severe odynophagia and dysphagia are the usual presenting symptoms. Many immunocompetent patients give a history of an upper respiratory infection 6 to 17 days prior to the onset of the swallowing problems, and most present with either skin or oral lesions suggestive of herpes simplex.[5] A high antibody titer to herpes simplex is found in these patients, but it is not diagnostic.

A double-contrast barium swallow can be helpful by showing ulcerations (punctate, linear, or stellate), plaques, a cobblestone pattern, or a diffusely shaggy mucosa.[37] Unfortunately, most of these findings are very similar to those seen with *Candida* esophagitis. Endoscopy is a better way to confirm the diagnosis. If the patient undergoes endoscopy very early in the course of the infection, one can see vesicular lesions in herpes esophagitis; however, since these are so short-lived, one is more likely to find only ulcerations. The ulcers may be confluent in the lower esophagus. The isolated ulcer can have a characteristic appearance with a raised yellow border (so-called volcano ulcers).[30] The primary reason endoscopy is better at diagnosis is that it allows one to obtain tissue for culture and histology. Although the culture positivity rate drops dramatically after the vesicular phase in herpes, the tissue still has characteristic histology. Herpes infections have multinucleated giant cells and eosinophilic intranuclear inclusions found in epithelial cells, whereas CMV causes basophilic intranuclear inclusions and periodic acid–Schiff–positive cytoplasmic inclusions in endothelial cells (Figs. 4 and 5).[1] These findings are most commonly located at the edge of the ulcers created by the infecting virus.

Complications from viral esophagitis include hemorrhage, fistula formation, dissemination, and superinfection.[38,39] Late complications, such as stricture, seem to be rare or nonexistent. *Candida* has been commonly described in association with herpes simplex.[4] The *Candida* is usually in the base of esophageal ulcerations with histologic evidence of herpes at the margin of the ulcers. It is believed by most investigators that the herpes virus is the primary infection and that the *Candida* has colonized the ulcer base in those with both organisms present.

Treatment for viral esophagitis is less clear than for *Candida* and probably less effective. Immunocompetent patients require no specific antiviral therapy, only symptomatic treatment with antacids and analgesics. The immunosuppressed patient with herpes simplex can be treated with either intra-

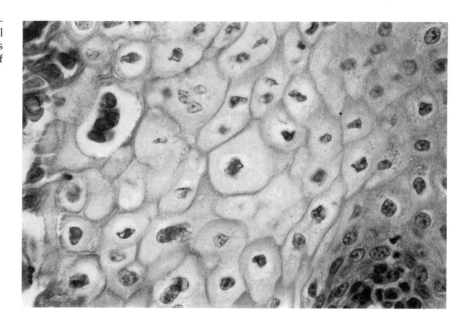

FIGURE 4 High-power view of esophageal biopsy showing multinucleated squamous cells and nuclear inclusions typical of herpes.

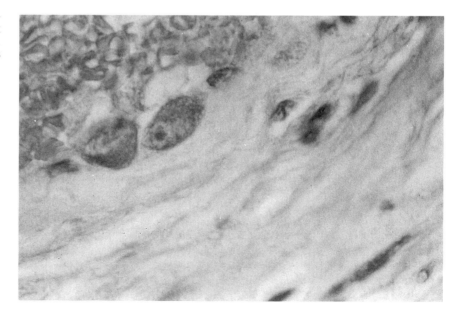

FIGURE 5 Esophageal biopsy showing the typical nuclear inclusion bodies and cytoplasmic granules of cytomegalovirus in an endothelial cell.

venous adenine arabinoside (Ara-A, vidarabine), acyclovir (9-[(2-hydroxyethoxy)methyl]guanine), or foscarnet (trisodium phosphonoformate). These agents are effective for visceral herpes infections, but the minimal side effects seen with acyclovir compared with vidarabine make it the agent of choice.[40-43] The treatment of herpes esophagitis with acyclovir has been quite successful.[30,39] The usual dose of acyclovir is 750 mg per square meter per day intravenously in divided doses. Resistance to acyclovir has been thought to be of little consequence until recently. Acyclovir-resistant herpes simplex virus infections have been described in patients with AIDS.[44,45] The resistance is caused by mutants that are either thymidine kinase deficient, have a thymidine kinase with an altered substrate specificity, or have an altered DNA polymerase. It appears that these cases of acyclovir-resistant herpes can be treated successfully with foscarnet.[45]

Until recently, there has been no effective therapy for CMV infections. A new agent, ganciclovir (DHPG, 9-[2-hydroxy-1-(hydroxymethyl)ethoxymethyl]guanine), has been developed and appears to be very effective for CMV infections.[46] In vitro ganciclovir appears to be approximately 50-fold more effective against CMV than acyclovir.[47] The dose of DHPG should be at least 3.0 mg per kilogram per day in three divided doses intravenously, but no more than 7.5 mg per kilogram per day because of neutropenia at higher doses. Ganciclovir can eradicate CMV from some immunocompromised patients.[48] Unfortunately, many immunocompromised patients relapse, and it is likely that these patients will require long-term, low-dose therapy as long as they remain immunodeficient.[49,50] Acyclovir has been used for prophylaxis of herpes virus and CMV with little or no benefit in most studies.[48] Ganciclovir is more toxic than acyclovir, especially with regard to bone marrow suppression, and thus may not prove to be useful for prophylaxis because of its toxicity.[48] Foscarnet has also been used to suppress CMV infections in patients with AIDS, but like ganciclovir it is not capable of clearing the virus from the host in most cases.[51]

Bacterial Esophagitis

Bacteria as a cause of esophagitis has probably been overlooked. Most investigators have thought that bacteria were secondary invaders after the primary infection by the more common organisms that have been discussed above. However, if one defines bacterial esophagitis as finding bacteria invading the mucosa or deeper layers of the esophagus, without any evidence for *Candida*, viral, or other fungal infections, one can find patients with purely bacterial esophagitis. One series found that 11 percent of their endoscopic biopsy series and 16 percent of their autopsy series fulfilled these criteria.[7] The diagnosis is made by doing special stains on the biopsy specimens and by examining them carefully for organisms and signs of invasion. The patients with bacterial esophagitis are usually immunocompromised. The significance of bacterial esophagitis is that it can be a source of bacterial sepsis, and it clearly requires different therapy (antibiotics) than the other forms of infectious esophagitis.

Another bacterial organism that may infect the esophagus is *Campylobacter pylori*. *C. pylori* is a bacterium that has recently been described in association with gastritis and peptic ulcer disease. It is found exclusively in gastric mucosa. Barrett's epithelium is a metaplastic change that occurs in the distal esophagus in some patients with severe gastroesophageal reflux. Since the Barrett's epithelium is gastric-like, one might expect to find these organisms, and indeed they have been identified in adults and children.[52-54] In one series, approximately 40 percent of patients with Barrett's epithelium had *C. pylori* in their gastric mucosa, but a similar frequency was found in age- and sex-matched controls.[52] They also found *C. pylori* in the Barrett's epithelium in 4 of 10 patients with *C. pylori* in the stomach, while 0 of 16 were found to have *C. pylori* in their Barrett's epithelium when there was no *C. pylori* in the gastric mucosa. Another group found that 52 percent of 23 patients with Barrett's epithelium had positive staining for *C. pylori* on biopsy specimens.[53] A child has been described whose *C. pylori*–positive Barrett's ulcer healed only after the addition of amoxicillin to his antireflux regimen.[54]

Other Infections

Cryptosporidium is an intestinal protozoon that can cause severe opportunistic infections in immunocompromised patients. Recently this organism has been identified in the esophagus of a child with AIDS.[55] *Torulopsis glabrata*, a fungus related to *Candida*, has been identified as a cause of esophageal ulcers in a patient with AIDS.[56]

CHAGAS' DISEASE

American trypanosomiasis, or Chagas' disease, is caused by the flagellate protozoon *Trypanosoma cruzi*.[57] The vectors for the spread of this disease are the *Triatoma* bugs. Infected *Triatoma* bugs suck blood from man and animals, after which they defecate on the wound and thus inoculate the host. Dogs, cats, opossums, rats, armadillos, and other rodents serve as the domestic and sylvatic reservoirs for *T. cruzi*. Chagas' disease is found only in the Western Hemisphere from southern Texas to southern Argentina.

Many (10 or more) years after the acute infection with *T. cruzi*, cardiomyopathy, megaesophagus, and megacolon develop secondary to destruction of the nerve plexuses and muscles in these organs. Not all of these complications are seen in every patient. Up to 40 percent of patients with megaesophagus have cardiomyopathy. The megaesophagus is clinically indistinguishable from achalasia. The lower esophageal sphincter pressure is normal to elevated, and there is poor relaxation with deglutition. The esophageal body loses its peristaltic activity and dilates (Fig. 6). The treatment is similar to that used for achalasia. Pneumatic dilatation of the lower esophageal sphincter is as successful for Chagas' disease as it is for achalasia.[58] If dilatation fails, then a Heller myotomy is used to relieve symptoms.

Although the megaesophagus is primarily a late development (less than 2 percent of patients with megaesophagus are under 9 years old), it can be found in infants with what is believed to be a congenital form of Chagas' disease. Only a few cases of infants with megaesophagus have been described, and most have died very young.[59]

a patient who might aspirate because the hypertonicity of the contrast will cause severe pulmonary problems. Barium aspiration is not a major problem unless the volume is large.

Once an abscess is identified, treatment must include (1) elimination of any further soilage of the site of perforation (if this is the cause of the abscess), (2) surgical drainage, (3) broad-spectrum antibiotic coverage (including anaerobes in many cases), and (4) provision of adequate nutrition enterally or parenterally.[65]

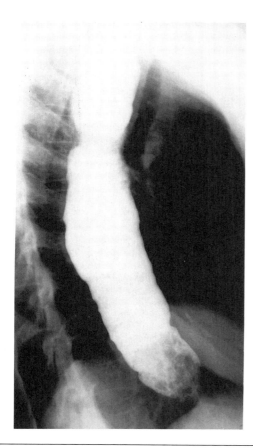

FIGURE 6 Megaesophagus of Chagas' disease. Barium swallow shows dilated, food-filled esophagus with sharp tapering at the gastroesophageal junction. The appearance is grossly indistinguishable from that of achalasia.

RETROESOPHAGEAL ABSCESS

Abscesses adjacent to the esophagus can occur at any level from the pharynx to the gastroesophageal junction. They develop in the majority of cases secondary to perforation of the esophageal wall, although blood-borne infection, complications of surgical procedures, extension from paravertebral abscesses, osteomyelitis of the sternum or ribs, and infected adjacent lymph nodes contribute to the list of potential causes of periesophageal abscesses. Over half of all esophageal perforations are iatrogenic (endoscopy, bronchoscopy, dilatation). The remainder are secondary to external trauma, foreign body ingestion, barogenic rupture (Boerhaave's syndrome), and spontaneous rupture.[60-63]

The diagnosis of periesophageal abscesses or perforations is made with a combination of clinical history, physical examination, standard chest radiographs, water-soluble or barium-contrast esophagrams, and computed tomographic scans of the chest. Careful consideration must be given to the choice of contrast used to evaluate the esophagus. Water-soluble contrast is preferable for diagnosing perforations, since it is better tolerated in an infected mediastinum than barium, but it is less reliable in making an accurate diagnosis.[64] Also, one must never give water-soluble contrast to

REFERENCES

1. MacDonald GB, Sharma P, Hackman RC, Meyers JD, Thomas ED. Esophageal infections in immunosuppressed patients after marrow transplantation. Gastroenterology 1985; 88:1111–1117.
2. Mathieson R, Dutta SK. Candida esophagitis. Dig Dis Sci 1983; 28:365–370.
3. Villar LA, Massanari RM, Mitros FA. Cytomegalovirus infection with acute erosive esophagitis. Am J Med 1984; 76:924–928.
4. Nash G, Jeffrey SR. Herpetic esophagitis. A common cause of esophageal ulceration. Hum Pathol 1974; 5:339–345.
5. Springer DJ, DaCosta LR, Beck IT. A syndrome of acute self-limiting ulcerative esophagitis in young adults probably due to herpes simplex virus. Dig Dis Sci 1979; 24:535–544.
6. Deshmukh M, Shah R, McCallum RW. Experience with herpes esophagitis in otherwise healthy patients. Am J Gastroenterol 1984; 79:173–176.
7. Walsh TJ, Beltisos NJ, Hamilton SR. Bacterial esophagitis in immunocompromised patients. Arch Intern Med 1986; 146:1345–1348.
8. Levine MS, Macones AJ, Laufer I. Candida esophagitis: accuracy of radiographic diagnosis. Radiology 1985; 154:581–587.
9. Wheeler RR, Peacock JE, Cruz JM, Richter JE. Esophagitis in the immunocompromised host: role of esophagoscopy in diagnosis. Rev Infect Dis 1987; 9:88–96.
10. Kodsi BE, Wickeremesinghe PC, Kozinn PJ, Iswara K, Goldberg PK. Candida esophagitis. A prospective study of 27 cases. Gastroenterology 1984; 71:715–719.
11. Trier JS, Bjorkman DJ. Esophageal, gastric, and intestinal candidiasis. Am J Med 1984; 76:39–43.
12. Tavitian A, Raufman JP, Rosenthal LE. Oral candidiasis as a marker for esophageal candidiasis in the acquired immunodeficiency syndrome. Ann Intern Med 1986; 104:54–55.
13. Porro GB, Parente F, Cernuschi M. The diagnosis of esophageal candidiasis in patients with acquired immune deficiency syndrome: is endoscopy always necessary? Am J Gastroenterol 1989; 84:143–146.
14. Klein RS, Harris CA, Small CB, et al. Oral candidiasis in high-risk patients as the initial manifestation of the acquired immunodeficiency syndrome. N Engl J Med 1984; 311:354–357.
15. Raufman JP, Tavitian A, Straus EW. Diagnostic, therapeutic, and prognostic implications of oral candidiasis in patients with AIDS and AIDS-related complex. Dig Dis Sci 1986; 31:476S.
16. DeGregorio MW, Lee WMF, Ries CA. Candida infections in patients with acute leukemia: ineffectiveness of nystatin prophylaxis and relationship between oropharyngeal and systemic candidiasis. Cancer 1982; 50:2780–2784.
17. Young JA, Elias E. Gastro-oesophageal candidiasis: diagnosis by brush cytology. J Clin Pathol 1985; 38:293–296.
18. Levine MS, Macones AJ, Laufer I. Candida esophagitis: accuracy of radiographic diagnosis. Radiology 1985; 154:581–587.
19. Sheft DJ, Shrago G. Esophageal moniliasis. The spectrum of the disease. JAMA 1970; 213:1859–1862.
20. Farman J, Tavitian A, Rosenthal LE, Schwartz GE, Raufman J. Focal esophageal candidiasis in acquired immunodeficiency syndrome (AIDS). Gastrointest Radiol 1986; 11:213–217.
21. Jones JM. Necrotizing candida esophagitis. Failure of symptoms and roentgenographic findings to reflect severity. JAMA 1980; 244:2190–2192.
22. Agha FP. Candidiasis-induced esophageal strictures. Gastrointest Radiol 1984; 9:283–286.
23. Orringer MB, Sloan H. Monilial esophagitis: an increasingly frequent cause of esophageal stenosis? Ann Thorac Surg 1978; 26:364–376.

24. Kantrowitz PA, Fleischli DJ, Butler WT. Successful treatment of chronic esophageal moniliasis with a viscous suspension of nystatin. Gastroenterology 1969; 57:424–430.

25. Fazio RA, Wickremesinghe PC, Arsura EL. Ketoconazole treatment of candida esophagitis—a prospective study of 12 cases. Am J Gastroenterol 1983; 78:261–264.

26. Ginsburg CH, Braden GL, Tauber AI, Trier JS. Oral clotrimazole in the treatment of esophageal candidiasis. Am J Med 1981; 71:891–895.

27. Eras P, Goldstein MJ, Sherlock P. Candida infection of the gastrointestinal tract. Medicine 1972; 51:367–369.

28. Medoff G, Dismukes WE, Meade RH III, Moseo JM. A new therapeutic approach to candida infections. Arch Intern Med 1972; 130:241–249.

29. Buss DH, Scharyj M. Herpes virus infection of the esophagus and other visceral organs in adults. Incidence and clinical significance. Am J Med 1979; 66:457–462.

30. Agha FP, Lee HH, Nostrant TT. Herpetic esophagitis: a diagnostic challenge in immunocompromised patients. Am J Gastroenterol 1986; 81:246–253.

31. Gill RA, Gebhard RL, Dozeman RL, Sumner HW. Shingles esophagitis: endoscopic diagnosis in two patients. Gastrointest Endosc 1984; 30:26–27.

32. Matsumoto J, Sumiyoshi A. Herpes simplex esophagitis—a study in autopsy series. Am J Clin Pathol 1985; 84:96–99.

33. Alexander JA, Brouillette DE, Chien M-C, et al. Infectious esophagitis following liver and renal transplant. Dig Dis Sci 1988; 33:1121–1126.

34. Quinnan GV Jr, Masur H, Rook AH, et al. Herpes virus infections in the acquired immune deficiency syndrome. JAMA 1984; 252:72–77.

35. Macher AM, Reichert CM, Straus SE, et al. Death in the AIDS patient: role of cytomegalovirus. N Engl J Med 1983; 103:1454.

36. Freedman PG, Weiner BC, Balthazar EJ. Cytomegalovirus esophagitis in a patient with acquired immunodeficiency syndrome. Am J Gastroenterol 1985; 80:434–437.

37. Meyers C, Durkin MG, Love L. Radiographic findings in herpetic esophagitis. Radiology 1976; 119:21–22.

38. Rattner HM, Cooper DJ, Zaman MB. Severe bleeding from herpes esophagitis. Am J Gastroenterol 1985; 80:523–525.

39. Fishbein PG, Tuthill R, Kressel H, Friedman H, Snape WJ Jr. Herpes simplex esophagitis. A cause of upper-gastrointestinal bleeding. Dig Dis Sci 1979; 24:540–544.

40. Alford CA. Acyclovir treatment of herpes virus infections in immunocompromised humans. Am J Med 1982; 73:225–228.

41. Meyers JD, Wade JC, Mitchell CD, Saral R, Lietman PS, Durack DT, Levin MJ, Segreti AC, Balfour HH. Multicenter collaborative trial of intravenous acyclovir for treatment of mucocutaneous herpes simplex virus infection in the immunocompromised host. Am J Med 1982; 73:229–233.

42. Van Der Meer JWM, Versteeg J. Acyclovir in severe herpes infections. Am J Med 1982; 73:271–274.

43. Spector SA, Hintz M, Wyborny C, Connor JD, Keeney RE, Liao S. Treatment of herpes virus infections in immunocompromised patients with acyclovir by continuous intravenous infusion. Am J Med 1982; 73:275–280.

44. Erlich KS, Mills J, Chatis P, et al. Acyclovir-resistant herpes simplex virus infection in patients with the acquired immunodeficiency syndrome. N Engl J Med 1989; 320:293–296.

45. Chatis P, Miller CH, Schrager LE, Crumpacker CS. Successful treatment with Foscarnet of an acyclovir-resistant mucocutaneous infection with herpes simplex virus in a patient with acquired immunodeficiency syndrome. N Engl J Med 1989; 320:296–300.

46. Collaborative DHPG Treatment Study Group. Treatment of serious cytomegalovirus infections with 9-(1,3-dihydroxy-2-propoxymethyl) guanine in patients with AIDS and other immunodeficiencies. N Engl J Med 1986; 314:801–805.

47. Stein DS, Verano AS, Levandowski RA. Successful treatment with ganciclovir of disseminated cytomegalovirus infection after liver transplant. Am J Gastroenterol 1988; 83:684–686.

48. Meyers JD. Management of cytomegalovirus infection. Am J Med 1988; 85(suppl 2A):102–106.

49. Laskin OL, Stahl-Bayliss CM, Kalman CM, Rosecan LR. Use of ganciclovir to treat serious cytomegalovirus infections in patients with AIDS. J Infect Dis 1987; 155:323–327.

50. Jacobson MA, Mills J. Serious cytomegalovirus disease in the acquired immunodeficiency syndrome (AIDS). Ann Intern Med 1988; 108:585–594.

51. Weber JN, Thom S, Barrison I, et al. Cytomegalovirus colitis and oesophageal ulceration in the context of AIDS: clinical manifestations and preliminary report of treatment with Foscarnet (phosphonoformate). Gut 1987; 28:482–487.

52. Paull G, Yardley JH. Gastric and esophageal *Campylobacter pylori* in patients with Barrett's epithelium. Gastroenterology 1988; 95:216–218.

53. Talley NJ, Cameron AJ, Shorter RG, Zinmeister AR, Phillips SF. *Campylobacter pylori* and Barrett's esophagus. Mayo Clin Proc 1988; 63:1176–1180.

54. DeGiacomo C, Fiocca R, Villani L, Bertolotti L, Maggiore G. Barrett's ulcer and *Campylobacter*-like organisms infection in a child. J Pediatr Gastroenterol Nutr 1988; 7:766–768.

55. Kaslow PG, Shah K, Benkov KJ, Dische R, LeLeiko NS. Esophageal cryptosporidiosis in a child with acquired immune deficiency syndrome. Gastroenterology 1986; 91:1301–1303.

56. Tom W, Aaron JS. Esophageal ulcers caused by *Torulopsis glabrata* in a patient with acquired immunodeficiency syndrome. Am J Gastroenterol 1987; 82:766–769.

57. Marsden PD. South American trypanosomiasis (Chagas' disease). Int Rev Trop Med 1971; 4:97–121.

58. Raizman RE, De Rezende JM, Neva FA. A clinical trial with pre- and post-treatment manometry comparing pneumatic dilatation with bougienage for treatment of Chagas' megaesophagus. Am J Gastroenterol 1980; 74:405–409.

59. Bittencourt AL, Vieira GO, Tavares HC, Mota E, Maguire J. Esophageal involvement in congenital Chagas' disease. Am J Trop Med Hyg 1984; 33:30–33.

60. Morrison JE, Pashley NR. Retropharyngeal abscesses in children: a 10-year review. Pediatr Emerg Care 1988; 4:9–11.

61. Curci JJ, Horman MJ. Boerhaave's syndrome: the importance of early diagnosis and treatment. Am J Surg 1976; 183:401–408.

62. Bladergroen MR, Lowe JE, Postlewait RW. Diagnosis and recommended management of esophageal perforation and rupture. Ann Thorac Surg 1986; 42:235–239.

63. James AE Jr, Montali RJ, Chaffee V, Strecker E-P, Vessal K. Barium or Gastrografin: which contrast media for diagnosis of esophageal tears. Gastroenterology 1975; 68:1103–1113.

64. Mayer JE Jr, Murray CA III, Varco RL. The treatment of esophageal perforation with delayed recognition and continuing sepsis. Ann Thorac Surg 1977; 23:568–573.

65. Murray PA, Finegold SM. Anaerobic mediastinitis. Rev Infect Dis 1984; 6(suppl 1):S123–S127.

Motor Disorders

Samuel Nurko, M.D.

Abnormalities of esophageal function occur frequently and can be primarily confined to the esophagus or can be secondary to systemic illnesses (Table 1; see Tables 2 and 3). By interfering with the normal progression of food transit from the mouth into the stomach or by failing to provide adequate protection from gastric acid, esophageal motor disorders can be debilitating and even life-threatening. Since the major esophageal functions are to transport food from the mouth to the stomach and to prevent reflux of gastric contents, the main manifestations of disease in this organ are either feeding difficulties or regurgitation. An earlier chapter discusses normal esophageal function and development and presents a general approach to the patient in whom an esophageal motor disorder is suspected. This chapter provides an in-depth discussion of the clinical manifestations of specific disorders in esophageal motility from the perspective of pathophysiology, diagnosis, and management. Because disorders of the oral and pharyngeal phase of swallowing have been described elsewhere in this volume, the following discussion relates mainly to clinical problems of the esophagus and the esophageal phase of swallowing (Table 1). It first focuses on the disorders that affect the upper esophagus (see Table 2) and later on those that affect the rest of the esophageal body and the lower esophageal sphincter (LES) (see Table 3).

TABLE 1
Esophageal Motility Disorders

Disorders that affect the striated muscle predominantly
Cricopharyngeal dysfunction
  Abnormalities of resting tone
  Abnormalities in relaxation
Neuromuscular disorders
  Neurologic disorders
  Muscular disorders
  Neuromuscular disorders
Structural lesions

Disorders that affect the smooth muscle predominantly
Primary esophageal motor disorders
Secondary esophageal motor disorders
  Gastrointestinal disorders
  Congenital malformations
  Collagen vascular diseases
  Neuromuscular disorders
  Infectious diseases
  Exogenous factors
  Other

DISORDERS OF THE CRICOPHARYNGEAL MUSCLE

Problems with the cricopharyngeal muscle usually present like those of the pharyngeal phase and are therefore difficult to differentiate. When there is cricopharyngeal dysfunction the symptoms usually appear shortly after birth or during the first months of life.[1] Repeated aspirations and choking are usual symptoms and can be life-threatening. Cricopharyngeal dysfunction should be suspected in children with pooling of saliva at the back of the pharynx, holding up of barium at the upper esophageal sphincter, and a shelf-like impression at the cricopharyngeal level.[1]

Evaluation of motor dysfunction of the pharyngoesophageal junction suggests two main defects of upper esophageal sphincter motility: (1) abnormalities in the sphincter resting pressure, and (2) abnormalities in the upper esophageal sphincter relaxation.[2]

Abnormalities of Resting Upper Esophageal Sphincter Pressure

Cricopharyngeal Hypertension. The term *cricopharyngeal spasm* was initially introduced after prominent cricopharyngeal impressions were seen by barium swallow.[2,3] Later it was found that clinically or radiographically diagnosed "esophageal spasm" did not correlate with elevated upper esophageal sphincter (UES) pressure measured by manometry.[2] It has been reported that a horizontal esophageal bar can be found in up to 5 percent of adult patients undergoing a barium swallow for all indications[1] and is a frequent radiologic sign in infants.[1,4] There are, however, reports in which the resting pressure of the UES was found to be elevated in patients with globus sensation in the pharynx,[3] although this finding has not been replicated in all patients.[2]

Cricopharyngeal Hypotension. Since tonic closure of the cricopharyngeus is due to tonic myoneural activity, a variety of myoneural disorders may lead to a decreased pressure in the UES. This includes amyotrophic lateral sclerosis, myasthenia gravis, oculopharyngeal muscular dystrophy, dystrophia myotonica, and polymyositis.[5] This hypotension can be diagnosed manometrically but will not be seen by radiography unless the UES weakness is extreme.[2] The clinical significance of UES hypotension is not clearly defined. It is possible that it allows air to enter the gastrointestinal (GI) tract during respiration and also predisposes to tracheobronchial aspiration of the esophageal contents.

Abnormalities of Cricopharyngeal Relaxation

Three types of abnormalities of cricopharyngeal relaxation have been described: (1) incomplete relaxation, (2) premature contracture, and (3) delayed relaxation.[2,6] All these abnormalities may result in dysphagia, and I will consider them separately.

Incomplete Cricopharyngeal Relaxation. Patients with cricopharyngeal achalasia show incomplete UES relaxation after the majority of swallows. Radiographically cricopharyngeal achalasia is characterized by a horizontal indentation on the posterior esophageal wall, with the barium passing the muscle very slowly and the cricopharyngeal muscle appearing to relax poorly.[7] At times there is complete functional obstruction, and no barium passes into the esophagus.[8] Manometric studies have confirmed this incomplete cricopharyngeal relaxation in some patients,[8-10] whereas in others the UES has been shown to relax normally.[1,2] The reason for this discrepancy between radiologic and manometric findings is not clear, although it may relate to the difficulty in studying this region. In children most studies have documented abnormal relaxation by cinefluoroscopy,[7,11,12] although manometric abnormalities have also been described.[13] The largest series in children was reported by Reichert et al[13] in 1977, who described the findings in 15 children. The onset of symptoms began at birth or shortly thereafter in 12 of 15, and the presenting symptoms were complaints of poor eating, throat congestion, choking, coughing, and nasal reflux. Because of lack of suspicion, the diagnosis was usually made at the end of the first year. All patients were diagnosed radiographically, and esophageal motility studies were performed in five, documenting the lack of cricopharyngeal relaxation in all. Abnormal esophageal motility was also noted. It is interesting to note that 10 of 15 patients had an associated disease: four myelomeningoceles and six congenital anomalies associated with CNS involvement. Cricopharyngeal achalasia has also been confirmed manometrically in other studies.[9] Dinari et al,[1] however, reported a child with cricopharyngeal achalasia in which there were radiologic abnormalities but a normal manometry. It has also been reported that cricopharyngeal achalasia may occur in children with Down's syndrome.[14]

Premature Cricopharyngeal Closure. It had been suggested that premature closure of the cricopharyngeal sphincter following deglutition plays a role in the pathogenesis of Zenker's diverticulum.[2] Recent studies, however, have found manometric abnormalities in only some[15] or none of the patients studied.[2] According to the recent manometric data, the universal acceptance of cricopharyngeal myotomy in the management of Zenker's diverticulum has little justification.[16]

In a recent manometric study in children, two patients were found to have delayed pharyngeal contraction with respect to cricopharyngeal relaxation, two were found to have incomplete cricopharyngeal relaxation, and one had both cricopharyngeal inco-ordination and failure to relax.[9] All had gastroesophageal reflux (GER), and one also had incomplete UES relaxation. In all cases of incomplete relaxation, the barium swallow was reported to be abnormal; all five patients had severe swallowing difficulties, and three had an associated syndrome with mental retardation (Russel-Silver

syndrome, 5p⁻ [cri-du-chat] syndrome, and minimal change myopathy).

Other case reports of cricopharyngeal inco-ordination in children have been published.[1,7,17] Some authors have described a "transient cricopharyngeal inco-ordination" that may occur in the newborn period.[18-20] The clinical features resemble tracheoesophageal fistula or laryngotracheoesophageal cleft, and the diagnosis has been made radiographically.[2,18] This "inco-ordination" is usually manifest from birth, and even though sucking is normal, infants may choke or even aspirate. The nature of the problem, however, has not been defined manometrically, although there is a case report in which the manometry was normal.[1]

Repeated aspirations and choking can be life-threatening. The clinical course is variable, and even though it tends to be progressive, with increasing severity in the respiratory complications and increasing nutritional problems, spontaneous improvement has been described, particularly in those in whom no associated anomalies were found.[1,7] Because it is known that some of these infants "outgrow" their inco-ordination, careful attention should be paid to the nutritional state of the infants, and feedings by spoon or gavage may be required until the patients are about 6 months of age, when symptoms usually disappear.[1,18] It should be mentioned, however, that fatal aspiration has been reported.[17,18] In one infant who died, the autopsy showed marked dilatation of the pharynx above the area of obstruction and hypertrophy of the pharyngeal constrictors. Aganglionosis of the proximal third, but not of the distal third, of the esophagus was noted,[18] but no further information is provided.

Delayed Cricopharyngeal Relaxation. If reflex cricopharyngeal relaxation is delayed, pharyngeal contents are propelled toward the upper esophagus before the UES is opened. It has been suggested that a delay in cricopharyngeal opening of more than one-third of a second[2] is associated with pulmonary aspiration. In children with familial dysautonomia (Riley-Day syndrome) the cricopharyngeal opening is delayed,[21] but once the sphincter opens, its opening is complete (unlike patients with cricopharyngeal achalasia).[2] Careful radiologic studies in 11 patients with Riley-Day syndrome have also demonstrated that they have disordered esophageal motility,[22] although it was suggested that the major cause of the disability was the cricopharyngeal abnormality, and others have suggested that the impaired pharyngeal muscle co-ordination creates the problem.[23] No manometric studies of these patients exist.

Delayed cricopharyngeal relaxation had not been shown manometrically until Wyllie et al[6] described two children whose drooling observed with the administration of nitrazepam proved to be secondary to delayed cricopharyngeal relaxation (Fig. 1), providing direct evidence that cricopharyngeal inco-ordination can be secondary to drug administration. They suggest that manometry should be considered in the evaluation of patients taking nitrazepam who have eating difficulties or aspiration pneumonia.

Treatment of Cricopharyngeal Disorders

The treatment of children with swallowing problems has to be directed on the one hand to control the primary problem and on the other to improve the nutritional status.[7]

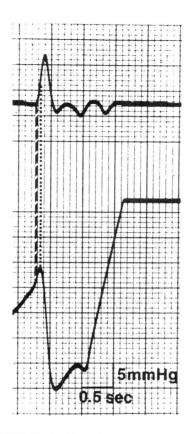

FIGURE 1 Delayed cricopharyngeal relaxation in a patient taking nitrazepam. The upper tracing represents hypopharyngeal contraction (onset at broken line); the lower tracing represents cricopharyngeal relaxation (onset at dotted line). Note that the hypopharyngeal contraction preceded the cricopharyngeal relaxation by 0.3 sec. (From Wyllie et al[6]; with permission of the New England Journal of Medicine.)

The treatment of cricopharyngeal achalasia in adults has ranged from bougienage to surgery.[1,2] The results with bougienage have been unsatisfactory owing to short-lasting effect, so for severe cases cricopharyngeal myotomy has been advocated.[2,24] Decrease in cricopharyngeal pressure occurs,[25] and most patients have relief of the dysphagia.[24] Major complications can occur, since the protective mechanism of the UES is taken away, and in fact deaths from aspiration have been described following myotomy.[24] The experience in children is very limited.[7] Successful dilatation with bougienage has been accomplished both in cases of achalasia[1,12] and in cricopharyngeal inco-ordination.[7,11] Some authors make the observation that, in contrast to adults, even one dilatation in infants and children may be successful in relieving the symptoms.[11] In the largest pediatric series of 15 patients with cricopharyngeal achalasia,[13] six were managed conservatively with nutrition and positioning, four with myelomeningocele had shunt revisions with subsequent improvement in three, four had gastrostomies, and two had tracheostomies. Only two patients underwent cricopharyngeal myotomy, and only moderate improvement was observed.

The smallest patient reported with cricopharyngeal achalasia treated with dilatations was 5 months old at the time of the treatment, and she responded well, without any evidence of obstruction 1.5 years after the procedure.[11] The smallest patient with cricopharyngeal inco-ordination treated with dilatations was 2.5 years and has remained symptom-free for 6 months after the dilatation.[1] There are also case reports of successful cricopharyngeal myotomy performed in children with either cricopharyngeal achalasia[9,12,13] or cricopharyngeal inco-ordination,[9] with good results reported at short-term follow-up. Because of the possibility of spontaneous improvement[1] and the good response reported after dilatation in infants and children,[1,7,11,12] a conservative approach should be undertaken, with aggressive nutritional support[7] and dilatations in those patients with severe compromise,[1] reserving surgery for the difficult patients who do not respond to the above-mentioned management.[1,7,11]

DISEASES THAT AFFECT THE STRIATED MUSCLE PORTION OF THE ESOPHAGUS

Many diseases can produce dysphagia secondary to buccopharyngeal involvement (Table 2). These illnesses can produce abnormalities of the tongue, pharyngeal muscles, cricopharyngeal muscle, upper esophagus, and even at times the lower esophageal body. Therefore, the precise genesis of the difficulty in swallowing may be very complex, involving multiple factors rather than a single one.[2,7] Some selected diseases that cause this type of dysphagia with impact in the pediatric age group will now be described.

Myopathic Disease

Muscular Dystrophies. Dysphagia is rare in most forms of muscular dystrophy, except for two relatively rare types of muscular dystrophies: (1) myotonic muscular dystrophy, and (2) oculopharyngeal dystrophy. The former is the one that can present in the pediatric age group.

Even though myotonic muscular dystrophy usually has its onset in the adult, it begins in infancy or childhood with considerable frequency.[26] It is characterized by myotonia, "myotonic facies," muscle wasting, frontal baldness, testicular atrophy, and cataracts. Pharyngeal muscle weakness is very frequently found in these patients,[23,27,28] although symptomatic involvement occurs in less than half.[2,27] Usually, however, myotonia or other evidence of disease is present for 2 to 15 years before the onset of dysphagia, and in addition to dysphagia these patients also have involvement of the striated as well as the smooth esophageal muscle.[2,23] Pharyngeal weakness of contraction is the predominant finding[2] and reveals itself as barium stasis and hypomotility in the radiograph. The UES may be incompetent and is responsible for the appearance of a continuous column of barium in the pharynx and the upper esophagus.[2,28] Manometric studies reveal reduction in the basal UES pressure and in the amplitude of pharyngeal and cricopharyngeal contractions.[2,23,28]

Inflammatory Myopathies. Systemic diseases in which there is inflammation of the skeletal muscle usually also affect the striated muscle of the pharynx and esophagus. Dysphagia is a frequent symptom in these patients.[2] In a series of 152 patients, dysphagia was present in 54 percent,[29] and

TABLE 2
Esophageal Motor Disorders that Affect the
Striated Muscle Predominantly

Cricopharyngeal dysfunction
   Abnormalities of resting tone
      Hypertension
      Hypotension
   Abnormalities in relaxation
      Incomplete relaxation (achalasia)
      Premature contraction
      Delayed relaxation

Nonesophageal diseases
   Neurologic diseases
      Disorders of the autonomic nervous system
         Familial dysautonomia
      Cerebral palsy
      Motor neuron disease
         Bulbar palsy
         Paralysis of the laryngeal nerve
      Demyelinating diseases
         Multiple sclerosis
      Cerebrovascular accidents
      Poliomyelitis
   Neuromuscular diseases
      Myasthenia gravis
      Botulism
   Muscular diseases
      Muscular dystrophies
         Myotonic muscular dystrophy
         Oculopharyngeal muscular dystrophy
      Inflammatory myopathies
         Dermatomyositis
         Polymyositis
      Metabolic
         Thyrotoxicosis
         Myxedema
   Structural lesions
      Foreign body
      Tumors
      Inflammatory disorders
      Congenital webs
      Extrinsic compression

in about 2 percent it may be the initial symptom.[2] The dysphagia is related to pharyngeal muscle weakness. In one study of six patients with polymyositis and dysphagia, barium appeared to pass the oropharynx with difficulty, and all patients showed retained barium in the vallecula and pyriform sinuses. Transport seemed to be affected only by gravity.[30] Manometric studies have revealed decreased cricopharyngeal pressure, with normal relaxation of the sphincter and poor amplitude of contractions in the pharynx and upper third of the esophagus.[31] It has been suggested that these abnormalities respond to the administration of steroids.[29] Recently it has been reported that these patients may also have abnormalities in the distal esophagus.[32]

Neurologic Diseases

Motor Neuron Disease. This is characterized by degeneration of the upper and/or lower motor neurons. Involvement of the bulbar neurons leads to paralysis of the tongue and the pharynx, which produces abnormalities in the buccal as well as in the pharyngeal phase of swallowing.[2] A recent survey in adults found that 73 percent of patients with motor neuron disease had difficulty in chewing and swallowing, with most problems being related to solid food rather than liquids.[33] Cricopharyngeal abnormalities have been found in adults with motor neuron disease.[23]

Bulbar palsy can occur in children. In the infant this is usually supranuclear, with difficulty in sucking or swallowing and prominent drooling being the frequent symptoms.[18] The jaw jerk tends to be exaggerated, which is a diagnostic clue,[18] and usually a picture of diffuse cerebral palsy and spasticity develops. In the lower motor neuron form of bulbar palsy, there are usually poor suck and nasal regurgitation of the formula. If facial bulbar paralysis is associated with facial diplegia, it constitutes the syndrome of Möbius.

Selective paralysis of the laryngeal nerve has been reported. Dysphagia and altered esophageal motility have been reported, and recovery usually occurs at the end of the first year.[18] Other processes that may induce motor neuron disease, with secondary problems in the pharyngeal and esophageal phases of swallowing, include neurosurgical procedures and tumors that involve the brain stem.[7]

Other Neurologic and Neuromuscular or Muscular Diseases

Myasthenia Gravis. This disease affects the end motor plate of the striated muscle, including the one situated in the esophagus. In children it can present in three clinical forms: (1) transient neonatal myasthenia gravis, (2) persistent neonatal myasthenia gravis, and (3) juvenile myasthenia gravis, which is the most common form.[18] Dysphagia, choking, and aspiration of food are frequent clinical manifestations of the disease.[2] The description of the swallowing difficulty is characteristic: The patient is able to swallow normally at the beginning of the meal, but progressive difficulty appears with each swallow. Manometrically these patients have been shown to have a decrease in the amplitude of peristaltic contractions, mainly in the upper esophagus, with the amount of decrease dependent upon how severely each particular patient is affected.[34] At times the proximal esophageal weakness may be apparent only with repetitive swallows, and cricopharyngeal dysfunction almost never occurs in these patients.[2] The distinguishing feature of this disease is the recovery of the manometric and clinical abnormalities with rest or the administration of anticholinesterase drugs. The intravenous administration of edrophonium chloride (Tensilon) in a dose of 0.2 mg per kilogram, up to 10 mg, produces prompt but transient relief in symptoms and radiographic and manometric abnormalities,[2,23] and it has been suggested that this diagnostic test should be employed in patients who show pharyngeal weakness without any obvious cause, particularly when ptosis is present.[2]

Other Neurologic Diseases. Swallowing difficulties are common in patients with multiple sclerosis.[2] In one study they were reported to occur in 55 percent of the patients, and cricopharyngeal dysfunction has been reported.[35] Even though cerebrovascular accidents are rare conditions in childhood, transient or persistent dysphagia is a frequent manifestation.[2] These problems occur when the lesions involve the swallowing center or the motor nuclei that control the hypopharynx, and the dysphagia may be one of the predominant symptoms.

Poliomyelitis. Bulbar poliomyelitis may cause dysphagia, which is thought to be due to pharyngeal paralysis.[2] There are manometric and radiographic studies in which cricopharyngeal function has been reported to be normal,[36] although other studies, relying mainly on radiographic observations, have reported cricopharyngeal abnormalities and cricopharyngeal achalasia in some of these patients.[2,23] The swallowing problems of these patients have been treated with prolonged nasogastric intubation, cricopharyngeal dilatations, cricopharyngeal myotomy, and even cricopharyngeal denervation, all with good results.[2]

Poliomyelitis is a disease that has been eradicated from many parts of the developed world, but late postpolio sequelae have been reported recently in patients who suffered from the disease many years ago. These late sequelae may occur more than 30 years after the original illness, and new symptoms include unaccustomed fatigue, new joint or muscle pain, new weakness in both muscles affected and those unaffected by polio, and new respiratory difficulties. Recently dysphagia has been noted in nearly 18 percent of polio survivors.[37,38] This new dysphagia is worse for solids, and radiographically it seems to be related to decreased pharyngeal peristalsis.[38]

Botulism. The syndrome of infant botulism is characterized by peripheral muscle weakness, hypotonia, respiratory depression, and diminished suck and swallow.[39,40] Although descending flaccid paralysis of striated muscles is the most striking clinical feature of the syndrome, difficulty in swallowing and delayed evacuation of stool are often initial findings and are often overlooked.[40] The symptoms in this disease result from the irreversible binding of the botulinum toxin to peripheral cholinergic terminals, with the subsequent prevention of the release of acetylcholine at the neuromuscular junctions, as well as preganglionic and postganglionic synapses.[40] In a recent study of four infants with this disease, Cannon[39] reported the results of esophageal motility in these infants. The major effect of the toxin on esophageal motility was the disruption of the UES function and peristalsis in the proximal esophagus. There was a reduction in UES pressure, and a marked reduction in percentage of UES relaxation after swallowing (1 to 20 percent in patients, as compared with 80 to 100 percent in controls). The hypopharyngeal and proximal esophageal contractions were of low amplitude and poorly co-ordinated. Gradual return of esophageal motor function accompanied improvement in peripheral muscle strength and return of the gag and suck reflexes. Interestingly, the botulinum toxin had no significant effect on the LES and the distal esophagus.

DISORDERS THAT AFFECT THE SMOOTH MUSCLE OF THE ESOPHAGUS

Achalasia

Achalasia is a motor disorder of the esophagus that presents as a functional obstruction at the esophagogastric junction (Table 3).[41] It is characterized by the following abnormali-

TABLE 3
Disorders that Affect the Smooth Muscle Predominantly

Primary esophageal motility disorders
Achalasia
Diffuse esophageal spasm
Nutcracker esophagus
Nonspecific esophageal motility disorders

Secondary esophageal motility disorders
Gastrointestinal problems
  Gastroesophageal reflux
  Chronic intestinal pseudo-obstruction
Congenital malformations
  Tracheoesophageal fistula
Collagen vascular diseases
Metabolic disorders
  Diabetes mellitus
  Thyroid problems
Neuromuscular disorders
  Muscular dystrophies
  Myasthenia gravis
  Degenerative disorders
  Autonomic nervous system problems
Infectious disorders
  Chagas' disease
Exogenous factors
  Drugs
  Food
Other illnesses
  Anorexia nervosa
  Graft vs host disease
  Iatrogenic
    Sclerotherapy
    Surgery

ties: (1) increased LES pressure, (2) partial or incomplete LES relaxation, and (3) loss of esophageal peristalsis.[41-43]

The illness is uncommon, with an estimated incidence of one case per 10,000 people.[44] It has been estimated that from all patients with achalasia fewer than 5 percent manifest symptoms before the age of 15.[41,45-49] Moersch[45] reported that out of 690 cases seen in the Mayo Clinic, only 12 (1.7 percent) presented in the pediatric age group. Olsen et al[47] reported that there were only 17 children (2.8 percent) out of 601 patients treated by him. In a recent epidemiologic study of achalasia in English children, Mayberry and Mayell,[50] based on a study of 129 children, determined that in Eire the incidence was 0.31 cases per 10^5 children per year and in England it was 0.11 per 10^5 children per year. No such epidemiologic information is currently available about children in the United States.

Etiopathogenesis

Numerous theories exist regarding the pathogenesis of the condition. Theories suggesting that the defect is neurogenic, myogenic, or hormonal have been postulated.[51] In the United States the great majority of cases have no known cause,[52] although in certain parts of the world Chagas' disease of the esophagus can give achalasia,[53,54] and achalasia has also been diagnosed in certain cases of carcinoma.[55,56]

In idiopathic cases of achalasia the incomplete relaxation of the LES is believed to be secondary to the fact that the postganglionic inhibitory nerves are either absent, reduced in number, functionally impaired, or lacking in central connections.[57,58] The disease seems to involve the Auerbach's plexus,[52] and absence of ganglion cells from the myenteric plexus in the dilated portion of the esophagus with normal ganglion cells in the distal nondilated segment has been described.[52,59] Ganglion cell degeneration appears to be prominent in the early years of the disorder, with progressive loss of neurons detected after a decade or more.[60] This progressive lesion of the plexus is accompanied by progression of the disease.[52] Even though the most consistent neuropathologic lesion has been the ganglion cell degeneration or loss in the esophageal myenteric plexus, these findings are not a constant feature, and multiple instances of normal ganglion cells have been described.[51] In a prospective study of 17 patients with achalasia who underwent surgical myotomy, Csendes et al[54] reported complete disappearance of ganglion cells in 94 percent and a decrease in the number of neurons with marked inflammatory infiltrate in 6 percent.

Many reports in children have found absent ganglion cells in the distal esophagus.[61-63] However, some other authors have described normal histology in some children with achalasia,[51,64] or adequate numbers of ganglion cells but extensive perineural fibrosis.[65]

Other neuropathologic findings that are frequently although inconstantly described include chronic inflammatory infiltrates in the myenteric plexus and degenerative changes in the smooth muscle or nerve fibers.[60] These findings could be secondary to neuronal degeneration and loss or to confounding variables.[60]

Most studies have noted no changes at the light microscopic level in the vagus nerves,[60] although other authors show evidence of nerve fiber degeneration at the electron microscopic level[52,66,67] in the vagus nerve and its dorsal motor nuclei. Electron microscopic studies on the muscle wall of achalasic LES[67,68] have confirmed the specific nerve tissue damage, which light and electron microscopic studies on the intrinsic and vagal innervation of the LES had previously demonstrated.[66,68,69] The evidence of histopathologic studies points then to a primary neurogenic abnormality in patients with achalasia.[52,66,67]

Indirect evidence for the lack of inhibitory innervation in patients with achalasia has also been provided by recent hormonal studies. It was initially shown that in the cat[70] the effect of cholecystokinin-octapeptide (CCK-OP) on the LES involves two different opposing mechanisms: On the one hand, it elicits an indirect inhibitory effect by stimulating inhibitory nerves that mediate physiologic LES relaxation, and, on the other, it also has a direct excitatory effect by stimulating excitatory receptors located on the LES smooth muscle. In intact cats the net effect of CCK-OP administration is LES relaxation, but after pharmacologic denervation with tetrodotoxin, CCK-OP produced LES contraction. In normal human volunteers the administration of CCK-OP results in LES relaxation.[58,70,71] Dodds et al[57] showed that when CCK-OP is administered to patients with achalasia there is a paradoxic LES contraction in 90 percent of the patients, in contrast to the normal LES relaxation obtained in normal people, suggesting that this LES contraction in the patient with achalasia may be the result of the postganglionic inhibitory denervation of the LES that has been described in the cat.[58,67]

Most indirect evidence comes from the observation that vasoactive intestinal peptide (VIP), which is considered a prime candidate as one of the inhibitory neurotransmitters involved in LES relaxation,[72] has been found to be reduced or completely lacking in patients with achalasia.[73,74] It has also been shown[67] that the nerve endings in patients with achalasia are rare, contain few synaptic vesicles, and are particularly lacking in the large granular ones, which are those considered to contain VIP.

It is important to stress that all the alterations described above may represent a primary event or may be secondary to defects in synaptic or neuromuscular transmission owing to defective transmitter synthesis, release, or metabolism, and further studies are necessary to delineate these possibilities.

Even though the main problem seems to be neurogenic in origin, minor changes in the smooth muscle of the esophagus have also been noted.[52,75] These changes seem to be secondary to neurogenic problems.[75] It has recently been suggested that the interstitial cell of Cajal (ICC) could also be involved in the pathogenesis of achalasia.[68] These authors found that the ICCs present in patients with achalasia are fewer in number and more highly modified than those in normal patients or patients with other esophageal disorders. Because their function is not known, it is difficult to know which role they play, if any, in the pathogenesis of achalasia.

It has usually been considered that the denervation is confined to the esophagus in patients with achalasia. Dooley et al,[52] however, found that in 7 of 13 patients with achalasia, there was also evidence of gastric (decreased acid production) and pancreatic (decreased pancreatic polypeptide release) denervation.

Genetics

The etiology of achalasia is unknown. The influence of genetic factors remains to be assessed, but the clustering of esophageal motor disorders in families has led to the suggestion that genetic factors may play an important role in the etiology of the disease. Many cases of achalasia in siblings have been reported, and inheritance as an autosomal recessive trait has been suggested because of the lack of consistent vertical transmission, the clustering of cases in families, and the occurrence of the disease in father and son.[76-78] There is one report in which lack of concordance of achalasia in monozygotic twins was described,[79] although the follow-up was only 3 years. In a later report the first documented cases of achalasia in monozygotic twins were described; the interval between the development of the disease in both was 12 years.[78] Although some of these findings point to genetic influence, no precise mode of inheritance is evident.

Associated Conditions

Achalasia has been associated with ACTH insensitivity and alacrima.[80-82] Usually the first manifestation is alacrima since birth, with the adrenal insufficiency manifesting after the first year and the achalasia presenting later (in one case at 6 years of age).[80] Different explanations have been suggested for these associations. It has been shown that the adrenal defect appears to be due to a receptor abnormality, with ACTH resistance in the zonae fasciculata and reticularis but normal response in the zona glomerulosa.[80] The neurologic defect responsible for the association between the alacrima and achalasia and its relationship with the adrenal defect remain unclear, although it has been postulated that an abnormality in the parasympathetic function is responsible.[80,82] Achalasia has also been associated with an autosomal recessive syndrome consisting of deafness, vitiligo, short stature, and muscle weakness.[83]

It has also been suggested that achalasia may be associated with pyloric stenosis, Hodgkin's disease, and Hirschsprung's disease. However, in a survey of 126 patients with achalasia and their first-degree relatives, it was found that there was no increased incidence of these conditions in either the patients or their relatives.[84]

Clinical Presentation

The usual age of presentation in adults is during the third and fourth decades of life. In a literature review of 167 patients, 57 percent were older than 6 years, with only 22 percent between 1 and 5 years, 15 percent between 30 days and 1 year, and 5.3 percent less than 30 days.[41] Even though it is a rare occurrence, the condition can present in the neonatal period[51,63,85-88] with the youngest patient reported being a 900-g, 14-day-old premature infant.[87,89] The mean age at the time of diagnosis in the pediatric patients, taken from a recompilation of all the pediatric series available (Tables 4 and 5) was 8.8 years (range: neonate to 17 years). The mean duration of symptoms prior to diagnosis was 23 months (range: 1 month to 8 years). It has been suggested that in adults there is a female preponderance, although in children there is conflicting information, with authors describing a preponderance of males,[49,50] no difference,[48] and a female preponderance.[41] From the review, the female-to-male ratio was 1.1 to 1.

Table 4 presents the symptoms of presentation of achalasia in children, taking the 12 pediatric series in which symptoms were reported.[41,48,49,51,61,62,65,76,90-93] There are a total of 159 children. The most prominent symptoms on presentation are dysphagia and vomiting. The dysphagia occurs initially with solids, but as the disease progresses it occurs also with liquids.[46] Patients describe the sensation of food getting caught in the middle to lower chest,[41,49] and the children are usually noted to be very "slow eaters" and to swallow repeatedly in order to get food passed into the stomach.[49,62] Vomiting may manifest initially as food remnants on the child's pillow and progresses to severe vomiting and inability to eat, with consequent weight loss.[41,46,90] The regurgitated food usually looks much like it did when it was swallowed and is not mixed with gastric juice.[45]

In contrast to adults, retrosternal pain does not seem to be a common complaint in children, having been reported in 1 to 50 percent of cases. When present, it is described as sharp and retrosternal and can be aggravated by the passage of food. Weight loss can be severe,[41] and particularly in younger children failure to thrive, aspiration, and recurrent pneumonia dominate the clinical history.[46,62,76] Sudden death from aspiration of esophageal contents has been report-

TABLE 4
Clinical Symptoms in 159 Children with Achalasia

Vomiting	86.2%
Dysphagia	79.8%
Weight loss	68.3%
Failure to thrive	56.2%
Nocturnal regurgitation	52.0%
Substernal pain	36.5%
Nocturnal cough	33.1%
Recurrent pneumonias	27.1%
Odynophagia	16.5%

This table is a recompilation of 12 pediatric series in which symptoms were reported.[41,48,49,51,61,62,65,76,90-93]

ed,[46,85] and overall the respiratory complications in children are more prominent than in adults.[41,46] The diagnosis in young infants can be difficult. The primary manifestations tend to be regurgitation and respiratory problems, so there is an overlap with infants who have other more common conditions like GER.[88]

Methods of Diagnosis

Radiography. A plain chest radiograph may show a widened mediastinum and an air-fluid level and should be a clue to the diagnosis. Another feature that may be present is lack of air in the stomach.[41] Radiographic features in a barium swallow include variable degrees of esophageal dilatation with tapering at the esophageal junction, which is sometimes referred to as beaking (Fig. 2).[41,76,90] The esophageal dilatation may be severe, with the esophagus occupying the whole mediastinum, and it may assume an S-shape, a form that some authors have called the sigmoid esophagus.[46] There may also be absence of peristalsis, tertiary contractions, and failure of LES relaxation.[90] Occasionally an epiphrenic diverticulum may be observed.

Endoscopy. The main clinical use of upper endoscopy in these patients is to exclude a malignancy or another cause of secondary achalasia, so the esophagogastric junction should be carefully examined. Berquist et al[41] reported that all the children with achalasia who underwent endoscopy had esophageal dilatation and that the gastroesophageal junction did not distend with air insufflation. They were able to get into the stomach in all patients. Endoscopy also provides information about the esophageal mucosa before treatment is undertaken, particularly to assess the presence of inflammation or infection.

Esophageal Motility. Esophageal motility remains the study of choice to make the diagnosis, and it provides quantitative information about the severity of the condition and the response to treatment (Fig. 3).[54] Four manometric findings are characteristic of achalasia:

Increased LES Pressure. LES pressure has been described as being elevated, usually twice normal, in the majority of patients.[43,94] It is important to point out that even though as a group patients with achalasia have higher LES pressure, there is enough overlap with normal people that a normal LES pressure does not exclude the diagnosis.

TABLE 5
Treatment of Achalasia in Children*

Author	Procedure	No. of Patients	Complications	Late Results Excellent	Good	Fair	Poor	Late Complications	Comments
Moersch[45]	Hydrostatic dilatation	12	0	12	0	0	0	NR	
Olsen et al[47]	Hydrostatic dilatation	11	0	7	0	0	4	NR	All poor results were in children <9 years old.
Payne et al[91]	Hydrostatic dilatation	17	0	1	1	5	10	Dysphagia 58.8%	Multiple repeat dilatations needed (2–12).
	Modified Heller	5	1 lung empyema	4	1	0	0	0	4 of the 5 failed dilatations.
Paul and Pahlawella[132]	Dilatation with nagus bag	1		0	0	0	1	NR	
	Modified Heller	4	1 perforation	2	2	0	0	NR	
Swenson and Oeconomopoulos[62]	Pneumatic dilatation	6	0	4	0	0	2	NR	All required redilatation after 6 months (mean no. of dilatations 2 [1–3])
	Heller	2	0	2	0	0	0	NR	
Redo and Bauer[131]	Pneumatic dilatation	2	0	2	0	0	0	NR	
	Heller	2	0	2	0	0	0	NR	
Polk and Burford[89]	Modified Heller	5	0	5	0	0	0	0	
Cloud et at[65]	Heller	7	0	6	1	0	0	Dysphagia (1)	1 required dilatation 4 years after surgery.
Tachovsky et al[92]	Modified Heller	14	1 empyema	12	1	1	0	Dysphagia (1) Reflux (1)	All patients had dilatations before surgery. One patient required dilatations after surgery.
Desai et al[61]	Modified Heller	6	1 perforation 1 atelectasis	6	0	0	0	NR	
Ballantine et al[93]	Modified Heller	9	1 intussusception 1 adhesion	7	0	2	0	Reflux (2)	Of the 9 patients, 3 also had a fundoplication. The 2 patients with reflux required a fundoplication.
Azizkhan et al[48]	Pneumatic dilatation (Mosher bag)	20	1 aspiration	2	3	2	13	Dysphagia (15) Reflux (2)	The 5 that improved required an average of 2 dilatations each.
	Modified Heller	12	1 bleeding	11	0	0	1	Dysphagia (1) Reflux (1)	1 required a postoperative dilatation and eventually repeat myotomy.
Accumulated case reports[48]	Modified Heller	20	NR	18	1	1	0	NR	
Boyle et al[49]	Hydrostatic dilatation	10	1 severe pain 2 fever	6	2	0	2	NR	Some of these patients are probably also included in the study by Nakayama.
Berquist et al[41]	Pneumatic dilatation	10	1 oropharyngeal hematoma	6	0	0	4	NR	2 of the patients required more than 1 dilatation. 11 required postoperative dilatations. 4 had myotomy and fundoplication.
	Modified Heller	12	0	1	0	0	11	Dysphagia (8)	
Koch et al[133]	Modified Heller	1	1 paraesophageal hernia	5	2	0	0	Dysphagia (2)	All also had fundoplications.
Buick and Spitz[51]	Modified Heller	15	0	9	3	2	1	Reflux (3)	6 had myotomy and fundoplication. 3 without fundoplication developed GER, and 1 required a fundoplication.
Lemmer et al[76]	Modified Heller	6	0	6	0	0	0	0	3 had myotomy and fundoplication.
Nakayama et al[90]	Pneumatic dilatation	15	1 severe pain 2 fever	11	0	0	4	Dysphagia (4)	4 required myotomy. 7 required 2 dilatations. 1 required 4 dilatations. 1 developed a peptic stricture.
	Modified Heller	8	1 epiphrenic diverticulum	6	2	0	0	Reflux (2)	
Seo and Winter[123]	Pneumatic dilatation	10		4	0	0	6	Reflux (1)	Only study where reflux was with pH probe. 1 developed a peptic stricture.
	Modified Heller	6		4	0	0	2	Reflux (2)	

TABLE 5
Treatment of Achalasia in Children (*Continued*)

Author	Procedure	No. of Patients	Complications	Late Results				Late Complications	Comments
				Excellent	Good	Fair	Poor		
Summary	Pneumatic dilatation	114	8 (7%)	55 (48.2%)	6 (5.2%)	7 (6.14%)	46 (40.3%)	Dysphagia (18) Reflux (3)	Many patients required more than 1 dilatation.
	Modified Heller	140	10 (7.1%)	106 (75.7%)	13 (9.2%)	6 (4.2%)	15 (10.7%)	Dysphagia (13) Reflux (11)	The performance of a fundoplication does not seem to offer a greater benefit.

*This represents a recompilation of all the pediatric series. Note the summary at the bottom.
NR = not reported.

Absence of Esophageal Peristalsis. This lack of esophageal peristalsis is the hallmark of the disease (Fig. 3).[42,43] Usually the aperistalsis involves the entire length of the esophagus, and tertiary waves of low amplitude have been described.[43] If the amplitude of these tertiary contractions is greater than 50 or 60 mm Hg or if three or more pressure waves appear in response to a single swallow, the condition is usually known as vigorous achalasia.[42]

Incomplete or Abnormal LES Relaxation. In normal individuals LES relaxation is usually 100 percent, but in patients with achalasia it usually represents less than 30 percent (Fig. 3).[43] However, the LES may also show complete relaxation. In a study of 23 patients with clinical and radiologic manifestations of achalasia, 30 percent had aperistalsis but complete LES relaxation.[95] This relaxation was of shorter duration than the duration in normal controls, and esophageal emptying in these patients was delayed. It was suggested that they represent early stages of the disease, and one patient had

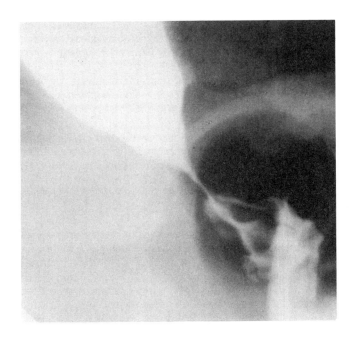

FIGURE 2 Barium swallow in a child with achalasia. Note esophageal dilatation and beaking.

progression from complete LES relaxation to incomplete relaxation over a period of 2 years. In another study of 135 patients without peristalsis, Vantrappen et al noted that 81 percent had incomplete LES relaxation and 19 percent had intermittent normal LES relaxation.[42]

Elevated Intraesophageal Pressure as Compared with Intragastric. This is the result of the functional obstruction at the level of the LES, and it is usually a useful clue to the diagnosis. In a study of 50 patients with achalasia, the esophageal pressure was 6.1 ± 0.7 mm Hg higher than the fundic pressure in 45.[94] There was also no correlation between LES pressure and intraesophageal pressure.[94]

It has become apparent that to make the diagnosis of achalasia, absence of esophageal body peristalsis is necessary; other criteria are often fulfilled but are not required.

Manometric abnormalities have been found in even the youngest patients. Asch et al[86] reported an infant who became symptomatic at 2 weeks of age in whom there was no esophageal peristalsis and the LES pressure ranged between 25 and 40 mm Hg.

Repeat manometry is usually not necessary after therapy as long as the symptoms disappear. If manometry is done after treatment, the following changes can be expected: The LES pressure is low. LES relaxation remains incomplete, although it is possible to see complete relaxation following a swallow. It is still controversial whether peristalsis returns after successful treatment. Because treatment fails to correct the underlying motility disorder, it has always been assumed that the therapy is palliative at best and that the peristaltic defect is a permanent one.[96] There are case reports in which return of peristalsis has been documented after pneumatic dilatation (PD).[42,96-99] In one study it was found that aboral peristalsis returned in 22 of 69 patients with achalasia after PD.[42] In another study of 34 patients treated successfully with PD, it was found that in 20 percent there was return of distally progressive contraction waves following therapy.[96] There are also reports of return of peristalsis after successful myotomy,[99] and there is one report of a 14-month-old child with achalasia in whom esophageal peristalsis returned 6 months after she underwent a Heller myotomy.[97] This "return of peristalsis" has been explained as secondary to a reduction in the diameter of the esophagus (allowing the perfusion catheter to detect the pressure waves) as a result of dilatation or surgery, rather than to a reversal of the degenerative process of the esophageal neurogenic structures.[42,99] Recent studies, however, have found that there was no correlation between the return of peristalsis and clinical

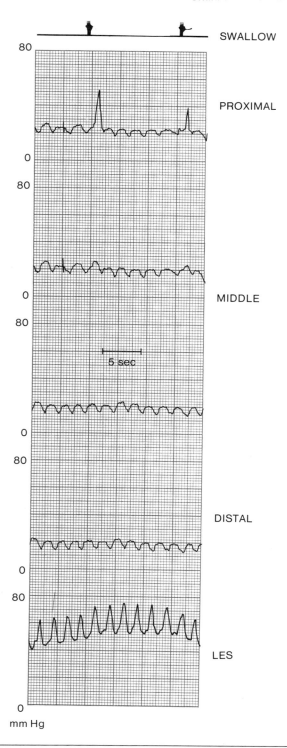

FIGURE 3 Esophageal manometry in a patient with achalasia. Note the high LES pressure, the lack of LES relaxation, and the lack of peristalsis.

status, the decrease in LES pressure, or the radiographically measured diameter of the esophagus.[96]

Radionuclide Tests. Recently radionuclide tests have been used as a screening tool to assess esophageal emptying, particularly before and after therapy. The most commonly used method involves the ingestion of a solid meal labeled with ^{99m}Tc-sulfur colloid,[100] although it can also be done with the ingestion of liquid. They have also been useful in the differential diagnosis of achalasia and other conditions like scleroderma because the pattern of retention is different, with the patients with achalasia retaining the tracer even in the upright position.[101] It is becoming clear that esophageal emptying studies using radionuclide techniques are a simple and noninvasive way to evaluate these patients and the result of the operation.[100] The value of radionuclide esophageal emptying studies in the clinical follow-up of these patients remains to be determined. They do not, however, provide a way accurately to predict eventual success in individual patients, and they do not seem to be better than the symptom scores.[100] They do remain a useful, objective way to study esophageal function that may have an important future role in the objective outcome when comparing different treatments.

Provocative Tests. Two provocative tests have been used in the past to diagnose achalasia: the Mecholyl test and the adminstration of CCK-OP.

The adminstration of acetyl-beta-methacholine (Mecholyl) in patients with achalasia produces a rise in esophageal baseline pressure and the occurrence of high-amplitude, repetitive contractions in the esophageal body. Dodds considers the Mecholyl test abnormal if there is a rise in esophageal pressure of greater than 25 mm Hg lasting for at least 30 seconds within 8 minutes after methacholine chloride (5 to 10 mg subcutaneously).[58,102] It is contraindicated in patients with asthma or heart disease, and the unpleasant cholinergic side effects and pain do not justify its routine use.

The administration of CCK-OP (see above) has been shown to produce paradoxical contraction in 90 percent of patients with achalasia.[58] In a study of 24 patients, CCK-OP produced paradoxical contraction in 21 and LES relaxation in six of seven controls. They compared these results with those obtained after the Mecholyl test and found that they both gave a similar percentage of positive responses (90 percent of patients with achalasia had abnormal contraction). If both tests are combined, in 94 percent of patients either one or the other was abnormal.[58] The CCK-OP paradoxical response is not specific for achalasia, because it might be expected to induce LES contraction in any condition in which the innervation to the LES is impaired, as in Chagas' disease, diabetic neuropathy, and the neuronal form of pseudo-obstruction.[58] This test has not been used in children, and the exact clinical role of both provocative tests in children remains to be determined, so their routine use should be avoided.

Differential Diagnosis

Achalasia has to be differentiated from other organic causes of esophageal obstruction, particularly benign or malignant neoplasms and benign strictures.[46] Payne et al[91] mention two children with clinical diagnosis of achalasia who underwent surgical exploration and were found to have leiomyomas of the distal esophagus. Usually endoscopy and biopsy are the methods of choice to exclude this condition. In adults, a condition mimicking manometrically proven achalasia secondary to carcinoma has been described,[55,103] but this has not been found in children. Even though adenocarcinoma of the stomach is the most common tumor presenting as achalasia, even extraintestinal tumors like oat-cell carcinoma of the lung and pancreatic carcinoma have been reported.[55]

Chagas' disease has to be part of the differential diagnosis in areas where it is endemic, particularly in South America.[104] The disease occurs from neuronal damage by the parasite *Trypanosoma cruzi*. The pathologic description of the megaesophagus seen in Chagas' disease consists of neuronal destruction of Auerbach's plexus, and this can also be seen in other parts of the GI tract and can also manifest as megacolon.[53] The LES of patients with Chagas' disease has been studied by esophagomyotomy (EM), and the denervation has been attributed to direct infection by the trypanosoma, and the changes observed in the smooth muscle and nerve endings are very similar to those reported in patients with idiopathic achalasia.[68] Usually the damage to the neural plexus of the esophagus occurs late in the disease, and there seems to be a correlation between the severity of the ganglion cell destruction and the symptoms.[104]

Recently patients originally diagnosed as having anorexia nervosa were shown manometrically to have achalasia.[49,105] In one study,[105] esophageal motor activity was investigated in 30 consecutive patients meeting standard criteria for the definition of anorexia nervosa, and it was found that seven had achalasia instead of primary anorexia nervosa. Analysis of their data shows that dysphagia for solids and liquids, as well as spontaneous vomiting and regurgitation, was more common among patients with abnormal esophageal motor function. Of interest is the fact that four of the seven patients with achalasia underwent mechanical dilatation with subsequent disappearance of the symptoms. Two other patients with achalasia were successfully treated with nifedipine. It is important to emphasize that the evaluation of the patients suspected of having primary anorexia nervosa should always include careful assessment of upper GI function and, when clinically indicated, of esophageal motor activity.

Treatment

The goal of therapy is to relieve the functional obstruction at the level of the LES. Table 5 shows the published reports of treatment of achalasia in children. Diet has no role in the primary treatment of the disease,[62] although a soft diet encourages more rapid esophageal emptying,[106] and elevation of the head of the bed helps prevent nocturnal regurgitation.[106] Nutritional rehabilitation, on the other hand, has to be an important part of the overall management of the patient.

Pharmacologic Treatment. Anticholinergic drugs have been found to be of no value.[62]

The manipulation of esophageal motility disorders using pharmacologic therapy was unsuccessful until reports on the use of isosorbide dinitrate and nifedipine[107] appeared. Nitrates have the effect of relaxing the smooth muscle,[107,108] and nifedipine is a calcium entry blocker; since Ca^{2+} is directly responsible for the activity of the myofibrils and consequently the tension generated, their use in reducing the LES pressure seems logical. Their usefulness, however, remains limited.[51]

Isosorbide dinitrate (5 to 10 mg) has been shown to cause a significant LES relaxation in patients with achalasia and

has allowed most patients to eat normal meals.[107] This improvement has been confirmed manometrically and with radionuclide esophageal transit measurements.[107] In one study the mean LES pressure fell from 47.3 ± 2.7 mm Hg to 15.3 ± 1.8 mm Hg.[109] The LES began to drop almost immediately, reaching its lowest level after 15 minutes and lasting for 60 minutes, although the clinical improvement lasted for 2 or 3 hours, permitting the ingestion of a meal. Long-term use of the drug is associated with a high incidence of either side effects, particularly headache in up to one-third, or early or late failure to respond, raising to 50 percent the number of patients who have some problems with this drug.[109] In a report of 15 adult patients, five received isosorbide dinitrate therapy successfully for 8 to 15 months.[107]

Nifedipine has been shown to decrease LES pressure and the amplitude of the esophageal contractions in normal volunteers.[110] Studies in patients with achalasia[107,110-113] have shown that nifedipine (10 to 20 mg) significantly decreases LES pressure and improves esophageal emptying. The 10-mg dose decreased LES pressure maximally about 19 minutes after administration, and the average decrease in LES pressure was 18 mm Hg, as compared with 16 minutes and a drop of 32 mm Hg after a 20-mg dose.[111] Nifedipine also decreases the amplitude of esophageal contractions.[114] A report of long-term use of nifedipine[111] from 6 to 18 months showed excellent response in two-thirds of the patients, and rare side effects that included venous dilatation, ankle swelling, heat, and systemic hypotension in one case, all appearing soon after ingestion of the drug. In all cases, with continued use the side effects either disappeared or decreased in severity. A comparison between isosorbide dinitrate and nifedipine[107] in adults showed that isosorbide had a more pronounced effect on symptomatic relief, early LES pressure fall (63.5 percent versus 46.7 percent), and improvement of esophageal emptying, as compared with nifedipine. These aspects, however, become blunted because of the higher incidence of side effects and of failure to respond with isosorbide.

The experience in children is limited, consisting mainly of case reports.[51,112,113] In the largest report four adolescents were administered 10 mg of nifedipine 15 minutes before each meal and before esophageal manometry.[112] In all cases there was a good clinical response and a manometrically proven fall in LES pressure. Two children developed mild transient headaches, and it was noted that they all experienced a recurrence of their symptoms if the medication was not taken.

The role of long-term pharmacologic therapy remains to be determined. It clearly has a role in patients in whom pneumatic dilatation or myotomy is contraindicated,[115] to achieve some weight gain before more aggressive therapy,[107] and for various reasons when definitive therapy has to be postponed, such as to wait for school vacation.[112]

Nonpharmacologic Treatment. There have been two main successful modalities to decrease the high pressure in the LES and to relieve the functional obstruction. One is surgical, with an esophagomyotomy (EM) and the other involves forceful pneumatic dilatation (PD). In a simple way they can be thought of as an approach that tries to relieve the obstruction from the exterior of the esophagus (surgery) and as an approach to do it from within the lumen (PD).

Dilatation. The use of bougienage has been uniformly disappointing,[41,48,90,91] and in one series an incidence of 6 percent of esophageal perforation was described.[116] Payne reported the use of bougienage in eight children, in whom it rarely provided more than very temporary relief.[91] Because of the short-term benefits and the complication rate, this type of therapy is no longer advocated.

PD consists of positioning a dilating device at the level of the LES, with the purpose of inflating it to apply direct pressure on the esophageal muscle to the muscle fibers of the LES.[41,51] It is interesting, however, that in experimental animals there is no evidence that the muscle fibers actually tear and not just stretch. Vantrappen and Janssen[117] have subjected dogs and monkeys to balloon dilatation of the LES, and histologic examination failed to distinguish sphincter segments of treated animals from those of controls.

The method that we currently employ uses the recently introduced microvasive balloons, which have a predetermined maximum diameter of inflation. To determine the size of the balloon to use, first the diameter of the esophagus is measured from the barium swallow. Three-fourths of that distance is usually the size of the first dilator used. In young children, general anesthesia is used. To introduce the dilator, a guide wire is placed through the biopsy channel of the endoscope into the stomach. The endoscope is then removed, leaving the guide wire across the esophageal junction. The position is then checked fluoroscopically. The dilating bag is introduced over the guide wire, and the bag is placed so that it is across the LES. The bag is then inflated rapidly with contrast so that it can be observed fluoroscopically. It is then maintained inflated for 1 minute and then deflated. The procedure is repeated, the dilator is removed, and a repeat endoscopy is performed. Other methods employed have included the use of the Mosher bag, the Browne-McHardy dilator, and others. These dilators increase in size depending on the pressure applied and do not have a predetermined diameter. The Browne-McHardy bag, however, has a nylon sac that limits the amount of distention. The pressure and the duration of the distention vary from center to center.[106,118] In adults[118-120] and in many pediatric centers, the PD is performed under intravenous sedation.[49,90] In younger children it is difficult to ensure that movement will be restricted, so general anesthesia may be safer.

The results of PD in adults have been satisfactory, with an overall response rate that varies from 60 to 95 percent,[118,121] depending on the technique used. It has also been reported that if the first dilatation is unsuccessful, 38 and 19 percent improve after a second or third dilatation.[47] It has been observed, however, that patients who have poor results originally or a rapid recurrence of their symptoms respond less to subsequent dilatations.[47] In a report of their experience with 455 dilatations Vantrappen and Hellemans[118] found that 77 percent of patients had excellent results, 8.7 percent had moderate results, and 14.4 percent had poor results. There was an overall improvement in 93 percent of the patients. In 41 of the patients symptoms recurred and another series of dilatations had to be performed, and approximately 50 percent of those had a good or excellent result.

The results of dilatation in children have been variable and are difficult to compare because of the different techniques used. PD has been used successfully in children for a variety of conditions other than achalasia, particularly for peptic strictures, anastomotic strictures, and restrictive Nissen repairs.[122] The use of PD for achalasia in children was first reported by Moersch in 1929.[45] As can be seen in Table 5, many authors have used PD with varying results. Overall there are approximately 114 children reported, in whom there was an overall improvement rate of 53.4 percent (61 patients). Of course, it is difficult to compare different studies and techniques, and the rate of improvement after PD among the different series varies from only 35 percent[48] to 100 percent.[45] Moreover, like adults, many children require more than one dilatation to respond. Nakayama[90] reported that of his 15 patients, seven responded to one dilatation, seven required two, and one required four, and in the patients who failed, the duration of symptom relief was much shorter than in patients with good response (6 weeks versus 18 months). It has also been suggested that if symptoms recur after PD in the first 6 months, the patient is likely to require a second dilatation[41] or eventually surgery.[123] Some authors have suggested that children who respond to PD are older than 9 years,[48] although many reports of successful PD in children younger than 5 have appeared.[41,124]

In a prospective manometric study in children, Seo and Winter[123] found that the mean LES pressure before therapy was 93 mm Hg, and after PD it was 46 mm Hg, as compared with 8 mm Hg after myotomy. Originally it was also suggested that after a failed myotomy a PD had a prohibitive risk. This, however, has not been the recent experience even in children,[41] five of whom underwent successful PD without complications after myotomy. Although both PD and EM are safe procedures with very low complication rates, both are potentially dangerous.[90]

Esophageal perforation after PD has been described in 1 to 5 percent of the cases.[51,121] Okike et al,[125] in their study of 899 patients with achalasia, found that the rate of esophageal perforation following PD was 4 percent, and following myotomy it was 1 percent. Reviewing their own experience Vantrappen and Hellemans[118] report an incidence of perforation of 2.6 percent of esophageal perforation and 4.3 percent of other complications (fever, pain, or pleural effusion) in a total of 537 patients with three or four dilatations each. A survey of 1,224 instances of PD for achalasia completed by the American Society of Gastrointestinal Endoscopy noted a 1.8 percent incidence of esophageal perforation.[126] The perforation usually occurs at the anterolateral esophageal wall. The symptoms include severe and persistent chest pain, usually fever, and unexplained tachycardia. Dysphagia and subcutaneous emphysema may also be seen.[127] A plain chest radiograph may reveal subcutaneous or mediastinal emphysema or a left-sided pleural effusion.[127] A definitive diagnosis is made with the use of a water-soluble contrast esophagogram. Some centers recommend the routine use of a postdilatation esophagogram,[128] because there are case reports of an esophageal perforation that was missed because of the paucity of symptoms, resulting in the patients' death.[127] In a prospective series of 41 patients undergoing PD and an early postprocedure esophagogram,[128] it was found that there were two immediate and two delayed esophageal perforations, for a perforation rate of 9.5 percent. This illustrates the fact that delayed perforations of the esophagus can occur and may not be present after the first study, emphasizing the need to closely observe all the patients and to obtain or repeat contrast studies if symptoms develop. By performing early contrast studies they also found six intramural hematomas, one of which progressed to a free perforation and the other five resolved spontaneously. They also showed that there is no correlation between the postdilatation appearance of the esophagus and the clinical outcome, suggesting that the esophagogram should be performed only to exclude complications and not to assess the adequacy of the forceful dilatation or to predict clinical outcome.

The mortality after a perforation has been reported to range from 0 to 50 percent.[118,125,127] Some authors prefer a nonoperative management of esophageal perforations,[118,119] but others continue to advocate aggressive surgical management.[127] In a recent report, Miller and Tiszenkel[127] describe their surgical management of six patients with esophageal perforation after PD. They advocate suturing the perforation followed by a modified Heller procedure, with excellent results. Vantrappen and Hellemans[118] report that 10 of 13 patients with esophageal perforation healed with TPN and broad-spectrum antibiotics for 2 weeks. In four of them a pleural effusion was evacuated by puncture or drainage under local anesthesia. Two other patients needed surgical drainage, and the last patient died. In a summary of the literature, Wong and Johnson[129] found 53 perforations reported, with only 17 patients having undergone surgery. A mortality of 4 percent was noted, and overall 68 percent of the patients were treated conservatively.

The other complication that has been rarely reported after PD is bleeding. In a review of 1,261 cases there was an incidence of 1.1 percent of moderate hemorrhages.[118] There have been no reports of perforation after PD in children. There were eight (7 percent) complications, which included one aspiration pneumonia (0.87 percent),[48] two children with severe pain (1.75 percent),[49,90] four children with fever (3.5 percent),[49,90] and one child with an oropharyngeal hematoma.[41]

Careful attention to placement of the dilator under fluoroscopy and pressure applied to the bag distending the esophagus minimizes complications after PD.[90] Fever or excessive pain in the chest or back following the procedure demands more careful evaluation. An esophagogram with water-soluble contrast should be performed, and if there is a major leak, thoracotomy should be employed, but if it is small most authors would treat conservatively with intravenous antibiotics and parenteral nutrition.[118,119]

GER can be a late complication of PD. This complication has been described in adults to range from 1 to 9 percent.[119] In one series of children, it was reported that two developed disabling reflux after PD,[48] and another reports an incidence of 12 percent, compared with 36 percent after myotomy.[123]

The successful dilatation of two children older than 8 years with achalasia has been reported with the use of a new method of transendoscopic dilatation. The results obtained were satisfactory and the follow-ups reported were of 4 months and 1 year, respectively.[130] The role that this method will play in the future remains to be determined, and clinical trials are needed.

Surgery. The surgical treatment varies, but the most common myotomy employed is the Heller myotomy and its variants, which consist in either a thoracic or an abdominal approach and a vertical incision of the esophagus extending along the serosal surface of the distal esophagus and tran-

secting the circular muscle fibers that make up the LES. Most of the different variations have to do with the length of the myotomy.[120]

Good to excellent results have been obtained after myotomy in 64 to 94 percent of adult patients.[113,125] In their report of 468 patients with achalasia who underwent myotomy, Okike et al[125] reported excellent to good long-term results in 85 percent of the surgically treated patients, as compared with 65 percent of a group of 431 patients treated by PD.

As can be seen in Table 5, from 140 children reported, 75.7 percent had excellent results and 9.2 percent had good results, giving an overall improvement rate of 84.9 percent. The improvement rate varies among series, going from as low as 10 percent[41] to as high as 100 percent.[89,92,131–133] The youngest patient reported after a successful myotomy was 6 weeks old,[63] and there are numerous reports of infants less than 6 months old with satisfactory results after myotomy.[88] The results after surgery are not uniformly good. In the series of Berquist et al[41] of five patients who underwent a myotomy as primary therapy, four had recurrence of symptoms 1 month to 5 years following surgery, and either repeat dilatation or surgical intervention was necessary to relieve the symptoms.

When surgery has been performed after failed PD, the results have been satisfactory, and previous dilatation does not seem to alter the response to surgery. Furthermore, the literature shows that after a failed dilatation, surgery is usually successful.[90,125] It has been reported, however, that when surgery is performed after dilatation the distal esophagus is firm and fibrous, making the separation of the muscular layer more difficult, and usually requiring opening of the mucosal layer.[120]

Esophageal perforation can also be a complication of myotomy. Most commonly it is secondary to inadvertent perforation of the mucosa at the time of the myotomy, which occurred in 14 percent of 502 collected cases.[118] Such a perforation can be closed with one or two sutures. Nevertheless, in 2 percent of those 502 patients and 1.7 percent of other series, it resulted in a fistula formation.[117,118,125] As can be seen in Table 5, there was a 1.42 percent incidence of perforation in the pediatric series.

Other rare complications include phrenic nerve paralysis, massive hemorrhage, and necrosis of the stomach and esophagus due to herniation.[118] The overall rate of severe complications after myotomy is said to be 3 to 4 percent.[118]

As can be seen in Table 5, there was an incidence of 7.1 percent of complications after EM. There were two perforations (1.42 percent)[61,132] and one of each of the following: lung empyema,[91] atelectasis,[61] intussusception,[93] adhesion,[93] bleeding,[48] paraesophageal hernia,[133] and epiphrenic diverticulum.[90] There was no mortality.

There are two main long-term complications after myotomy[76]: failure to relieve the obstructive symptoms and GER. Failure to relieve the obstruction is usually secondary to an inadequate myotomy, usually due to failure to carry the muscle division distally enough to divide all of the obstructing circular muscle fibers.[76,134] This has made some authors recommend that the myotomy should include the entire length of the gastroesophageal junction, thus requiring extension onto the stomach cardia for about 1 to 1.5 cm,[76] although different authors recommend different distances,[118] because excessive distal extension of the myotomy onto the stomach contributes to the major long-term complication of myotomy, which is GER.

Significant dysphagia after the operation has been reported in 1 to 9 percent of the patients, although mild dysphagia may be found in up to 20 percent.[129] This dysphagia is most frequently due to incomplete myotomy, and it represents the most frequent indication for reoperation in up to 58 percent of patients.[118,134] In the evaluation of those patients manometry and endoscopy are important to permit the differentiation between an inadequate myotomy (high LES pressure still present) and a complication from the operation (e.g., severe esophagitis and a stricture).[134]

The true incidence of GER is unknown. Most authors' estimates vary from 3 to 21 percent (mean 10 percent) of the cases,[125,134,135] although one suggested that it can be as high as 62 percent.[136] In a long-term study,[137] it was estimated that 52 percent of patients suffered from it. This latter report is important because of the long follow-up, with an average of 7 years. They also report that the incidence of reflux increases with the passage of time, 24 percent after 1 year and 48 percent after 10 years, and becomes stable only after 13 years. In a study of 70 patients after EM, asymptomatic GER was detected in 14.3 percent, symptomatic GER in 8.6 percent, peptic strictures in 5.7 percent, and Barrett's esophagus in 4.5 percent.[135] It is thought that the incidence of GER is related to the surgical technique. The authors with the largest experience have suggested that the anterior myotomy should not extend more than a few millimeters beyond the gastroesophageal junction, as further dissection into the anterior wall of the stomach results in an incompetent gastroesophageal junction.[125,134] In general, less GER is noted in studies which specified that the anterior myotomy extended up to or less than 1 cm from the gastroesophageal junction.[125,134]

The scope of this problem in the pediatric patient is unknown. In a pediatric series of 10 patients studied by pH monitoring, it was reported that GER was present in 36 percent of children post myotomy, as compared with 12 percent after PD,[123] and other series have reported severe and disabling reflux after EM[38,51,90,91] (Table 5).

Peptic strictures can develop as a complication of GER in 3 to 6 percent of the patients.[118,135] Two peptic strictures secondary to disabling GER after myotomy have been described in the pediatric literature.[90,123] Barrett's esophagus has also been described as complication of the GER that can occur after myotomy.[135,138] In one series of 70 patients treated with EM, three cases of Barrett's esophagus (4.3 percent) were found 5, 8, and 15 years after the procedure.[135] In one case an adenocarcinoma was reported to have developed in a Barrett's esophagus many years after Heller's myotomy,[138] and in another two, dysplastic changes were found.[135]

Because of the development of postoperative GER and the severe sequelae that can accompany it, the need to perform an antireflux procedure at the time of the myotomy has been argued by some. This is also controversial and depends on the experience and results of the different surgeons.[118] The point merits careful consideration, particularly if one considers that overall the results from surgical therapy tend to be better, but the long-term outcome can be dramatically affected by GER complications.

One side of the discussion[125,139,140] claims that a precise myotomy carried just onto the stomach relieves dysphagia effectively and does not cause reflux. They also mention that the additional dissection necessary to do an antireflux repair is meddlesome, and the fundoplication runs the additional risk of causing a distal obstruction, thereby defeating the purpose of the myotomy. They suggest that the only indication for an antireflux procedure is the presence of a hiatal hernia. In their long-term follow-up from the Mayo Clinic, Okike et al[125] reported a 3 percent incidence of GER-related complications and suggested that an antireflux procedure is not routinely necessary.

Others[140,141] have recommended the routine use of a fundoplication. They argue that to perform an adequate myotomy a greater area of exposure is necessary and that the use of fundoplication does not change the long-term effectiveness of the surgery but avoids the GER complications. Nissen fundoplications, Belsey and Collins repairs, and anterior gastropexy of Boeremia have been reported with varying degrees of success.[118] Recently it has been suggested that an antireflux procedure should be performed only in certain circumstances: presence of hiatal hernia, presence of pretreatment esophagitis and GER, or when the integrity of the esophageal mucosa is compromised (excision of diverticulum or perforation).[140,142]

The presence of preoperative GER has recently been studied, and it has been suggested that if there is pathologic GER an antireflux procedure should be done at the time of the myotomy.[143] In a prospective study of five patients, it was found that in two reflux occurred 16.8 percent and 53.3 percent of the total time, with prolonged episodes in the supine position. They suggest that an antireflux procedure should be added in patients with prolonged supine reflux. Smart et al[144] caution that the use of preoperative 24-hour pH monitoring may be altered by the presence of food residue. In a prospective study of 17 patients with achalasia before PD, they found that one had evidence of typical episodes of GER by 24-hour pH monitoring, and nine had increased times of acid exposure. They showed that this increased exposure was secondary to lactic acid from food residue and not from refluxed acid, so they conclude that preoperative esophageal pH studies do not offer a valid means for the selection of patients in whom an antireflux procedure should be combined with the cardiomyotomy.

It is difficult to draw conclusions, because it is usually difficult to compare one surgical technique with another. However, in one adult series they compared patients after EM with or without a Nissen fundoplication. Symptoms of GER were present in 10 of 12 patients after EM alone and in none of the Nissen patients, although one developed dysphagia, suggesting that an antireflux procedure should have been done.[145] Recently, however, 24-hour pH determinations were done in a prospective study of five patients who underwent a successful myotomy for achalasia,[146] and they found that even though in two of five patients there was more GER while supine, there was no difference between the patients and the controls in the total amount of reflux or total number of reflux episodes, supporting again the notion that a fundoplication is not routinely necessary.

Some authors have not considered fundoplication necessary when children undergo a myotomy.[48,65,91,92] In some series, however, GER has developed when a myotomy was performed without a fundoplication. Buick and Spitz[51] report nine children who had a myotomy without an antireflux procedure. In six a postoperative barium swallow was obtained, and in three there was symptomatic and radiologic GER, suggesting that a fundoplication might have been useful. Koch et al[133] performed cardiomyotomy and fundoplication in seven children and reported mild intermittent dysphagia in two and excellent results in the rest, with a follow-up of 7 to 18 years. Ballantine et al[93] reported nine children in whom an esophagomyotomy was performed. In three an antireflux procedure was also performed, and of the remaining six, two developed reflux that required surgical correction. They suggest that there is an increased risk for the appearance of reflux with the passage of time. It is not clear how these factors are going to be altered now that potent H_2 blockers are being used and will probably reduce the severity of this complication. It is clear, then, that the argument for the need for antireflux surgery following myotomy centers on the small percentage of patients who develop the complications from GER. Because this percentage is so small and because it is not possible to predict reliably who those patients are going to be, it is probably not necessary to subject all patients to a longer and more difficult procedure to prevent the few cases of troublesome reflux; this is also the latest recommendation from most of the adult series.[139,147]

Obstructive symptoms after a wrap have also been reported as a complication.[134] This could result from the effect of the wrap around an atonic esophagus[41] and may need an additional surgical procedure for its correction.[148] In children this complication has also been described.[41,48,133] This potential complication has led to the recommendation of a partial fundoplication.[51]

Medical Versus Surgical Therapy. The results obtained with either of the two main treatments vary from center to center, and the most extensive experience comes from the adult literature. In one of the largest adult series, the Mayo Clinic[125] reported the results on 899 patients and compared the late results of treatment with dilatation and EM. They concluded that myotomy was more successful and safer than dilatation, with poor results being obtained twice as often with dilatation as with myotomy. Overall the adult experience reports a success rate of 65 to 75 percent after PD, and of 85 to 90 percent after EM.[125] Other series[121] report better results after PD. They report that only 10 percent of patients with achalasia required cardiomyotomy after PD. In deciding the type of treatment to be used one has to understand that it is difficult to compare the results reported from different studies, because usually the techniques used vary among them.[118] There is, however, one randomized prospective study in 38 adults trying to compare both treatments.[120] After a 3.5-year follow-up, 61 percent of the patients in the PD group were free of dysphagia, as compared with all the patients in the surgical group. Thirty-one percent of patients in the surgical group and 7 percent of the patients in the PD group had GER (as defined by positive acid reflux test). The LES pressure after treatment was lower in the surgical group (8.4 versus 15.2 mm Hg). They conclude that because surgical treatment is accompanied by longer symptom relief, it should be the primary treatment, although they do not comment on the pos-

sible long-term problems related to GER in their surgical patients.

As can be seen in Table 5, the experience in children also varies from center to center. Grouping all the studies, with an understanding of the problems inherent in doing so, a few things become apparent. The percent improvement was higher after EM than after PD (84.9 percent versus 53.4 percent), and the complication rate was highly similar (7 percent). It can be noted, however, that the short- and long-term complications after EM were of major severity (including two perforations), compared with the complications after PD.

Both medical and surgical therapies are effective. On the one hand, PD is safe and, unless repeated dilatations are necessary, requires a shorter stay in the hospital. The risk of perforation is always present, and improvement of the dysphagia varies among studies but is probably not as great as that occurring after myotomy. On the other hand, EM generally results in a more complete and longer duration relief of the dysphagia, but GER is a major complication, and a thoracotomy is needed. The cost and morbidity associated with thoracotomy are significant.

Some authors continue to recommend Heller myotomy as the primary treatment of achalasia in children.[51,76,92,93] In contrast, other authors have suggested that because results after PD and EM in children are similar and PD is effective and safe, particularly in older children, PD should be attempted first.[41,48,90]

We recommend that PD be performed first, because it is effective in more than 50 percent of the patients, avoids a thoracotomy, and has a low rate of short- and long-term complications, with a nearly absent mortality. If after two dilatations there is no response, surgery should be done. If after a first successful dilatation symptoms recur, a second dilatation should be performed, and if it fails surgical management is indicated. On the other hand, if the second dilatation is successful and symptoms recur some time later, a third dilatation may be considered first unless the time to recurrence is short. When surgery is indicated, it should be performed without an antireflux procedure unless there is significant GER preoperatively or the presence of a hiatal hernia. Pharmacologic therapy with nifedipine can be used to buy time to prepare for the definitive treatment and to adjust to the child's school schedule.

Long-Term Follow-Up

After successful therapy a recurrence of symptomatic achalasia may develop, even after a symptom-free period of many years.[118] This may occur after either PD or myotomy without any evidence of peptic or stenosing esophagitis. The reason for this is unknown. It may be due to slow progression of the degenerative process of the myenteric plexus and other nervous structures. Some patients seem to be resistant to therapy, and it has been noted that some patients who fail PD respond poorly to myotomy and that forceful dilatations are less successful in patients with previous PD or myotomy.[118]

Esophageal cancer, particularly squamous cell carcinoma, has been considered by some authors to be a late complication of achalasia.[149] Numerous case reports and retrospective reviews have appeared to substantiate the association between achalasia and esophageal carcinoma,[149] with most series estimating an incidence of 5 percent of esophageal carcinoma in these patients.[149-151] Esophageal cancer arises at a younger age in these patients with a mean of 48 years,[149,151] and the mean time from diagnosis of the achalasia to the occurrence of the malignancy is 17 years. In a population-based study,[150] it was estimated that the prevalence of this complication was 1 percent, and an autopsy study reported a prevalence of 1.5 percent.[152] It has been suggested that this complication is more likely in patients who have had a long course without treatment or have failed therapy, raising the possibility that mucosal irritation from stasis of different substances may be an important factor. Because of this possibility, some authors have advocated frequent endoscopy with cytology and biopsy every 3 to 5 years,[153] particularly because any warning symptoms are more likely to occur late as a result of the dilated esophagus. It is also not known what role other risk factors (e.g., alcohol, tobacco) play in the development of this complication.

Recently, however, a prospective study of 100 patients with manometrically proven achalasia was undertaken, and no cases of esophageal carcinoma were identified, although the follow-up was for a mean of 77.6 months (range 6 to 276 months). In the same paper they also describe their retrospective experience with 153 cases of esophageal carcinoma; they found no association with achalasia.[149]

There is currently no information about the incidence of this complication in patients who developed achalasia as children, although so far as we can tell there are no cases of esophageal carcinoma that have arisen in adults who had achalasia as children. At this time, with our current knowledge, it is believed that a surveillance program in adults would not be cost-effective, not only for the amount of psychological trauma that would be inflicted, but also because there are no data showing that such an approach can alter the outcome.[149] It is recommended that diagnostic tests in treated achalasia patients rely on clinical criteria, with particular attention paid to recurrence of symptoms or newly developed dysphagia or pain.[149] Because there is no information about the long-term prognosis of children with achalasia, these children should be followed closely, and the threshold for initiating an evaluation should be low.

Other Primary Motility Disorders

Advances in esophageal manometry and more widespread use of this technique in the evaluation of patients with noncardiac chest pain or dysphagia have shown that patients with primary esophageal motor disorders do not fit into the simple classification of achalasia and diffuse esophageal spasm.[42] A variety of motor alterations have been described in the adult literature, and even though some distinct clinical entities like diffuse esophageal spasm (DES) and nutcracker esophagus have been identified, a larger proportion of patients remain in the category of nonspecific esophageal motility disorders (NEMD).[154]

DES is a primary disorder of the motor activity in the smooth muscle portion of the esophagus.[155] It represents a group of disorders in which there are high-amplitude, repetitive nonperistaltic esophageal contractions. DES is a distinct clinical entity in adults, but its incidence in children is unknown, and there are only case reports.[156] The pathophysiology is still unknown, although it has been suggested that it is the result of damage to the inhibitory esophageal nerves and the consequent increase in excitatory input. In adults this syndrome is characterized by chest pain and/or dysphagia that is usually not progressive or associated with weight loss.[157] Because of the predominance of the chest pain, these patients are usually evaluated first for coronary artery disease.[154] The pain may be initiated by the ingestion of very cold or very hot meals, and dysphagia is usually present in 30 to 60 percent of the patients and, in contrast to the pain in achalasia, it is not constant.[155] The barium swallow may show frequent nonpropulsive contractions indenting the barium column, usually only in the lower third. There may also be delayed transit documented either by radiography or emptying scans. The diagnosis, however, is established manometrically using the following criteria: (1) repetitive simultaneous (nonperistaltic) contractions, at least 10 percent of wet swallows; (2) periods of normal peristaltic sequences; (3) alterations in the contraction waves (increased duration and amplitude), although there are patients who can have normal amplitude; (4) a normal LES in most patients, although incomplete LES relaxation or a hypertensive sphincter has been described.[158] This alteration in the LES and some long-term follow-up of patients with DES confirming the rare evolution of some cases of DES into achalasia suggest that the two disorders may represent points on a continuum of esophageal motility dysfunction.[42,158,159]

In children this is an extremely rare entity.[156,160] In infants the presentation is usually with apnea and bradycardia, and in older children the presentation is similar to that in adults. There is a particularly well-documented case reported by Fontan et al[156] in which a newborn was found to have bradycardia, obstructive apnea, and central apnea, all of which were consistently associated with manometric findings typical of diffuse esophageal spasm. They suggested that the symptoms in this infant were secondary to vagally induced responses because the infant showed immediate decrease in heart rate after esophageal spasms, with lack of a temporal relationship between the apnea and bradycardia, and subsequent good clinical response to the use of anticholinergic medication.

Using the above-mentioned criteria, it is estimated that only 10 percent of adult patients referred for esophageal motility because of chest pain have DES.[157] The most frequent finding is what is now called nutcracker esophagus. This is a clinical entity presenting as noncardiac chest pain and occasionally dysphagia. The barium swallow and radionuclide emptying scans are usually normal, and the diagnosis is made manometrically, with high-amplitude peristaltic waves being the hallmark of the disease.[19,157] The mean peristaltic amplitude is usually greater than 120 mm Hg, and there is usually increased duration of the wave.

A large number of patients with noncardiac chest pain have been shown to have manometric abnormalities that cannot be classified as one of the above disorders. These patients are now classified as having NEMD, and the manometric findings can vary from a "hypertensive LES" with normal relaxation and peristalsis to minor abnormalities in the peristaltic sequences with repetitive contractions or isolated prolonged contractions.[19] The incidence of these esophageal disorders in children is not known at this time.

Esophageal dysmotility in infants has also been linked to the "near-miss" sudden infant death syndrome in a report of four infants with radiographically proven esophageal dysmotility.[160] The alterations consisted of distal esophageal spasm and esophageal strictures. No manometric studies were performed, so it is difficult to know the type of motor alterations. They were all born prematurely, the symptoms occurred after feeding, and they all had esophageal strictures, suggesting that they all had long-term GER. Of interest is the fact that two patients developed apnea during the barium study in relation to esophageal dysmotility, and that they all improved after aggressive antireflux treatment was undertaken.

The therapeutic armamentarium for the primary motility disorders, with the exception of achalasia, is greatly limited. Treatment is directed toward symptom reduction. Calcium-channel blockers and nitrates have been shown in uncontrolled trials to improve the symptoms of patients with spastic disorders.[19,161] Of interest is the recent observation in a double-blind study that trazodone hydrochloride (an antidepressant drug) produced global improvement and reduced distress from esophageal symptoms. This improvement was not related to manometric changes, emphasizing that manometric abnormalities may not be solely responsible for the symptoms.[162] The fact that an antidepressant has such a marked influence over these disorders raises the issue of the importance of psychiatric alterations in these patients and their relationship to esophageal motor disorders. Previous studies have revealed that a psychiatric disorder at some point in the patient's lifetime is present in approximately 80 percent of patients with esophageal contraction abnormalities.[163]

If conservative treatment fails, the use of PD or surgery has been advocated to treat patients with spastic esophageal disorders. PD has been reported to improve the dysphagia of 40 percent of the patients with severe manometric abnormalities, particularly if there is incomplete LES relaxation.[118] Surgery should be the last resort[157]; a long myotomy is generally advocated for intractable cases, and good results have been reported.[164]

MOTOR DISORDERS IN ESOPHAGEAL ATRESIA AND TRACHEOESOPHAGEAL FISTULA

A complete consideration of esophageal atresia is beyond the scope of this discussion. I will therefore describe only the aspects that are related to esophageal motility. Primary repair of esophageal atresia permits the restoration of GI continuity but does not ensure normal esophageal function. Early surgical intervention allows the neonate to survive, but it has become clear that many children surviving the repair of esophageal atresia frequently have symptoms related to esophageal motor dysfunction, including regurgitation, vomiting, heartburn, dysphagia, and chronic respiratory symptoms, such as nocturnal wheezing and recurrent pneumonias.[165–167] Some patients also develop strictures near the anastomotic site, which have been attributed by some authors to reflux

esophagitis.[168] Long-term follow-up of these children with esophageal atresia repair has revealed disordered esophageal motility in almost all the children studied.[165–170] Manometric tests and long-term pH monitoring have proved to be the most sensitive indicators of esophageal abnormalities in these patients.[165–167] Most series have shown almost universal alterations in the peristalsis of the esophagus, with rare reports of normal esophageal function (1 of 22 patients).[166] The alterations described have been lack of peristalsis, with esophageal contractions that tend to be simultaneous and weak although at times of normal amplitude.[166,169] The most frequent abnormality has been absent peristalsis in the proximal esophagus, with frequent simultaneous contractions and prolongation of acid clearance.[165,168] In the study of Winter et al,[168] the LES pressure was found to be absent in 5 of 22 patients or very low (9 mm Hg) in 17 of 22,[103] whereas more recent series found a mean of 22 ± 14 mm Hg (range 1 to 52) in one study and normal LES in 7 of 10 patients.[165] It has been suggested that a low LES pressure in these patients correlates with the development of aspiration pneumonia,[167] although two recent studies[171,172] found no correlation between abnormalities in pulmonary function tests in these patients and the presence of GER, esophagitis, or esophageal dysfunction.

The long-term esophageal function has been recently described by Biller et al, who studied 12 adult patients who had their original repair in the first week of life.[171] The mean age was 26 at the time of the evaluation. During manometry they found a mean LES pressure or 21.3 ± 2.8 mm Hg, with only two patients having LES pressure less than 15 mm Hg (both had esophagitis). Ten had complete LES relaxation after swallowing, and the amplitude of the contraction was also low throughout the esophagus, although the duration was normal. All patients had at least one portion of aperistalsis, with most patients showing a diffuse abnormality. The UES pressure and function were normal.

This abnormal motor function seems to hamper the ability of the esophagus to provide an efficient acid clearance and at times an effective barrier, which probably predisposes these patients to complications from GER.[165,168]

The etiology of the abnormal esophageal motor dysfunction is unclear. Some authors have suggested that there is damage to the esophageal branches of the vagus during the surgical repair,[166,173] although recently most studies have documented normal function of the LES[165,168] and in one instance a normal methacholine (Mecholyl) test was found in the two patients in whom this test was performed, suggesting that the motor impairment is not due to simple denervation.[165] They suggest that the alterations may be secondary to ischemia, and because motor problems are also found in children with tracheoesophageal fistula without esophageal atresia,[174] it is likely that the motor disorder is part of the congenital anomaly.[165] To further support this view, there is experimental evidence in dogs that even though cervical vagotomy produces low LES pressure, thoracic procedures including vagotomy, resection of the esophageal branches of the vagus, phrenic nerve resection, and midesophageal resection have no significant effects on the LES.[175,176] To further support the theory that the esophageal motility alterations are present since birth, before the operation, Romeo et al recently reported esophageal motility studies of both the proximal and the distal segments in 20 newborns with esophageal atresia before surgical repair.[177] They found that the LES length varied from 8 to 14 mm, and the pressure was between 22 and 35 mm Hg in 84 percent. The LES pressure was low in 16.7 percent of the patients, and there was incomplete relaxation in 8.4 percent. There was also incomplete relaxation of the UES in 12.5 percent of the patients. The esophageal body in the proximal and distal segments showed a positive basal tone with total motor inco-ordination. In summary, their study supports the concept that the esophageal motor inco-ordination is an intrinsic part of the congenital malformation, and they suggest that, because the LES pressure was almost always normal, in the cases where it is low postoperatively it could be secondary to surgical trauma.

Acid-Induced Motility Disorders

Patients with chronic GER often have nonspecific distal esophageal motility problems.[157,178,179] Multiple studies have suggested that esophageal acid clearance is usually prolonged in patients with peptic esophagitis,[178-180] and it has been suggested that the acid clearance improves with medical therapy.[180] Such findings led to the hypothesis of a vicious circle in which reflux leads to esophagitis, which in turn decreases acid clearance, which in turn aggravates the esophagitis.[178]

It is known that normal acid clearance involves clearance of the acid by esophageal peristalsis and then neutralization of the residual acid by saliva.[178,181] It has been shown that when there is failed peristalsis there is abnormal esophageal acid clearance.[182] In a recent study Kahrilas et al[178] showed that the fraction of patients with GER with an abnormally high peristaltic failure rate increased with increasing severity of the reflux disease; 3 percent of patients with non-inflammatory GER disease, 11 percent with mild esophagitis, and 30 percent with severe esophagitis. They found that complete absence of peristalsis after deglutition was the most common alteration, and they also suggested that an abnormal amplitude in the esophageal contractions may also contribute. They described regional peristaltic hypotension in 25 percent of patients with mild esophagitis, and 48 percent of patients with severe esophagitis.

Esophageal motor alterations have also been described in children. Hillemeier et al[183] showed that infants with GER and failure to thrive or pulmonary disease had significantly lower peristaltic amplitude in the distal body of the esophagus (28.3 ± 4.8 and 23.2 ± 5.5 mm Hg) than a group of infants with reflux but without serious sequelae (50.2 ± 3.2 mm Hg). They found an increased number of nonperistaltic sequences in the two complicated groups, but the LES pressure was not different between the infants with and without severe GER. They also found a correlation between abnormal esophageal peristalsis and delayed gastric emptying, suggesting that children with GER have a diffuse abnormality of upper GI function. Recently Cucchiara et al[179] tried to address the question of whether the motor abnormalities in GER are a primary defect or secondary to esophagitis.[179,184] They compared the esophageal motility in children with proven severe esophagitis with that in children with mild or no microscopic esophagitis and children with emesis secondary to other conditions. They found that there was no difference in LES pressure or duration and velocity of the contractions among the three groups. The children with severe esophagitis had significantly decreased peristaltic amplitude (mean of 30.3 ± 5.4 mm Hg) and more nonspecific motor disorders such as simultaneous contractions, double peaked waves, and broad-based waves. The manometric studies were repeated after medical therapy and endoscopic follow-up; the peristaltic amplitude increased to 55.8 ± 11.6 mm Hg, and there was a significant reduction in the number of nonspecific motor abnormalities (6.36 ± 6.7 percent versus 29.1 ± 24.6 percent before treatment) suggesting that the esophageal motor alterations are secondary to the inflammation.

The effects of surgical correction of GER on esophageal motility have also been examined. In a recent report comparing 18 healthy controls and 32 adults with GER before and after Nissen fundoplication, Gill et al[185] found that the GER patients had a lower mean LES pressure and amplitude of esophageal peristalsis before the operation. After the fundoplication the mean amplitude of esophageal peristalsis increased significantly, and the LES pressure increased significantly and was not different from that of controls. Euler et al[186] studied nine children before and after the performance of a Nissen fundoplication and showed a mean LES pressure increase of 10.9 mm Hg (range: 5.3 to 22 mm Hg). Recently in another study of eight children it was found that the LES pressure and the length increased from 10.7 ± 3.9 cm H_2O and 1.1 ± 0.5 cm H_2O before to 26.7 ± 7.7 cm H_2O and 2.3 ± 0.8 cm H_2O after the operation.[187]

The question that remains to be answered is whether these motility alterations were the primary predisposing factor in the development of the esophagitis or were secondary to the esophagitis.[178,183] Recent literature seems to suggest that the esophageal motility alterations found in these children are secondary to esophagitis, reversible with therapy, and not a primary event.[179]

Even if we assume that the esophageal motor alterations in children with esophagitis are secondary to the inflammation, it is possible that an abnormal LES function and pressure could predispose the patient to develop esophagitis.[187] It has been demonstrated in the cat that acute experimental esophagitis has a deleterious effect on the mechanical properties of the LES, with recovery taking 4 to 6 weeks.[188] However, it has been shown that a minority of patients with esophagitis exhibit hypotension LES[157] and that there is no correlation between impaired motor function in the esophageal body and hypotensive LES.[178] Most manometric studies in adults[178] and children[179,183] have failed to demonstrate a difference in the LES pressure between normal controls and patients with GER, and it has also been reported that most of the reflux episodes are secondary to transient inappropriate relaxations of a normal-pressure LES and not to a chronically hypotensive sphincter.[189,190] It has been shown, however, that if the LES pressure is low, the patient will have a higher incidence of complications and a worse response to medical therapy.[191]

Chronic Idiopathic Intestinal Pseudo-obstruction

This syndrome is characterized by intermittent symptoms and signs of intestinal obstruction without evidence of actual mechanical blockage. Various motility abnormalities throughout the body have been described; besides the small bowel, the esophagus is frequently involved.[192-194] At least 85 percent of patients have abnormal esophageal motility. Most patients exhibit aperistalsis and often decreased or absent LES.[192] In the recent national survey reported by Vargas et al,[194] esophageal motility studies were performed in 14 children. All patients had a low LES, with failure to relax with swallowing. Low-amplitude waves occurred in the esophageal body, with lack of propagation and the presence of tertiary contractions in all 14 patients. Because none of the patients had histologic studies done to correlate whether they had a myopathic or a neuropathic form, no further conclusions can be reached. It can be concluded, however, that because of the high incidence of esophageal motor abnormalities in these patients, esophageal motility can be used as an initial screening test, particularly if small bowel motility studies are not available where the patient is located.

Endoscopic Injection Sclerotherapy

Endoscopic injection sclerotherapy (EIS) of esophageal varices is an effective treatment modality for patients who have had variceal hemorrhage.[195] It has also been successfully used in children. Following EIS the histologic changes in the esophageal wall include thrombosis of the submucosal vessels, esophagitis, ulceration, and subsequently fibrosis.[196] Persistent dysphagia after EIS has been uncommon despite extensive damage to the esophageal mucosa, although there are reports of esophageal strictures following the procedure.[197] The results of esophageal motility studies in patients undergoing EIS have varied. It was originally reported that EIS caused a reduction in LES and in the amplitude of contraction and diminished acid clearance.[198] Others also noted an increase in nonperistaltic contractions in those patients with difficulty swallowing.[199] Schade[200] reported that EIS had no effect on LES pressure, acid reflux, or the velocity of peristalsis. Esophageal motility was studied prospectively in 25 patients undergoing sclerotherapy.[195] They found that the esophageal motility of these patients was not different from that of controls. However, in a retrospective study of four patients with esophageal strictures as a result of the procedure, they found repetitive nonperistaltic contractions and dysphagia. The differences in these studies may be related to differences in EIS techniques, and it can be concluded that the onset of dysphagia usually signifies the presence of complications, particularly stricture formation, and that esophageal motility is usually markedly altered in those cases.[195]

Collagen Vascular Disorders

Of all the collagen vascular disorders, scleroderma shows the most marked esophageal abnormalities.[201-204] Scleroderma is a systemic disease of unknown etiology characterized by excessive deposition of collagen and other connective tissue components in skin and other target organs, most notably the GI tract.[201,202] Esophageal abnormalities are present in one-half to three-fourths of patients with scleroderma, a much higher frequency than in patients with other collagen vascular disorders.[204-206] Prominent digestive symptoms in these patients are dysphagia, weight loss, and diarrhea alternating with constipation.[202] In advanced cases the esophageal involvement can be easily diagnosed by cinefluoroscopy, whereas at an early stage it can be detected by esophageal manometry[202] or more recently by the use of scintigraphic techniques.[203] The manometric findings are quite suggestive of the diagnosis, although not pathognomonic, as severe reflux esophagitis can have the same manometric appearance.[178] The scintigraphic findings are nonspecific, usually showing poor esophageal and gastric emptying,[203] and it is now considered a good screening technique. The characteristic esophageal manometric findings are (1) incompetent lower esophageal sphincter, (2) low-amplitude esophageal contractions in the smooth portion of the esophagus, and (3) late alterations in the striated muscle section.[205,206] The incompetent LES fails to provide an effective barrier against the gastric acid, and the abnormal peristalsis provides an inadequate acid clearance, predisposing the patients to severe complications from GER.[205] It is then not surprising that patients with scleroderma may have heartburn as a prominent symptom.[205]

The severity of the esophageal motor dysfunction in scleroderma varies.[202,205] It has been shown that alterations are more severe in patients with progressive systemic sclerosis (PSS) than in those with localized scleroderma (LS).[202] When comparing patients with PSS to patients with LS and controls, Hamel-Roy et al[202] found that only the patients with PSS had marked functional abnormalities of esophageal motility. In the distal esophagus they found tertiary contractions in 58 percent of patients with PPS, compared with 5 percent of LS patients and 4 percent of controls. The amplitude of the contractions in both the proximal and distal esophagus was also significantly decreased in PSS, and 10 of 11 patients with PSS had a decreased LES pressure, with a mean of 6 ± 2 mm Hg, as compared with 17 ± 2 in LS patients and 24 ± 1 in controls. Some patients with LS also had a decreased LES pressure, suggesting that they could evolve toward a more systemic form of the disease.[202,207] Nine patients with PSS also had inco-ordination between the LES and the peristalsis, and all 11 had incomplete relaxation, whereas LS patients did not show any difference from controls in these respects.[202] In advanced cases there was no detectable sphincter, with the stomach and esophagus functioning as a common cavity. As reported by previous authors, they also found that Raynaud's phenomenon is closely associated with the loss of esophageal peristalsis.[202,205,207,208]

In a recent study of children with scleroderma, Flick et al[209] studied seven children with PSS and two with LS. The most frequent symptoms in patients with PSS were regurgitation, heartburn, and dysphagia. They showed that in 72 percent of the patients with PSS (mean age 15; range 10 to 18) there was either a decreased LES pressure, tertiary waves, or feeble contractions. They found a strong correlation between the presence of Raynaud's phenomenon and esophageal symptoms but no correlation with disease duration. There was a correlation between dysphagia and the presence of esophageal motor abnormalities. In contrast to adults, they also did not find any correlation between the presence of esophageal motor abnormalities and Raynaud's phenomenon. Both patients with LS had no esophageal symptoms and minimal nonspecific alterations in the esophageal motility (tertiary waves and variability in amplitude). Of interest is the fact that after 4 years follow-up none of the patients with LS had either progression of their motor abnormalities or the appearance of symptoms, challenging the suggestion that nonspecific esophageal abnormalities may indicate which patients will develop a more progressive illness.

The pathogenesis of the esophageal motor disorder in these patients remains unknown.[209] In some pharmacologic studies, Cohen et al[207] showed that the LES pressure in patients with intact peristalsis is higher and demonstrates an increase in sphincter pressure after the administration of methacholine (a cholinergic agonist) or edrophonium (a cholinesterase inhibitor). In patients with reduced or absent peristalsis, the sphincter responds to methacholine but shows a diminished response after the administration of edrophonium. Some patients with absence of peristalsis do not show any response to methacholine, suggesting extensive muscle atrophy. All patients with scleroderma showed a diminished response of the LES to gastrin injection. They suggested that patients with scleroderma have an early abnormality in cholinergic neuronal function which later is compounded by smooth muscle atrophy. It is possible that a neural lesion occurs early in scleroderma and disrupts esophageal motor function before the development of significant smooth muscle disease.[202,207] Studies of motility abnormalities in the small bowel, colon, and anorectal area seem to support this hypothesis.[202,207] Other authors suggest that the LES hypotension is secondary to a primary muscle defect,[210] although the finding of abnormal motor function in areas of normal muscle in several studies suggests that atrophy is a later stage of the disorder.[69,209]

At present there is no specific treatment for the esophageal alterations secondary to scleroderma. The treatment is symptomatic, trying to prevent the complications from GER. Cimetidine,[211] metoclopramide,[212] and cisapride[213] have been shown to cause symptomatic improvement.

Even though the esophageal motor abnormalities of scleroderma have been well characterized, other connective tissue diseases also have motor alterations,[204] particularly in patients with systemic lupus erythematosus (SLE) and those with mixed connective tissue diseases (MCTD), which is a disorder that has overlapping features of PSS, SLE, and polymyositis and is characterized serologically by the presence of high titers of hemagglutinating antibody to ribonucleoprotein.

In a study of 17 adults with MCTD, Gutierrez et al[204] showed that 82 percent of patients had abnormal esophageal motility. The mean LES and UES pressures were lower than in controls, and the amplitude of esophageal contractions was significantly decreased. In 53 percent of patients there was total aperistalsis of the esophagus, including the upper third, reflecting involvement of the striated muscle. They suggest that the diagnosis of MCTD should be entertained when total aperistalsis in the esophageal body is found, although this pattern can be seen occasionally in patients with PSS and SLE.[201,204] In a recent study of four children with MCTD,[209] three had low LES pressure, two had tertiary waves, and two had feeble contractions. They found no evidence of aperistalsis, in contrast to the findings in the above-mentioned study.

The question of whether steroids will improve the esophageal motility problems remains unanswered. It has been suggested that the abnormal peristalsis in MCTD returns to normal after steroid treatment, although in the study by Gutierrez et al[204] 14 patients had been receiving steroids for a mean of 6.9 years, and all had abnormal peristalsis. This question needs to be addressed with a prospective study.

Esophageal symptoms and aperistalsis are not prominent manifestations of SLE. Patients with SLE can also have esophageal motor abnormalities (approximately 50 percent).[201,204] In a series of 14 patients, three had low LES, one had aperistalsis, two had changes similar to PSS, and four had minor esophageal abnormalities.[204] Even though heartburn was a very common symptom, no correlation between motility abnormalities and symptoms could be established.

Sjögren's syndrome, which is characterized by xerostomia and keratoconjunctivitis, can have involvement of other organs, including the GI tract.[214] Esophageal function has been recently studied in these patients, and it was shown that they have minor motor differences with controls (shorter peristaltic contraction time and faster peristaltic velocity in the distal part of the esophagus).[214] Webs were found in 10 percent, and it was concluded that the dysphagia that was reported by 73 percent of the patients is probably related to the lack of saliva, making the solid bolus passage difficult.

Graft-Versus-Host Disease (GVHD)

Dysphagia, painful swallowing, and severe retrosternal pain can develop in patients with chronic GVHD. In one series 8 of 63 patients developed this problem, including a 12-year-old and a 19-year-old patient.[215] No infectious pathogens were identified, and in all an endoscopy showed desquamative esophagitis in the upper and middle esophageal third, and frequently webs. The distal esophagus was described as normal in all but two patients. Seven underwent esophageal manometry and five had abnormalities, including two with aperistalsis, one with simultaneous contractions and aperistalsis after swallowing, and two with high-amplitude, long-duration peristaltic contractions. They suggested that reflux esophagitis was present in at least three patients, including two with distal strictures, and that the esophageal motor disorder is secondary to the immunologic response to GVHD, and that as a result of delayed acid clearance these patients are prone to develop complications from acid reflux. It is interesting that the pathologic description of the esophagus of those symptomatic patients who died did not indicate any abnormalities of the myenteric plexus or the smooth muscle, with only severe mucosal abnormalities, further reinforcing the impression that the motility disorder is secondary to the mucosal lesion. Whether the abnormal motility is secondary to the mucosal lesion that occurs with GVHD or to reflux esophagitis or to both is not known, but these esophageal motor alterations are of interest because they seem to be secondary to immunologic phenomena.

SUMMARY

This discussion is the clinical extension of that in Chapter 15, Esophageal Motility. In it, the pathophysiology and clinical manifestations of specific motor disorders of the esophagus, including achalasia are discussed. In addition, a detailed approach to the treatment of these conditions affecting the esophagus is provided.

REFERENCES

1. Dinari G, Danzinger Y, Mimouni M, Rosenbach Y, Zahavi I, Grunebaum M. Cricopharyngeal dysfunction in childhood: treatment by dilatations. J Pediatr Gastroenterol Nutr 1987; 6:212–216.
2. Kilman WJ, Goyal RK. Disorders of pharyngeal and upper esophageal sphincter motor function. Arch Intern Med 1976; 136:592–601.
3. Watson WC, Sullivan SN. Hypertonicity of cricopharyngeal sphincter: cause of globus sensation. Lancet 1974; ii:1417–1418.
4. Gideon A, Nolte K. The non-obstructive pharyngeo esophageal cross roll. Ann Radiol 1973; 16:129–135.
5. Vantrappen G, Hellmans J. Diseases of the esophagus. New York: Springer-Verlag, 1974:399.
6. Wyllie E, Wyllie R, Cruse RP, Rothner DA, Erenberg G. The mechanism of nitrazepam-induced drooling and aspiration. New Engl J Med 1986; 314:35–38.
7. Fisher SE, Painter M, Milmore G. Swallowing disorders in infancy. Pediatr Clin North Am 1981; 28:845–853.
8. Parrish RM. Cricopharyngaeus dysfunction and acute dysphagia. Can Med Assoc J 1968; 99:1167–1171.
9. Staiano A, Cucchiara S, Vizia B, Andreotti M, Auricchio S. Disorders of upper esophageal sphincter motility in children. J Pediatr Gastroenterol Nutr 1987; 6:892–898.
10. Hurwitz AL, Nelson JA, Haddad JK. Oropharyngeal dysphagia: manometric and cine-esophagographic findings. Am J Dig Dis 1975; 20:313–324.
11. Lernau OZ, Sherzer E, Mogle P, Nissan S. Congenital cricopharyngeal achalasia. Treatment by dilatations. J Pediatr Surg 1984; 19:202–203.
12. Bishop HC. Cricopharyngeal achalasia in childhood. J Pediatr Surg 1974; 9:775–778.
13. Reichert TJ, Bluestone CD, Stool SE. Congenital cricopharyngeal achalasia. Ann Otol Rhinol Laryngol 1977; 86:603–610.
14. Gelfand M. Dysphagia due to esophageal motility disorder in Down's syndrome. Gastroenterology 1981; 80:1154.
15. Duranceau A, Rheault MJ, Jamieson GC. Physiologic response to cricopharyngeal myotomy and myotomy suspension. Surgery 1983; 94:655–662.
16. Green RE, Castell DO. The upper esophageal sphincter. In: Castell DO, Richter JE, Dalton CB, ed. Esophageal motility testing. New York: Elsevier, 1987:183.
17. Utian HL, Thomas RG. Cricopharyngeal incoordination in infancy. Pediatrics 1969; 43:402–406.
18. Suck and swallow. In: Gryboski J, Walker WA, eds. Gastrointestinal problems in the infant. 2nd ed. Philadelphia: WB Saunders, 1983:12.
19. Ardan GM, Benson PF, Butler NR. Congenital dysphagia resulting from dysfunction of the pharyngeal musculature: a clinical and a radiological study. Dev Med Child Neurol 1965; 7:157–166.
20. Frank MM, Baghdassarian L, Gatewood OM. Transient pharyngeal incoordination in the newborn. Am J Dis Child 1966; 111:178–181.
21. Riley CM. Familial dysautonomia. Adv Pediatr 1957; 5:157–190.
22. Margulies SE, Brunt PW, Donner MW. Familial dysautonomia, a cineradiographic study of the swallowing mechanism. Radiology 1968; 90:107–112.
23. Silbiger ML, Pikielney R, Donner MW. Neuromuscular disorders affecting the pharynx. Cineradiographic analysis. Invest Radiol 1967; 2:442–448.
24. Hurwitz AL, Duranceau A. Upper esophageal sphincter dysfunction. Pathogenesis and treatment. Am J Dig Dis 1978; 23:275–281.
25. Henderson RD, Marryat G. Cricopharyngeal myotomy as a method of treating cricopharyngeal dysphagia secondary to gastroesophageal reflux. J Thorac Cardiovasc Surg 1977; 74:721–725.
26. Huttenlocher PR. Disease of muscle. In: Behrman RE, Vaughan VC, eds. Nelson textbook of pediatrics. 13th ed. Philadelphia: WB Saunders, 1987:1337.
27. Eckardt VF, Nix W, Kraus W, Bohl J. Esophageal motor function in patients with muscular dystrophy. Gastroenterology 1986; 90:628–635.
28. Nowak TV, Ionasecu V, Anuras S. Gastrointestinal manifestations of the muscular dystrophies. Gastroenterology 1982; 82:800–810.
29. Pearson CM, Currie S. Polymyositis and related disorders. In: Walton JN, ed. Disorders of voluntary muscles. New York: Churchill-Livingstone, 1974:614.
30. Grunebaum M, Salinger H. Radiologic findings in polymyositis-dermatomyositis involving the pharynx and the upper esophagus. Clin Radiol 1971; 22:97–100.
31. Strobel CT, Byrne WJ, Ament ME, Euler AR. Correlation of esophageal lengths in children with height. Application to the Tuttle test without prior esophageal manometry. J Pediatr 1979; 94:81.
32. Horowitz M, McNeil JD, Maddern GJ, Collins PJ, Sherman DJ. Abnormalities of gastric and esophageal emptying in polymyositis and dermatomyositis. Gastroenterology 1986; 90:434–439.
33. Mayberry JF, Atkinson M. Swallowing problems in patients with motor neuron disease. J Clin Gastroenterol 1986; 8:233–234.
34. Fischer RA, Ellison GW, Thayer WR. Esophageal motility in neuromuscular disorders. Ann Intern Med 1965; 63:229–248.
35. Daly DD, Code CF, Anderson HA. Disturbances of swallowing and esophageal motility in patients with multiple sclerosis. Neurology 1962; 12:250–256.
36. Kramer P, Atkinson M, Wyman SM. The dynamics of swallowing. II. Neuromuscular dysphagia of the pharynx. J Clin Invest 1957; 36:589–595.
37. Coelho CA, Ferrante R. Dysphagia in postpolio sequela: report of three cases. Arch Phys Med Rehabil 1988; 69:634–636.
38. Cosgrove SL, Alexander MA, Kitts EL, Swan BE, Klein MV, Bauer RE. Late effects of poliomyelitis. Arch Phys Med Rehabil 1987; 68:4–7.
39. Cannon RA. Differential effect of botulinal toxin on esophageal motor function in infants. J Pediatr Gastroenterol Nutr 1985; 4:563–567.
40. Brown LW. Infant botulism. Adv Pediatr 1981; 28:141–157.
41. Berquist WE, Byrne WJ, Ament ME, Fonkalsrud EW, Euler AR. Achalasia: diagnosis, management and clinical course in 16 children. Pediatrics 1983; 71:798–805.
42. Vantrappen G, Janssens H, Hellemans J, et al. Achalasia, diffuse esophageal spasm, and related motility disorders. Gastroenterology 1979; 76:450–457.
43. Cohen S. Motor disorders of the esophagus. N Engl J Med 1979; 301:184–192.
44. Earlam RJ, Ellis FH, Nobrega FT. Achalasia of the esophagus in a small urban community. Mayo Clin Proc 1969; 44:478–482.
45. Moersch HJ. Cardiospasm in infancy and childhood. Am J Dis Child 1929; 38:294–298.
46. Singh H, Sethi RS, Gupta HL, Khetargal SK. Cardiac achalasia in childhood. Postgrad Med J 1969; 45:327–335.
47. Olsen AM, Harrington SW, Moersch HJ, Andersen HA. The treatment of cardiospasm: analysis of a twelve year experience. J Thorac Surg 1951; 22:164–187.
48. Azizkhan RG, Tapper D, Eraklis A. Achalasia in childhood: a 20 year experience. J Pediatr Surg 1980; 15:452–456.
49. Boyle JT, Cohen S, Watkins JB. Successful treatment of achalasia in childhood by pneumatic dilatation. J Pediatr 1981; 99:35–40.
50. Mayberry JB, Mayell MJ. Epiodemiological study of achalasia in children. Gut 1988; 29:90–93.
51. Buick RG, Spitz L. Achalasia of the cardia in children. Br J Surg 1985; 72:341–343.
52. Dooley CR, Taylor IL, Valenzuela JE. Impaired acid secretion and pancreatic polypeptide release in some patients with achalasia. Gastroenterology 1983; 84:809–813.
53. Martin S, Campos JV, Tafuri WL. Chagas enteropathy. Gut 1973; 14:910–919.
54. Csendes A, Smok F, Braghetto I, Ramirez C, Velasco N, Henriquez A. Gastroesophageal sphincter pressure and histological changes in distal esophagus in patients with achalasia of the esophagus. Dig Dis Sci 1985; 30:941–945.
55. Tucker HJ, Snape WJ, Cohen S. Achalasia secondary to carcinoma: manometric and clinical features. Ann Intern Med 1978; 89:315–318.
56. McCallum RW. Esophageal achalasia secondary to gastric gastrinoma. Am J Gastroenterol 1979; 72:24–29.
57. Dodds WJ, Dent J, Walter JH, Patel GK, Toouli J, Arndorfer RC. Paradoxical lower esophageal sphincter contraction induced by cholecystokinin-octapeptide in patients with achalasia. Gastroenterology 1981; 80:327–333.
58. Holloway RH, Dodds WJ, Helm JF, Hogan WJ, Dent J, Arndorfer RC. Integrity of cholinergic innervation to the lower esophageal sphincter in achalasia. Gastroenterology 1986; 90:924–929.
59. Gallone L, Peri G, Galliera M. Proximal gastric vagotomy and anterior fundoplication as complementary procedures to Heller's operation for achalasia. Surg Gynecol Obstet 1982; 155:337–341.
60. Qualman SJ, Haupt HM, Yang P, Hamilton SR. Esophageal Lewy bod-

ies associated with ganglion cell loss in achalasia. Gastroenterology 1984; 87:848–856.

61. Desai JR, Vyas PN, Desai NR. Cardiospasm in the younger age group. Indian J Pediatr 1967; 34:31–33.

62. Swenson O, Oeconomopoulos CT. Achalasia of the esophagus in children. J Thorac Cardiovasc Surg 1961; 41:49–59.

63. Elder JB. Achalasia of the cardia in childhood. Digestion 1970; 3:90–96.

64. Rickham PP, Boekman CR. Achalasia of the esophagus in young children. Clin Pediatr 1963; 2:676–681.

65. Cloud DT, White RF, Likner LM, Taylor LC. Surgical treatment of esophageal achalasia in children. J Pediatr 1966; 1:137–144.

66. Casella RR, Ellis FH, Brown AL. Fine structure changes in achalasia of the esophagus. I. Vagus nerves. Am J Pathol 1965; 46:279–288.

67. Friesen DL, Henderson RD, Hanna W. Ultrastructure of the esophageal muscle in achalasia and diffuse esophageal spasm. Am J Clin Pathol 1983; 79:319–325.

68. Faussone-Pellegrini MS, Cortesini C. The muscle coat of the lower esophageal sphincter in patients with achalasia and hypertensive sphincter. An electron microscopy study. J Submicroc Cytol 1985; 17:673–685.

69. Gryboski JD. The swallowing mechanism of the neonate. I.Esophageal and gastric motility. Pediatrics 1965; 35:445–452.

70. Behar J, Biancani P. Effect of cholecystokinin octapeptide on lower esophageal sphincter. Gastroenterology 1977; 73:57–61.

71. Resin H, Stern DH, Sturdevant RA, Isenberg JI. Effect of the C-terminal octapeptide of cholecystokinin on lower esophageal sphincter pressure in man. Gastroenterology 1973; 64:946–949.

72. Goyal RK, Rattan S, Said S. VIP as a possible neurotransmitter of non-cholinergic, non-adrenergic inhibitory neurons. Nature 1980; 288:378–380.

73. Aggestrup S, Uddman R, Jensen SL, Undler F, Schaffalitzky O, Holst JJ, Hakanson R, Ekman R, Sorensen HR. Regulatory peptides in the lower esophageal sphincter of man. Regul Pept 1985; 10:167–178.

74. Aggestrup S, Uddman R, Sundler F, Fahrenkrug J, Hakanson R, Sorensen HR, Hambraeus G. Lack of vasoactive intestinal polypeptide nerves in esophageal achalasia. Gastroenterology 1983; 84:924–927.

75. Casella RR, Ellis FH, Brown AL. Fine structure changes in achalasia of the esophagus. II. Esophageal smooth muscle. Am J Pathol 1965; 46:467–475.

76. Lemmer JH, Coran AG, Wesley JR. Achalasia in children: treatment by anterior esophageal myotomy (modified Heller operation). J Pediatr Surg 1985; 20:333–338.

77. Bosher LP, Shaw A. Achalasia in siblings. Am J Dis Child 1981; 135:709–710.

78. Stein DT, Knauer M. Achalasia in monozygotic twins. Dig Dis Sci 1982; 27:636–640.

79. Eckrich JD, Winans CS. Discordance of achalasia in identical twins. Dig Dis Sci 1979; 24:221.

80. Geffner ME, Lippe BM, Kaplan SA, Berquist WE, Bateman B, Paterno VI, Seegan R. Selective ACTH insensitivity, achalasia and alacrima: a multisystem disorder presenting in childhood. Pediatr Res 1983; 17:532–536.

81. Illgrove H, Clayden GS, Grant DB, McCaulay JC. Familial glucocorticoid deficiency with achalasia of the cardia and deficient tear production. Lancet 1978; i:1284.

82. Pombo M, Devesa J, Taborda A, Iglesias M, Garcia-Moreno F, Gaudiero GJ, Martinon JM, Castro-Gago M, Pena J. Glucocorticoid deficiency with achalasia of the cardia and lack of lacrimation. Clin Endocrinol 1985; 23:237–243.

83. Rozychi DL, Ruben RJ, Ralpin I, Spiro AJ. Autosomal recessive deafness associated with short stature, vitiligo, muscle wasting and achalasia. Arch Otorynolaryngol 1971; 93:194–197.

84. Mayberry JF, Atkinson MA. Achalasia and other diseases associated with disorders of gastrointestinal motility. Hepatogastroenterology 1986; 33:206–207.

85. Badrawy R, Abou-Bieh A. Congenital achalasia of the esophagus in children. J Laryngol Otol 1975; 89:697–706.

86. Asch MJ, Liebman W, Lechman RS, Mogre T. Esophageal achalasia: diagnosis and cardiomyotomy in a newborn infant. J Pediatr Surg 1974; 9:911–912.

87. The esophagus. In: Gryboski J, Walker WA, eds. Gastrointestinal problems in the infant. Philadelphia: WB Saunders, 1983:183.

88. Moazam F, Rodgers BM. Infantile achalasia. Brief clinical report. J Thorac Cardiovasc Surg 1976; 72:809–812.

89. Polk HC, Burford TH. Disorders of the distal esophagus in infancy and childhood. Am J Dis Child 1964; 108:243–251.

90. Nakayama DK, Shorter NA, Boyle T, Watkins JB, O'Neill JA. Pneumatic dilatation and operative treatment of achalasia in children. J Pediatr Surg 1987; 22:619–622.

91. Payne WS, Ellis FH, Olsen AM. Treatment of cardiospasm (achalasia of the esophagus) in children. Surgery 1961; 50:731–735.

92. Tachovsky TJ, Lynn HB, Ellis FH. The surgical approach to esophageal achalasia in children. J Pediatr Surg 1968; 3:226–231.

93. Ballantine TN, Fitzgerald JF, Grosfield JL. Transabdominal esophagomyotomy for achalasia in children. J Pediatr Surg 1980; 15:457–461.

94. Uribe P, Csendes A, Larrain A, Ayala M. Motility studies in fifty patients with achalasia of the esophagus. Am J Gastroenterol 1974; 62:333–336.

95. Katz PO, Richter JE, Cowan R, Castell DO. Apparent complete lower esophageal sphincter relaxation in achalasia. Gastroenterology 1986; 90:978–983.

96. Lamet M, Flesher B, Achkar E. Return of peristalsis in achalasia after pneumatic dilatation. Am J Gastroenterol 1985; 80:602–604.

97. Cucchiara S, Staiano C, Di Lorenzo C, Ambrosio D, Anderotti MR, Auricchio S. Return of peristalsis in a child with esophageal achalasia treated by Heller's myotomy. J Pediatr Gastroenterol Nutr 1986; 5:150–152.

98. Mellow MH. Return of peristalsis in idiopathic achalasia. Gastroenterology 1976; 70:1148–1151.

99. Bianco A, Cagossi M, Scrimieri D, et al. Appearance of esophageal peristalsis in treated idiopathic achalasia. Dig Dis Sci 1986; 31:40–48.

100. Holloway RH, Krosin G, Lange RC, Baue AE, McCallum RW. Radionuclide esophageal emptying of a solid meal to quantitate results of therapy in achalasia. Gastroenterology 1983; 84:771–776.

101. Russell CO, Hill LD, Holmes ER, Hull DA, Gannon R, Pope CE. Radionuclide transit: a sensitive screening test for esophageal dysfunction. Gastroenterology 1981; 80:887–892.

102. Kramer P, Ingelfinger FJ. Esophageal sensitivity to Mecholyl in cardiospasm. Gastroenterology 1968; 54:771–773.

103. Helm JF, Dodds WJ, Hogan WJ, Arndorfer RC. Carcinoma of the cardia masquerading as idiopathic achalasia. Gastroenterology 1982; 82:1082A.

104. Betarrello A, Pinott HW. Esophageal involvement in Chagas' disease. Clin Gastroenterol 1976; 5:103–109.

105. Stacher G, Kiss A, Wiesnagrotki S, Bergmann H, Hobart J, Schneider C. Oesophageal and gastric motility disorders in patients categorised as having primary anorexia nervosa. Gut 1986; 27:1120–1126.

106. McCallum RW. The management of esophageal motility disorders. Hosp Practice 1988; Feb:131–142.

107. Gelfond M, Rosen P, Gilat T. Isosorbide dinitrate and nifedipine treatment of achalasia: a clinical, manometric and radionuclide evaluation. Gastroenterology 1982; 83:963–969.

108. Dodds WJ, Stewrat ET, Kishk SM, Kahrilas PJ, Hogan WJ. Radiological amyl nitrate test for distinguishing pseudoachalasia from idiopathic achalasia. AJR 1986; 146:21.

109. Gelfond M, Rozen P, Keren S, Ghat T. Effects of nitrates on LOS pressure in achalasia: a potential therapeutic aid. Gut 1981; 22:312–318.

110. Hongo M, Traube M, McAllister RG, McCallum RW. Effects of nifedipine on esophageal motor function in humans: correlation with plasma nifedipine concentration. Gastroenterology 1984; 86:8–12.

111. Bortolloti M, Labo G. Clinical and manometric effects of nifedipine in patients with esophageal achalasia. Gastroenterology 1980; 80:39–44.

112. Maksimak M, Perlmutter DH, Winter HS. The use of nifedipine in the treatment of achalasia in children. J Pediatr Gastroenterol Nutr 1986; 5:883–886.

113. Smith H, Buick R, Booth I, Campbell C. The use of nifedipine for treatment of achalasia in children. (Letter) J Pediatr Gastroenterol Nutr 1988; 7:146.

114. Richter JE, Dalton CB, Buice RG. Nifedipine, a potent inhibitor of contractions in the body of the human esophagus. Gastroenterology 1985; 89:549–554.

115. Thomas E, Lebow RA, Gubler RJ, Bryant LR. Nifedipine for the poor risk elderly patient with achalasia: objective response demonstrated by solid meal study. South Med J 1984; 77:394–401.

116. Yon J, Christensen J. An uncontrolled comparison of treatments of achalasia. Ann Surg 1975; 182:672–676.

117. Vantrappen G, Janssen S. To dilate or to operate? That is the question. Gut 1983; 24:1013–1019.
118. Vantrappen G, Hellemans J. Treatment of achalasia and related motor disorders. Gastroenterology 1980; 79:144–154.
119. Dellipiani AW, Hewetson KA. Pneumatic dilatation in the management of achalasia: experience of 45 cases. Q J Med 1986; 58:253–258.
120. Csendes A, Velasco N, Braghetto I, Henriquez A. A prospective randomized study comparing forceful dilatation and esophagomyotomy in patients with achalasia of the esophagus. Gastroenterology 1981; 80:789–795.
121. Fellows JW, Ogilvie AL, Atkinson MP. Pneumatic dilatation in achalasia. Gut 1983; 24:1020–1023.
122. Sato Y, Frey EE, Smith WL, Pringle KC, Soper RT, Franken EA. Balloon dilatation of esophageal stenosis in children. AJR 1988; 150:639–642.
123. Seo JK, Winter HS. Esophageal manometric and clinical response to treatment in children with achalasia. (Abstract) Gastroenterology 1987; 92:1634.
124. Liebman WM, Appelbaum M, Thaler MM. Achalasia of the esophagus. Pneumatic dilatation in a 4 year old. Am J Gastroenterol 1978; 70:73–75.
125. Okike N, Payne SW, Newfeld DM, Bernatz PE, Pairolero PC, Sanderson DR. Esophagomyotomy versus forceful dilatation for achalasia of the esophagus: results in 899 patients. Ann Thorac Surg 1979; 28:119–125.
126. Mandelstam P, Sugawa C, Silvis SE, et al. Complications associated with esophagogastroduodenostomy and duodenoscopy and with esophageal dilatations. Gastrointest Endosc 1976; 23:16–19.
127. Miller RE, Tiszenkel HI. Esophageal perforation due to pneumatic dilatation for achalasia. Surg Gynecol Obstet 1988; 166:458–460.
128. Ott DJ, Richter JE, Wu WC, Men Chen Y, Castell DO, Gelfand DW. Radiographic evaluation of esophagus immediately after pneumatic dilatation for achalasia. Dig Dis Sci 1987; 32:962–967.
129. Wong RK, Johnson LF. Achalasia. In: Castell DO, Johnson LE, eds. Esophageal function in health and disease. New York: Elsevier Biomedical, 1983:99.
130. Perisic VN. Achalasia in children. Am J Dis Child 1988; 142:16.
131. Redo FS, Bauer CH. Management of achalasia in infancy and childhood. Surgery 1963; 53:263–269.
132. Paul AT, Pahlawella GDS. Unusual forms of achalasia cardia and associated neuromuscular disorders of the esophagus. Postgrad Med J 1961; 37:514–522.
133. Koch A, Bettex M, Tschappeler H, Konig W. The function of the esophagus following cardiomyotomy in childhood achalasia. Z Kinderchir 1983; 38:206–214.
134. Ellis FH, Gibb SP. Reoperation after esophagomyotomy for achalasia of the esophagus. Am J Surg 1975; 129:407–412.
135. Agha FP, Keren DF. Barrett's esophagus complicating achalasia after esophagomyotomy. J Clin Gastroenterol 1987; 9:232–237.
136. Acheson ED, Hadley GD. Cardiomyotomy for achalasia of the cardia. Br J Med 1958; 1:549–553.
137. Jara FM, Toledo-Pereyra LH, Lewis JW, Magilligan DJ. Long term results of esophagomyotomy for achalasia of the esophagus. Arch Surg 1979; 114:935–936.
138. Feczko PJ, Ma CK, Halpert RD. Barrett's metaplasia and dysplasia in postmyotomy achalasia patients. Am J Gastroenterol 1983; 78:265–268.
139. Ellis HF, Gibb PS, Crosier RE. Esophagus. Ann Surg 1980; 192:157–161.
140. Skinner DB. Myotomy and achalasia. (Editorial) Ann Thorac Surg 1984; 37:183–184.
141. Belsey R. Functional disease of the esophagus. J Thorac Cardiovasc Surg 1966; 52:164.
142. Murray GF, Battaglini JW, Blair AK, Starek PJ, Wilcox BR. Selective application of fundoplication in achalasia. Ann Thorac Surg 1984; 37:185–188.
143. Shoenut PJ, Trenholm BG, Eng M, Micflikier AB, Teskey JM. Reflux patterns in patients with achalasia without operation. Ann Thorac Surg 1988; 45:303–305.
144. Smart HL. Foster PN, Evans DF, Slevin B, Atkinson M. Twenty four hour esophageal acidity in achalasia before and after pneumatic dilatation. Gut 1987; 28:883–887.
145. Donahue PE, Schlesinger PK, Bombeck CT, et al. Achalasia of the esophagus. Ann Surg 1986; 203:505–511.

146. Thomson D, Shoenut JP, Trenholm BG, Teskey JM. Reflux patterns following limited myotomy without fundoplication for achalasia. Ann Thorac Surg 1987; 43:550–553.
147. Goulbourne JA, Walbaum PR. Long term results of Heller's operation for achalasia. J R Coll Surg Edinburgh 1985; 30:101–103.
148. Mercer CD, Hill LD. Reoperation after failed esophagomyotomy for achalasia. Can J Surg 1986; 29:177–181.
149. Choung JJ, Dubovik S, McCallum RW. Achalasia as a risk factor for esophageal carcinoma. A reappraisal. Dig Dis Sci 1984; 29:1105–1108.
150. Norton GA, Postkehwat RW, Thompson WM. Esophageal carcinoma: a summary of populations at risk. South Med J 1980; 73:23–27.
151. Just-Viera JO, Haight C. Achalasia and carcinoma of the esophagus. Surg Gynecol Obstet 1967; 128:1081–1095.
152. Khan MV, Maltzman B, Jonnard R. Carcinoma of esophagus: autopsy reports. NY State J Med 1980; 4:575–579.
153. Heiss FW, Tarshis A, Ellis FH. Carcinoma associated with achalasia. Occurrence 23 years after esophagomyotomy. Dig Dis Sci 1984; 29:1066–1069.
154. Benjamin SB, Richter JE, Cordova CM, Knuff TE, Castell DO. Prospective manometric evaluation with pharmacological provocation of patients with suspected esophageal motility dysfunction. Gastroenterology 1984; 84:893–901.
155. McCallum RW. The spectrum of esophageal motility disorders. Hosp Pract 1987; Dec:51–63.
156. Fontan JP, Heldt GP, Heyman MB, Marin MM, Tooley WH. Esophageal spasm associated with apnea and bradycardia in an infant. Pediatrics 1984; 73:52–55.
157. Katz PO, Castell DO. Review: esophageal motility disorders. Am J Med Sci 1985; 290:61–69.
158. Richter JE. Diffuse esophageal spasm. In: Castell DO, Richter JE, Dalton CB, eds. Esophageal motility testing. New York: Elsevier Biomedical, 1987:118.
159. Longstreth JF, Foroozan P. Evolution of symptomatic diffuse esophageal spasm to achalasia. South Med J 1982; 75:217–220.
160. Schey WL, Replogie R, Campbell C, Meus P, Levinsky RA. Esophageal dysmotility and the sudden infant death syndrome. Radiology 1981; 140:67–71.
161. Richter JE, Dalton CB, Bradley LA, Castell DO. Oral nifedipine in the treatment of noncardiac chest pain in patients with the nutcracker esophagus. Gastroenterology 1987; 93:21–26.
162. Clouse RE, Lustman PJ, Eckert TC, Ferney DM, Griffith LS. Low dose trazodone for symptomatic patients with esophageal contraction abnormalities: a double blind placebo-controlled trial. Gastroenterology 1987; 92:1027–1036.
163. Clouse RE, Lustman PJ. Psychiatric illness and contraction abnormalities of the esophagus. N Engl J Med 1983; 309:1337–1342.
164. Jamieson WE, Miyagishima RT, Carr DM, Stordy SN, Sharp FR. Surgical management of primary motor disorders of the esophagus. Am J Surg 1984; 148:36–42.
165. Werlin SL, Dodds WJ, Hogan WJ, Glicklich M, Arndorfer R. Esophageal function in esophageal atresia. Dig Dis Sci 1981; 26:796–800.
166. Orringer MB, Kirsh MM, Sloan H. Long term esophageal function following repair of esophageal atresia. Ann Surg 1977; 186:436–443.
167. Whitington PF, Shermeta DW, Seto DS, Jones L, Hendrix TR. Role of lower esophageal sphincter incompetence in recurrent pneumonia after repair of esophageal atresia. J Pediatr 1977; 91:550–554.
168. Winter HS, Madara JL, Stafford RJ, Tapper D, Goldman H. Delayed acid clearance and esophagitis after repair of esophageal atresia. (Abstract) Gastroenterology 1981; 80:1317.
169. Lind JF, Blanchard RJ, Guhda H. Esophageal motility in tracheoesophageal fistula and esophageal atresia. Surg Gynecol Obstet 1966; 123:557.
170. Takano K, Iwafuchi M, Uchiyama M, Yagi M, Ueno A, Iwasaki M. Evaluation of lower esophageal sphincter function in infants and children following esophageal surgery. J Pediatr Surg 1988; 23:410–414.
171. Biller JA, Allen JL, Schuster SR, Treves ST, Winter HS. Long-term evaluation of esophageal and pulmonary function in patients with repaired esophageal atresia and tracheo-esophageal fistula. Dig Dis Sci 1987; 32:985–990.
172. LeSouef PN, Myers NA, Landau LI. Etiologic factors in long term respiratory function abnormalities following esophageal atresia repair. J Pediatr Surg 1987; 22:918–922.
173. Burges JN, Carlson HC, Ellis FH. Esophageal function after successful

repair of esophageal atresia and tracheo esophageal fistula. J Thorac Cardiovasc Surg 1968; 56:667–682.

174. Johnston PW, Hastings H. Congenital tracheoesophageal fistula without esophageal atresia. Am J Surg 1966; 112:232–240.

175. Haller JA, Brooker AF, Talbert JL, Baghjdassarian O, Vanhoutte J. Esophageal function following resection: studies in newborn puppies. Ann Thorac Surg 1966; 2:180–184.

176. Carveth SW, Schlegel FJ, Code CF, Ellis FH. Esophageal motility after vagotomy, phrenicotomy, myotomy and myomectomy in dogs. Surg Gynecol Obstet 1962; 114:31–37.

177. Romeo G, Zuccarello B, Proietto F, Romeo C. Disorders of the esophageal motor activity in atresia of the esophagus. J Pediatr Surg 1987; 22:120–124.

178. Kahrilas PJ, Dodds WJ, Hogan WJ, Kern M, Arndorfer RC, Reece A. Esophageal peristaltic dysfunction in peptic esophagitis. Gastroenterology 1986; 91:897–904.

179. Cucchiara S, Stalano A, DiLorenzo C, D'Ambrosio R, Anderotti MR, Prato M, DeFilippo P, Auricchio S. Esophageal motor abnormalities in children with gastroesophageal reflux and peptic esophagitis. J Pediatr 1986; 108:907–910.

180. Stanciu C, Bennett JR. Oesophageal acid clearing: one factor in the production of reflux esophagitis. Gut 1974; 15:852–857.

181. Helm JF, Dodds WJ, Pelc LR, Palmer DW, Hogan WJ, Teeter BC. Effect of esophageal emptying and saliva on clearance of acid from the esophagus. N Engl J Med 1983; 310:284–288.

182. Helm JF, Dodds WJ, Reidel DR, Teeter BC, Hogan WJ, Arndorfer RC. Determinants of esophageal acid clearance in normal subjects. Gastroenterology 1983; 85:607–612.

183. Hillemeier CA, Grill BB, McCallum R, Gryboski J. Esophageal and gastric motor abnormalities in gastroesophageal reflux during infancy. Gastroenterology 1983; 84:741–746.

184. Dodds WJ, Hogan WJ, Helm JF, Dent J. Pathogenesis of reflux esophagitis. Gastroenterology 1981; 81:378–394.

185. Gill RC, Bowes KL, Murphy PD, Kingma YJ. Esophageal motor abnormalities in gastroesophageal reflux and the effects of fundoplication. Gastroenterology 1986; 31:364–369.

186. Euler AR, Fonkalsrud EW, Ament ME. Effect of Nissen fundoplication on the lower esophageal sphincter pressure of children with gastroesophageal reflux. Gastroenterology 1977; 72:260–262.

187. Opie JC, Chaye H, Fraser GC. Fundoplication and pediatric esophageal manometry: actuarial analysis over 7 years. J Pediatr Surg 1987; 22:935–938.

188. Biancani P, Dodds J, Story E, Selling J, McCallum RW. Gastrointestinal motility. In: Christensen J, ed. In: Gastrointestinal motility. New York: Raven Press, 1980; 75.

189. Dodds WJ, Dent J, Hogan WJ, Helm JF, Hauser R, Patel GK, Egide MS. Mechanisms of gastroesophageal reflux in patients with reflux esophagitis. N Engl J Med 1982; 307:1547–1552.

190. Baldi F, Ferrarini F, Balestra D, Barioni D, Longanesi A, Miglioli M, Barbara L. Oesophageal motor events at the occurrence of acid reflux and during endogenous acid exposure in healthy subjects and in patients with esophagitis. Gut 1985; 26:336–344.

191. Behar J, Sheahan DG, Biancani P, Spiro HM. Medical and surgical management of reflux esophagitis. N Engl J Med 1975; 293:263–268.

192. Schuffler MD, Rohrmann CA, Chafle RG. Chronic intestinal pseudo-obstruction. A report of 27 cases and a review of the literature. Medicine 1981; 60:173–196.

193. Schuffler MD, Pope CE II. Esophageal motor dysfunction in idiopathic intestinal pseudo-obstruction. Gastroenterology 1976; 70:677–682.

194. Vargas JH, Sachs P, Ament ME. Chronic intestinal pseudo-obstruction syndrome in pediatrics. Results of a national survey by members of the North American Society of Pediatric Gastroenterology and Nutrition. J Pediatr Gastroenterol Nutr 1988; 7:323–332.

195. Cohen LB, Simon C, Korstein MA, Scherl EJ, Skorniky J, Guelrud MB, Waye JD. Esophageal motility and symptoms after endoscopic injection sclerotherapy. Dig Dis Sci 1985; 30:29–32.

196. Evan DM, Jones DB, Cleary BK, Smith PK. Esophageal varices treated by sclerotherapy: a histopathologic study. Gut 1982; 23:615–620.

197. Haynes WC, Sanowski RA, Foutch PG, Bellapravalu S. Esophageal strictures following endoscopic variceal sclerotherapy: clinical course and response to dilation therapy. Gastrointest Endosc 1986; 32:202–205.

198. Ogle SJ, Kirk CJ, Bailey RJ, Johnson AG, Williams R, Murray-Lyon IM. Oesophageal function in cirrhotic patients undergoing injection sclerotherapy for oesophageal varices. Digestion 1978; 18:178–185.

199. Sauerbruch T, Wirsching R, Leisner B, Weinzierl M, Pfahler M, Baumgartner G. Esophageal function after sclerotherapy of bleeding varices. Scand J Gastroenterol 1982; 17:745–751.

200. Schade RR, Reilly JJ, Gavalewr JS, Van Thiel DH. Variceal sclerosis: does it have long term adverse effects upon the esophagus? (Abstract) Hepatology 1982; 2:712.

201. Hoffman BI, Katz WA. The gastrointestinal manifestations of systemic lupus erythematosus: a review of the literature. Semin Arthritis Rheum 1980; 9:227–247.

202. Hamel-Roy J, Devroede C, Arhan P, Tetreault L, Duranceau A, Menard HA. Comparative esophageal and anorectal motility in scleroderma. Gastroenterology 1985; 88:1–7.

203. Maddern GJ, Horowitz M, Jamieson GG, Chatterton BE, Collins PJ, Roberts-Thomson P. Abnormalities of esophageal and gastric emptying in progressive systemic disorders. Gastroenterology 1984; 87:922–926.

204. Gutierrez F, Valenzuela M, Ehresmann GR, Quismorio FP, Kitridou RC. Esophageal dysfunction in patients with mixed connective tissue diseases and systemic lupus erythematosus. Dig Dis Sci 1982; 27:592–597.

205. Cohen S, Laufer I, Snape WJ, Shiau YF, Levine GM, Jimenez S. The gastrointestinal manifestations of scleroderma: pathogenesis and management. Gastroenterology 1980; 79:155–166.

206. Turner R, Lipshutz W, Miller W. Esophageal dysfunction in collagen diseases. Am J Med Sci 1973; 265:191–199.

207. Cohen S, Fisher R, Lipshutz W, Turner R, Myers A, Schumacher R. The pathogenesis of esophageal dysfunction in scleroderma and Raynaud's disease. J Clin Invest 1972; 52:2663–2668.

208. Hurwitz AL, Duranceau A, Postlethwait RW. Esophageal dysfunction and Raynaud's phenomenon in patients with scleroderma. Am J Dig Dis 1976; 21:601–606.

209. Flick JA, Boyle JT, Tuchman DN, Athreya BH, Doughty RA. Esophageal motor abnormalities in children and adolescents with scleroderma and mixed connective tissue disease. Pediatrics 1988; 82:107–111.

210. Weihrauch TR, Korting GW, Ewe K, Vogt G. Esophageal dysfunction and its pathogenesis in progressive systemic sclerosis. Klin Wochenschr 1978; 56:963–970.

211. Petrokubi RJ, Jeffries GH. Cimetidine versus antacids in scleroderma with reflux esophagitis. Gastroenterology 1979; 77:691–696.

212. Ramirez-Mata M, Ibanez G, Alarcon-Segovia D. Stimulatory effect of metoclopramide on the esophagus and lower esophageal sphincter of patients with PSS. Arthr Rheumatol 1977; 20:30–35.

213. Horowitz M, Maddern GJ, Maddox A, Wishart J, Chatterton BE, Shearman DJ. Effects of cisapride on gastric and esophageal emptying in progressive systemic sclerosis. Gastroenterology 1987; 93:311–315.

214. Kjellen G, Fransson SG, Lindstrom F, Sokjer H, Tibbling L. Esophageal function, radiography and dysphagia in Sjogren's syndrome. Dig Dis Sci 1986; 31:225–229.

215. MacDonald GB, Sullivan KM, Schuffler MD, Shulman MS, Thomas ED. Esophageal abnormalities in chronic graft versus host disease in humans. Gastroenterology 1981; 80:914–921.

PART 5

Reflux and Esophagitis

A. Craig Hillemeier, M.D.

It is common for infants to have recurrent problems with "spitting up" or "vomiting" during the first year of life. The severity of symptoms varies from an occasional burp to persistent emesis. Evaluation of most of these infants reveals no definable anatomic, metabolic, infectious, or neurologic etiology, and they are labeled with the descriptive term *gastroesophageal reflux* (GER), which refers to the presence of gastric contents proximal to the stomach. Current diagnostic tests are able to detect and quantitate GER in large numbers of infants, including many who are not overtly symptomatic. The pervasive nature of GER during infancy results in its presence in many infants who have other, possibly related health problems such as growth failure, respiratory disease, apnea, and behavioral problems. The clinical determination of a cause-and-effect relationship between GER and other disorders is often difficult and must be approached with caution.

PHYSIOLOGY

The upper gastrointestinal (GI) tract distal to the midesophagus is composed of smooth muscle and is therefore not under voluntary control. The esophagus functions as a muscular tube, and a peristaltic wave of contraction involving the external circular muscle layer is responsible for the mechanical forces that transport ingested food through the esophagus into the stomach.

The distal end of the esophagus has an area of tonically contracted circular smooth muscle known as the lower esophageal sphincter (LES). This tonically contracted smooth muscle relaxes, allowing the peristaltic wave in the esophagus to propel the ingested food into the stomach. Abnormalities of this high pressure zone of tonically contracted muscle have long been suspected of being the factor responsible for GER during infancy. The concept that abnormally low resting pressure in the LES during infancy is responsible for GER has not been supported by studies, which have shown LES pressures in infants to be similar to those in older children or adults.

The possibility that the LES might undergo episodes of transient relaxation unassociated with a normal esophageal peristaltic mechanism, allowing gastric contents to reflux into the esophagus, has had increasing support. Relaxation of the LES occurs through release of a neurotransmitter by a system of enteric neurons. This transmitter is not a classic adrenergic or cholinergic transmitter, and there is strong evidence to suggest a neurotransmitter such as vasoactive intestinal peptide. Possible explanations for inappropriate relaxation of the LES may be related to the central nervous system or a developmentally exaggerated enteric reflex. The origin of this enteric reflex could be either proximal (i.e., esophageal) or distal (i.e., gastric distention) in origin.

DIAGNOSTIC EVALUATION

It is important to realize that the term *GER during infancy* refers to a group of symptoms without a defined etiology, and any process that interrupts normal gastrointestinal motility may result in GER. Therefore, a test that attempts to quantitate the presence of GER does not necessarily give any information as to the pathogenesis of the reflux. In addition to the previously mentioned systemic processes that may present with GER, specific intestinal causes of GER include gastric outlet obstruction associated with duodenal or gastric ulcer, pyloric ulcer, pyloric stenosis, or even more distal intestinal obstruction. GER may also be seen in the numerous disorders of intestinal motility that may involve enteric neural or muscle function.

Barium Swallow

Contrast radiographic studies of the esophagus during and after ingestion of barium have long been used to study GER during infancy (Fig. 1). While it was initially believed that most infants with GER might have hiatal hernias demonstrable by barium swallow, further experience has shown that although occasional infants and children with GER do have hiatal hernias (especially those with CNS impairment), most do not. While there is considerable disagreement over the role of the barium swallow or upper GI studies in evaluating the severity of GER in a given infant, it is important that an infant with severe symptoms suggestive of GER have such a study to rule out the presence of a large hiatal hernia, esophageal stricture, atypical pyloric stenosis, duodenal web, gastric web, or other anatomic cause of recurrent vomiting.

Attempts have been made to quantitate the degree of reflux that occurs during a conventional contrast study and have proven somewhat successful in spite of the limited time duration of a barium swallow. However, if valuable information is to be obtained from this test, it must be performed in a standard manner by an experienced observer.[1] Although the sensitivity of the barium swallow in detecting GER can be quite high, it has a fairly low specificity, as many infants with few or no clinically significant symptoms of GER reflux some barium into the esophagus.[2,3] Because barium is an inert substance that does not activate the various receptors in the

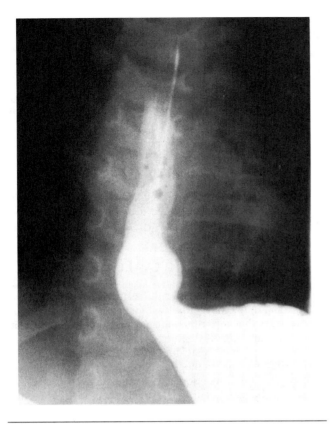

FIGURE 1 Contrast radiography demonstrating an episode of gastric reflux into the distal esophagus.

duodenum that co-ordinate motor activity, a barium contrast study provides little useful information regarding a physiologically regulated process such as rate of gastric emptying.

pH Probe

The development of thin flexible pH probes that can be placed in the esophagus for considerable lengths of time and still allow the infant or child the opportunity to function in a relatively "normal" fashion has added considerable data to our understanding of GER and what therapies may be most effective. Although restricted by their ability to determine only those episodes of reflux that cause a change in esophageal pH and their inability to determine the volume of refluxed material, pH probe studies are able to determine how frequently episodes of acid reflux occur, how long it takes the acid to be cleared, and how often over a given period of time there is acid in the distal esophagus (Fig. 2). These studies can then be used to examine such issues as the effect of feeding, body position, or state of consciousness on GER and whether pharmacologic or medical therapies are effective in reducing total reflux time.

Initial reports of pH probe studies utilized a variation of the Tuttle test,[4] in which a volume of 0.1N HCl was instilled into the stomach of a fasting infant or child, and after a pH probe was placed in the esophagus various maneuvers were performed in an attempt to raise intragastric pressure. A decrease in intraesophageal pH to less than 3.0 on two different occasions was considered confirmation of GER.[5] This test showed some ability to detect infants who were having significant problems from GER,[6] but many infants with typical reflux symptoms have a negative acid reflux test, and the repetitive nasogastric intubations to instill the HCl and then place the pH probe are uncomfortable for the patient.

Prolonged pH probe studies with the installation of a flexible pH probe and observation of the infant or child in a more physiologic setting have proven to be more sensitive and reliable indicators of the severity of GER. Recent development of a pediatric-sized ambulatory pH probe allows monitoring of intraesophageal pH while the child carries on daily activities free of the attachment to a stationary pH meter and strip-chart recorder.[7]

While prolonged 24-hour pH probe studies have the ability to monitor a child in a nearly physiologic setting with a normal dietary intake, they suffer from an inability to accurately detect reflux in the postprandial period. After a feeding, ingested foodstuffs buffer the gastric acidity for varying periods of time and alter the ability of the pH probe to accurately detect reflux episodes. The use of a relatively acidic, low-buffering food (e.g., apple juice) for at least one feeding during a prolonged pH probe allows a more accurate determination of GER during the postprandial period.[8] It is possible that pH probe studies that do not cover a sleep period may miss significant episodes of reflux, which tend to occur during this time period in patients who have chronic respiratory disease. Ambulatory and computerized telemetry systems for extended esophageal pH monitoring have been shown to be practical for infants and children.[7,9] Such systems have the advantage of allowing pH probes to be performed in a more physiologic setting, with the data then transmitted to a central data collection facility.

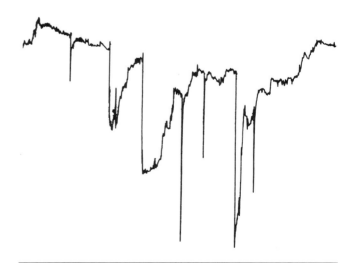

FIGURE 2 Time chart recording of a pH probe in the distal esophagus. Episodes of acid reflux into the esophagus are denoted by downward deflections.

Endoscopy and Esophageal Biopsy

Although direct visualization of macroscopic evidence of esophageal ulceration or inflammation is strongly suggestive of esophagitis secondary to the reflux of gastric contents, these changes are often not seen even in situations of severe GER. Esophageal mucosal biopsy has been used to assess the severity of esophagitis that results from GER (Fig. 3), and the emergence of small flexible fiberoptic endoscopes over the last 10 to 15 years has greatly increased the number of biopsies performed in the pediatric patient. Basal cell hyperplasia of the esophageal mucosal epithelium and increased length of the stromal papillae have long been established as histologic criteria of reflux esophagitis in adults,[10] but normal thickening of the basal zone in the distal esophagus has led to caution in interpreting these changes in the distal esophagus of the human infant. The presence of intraepithelial eosinophils has been shown to correlate with the clinical presence of GER during infancy.[11] Other infiltrates of the esophageal tissue such as lymphocytes and polymorphonuclear leukocytes are seen in reflux esophagitis, although mild to moderate infiltrates of these cells are seen under normal conditions. Eosinophilic infiltrates have been found to be far more specific indicators of reflux esophagitis,[12,13] with one or more intra-epithelial eosinophilic infiltrates being sufficient to establish the presence of GER in an infant.

As more esophageal biopsies are performed in pediatric-aged patients, a histologic condition called Barrett's esophagus is being seen with greater frequency. Barrett's esophagus is a condition in which the normal stratified squamous epithelium of the esophagus is converted to columnar epithelium with occasional glandular elements. Previously this condition was thought to occur almost exclusively in adults who have chronic GER, and when it was seen in children it was thought to represent a congenital anomaly.[14] However, it has now been described in a large series of children with GER. Histologic changes compatible with Barrett's esophagus have been described in as many as 13 percent of children with endoscopically documented esophagitis, and it has been proposed that GER is often responsible for these changes in the esophageal mucosa and that they are often not congenital phenomena.[15] Children with Barrett's esophagus often have associated esophageal strictures. It is hoped that future studies will address the concerns raised about the malignant potential of the mild dysplasia that is often noted in these ectopic areas of intestinal glandular epithelium.[16]

Manometrics

The ability to measure the pressure profiles and their dynamic changes in the body of the esophagus has not proven very helpful in determining either the etiology or the severity of GER during infancy and today remains primarily a research tool, often providing little clinically useful information in the individual patient. Initial reports suggested that many infants with GER had decreased LES pressures,[17] but later studies have shown that most fall within the normal range.[18] Although it appears that a small subset of patients with GER have markedly decreased resting LES pressures, some infants with GER have actually been shown to have increased LES pressure.[19]

With the advent of esophageal manometrics in the 1960s came the potential to determine what pressures exist in the lower esophageal sphincter during normal infant development and in infants who suffer from GER. The issue of whether or not LES tone is reduced in the period of infancy has been the subject of many investigators, with some finding LES pressures reduced in the newborn period[20] while others have found no differences.[21,22] One reason that it may be difficult to accurately and reproducibly measure LES pressure in infants of markedly different sizes and ages is that the relative amount of stretch that the manometric catheter provides to the LES area affects the measurement of the pressure because it affects the laplacian relationship that determines LES pressure.[23]

With the realization that reduced steady-state LES pressure may not explain GER during infancy, attention has turned to abnormal relaxation of the LES as the possible pathogenetic agent for GER. In adult populations, so-called inappropriate relaxation of the LES has been shown to be a primary etiologic event for GER, and there is some indication that similar events occur during some episodes of GER in infancy.[24] Although little follow-up work has been performed on this potentially fruitful line of investigation in pediatric patients,

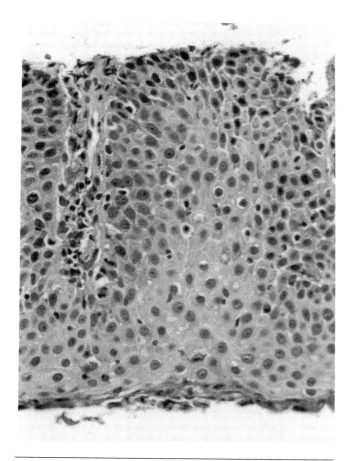

FIGURE 3 Biopsy of the distal esophagus demonstrating inflammatory cells in the squamous mucosa.

recent data suggest that inappropriate relaxation may be the result of nonperistaltic swallowing events[25] or gastric distention postprandially.[26]

Peristalsis, or the timely sequence of pressure wave down the esophagus, may be of importance in both the primary swallowing sequence and the clearance of acid during an episode of reflux. Manometric evaluation of swallowing and the peristaltic response to physiologic stimuli such as acid reflux or volume distention in the infant's esophagus has not been extensive. It has been reported that some infants with large amounts of GER have a decreased amplitude of peristalsis in the body of the esophagus,[27] but it is not clear what role this decreased amplitude of peristalsis plays in GER. Pharmacologic therapy with cholinergic agonists such as bethanechol may increase peristaltic amplitude in the esophagus of infants,[27] although the impact of this increase on delayed acid clearance is uncertain.

Scintigraphy

A radionuclide such as ^{99m}Tc can be added to the infant's diet and allow the performance of a gastroesophageal scintiscan. The location of the formula can be monitored under a gamma counter, and time and amount of radionuclide refluxed to the esophagus or lungs as well as the rate of emptying from the stomach can be determined. The gastroesophageal scintiscan has the advantage of being noninvasive, low in radiation, and potentially available wherever a gamma counter is available. In practice, however, the test requires considerable experience before reproducible results can be obtained and also requires the infant to maintain a stationary position for relatively long periods of time if data such as the quantification of reflux time are to be obtained. The esophageal scintiscan has an advantage over a traditional pH probe in that it is able to detect reflux in the postprandial period when the gastric contents may be alkalized and GER undetectable by pH probe. While the gastroesophageal scintiscan has been shown to be useful in evaluating the severity of GER,[28] it has not become widely used because it is not as sensitive as an upper GI study in ruling out anatomic obstruction and does not allow the amount of ambulation or mobility that a prolonged pH probe study does in quantitating the amount of reflux.

The ability of the gastroesophageal scintiscan to detect in a relatively physiologic manner the rate of gastric emptying does offer something that is not obtainable by other diagnostic tests. However, it is not at present clear how valuable it is to determine the rates of gastric emptying in a child with reflux. While it has been shown that some infants with severe GER have delayed gastric emptying,[29] the vast majority of infants with GER have gastric emptying rates that fall within the normal range.[30]

The gastroesophageal scintiscan may document the pulmonary aspiration of gastric contents by demonstrating the presence of radionuclide in the lungs after it is ingested. Attempts to document the aspiration of gastric contents with ingested radionuclide have proven to be variably successful because of inherent limitations of the technique,[31] and many have not found the so-called milk scan to be helpful, although in the right hands it is claimed to have sufficient sensitivity to be clinically useful.[32] The use of bronchial lavage to determine the presence of intratracheal lipid-laden macrophages has shown some promise in detecting those children who may be aspirating ingested foodstuffs into their lungs.[33]

THERAPY

The traditional therapy of placing a child in an infant seat to reduce the amount of GER has been evaluated with pH probe studies and has not been shown to be effective in reducing GER. A controlled, prospective comparison of the use of the infant seat versus head-elevated prone positioning in a harness has shown that the head-elevated prone positioning resulted in both fewer and briefer episodes of GER.[34]

Many infants can be effectively treated with smaller, more frequent feedings. This presumably reduces the amount of formula in the stomach that is available for reflux. The institution of continuous drip nasogastric tube feedings has also been shown to be a successful means of getting adequate weight gain and may allow surgical intervention to be avoided.[35] If the infant does not begin to show catch-up growth during the first 7 days of nasogastric feeding, he does not benefit from longer periods.

Thickened Feedings

Traditionally the mother of the child with symptomatic GER has been advised to thicken the child's feedings in an attempt to reduce the child's symptoms. This assumption has been tested with the pH probe, and thickened feedings (apple juice thickened with rice cereal) were found to have no effect on reflux time unless the infant was in the head-elevated prone position after the feeding.[36] However, it is possible that infants with GER who are given thickened feedings may not have significantly reduced reflux time, but the number of episodes of emesis, the time spent crying, and the time spent awake are all reduced.[37]

Surgical Correction

Surgical procedures to tighten the LES and prevent the reflux of gastric contents into more proximal areas have become increasingly more common, with fundoplications becoming one of the most common surgical procedures in many pediatric surgery centers. For the child in whom GER is thought to be the cause of an unacceptable symptom, there is little doubt that surgical intervention can terminate the GER. Long-term follow-up has shown efficacy rates ranging from 60 to greater than 90 percent.[38,39] The Nissen fundoplication, which involves a 360-degree wrap of the fundus around the distal 3.5 cm of the esophagus, is the most common procedure, and a recent comprehensive follow-up of a minimum of 5 years shows that 88 percent of infants and children had a good clinical outcome[40] and that neurologically impaired children had results as good as those of neurologically normal children. It has been suggested that fundoplications be combined with pyloroplasty in those patients with GER and delayed gastric emptying.[41]

Unfortunately, the incidence of complications following this procedure is not insignificant and, therefore, the decision to use the procedure should not be made lightly. The incidence of reoperation because of small intestinal obstruction secondary to adhesions ranges from 5 to 10 percent in most large series,[38,42,43] compared with approximately 1 percent for other causes of laparotomy. This complication can be particularly unfortunate in the patient who has been made unable to vomit, and in one series of patients with obstruction secondary to intestinal adhesions following fundoplication, less than 20 percent of children with obstruction presented with vomiting. It is therefore important that patients who have had a fundoplication be evaluated by radiography if obstruction secondary to adhesions is suspected.

The placement of a gastrostomy tube has been shown to either initiate GER or worsen pre-existing GER. It has been shown that as many as 25 percent of neurologically impaired patients who are not symptomatic prior to gastrostomy tube placement will become symptomatic for GER after the procedure.[44] It has been speculated that these patients had GER prior to surgery, but others have shown that the placement of a gastrostomy tube can reduce either the length of the high-pressure zone at the LES or the actual pressure at this area.[45]

Pharmacotherapy

Since GER during infancy is such a widespread symptom, there has been a diligent search to determine if a drug will be effective in treating it. Antacids or H_2 antagonists such as cimetidine have been shown to be effective in reducing the amount of acid present in gastric contents and may reduce the peptic esophagitis that may be present.[46] Although this therapy and the others described here often effectively treat GER, many patients (particularly older children) continue to be symptomatic while on this therapy or relapse when it is discontinued.

Metoclopramide has been found to mildly increase resting LES pressure and to increase rates of gastric emptying under many conditions. Unfortunately, metoclopramide has side effects that range from 11 to 34 percent. Drowsiness and restlessness are the most common side effects, but the most troublesome is the extrapyramidal reaction that seems to occur with increased frequency in children. This is an acute dystonic type of extrapyramidal reaction that manifests as neck pain and rigidity, trismus, and oculogyric crisis.[47] Although some have reported efficacy of metoclopramide in treating GER in the pediatric age group, others argue that either metoclopramide is ineffective or high doses (which may increase the incidence of side effects) are necessary to see therapeutic results.[48,49]

Bethanechol, a muscarinic agonist, has been shown to greatly increase LES pressure in more than 90 percent of the patients to whom it is given, but many investigators have not been able to show that it is effective in reducing GER measured by pH probe,[49] and it has a high frequency of undesirable side effects.[50] Domperidone, an agent similar to metoclopramide, reportedly has fewer central nervous system side effects, and there is some suggestion that it may improve symptoms of GER.[51] Cisapride, which has recently been developed, probably is the most promising of the pharmacologic agents in its potential to treat GER,[52,53] although it is not yet widely available.

RESPIRATORY DISEASE

The role of GER in the pathogenesis of respiratory disease in both the infant and older child has been one of the most interesting areas of GER, with GER being suggested as an etiologic factor in children with apnea, SIDS, asthma, recurrent pneumonia, and bronchopulmonary dysplasia. The experience with children who have cystic fibrosis has suggested that chronic lung disease predisposes to GER[54] and serves to draw into question much of the data that purport to show that GER is the cause of chronic lung disease.

Studies of infants affected with chronic bronchopulmonary dysplasia have shown a significant amount of GER.[55] Fundoplication and gastrostomy have been found to be effective in facilitating growth and feeding in addition to decreasing oxygen requirements in infants with severe bronchopulmonary dysplasia and GER,[56] although it is not clear whether the improvement in pulmonary function is due to an improvement in nutritional status from the gastrostomy or prevention of reflux from the fundoplication.

REFERENCES

1. McCauley RG, Darling DB, Leonidas JC, Schwartz AM. Gastroesophageal reflux in infants and children. A useful classification and reliable physiologic technique for its demonstration. AJR 1978; 130:47–50.
2. Cleveland RH, Kushner DC, Schwartz AN. Gastroesophageal reflux in children. Results of a standardized fluoroscopic approach. AJR 1983; 141:52–56.
3. Siebert JJ, Byrne WJ, Culer AR, Latture T, Leach M, Campbell M. Gastroesophageal reflux—the acid test. Scintigraphy or the pH probe? AJR 1983; 140:1087–1090.
4. Tuttle SG, Grossman MI. Detection of gastroesophageal reflux by simultaneous measurement of intraluminal pressure and pH. Soc Exp Biol Med 1958; 98:225.
5. Euler AR, Ament ME. Detection of gastroesophageal reflux in the pediatric age patient by esophageal intraluminal pH probe measurement (Tuttle test). Pediatrics 1977; 60:65–68.
6. Christie DL. The acid reflux test for gastroesophageal reflux. J Pediatr 1979; 94:78–81.
7. Haase GM, Meagher DP, Goldson E, Falor WH. A unique teletransmission system for extended four channel esophageal pH monitoring in infants and children. J Pediatr Surg 1987; 22:68–74.
8. Sondheimer JM. Continuous monitoring of distal esophageal pH: a diagnostic test for gastroesophageal reflux in infants. J Pediatr 1980; 96:804–807.
9. Newman LJ, Berezin S, San-Filippo JA, Halata M, Medow MS, Schwars SM. A new ambulatory system for extended esophageal pH monitoring. J Pediatr Gastroenterol Nutr 1985; 4:707–710.
10. Ismail-Beigi F, Horton CE, Pope CE. Histologic consequences of gastroesophageal reflux in man. Gastroenterology 1970; 58:163–174.
11. Winter HS, Madara JL, Stafford RJ, Grand RJ, Quinlan JE, Goldman H. Intraepithelial eosinophils. A new diagnostic criterion for reflux esophagitis. Gastroenterology 1982; 83:818–823.
12. Groben PA, Siegal GP, Shub MD, Ulshen MH, Askin FB. Perspectives in pediatric pathology, Vol 11. Basel: Karger, 1987: 124.
13. Shub MD, Ulshen MH, Hargrove CB, Siegal GP, Groben PA, Askin FB. Esophagitis: a frequent consequence of gastroesophageal reflux in infancy. J Pediatr 1985; 107: 881–884.
14. Rector LE, Connerley ML. Aberrant mucosa in the esophagus in infants and children. Arch Pathol Lab Med 1941; 31:285–294.

15. Dahms B, Rothstein FC. Barrett's esophagus in children. A consequence of chronic gastroesophageal reflux. Gastroenterology 1984; 86:318–323.
16. Cooper JE, Spits L, Wilkins BM. Barrett's esophagus in children: a histologic and histochemical study of 11 cases. J Pediatr Surg 1987; 22:103–108.
17. Euler AR, Ament M. Value of esophageal manometric studies in the gastroesophageal reflux of infancy. Pediatrics 1977; 59:58–62.
18. Arasu TS, Wyllie J, Fitzgerald JR. Gastroesophageal reflux in infants and children—comparative accuracy of diagnostic methods. J Pediatr 1980; 96:798–802.
19. Herbst J, Book L, Johnson D, Jolley S. The lower esophageal sphincter in gastroesophageal reflux in children. J Clin Gastroenterol 1979; 1:119–122.
20. Boix-Ochoa J, Lafuente JM, Gil-vernet JM. Maturation of the lower esophagus. J Pediatr Surg 1976; 11:749–754.
21. Vanderhoof JA, Rapoport PJ, Paxson CL. Manometric diagnosis of lower esophageal sphincter incompetence in infants: Use of a small, single-lumen perfused catheter. Pediatrics 1978; 62:805–808.
22. Moroz S, Espinoza J, Cumming W, Diamant N. Lower esophageal sphincter function in children with/without gastroesophageal reflux. Gastroenterology 1976; 71:236–242.
23. Hillemeier C, Grybosk J, McCallum R, Biancani. Developmental characteristics of the lower esophageal sphincter in the kitten. Gastroenterology 1985; 89:760–766.
24. Werlin S, Dodds W, Hogan W, Arndorfer R. Mechanisms of gastroesophageal reflux in children. J Pediatr 1980; 97:244–248.
25. Paterson WG, Rattan S, Goyal RK. Pathophysiology of inappropriate lower esophageal relaxation. Gastroenterology 1985; 88:1533.
26. Holloway RH, Hongo M, Berger K, McCallum RW. Gastric distention: a mechanism for postprandial gastroesophageal reflux. Gastroenterology 1985; 89:779–784.
27. Sondheimer JM, Arnold G. Effect of bethanechol on esophageal peristalsis of infants with gastroesophageal reflux. Pediatr Res 1985; 19(4):731A.
28. Blumbrogen JD, Rudd TG, Christie DL. Gastroesophageal reflux in children: radionuclide gastroesophagography. AJR 1980; 135:1001–1004.
29. Hillemeier AC, Lange R, McCallum R, Seashore J, Gryboski JD. Delayed gastric emptying in infants with gastroesophageal reflux. J Pediatr 1981; 98:190–193.
30. Rosen PR, Treves S. The relationship of gastroesophageal reflux and gastric emptying in infants and children: concise communication. J Nucl Med 1984; 25:571–574.
31. Paton JY, Cosgriff PS, Nanayakkara CS. The analytical sensitivity of Tc99m radionuclide 'milk' scanning in the detection of gastro-oesophageal reflux. Pediatr Radiol 1985; 15:381–383.
32. McVeagh P, Howman GR, Kemp A. Pulmonary aspiration studied by radionuclide milk scanning and barium swallow roentgenography. Am J Dis Child 1987; 141:917–921.
33. Nussbaum E, Magi JC, Mathis R, Galant SP. Association of lipid-laden alveolar macrophages and gastroesophageal reflux in children. J Pediatr 1987; 110:190–194.
34. Orenstein DR, Whitington PF. Positioning for prevention of infant gastroesophageal reflux. J Pediatr 1983; 103:534–537.
35. Ferry GD, Selby M, Pietro TJ. Clinical response to short-term nasogastric feeding in infants with gastroesophageal reflux and growth failure. J Pediatr Gastroenterol Nutr 1983; 2:57–61.
36. Bailey DJ, Andres JM, Danek GD, Pineiro-Carrero VM. Lack of efficacy of thickened feeding as treatment for gastroesophageal reflux. J Pediatr 1987; 110:187–189.
37. Orenstein SR, Magill LH, Brooks P. Thickening of infant feedings for therapy of GER. J Pediatr 1987; 110:181–186.
38. Dedinsky GK, Vane DW, Black T, Turner MK, West KW. Complications and reoperation after Nissen fundoplication in childhood. Am J Surg 1987; 153:177–183.
39. Opie JC, Chaye H, Fraser GC. Fundoplication and pediatric esophageal manometry: actuarial analysis over 7 years. J Pediatr Surg 1987; 22:935–938.
40. Turnage RH, Oldham KT, Coran AG, Blane C. Late results of fundoplication for gastro esophageal reflux in infants and children. Surgery; in press.
41. Fonkalsrud EW, Berquest W, Vargas J, Ament ME, Foglia RP. Surgical treatment of the gastroesophageal reflux syndrome in infants and children. Am J Surg 1987; 154:11–18.
42. Wilkins BM, Spitz L. Adhesion obstruction following Nissen fundoplication in children. Br J Surg 1987; 74:777–779.
43. Jolley SG, Tunell WP, Hoelzer DJ, Smith EI. Postoperative small bowel obstruction in infants and children: a problem following Nissen fundoplication. J Pediatr Surg 1986; 21:407–409.
44. Mollitt DL, Golladay ES, Seibert JJ. Symptomatic gastroesophageal reflux following gastrostomy in neurologically impaired patients. Pediatrics 1985; 76:124–126.
45. Jolley SG, Tunell WP, Hoelzer DJ, Thomas S, Smith EI. Lower esophageal pressure changes with tube gastrostomy: a causative factor of gastroesophageal reflux in children? J Pediatr Surg 1986; 21:624–627.
46. Cucchiara S, Staiano A, Romaniello G, Capobianco S, Auricchio S. Antacids and cimetidine treatment for gastro-oesophageal reflux and peptic oesophagitis. Arch Dis Child 1984; 59:842–847.
47. Harrington RA, Hamilton CW, Brogden RN, Linkowick JA, Romankiewicz JA, Hiel RC. Metoclopramide—an updated review of its pharmacologic properties and clinical use. Drugs 1983; 25:451–494.
48. Hyams JS, Leichtner AM, Zamett LO, Walters JK. Effect of metoclopramide on prolonged intraesophageal pH testing in infants with gastroesophageal reflux. J Pediatr Gastroenterol Nutr 1986; 5:716–720.
49. Orenstein SR, Lofton SW, Orenstein DM. Bethanechol for pediatric gastroesophageal reflux: a prospective, blind, controlled study. J Pediatr Gastroenterol Nutr 1986; 5:549–555.
50. Levi P, Marmo F, Saluzzo C, DellOlio D, Ansaldi N, Guiliani L, Guardamagna O, Mostert M, Ponzone A. Bethanechol versus antacids in the treatment of gastroesophageal reflux. Helv Paediatr Acta 1985; 40:349–359.
51. Grill BB, Hillemeier AC, Semeraro LA, McCallum RW, Gryboski JD. Effects of domeperidone therapy on symptoms and upper gastrointestinal motility in infants with gastroesophageal reflux. J Pediatr 1985; 106:311–316.
52. Cucchiara S, Staiano A, Capozzi C, Di-Lorenzo C, Boccieri A, Auricchio S. Cisapride for gastro-esophageal reflux and peptic oesophagitis. Arch Dis Child 1987; 62:454–457.
53. Saye AN, Forget PP, Geubelle F. Effect of Cisapride on gastroesophageal reflux in children with chronic bronchopulmonary disease: a double-blind cross-over pH-monitoring study. Pediatr Pulmonol 1987; 3:8–12.
54. Scott RB, Oloughlin EV, Gall DG. Gastroesophageal reflux in patients with cystic fibrosis. J Pediatr 1985; 106:223–227.
55. Hoyoux D, Forget P, Lambrechts L, Geubelle F. Chronic bronchopulmonary disease and gastroesophageal reflux in children. Pediatr Pulmonol 1985; 1:149–153.
56. Giuffre RM, Rubin S, Mitchell I. Antireflux surgery in infants with bronchopulmonary dysplasia. Am J Dis Child 1987; 141:648–651.

CHAPTER 26

The Stomach and Duodenum

PART 1

Congenital Anomalies

Vanessa M. Wright, M.B., B.S., F.R.C.S., F.R.A.C.S.

Like congenital anomalies of the esophagus, congenital anomalies of the stomach, although present at birth, may not produce symptoms until well beyond infancy.

ANTRAL DIAPHRAGM

An antral diaphragm is a rare anomaly. It is composed of a submucosal web covered by gastric mucosa. Obstruction may be complete, or partial if the web has a perforation. Synonyms for this disorder are antral mucosal membrane, prepyloric septum, gastric antral web or diaphragm, antral web, and prepyloric mucosal diaphragm.

Clinical Presentation

A complete web produces symptoms identical to those of pyloric atresia—persistent non–bile-stained vomiting commencing shortly after birth. The much more common incomplete web presents with a spectrum of symptoms depending on the size of the perforation in the web. Prominent symptoms in the early months of life are vomiting and failure to thrive. In later childhood, epigastric pain and fullness after eating with vomiting and flatulence are presenting symptoms. Frequently in these children the history goes back to infancy, and other diagnoses including peptic ulcer and recurrent viral gastroenteritis will have been entertained, resulting in delay in making the correct diagnosis.[1] In addition, the radiologic diagnosis of an incomplete antral web may be difficult.[2] The presence of a large perforation in the antral web may result in few troublesome symptoms, and the diagnosis may not be made until well into adult life.[3]

Diagnosis

The complete web appears on a plain abdominal radiograph as an air-filled stomach with no distal gas. In the infant and older child with an incomplete web, the plain radiograph may be normal or may reveal a distended stomach. Careful contrast studies demonstrate a lucent line across the gastric

antrum, often associated with poor antral filling (Fig. 1). Where the orifice in the web is small, delayed gastric emptying is obvious. However, in many cases the liquid barium may pass through the web relatively unhindered. The key to successful radiologic diagnosis is a high index of suspicion of the diagnosis on clinical grounds. Upper gastrointestinal (GI) endoscopy now plays an invaluable role in the diagnosis of an antral web and would be employed in every suspected case irrespective of the radiologic findings. The endoscopic appearances of the antral web are the following:

1. A small, fixed antral aperture surrounded by smooth gastric mucosa

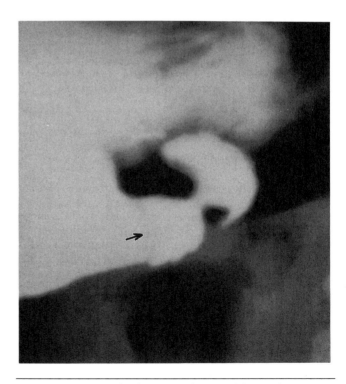

FIGURE 1 Antral diaphragm with typical lucent line.

423

2. Constant size of the web with gastric peristalsis
3. Normal peristalsis in the gastric wall proximal and distal to the web[4,5]

Management

The complete web in the neonate is treated by early surgical excision with careful inspection of the remainder of the GI tract for further atresias. In the older child with significant symptoms and a web with a small orifice, excision of the web is followed by a rapid resolution of symptoms in the majority of cases. Endoscopic transection of the web has been described.[6]

Conservative management in those infants diagnosed radiologically as having an antral web but little delay in gastric emptying has been advocated.[7] Management includes a low-residue formula, drugs to enhance gastric emptying, and a careful feeding regimen. Conservative management is justified if the radiologic findings suggest little hold-up of barium and endoscopically the orifice in the diaphragm is not highly stenotic. However long-term follow-up is essential to ensure early recognition of further symptoms.

GASTRIC DUPLICATION

Duplications of the stomach are rare. Several series report a higher incidence in females than males.[8,9] Complete duplication of the stomach extending from the esophagus to the pylorus is very unusual. Cystic duplications closely applied to the pyloric region occur,[10,11] as do cysts on a pedicle containing branches of the gastroepiploic vessels. Cysts closely applied to the pancreas but with a blood supply from the gastroepiploic vessels have also been described.[12] Other sites of origin include the greater curve of the stomach and the posterior wall. The majority of gastric duplications do not communicate with the lumen of the GI tract unless ulceration of the common wall occurs.

Clinical Presentation

A large cyst may present as an abdominal mass. If the cyst impedes gastric emptying, vomiting occurs with consequent failure to thrive if the diagnosis is delayed. A cyst confined to the pyloric region may masquerade as pyloric stenosis.[10] Gastric duplications are lined by gastric mucosa, and it is assumed that the acid and/or pepsin-containing cyst fluid causes ulceration and inflammation of the cyst wall. Ulceration through the adjacent stomach wall produces bleeding manifested by hematemesis and/or melena. Ulceration into the peritoneal cavity may produce an inflammatory mass or peritonitis. A fistula into the colon has also been described.[8,12] A cyst on a long pedicle may undergo torsion. Occasionally the cyst is discovered as an incidental finding at laparotomy. A gastric duplication cyst may present at any time from the early neonatal period into adult life.

Diagnosis

The duplication cyst may be palpable. Barium studies may reveal indentation of the gastric wall and, in the case of a pyloric duplication cyst, gastric outlet obstruction. Ultrasound examination of the upper abdomen should reveal a cystic lesion and define its relationship to adjacent structures.

Management

Excision of a gastric duplication is always advisable. Conservative surgery is usually possible, sacrificing only a small area of adjacent stomach. In those cases that present with an inflammatory mass, actual identification of the cause of the problem may be difficult,[8,12] and repeated surgery is not unusual. In complete duplications, excising the bulk of the cyst and stripping the residual mucosa from the adjacent stomach wall has been described[13] and allows the duplication to be excised without sacrificing normal stomach. The prognosis following surgery is excellent.

MICROGASTRIA

This extremely rare condition has been described in association with other intra-abdominal malformations, including pyloric atresia, malrotation, situs inversus, transverse liver, absence of the gallbladder, and asplenia.[14,15] Skeletal anomalies may also occur, in particular spinal and upper limb anomalies.[16,17] In a patient in whom microgastria was associated with pyloric atresia, anophthalmia, micrognathia, and a porencephalic cyst also occurred.[18]

Clinical Presentation

Most infants with microgastria present with failure to thrive and symptoms of gastoesophageal reflux. Depending upon the severity of the symptoms, the diagnosis may be made shortly after birth or may be delayed for some months.[19] Aspiration pneumonia secondary to gastroesophageal reflux is a common problem in these children.

Diagnosis

A contrast study of the upper GI tract shows the small tubular stomach (Fig. 2) and in most cases a megaesophagus with gastroesophageal reflux. Malrotation can also be demonstrated if it is present.

Management

The principal problem appears to be an absence of the normal gastric reservoir; dilation of the esophagus therefore occurs to provide a reservoir. The consequences of this may be frequent vomiting, aspiration pneumonia, and esophagitis. Increasing the capacity of the stomach by anastomosing a double-lumen jejunal pouch to the stomach with a distal

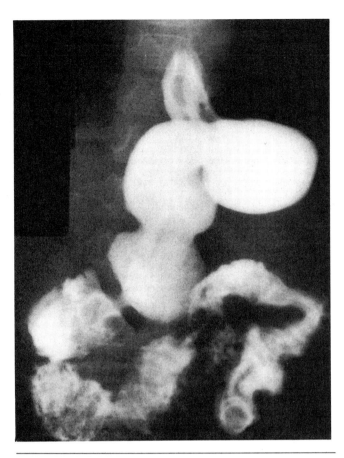

FIGURE 2 Microgastria without malrotation.

Roux-en-Y jejunojejunostomy (Hunt-Lawrence) has reversed the changes in the esophagus[20] and allowed satisfactory feeding and weight gain.[18,20] In those cases in which symptoms are not severe, it is possible to achieve steady weight gain by a strategy of frequent small-volume, high-calorie meals. A nonsurgical approach should be tried after the diagnosis is first established, with repeat contrast studies to assess the effect on the esophagus.[15,19]

PYLORIC ATRESIA

Atresia of the pylorus represents less than 1 percent of all atresias of the alimentary tract.[21] Although it is usually a solitary atresia, it has been described in association with multiple atresias of the small and large intestine.[22-24]. A familial incidence in both solitary pyloric atresia and pyloric atresia with multiple atresias is reported[22-25] and suggests the possibility of a genetic factor in the etiology of this rare condition. The association between pyloric atresia and epidermolysis bullosa letalis is well recognized as an autosomal recessive syndrome.[26]

Clinical Presentation

The pregnancy may be complicated by polyhydramnios, as in other high intestinal atresias. Low birth weight is common. Vomiting is persistent and non–bile-stained and starts in the first days of life. Examination may reveal upper abdominal distention and visible peristalsis. Rupture of the stomach may be the presenting feature and can occur very early.[27] With the advent of widely available prenatal ultrasound scanning, pyloric atresia may be diagnosed on a routine scan. When a family has already had a baby with pyloric atresia, prenatal ultrasound scans of subsequent pregnancies should enable a prenatal diagnosis in further affected siblings. In the family in which pyloric atresia has been associated with epidermolysis bullosa letalis, the one in four risk of recurrence dictates early ultrasound scan and skin biopsy,[28] since epidermolysis bullosa letalis is a lethal condition.

Diagnosis

A plain abdominal radiograph shows air confined to the stomach. The presence of calcification in the abdomen on a radiograph suggests the likelihood that the pyloric atresia is associated with multiple atresias.

Management

Decompression of the stomach using a nasogastric tube should be commenced as soon as the diagnosis is established. If the diagnosis is delayed and vomiting is copious, a metabolic alkalosis with hypochloremia and hypokalemia requires correction prior to surgery.

The surgical procedure carried out depends upon the precise nature of the pyloric lesion. A simple membrane may be excised and a Heinike-Mikulicz pyloroplasty performed. Where there is complete loss of bowel continuity or a thick fibrous mass of tissue connecting the two ends of the bowel, a gastroduodenostomy is the treatment of choice.[29] Rarely, a gastrojejunostomy may be the only option.

Postoperatively the stomach is decompressed with a nasogastric tube until the anastomosis functions. Nutrition and fluid balance are maintained with total parenteral nutrition. The prognosis for isolated pyloric atresia is excellent. When pyloric atresia is associated with multiple small and large bowel atresias, the outcome is uniformly fatal, as in cases of pyloric atresia associated with epidermolysis bullosa letalis.

REFERENCES

1. Blazek FD, Boeckman CR. Prepyloric antral diaphragm. Delays in treatment. J Pediatr Surg 1987; 22:948–949.
2. Campbell DP, Vanhoutte JJ, Ide Smith E. Partially obstructing antral web—a distinct clinical entity. J Pediatr Surg 1973; 8:723–728.
3. Woolley MM, Gwinn JL, Mares A. Congenital partial gastric antral obstruction, an elusive cause of abdominal pain and vomiting. Ann Surg 1974; 180:265–273.
4. Banks PA, Wayne ID. The gastroscopic appearance of antral web. Gastrointest Endosc 1969; 15:228–229.
5. Schwartz SE, Rowden DR, Dudgeon DL. Antral mucosal diaphragm. Gastrointest Endosc 1977; 24:33–34.
6. Berr F, Rienmueller R, Sauerbruch T. Successful endoscopic transection of a partially obstructing antral diaphragm. Gastroenterology 1985; 89:1147–1151.
7. Tunnell WP, Ide Smith E. Antral Webb in infancy. J Pediatr Surg 1980; 15:152–155.

8. Krenier RM, Lepoff RB, Izant RJ. Duplication of the stomach. J Pediatr Surg 1970; 5:360–364.
9. Abrami G, Dennison WM. Duplication of the stomach. Surgery 1961; 49:794–801.
10. Anas P, Miller RC. Pyloric duplication masquerading as hypertrophic pyloric stenosis. J Pediatr Surg 1971; 6:664.
11. Grosfeld J, Boles ET, Reiner C. Duplication of pylorus in the newborn: a rare cause of gastric outlet obstruction. J Pediatr Surg 1970; 5:365–369.
12. Parker BC, Guthrie J, France NE, Atwell JD. Gastric duplication in infancy. J Pediatr Surg 1972; 7:294–298.
13. Lister J, Vaos GC. Duplication of the alimentary tract In: Rob & Smith's operative surgery. Paediatric surgery. London: Butterworths, 1988.
14. Blank E, Chisolm AJ. Congenital microgastria, a case report with a 26 year follow-up. Pediatrics 1973; 51:1037–1041.
15. Hochberger O, Swoboda W. Congenital microgastria. A follow-up observation over six years. Pediatr Radiol 1974; 2:207–208.
16. Schulz RD, Niemann F. Congenital microgastria occurring in combination with skeletal malformations—new syndrome. Helv Paediatr Acta 1971; 26:185–191.
17. Aintablian NH, Slim MS, Antoun BW. Congenital microgastria. Case report and review of the literature. Pediatr Surg Int 1987; 2:307–310.
18. Anderson KD, Guzzetta PC. Treatment of congenital microgastria and dumping syndrome. J Pediatr Surg 1983; 18:747–750.
19. Gorman B, Shaw DG. Congenital microgastria. Br J Radiol 1984; 57:260–262.
20. Neifeld JP, Berman WF, Lawrence W, Kodroff MB, Salzberg AM. Management of congenital microgastria with a jejunal reservoir pouch. J Pediatr Surg 1980; 15:882–885.
21. Thompson NW, Parker W, Schwartz S, Holt JF. Congenital pyloric atresia. Arch Surg 1968; 97:792–796.
22. Guttman FM, Braun P, Garance PH, Blanchard PPC, Dollaire L, Des Jardins JG, Perreault G. Multiple atresias and a new syndrome of hereditary multiple atresias involving the gastrointestinal tract from stomach to rectum. J Pediatr Surg 1973; 8:633–640.
23. Hendren W. Multiple atresias and a new syndrome of hereditary multiple atresias involving the gastrointestinal tract from stomach to rectum. J Pediatr Surg 1973; 8:640.
24. Puri P, Guiney EJ, Carroll R. Multiple gastrointestinal atresias in three consecutive siblings: observations on pathogenesis. J Pediatr Surg 1985; 20:22–24.
25. Keramidas DC. Congenital pyloric atresia in siblings. Arch Surg 1974; 108:123.
26. Rosenbloom MS, Ratner M. Congenital pyloric atresia and epidermolysis bullosa letalis in premature siblings. J Pediatr Surg 1987; 22:374–376.
27. Burnett HA, Halpert B. Perforation of the stomach of a newborn infant with pyloric atresia. Arch Pathol 1947; 44:318.
28. Rodeck CH, Eady RAJ, Gosden CM. Prenatal diagnosis of epidermolysis bullosa letalis. Lancet 1980; i:949–952.
29. Bronsther B, Nadeau MR, Abrams MW. Congenital pyloric atresia—a report of three cases and a review of the literature. Surgery 1971; 69:130–136.

PART 2

Gastritis in Childhood

Brendan Drumm, M.B., Ch.B., FRCPC
Philip Sherman, M.D., FRCPC

Gastritis is generally divided into two categories, primary and secondary, on the basis of the underlying etiology of mucosal inflammation. This division is especially relevant because the natural history of primary gastroduodenal inflammation is different from that due to secondary causes.[1] Secondary gastritis is an acute inflammatory process that is associated with an acute stress, systemic illnesses, or the ingestion of ulcerogenic agents. On the other hand, primary gastritis is of uncertain etiology, although recent studies (which are summarized in more detail below) indicate that many cases of primary gastritis are caused by a bacterial infection of the stomach and that other cases may be due to reflux of bile acids from the duodenum into the gastric lumen. Primary gastritis is more often a chronic inflammatory process that is associated with peptic ulcer disease, particularly duodenal ulcers.[2]

Gastritis is defined as microscopic evidence of inflammation affecting the gastric mucosa. Gastritis does *not* specifically refer to mucosal lesions that are demonstrated by either radiographic studies or endoscopic visualization. In fact, there is a poor correlation between gastritis diagnosed by either barium meal[3] or endoscopy[4,5] and histologic evidence of mucosal inflammation. Endoscopists should, therefore, refer to abnormalities that are visualized through the endoscope in descriptive terms—for example, evidence of erythema, granularity, nodularity, subepithelial hemorrhages, and mucosal friability.[5,6] Histologically normal mucosa may appear erythematous at the time of endoscopy (often erroneously referred to as gastritis). Conversely, endoscopically normal-appearing gastric mucosa may have histologic evidence of inflammation.[4,5] Therefore, it appears prudent to recommend that mucosal biopsies be obtained from all children undergoing diagnostic esophagogastroduodenoscopy who do not have evidence of a bleeding diathesis.[5,7,8]

A pathologic diagnosis of gastritis is not clear-cut, however, since there are normally a limited number of chronic inflammatory cells present in the lamina propria. Mild mucosal inflammation is frequently difficult to distinguish from normal mucosa and often requires review by experienced pathologists.[5,9,10] Evidence of associated mucosal ulceration, mucin depletion, and infiltration of surface epithelial cells by acute inflammatory cells is observed in cases of more severe gastritis.[9–11] However, there are no universally accepted criteria to characterize the presence and severity of gastritis. Existing definitions and nomenclature are variable and confusing. Some investigators[9,10] divide histologic evidence of gastritis into active (presence of polymorphonuclear leukocytes), chronic (presence of chronic inflammatory cells without polymorphonuclear leukocytes), chronic-active (increased numbers of both acute and chronic inflammatory cells), and atrophic (or autoimmune) gastritis which, in turn, is associated with the presence of systemic antiparietal cell antibodies. More detailed definitions of gastritis also consider secondary causes of mucosal inflammation.[12]

The underlying mechanisms that result in gastric inflammation are not yet clearly delineated. However, recent research has identified a number of mediators of mucosal inflammation which could play a role in the development of gastritis. These include, for example, platelet-activating factor, cachectin, leukotrienes, free oxygen radicals, lymphokines, and monokines. The relative contribution and role of each of these inflammatory mediators in the pathogenesis of primary and secondary cases of gastritis require clarification. Current understanding of gastric inflammation suggests that an imbalance exists between mucosal defenses that normally protect mucosal surfaces and aggressive factors that compromise mucosal integrity (Fig. 1). Mucosal defenses include the surface mucous layer overlying epithelial cells,[13] an unstirred water layer,[14] locally produced and pancreaticobiliary sources of bicarbonate,[15,16] mucosal blood flow,[17] rapid cell turnover (also referred to as restitution),[18] surface-active hydrophobic phospholipids present on the apical membranes of surface epithelial cells,[19] and epidermal growth factor.[20] A deficiency in one or more of these components, which together constitute a "cytoprotective" barrier,[21,22] may result in gastric inflammation even when there are normal levels of aggressive factors. Normal host defenses are confronted by a number of aggressive agents, many of which are present in the lumen as substances necessary for the normal process of digestion. Acid and pepsins are both normally active in the lumen of the stomach, and bile acids are present in the lumen of the small intestine. However, in certain circumstances acid, pepsin, and bile acids (either alone or in combination) may cause mucosal inflammation. Experimental work clearly indicates, for example, that exogenous acid can induce mucosal inflammation and ulceration in the stomach.[23] In children with gastric inflammation or ulceration, however, both basal and hormonally (pentagastrin) stimulated gastric acid levels are often comparable to levels in controls.[24] Therefore, interest has also focused on other potential aggressive factors that could predispose to mucosal inflammation and ulceration in the stomach. These include pepsinogens I and II[25] and inappropriate release of gastrin,[26] an endogenous hormone that stimulates proton release from parietal cells in the stomach. Most recently, attention has also been directed to a bacterium, currently referred to as *Campylobacter pylori*,[27] which appears to play an etiologic role in many cases of primary gastritis.[4]

CLINICAL SYMPTOMS OF GASTRIC INFLAMMATION

The most common symptoms of gastritis are abdominal pain and upper gastrointestinal (GI) blood loss. Localization of crampy abdominal pain to the epigastrium and a relationship of the abdominal pain to meals, which frequently accompanies gastritis in adults, are less common in children. In young children abdominal pain may manifest solely as increased irritability and a change in the normal feeding pattern. We have recently observed that primary gastritis is associated with more severe clinical symptoms when there is endoscopic evidence of associated ulceration.[28] Gastritis without evidence of ulcer disease is associated with vague symptoms, usually abdominal pain alone. In addition, abdominal pain is not invariably alleviated by resolution of the gastric inflammation.[28] Therefore, identification of mucosal inflammation does not establish gastritis as the underlying etiology of abdominal symptoms in all instances. In fact, with advancing age histologic evidence of gastritis is increasingly common among an asymptomatic population.[29]

Gastritis can present with fatigue due to iron deficiency anemia resulting from chronic occult blood loss. Alternatively, acute hemorrhage may occur with hematemesis and/or melena. Because the presenting symptoms of gastritis are not specific, a variety of other diagnostic entities giving rise to abdominal pain and GI blood loss must also be considered (Table 1).

CAUSES OF GASTRITIS

As outlined in Table 2, gastric inflammation can result from a wide variety of causes. We will review the various causes of gastric inflammation in children under two main categories, primary gastritis and secondary gastritis.

Primary Gastritis

Campylobacter pylori–Associated Gastritis

In 1983, Warren and Marshall[30] described the presence of spiral-shaped organisms on the antral mucosa in patients with histologic evidence of chronic-active gastritis. They referred

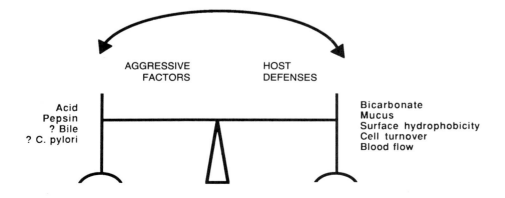

FIGURE 1 Pathogenesis of gastritis. Under normal circumstances there exists a balance between aggressive factors and host defenses. Either an increase in aggressive factors or a decrease in mucosal defenses can tip the "scale" to the right, resulting in gastric inflammation. Conversely, therapy is directed at tipping the "scale" to the left, either by neutralizing aggressive factors or by promoting mucosal defenses.

TABLE 1
Differential Diagnosis of Gastritis

Presenting as Upper Gastrointestinal Hemorrhage
Non-GI sources
  Nasopharynx
  Chest
  Maternal blood (newborn)
GI sources
  Erosions
  Ulceration
  Esophagitis
  Duodenitis
  Varices
  Mallory-Weiss tear
Rare: Hematobilia
      Structural lesions
        Ectopic pancreas
        Duplication
        Polyp
        Angiodysplasias
          (arteriovenous malformation, telangiectasia)
      Bleeding diathesis
      Disorder of collagen synthesis—Ehlers-Danlos
        syndrome

Presenting as Epigastric Abdominal Pain
  Biliary tract disorders
  Pancreatitis
  Genitourinary pathology—renal stones, infection
  Duplication or other congenital anomalies
  Idiopathic (nonulcer dyspepsia)
  Functional

TABLE 2
Causes of Gastritis

A. Primary
  1. Associated with *Campylobacter pylori*
  2. Associated with bile acid reflux

B. Secondary
  1. Stress
    a. Major systemic illness
    b. Sepsis
    c. Burns
    d. Head trauma
  2. Ingested exogenous agents
    a. Corticosteroids
    b. Nonsteroidal anti-inflammatory drugs
    c. Ethanol
    d. Corrosives
  3. Infections
    a. Viral—cytomegalovirus, herpes simplex
    b. Fungal—*Candida*
  4. Others
    a. Crohn's disease
    b. Eosinophilic gastritis
    c. Ménétrier's disease (hypertrophic gastritis)
    d. Varioliform (chronic erosive gastritis)
    e. Autoimmune (atrophic)
      i. Pernicious anemia
      ii. Immunodeficiencies

to these bacteria as *Campylobacter*-like organisms because they showed morphologic similarities to members of the *Campylobacter* genus. Some years earlier Steer and Colin-Jones[31] had made a similar observation, but the significance of their findings was questioned because attempts to culture the organisms resulted in the growth of *Pseudomonas aeruginosa*. However, Marshall et al[32] were able successfully to culture the bacteria from endoscopic biopsies of antral mucosa. The organisms were initially referred to as *Campylobacter pyloridis,* but subsequently the grammatically correct name *Campylobacter pylori* was assigned.[27] Since then, numerous reports from many parts of the world have confirmed an association between the presence of these organisms and antral gastritis.[33] This bacterium has been identified in the antrum by microscopy or culture in approximately 80 percent of patients with primary gastritis. There is also a strong association between the presence of *C. pylori*

organisms in the antrum and duodenal ulcer disease.[4,33,34] It is of interest that prior to the identification of this organism in the gastric antrum, an association between the presence of antral gastritis and duodenal ulcer disease had been observed.[2]

There remains a possibility that these organisms exist as commensals on the gastric antrum or that bacterial colonization of the stomach occurs simply as a result of gastric inflammation. However, we have provided evidence to support a pathogenic role for *C. pylori*, since the bacteria were present only on the antral mucosa of children with primary gastritis (Table 3). Organisms were not identified on inflamed gastric mucosa in cases of secondary gastritis.[4,35] In addition, *C. pylori* was not present in normal gastric biopsies obtained from a relatively large number of children and adolescents. Further evidence to support the pathogenicity of these bacteria is provided by case reports of human volunteer studies in which two volunteers ingested a pure culture of *C. pylori*.[36,37] Each subject then developed evidence of inflammation in what was previously normal gastric mucosa. Con-

TABLE 3
Results of Silver Staining, Culture, and Urease
Testing for *C. pylori* in Antral Biopsy Specimens
from 67 Children

Group	No. of Subjects	Positive on Silver Staining	Positive Culture	Positive Urease Test
Normal children	49	0	0	0
Children with primary gastritis	10	7	7	3
Children with secondary gastritis	8	0	0	0

From Drumm et al[4]; with permission of the New England Journal of Medicine.

versely, there is marked improvement or complete healing of gastritis following clearing of *C. pylori* from the antrum.[28]

C. pylori is a gram-negative, spiral or curved-shaped rod 3 to 5 μm in length. The organism grows only under microaerophilic conditions in vitro and, as it appears to require blood or heme as a nutrient source, grows optimally on blood agar plates. The organism has multiple unipolar flagella and, when viewed under phase-contrast microscopy, it moves in a darting fashion typical of other *Campylobacter* species. Several features distinguish *C. pylori* from most other *Campylobacter*.[33,34] These include high levels of urease production and optimal growth at 37 °C rather than at 42 °C. In addition, *C. pylori* has multiple sheathed flagella, in contrast to the single unsheathed flagellum that is typical of other members of the genus. The outer membrane protein and cellular fatty acid profiles of *C. pylori* are also distinct from those of most other *Campylobacter*. Most importantly, partial analysis of 16S ribosomal RNA sequences indicate that *C. pylori* is phylogenetically more closely related to *Wolinella succinogenes* strains than it is to organisms of the *Campylobacter* genus.[38]

Bile Acid Reflux

Duodenogastric reflux of bile acids has also been suggested as a possible cause of primary gastritis.[39] However, considerable skepticism persists regarding the etiologic role of bile acids in most cases of primary gastritis. The diagnosis is usually considered in adults who have previously undergone either a partial gastrectomy or a gastric drainage procedure.[39] Patients frequently present with abdominal pain and bile-stained vomiting. Dixon et al[40] suggested that there are unique histopathologic features of gastric tissue obtained from patients with bile acid–induced gastritis. These pathologic changes include foveolar hyperplasia, edema, and vasodilatation in the lamina propria, and a paucity of acute and chronic inflammatory cells. The frequency of such changes and their etiologic relevance to gastric inflammation in children have not been established.

Secondary Gastritis

Stress

Stress gastritis is also referred to as acute gastritis and erosive gastritis.[29] Many clinical conditions are associated with stress gastritis, but most commonly it is associated with severe stress in an acutely ill patient.[41] Some patients develop isolated gastroduodenal erosions, and, in severe cases, mucosal ulcerations occur in multiple sites within the stomach and duodenum. Frequently cited stresses include burns, severe head injury, major surgical procedures, sepsis, multiple trauma (including fractures), and respiratory failure.[42]

The underlying cause of stress-associated erosions and ulceration in the stomach is not known, but it is likely multifactorial in etiology. For example, local mucosal ischemia due to impaired blood flow is implicated as a cause of stress erosions in GI mucosa.[43] Other potential pathogenic mechanisms include increased secretion of acid and pepsin, decreased production of mucus, decreased gastric somatosta-

tin level, alterations in levels of adrenal steroids and catecholamines, and an impairment in the local production of prostaglandins.[44] An excellent review by Hernandez[45] cites experimental data showing that some of these lesions are mediated via peptides produced in the central nervous system. For example, thyrotropin-releasing hormone, which promotes vagus nerve–dependent increases in acid and pepsin secretion, accentuates the gastric pathology associated with stress in experimental animals.

In a prospective study of adults who had suffered burns involving more than a quarter of their body surface area, 78 percent of subjects had endoscopic evidence of mucosal abnormalities in the stomach or duodenum.[46] In another study of adults who had suffered severe trauma, gastric erosions were present in all 42 patients who were evaluated.[47] Although the majority of adults with severe stress develop gastric erosions, up to 75 percent remain clinically asymptomatic.[46] In those who are symptomatic, the common presenting features are hematemesis and melena rather than abdominal pain.[46]

Exogenous Agents

Corticosteroids. There has been considerable debate as to the role of exogenous steroids in the etiology of upper GI pathology.[48] A meta-analysis of 71 controlled trials by Messer et al[49] did show an increased risk of ulcer disease and GI hemorrhage among patients who had received corticosteroids. The mechanism by which exogenous steroids might cause gastric ulceration is not known. However, an inhibitory effect on local production of prostaglandins and gastric mucus is postulated.[50]

Nonsteroidal Anti-inflammatory Drugs. Nonsteroidal anti-inflammatory drugs (NSAIDs) such as acetylsalicylic acid, phenylbutazone, indomethacin, ibuprofen, flufenamic acid, mefenamic acid, and naproxen are known to cause both gastritis and mucosal ulceration.[50] In 1938 initial reports suggested an association between acetylsalicylic acid ingestion and gastritis.[51] Subsequent studies support an increased incidence of gastritis, ulcers, and upper intestinal blood loss among subjects receiving the drug.[52] NSAIDs are believed to damage the gastric mucosa through an impairment in the function of normal host mucosal defences by inhibiting mucosal bicarbonate secretion, causing focal loss of the surface mucous layer and reducing the surface hydrophobicity of apical membranes on surface epithelial cells.[53,54]

Ethanol. In experimental animals, administration of alcohol induces gastric erosions and hemorrhage.[55] Tarnawski et al[56] demonstrated that a single dose of 40 percent alcohol induces focal hemorrhage and edema of human gastric mucosa within 5 minutes of ingestion. Clinical studies also indicate that ethanol induces gastric pathology. For example, Laine and Weinstein[6] observed subepithelial gastric hemorrhages at endoscopy in 20 of 125 adults who regularly consumed alcohol. Mucosal histology showed areas of subepithelial hemorrhage surrounded by regions of mucosal edema, but inflammatory cell infiltrate was minimal. The lesions rapidly disappeared upon the discontinuation of ethanol intake.

Corrosives. Although ingestion of corrosives is commonly associated with lesions of the esophagus, gastric lesions can also occur.[57] Gastric outlet obstruction, or corrosive pyloric stenosis, can develop as a complication some 4 to 8 weeks after the ingestion of either acid or lye.[58,59]

Other Exogenous Agents. Agents also reported as causes of gastritis include iron,[60] potassium chloride, calcium salts, and antibiotics such as penicillin, chloramphenicol, sulfonamides, tetracyclines, and cephalosporins.[50] The frequency of their association among cases of symptomatic gastritis in children is not known.

Infectious Agents (other than C. pylori)

Isolated reports associate gastric infection with pathogenic organisms such as cytomegalovirus,[61] herpes simplex virus,[62] and *Candida albicans*[63] with gastritis. The infections occur mainly in patients with primary and secondary immunodeficiencies. Other infectious agents that may be rare causes of gastritis have been reviewed in detail by Weinstein.[29]

Other Causes

Crohn's Disease. In adults, up to 40 percent of patients with Crohn's disease have gastroduodenal involvement.[64] Lenaerts et al[65] obtained gastroduodenal biopsies from 228 children with Crohn's disease and found evidence of gastroduodenal inflammation in 32 percent. Symptoms such as epigastric pain and a feeling of fullness, which may be accompanied by nausea and vomiting, may help to identify those children with Crohn's disease who have significant inflammation in the proximal GI tract. As these symptoms are nonspecific and equally suggestive of primary ulcer disease, many of these children may initially be misdiagnosed as having peptic ulcers.[66] The presence of chronic perianal lesions, such as fissures and tags, should raise the possibility of Crohn's disease as a diagnostic consideration.[66]

Eosinophilic Gastritis. Eosinophilic gastritis is a rare intestinal disorder of unknown etiology which is characterized by an intense eosinophilic infiltration of the gastric mucosa.[67] Often accompanied by a peripheral eosinophilia, it can involve the stomach alone or together with more distal intestinal inflammation (eosinophilic gastroenteritis). Vomiting, abdominal pain, and weight loss are the major presenting symptoms in subjects with gastric involvement.[67] A quarter of the patients also have a significant protein-losing enteropathy with hypoproteinemia and clinical evidence of pitting edema. At present, the diagnosis is based upon the identification of a marked increase in the number of eosinophils in the mucosal biopsies.

Ménétrier's Disease. Also referred to as hypertrophic gastritis, this rare condition of unknown etiology is characterized by giant hypertrophy of the mucosal folds in the stomach. It is frequently associated with symptoms related to massive protein losses from the stomach. There is uncertainty as to whether or not childhood hypertrophic gastritis is the same disease as that described in adults.[68,69] In children, Ménétrier's disease tends to resolve spontaneously, whereas in adults it has a more chronic and debilitating clinical course.[70] In children, vomiting is the most common presenting clinical symptom. It is usually associated with abdominal pain, anorexia, and edema resulting from hypoproteinemia.[68,69] Studies confirm the presence of increased protein loss from the stomach[71] and widening of gap junctions between gastric epithelial cells,[72] a finding which suggests that fluid and protein losses occur primarily via a paracellular pathway. An infectious etiology for childhood-onset Ménétrier's disease has been proposed because of its acute presentation and self-limited course.[68,69] Cytomegalovirus has been implicated in three childhood cases in which characteristic inclusion bodies were observed in gastric mucosa and the virus was recovered from either gastric juice or urine.[69] Hill et al[73] recently reported the isolation of *C. pylori* from the antrum of three children with transient protein-losing gastropathy.

Varioliform Gastritis. Varioliform gastritis, also variously referred to as chronic erosive gastritis and lymphocytic gastritis,[12] is an uncommon cause of gastritis which affects predominantly male adults.[74] To date, only two cases have been reported in the pediatric literature.[4,75] Although suggested to have an allergic basis, the underlying cause of varioliform gastritis is unknown. Among adults, isolation of *C. pylori* is lower among subjects with this disease compared with those with primary gastritis.[76] In the one adolescent we examined,[4] there was no evidence of *C. pylori* colonization of the antrum in association with endoscopic, radiologic, and histologic evidence of varioliform gastritis.

Autoimmune Causes of Gastritis (Atrophic Gastritis). Autoimmune gastritis is characterized by the presence of systemic autoantibodies directed against either gastric parietal cells[77] or gastrin-producing cells in the antrum of the stomach.[78] Recent evidence indicates that the autoantibodies are specifically directed against the acid-producing proton pump on the apical membrane surface of parietal cells.[79] The association of autoimmune gastritis with intrinsic factor antibodies, achlorhydria, and manifestations of cobalamin malabsorption (pernicious anemia) is rare in children. However, the frequency of circulating autoantibodies among a group of children with histologic evidence of gastritis has not, to our knowledge, been formally evaluated. Subjects with primary immunodeficiency disorders—in particular, hypogammaglobulinemia—are at increased risk of autoimmune gastritis and absent[80] or depressed[81] secretion of gastric acid. Gastric colonization with *C. pylori* does not appear to be associated with atrophic gastritis.[82]

DIAGNOSIS OF GASTRITIS

Histologic evidence of mucosal inflammation is essential to establish definitively a diagnosis of gastritis, and it frequently aids in the differentiation of various etiologic considerations.[4,12,40,50] Therefore, biopsies of the antrum, as well as the esophagus and duodenum, should be obtained from all children who undergo upper endoscopy. In contrast to subjects with primary gastritis in whom the gastric mucosa is frequently macroscopically normal, endoscopy in patients with secondary gastritis frequently shows multiple areas of florid inflammation with or without hemorrhage (Fig. 2).

Patients should be carefully selected to determine the need for upper endoscopy and mucosal biopsies. A detailed clinical history and complete physical examination will frequently differentiate the various diagnostic considerations listed in Table 1. If a positive history of drug ingestion (NSAIDs,

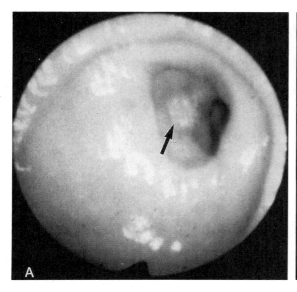
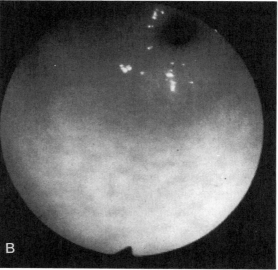

FIGURE 2 *A*, Endoscopic photograph showing normal-appearing antral mucosa; histologic examination of an antral biopsy, however, revealed evidence of acute gastritis and colonization with *C. pylori*. A duodenal ulcer (*arrow*) is visible through a patent but irregular pyloric channel. *B*, Endoscopic evidence of erythema and granularity in the gastric antrum in an adolescent with radiologic evidence of terminal ileitis due to Crohn's disease. Histology of mucosal biopsies demonstrated acute and chronic inflammation and the presence of a noncaseating granuloma. *C. pylori* colonization of the antrum was not demonstrated by culture, silver stain, urease testing, or serology.

corticosteroids) is obtained, it should raise the possibility of secondary gastric inflammation. In certain clinical situations, such as the presence of melena, placement of a nasogastric tube may establish the presence of proximal GI hemorrhage and justify proceeding with specific investigations.

Barium meal, particularly a double-contrast study,[83] may be helpful to exclude other upper GI disorders that may overlap in their clinical presentation with gastritis (i.e., ulceration, varices). Newer radiographic techniques may also prove useful as screening methods in the future. For example, imaging of the abdomen after oral administration of sucralfate labeled with ^{99m}Tc may prove useful as a diagnostic aid because prolonged adherence of the sucralfate-tagged marker to inflamed gastric mucosa occurs after the induction of gastritis in experimental animals.[84]

Diagnosis of *C. pylori* Infection

Endoscopy. At present, the definitive diagnosis of *C. pylori*–associated gastritis requires that mucosal biopsies of the gastric antrum be obtained at the time of upper endoscopy. Colonization of the antrum can be identified by both histologic examination and culture.[4] As shown in Figure 2*A*, the gastric mucosa in children with primary, *C. pylori*–associated gastritis often appears normal to the endoscopist. Efforts to establish noninvasive methods to detect the presence of *C. pylori* are currently under way, and some of the approaches discussed below may lead to less invasive screening tests in the near future.

Histology. Wyatt and Dixon[12] recently published a detailed report outlining the histologic features of *C. pylori*–

associated gastritis. Antral mucosal biopsies show an increase in the number of mononuclear cells, and, in most cases, the number of neutrophils is also increased (Fig. 3). In addition, there is depletion of intracellular mucin content. The organisms colonize only gastric tissue. However, *C. pylori* is occasionally demonstrated in the esophagus and duodenum, but only in areas of gastric metaplasia. The bacteria are demonstrated on the surface of the gastric mucosa using either Giemsa or modified silver stain (Fig. 4). When present in large numbers, they can also be seen by experienced pathologists on sections stained with hematoxylin and eosin. *C. pylori* occupies a unique location because it is present within and underneath the surface mucous layer. Histologic identification of spiral-shaped organisms in gastric mucus and on the surface of gastric mucosa correlates strongly with positive primary culture of *C. pylori* from mucosal biopsy specimens.[4] Ultrastructural studies show the spiral morphology of organisms present on gastric epithelium (Figs. 5 and 6). The underlying gastric epithelial cells may show loss of their apical microvillous membrane surface structure.[34] Intimate attachment of *C. pylori* to surface epithelial cells in regions of pedestal formation, similar to that observed during attachment of enteropathogenic *Escherichia coli* to intestinal enterocytes,[85] has been reported.[34]

Culture. For culture of *C. pylori*, antral biopsies should be placed directly into a sterile container and delivered to the microbiology laboratory within 1 hour. If biopsies are held in room air for a longer period of time, the organisms become nonviable. Culture of *C. pylori* is performed by inoculation of minced biopsy specimens onto blood agar plates, which are held under microaerophilic conditions at 37°C. Media that contain nalidixic acid or vancomycin (i.e., Skirrow's

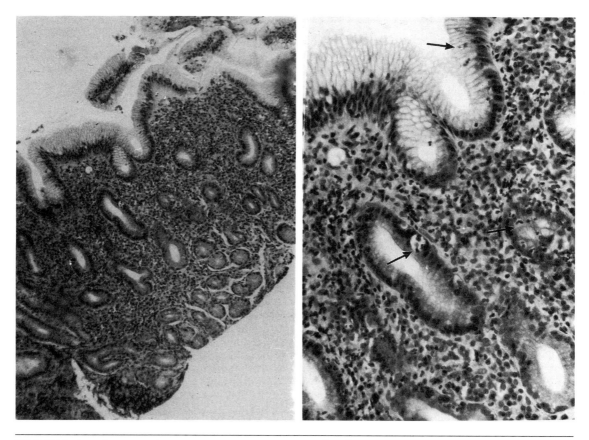

FIGURE 3 Antral mucosa demonstrating active gastritis with polymorphonuclear leukocytes (*arrows*) invading the surface epithelium (hematoxylin and eosin). (From Drumm et al[4]; with permission of the New England Journal of Medicine.)

medium) are frequently used to minimize overgrowth of organisms from the oropharyngeal flora. *C. pylori* is slow to grow in comparison with other *Campylobacter* species, and visible colonies commonly require 5 to 7 days of culture.[34]

Urease Activity. As *C. pylori* produces high levels of the enzyme urease,[33,86] this property can be used to screen for the presence of bacteria in antral biopsy specimens. A portion of the biopsy is placed on urea medium,[87] and hydrolysis of urea leads to a color change of the medium from tan to pink. The color change may occur as soon as 30 minutes after inoculation, but in the presence of small numbers of bacteria the color reaction may take up to 24 hours. The sensitivity of urease testing varies from 50 to 90 percent.[4,87] Commercial kits, which are based on similar principles, are available for use in the endoscopy suite. Initial reports indicate that these kits appear to be of value as screening tests,[88,89] but false-positive reactions due to the presence of other urease-producing organisms can occur.[90]

Breath Tests. The ^{14}C-urea breath test has been shown to be a sensitive screening test.[91] As this test employs a radioactive label, it is not acceptable for routine use in children. Graham et al[92] described a ^{13}C-urea breath test to screen for the presence of urease-producing organisms. Subjects were fasted overnight and then administered oral urea labeled with carbon-13, a stable, naturally occurring, nonradioactive isotope. In the presence of urease-producing organisms, elevated levels of ^{13}C-labeled CO_2 are detected in expired breath samples. The test results correlate well with both histology and culture of antral biopsies in the identification of *C. pylori*.[92] This substrate is expensive and analysis requires mass spectrometry, but further studies may demonstrate its usefulness as a screening test in childhood.

Serology. Measurement of *C. pylori*–specific serum antibodies may also prove useful as a screening test in children. Positive serology for *C. pylori* is extremely rare among children,[93] and when present it is invariably associated with both active *C. pylori* colonization of the stomach and histologic evidence of gastritis.[94,95]

Diagnosis of Secondary Causes of Gastritis

The role of diagnostic upper endoscopy in the assessment of patients with stress-associated upper GI bleeding remains controversial.[50] A presumptive diagnosis can usually be made without direct visualization of the bleeding lesion. Endoscopy may, however, be useful in the localization of lesions if the diagnosis is in doubt or if either therapeutic endoscopy or surgical intervention is considered. When obtained, mucosal biopsies usually demonstrate acute inflammation with a predominance of polymorphonuclear leukocytes.[29]

Following ingestion of corrosives, endoscopy may be considered to define the anatomic site of mucosal damage but

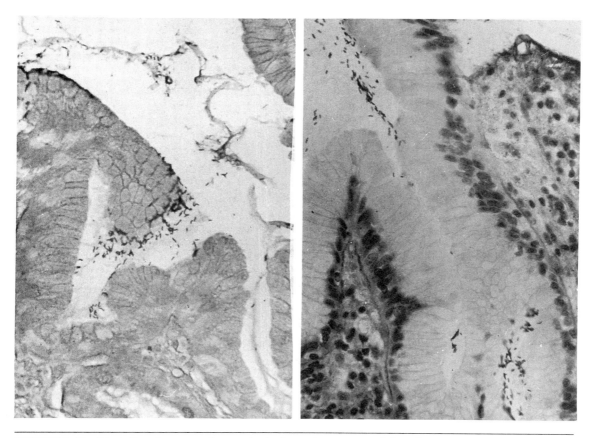

FIGURE 4 Modified silver impregnation method of antral mucosa (with histologic evidence of active gastritis) demonstrates gastric *Campylobacter*-like organisms. (From Drumm et al[4]; with permission of the New England Journal of Medicine.)

should be performed with extreme caution under general anesthesia. Owing to a high risk of perforation, no attempt should be made to pass an endoscope through regions of ulcerated esophageal mucosa. Mucosal histology shows edema and submucosal hemorrhage, but, in contrast to primary gastritis, the inflammatory cell infiltrate within the stomach is mild.

Double-contrast barium meal may suggest the possibility of gastroduodenal Crohn's disease (Fig. 7). However, definitive diagnosis should be made using upper endoscopy and mucosal biopsies. At endoscopy, symptomatic children demonstrate red, granular gastroduodenal mucosa (see Fig. 2*B*). Mucosal biopsies show noncaseating, granulomatous inflammation in approximately 30 percent of patients with gastroduodenal Crohn's disease.[64–66]

In eosinophilic gastritis upper endoscopy demonstrates nodularity, increased friability, and erosions of the gastric mucosa.[67] In Ménétrier's disease, both barium meal and upper endoscopy demonstrate large, irregular mucosal folds. (Fig. 8); the changes are frequently more prominent in the upper portions of the stomach. Gastric mucosal biopsies show hypertrophy and hyperplasia of the gastric glands, cyst formation, and edema of the lamina propria. There is an inflammatory cell infiltrate that consists of a mixture of eosinophils, lymphocytes, and plasma cells.

The diagnosis of varioliform gastritis is established by classic findings following barium meal or upper endoscopy. Bar-

ium studies demonstrate discrete radiolucent halos with central deposits of barium throughout the stomach. At endoscopy, the gastric mucosal pattern is abnormal with multiple small "volcano-like" elevations that contain a central erosion.[96,97] Mucosal histology demonstrates hyperplasia of gastric pits in the antrum and epithelial cell hypertrophy in the body of the stomach. In the region of the aphthoid nodules the lamina propria contains an inflammatory cell infiltrate that consists primarily of lymphocytes and plasma cells,[76] although polymorphonuclear cells can also be evident.[74]

Mucosal biopsies in cases of autoimmune gastritis show a mild lymphocytic infiltration in either the fundus or the antrum.[77] With inflammation of fundic tissue a decrease in the number of parietal cells is also noted.[98]

THERAPY OF GASTRITIS

General Principles

All patients with massive upper GI hemorrhage must first have their intravascular volume restored and then maintained. Establishment of large-bore intravenous catheters, infusion of normal saline, and access to cross-matched blood are the immediate priorities. The efficacy of pharmacologic treatment of acute gastritis that is associated with hemorrhage remains controversial. There is little information available on

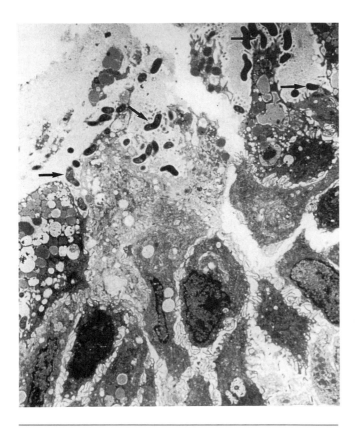

FIGURE 5 Transmission electron photomicrograph of antral mucosa shows spiral-shaped *Campylobacter*-like organisms (*arrows*) adherent to surface epithelial cells and contained in the overlying mucous layer. (Courtesy of Dr. Ernest Cutz, Department of Pathology, The Hospital for Sick Children, Toronto, Ontario.)

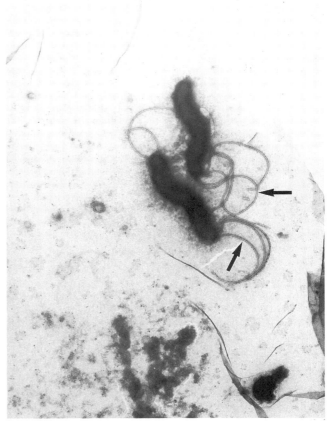

FIGURE 6 Transmission electron photomicrograph after negative staining of *Campylobacter pylori*. Note the spiral shape of the organism (comparable to intestinal *Campylobacter*) and the presence of flagellae (*arrows*).

the treatment of childhood gastritis; therefore, we have to rely largely on the results of studies in adults to indicate optimal methods of treatment. The primary goal of medical therapy has been to raise intragastric pH. Antacids, administered via a nasogastric tube, are frequently used for this purpose.[99] H_2-receptor antagonists have also been used to treat acute, stress-related gastritis and hemorrhage, but there are conflicting reports regarding efficacy.[100-103] The role for therapeutic endoscopy to control massive blood loss arising from gastritis appears promising, at least when performed by experienced therapeutic endoscopists to control bleeding arising from localized lesions.

C. pylori–Associated Gastritis

Raws et al[104] examined the effects of several medications on both the healing of antral gastritis and the clearing of *C. pylori* colonization. Both sucralfate and the H_2-receptor antagonist cimetidine had no effect on the severity of gastritis or *C. pylori* colonization. In contrast, in the majority of subjects tested, both amoxicillin and colloidal bismuth subcitrate resulted in an improvement in the severity of gastritis and

in the apparent eradication of *C. pylori*. It should be emphasized that gastritis resolved only in those patients in whom *C. pylori* colonization was cleared. We recently examined the effects of oral ampicillin taken in combination with liquid bismuth subsalicylate on *C. pylori* colonization and antral gastritis in 16 children.[28] Combination therapy successfully cleared *C. pylori* colonization of the antrum in 75 percent of the patients. In each instance, clearing of *C. pylori* was associated with either improvement or complete clearing of antral gastritis. Although bismuth subcitrate is not commercially available at present in North America, it may be preferable to bismuth subsalicylate for use in children because of the reported association between salicylate therapy and Reye's syndrome. Reye's syndrome has not been reported in a child receiving bismuth subsalicylate.

Secondary Gastritis

Stress-Associated Gastritis. Lacroix et al[105] examined the effects of cimetidine prophylaxis on the development of upper GI hemorrhage in a placebo-controlled study of a group of patients in a pediatric intensive care unit. While cimeti-

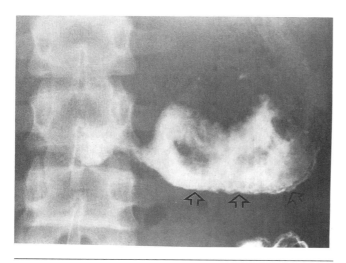

FIGURE 7 Double-contrast barium meal demonstrates mucosal irregularity in the antral and fundic regions of the stomach (*arrows*). The study was performed in an adolescent with radiologic evidence of segmental ileocolitis due to Crohn's disease.

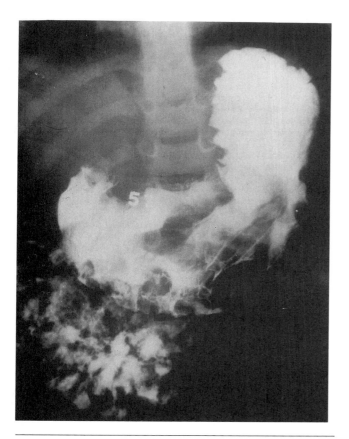

FIGURE 8 Barium meal shows large filling defects in the wall of the stomach of a 3-year-old boy who presented with an 11-day history of vomiting and peripheral edema. The serum albumin was 18 g per liter. At endoscopy, prominant gastric rugae were seen and mucosal biopsies showed typical changes of Ménétrier's disease (see text). Silver stain of antral biopsies did not demonstrate the presence of *Campylobacter*-like organisms.

dine significantly increased the pH of gastric fluid, there was no significant decrease in the rate of upper GI bleeding. The efficacy of gastric acid neutralization in the prevention of stress-associated hemorrhage in adults has produced conflicting results. However, recent meta-analysis of data from 16 previous studies concluded that prophylaxis with antacids and cimetidine both significantly reduced the frequency of mucosal bleeding in comparison with placebo.[106] Cannon et al[107] recently reported that sucralfate is just as effective as either H[2] antagonists or antacids in the prevention of stress ulceration.

Exogenous Agents. Specific therapy is usually not required for the treatment of drug- and alcohol-induced gastritis. In adults, both endoscopic and histologic changes associated with ingestion of these agents show resolution within 4 weeks of discontinuation of the ingestion of these medications.[50] There is increasing evidence to show that concomitant administration of exogenous prostaglandins prevents GI inflammation in adults who continue to receive NSAIDs.[108]

Immediately following ingestion of a corrosive agent, close clinical observation is required because of the risk of gastric perforation. To prevent further damage to the esophageal mucosa, vomiting should not be induced. The treatment of corrosive gastritis includes corticosteroid and antibiotic therapy, as is the case for corrosive esophagitis. Antacids are frequently used, but their therapeutic efficacy is not proven.

Other Causes. The treatment of Crohn's disease, eosinophilic gastritis, and Ménétrier's disease is described in detail in other chapters. Gastric inflammation due to Crohn's disease responds to antiulcer medications such as sucralfate and administration of exogenous corticosteroids.[66] The optimal treatment of eosinophilic gastritis is not defined. Oral corticosteroids are currently the primary mode of therapy,[50] as trials of dietary manipulations and cromolyn sodium are usually without benefit. A new mast cell stabilizer, ketotifen, may prove useful in selected cases.[109]

In children, with Ménétrier's disease, gastric inflammation is a self-limited disorder lasting 4 to 6 weeks, which responds to supportive care. Maintenance of intravascular volume and a high-protein diet are useful adjuncts in those subjects with significant hypoalbuminemia arising from massive gastric protein loss. Treatment of autoimmune gastritis is focused on complications arising from reduced gastric acidity. For example, proliferation of bacteria in the proximal small intestine[110] is treated with broad-spectrum oral antibiotics. In those cases in which cobalamin deficiency is documented, parental vitamin B[12] supplementation is necessary.

Acknowledgment

P. Sherman is the recipient of a Career Scientist Award from the Ontario Ministry of Health, Research Personnel Development Program.

REFERENCES

1. Drumm B, Rhoads JM, Stringer D, Sherman P, Ellis L, Durie P. Peptic ulcer disease in children: etiology, clinical findings and clinical course. Pediatrics 1988; 82:410–414.

2. Schrager S, Spink R, Mitra S. The antrum in patients with duodenal and gastric ulcers. Gut 1967; 8:497–508.
3. Dooley CP, Larson AW, Stace NH, Renner IG, Valenzuela JE, Eliasoph J, Colletti PM, Halls JM, Weiner JM. Double contrast barium meal and upper gastrointestinal endoscopy. A comparative study. Ann Intern Med 1984; 101:538–545.
4. Drumm B, Sherman P, Cutz E, Karmali M. Association of *Campylobacter pylori* on the gastric mucosa with antral gastritis in children. N Engl J Med 1987; 316:1557–1561.
5. Black DB, Haggitt RC, Whitington PF. Gastroduodenal endoscopic-histologic correlation in pediatric patients. J Pediatr Gastroenterol Nutr 1988; 7:353–358.
6. Laine L, Weinstein WM. Histology of alcoholic hemorrhagic "gastritis": a prospective evaluation. Gastroenterology 1988; 94:1254–1262.
7. Ament ME, Berquist WE, Vargas J, Perisic V. Fiberoptic upper intestinal endoscopy in infants and children. Pediatr Clin North Am 1988; 35:141–155.
8. Colin-Jones DG. Endoscopy or radiology for upper gastrointestinal symptoms? Lancet 1986; i:1022–1023.
9. Blackstone MO. Endoscopic interpretation: normal and pathologic appearances of the gastrointestinal tract. New York: Raven Press, 1984.
10. Whitehead R, Truelove SC, Gear MWL. The histological diagnosis of chronic gastritis in fiberoptic gastroscope biopsy specimens. J Clin Pathol 1972; 25:1–11.
11. Marshall BJ, Armstrong JA, Francis GJ, Nokes NT, Wee SH. Antibacterial action of bismuth in relation to *Campylobacter pyloridis* colonization and gastritis. Digestion 1987; 37(suppl 2):16–30.
12. Wyatt JL, Dixon MF. Chronic gastritis—a pathogenetic approach. J Pathol 1988; 154:113–124.
13. Allen A, Hutton DA, Leonard AJ, Pearson JP, Sellers LA. The role of mucus in the protection of the gastroduodenal mucosa. Scand J Gastroenterol 1986; 21(suppl 125):71–77.
14. Duane WC, Levitt MD, Staley NA, McHale AP, Wiegand DM, Fetzer CA. Role of the unstirred layer in protecting the murine gastric mucosa from bile salts. Gastroenterology 1986; 91:913–918.
15. Wenzl E, Feil W, Starlinger M, Schiessel R. Alkaline secretion. A protective mechanism against acid injury in rabbit duodenum. Gastroenterology 1987; 92:709–715.
16. Isenberg JI, Selling JA, Hogan DL, Koss MA. Impaired proximal duodenal mucosal bicarbonate secretion in patients with duodenal ulcers. N Engl J Med 1987; 316:374–379.
17. Cheung LY, Ashley SW. Gastric blood flow and mucosal defense mechanisms. Clin Invest Med 1987; 10:201–208.
18. Lacy ER, Ito S. Rapid epithelial restitution of the rat gastric mucosa after ethanol injury. Lab Invest 1984; 51:573–583.
19. Lichtenberger LM. Membranes and barriers: with a focus on the gastric mucosal barrier. Clin Invest Med 1987; 10:181–188.
20. Poulsen SS. On the role of epidermal growth factor in the defence of the gastroduodenal mucosa. Scand J Gastroenterol 1987; 22(suppl 128):20–21.
21. Silen W. What is cytoprotection of the gastric mucosa? Gastroenterology 1988; 94:232–235.
22. Miller TA. Gastroduodenal mucosal defense: factors responsible for the ability of the stomach and duodenum to resist injury. Surgery 1988; 103:389–397.
23. Silen W, Walsh JH, Garner A, Robert A, Pfeiffer CJ, Szabo S. Lessons from experimental ulcers. "Take-Home Messages" from the 5th International Conference on Experimental Ulcer. Dig Dis Sci 1986; 31:1265–1268.
24. Euler AR, Byrne WJ, Campbell MF. Basal and pentagastrin-stimulated gastric acid secretory rates in normal children and in those with peptic ulcer disease. J Pediatr 1983; 103:766–768.
25. Defize J, Meuwissen SGM. Pepsinogens: an update of biochemical, physiological, and clinical aspects. J Pediatr Gastroenterol Nutr 1987; 6:493–508.
26. Taylor IL. Gastrointestinal hormones in the pathogenesis of peptic ulcer disease. Clin Gastroenterol 1984; 13:355–382.
27. Marshall BJ, Goodwin CS. Revised nomenclature of *Campylobacter pyloridis*. Int J Syst Bacteriol 1987; 37:68.
28. Drumm B, Sherman P, Chiasson D, Karmali M, Cutz E. Treatment of *Campylobacter pylori*-associated antral gastritis in children with bismuth subsalicylate and ampicillin. J Pediatr 1988; 113:908–912.
29. Weinstein WM. Gastritis. In: Sleisenger MH, Fordtran JS, eds. Gastrointestinal Disease. Pathophysiology, Diagnosis, Management, 3rd ed. Philadelphia: WB Saunders, 1983:559.
30. Warren JR, Marshall BJ. Unidentified curved bacilli on gastric epithelium in active chronic gastritis. Lancet 1983; i:1273–1275.
31. Steer HW, Colin-Jones DG. Mucosal changes in gastric ulceration and their response to carbenoxolone sodium. Gut 1975; 16:590–597.
32. Marshall BJ, Royce H, Annear DI, Goodwin CS, Pearman JW, Warren JR, Armstrong JA. Original isolation of *Campylobacter pyloridis* from human gastric mucosa. Microbios Lett 1984; 25:83–88.
33. Blaser MJ. Gastric *Campylobacter*-like organisms, gastritis and peptic ulcer disease. Gastroenterology 1987; 93:371–383.
34. Goodwin CS, Armstrong JA, Marshall BJ. *Campylobacter pyloridis*, gastritis, and peptic ulceration. J Clin Pathol 1986; 39:353–365.
35. Drumm B, O'Brien A, Cutz E, Sherman P. *Campylobacter pyloridis*-associated primary gastritis in children. Pediatrics 1987; 80:192–195.
36. Marshall BJ, Armstrong JA, McGechie DB, Glancy RJ. Attempt to fulfil Koch's postulates for pyloric *Campylobacter*. Med J Aust 1985; 142:436–439.
37. Morris A, Nicholson, G. Ingestion of *Campylobacter pyloridis* causes gastritis and raised fasting gastric pH. Am J Gastroenterol 1987; 82:192–199.
38. Romaniuk PJ, Zoltowska B, Trust TJ, Lane DJ, Olsen GJ, Pace NR, Stahl DA. *Campylobacter pylori*, the spiral bacterium associated with human gastritis, is not a true *Campylobacter* sp. J Bacteriol 1987; 169:2137–2141.
39. Ritchie WP. Alkaline reflux gastritis: a critical reappraisal. Gut 1984; 25:975–987.
40. Dixon MF, O'Connor HJ, Axon A, King RFJG, Johnston D. Reflux gastritis: distinct histopathological entity? J Clin Pathol 1986; 39:524–530.
41. Silen W. The clinical problem of stress ulcers. Clin Invest Med 1987; 10:270–274.
42. Brooks FP. Stress ulcer: etiology, diagnosis and treatment. Med Clin North Am 1966; 50:1447–1455.
43. Menguy R. The prophylaxis of stress ulceration. N Engl J Med 1980; 302:461–462.
44. Szabo S, Gallagher GT, Horner HC, Frankel PW, Underwood RH, Konturek SJ, Brzozowski T, Trier JS. Role of the adrenal cortex in gastric mucosal protection by prostaglandins, sulphydryls, and cimetidine in the rat. Gastroenterology 1983; 85:1384–1390.
45. Hernandez DE. Neuroendocrine mechanisms of stress ulceration: focus on thyrotropin-releasing hormone (TRH). Life Sci 1986; 39:279–296.
46. Czaja AJ, McAlhany JC, Pruitt BA. Acute gastroduodenal disease after thermal injury. An endoscopic evaluation of incidence and natural history. N Engl J Med 1974; 291:925–929.
47. Lucas CE, Sugawa C, Riddle J, Rector F, Rosenberg B, Walt AJ. Natural history and surgical dilemma of "stress" gastric bleeding. Arch Surg 1971; 102:266–273.
48. Conn HO, Blitzer BL. Nonassociation of adrenocorticosteroid therapy and peptic ulcer. N Engl J Med 1976; 294:473–479.
49. Messer JM, Reitman D, Sacks HS, Smith H, Chalmers TC. Association of adrenocorticosteroid therapy and peptic-ulcer disease. N Engl J Med 1983; 309:21–24.
50. Cheili R, Perasso A, Giacosa A. Gastritis. A critical review. Berlin: Springer-Verlag, 1987.
51. Douthwaite AH, Lintott GAM. Gastroscopic observation of the effect of aspirin and certain other substances on the stomach. Lancet 1938; ii:1222.
52. Levy M, Miller DR, Kaufman DW, Siskind V, Schwingl P, Rosenburg L, Strom B, Shapiro S. Major upper gastrointestinal tract bleeding. Relation to the use of aspirin and other non-narcotic analgesics. Arch Intern Med 1988; 148:281–285.
53. Fromm D. How do non-steroidal anti-inflammatory drugs affect gastric mucosal defenses? Clin Invest Med 1987; 10:251–258.
54. Lichtenberger LM, Richards JE, Hills BA. Effect of 16, 16-dimethyl prostaglandin E_2 on the surface hydrophobicity of aspirin-treated canine gastric mucosa. Gastroenterology 1985; 88:308–314.
55. Valencia-Parparcén J. Alcoholic gastritis. Clin Gastroenterol 1981; 10:389–399.
56. Tarnawski A, Hollander D, Stachura J, Klimczyk B, Mach J, Bogdal J. Alcohol injury to the normal human gastric mucosa: endoscopic, histologic and functional assessment. Clin Invest Med 1987; 10:259–263.
57. Allen RE, Thoshinsky MJ, Stallone RJ, Hunt TK. Corrosive injuries of the stomach. Arch Surg 1970; 100:409–412.
58. Poteshman NL. Corrosive gastritis due to hydrochloric acid ingestion.

Am J Roentgenol 1967; 99:182–185.

59. Chong GC, Beahrs OH, Payne WS. Management of corrosive gastritis due to ingested acid. Mayo Clin Proc 1974; 49:861–865.

60. Covey TJ. Ferrous sulphate poisoning. J Pediatr 1964; 64:218–226.

61. Henson D. Cytomegalovirus inclusion bodies in the gastrointestinal tract. Arch Pathol 1972; 93:477–482.

62. Howiler W, Goldberg HI. Gastroesophageal involvement in herpes simplex. Gastroenterology 1976; 70:775–778.

63. Cronan J, Burrell M, Trepeta R. Aphthoid ulcerations in gastric candidiasis. Radiology 1980; 134:607–611.

64. Fielding JF, Toye DKM, Beton DC, et al. Crohn's disease of the stomach and duodenum. Gut 1970; 11:1001–1006.

65. Lenaerts C, Roy CL, Vaillancourt M, Weber AM, Morin CL, Seidman EG. Upper GI tract involvement in children with Crohn's disease. (Abstract) Gastroenterology 1987; 92:1499.

66. Griffiths AM, Alemayehu E, Sherman P. Clinical features of gastroduodenal Crohn's disease in adolescents. J Pediatr Gastroenterol Nutr 1989; 8:166–171.

67. Whitington PF, Whitington GL. Eosinophilic gastroenteropathy in childhood. J Pediatr Gastroenterol Nutr 1988; 7:379–385.

68. Chouraqui JP, Roy CC, Brochu P, Gregoire H, Morin CL, Weber AM. Ménétrier's disease in children: report of a patient and review of sixteen other cases. Gastroenterology 1981; 80:1042–1047.

69. Stillman AE, Manthei U, Pinnas J. Transient protein-losing enteropathy and enlarged gastric rugae in childhood. Am J Dis Child 1981; 135:29–33.

70. Scharschmidt BF. The natural history of hypertrophic gastropathy (Ménétrier's disease). Report of a case with 16-year follow-up and review of 120 cases from the literature. Am J Med 1977; 63:644–652.

71. Florent C, Vidon N, Flourié B, Carmentrand A, Zerbani A, Maurel M, Bernier JJ. Gastric clearance of alpha-1-antitrypsin under cimetidine perfusion. New test to detect protein-losing gastropathy? Dig Dis Sci 1986; 31:12–15.

72. Kelly DG, Miller LJ, Malagelada JR, Huizenga KA, Markowitz H. Giant hypertrophic gastropathy (Ménétrier's disease): pharmacologic effects on protein leakage and mucosal ultrastructure. Gastroenterology 1982; 83:581–589.

73. Hill ID, Sinclair-Smith C, Lastovica AJ, Bowie MD, Emms M. Transient protein losing enteropathy associated with acute gastritis and *Campylobacter pylori*. Arch Dis Child 1987; 62:1215–1219.

74. Gallagher CG, Lennon JR, Crowe JR. Chronic erosive gastritis: a clinical study. Am J Gastroenterol 1987; 82:302–306.

75. Caporali R, Luciano S. Diffuse varioliform gastritis. Arch Dis Child 1986; 61:405–407.

76. Dixon MF, Wyatt JI, Burke DA, Rathbone BJ. Lymphocytic gastritis—relationship to *Campylobacter pylori* infection. J Pathol 1988; 154:125–132.

77. De Aizpurua HJ, Cosgrove LJ, Ungar B, Toh BH. Autoantibodies cytotoxic to gastric parietal cells in serum of patients with pernicious anemia. N Engl J Med 1983; 309:625–629.

78. Vandelli C, Bottazzo GF, Doniach D, Franceschi F. Autoantibodies to gastrin-producing cells in antral (type B) chronic gastritis. N Engl J Med 1979; 300:1406–1410.

79. Karlsson FA, Burman P, Loof L, Mardh S. Major parietal cell antigen in autoimmune gastritis with pernicious anemia is the acid-producing H$^+$, K$^+$-adenosine triphosphate of the stomach. J Clin Invest 1988; 81:475–479.

80. Borriello SP, Reed PJ, Dolby JM, Barclay FE, Webster ADB. Microbial and metabolic profile of achlorhydric stomach: comparison of pernicious anemia and hypogammaglobulinemia. J Clin Pathol 1985; 38:946–953.

81. Den Hartog G, Van Der Meer JWM, Jansen JBMJ, Van Furth R, Lamers CBHW. Decreased gastrin secretion in patients with late-onset hypogammaglobulinemia. N Engl J Med 1988; 318:1563–1567.

82. Siurala M, Sipponen P, Kekki M. *Campylobacter pylori* in a sample of Finnish population: relations to morphology and function of the gastric mucosa. Gut 1988; 29:909–915.

83. Levine MS, Rubesin SE, Herlinger H, Laufer I. Double-contrast upper gastrointestinal examination: technique and interpretation. Radiology 1988; 168:593–602.

84. Vasquez TE, Bridges RL, Braunstein P, Jansholt AL, Meshkinpour H. Gastrointestinal ulcerations: detection using a technetium-99m–labeled ulcer avid agent. Radiology 1983; 148:227–231.

85. Boedeker EC, Sherman P. Mechanisms of *Escherichia coli* enteritis. Front Gastrointest Res 1986; 13:309–330.

86. Mobley HCT, Cortesia MJ, Rosenthal LE, Jones BD. Characterization of urease from *Campylobacter pylori*. J Clin Microbiol 1988; 26:831–836.

87. McNulty CAM, Wise R. Rapid diagnosis of *Campylobacter*-associated gastritis. Lancet 1985; i:1443–1444.

88. Morris A, McIntyre D, Rose T, Nicholson G. Rapid diagnosis of *Campylobacter pyloridis* infection. Lancet 1986; i:149.

89. Borromeo M, Lambert JR, Pinkard KJ. Evaluation of "CLO-test" to detect *Campylobacter pyloridis* in gastric mucosa. J Clin Pathol 1987; 40:462–468.

90. Vaira D, Holton J, Cairns S, Polydoron A, Falzon M, Dowsett J, Salmon PR. Urease tests for *Campylobacter pylori*: care in interpretation. (Letter) J Clin Pathol 1985; 41:812–813.

91. Bell GD, Weil J, Harrison G, et al. ^{14}C-urea breath analysis: a noninvasive test for *Campylobacter pylori* in the stomach. Lancet 1987; i:1367–1368.

92. Graham DY, Klein PD, Evans DJ Jr, et al. *Campylobacter pyloris* detected noninvasively by the ^{13}C-urea breath test. Lancet 1987; ii:1174–1177.

93. Jones DM, Eldridge J, Fox AJ, et al. Antibody to the gastric Campylobacter-like organism ("*Campylobacter pyloridis*")—clinical correlations and distribution in the normal population. J Med Microbiol 1986; 22:57–62.

94. Mitchell HM, Bohane TD, Berkowicz J, Hazell ST, Lee A. Antibody to *Campylobacter pylori* in families of index children with gastrointestinal illness due to *C. pylori* (Letter) Lancet 1987; ii:681–682.

95. Drumm B, Perez-Perez G, Blaser M, Sherman P. Intrafamilial clustering of *Campylobacter pylori* infection. (Abstract) Gastroenterology 1989; 96:130.

96. Cappell MS, Green PHR, Merboe C. Neoplasia in chronic erosive (varioliform) gastritis. Dig Dis Sci 1988; 33:1035–1039.

97. Haot J, Hamichi L, Wallez L, Mainguet P. Lymphocytic gastritis: a newly described entity: a retrospective endoscopic and histological study. Gut 1988; 29:1258–1264.

98. Strickland RG, Mackey IR. A reappraisal of the nature and significance of chronic atrophic gastritis. Am J Dig Dis 1973; 18:426–440.

99. Simonian SJ, Curtis LE. Treatment of hemorrhagic gastritis by antacids. Surg 1976; 184:429–434.

100. Hoare A, Bradby GVH, Hawkins CF, Kang JY, Dykes PW. Cimetidine in bleeding peptic ulcer. Lancet 1979; ii:671–673.

101. Pickard RG, Sanderson I, South M, Kirkham JS, Northfield TC. Controlled trial of cimetidine in acute upper gastrointestinal bleeding. Br Med J 1979; i:661–662.

102. Teres J, Bordas JM, Rimola A, Bru C, Rodes J. Cimetidine in acute gastric mucosal bleeding. Results of a double-blind randomized trial. Dig Dis Sci 1980; 25:92–96.

103. Nowak A, Sadlinski CZ, Gorka Z. Nowakowska E, Rudzki J, Gibinski K. Ranitidine in the treatment of acute gastrointestinal hemorrhage—a comparative study. Hepatogastroenterology 1981; 28:267–269.

104. Rauws EA, Langenberg W, Houthoff HJ, Zanen HC, Tytgat GNJ. *Campylobacter pyloridis*–associated chronic active antral gastritis. Gastroenterology 1988; 94:33–40.

105. Lacroix J, Infante-Rivard C, Gauthier M, Rousseau E, van Doesburg N. Upper gastrointestinal tract bleeding acquired in a pediatric intensive care unit: prophylaxis trial with cimetidine. J Pediatr 1986; 108:1015–1018.

106. Shuman R, Schuster DP, Zuckerman GR. Prophylactic therapy for stress ulcer bleeding: a reappraisal. Ann Intern Med 1987; 106:562–567.

107. Cannon LA, Heiselman D, Gardner W, Jones J. Prophylaxis of upper gastrointestinal tract bleeding in mechanically ventilated patients. Arch Intern Med 1987; 147:2101–2106.

108. Graham DY, Agrawal NM, Roth SH. Prevention of NSAID-induced gastric ulcer with misoprostol: multicentre, double-blind, placebo-controlled trial. Lancet 1988; ii:1277–1280.

109. Moore D, Lichtman S, Lentz J, Stringer D, Sherman P. Eosinophilic gastroenteritis presenting in an adolescent with isolated colonic involvement. Gut 1986; 27:1219–1222.

110. Sherman P, Lichtman S. Small bowel bacterial overgrowth syndrome. Surv Dig Dis 1987; 50:157–171.

Peptic Ulcer

Edmund J. Eastham, M.B., B.S., F.R.C.P.

Peptic ulcer is among the most common of chronic diseases, occurring in 5 to 10 percent of the population in their lifetime.[1] It is probably many different diseases with diverse genetic and environmental causes, all leading to a common clinical manifestation—a sharply circumscribed loss of tissue involving mucosa, submucosa, and muscular layer, occurring in areas of the digestive tract exposed to acid-pepsin gastric juices, chiefly the stomach and duodenum. As with any common adult condition, it would not be surprising for cases to present in childhood; indeed, childhood peptic ulceration is no longer considered a rare disease, and today's pediatrician is certainly more aware of its possibility and requires insight into optimal techniques of diagnosis and management. By convention, ulcers are described as primary or secondary, gastric or duodenal. Primary duodenal ulceration in clinical practice is the most important and has generated the largest interest in terms of research and publications.

PRIMARY DUODENAL ULCERATION

Incidence

The true incidence is unknown, but, as with adult studies, it varies considerably from one country to another and indeed from different geographic areas within each country. In Britain, for example, most case reports are from the north,[2-9] with an almost fourfold difference in prevalence between Newcastle-upon-Tyne (110 cases) and London (30 cases) seen over the same time period.[7,9] Ulcers are relatively common in Anglo-Saxon and Scandinavian countries by comparison with Mediterranean lands, and several large series have also been reported from North America[10-13] and from Eastern Europe. In a review of 417,251 children treated in the pediatric departments in Sweden during the years 1953 to 1962, Karlstrom found 184 with peptic ulcers—an incidence of 4.4 per 10,000 patients.[14] This figure is probably an underestimate of the true incidence, as the diagnosis was not made by upper gastrointestinal (GI) endoscopy. The number of new cases seen each year depends on a variety of factors, including interest of the department, their indications for investigations, and the different methodologies available to them. Reviewing some 16 publications involving 1,000 cases indicates that the average number of new cases seen each year by each center is 3.5. It is of interest that in our own unit the more liberal policy adopted in the late 1970s for selecting patients for investigations has had a strong impact on the numbers: The average annual detection rate has risen from 1.5 to 5.4.

It is well reported that the incidence and virulence of adult peptic ulcer disease have been declining for the past few decades. Hospital admissions have been declining both in the United States and in England and Wales[15] for the past 20 years. In parallel, the number of surgical operations for peptic ulcer disease has also declined, even before the introduction of the H_2-receptor antagonists.[16,17] There are many hypotheses advanced to account for this decreased incidence, severity, and mortality, but in children these trends do not appear to be occurring. Indeed, it is believed by some that the incidence may be increasing and that this is real and not simply attributable to better diagnosis.[3,4]

As with adults, the incidence of ulcers in boys is two to three times that seen in girls.[3-5,9,12] This difference tends to be less with younger age.

Pathogenesis

Despite literally hundreds of adult and animal studies, we still do not know the cause of duodenal ulceration. Table 1 lists the factors involved, many of them being closely interlinked and having advocates of equal verbosity. Very little of our understanding comes from work in children, perhaps because numbers are relatively small and investigative techniques are highly invasive. As long ago as 1910, Schwartz postulated the following[18]:

1. "Ohne Säure, Kein Geschwür" (No acid, no ulcer)
2. The ulcer formula is one of autodigestive power (attacking forces) versus resistance of mucus (defending forces).
3. An ulcer is only a symptom of underlying ulcer diathesis.

These three postulates are still the foundations upon which we build. The relapsing nature of the disease suggests that at times the attacking forces dominate, resulting in an active ulcer, and that after a variable interval the balance is re-

TABLE 1
Factors Involved in Pathogenesis of
Duodenal Ulceration

Hydrochloric acid
Pepsin
Mucous barrier
Bicarbonate
Hormones
Bile
Prostaglandins
Genetic inheritance
Diet
Drugs
Infection
Psychological factors

established and the ulcer heals. However, there is no ready explanation for why the imbalance occurs initially or why such episodes often become more frequent in many patients whereas they disappear altogether in others.

Acid

The complex mechanisms involved in acid secretion and its regulation are dealt with elsewhere in this volume. Although it is recognized that the maxim "no acid, no ulcer" holds true for treatment of duodenal ulceration, it may not be true to say that acid per se causes duodenal ulcer. For example, it is now appreciated that although 30 to 40 percent of adult patients have hypersecretion of acid (as evidenced by an elevated peak acid output), there are a considerable number of people with acid hypersecretion who do not develop ulcers.[19] Conversely, ulcers can develop in individuals with normal or even diminished gastric acid output. Pediatric studies, although few, have tended to find a similar pattern of hypersecretion. Basal acid output, peak acid output, and maximal acid output values are all higher in children with duodenal ulcers than in controls, although there is a considerable overlap. Table 2 shows values of maximal acid output from six sources with a mean of 0.293 mmol H^+ per kilogram per hour for controls and 0.393 mmol H^+ per kilogram per hour for ulcer patients. In our own series,[9] studies of acid production have been performed on 26 children. In seven of these betazole was used, and in the remainder pentagastrin. Both of these agents produce comparable levels of acid secretion.[23] In nine (35 percent) of the 26 investigated, there was evidence of hypersecretion. This is thought to reflect an increased parietal cell mass, but recent data suggest that it may be an acquired phenomenon: When the ulcer first develops, the acid secretion is probably normal but increases in relation to the length of the disease. A further possibility for the hypersecretion is an increased drive (vagal and/or hormonal) on the parietal cell, but as yet there are no convincing data in adults and none at all in children.[24]

Maximal acid output (MAO) determination in adults is generally considered of little value in predicting ulcer outcome and has not identified patients subject to more frequent complications or symptomatic recurrences. One recent study, however, in a group of 94 patients did show significantly more relapses (72 percent versus 28 percent) in subjects with a particularly high MAO, greater than 60 mmol per hour.[25] This may represent a particular subgroup with different pathogenetic mechanisms, and alternative therapeutic regimens may prove effective in preventing ulcer recurrence. Whether a similar subgroup occurs in children is not known. A further way of looking at acid output is in terms of the amount secreted throughout the entire 24-hour period. Again, data pertinent to children are lacking, but it is clear that adult patients with duodenal ulcer secrete a greater amount of acid over a 24-hour period. Recent interest has centered on the evidence that nocturnal acid secretion may be the predominant pathogenetic mechanism, and this has formed the basis for the use of H^2-receptor antagonists given once at night for both ulcer healing and long-term maintenance. This concept, however, has recently been challenged in a study showing that ulcer healing rates were identical at 4 and 8 weeks in patients taking famotidine (with a 12-hour action) as a single dose taken either in the morning or at bedtime.[26]

Pepsin

Although most studies have concentrated on the role of hydrochloric acid in the pathogenesis of ulcer disease, this emphasis has tended to obscure the fact that acid has never on its own been shown to induce an ulcer! The role of secretion of pepsin in ulcer disease has received intermittent attention over the years, but there now appears to be a substantial amount of data to support its importance in the ulcer diathesis. For a full account of the subject, the reader is referred to an excellent recent review article.[27] Pepsin is active only in an acid milieu and is stored in the gastric mucosa as an inactive proenzyme, called pepsinogen, prior to secretion. Both pepsin and pepsinogen exist in more than one form, but unfortunately progress in this area of research has been frustrated by confusion over the terminology used to distinguish one enzyme from another.[28]

The serum pepsinogens (Pg) have received most attention because radioimmunoassay techniques exist for their measurement. They can be divided into three major groups—pepsinogen I or A (Pg I), pepsinogen II or C (Pg II), and "slow-migrating protease" (SMP). The Pg I group has been most studied in relationship to peptic ulceration and can exist in five different isozymogen forms.[29] These are found in the chief and mucous neck cells of the mucosa of the gastric fundus and body but not in antral mucosa. Serum Pg I is raised above the normal range in one-half to two-thirds of adult patients with ulcers, is higher in those with the more severe forms of the disease, and has been shown to correlate with the acid secretory capacity of the stomach. Tam has recently reported a small study from Hong Kong in which Pg I was measured in 14 children with ulcers and their parents[30]: 43 percent of children and 46 percent of parents were hyperpepsinogenemic, and it was believed that the inheritance was autosomal dominant with incomplete penetrance. Measurement of Pg I can therefore be used as a marker for the ulcer diathesis in some families[31] and may be useful in identifying patients at risk. It does not, however, tell us how these enzymes are responsible for the disease process.

Pepsin itself exists in four isomer forms—pepsins 1 to 4. Each has different mucolytic activities, pepsin 1 being the

TABLE 2
Maximal Acid Output (MAO) in Control and Duodenal Ulcer (DU) Patients*

Authors	MAO (Controls)	MAO (DU)
Ghai et al[20]	0.202	0.300
Habbick et al[4]	None	0.330
Robb et al[5]	0.350	0.330
Fieber et al[21]	0.372	None
Murphy et al[9]	None	0.520
Christie and Ament[22]	0.238	0.486
MEAN	0.298	0.393

* mmol of H^+ per kilogram per hour.

most active. Although the mucous layer adherent to the gastroduodenal epithelium is impermeable to pepsin, the surface of this barrier is being continually eroded by this agent in the gastric juice. Once the mucous barrier has been removed, this enzyme is able to come into contact with the surface of the cell membrane and may then be allowed to initiate proteolytic effects. Increased concentrations of pepsin have been found in the gastric juice of adult patients with duodenal ulcer and usually with a mucolytic profile compatible with pepsin 1.[32] It has therefore recently been suggested that pepsin may be the "missing" aggressive factor for the etiology of peptic ulcers. Further studies on this substance and its relationship to the healing and recurrence of ulcers are awaited with interest.

Mucus-Bicarbonate Barrier

The gastroduodenal epithelium secretes a layer of water-insoluble mucous gel that forms a continuous coat of 180 μm thickness and serves various protective functions. It acts as a diffusion barrier to luminal pepsin, preventing its access to the epithelial surface, and it also provides a barrier to hydrogen ions, which are neutralized by the bicarbonate within the mucus, thus establishing a pH gradient at the epithelial surface. Bicarbonate production by the mucosa is stimulated by prostaglandins and calcium but is inhibited by alcohol, noradrenaline, taurocholate, and nonsteroidal anti-inflammatory drugs.[33] The mucous layer also protects the mucosa from mechanical damage, which may occur during the motile process of digestion, and it also provides protection for rapid re-epithelialization by surface mucous cells following acute damage.

The structure of adherent gastric mucus has been found to be deficient in adult patients with ulcer disease, with a decreased polymerization of the component glycoproteins.[34] This impairment of the barrier is associated with raised amounts of pepsin 1, which digests the mucous layer more aggressively than the major pepsin, pepsin 3, under conditions that pertain both in the stomach (pH 2) and duodenum (pH 4-5).[35] In addition, in ulcer disease, the bicarbonate response to an acid load may be defective,[36] and an abnormal pH gradient in response to luminal acid has also been demonstrated, indicating a deficit in the ability of these patients to maintain juxtamucosal neutrality in the face of luminal acidity. Although this evidence points to a link between abnormalities of the mucus-bicarbonate barrier and ulcer pathogenesis, there is as yet no direct evidence for such a causal relationship. No data exist within the pediatric age range with regard to mucus, pepsins, or bicarbonate secretion either in normal controls or in ulcer patients. This is a potential area for future research.

Hormones

As gastrin is a potent stimulant of gastric secretion, it was originally thought that the hypersecretion of acid in duodenal ulcer might partly be accounted for by hypergastrinemia. However, the development of a specific radioimmunoassay for serum gastrin showed that this was not the case. Gastrin is released from G cells in the antrum and duodenal mucosa. When acid secretion increases and the pH falls below a critical point, gastrin release is "switched off." In response to a protein meal, blood gastrin levels in adults (the integrated gastrin response) were found not only to be higher but also to remain elevated longer in ulcer patients than in controls. There are conflicting results in the proportions of the G17 and G34 components which are in excess in these patients. Nevertheless, the excess itself may be a result of increased G-cell activity, or G-cell hyperplasia, or a defect in the gastrin feedback mechanism. Whether any of this relates to children is not known. Other hormones such as secretin, cholecystokinin, gastric inhibitory peptide, vasoactive intestinal peptide, somatostatin, and bombesin have been investigated in adults and to date it seems unlikely that any of them has a direct role in the etiology of peptic ulceration.

Bile

If gastric mucosa is exposed to bile salts, there is a breakdown in the adherent mucous structure, and this mucolytic effect may therefore expose the mucosa to acid and other damaging factors, resulting in ulcer formation. It has been speculated, therefore, that bile salts may play a role in ulcer formation, although as yet there is no firm evidence to support this proposition.

Prostaglandins

Exogenous prostaglandins have been shown to protect gastric mucosa from the effects of a variety of damaging agents such as nonsteroidal anti-inflammatory drugs, bile, serotonin, alcohol, boiling water, and 0.6 N hydrochloric acid.[37,38] Local (endogenous) generation of these substances within gastric mucosa has been considered responsible for mucosal adaptation to attack by mild irritants—so-called cytoprotection. This is accomplished by mechanisms other than inhibition of gastric acid secretion. Direct endoscopic studies in normal volunteers with simultaneous assessment of mucosal histology have demonstrated that prostaglandin E_2 effectively protects the gastric and duodenal mucosa against injury produced by 60 percent alcohol. A protective effect has similarly been found against aspirin, indomethacin, and even laser beams. It has been suggested that one mode of action of prostaglandins is to enhance the mucus-bicarbonate barrier, and there is evidence that both the mucous gel and bicarbonate secretion components are influenced by these agents. Nonsteroidal anti-inflammatory drugs are prostaglandin synthetase inhibitors and as such probably account for the inhibition of bicarbonate secretion produced by these drugs. Recent studies have also demonstrated that a number of currently used ulcer-healing drugs (aluminum-containing antacids, colloid bismuth, and sucralfate) are capable of enhancing both gastroduodenal prostaglandin synthesis and bicarbonate secretion. Prostaglandins influence a number of other protective mechanisms such as blood flow and surface active phospholipids. They are synthesized from their precursors—essential fatty acids—by all nucleated cells. Deficiency of mucosal prostaglandins and resultant impaired mucosal defensive mechanisms have been implicated as possible factors involved in the pathogenesis of ulcer disease.[39]

Genetic Factors

Like many common diseases, genetic studies of peptic ulcer have suffered from confusion engendered by the varying definitions of "affected" used by different investigators. "Affected" has been applied to a range of people, from one who has abdominal pain to one with an endoscopically demonstrated crater. Some studies also fail to separate out gastric from duodenal disease. Despite these difficulties, it has been known for many years that genetic factors play a role in the etiology of peptic ulcer, based on three lines of evidence: family studies, twin studies, and blood group studies.

Family Studies. Family aggregation was noted in the late 1800s, and most adult reports indicate a positive family history in 20 to 50 percent of individuals with peptic ulcer, compared with 5 or 15 percent of controls, i.e., a two to three times greater incidence in first-degree relatives.[40,41] This increased incidence is particularly well marked in the case of children—ranging from 33 to 62 percent in different series.[4,9,42,43]

Some years ago in our department, a survey was performed of 50 children with radiologically or surgically confirmed duodenal ulcers. All families were visited, and full histories were taken; whenever there was a suspicion that a relative was also affected, their family doctor was contacted, hospital notes followed up, and details of site and age at diagnosis obtained. For each propositus, a control child was identified by the family doctor who matched for age, sex, social status, family size, and locality. Table 3 shows some of the results. There was a greater proportion of positive relatives of each category in the families of the propositi than in those of the controls—25.3 percent of first-degree relatives in the families of propositi, but only 8.7 percent in control families. The proportion of positives diminished from the first to the second to the third degree of relationship in both propositi and control families. In addition, in male relatives of propositi, the proportion was higher than in females for each degree of relationship, e.g., 31 percent and 20 percent in first-degree relatives.

Using these data, Jackson[44] was able to calculate the heritability of childhood ulcers and found a figure of 0.91, which is considerably higher than the heritability of 0.37 derived for adults[45] and, of interest, even higher than that for hypertrophic pyloric stenosis.

Twin Studies. Twin studies help to resolve the question of whether familial aggregation is due to common genes or to a common environment. Traditional studies compare the frequency of concordance (both members of the twin pair affected) for monozygotic (identical) twins with that for dizygotic twins. As monozygotic twins share all genes, they should be concordant for purely genetically caused disorders. Dizygotic twins are no more alike genetically than a pair of siblings. If the characteristic studied is purely genetically determined with no environmental influence, there should be 100 percent concordance in dizygotic twins. For a disorder entirely determined by environmental factors, the concordance in monozygotic twins should equal that in dizygotic twins. If clinical expression of the disorder requires interaction between a genetic predisposition and an environmental agent, one would expect a higher concordance among monozygotic twins (although less than 100 percent). Although the reported percentage varies in different studies, concordance in monozygotic twins is always higher than that in dizygotic twins[40,46] and probably about 50 percent. These studies show that a large part of the familial aggregation is due to genetic factors.

Blood Group Studies. It is well known that the incidence of duodenal ulcer in persons with blood group O is about 1.3 times that of persons with the other blood groups. Likewise, there is a 1.5 times higher incidence in salivary blood group nonsecretors. A number of other less well-studied genetic traits have also been reported to be associated with peptic ulcer; these include alpha^1-antitrypsin deficiency, cystic fibrosis, phenylketonuria, G6PD deficiency, and certain HLA antigens.

An excess of group O has also been noted in children,[4,5,44,47] but no excess of nonsecretors.[44] The mechanism whereby blood group O predisposes to ulcer formation is unknown even after two decades of study, probably because the magnitude of the association is so small.

The actual mode of inheritance of the genetic predisposition to develop ulcer disease has still to be resolved. There are those who believe it to be polygenic or multifactorial—due to the interaction of several genes with environmental factors.[48] While there may be such a contribution, there is more compelling evidence that the major genetic factors and the differing physiologic observations can be best accounted for by genetic heterogeneity.[46]

An ulcer crater is the final common pathway of a group of disorders. Several lines of evidence support this hypothesis of heterogeneity:

1. Genetic separation of gastric and duodenal ulcers.
2. Rare genetic syndromes with peptic ulceration.

TABLE 3
Genetics of Ulcer Disease: Relatives with Positive Histories by Degree of Relationship

Degree of Relationship	50 Families of Children with Ulcers			50 Control Families		
	No.	No. Positive	Percentage	No.	No. Positive	Percentage
First degree	217	55	25.3	231	20	8.7
Second degree	561	84	15.0	553	41	7.4
Third degree	713	38	5.3	653	15	2.3

3. Variable incidence and types of ulcer in different ethnic groups.
4. Physiologic differences between ulcer patients.
5. Family studies that demonstrate the genetic basis of certain physiologic abnormalities.

The implication of the genetic heterogeneity theory is that the pathophysiology, and therefore optimal treatment, may well differ among different types of ulcer patients. In the future, therefore, with a better understanding of the factors involved, there may be different specific modes of therapy, prevention, and genetic counseling.

Diet

One factor, until recently little considered, accounting for the decreased incidence of ulcer disease in adults could be the increased consumption of, and interaction between, dietary essential fatty acids and the natural defense mechanisms of the gastroduodenal mucosa. As has already been stated, prostaglandins are involved in the intrinsic defense of the mucosa. They are synthesized from arachidonic or linoleic acids—both essential fatty acids of the polyunsaturated type. Vegetable oil is the major dietary source of these fatty acids, and their ingestion in western countries has been increasing since the beginning of this century. For example, the daily intake of vegetable oils has increased in the United States from 21 g per day per person in 1910 to 68 g per day per person in 1980.[49] This enormous increase could account in part for the current improved trends in adults.[50]

In other mammals, the mucosal defenses are very effective, so peptic ulcer disease in the wild is rare. Only when animals receive food with which they are unfamiliar do peptic ulcers develop. This has been seen in pigs, foals, and dolphins. High-fiber diets may also play a role in ulcer prevention, and one review noted that the lipid-soluble fraction of wheat bran and unrefined wheat may have a protective effect related to reduced duodenal ulcer incidence in northern India.[51] Duodenal ulcer patients on low-fiber diets relapse more quickly than those on bran-supplemented diets in Norway.[52] The excess use of spices or peppers may also be related to a high incidence of ulcer disease in southern India. This recent rekindled interest in dietary factors has yet to coalesce into a coherent body of data. A study on dietary habits of children with duodenal ulcers would be of interest, but meanwhile suggesting a diet high in fiber and polyunsaturated oils and low in spices would seem to be prudent and healthy. Finally, apart from its antacid properties, bovine milk also appears to exert an antiulcer effect in the lipid fraction, perhaps because the active components protect the gastric mucosa through the action of surface-active lipids.[53]

Drugs

The long lists of drugs known to affect the gastroduodenal mucosa adversely appear to have little importance in pediatric ulcer disease. These include aspirin, nonsteroidal anti-inflammatory agents, indomethacin, alcohol, and smoking. Certainly in the older child with an ulcer who does smoke, this should be strongly discouraged for many reasons, not the least of which is that smoking certainly delays ulcer healing.

Infection

It is nearly a century since spiral organisms were found in the stomachs of humans, but they were always believed to be contaminants. In 1983, Warren and Marshall in Australia isolated a new bacterium, now called *Campylobacter pylori*, and found that the gastric antrum of nearly all adult patients with duodenal ulcers were colonized with this organism, which was also causing an active chronic gastritis.[54,55] The association between this organism and peptic ulcer disease is of great clinical interest. It may play a role in the pathogenesis by weakening the gastric mucosal barrier and allowing acid to injure the mucosa. Patients with a high gastric output or a propensity to ulcer formation in the duodenum first develop gastric metaplasia, which is then colonized by *C. pylori*.[56] In non-iatrogenic cases, the association between this bacterium and duodenal ulceration approaches 100 percent in adults and has been confirmed world-wide. However, not everyone with antral colonization develops an ulcer, and indeed serologic studies have revealed an increasing exposure to this bacterium with increasing age, as judged by the presence of specific IgG antibody titers.

The presence of *C. pylori* in antral biopsies has been confirmed in children, some of whom had duodenal ulcers.[57-60] Using a sensitive ELISA assay to measure specific IgG *C. pylori* antibodies, we have found a close association between high titers and the presence of histologically proven gastritis and positive *C. pylori* cultures. Using these titers as an indicator of active infection, we have examined sera from 200 normal school children aged 5 to 16 years and have found an incidence of 5 percent. In contrast, 25 percent of 100 consecutive children examined endoscopically had positive titers and proven active chronic gastritis with organism identification. In 12 patients a duodenal ulcer was present, but, unlike adult studies, only 50 percent of these had gastritis secondary to *C. pylori*.

Adult ulcer patients treated with H_2-receptor antagonists experience healing of their ulcer after 2 months treatment in 90 percent of cases. The relapse rate, however, is high, with 70 percent of patients developing active ulcers again within the next year.[61-63] Although treatment with such drugs heals the ulcer, it does not eradicate the *C. pylori* if present nor heal the active chronic gastritis. This is significant, since the available evidence from diverse sources suggests that antimicrobial agents and bismuth compounds reduce *C. pylori* infection, and this is accompanied by healing rates comparable to those achieved with suppression of gastric acid. More importantly, these agents may reduce the incidence of duodenal ulcer relapse.[64] In a study from Yugoslavia, Perisic and Sarjanovic[65] have reported 9 of 32 children with endoscopically proven ulcers to be resistant to treatment with cimetidine, ranitidine, and sucralfate. Re-examination of these children, including antral biopsies, revealed *C. pylori* in all cases, and treatment with amoxicillin, 250 mg three times a day for 6 weeks, resulted in complete healing in six of these children and eradication of the organism. A 3-month follow-up demonstrated sustained remission. Clearly, further work in this area is needed to clarify the association between *C. pylori*, antral gastritis, and duodenal ulceration in children. This may not only have implications for treatment regimens but may also lead to further understanding of their pathogenesis.

Psychological Factors

The importance of emotional disturbances in the pathogenesis of peptic ulcer disease was once widely accepted. At one time it was believed that ulcer patients had a distinct and predictable personality, characterized by a hard-driving stereotype and an internal conflict resulting from strong dependency needs. However, early studies were often uncontrolled and not designed in such a way as to eliminate subjective bias. As a result, in the last decade, many doctors have come to believe that emotional factors may be unimportant in the pathogenesis of ulcer disease because most studies reported that neither the frequency nor the apparent severity of stressful life events differed between patients and controls. In a recent survey, however, Feldman et al[66] examined both "internal" personality attributes and "external" environmental factors in a case-controlled study involving 49 men and found a strong association between life events stress, psychosocial factors, and peptic ulcer disease. Hypochondriasis, a negative perception of their life events, dependency, and a lowered ego strength were the four variables that best discriminated ulcer patients from controls.

Well-designed studies with adequate controls have not been performed in children with ulcers. Authors briefly mention emotional stress, e.g., Robb et al[5] (58 percent) and Chiang et al[67] (39 percent), without defining the parameters measured and without any controls. Like others[68] we certainly have been impressed in a few children with identifiable events responsible for exacerbations of ulcer disease and its complications, but we are less certain about their role in the genesis of the original ulcer.

Clinical Features

A high index of suspicion should be maintained at all times when evaluating children with abdominal pain. Even so, the diagnosis of duodenal ulceration on a routine basis in a clinic is still difficult.[69,70]

Age

In young infants, the most common modes of presentation are perforation and hematemesis, although vomiting has often also been prominent. The diagnosis in these cases is usually therefore relatively straightforward. In the older age group, the mean age at diagnosis is 11 to 12 years, but symptoms are reported to have been present in 46 percent before the age of 10 and in 15 percent before 6 years of age.[9] The mean interval from the reported onset of symptoms to the time of diagnosis was 1.8 years. When symptoms began in early childhood, the delay was considerably longer—4.8 years. Ulcers, therefore, are not confined to teenagers.

Pain

This is the most prominent mode of presentation in 90 percent of children. A clear-cut history of periodicity can usually be obtained in two-thirds, and this may last from a few weeks to 6 months or more. As night-time pain is often said to be a feature of ulcer, being present in up to 60 percent of cases,

a direct inquiry should therefore always be made. Nonspecific recurrent abdominal pain in childhood occurs in up to 10 percent of children, and Apley's detailed studies revealed organic disease in less than 10 percent.[71] It is pertinent to point out that nocturnal pain was present in only 7 percent of the 118 children he studied.

The character, quality, and severity of ulcer pain is very variable and of little help. A temporal relationship to meals and relief by antacids is present in about half of patients. The most common site of the pain is the epigastrium (50 percent), although in one-third of cases it is consistently central.

Vomiting

Episodes of vomiting occur in about 40 percent of patients, usually preceded by pain. The younger patients (less than 6 years) tend to vomit more frequently and the older adolescent less so. Changes in appetite have not been a notable feature.

Hematemesis and Melena

Either or both of these are noted in approximately 50 percent of reported cases, and since this usually prompts a hospital admission, the decision for further urgent investigation usually follows. Bleeding does not necessarily occur early in the illness; more than half of our patients have symptoms consistent with peptic ulcer disease for at least 1 year before the episode of bleeding. Earlier diagnosis should thus reduce the incidence of bleeding, which at 50 percent is unacceptable. As a presenting symptom, upper GI bleeding accounted for 36 percent of new cases in our department in the 1960s. This figure had fallen to 15 percent by 1979, almost certainly as a result of the policy of investigating larger numbers of children with abdominal pain.

Occult Bleeding and Perforation

Both of these have been reported in up to 10 percent of cases,[67,68,72] although we ourselves have seen only one perforation outside of the neonatal period.

Tenderness

Epigastric tenderness may be absent, mild, or quite striking, depending on the activity of the disease at the time. If absent it may be prudent to arrange to see and investigate a child during an attack to maximize this finding.

The first decision to make when faced with children with recurrent abdominal pain is which to investigate. Those presenting with bleeding automatically qualify, but we also firmly believe that those with nocturnal pain and/or a positive immediate family history should also be investigated further—irrespective of the site of pain. We adopted this policy in the late 1970s, and it resulted not only in a threefold increase in the number of endoscopies performed but also a threefold increase in ulcer detection.

Some adult physicians have devised computer-based discriminant function by multivariate analysis to aid them in the diagnostic process. Recently, Tomomasa et al[73] from Japan have utilized such a system in a small group of 29 children with either gastric or duodenal ulceration and have examined 13 ulcer-related signs and symptoms. The multivariant analysis revealed that family history, bleeding, and the relation between the time of pain and that of eating had relatively high predictive values. They devised a cumulative score and found that their cut-off value of 1.4 for sensitivity, specificity, and positive and negative predictability was 89 percent, 85 percent, 63 percent and 96 percent respectively; this is an exciting area that deserves further research.

Diagnostic Tests

The availability of modern fiberoptic instruments suitable for use in all ages in childhood has resulted in a swing away from barium studies and a firm belief that upper GI endoscopy is the investigation of choice. The procedure is dealt with in more detail elsewhere but is well tolerated and safe.[74-76] Studies comparing radiologic and endoscopic techniques have shown the former to be diagnostic in 50 to 89 percent of duodenal ulcers demonstrated endoscopically.[76] The risk of false-positive radiologic diagnosis may also be especially high in pediatric populations, as Miller and Doig[77] failed to demonstrate any abnormality on endoscopy in 63 percent of 89 children with abdominal pain and a barium meal diagnosis of peptic ulcer. Further advantages of endoscopy are the ability to take biopsy samples, e.g., gastric antrum for histologic and microbiologic (*C. pylori*) analysis, and the fact that

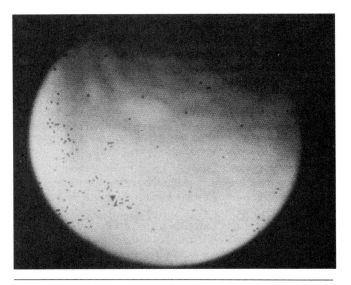

FIGURE 1 Endoscopic view of gastric antrum showing diffuse nodularity, typical of *Campylobacter pylori* gastritis.

other diagnoses, which would not be proven radiologically, are now being frequently encountered—e.g., mild esophagitis, gastritis, bile reflux.

At endoscopy, specific attention should be paid to the gastric antrum looking for changes of active chronic gastritis.

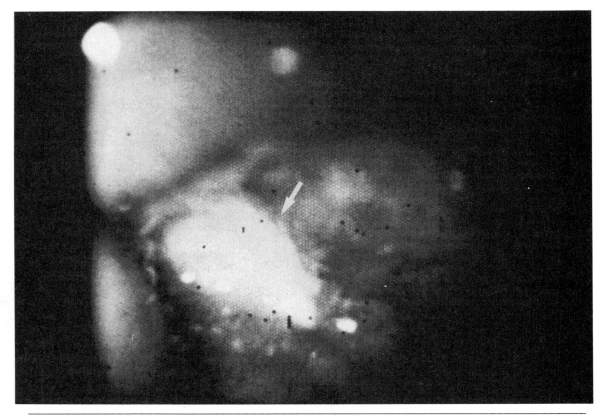

FIGURE 2 Endoscopic view of a single ulcer in the duodenal cap. There is associated mild deformity and surrounding duodenitis.

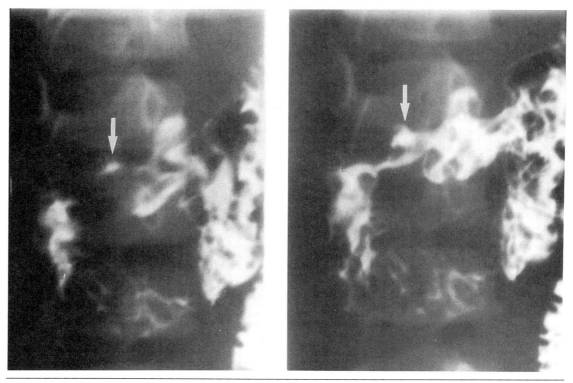

FIGURE 3 Barium meal showing a persistent filling defect (*arrow*) caused by a postbulbar duodenal ulcer in a 5-year-old girl. Endoscopy confirmed the ulcer and the presence of *C. pylori* gastritis.

Unfortunately, visual inspection fails to diagnose up to 80 percent of cases in adults, and thus antral biopsies should be undertaken routinely at any diagnostic endoscopy. They should be sent either to microbiology for *C. pylori* culture or to histology for routine examination including special staining techniques, e.g., Giemsa stain and Warthin Starry silver stain, again to identify this organism. Of the 25 cases of *C. pylori*–proven gastritis that we have seen, 50 percent have had a characteristic diffuse fine nodularity (Fig. 1) of the antrum. We have not encountered this finding in any other condition to date.

Examination of the duodenum may reveal scarring with deformity, duodenitis, and an active ulcer(s) (Fig. 2) that may or may not show evidence of bleeding. Large endoscopically diagnosed pediatric series do not yet exist, but of the last 40 cases we have seen, 15 percent had multiple ulcers, duodenitis was present in 50 percent, and 70 percent had obvious duodenal deformity, often severe and associated with scarring, suggesting longstanding disease. Although the numbers are relatively small, it is our distinct impression that those patients with deformity and scarring at initial diagnosis are the ones who have long-term problems in comparison to the teenage girl with an isolated single ulcer who heals quickly and has a low recurrence rate.

When endoscopy cannot be performed, a radiologic opinion should be sought, either with an experienced pediatric radiologist or with someone with an interest in GI diseases. The hallmark of an ulcer is a persistent filling defect (Fig. 3) with or without deformity and with visible radiating mucosal folds (Fig. 4). Duodenal irritability and a nondisten-

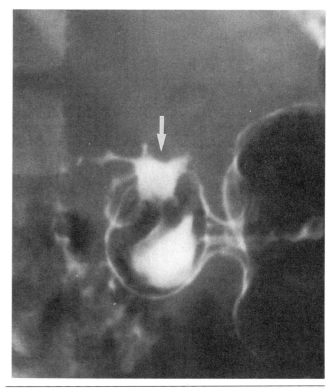

FIGURE 4 Barium meal showing large ulcer crater (*arrow*) in the duodenum of a 12-year-old boy. The ulcer crater is seen head on with radiating mucosal folds.

sible cap are frequent findings in normal anxious children. Deformity by itself does not indicate active disease and may simply reflect healing with scar formation.

Other investigations that may be necessary are a full blood count and fecal occult blood analysis. Where available, *C. pylori* antibody titers should be sought, as should Pg I estimation, as there is recent evidence that a normal value at diagnosis carries a favorable prognosis.[78] In children with multiple and refractory ulcers, a serum gastrin level should be measured to exclude Zollinger-Ellison syndrome, remembering to discontinue any H[2]-receptor antagonist for 48 hours, as these cause elevated levels by virtue of the negative feedback mechanism. Finally, although much has been made of basal, maximal, and peak acid outputs, in clinical practice these measurements do not alter the subsequent management and should not therefore be routinely performed.

Management

The short-term treatment of duodenal ulcers in adults can readily be achieved by a wide variety of drugs (Table 4), all of which have remarkably similar healing rates—70 to 80 percent at 4 weeks and 85 to 95 percent at 8 weeks.[79] The choice, therefore, for the prescribing doctor is wide, and other factors such as drug safety, speed of symptom relief, convenience of the therapy, and prevention of recurrence all have to be borne in mind.

The natural history of untreated duodenal ulceration in children is still not known, although recorded series before the advent of the H[2]-receptor antagonists show that 25 to 40 percent required surgery because of complications or disabling pain.

Antacids

These are the conventional and still widely used drugs in the treatment of ulcers. Low-dose aluminum and magnesium antacids are given for up to 6 weeks in a dose of 30 ml per 1.73 m^2 at 1 hour and 3 hours after each meal and at bedtime.[68] It is known that such antacid therapy can be as effective as H[2]-antagonists in ulcer healing, but the regimen to be employed must involve very frequent intake of large amounts of antacids, which is often associated with side effects such as diarrhea.[80]

TABLE 4
Drugs for the Medical Treatment of
Duodenal Ulcers*

Acid-Controlling Agents	Mucosal Protectives
Antacids	Sucralfate
H[2] receptor antagonists	Colloidal bismuth
Cimetidine	Prostaglandins
Ranitidine	Misoprostol
Nizatidine	Enprostol
Famotidine	Aluminum antacids
Pirenzepine	
Omeprazole	

* Some of these agents may not be available in all countries.

TABLE 5
Endoscopically Proven Healing Rates of
Duodenal Ulceration in Children Treated
with H[2]-Antagonists

Source	Treatment	Length	Healing
Denavit et al[85]	Cimetidine	8 weeks	88%
Chiang et al[67]	Cimetidine	8 weeks	87%
Oderda et al[78]	Ranitidine	8 weeks	94%
Tam and Saing[86]	Ranitidine	6 weeks	76%

H[2]-Receptor Antagonists

These were introduced for clinical use over a decade ago and have become the most popular choice in present-day ulcer therapy. Cimetidine and ranitidine have both been used in children, although reported experience in this area is still very limited, and in the few studies available[9,67,81-86] patient populations were usually small, there was often no consistent protocol of drug treatment, and conclusions regarding incidence of healing and recurrence were sometimes reached without objective confirmation. Symptomatic relief could be obtained in 63 to 88 percent of patients,[9,81] but higher figures of 76 to 94 percent were obtained in those subjected to endoscopy (Table 5). We currently give cimetidine (25 mg per kilogram per day in divided dosage up to 400 mg twice a day) or ranitidine (6 mg per kilogram per day in divided dosage up to 150 mg twice a day) for 8 weeks. Those children who relapse within the next year are given a further full course and then put onto nocturnal maintenance (10 mg per kilogram of cimetidine or 3 mg per kilogram of ranitidine) for 6 months. If they relapse further, the cycle is repeated but with nocturnal maintenance extending to 2 years. In a small number this may need to be increased even further on an individual basis. Because of our increasing use of these agents both in terms of patient numbers and time on treatment, we currently prefer ranitidine, which appears to be free of side effects. Although apparently rare, cimetidine has been known to cause gynecomastia, cerebral toxicity, and cholestatic jaundice[87-89] in children.

There are no data in children with regard to the use of the newer H[2]-antagonists nizatidine and famotidine, nor with the other acid-controlling agents, pirenzepine (a muscarinic receptor antagonist) and omeprazole (a gastric secretory inhibitor).

Sucralfate

This is a chemical complex of sucrose actasulfate and aluminum hydroxide and has the potential to neutralize hydrogen ions and absorb pepsin. It also increases the output of soluble mucus by a prostaglandin-independent mechanism and in addition binds intraluminal epidermal growth factor, enabling it to be available for longer periods for wound healing. Healing rates have been reported in adult studies, similar to those achieved with H[2]-antagonists, but significantly relapse rates were less both after an initial 6-week course and also on maintenance therapy for 1 year.[90] Chiang et al[67] treated 17 children with 1 g four times a day for 8 weeks and reported a healing rate of 92 percent. Of the 16 given maintenance nocturnal therapy of 1 g for 1 year, only 12.5 percent relapsed. Further trials are needed in children to evaluate this compound.

Colloidal Bismuth

Although bismuth compounds have been used for the relief of gastric disorders for over 200 years, the basis of their activity is poorly understood. Bismuth salts have a wide variety of actions that include an antacid effect, coating of the gastric mucosa, decreasing gastric and intestinal motility, increasing mucus secretion, and inhibiting the growth of a variety of microorganisms.[91] Their primary ulcer healing rates are almost equal to the H_2-antagonists, but more importantly there is now convincing evidence that the relapse rate is reduced following a healing course.[64,92] This is believed to be due to concomitant eradication of the organism *C. pylori* in the gastric antrum.[64] It is this eradication that has generated many studies in the past few years in adults, and the current "best-bet" therapy is to use a combination of ampicillin (for 2 weeks) and a bismuth compound (for 2 months). This does not eradicate the organism in all cases, relapse rates tend to be high (50 percent in the next year), and there remains the worry of repeated courses of therapy and the possible dangers of the absorbed bismuth. Nevertheless, in children with duodenal ulcers in whom the organism is identified on gastric biopsy, it is our current policy to use this therapy instead of H_2-antagonists. No data yet exist with regard to large trials or subsequent relapse rates.

Surgery

The surgical treatment of primary peptic ulcer disease concerns basically the management of a complication (hemorrhage, perforation, or obstruction), although it is anticipated that a percentage of all patients ultimately require surgical treatment at a later stage. When surgical treatment is required, a combination of vagotomy, pyloroplasty, and ligation of the bleeding point or closure of a perforation is the most commonly performed procedure.[6,75,93] Others have preferred vagotomy and gastroenterostomy.[94] If the patient has not previously received an H_2-antagonist, however, it would now seem logical for the surgeon to perform only the life-saving procedure—ligation or closure—and for the patient then to be treated medically.

More definitive surgery may be necessary at a later date for refractory or frequently relapsing ulcers despite intensive medical therapy. The decision for the clinician between long-term drug therapy (either continuously or intermittently) and surgery is a difficult one. The right decision can be made only if the clinician is clear what surgery can offer. Suitable data from large adult series are available. Truncal vagotomy was introduced in place of partial gastrectomy in order to have an operation with a low mortality that could be performed by most general surgeons. The long-term follow-up (16 years), however, gave recurrence rates of 10 percent and thus the combination of vagotomy and antrectomy became popular and, while giving a very high cure rate, undoubtedly left a few patients with significant side effects.[95] The aim of proximal gastric (highly selective) vagotomy was to achieve the same cure rate with minimal side effects. This aim has been real-

ized in centers where there is considerable experience and training, but proximal gastric vagotomy is a far more difficult operation than truncal vagotomy and probably not a procedure that is successful in the hands of a surgeon doing a few a year. This therefore excludes most pediatric surgeons.

Long-Term Prognosis

Some reports[2,94] have suggested that the prognosis for peptic ulcer disease diagnosed in childhood may be good, although others have been more cautious in their views.[3,10,13] These opinions were based on relatively short-term studies, however. Puri et al[6] supported the less optimistic view by reporting a high incidence of recurrence in a group of 31 patients followed up for 3 to 18 years. Collins et al[96] recently reported a 20-year follow-up of 31 subjects, only three of whom had a proven ulcer recurrence after the age of 16 years, although two of these had developed GI hemorrhage and one a perforation.

Shortly before the introduction of the H_2-antagonists, we analyzed the follow-up data of 75 children with radiologically proven ulcer craters. The results are shown in Figure 5. Overall, the figures suggest that rather more than 50 percent were symptom-free at the time their observations ended, even though 16 percent had undergone a surgical procedure. This study was not endoscopically controlled, and the follow-up was relatively short in the majority. In a separate study, Murphy et al[97] followed up 19 individuals in whom the diagnosis had been made in childhood 14 to 27 years previously. A high incidence of morbidity persisting into adult life was

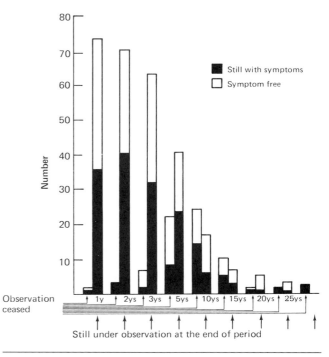

FIGURE 5 Follow-up of 75 children with radiologically proven duodenal ulcer. Numbers with and without symptoms at different observation periods.

found. Forty-seven percent had had a proven ulcer since entering adult life, and 37 percent had undergone surgery. Serious complications had occurred at some time in the past in 53 percent, in the majority after the age of 21 years. These findings firmly reinforce the opinion that the disorder frequently persists into adult life if not treated with H_2-antagonists or sucralfate. It remains to be established whether or not these agents reduce the significant long-term morbidity when used as a maintenance therapy, and proof will have to come from well-matched, placebo-controlled, double-blind studies, which will probably require multicenter trials.

PRIMARY GASTRIC ULCERATION

Primary gastric ulcers are rare in childhood, their etiology is unclear, and a hereditary predisposition has not been established. We have seen only one case during 500 upper GI endoscopies in the past 10 years. Studies exclusively devoted to this entity are lacking, small numbers being quoted as part of overall "peptic-ulcer" series. The position of the ulcer is often not stated, and this is important, since there appears to be a distinction between those occurring in the acid-secreting portion of the stomach (e.g., lesser curve) and those occurring in the non–acid-secreting portion (i.e., the prepyloric antral region). The latter are associated with high levels of acid secretion and blood group O status and occur in association with duodenal ulceration.[98,99] They probably have a similar etiology and natural history. True gastric ulcers, however, occur in the presence of acid hyposecretion and blood group status A and are usually found on the border zone between the parietal cell area and pyloric mucosa.[101]

A review of seven series involving 317 cases of peptic ulceration reveals a gastric ulcer in 43 (ratio of 1:7). Drumm et al,[100] for example, found only four gastric ulcers in 36 patients diagnosed surgically or endoscopically over a 5-year period. Kumar et al[7] found only two cases in 84 peptic ulcer patients. Nord et al,[82] however, found that primary gastric ulcers outnumbered duodenal in their series of 32 children, but of the 17 cases, 14 were said to be antral.

Ulcers occur when the mucosal barrier is breached by acid and peptic digestion of the mucosa ensues. The many factors controlling these aspects have not been studied in children, but in adults there is current interest in duodenogastric reflux as a major contributory factor.[102,103] Others believe that antral stasis is important, and this is believed to produce prolonged stimulation of gastric secretion, which overrides the normal tendency for gastrin release to cease when the antral pH becomes sufficiently acid.[104]

Clinically, as with duodenal ulcers, the diagnosis can be difficult, and a high index of suspicion and a low threshold to undertake endoscopy are needed. In young children, food refusal, pain, and crying may suggest the diagnosis. Hematemesis and/or melena may be a more dramatic presentation at this age, although perforation is rare. In the older child, pain predominates, but a temporal relationship to meals is unusual. Serious hemorrhage becomes less common with advancing age.

The investigation of choice is again upper GI endoscopy, taking particular notice of the lesser curve and the prepyloric region. Barium studies fail to demonstrate many gastric ulcers and are probably less accurate than for duodenal ulcers. Nord et al[82] reported that only 50 percent of their series were identified radiologically.

Data on treatment of gastric ulcers are scant. There is no good evidence that dietary regimens play a significant role. Antacids relieve pain, and indeed Nord et al found that cimetidine offered no advantage over conventional antacids in the treatment of antral ulcers. Most clinicians, however, would currently choose an H_2-antagonist as their first line of management. Chronicity does not appear to be a feature of gastric ulcers, and thus one 8-week course should be sufficient to safely heal the majority, without the need to consider maintenance therapy.

SECONDARY PEPTIC ULCERATION

Occasionally peptic ulceration may be due to another underlying disease such as Crohn's disease, and in this situation there are usually extensive mucosal disease and multiple ulcers. Endoscopic biopsies should be taken in a search for granulomata, although these may not always be seen in the superficial biopsy material obtained.

Stress

The majority of secondary ulcers are believed to be due to some form of stress. They occur with equal frequency in both sexes and tend to be acute, superimposed on a background of hemorrhagic gastritis or duodenitis and acute erosions. In many people's experience they are largely a terminal event in an otherwise seriously ill child and are often found for the first time at autopsy.[7,101] They tend to present as an acute medical emergency with bleeding and perforation and appear with equal frequency in the stomach and duodenum regardless of age.[13,105,106] With the exception of those associated with intracranial lesions (Cushing's ulcers), gastric hypersecretion has rarely been observed. Thus, if surgery is necessary the simplest operative procedure is ligation and plication.

Curling's Ulcers

In 1842, Curling reported four cases of duodenal ulceration in a series of 10 with widespread burns and suggested a causal relationship. Since then this phenomenon has been widely accepted, and many severely burned patients are treated prophylactically with antacids or later with an H_2-antagonist. In one series of 316 burned children, Dimick[107] reported 7 percent who developed Curling's ulcers, although higher figures of 13 percent have been quoted.[108] In the first few days following a major burn, gastric fundal acute stress ulcers are common, and it is probably this disruption of the physiology that leads to the acute duodenal ulcer, classically developing 2 or more weeks later.

Cushing's Ulcers

More accurately called Cushing-Rokitansky ulcers, these develop in children following cerebral trauma or surgery or hypertensive encephalopathy. They present usually with bleeding, characteristically about 1 week later. Although thought by Cushing to be secondary to a hypothalamic disturbance, Schlumberger[109] suggested that parasympathetic stimulation first produces vascular and secretory effects in the stomach and that ACTH and cortisol secretion resulting from stimulation of the supraoptic nuclei further increases acid secretion and impairs mucosal healing. Steroids, of course, also suppress prostaglandin synthesis and alter gastric mucus. It is further possible that one of the neuroendocrine hormones may also play a role, although data in children are lacking.

Many clinicians now utilize prophylactic cimetidine or ranitidine for a few weeks in children with extensive central nervous system lesions of diverse etiology. Published well-controlled series are, however, lacking, although this practice would appear to be safe and sensible. For a much more comprehensive review of stress ulceration based largely on adult data but examining the factors involved in pathogenesis, the reader is referred to a recent large review by Wilcox and Spenney.[110]

Zollinger-Ellison Syndrome

In 1955, Zollinger and Ellison described a syndrome consisting of peptic ulceration, marked gastric hypersecretion, and non–beta islet cell tumor of the pancreas.[111] It is now known that all patients with this syndrome have high levels of circulating gastrin originating from a gastrinoma that is usually pancreatic but, on occasion, can be gastric or duodenal. The hypersecretion of gastric acid, as a result of the greatly expanded parietal cell mass, leads not only to peptic ulcer disease but to duodenitis, jejunal mucosal erosions, stunting of villi, and acute inflammatory changes.

Clinical Features

The syndrome is rare in the pediatric population, with about 50 case reports now in the literature. It occurs more commonly in boys than girls (4:1). The outstanding symptom is abdominal pain, commonly accompanied by vomiting and GI bleeding.[112] Although gastrin has a stimulatory effect on motility and pancreatic secretion, the presence of diarrhea is much less common than in adults. Ulcers may be multiple and are usually duodenal, although a few are located in the jejunum and stomach. Tumor metastases may be found in the liver. The stomach may show pronounced hypertrophy of the gastric rugae, and the duodenum may be dilated. However, everything may appear typical of an ordinary peptic ulcer, but multiple recurrences, refractory ulcers, and the development of diarrhea should alert the clinician to measure the serum gastrin.

Investigations

In adults a fasting serum gastrin level of greater than 100 pg per milliliter is suggestive of this entity, although some children with duodenal ulcers have values higher than this.[68]

In the Zollinger-Ellison syndrome, however, values in the thousands can usually be expected. When the diagnosis is in doubt, two provocative tests may be employed: the calcium infusion test and the secretin infusion test.

Calcium Infusion Test. Calcium is infused at a dosage of 15 mg per kilogram for a 3-hour period. Gastrin levels in normal subjects show little change over this period, but those with Zollinger-Ellison syndrome show a two- to threefold increase over basal values or a peak of over 500 pg per milliliter.

Secretin Infusion Test. Whereas secretin inhibits acid output in "ordinary" duodenal ulcer patients, it causes paradoxical stimulation in those with Zollinger-Ellison syndrome. Norton et al in adults found this test to be more reliable than the calcium test.[113] Not only serum gastrin but also gastric acid output will increase following a provocation dose of 3 μg per kilogram per hour, whereas it drops sharply in ulcer patients.

Tumor Localization

The tumor cannot be located, even by exploratory laparotomy, in up to 50 percent of cases. Preoperative ultrasound scan was of little use (20 percent positive) in one adult series, although it should be better in cases of liver metastases. Computed tomography did a little better (40 percent positive), but angiography had the greatest individual sensitivity (60 percent).[113] Other highly invasive procedures that have been attempted are selective arterial secretin infusions and measurement of the immediate release of gastrin and transhepatic portal venous sampling for gastrin assay. These have not been employed in children.

Medical Treatment

Given in sufficient dosage, H$_2$-receptor antagonists can often relieve the patient's symptoms, and in adults, the newer agent, omeprazole, appears to be a potent alternative. Perhaps more exciting is the use of the somatostatin analogue SMS 201-995, which is administered by twice-daily subcutaneous injection. Although painful and causing local irritation, it has been shown to control symptoms and reduce gastrin levels and gastric acid secretion.[114] The relative lack of side effects makes this analogue a very promising agent in patients with surgically incurable disease, i.e., some 70 percent of those with Zollinger-Ellison syndrome. Reports of its use in children are awaited.

Surgical Treatment

The increasing availability of drugs to control the symptoms has deflected surgical attention away from total gastrectomy and toward attempts to extirpate the tumor. Approximately half of gastrinomas are malignant, but they generally pursue an indolent course. Gastrectomy has been shown to induce regression of both primary and secondary tumors, with a return of serum gastrin levels to normal. However, excision of the gastrinoma, where possible, still leaves the patient hypergastrinemic with the need for long-term H$_2$-antagonist therapy. Enucleation of a tumor in the pancreatic head may be possible, although partial pancreatoduodenectomy is indicated for lesions in the body and tail.

Metastatic Disease

Hepatic metastases are present at the time of diagnosis in up to 37 percent of adults.[113] Since these secondary tumors are generally detectable by initial imaging, operation can often be avoided. Streptozotocin and 5-fluorouracil prolong life, but the overall 5-year survival is less than 20 percent.

REFERENCES

1. Langman MJS. Epidemiology of peptic ulcer. In: Bockus HL, ed. Gastroenterology. London: WB Saunders, 1974:611.
2. Goldberg HM. Duodenal ulcers in children. Br Med J 1957; 1:1500–1502.
3. Milliken JC. Duodenal ulceration in children. Gut 1965; 6:25–28.
4. Habbick BF, Melrose AG, Grant JC. Duodenal ulcer in childhood. Arch Dis Child 1968; 43:23–28.
5. Robb JDA, Thomas PS, Orszulok J, Odling-Smee GW. Duodenal ulcer in children. Arch Dis Child 1972; 47:688–696.
6. Puri P, Boyd E, Blake N, Guiney EJ. Duodenal ulcer in childhood: a continuing disease in adult life. J Pediatr Surg 1978; 13:525–526.
7. Kumar D, Spitz L. Peptic ulceration in children. Surg Gynecol Obstet 1984; 159:63–66.
8. White A, Carachi R, Young DG. Duodenal ulceration presenting in childhood: longterm follow-up. J Pediatr Surg 1984; 19:6–8.
9. Murphy MS, Eastham EJ, Jimenez M, Nelson R, Jackson RH. Duodenal ulceration: review of 110 cases. Arch Dis Child 1987; 62:544–558.
10. Michener WM, Kennedy RLJ, Dushane JW. Duodenal ulcer in childhood. Am J Dis Child 1960; 100:814–817.
11. Singleton EB, Faykus MH. Incidence of peptic ulcer as determined by radiological examination in the pediatric age group. J Pediatr 1964; 65:858–862.
12. Sultz HA, Schlesinger ER, Feldman JG, Mosher WE. The epidemiology of peptic ulcer in childhood. Am J Publ Health 1970; 60:492–498.
13. Deckelbaum RJ, Roy CC, Lussier-Lazaroff J, Morin CL. Peptic ulcer disease: a clinical study in 73 children. Can Med Assoc J 1974; 111:225–228.
14. Karlstrom F. Peptic ulcer in children in Sweden during the years 1953–1962. Ann Paediat 1964; 202:218–222.
15. Coggon D, Lambert P, Langman MJS. 20 years of hospital admissions for peptic ulcer in England and Wales. Lancet 1981; i:1302–1304.
16. Fineberg HV, Pearlman LA. Surgical treatment of peptic ulcer in the United States. Trends before and after the introduction of cimetidine. Lancet 1981; i:1305–1307.
17. Wyllie JH, Clark CG, Alexander-Williams J, Bell PRF, Kennedy TL, Kirk RM, Mackay C. Effect of cimetidine on surgery for duodenal ulcer. Lancet 1981; i:1307–1308.
18. Schwartz K. Ueber penetrierende magenund jejunal-geschwüre. Beitr Klin Chir 1910; 67:96–128.
19. Feldman M. Peptic ulcer disease: pathophysiology and strategies for drug therapy. Curr Concepts Gastroenterol 1985; 3:13–19.
20. Ghai OP, Singh M, Walia BNS, Gadekar NG. An assessment of gastric secretory response with "maximal" augmented histamine stimulation in children with peptic ulcer. Arch Dis Child 1965;40:77–79.
21. Fieber M, Meschede R, Tolckmitt W. Aciditat und peptische aktivitat des magensafts bei gesunden und mucoviscidosis kranken kindern. Z Zinkerkeilkd 1975; 120:199–209.
22. Christie DL, Ament ME. Gastric acid hypersecretion in children with duodenal ulcer. Gastroenterology 1976; 71:242–244.
23. Isenberg JI. Peptic ulcer disease. In: Sleisenger MH, Fordtran JS, eds. Gastrointestinal disease. Pathophysiology, diagnosis, management. Philadelphia: WB Saunders, 1978:717.
24. Baron JH. Current views on pathogenesis of peptic ulcer. Scand J Gastroenterol 1982; 17(suppl 80):1–10.
25. Battaglia G, Farini R, Di Mario F, Vianello F, Piccoli A, Plebani M, Naccarato R. Is maximal acid output useful in identifying relapsing duodenal ulcer patients? J Clin Gastroenterol 1985; 7:375–378.
26. De Pretis G, Dobrilla G, Ferrari A, Fontana G, Maiolo P, Marenco G, Menardo G, Pallini P, Rossini FP, Saggioro A. Comparison between single morning and bedtime doses of 40 mg famotidine for the treatment of duodenal ulcer. Aliment Pharmacol Ther 1989; 3:285–291.
27. Venables CW. Mucus, pepsin and peptic ulcer. Gut 1986;27:233–238.
28. Foltmann B. Gastric proteases—structure, function, evolution and mechanism of action. Essays Biochem 1983; 52–84.
29. Defize J, Meuwissen SGM. Pepsinogens: an update of biochemical, physiological and clinical aspects. J Pediatr Gastroenterol Nutr 1987; 6:493–508.
30. Tam PKH. Serum pepsinogen I in childhood duodenal ulcer. J Pediatr Gastroenterol Nutr 1987; 6:904–907.
31. Rotter JL, Sones JQ, Samloff IM, Richardson CT, Gursky JM, Walsh JH, Rimoin DL. Duodenal ulcer disease associated with elevated serum pepsinogen I. An inherited autosomal dominant disorder. N Engl J Med 1979; 300:63–66.
32. Pearson JP, Ward R, Allen A, Roberts NB, Taylor WH. Mucus degradation by pepsin: comparison of mucolytic activity of human pepsin 1 and pepsin 3: implications in peptic ulceration. Gut 1986; 27:243–248.
33. McQueen S, Hutton DA, Allen A, Garner A. Gastric and duodenal surface mucus gel thickness in the rat: effect of prostaglandins and damaging agents. Am J Physiol 1983; 8:388–394.
34. Younan F, Pearson J, Allen A, Venables C. Changes in the structure of the mucus gel on the mucosal surface of the stomach in association with peptic ulcer disease. Gastroenterology 1982; 82:827–831.
35. Shorrock CJ, Rees WDW. Gastroduodenal bicarbonate secretion. In: Salmon PR, ed. Key developments in gastroenterology. New York: John Wiley & Sons, 1988:171.
36. Isenberg JI, Hogan DL, Selling JA, Koss MA. Duodenal bicarbonate secretion in normal subjects and duodenal ulcer patients. Dig Dis Sci 1985; 30:A–17.
37. Robert A, Nezamis JE, Lancaster C, Hanchar AJ. Cytoprotection by prostaglandins in rats. Prevention of gastric necrosis produced by alcohol, HCl, NaOH, hypertonic NaCl and thermal injury. Gastroenterology 1979; 77:433–443.
38. Miller T. Protective effects of prostaglandins against gastric mucosal damage: current knowledge and proposed mechanisms. Am J Physiol 1983; 245:601–623.
39. Smith CL, Hillier K. Duodenal mucosa synthesis of prostaglandins in duodenal ulcer disease. Gut 1985; 26:237–240.
40. Rotter JI. Peptic ulcer disease—more than one gene, more than one disease. Prog Med Genet 1980; 4:1–58.
41. McConnell RB. Heredity in gastroenterology: a review. Gut 1960; 1:273–284.
42. Blodgett MD, Morris N, Lurie HJ. Children with peptic ulcers and their families. J Pediatr 1963; 62:280–281.
43. Netakhata ZN. Clinical picture and diagnosis of peptic ulcer in children. Pediatriya 1970; 72:67–71.
44. Jackson RH. Genetic studies in peptic ulcer disease in childhood. Acta Paediatr Scand 1972; 61:493–494.
45. Falconer DS. The inheritance of liability to certain diseases, estimated from the incidence among relatives. Ann Hum Genet 1965; 29:51–76.
46. Rotter JI. Genetic aspects of ulcer disease. Comp Ther 1981; 7:16–25.
47. Fällström SP, Reinand T. Peptic ulcer in children. Acta Paediatr 1961; 50:431–436.
48. Cowan WK. Genetics of duodenal and gastric ulcer. Clin Gastroenterol 1973; 2:539–546.
49. Nutrient content of the national food supply. Washington, DC: Department of Agriculture, Human Nutrition Information Service, 1984.
50. Hollander D, Tarnawski A. Dietary essential fatty acids and the decline in peptic ulcer disease—a hypothesis. Gut 1986; 27:239–242.
51. Tovey FI, Javaraj AP, Clark CG. Diet and peptic ulcer. Lancet 1987; ii:398.
52. Editorial. Diet and peptic ulcer. Lancet 1987; ii:80–81.
53. Dial EJ, Lichtenberger LM. The extraction of antiulcer activity from bovine milk and a possible explanation for its mechanism of action. Gastroenterology 1986; 90:1394.
54. Warren JR. Unidentified curved bacilli on gastric epithelium in active chronic gastritis. Lancet 1983; i:1273–1275.
55. Rathbone BJ, Wyatt J, Heatley RV. *Campylobacter pyloridis*—a new factor in peptic ulcer disease? Gut 1986; 27:635–641.
56. Steer HW. Surface morphology of the gastroduodenal mucosa in duodenal ulceration. Gut 1984; 25:1203–1210.
57. Czinn SJ, Dahms BB, Jacobs GH, Kaplan B, Rothstein FC. Campylobacter-like organisms in association with symptomatic gastritis in children. J pediatr 1986; 109:80–83.
58. Drumm B, Sherman P, Cutz E, Karmali M. Association of *Campylobacter pylori* on the gastric mucosa with antral gastritis in children. New Engl J Med 1987; 316:1557–1561.

59. Kilbridge P, Dahms BB, Czinn SJ. *Campylobacter pylori*–associated gastritis and peptic ulcer disease in children. Am J Dis Child 1988; 142:1149–1152.

60. Eastham EJ, Elliott TSJ, Berkeley D, Jones DM. *Campylobacter pyloridis* gastritis in children. J Infect 1988; 16:77–79.

61. Bardhan KD. Intermittent treatment of duodenal ulcer with cimetidine. Br Med J 1980; 281:20–22.

62. Rune SJ, Mollman KM, Rahbek I. Frequency of relapses in duodenal ulcer patients treated with cimetidine during symptomatic periods. Scand J Gastroenterol 1980; 15(Suppl 58):85–92.

63. Hetzel DJ, Hecker R, Shearman DJC. Long-term treatment of duodenal ulcer with cimetidine. Intermittent or continuous therapy? Med J Aust 1980; 2:612–614.

64. Coughlan G, Gilligan D, Humphries H, McKenna D, Dooley C, Sweeney E, Keane C, O'Morain C. *Campylobacter pylori* and recurrence of duodenal ulcers—a 12-month follow-up study. Lancet 1987; ii:1109–1111.

65. Perisic VN, Sarjanovic L. *Campylobacter pylori*, resistant duodenal ulcers, and antibiotic treatment. J Pediatr Gastroenterol Nutr 1988; 7:934–935.

66. Feldman M, Walker P, Green J, Weingarden K. Life events stress and psychosocial factors in men with peptic ulcer disease. Gastroenterology 1986; 91:1370–1379.

67. Chiang BL, Chang MH, Lin MI, Hsu JY, Wang CY, Wang TH. Chronic duodenal ulcer in children: clinical observation and response to treatment. J Pediatr Gastroenterol Nutr 1989; 8:161–165.

68. Silverman A, Roy CC. Pediatric clinical gastroenterology. London: CV Mosby, 1983.

69. Grybosky JD. Pain and peptic ulcer disease in children. J Clin Gastroenterol 1980; 2:277–279.

70. Nord KS. Peptic ulcer disease in children and adolescents: evolving dilemmas. J Pediatr Gastroenterol Nutr 1983; 2:397–399.

71. Apley J. The child with abdominal pain. Oxford: Blackwell Scientific Publications, 1975.

72. Tam PKH, Saing H, Lau JTK. Diagnosis of peptic ulcer in children: the past and present. J Pediatr Surg 1986; 21:15–16.

73. Tomomasa T, Hsu JY, Shigeta M, Itoh K, Ohyama H, Terashima N, Kambe Y, Aoki S, Kuroume T. Statistical analysis of symptoms and signs in pediatric patients with peptic ulcer. J Pediatr Gastroenterol Nutr 1986; 5:711–715.

74. Gans SL, Ament M, Christie DL, Liebman WB. Pediatric endoscopy with flexible fiberscopes. J Pediatr Surg 1975; 10:375–380.

75. Tedesco FJ, Goldstein PD, Gleason WA, Keating JP. Upper gastrointestinal endoscopy in the pediatric patient. Gastroenterology 1976; 70:492–494.

76. Ament ME, Christie DL. Upper gastrointestinal fiberoptic endoscopy in pediatric patients. Gastroenterology 1977; 72:1244–1248.

77. Miller V, Doig CM. Upper gastrointestinal tract endoscopy. Arch Dis Child 1984; 59:1100–1102.

78. Oderda G, Altare F, Dell'Olio D, Ansaldi M. Prognostic value of serum pepsinogen I in children with peptic ulcer. J Pediatr Gastroenterol Nutr 1988; 7:645–650.

79. Colin-Jones DG. Medical treatment of peptic ulcer. In: Misiewicz JJ, Pounder RE, Venables CW, eds. Diseases of the gut and pancreas. Edinburgh, Blackwell Scientific Publications, 1987.

80. Ippoliti AF, Sturdevant RAC, Isenberg JI, Binder M, Camacho R, Cano C, Cooney C, Kline MM, Koretz RL, Meyer JH, Samloff IM, Schwabe AD, Strom EA, Valenzuela JE, Wintroub RH. Cimetidine versus intensive acid therapy for duodenal ulcer. Gastroenterology 1978; 74:393–395.

81. McNeish AS, Aytron CA. Cimetidine treatment of duodenal ulcer in children—a controlled trial. In: Torsoli A, Lucchelli PE, Brimblecombe RW, eds. H₂-antagonists. Capri: Excerpta Medica, 1980:108.

82. Nord KS, Rossi TM, Lebenthal E. Peptic ulcer in children. Am J Gastroenterol 1981; 75:153–157.

83. Harms HK, Bertele RM. Diagnostik und therapie der akuten magenerosionen und des gastroduodenalen ulcus. Gastroenterol Reiche 1980; 10:53–58.

84. Thomson RB, Attenburrow AA, Goel KM. Cimetidine in primary duodenal ulcer in children. Scott Med J 1983; 28:164–167.

85. Denavit MF, Guerin J, Caldera R, Rossier A. Ulcere duodenal chez un nourveaune. Ann Pediatr 1978; 25:494–498.

86. Tam PKH, Saing H. The use of H₂-receptor antagonist in the treatment of peptic ulcer disease in children. J Pediatr Gastroenterol Nutr 1989; 8:41–46.

87. Bale JF, Roberts C, Brook L. Cimetidine-induced cerebral toxicity in children. Lancet 1979; i:725–726.

88. Lilly TR, Hitch DC, Javitt NB. Cimetidine cholestatic jaundice in children. J Surg Res 1978; 24:384–387.

89. Ranitidine versus cimetidine in peptic ulcer. Drug Ther Bull 1982; 20:57–59.

90. Bolin TD, Davis AE, Duncombe VM, Billington B. Role of maintenance sucralfate in prevention of duodenal ulcer recurrence. Am J Med 1987; 83:91–94.

91. Wilson TR. The pharmacology of tri-potassium di-citrate bismuthate (TDB). Postgrad Med J 1975; 51:18–21.

92. Miller JP, Faragher EB. Relapse of duodenal ulcer—does it matter which drug is used in initial treatment? Br Med J 1986; 293:1117–1118.

93. Ravitch MM, Duremdas GD. Operative treatment of chronic duodenal ulcer in childhood. Ann Surg 1970; 171:641–646.

94. Curci MR, Little K, Sieber WK, Kiesewetter WB. Peptic ulcer disease in childhood reexamined. J Pediatr Surg 1976; 11:329–335.

95. Johnson AG. The management of peptic ulcer disease. Roy Soc Med Curr Med Lit 1984; 3:153–157.

96. Collins JSA, Glasgow JFT, Trouton TG, McFarland RJ. Twenty year review of duodenal ulcer. Arch Dis Child 1986; 61:407–408.

97. Murphy MS, Eastham EJ. Peptic ulcer disease in childhood: long-term prognosis. J Pediatr Gastroenterol Nutr 1987; 6:721–724.

98. Johnson HD, Love AHG, Rogers NG, Wyatt AP. Gastric ulcers, blood groups and acid secretion. Gut 1964; 5:402–411.

99. Langman MS, Doll R. ABO blood groups and secretor status in relation to clinical characteristics of peptic ulcers. Gut 1965; 6:270–273.

100. Drumm B, Rhoads JM, Stringer DA, Sherman PM, Ellis LE, Durie PR. Peptic ulcer disease in children: etiology, clinical findings and clinical course. Pediatrics 1988; 82:410–414.

101. Anderson CM, Burke V. Paediatric gastroenterology. Oxford: Blackwell Scientific Publications, 1975.

102. Ilci T, Whitfield PF, Boulos PB, Hobsley M. Gastric outlet loss and enterogastric reflux after gastrectomy. Br J Surg 1988; 75:272–274.

103. Niemelä S, Heikkilä J, Lehtola J. Duodenogastric bile reflux in patients with gastric ulcer. Scand J Gastroenterol 1984; 19:896–898.

104. Dragstedt LR. Gastrin and peptic ulcer. Arch Surg 1965; 91:1005–1010.

105. Nord KS, Lebenthal E. Peptic ulcer in children: a review. Am J Gastroenterol 1980; 73:75–80.

106. Kirschner BS. Peptic ulcer disease in children. Compr Ther 1976; 2:53–60.

107. Dimick S. Sixth national burn seminar: gastrointestinal ulceration. Bleeding in children. J Trauma 1967; 7:119–120.

108. Bruck HM, Pruitt BA. Curling's ulcer in children: a 12 year review of 63 cases. Trauma 1972; 12:490–496.

109. Schlumberger HG. Coexistent gastroduodenal and cerebral lesions in infancy and childhood. Arch Pathol 1951; 52:43–66.

110. Wilcox CM, Spenney JG. Stress ulcer prophylaxis in medical patients; who, what and how much? Am J Gastroenterol 1988; 83:1199–1211.

111. Zollinger RM, Ellison EH. Primary peptic ulcerations of the jejunum associated with islet cell tumors of the pancreas. Ann Surg 1955; 142:709–713.

112. Buchta RM, Kaplan JM. Zollinger-Ellison syndrome in a nine year old child: case report and review of this entity in childhood. Pediatrics 1971; 47:594–598.

113. Norton JA, Doppman JL, Collen MJ, Harmon JW, Maton PN, Gardner JD, Jensen RT. Prospective study of gastrinoma and resection in patients with Zollinger-Ellison syndrome. Ann Surg 1986; 204:468–479.

114. Williamson RCN. Endocrine and other unusual pancreatic tumors. Curr Opin Gastroenterol 1987; 3:749–755.

PART 4

Trauma and Foreign Substances

John A. Dodge, M.D., F.R.C.P. (Lon., Edin. Ire.), D.C.H.

TRAUMA TO THE STOMACH AND DUODENUM

Hollow abdominal viscera are less susceptible than solid organs to damage by blunt trauma or crush injuries to the abdomen. Penetrating wounds of the stomach are likely to cause peritonitis and may be associated with pancreatic injury.

Hematoma of the duodenum is a well-recognized consequence of blunt trauma to the abdomen in children.[1] An intramural hematoma in a child without an appropriate history of injury raises a serious question of child abuse.[2] A "coiled spring" appearance from a large obstructing mass is seen on contrast radiography in the acute phase. As the hematoma resolves, an indentation of the lateral wall of the second part of the duodenum is seen, which represents mucosal fold thickening. Newer methods of imaging (computed tomography and magnetic resonance imaging) show similar appearances. A well-defined concentric ring configuration on magnetic resonance imaging may be due to hemosiderin-laden macrophages.[3]

Iatrogenic Trauma

Iatrogenic injury to the stomach can be caused by intubation, endoscopy, and surgical procedures such as dilatation of esophageal or gastric strictures. Perforation of the stomach in critically ill neonates is usually attributed to local hypoxia-ischemia, but "spontaneous" gastric rupture is also described.[4] An increased risk of perforation has been found in neonates mechanically ventilated via face mask or nasal prongs but not when endotracheal intubation was used.[5]

Damage to the stomach and duodenum may also result from the use of certain drugs. Gastritis and ulceration related to aspirin, indomethacin, and corticosteroids are well known, and many other drugs produce upper gastrointestinal (GI) symptoms of varying severity. A particular risk of GI perforation occurs with the oral[6] or intravenous[7] use of indomethacin for pharmacologic closure of a patent ductus arteriosus in very low birth weight infants. In one series of 82 such infants, eight developed focal perforation of the gut without evidence of necrotizing enterocolitis, including two in whom the stomach was involved.[6] Tolazoline used in the management of pulmonary hypertension has also caused duodenal perforation[8] and gastric hemorrhage[9] in neonates. Intravenous ranitidine was used in one extremely sick anuric preterm neonate in the successful management of severe blood loss that followed tolazoline therapy.[10]

CORROSIVE GASTRITIS

In contrast to its effect on the esophagus, ingestion of strong alkalis rarely causes serious injury to the stomach, perhaps because they are at least partly neutralized by gastric acid. In one large series of patients with corrosive esophagitis from alkalis, only 1.7 percent had associated gastritis, and the majority of these were adults.

Conversely, and perhaps surprisingly, ingestion of strong acids usually causes relatively little damage to the esophagus but is likely to produce severe corrosive gastritis. The acid passes rapidly through the esophagus but is held up at the pylorus, where it induces pyloric (and antral) spasm and therefore remains in contact with the gastric mucosa. A "coagulation necrosis" ensues in which inflammation and edema are followed by lymphatic and vascular obstruction. The antral mucosa is sloughed, and varying degrees of necrosis occur with eventual healing, fibrosis, and antral deformity.[11]

Clinical Features. Most pediatric cases occur in adolescents, who have taken the acid with suicidal intent. A child who has swallowed a strong acid is likely to be given copious amounts of water, and vomiting may or may not be induced. There is often severe abdominal pain, perforation may occur, and the patient may be in circulatory shock. Hematemesis, if present, can be life threatening. If the child survives, recurrence or persistence of vomiting denotes developing antral obstruction, which may occur after an interval of several weeks or months.[11,12]

Radiologic investigation of early cases shows enlarged mucosal folds with filling defects representing hematomas and varying degrees of ulceration.[13] Subsequently fibrosis may lead to complete or partial antral obstruction. The severity of mucosal injury should be evaluated initially by careful gastroscopy, although there is a danger of instrumental perforation.[14]

Management. The immediate management of the child once he has reached the hospital consists of large doses of dilute antacids, and, as necessary, intravenous fluid, plasma, or blood replacement. Nasogastric suction is contraindicated if investigations reveal severe mucosal damage and a consequent danger of perforation, but if this is not thought likely a flexible, double-lumen tube can be used. Corticosteroids have been prescribed in an attempt to prevent stricture formation, but there is no published evidence that they do any good.

Progress can be monitored by repeated endoscopy. Massive hemorrhage, perforation, or a black appearance on endoscopy, indicating gangrene with full-thickness necrosis, requires early surgical intervention in the form of total or partial gastrectomy. If antral obstruction occurs, elective surgery is required and a Billroth I operation is the procedure of choice. Extensive fibrosis may require total gastrectomy.[12] One boy who developed a severe pyloric stricture following ingestion of (unnamed) alkali three weeks previously, without apparent immediate symptoms, has been successfully treated by balloon dilatation of the stricture.[15]

FOREIGN BODIES

Most foreign bodies reaching the stomach can be allowed to pass through the GI tract without intervention, although for larger objects such as coins this may take several weeks.[16] Delay in transit is likely to occur at the sphincter zones (pylorus, ileocecal valve) or points of constriction (ligament of Treitz).

Children under 2 years of age are particularly at risk, and an enormous variety of objects are swallowed, including marbles, coins, screws, and small toys. Occasionally sharp objects such as open safety pins or even razor blades have been swallowed by older, emotionally disturbed children, and these pose an obvious risk of perforation.

Small, blunt foreign bodies in the stomach require no active intervention unless there is a co-existing stenosis or stricture.[17] Removal of sharp objects needs to be carried out through a gastrotomy, but large blunt objects that cannot traverse the pylorus can be recovered using a flexible endoscope.

BEZOARS

Bezoars are intraluminal masses found in the upper GI tract, mainly the stomach. The name is derived from the Persian language and means an antidote to poison. Concretions in stomachs of animals, particularly goats, were prized in ancient times for their alleged magical and protective properties. Today the term has purely medical usage and denotes gastric accumulations of exogenous matter. An early paper by de Bakey and Ochsner (1938) reviewed 311 cases, including 8 of their own, and remains the most comprehensive reference.[19] Most other reports in the literature describe single cases. Bezoars are composed of undigested material, which may be milk curds (*lactobezoars*), exclusively found in young infants; *trichobezoars*, in which the main constituent is hair; and *phytobezoars*, consisting of undigested vegetable matter and almost always found in adult subjects who have had gastric surgery with vagotomy, treatment with H_2-receptor antagonists, or abnormal gastric function secondary to diabetes mellitus. *Antacid bezoars*, which are essentially concretions of dehydrated antacid, occur sometimes in patients given high doses of antacids during treatment of gastric bleeding. One such case has been described in a neonate.[18] *Trichophytobezoars*, as the name suggests, are composed of a mixture of hair and vegetable fibers.

Trichobezoars

These very rare masses are characteristically found in children or young adults with mental disturbance or retardation. The majority of patients are female. Eighty percent are less than 30 years of age, the youngest on record being only 1 year old.[19]

Clinical Features. Symptoms vary considerably and may be difficult to elicit if the patient suffers from mental subnormality or emotional disturbance. The child may be known to eat hair, and patchy baldness from hair pulling (trichotillomania) may be present.[20,21] Sometimes fibers from carpets or clothes, dolls' hair, raffia, or animal hair are ingested. There is usually weight loss, anorexia, and vomiting. Abdominal distention may have been noted, and 70 percent of patients complain of abdominal pain.[19]

Physical examination may disclose marked halitosis. Abdominal palpation nearly always reveals a firm mass in the left upper quadrant which may or may not be tender or indentible. Crepitus may be noted on palpation. The differential diagnosis includes gastric outlet obstruction, pancreatic pseudocyst, and gastric duplication.

Numerous complications are associated with trichobezoars. Iron deficiency anemia is nearly always present and is generally attributed to chronic blood loss from erosions or ulceration of the gastric mucosa, characteristically on the lesser curve. Megaloblastic anemia due to vitamin B_{12} deficiency is also described.[4] However, there is also good evidence that iron deficiency, which is a known cause of pica, may precede the eating of hair.[21]

The intragastric mass sometimes extends through the pylorus, and satellite bezoars can be found in the small intestine. One child with several such bezoars required four laparoto-

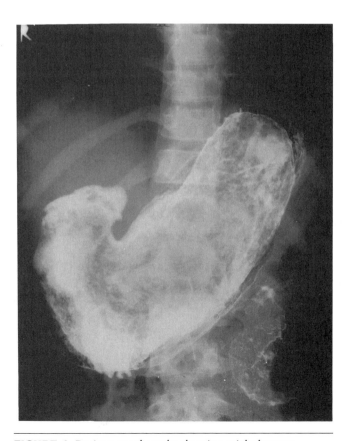

FIGURE 1 Barium meal study showing trichobezoar.

mies between the ages of 5 and 10 years. On two occasions small bowel intussusceptions were found.[22,23] Ulceration by bezoars in either the stomach or intestine may be followed by perforation and peritonitis.[20] Altered and increased bacterial content of the stomach and small bowel lumen may be the cause of a reported association of steatorrhea,[24] and hypoproteinemia due to excessive GI protein loss has also been described.[25] Extension of a gastric trichobezoar into the duodenum has resulted in biliary obstruction and jaundice.[26] There is a single case report of a girl with colicky upper abdominal pain who was found to have pancreatitis, which was believed to be secondary to irritation of the ampulla of Vater by the tail of a gastric trichobezoar that extended to the midileum.[27]

Psychiatric disturbance is often overt,[28] and despite the visible evidence to the contrary (alopecia and a bezoar) affected children often deny eating hair.

Investigations. The bezoar may be seen on a plain radiograph or as an echogenic dense solid mass with "clean" sonic shadowing posteriorly on ultrasonography.[19,20] It can also be visualized endoscopically. In most reported cases the diagnosis has been confirmed by a barium meal (Fig. 1).

Management. Surgical removal through a longitudinal incision is the standard treatment for an uncomplicated bezoar, and a thorough search should be made for satellite masses in the small intestine at the time of operation. Obstruction, perforation, and peritonitis require appropriate surgical management. No attempt should be made to disrupt the bezoar endoscopically because of the risk of detaching fragments and forming satellite intestinal lesions. Psychiatric care is often indicated. Recovery is usually rapid and uneventful but recurrence may follow, particularly if there are continuing psychological problems.[23]

Lactobezoars

The apparent incidence of these masses varies considerably among different neonatal units. Numerous reports of increasing incidence of lactobezoars in low birth weight infants

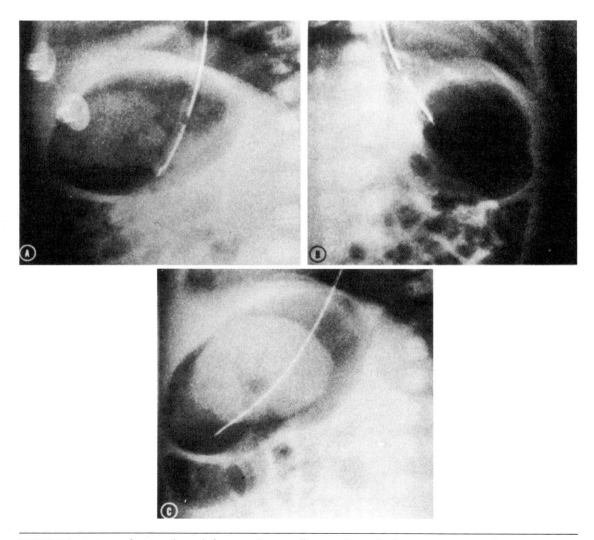

FIGURE 2 A, Lateral view of an abdomen after instillation of 10 ml of air into stomach demonstrates intragastric mass typical of lactobezoar. B, Bezoar no longer visible after feedings withheld for 48 hours. C, Recurrence of bezoar 7 days after onset of feedings of human milk. (From Yoss.[35])

appeared about 10 years ago,[31] but the incidence seems to have waned recently. It is believed that these temporal and geographic variations relate to differences in feeding practice.

Lactobezoars are composed mainly of casein, fat, and calcium.[32] One report quoted an incidence of 29 of 442 infants weighing less than 2,000 g who were fed a casein-predominant formula, whereas none of 223 fed whey-predominant formulae developed lactobezoars[33] and none has since been reported in infants so fed.[34] However, they have also been seen, albeit rarely, in infants fed human milk.[35] Other associated factors include very low birth weight, respiratory distress syndrome, and birth asphyxia. Factors that delay gastric emptying such as immaturity and the supine position may also contribute.

Clinical Features. Lactobezoars may be clinically silent and discovered incidentally as a radiographic shadow. Symptoms include abdominal distention, regurgitation, vomiting, and increased gastric residue during nasogastric feeding. A palpable mass may be present in the left upper quadrant. Gastric perforation has been described.[36,37]

The diagnosis is confirmed by the radiologic demonstration of an intragastric mass, which may be more easily seen after air has been injected through a feeding tube (Fig. 2).[31]

Management. Unless perforation has occurred, surgery is not necessary. Oral feeds are withheld for 1 to 2 days during which the baby is kept well hydrated with intravenous fluids. Resolution is usually prompt and recurrence rare.

REFERENCES

1. Winthrop AL, Wesson DE, Filler RM. Traumatic duodenal hematoma in the pediatric patient. J Pediatr Surg 1986; 21:757–760.
2. Kleinman PK, Brill PW, Winchester P. Resolving duodenal-jejunal hematoma in abused children. Radiology 1986; 160:747–750.
3. Hahn PF, Stark DD, Vivi LC, Ferrucii JT. Duodenal hematoma: The ring sign in MR imaging. Radiology 1986; 159:379–382.
4. James EA, Heller RM, White JJ, Schaffer JA, Shaker IJ, Haller JA Jr, Dorst JP. Spontaneous rupture of the stomach in the newborn: clinical and experimental evaluation. Pediatr Res 1976; 10:79–82.
5. Garland JS, Nelson DB, Rice T, Neu J. Increased risk of gastrointestinal perforations in neonates mechanically ventilated with either face mask or nasal prongs. Pediatrics 1985; 76:406–410.
6. Nagaray HS, Sandhu AS, Cook LN, Buchino JJ, Groff DB. Gastrointestinal perforation following indomethacin therapy in very low birth weight infants. J Pediatr Surg 1981; 16:1003–1007.
7. Scholz TD, McGuinness GA. Localised intestinal perforation following intravenous indomethacin for patent ductus arteriosus. J Pediatr Gastroenterol Nutr 1988; 7:773–775.
8. Wilson RG, George RJ, McCormick WJ, Raine PAM. Duodenal perforation associated with tolazoline. Arch Dis Child 1985; 60:878–879.
9. Dillard RG. Fatal gastrointestinal haemorrhage in a neonate treated with tolazoline. Clin Pediatr (Phila) 1982; 21:761–762.
10. Rosenthal M, Miller PW. Ranitidine in the newborn. Arch Dis Child 1988; 63:88–89.
11. Cochran ST, Fonkalsrud EW, Gyepes MT. Complete obstruction of the gastric antrum in children following acid ingestion. Arch Surg 1978; 113:308–310.
12. Zivkovic SM, Rakic D, Milosevic V, Stojanovic L. Total gastrectomy in an infant with corrosive gastritis. Z Kinderchir 1983; 39:141–142.
13. Kleinhaus U, Rosenberger A, Adler O. Early and late radiological features of damage to the stomach caused by acid ingestion. Radiol Clin 1977; 46:26–37.
14. Lowe JE, Graham DY, Boisanbin EV, Lanza FL. Corrosive injury to the stomach. The natural history and role of fiberoptic endoscopy. Am J Surg 1979; 137:803–806.
15. Treem WR, Long WR, Friedman D, Watkins JB. Successful management of an acquired gastric outlet obstruction with endoscopy guided balloon dilatation. J Pediatr Gastroenterol Nutr 1987; 6:992–996.
16. Pellerin D, Fortier-Beaulieu M, Guegan J. The fate of swallowed foreign bodies: experience of 1250 instances of sub-diaphragmatic foreign bodies in children. Prog Pediatr Radiol 1969; 2:286.
17. Fleisher AG, Holgersen LO, Stanley-Brown EG, Mones R. Prolonged gastric retention of a swallowed coin following pyloromyotomy. J Pediatr Gastroenterol Nutr 1986; 5:811–813.
18. Portugeuz-Malavasi A, Aranda JV. Antacid bezoar in a newborn. Pediatrics 1979; 63:679–680.
19. De Bakey M, Ochsner A. Bezoars and concretions. A comprehensive review of the literature with an analysis of 303 collected cases and a presentation of 8 additional cases. Surgery 1938; 4:934–963 and Surgery 1939; 5:132–160.
20. Beck AR, Leichteting JJ. Multiple small bowel perforations: an unusual complication of trichobezoar. Mt Sinai J Med (NY) 1972; 39:293–300.
21. McGehee FT, Buchanan GR. Trichophagia and trichobezoar: etiologic role of iron deficiency. J Pediatr 1980; 97:946–948.
22. Dasgupta HK, Chandra SS, Gupta M, Sanwal BL, Bhargawa SC, Vaid RL. Trichobezoar: clinical diagnosis. Postgrad Med J 1979; 25:181–182.
23. Booth IW, Harries JT, Glaser DR, Graham PJ. Multiple bezoars and laparotomies. J Roy Soc Med 1981; 74:691–692.
24. Hossenbocus A, Colin-Jones DG. Trichobezoar, gastric polyposis, protein-losing gastroenteropathy and steatorrhoea. Gut 1973; 14:730–732.
25. Valberg LS, McCorriston JR, Partington MW. Bezoar: an unusual cause of protein-losing gastroenteropathy. Can Med Assoc J 1966; 94:388–392.
26. Schreiber H, Filston HC. Obstructive jaundice due to gastric trichobezoar. J Pediatr Surg 1976; 11:103–104.
27. Shawis RN, Doig CM. Gastric trichobezoar associated with transient pancreatitis. Arch Dis Child 1984; 59:994–995.
28. Aleksandrowicz MK, Mares AJ. Trichotillomania and trichobezoar in an infant. J Am Acad Child Psychiatry 1978; 17:533–539.
29. Ratcliffe JF. The ultrasonic appearance of a trichobezoar. Br J Radiol 1982; 55:166–167.
30. McCracken S, Jongeward R, Silver TM, Jafri SZH. Gastric trichobezoar: sonographic findings. Radiology 1986; 161:123–124.
31. Schreiner RL, Brady MS, Franken EA, Stevens DC, Lemons JA, Gresham EL. Increased incidence of lactobezoars in low birth weight infants. Am J Dis Child 1979; 133:936–940.
32. Jenness R. The composition of milk. In: Larson BL, Smith VR, eds. Lactation: a comprehensive treatise. New York, Academic Press, 1974:1.
33. Schreiner RL, Brady MS, Ernst JA, Lemons JA. Lack of lactobezoars in infants given predominantly whey protein formulas. Am J Dis Child 1982; 136:437–439.
34. Silverio J. Lactobezoar risk. Pediatrics 1988; 81:177–178.
35. Yoss BS. Human milk lactobezoars. J Pediatr 1984; 105:819–822.
36. Laukoff AH, Gadsden RH, Hennigar GR, Weff CM. Lactobezoar and gastric perforation in a neonate. J Pediatr 1970; 77:875–877.
37. Erenberg A, Shaw RD, Yousefzadeh D. Lactobezoar in the low birth-weight infant. Pediatrics 1979; 63:642–646.

Esophageal and Gastric Neoplasms

Alan M. Leichtner, M.D.

ESOPHAGEAL NEOPLASMS

Not only are neoplasms of the gastrointestinal (GI) tract quite rare in children, but among the various sites of involvement, esophageal neoplasms are especially unusual. Nevertheless, tumors of the esophagus are worthy of discussion for at least two reasons. First, the cost of misdiagnosis is high in that delay may adversely affect the already poor prognosis for esophageal malignancies. Second, a number of conditions of childhood may predispose individuals to develop esophageal cancer in adulthood. Thus, it is important for the pediatrician and pediatric gastroenterologist to be aware of the pathogenesis of esophageal carcinoma so that high-risk individuals may be identified and monitored for the development of cancer.

Incidence

Both benign and malignant neoplasms of the esophagus are rarely reported in the pediatric literature, and most series of esophageal tumors include only adult patients. Overall, esophageal carcinoma is identified more frequently than benign tumors; in one large autopsy series, benign lesions accounted for only 17.8 percent of esophageal tumors.[1] The most common benign tumor of the esophagus is the leiomyoma,* followed in frequency by esophageal polyps. Although an extensive review of 163 benign tumors and cysts of the esophagus in all age groups reported no tumors in the pedi-

TABLE 1
Benign Tumors of the Esophagus

Epithelial tumors
1. Polyps
2. Squamous cell papillomas
3. Other epithelial, including cysts, adenomas

Nonepithelial tumors
1. Leiomyoma
2. Other mesenchymal, including lipomas, fibromas
3. Vascular
4. Granular cell tumors

Heterotopic tumors, e.g., pancreatic rests, thyroid nodules

Modified from Nemir et al.[6]

---

* The terms *leiomyoma* and *leiomyosarcoma* are still used here because of their clinical implications, although recent evidence suggests that these lesions should more correctly be designated undifferentiated mesenchymal tumors.

atric age group,[2] there have been reports of leiomyoma,[3] rhabdomyoma,[4] and squamous cell papilloma[5] in children. A classification of benign tumors of the esophagus is presented in Table 1.

Of the malignant esophageal tumors, by far the most common form in adults is squamous cell carcinoma, which, depending on the population studied, may account for more than 90 percent of malignant esophageal tumors.[7] The incidence of this neoplasm demonstrates remarkable world-wide variation. In central Asia, there is a hyperendemic belt and in regions of France, Iran, the Soviet Union, China, Singapore, Kenya, Zimbabwe, and South Africa, the reported incidence is extremely high.[8] Even within the United States, there is significant variation in incidence from region to region, although overall the incidence appears to be highest in black males.[9] Reports of esophageal squamous cell carcinoma in the pediatric age group are few. In the 1958 review of visceral squamous cancer in children by Moore, only one of 48 cancers occurred in the esophagus.[10] More recently, Soni and Chatterji reported the occurrence of such a tumor in the esophagus in an 8-year-old girl who presented with progressive dysphagia.[11]

Adenocarcinoma of the esophagus accounts for up to 15 percent of all esophageal malignancies in adults.[12] Most adenocarcinomas are thought to arise in areas of columnar-lined or Barrett's esophagus.[13] A case of adenocarcinoma of the middle third of the esophagus has been reported in a 15-year-old boy with dysphagia.[14] In another report of a 14-year-old, an adenocarcinoma of the gastroesophageal junction was found, but it was unclear whether the lesion originated in the stomach or esophagus.[15]

Secondary involvement of the esophagus by tumors arising in other sites is rare in childhood. However, suspected leukemic infiltration of the esophagus has been reported in a boy with acute lymphocytic leukemia.[16]

Etiology

Although it is clear that most pediatricians and even pediatric gastroenterologists never see a child with an esophageal tumor, many of the conditions that predispose adults to the development of esophageal malignancies begin in childhood. The predisposing factors hypothesized to play a role in the development of squamous cell carcinoma of the esophagus include the ingestion of carcinogens in soil, water, or foodstuffs, exposure to physical insults, nutritional deficiencies, and the presence of a number of underlying conditions (Table 2).[8]

TABLE 2
Putative Factors Predisposing to Squamous
Cell Carcinoma

Ingested carcinogens
Nitrosamines, alcohol, opiates, tobacco, fermented foods

Physical insults
Hot foods and drinks, caustics

Nutritional deficiencies
Zinc, vitamin A

Predisposing conditions
Achalasia, esophageal webs or other obstructing lesions, celiac
disease, tylosis plantaris et palmaris

Of greatest relevance to those caring for children is the demonstrated association of this cancer with previous physical insults resulting from the ingestion of caustic substances. Although the length of the follow-up of their patients was not noted, Bigger and Vinson reported the development of esophageal carcinoma in seven of 200 patients who had a history of caustic burns of the esophagus.[17] Given the estimate of 5,000 caustic ingestions per year in children under 5 years of age in the United States, the potential significance of such injuries to the later development of esophageal cancer is clear.[18] In a large series of patients with squamous cell carcinoma of the esophagus, 63, or 2.6 percent, were noted to have a history of lye injury.[19] The latency period between ingesting the lye and the subsequent diagnosis of carcinoma ranged between 13 and 71 years, with a mean of 41 years. The carcinoma usually appeared to arise in an area of stricture, commonly at the level of the tracheal bifurcation.

Achalasia of the esophagus also seems to predispose individuals to the development of squamous cell carcinoma. Approximately 3 to 7 percent of patients with achalasia eventually develop esophageal cancer.[20] The average duration of achalasia at the time of diagnosis of malignancy is 17 years. As is the case with patients who develop carcinoma of the esophagus after caustic injury, patients with esophageal cancer and achalasia present at a relatively younger age than do patients without these predisposing conditions. The lesions typically occur in the middle third of the esophagus and are often exophytic. Joske and Benedict hypothesized that the key factor in the association between esophageal strictures, achalasia, and esophageal webs and esophageal cancer was the presence of esophageal obstruction.[21] Whether obstruction increases the contact time between luminal carcinogens and the mucosa or whether a different mechanism is important remains to be established.

Adenocarcinoma of the esophagus could potentially arise in esophageal mucous glands, in areas of heterotopic gastric mucosa, or in Barrett's epithelium. Although previously reported to be quite unusual, gastric heterotopia has been observed in 21 percent of specimens of esophagus prospectively examined at autopsy of children from 0 to 14 years of age.[22] Nevertheless, since this finding was most frequent in the upper esophagus where adenocarcinoma is unusual and its prevalence decreased with increasing age of the patient, it seems unlikely that gastric heterotopia is associated with the development of adenocarcinoma. On the other hand,

adenocarcinoma in adults is strongly associated with the presence of columnar-lined (Barrett's) esophagus, found in more than 80 percent of cases. In one series of patients with Barrett's esophagus, 15 percent of symptomatic patients had a co-existing adenocarcinoma arising from their Barrett's mucosa.[23] In recent years, better techniques of endoscopy and esophageal biopsy have permitted identification of a number of children with chronic esophagitis beginning even in infancy. Furthermore, Barrett's esophagus has been reported to occur in patients as young as 6 years of age.[24] Whether this subset of patients is at risk for development of adenocarcinoma in adulthood has not yet been determined.

Pathology

Leiomyomas usually present as rounded intramural masses that do not involve the overlying mucosa. They may be found at any level in the esophagus and, in one case report of a child, the entire length of the esophagus was thought to be involved.[3] Esophageal polyps, on the other hand, are most frequent in the proximal esophagus. Most are pedunculated, have stroma consisting of a variety of cells of mesenchymal origin, and probably should be designated fibroepithelial polyps.

Usually, squamous cell carcinomas are found in the midthoracic esophagus. The gross appearance is most frequently a fungating mass; ulcerative or infiltrative forms are less common. The tumor extends locally be direct invasion and by intramural lymphatic spread. Unfortunately, metastases via lymphatics to various mediastinal structures occur early. Distant blood-borne metastases tend to involve lungs and liver. Recently, a superficially invasive form of squamous cell carcinoma has been recognized and appears to carry a much better prognosis, with 5-year survival rates as high as 90 percent.[25]

In contrast, most adenocarcinomas occur in the distal esophagus and must be differentiated from adenocarcinoma of the stomach arising in the cardia. As with squamous cell carcinoma, esophageal adenocarcinomas may present as polypoid, ulcerated, or infiltrating lesions, although the first two are more common. Again, spread via lymphatics occurs early, and distant metastases are likely to be present at the time of diagnosis.

Clinical Features

Benign esophageal tumors frequently cause no symptoms and are found incidentally during radiographic or endoscopic procedures.

In adults with esophageal cancer, no symptoms accurately predict the presence of early lesions. When dysphagia, the classic symptom in older patients, is present, significant spread of the tumor is likely to have occurred. In the case reports of benign and malignant esophageal tumors in children, dysphagia is frequently the presenting symptom.[3,11,14,15] Other reported symptoms include regurgitation or vomiting, hematemesis, odynophagia, chest pain, weight loss, and respiratory difficulties. The latter may result either from aspiration of food or secretions in an obstructed esophagus or from compression or invasion of respiratory structures by tumor.

Physical examination is unlikely to aid significantly in the diagnosis. Occasionally, evidence of poor nutrition, dehydration, or anemia may be present. Drooling, stridor, tachypnea, and an abnormal chest examination suggest respiratory complications.

Diagnosis

Although a chest radiograph may occasionally show evidence of a pulmonary complication or underlying esophageal disease, the primary radiographic study is the barium swallow. This study may demonstrate an exophytic or ulcerated lesion or reveal rigidity and decreased distensibility suggestive of an infiltrating tumor (Fig. 1). At times, certain esophageal tumors may be confused radiographically with foreign bodies, benign strictures, severe esophagitis, esophageal varices, and achalasia.[26]

Esophagogastroscopy is the preferred technique for definitive diagnosis of most esophageal tumors. The gross appearance and extent of the lesion can be noted, and biopsies or brushings for histologic and cytologic examination can be performed. (Color Plate II*E* is an endoscopic view of the lesion shown in Fig. 1.) Occasionally, the findings may be subtle and mimic other benign conditions such as esophagitis. Multiple forceps biopsies should be done to provide maximal yield for accurate diagnosis of esophageal malignancies.[27] Brushings for cytologic examination have the advantage of sampling a greater surface area of mucosa than does biopsy, and combining the techniques can further increase the diagnostic yield to more than 95 percent.[28]

Further evaluation of esophageal tumors, particularly cancers, is aided by newer imaging techniques such as computed tomography, magnetic resonance imaging, and endoscopic ultrasonography. These modalities can help define the extent and nature of the primary tumor as well as detect sites of spread. Bronchoscopy to detect invasion of the trachea and bronchi and laparoscopy to detect liver and peritoneal metastases may be useful in staging malignant lesions.

Treatment

Because of the limited clinical information available, the approach to any esophageal tumor in a child must be individualized. Symptomatic benign tumors of the esophagus may be cured by simple excision. Although many polypoid lesions may be removed at endoscopy, other lesions may require a surgical approach. Typically, esophagectomy with primary anastomosis is performed. However, on occasion colon interposition or another esophageal replacement procedure may be required.

The treatment of esophageal cancer in adult patients is tempered by the very poor prognosis of both squamous cell carcinoma and adenocarcinoma. In childhood, however, the young age of the patient and absence of information regarding prognosis in this age group justify an aggressive approach. When possible, surgical resection of esophageal cancer should

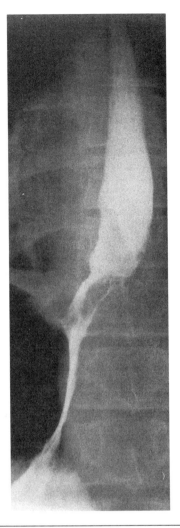

FIGURE 1 A 21-year-old female who presented with dysphagia had a barium swallow. She had undergone surgical repair of a tracheoesophageal fistula in the neonatal period. A luminal mass is noted in the midesophagus. Endoscopic biopsies demonstrated adenocarcinoma. Note that this is a prone film, and hence the heart is to the left of the figure. (Courtesy of Richard Sandler and Harland Winter.)

be attempted. Although for squamous cell carcinoma the use of radiation alone may be as effective as surgery, it appears to be less effective in the treatment of adenocarcinoma. The role of chemotherapy is not established for either malignancy. The utility of combination therapy must also await further study.

Although treatment for esophageal cancer rarely effects a cure, major strides have been made in providing palliation. Dilatation of the esophageal lumen, placement of esophageal prostheses, and decreasing tumor bulk with electrocoagulation or laser treatment may restore patency of the esophageal lumen enough to permit oral nutrition. Early aggressive nutritional rehabilitation via oral, enteral feeding tube, or central venous hyperalimentation routes is extremely important.

Prognosis

The 5-year survival for squamous cell carcinoma is less than 5 percent and that for adenocarcinoma is only slightly better. Patients with squamous cell carcinoma arising in areas of stricture following caustic ingestions appear to have a somewhat improved prognosis,[19] whereas patients with co-existing achalasia do more poorly, despite also presenting at a relatively early age.[20] Reported cases of children with esophageal cancer are too few to permit useful determination of prognosis.

Conclusions

Clearly, the role of the pediatrician or pediatric gastroenterologist with regard to tumors of the esophagus is one of identification and, when possible, prevention of the predisposing conditions. World-wide, more epidemiologic studies are required so that the pathogenesis of esophageal cancer in hyperendemic areas can be understood. Efforts to eliminate caustic ingestions by better packaging of caustic agents and improved education of the consumer must continue. Patients with longstanding esophageal obstruction or chronic esophagitis and columnar-lined (Barrett's) esophagus should be treated aggressively, and surveillance for complicating esophageal carcinoma should be considered in adolescents and young adults. Recommendations for surveillance of adult patients with identified Barrett's esophagus are much debated, and further studies are required before the cost-effectiveness of surveillance and appropriate interval for endoscopic procedures can be established.[29]

GASTRIC NEOPLASMS

Although the stomach is a more frequent site for tumors in childhood than is the esophagus, gastric neoplasms are still exceedingly rare. A number of benign tumors do occur in the stomach and include teratomas, which are diagnosed almost exclusively in infancy. In contrast to the situation in adults, in whom approximately 95 percent of gastric malignancies are adenocarcinomas,[30] in children the most common cancers are non-Hodgkin's lymphomas and leiomyosarcomas. General GI aspects of carcinoid tumors, lymphomas, and leiomyosarcomas are reviewed in a later chapter. Therefore, the main focus of the following discussion is gastric carcinoma and certain benign tumors of the stomach.

Incidence and Etiology

Unlike the incidence of colon cancer, which is steadily rising, gastric cancer has demonstrated a striking decrease in rate of occurrence in the United States. Nevertheless, this malignancy remains a significant problem world-wide. A marked variation in the incidence of gastric cancer exists between different regions, with Japan and several other countries such as Costa Rica, Chile, Columbia, Iceland, Finland, Hungary, and Poland having very high rates. Interestingly, Japanese who have migrated to Hawaii, a low incidence area,

experience decreasing occurrence rates of gastric cancer over subsequent generations.[31]

Epidemiologic studies have demonstrated that a diet rich in pickled, salted, or smoked foods may be associated with the high occurrence of the intestinal type of gastric cancer. It is hypothezised that ingested nitrates and nitrites may combine with amines, amides, or other compounds to form carcinogenic substances.[32]

Several lines of evidence have suggested that genetic factors may also play a role in the etiology of gastric cancer. Blood group A has been shown to be more frequent in patients with gastric cancer.[33] Moreover, there appears to be a two- to threefold greater incidence of this cancer in relatives of persons similarly affected.

The incidence of gastric carcinoma increases with age, and only a small percentage of cases occur in young individuals. Furthermore, in McNeer's classic series of 501 cases of gastric cancer in individuals under 31 years of age, only 0.4 percent of cases occurred in children 10 years or younger, 3.4 percent occurred in children between 11 and 15 years, and 11.8 percent occurred in children between 16 and 20 years.[34] In this study, there were approximately equal numbers of males and females affected, although other reports of older individuals note a preponderance of cases in males, especially for the intestinal type of carcinoma.

Conditions predisposing adults to develop gastric cancers include chronic atrophic gastritis, certain types of intestinal metaplasia of the stomach, pernicious anemia, hypertrophic gastropathy, and a previous gastrectomy (Table 3). Because of the rarity of this tumor in childhood, the significance of these factors for the pediatric age group is not clear. However, an association between gastric neoplasms and immunodeficiency diseases, including isolated IgA deficiency,[35] ataxia telangiectasia,[36] and other conditions, has been noted. Both the adenomatous polyposis syndromes, familial polyposis and Gardner's syndrome, and Peutz-Jeghers syndrome, in which hamartomatous polyps are found, are associated with the development of adenomas and adenocarcinoma of the stomach and duodenum, obligating surveillance of children with these syndromes. Finally, gastric adenocarcinoma has also developed as a late complication in individuals previously treated for abdominal lymphoma.[37]

Pathology

Carcinomas of the stomach are classified on the basis of a variety of characteristics, including the degree of differentiation, ability to secrete mucus, pattern of the cellular ar-

TABLE 3
Conditions Predisposing to Gastric Cancer

Chronic atrophic gastritis
Intestinal metaplasia of the stomach
Pernicious anemia
Hypertrophic gastropathy
Immunodeficiency
Polyposis syndromes—familial polyposis, Gardner's syndrome, Peutz-Jeghers syndrome
Previous partial gastrectomy
Previous treatment for abdominal lymphoma

rays (e.g., medullary or papillary), and whether the cells are cohesive (intestinal or expanding type) or infiltrate independently (diffuse or infiltrating type). In childhood, the mucinous type of gastric adenocarcinoma appears to be the most common pattern.[38] Grossly, the lesions may appear polypoid or ulcerative or may infiltrate the wall of the stomach diffusely (linitis plastica). Most tumors are located in the antrum, along the lesser curvature. A potentially curable form of gastric cancer in which disease is limited to the mucosa or submucosa has been described and termed "early gastric cancer."[39]

Gastric carcinoma is a rather aggressive malignancy and has a tendency to spread early via lymphatics to regional lymph nodes and by direct extension into contiguous structures. Lesions may spread great distances along the intramural lymphatics, necessitating wide resection margins at the time of surgery.[30] Distant blood-borne metastases occur in the liver, lungs, brain, and bones. Aggressive behavior of the tumor has been noted in cases occurring in childhood.[34,40]

Clinical Features

The clinical manifestations of gastric carcinoma include epigastric pain, anorexia, early satiety, weight loss, GI bleeding, and vomiting or other symptoms of gastric obstruction.

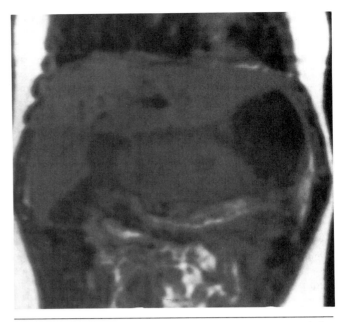

FIGURE 3 Magnetic resonance imaging of the upper abdomen of the same patient depicted in Figure 2. Below the liver, a central mass is seen replacing the distal stomach. (Courtesy of the Teaching Collection, Department of Radiology, The Children's Hospital, Boston.)

In younger individuals, severe inanition is uncommon.[34] Anemia, an elevated erythrocyte sedimentation rate, and occult blood in the stools are frequently noted in both adults and children with gastric carcinoma. Although a palpable mass was noted in only 30 percent of older adults, McNeer noted that finding in more than 70 percent of individuals 30 years old or younger.[34] Signs of advanced gastric cancer include ascites, characteristic palpable adenopathy, a cul-de-sac mass, and other classic features.

Diagnosis

In the diagnosis of a child suspected of having a gastric malignancy, a barium upper GI series may demonstrate a polypoid mass, ulceration lacking the characteristics of benign gastric ulceration, or poor distensibility suggestive of intramural tumor. As an example of such a study, Figure 2 shows an upper GI series in a child with gastric lymphoma. Abdominal ultrasonography, computed tomography, and magnetic resonance imaging may permit detection of metastasis (Fig. 3). Endoscopy frequently affords accurate histologic diagnosis of gastric lesions. Specifically in the diagnosis of carcinoma, the best yield is provided by multiple biopsies[27] or a combination of biopsy and cytologic techniques. To date, the significance of gastric secretory studies demonstrating achlorhydria, low serum pepsinogen levels as found in adults with atrophic gastritis, and elevated levels of carcinoembryonic antigen in the diagnosis and management of children with gastric carcinoma remains to be determined.

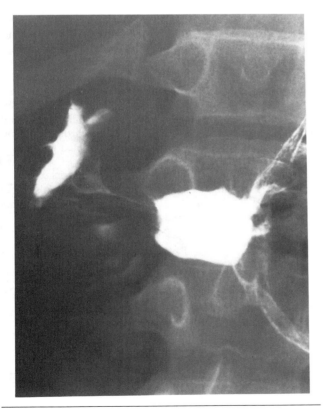

FIGURE 2 Selective view of the antrum from an upper GI series in a 15-year-old boy who presented with hematemesis, weight loss, and right upper quadrant abdominal pain. A mass is seen encircling the antrum and almost completely obstructing it. Endoscopic biopsies revealed a large cell immunoblastic lymphoma. (Courtesy of the Teaching Collection, Department of Radiology, The Children's Hospital, Boston.)

Treatment

For local disease without metastases, surgery emphasizing wide resection margins to ensure total excision of the tumor is the primary therapy. Adjuvant treatment with chemotherapy or radiation has sometimes been recommended, but more controlled studies are necessary to evaluate its utility. With disseminated disease, surgery is mainly palliative, and chemotherapy or radiation is offered. Combined chemotherapy with 5-fluorouracil, mitomycin C, and doxorubicin or a similar combination seems to show some promise.[41] In childhood, the accumulated data are not sufficient to suggest that a different therapeutic approach is required. Therefore, until multicenter trials can be undertaken, treatment programs should be individualized, using the experience in adults as a model.

Prognosis

The prognosis of gastric cancer in adults appears to be related to the degree of invasion of the gastric wall and the presence of lymph node involvement and peritoneal and distal metastases. Overall, the 5-year survival rate is an extremely poor 16 percent.[42] Although no series of children with gastric carcinoma is large enough to allow reasonable calculation of prognosis, anecdotal evidence suggests that delay in diagnosis frequently contributes to poor patient survival.

Other Gastric Cancers

GI carcinoid tumors, lymphomas, and leiomyosarcomas are discussed elsewhere in this book. The stomach is an unusual site for carcinoid tumors and lymphoma in childhood, but pediatric cases have been reported.

In contrast, the stomach is the most common site for malignant smooth muscle tumors of the GI tract in childhood. In 1973, Wurlitzer collected 34 cases for review.[43] Twenty of the tumors were judged to be leiomyosarcomas and 14 were benign leiomyomas. Frank hematemesis was the most frequent symptom in these children, although some evidence of GI bleeding was noted in more than 80 percent of cases. Leiomyosarcoma of the stomach appears to be a very aggressive tumor with a tendency for early metastases, and the prognosis is guarded.[44] Since it may be difficult to differentiate benign from malignant lesions, a wide surgical excision is recommended.

In 1977, Carney et al reported an association of gastric leiomyosarcoma and two other tumors, functioning extraadrenal paraganglioma and pulmonary chondroma.[45] This association obligates a careful search for other tumors in children found to have leiomyosarcomas of the stomach.

Benign Neoplasms of the Stomach

Benign neoplasms of the stomach are uncommon in children. They include adenomatous and hyperplastic polyps, leiomyomas, lipomas, and other lesions.[46] As noted above, benign smooth muscle tumors are identified less frequently in children than are leiomyosarcomas. Although rare, the gastric teratoma appears to occur exclusively in childhood. In 1981, Cairo et al described what they calculated to be only the fifty-first reported case of gastric teratoma in childhood.[47] Virtually all patients with gastric teratomas have been male, and the vast majority have been less than 1 year of age at the time of diagnosis.[47,48]

Teratomas are thought to arise from pluripotential cells and contain tissue originating from more than one germ cell layer (i.e., endoderm, ectoderm, and mesoderm) in an area in which the structures are not usually found. The most common site for teratomas in childhood is the sacrococcygeal region, which accounts for approximately 60 to 65 percent of all such lesions. In the stomach, more than 90 percent of teratomas occur along the greater curvature. Moriuchi found no malignant lesions in his review of reported cases.[48]

Clinically, gastric teratomas usually present as large intraabdominal masses. Women giving birth to newborns with gastric teratomas may experience premature labor or dystocia. The infant may suffer from respiratory insufficiency associated with a large abdominal mass and limitation of movement of the diaphragm. Upper GI bleeding is occasionally noted as a result of intramural growth of the tumor and ulceration of the overlying mucosa.[47,49] Radiographic studies of the abdomen may demonstrate calcifications corresponding to bony structures or teeth within the teratoma. Preoperative diagnosis can be further aided by ultrasonography and computed tomography.[50] Since gastric teratomas tend to be benign, successful excision should result in cure.

Conclusions

Given their rarity, gastric tumors in childhood are almost always unexpected findings. Nevertheless, the differential diagnosis of upper GI symptoms in childhood must include these rare lesions if timely treatment, especially for gastric malignancies, is to be instituted.

Acknowledgments

The author is grateful to Dr. Antonioli for his review of this chapter.

REFERENCES

1. Plachta A. Benign tumors of the esophagus: review of literature and report of 99 cases. Am J Gastroenterol 1962; 38:639–652.
2. Totten RS, Stout AP, Humphreys GH, Moore RL. Benign tumors and cysts of the esophagus. J Thorac Surg 1953; 25:606–619.
3. Nahmad M, Clatworthy HW. Leiomyoma of the entire esophagus. J Pediatr Surg 1973; 8:829–830.
4. Pai GK, Pai PK, Kamath SM. Adult rhabdomyoma of the esophagus. J Pediatr Surg 1987; 22:991–992.
5. Arima T, Ikeda K, Satoh T, Hayashida Y, Matsuo S, Ueda K. Squamous cell papilloma of the esophagus in a child. Int Surg 1985; 70:177–178.
6. Nemir P, Wallace HW, Fallahnejad M. Diagnosis and surgical management of benign disease of the esophagus. Curr Probl Surg 1976; 13:1.
7. Turnbull ADM, Goodner JT. Primary adenocarcinoma of the esophagus. Cancer 1968; 22:915–918.
8. Sales D, Levin B. Incidence, epidemiology, and predisposing factors. In: DeMeester TR, Levin B, eds. Cancer of the esophagus. Orlando: Grune & Stratton, 1985:1.
9. Maram ES, Kurland LT, Ludwig J, Brian DD. Esophageal carcinoma in Olmsted County, Minnesota, 1935–1971. Mayo Clin Proc 1977; 52:24.
10. Moore C. Visceral squamous cancer in children. Pediatrics 1958; 21:573–581.
11. Soni NK, Chatterji P. Carcinoma of the esophagus in an eight-year-old child. J Laryngol Otol 1980; 94:327–329.
12. Faintuch J, Shepard KV, Levin B. Adenocarcinoma and other unusual variants of esophageal cancer. Semin Oncol 1984; 11:196–202.

13. Haggitt RC, Tryzelaar J, Ellis FH, Colcher H. Adenocarcinoma complicating columnar epithelium-lined (Barrett's) esophagus. Am J Clin Pathol 1978; 70:1–5.
14. Al Hilou R, Atkins J, Matthews HR. Oesophageal adenocarcinoma in a boy of fifteen years. J Laryngol Otol 1984; 98:643–646.
15. Elliott MJ, Ashcroft T. Primary adenocarcinoma of the gastro-oesophageal junction in childhood: a case report. Scand J Thorac Cardiovasc Surg 1983; 17:65–66.
16. Al-Rashid RA, Harned RK. Dysphagia due to leukemic involvement of the esophagus. Am J Dis Child 1971; 121:75–76.
17. Bigger IA, Vinson PP. Carcinoma secondary to burn of the esophagus from ingestion of lye: report of a case. Surgery 1950; 28:887–889.
18. Leape LL, Ashcraft KW, Scarpelli DG, Holder TM. Hazard to health-liquid lye. N Engl J Med 1971; 284:578–581.
19. Appelqvist P, Salmo M. Lye corrosion carcinoma of the esophagus: a review of 63 cases. Cancer 1980; 45:2655–2658.
20. Carter R, Brewer LA. Achalasia and esophageal carcinoma: studies in early diagnosis for improved surgical management. Am J Surg 1975; 130:114–118.
21. Joske RA, Benedict EB. The role of benign esophageal obstruction in the development of carcinoma of the esophagus. Gastroenterology 1959; 36:749–755.
22. Variend S, Howat AJ. Upper oesophageal gastric heterotopia: a prospective necropsy study in children. J Clin Pathol 1988; 41:742–745.
23. Sarr MG, Hamilton SR, Marrone GC, Cameron JL. Barrett's esophagus: its prevalence and association with adenocarcinoma in patients with symptoms of gastroesophageal reflux. Am J Surg 1985; 149:187–193.
24. Hassall E. Weinstein WM, Ament ME. Barrett's esophagus in children. Gastroenterology 1985; 89:1331–1337.
25. Schmidt LW, Dean PJ, Wilson RT. Superficially invasive squamous cell carcinoma of the esophagus: a study of seven cases in Memphis, Tennessee. Gastroenterology 1986; 91:1456–1461.
26. Wiot JW, Felson B. Cancer of the gastrointestinal tract. I. Esophagus: radiographic differential diagnosis. JAMA 1973; 226:1548–1552.
27. Graham DY, Schwartz JT, Cain CD, Gyorkey F. Prospective evaluation of biopsy number in the diangosis of esophageal and gastric carcinoma. Gastroenterology 1982; 82:228–231.
28. Winawer SJ, Sherlock P, Belladonna JA, Melamed M, Beattie EJ. Endoscopic brush cytology in esophageal cancer. JAMA 1975; 232:1358.
29. Acker E, Carey W. The cost of surveillance for adenocarcinoma complicating Barrett's esophagus. Am J Gastroenterol 1988; 83:291–294.
30. Hendricks JC. Malignant tumors of the stomach. Surg Clin North Am 1986; 66:638–693.
31. Haenzel W, Kurihara M, Segi M, Lee RKC. Stomach cancer among Japanese in Hawaii. J Natl Cancer Inst 1972; 49:969.
32. Mirvish SS. The etiology of gastric cancer. Intragastric nitrosamide formation and other theories. J Nat Cancer Inst 1983; 71:631.
33. Aird I, Bentall HH, Roberts JAF. A relationship between cancer of the stomach and the ABO blood groups. Br Med J 1953; 1:799.
34. McNeer G. Cancer of the stomach in the young. AJR 1941; 45:537–543.
35. Fraser KJ, Raubin JG. Selective deficiency of IgA immunoglobulins associated with carcinoma of the stomach. Aust Ann Med 1970; 19:165–167.
36. Haerer AF, Jackson JF, Evers CG. Ataxia-telangiectasia with gastric adenocarcinoma. JAMA 1969; 210:1884–1887.
37. Sellin J, Levin B, Reckard C, Riddell R. Gastric adenocarcinoma following gastric lymphoma. Cancer 1980; 45:996–1000.
38. Mulligan RM, Rewber RR. Histogenesis and biological behavior of gastric carcinoma. Arch Pathol 1954; 58:1–25.
39. Qizilbash AH, Stevenson GW. Early gastric cancer. Pathol Ann 1979; 14:317.
40. Siegel SE, Hays DM, Romansky S, Isaacs H. Carcinoma of the stomach in childhood. Cancer 1976; 38:1781–1784.
41. The Gastrointestinal Tumor Study Group. Randomized study of combination chemotherapy in unresectable gastric cancer. Cancer 1984; 53:13–17.
42. The Gastrointestinal Tumor Study Group. Controlled trial of adjuvant chemotherapy following curative resection for gastric cancer. Cancer 1982; 49:1116–1122.
43. Wurlitzer FP, Mares AJ, Isaacs H, Landing BH, Wooley MM. Smooth muscle tumors of the stomach in childhood and adolescence. J Pediatr Surg 1973; 8:421–427.
44. Johnson E, Hutter Jr JJ, Paplanus SH. Leiomyosarcoma of the stomach: results of surgery and chemotherapy in an eleven-year-old girl with liver metastases. Med Pediatr Oncol 1980; 8:137–142.
45. Carney JA, Sheps SG, Go VL, Gordon H. The triad of gastric leiomyosarcoma, functioning extra-adrenal paraganglioma and pulmonary chondroma. N Engl J Med 1977; 296:1517–1518.
46. Fevre M, Huguenin R. Malformations tumorales et tumeurs de l'enfant. Paris: Masson & Cie, 1954.
47. Cairo MS, Grosfeld JL, Weetman RM. Gastric teratoma: unusual cause for bleeding of the upper gastrointestinal tract in newborn. Pediatrics 1981; 67:721–724.
48. Moriuchi A, Nakayama M, Muta H, et al. Gastric teratoma of children: a case report and review of the literature. Acta Pathol Jpn 1977; 27:749–758.
49. Matias IC, Huang YC. Gastric teratoma in infancy: report of a case and review of world literature. Ann Surg 1973; 178:631–636.
50. Bowen B, Ros PR, McCarthy MJ, Olmsted WW, Hjermstad BM. Gastrointestinal teratomas: CT and US appearance with pathologic correlation. Radiology 1987; 162:431–433.

6

Motor Disorders Including Pyloric Stenosis

Peter J. Milla, M.Sc., M.B.B.S., F.R.C.P.

The movement of bowel contents from one specialized region of the gut to another occurs as a result of the co-ordinated contraction of the smooth muscle coats. In this chapter the present state of knowledge of motor activity of the stomach and duodenum in the infant and child is summarized, and conditions in which motor activity is disordered are discussed. Despite investigation spanning the last century, knowledge derived from systematic scientific observation in this area remains scarce, and our understanding of the pathophysiology of human gastroduodenal motility in the infant and child is far from complete. However, the practical application of such knowledge as exists is beginning to affect the practice of clinical pediatric medicine.

NORMAL MOTOR ACTIVITY OF THE STOMACH AND DUODENUM

The pattern of contractions that occur in a particular region of the gut is related to and integrated with the function of that region of the gastrointestinal (GI) tract. In the case of the stomach, the organ acts as a reservoir where the process of digestion is initiated, tonicity is reduced by gastric secretion, and the food is then ground into a slurry—the chyme—which is discharged intermittently into the duodenum. In the duodenum the process of digestion is continued with the discharge of pancreatic enzymes and bile salts, and the absorption of nutrients is begun. In order to accommodate these activities, the contractile activity of the stomach is regulated to produce at least four functions and the duodenum two functions.

Stomach

The four functions of the stomach are as follows:

1. When a meal is ingested, the muscle of the proximal stomach (the fundus and upper half of the body of the stomach) relaxes to accommodate the meal. Thus, large volumes can be stored with little increase in intragastric pressure, allowing large meals to be taken irregularly.
2. Digestion is initiated by secreting acid and pepsin, and gastric contractions mix food with gastric secretions; in addition, the distal corpus and antrum act as a muscular pump to break up food into small particles.
3. Gastric contractions are co-ordinated with contractions in the duodenum in the digestive phase to allow the gastric contents to be emptied through the pylorus into the duodenum in a controlled and orderly manner.

4. After the digestible food is emptied into the duodenum, the digestive phase ends and the remaining gastric contents are swept into the duodenum periodically by bursts of forceful rhythmic contractions that are characteristic of the interdigestive phase in both the gastric antrum and duodenum.

Function and Anatomy. The smooth muscle cells of the stomach are arranged in three layers: an outer longitudinal layer, a middle circular layer, and an inner oblique layer. None of these layers covers the entire stomach, and the oblique layer is the least complete, being formed by two bands on the anterior and posterior surfaces. The circular and longitudinal layers thicken as they approach the duodenum. At the junction of the stomach and duodenum a thickening is prominent and forms the pylorus.[1]

As far as motor function is concerned, the organ can be divided into two major areas (Fig. 1). The proximal half exhibits mainly tonic activity and allows for large changes in intragastric volume. The distal region includes the lower half of the body, the antrum, and the pylorus. Contraction in this region is phasic and organized to impart movement to the intragastric contents. The activities of the two areas are controlled by a variety of mechanisms, and the function of one area may influence that of the other.

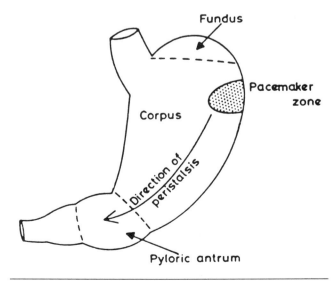

FIGURE 1 Regions of the stomach.

Duodenum

The process of digestion is continued in the duodenum, where pancreatic and biliary secretions are added to the chyme. Two patterns of motor activity occur: (1) when the duodenum is receiving chyme after feeding, continuous segmenting activity occurs to ensure maximal mixing of the intraluminal contents and exposure to the mucosa; (2) in the fasting or interdigestive state, when the lumen is devoid of nutrients, a band of forceful contractions is propagated in an aboral direction, sweeping exhausted chyme down the gut. As in the stomach, there are three muscle layers—an outer longitudinal layer, an inner circular layer, and the muscularis mucosae.

Control of Gastroduodenal Motor Activity

The regulatory processes that co-ordinate these different but mutually related functions and match them to the needs of digestion are complicated by a hierarchical arrangement of controls that act upon the smooth muscle cells of the muscularis propria at many different levels to produce the required effect. The operation of these control mechanisms remains the major unsolved problem of GI physiology today. Recent years have shown that the properties of the smooth muscle itself, an intrinsic network of nerves, the enteric nervous system with multiple neurotransmitters modulated by extrinsic nerves, and paracrine and endocrine polypeptide hormone controls are the major constituents of such control mechanisms.

Muscle

Contractile Power. The power for motility is derived from the smooth muscle of the stomach and duodenum. The smooth muscle cells are closely attached to one another by tight junctions, or nexi, which allow low-resistance electrical connections and thus produce a functional syncytium, in which depolarization can spread and take place synchronously throughout the muscle mass.

The duodenal and distal gastric smooth muscle cells also possess the property of rhythmic variation of transmembrane potential, which is present even during complete motor quiescence. The variation in membrane potential results in depolarization and repolarization of the muscle cell membrane and is probably due to rhythmic changes in activity of membrane ion pumps. Like skeletal muscle, intestinal smooth muscle has the ability to shorten and generate force. This contractile component is analogous to that in skeletal muscle but is modified for particular purposes in different parts of the gut, e.g., the lower esophageal sphincter. Intestinal smooth muscle, however, also has an elastic component that accommodates transient behavior. The molecular basis of these properties is poorly understood, but current evidence suggests that a cross-bridge cycle, i.e., a cyclic interaction between actin and myosin of sliding filaments involving modification of actin-myosin ATPase, is adequate to explain smooth muscle mechanochemistry. It is also clear that

although less efficient than skeletal muscle under conditions of shortening, smooth muscle is adapted to operate under much lower input and output power requirements. For further details, readers are referred to excellent recent reviews of this area.[2,3]

The muscle cells of the proximal stomach have somewhat different properties: They do not exhibit rhythmic oscillation of the resting membrane potential, and at their resting membrane potential they are partially contracted. Thus, hyperpolarization of these cells allows them to relax and fulfill the reservoir function of this part of the stomach. In addition, cells in this region of the stomach are adapted to this role by virtue of their length-tension properties.[4]

The pattern of contractions of both stomach and duodenum and their response to different meals suggest the presence of very versatile control mechanisms that can integrate sensory information from different sources and control both the spatial and temporal pattern of contractions. The control mechanisms are present in the wall of the stomach and duodenum and utilize interactions between smooth muscle cells, the intrinsic enteric nervous system, and chemicals released by endocrine cells. Because of the system's ability to receive an input, process it, and elaborate an output, it is often referred to as the "little brain" or "gut brain."

Myogenic Control

The myogenic control of contraction is related to the electrical activity generated in the distal gastric and duodenal smooth muscle.[5] Two types of activity can be detected—electrical control activity (ECA) or slow wave activity or the basic electrical rhythm, and electrical response activity (ERA) or spike activity. ECA is always present and is a rhythmic oscillation of membrane potential that controls smooth muscle contractions (Fig. 2). If the amplitude of the oscillating membrane potential does not reach the excitation threshold, then contraction does not occur. If, however, following the release of neurotransmitters or polypeptide hormones from endocrine cells, the membrane potential depolarizes beyond the threshold, then a burst of rapid oscillating spike potentials occurs and the smooth muscle contracts. It is important to note that, as a consequence of this arrangement, smooth muscle cells contract only once during one cycle of ECA and contraction occurs only during the depolarized phase of the cycle. It also follows that the maximal frequency of contraction in any part of the gut is at the frequency of the ECA, and that if the required neurochemical stimulus is not present the frequency of contraction is less than the maximal frequency. The above represents the temporal control of contractions at a given site.

For mixing and propulsive movements to occur, the temporal relationship between contractions occurring at adjacent sites is important—that is, the spatial control of contractions. For propulsion to occur, sequential contractions at adjacent sites in the stomach and duodenum are necessary rather than those that occur in a disorderly fashion that would tend to have a mixing effect with little or no transit. Although it may appear that the former is due to propagation of contractions, it is the sequential occurrence of contractions at adjacent sites

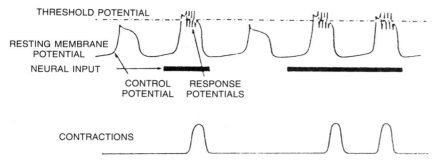

THRESHOLD POTENTIAL

RESTING MEMBRANE POTENTIAL

NEURAL INPUT

CONTROL POTENTIAL

RESPONSE POTENTIALS

CONTRACTIONS

FIGURE 2 The temporal control of electrical response activity. Upper trace is of an intracellular recording from smooth muscle cells and lower trace is contraction of the gut muscle coat.

which gives this appearance and is due to the syncytial nature of gastric intestinal smooth muscle, ECA, and the ordered release of neurotransmitters at adjacent sites. By controlling the release of neurochemicals, the control mechanism determines the lengths of gut that are stimulated to contract at different times. The spatial organization of ECA thus determines the sequence of contractions that occurs in each segment.

In summary, therefore, the ECA determines the timing of each contraction, and the ECA frequency determines the maximal frequency of contraction. Whether contraction occurs, however, depends not upon the smooth muscle but upon the local environment created by the control mechanism.

Intrinsic Nervous Control

Exact details of the mechanisms of control of the action potential and hence muscular contraction remain uncertain. That neural input from the myenteric plexus is of major importance and that this input is predominantly inhibitory are clear. Blocking the myenteric plexus with tetrodotoxin results in contraction at the slow wave frequency. Such an arrangement suggests that patterns of varying muscle contraction occur as a result of varying the underlying background inhibitory neural input.

The myenteric plexus serves as the immediate level of control and links receptors with the effector organ—the smooth muscle coats. Recent work has shown that the plexus is not just a simple relay station co-ordinating muscle contraction and conveying instructions from higher centers but that it contains programs of integrated and purposeful movements and is the main level of control of motor activity. The myenteric plexus responds to neural input from both local receptors and higher cortical centers by selecting the appropriate program. Our knowledge of the organization of the myenteric and submucous plexuses is increasing, and we now know that in addition to the classic cholinergic and adrenergic nerves a third class, nonadrenergic noncholinergic (NANC) nerves, is present. Cholinergic nerves are predominantly excitatory adrenergic, and NANC nerves are predominantly inhibitory. The neurotransmitter for the NANC nerves is uncertain, but ATP, vasoactive intestinal peptide (VIP), and serotonin are all candidates. The inhibitory input is almost certainly applied to neurons of the intrinsic plexus rather than directly to the smooth muscle cells. For further information, readers are referred to an excellent review by Furness and Costa.[6]

Extrinsic Nervous Control

Extrinsic nerves exert a major influence on gastric and duodenal motility. The gastric motor effect of vagotomy has been recognized for years, confirming that the stomach has a rich vagal innervation in addition to fibers passing through the celiac plexus. Vagotomy produces a decrease in gastric contraction, in gastric distensibility, and in gastric emptying of solids and semisolids which is believed to be due to loss of extrinsic cholinergic excitatory and NANC inhibitory innervation. The vagus nerve contains both efferent and afferent fibers, and in the human up to 80 percent are of the latter type. Vagal receptors have been identified which discharge in response to antral contractions,[3] and neurons in dorsal vagal nuclei have been identified which respond to gastric distention.[7] The responses of such neurons are complex and can be altered by enkephalin or cholecystokinin octapeptide,[8] suggesting that much processing of the information from the stomach must take place. Vagal efferent fibers are of two main types: cholinergic excitatory and NANC inhibitory. Little is known of the latter, but the former have their cell bodies in the dorsal vagal nuclei and their axons synapse with cell bodies of the myenteric plexus. Thus, the complex extrinsic innervation allows the central nervous system to modulate gastroduodenal motor function not only in response to stimuli from the GI tract but also from higher centers[9] such as labyrinthine stimuli. In addition, it is important in the vomiting reflex[10] and in the senses of appetite and satiety.[11]

Gastrointestinal Polypeptides

A variety of polypeptides originating from the gut and capable of affecting smooth muscle have now been described, although their physiologic role is far from clear. Such agents in the GI tract may act in three ways: endocrine—as distantly activating humoral agents; paracrine—as locally active agents; neurocrine—as neurotransmitters. Although nearly all the evidence regarding these agents and their roles has been derived indirectly, it seems likely that it is the paracrine and neurocrine modes of action which are important in the gut and may act as an additional control system. Five peptides seem to be important: Motilin has been implicated in the initiation of phase III activity in the foregut. Gastrin and cholecystokinin (CCK) both disrupt the fasting pattern, and enkephalins abolish irregular contractile activity. Recently peptide tyrosine tyrosine (PYY) has been shown to have a marked effect on GI motor activity, but its role remains to be defined.

Specific Patterns of Gastroduodenal Motility

Proximal Stomach

Proximal Receptive Relaxation. Little contractile activity occurs in proximal regions of the stomach, where the predominant activity is receptive relaxation[1]: On swallowing, the proximal muscle relaxes to accommodate the ingested food. This mechanism is so efficient that the average full-term infant can accommodate 60 to 70 ml of feed with a rise in intragastric pressure of only 5 mm Hg. Receptive relaxation is mediated by the vagal reflex, as outlined above. A number of putative neurotransmitters have been studied, and most recent evidence favors VIP as the NANC inhibitory transmitter in this region of the stomach.

Tonic Contraction. Following ingestion of a meal, the proximal region of the stomach exhibits weak tonic contractions, which may play a role in passing intragastric contents to the antrum and pylorus. Vagal and intrinsic cholinergic factors are believed to be important in stimulating such a response.[4]

Distal Stomach and Duodenum

Postprandial or Digestive Activity. The caudal or distal region of the stomach behaves quite differently from the proximal region, and together with the duodenum a separate pattern of activity occurs according to whether a meal has just been eaten or the individual is fasting. After a meal, rhythmic phasic contractions begin near the middle of the stomach and are propagated toward the duodenum. The antral waves (about three per minute in humans) are constant in terms of frequency and propagation velocity and are determined by a pacemaker region on the greater curvature of the stomach (see Fig. 1). The timing and spread of the contractions are regulated by the ECA of the smooth muscle cells, as discussed previously. Those cells that have the fastest intrinsic frequency serve as the pacemaker. Action potentials spread from the midstomach to the duodenum but not to the fundal region of the stomach, ensuring that propagation of contractions with a maximal frequency and velocity of the action potentials occurs only in the aboral direction. The occurrence, timing, amplitude, and spread of gastric contractions depend upon the integrity of the gastric muscle, its innervation, and the endocrine balance.

These seemingly simple peristaltic contractions of the gastric body and antrum cause fairly complex movements of the intragastric contents, which result in mixing of the contents, mechanical breakdown of food particles, and gastric emptying. The antrum and pylorus are the sites of regulation for the emptying of solids. When a mixed meal is consumed, liquids empty more rapidly than solids, which are retained by antral contractile activity and are passed through the pylorus only when they have been broken down into particles approximately 1 mm square.[12,13]

When contraction begins, gastric contents are propelled toward the duodenum, but only a small amount enters the duodenum. As a consequence, pressure rises in the antrum and provides a continued driving force across the pylorus. As the pressure falls, retropulsion may occur and the consequent mixing and shearing of flows that take place cause food particles to be broken down. Gastric emptying also occurs during the contractions, but the amount emptied depends upon the force of peristaltic contractions, tone of the proximal stomach, and the contractile activity of the pylorus and duodenum. In the digestive phase, contraction of the pylorus and proximal duodenum is highly co-ordinated, up to 70 percent of antral contractions being linked to groups of one to three sequential duodenal contractions separated by periods of relative quiescence. This pattern of activity seems to be important for gastric emptying and is modulated not only by neural factors but also by nutrients via paracrine and endocrine polypeptide hormones.[1] That both the nature of a meal and polypeptide hormones influence gastric emptying seems to be beyond doubt from a number of experimental studies in animals[1] and the human infant.[14,15] In the infant it is clear that increasing calorie density of feeds, with either carbohydrate in the form of glucose polymers versus monosaccharides, or lipids in the form of long-chain triglycerides versus medium-chain triglycerides, results in slower emptying.

Fasting or Interdigestive Activity. Toward the end of fed activity, contractions become more forceful and propel any remaining undigested food into the duodenum, leaving the stomach empty. The pattern of activity then changes to that seen in the fasted state in both stomach and duodenum. In the interdigestive period the motor activity of several regions of the GI tract has a characteristic specific integrated and cyclic pattern. This cyclic pattern of fasting activity was first shown in dogs by Szurszewski in 1969,[16] and for the most part co-ordination of contractions between antrum and duodenum does not occur. The pattern is characterized by what he termed a "migrating myoelectric complex" (MMC).

It was not until 1975 that the first demonstration of the MMC in humans was published.[17] At intervals of approximately 100 minutes, brief periods (about 5 min) of rhythmic contraction recur at the frequency of the ECA of three cycles per minute in the antrum and 11 cycles per minute in the duodenum (Fig. 3). These episodes of rhythmic contraction, phase III activity, are preceded by a period of irregular contraction (phase II activity) in which about 10 percent of antral contractions are co-ordinated with those in the duodenum and are followed by a period of quiescence (phase I activity). Phase III activity migrates relatively slowly down the entire small intestine from the antrum and duodenum to the terminal ileum, taking about 90 to 120 minutes to migrate; a new complex usually arises proximally as one dies away distally. However, some cycles may begin distal to the duodenum and others may fail to progress down the complete length of the small intestine. Fenton et al[18] have demonstrated similar patterns in children (Fig. 3); these differ from those in adults only in the very young, in whom propagation velocity is slower and duration of phase III activity longer.[19] The purpose of the MMC is obscure, although it has been suggested that it may have a role in preventing the aboral migration of colonic bacteria[20] or in cleansing the intestine of

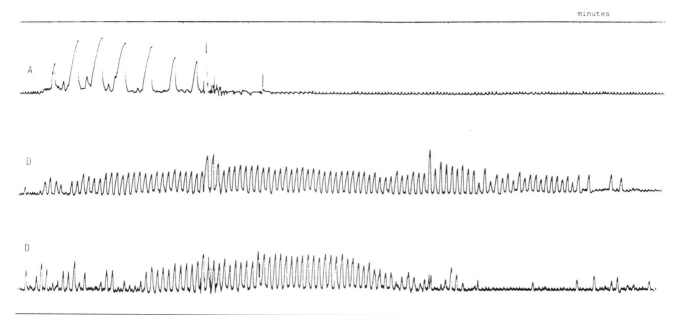

minutes

FIGURE 3 Pressure changes in the antrum and duodenum in the fasting state during phase III activity.

cellular debris, residual food, and secretions, which is aided by the increased gastric acid and biliary and pancreatic secretion at the start of phase III activity. Studies in both humans and the experimental animals have shown phase III activity to be highly propulsive.

Like fed activity, fasting activity requires the integrity of smooth muscle, innervation, and humoral secretion. In the stomach extrinsic innervation seems to be much more important than in the jejunum or ileum, and motilin surges are associated with phase III activity.

DISORDERS OF GASTRODUODENAL MOTOR ACTIVITY

Motility disorders result in alterations of motor activity which are clinically significant and interfere with normal receptive relaxation[21] and propulsive functions of the stomach and duodenum. Most often no obvious anatomic abnormality is present, although clearly hypertrophic pyloric stenosis is an exception to this. Some disorders may be acute owing to transient metabolic changes or immunologic responses: in this chapter only chronic conditions are considered. Motor dysfunction may be restricted to the stomach or duodenum or may be part of a more diffuse disease. Commonly the clinical presentation is regional, e.g., recurrent vomiting, yet investigation reveals dysfunction in other regions of the gut.

Mechanisms of Disordered Motility

Motility disorders result from a disturbance of the complex control mechanisms which may occur at many different levels—end organ, intermediate regulating pathways, and higher centers—with smooth muscle, nerves, or endocrine cells involved.

Smooth Muscle

Damage to smooth muscle cells results in reduced intraluminal pressure generated in the intestine and delayed transit. Manometric recordings might be expected to show either a normal pattern of contractions of reduced amplitude or virtually no contractile activity at all.[22] Such a pattern of activity results in delayed transit and may cause bacterial overgrowth and thus malabsorption. In childhood, some cases of gastric stasis and duodenal pseudo-obstruction are due to smooth muscle disease (see below).

Nerve

Damage to the myenteric plexus results in disruption of normal patterns of contractile activity. Although denervation might be expected to release the smooth muscle from its customary inhibition, resulting in increasing contractility, this is unlikely to result in purposeful propagated movements. Some processes are restricted to one type of neuron, whereas others are completely unselective, resulting in damage to both inhibitory and excitatory networks. Disorders due to myenteric plexus disease include chronic idiopathic pseudo-obstruction, toxins from intestinal bacterial pathogens as well as ingestion of environmental toxins, infection by viruses such as cytomegalovirus and protozoans as in Chagas' disease, and developmental disorders. Disorders such as diabetes mellitus, amyloidosis, vasculitic and ischemic disease, and infiltrative disorders, e.g., lymphomas, which might be expected to affect enteric nerves, do so extremely rarely in childhood but with much greater frequency in adult life.

There is increasing evidence to suggest that disease outside the gut affecting the extrinsic innervation can disrupt normal patterns of activity, varying with the level of nervous involvement. This is particularly well illustrated by the effect of vagotomy on motor activity, which may occur accidently following esophageal surgery in infants and is discussed below. The central nervous system may also disturb normal patterns of activity through the autonomic nervous system. In general, parasympathetic activity stimulates motor activity and sympathetic activity suppresses it. Increased sympathetic activity is well recognized in stress, in which it has been shown to disturb small intestinal motility and result in vomiting.

Gastrointestinal Hormones

Disturbance of polypeptide hormone and neuroamine metabolism may also produce effects on GI nerves and smooth muscle and hence motility. An increase in slow wave frequency occurs in conditions in which catecholamines are secreted excessively, such as hyperthyroidism, or produced ectopically, such as pheochromocytoma and some neuroblastomas and ganglioneuromas. Decreased slow-wave frequency may conversely occur in hypothyroidism. Ectopic production of VIP in childhood, usually from tumors of the neural crest such as ganglioneuromas but very occasionally from pancreatic tumors, is associated with gastric stasis and ileus. The effect of VIP is one of inhibition, and this may account for the abnormalities of both fasting and postprandial activity which have been described.[23]

Clinical Manifestations of Disordered Gastroduodenal Motility

Many parents consult pediatricians and pediatric gastroenterologists because their children vomit or suffer from epigastric discomfort. Despite careful investigation, a diagnosis of organic disease is often not made. Table 1 lists the symptoms that may be complained of; none is very specific. In most cases a diagnosis cannot be made on clinical history alone. The symptoms of delayed and accelerated gastric emptying have much in common, and the typical symptoms of dumping due to hypovolemia and hypoglycemia occur in only a minority of cases. It is only when food from the previous day is vomited that seriously delayed gastric emptying is certain. Thus, gastroduodenal motor disorders often present with nonspecific clinical signs and symptoms. The obvious exception is hypertrophic pyloric stenosis, in which the character of the vomiting, the presence of visible gastric peristalsis, and a palpable pyloric tumor (see below) enable the clinician to diagnose the condition with sufficient certainty for surgery to be undertaken in a large proportion of patients.

Rapid Gastric Emptying

Rapid emptying of liquids most frequently occurs following surgical procedures and in some patients with peptic ulcer. After both proximal and distal gastric resection, increased liquid emptying rates are seen. After proximal resection the accommodating reservoir is lost, and after a meal intragastric pressure rises. Following distal resection, resistance from the antropyloric region is lost.

TABLE 1
Symptoms of Disordered Gastroduodenal Motility

Rapid Emptying/Dumping	Delayed Emptying
Nausea, vomiting	Epigastric fullness
Abdominal cramps, diarrhea	Early satiety
Early satiety	Nausea, vomiting
Epigastric fullness	Pyrosis
Faintness	Belching
Pallor	
Sweating	

Vagotomy is not commonly performed in childhood, but damage to the vagus may occur following esophageal surgery and have similar effects, which are discussed below.

Delayed Emptying

There are many causes of delayed gastric emptying, as shown in Table 2. Of course, it is always important to exclude anatomic causes such as hypertrophic pyloric stenosis, duodenal stenosis—both intrinsic and extrinsic, duodenal web, and malrotation of the small intestine causing duodenal obstruction. Some of these conditions are associated with disordered motor activity other than that caused by the obstruction in which either the smooth muscle or the innervation is diseased or they are operating in an abnormal environment.

Duodenogastric Reflux

Bile-stained vomiting occurs in conditions in which there is obstruction beyond the second part of the duodenum and in conditions causing pseudo-obstruction of the duodenum and upper jejunum. Usually when there is severe bilious vomiting and no anatomic obstruction is found, the pseudo-obstruction is neuropathic in origin.

TABLE 2
Conditions Causing Delayed Gastric Emptying

Anatomic obstruction	Pyloric stenosis, duodenal stenosis, duodenal web
Metabolic or electrolyte disorder	Hypokalemia, acidosis, hypothyroidism
Drugs	Opioids, anticholinergics
Neuronal dysfunction	Central nervous system disease, vagotomy, intestinal pseudo-obstruction
Muscle disease	Visceral myopathy, systemic lupus erythematosus, myotonic dystrophy
Infection	Viral, bacterial toxins
Idiopathic	Electrical control activity arrhythmias

DISEASES OF THE STOMACH AND DUODENUM

Structural and Metabolic Disorders

Hypertrophic Pyloric Stenosis

The grossly thickened circular muscle of hypertrophic pyloric stenosis results in a well-recognized clinical presentation of projectile vomiting and failure to thrive. The muscular hypertrophy is usually not present at birth but starts in the first few weeks of life.[24] The natural history of the condition is for vomiting to continue into the third month of life and for survivors to recover after this. The condition is more common in first-born children, and males are affected five times more frequently than females. Inheritance is polygenic, and there is thus an increased risk in siblings and the offspring of affected children. The risk is highest (approximately 20 percent) in the first-born male of a mother who herself was affected.

Although the etiology is not known and the nature of the pathologic process is not clear, it is now known that this is not a congenital disorder.[24] Most evidence suggests that the local enteric innervation is involved[25] and that primarily argyrophilic neurons are affected.[26] In the majority of cases hypertrophic pyloric stenosis can be thought of as an isolated pseudo-obstructive lesion. In some, however, it is part of a more generalized pseudo-obstructive condition and may be associated with a malrotation and short small intestine.[27] It is also increasingly recognized in association with other gut anomalies such as esophageal and duodenal atresia and anorectal anomalies. In about 15 percent of cases of pyloric stenosis a hiatal hernia and gastroesophageal reflux are present.[28] Whether this is a consequence of the obstruction or whether the neural abnormality is not restricted to the pylorus is not clear.

Clinical Features. The infants present with vomiting, which is never bile-stained but frequently contains stale milk; it usually starts in the second or third week of life but may present earlier or much later. The vomiting becomes increasingly forceful and copious until it is projectile. At the beginning the infant is irritable and hungry; with increasing malnutrition, however, the baby becomes miserable and lethargic. Characteristically the early part of the feed is taken eagerly; as the stomach fills, the baby starts to become anxious and fretful, visible peristalsis may be easily seen (it is presumed that the baby perceives this prior to vomiting), and then vomiting occurs, which is often projectile in nature. A pyloric tumor is then usually easily palpable. The other features are the consequence of gastric outlet obstruction and loss of gastric secretions; these include constipation, dehydration, and metabolic alkalosis.

When there is doubt about the diagnosis, radiologic or ultrasound studies should be undertaken. A plain film often shows pyloric hold-up and a dilated stomach with absent gas distal to the pylorus. Ultrasound studies confirm the presence of a pyloric tumor and barium studies the long, narrow pyloric canal. The presence of gastroesophageal reflux should be sought, as it may influence postoperative management.

Management and Prognosis. There is universal agreement that pyloromyotomy is the treatment of choice. Most infants are referred for surgery before any significant biochemical disturbances have occurred and require no special preparation other than a gastric washout 2 to 3 hours prior to operation. However, if dehydration and metabolic alkalosis are present, they must be corrected first and surgery delayed for 24 to 48 hours. There are two well-recognized postoperative problems: continued signs of pyloric obstruction due to an incomplete myotomy, and wound dehiscence. The former frequently settles with conservative management, so several days should elapse before re-exploration. The latter is probably due to malnutrition rather than surgical technique. In about 15 percent of patients, vomiting continues owing to the associated gastroesophageal reflux; usually only a small proportion require further surgery and fundoplication.[29]

Duodenal Obstruction

Obstructive lesions of the duodenum may be classified as intrinsic or extrinsic. Intrinsic lesions may be due to atresia, stenosis, or a web that may be complete or contain a perforation. The second part of the duodenum is the most common site, and its relationship to the ampulla of Vater determines whether the vomit is bile-stained. Extrinsic obstructions are most commonly associated with malrotation and Ladd's bands. An annular pancreas is of significance only if there is an associated intrinsic lesion.

Clinical Features and Diagnosis. Maternal hydramnios is very uncommon, and the diagnosis may be suspected from prenatal ultrasound scans. The infant presents with vomiting during the first day of life, which often precedes the first feed and is bile-stained in more than half. The lack of bile often leads to a serious delay in diagnosis. Plain abdominal radiographs may reveal the characteristic "double bubble," but if vomiting or gastric aspiration has taken place immediately before the films are exposed, this may not be seen; 10 ml of air injected down a nasogastric tube provides the necessary contrast.

Management. Initially the stomach and proximal duodenum must be decompressed via a freely draining nasogastric tube. Continuous or frequent aspiration is essential to prevent inhalation of gastric contents. If diagnosis is delayed, subsequent dehydration and metabolic alkalosis must be corrected before surgery. At surgery either a duodenoduodenostomy or a duodenojejunostomy is done to bypass the obstruction. Often the proximal duodenum is dilated and hypertrophied and may take some time to function normally following operation. As a consequence, a temporary gastrostomy may be required to control vomiting. A transanastomotic tube of silicon rubber allows early feeding and may be left in situ for several weeks if necessary. In most cases oral feeding can be instituted after 1 week and the gastrostomy tube removed at about 12 days.

Idiopathic Gastroparesis

Gastroparesis may develop in apparently healthy children without evidence of systemic disease. Sometimes the symptoms are acute, may be preceded by a flu-like illness, or may be part of a gastroenteric infection. The abnormality may be confined to the antrum with impairment of emptying of solids but not liquids. There have also been several case reports of patients with arrhythmias of gastric ECA and idiopathic gastroparesis. Symptoms may be mild, with early satiety, nausea, and occasional vomiting, or severe, with uncontrollable nausea and vomiting.

Gastric Antral Dysrhythmias. In 1978 Telander et al[29] described an unusual case of persistent vomiting in an infant associated with marked impairment of gastric emptying. A series of elegant investigations showed marked dysfunction of antral smooth muscle due to a disturbance of ECA. ECA increased from its customary frequency of three cycles per minute to six cycles per minute. The authors coined the term "tachygastria." In this patient normal depolarization frequencies occurred in vitro when indomethacin was added to the bathing medium, suggesting that an abnormality of the local synthesis of prostaglandins was involved. In another infant antrectomy was curative.[30] You et al[31] found that 50 percent of a group of patients with functional upper abdominal discomfort had abnormalities of antral ECA. Diagnosis of these infants, however, relied upon highly invasive and difficult methods for recording intraluminal myoelectric activity. More recently, attempts to measure antral ECA by surface electrodes have been more successful owing to the application of sophisticated signal processing techniques, and now a noninvasive way of investigating these patients exists. In a group of patients with intestinal pseudo-obstruction investigated in the author's laboratory using surface electrogastrography, a variety of dysrhythmias were seen in addition to a tachygastria; these are shown in Figure 4. In a patient with smooth muscle disease, no dominant frequency could be found, and in another only a bradyarrhythmia was present.[32]

Migraine. Nausea and vomiting are frequent symptoms in classic migraine. There is some indirect evidence—delayed absorption of salicylate which is corrected by metaclopramide—to suggest that gastric emptying is delayed in migraine. Clinically it may be difficult to differentiate patients with migraine and idiopathic gastroparesis from those with psychogenic vomiting and anorexia nervosa.

Lesions of the Extrinsic Innervation

Central Nervous System

Local lesions of the vagal and vestibular nuclei and of the labyrinth, as well as raised intracranial pressure, may result in disordered gastroduodenal motility and thus vomiting. Tumors and congenital abnormalities are the most common chronic disorders and interfere either directly with the dorsal vagal nuclei or, more likely in the case of raised pressure, by stimulating the chemoreceptor trigger zone in the area postrema in the floor of the fourth ventricle. The chemoreceptor trigger zone is an important sensory input to the vomiting reflex and thus may initiate vomiting when stimulated.

Autonomic Nervous System

Infectious, Metabolic, and Degenerative Causes. A number of infectious organisms have been reported to cause autonomic dysfunction resulting in nausea, vomiting, and even pseudo-obstruction. These include varicella[33] and Epstein-Barr virus.[34] Autonomic dysfunction also occurs in the Guillain-Barré syndrome and may be unrelated to the degree of sensory and motor disturbances.

The common metabolic causes of gastroparesis in the adult population—diabetes mellitus and amyloidosis—occur extremely rarely in childhood. However, degenerative conditions clearly occur and may be familial. The most common of these is the pandysautonomia of the Riley-Day syndrome, in which there are abnormalities of both cholinergic and NANC nerves. Vomiting is very common and may be associated with constipation, internal ophthalmoplegia, lack of tears and sweating, and orthostatic hypotension. With the exception of orthostatic hypotension these features were also present in four children reported to have a postganglionic cholinergic dysautonomia.[35] In one patient with this condition studied by the author, it was possible to arrive at a diagnosis by studying the innervation of the sweat glands involved. These patients all demonstrate denervation hypersensitivity, particularly in relation to cholinergic agonists. Waterfall et al[36] described one patient with GI dysmotility in whom, on the basis of in vitro studies of antral muscle, they demonstrated defects proximal to smooth muscle and enteric nerves; they speculated that the condition was due to a failure of nonadrenergic inhibitory innervation.

Vagotomy. Although vagotomy is not a common purposeful operation in children, it is used in the treatment of severe peptic ulcer disease and may occur as a consequence of difficult surgery for congenital esophageal anomalies. After a highly selective vagotomy, relaxation of the proximal stomach is impaired. As a consequence, rapid initial emptying of liquids may occur, with about 25 percent of patients complaining of early satiety and epigastric fullness. These symptoms tend to improve with time.[37] With truncal and total vagotomy the entire stomach loses its vagal innervation. In addition to impaired relaxation of the proximal stomach, disturbances of ECA occur more frequently after these types of vagotomy and there is thus defective antral motility and emptying of solids.[38]

Interdigestive motor complexes are less regular and less frequent, which may also contribute to the stasis of solids. The combination of very fast liquid and slow solid emptying can be extremely difficult to manage. One group has proposed the use of uncooked starch to control the dumping, which is very troublesome in infants.[39] Drainage procedures such as pyloroplasty, although helpful in controlling the stasis of solids, do nothing to control the dumping and diarrhea.

Enteric Nervous System

Primary disorders of gut motor activity may be either diffuse or regional in their presentation. In this section we are concerned with those disorders that result in abnormal gastroduodenal motility and present with early satiety, postprandial epigastric fullness, nausea, vomiting, and failure to thrive. Their etiology remains obscure. Some are congenital and may be inherited, others acquired and potentially reversible. It is likely that the so-called superior mesenteric artery syndrome is in fact a duodenal pseudo-obstructive disorder rather than a mechanical obstruction.

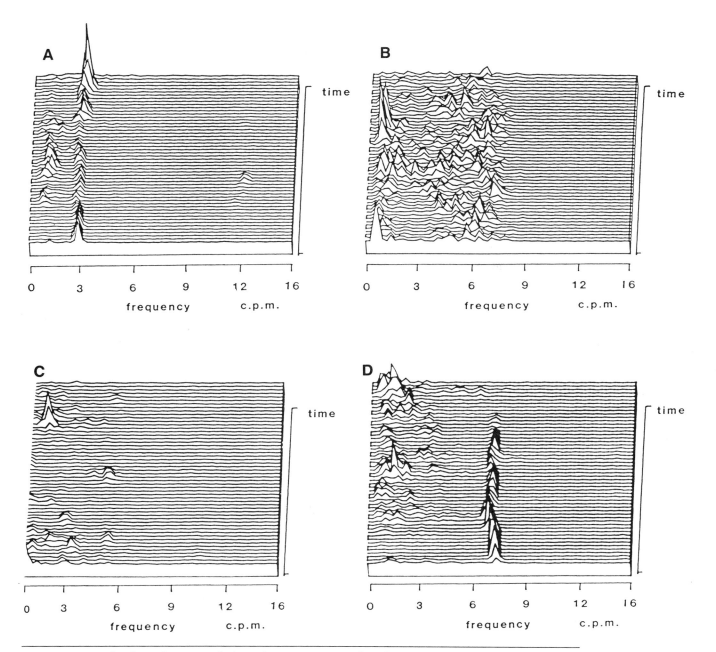

FIGURE 4 Pseudo–three-dimensional plots of a running spectral analysis of surface electrogastrograms of *A*, control children, *B* and *C*, myopathic pseudo-obstruction–hollow visceral myopathy, and *D*, neuronal pseudo-obstruction.

When the primary disease appears to be of the stomach and/or duodenum, the terms *idiopathic gastroparesis* and *duodenal pseudo-obstruction* are used. They are uncommon but usually present during the first few years of life, and it is in this age group that there is the highest mortality rate.[40] In the majority distinctive abnormalities can be found either in the smooth muscle or in the myenteric plexus.

Disease of enteric nerves may be familial and limited entirely to the gut, as in congenital absence of argyrophil nerves (which is inherited as an X-linked or perhaps an autosomal recessive trait[27]) and familial megaduodenum,[41] or as part of a familial peripheral and autonomic neuropathy, such as familial visceral neuropathy. Sporadic cases have also been reported with a peripheral neuropathy in which enteric nerves have been involved. The pathogenesis of the neural disease is unknown.

Disorders Affecting Gastroduodenal Smooth Muscle

In adult life, most gastroduodenal muscle disease occurs secondary to a number of different conditions, including dystrophia myotonica, systemic sclerosis, Ehlers-Danlos syndrome, dermatomyositis, and systemic lupus erythematosus. In only a minority is there smooth muscle disease restricted to the gut. The reverse is true in children; smooth muscle disease as part of a systemic disease occurs extremely rarely and the majority suffer from two syndromes, the pathogenesis of which is not understood.

Hollow Visceral Myopathy Syndrome

In adult life the hollow visceral myopathy syndrome appears to account for most of the reported cases and may be inherited as either an autosomal dominant or an X-linked dominant trait.[42] This disease is a purely smooth muscle disorder that has now been described in childhood, but whether it is a myopathic or a dystrophic process remains to be determined.[43] The affected muscle cells show a variety of abnormalities, with cell fragmentation, collagen deposition, and central vacuolar degeneration of the fibers, giving the muscle a honeycombed appearance. The longitudinal muscle is more affected than the circular muscle. The disease process is not restricted to any particular regions of the gut and may affect esophagus, stomach, and small or large intestine. The urinary tract may also be affected, with hydroureter and a large bladder.

Megacystis-Microcolon-Hypoperistalsis Syndrome

A similar but different disease occurring sporadically is the megacystis-microcolon-hypoperistalsis syndrome described in neonates by Berdon et al.[44]

Drugs

A variety of drugs have been found to affect gastroduodenal motility and a number of others may be expected to do so.

Cholinergic Agents. The agonist bethanechol enhances gastric motor activity, whereas antagonists inhibit contractile activity and delay gastric emptying. Some tricyclic antidepressants and imipramine also have anticholinergic activity.[45] The new prokinetic agent cisapride is included here, as it is clear that at least part of its action relates to the release of acetylcholine from preganglionic fibers. Cisapride may thus be helpful in delayed gastric emptying and duodenal dysmotility.

Adrenergic Agents. Adrenergic agonists tend to delay gastric emptying, especially beta-agonists such as salbutamol and alpha-agents like clonidine. Beta-blocking agents enhance gastric emptying.[46]

Dopaminergic Agents. Dopamine D_2 agonists such as apomorphine, bromocriptine, and L-dopa are potent emetic agents that exert their effects both centrally and peripherally.[47] There are two commonly available D_2 antagonists—metoclopramide and domperidone—both of which stimulate gastric antral contractility and gastric emptying. As it crosses the blood-brain barrier poorly, domperidone is less likely than metoclopramide to cause central side effects.

Opioids. The effects of exogenous opiates on the stomach depend upon the dose given; at low to moderate dose contractile activity is enhanced, whereas at high dose there is diminished activity.[48] Endogenous opiates may act as hormones (endorphins) or as paracrine neurotransmitters (enkephalins). They inhibit antral motility, and beta-endorphins may be responsible for the inhibitory effects of stress on fed antral motility.[49]

Ca^{2+}-Channel Blockers. These agents block the movement of Ca^{2+} across smooth muscle cell membranes, nifedipine and verapamil being the two most commonly used. They may thus affect contractile activity, and they can be expected to have an effect on gastroduodenal motility, although this has not yet been described.

Chemotherapeutic Agents. A number of cytotoxic drugs used in the treatment of leukemia and solid tumors induce severe nausea and vomiting that respond poorly to treatment. The agents that are most commonly troublesome include cisplatin, mustine, cyclophosphamide, doxorubicin, and vincristine. No one antiemetic therapy seems to be wholly effective, and treatment consists of trials of high-dose steroids, metoclopramide, domperidone, nabilone, and phenothiazines alone or in combination.

Gastroduodenal Motility in Other Gastrointestinal Disorders

Gastroesophageal Reflux

Although the motor mechanisms of gastroesophageal reflux (GER) are relatively well described in children, the association with disease elsewhere in the GI tract is less well defined. It is clear that clinically it may occur with obstructive lesions (see above) such as pyloric stenosis and malrotation and that it may be part of a generalized pseudo-obstructive disease that also affects the stomach and duodenum, but it is not clear whether gastric emptying is affected in those who present with GER alone. Studies in adults are confused owing to the investigation of different patient groups and widely differing methodologies.

In patients treated surgically by fundoplication a proportion may develop acute gas-bloat or a more chronic syndrome of early satiety, bloating, nausea, and vomiting. Manometric studies show antral hypomotility, and it is likely that inadvertent damage to the vagi occurs at the time of surgery.

Small Intestinal Malrotation

The majority of children who develop symptoms related to malrotation do so within the neonatal period and present with features of complete or incomplete upper intestinal obstruction. A proportion of children postoperatively have prolonged feeding difficulties and recurrent vomiting. Investigation of a group of such children showed antroduodenal dysmotility compatible with a neuropathic pseudo-obstruction.[50] It is of interest that malrotation is a common feature of pseudo-obstructive disorders. The authors speculate that the underlying disease process is responsible for the disordered movement of the intestine around the superior mesenteric artery during the course of embryologic development.

DIAGNOSTIC TECHNIQUES

In order to understand the gastroparetic or pseudo-obstructive disorder and plan rational treatment, the involved areas must be defined and the physiology and pathology of the affected areas studied.

Radiology/Transit Studies

Conventional contrast radiography is used to delineate anatomic abnormalities and, together with studies of transit either by isotope (where permitted in children) breath H_2 mouth-to-cecal transit or radiopaque pellets, they provide a limited description of the disease but no clues to the nature of the disorder.

Manometry

Studies of motility are helpful in delineating both the extent of the disease and the disease process causing the disorder. In patients with suspected pseudo-obstruction, at least three areas of the GI tract—the esophagus, the upper small intestine, and the rectosigmoid colon—should be studied, as the disease process may not be restricted to the stomach and duodenum. In these areas, swallow-induced peristalsis, fasting activity, and the gastrocolonic response to food can be used as tests of the integrity of the enteric nervous system and of the contractile activity of the smooth muscle. In addition, postprandial activity provides information regarding the humorally mediated response to food and whether entero-enteric reflexes are intact.

In the esophagus, swallow-induced peristalsis and the associated relaxation of the lower esophageal sphincter can be studied using a Dent sleeve assembly modified for use in infants and young children. Particular attention should be paid to the nature of the primary peristaltic sequence, whether secondary peristalsis occurs in response to reflux, and the presence of tertiary contractions. The amplitude and form of the contractile waves are also noted.

The cyclic nature of the fasting gastric and duodenal motor activity is determined by the inherent activity of the enteric nervous system. This can be utilized to test whether the enteric nervous system is intact and whether extrinsic nervous modulation is present. Observation of the disruption of fasting activity and the establishment of postprandial activity provides information regarding the humorally mediated response to food and clarifies whether entero-enteric reflexes are intact. In order to test these motor functions, the author observes three cycles of fasting activity and then administers a standardized age-appropriate meal.

Manometric studies have shown that myopathic processes produce low-amplitude, poorly propagated contractions,[22,42] whereas neuropathic processes are associated with contractions of normal amplitude that are often bizarre in waveform, abnormally propagated, and, in phase III activity, ill formed.[22,51] Disturbance of the neuroendocrine environment may also be detected with increased ECA frequency in conditions in which catecholamines are secreted in excess, such as hyperthyroidism, pheochromocytoma, and ganglioneuroma and with decreased ECA frequency in preterm infants and hypothyroidism.

At the same time that a feed is given to induce postprandial activity, rectosigmoid motility can be measured and the increased activity studied. Another useful test is to observe the response to a few milliliters of bisacodyl instilled rectally. In addition to changes in the motility index, the amplitude and form of contractile waves are studied. Thus, information regarding both smooth muscle, local enteric nerves, and those involved in the gastrocolonic response and entero-enteric reflexes can be obtained.

Gastric Emptying

Methods that have been used to measure gastric emptying in infants have all involved either invasive intubation studies or the use of radioisotopes. The former methods have until recently been most used, either the serial test meal or a modified version of the George method.[52] The George method and its modifications allow a single meal to be followed.

For those with access to a gamma camera, emptying of milk or solids[53] can be studied by labeling the test meal with indium diethylenetriamine pentacetic acid for the fluid phase or ^{99m}Tc attached to a number of different stable substances, such as aggregated ferrous hydroxide or tin colloid, which are not adsorbed onto the gastric mucosa or absorbed. Successive 90-second images over a 60- to 90-minute period are obtained, the counts in each image computed, and emptying curves and half-empty times calculated. This method suffers from the difficulty of relating planar changes to a three-dimensional organ; in small infants especially, superimposition of parts of the stomach over the small intestine makes separation of emptied and retained meal difficult.

Electrogastrography

Electrogastrography (EGG)[54] can be defined as the recording of myoelectric activity of the smooth muscle of the stomach by means of electrodes attached to the abdominal skin. The first EGG was recorded by Alvarez in 1921, but the advent of powerful personal microcomputers has revived interest in it. This method has the great advantage of permitting the study of gastric myoelectric activity in both the fasted and fed state totally noninvasively and readily detects disturbance of ECA.

Histology

Although some cases of pseudo-obstruction have been described with no apparent lesion of either muscle or nerve, usually adequate full-thickness biopsies of an appropriate region of the gut have not been taken or have not been rigorously examined. To demonstrate disease of smooth muscle or enteric nerves in the majority of patients with pseudo-obstructive disorders, routine paraffin-embedded material stained with hematoxylin and eosin or a trichrome stain is completely inadequate. Only if there is widespread severe fibrosis can a defect of muscle be detected. Ultrastructural studies are necessary for both muscle and nerve. In addition to electron microscopy, enteric nerves must be studied by silver staining and by immunocytochemistry and histochemistry.[55,56] Studies such as those described above define the nature as well as the extent of the disease and in some instances are helpful in understanding the etiology of the disorder.

MANAGEMENT

Surgery

In patients with a clearly defined anatomic abnormality, surgery is indicated and is often curative. In those whose disease has made them severely malnourished, who are dehydrated, or whose biochemistry is disturbed, appropriate treatment prior to surgery should be carried out.

However, in patients in whom there is not an anatomic abnormality it is usually not possible to treat a primary motility disorder by these means. It is hoped that this discussion dispels the naive view that all problems of delayed gastric emptying can be resolved by cutting the pylorus.

In those patients with an isolated tachygastria, antrectomy has been successful.[30] However, this step should be embarked upon only after a thorough evaluation and the elimination of a more generalized pseudo-obstructive disorder by the careful investigations described above. In some children with the superior mesenteric artery syndrome or duodenal pseudo-obstruction a gastroenterostomy has proved successful.

In those with generalized pseudo-obstructive disease, adhesional obstruction commonly occurs after laparotomy, and the risk increases with repeated laparotomy. Adhesional obstruction should be treated conservatively, surgery being employed only when there are localizing signs or incipient peritonitis.

Medical Management

Usually little can be done directly to treat the underlying disease process even when it is clearly an acquired process. However, much can be done to treat the consequence of the secondary effects of malnutrition and primary disease exacerbation. The majority of patients who die from gastroduodenal motor disorders do so from malnutrition and its consequence or serious electrolyte imbalance.

Primary Disease Exacerbation

Although the nature of the pathologic process is often not known, it is common for exacerbation to be associated with factors such as infection, anesthetics, drugs, and procedures involving gut handling that may normally adversely affect gut motility.

Malnutrition

Many patients die from malnutrition. This is totally avoidable with the judicious use of parenteral nutrition. Many episodes subside completely provided that nutrition is maintained. Only the most severely affected need to be considered for home parenteral nutrition. Others tolerate modern enteral formulas but not normal food.

Pharmacologic Agents

Most attempts at treatment with prokinetic agents (metoclopramide, domperidone, or cisapride) in patients with neuromuscular disease of the gut are unsuccessful, yet occasionally one of these agents is helpful. Some tachygastrias have been associated with disturbed prostaglandin metabolism.[29] In such patients treatment with a prostaglandin synthetase inhibitor such as indomethacin may be successful. Until an understanding of the disease process itself is obtained, drugs will provide only marginal relief at best.

PROGNOSIS

The prognosis for patients with uncomplicated pyloric stenosis or malrotation is excellent, and only a success rate of 100 percent is acceptable. However, in those patients in whom the stomach and duodenum are involved in a pseudo-obstructive disorder, either restricted to the region or as part of a more generalized disease of the GI tract, the prognosis is more uncertain. In conditions in which the extrinsic innervation is affected, the prognosis is that of the underlying condition. In those patients in whom there is intrinsic neuromuscular disease, particularly when it is part of a diffuse condition of the gut, the overall mortality rate may be as high as 25 percent, with the highest rate in the first few years of life. The majority of patients die from sepsis, malnutrition, electrolyte imbalance, or aspiration.

Only in the last 10 years have many of the diseases that cause gastroduodenal motor disorders been recognized. However, effective treatment for many will ensue only when a much greater understanding of the disorders is achieved.

REFERENCES

1. Kelly KA. Motility of the stomach and gastroduodenal junction. In: Johnson LR, ed. Physiology of the gastrointestinal tract. 2nd ed. New York: Raven Press, 1987:393.
2. Hartshorne DJ. Biochemistry of contractile processes in smooth muscle. In: Johnson LR, ed. Physiology of the gastrointestinal tract. 2nd ed. New York: Raven Press, 1987:423.
3. Paul RJ. Mechanochemical energy conversion relations between metabolism and contractability. In: Johns LR, ed. Physiology of the gastrointestinal tract. 2nd ed. New York: Raven Press, 1987:483.
4. Andrews PLR, Grundy D, Scratcherd T. Vagal afferent discharge from mechanoreceptors of the ferret stomach. J Physiol 1980; 298:513.
5. Sarna SK. Gastrointestinal electrical activity. Gastroenterology 1975; 68:1631.
6. Costa M, Furness JB, Llewellyn-Smith IJ. Histochemistry of the enteric nervous system. In: Johnson LR, ed. Physiology of the gastrointestinal tract. 2nd ed. New York: Raven Press, 1987:1.
7. Ewart WR, Wingate DL. Central representation and opioid modulation of gastric mechanoreceptor activity in the rat. Am J Physiol 1983; 244:G27–G32.
8. Ewart WR, Wingate DL. Cholecystokinin octapeptide and gastric mechanoreceptor activity in the rat brain. Am J Physiol 1983; 244:G613–G617.
9. Stern RM, Koch KL, Stewart WR, Lindblad IM. Spectral analysis of tachygastria recorded during motion sickness. Gastroenterology 1987; 92:92–97.
10. Andrews PLR, Hawthorn J. The neurophysiology of vomiting. Bailliere's Clin Gastroenterol 1988; 2:141–168.
11. Stricker EM. Biological bases of hunger and satiety; therapeutic implications. Nutr Rev 1984; 42:333–340.
12. Hinder RA. Individual and combined roles of the pylorus and antrum in the canine gastric emptying of a liquid and digestible solid. Gastroenterology 1983; 84:281–286.
13. Meyer JH, Ohashi H, Jehn D, Thomson JB. Size of liver particles emptied from the human stomach. Gastroenterology 1981; 80:1489–1496.
14. Cavell B. Effect of feeding an infant formula with high energy density on gastric emptying in infants with congenital heart disease. Acta Paediatr Scand 1981; 70:517–520.
15. Siegel M, Lebenthal E, Krantz B. Effect of calorie density on gastric emptying in premature infants. J Pediatr 1984; 804:108–112.
16. Szurszewski JH. A migrating electric complex of the canine small intestine. Am J Physiol 1969; 217:1757–1763.
17. Stanciu C, Bennett JR. The general pattern of gastroduodenal motility: 24 hr recordings in normal subjects. Rev Med Chir Soc Med Nat Iasi 1975; 79:31–36.
18. Fenton TR, Harries JT, Milla PJ. Disordered small intestinal motility: a rational basis for toddler's diarrhoea. Gut 1983; 24:897–903.
19. Fenton TR, Milla PJ. Age related differences of MMC. Pediatr Res 1984; 18:1061.
20. Vantrappen G, Janssens J, Hellemans J, Shoos Y. The interdigestive motor complex of normal subjects and patients with bacterial overgrowth of the small intestine. J Clin Invest 1977; 59:1158–1166.
21. Smout AJPM. Gastric emptying. In: Wood C, ed. Motility: a forgotten factor in gastrointestinal diseases. R Soc Med London 1985; 21–32.
22. Wozniak ER, Fenton TR, Milla PJ. Fasting small intestinal motor activity in chronic idiopathic intestinal pseudo-obstruction. Pediatr Res 1984; 18:1060.
23. Booth IW, Fenton TR, Milla PJ, Harries JT. A pathophysiological study of the intestinal manifestations of a vasoactive intestinal peptide calcitonin and catecholamine secretory tumor. Gut 1983; 24:954–959.
24. Okorie NM, Dickson JS, Carver RA, Steiner GM. What happens to the pylorus after pyloromyotomy. Arch Dis Child 1988; 63:1339–1340.
25. Friesen SR, Pearse ASE. Pathogenesis of congenital pyloric stenosis: histochemical analyses of pyloric ganglion cells. Surgery 1963; 53:604–607.
26. Rintoul JR, Kirkman NF. The myenteric plexus infantile pyloric stenosis. Arch Dis Child 1961; 36:474–480.
27. Tanner MS, Smith B, Lloyd JK. Functional intestine obstruction due to deficiency of argyrophil neurones in the myenteric plexus. Arch Dis Child 1978; 51:837–841.
28. Scharli A, Sieber WK, Kiesewether WB. Hypertrophic pyloric stenosis at the Children's Hospital of Pittsburgh from 1912–1967. J Pediatr Surg 1969; 4:108–114.
29. Telander RL, Morgan KG, Kreulen DL, Schmalz PF, Kelly KA, Syurszewski JH. Human gastric atopy with tachygastria and gastric ventilation. Gastroenterology 1978; 75:497–501.
30. Cucchiara S, Janssens J, Vantrappen G, Geboes K, Ceccatelli P. Gastric electrical dysrhythmia (tachygastria) in a girl with intractable vomiting. J Pediatr 1986; 108:264–267.
31. You CH, Lee KY, Chey WY, Menguy R. Electrogastrographic study of patients with unexplained nausea, bloating and vomiting. Gastroenterology 1980; 79:311–314.
32. Bissett WM, Devane S, Milla PJ. Gastric antral dysrhythmias—a cause of vomiting. Pediatr Res 1988; 24:409.
33. Wyburn-Mason M. Visceral lesions in herpes zoster. Br Med J 1959; i:678–681.
34. Yarh MD, Frontena AT. Acute autonomic neuropathy: its occurrence in infectious mononucleosis. Arch Neurol 1975; 32:132–133.
35. Harik SI, Ghandour MH, Farah FS, Afifi AK. Postganglionic cholinergic dysautonomia. Am Neurol 1977; 1:393–396.
36. Waterfall WE, Cameron GS, Sarna SK, Lewis TD, Daniel EE. Disorganized electrical activity in a child with idiopathic intestinal pseudo obstruction. Gut 1981; 22:77–83.
37. Sinnett HD, Johnson AG. The effect of highly selective vagotomy on gastric adaptive relaxation. Br J Surg 1982; 69:686.
38. Mroz CT, Kelly KA. The role of the extrinsic antral nerves in the regulation of gastric emptying. Surg Gynecol Obstet 1977; 145:369–377.
39. Gitzelmann R, Hirsig J. Infant dumping syndrome: reversal of symptoms by feeding uncooked starch. Eur J Pediatr 1986; 145:504–506.
40. Vargas JH, Sachs P, Ament ME. Chronic intestinal pseudo obstruction syndrome in pediatrics. J Pediatr Gastroenterol Nutr 1988; 7:323–332.
41. Law DH, Ten Eyck EA. Familial megaduodenum and megacystis. Am J Med 1962; 33:911–922.
42. Schuffler MD, Lowe MC, Bill AH. Chronic idiopathic intestinal pseudo obstruction. 1. Hereditary hollow visceral myopathy. Clinical and pathological studies. Gastroenterology 1977; 73:339–344.
43. Milla PJ, Lake BD, Spitz L, et al. Chronic idiopathic intestinal pseudo obstruction in infancy: smooth muscle disease. In: Labo G, Bortolotti M, eds. Gastrointestinal motility. Verona: Cortina International, 1983:125.
44. Berdon WE, Baker DH, Blane WA, Gay B, Santulli TV, Donovan G. Megacystis-microcolon-intestinal hypoperistalsis syndrome: a new cause of intestinal obstruction in the newborn. AJR 1976; 126:957–964.
45. Consolo S, Morselli PL, Zaccala M, Garattini S. Delayed absorption of phenylbutazone caused by desmethyl-imipramine in humans. Eur J Pharmacol 1970; 10:239–242.
46. Bear R, Steer K. Pseudo obstruction due to clonidine. Br Med J 1976; i:197.
47. Kebanian JW, Calne DB. Multiple receptors for dopamine. Nature 1979; 277:93–96.
48. Sullivan SN, Lamki L, Corcoran P. Inhibition of gastric emptying by enkephalin analogue. Lancet 1981; ii:86–87.
49. Stanguellini V, Malagelada J-R, Zinsmeister A, Go VLW, Kao PC. Stress induced gastrointestinal motor disturbances in humans: possible humoral mechanisms. Gastroenterology 1983; 85:83–91.

50. Devane SP, Bisset WM, Milla PJ. Persistent feeding problems after correction of intestinal malrotation: a manometric assessment. Pediatr Res 1988; 24:409.

51. Stanguellini V, Camilleri M, Malayelada JR. Chronic idiopathic pseudo-obstruction: clinical and intestinal manometric findings. Gut 1987; 28:5–12.

52. Hurwitz A. Measuring gastric volumes by dye dilution. Gut 1981; 22:85–93.

53. Di Lorenzo C, Piepsz A, Ham H, Cadronel S. Gastric emptying with gastro esophageal reflux. Arch Dis Child 1987; 62:449–453.

54. Volkers ACW, Van der Schee EJ, Grashuis JL. Electrogastrography in the dog: waveform analysis by a coherent averaging technique. Med Biol Eng Comput 1983; 21:56–60.

55. Krishnamurthy S, Schuffler MD. Pathology of neuromuscular disorders of the small intestine and colon. Gastroenterology 1987; 93:610–639.

56. Lake BD. Observations on the pathology of pseudo obstruction. In: Milla PJ, ed. Disorders of gastrointestinal motility in childhood. Chichester: Wiley and Sons, 1988:81.

CHAPTER 27

The Intestines

PART 1

Congenital Anomalies

David Wesson, M.D.

EMBRYOLOGY

This subject has been reviewed recently by Moore.[1] The primitive gut, which arises from the dorsal part of the yolk sac during the fourth week of human development, gives rise to the digestive system. The endothelium of the gut derives from the endoderm of the primitive gut and the ectoderm of the stomodeum and proctodeum at its proximal and distal ends. Most of the epithelial attachments to the gut, including the liver and the pancreas, arise from the endoderm of the primitive gut. The connective tissue elements of the wall of the digestive tract, including the smooth muscle coat, arise from splanchnic mesenchyme.

The primitive gut is divided into three parts: foregut, midgut, and hindgut. The foregut gives rise to the pharynx, lower respiratory system, esophagus, stomach, and upper portion of the duodenum down to the opening of the bile duct, in addition to the liver, pancreas, and biliary system. All the abdominal components receive their blood supply from the foregut artery, which later becomes the celiac artery. The midgut gives rise to the small intestine beyond the opening of the bile duct, plus the cecum, appendix, ascending colon, and most of the transverse colon. These structures receive their blood supply via the artery of the midgut, which becomes the superior mesenteric artery. The midgut is attached to the posterior abdominal wall by the dorsal mesentery. It communicates ventrally with the yolk sac through the yolk stalk.

As it grows, the midgut lengthens and forms a loop that protrudes into the umbilical cord. Its cranial limb forms the small bowel, and its caudal limb forms the cecum and proximal colon. As it moves back into the peritoneal cavity, the midgut rotates counterclockwise. The cranial limb or small intestine returns first, passing posterior to the superior mesenteric artery. The caudal limb or colon returns last to lie anterior to the superior mesenteric artery and small intestine. Further counterclockwise rotation brings the midgut to its final position. The dorsal mesentery of the midgut attaches to the posterior abdominal wall close to the duodenum and ascending colon so that these structures become retroperitoneal.

The hindgut gives rise to the left part of the transverse colon, descending colon, sigmoid colon, rectum, and superior portion of the anal canal. These structures are supplied by the artery of the hindgut, which becomes the inferior mesenteric artery. The caudal part of the hindgut, the cloaca, contacts the proctodeum or surface ectoderm throughout the cloacal membrane. The cloaca is divided into dorsal and ventral parts by a sheet of mesenchyme that lies in the coronal plane called the urorectal septum. This septum gradually extends caudally and divides the hindgut into the ventral urogenital sinus and the dorsal anorectal canal. This process is complete by the end of the seventh week of human development. The epithelium of the anal canal is derived from the endoderm of the hindgut superiorly and the ectoderm of the proctodeum inferiorly. The two meet at the pectinate line.

Common malformations of the midgut include Meckel's diverticulum, abnormalities of rotation and fixation, duplication, and stenosis and atresia of the small bowel. Abnormalities of the hindgut include various types of imperforate anus, duplication, and stenosis and atresia of the colon.

DEVELOPMENTAL ANOMALIES OF THE INTESTINE

Atresia and Stenosis

Classification

An atresia is a complete obstruction of the lumen of a hollow viscus. There are several types of intestinal atresia.[2] In type I, an intact diaphragm or membrane composed of mucosa and submucosa obstructs the lumen. The muscularis and serosa are intact. Externally, there is no evidence of obstruction apart from a change in diameter of the bowel, which may be seen distal to the actual lesion if the membrane stretches, as in a wind sock anomaly. Type II atresias are more obvious gaps in bowel continuity in which a short fibrous band connects proximal and distal segments. In type III, there is no connecting tissue between the blind ends, and there is usually an associated V-shaped gap in the mesentery.

Two other types of atresia have been described. In type IIIB, there is a proximal small bowel atresia and an absence of the distal superior mesenteric artery and dorsal mesentery. The small bowel distal to the atresia is coiled like an apple peel and foreshortened; it receives its blood supply in a retrograde fashion from the ileocolic, right colic, or inferior mesenteric artery. This deformity may be due to a volvulus of all or part of the midgut during fetal life. Much of the gut supplied by the superior mesenteric artery disappears, leaving a high jejunal or occasionally even a distal duodenal atresia. The distal ileum winds around a thin vascular stalk, which usually consists of the left branch of the ileocolic artery. A large gap in the mesentery is present along with intestinal malrotation and a microcolon. The prognosis is worse in these latter cases because of the associated short gut. The apple peel type of intestinal atresia has been reported to affect more than one individual in the same family.[3]

Type IV atresias are multiple, like a string of sausages. Also, the bowel may be foreshortened. Multiple atresias have been reported in several families as well as in sporadic cases.[4] Because of the proximal obstruction, distal atresias may be overlooked at operation, especially if they are not associated with a gap in the bowel or mesentery. The possibility of a second or even multiple distal atresias must be kept in mind in every case of intestinal atresia; air or saline always should be flushed from the most proximal obstruction into the colon at the time of repair.

Pathophysiology

Jejunal and ileal atresias result from ischemic necrosis of the fetal intestine,[5] usually acquired in utero and not genetically determined. Specific causes include volvulus, intussusception, internal hernia, and interruption of the segmental mesenteric blood supply leading to intestinal necrosis. Because the bowel is sterile in the fetus, necrotic tissue is resorbed, leaving blind proximal and distal ends, often with a gap in the mesentery. Peristalsis causes increasing dilation of the upper end, which is most marked when the obstruction is in the proximal jejunum. In addition to causing technical difficulties with the anastomosis, this dilated segment can also lead to functional obstruction after repair because of ineffective peristalsis, partly because the dilation prevents apposition of the mucosa of the bowel as peristaltic waves pass through it and partly because the normal co-ordinated muscle activity is disturbed.

Incidence

Duodenal atresia occurs in from 1 in 20,000 to 1 in 40,000 births. Approximately 30 percent of babies with duodenal atresia have Down's syndrome. Duodenal atresia is also associated with esophageal atresia, malrotation of the midgut, annular pancreas, imperforate anus, congenital heart disease, and intrauterine growth retardation. The degree of obstruc-

tion varies from partial in duodenal stenosis to complete in duodenal atresia. However, apart from the fact that diagnosis may be delayed for days or weeks, duodenal stenosis is highly similar to duodenal atresia and requires essentially the same treatment.

Duodenal atresia and stenosis may be associated with malrotation. Therefore, malrotation should be ruled out whenever operation for duodenal atresia or stenosis is to be delayed. On the other hand, intrinsic obstruction should always be ruled out in cases of malrotation at operation by passing saline or a catheter through the duodenum into the upper jejunum.

Jejunal and ileal atresias are more common than duodenal atresia. The reported incidence varies from as high as 1 in 332 to as low as 1 in 5,000 births.[2] They are thought to be acquired in utero as the result of some intrauterine event (arterial occlusion, volvulus, intussusception) rather than failure of initial canalization of the gut. Associated anomalies, including Down's syndrome and malrotation, are less common than with duodenal atresia.

Colonic atresias account for approximately 10 percent of intestinal atresias and occur at a rate of approximately 1 in 40,000 live births.[2] Colonic atresias are more likely to be type I and may be difficult to diagnose at operation if the external surface of the bowel looks normal. This feature is an added reason for obtaining a contrast examination of the colon before operating on any baby with intestinal obstruction. The rare association between colonic atresia and Hirschsprung's disease must also be remembered.

Diagnosis

Fifteen to 20 percent of cases of polyhydramnios are associated with gastrointestinal (GI) obstruction in the fetus, and over 50 percent of cases of esophageal and duodenal atresia are associated with polyhydramnios. Often the exact anatomic cause can be confirmed in utero by ultrasonographic examination, allowing for prompt treatment after birth and thereby reducing the risk of complications such as dehydration, electrolyte imbalance, and aspiration pneumonia. However, prenatal ultrasonography is not always accurate and the diagnosis should always be confirmed by plain films and contrast examinations after birth. Choledochal cyst is particularly difficult to distinguish from duodenal atresia by antenatal ultrasonography.

Clinical manifestations of neonatal intestinal obstruction include bilious vomiting, abdominal distention, and failure to pass meconium. The incidence of jaundice is increased. The abdomen may be grossly distended with visible or palpable loops of intestine if the obstruction is distal.

Duodenal atresia causes a classic "double bubble" sign with absence of distal gas on a plain upright abdominal radiograph. This sign may be obscured by excessive fluid in the stomach. However, simple aspiration of the stomach through a nasogastric tube and injection of 30 to 60 ml of air confirm the diagnosis; barium or other contrast agents are unnecessary. If immediate operation is not planned (because of extreme prematurity, metabolic disturbance, or another anomaly), a barium enema should be done to rule out malrotation and potential midgut volvulus.

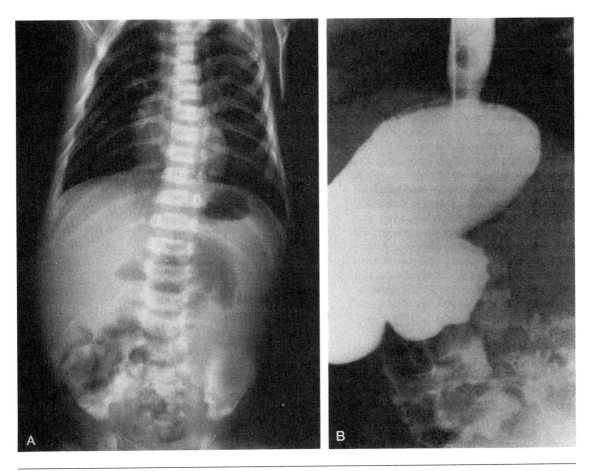

FIGURE 1 *A*, Plain upright radiograph in a 3-week-old baby with Down's syndrome and bilious vomiting. Note the air-fluid level in the duodenum. *B*, Barium contrast study of the upper gastrointestinal tract of the same baby as in *A*. Note the dilated stomach and proximal duodenum with collapsed distal bowel. The baby had duodenal stenosis and did well after duodenoduodenostomy.

Duodenal stenosis usually causes only partial obstruction, but plain abdominal radiographs often show an air-fluid level in the duodenum (Fig. 1).

The diagnosis of jejunal or ileal atresia also can be confirmed by radiologic examinations. Plain abdominal radiographs reveal dilated loops of small bowel with air-fluid levels. The more distal the atresia, the more obvious the distention. Intraperitoneal calcification suggests prenatal perforation of the gut and meconium peritonitis. The differential diagnosis of small bowel atresia includes Hirschsprung's disease, colonic atresia, meconium ileus, and malrotation with volvulus. A barium enema should be performed in all of these cases to rule out Hirschsprung's disease and malrotation. Microcolon is observed in cases of ileal atresia, and it will not be possible to reflux contrast medium into dilated loops of more proximal bowel. In meconium ileus, there is microcolon too, but often contrast medium can be injected retrogradely into the proximal dilated ileum to demonstrate typical intraluminal filling defects caused by abnormal meconium. The latter maneuver may be therapeutic as well as diagnostic (see below).

Treatment

Treatment is divided into two stages. Preoperative care involves establishment of an intravenous line, nasogastric suction, and correction of any fluid and electrolyte imbalance. If malrotation and volvulus have been excluded, operation can be postponed until the patient is in optimal condition and other metabolic, cardiac, and respiratory conditions have been treated.

At operation duodenal atresia is best approached through a transverse right upper quadrant incision. After the right colon is mobilized off the duodenum and the entire duodenum inspected, the best and safest procedure is an end-to-side or side-to-side duodenoduodenostomy. A duodenojejunostomy is also acceptable. Even in cases of duodenal stenosis due to a persistent membrane, it is unwise to try to resect the obstructing membrane because of the possibility of damaging the bile duct or pancreatic duct. In cases of duodenal atresia, a small catheter should be passed into the distal bowel and either air or saline injected through the entire small bowel to rule out additional stenoses or atresias. Duodenal atresia may be associated with a preduodenal portal vein, but this lesion can be treated by duodenoduodenostomy also, provided that care is taken to avoid damaging the vein. Postoperative nasogastric drainage is usually satisfactory, but in some cases a gastrostomy may be indicated.

Jejunal and ileal atresias can be approached through a transverse incision below or just above the umbilicus. In most, a simple end-to-end anastomosis can be made. This procedure usually requires a back cut on the antimesenteric border of the distal bowel and either resection or tapering of the bulbous proximal end. Some authorities have advised tapering in every case to reduce the incidence of anastomotic dysfunction. Postoperatively, nasogastric drainage is continued until intestinal function resumes. Multiple atresias must be repaired primarily, while great care is taken to preserve intestinal length. In cases with short segments between atretic lesions, it may be preferable to resect the entire section of involved bowel rather than perform multiple anastomoses, provided that this will leave an adequate length of bowel (at least 30 cm of jejunum and ileum with an intact ileocecal sphincter, but ideally more than 75 cm).

In most cases of neonatal intestinal obstruction, total parenteral nutrition (TPN) is started within 24 to 48 hours of surgery and continued until oral feeding is established. Delayed emptying of the duodenum may occur after repair of a duodenal atresia, but reoperation should not be attempted for at least 3 weeks and only when radiologic studies show obstruction. In some cases of jejunal and ileal atresia, especially types IIIB and IV, the short bowel syndrome may complicate the postoperative phase. Most babies without serious other problems such as prematurity, respiratory distress syndrome, or short gut survive. The prognosis for babies with multiple atresias depends on the amount of bowel present.

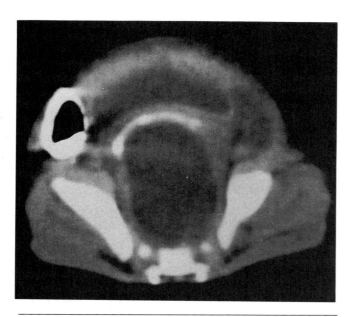

FIGURE 2 CT scan in a newborn boy with a pelvic mass obstructing the bowel and bladder. Note the cystic mass anterior to sacrum displacing colon to the right. The cyst was drained into the rectum by cystoproctostomy, and there was no recurrence at 2-year follow-up.

The overall survival for jejunal, ileal, and colonic atresia is approximately 90 percent. In most patients, death is caused by associated anomalies. Sepsis and TPN-associated liver failure may complicate cases, particularly those with associated short gut syndrome. Late problems include recurrent obstruction from anastomotic dysfunction, stricture, and adhesions.[6]

Duplications

A duplication is a cystic or tubular malformation of the gut, lined by intestinal mucosa and having a smooth muscle coat, which shares a common blood supply with the adjacent gut. Typically, a tubular duplication communicates with the adjacent intestinal lumen. Duplications, which may occur at any level from mouth to anus, are most commonly found in the small bowel.[7] They may be multiple.

Duplications are important because they can enlarge, causing compression of neighboring bowel, or lead to the development of a volvulus or intussusception. Most present in early childhood, but some are not recognized until adult life. Frequently they contain ectopic gastric mucosa that secretes acid-peptic juice and can cause ulceration, inflammation, pain, bleeding, or perforation within the duplication cyst itself or in the adjacent intestine.

In infants, rectal duplication cysts may produce obstruction to both the gut and the urinary tract at the level of the bony pelvis (Fig. 2).

Duplication must be considered in the differential diagnosis of obscure abdominal pain, cystic abdominal masses, and GI hemorrhage. Ultrasonography and CT scan help localize the cyst. A Meckel's scan is positive if the duplication contains ectopic gastric mucosa.

Although duplications share a common wall and blood supply with the adjacent bowel, they have separate mucosal linings. Generally, the cystic type involves short segments of the bowel, whereas the tubular type involves longer segments and occasionally the entire intestine. Unlike Meckel's diverticula, duplications occur on the mesenteric border, making it difficult to excise them without removing attached bowel.

Because of their complications, all duplications should be removed. Most can be excised along with the entire segment of adjacent attached bowel, which is repaired by primary end-to-end anastomosis. When this approach would involve resecting an excessive amount of bowel, the duplication can be opened in several places to allow excision of the mucosal lining, leaving the seromuscular layers in situ. This technique is preferred to multiple side-to-side anastomoses because the offending gastric mucosa is removed. Cystic duplications of the rectum can be treated by the creation of a wide cystoproctostomy. The prognosis is excellent in most cases. The overall survival exceeds 90 percent.[7,8]

Meckel's Diverticulum

Meckel's diverticulum, first described by Meckel in 1809, is a remnant of the vitellointestinal or omphalomesenteric duct, which arises from the ileum proximal to the ileocecal sphincter. Meckel's diverticula are present in 1 to 2 percent of the general population. The male-to-female ratio is 3:1.

Ectopic tissue (pancreatic, gastric) is present in more than half. They are true diverticula because they contain all layers of the gut wall. Other related anomalies of the omphalomesenteric duct include Meckel's bands (remnants of the vitelline vessels), umbilical cysts, and patent omphaloileal fistulas.

Abnormal Rotation and Fixation

As the intestines return to the abdomen from the umbilical cord at about the tenth week of gestation, they undergo counterclockwise rotation about the axis of the superior mesenteric artery, followed by fixation to the posterior abdominal wall as described in greater detail above. Both the duodenal-jejunal loop and the cecal-colic loop of the midgut rotate approximately 270 degrees about the axis of the superior mesenteric artery. The duodenal-jejunal loop rotates behind the artery, and the cecal-colic loop rotates anterior to it. Finally, the duodenum and ascending colon become fixed to the posterior abdominal wall. In this way the intestines assume their normal postnatal position. When this process of rotation and fixation goes awry, the intestine is predisposed to obstruction and volvulus with secondary ischemia and infarction.[9]

Nonrotation occurs when this process fails completely. The duodenal-jejunal loop ends up on the right side of the abdomen and the cecal-colic loop on the left. The base of the mesentery is reasonably broad, and the duodenum is separated from the cecum. Nonrotation, which rarely results in obstruction or volvulus, is associated with congenital diaphragmatic hernia, omphalocele, and gastroschisis.

In malrotation, the most common and potentially dangerous abnormality of rotation, the normal process is arrested with the cecum in the right upper quadrant near the duodenum. The duodenal-jejunal loop remains to the right of the midline. The base of the mesentery is a very narrow pedicle centered on the superior mesenteric artery and vein. Obstruction of the duodenum may result from peritoneal bands (Ladd's bands) extending from the cecum to the right upper quadrant. A very serious and at times sinister complication of malrotation is intestinal volvulus with subsequent necrosis of the entire midgut around its narrow vascular pedicle. Lymphatics also may be obstructed by the volvulus, leading to chylous ascites. Malrotation is associated with diaphragmatic hernia, omphalocele, mesenteric cysts, Hirschsprung's disease, and occasionally intussusception.

Volvulus of the midgut from malrotation is most common during infancy, but it can occur at any age. Typically the child feeds well at birth and then develops anorexia, bilious vomiting, vague fullness in the right upper quadrant with or without distention, and the passage of blood-tinged mucus per rectum. When treatment is delayed, total cardiovascular collapse may ensue. The diagnosis of volvulus of the midgut must be suspected in all cases of obstruction to the upper intestine in infants. After initial resuscitation the diagnosis can be confirmed by barium enema, which reveals the cecum in the right upper quadrant, or upper barium contrast films via nasogastric tube, which show absence of the normal ligament of Treitz to the left of the midline and a corkscrew obstruction in the distal duodenum. Emergency operation is indicated to relieve

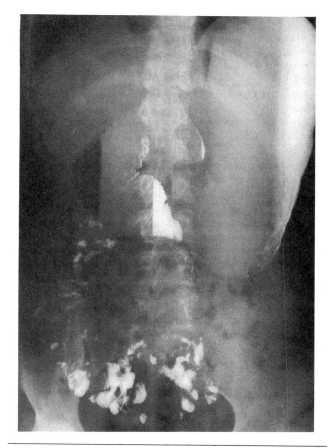

FIGURE 3 Barium contrast study of the upper gastrointestinal tract in a 12-year-old girl with a long history of recurrent abdominal pain and bilious vomiting. Note the dilated stomach and proximal duodenum with air-fluid levels, absence of the ligament of Trietz, and collapsed small bowel, all on the right. At operation she had malrotation with partial midgut volvulus but no ischemia. She did well after undergoing a Ladd's procedure.

the volvulus, broaden the base of the mesentery, and place the bowel in the position of nonrotation (Ladd's procedure). Intrinsic obstruction of the duodenum should be ruled out at operation.

Patients with abnormalities of rotation can present with duodenal obstruction, usually in the neonatal period. The infant may have fed for a brief period and passed meconium normally. Jaundice is common. The main clinical manifestations are anorexia and bilious vomiting. Plain films may reveal a typical "double bubble" appearance of duodenal obstruction, with some distal gas, but the diagnosis is confirmed by barium enema or upper GI series as described above (Fig. 3).

Rare abnormalities of rotation, including reversed rotation in which the transverse colon ends up dorsal to the superior mesenteric artery, can result in internal herniation and other unusual forms of obstruction. These include mesocolic hernias, paraduodenal hernias, and obstruction to the midtransverse colon by the superior mesenteric artery. These conditions present as partial bowel obstructions, occasionally associated with acute abdominal pain, but rarely are they diagnosed preoperatively. However, any patient with abdominal symptoms, particularly bilious vomiting and recurrent abdominal cramps associated with an abnormality of rotation, should undergo laparotomy.

The patient should be prepared for surgery with intravenous fluids to restore fluid and electrolyte balance, nasogastric suction, and intravenous antibiotics because a bowel resection may be necessary. The abdomen is explored through an upper transverse incision. The bowel should first be untwisted, usually by counterclockwise rotation around the axis of the superior mesenteric artery and vein. Often, three full turns are required. The cecal bands between the cecum and paraduodenal region should be divided. The dissection is continued between the cecum and right colon on the left and the duodenum on the right, the mesentery being broadened around the superior mesenteric artery and vein. The duodenal loop should be straightened out somewhat, although it is not usually possible to straighten it completely. The duodenum then descends on the right side of the abdomen, and the colon is placed on the left side. The appendix should be removed. In cases of volvulus with ischemia of the gut, a period of observation may be necessary before closing the abdomen. Usually obviously nonviable intestinal segments should be resected, but if the entire midgut is severely ischemic, it may be wiser to close the abdomen and plan for a second operation in 12 to 24 hours to allow recovery of at least some of the affected bowel and thus minimize the amount that requires resection. It is not usually necessary to fix the bowel to prevent recurrent volvulus.

Meconium Ileus

Meconium ileus is a type of mechanical obstruction of the distal small bowel and colon caused by thickened intraluminal meconium, a condition unique to cystic fibrosis. The exact cause is not known, but two factors have been implicated: pancreatic exocrine insufficiency and abnormal intestinal secretions. The differential diagnosis includes meconium plug syndrome, in which the distal colon and occasionally the small bowel are obstructed by thickened meconium and which can be cured by enemas. The differential diagnosis also includes ileal atresia and Hirschsprung's disease.

The incidence of cystic fibrosis among Caucasians is approximately 1 in 2,000 live births. The reported incidence of meconium ileus in cases of cystic fibrosis ranges from 7 to 25 percent, with a mean of approximately 15 percent. Meconium ileus has been reported in a few patients who did not have cystic fibrosis, but for all practical purposes, meconium ileus does not occur in the absence of that disease. Meconium ileus accounts for 9 to 33 percent of neonatal small bowel obstructions.[10]

Clinically, meconium ileus is subdivided into two forms: simple (uncomplicated) and complicated. In simple meconium ileus, the distal small bowel is obstructed by thickened meconium. The proximal small bowel is dilated and thick-walled. The distal colon is narrow and empty (microcolon). Complicated cases have additional features including intes-

tinal volvulus, atresia, necrosis, perforation, meconium peritonitis, and meconium pseudocyst. All these result from the mass effect of the inspissated meconium in the bowel, which acts as a fulcrum for volvulus of the bowel, leading to secondary necrosis and perforation.

The histologic hallmark of meconium ileus is distention of the goblet cells of the intestinal mucosa.

Clinically, simple meconium ileus presents clinical features similar to other types of distal intestinal obstruction in the newborn infant. The differential diagnosis includes ileal atresia, colonic atresia, and Hirschsprung's disease. However, a family history of cystic fibrosis is highly suggestive of the diagnosis. On physical examination, the baby is usually normal, apart from the presence of abdominal distention. The rectum, usually empty on digital examination, may be narrower than normal. Complicated meconium ileus tends to cause more abdominal distention owing to excessive fluid in the peritoneal cavity and occasionally to cystic collections of meconium, which may be palpable.

The radiologic features of simple meconium ileus are difficult to distinguish from those of ileal atresia, but there may be a soap bubble appearance in the right lower quadrant and a lack of air-fluid levels on the upright film. A microcolon is seen on contrast enema in meconium ileus. Occasionally, it is possible to reflux the contrast into the distal ileum, outlining the meconium pellets and the proximal dilated bowel as well. In complicated meconium ileus, there is a suggestion of free fluid on the plain films and occasionally calcification within the peritoneal cavity. Pneumoperitoneum may develop if there is a perforation. A contrast enema also reveals a microcolon.

A definitive diagnosis of meconium ileus rests on the diagnosis of cystic fibrosis by finding a sweat chloride concentration greater than 60 mEq per liter. Often, an initial diagnosis is based on the clinical, radiologic, and operative findings because it may be 1 month before reliable sweat electrolyte results can be obtained.

In addition to ileal atresia, the differential diagnosis includes total colonic aganglionosis. However, in total colonic aganglionosis, the contrast agent can usually be refluxed into the dilated bowel without outlining inspissated meconium.

In simple cases, nonoperative treatment is attempted first by the radiologist at the time of the contrast enema. Mildly hypertonic agents such as dilute Gastrografin or Hypaque with acetylcysteine can be used to break up the meconium that is obstructing the distal ileum. If this fails, operative treatment is required. At operation, the options include opening the bowel, to remove the meconium, performing an ileostomy at the proximal end of the obstructed segment, and inserting a T-tube into the bowel for postoperative irrigation with acetylcysteine. All cases of complicated meconium ileus require surgical treatment. The procedure depends on the operative findings, but an enterostomy of some kind is usually required.

Extra attention must be given to the child's nutritional requirements and pulmonary function in the postoperative period. TPN is commenced shortly after the surgery, and the child may require a modified diet such as Pregestimil along with pancreatic enzyme supplements once oral feeds begin. Chest physiotherapy should be given.

The overall prognosis depends on the rate of progression of the underlying pulmonary disease. Children with cystic fibrosis who recover from meconium ileus have the same prognosis as those who do not have this complication.

Aganglionosis (Hirschsprung's Disease)

Hirschsprung's disease is the congenital absence of ganglion cells in the submucosal and myenteric plexuses of the distal intestine. The aganglionic segment always begins in the distal rectum and extends proximally to the so-called transition zone, where it blends into normal bowel. In most cases, the transition zone is in the rectosigmoid colon, but occasionally it is in the more proximal colon or ileum. A few isolated cases of total intestinal aganglionosis have been described.

Malformations of the Anus and Rectum

Imperforate Anus

The term *imperforate anus* embraces a myriad of anomalies without an obvious anal opening. Most have a fistula from the distal rectum to the perineum or genitourinary system. The incidence is approximately 1 in 5,000 births. Anorectal anomalies may occur in isolation or as part of the VACTERL (*vertebral, anorectal, cardiovascular, tracheoesophageal, renal, and limb*) syndrome.[11]

From a clinical perspective, these lesions are divided into high and low types, depending on whether they end above or below the puborectal component of the levator ani complex. Low defects can be handled by simple dilatation or a minor perineal operation. High defects require a temporary colostomy and formal pull-through procedure. Most high lesions end with a fistula from the bowel to bladder, urethra, or vagina. Often there are associated anomalies in the genitourinary tract, spine, and heart.

The most widely accepted classification, the Wingspread classification, distinguishes two main types—supralevator and translevator. The supralevator type is divided into high and intermediate subgroups. A rare group is also recognized, which includes cloacal malformations in which the urinary system, genital system, and GI system drain into a common channel that communicates with the perineum. Clinically, these cases are almost always recognized at birth by the absence of a normal anus. The usual signs and symptoms of a low intestinal obstruction develop. The most important point is to distinguish high lesions from low lesions; this can almost always be done on the basis of clinical evidence.

The high lesions are more common in boys, but there are no other known genetic factors. Associated anomalies include esophageal atresia, intestinal atresia, malrotation, renal agenesis, hypospadias, vesicoureteral reflux, bladder exstrophy, and cardiac and skeletal anomalies.

In boys, if meconium appears anywhere in the perineum, either through an anocutaneous fistula or in the median raphe of the scrotum, the lesion is a low one that can be treated by either simple dilatation or perineal anoplasty. On the other hand, if meconium is passed in urine but is not visible elsewhere in the perineum, the lesion is almost certainly a high one and a diverting colostomy is indicated.

In girls, an anocutaneous or anovestibular fistula to the posterior fourchette or the vagina is almost always visible in low lesions. These can both be treated by simple dilatation. If the opening of the bowel cannot be seen, it is likely that there is a high rectovaginal fistula, which requires a temporary diverting colostomy and formal reconstruction at a later date.

Lateral upside-down radiographs are no longer considered accurate enough to help determine the level of lesion. Ultrasonography and CT have been recommended for the same purpose, but neither has been proven to be reliable in practice.

In high lesions, the internal anal sphincter is absent for all practical purposes, although it may be represented by a small thickening of the distal circular muscle at the end of the bowel. The external sphincter is almost always present at least in part, although its normal relationship to the bowel is obviously lost if the anus is ectopic or if there is no perineal opening from the bowel. The levator ani muscles, and in particular the puborectal muscle, are almost always present, although in high lesions the puborectal muscle is quite small and tightly applied to the urethra or vagina. As a rule, patients with defects in the sacrum have less well-developed sphincter muscles.

A radiograph of the spine and ultrasonography of the urinary system should be obtained in all cases. If there is doubt as to the level of the fistula in boys, a retrograde urethrogram can be done to identify the level of the fistula.

In high lesions requiring a pull-through procedure, a diverting colostomy is performed in the neonatal period and pull-through at 3 to 9 months of age. At the moment, the most favored procedure is the Pena midsagittal anorectoplasty.[11] The colostomy is closed after the anoplasty has healed and any necessary dilatations have been completed. The Mollard procedure is favored by some authorities.[12]

Complications include stricture of the anocutaneous anastomosis, recurrent rectourinary fistula, mucosal prolapse, constipation, and incontinence. Incontinence is by far the most troublesome. The most important determinant of continence is the level of the initial lesion. In general, all children with low lesions achieve normal continence, whereas only a minority of those with high lesions achieve normal continence before school age. Most continue to improve to the point where they achieve socially acceptable continence by adolescence.

Cloacal Exstrophy

This is a rare form of imperforate anus, also called vesicointestinal fissure, in which the bowel (usually the ilecocecal region) and the bladder open onto the lower abdominal wall in a common mucosal field composed of transitional bladder epithelium in the midline and intestinal epithelium on either side.[13] The genitalia are ambiguous, but there is seldom an adequate phallus. Most of these children are raised as females. The small bowel may be shorter than normal, occasionally to the point of causing symptoms. The distal bowel beyond the exstrophy is colon, which is also shorter than normal and in most cases ends blindly above the levator ani.

In these cases the best way to establish adequate GI function is to bring out a permanent enterostomy, either an ileostomy—leaving the colon for later reconstruction—or a colostomy after separating the bowel from the bladder and anastomosing the ileum to the colon. The prognosis has improved considerably in recent years with supportive measures including TPN; in the past most babies died, but now most survive.

REFERENCES

1. Moore KL. Digestive system. In: Essentials of human embryology. Toronto: BC Decker, 1988.
2. Grosfeld JL. Jejunoileal atresia and stenosis. In: Welch KJ, Randolph JG, Ravitch MM, O'Neill JA Jr, Rowe MI, eds. Pediatric surgery. Chicago: Year Book, 1986.
3. Seashore JH, Collins FS, Markowitz RI, Seashore MR. Familial apple peel. Jejunal atresias: surgical, genetic and radiographic aspects. Pediatrics 1987; 80:540–544.
4. Guttman FN, Brown P, Garance PH, et al. Multiple atresias and a new syndrome of hereditary multiple atresias involving the gastrointestinal tract from the stomach to rectum. J Pediatr Surg 1973; 8:633.
5. Haller JA Jr, Tepas JJ, Richard L, Shermeta DW. Intestinal atresia: current concepts of pathogenesis, pathophysiology and operative management. Am Surg 1983; 49:385–391.
6. Rescoria FJ, Grosfeld JL. Intestinal atresia and stenosis: analysis of survival in 120 cases. Surgery 1985; 98:688–676.
7. Hocking M, Young DG. Duplications of the alimentary tract. Br J Surg 1981; 68:92–96.
8. Ildstad ST, Tollerud DJ, Weiss RG, Ryan DP, McGowan MA, Martin LW. Duplications of the alimentary tract: clinical characteristics, preferred treatment and associated malformations. Am Surg 1988; 208:184–189.
9. Bernardi RS. Anomalies of midgut rotation in the adult. Surg Gynecol Obstet 1980; 151:113–124.
10. Lloyd DA. Meconium ileus. In: Welch KJ, Randolph JG, Ravitch MM, O'Neill JA Jr, Rowe MI, eds. Pediatric surgery. Chicago: Year Book, 1986.
11. Templeton JM, O'Neill JA Jr. Anorectal malformations. In: Welch KJ, Randolph JG, Ravitch MM, O'Neill JA Jr, Rowe MI, eds. Pediatric surgery. Chicago: Year Book, 1986.
12. Mollard P, Marechal JM, de Beanjeu MJ. Surgical treatment of high imperforate anus with definition of the puborectalis sling by an anterior perineal approach. J Pediatr Surg 1978; 13:499.
13. Ziegler MM, Duckett JW, Howell CG. Cloacal exstrophy. In: Welch KJ, Randolph JG, Ravitch MM, O'Neill JA Jr, Rowe MI, eds. Pediatric surgery. Chicago: Year Book, 1986.

PART **2**

Trauma and Foreign Bodies

David Wesson, M.D.

EPIDEMIOLOGY

Injuries to the intestines, fortunately quite rare in children, can be caused by blunt or penetrating forces. In civilian practice, blunt trauma is much more common. Although reliable data on the actual incidence in defined populations are not available, frank perforations occur in less than 1 percent of all cases of blunt abdominal trauma in children.[1] Cases in boys outnumber those in girls. The causes include motor vehicle accidents (passengers or pedestrians), assault (including child abuse), and accidental gunshot wounds. The most common cause is a lap belt injury, which typically occurs in rear seat passengers of cars involved in head-on collisions.[1,2] If the belt is worn above the bony pelvis, the bowel may be caught between the belt and spine and torn by the forces of deceleration. Such injuries are associated often with unstable fractures or dislocations of the lumbar spine, some-times with spinal cord damage. This association should always be ruled out by careful clinical examination and anteroposterior and lateral spine radiographs.[2]

PENETRATING WOUNDS

Penetrating wounds to the intestines in children are quite rare in most Western countries, with the exception of a few large cities in the United States where crime, particularly drug-related crime, has exposed older children and adolescents to knives and guns.[3]

A penetrating injury through the peritoneum is usually quite obvious on clinical grounds. It must be kept in mind that any penetrating injury below the nipples may involve the abdomen.

Treatment begins with a primary survey to detect other life-threatening injuries followed by initial resuscitation. Usually, this approach requires oxygen by mask, nasogastric suction, establishment of two peripheral intravenous lines, and infusion of lactated Ringer's solution and/or blood to maintain the vital signs. Broad-spectrum antibiotics should be given intravenously.

Most authorities recommend laparotomy for all penetrating wounds that breach the peritoneum.[4] Recently, some have advised a selective approach, especially for knife wounds, reserving operation for patients who develop peritonitis.[5] Small bowel injuries are repaired primarily, but most colonic injuries, especially those with fecal contamination of the peritoneum or devitalized bowel, require resection and colostomy.

BLUNT INJURIES

Blunt injuries are more difficult to diagnose. Only a small minority of all children who suffer blunt abdominal trauma have significant intestinal injuries, but the consequences of missing one can be devastating. Contusions and hematomas are not of much clinical importance except when they may obstruct the bowel.

Blunt intestinal injuries include contusions, serosal tears, frank perforations, and lacerations of the mesentery with or without intestinal ischemia. Most are caused by direct impalement of the bowel against the spine. Perforations result in chemical and bacterial peritonitis; mesenteric tears may cause infarction of the bowel with subsequent perforation and peritonitis.

Frank perforations are the most important type of blunt injury. They may be retroperitoneal (duodenum, colon, or rectum) or intraperitoneal (small bowel, colon, or rectum). They may be clinically occult, especially in the first 12 to 24 hours.

Diagnosis is mainly by history and physical examination. Any injury of the abdominal wall should suggest the possibility of an intestinal injury. Obvious transverse, linear seatbelt contusions, tire marks, or bruises are helpful, but the essential diagnostic features of intestinal trauma are abdominal pain exacerbated by movement, abdominal tenderness, guarding, and absence of bowel sounds. For such patients with clear signs of peritonitis, immediate laparotomy is indicated after initial resuscitation as described above for penetrating injuries. The late manifestations of intestinal perforation include fever, tachycardia, and ascites. In equivocal cases, careful repeated examination is the best way to reach a diagnosis.

Plain radiographs are notoriously unreliable because less than 50 percent of cases have pneumoperitoneum. Computed tomography (CT) with contrast may reveal free air, extravasation of contrast medium, or free fluid in the abdomen, but the sensitivity and specificity of CT have not been established. Diagnostic peritoneal lavage is quite sensitive but not specific; it is positive if there are more than 500 WBCs per square millimeter, food particles, or bacteria in the fluid.

A devascularizing or serosal injury may cause obstruction by producing an adynamic segment or fibrous stricture.

Delayed perforations of the bowel have also been reported.[6] They probably result from a devascularizing injury to the mesentery that leads to infarction and perforation some days later. Late complications of intestinal injuries include intra-abdominal abscess, bowel obstruction (adhesive, anastomotic), enterocutaneous fistula, and stricture.

FOREIGN BODIES

About 1,500 people die each year in the United States from ingested foreign bodies (FBs). Almost all ingested FBs pass spontaneously, but a few lodge in the pharynx, esophagus, or stomach. Very few lodge in the intestine. In fact, almost all FBs that pass the cricopharyngeal muscle pass through the rest of the gut quite easily. Less than 1 percent require surgery.

Children most often ingest coins, batteries, toys, pins, crayons, and caps from ball-point pens. The diagnosis should be suggested by history and confirmed by plain radiographs. As long as there is no compromise of the airway or sign of perforation, there is never any hurry to remove FBs from the intestine. Patients with esophageal FBs should be admitted for urgent removal. All others can be followed on an outpatient basis unless symptoms develop. Asymptomatic FBs in the stomach should be allowed to pass spontaneously. Those that cause symptoms should be removed, preferably endoscopically.

It is safe to follow patients with coins and other blunt FBs in the gut clinically and by plain radiographs monthly until spontaneous passage occurs. In cases of sharp FBs such as straight pins, more frequent assessments at weekly intervals are indicated. Surgical extraction is indicated if the patient develops symptoms or signs of perforation or if the FB fails to progress for several weeks.

Button batteries for cameras, hearing aids, and other small devices have caused much concern lately. They contain potentially caustic chemicals that can damage tissue. Also they generate electrical current and at least theoretically can cause low-voltage electrical burns to intestinal tissue. Most authorities agree that button batteries in the esophagus should be removed urgently; the correct management of batteries in the bowel is less clear. The only significant complication reported to date is a perforation of a Meckel's diverticulum by a battery.[7] Patients with batteries in the intestines should be managed as patients with sharp FBs described above. The results of the National Button Battery Ingestion Study, which started in 1982, confirm that "the vast majority of battery ingestions are benign and can be managed without endoscopic or surgical intervention."[8] Esophageal lodgment is the only indication for urgent removal. Endoscopic retrieval failed in two-thirds of attempts. Ninety percent passed spontaneously through the gut, almost always within 2 weeks.[8]

No evidence supports the use of special diets or laxatives in patients with intestinal FBs. The most important part of treatment is simply to reassure the parents and family doctor that almost all FBs pass harmlessly through the gut and that as long as the child remains asymptomatic, there is no cause for alarm.

REFERENCES

1. Cobb LM, Vinocur CD, Wagner DW, Weintraub WH. Intestinal perforation due to blunt trauma in children in an era of increased non-operative treatment. J Trauma 1986; 26:461–463.
2. Taylor GA, Eggli KD. Lap belt injuries of the lumbar spine in children: a pitfall in CT diagnosis. AJR 1988; 150:1355–1358.
3. Barlow B, Niemirska M, Gandhi RP. Ten year's experience with pediatric gunshot wounds. J Pediatr Surg 1982; 17:927–932.
4. Blaisdell FW. General assessment, resuscitation and exploration of penetrating and blunt abdominal trauma. In: Blaisdell FW, Trunkey DD, eds. Trauma management. New York: Thieme Stratton, 1982:1.

5. Hill AC, Schecter WP, Trunkey DD. Abdominal trauma and indications for laparotomy. In: Mattox KL, Moore EE, Feliciano D, eds. Trauma. East Norwalk, CT: Appleton and Lange, 1988.
6. Winton TL, Girotti MJ, Manley PN, Sterns EE. Delayed intestinal perforation after non-penetrating abdominal trauma. Can J Surg 1985; 28:437–439.
7. Willis GH, Ho WC. Perforation of Meckel's diverticulum by an alkaline hearing aid battery. Can Med Assoc J 1982; 126:497–498.
8. Litovitz TL. Battery ingestions: product accessibility and clinical course. Pediatrics 1985; 75:469–476.

PART 3

Acute Intestinal Obstruction

David Wesson, M.D.

Intestinal obstruction is the pathologic blockage of aboral progression of intestinal contents. The blockage may be mechanical or paralytic. The latter, commonly called paralytic ileus, is caused by failure of the motor function of the gut.

Mechanical obstructions can be either simple or strangulating. Strangulating obstructions impair intestinal blood flow and may cause necrosis of the bowel from increased intraluminal pressure, as in a closed loop obstruction when the intestinal lumen is obstructed at two points, or from occlusion of mesenteric blood vessels, as in an incarcerated hernia, volvulus, or intussusception. Direct pressure necrosis can occur also where the bowel is held by a fibrous band or a tight hernial ring. Strangulating obstructions have much higher morbidity and mortality than simple obstructions.

GENERAL MANIFESTATIONS

The clinical manifestations of intestinal obstruction vary with the site and cause. Optimal treatment depends on early diagnosis and on an understanding of the pathophysiology of obstruction. The first and most important pathophysiologic change is loss of fluid and electrolytes into the gut, which results in hypovolemia or shock if neglected. In addition, bacteria proliferate in the gut lumen. If the mucosal barrier fails, these bacteria and their toxins may enter the peritoneum or circulation and cause local or systemic sepsis and toxicity. In strangulating obstructions, blood flow is impaired, and frank necrosis of the gut with perforation and peritonitis may ensue. Perforations may result too from overdistention or pressure necrosis by adhesive bands or hernial rings.

Pain is one of the cardinal manifestations of intestinal obstruction. There are two types of such pain:

1. Splanchnic or visceral pain from the gut itself that is deep and poorly localized (periumbilical from small bowel and suprapubic from the colon). Although the bowel can be cut, burned, or crushed without pain, distention and traction on the mesentery cause visceral pain. The autonomic response to this type of pain includes sweating, nausea, and hypotension.
2. Parietal pain from the body wall, which is better localized and is associated with tenderness and rigidity. This type of pain occurs in the presence of peritonitis.

The afferent pain pathways from the gut itself travel via splanchnic sympathetic fibers from the stomach and duodenum to T7 and T8, from the small bowel to T8, T9, and T10, and from the colon to the sacral nerves. Visceral sensations other than pain travel via parasympathetic fibers.[1] Parietal pain from peritonitis may also occur. This sensation is carried via peripheral nerves to the spinal cord nerve roots T7 to L1.

Intestinal obstruction causes intermittent central abdominal pain with vomiting that is typically bilious or feculent and is followed by obstipation. The patient may pass gas and stool from the distal bowel in the first few hours. In cases of intussusception or volvulus, bloody stool or mucus may be passed. Steady unremitting pain made worse by movement suggests strangulation of the involved gut with secondary peritonitis. There may be a history of previous abdominal surgery or a family history of pyloric stenosis, cystic fibrosis, or polyposis.

Physical examination begins with a general assessment of the patient, emphasizing the vital signs, hydration, and nutrition. Abdominal examination includes inspection for old incision scars, hernias, distention, and visible peristalsis. Palpation may reveal distended loops of bowel, a hernia, or a mass (intussusception, feces, or tumor being the most common) and localized or generalized tenderness and rigidity. Although tenderness may be elicited over distended, obstructed loops of bowel without ischemia, it should be regarded as a sign of necrosis or perforation, especially when accompanied by muscular rigidity. Rectal examination is essential in all cases of acute abdominal pain. It may reveal impacted stool, occult or frank blood, or an intraluminal mass such as a polyp or intussusceptum.

Any acute abdominal disease, including intestinal obstruction, may be difficult to diagnose in mentally handicapped children. Timely diagnosis of any bowel obstruction depends mainly on a clear history, which may be difficult to obtain in such cases. Mentally handicapped children also have an increased risk of developing intestinal obstruction because of drug-induced autonomic dysfunction, congenital malformations (e.g., duodenal stenosis in Down's syndrome), CSF shunts, dietary imbalance or indiscretion, aerophagia, and chronic constipation.

The clinical findings vary with the level of obstruction. In high or proximal obstructions to the stomach, duodenum, and upper jejunum, the cramps are more frequent and the vomiting occurs earlier and is also more frequent. There is less abdominal distention; in fact, the abdominal examination may be normal. However, loss of water and Na^+, H^+, K^+, and Cl^- soon leads to dehydration, hypokalemia, and hypochloremic metabolic acidosis. Plain radiographs may also be normal. This pattern, with the lack of obvious signs on abdominal examination, makes diagnosis of high obstructions difficult.

In contrast to the above, when the obstruction is low or distal in the jejunum, ileum, or colon, the vomiting occurs later and is less frequent. Bacterial overgrowth may result in feculent vomitus. The abdomen becomes distended, often with palpable loops of dilated bowel. Large volumes of water may accumulate in the gut lumen, but electrolyte imbalance is less likely because less H^+ and Cl^- are lost.

A tentative diagnosis of intestinal obstruction can almost always be made on the history and physical examination. In most cases, a specific cause can be identified or at least suspected when the patient's age, past history, and physical examination are taken into account. The differential diagnosis includes perforating peptic ulcer, pancreatitis, sickle cell crisis, Henoch-Schönlein purpura, biliary colic, lead poisoning, familial Mediterranean fever, lower lobe pneumonia, acute adrenal insufficiency, acute cholecystitis, renal colic, torsion of the testicle or ovary, diabetic ketoacidosis, and acute intermittent porphyria.

Diagnostic imaging studies are needed to confirm the diagnosis and possibly reveal the exact cause and site of obstruction. Direct communication between the surgeon and radiologist is essential when planning these studies and interpreting the results.

Plain anteroposterior radiographic examinations in the supine and erect positions are the most useful diagnostic tests. In small bowel obstruction, these reveal dilated bowel with air-fluid levels with or without gas or stool in the colon (Fig. 1). Multiple distended loops suggest a distal obstruction. Occasionally, patients with duodenal or high small bowel obstructions or short closed-loop obstructions have normal or

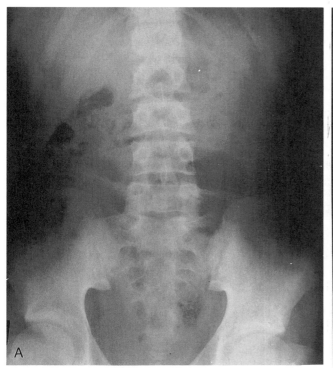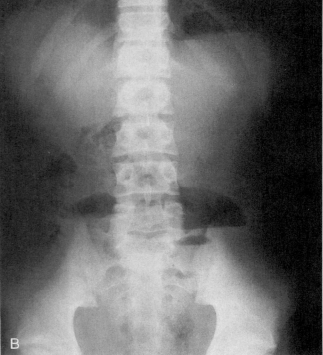

FIGURE 1 Plain AP supine (A) and erect (B) examination in an adolescent with adhesive small bowel obstruction after appendectomy for acute appendicitis. Note distended loops of bowel with gas and air-fluid levels.

nearly normal plain radiographs. In a recent series from the Mayo Clinic, one-half of the cases of strangulating obstruction lacked definite radiologic evidence of obstruction.[2] Patients with paralytic ileus typically have dilated small bowel and colon down to the rectum.

Ultrasonography has been used when a mass is palpable to confirm its location and composition. A recent report by Meiser and Meissner suggests that ultrasonography may have even greater use in diagnosing bowel obstructions.[3] These authors found it to be diagnostic in cases of high duodenal or small bowel obstruction (especially those with normal plain examinations), concealed femoral hernia, and early postoperative obstruction when it can separate mechanical causes from paralytic ileus. For example, ultrasonography may reveal a small bowel intussusception in the early postoperative period after laparotomy when it is difficult to distinguish from paralytic ileus.

Although contraindicated in high-grade or complete obstructions, contrast examinations may be helpful in selected cases. Metrizamide is highly useful for upper gastrointestinal (GI) contrast studies because it is nearly isotonic, it is not absorbed or diluted significantly in the gut, it is not toxic, and it is quickly absorbed when it escapes into the peritoneum through a perforation. Contrast barium studies may be indicated in high partial obstructions to rule out malrotation with volvulus or duodenal obstruction by Ladd's bands. Barium enema examinations may be helpful in distal obstructions to rule out malrotation and/or volvulus, intussusception, or Hirschsprung's disease. More recently, air has been used as a contrast medium to diagnose and treat ileocolic intussusception in infants.

Blood tests including complete blood count (CBC), blood urea nitrogen (BUN), creatinine, and electrolytes should be done routinely as a guide to proper resuscitation. However, no blood test is a reliable indicator of the need for operation.

The treatment of intestinal obstruction includes two separate phases, resuscitation and definitive treatment, always in that order. The essential features of resuscitation are outlined in Table 1.

With a few notable exceptions, definitive treatment requires urgent operation, and every effort should be made to avoid unnecessary delays in getting the patient to the operating room. The exceptions to this rule include early postoperative, partial, and recurrent adhesive obstructions, pyloric stenosis, intussusceptions, meconium ileus, and duodenal hematomas. Prompt recognition of the need for operation is the cornerstone of treatment, keeping in mind the fact that operation has some morbidity of its own and that some cases resolve spontaneously. Nevertheless, it is often said that the sun should never set or rise on a case of bowel obstruction.

TABLE 1
Essential Features of Resuscitation

Hold all oral intake.
Decompress the stomach by nasogastric tube.
Establish an intravenous line, and replace fluid and electrolyte deficits and continuing losses.
Type and crossmatch blood if operation is anticipated.

TABLE 2
Etiologic Classification of Acquired Mechanical Intestinal Obstruction

Intraluminal
Polyp
Tumor
Feces (impaction, meconium ileus equivalent)
Bezoar
Intussusception
Foreign body
Parasites

Intramural
Stricture (anastomotic, Crohn's disease, necrotizing enterocolitis)
Tumor
Pyloric stenosis
Hematoma

Extrinsic
Postoperative adhesions
Adhesions from other causes (appendicitis, primary peritonitis)
Hernia (internal, external)
Volvulus (gastric, midgut, colonic)
Tumor

The decision to operate is based on clinical judgment and cannot be made on the basis of radiographs or blood tests alone. The consequences of delay include necrosis and perforation and may necessitate a massive bowel resection and lead to local or systemic sepsis. Immediate operation is indicated if strangulation is suspected by fever, tachycardia, or signs of peritonitis. Perhaps the most reliable indication of strangulation is severe, unremitting pain that persists in spite of nasogastric tube decompression.

Conservative or nonoperative therapy can be attempted for 6 to 12 hours in early, simple mechanical obstructions, especially partial or early postoperative obstructions (within 3 weeks of a previous laparotomy) and in children with recurrent small bowel obstructions. Operation can be delayed in pyloric or duodenal obstructions provided that malrotation and volvulus can be ruled out. Operation can be avoided completely in most infants with ileocolic intussusception provided that it is completely reduced by air or hydrostatic pressure.

MECHANICAL OBSTRUCTION

Classification

Mechanical obstructions may have congenital or acquired causes. Congenital causes may present in the neonatal period, as in duodenal or jejunal atresia, or later, as in malrotation, duodenal web, or Hirschsprung's disease.

The acquired mechanical intestinal obstructions are classified by etiology in Table 2.

Pathophysiology

Simple Obstruction

In all forms of mechanical obstruction, intestinal contents accumulate proximal to the site of obstruction. The bowel distends with swallowed air, ingested liquids and solids, GI secretions, CO_2 from neutralized HCO^-, and other gases produced by bacterial fermentation. Vomiting ensues because of retrograde flow of gas and fluid into the stomach or by reflux from distention of the distal gut. The combination of these external and internal losses of water and electrolytes results in hypovolemia, tachycardia, decreased central venous pressure, oliguria, azotemia, and hemoconcentration. Gut distention may also impair normal ventilation by limiting diaphragmatic excursion. However, provided that gut ischemia and necrosis do not develop, a patient may survive with a complete bowel obstruction for many days or even weeks as long as maintenance and replacement water and electrolytes are given intravenously.

Although the small bowel normally contains few bacteria, these proliferate rapidly in the presence of obstruction and the small bowel contents become feculent. In simple obstructions, this is of little clinical significance.

Strangulating Obstruction

In strangulating obstructions, all of the sequelae of simple obstruction occur. In addition, there is loss of blood, especially plasma, into the compromised bowel, leading more rapidly to shock. When strangulation progresses to gangrene, local peritonitis develops; if free perforation ensues, peritonitis becomes generalized.

The normal gut mucosal barrier may be damaged and toxins from the intraluminal bacteria and from the ischemic or gangrenous bowel itself enter the peritoneal fluid and circulation.

Specific Causes of Intestinal Obstruction

Gastric Volvulus

Gastric volvulus is most common in newborn infants, although it may occur in later childhood, especially in the mentally retarded. It may occur in association with a diaphragmatic hernia (Morgagni's or Bochdalek's) or paraesophageal hiatal hernia. The stomach twists, either on its long axis (organoaxial) or its mesentery (mesenteroaxial). If the diagnosis is delayed, gangrene and perforation of the stomach may ensue.

The clinical picture may be acute or chronic. It includes vomiting, respiratory distress, and occasionally difficulty in passing a nasogastric tube. In plain radiographs there is massive distention of the stomach and an abnormal stomach bubble that may be partly within the thorax. Contrast studies may reveal a bird's beak deformity just below the diaphragm. The definitive treatment is emergency surgical reduction and gastropexy with repair of any associated diaphragmatic hernia.

Duodenal Hematoma

Duodenal hematoma results from bleeding into the bowel wall, usually in the second or third part of the duodenum. The most common cause is a direct blow from a blunt object

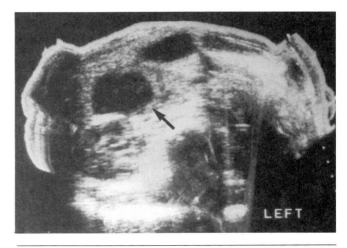

FIGURE 2 Abdominal ultrasonogram from a 7-year-old-boy who fell on his bicycle handlebars. The duodenal hematoma is the lucent area anterior to the right kidney indicated by the arrow.

such as a bicycle handlebar, fist, or hockey stick. The blood clot that accumulates in the bowel wall obstructs the lumen. The diagnosis can be confirmed by ultrasonography (Fig. 2) or upper intestinal contrast radiography (Fig. 3). Treatment includes gastric decompression and intravenous fluids. Most cases will resolve spontaneously in a few days. Total parenteral nutrition may be needed if the obstruction does not resolve in 2 or 3 days. Operation is seldom, if ever, required.

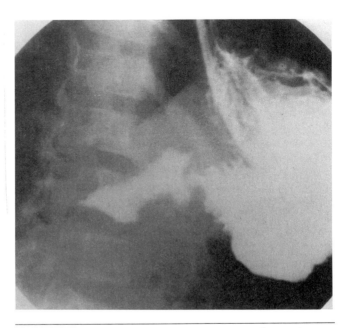

FIGURE 3 Upper gastrointestinal contrast radiography series from the patient shown in Figure 2. Note complete obstruction in the second part of the duodenum.

Superior Mesenteric Artery Syndrome

Superior mesenteric artery (SMA) syndrome, also called cast syndrome, Wilkie's syndrome, duodenal ileus, and arteriomesenteric duodenal compression syndrome, is an uncommon but important cause of extrinsic duodenal obstruction in children. The point of obstruction is in the third part of the duodenum where it sweeps anteriorly over the spine at L2 posterior to the SMA.

The SMA syndrome usually occurs in older children and adolescents. Predisposing factors include rapid linear growth without weight gain, scoliosis, spinal surgery (especially for scoliosis), weight loss, the supine position, confinement to bed (especially in a body cast), and an abnormally high position of the ligament of Treitz. The exact mechanism is unknown.

Symptoms may be acute or chronic. Typically, there is mild abdominal pain, anorexia, nausea, and voluminous but infrequent bilious vomiting. Abdominal examination may reveal a succussion splash. The differential diagnosis includes anorexia nervosa and bulimia.

Plain radiographs may be normal, especially after the patient has vomited, but they may show a distended stomach with food residue and an air-fluid level. The diagnosis can be confirmed by upper intestinal contrast films (Fig. 4).

Treatment begins with nasogastric decompression and intravenous fluids. The patient should be encouraged to remain upright or lie prone or semiprone with the left side down. Metoclopramide may help. If this treatment fails, a soft nasojejunal feeding tube can be placed beyond the ligament

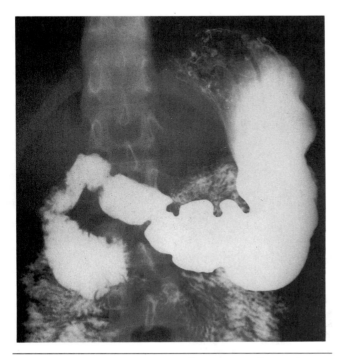

FIGURE 4 Upper gastrointestinal contrast radiography series from a 15-year-old girl with superior mesenteric artery (SMA) syndrome. Note partial obstruction in the third part of the duodenum.

TABLE 3
Causes of Intestinal Obstruction in Children

Pyloric stenosis	25%
Intussusception	18%
Atresia	15%
Incarcerated hernia	11%
Imperforate anus	8%
Hirschsprung's disease	6%
Postoperative adhesions	5%
Malrotation	5%
Meconium plug	3%
Meconium ileus	3%
Annular pancreas	1%
Meckel's diverticulum	1%

From Janik JS, et al.[4]

of Treitz under fluoroscopic control and a standard liquid diet started. Nasogastric losses can be replaced via the nasojejunal tube, but total parenteral nutrition is seldom indicated. This treatment may be continued at home until the obstruction resolves spontaneously.

Very rarely operative treatment by Ladd's procedure to move the duodenum out from under the SMA is required.

Postoperative Adhesions

Adhesions form within the peritoneal cavity after almost any laparotomy, especially for inflammatory conditions such as appendicitis, ulcerative colitis, and Crohn's disease. They tend to occur in areas of ischemia or serosal damage. There is no reliable way of preventing them. In 5 percent or less of cases, adhesions cause a postoperative bowel obstruction. Janik et al reviewed a series of adhesive obstructions treated by operation at a large children's hospital over an 11-year period.[4] Adhesions ranked seventh in the list of causes of intestinal obstruction (Table 3).

In the report of Janik et al, 80 percent of adhesive obstructions occurred within 2 years of the previous laparotomy. Wilkins and Spitz followed up a large series of children who had undergone laparotomy in the newborn period.[5] Postoperative adhesive obstructions occurred in 8 percent of cases, 75 percent within 6 months and 90 percent within 12 months of the initial surgery. Because of the apparently high incidence, these authors warn parents and general practitioners of this possibility for all neonates who undergo laparotomy.

In Janik's series, the most common preceding procedures were for appendicitis, ulcerative colitis, Wilms' tumor and other neoplasms, intussusception, Meckel's diverticulum, gastroesophageal reflux, malrotation, congenital diaphragmatic hernia, and gastroschisis, in that order. In the neonatal follow-up report by Wilkins and Spitz, the most common previous operations were for gastroschisis and malrotation.

Most cases can be diagnosed clinically and confirmed by plain radiographs. Initial treatment is resuscitation as outlined above. The most difficult point in managing patients with adhesive obstructions is to decide if and when operation is indicated. Many, perhaps the majority, resolve without operation.[4] On the other hand, the morbidity and mortality

TABLE 4
Guide to Therapy of Adhesive Bowel Obstruction

Factors Favoring Early Operation	Factors Favoring Nonoperative Therapy
Severe pain	Early presentation
Late presentation (>3 weeks postop)	Multiple previous obstructions
Tachycardia, fever	Pain relieved by nasogastric drainage
Localized tenderness, guarding	Partial obstruction
Leukocytosis	Crohn's disease

rise sharply if strangulation, for which there is no reliable marker, occurs. If operation is delayed, the morbidity and mortality rise even higher. In the end, the decision to operate depends on the judgment of the surgeon.

Several clinical and radiologic factors summarized in Table 4 can be used as a guide to treatment even though none is foolproof.

Operation is indicated if the patient does not improve significantly in 6 to 12 hours. Because the bowel may be opened during the operation (deliberately or inadvertently), prophylactic antibiotics, such as gentamicin and clindamycin or metronidazole in combination or cefoxitin, which are effective against intestinal flora, should be given before operation to reduce the risk of postoperative infections.

The operations performed and wound infection rates from Janik's series are summarized in Table 5. These data reinforce the increased morbidity associated with strangulation and the need for bowel resection.

Intussusception

Intussusception is the invagination of a part of the intestine into itself. It is the second most common cause of intestinal obstruction in children after pyloric stenosis. Most intussusceptions start near the ileocecal junction, but a few begin elsewhere in the small bowel or colon. The male-to-female ratio is about 3:2. The peak incidence is in early infancy; about two-thirds of cases occur in the first year, but it can present in older children.[6] It can also occur in the fetus and may present as an atresia in the newborn.

Most cases are called idiopathic because there is no obvious predisposing lesion or lead point. Some may be due to hypertrophied Peyer's patches in the ileum caused by viral infections (most often adenovirus) that act as lead points. There are many other specific causes, which are listed in Table 6. Lead points are more common in older children.[6]

The most common type of intussusception is ileocolic, but some are ileoileocolic, jejunojejunal, jejunoileal, or colocolic. More than 90 percent occur near the ileocecal valve. Intussusceptions cause compression of the intramural and mesenteric veins, leading to edema and hemorrhage in the bowel wall. Eventually, arterial inflow is impaired and ischemia and infarction follow.

The typical patient is a previously healthy infant who develops severe abdominal colic, at 15- to 20-minute intervals with drawing up of the legs and pallor, separated by periods of apathy and followed by vomiting, passage of "currant-jelly" stool, and a sausage-shaped abdominal mass. However, by no means are all cases typical. Almost all older patients present with pain, but some younger infants (up to 20 percent) have no obvious pain at all. About one-third do not pass blood or mucus, and one-third have no palpable abdominal mass. Many older children have pain alone without other symptoms or signs.[6] The differential diagnosis includes gastroenteritis and other forms of obstruction, including malrotation with volvulus. Henoch-Schönlein purpura should be considered in older children.

When the diagnosis of intussusception is suspected, the first step is to resuscitate the patient with intravenous fluids and drain the stomach with a nasogastric tube. Occasionally, children present with symptoms of only 1 or 2 hours' duration without any vomiting. The intravenous and nasogastric tube can be omitted in such cases. Plain radiographs are not required. When the child is considered fit for operation, should

TABLE 5
Procedures and Morbidity in Adhesive Obstruction

Procedure	Wound Abscess Rate
Enterolysis only (74%)	4%
Enterolysis and resection (16%)	22%
Enterolysis and enterotomy (<8%)	30%
Enterolysis and repair of perforation (<3%)	50%

From Janik et al.[4]

TABLE 6
Specific Causes of Intussusception

Meckel's diverticulum
Lymphoma or other neoplasm
Henoch-Schönlein purpura
Polyps (Peutz-Jeghers syndrome, juvenile polyps)
Ectopic pancreas
Duplication
Intramural hematoma (hemophilia)
Cystic fibrosis (inspissated stool)
Hemangioma
Ventriculoperitoneal shunt
Intestinal parasites

that be necessary, he or she is taken to radiology for a contrast enema under fluoroscopic guidance to confirm the diagnosis and attempt nonoperative reduction by hydrostatic pressure through a barium column or air pressure.[7,8] The surgeon should attend. Recently, we have switched to pneumatic reduction because it is quicker (requires less fluoroscopy time), less messy, and possibly safer if a perforation should occur. Manometric control of pneumatic reduction is essential. Nonoperative reduction should be attempted in older children as well, because most cases are still idiopathic even though a lead point is more common than in infants.

The main risk of hydrostatic or pneumatic reduction is perforation of the bowel, which occurs in 1 percent or less of cases, usually in the intussuscipiens and often in the transverse colon. The risk of perforation is greatest in infants less than 6 months of age with histories of 3 days or longer. A successful reduction is indicated by the free flow of contrast into the small bowel, a "whooshing" sound on auscultation during pneumatic reduction, relief of symptoms, or disappearance of the abdominal mass.

Nonoperative reduction is successful in more than 75 percent of cases. The risk of recurrence after such a reduction is about 10 percent. Successful nonoperative reduction usually means there is no lead point, although there have been a few cases of successful hydrostatic reduction in patients who were found later to have a lead point. Each recurrence should be treated as if it were the first episode; multiple occurrences are not an indication for operation, provided that each reduction is complete.

Following successful reduction, the patient should be admitted to hospital for 12 to 24 hours of observation. Prior to discharge, the parents should be told of the risk of recurrence. When the reduction is incomplete or when a persistent filling defect indicating a mass lesion is noted, operation is indicated. An exception to this rule may be made when the filling defect is thought to be due to edema in the area of the ileocecal valve. In such cases, an ultrasonographic or repeat colon examination in a few days should be done; if normal, operation can be omitted.

Intravenous antibiotics should be given before operation. We attempt manual reduction at operation in most cases but perform resection and primary anastomosis if that is not possible or if a lead point is seen or palpated in the involved bowel. The risk of recurrence is about 1 percent after manual reduction and virtually nonexistent after resection.

Ein reviewed 1,200 cases of intussusception treated at a single institution over 40 years.[9] Sixty-five had pathologic lead points, of which only 11 were lymphomas. All of these were more than 3 years of age; nine of the 11 had been ill for more than 1 week, had lost weight, and had palpable abdominal masses. Only one underwent reduction hydrostatically, but there was a residual filling defect in the cecum. This report suggests that there is no reason to fear missing a lymphoma in cases that are reduced completely without any residual radiologic abnormality.

Postoperative Intussusception

Postoperative small bowel intussusception (usually jejunojejunal) is an uncommon but insidious cause of intestinal obstruction. It usually involves the small bowel alone and occurs within 2 weeks of a previous laparotomy. Typically, the patient does well for several days and may even resume oral intake. Abdominal cramps, anorexia, vomiting, and distention develop, suggesting a mechanical obstruction. It is difficult to diagnose a postoperative intussusception because it blends into the usual period of postoperative paralytic ileus; even when it is suspected, it is difficult to prove radiologically. The best diagnostic procedure is an upper intestinal contrast series, although ultrasonography may help also. Treatment is by reoperation. Fortunately, strangulation is uncommon and most cases can be reduced manually.

Necrotizing Enterocolitis

This is a disease of newborns that results in inflammation and occasionally full-thickness necrosis of the bowel. In some cases, the bowel heals with fibrosis, which can produce one or more strictures, usually in the colon (70 percent) or distal ileum (15 percent). Most often, strictures form in defunctioned bowel distal to a previously constructed enterostomy, but they may develop slowly over some weeks or months in cases not previously operated upon. The diagnosis is usually confirmed by contrast enema examination of the bowel. Such a study of the defunctioned bowel is mandatory prior to closing a diverting ileostomy or colostomy.

The best treatment is elective resection and anastomosis, which can be combined with closure of the enterostomy.

Meconium Ileus Equivalent

Meconium ileus equivalent (MIE), sometimes called distal intestinal obstruction syndrome, is a type of intestinal obstruction that occurs only in patients with cystic fibrosis. Rubinstein distinguished MIE from constipation and defined the two conditions as follows[10]:

Constipation: An episode of abdominal cramps and decreased stool frequency that responds to laxatives.
MIE: A postneonatal partial or complete bowel obstruction characterized by severe abdominal pain and radiologic signs of obstruction.

MIE occurs in up to 15 percent of all cystic fibrosis patients, mainly in adolescents and adults. It may be acute, subacute, or chronic and recurring. Caused in part by pancreatic exocrine insufficiency, MIE is more common in patients with poorly controlled steatorrhea. It may be precipitated by eating binges. A thick layer of mucus forms over the small bowel mucosa to which the luminal contents adhere. MIE is not more common in patients who were born with true meconium ileus.

The clinical features of MIE include crampy abdominal pain, a change in stooling habit, abdominal distention, and a right lower quadrant abdominal mass. There may be a history of excess fluid loss from a respiratory infection, exercise, or hot weather. The patient may have failed to take his or her pancreatic enzymes as prescribed. Radiographs show increased amounts of gas and stool in the small bowel and a ground glass appearance or bubbly mass of stool, usually in the right lower quadrant. The differential diagnosis includes appendicitis, intussusception, and volvulus.

The incidence of MIE can be minimized by taking large quantities of fluids by mouth, a high-residue diet including bulk-forming laxatives as required, plenty of physical exercise, and optimal doses of pancreatic enzymes.

When MIE occurs, conventional treatment regimens include nasogastric drainage, intravenous fluids, and enemas. Some authorities recommend instillation of 10 percent acetylcysteine (30 ml of a 20 percent solution in normal saline every 4 to 8 hours), pancreatic enzymes, Gastrografin,[11] and polyethylene glycol (PEG)[12] down the nasogastric tube. Between 50 and 100 ml of Gastrografin diluted fourfold in water or juice is given.[11] This method is contraindicated in the presence of dehydration, prolonged or complete obstruction, peritonitis, or iodine sensitivity, and in children less than 5 years of age. PEG is given after an intravenous dose of metaclopramide (5 to 10 mg) at a rate of 750 to 1,000 ml per hour to a total of 5 to 6 liters.[12] It, too, is contraindicated in the face of prolonged or complete obstruction or signs of peritonitis.

Colonic Volvulus

Volvulus, or twisting of the colon, usually the transverse or sigmoid, may cause acute or subacute colonic obstruction. It occurs in mentally retarded children, often in association with aerophagia and chronic constipation. In fact, colonic volvulus is a significant cause of death in the mentally handicapped. Roy and Simon recently reported that acute obstruction caused approximately 6 percent of 260 deaths in a series of mentally handicapped patients in England.[13] Of these, sigmoid volvulus was the single most common cause. Excessive length of the colon may be a contributing factor. Because the colon twists, strangulation and perforation may develop. Typically, the patient develops bilious vomiting and marked gaseous abdominal distention.

Plain radiographs show massively dilated loops of bowel. Contrast enema examination of the colon reveals a "beak" deformity at the site of the twist.

The best treatment is endoscopic decompression by flexible or rigid sigmoidoscopy or colonoscopy, followed by elective resection of the bowel; if decompression is unsuccessful, emergency colectomy usually with a temporary colostomy is required.

Roundworms

Roundworm (*Ascaris lumbricoides*) infestation, usually of the ileum, is common in pediatric practice in tropical and subtropical countries. It is a frequent cause of intestinal colic. At the Pediatric Surgery Department of the Medical College of Calcutta, roundworm boluses are the most common cause of small bowel obstruction.[14]

Treatment is controversial. Some authorities advocate immediate operation, whereas others advise medical therapy, reserving surgery for those who fail to improve. Sarkar et al[14] treated 34 cases with antispasmodics, intravenous fluids, nasogastric suction, and anthelmintics (piperazine citrate 75 mg per kilogram intravenously once daily on days two and

three). Twenty-nine were relieved on this regimen with passage of the worms per rectum. Five required surgery, two of whom died. Other factors such as bands or adhesions contributed to failure of medical therapy.

PARALYTIC ILEUS

Paralytic ileus is a type of intestinal obstruction caused by failure of the normal peristaltic motor function of the small intestine. It occurs to at least some degree after most abdominal operations, but in the absence of peritonitis the small bowel is not usually affected. It may be caused by local factors such as peritonitis, ischemia or surgical manipulation of the bowel, retroperitoneal hemorrhage, operation or inflammation, fractures of the spine, pneumonia, or systemic factors including hypokalemia, drugs (vincristine), systemic sepsis, uremia, diabetic ketoacidosis, and myxedema.

Paralytic ileus is an acute, usually self-limiting, condition; it should be distinguished from chronic intestinal pseudo-obstruction. The latter is a rare disorder also caused by abnormal gut motility of unknown cause and characterized by recurrent attacks of abdominal pain, distention, vomiting, weight loss, and a tendency to wax and wane. Although the causes differ, the pathophysiologic effects are similar to those of mechanical obstruction except that strangulation is rare. The diagnosis is usually made on clinical grounds. The problem is to differentiate it from a mechanical obstruction. A key feature of paralytic ileus is the absence of bowel sounds.

Radiologic studies may help to distinguish mechanical obstruction from paralytic ileus. Typically, there is gas throughout the bowel, including the colon and rectum in paralytic ileus. Mechanical obstructions cause progressive bowel distention, with distended proximal and collapsed distal segments. Ultrasound may also help to differentiate the two.[3]

Paralytic ileus usually resolves spontaneously on conservative therapy, which should include intravenous fluids and nasogastric decompression.

REFERENCES

1. Diethelm AG. The acute abdomen. In: Sabiston DC Jr, ed. Textbook of surgery. 13th ed. Philadelphia: WB Saunders, 1986: 790.
2. Mucha P Jr. Small intestinal obstruction. Surg Clin North Am 1987; 67:597–620.
3. Meiser G, Meissner K. Ileus and intestinal obstruction— ultrasonographic findings as a guideline to therapy. Hepatogastroenterology 1987; 34:194–199.
4. Janik JS, Ein SH, Filler RM, et al. An assessment of the surgical treatment of adhesive small bowel obstruction in infants and children. J Pediatr Surg 1981; 16:225–229.
5. Wilkins BM, Spitz L. Incidence of postoperative adhesion obstruction following neonatal laparotomy. Br J Surg 1986; 73:762–764.
6. Schuh S, Wesson DE. Intussusception in children two years of age and older. Can Med Assoc J 1987; 136:269–272.
7. Tamanaha K, Wimbish K, Talwalka YB, Ashimine K. Air reduction of intussusception in infants and children. J Pediatr 1987; 3:733–736.
8. She YX. Treatment of intestinal intussusception with particular emphasis reduction by colonic insufflation. Report of 5110 cases. Chir Pediatr 1982; 23:373–378.
9. Ein SH, Stephens CA, Shandling B, Filler RM. Intussusception due to lymphoma. J Pediatr Surg 1986; 21:786–788.

10. Rubinstein S, Moss R, Lewiston N. Constipation and meconium ileus equivalent in patients with cystic fibrosis. Pediatrics 1986; 78:473–479.
11. O'Halloran SM, Gilbert J, McKendrick OM, et al. Gastrograffin in acute meconium ileus equivalent. Arch Dis Child 1986; 61:1128–1130.
12. Cleghorn GJ, Stringer DA, Forstner GG, Durie PR. Treatment of distal intestinal obstruction syndrome in cystic fibrosis with a balanced intestinal lavage solution. Lancet 1986; i:8–10.
13. Roy A, Simon GB. Intestinal obstruction as a cause of death in the mentally handicapped. J Ment Defic Res 1987; 31:193–197.
14. Sarkar PK, Pan GD, Bhowmick PK. Management of roundworm obstruction in light of pathogenesis. J Indian Med Assoc 1987; 85:5–8.

PART

4

Hernias

David Wesson, M.D.

A hernia is an abnormal protrusion of an organ or part of an organ through structures that normally contain it. The types of hernias that involve the intestine are listed in Table 1. Of the external hernias, the most common are indirect inguinal hernias; these are especially common in boys. An incarcerated hernia is one that cannot be reduced easily. Incarceration often leads to strangulation. In a strangulated hernia, the blood supply to the herniated organ is impaired. This leads to infarction if the hernia is not reduced promptly by either taxis or surgery. The risk of incarceration and strangulation of inguinal hernias is greatest in the first few months of life. Femoral hernias are relatively more common in girls than in boys. Although commonly observed in black children, umbilical hernias in childhood are of cosmetic significance only.

DIAPHRAGMATIC HERNIA

Of the internal hernias, diaphragmatic hernias that occur through a patent foramen of Bochdalek, usually on the left, are the most important.[1] Because they are associated often with pulmonary hypoplasia, they have a significant mortality rate. The herniated viscera usually include the small bowel, colon, stomach, spleen, and part of the liver. The most common presentation is acute respiratory failure in the newborn. The mortality rate is around 50 percent, largely because of the underlying pulmonary hypoplasia. In later childhood, Bochdalek hernias are often asymptomatic, but they may present with dyspnea, intermittent abdominal pain, or vomiting if the bowel becomes obstructed at the site of herniation or if it undergoes volvulus. Physical examination may reveal decreased breath sounds over the involved thorax and dullness to percussion. Congenital diaphragmatic hernias (CDH) may even be detected serendipitously by chest radiography.

Plain radiographic examinations usually suggest the diagnosis, although congenital diaphragmatic hernia may be difficult to distinguish from an eventration of the diaphragm or an adenomatoid malformation of the lung. In such cases, contrast studies of the gastrointestinal (GI) tract from either above or below may be helpful in confirming the diagnosis.

In all cases of congenital posterolateral diaphragmatic hernia, the treatment is surgical repair, usually through an abdominal incision after the patient has been stabilized. No longer is the patient rushed to the operating room. The viscera are reduced into the abdomen, and the diaphragm is repaired with interrupted sutures. Malrotation of the midgut occurs in all cases but does not require any specific treatment.

Hernias through the foramen of Morgagni, which is a defect in the diaphragm between the xiphisternal and costal parts of the diaphragm, are very rare. They account for only 1 to 2 percent of all CDH. The sac may contain part of the colon, small bowel, or, less often, the liver. They are often asymptomatic and may be recognized incidentally on chest radiography. They may cause acute obstruction and even strangulation of the involved bowel, and rarely they may cause cardiac tamponade by compressing the heart. For these reasons, this type of anterior CDH should also be repaired operatively.

Some diaphragmatic hernias are acquired as the result of blunt trauma from automobile accidents, blows to the abdo-

TABLE 1
Classification of Hernias of the Intestines

External	Internal
Inguinal	Diaphragmatic
Indirect	Bochdalek
Direct	Morgagni
Femoral	Abdominal wall
Umbilical	Spigelian
Incisional	Other
Obturator	Mesenteric
Lumbar	Paraduodenal

men, and falls. This type of hernia, which occurs more often on the left than on the right, usually is evident on plain radiography, although it may be difficult to recognize in the early postinjury period. Any opacity above the left diaphragm that appears after blunt abdominal trauma should be viewed with suspicion. The risk of strangulation in post-traumatic diaphragmatic hernias is considerably greater, so they should be repaired promptly.

Hiatal hernias are another subgroup of diaphragmatic hernia. They can be divided into sliding and rolling hernias. The latter are also called paraesophageal hernias. This type of hernia may be associated with gastroesophageal reflux, but, perhaps more important, the paraesophageal type may cause gastric volvulus or become incarcerated and present with obstruction to swallowing and occasionally gangrene and perforation of the involved portion of the stomach. These hernias are discussed elsewhere in this book.

UMBILICAL HERNIA

Umbilical hernias are common in otherwise healthy newborns, especially prematures.[2] They are 5 to 10 times more common in blacks than in whites. Also they are more common in children with Beckwith-Wiedemann syndrome, in those with Hurler's syndrome, and in patients with trisomy 13 or 18. They occur through a defect in the fascia at the umbilical ring. Often they are apparent only when the baby cries or strains; even a small fascial defect will allow a large amount of bowel to protrude through it, causing a significant swelling that is covered only by the skin of the umbilicus. Most umbilical hernias close spontaneously during the first 12 to 24 months of life. The risk of incarceration or strangulation in infancy is negligible. Although umbilical hernias are more prominent when the baby cries, they rarely cause pain. Rupture of the overlying skin is virtually unheard of. For these reasons, observation alone is appropriate in the first 2 or 3 years of life. If an umbilical hernia persists beyond that age, it is unlikely to resolve and should be repaired for cosmetic reasons and to prevent incarceration later in life.

INGUINAL HERNIA

In inguinal hernias, the most common condition requiring surgery in childhood, the involved viscus, which is usually the bowel or omentum in boys but often the ovary or fallopian tube in girls, protrudes into a patent processus vaginalis testis along the inguinal canal.[3-5] In indirect inguinal hernias, which are far more common in children than direct hernias, the bowel follows the course of the processus vaginalis testis through the internal ring, lateral to the inferior epigastric vessels. In direct hernias, the bowel enters the canal through its posterior wall medial to the inferior epigastric vessels.

Among patients with inguinal hernias, boys outnumber girls 6 to 1. The incidence is higher in premature infants, those with connective tissue disorders (e.g., Ehlers-Danlos syndrome), bladder exstrophy, ascites, and ventriculoperitoneal shunts and those undergoing peritoneal dialysis. The incidence

is approximately 1 in every 50 live male births. There is a familial tendency for hernia formation. Sixty percent are on the right, 25 percent on the left, and 15 percent bilateral.

If the processus vaginalis testis fails to obliterate after the testis descends at approximately the eighth month of fetal life, a potential hernia exists, although, strictly speaking, the diagnosis of hernia can be made only when something protrudes into the sac. The incidence of patent processus vaginalis is much higher than the incidence of inguinal hernia. Whether a hernia develops depends in part on the diameter of the patent processus. If it is large enough to accept an abdominal viscus, a hernia is likely; when it is too narrow for this, it may accept some fluid, which can lead to the formation of a hydrocele of the tunica vaginalis testis or of the spermatic cord. Hydroceles, in contrast to hernias, do not come and go, have no mass or swelling proximally along the spermatic cord, and are not easily reducible. Complete hernias extend down to the tunica vaginalis testis in the scrotum, whereas incomplete hernias extend only part way along the cord. However, incarceration can occur with either type.

Typically, there is a history of an intermittent swelling in the groin, which extends toward or into the scrotum and tends to appear when the baby cries or strains. Most often, there is no apparent discomfort associated with the presence of the bulge. The best way to confirm the diagnosis on physical examination is to see and feel the herniated viscus or fluid in the sac and to feel its reduction by gentle taxis. The silk glove sign and thickening of the cord by palpation are unreliable diagnostic signs.

The differential diagnosis includes hydrocele, femoral hernia, an undescended testicle in the inguinal canal (always check the position of the ipsilateral testicle when examining a child for a hernia), and an inflamed lymph gland above the inguinal ligament. In the latter situation, there may be an irreducible mass in the groin that is very difficult to distinguish from an incarcerated inguinal hernia. Typically, this type of lymphadenitis occurs early in infancy. There may be a history of previous or co-existent infection of the umbilical cord stump. There is no history of anorexia or vomiting and no thickening or swelling of the spermatic cord or testicle on the ipsilateral side.

If it is not possible to demonstrate the hernia on examination, it is better to re-examine the baby than to operate on the basis of the history alone. Herniography is an alternative diagnostic test that is seldom used except in older children in the differential diagnosis of obscure inguinal pain.

Once the diagnosis is confirmed, the treatment is surgical repair under general anesthesia. Because the risk of incarceration is greatest in early infancy, there is no reason to delay operation in otherwise healthy children even in the first week or two of life. Most often, the surgery can be performed on an outpatient basis. The only exceptions to this recommendation are patients with other medical conditions that make anesthesia risky, including extreme prematurity and severe cardiac or respiratory disease. In such patients, repair of asymptomatic hernias may be delayed.

The symptoms of incarceration include irritability, loss of appetite, abdominal pain, and vomiting. On examination, there is a tender mass in the inguinal canal, which may transilluminate. Often, there is edema of the distal spermatic cord and testis. On rectal examination, the herniated viscus may be palpable entering the inguinal canal. In most infants, an incarcerated hernia strangulates in a matter of hours, leading to infarction of the ipsilateral testis and the contained viscus. The testis is at risk because the spermatic vessels run along the cord beside the sac and may be obstructed by the hernia. Necrosis of the incarcerated bowel in children is quite rare. In girls, the ovary may be chronically incarcerated without strangulation.

The initial treatment of an incarcerated hernia is reduction by taxis after sedating the baby in the Trendelenburg position for 1½ to 2 hours. If reduction is successful, the baby should be admitted to hospital for repair in approximately 48 hours when the edema has partially resolved. If reduction is unsuccessful, the baby should be taken to the operating room immediately for surgical repair.

OTHER HERNIAS

Femoral hernias are the next most common type of groin hernia after indirect inguinal hernias. They occur through the femoral canal medial to the femoral vein, posterior to the in-guinal ligament, and lateral to the lacunar ligament. Clinically, the swelling appears below the inguinal ligament.

Direct inguinal hernias are even rarer in children. I have seen two cases personally, one in a boy with chronic cough due to cystic fibrosis.

REFERENCES

1. Anderson KD. Congenital diaphragmatic hernia. In: Welch KJ, et al, eds. Pediatric surgery. 4th ed. Chicago: Year Book Medical Publishers, 1986: 589.
2. Shaw A. Disorders of the umbilicus. In: Welch KJ, et al, eds. Pediatric surgery. 4th ed. Chicago: Year Book Medical Publishers, 1986: 735.
3. Rowe MI, Lloyd DA. Inguinal hernia. In: Welch KJ, et al, eds. Pediatric surgery. 4th ed. Chicago: Year Book Medical Publishers, 1986: 735.
4. Solomon JR. Inguinal hernias and hydroceles. In: Jones PG, Woodward AA, eds. Clinical pediatric surgery. 3rd ed. London: Blackwell, 1986: 305.
5. Leape LL. Inguinal hernia. In: Leape LL. Patient care in pediatric surgery. Boston: Little, Brown & Co, 1987: 373.

PART 5

Peritonitis

Barry Shandling, M.B., Ch.B., F.R.C.S.(Eng.), FRCSC, F.A.C.S.

MECONIUM PERITONITIS

Pathophysiology

Meconium peritonitis results from an antenatal escape of meconium into the peritoneal cavity, usually as a consequence of a malformation leading to intestinal obstruction.[1,2] The condition is not likely to develop before the 3rd month of gestation, but it has been documented at as early as 24 weeks of fetal life. Histologic evidence supports the hypothesis that vascular insufficiency may result in bowel wall perforation without prior intestinal obstruction.[1] A temporary decrease of mesenteric blood flow could lead to intestinal atresia and/or meconium peritonitis. Causes of intestinal obstruction that may result in peritonitis in utero include atresia (10 to 25 percent),[3] volvulus, stenosis, cystic fibrosis (15 percent) with meconium ileus, and Hirschsprung's disease. The condition also has been associated with intussusception, vascular insufficiency, duplication, and Meckel's diverticulum,[4] but in up to 28 percent there is no detectable cause.[3]

Meconium consists of liquor amnii, which contains squamous cells from the skin and even hair, bile salts and pig-ments, pancreatic and intestinal secretions, mucus, cholesterol, uric acid, ions, and glucose. The enzymes and bile salts are particularly irritating, causing inflammation of the peritoneal cavity that will vary in severity depending on the amount of the leak and its duration. Hilgier[5] has shown in newborn guinea pigs a rapid proliferative fibroblastic reaction to meconium. A localized pseudocyst may form around the perforation and meconium, or inflammation may be generalized.[6] These cysts, which may be small or huge, can contain gas if the perforation persists after birth, or there may be free intraperitoneal air. As the lesion progresses, granulomas and calcification may develop; if the processus vaginalis is not obliterated, leading to unilateral or bilateral scrotal masses, the inflammatory process together with meconium may surround the testis.

Calcification is found in 65 percent of cases, with calcified areas surrounded by foreign body giant cells and phagocytic histiocytes. The loose, myxoid surrounding fibroconnective tissue may contain scattered fibroblasts, histiocytes, and chronic inflammatory cells. Patients with meconium peritonitis without cystic fibrosis are more likely to have calcification present.[7]

Clinical Features

Associated anomalies were reported in less than 10 percent of Santulli's series of 77 patients, 13 of whom weighed less than 2,000 g.[8] There may be prenatal polyhydramnios, depending on the level of the intestinal obstruction, and in most newborn infants clinical features of intestinal obstruction, bilious vomiting, abdominal distention, and failure to pass meconium are apparent. One has operated upon children beyond the newborn period with dense adhesive intestinal obstruction but without an illness during postnatal life to account for this finding. Probably these patients had meconium peritonitis. When there is scrotal or inguinal swelling, the diagnoses of testicular teratoma, gonadoblastoma, Leydig cell tumors, fibrous pseudotumors, calcinosis, and endodermal sinus tumors must be considered.

Plain films of the abdomen may show localized or diffuse intra-abdominal calcification with or without free air. In the presence of intestinal obstruction there will be distention of loops of bowel with multiple air-liquid levels. Prenatal ultrasonography may demonstrate dilated bowel cysts or hydrops fetalis.[7,10]

Management

Without intestinal obstruction meconium peritonitis may not require surgical intervention. If there is bowel obstruction but no concomitant unsealed perforation, there is no urgency but probably an operation will be necessary. Nasogastric suction must be commenced, electrolyte and fluid imbalance corrected, and the patient rendered fit for operation. If there is evidence of free intraperitoneal air there is somewhat more urgency to operate, but more will be lost by operating too soon than by preparing the patient adequately. The operation may be exceedingly difficult, with innumerable dense adhesions accompanied by considerable blood loss. Antibiotics should be given preoperatively. Operative treatment is aimed at sealing any perforation and relieving intestinal obstruction. In the absence of infection, primary resection and anastomosis may be feasible. With the presence of secondary bacterial peritonitis, especially in the case of premature infants, the establishment of temporary stomas coupled with total parenteral nutrition is well tolerated and advisable. Cysts may be evacuated, but heroic attempts at complete or partial excision are dangerous and unnecessary. Tibboel and Molenaar, in a review of 1,084 patients, have reported a constant mortality over the past 15 years of 55 percent.[1]

PRIMARY PERITONITIS

This condition is a highly uncommon cause of "acute abdomen" in childhood. Inflammation occurs within the peritoneal cavity in the absence of a demonstrable cause other than the microorganism involved. Most cases occur among children with chronic renal disease with or without ascites. Occasionally, a healthy child, usually a girl, may develop primary peritonitis, with the diagnosis usually being made at laparotomy. Pneumococci or streptococci are the usual causative organisms, but gram-negative bacilli and viruses may play a part. These latter cases of apparent spontaneous primary peritonitis usually occur in children less than 7 years of age.

The condition develops rapidly, within 48 hours, with symptoms of diffuse abdominal pain, vomiting, and abdominal distention. Pyrexia is greater than that found in appendicitis. On examination severe abdominal tenderness is either generalized or confined to the lower abdomen. There is no localized tenderness as a rule. Rigidity may be present with signs of adynamic ileus.

A polymorphonuclear cell leukocytosis is almost invariable. In children with renal disease the urinalysis and serum chemistry are appropriately abnormal.

Bacterial culture of a needle aspirate from the peritoneal cavity is safe and may save an ill child from an unnecessary operation. If gram-positive organisms are found, specific antibiotic treatment should be instituted and an operation is not necessary. Finding gram-negative bacteria, however, may not negate the necessity for laparotomy. At operation there is free fluid in the peritoneal cavity; this fluid may be clear or turbid. Inflammation of the peritoneal contents varies in severity. Examination of the appendix (which is usually removed) shows periappendicitis. With treatment of intravenously administered antibiotics the prognosis is excellent, and recovery takes place within a few days.

SECONDARY PERITONITIS

In the newborn infant the umbilicus may be the portal of entry of organisms into the peritoneum. Omphalitis may spread by contiguity to involve the parietal peritoneum. More often peritonitis results from gangrenous bowel, whether due to volvulus, necrotizing enterocolitis, or idiopathic gastric or intestinal perforation. In older children, by far the most common cause of peritonitis is a perforated appendix; less common causes are bowel perforation from peptic ulceration or inflammatory bowel disease, for example, and perforation of the extrahepatic biliary ducts, leading to the development of bile peritonitis.[3] Peritonitis can complicate ventriculoperitoneal or lumboperitoneal shunts in children with hydrocephalus.[1,2,4,11] With the increasing use of chronic ambulatory peritoneal dialysis, *Staphylococcus epidermidis* is a frequent contaminant of the peritoneal cavity, but any organism may be involved.[12]

The clinical picture of secondary peritonitis is similar to that of primary peritonitis, except that in cases of intestinal perforation there may be free air within the peritoneal cavity with hyper-resonance and decreased liver dullness. Roentgenograms of the abdomen show the presence of free air.

Management

All patients with generalized peritonitis must be adequately prepared for operation before and not during any operative treatment. Such preparation includes rapid rehydration and correction of electrolyte imbalance. The child with severe dehydration requires replacement of 10 to 15 percent of the body weight; it is wise to correct half this loss before embarking on any surgery. Several hours of preoperative preparation will reduce the incidence of major postoperative complications, especially acute tubular necrosis. Frequently the degree of underhydration is underestimated, with potentially disastrous complications. Preoperative resuscitation should include the administration of antibiotics. Those recommended are a combination of ampicillin, aminoglycoside, and metronidazole or clindamycin or one of the cephalosporins, e.g., cefoxitin.

ABSCESS

When the peritoneal inflammation is not generalized, it may take the form of a localized abscess or abscesses. Pus may collect around a perforated appendix, in the pelvis, or within the peritoneal cavity between loops of bowel or against the abdominal wall. Most dangerous are subphrenic abscesses, which can rupture through the diaphragm into the pleural space and lung.

The most frequently encountered abscess is associated with perforation of an inflamed appendix,[8] when the inflammation is walled off and confined to the immediate vicinity of the appendix. Usually the history in such patients is of symptoms of more than 48 hours' duration. In addition to abdominal pain, initially central and then radiating to the right lower quadrant, with or without anorexia, nausea, and vomiting, there may be high fever.

In some cases an obvious palpable tender mass in the right lower quadrant and even redness and edema of the overlying skin are found.

Pelvic abscess causes diarrhea with tenesmus, fever, ileus, and sometimes urinary symptoms including frequency and dysuria. On rectal examination there is a tender mass that may be indurated or soft and fluctuant.

Subphrenic suppuration may be accompanied by edema of the overlying skin and elevation of the hemidiaphragm, often with a "sympathetic" effusion in the ipsilateral pleural cavity. The liver may be displaced downward.

Localization of these subphrenic collections is difficult; ultrasonography and/or computed tomography is the most useful diagnostic modality, but gallium scan may be necessary to locate the lesion.

Management

Appendiceal Abscess. There is some controversy regarding the best treatment. The more conservative approach, to which I subscribe, is initially to keep the patient under close observation. If there are signs of bacteremia and/or high fever, it is best to give antibiotics by intravenous injection. Usually improvement follows with gradual remission of symptoms and signs, including shrinkage and finally disappearance of the mass. About 3 months later an interval appendectomy can be done with a minimum of morbidity.

If, under observation, the mass increases in size or if signs of generalized peritonitis develop, it is necessary to intervene surgically; however, this is rarely the case. The very fact that

an abscess did develop instead of generalized peritonitis is indicative of the body's ability to wall off and deal with the infection. More aggressive surgeons operate as soon as the abscess is diagnosed. They drain the abscess and attempt to remove the appendix at the same operation.

Pelvic Abscess. Here too, there is controversy. These abscesses either resolve or drain spontaneously. Often an episode of "diarrhea" is reported; actually this represents the spontaneous drainage of the abscess via the rectum. With drainage the high temperature plummets and the patient is relieved of all symptoms and signs. More aggressive surgeons drain the abscess via the rectum.

Intraperitoneal and Subphrenic Abscess. The advent of ultrasonographic imaging with its interventional potential has radically changed the management of intraperitoneal suppuration. The best current choice is needle aspiration of the contents of the abscess, which is done under ultrasonographic guidance, followed, if necessary, by a period of drainage via a catheter inserted into the abscess cavity.[9] Often, it is not necessary to operate in order to drain a subphrenic abscess.

ADHESIONS

Adhesions are of two types. Generalized adhesions are presumed to follow meconium peritonitis and may be so widespread and dense as to obliterate the peritoneal cavity. The most common localized congenital adhesion to be encountered is that which is found in association with a Meckel's diverticulum. It may even result in an attachment of the terminal ileum or Meckel's diverticulum to the parietal peritoneum at the back of the umbilicus. Around such an isolated band crossing the peritoneal cavity the intestine may become twisted with a volvulus with or without gangrene.

Ladd's bands are the condensation of peritonitis which are seen only in cases of malrotation of the midgut and may give rise to duodenal obstruction where they cross that organ. Familial Mediterranean fever, a form of polyserositis, can result in a peritoneal cavity laced with adhesions, a potential cause of adhesive intestinal obstruction. Chronic peritoneal dialysis and ventriculoperitoneal shunts, particularly those complicated by infection, may also eventually lead to the formation of fibrous adhesions in the peritoneal cavity.

As a rule, intraperitoneal adhesions are either innocuous and quite asymptomatic or give rise to intestinal obstruction with or without intestinal ischemia. Frequently physicians diagnose "adhesions" as the cause of chronic abdominal pain or constipation in children who have had previous abdominal operations. However, surgeons are convinced that adhesions rarely, if ever, cause chronic or recurrent abdominal pain.

Management

The extent of intraperitoneal inflammation should be minimized whenever possible. For example, whereas an appendectomy for nonperforated appendicitis may give rise to localized adhesion formation, a perforated appendix with generalized peritonitis may result in the generalized formation of adhesions. All forms of intraperitoneal inflammation should be vigorously and adequately treated. Rough handling by the operating surgeon only causes more inflammation of the delicate serous surfaces and guarantees that more adhesions will follow. It was hoped that corticosteroids might minimize the effects of inflammation within the peritoneal cavity, but this has never been shown to be the case.

If acute adhesive intestinal obstruction develops, an operation is necessary; the appropriate procedure is division (or lysis) of adhesions, with or without resection of nonviable intestine, and end-to-end anastomosis or an enterostomy.

REFERENCES

1. Tibboel D, Molenaar JC. Meconium peritonitis—a retrospective, prognostic analysis of 69 patients. Z Kinderchir 1984; 39:25–28.
2. Forouhar F. Meconium peritonitis. Pathology, evolution, and diagnosis. Am J Clin Pathol 1982; 78:208–213.
3. Daum R, Schutze U, Hill E, Hoffman H. Mortality of preoperative peritonitis in newborn infants without intestinal obstruction. Prog Pediatr Surg 1979; 13:267–271.
4. Chattergee SK. Distal esophageal atresia with meconium peritonitis. J Pediatr Surg 1981; 16:517–518.
5. Hilgier A. Observations on the reactions of the peritoneum in newborn guinea pigs to the introduction of meconium and bacterial infection. Prob Med Wieku Rozwoj 1975; 4:129.
6. Lorimer WS, Ellis DH. Meconium peritonitis. Surgery 1966; 60:470–475.
7. Finkel LI, Slovis TL. Meconium peritonitis, intraperitoneal calcifications and cystic fibrosis. Pediatr Radiol 1982; 12:92–93.
8. Santulli TV. Meconium peritonitis. In: Holder TM, Ashcroft KW, eds. Pediatric surgery. Philadelphia: WB Saunders 1980: 367.
9. Shandling B, Ein SH, Simpson JS, Stephens CA, Bandi SK. Perforating appendicitis and antibiotics. J Pediatr Surg 1974; 9:79.
10. Baeckert P, Mieth D, Schneider H, Schwobel M. Meconium peritonitis: description of 3 cases with abnormal prenatal ultrasound findings. Helv Paediatr Acta 1987; 41:539–544.
11. Lortat JS, Pierre-Khan A, Renier D, Hirsch JF, Martelli H, Pellerin D. Abdominal complications of ventriculo-peritoneal shunts in children. 65 cases. Chir Pediatr 1984; 25:17–21.
12. McAllister TA, Mocan H, Murphy AV, Beattie TJ. Antibiotic susceptibility of staphylococci from CAPD peritonitis in children. J Antimicrob Chemother 1987; 19:95–100.

P A R T **6**

Perianal Lesions

Barry Shandling, M.B., Ch.B., F.R.C.S.(Eng.), FRCSC, F.A.C.S.

FISSURE-IN-ANO

Pathophysiology

An anal fissure is an ulcer in the form of a crack or split in the skin of the anus. Usually the consequence of the painful passage of a hard stool, this lesion has a tendency to be self-limiting and to heal, provided that the inciting cause is corrected and not allowed to recur. The abnormal stretching of the anus when a particularly large and hard stool traverses it literally tears the skin. The location is almost always in the midline, either in a posterior or an anterior position. It is postulated that in these two positions the anus is least well supported by the external anal sphincter mechanism. The resultant ulcer (for that is what it is) is traumatized by the passage of hard stools and is perforce contaminated and bleeds easily. Blood usually is evident on the toilet paper but may be seen as blood on the surface of the hard stool or even as blood dripping from the anus into the toilet bowl. Occasionally the child may pass blood unrelated to passage of stool—presumably blood that has collected within the rectal ampulla. Accompanying the development of the fissure there may be severe anal pain. Such painful defecation leads to a reluctance to defecate and to fecal retention. More stool accumulates, resulting in even more painful defecation. Thus the stage is set for the development of chronic constipation, encopresis, and the socially disruptive effects thereof.

In the depths of the fissure are transversely oriented muscle fibers, those of the internal anal sphincter.[1] It is thought that severe spasm of this muscle results in severe anal pain. The ulcer that is the fissure tends to heal provided that the skin does not close over the (infected) base prematurely. In the latter case breakdown and recurrence of the lesion are likely. With an established infected fissure there are the changes of chronic inflammation. The consequent edema results in the development of an anal tag or external hemorrhoid, resembling an anal polyp, and is often referred to as a "sentinel pile." These are usually seen in relation to the anteriorly located fissure.

Clinical Findings

Most patients with fissures are infants, and usually a history can be elicited of the passage of a constipated stool at the onset. The parent often describes the actual precipitating bowel movement in stark detail, being able exactly to pinpoint the date and time. After the initial episode there is often a history of screaming with bowel movements and the appearance, intermittently, of blood on the diaper, stool, or both.[2] In the older child there may be great apprehension in relation to incipient bowel movements, leading to attempts at fecal retention. The patient may cross the legs, run off into a corner, or refuse to use the potty or toilet, and many days may elapse between bowel movements. Occasionally the onset of the condition is related to diarrhea. This may be the consequence of gastroenteritis or of the ingestion of antibiotics, usually ampicillin. Crohn's disease may present as an anal fissure, usually accompanied by rather more perianal infection with edema and discharge than is seen with a simple fissure. These patients are not infants but usually teenagers.[3]

In chronically affected patients cultures of swabs of the area may show infestation by *Candida*. With multiple fissures, usually associated with excoriation and edema of the entire perianal area, a hemolytic streptococcal infection may be found.[4]

Physical examination should be confined to inspection. In the infant the supine position with hips flexed is preferred, and by parting the buttocks with each hand the fissure may be seen readily. It is not necessary to insert a finger into the anus, as there is nothing to be palpated, and such an examination may well cause excruciating pain. By gently parting the buttocks and stretching the anal skin laterally any fissure will become evident. Insertion of an anal speculum, proctoscope, or glass tube is not necessary when examining a child for an anal fissure. If Crohn's disease is suspected, investigation should be instituted to confirm or negate this diagnosis.

Management

Treatment is directed at the almost invariable concomitant constipation. The aim is to ensure that the stools are soft and passed regularly. Modification of the diet with or without the addition of laxatives ensures the proper consistency of the stools. In older children the judicious use of fiber additives usually accomplishes the desired objective. If there is no stool for 48 hours it is wise to administer a suppository or enema to prevent massive accumulation of stool that would further inhibit the healing process or cause the recurrence of a fissure. When diarrhea is present this should similarly be dealt with.

An important aspect of treatment is to instruct the parents not just to clean the anus with toilet paper after every bowel movement but actually to wash the anus with soap and water in a bath after every stool. Failure to do so results in the continued presence of fecal matter within the fissure, inhibiting healing and promoting continued sphincter spasm causing pain.

In infants with recalcitrant fissures, the daily insertion of a well-lubricated index finger (by a parent) will abolish the spasm and pain and promote healing. The application of local anesthetic ointment is frequently advised to decrease pain; however, it is of little or no value in abolishing muscle spasm, and I have never known it to be useful.

Rarely, is it necessary to operate on infants and children with fissures.[5] In the rare instance in which this may be required, the patient is more likely to be an older child with a chronic fissure of many months' or even years' duration. Forcible stretching of the sphincter, wide excision of the fissure, or internal anal sphincterotomy usually suffices. As a general anesthetic is necessary, I use all three modalities; instead of a lateral sphincterotomy the fissure is excised and the muscle divided in the depths of the site of the excised fissure. No postoperative dressings are required. Scrupulous perineal hygiene is paramount.

RECTAL PROLAPSE

Pathophysiology

Prolapse of the rectum was more common 50 years ago than now, perhaps owing to improved nutrition in industrialized countries.[6] The condition is seen with greater frequency in tropical and underdeveloped countries and occurs in the second and third years of life. There are several predisposing factors. Probably the likeliest in North America and Europe is prolonged time spent on a potty, sometimes in association with constipation. In tropical countries diarrhea is a more frequent association.[7] Less common predisposing factors include cystic fibrosis. Of 605 cases of this disease there were 48 patients in whom prolapse preceded the diagnosis of pancreatic insufficiency.[8-11] Infestation with parasites,[7] e.g., *Trichuris*, *Entamoeba histolytica*,[10] *Giardia lamblia*, and *Schistosoma*, has also been implicated. Other factors include vomiting, constipation with straining, whooping cough, vesical or urethral calculus, rectal polyps, spinal cord lesions, and malnutrition—the latter in association with loss of the ischiorectal fat pad. In cases of anal stenosis with severe straining, some mucosal prolapse may occur. Curiously, considering the total lack of tone in the pelvic floor, the condition occurs infrequently with spinal dysraphism. However, there is an association with ectopia vesicae. Rectal prolapse may also complicate certain anorectal operations, especially procedures to correct imperforate anus.[12] Placing a toddler on a potty with the hips and knees flexed for protracted periods facilitates prolapse of the rectum. The rectum (indeed many feet of intestine) has also been sucked out of the anus by inadvertent contact with the vacuum extraction of water from swimming pools.

Rectal prolapse may be of two varieties. The less serious type is only mucosal (or partial) prolapse, and the protrusion is only intermittent and less pronounced.[13] Most cases are of this variety, and almost all require minimal conservative treatment. The second variety is more pronounced (5 cm or more) prolapse of protracted duration,[14] frequently requiring manual reduction by the parents. It is considered to be complete, consisting of all coats of the bowel wall,[15] and may be a consequence of neglecting to treat a minor degree of mucosal prolapse. Solitary ulcer of the rectum may complicate the condition.[16] This type of prolapse may be associated with fecal incontinence that may be due to stretching of the pudendal nerves in association with the prolapse. The term *procidentia* includes prolapse of the perirectal supporting tissue and bladder and perirectal herniation of abdominal viscera.

Clinical Findings

The parents make the diagnosis, as it is usually neither possible nor convenient to recreate in the office the conditions under which the prolapse presents.[17] The condition is a harrowing one for lay people, especially as some rectal bleeding may accompany the prolapse. There are usually no concomitant symptoms, and parents often relate with amazement that the condition is painless. Frequently, the bowel returns to the pelvis spontaneously with resumption of the upright position, but if there is a considerable amount of bowel protruding its reduction may be difficult even by manual pressure. After reduction, especially if the rectum is edematous as a consequence of venous engorgement, the tone in the anorectal muscle complex seems absent. However, within hours it returns to normal. Thus rectal examination, if prolapse has not immediately preceded, reveals no abnormality.

Rectal prolapse must be distinguished from a prolapsing rectal polyp. The latter looks plum-colored and does not involve the entire anal circumference. Otherwise it may mimic prolapse, appearing with defecation and reducing spontaneously. An intussusception may be extruded via the anus and may be mistaken for a rectal prolapse. An examining finger will readily differentiate between the two; with the former it is possible to insert the finger around the prolapsing apex of the intussusception, between it and the lining of the anal canal.

Investigations such as defecography have not proved useful. In all cases of rectal prolapse sweat chlorides should be measured.[8,11]

Management

Most children with rectal prolapse are successfully managed by simple nonoperative means. Constipation should be treated by dietary modification (fiber) with or without the additional use of laxatives. If diarrhea is the precipitating cause, its correction may be all that is required. Co-existing conditions such as anal stenosis and parasitic infestations need to be treated at the outset. It is advisable to recommend abandonment of the potty. The child should defecate sitting on an adult toilet on a special seat with a small hole so that accidental immersion may be avoided. In this way, too, the feet are off the floor and the knees are not pressed up against the abdomen to try to expel the abdominal contents via the anus. It is not my practice to recommend defecation in the lateral recumbent position or to tape the buttocks together, as recommended by some. Both are somewhat aesthetically repellent and complicate matters for the parents.

If such simple measures are unsuccessful then I proceed to submucosal injection of sclerosant. It does not matter what is used, and several solutions are available, including quinine, 30 percent saline, 1 percent sodium morrhuate, and 5 percent phenol in almond oil. I prefer ethanolamine oleate. The injection is done under a general anesthetic; just enough solution is injected into the submucosa to cause blanching. Usually this amounts to less than 2 ml and the injections are made circumferentially in four sites about 7 to 8 cm proximal to the mucocutaneous junction.[14,18-23]

If injection treatment is unsuccessful (it may be necessary to repeat the injections several times), then I proceed to the insertion of a monofilament nonabsorbable perianal suture, the operation of cerclage, or the Thiersch procedure. I have never found it necessary to do any procedure of greater complexity. Presacral packing[21] and the recently described presacral insertion of a polygalactin mesh[24] are popular current procedures. Results generally are good, probably because the condition is self-limiting.

Prolapse as a complication of anorectal surgery requires specialized procedures for its correction.[15,18,25,26]

Others have described various procedures including linear cauterization of the rectum,[27] Ivalon sponge rectopexy,[28] Wells rectopexy,[29] trans-sacral rectopexy, rectosigmoidectomy, anterior resection,[30] and stripping and plication.[12]

HEMORRHOIDS

Pathophysiology

Hemorrhoids are of two varieties: internal and external. Internal hemorrhoids, varicose dilations of the tributaries of the superior rectal vein, manifest in the left lateral, right anterolateral, and right posterolateral positions. Such hemorrhoids may bleed, prolapse, or become strangulated as a consequence of longstanding prolapse. Constipation may be a factor in the pathogenesis of the condition, usually the consequence of a diet lacking adequate quantities of fiber. In the pediatric age groups primary internal hemorrhoids are virtually unknown. However, in conditions in which portal vein obstruction exists, either intrahepatic or extrahepatic, hemorrhoids may become evident, representing (as in the esophagus) a site of portosystemic anastomosis. Indeed, the development of massive rectal variceal bleeding has been described following sclerotherapy for bleeding esophageal varices.[31] For a detailed description of the pathogenesis of hemorrhoids, readers are referred to papers by Haas et al[32] and Shafik.[33]

External hemorrhoids have already been referred to in a preceding section.

Clinical Findings

In the absence of prolapse and/or strangulation, the presenting symptom is rectal bleeding. In association with portal vein obstruction one should seek other stigmata, e.g., splenomegaly, icterus, anemia, ascites. Diagnosis is made by proctoscopy if bleeding is the only symptom.

Management

If symptomatic, internal hemorrhoids are best, least painfully, and most conveniently treated by rubber band ligation.[34-37] Careful consideration should be given to patients with portal vein obstruction, as hemorrhoidectomy may aggravate portal hypertension.

External hemorrhoids, in the absence of symptoms representing an anal fissure, require no treatment. With advancing age there are increasing incidence and number of anal tags.[34]

ANAL ABSCESS/FISTULA

Pathogenesis

Perianal suppuration in children is usually encountered in infants who are in diapers. The infection may be the consequence of the deeper spread of infection from a diaper rash. A small perianal pustule, instead of spontaneously rupturing and draining, spreads in the plane between the internal and external anal sphincters. More often the source of the abscess is an infected anal gland. These glands drain into the anal crypts, between the columns of Morgagni, at the level of the pectinate line. If drainage is inadequate, or if infected material lodges in a crypt, leading to cryptitis, a fistulous abscess results.[38,39] The caudally directed portion of the anal gland, which occupies the intermuscular plane, becomes infected, and the infection continues to spread toward the perineum. It has been suggested that fistula-in-ano in childhood may be congenital, the result of an abnormal formation of anal glands.[40]

In adults the internal opening of a fistula is often in the midline, but in infants it is radially opposite the external opening. Rarely there may be two anal fistulae present. An anteriorly placed abscess may appear to be a periurethral abscess. These turn out to be lower intermuscular abscesses, "pointing" at somewhat more of a distance from the anus than the more common lateral infection.

At least 50 percent of perianal abscesses recur as fistulae. An abscess represents the acute stage of the infective process, and the fistula represents the chronic stage. When a fistulous abscess ruptures spontaneously, it becomes a fistula. Similarly, when a surgeon drains or deals ineffectually with such an abscess, a fistula results. Thus a fistula complicates a low intermuscular abscess (from an infected anal gland), whereas a perianal abscess (with penetrating infection from the skin) may not be complicated by development of a fistula following drainage.

The more complex forms of abscess (e.g., ischiorectal) and fistula (high intermuscular and pelvirectal) are rarely encountered in children.[41] In older children there is greater likelihood of such suppuration being a complication of inflammatory bowel disease, especially Crohn's disease.

Pruritus ani, perianal cellulitis, and blood streaking of stools may on occasion be due to group A beta-hemolytic streptococci.[42]

Clinical Findings

An indurated tender area of the perianal skin, with or without overlying redness, is the earliest sign of perianal suppuration; it may occur at any site around the circumference of the anus, in contrast to the condition in adults. When located at a distance from the anus, anteriorly in the midline, the lesion may be confused with a periurethral abscess. There are no urinary symptoms, however, and in the absence of urethral obstructive disease, periurethral suppuration need not be considered.

When a fistula is present there is usually a history of repeated cycles of healing, followed by the development of a small localized area of suppuration (like a "pimple"). This pustular lesion discharges some pus and/or blood and proceeds to heal and remain healed until the next episode of inflammation, culminating once more in spontaneous drainage.

When perianal suppuration complicates inflammatory bowel disease, usually there are appropriate clinical findings, and further radiologic and/or endoscopic investigation may be indicated.

Cultures of discharged material as well as of the perianal skin should be done so as to employ appropriate antibiotics where indicated.

Management

When treating perianal suppuration in children, to wait for fluctuation before instituting drainage is to wait too long and perhaps to facilitate the subsequent development of anal fistula. The abscess should be adequately drained and lightly "packed" in order to ensure drainage for 48 hours postoperatively.

When a fistula is being treated, a probe is inserted into the external opening. The internal opening of the fistula in children is on the pectinate line radially opposite the external orifice. The probe is gently passed out of the internal opening, and the fistula is then unroofed by incising down onto the probe with the electrocautery. Other than keeping the area scrupulously clean by washing with soap and water there is no special aftertreatment, and the patients are remarkably symptom-free.

REFERENCES

1. Duthie HL. Defaecation and the anal sphincters. Clin Gastroenterol 1982; 11:621–631.
2. Levene MI. Rectal bleeding in the first month of life. Postgrad Med J 1979; 55:22–23.
3. Sainio P. Fistula-in-ano in a defined population. Incidence and epidemiological aspects. Ann Chir Gynaecol 1984; 73:219–224.
4. Farmer G. Perianal infection with group A streptococcus. Arch Dis Child 1987; 62:1169–1170.
5. Shub HA, Salvati EP, Rubin RJ. Conservative treatment of anal fissure: an unselected, retrospective and continuous study. Dis Colon Rectum 1978; 21:582–583.
6. Duhamel J, Pernin P. Anal prolapse in the child. Ann Gastroenterol Hepatol 1985; 21:361–362.
7. Eriksen CA, Hadley GP. Rectal prolapse in childhood—the role of infections and infestations. S Afr Med J 1985; 68:790–791.
8. Stern RC, Izant RJ Jr, Boat TF, Wood RE, Matthews LW, Doershuk CF. Treatment and prognosis of rectal prolapse in cystic fibrosis. Gastroenterology 1982; 82:707–710.
9. Olsen MM, Gauderer MW, Girz MK, Izant RJ Jr. Surgery in patients with cystic fibrosis. J Pediatr Surg 1987; 22:613–618.
10. Gilman RH, Davis C, Fitzgerald F. Heavy Trichuris infection and amoebic dysentery in Orang Asli children. A comparison of the two diseases. Trans R Soc Trop Med Hyg 1976; 70:313–316.
11. Morris LJ, Mascia AV, Farnsworth PB. Cystic fibrosis: making a correct and early diagnosis. J Fam Pract 1978; 6:749–756.
12. Momoh JT. Quadrant mucosal stripping and muscle pleating in the management of childhood rectal prolapse. J Pediatr Surg 1986; 21:36–38.
13. Qvist N, Rasmussen L, Klaasborg KE, Hansen LP, Pedersen SA. Rectal prolapse in infancy: conservative versus operative treatment. J Pediatr Surg 1986; 21:887–888.
14. Wyllie GG. The injection treatment of rectal prolapse. J Pediatr Surg 1979; 14:62–64.
15. Freeman NV. Rectal prolapse in children. J R Soc Med 1984; 77(suppl 3):9–12.

16. Du Boulay CE, Fairbrother J, Isaacson PG. Mucosal prolapse syndrome—a unifying concept for solitary ulcer syndrome and related disorders. J Clin Pathol 1983; 36:1264–1268.

17. White CM, Finlay JM, Price JJ. The occult rectal prolapse syndrome. Br J Surg 1980; 67:528–530.

18. Freeman NV. The foreskin in anoplasty. Dis Colon Rectum 1984; 27:309–313.

19. Engels M. Anorectal prolapse. Padiatr Padol 1987; 22:123–129.

20. Burger P, Reppin G, Klaer U, Romer KH, Franke B. Therapy of pediatric anorectal prolapse. Zentralbl Chir 1986; 111:482–487.

21. Corman ML. Rectal prolapse in children. Dis Colon Rectum 1985; 28:535–539.

22. Dekhkanov ID, Alimov RI, Abdufataev T. Sclerotherapy of rectal prolapse in children. Vestn Khir 1980; 124:112–114.

23. Dutta BN, Das AK. Treatment of prolapsed rectum in children with injections of sclerosing agents. J Indian Med Assoc 1977; 69:275–276.

24. Scheye T, Marouby D, Vanneuville G. Total rectal prolapse in children. Modified Lockhart-Mummery operation. Presse Med 1987; 16:123–124.

25. Nixon HH, Puri P. The results of treatment of anorectal anomalies: a thirteen to twenty year follow-up. J Pediatr Surg 1977; 12:27–37.

26. Caouette-Laberge L, Yazbeck S, Laberge JM, Ducharme JC. Multiple-flap anoplasty in the treatment of rectal prolapse after pull-through operations for imperforate anus. J Pediatr Surg 1987; 22:65–67.

27. Hight DW, Hertzler JH, Philippart AI, Benson CD. Linear cauterization for the treatment of rectal prolapse in infants and children. Surg Gynecol Obstet 1982; 154:400–402.

28. Boulos PB, Stryker SJ, Nicholls RJ. The long-term results of polyvinyl alcohol (Ivalon) sponge for rectal prolapse in young patients. Br J Surg 1984; 71:213–214.

29. Atkinson KG, Taylor DC. Wells procedure for complete rectal prolapse. A ten-year experience. Dis Colon Rectum 1984; 27:96–98.

30. Schlinkert RT, Beart RW Jr, Wolff BF, Pemberton JH. Anterior resection for complete rectal prolapse. Dis Colon Rectum 1985; 28:409–412.

31. Azmy AA. Bleeding rectal varices following injection sclerotherapy of oesophageal varices in a child. Z Kinderchir 1987; 42:252.

32. Haas PA, Fox TA Jr, Haas GP. The pathogenesis of hemorrhoids. Dis Colon Rectum 1984; 27:442–450.

33. Shafik A. A new concept of the anatomy of the anal sphincter mechanism and the physiology of defecation. X. Anorectal sinus and band: anatomic nature and surgical significance. Dis Colon Rectum 1980; 23:170–179.

34. Wienert V, Albrecht O, Gahlen W. Results of incidence analyses in external hemorrhoids. Hautarzt 1978; 29:536–540.

35. Wienert V. Ambulatory hemorrhoidectomy through rubber band ligation—review of the literature. Fortschr Med 1977; 95:1619–1622.

36. Ruiz-Moreno F. Hemorrhoidectomy—how I do it: semiclosed technique. Dis Colon Rectum 1977; 20:177–182.

37. Lau WY, Chow HP, Poon GP, Wong SH. Rubber band ligation of three primary hemorrhoids in a single session. A safe and effective procedure. Dis Colon Rectum 1982; 25:336–339.

38. Eisenhammer S. The internal sphincter and the anorectal abscess. Surg Gynecol Obstet 1956; 103:501–506.

39. Parks AG. Pathogenesis and treatment of fistula-in-ano. Br Med J 1961; 1:463–469.

40. Fitzgerald RJ, Harding B, Ryan W. Fistula-in-ano in childhood: a congenital etiology. J Pediatr Surg 1985; 20:80–81.

41. Duhamel J. Anal fistulae in childhood. Am J Proctol 1974; 26:40–43.

42. Kokx NP, Comstock JA, Facklam RR. Streptococcal perianal disease in children. Pediatrics 1987; 80:659–663.

PART 7

Gastrointestinal Manifestations of Immunodeficiency States

Cova Gurbindo, M.D., Ph.D.

Ernest G. Seidman, M.D.

The fetal intestine plays an important role in the ontogeny of both the cellular and humoral immune systems. Postnatally, the human intestine develops histologic characteristics of a secondary lymphoid organ. Lymphoid follicles, germinal centers, small lymphocytes, and plasma cells are abundant. The importance of the intestine as an immune barrier is highlighted by the intimate proximity of the gut-associated lymphoid tissue (GALT) to the luminal surface of the gastrointestinal (GI) tract, an external environment rich in microbial pathogens and dietary antigens.

It is thus perhaps not surprising that there is a strong clinical relationship between immunodeficiency states, either primary or secondary, and significant GI disorders. This association demonstrates the critical role of the immune system in maintaining GI homeostasis. Not only are GI abnormalities frequently noted in patients with immunodeficiency syndromes, but they are occasionally severe enough

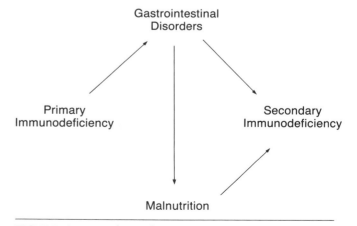

FIGURE 1 Inter-relationships among immune competence, nutritional status, and gastrointestinal disorders.

to become the patient's presenting complaint. Furthermore, primary intestinal diseases may secondarily cause substantial losses of immune system components so as to simulate a primary immunodeficiency (Fig. 1).

Nonimmune host defense factors, in addition to the major contribution by the GALT, are known to play an important role in mucosal protection against an external environment rich in potentially noxious antigens and pathogens. These nonimmune factors include gastric acidity, luminal proteases, intestinal motility, the mucus-glycocalyx, and the normal intestinal flora. These additional mucosal defense mechanisms may explain the fact that major deficiencies in either the humoral or cell-mediated immune system exist in certain patients without the presence of significant GI symptoms.

Repeated bacterial or severe viral and fungal infections are the hallmark of immunodeficiency states. Chronic diarrhea, often with malabsorption and concomitant failure to thrive, is characteristic of several of the immunodeficiency syndromes (Fig. 1). In this discussion, we shall review the GI manifestations of primary and secondary immunodeficiency states.

GASTROINTESTINAL MANIFESTATIONS OF PRIMARY IMMUNODEFICIENCY SYNDROMES

The primary immunodeficiency syndromes are a heterogeneous group of diseases that result in failure to manifest an efficient immune-mediated inflammatory response,

accompanied by repeated bacterial, fungal, and viral infections of variable severity. An immunodeficiency may involve any of the components of the immune system, including lymphocytes, phagocytic cells, and complement proteins.

The progenitors of immunocompetent cells are derived from multipotent hematopoietic stem cells. Within the thymus, bone marrow precursor cells are induced to express T-cell characteristics, including the surface glycoproteins that serve as differentiation markers as well as antigen receptors. The T-lymphocyte subpopulations can thereby be classified into helper (T_H) and suppressor or cytotoxic (T_S) groups. Other functionally distinct subsets of T cells also exist and may be similarly identified by their surface antigens.

Antigen-presenting cells, including those of the monocyte-macrophage series, Langerhans cells, dendritic cells, and Kupffer cells are important collaborators in the immune responses of T and B lymphocytes. Following the interaction of the T-cell receptor with antigen presented in association with major histocompatibility complex (MHC) molecules, T cells become activated to produce lymphokines, such as interleukin-2 (IL-2), and to express IL-2 receptors. The subsequent interaction of IL-2 with its receptor is a critical step in immune regulation and is required for many effector and regulatory T-cell functions (Fig. 2).

B-lymphocyte development begins within the fetal liver and subsequently continues in the bone marrow. Precursor cells give rise to a rapidly dividing population of pre-B cells that lack immunoglobulin receptors but do produce cytoplasmic heavy chains. The next stage of differentiation is character-

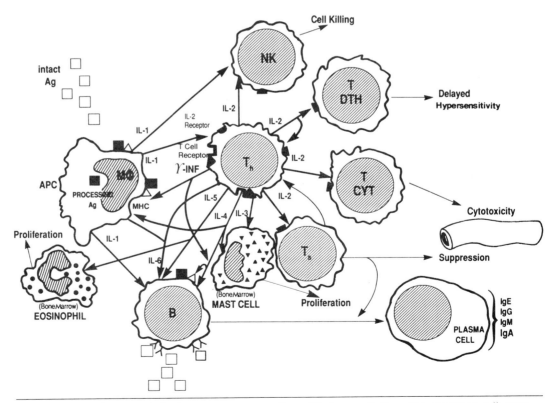

FIGURE 2 Cytokines and the immune response. T_H = T-helper cell; T_S = T-suppressor cell; DTH = delayed hypersensitivity; CYT = cytotoxicity; IL = interleukin; γ-INF = gamma interferon; NK = natural killer cell; B = bursal cell; Mφ = macrophage.

ized by immature surface-immunoglobulin–bearing B lymphocytes that express IgM, which are already committed to the specificity of the antibodies that they and their plasma cell progeny will secrete. Most B lymphocytes then further mature and acquire surface IgD. During subsequent development of isotype diversity, one of the subclasses of IgG (1 to 4) or IgA (1 to 2) is expressed by separate subpopulations of B cells, which then lose their surface IgM and IgD. During this diversification process, B lymphocytes acquire other cell-surface receptors that allow them to respond to antigens and to T-cell help by proliferation and differentiation to plasma cells.

The initiation and completion of specific immune responses involve a complex series of genetically restricted interactions between antigen-presenting cells and T-cell subpopulations for cell-mediated immunity (CMI), and between these cells and B cells for antibody response. The T_H and T_S lymphocytes exert positive and negative regulatory effects, respectively, on B-cell responses. Similarly, B cells and antibodies can affect the activities of functionally distinct subpopulations of T cells through specific receptors. Primary immunodeficiency diseases may be attributable to a wide variety of defects in the development and function of the immune system. On the basis of considerable advances in the understanding of the cellular and molecular components of the normal immune system, the primary immunodeficiencies (ID) have been reclassified (Table 1) by the World Health Organization Scientific Group on ID.[1]

Predominantly Antibody Defects

Mucosal Humoral Immunity

The mucosal surface of the GI tract represents an extensive and efficient barrier protecting the host internal milieu, preventing penetration by pathogenic organisms and potentially noxious luminal antigens and toxins. An important component of the host mucosal defense at the epithelial surface is the presence of intestinal antibodies, most notably secretory IgA (sIgA).[2] A deficiency in secretory intestinal antibody may impair mucosal barrier function, resulting in increased uptake of macromolecular antigens that could then contribute to the pathogenesis of intestinal or systemic disease states.[3] The interaction of intestinal antibodies with antigens, enterotoxins, or bacteria can prevent their attachment to epithelial cell membranes, inhibiting antigen uptake by the enterocyte. The formation of antigen-antibody complexes on the surface of the small intestine may also facilitate the operation of other nonimmunologic host defense mechanisms, thereby clearing potential pathogens from the intestine.[3] Thus, under normal conditions, the mature mucosal immune system limits antigen uptake and eliminates pathogens.

These theories have been supported by studies in patients with common variable hypogammaglobulinemia, who were shown to have markedly increased absorption of dietary antigens.[4] Other investigators have noted an increased incidence of intestinal infections in immunodeficient children, such as *Campylobacter jejuni* enteritis in patients with a defect of the humoral system.[5] Although symptoms in such cases were similar to those seen in normal children, the clinical

TABLE 1
Classification of Primary Immunodeficiency Diseases

A. Predominantly Antibody Defects
X-linked agammaglobulinemia
X-linked hypogammaglobulinemia with growth hormone deficiency
Autosomal recessive agammaglobulinemia
Ig deficiency with increased IgM (and IgD) ("hyper-IgM syndrome")
IgA deficiency
Selective deficiency of other Ig isotypes
K-chain deficiency
Immunodeficiency with thymoma
Transient hypogammaglobulinemia of infancy

B. Combined Immunodeficiency
Common variable immunodeficiency
Predominant antibody deficiency
Predominant cell-mediated immunity defect

Severe combined immunodeficiency
Reticular dysgenesis
Low T- and B-cell numbers
Low T-, normal B-cell numbers
Adenosine deaminase deficiency
Purine nucleoside phosphorylase deficiency
Major histocompatibility complex Class I deficiency ("bare lymphocyte syndrome")
Major histocompatibility complex Class II deficiency

C. Immunodeficiency Associated with Other Major Defects
Wiskott-Aldrich syndrome
Ataxia-telangiectasia
Third and fourth pouch/arch syndrome (DiGeorge)
Transcobalamin-2 deficiency
Immunodeficiency with partial albinism
Immunodeficiency following hereditary defective response to Epstein-Barr virus

D. Defects of Phagocytic Function
X-linked chronic granulomatous disease
Autosomal recessive chronic granulomatous disease
Phagocyte membrane defect beta-95 deficiency
Chediak-Higashi syndrome
Neutrophil G6PD deficiency
Myeloperoxidase deficiency
Secondary granule deficiency
Schwachman's disease

E. Complement Deficiency
C1q
C1r
C4
C2
C3
C5
C6
C7
C8 alpha-gamma
C8 beta
C9
C1 inhibitor
Factor I
Factor H
Properdin

course of immunodeficient patients tended to be prolonged and unaffected by antibiotic therapy. Chronic diarrhea is the second most common infectious complication of antibody deficiency syndromes.[1]

X-Linked Agammaglobulinemia

This congenital disorder, first described by Bruton,[6] is characterized by absent or very low levels of all immunoglobulin classes as well as absent secretory immunoglobulin. The infants afflicted with this disease remain well during the first 6 to 9 months of life, by virtue of maternally transmitted immunoglobulin.[7] The typical patient is a male presenting at about 6 months of age with severe respiratory infection or meningitis. IgG, IgA, and IgM are far below the 95 percent confidence limits for appropriate age- and race-matched controls (usually less than 100 mg per deciliter total immunoglobulin). Polymorphonuclear functions are usually normal if IgG antibodies with intact Fc functions are provided, but some patients with this condition have had transient, persistent, or cyclic neutropenia.[8]

In addition to a virtual absence of serum immunoglobulins of all classes, an inability to make antibody after stimulation with potent antigen and the absence of plasma cells in lymphoid tissues are noted. The current evidence suggests that the underlying defect lies within the B cell itself, reflecting an intrinsic maturation block in pre–B-cell to B-cell differentiation.[9] Cell-mediated immunity is normal, and a normal number of pre-B cells are found in the bone marrow.[7] However, plasma cells and blood lymphocytes bearing surface immunoglobulin or the Epstein-Barr virus (EBV) receptor or reacting with anti–B-cell monoclonal antibodies are absent or present only in very low number.[7]

In addition to recurrent bacterial infections, patients often have persistent viral or parasitic infections. The child may present with chronic diarrhea or a malabsorptive syndrome with associated protein-losing enteropathy. Giardiasis, bacterial overgrowth syndrome (not correlating with diarrhea), nonspecific colitis, and chronic rotavirus infection are well-described complications of this disorder.[10,11] The important role of antibody in protecting against these infectious agents is made obvious by their frequent occurrence in X-linked agammaglobulinemia and by the favorable response of these patients to replacement therapy with immunoglobulin.[11] In general, GI manifestations are much less notable than those encountered in patients with late-onset type common variable immunodeficiency (discussed below).

IgA Deficiency

Selective IgA deficiency is the most common primary immunodeficiency disorder, with prevalence among healthy adults reported to be as high as 1 in 300.[8,12] While the majority of patients are entirely well, the literature is replete with reports associating IgA deficiency with many conditions, including recurrent infections and various autoimmune diseases.[13]

The basic defect leading to selective IgA deficiency is unknown. Most IgA-deficient patients have immature B cells that express membrane-bound IgA, with IgM and IgD coexpression.[14] These B cells resemble those found in umbilical cord blood and are not easily induced to become mature IgA-secreting plasma cells, suggesting a B-cell maturation arrest.[14] In some patients, the defect involves a secretory component as well.[15] Of possible etiologic and significant clinical importance is the presence of antibodies to IgA in

TABLE 2
Secretory and Serum IgA

	Secretory	Serum
Molecular form	Polymeric	Monomeric
Subclasses	$IgA_1 \geq IgA_2$	$IgA_1 > IgA_2$
Origin	Mucosal tissues	Bone marrow
IgA deficiency	Decreased or normal	Decreased

the serum samples of as many as 44 percent of patients with selective IgA deficiency.[7,16,17] Patients deficient in IgA have had severe or even fatal anaphylactic reactions after intravenous administration of IgA-containing products.[16] For this reason, parenteral administration of blood or blood products, including immunoserum globulin, is potentially hazardous.

Normally, there is a differential distribution of IgA subclasses throughout the body (Table 2). IgA in bone marrow plasma cells and serum is predominantly IgA1. By contrast, IgA in secretions and intestinal plasma cells contain equal amounts of IgA1 and IgA2.[18] Most IgA-deficient patients do lack both serum and secretory IgA1 and IgA2. In some patients with serum IgA deficiency, IgA2-producing plasma cells may be plentiful in the bowel. IgG subclass deficiency and IgE deficiency may also be seen in patients with "selective IgA deficiency," thus reflecting a more generalized abnormality in the terminal differentiation of the B cell in such patients. This mixed defect is particularly characteristic of those patients with GI symptoms.[9] Susceptibility to infection among children with selective IgA deficiency is significantly associated with IgG subclass 2 or 4 deficiency.[19] The identification of an IgG subclass deficiency may theoretically lead to therapeutic options, in that an associated IgG subclass deficiency may benefit from replacement therapy. However, the risks of blood product administration in such patients, as mentioned above, preclude their routine use.[16]

As noted above, there is an association between IgA deficiency and a wide variety of GI disorders (Table 3). The majority of patients do not, however, suffer from significant clinical symptoms. Other host defense mechanisms likely compensate and protect the mucosal barrier, including an increase in IgM-secreting cells[20] and various nonimmune factors discussed earlier.[21]

TABLE 3
Gastrointestinal Manifestations of IgA Deficiency

None
Giardia lamblia infestation
Nodular lymphoid hyperplasia
Nonspecific enteropathy ± bacterial overgrowth ± disaccharidase deficiency
Increased incidence of circulating antibodies to food antigens
Gluten-sensitive enteropathy
Pernicious anemia/atrophic gastritis/increased risk of gastric cancer
Idiopathic inflammatory bowel disease (Crohn's disease, ulcerative colitis)

In addition to the high prevalence of chronic diarrhea and steatorrhea, there is a 10- to 12-fold increased incidence of celiac disease among IgA-deficient patients.[22] Celiac disease in the IgA-deficient patient cannot be distinguished clinically, radiologically, or by laboratory means from celiac disease in otherwise normal individuals. The only differentiating feature is found by immunohistochemical staining of small intestinal biopsy, which reveals a lack of IgA-producing plasma cells.[23] Patients with IgA deficiency may also have chronic diarrhea and villous atrophy on jejunal biopsy without concomitant celiac disease. The clinical differentiation depends upon response (symptoms and biopsy) to a gluten-free diet (Fig. 3).

Giardia lamblia infestation is a common problem in these patients.[24] The prevalence of IgA deficiency among patients with Crohn's disease also appears to be significantly increased, according to some authors.[25] Although there is an increased prevalence of both serum IgG antibodies against food antigens and circulating immune complexes in IgA-deficient patients, an association with food allergy is not clear-

FIGURE 3 Gluten-sensitive enteropathy in association with autosomal recessive agammaglobulinemia. The patient was a 13-year-old female who presented with chronic diarrhea and growth failure that responded to a gluten-free diet. *A,* Jejunal biopsy shows a moderate to severe villous atrophy, crypt hyperplasia, and chronic inflammatory changes (HPS stain, ×120). An abundance of IgM-containing plasmocytes (*B*) and an absence of IgA-containing plasmocytes (*C*) were noted (immunoperoxidase stain, ×300). (Courtesy of P. Russo, M.D.)

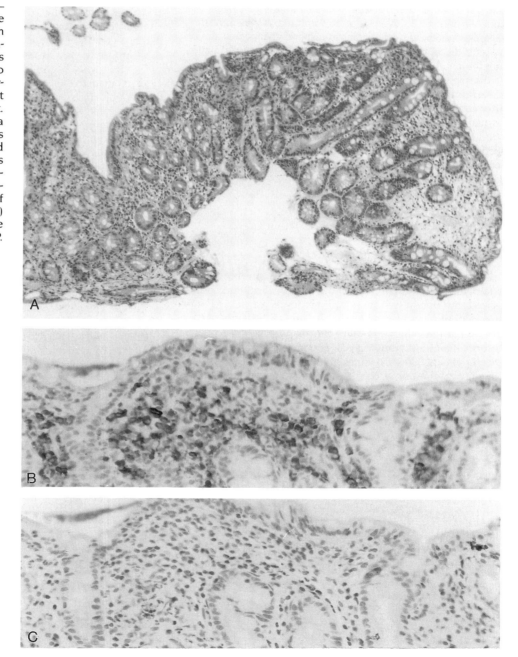

ly established in these patients.[26] Finally, an increased risk of GI malignancy has been associated with IgA deficiency.[27] Currently, there is no specific treatment for IgA deficiency beyond the vigorous treatment of infections with appropriate antimicrobial agents. Even if serum IgA were to be replaced, it could not be transported into external secretions, since the latter is an active process involving epithelial cells and locally produced IgA.[8]

Transient Hypogammaglobulinemia of Infancy

Postnatally, there is a physiologic decrease in the serum IgG concentration as the maternally derived IgG is catabolized. A nadir is reached between the third and sixth months. In premature infants, the amount of transplacentally acquired immunoglobulin is considerably less, and thus the serum IgG concentrations are lower. Intrinsic immunoglobulin synthesis follows as the neonate begins to respond to antigenic stimuli, with the appearance of IgM first, followed by IgG and, much later, IgA.

Transient hypogammaglobulinemia is primarily a deficiency of serum IgG. Normal antibody responses are demonstrable after antigenic stimuli such as tetanus. Circulating B cells are normal in number, but the B-cell response to T cell–dependent stimulation with pokeweed mitogen is decreased, probably secondary to a lack of T-cell help.[28] Infants with this uncommon disorder may present with chronic diarrhea and malabsorption and normally recover spontaneously between the ages of 1 and 2 years.[8]

Combined Immunodeficiency

Common Variable Immunodeficiency

Common variable immunodeficiency (CVI) represents a heterogeneous group of familial or sporadic diseases characterized by B-cell dysfunction, low levels of serum immunoglobulins, and a failure of B cells to differentiate to mature plasma cells.[29,30] T-cell abnormalities have also been described and are thought to either cause or exacerbate the B-cell defects.[31,32] A decreased proliferative response to phytohemagglutinin (PHA) or anti-CD$_3$ monoclonal antibody activation has been noted, as has a lower IL-2 secretion.[33] These abnormalities are restored by addition of exogenous IL-2 or by using phorbol myristate acetate (PMA) as a mitogen (protein-kinase activator).

IL-2 receptor expression is also impaired in CVI when patients' peripheral blood mononuclear cells (PBMC) are incubated with anti-CD$_3$ antibodies. However, IL-2 and IL-2

TABLE 4

Gastrointestinal Manifestations of Common Variable Immunodeficiency

---

Giardia lamblia infestation
Bacterial overgrowth syndrome
Infectious diarrhea (bacterial, viral)
Pernicious anemia/atrophic gastritis/gastric carcinoma
Nodular lymphoid hyperplasia
Gluten-sensitive enteropathy
Nonspecific enteropathy/colitis

---

receptor mRNA expressions by PBMC are normal, suggesting a possible defect at the post-transcriptional level.[34] The defective IL-2 production in CVI was also reversed by normal allogeneic macrophages, reflecting a potential defect of macrophage activation in selected patients with this disorder.[34]

Common Variable Immunodeficiency Plus Predominant Antibody Deficiency

This syndrome is similar clinically to X-linked agammaglobulinemia and is characterized by low levels of IgG as well as of the other immunoglobulin classes. It can occur sporadically at any age, but familial cases have been identified, primarily with autosomal recessive inheritance. Peripheral B cells do not synthesize immunoglobulin normally when stimulated by mitogens, as described above. Although CVI patients generally have a decreased number of Ig-secreting cells in GALT, this is not a consistent finding.

Children with this disorder typically present with a history of recurrent otitis media, bronchopulmonary infections, and chronic diarrhea.[30] A number of GI symptoms and signs are associated with CVI (Table 4). The majority of patients develop significant malabsorption,[35] often due to giardiasis.[36] Such patients usually have mild steatorrhea, and small bowel biopsy reveals mild to moderate villous atrophy. These abnormalities may sometimes respond favorably to treatment with metronidazole.

There is little evidence demonstrating an increased incidence of parasites other than *Giardia* in CVI patients from industrialized countries.[36] No information is available concerning such patients in less developed areas of the world. Although bacterial overgrowth is commonly recognized, its presence does not correlate with achlorhydria, diarrhea, steatorrhea, lactose intolerance, vitamin B$_{12}$ malabsorption, or the presence of *Giardia*.[37] Other specific pathogens noted in CVI patients include rotavirus,[11] *C. jejuni*,[38] and *C. fetus*.[39]

Patients with acquired agammaglobulinemia do have a high incidence of gastritis and pernicious anemia–like syndrome without antibodies to intrinsic factor, gastric parietal cells, or thyroglobulin.[40] Nodular lymphoid hyperplasia is often encountered in the bowels of CVI patients who do have B cells, and there is an increased incidence of GI tumors in these patients.[41,42] Nodular lymphoid hyperplasia is also seen in patients with selective IgA deficiency as well as in normal individuals. As noted with congenital X-linked agammaglobulinemia, CVI patients have an increased incidence of generalized lymphomas,[35] and those with gastritis carry an increased risk of gastric carcinoma.[43]

Of interest is a report that a subset of CVI patients with excessive suppressor cell activity benefited from therapy with cimetidine.[44] This H$_2$-receptor antagonist reduced suppressor cell activity, presumably allowing for endogenous immunoglobulin production.

Common Variable Immunodeficiency Plus Predominant Cell-Mediated Immunity Defect

This immunodeficiency is characterized by decreased or absent T-cell number and reflects a primary abnormality of T-cell development.[1] The presumed pathogenesis is either an excessively activated suppressor T-cell function, markedly reduced T-cell numbers, or autoantibodies to T cells.[1] Studies of cellular immune function have shown delayed cutaneous anergy to ubiquitous antigens and low to absent in vitro lymphocyte responses to mitogens and allogeneic cells. Such patients have profound deficiencies of total T cells and T-cell subsets. Despite the numerical deficiency, there is usually a normal helper (CD4) to suppressor (CD8) cell ratio, in contrast to AIDS, as described later. Peripheral lymphoid tissues are hypoplastic, with paracortical lymphocyte depletion. The thymus is typically very small, and no Hassall's corpuscles or thymic epithelium is present.[8]

There is a great deal of clinical variability in this syndrome, which may be transmitted in an autosomal recessive pattern. Patients may present late in infancy and childhood, whereas others are indistinguishable from those with severe combined immunodeficiency syndrome (SCID) who present earlier. As with SCID patients, respiratory tract infections are severe, and malnutrition is often secondary to diarrhea and malabsorption. The GI manifestations are primarily those of oral, esophageal, and perianal candidiasis. The entire small and large intestine may be involved by nonspecific enterocolitis (Fig. 4), contributing to the chronic diarrhea and malabsorption.[45] An underlying cause for the enterocolitis is not often determined, and patients frequently require nutritional support in the form of enteral elemental diets or total parenteral nutrition.

Severe Combined Immunodeficiency

SCID is a hereditary disorder characterized by a profound deficiency of both T- and B-lymphocyte function and by the onset of severe, life-threatening infections in the first months of life. A great diversity of genetic, enzymatic, hematologic, and immunologic features (see Table 1) characterize this large category of syndromes, all of which manifest clinically as a severe congenital immunodeficiency.[1,8]

The affected infant presents with severe infections, chronic diarrhea, malabsorption, and failure to thrive. There may be a history of a neonatal hyperpigmented rash secondary to graft-versus-host disease (GVHD), resulting from transplacentally acquired maternal lymphocytes. Intractable diarrhea and persistent oral thrush are common presentations. The diarrhea may begin slowly and become massive, watery, bloody, and mucopurulent. The pathophysiologic mechanisms underlying the intractable diarrhea are poorly understood. These patients are extremely susceptible to viral infections and often succumb to overwhelming varicella, herpes, or cytomegalovirus (CMV) infection. It is worthwhile investigating stools for viral particles in these patients, in that viruses—singly or in concert—may play an important role in the pathogenesis of the diarrhea.[11,46] These patients are also susceptible to systemic infections caused by organisms such as *Candida albicans, Pneumocystis carinii, Listeria monocytogenes,* and CMV. Some viral agents such as rotavirus, adenovirus, picornavirus, and parvovirus, which normally cause self-limited diarrhea, may cause a chronic enteropathy in SCID.[47] Enteropathogenic bacteria such as *Salmonella* and *Escherichia coli* can also cause chronic infections in these patients.[23]

Histologic features of the intestinal mucosa in SCID include the absence of plasma cells, blunted villi, and the presence of PAS-positive macrophages in the lamina propria (Fig. 5). Most patients with SCID have profound lymphopenia with few mature T cells and low levels of immunoglobulins. Cutaneous anergy and failure to reject transplants are noted. Peripheral eosinophilia is not uncommon. These patients are very susceptible to GVHD, and thus bone marrow

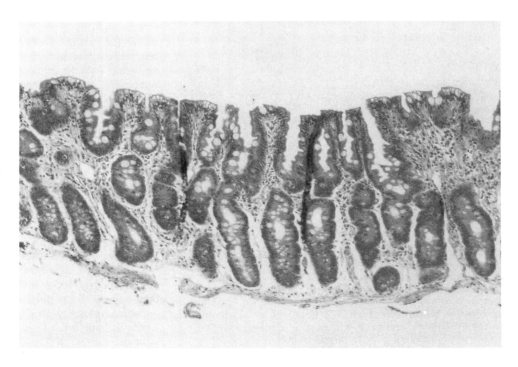

FIGURE 4 Nonspecific enteropathy of common variable immunodeficiency. Small bowel biopsy from a 3-year-old boy with chronic diarrhea and failure to thrive unresponsive to gluten-free diet or metronidazole. There is irregular, subtotal villous atrophy with acute and chronic inflammatory cell infiltrate of the lamina propria (HPS stain, ×120). (Courtesy of P. Russo, M.D.)

transplantation is best performed after removal of T cells from the donor marrow using monoclonal antibodies.[48] Analysis of lymphocyte subpopulations has demonstrated marked heterogeneity among SCID patients. Despite the uniformly profound lack of T- or B-cell function, many patients have an elevated percentage of B cells and extremely low percentages of T cells and subsets, but with surface marker characteristics of mature T cells.[8] Another phenotype has been characterized in two infants with SCID, in which lymphocytes are large and granular with natural killer (NK) cell phenotype and function.[49] Fontan et al[50] described two cases of SCID with normal T-lymphocyte numbers in which the patients' T cells retained some regulatory activities. Among SCID patients with autosomal recessive inheritance, approximately one-half have an enzyme defect: either adenosine deaminase (ADA) or purine nucleoside phosphorylase (PNP) deficiency (Fig. 5).[51,52] These patients are clinically similar to other

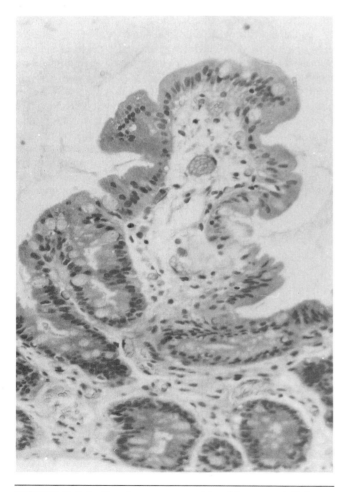

FIGURE 5 Intestine in severe combined immunodeficiency. The patient presented with intractable diarrhea, failure to thrive, and persistent oral candidiasis during infancy. Investigations confirmed adenosine deaminase deficiency. The jejunal and rectal biopsies (not shown) demonstrate a markedly hypocellular lamina propria with absence of plasmocytes (HPS stain, ×300). (Courtesy of P. Russo, M.D.)

SCID cases, and optimal treatment is bone marrow transplantation. In the absence of a suitable bone marrow donor, the ADA-deficient patient may be supported with transfusions of frozen, irradiated red blood cells as a source of ADA. Intravenous hyperalimentation is often an essential supportive therapy to prevent or treat secondary malnutrition.

Severe Combined Immunodeficiency with Defective Expression of Major Histocompatibility Complex Antigens

Two forms of SCID are associated with defective expression of major histocompatibility complex (MHC) antigens. MHC class I antigen deficiency is commonly referred to as the "bare lymphocyte syndrome" (BLS). In the second group, MHC class I antigen deficiency and absence of MHC class II antigens co-exist.

BLS is a rare immunodeficiency disease caused by or associated with the failure of expression of cell-surface antigens encoded for by the MHC. Since this disorder was first described, approximately 30 cases have been reported.[53-55] The group is heterogeneous with regard to defective cell-surface antigen expression. In some patients, there is defective expression only of class I MHC antigens encoded for by the HLA-A, B, and C genetic loci. In other patients, class II MHC antigens (HLA-DR, D2, and DP antigens) are not expressed.[54,55] Patients who fail to express both class I and class II MHC antigens have also been identified.[54]

Clinically, this syndrome is manifested as a combined immunodeficiency presenting early in life. Affected individuals are susceptible to a number of severe and/or opportunistic infections by a wide variety of pathogens. Oral candidiasis, bacterial pneumonia, *Pneumocystis* pneumonia, septicemia, and undue susceptibility to enteroviruses, herpes, and other viral agents are commonly noted.

There is variable hypogammaglobulinemia with decreased serum IgM and IgA and poor to absent antibody production. Severe, chronic diarrhea and malabsorption are also characteristic features of patients with the BLS. Death is common within the first few years of life. B-cell percentage is usually normal, but plasma cells are absent in tissues. Although lymphopenia is only moderate, T-cell function is decreased, although detectable both in vivo and in vitro. The thymus and other lymphoid organs are severely hypoplastic.

Because MHC antigens have an important role as recognition structures for interactions among immunocompetent cells, it has generally been assumed that the immune deficiency can be attributed to the inability of cells to recognize antigens in the context of self-MHC molecules. However, other possible mechanisms contribute to the defective immune responsiveness seen in individuals with BLS. For example, class II MHC antigens are directly involved in B-cell activation events that are independent of interactions between immunocompetent cells. Class II antigen-deficient B cells have a profound intrinsic defect in their response to stimuli that induce B-cell activation and proliferation. This defect is accompanied by a block in B-cell differentiation that results in the presence of a population of B cells that express the HB-4 antigen, a marker normally found only on a subset of B cells. These cells also fail to express a non-MHC encoded B-cell antigen, the CD21 (C3d/EBV receptor) molecule.[56]

A variety of regulatory gene defects could produce the MHC deficiency syndrome, and defective transcription of class II MHC gene has been demonstrated in cells from some BLS patients.[57] It appears that the heterogeneity of the molecular lesions may produce variability in the magnitude of both the class II deficiency and the B-cell function. The early maturational events leading to the production of B cells do not appear to be affected by the absence of class II antigens, since the numbers of Ig cells are normal in BLS. B cells are IgM+/IgD+, and expression of kappa and lambda light chains is normal. The most notable abnormality regarding surface Ig expression is the absence of detectable IgA+ B cells. This finding may reflect a disruption, at any level, of the co-ordinated events involved in heavy-chain isotype switching and Ig expression, or a defect in a helper T-cell function required for the expansion of IgA+ cells. There is an increased frequency of B cells expressing CD38 antigen, reflecting a population of relatively immature B cells,[58] and thus suggesting that B-cell maturation is delayed or arrested. The most striking phenotypic abnormality is the absence of CD21 antigens, which serve as the B-cell receptor for C3d complement fragment as well as for EBV. The slow initial growth that has been reported for EBV-transformed BLS B cells is consistent with these data. CD21 is expressed during the transition of pre-B cells to their surface Ig+ progeny, and it is normally present on the vast majority of Ig+ cells in both the neonate and adult. The absence of CD21 antigens indicates that pre-B to B maturation is incomplete in BLS.

Immunodeficiency Associated with Other Defects

Wiskott-Aldrich Syndrome

Wiskott-Aldrich syndrome is an X-linked recessive condition characterized by T-cell dysfunction, severe eczema, thrombocytopenia, and repeated opportunistic infections. Patients present in the first few months of life with the above clinical picture, often accompanied by bloody diarrhea.[59,60] Although other GI complications are not prominent, malabsorption and nonspecific colitis have been reported.[37]

The median survival has been shown to be less than 6 years, with more than 50 percent of patients dying of infection, 27 percent with hemorrhage, and 5 percent with tumors, almost all of which involve the lymphoreticular system.[61] In younger patients, infections are caused by pneumococci and other bacteria with polysaccharide capsules. They characteristically present with otitis media, pneumonia, meningitis, and/or sepsis. Later, infections with agents such as *P. carinii* and herpesvirus become more frequent.

These patients produce specific antibodies poorly but have normal numbers of B lymphocytes and plasma cells and normal or increased rates of globulin synthesis. Their T cells exhibit a progressive decrease in number and function. Patients with this defect have an impaired humoral immune response to polysaccharide antigens. Studies of immunoglobulin metabolism have shown an accelerated rate of synthesis as well as hypercatabolism of albumin, IgG, IgA, and IgM, resulting in highly variable immunoglobulin concentrations, even within the same patient. The predominant pattern is a low serum IgM, elevated IgA and IgE, and normal or slightly low IgG concentration. Lymphocyte responses to mitogens are depressed. There are low percentages of CD3 T cells, as well as CD4 and CD8 subsets. Optimal therapy requires bone marrow transplantation, which appears to correct all of the problems with the exception of thrombocytopenia.

Ataxia-Telangiectasia

This multisystem hereditary disease is associated with a complex immunodeficiency, impaired organ maturation, x-ray hypersensitivity, and a high incidence of neoplasia.[62] It is characterized by cerebellar ataxia apparent at the time the child begins to walk and progressing until he or she is confined to a wheelchair, usually by the age of 10 to 12 years. Oculomotor abnormalities consist of nystagmus and difficulty in initiating voluntary eye movements. Oculocutaneous telangiectasia first appears as dilated venules on the conjunctiva between the ages of 2 and 8 years. Patients present with repeated sinopulmonary infections and progressive bronchiectasis (80 percent of cases). Common viral exanthems and smallpox vaccination have not usually resulted in untoward sequelae, although fatal varicella infection has been described.[8]

GI disease is not a characteristic feature in these patients unless secretory IgA is also deficient. The patients are at increased risk of developing malignancies, including non-Hodgkin's lymphoma, lymphocytic leukemia, Hodgkin's disease, and adenocarcinoma of the stomach.

The synthesis of antibodies and certain immunoglobulin subclasses appears to be disrupted owing to abnormal B-cell and helper T-cell function in these patients. Individuals affected have various disorders of cell-mediated immunity, including the inability to produce antigen-specific cytotoxic lymphocytes against viral pathogens.[63] The most frequent humoral immunologic abnormality is the selective absence of IgA, found in 50 to 80 percent of these patients. Hypercatabolism of IgA is also known to occur. IgE concentrations are low, and IgG2 and total IgG may also be decreased. Moderately depressed proliferative responses to T- and B-cell mitogens are noted. Reduced percentages of total T cells and T cells of the helper phenotype, with normal or increased percentages of T-suppressor cells, are found. The thymus is very hypoplastic, with poor organization. This disease is considered a model of aberrant gene control, with persistently increased production of alpha$_1$-fetoprotein and carcinoembryonic antigen. No satisfactory treatment has yet been found.

Third and Fourth Pouch/Arch Syndrome (DiGeorge's Syndrome)

Congenital thymic aplasia, or third and fourth pouch/arch syndrome (DiGeorge's syndrome), is a rare syndrome resulting from the failure of formation of the third and fourth pharyngeal pouches during early embryogenesis. Other structures forming at the same time are also frequently affected, resulting in anomalies of the great vessels (right-sided aortic arch), esophageal atresia, bifid uvula, congenital heart disease (atrial and ventricular septal defects), and dysmorphic facial features. It has become apparent that a variable degree of hypoplasia is more frequent than total aplasia of the thymus and parathyroid glands. Some affected children may grow normally, and such patients are referred to as having partial DiGeorge's syndrome.

Clinically the syndrome is characterized by absent T-lymphocyte function, cardiovascular abnormalities, and hypoparathyroidism.[64] Patients present with hypocalcemic tetany early in life, a shortened philtrum, micrognathia, ear anomalies (low-set, notched lobes), an antimongoloid slant to the eyes, and hypertelorism.

Thymic hypoplasia or aplasia is associated with a cellular immune deficit and severe infections. Those with the complete syndrome may resemble patients with SCID in their susceptibility to infection with low-grade or opportunistic pathogens (fungi, viruses, and P. carinii) and to GVHD from nonirradiated blood transfusions.

Concentrations of serum immunoglobulins are nearly normal for age, but IgA may be diminished and IgE is sometimes elevated. T-cell percentages are decreased, with a relative increase in the percentage of B cells. Proliferative response of lymphocytes may be absent, reduced, or normal, depending on the degree of thymic deficiency. GI manifestations in the children who survive the hypocalcemic seizures include esophageal atresia, GI candidiasis, and intractable diarrhea.

Immunodeficiency Following Hereditary Defective Response to Epstein-Barr Virus

In this syndrome, also known as X-linked lymphoproliferative syndrome, the affected patient typically develops a chronic, often fatal infectious mononucleosis, progressive hypogammaglobulinemia, aplastic anemia, or malignant B-cell lymphoma following EBV infection.[65] Although at first this susceptibility to EBV appeared to be transmitted as a X-linked recessive trait, several cases have subsequently been reported in female patients.

These patients appear to be immunologically normal prior to EBV infection.[66] Subsequent to EBV infection, circulating B-cell population and immunoglobulins decrease. The predominant T cell in the peripheral circulation becomes the NK cell. Subsequently, a proliferative B-cell disorder (lymphoma) may develop in approximately 35 percent of patients.[67]

There is a marked impairment in the production of antibodies to the EBV nuclear antigens, whereas titers of antibodies to the viral capsid antigen have ranged from zero to markedly elevated. Antibody-dependent cell-mediated cytotoxicity against EBV-infected cells has been low in most affected individuals, and NK function is also depressed. There is also a deficiency in long-term T-cell immunity to EBV.[68] Studies of lymphocyte subpopulations have revealed elevated percentages of cells of the suppressor phenotype (CD8). Immunoglobulin synthesis in response to polyclonal B-cell mitogen stimulation in vitro is markedly depressed. Thus both EBV-specific and nonspecific immunologic abnormalities occur in these patients.[68]

The clinical spectrum is variable, as typified by the following cases. The first presented at age 6 with aplastic anemia. He subsequently developed a fulminant infectious mononucleosis with renal and hepatic failure, resulting in death within weeks. The second child presented at 8 years of age with a history of a fever of unknown origin of several years duration. Massive hepatosplenomegaly was noted on physical examination. Liver biopsy revealed microabscesses focally without granulomas, resembling a "septic" hepatitis. Multiple cultures were negative for bacterial, fungal, and viral pathogens. The patient eventually underwent elective splenectomy, which revealed a lymphoproliferative disorder and erythrophagocytosis. Specific antibody titers to EBV were demonstrated to increase significantly. The patient is being treated with antiviral agents, but the prognosis remains poor.

Defects of Phagocytic Function

Genetically determined defects of phagocytic function occur, affecting polymorphonuclear and/or mononuclear phagocytes (see Table 1). Neutrophil function is generally characterized as movement in response to chemotactic stimuli, adherence, endocytosis, and killing or destruction of ingested particles. Mobility depends on the integrity of the cytoskeleton and the contractile system, whereas directional mobility is receptor-mediated. Endocytosis depends on the expression of membrane receptors (for IgG, C3b, IC3b, etc.) and on the fluidity of the membrane.

Defects in intracellular killing of ingested microorganisms result from failure of the "respiratory burst," which is critical to production of superoxide radicals, oxygen singlets, hydroxyl radicals, and hydrogen peroxide. The organisms cultured from the lesions of patients with this type of defect are generally catalase producing, and include Staphylococcus, E. coli, fungi, and other opportunistic organisms. Patients with defective endocytosis and killing tend to have chronic infected granulomas, especially of lymph nodes, liver, and lung.

Patients whose neutrophils fail to adhere normally to surfaces have a biosynthetic defect of a 95-kDa chain glycoprotein (CD11/CD18). These molecules are present on the surfaces of all leukocytes and play a critical adhesive role in cell-microbe, cell-cell, and cell-surface interactions.

In the classic case, a patient with a neutrophil functional defect has had multiple invasive bacterial (especially Pseudomonas, Serratia, and Staphylococcus aureus) and fungal (Aspergillus and Candida species) infections beginning during the first year of life. The early infections involve primarily the skin and portals of entry: impetigo, paronychia, periodontitis, sinusitis, and perirectal abscesses. Later infections involve deeper structures: lymphadenitis, pneumonia, osteomyelitis, and splenic and hepatic abscesses. Tables 1 and 5 summarize the primary defects of phagocytic function (WHO classification).

Chronic Granulomatous Disease

Chronic granulomatous disease (CGD) is a group of genetic disorders characterized by recurrent pyogenic infections of the respiratory tract, skin, and soft tissues. Phagocytes from patients with CGD are unable to kill a wide variety of microorganisms effectively.

The neutrophils of patients with CGD demonstrate normal chemotaxis, engulfment, and degranulation, but their ability to kill microorganisms is impaired. Neutrophils from

TABLE 5
Defects of Phagocytic Function

Disease	Affected Cells*	Functional Defects
X-linked CGD[†]	N+M	↓ Oxidative metabolism
Autosomal recessive CGD	N	↓ Microbial activity
Phagocyte membrane defect CD11/CD18 leukocyte glycoprotein deficiency	N+M+L	↓ Adherence and ↓ phagocytosis
Chediak-Higashi syndrome	N+M	↓ Microbicidal activity ↓ Chemotaxis ↑ Oxidative metabolism Delayed degranulation
Neutrophil G6-PD deficiency	N	↓ Killing
Myeloperoxidase deficiency	N	↑ Oxidative metabolism ↓ Microbicidal activity
Secondary granule deficiency	N	↓ Microbicidal activity ↓ Chemotaxis ↓ Oxidative metabolism
Schwachman's disease	N	↓ Mobility and ↓ adherence

  * N = neutrophil; M = macrophage; L = lymphocyte.
  † CGD = chronic granulomatous disease.

these patients stimulated in vitro with a variety of particulate and soluble stimuli fail to consume oxygen needed for the production of superoxide anions, hydrogen peroxide, and hydroxyl radicals. NADPH-oxidase is found exclusively in phagocytes and is dormant unless activated: NADPH is the physiologic electron source; a flavin and a phagocyte b-cytochrome are also postulated to function in a short electron transport chain that transfers a single electron to molecular oxygen to form the superoxide anion. The failure to produce superoxide anions in CGD could result from abnormalities in the components of the oxidase itself as well as in its activation pathway. CGD is therefore heterogeneous at the genetic level. The CGD phenotype has two major forms of inheritance: X-linked recessive and autosomal recessive. There are at least three distinct genetic forms of CGD[69]: type I X-linked (cytochrome b–negative, the most common form), type II autosomal recessive (cytochrome b–positive, the next most common), and type III autosomal recessive (cytochrome b–negative). Another type has been described in only two cases: X-linked, cytochrome b–positive. Deficiencies of flavin have been also observed in some patients.

The *sine qua non* for the diagnosis of CGD is the demonstration of an absent or greatly diminished respiratory burst capacity. This defect is best determined by measuring superoxide (O_2^-) production in response to both soluble (PMA) and opsonized particulate stimuli (zymosan). In the majority of cases of CGD, there is either no detectable O_2^- generation or production at rates between 0.5 and 10 percent of control.[70] An alternative method for measuring respiratory burst activity is the nitroblue tetrazolium (NBT) test, which is normally reduced to its purple formazan crystals following stimulation of cells. In the most common forms of CGD, no NBT reduction is observed in any of the cells. In some of the variant forms, however, a high percentage of cells may contain small amounts of formazan. The NBT test

is invaluable in classifying variant forms of CGD. As detailed above, because the major classification criteria for CGD depend on the cytochrome b spectrum, its determination is essential. This can be accomplished using intact neutrophils or in subcellular fractions by Western blot analysis using antibodies to the two subunits of cytochrome b.[71]

The clinical CGD syndrome comprises recurrent infection, multifocal abscesses affecting the skin and liver, lymphadenopathy, hepatosplenomegaly, chronic lung disease, and persistent diarrhea. Steatorrhea and vitamin B_{12} malabsorption are commonly noted. Jejunal biopsy usually reveals normal villi, but lipid-filled, pigmented, foamy histiocytes are present in the lamina propria throughout the GI tract.[72]

Patients with CGD may present with an enterocolitis resembling Crohn's disease. The similarities include physical findings (most notably perianal abscesses and fistulae), sigmoidoscopic appearance, and radiographic abnormalities. Granulomas and giant cells are found quite frequently in rectal biopsies (Fig. 6). The mechanism of granuloma formation in CGD is unknown. It has been postulated that in view of the defective respiratory burst in CGD phagocytes, there is persistent inflammation because chemoattractants are not oxidatively inactivated. Delayed clearance of microorganisms also may explain these inflammatory changes. Similar hypotheses have been proposed to explain granuloma formation in Crohn's disease.

In addition to frequent hepatic and perirectal abscesses, patients with CGD may develop a granulomatous narrowing of the antrum, with symptoms suggestive of gastric outlet obstruction.[73] The NBT test is a useful diagnostic screen in patients presenting with an unexplained annular narrowing of the antrum.[74,75] Diagnosis may be confused with pyloric stenosis, peptic ulcer disease, eosinophilic gastroenteritis, or Crohn's disease. However, tissue examination and the NBT test are diagnostic.

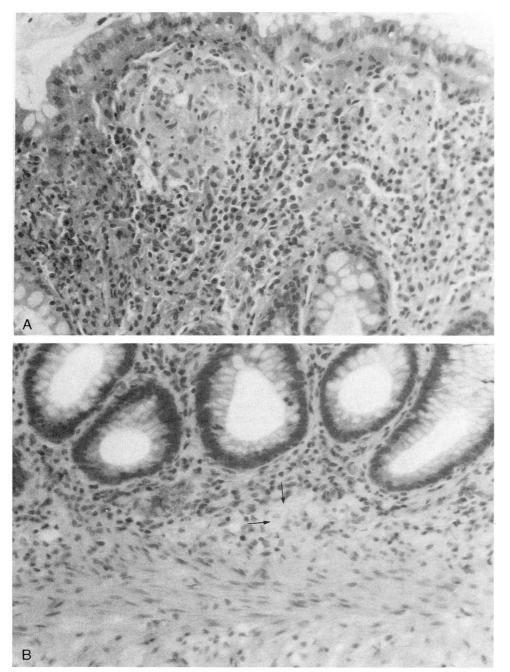

FIGURE 6 Longstanding colitis in a patient with chronic granulomatous disease. His severe colitis and perianal involvement resembling Crohn's disease were resistant to usual therapy (Salazopyrine, 5-ASA, prednisone, 6-mercaptopurine) but responded to total parenteral nutrition and complete bowel rest. *A*, Rectal biopsy shows two granulomas in the superficial part of the mucosa and a dense chronic inflammatory reaction peripherally. *B*, Foamy macrophages (*arrows*) are seen near the muscularis mucosae (HPS stain, ×300). (Courtesy of P. Russo, M.D.)

The gastric outlet obstruction often can be managed medically with broad-spectrum antibiotics and continuous enteral alimentation. Nutritional support and antimicrobials have been shown to obviate the need for surgery.[76] The symptomatic resolution of the obstruction occurred after 2 to 4 months of therapy. Adjunctive use of steroids may hasten the resolution of gastric outlet obstruction.[77] Recently, Ezekowitz and colleagues demonstrated the effect of gamma-interferon (IFN-gamma) on CGD phagocyte superoxide generation, NADPH-oxidase kinetics, and expression of the gene for the phagocyte cytochrome *b* heavy chain.[78] In vitro treatment with IFN-gamma increased the respiratory burst activity of PMN and macrophages from patients with CGD type IA variant (X-linked, A designates a form in which phagocytes exhibit decreased but detectable superoxide production). Phagocytes from classic type I, IIA, and II CGD did not respond to IFN-gamma. In vivo studies demonstrated similar responses. IFN-gamma appears to up-regulate expression of cytochrome *b* genes by increasing their transcription or through post-translational stabilization of mRNA.[78] These studies establish the potential efficacy of IFN-gamma in the treatment of these patients.

It is critically important for the clinician to consider the possibility of CGD in patients with a "Crohn's-like" disease in whom a history of recurrent infections and abscesses is noted. The intestinal and perianal manifestations are remarkably similar.

CD11/CD18 Leukocyte Glycoprotein Deficiency

CD11/CD18 leukocyte glycoprotein deficiency is a rare inherited disorder of leukocyte function that is manifested by recurrent infections. This impairment in immunity may be the result of absent or deficient expression of three plasma membrane glycoproteins: LFA-1 (CD11a/CD18), which serves as an adhesion-promoting molecule facilitating lymphocyte blastogenesis, cellular cytotoxicity (CTL, NK, and K), and lymphocyte-endothelial cell adhesion; Mol (CD11b/CD18) receptor for C3bl (CR3), which is an adhesion-promoting molecule facilitating PMN aggregation, PMN/macrophage (Mϕ) adhesion to substrates, and PMN/Mϕ chemotaxis; and P150,95 (CD11c/CD18), a poorly defined glycoprotein that may promote adhesion of PMN and Mϕ to substrates and also bind C3bi.[79]

There are at least two variants of CD11/CD18 leukocyte glycoprotein deficiency.[80] The degree of CD11/CD18 deficient expression (ranging from 10 percent of normal to totally absent) correlates closely with the severity of the clinical manifestations and the magnitude of the in vitro cellular abnormalities.

The clinical manifestations include delayed umbilical cord separation (2 to 3 weeks), leukocytosis, a neutrophil mobilization defect with the lack of neutrophils in inflammatory exudates arising from sites of active infection, and recurrent bacterial infections. Stomatitis/pharyngitis is present in 40 percent and gingivitis/periodontitis in 56 percent of patients. The oral manifestations of this disorder may be mistaken for Crohn's disease.

Bacterial septicemia is a common complication and may frequently result in the death of affected patients. Common bacterial pathogens include *Staphylococcus aureus*, group A beta-hemolytic *Streptococcus, Proteus mirabilis, Pseudomonas aeruginosa,* and *E. coli*. Severe viral infections (viral meningitis or fatal enteroviral infection) and oral candidiasis have also been described. We have also seen a patient presenting with an ischiorectal abscess resembling Crohn's disease.

In vitro leukocyte abnormalities include a defect in adhesion by unstimulated or PMA-stimulated cells. Neutrophils fail to demonstrate aggregation in response to stimulants (e.g., C5a, PMA). Impairment of directed motility is demonstrated in vitro in response to chemoattractants. A severe defect in CR3 aggregation activity is noted. The NBT for respiratory burst activity is impaired, as is secretion of granular contents by neutrophils and monocytes when induced by particulate stimuli. Lymphoid cells present a diminished blastogenic activity to mitogen (PMA). There is also an impairment in cytotoxic activity mediated by T lymphocytes, NK cells, and K cells.[80]

No specific therapy has been shown to ameliorate the clinical manifestations of the disorder. Antibiotic therapy has proved to be successful in most situations, but several patients have died from bacterial sepsis. Bone marrow transplantation may represent optimal therapy in patients with the severe form of the disease.

Other Disorders at Times Associated with Immunodeficiency

A number of other clinical disorders are associated with various forms of immunodeficiency (Table 6). In the majority of these disorders, the immune defect is usually secondary to a congenital or acquired disorder.

Chronic Mucocutaneous Candidiasis

Chronic mucocutaneous candidiasis is a syndrome characterized by *Candida* infection involving the esophageal and buccal mucosa, skin, and nails. It is frequently associated with an endocrinopathy (Addison's disease, hypoparathyroidism, hypothyroidism) and pernicious anemia. This condition may result from a variety of causes, including a primary defect in cell-mediated immunity to *Candida* (autosomal recessive). Patients may present with esophageal candidiasis in the presence or absence of oral involvement. Therefore, any patient with mucocutaneous candidiasis who has dysphagia, odynophagia, or hematemesis should be suspected of having *Candida* esophagitis even if oral involvement is not evident. These individuals are at risk for development of esophageal stricture and thus require aggressive treatment for chronic *Candida* infection. The use of antacids of H$_2$ antagonists may worsen the esophageal involvement with *Candida* by reducing gastric acidity.

We have followed an adolescent male with familial chronic mucocutaneous candidiasis who presented with a chronic indeterminate colitis. His colitis was unresponsive to medical management including sulfasalazine, steroids, elemental diet, parenteral nutrition, 6-mercaptopurine, and cyclosporine. His unrelenting colitis eventually required colectomy, and no recurrence of disease has been noted after 1 year. Interestingly, his mother, also affected by chronic mucocutaneous candidiasis, also has primary biliary cirrhosis.

TABLE 6
Selected Disorders Potentially Associated with Immunodeficiency

---

Chronic mucocutaneous candidiasis ($\pm$ endocrinopathy)
Chromosomal abnormalities
  Bloom syndrome
  Fanconi anemia
  Down's syndrome
Prematurity
Malnutrition
Malignancies
Autoimmunity
Immunosuppressive therapy
Metabolic diseases
  Type I orotic aciduria
  Biotin deficiency
Metal transport defects/deficiency
  Acrodermatitis enteropathica
  Calcium transport defect
  Trace metal deficiencies
Hypercatabolism of immunoglobulins
  Myotonic dystrophy
  Intestinal lymphangiectasia
  Inflammatory bowel disease
Viral infections
  Acquired immunodeficiency syndrome (AIDS)

GASTROINTESTINAL MANIFESTATIONS OF SECONDARY IMMUNODEFICIENCIES

Malnutrition and Cancer

In addition to the relatively rare congenital and primary immune deficiencies discussed above, various common clinical conditions may predispose to an acquired defect in host immune defense (Table 6). A temporary deficiency in secretory antibody is seen in conditions such as prematurity and protein-calorie malnutrition. Malignancies such as lymphoma are other notable examples of acquired immunologic function abnormalities. The undernourished host is immunodeficient, demonstrating several immunologic alterations: depression in the number of T cells, decreased T-lymphocyte responses,[81] and decreased IL-1 production[82]; a phagocytic dysfunction has also been reported including decreased chemotactic responses[83] and decreased bactericidal capacity of polymorphonuclear leukocytes.[84] Although immunoglobulin concentrations are normal or elevated and adequate antibody response to antigenic stimulation is generally produced, a reduced humoral response to measles has been reported, and some evidence exists that immunoglobulin function is deficient, including decreased concentration of secretory IgA.[85]

The depression of peripheral T-cell function is paralleled by a similar depression of T-cell function in the intestinal mucosa. This may contribute to the enhanced entry of luminal viruses, bacteria, parasites, or toxins across the mucosal barrier. Antigen presentation to macrophages and plasma cells in the lamina propria and stimulation by T-helper lymphocytes are likely to be deficient. A lack of normal intestinal cell function may well lead to altered macrophage microbicidal activity, and a reduction in IgA antibody activity leads to reduced secretory IgA production and to increased risk of enteric infections. The mucosa in malnutrition responds poorly to antigen presentation and places the patient at risk of excessive absorption of luminal antigens[86] and a higher frequency of mucosal infections.

In pediatric patients with lymphomas and leukemias, diarrhea is a frequent complication. This is partially secondary to infiltration of the intestinal wall by the neoplasm.[87] Other factors include the loss of the epithelial barrier, the severity and duration of the neutropenia, the immunologic deficiencies determined by the illness per se, and the immunosuppressive treatment administered. These factors in concert may result in severe intestinal infections due to constituents of the normal intestinal flora. Several studies have indicated that there is an enhanced susceptibility to *Salmonella* (principally *S. typhimurium* and *S. derby*) in cancer patients. This is especially true in patients suffering from leukemia. The GI disease usually resolves when cytotoxic therapy is discontinued. Patients with severe antibody deficiency secondary to chronic lymphatic leukemia or myeloma are not as prone to bowel infections as patients with primary hypogammaglobulinemia, probably because they retain some local antibody production.

Immunosuppressive Therapy

Another large category includes iatrogenically induced immune deficiency due to treatment with corticosteroids or other immunosuppressive drugs. Immunosuppressive agents are frequently used in the management of patients with autoimmune diseases, transplants (bone marrow, heart, kidney, liver), and cancer. The infectious complications of immunosuppressive therapy represent an important cause of morbidity and mortality in these patients.[88] Cyclosporine, azathioprine, antithymocyte globulin, and steroids have been used postoperatively to control rejection episodes and prolong graft survival but may put the patient at risk for acquiring life-threatening infectious illnesses. The influence of these drugs on the capacity to produce IL-1 and IL-2, IL-2 receptor expression, and suppression of local inflammatory response by decreasing monocyte adherence, polymorphonuclear chemotaxis, tissue kinin release, and decreased percentage of circulating T lymphocytes, explains the increased morbidity and mortality caused by intracellular microorganisms.

The GI tract in such an immunocompromised host is frequently involved by chronic fungal infections (particularly *Candida*), unusual parasites such as *Strongyloides*, and viral infections such as herpes and CMV.[89] In a recent report, Proujansky et al[90] described four children with CMV infection in the post-transplant period whose initial symptoms were of serious GI disease. One or more areas of the GI tract can be involved simultaneously, resulting in dysphagia, nausea, vomiting, delayed gastric emptying, abdominal pain, GI hemorrhage, or diarrhea. The authors thus recommend prompt endoscopic evaluation, including histologic examination and viral culture of mucosal biopsy specimens, in such immunosuppressed patients. Reduction in immunosuppression may be effective but must be weighed against the risk of graft rejection. Antiviral agents have some efficacy. Hyperimmune globulin has not been effective in treating active CMV infection but may prevent infection in selected patients.[91]

Acrodermatitis Enteropathica

Metabolic diseases such as acrodermatitis enteropathica result in hypogammaglobulinemia and abnormal cell-mediated immunity. This autosomal recessive disease, characterized by an eczematous rash, alopecia, chronic diarrhea, malabsorption, and recurrent sinopulmonary infections, can be mimicked by acquired conditions resulting in severe zinc deficiency, such as Crohn's disease and intractable diarrhea of infancy. The symptoms and immunologic abnormalities respond to zinc supplementation. It is unclear whether the diarrhea results from infection in the bowel or is related to the zinc deficiency itself. Hypogammaglobulinemia may occur in some patients with more advanced disease; it is not known whether this is due to a protein-losing enteropathy or a direct effect on lymphocytic function.

Protein-Losing Enteropathies

Excessive loss of proteins including immunoglobulins into the GI tract is common to many GI disorders, including chronic inflammatory bowel disease, hypertrophic gastritis (Ménétrier's disease), eosinophilic gastroenteropathy, and intestinal lymphangiectasia. Lymphocytes as well as immunoglobulins may be lost. The lymphopenia may lead to defects in cell-mediated immunity. Hypoalbuminemia is an important diagnostic feature, and it is likely that affected patients never develop hypogammaglobulinemia without hypoalbuminemia. However, this is theoretically possible in patients with particularly efficient hepatic synthesis of albumin but subnormal immunoglobulin synthesis.

It is often difficult to distinguish between the secondary hypogammaglobulinemia that complicates the chronic diarrhea of protein-losing enteropathies and the primary humoral immunodeficiency that is accompanied by chronic diarrhea. In the former, the relative molecular sizes favor the preferential loss of smaller albumin and IgG compared to IgA and IgM. Patients with protein-losing enteropathy produce antibodies when test immunized with antigens such as tetanus toxoid or pneumococcal polysaccharide vaccines, and this probably explains why they are not as susceptible to infections. This is in striking contrast to patients with primary hypogammaglobulinemia, who fail to make such antibodies. The diagnosis of primary hypogammaglobulinemia may be excluded by demonstrating normal numbers of plasma cells in the lamina propria of the intestinal mucosa and in bone marrow.

Intestinal Lymphangiectasia

The combination of lymphopenia and protein-losing enteropathy suggests the diagnosis of intestinal lymphangiectasia. T lymphocytes are lost from the intestine or into chylous effusions, and this may be associated with a failure to manifest delayed hypersensitivity skin reactions. Susceptibility to infections is variable but rarely severe. Diagnosis requires confirmation by intestinal biopsy. Lymphangiography may show other lymphatic abnormalities in familial cases. As with other protein-losing enteropathies, serum IgM tends to remain within normal limits while the serum IgG and IgA may fall to very low levels. This pattern may be seen in patients with primary hypogammaglobulinemia, although the serum IgA is usually much lower. However it differs from that seen in the hypogammaglobulinemia secondary to lymphoproliferative disease, in which the serum IgM is usually the first immunoglobulin class to fall.

There is usually a good response to a fat-restricted diet and supplementation with medium-chain triglycerides. This reduces the lymphatic flow in the intestine, thus reducing the pressure driving the gut losses. Steroids are helpful when the lymphangiectasia is due to local inflammation such as in Crohn's disease and may also have a short-term palliative effect in malignant infiltration.

Acquired Immunodeficiency Syndrome

The first cases of pediatric acquired immunodeficiency syndrome (AIDS) were reported in 1982, about 1 year following description of the first adult cases. Since then, nearly 1,000 cases have been reported, and this number is expected to increase 10-fold by 1991.[92] This highly lethal disorder is characterized by a profound derangement of cell-mediated immunity associated with a marked predisposition to opportunistic infections. Pediatric centers are increasingly faced with the challenge of caring for young patients with AIDS who present with many unusual GI and hepatic infections and severe malnutrition. In this chapter, we will concentrate on the GI manifestations commonly seen in pediatric AIDS patients. The hepatic complications are reviewed in Chapter 28, Part 22.

Etiopathogenesis of AIDS

AIDS is believed to be caused by the virus now known as human immunodeficiency virus (HIV). This virus was first reported by Barre-Sinoussi et al[93] in France and called lymphadenopathy-associated virus (LAV). Later, Gallo et al[94] reported finding the same virus, which they called the human T lymphotropic virus type III (HTLV-III), in AIDS patients from the United States. The virus was also referred to as the AIDS-associated retrovirus (ARV).[95] In 1986, the International Committee for the Taxonomy of Viruses suggested that the virus be called human immunodeficiency virus (HIV), and this term has now become widely accepted.[96]

The HIV uses a reverse transcriptase to transcribe DNA from the viral RNA. This DNA is then incorporated into the human cellular DNA, where it can remain latent for months to years. After some yet-to-be-identified activating event, viral proteins are made from the DNA using the cellular machinery. These proteins are assembled in the cellular cytoplasm, and viral particles then bud off from the cell. These free viral particles can then infect other cells, or cells can become infected via cell fusion.[97]

The recognition that the CD4 antigen on the surface of human helper T lymphocytes is a major cellular receptor for the HIV envelope protein gp 120 led to the inference that endocytosis of the virus by cells expressing the CD4 molecule is an initial step in the infection. However, HIV can also infect cells lacking CD4, including brain astrocyte cell lines, human fibroblasts, and endothelial and epithelial cells of seropositive individuals. Fusion of the target cell membrane with the HIV transmembrane envelope protein (gp 47) is one possible means of virus entry. Antibody-dependent enhancement of virus infection can mediate HIV infection of cells. Virus-antibody complexes permit HIV infection of macrophages and T cells, most likely via the complement and/or Fc receptor.

Immunopathology of HIV Infections

The immunologic abnormalities found in AIDS are those of a severe and profound cellular immune deficiency. The immune dysfunctions identified in HIV infection were at first linked to the cytopathic effects of HIV on helper T lymphocytes, which normally play a key role in regulating immune function (Fig. 2). HIV infection is known to cause epiphenomena including decreased expression of immunologic recognition sites, such as CD4 and the IL-2 receptor, and reduced production of cytokines such as IL-1, IL-2, and IFN-gamma.[98,99] HIV envelope proteins have been found to be toxic or inhibitory to immune cells. Circulating in the blood, these proteins may block the ability of lymphocytes to recognize or respond to foreign antigens and may interfere with the function of antigen-presenting cells.

HIV is also associated, often early in the infection, with a polyclonal activation of B cells, resulting in hypergammaglobulinemia. While producing elevated levels of immunoglobulins, B cells of HIV-infected individuals appear to be refractory to stimulation by mitogens, to polysaccharide antigens, and to newly encountered protein antigens. The resulting inability to produce the antibodies required for protective responses to many bacterial pathogens plays an important role in predisposing these patients to the development of bacterial infections. Other pathologic consequences include the production of autoantibodies and various circulating immune complexes, often associated with significant morbidity. The destruction of activated helper T cells by lymphocytotoxic autoantibodies directed against a normal cellular protein (pl8) has been suggested as one of the possible mechanisms for the substantial loss of CD4+ cells in advanced HIV disease. Positive tests for antinuclear antibodies and an increased frequency of B-cell malignancies occurs in AIDS patients and HIV-infected individuals. The B-cell activation may thus, in and of itself, amplify the immunoregulatory abnormalities in this disease.[100]

In general, helper T lymphocytes are most susceptible to the cytopathic effects of HIV, but macrophage killing has also been observed.[101] Cell death may result from direct membrane disruption involving calcium channels and/or phospholipid synthesis.

Transmission of HIV in Children

HIV is generally transmitted by one of three routes: (1) through sexual contact, (2) via parenteral exposure to infective blood or blood products, including exposure to contaminated materials in drug abusers, and (3) from infected mothers to their newborn infants. Perinatal transmission is the most common mode in prepubertal children, accounting for nearly 80 percent of patients under 13 years of age. AIDS has commonly been recognized in infants born to prostitutes and drug-addicted mothers. In certain centers, infants born to Haitian immigrants account for a large proportion of cases. The transmission can theoretically occur in utero (transplacental passage of the virus), during labor and delivery (exposure to infective maternal blood and secretions), or postnatally (breast-feeding).

Transfusion of HIV-infected blood or blood products has accounted for about 20 percent of cases in children. The majority of such cases have affected children with coagulation disorders, chronic anemias, or hematologic disorders requiring multiple transfusions. Sexual contact is the second most common mode of transmission in adolescents, following blood or blood product transfusions. There have been no reported cases of transmission within schools and no reports of casual transmission attributable to household contact.[102]

TABLE 7
Opportunistic Organisms Infecting the Gastrointestinal Tract in Acquired Immunodeficiency Syndrome

Viral	Bacterial	Fungal	Parasitic
Cytomegalovirus	*Salmonella*	*Candida*	*Cryptosporidium*
Rotavirus	*Campylobacter*-like organisms	*Aspergillus*	*Strongyloides*
Herpes simplex	*Listeria*		*Giardia*
Adenovirus	*Mycobacterium avium-intracellulare*		*Amoeba*
Coxsackie	*Plesiomonas shigelloides*		*Isospora belli*

Time Course and Latency

The time from infection with the virus to development of clinical symptoms is variable and may depend on the timing of infection, the dose of virus, the host's immune response, and other associated illnesses. In perinatally acquired disease, infants generally present clinical illness in the first 2 years of life. Those infected in utero generally develop symptoms earlier than infants infected via blood transfusion early in life (9 versus 14 months).[103] The adolescent age group appears more resistant to HIV virus than either adults or infants.

Levy, in a recent publication,[98] summarized the possible stages in the course of HIV infection and latency. Acute infection is characterized by the presence of free virus (or its antigen) in the blood with absence of antibodies to HIV. There is a rapid increase of CD8+ cells with a concomitant decrease in CD4+ cells. After a short period (2 to 12 weeks) a resistant state develops, and CD8+ cells return to normal levels, while CD4+ cells decrease at a slow rate, leading to an inversion of the helper:suppressor ratio. Free virus is not detected in blood because it is produced episodically. After a variable time lag, the resistant state wanes for reasons that remain unclear. It may be that concomitant viral or parasitic infections activate immune cells, produce more virus, or become more sensitive to HIV infection. The virus enters multiple replicative cycles, during which a variant strain can emerge that may be resistant to the immune response and highly cytopathic, further compromising the host's immune defense. Viremia is accompanied by enhanced destruction of CD4+ cells and progression of disease. During the latent period of retrovirus infection, very little viral protein or RNA is made.

General Clinical Manifestations

Infants with AIDS acquired during the pre- or perinatal period are often of low birth weight and have failure to thrive associated with chronic diarrhea and generalized lymphadenopathy. Severe interstitial pneumonia and asymptomatic hepatosplenomegaly with hypergammaglobulinemia are other modes of presentation.

Early symptoms may be nonspecific yet quite persistent and severe. Oral candidiasis refractory to therapy, with failure to thrive, is a common presentation. Common physical findings include lymphadenopathy, hepatosplenomegaly, and parotiditis (10 to 20 percent). Bacterial infection is more common than opportunistic infection. Viral infections such as stomatitis due to herpes simplex virus, persistent EBV infection, and fatal measles are other known infections. *P. carinii* pneumonia is the most frequent opportunistic infection seen in children with HIV infection.[103,104] Morbidity and mortality are high. Other severe opportunistic infectious complications include chronic infection with *Mycobacterium avium-intracellulare*, systemic CMV, progressive herpes simplex virus disease, and cerebral toxoplasmosis.

Recurrent diarrhea or severe intractable diarrhea with malabsorption is a common and difficult management problem in HIV-infected children. A wide variety of pathogens and opportunistic infections have been reported to involve the GI tract and liver in AIDS patients. For the clinician, the diversity of the organisms is further complicated by the unusual endoscopic and histologic findings. Involvement of the GI tract by opportunistic infections and a severe form of Kaposi's sarcoma are prominent features of this condition and contribute significantly to its morbidity and mortality. They are summarized in Table 7 and reviewed below in greater detail.

Lymphoid interstitial pneumonitis is the most frequent type of pulmonary involvement associated with HIV infection in children. Central nervous system dysfunction has been demonstrated in as many as 50 to 90 percent of children.[105] Cardiomyopathy is less well described in children than in adults. Nephropathy has been described, and various hepatic abnormalities have been encountered. Other manifestations of HIV infection in children include anemia, leukopenia, and thrombocytopenia. B-cell lymphomas are the most common malignancy. Kaposi's sarcoma is rare in children, but a form without skin lesions has been described. An embryopathy with craniofacial dysmorphic features has been reported in association with congenitally HIV-infected children.[106]

The prognosis for children with this disease is very poor. Survival analysis indicates that children in whom AIDS is diagnosed before 1 year of age have a more fulminant course than when the diagnosis is made later in life.[103] In children with HIV infection, the early mortality is approximately 61 percent. Survival may also vary depending on clinical presentation. Children with *P. carinii* pneumonitis tend to have a more fulminant course than those with other opportunistic infections.

Gastrointestinal Disease in AIDS

Enteric diseases are among the most common and devastating problems that affect patients with HIV infection (Table 8). The majority of AIDS patients (50 to 90 percent) suffer from chronic diarrheal illnesses.[107] There are three major mechanisms for the pathogenesis of GI disease: (1) opportunistic infection(s) of the gut in the context of cellular immune deficiency, (2) uncommon tumors: Kaposi's sarcoma or B-cell lymphoma, and (3) direct HIV effect on the gut.[108] Diarrhea, loss of weight, and malabsorption are the major manifestations in any form of gut disease in AIDS with the exception of Kaposi's sarcoma of the gut, which is commonly asymptomatic despite extensive infiltration. The severity and duration of symptoms associated with enteric pathogens are generally determined by the host's immunologic response to the organism. The virulence of the pathogen may also affect the clinical response to infection. The availability of effective anti-infective therapy is among the most decisive factors in determining the duration and outcome of enteric infections in AIDS patients. Defects in local GI immunity associated with AIDS, reviewed below, may be important in the progression of AIDS involving the GI tract and the numerous infections now associated with this disease.

Intestinal Mucosal Immunity in AIDS

Cell-mediated Immunity. Phenotypic analysis of small intestinal mucosal mononuclear cells in AIDS reveals a significant decrease in total T-cell number, and particularly in

TABLE 8
Gastrointestinal Manifestations of AIDS by Site of Involvement

Oral cavity	Candidiasis
	Herpes simplex virus
	Human papilloma virus
	Hairy leukoplakia
	Kaposi's sarcoma
	Lymphoma
Esophagus	Candidiasis
	Cytomegalovirus
	Herpes simplex virus
	Cryptosporidiosis
	Kaposi's sarcoma
	Lymphoma
Stomach	Cytomegalovirus
	Cryptosporidiosis
	Kaposi's sarcoma
Small intestine	Giardiasis
	Cryptosporidiosis
	Cytomegalovirus
	Salmonella/Shigella
	Mycobacteria
	Lymphoma
Colon	Cytomegalovirus
	Salmonella, Shigella
	Campylobacter
	Entamoeba
	Lymphoma
Anus/rectum	Kaposi's sarcoma
	Lymphoma
	Squamous cell carcinoma
	Papovavirus

the CD4-positive T-cell subset. CD8 lymphocytes comprise a significantly greater proportion of the total T-cell population in AIDS, and so the CD4/CD8 mucosal T-cell ratios are decreased. NK cells are described as normal.[109]

The CD2-positive T cells are decreased in the intraepithelial region of the small intestine in AIDS patients, but such changes have not been noted in rectal tissue. Expression of IL-2 receptors is not noted on T lymphocytes in the intestinal epithelium or lamina propria of AIDS or AIDS-related complex (ARC) patients.[109] Lymphoid follicles in the rectal mucosa of AIDS patients reveal a normal B-cell area surrounded by CD8, without CD4 positive cells in the perifollicular area. Abnormalities in the CD4 mucosal T cells likely reflect either the direct local infection or the systemic effect of HIV infection.

Local Humoral Immunity. Plasma cells in the lamina propria of the small intestine and rectal biopsies has been studied by Kotler et al.[110] They noted decreased IgA, increased IgM, and normal distribution of IgG-containing plasma cells. The number of IgA-containing plasma cells did not correlate with the presence of opportunistic infections, Kaposi's sarcoma, or GI symptoms. Decreased IgA plasma cells in the lamina propria may be a secondary effect of decreased CD4 regulation of B-cell differentiation.[109]

Such alterations in mucosal immunity and mucosal defense likely render AIDS and ARC subjects susceptible to enteric infections and systemic infections in which the intestinal tract is the portal of entry.

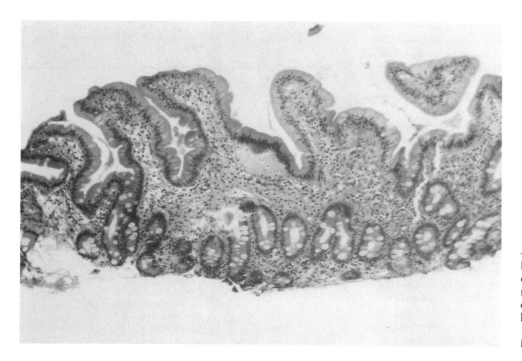

FIGURE 7 Nonspecific enteropathy of AIDS. Jejunal biopsy reveals mild villous atrophy and chronic inflammation of the lamina propria (HPS stain, ×120). (Courtesy of P. Russo, M.D.)

Nonspecific Enteropathy Associated with AIDS

In view of the multiple and unusual organisms involving the intestinal tract in AIDS (see Table 7), it is important for the clinician to realize that the morphologic expression of disease in these immunocompromised hosts may also differ drastically from the usual. Tuberculosis, for example, may not be associated with either caseous necrosis or granuloma formation but may present as a nonspecific colonic ulcer in AIDS.[111] Cytomegalovirus, a common cause of colitis in AIDS,[112,113] causes an unusual, patchy involvement requiring multiple biopsies for proper diagnosis.[111–113]

Observations on the GI structure and absorption in AIDS suggest that a nonspecific enteropathy with nutrient malabsorption and malnutrition is common.[114] This subgroup of patients has a severe enteropathy not attributable to a specific infection (Fig. 7). HIV infection of enterochromaffin cells in the intestinal mucosa, other crypt cells, and possibly columnar epithelial or goblet cells[115] might explain this chronic diarrhea in the absence of any known bowel pathogens. Aggressive nutritional support is often necessary for such patients. The isolation of infectious virus from the bowel emphasizes that this site should also be regarded as a potential source of viral transmission.

Opportunistic Gastrointestinal Infections In AIDS

Fungi. *Candida albicans* is frequently part of the normal oral flora and is the species most frequently found in oral *Candida* infections. Oral candidiasis is thus a sensitive clinical marker of immunosuppression and frequently the earliest and probably the most common of the opportunist infections seen in AIDS. Oral candidiasis may have different appearances in association with HIV infection, including pseudomembranous candidiasis, atrophic candidiasis, and angular cheilitis. Plaques of *Candida* may be demonstrated in the esophagus and are readily visualized by esophagoscopy and biopsy (Fig. 8). The presence of oral candidiasis in AIDS patients signals the likely co-existence of esophageal involvement and thus requires aggressive management. Significant strictures of the esophagus may result, even despite antifungal therapy.

Despite the remarkably high frequency of symptomatic candidiasis in the upper alimentary canal, mucosal disease in the lower GI tract of symptomatic AIDS patients has rarely been reported.[108,116,117] In terminally ill patients with AIDS and disseminated candidiasis, it has not been proven that oral or esophageal areas may serve as a nidus for dissemination of *Candida* to other organs.

Many antifungal agents have been used to treat oroesophageal candidiasis in AIDS. Nystatin tablets or suspension may be beneficial for treating oral cavity involvement. However, suboptimal response is not uncommonly seen in immunocompromised patients. Infants can be treated by clotrimazole vaginal tablets placed inside a pacifier. This treatment has been successful and well accepted. Ketoconazole is the mainstay of therapy for esophageal involvement. In some cases there is fungal resistance to the drug.[118] Malabsorption of this agent in patients with decreased gastric acid secretion may explain the failure of this agent to eradicate esophageal candidiasis in some patients. When esophageal candidiasis fails to respond to higher doses of ketoconazole, or hepatic dysfunction limits its use, the patients require low-dose intravenous amphotericin B to treat the disease.

Protozoa. Cryptosporidia are coccidial protozoan parasites of the subphylum sporozoa. Prior to 1982, there were only 12 reported cases of human infection with this predominant-

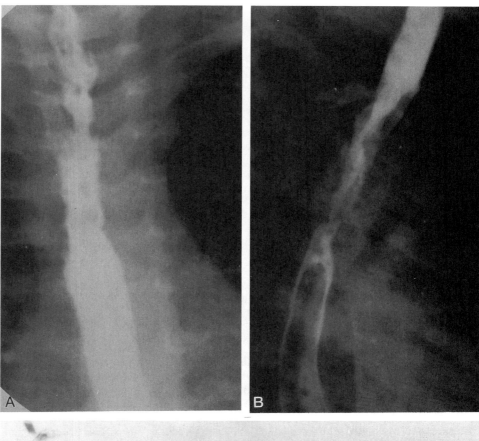

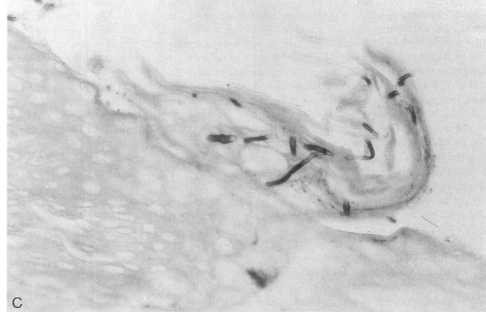

FIGURE 8 Severe esophageal candidiasis in a child with AIDS. Barium esophagogram showing an irregular narrowing in the proximal third of the esophagus (*A*), with irregular mucosa and *Candida* mycetoma (*B*). Endoscopy confirmed grade 4 *Candida* esophagitis, with confluent and nodular elevated plaques, superficial ulceration, and narrowing of the esophageal lumen. Biopsy revealed fungal spores and hyphae (*C*) invading the esophageal mucosa (Grocott stain, ×480). (Courtesy of P. Russo, M.D.)

ly animal protozoal parasite.[119] It is now widely recognized that this organism is a relatively common cause of persistent, severe secretory diarrhea in AIDS. A member of the Coccidia family, *Isospora belli*, causes disease similar to cryptosporidiosis.

Transmission of this parasite may occur from an animal reservoir, and via human-to-human spread.[120] *Cryptosporidium* infects the small bowel predominantly, where the parasite lies in the microvilli of the columnar cells in an intracellular fashion, causing villous atrophy (Fig. 9). It com-

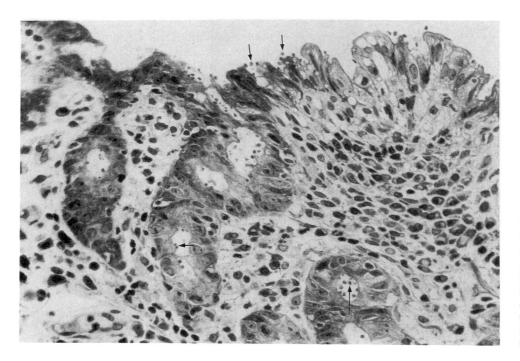

FIGURE 9 *Cryptosporidium*-induced enteritis in an infant with AIDS. Small bowel biopsy shows severe villous atrophy and chronic inflammation. Note the numerous cryptosporidial organisms (*arrows*) dotting the surface epithelium and crypts (trichrome stain, ×480). (Courtesy of P. Russo, M.D.)

pletes its life cycle on the microvillous surface and excretes many cysts into the bowel lumen. The stool of infected patients may be infectious for long periods of time.

In the immunosuppressed patient, there is a failure to eliminate the organism, and cysts are continually excreted. The parasite is associated with a persistent, often voluminous watery diarrhea in AIDS. The diarrhea is often accompanied by nausea, abdominal pain, anorexia and vomiting, and a low-grade fever. Weight loss is marked, and malabsorption rapidly becomes a clinical problem. Dysphagia associated with infection of the distal esophagus has been described in a 2-year-old girl.[121] *Cryptosporidium* may produce hepatobiliary disease in association with CMV in AIDS patients who may or may not have diarrhea.[122]

The diagnosis of cryptosporidiasis can be made by the finding of acid/alcohol-fast cysts in fresh stool specimens. Effective therapy for cryptosporidiosis is not currently available, although spiramycin has been useful in some cases.[123] The disease is often catastrophic for the patient, with debilitating, often fatal diarrhea. At present, supportive care including fluid replacement and enteral or parenteral nutrition is generally offered. There is no evidence that total parenteral nutrition is beneficial to survival in cryptosporidiosis.

The most common nonopportunistic protozoan parasite in AIDS patients is *Giardia lamblia*. This organism generally causes an acute diarrheal illness similar to that observed in immunocompetent persons.[124] A prolonged, debilitating diarrheal illness like that caused by *Cryptosporidium* is not observed. Therapy for *Giardia* is effective, and standard antimicrobial therapy can eradicate the parasite.[124]

Bacteria. Common bacterial pathogens such as *Salmonella, Shigella, Campylobacter,* and *Yersinia* may often cause gastroenteritis in AIDS. Diarrheal illness is accompanied by abdominal pain and fever, and in some cases bloody diarrhea and bacteremia are present.[125] *Salmonella* bacteremia may precede the onset of clinical AIDS and occur in the absence of intestinal symptoms. It is characterized by relapse

with multidrug-resistant organisms and may be life-threatening.[126,127] AIDS patients handle *Salmonella* abnormally, probably because these organisms are falcultative intracellular bacteria. In general, they do not seem to develop special problems from *Campylobacter* or other enterobacteria. Bacterial infections normally handled principally by the humoral or phagocytic immune system present little problem in most AIDS patients.

Mycobacteria, both *M. tuberculosis* (*M.tb*) and the atypical species, particularly *M. avium-intracellulare* (*M.ai*) are also well-documented as causes of infection in AIDS. The *M.tb* organism, a potential pathogen of the immunocompetent individual, tends to present at an earlier stage of AIDS. Patients infected with *M.tb* of the bowel at this stage may present with a typical pattern of ileocecal infection, a mass in the right lower quadrant, loss of weight, and bleeding per rectum. As noted above, however, histologic findings are usually atypical and require cultures for diagnosis.[111] *M.ai* is associated with later infection in AIDS. GI tract involvement is characterized by moderately severe diarrhea, fever, and weight loss.[128] The only histologic findings may be acid-fast bacilli. The lamina propria often shows massive numbers of foamy macrophages that are filled with bacilli, histologically resembling Whipple's disease.[129] Infections with atypical mycobacteria in patients with severe immunodeficiency frequently become disseminated. Acid-fast bacilli may be found in many organs. Liver involvement has been reported in children more often than small bowel involvement.[130] Unfortunately, antimicrobial therapy for *M.ai* requires multiple antibiotics and often fails to eradicate the organism.

Viruses. Herpes simplex virus often causes recurrent episodes of painful stomatitis. Intraorally, the lesions appear most commonly on the palate but may also occur on other keratinized surfaces, including the gingiva. The lesions may persist for several weeks, causing considerable pain and difficulty in eating. Esophageal involvement is heralded by odynophagia or dysphagia. In childhood AIDS, perioral lesions are seen commonly, suggesting an association between recurrence and length of time since primary infection.[131] Diagnosis can be confirmed by viral culture in the case of early lesions, by cytologic smears showing characteristic viral giant cells, or by use of monoclonal antibodies. Treatment with acyclovir is generally highly effective.

Persistent and unusual manifestations of EBV infection are common in children with AIDS, including oral hairy leukoplakia.[132] Virtually all patients with hairy leukoplakia are antibody positive for HIV. The lesion is occasionally seen on the buccal or labial mucosa as well as the tongue. The lesion is characteristically white, it does not rub off, and the surface may become so thick that hair-like projections appear. Microscopically, there are characteristic changes consisting of folds or hairs, hyperparakeratosis, acanthosis, vacuolation of bands, and little if any subepithelial inflammation.[133] The lesions may extend to the esophagus, where they appear as linear ulcerations in the midportion of the esophagus associated with marked dysphagia.

EBV is present in hairy leukoplakia tissue in prolific and fully replicating form. In cases in which biopsy is not possible, cytospin and filter in situ hybridization techniques have been developed.[134] The morphologic appearance of the esophageal lesion resembles closely that seen in the mouth. Acyclovir is effective treatment for hairy leukoplakia at high doses. An analogue of acyclovir, descyclovir, showed temporary elimination or almost complete resolution of the lesion.[133]

CMV infection is present in 70 percent of adult patients with AIDS but is less common in pediatric patients. The spectrum of GI manifestations of CMV in AIDS ranges from mild to moderate diarrhea with weight loss to severe gastroenterocolitis with intestinal or colonic perforation. In CMV colitis, the most common cause of colitis in AIDS,[112,113] patients present with fever, diarrhea that may be blood-streaked, and variable abdominal pain. Abdominal radiographs may show generalized dilatation of the large bowel with or without small bowel fluid levels. The natural history of this infection is spontaneous bouts of dilatation, which generally resolve in 3 to 8 days regardless of therapy. In some instances the infection may lead to massive bleeding. The endoscopic appearance ranges from nonspecific erythema or friability to ulcerated hemorrhagic or necrotic lesions.[135] Histology may allow for the identification of viral inclusion cells surrounded by mononuclear inflammatory changes. Cultures from biopsies, resected specimens, and urine are often positive for CMV, but the virus may not be recovered from stool. Often the cecum alone is involved, and immunohistochemical staining is required for diagnosis. Goodman et al considered CMV to be a secondary pathogen because they were unable to identify CMV infection in undamaged colonic mucosa.[136] CMV has also been demonstrated in uninflamed bowel from AIDS patients, and its role as a cause of primary colitis versus a secondary invader is disputed.[137] The exact role of CMV in the pathogenesis of colitis remains unclear. The known affinity of CMV for endothelial cells is intriguing in view of the association of Kaposi's sarcoma and CMV infection and because Kaposi's sarcoma may arise from endothelial cells.

Ganciclovir, an acyclic nucleoside analogue similar in structure to acyclovir, has been shown to be effective in several forms of CMV infection. Recurrent viremia was noted to occur in AIDS patients when treatment was discontinued. It appears that ganciclovir is most effective against active CMV infections but does not eradicate CMV in its latent phase.[138] Lim et al, using an antiviral agent plus hyperimmune plasma, coupled with partial ileocolic resection, achieved clinical response as well as disappearance of CMV from ileal and colonic tissue.[139]

Gastrointestinal Neoplasms in AIDS

Malignancy has rarely been reported in children with AIDS. B-cell lymphomas are most common, whereas Kaposi's sarcoma is relatively rare compared to its incidence in adults. Kaposi's sarcoma is thought to be a tumor of endothelial cell origin, and the gut lesions resemble highly vascular submucosal plaques or nodules. The lesions can occur in any part of the GI tract and are most frequently asymptomatic.

Intestinal Kaposi's sarcoma may often be the first clinical manifestation of AIDS in adults and requires biopsies to make a specific diagnosis.[140] Endoscopic biopsies frequently fail to make the diagnosis owing to the submucosal nature of lesions. The basic elements of the tumors are spindle cells and vascular clefts with extravasated red blood cells. The cell of origin of the sarcoma may be the lymphatic endothelial cell, as demonstrated by enzymatic markers and polyclonal and monoclonal antibodies specific for vascular/lymphatic endothelium.

The etiology of Kaposi's sarcoma remains unclear. Clinical manifestations are present if multiple lesions cause bowel obstruction due to tumoral masses or if perforation with peritonitis occurs. Mesenteric cyst formation and protein-losing enteropathy due to mesenteric lymphatic obstruction have also been observed.[141]

Enteric lesions have been treated by radiotherapy, chemotherapy, antiviral agents, and interferon. None of these strategies can guarantee better than a 50 percent response rate, and remissions are rarely permanent. In general, Kaposi's sarcoma is associated with a poor prognosis.

Non-Hodgkin's lymphomas have been reported in homosexual men, intravenous drug abusers, and hemophiliacs. Virtually all such patients with lymphomas have positive serology for HIV. Involvement of the GI tract by non-Hodgkin's lymphoma in AIDS is a common mode of presentation of these tumors. Any site in the GI tract may be involved, although rectal lesions are particularly common. The lesions are generally fungating, bulky, cauliflower-like masses. Hemorrhage or ulceration can occur. Circumferential involvement leading to obstruction has been seen.

Signs and symptoms of GI lymphoma in AIDS depend on its location (Table 8). Dysphagia and hematemesis are hallmarks of esophageal disease. Epigastric pain and upper GI bleeding suggest gastric involvement. Obstruction, perforation and peritonitis, or bleeding is seen with small bowel tumors. Pericecal perforation, rectal pain, mucoid anal discharge, rectal bleeding, and decreasing stool caliber suggest colonic disease.

The majority of lymphomas have been of B-cell origin. Polyclonal hyperglobulinemia accompanies the early nonmalignant lymphoid changes. The lymphoma probably arises from an initial multiclonal B-cell expansion. There is some evidence that lymphomas may arise from persistent viral infections such as EBV. However AIDS patients with lymphoma also demonstrate concurrent exposure to human T-cell leukemia virus I, suggesting a possible role for this virus as well.[142] Prognosis for non-Hodgkin's lymphoma in AIDS is extremely poor. Treatment is based on surgical resection and chemotherapy; agents that have been used include methotrexate or bleomycin, doxorubicin, cyclophosphamide, vincristine, and dexamethasone.[141]

REFERENCES

1. Rosen FS, Wedgwood RJ, Eibl M, Aititi F, Cooper MD, Good RA, Griscelli C, Hanson LA, Hitzig WH, Matsumoto S, Seligmann M, Soothill JF, Waldmann TA. Primary immunodeficiency diseases. Report of a World Health Organization Scientific Group on Immunodeficiency. Clin Immunol Immunopathol 1986; 40:166–196.

2. Walker WA, Isselbacher KJ. Intestinal antibodies. N Engl J Med 1977; 297:767–773.

3. Walker WA, Isselbacher KJ. Uptake and transport of macromolecules by the intestine: possible role in clinical disorders. Gastroenterology 1974; 67:531–550.

4. Cunningham-Rundles C, Carr RI, Good RA. Dietary protein antigenemia in humoral immunodeficiency. Correlation with splenomegaly. Am J Med 1984; 76:181–185.

5. Melamed I, Bujanover Y, Igra YS, Schwartz D, Zakuth V, Spirer Z. Campylobacter enteritis in normal and immunodeficient children. Am J Dis Child 1983; 137:752–753.

6. Bruton OC. Agammaglobulinemia. Pediatrics 1952; 9:722–738.

7. Buckley RH. Humoral immunodeficiency. Clin Immunol Immunopathol 1986; 40:13–24.

8. Buckley RH. Immunodeficiency diseases. JAMA 1987; 258:2841–2850.

9. Rosen FS, Cooper MD, Wedgwood RJP. The primary immunodeficiencies. N Engl J Med 1984; 311:235–242.

10. Ochs HE, Ament ME, Davis SD. Giardiasis with malabsorption in X-linked agammaglobulinemia. N Engl J Med 1972; 287:341–342.

11. Saulsbury FT, Winkelstein JA, Yolken RH. Chronic rotavirus infection in immunodeficiency. J Pediatr 1980; 97:61–65.

12. Rosen FS, Janeway CA. The gammaglobulins. III. The antibody deficiency syndromes. N Engl J Med 1966; 275:709–715.

13. Ammann AJ, Hong R. Selective IgA deficiency: presentation of 30 cases and a review of the literature. Medicine 1971; 50:223–236.

14. Conley ME, Cooper MD. Immature IgA B cells in IgA-deficiency patients. N Engl J Med 1981; 305:475–479.

15. Strober W, Krakauer R, Klaeveman HC, Reynolds HY, Nelson DL. Secretory component deficiency: a disorder of the IgA immune system. N Engl J Med 1976; 294:351–356.

16. Burks AW, Sampson HA, Buckley RM. Anaphylactic reactions following gammaglobulin administration in patients with hypogammaglobulinemia: detection of IgE antibodies to IgA. N Engl J Med 1986; 314: 560–564.

17. Ferreira A, Garcia MC, Lopez-Trascasa M, Pascual D, Fontan G. Anti-IgA antibodies in selective IgA deficiency and primary immunodeficient patients treated with gammaglobulin. Clin Immunol Immunopathol 1988; 47:199–207.

18. Mestecky J, Russell M, Jackson S, Brown T. The human IgA system: a reassessment. Clin Immunol Immunopath 1986; 40:105–114.

19. Ugazio AG, Out TA, Plebani A, Duse M, Monafo V, Nespoli L, Burgio GR. Recurrent infections in children with "selective" IgA deficiency: association with IgG$_2$ and IgG$_4$ deficiency. Birth Defects 1983; 19:169–171.

20. Savilahti E. IgA deficiency in children. Immunoglobulin containing cells in the intestinal mucosa, immunoglobulins in secretions, and serum IgA levels. Clin Exp Immunol 1973; 13:395–406.

21. Seidman E, Walker A. Gastroenterology and liver disorders. In: Stiehm R, ed. Immunologic disorders in infants and children. 3rd ed. Philadelphia: WB Saunders, 1989: 503.

22. Asquith P, Thompson RA, Cooke WT. Serum immunoglobulins in adult coeliac disease. Lancet 1969; i:129–131.

23. Ament M. Immunodeficiency syndrome and gastrointestinal disease. Pediatr Clin North Am 1975; 22:807–825.

24. Brown WR, Savage DC, Dubois RW, Alp MH, Mallory A, Kern F. Intestinal microflora of immunoglobulin-deficient and normal human subjects. Gastroenterology 1972; 62:1143–1152.

25. Ross IN, Asquith P, ed. Primary immune deficiencies. In: Asquith P. Immunology of the gastrointestinal tract. Edinburgh: Churchill-Livingstone, 1979: 152.

26. Cunningham-Rundles C, Brandeis WF, Good RA, Day NK. Milk precipitins, circulating immune complexes and IgA deficiency. Proc Natl Acad Sci 1978; 75:3387–3389.

27. Fraser KJ, Rankin JG. Selective deficiency of IgA immunoglobulins associated with carcinoma of the stomach. Australas Ann Med 1970; 19:165–167.

28. Siegel RL, Issekutz T, Schwaber J, Rosen FS, Geha RS. Deficiency of T helper cells in transient hypogammaglobulinemia of infancy. N Engl J Med 1981; 305:1307–1313.

29. Cunningham-Rundles S, Cunningham-Rundles C, Siegal FP, Gupta S, Smith E, Kosloff C, Good RA. Defective cellular immune response in vitro in common variable immunodeficiency. J Clin Immunol 1981; 1:65–72.

30. Hausser C, Virelizier JL, Buriot D, Griscelli C. Common variable hypogammaglobulinemia in children. Am J Dis Child 1983; 137:833–837.

31. Jones BM. Identification of B-cell and T-helper-cell defects and of suppressor cell hyperactivity in humoral immunodeficiency. Clin Immunol Immunopathol 1984; 32:41–51.

32. Lopez-Botet M, Fontan G, Garcia-Rodriguez M, Landazuri M. Relationship between IL-2 synthesis and the proliferative response to PHA in different primary immunodeficiencies. J Immunol 1982; 128:679–683.

33. Kruger G, Welte K, Ciobanu N, Cunningham-Rundles C, Ralph P, Venuta S, Feldmann S, Koziner B, Wang CY, Moore MA, Mertelsmann RJ. IL-2 correction of defective in vitro T-cell mitogenesis in patients with common varied immunodeficiency. Clin Immunol 1984; 4:295–303..

34. Fiedler W, Sykora KW, Welte K, Kolitz JE, Cunningham-Rundles C, Holloway K, Miller G, Sauza K, Merterlsmann R. T cell activation defect in common variable immunodeficiency: restoration by phorbol myristate acetate (PMA) or allogeneic macrophages. Clin Immunol Immunopathol 1987; 44:206–218.

35. Hermans PE, Diaz-Buxo JA, Stobo JD. Idiopathic late-onset immunoglobulin deficiency: clinical observations in 50 patients. Am J Med 1976; 61:221–237.

36. Webster ADB. Giardiasis and immunodeficiency diseases. Trans R Soc Trop Med Hyg 1980; 74:440–443.

37. Ochs HD, Ament ME, David SD. Structure and function of the gastrointestinal tract in primary immunodeficiency syndromes and in granulocyte dysfunction. Birth Defects 1975; 11:199–207.

38. Ahnen DJ, Brown WR. Campylobacter enteritis in immune-deficient patients. Ann Intern Med 1982; 96:187–188.

39. Henochowicz S. Chronic diarrhea and weight loss in a patient with common immunodeficiency. Ann Allergy 1986; 56:410–413.

40. Twomey JJ, Jordan PH, Laughter AH, Meuwissen HJ, Good RA. The gastric disorder in immunoglobulin-deficient patients. Ann Intern Med 1970; 72:499–504.

41. Webster ADB, Kenwright S, Ballard J, Shiner M, Slavin G, Levi AJ, Loewi G, Asherson GL. Nodular lymphoid hyperplasia of the bowel in primary hypogammaglobulinaemia: study of in vivo and in vitro lymphocyte function. Gut 1977; 18:364–372.

42. Johnson BL, Goldberg LS, Pops MA, Weiner M. Clinical and immunological studies in a case of nodular lymphoid hyperplasia of the small bowel. Gastroenterology 1971; 61:369–374.

43. Hermans PE, Huizenga KA. Association of gastric carcinoma with idiopathic late-onset immunoglobulin deficiency. Ann Intern Med 1972; 76:605–609.

44. White WB, Ballow M. Modulation of suppressor-cell activity by cimetidine in patients with common variable hypogammaglobulinemia. N Engl J Med 1985; 312:198–202.

45. Lawlor GJ, Ammann AJ, Wright WC, La Franchi SH, Bilstrom D, Stiehm ER. The syndrome of cellular immunodeficiency with immunoglobulins. J Pediatr 1974; 84:183–192.

46. Levinsky RJ, Marshall WC, Pincott J, Harries JT. Protracted diarrhea, immunodeficiency and viruses. Eur J Pediatr 1982; 138:271–272.

47. Jarvis W, Middleton P, Gelfan E. Significance of viral infections in severe combined immunodeficiency disease. Pediatr Infect Dis 1983; 2:187–192.

48. Reinherz EL, Geha R, Rappaport JM, Wilson M, Penta AC, Hussey RE, Fitzgerald KA, Daley JF, Levine H, Rosen FS, Schlossman SF. Reconstitution after transplantation with T lymphocyte depleted, HLA-

haplotype-mismatched bone marrow for severe combined immunodeficiency. Proc Natl Acad Sci USA 1982; 79:6047–6051.

49. Sindel LJ, Buckley RH, Schiff SE. Severe combined immunodeficiency with natural killer cell predominance: abrogation of graft versus host disease and immunological reconstitution with HLA identical bone marrow cells. J Allergy Clin Immunol 1984; 73:829–836.

50. Fontan G, Garcia ME, Carrasco S, Zabay JM, Gomez de la Concha E. Severe combined immunodeficiency with T lymphocytes retaining functional activity. Clin Immunol Immunopathol 1988; 46:432–441.

51. Morgan G, Levinsky RJ, Hugh-Jones K, Fairbanks LD, Morris GS, Simmonds HA. Heterogeneity of biochemical, clinical and immunological parameters in severe combined immunodeficiency due to adenosine deaminase deficiency. Clin Exp Immunol 1987; 70:491–499.

52. Hirschhorn R. Inherited enzyme deficiencies and immunodeficiency: adenosine deaminase (ADA) and purine nucleoside phosphorylase (PNP) deficiencies. Clin Immunol Immunopathol 1986; 40:157–165.

53. Touraine JL, Betuel H, Gouillet G, Jeune M. Combined immunodeficiency disease associated with absence of cell surface HLA-A and B-antigens. J Pediatr 1978; 93:47–51.

54. Touraine JL, Marseglia GL, Betuel H. Thirty international cases of bare lymphocyte syndrome. Biological significance of HLA antigens. Exp Hematol 1985; 13(Suppl 17):86–87.

55. Adam MR, Dopfer Q, Dammer G, Peter HH, Schleter MG, Muller C, Niethammer D. Defective expression of HLA-DR region determinants in children with congenital agammaglobulinemia and malabsorption: a new syndrome. In: Albert ED, Paur MP, Mayr WR, eds. Histocompatibility testing. Heidelberg: Springer-Verlag, 1984: 645.

56. Clement L, Plaeger-Marshall S, Haas A, Saxon A, Martin A. Bare lymphocyte syndrome: consequences of absent Class II major histocompatibility antigen expression for B lymphocyte differentiation and function. J Clin Invest 1988; 81:669–675.

57. Lisowska-Grospierre B, Charron B, Preval C, Durandy G, Griscelli C, Mach B. A defect in the regulation of major histocompatibility complex Class II gene expression in human HLA-DR negative lymphocytes from patients with combined immunodeficiency syndrome. J Clin Invest 1985; 76:381–385.

58. Teeder T, Clement L, Cooper M. Discontinuous expression of a membrane antigen HB-7 during B cell differentiation. Tissue Antigens 1984; 24:140–151.

59. Aldrich RA, Steinberg AG, Campbell DC. Pedigree demonstrating a sex-linked recessive condition characterized by draining ears, eczematoid dermatitis and bloody diarrhea. Pediatrics 1954; 13:133–139.

60. St. Geme JW, Prince JT, Burke BA, Good RA, Krivit W. Impaired cellular resistance to herpes-simplex virus in Wiskott-Aldrich syndrome. N Engl J Med 1965; 273:229–234.

61. Perry GS, Spector BD, Schuman LM, Mandell JS, Anderson E, McHugh RB, Hanson MR, Fahlstrom SM, Krivit W, Kersey JH. The Wiskott-Aldrich syndrome in the United States and Canada, 1892–1979. J Pediatr 1980; 97:72–78.

62. Waldmann TA, Misiti J, Nelson DL, Kraemer KH. Multisystem hereditary disease with immunodeficiency, impaired organ maturation. X-ray hypersensitivity and a high incidence of neoplasia. Ann Intern Med 1983; 99:367–379.

63. Boder E. Ataxia telangiectasia: some historic clinical and pathologic observations. Birth Defects 1975; 11:255–270.

64. DiGeorge AM. Congenital absence of the thymus and its immunologic consequences. Concurrence with congenital hypoparathyroidism. Birth Defects 1968; 4:116–121.

65. Purtillo DT, Sakamoto K, Barnabei V, Seeley J, Bechtold T, Rogers G, Yetz J, Harada S. Epstein-Barr virus–induced disease in boys with the X-linked lymphoproliferative syndrome (XLP). Am J Med 1982; 73:49–56.

66. Sullivan JL, Byron KS, Brewster FE, Baker SM, Ochs HD. X-linked lymphoproliferative syndrome: natural history of the immunodeficiency. J Clin Invest 1983; 71:1765–1768.

67. Purtillo DT. Abnormal lymphocyte subsets in X-linked lymphoproliferative syndrome. J Immunol 1981; 127:2618–2620.

68. Purtillo DT. Epstein-Barr virus–induced diseases in the X-linked lymphoproliferative syndrome and related disorders. Biomed Pharmacother 1985; 39:52–58.

69. Curnutte JT. Classification of chronic granulomatous disease. Hematol Oncol Clin North Am 1988; 2:241–252.

70. Curnutte JT, Whitten DM, Babior BM. Defective superoxide production by granulocytes from patients with chronic granulomatous disease. N Engl J Med 1974; 290:593.

71. Segal AW. Absence of both cytochrome b-245 subunits from neutrophils in X-linked chronic granulomatous disease. Nature 1987; 326:88.

72. Ament ME, Ochs HD. Gastrointestinal manifestations of chronic granulomatous disease. N Engl J Med 1983; 288:382–387.

73. Mulholland MW, Delaney JP, Simmons RL. Gastrointestinal complications of chronic granulomatous disease: surgical implications. Surgery 1983; 94:569–575.

74. Griscom NT, Kirkpatrick JA Jr, Girdany BR, Berdon WE, Grand RJ, Mackie GG. Gastric antral narrowing in chronic granulomatous disease of childhood. Pediatrics 1974; 54:456–460.

75. Johnson FE, Humbert JR, Kuzela DC, Todd JK, Lilly JR. Gastric outlet obstruction due to X-linked chronic granulomatous disease. Surgery 1975; 78:217–223.

76. Dickerman JD, Colletti RB, Tampas JP. Gastric outlet obstruction in chronic granulomatous disease of childhood. Am J Dis Child 1986; 140:567.

77. Chin TW, Stiehm ER, Falloon J, Gallin JI. Corticosteroids in the treatment of obstructive lesions of chronic granulomatous disease. J Pediatr 1987; 3:349.

78. Ezekowitz RAB, Orkin SH, Newburger PE. Recombinant interferon gamma augments phagocyte superoxide production and X-chronic granulomatous disease gene expression in X-linked variant chronic granulomatous disease. J Clin Invest 1987; 80:1009.

79. Tood RF III, Freyer DR. The CD11/CD18 leukocyte glycoprotein deficiency. Hematol Oncol Clin North Am 1988; 2:13–31.

80. Anderson DC, Schnakstiec FC, Finegold MJ. The severe and moderate phenotype of heritable Mac-1, LFA-1 deficiency: their quantitative definition and relation to leukocyte dysfunction and clinical features. J Infect Dis 1985; 152:668.

81. Corman L. The relationship between nutrition, infection and immunity. Med Clin North Am 1985; 69:519–531.

82. Bhaskaram P, Sivakumar B. Interleukin-1 in malnutrition. Arch Dis Child 1986; 61:182–185.

83. Schoper K, Douglas S. Neutrophil function in children with kwashiorkor. J Lab Clin Med 1976; 88:450–461.

84. Arbo A, Santos JI. Diarrheal diseases in the immunocompromised host. Pediatr Infect Dis J 1987; 6:894–906.

85. Srisinba S, Suskind R, Edelman R, Asvapaka C, Olsen RE. Secretory and serum IgA in children with protein-calorie malnutrition. Pediatrics 1975; 55:166–170.

86. Shiner M. Immune mechanisms in the small bowel mucosa of children with malnutrition. In: Rozen P, ed. Frontiers in gastrointestinal research. Vol 13. Basel: Karger, 1986: 172.

87. Prolla J, Kirsner J. The gastrointestinal lesions and complications of leukemias. Ann Intern Med 1964; 61:1084–1103.

88. Engelhard D, Marks M, Good R. Infections in bone marrow transplant recipients. J Pediatr 1986; 108:335–346.

89. Boulton AJM, Slater DN, Hancock BW. Herpes virus colitis. A new cause of diarrhea in a patient with Hodgkins disease. Gut 1982; 23:247–249.

90. Proujansky R, Orenstein SR, Kocoshis SA, Yunis EJ, Starzl TE. Cytomegalovirus gastroenteritis after liver transplantation. J Pediatr 1988; 113:700–703.

91. Raklla J, Wiesner RH, Taswell HF. Incidence of cytomegalovirus infection and its relationship to donor-recipient serologic status in liver transplantation. Transplant Proc 1987; 19:2399–2402.

92. Morgan WM, Curran JW. Acquired immunodeficiency syndrome: current and future trends. Public Health Rep 1986; 101:459–465.

93. Barre-Sinoussi F, Cherman JC, Rey F, Nugeyre M, Chamaret S, Gruest J, Dauguet C, Axter-Blin C, Vezinet F, Rouzioux C, Rozenbaum W, Montaignier L. Isolation of a T-lymphotropic retrovirus from a patient at risk for acquired immunodeficiency syndrome (AIDS). Science 1983; 220:868–871.

94. Gallo RC, Salahuddin SZ, Popovic M, Shearer GM, Kaplan M, Haynes B, Palker T, Redfield R, Oleske J, Safai B, White G, Foster P, Markham P. Frequent detection and isolation of cytopathic retrovirus (HTLV-III) from patients with AIDS and at risk for AIDS. Science 1984; 224:500–503.

95. Levy JA, Hoffman AD, Kramer SM, Landis JA, Shimabukuro JM. Isolation of lymphocytopathic retrovirus from San Francisco patients with AIDS. Science 1984; 225:840–842.

96. Coffin J, Haase A, Levy AJ, Montagnier L, Oroszlar S, Teich N, Temin H, Toyoshimak, Varmus H. Human immunodeficiency viruses. Science 1986; 232:697.

97. Gallo RC, Streicher HZ. Human T-lymphotropic retroviruses (HTLV-

I, II and III): the biological basis of adult T-cell leukemia/lymphoma and AIDS. In: Broder S, ed. AIDS: Modern concepts and therapeutic challenges. New York: Marcel Dekker, 1987: 1.

98. Levy JA. Mysteries of HIV: challenges for therapy and prevention. Nature 1988; 333:519–522.

99. Koening S, Rosenberg ZF. Immunology of infection with the human immunodeficiency virus (HIV): a view from the III International Conference on AIDS. Ann Intern Med 1987; 107:409–411.

100. Mizuma H, Litwin S, Zolla-Pazner S. B-cell activation in HIV infection: relationship of spontaneous immunoglobulin secretion to various immunological parameters. Clin Exp Immunol 1988; 71:410–416.

101. Fauci AS. The human immunodeficiency virus: infectivity and mechanisms of pathogenesis. Science 1988; 239:617–622.

102. Rogers MF. Pediatric HIV infection: epidemiology, etiopathogenesis, and transmission. Pediatr Ann 1988; 17:324–331.

103. Roger MF, Thomas PA, Starcher ET, Thomas P, Starcher E, Noa M, Bush T, Jaffe H. Acquired immunodeficiency syndrome in children: report of the Centers for Disease Control National Surveillance, 1982–1985. Pediatrics 1987; 79:1008–1014.

104. Rubinstein A, Morecki R, Silverman B, Charytan M, Krieger B, Andiman W, Ziprkowski M, Goldman H. Pulmonary disease in children with acquired immunodeficiency syndrome and AIDS-related complex. J Pediatr 1986; 108:498–503.

105. Belman AL, Diamond G, Dickson D. Pediatric acquired immunodeficiency syndrome. Am J Dis Child 1988; 142:29–35.

106. Marion RW, Wiznia AA, Hutcheon G, Rubinstein A. Correlation between severity of dysmorphism and age at diagnosis of immunodeficiency. Am J Dis Child 1987; 141:429–431.

107. Quinn TC, Piot P, McCormick JB. Serologic and immunologic studies in patients with AIDS in North America and Africa. JAMA 1987; 257:2617–2621.

108. Weber J. Gastrointestinal disease in AIDS. Clin Immunol Allergy 1986; 6:519–541.

109. Rodgers VD, Kagnoff MF. Abnormalities of the intestinal immune system in AIDS. Gastroenterol Clin North Am 1988; 17:487–494.

110. Kotler DD, Sholer JV, Tiernay AR. Intestinal plasma cell alterations in acquired immunodeficiency syndrome. Dig Dis Sci 1987; 32:129.

111. Rotterdam H. Contributions of gastrointestinal biopsy to an understanding of gastrointestinal diseases. Am J Gastroenterol 1983; 78:140–148.

112. Knapp AB, Horst DA, Eliopoulos G, Gramm HF, Gaber LW, Falchuk KR, Falchuk ZM, Trey C. Widespread cytomegalovirus gastroenterocolitis in a patient with acquired immunodeficiency syndrome. Gastroenterology 1983; 85:1399–1402.

113. Gertler SL, Pressman J, Price P, Brozinsky S, Miyai K. Gastrointestinal cytomegalovirus infection in a homosexual man with severe acquired immunodeficiency syndrome. Gastroenterology 1983; 85:1403–1406.

114. Kotler DP, Gaetz HP, Lange M, Klein EB, Hoh PR. Enteropathy associated with acquired immunodeficiency syndrome. Ann Intern Med 1984; 101:421–428.

115. Nelson JA, Wiley CA, Reynolds-Kholer C, Reese CE, Margaretten W, Levy JA. Human immunodeficiency virus detected in bowel epithelium from patients with gastrointestinal symptoms. Lancet 1988; i:259–262.

116. Chandrasekar PH, Molinari JA. Oral candidiasis: forerunner of acquired immunodeficiency syndrome (AIDS). Oral Surg 1985; 60:532–534.

117. Eras P, Goldstein MJ, Sherlock P. Candida infection of the gastrointestinal tract. Medicine 1972; 51:367–378.

118. Tavitian A, Raufman JP, Rosenthal LE, et al. Ketoconazole-resistant Candida esophagitis in patients with AIDS. Gastroenterology 1986; 90:443.

119. Tzipori S. Cryptosporidiosis. Microbiol Rev 1983; 47:84–96.

120. Casemore DP, Sands RL, Curry A. Cryptosporidium species: a "new" human pathogen. J Clin Pathol 1985; 38:1321–1336.

121. Kazlow PG, Shah K, Benkov KJ. Esophageal cryptosporidiosis in a child with acquired immune deficiency syndrome. Gastroenterology 1986; 91:1301.

122. Dowsett JF, Weller IV. AIDS and the liver. Gastroenterology 1988; 4:444–451.

123. Whiteside M, MacLeod C, Fischl M, et al. Update: Treatment of cryptosporidiosis in patients with AIDS. JAMA 1984; 251:1661.

124. Janoff EN, Smith PD, Blaser MJ. Acute antibody response to *Giardia lamblia* are depressed in patients with AIDS. J Infect Dis 1988; 157:798–804.

125. Jacobs JL, Gold JW, Murray HW, Roberts RB, Armstrong D. Salmonella infections in patients with the acquired immunodeficiency syndrome. Ann Intern Med 1985; 102:186–188.

126. Glaser JB, Morton-Kutel L, Berger SR, Weber J, Siegal FP, Lopez C, Robbins W, Landesman H. Recurrent *Salmonella typhimurium* bacteremia associated with the acquired immunodeficiency syndrome. Ann Intern Med 1985; 102:189–193.

127. Smith PD, Macher AM, Bookman MA, Boccia RV, Steis RG, Gill V, Manischewitz J, Gelmann EP. *Salmonella typhimurium* enteritis and bacteremia in the acquired immunodeficiency syndrome. Ann Intern Med 1985; 102:207–210.

128. McLoughlin LC, Nord KS, Joshi VV, Oleske JH, Connoz EM. Severe gastrointestinal involvement in children with the acquired immunodeficiency syndrome. Gastroenterol Nutr 1987; 6:517–524.

129. Roth RI, Owen RL, Keren DF. Intestinal infection with *Mycobacterium avium* in acquired immune deficiency syndrome (AIDS). Histological and clinical comparison with Whipple's disease. Dig Dis Sci 1985; 30:497–504.

130. Collins JC, Rubinstein A, Morecki R. *Mycobacterium avium- intracellulare* (M.ai) infection in readily diagnosed by liver biopsy in children with AIDS. Gastroenterology 1985; 88:1654.

131. Scott GB, Buck BE, Leterman JG, Bloom FL, Parks WP. AIDS in infants. N Engl J Med 1984; 310:76–81.

132. Greenspan JS, Mastrucci MT, Leggott PJ, et al. Hairy leukoplakia in child. (Letter) AIDS 1988;2.

133. Greenspan D, Greenspan JS. The oral clinical features of HIV infection. Gastroenterol Clin North Am 1988; 17:535–543.

134. Greenspan JS, Greenspan D, De Souza Y, Freese UK. Diagnosis and investigation of hairy leukoplakia using non invasive techniques. Third International Conference of HIV. Washington, DC, 1987.

135. Meiselman MS, Cello JP, Margatten W. Cytomegalovirus colitis: report of the clinical, endoscopic and pathologic findings in two patients with the acquired immune deficiency syndrome. Gastroenterology 1985; 88:171–175.

136. Goodman ZD, Boitnott JK, Yardley JM. Perforation of the colon associated with cytomegalovirus infection. Dig Dis Sci 1979; 24:376–380.

137. Gottlieb MS, Groopman JE, Weinstein WM, Fahey JL, Detels R. The acquired immunodeficiency syndrome. Ann Intern Med 1983; 99:208–220.

138. Erice A, Jordan C, Chace BA, et al. Ganciclovir treatment of cytomegalovirus disease in transplant recipients and other immunocompromised hosts. JAMA 1987; 257:3082–3087.

139. Lim W, Kahn E, Gupta A, Slade H, Fagin J, Kaplan M, Daum F, Pahwa S. Treatment of cytomegalovirus enterocolitis with ganciclovir in an infant with acquired immunodeficiency syndrome. Pediatr Infect Dis J 1988; 7:354–357.

140. Friedman-Kiem AE, Laubenstein LJ, Rubinstein P, Buimovici-Klein E, Marmor M, Stalil R, Spigland I, Soo Kim K, Zolla-Pazner S. Disseminated Kaposi's sarcoma in homosexual men. Ann Intern Med 1982; 96:693–700.

141. Friedman SL. Gastrointestinal and hepatobiliary neoplasms in AIDS. Gastroenterol Clin North Am 1988; 17:465–486.

142. Kaplan LD. Volderding PA, Abrams DT. Update on AIDS-associated non-Hodgkin's lymphoma in San Francisco. Third International Conference on AIDS. Washington, DC, 1987:9.

PART 8

Bacterial Infections

John D. Snyder, M.D.

Diarrheal disease continues to be one of the leading health problems in the world and may account for as many as 4.5 to 5 million deaths per year in children less than 5 years old in developing countries.[1] The magnitude and severity of the problem are less in the developed world, but costly hospital admissions still occur frequently (13.8 per 1,000 infants in the United States in 1984),[2] and nearly 400 infants die each year in the United States from diarrhea.[3] The rates of diarrhea in developing countries are very similar to those in the United States at the turn of the twentieth century.[4]

This chapter deals primarily with the bacterial causes of diarrhea, and a list of the bacterial pathogens is included in Table 1. Most bacterial pathogens found in developed countries are also found in developing countries, but the incidence of illness caused by these organisms varies greatly. Approximately 15 percent of diarrheal episodes in children in developed countries are caused by bacterial agents,[5,6] while as many as 45 percent of episodes in developing countries are caused by bacterial agents.[6,7] Although almost all of the bacterial enteric pathogens are found throughout the world, their impact on health varies greatly. For example, *Vibrio cholerae* and enterotoxigenic *Escherichia coli* (ETEC) cause far more illness in the developing than in the developed world.[8] In contrast, *Campylobacter jejuni* is the most common bacterial cause of acute diarrhea in the United States and the United Kingdom[9,10] but does not appear to be an important pathogen in persons older than 2 years in developing countries.[11]

The mechanisms associated with the spread of bacterial enteric infections are similar throughout the world. Most of the pathogens listed in Table 1 are transmitted primarily by the fecal-oral route, with contaminated food or water serving as the vehicle.[12] A large innoculum is usually required except for *Shigella*, for which less than 100 organisms have been shown to cause illness in volunteers.[12]

Several risk factors appear to be of particular importance in the spread of bacterial enteric infections. Socioeconomic factors that influence access to potable water, hygienic practices, and sanitation conditions play a major role in transmission of enteric infections.[4,13] The single most important of these risk factors appears to be the educational level of the mother.[14]

In developed countries, exposure to daycare facilities and travel to less developed countries increase the risk for enteric infections. The likelihood of contamination of toys and clothing is great in daycare centers where many children are still in diapers and are not yet toilet trained.[15] Travelers are at risk of a rapid change in intestinal flora, which often includes enterotoxigenic *E. coli*, the most common agent causing traveler's diarrhea.[16] Exposure to animals may also increase the risk for enteric infection.[17]

TABLE 1

Mechanisms of Disease Caused by the Most Frequently Recognized Bacterial Enteric Organisms

Invasion
Campylobacter jejuni
Escherichia coli (enteroinvasive)
Salmonella enteritidis
Shigella
Yersinia enterocolitica

Enterotoxin Production
Vibrio species
Escherichia coli (enterotoxigenic)
Aeromonas hydrophila
Plesiomonas shigelloides
Clostridium difficile

Cytotoxin Production
Shigella
Escherichia coli (enterohemorrhagic, enteropathogenic)
Clostridium difficile

Adherence
Escherichia coli (enteropathogenic)

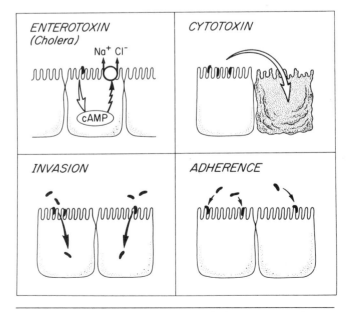

FIGURE 1 Pathogenesis of bacterial diarrhea. Diarrhea is caused by one of four mechanisms: invasion, enterotoxin or cytotoxin production, or mucosal adherence.

MECHANISMS OF INFECTIONS

Bacterial enteric pathogens cause illness by one of four major mechanisms: invasion, enterotoxin or cytotoxin production, and mucosal adherence with damage to the microvillous membrane (Fig. 1). The majority of these organisms act primarily by invading the bowel mucosa. The first step in invasion is adherence of the organism to the mucosal surface. A number of structural properties of organisms aid in adherence, including pili, motility devices, chemotactic factors, and adhesions.[18] These properties help the organism compete against the body's host defense system, made up of the gastric acidity barrier, intestinal motility, the indigenous intestinal flora, the mucous gel covering the mucosa, the secretory, humoral, and cell-mediated immune systems, and the gut-associated lymphoid tissues.[19]

The invasive organisms generally infect the distal small intestine and colon, often resulting in dysentery.[20] The illness caused by these organisms is often characterized by frequent small bowel movements containing mucus, blood, or pus. The diarrhea may be associated with fever and tenesmus and pain on defecation.[20]

Enterotoxin-producing organisms neither invade nor damage the gut mucosa. The prototype of these organisms, V. cholerae, acts through an enterotoxin that can cause massive secretion of electrolytes and water by stimulating cyclic AMP in small intestinal mucosal cells.[21] The diarrhea is often watery and can be associated with vomiting. Blood and pus are not typically found in the stools.[20]

In contrast, cytotoxin-producing organisms cause cell damage and death. Cytotoxins cause cell injury, inflammation, and intestinal secretion by inhibiting protein synthesis as well as by elaborating inflammatory mediator substances. The Shiga toxin of Shigella organisms is the classic example of a powerful cytotoxin. Clostridium difficile acts by producing two toxins, an enterotoxin and a cytotoxin.[21] The enterotoxin causes secretion by damaging the mucosa, and the cytotoxin causes tissue destruction after previous mucosal damage has occurred.[22]

The final mechanism, adherence, is exemplified by enteropathogenic E. coli (EPEC). In this form, E. coli organisms adhere intimately to enterocytes, resulting in dissolution of the microvilli, cupping of the enterocyte outer membrane around the bacterium, and round cell inflammation of the lamina propria.[23] The precise mechanism for tissue injury is not known but may involve the elaboration of a cytotoxin similar to the Shigella cytotoxin.[23]

Regardless of the mechanism of action, the majority of bacterial enteric infections cause self-limited loss of electrolytes and water. Although the invasive organisms can potentially cause dysentery, they also produce a range of symptoms from asymptomatic infection to mild, moderate, or severe dehydration. Approximately 10 percent of all diarrheal episodes are severe enough to result in dehydration, and 0.5 to 1 percent can result in severe, life-threatening dehydration.[24]

In general, children are at greater risk for acquiring and suffering more from diarrhea than are adults.[1] Several factors combine to play an important role in the increased risk of diarrhea in children, including immunologic mechanisms, breast-feeding, development of normal flora in the bowel, and development of intestinal host defenses including receptor sites, gastric acidity and mucus, and the greater difficulty in maintaining standards of personal hygiene and sanitation.

The indigenous intestinal flora, an important component of the body's ability to resist infection, develops over the first few months of life.[25] This flora is remarkably stable and is altered only under unusual circumstances, such as the ingestion of a large quantity of an enteric pathogen or antibiotic administration.[25] Antibiotic administration resulting in reduction of normal enteric flora can greatly reduce the infective dose of a pathogen.[26,27] These studies indicate that the intact flora is a major factor interfering with colonization of the intestinal tract by pathogenic bacteria.[25]

Gastric acidity is not fully developed at birth and requires 1 or more months to reach adult levels.[28] When the pH of the gastric juice is greater than 4.0, bacteria can survive passage through the stomach, but a pH of less than 4.0 is bactericidal.[29]

The mucosal barriers encountered by organisms vary with age. The composition of intestinal mucus, an important component of the physical barrier, is different in infant and adult animals.[30] Preliminary studies indicate that binding capabilities may have similar age-specific differences.[31] In addition, the binding characteristics of receptors for organisms and their toxins have been shown to vary with age.[32,33]

Immune factors, both systemic and mucosal, also play an important role in the susceptibility of infants to enteric infection.[34] Significant immunoglobulin production does not usually occur until the neonatal period and is initiated by antigenic stimulation of B cells.[35] IgM production occurs rapidly after birth, but protective levels of IgG can take 4 to 6 months to develop.[36] While the capacity for IgG production is being developed, maternal antibodies acquired transplacentally help provide protection. The mucosal immune system also has important developmental differences.

Feeding practices also appear to be critical factors in the development of enteric infections in children of different ages. Breast-fed infants have fewer episodes of diarrhea than their artificially fed counterparts for several reasons. Breast milk, especially colostrum, is rich in protective immunologic factors. Maternal antibodies to specific enteric pathogens can be transmitted in breast milk.[32] Beyond the immune properties, breast milk provides a safer, hygienic food source with lower risk of contamination than bottled milk or prepared foods, especially in areas with poor sanitation.

Weaning practices also appear to play an important role in enteric infections. The age group most at risk for diarrhea is the 6- to 12-month-old group, which corresponds to the weaning period in many cultures.[1] Factors related to this increased risk include cessation of the relatively safe and protective breast milk, institution of nutritionally marginal feeding practices, especially in less developed countries, and the increased risk of environmental contamination of prepared food.

The final risk factor related to increased susceptibility to enteric infection is greater exposure to fecal contact in infants and young children. Hygienic practices must be learned; before these practices can be learned, young children are often exposed to their own feces as well as to those of other children in child care situations.

CLINICAL DISEASE

Regardless of the pathogenic mechanism or the age of the individual, the great majority of diarrheal episodes share several features. Although the definition of diarrhea varies by culture and convention, most definitions include increased frequency and altered form of stool in their criteria.[1] Regardless of the pathogen involved, enteric infections can range from asymptomatic to mild, moderate, or severe dehydration. Invasive organisms may be associated with pussy or bloody stools, whereas enterotoxigenic organisms by nature do not result in dysentery. Less than 10 percent of acute diarrheal episodes are associated with measurable dehydration.[24]

The following section deals with the characteristic features of the illness caused by the important bacterial enteric pathogens listed in Table 1.

Campylobacter

C. jejuni and the related species, including *C. coli* and *C. laridis*, cause diarrheal illness ranging in severity from mild diarrhea to fulminant colitis.[37] The organisms are gram-negative curvilinear rods.

C. jejuni infects either the colon or the distal small intestine[17] and is presumed to be an invasive organism because it causes an inflammatory tissue response and can cause bacteremia.[17] It also produces an enterotoxin similar to cholera toxin, but the biologic relevance of the toxin is questionable.[37]

Clinical illness follows ingestion of organisms, with undercooked chicken and untreated water having been identified as important vehicles of infection.[38,39] Most episodes are sporadic, with no easily demonstrable source.[13]

The symptoms of an episode often begin with fever and malaise, followed within 24 hours by nausea, diarrhea, and abdominal pain.[13] The diarrhea can be profuse and watery and may contain blood and white blood cells. The majority of cases are self-limited, but recurrent or chronic episodes can occur.[17] Complications include meningitis, abscesses, pancreatitis, Reiter's syndrome, and Guillain-Barré syndrome.[37]

Atypical *Campylobacter*-like organisms have been isolated from asymptomatic and ill homosexual men.[40] These organisms cause disease which resembles that caused by *C. jejuni*.[41]

In developing countries *C. jejuni* appears to be associated with illness only during the first 2 years of life.[42] Illness in adults is limited primarily to travelers to these countries who usually develop self-limited, watery diarrhea.[43] The low rate of illness in developing countries is directly related to antibody levels. Significantly higher *C. jejuni*–specific serum IgA, IgG, and IgM antibody levels have been reported in Bangladeshi than in American children in several age groups.[44]

Several methods of detection of *Campylobacter* organisms are available. A simpler method for producing the lower oxygen, higher carbon dioxide content environment required for *Campylobacter* growth has recently been described.[45] Direct visualization of the organism from Gram's stained fecal specimens can permit a rapid presumptive diagnosis.[46]

Campylobacter pylori

The first report of the association of *C. pylori* and inflammation of the gastric antrum occurred in 1983.[47] Since then numerous reports have confirmed the association of *C. pylori* with gastric and duodenal ulcers.[48] When gastritis is present, the rate of recovery of *C. pylori* has routinely exceeded 60 percent in studies in adults.[49-52] In children, the rate of recovery when histologic evidence of inflammation is present approaches 70 percent.[53] *C. pylori* has not been reported in normal biopsies or in biopsies from patients with gastritis secondary to medications or inflammatory bowel disease.[53] The strongest evidence for a causative role of *C. pylori* in peptic disease is the production of disease by inoculation of volunteers.[54,55]

Symptoms of *C. pylori* infection are identical to those of peptic disease and include epigastric pain, nausea, and vomiting.[47] The suspicion of *C. pylori* infection should be raised in patients who do not respond to standard antacid or H$_2$-blocker therapy.[48]

The diagnosis of *C. pylori* infection is made by culture of biopsy specimens, identification of urease activity from biopsy specimens, or identification of organisms on silver stain of biopsy specimens.[47] Serologic confirmation utilizing enzyme-linked immunosorbent assay (ELISA) techniques is currently being studied.

Salmonella

Salmonellae are gram-negative, motile, aerobic bacilli that do not ferment lactose and sucrose but produce acid in the presence of glucose, maltose, and mannitol. Salmonellae are classified into three species: *S. enteritidis, S. typhi,* and *S. choleraesuis. S. enteritidis,* which will be discussed in this section, is by far the largest *Salmonella* species and includes over 1,500 serotypes, which are identified on the basis of lipopolysaccharide components of the cell wall and flagellar protein.[12] The dose of *S. enteritidis* required to cause infection may be less than 1,000 colony-forming units for some individuals, but larger doses are likely to be the cause of large outbreaks.[56] The usual incubation period is 12 to 72 hours, but an incubation period of 10 days has been reported in an outbreak in a neonatal nursery.[57] The peak incidence of disease occurs in infancy and early childhood.[58] The organisms are acquired by ingesting contaminated food or drink, although contaminated marijuana was the cause of one large multistate outbreak.[59] Risk factors for acquiring infection include exposure to penicillins within 4 weeks of infection and achlorhydria or antacid use.[60]

A typical episode of *Salmonella* gastroenteritis is accompanied by fever and nausea and can be associated with bloody or watery diarrhea.[61] Episodes are usually self-limited. Bacteremia is a fairly common occurrence and can lead to systemic complications in infants.[62] *S. enteritidis* bioserotypes, *S. paratyphi* A, B, and C, can cause enteric fever similar to typhoid fever[12] (see below).

The median duration of excretion of organisms is about 3 weeks but may be prolonged with antibiotic treatment.[63] Excretion appears to be more often prolonged in children less than 5 years old and in those with symptomatic as opposed to asymptomatic infections.[63] Since excretion of organisms almost always stops spontaneously, follow-up stool cultures are rarely required.[63]

Standard stool cultures will isolate *Salmonella* organisms, but plasmid analysis has proved to be an important new tool in investigation of epidemics. Plasmid analysis permits identification of organisms that cannot be typed by other techniques and has been used successfully for tracing pathogens involved in outbreaks of illness.

Typhoid Fever

S. typhi is a species of *Salmonella* which contains only one serotype, in contrast to more than 1,500 serotypes of *S. enteritidis*, and is found only in humans.[12] The incidence of disease continues to decline in the United States, with more than 60 percent of infections having been acquired by travelers to developing countries.[64]

As with paratyphoid, the severity of typhoid fever ranges from mild fever and malaise to high spiking fever, toxemia, intestinal ulcerations, and perforation.[12] The classic presentation of typhoid fever consists of fever, headache, abdominal distress and distention, mild bronchitis, and rose spots. Diarrhea, constipation, and vomiting have also been reported.[65] Children are less likely to develop typhoid facies, which are marked by lack of expression, slack jaw, dilated pupils, and dry skin and lips. Intestinal perforation, the most serious complication, is more likely to occur during the third or fourth week of illness. Fortunately, perforation is rare in children.[65] Despite antibiotic therapy, the hospital case-fatality rates for severe typhoid fever are still between 12 and 32 percent.[37]

Shigella

Shigellae are gram-negative, nonmotile rods that are divided into four major serologically different species: *S. dysenteriae* (group A), *S. flexneri* (group B), *S. boydii* (group C), and *S. sonnei* (group D). *S. sonnei* accounts for the majority of isolates reported in the United States, while *S. dysenteriae* and *S. flexneri* cause the majority of infections in developing countries.[66] All four species can cause a spectrum of illness, but in general *S. dysenteriae* causes the most severe and *S. sonnei* the least severe episodes.[67] In contrast to increasing numbers of *Campylobacter* and *Salmonella* infections, the incidence of shigellosis is declining in the United States.[68]

Shigella organisms cause disease by invading epithelial cells, and plasmids play an important role in mediating the invasiveness.[69] Exotoxin (Shiga toxin) elaborated by *Shigella* organisms is important in their virulence and has neurotoxic, enterotoxic, and cytotoxic properties.[70] The infective dose is small; as few as 10 organisms can cause disease.[71] Spread of disease is often through interpersonal contact.

The spectrum of clinical illness of shigellosis ranges from asymptomatic infection to severe dysentery or toxic manifestations. The majority of patients will have mild, self-limited diarrhea, which may be associated with low-grade fever. Mild vomiting is not uncommon. Anal sphincter tone may be lax, and rectal prolapse may occur. The dysentery form often includes an initial phase of watery diarrhea, high fever, and malaise, which is followed within 24 hours by tenesmus and colitis.[13] Invasion of the colonic mucosa can result in profuse loss of blood and serum proteins.[72]

Shigella can also cause systemic toxicity, especially in less well-cared-for or undernourished children.[73] The onset of symptoms is usually abrupt and may be accompanied by high fever and convulsions. Vasomotor collapse can occur, and mortality may be high without aggressive therapy for shock.

Yersinia

Y. enterocolitica is an invasive pathogen that can cause acute and chronic diarrhea in children.[74] In older children and adults, it can also cause mesenteric adenitis, which can mimic appendicitis. *Y. enterocolitica* is commonly isolated in Europe and Canada but is identified less commonly in the United States.[75] In Wisconsin, infection showed a summertime peak and was more common in rural counties.[75] Outbreaks have been associated with contaminated milk and food items.[76]

Acute self-limited diarrhea is usually seen in *Y. enterocolitica* infections, but fever and crampy abdominal pain also occur. The pain can mimic acute appendicitis, and *Y. enterocolitica* was identified as the cause of an outbreak of appendicitis in New York state.[77] The illness is usually mild in children,[78] but chronic diarrhea has been reported.[75] Erythema nodosum and arthritis have been reported more commonly in older patients.[79] *Y. enterocolitica* can also mimic Crohn's disease, including nodularity, mucosal thickening of the terminal ileum and colon, and the presence of aphthous ulcers.

Isolation of *Y. enterocolitica* has been simplified by the development of a new enrichment medium.[80] Previously, isolation often required long periods of cold enrichment.

Escherichia coli

E. coli is among the most common flora that inhabit the healthy colon, but it can also cause a variety of disease states. The organism is a gram-negative bacillus that is motile and may form chains. The strains that cause disease are primary pathogens that possess specific virulence properties not found in normal flora.[23] These properties allow *E. coli* strains to cause illness by one of four mechanisms: enterotoxin or cytotoxin production, adherence, and invasion. *E. coli* is divided into classes that have a fairly small and distinct group of O serogroups, O:H serotypes, and capsular antigens with specific virulence properties. Several of these classes have similar mechanisms of adhesion to gut epithelium.[23]

Although *E. coli* is an important pathogen in the developing world, it causes disease much less frequently in developing countries.[81] However, a recent study of hemorrhagic colitis indicates that enterohemorrhagic *E. coli* (EHEC) may be widely distributed in the United States and should be considered especially in a patient with bloody diarrhea but no white blood cells in the stool.[82]

The enterotoxigenic strains of *E. coli* (ETCE) produce either a heat-labile or heat-stable toxin and must produce surface colonization factors (pili) to promote adherence.[83] The production of toxins and colonization factors is plasmid mediated. ETEC strains cause traveler's diarrhea and infantile diarrhea in developing countries. Enteropathogenic *E. coli* (EPEC) does not invade the mucosa but adheres to the intestinal surface and causes damage to the brush border. The illness is usually self-limited but can become chronic.[23] Enteroinvasive *E. coli* (EIEC) acts by invading the intestinal mucosa and can cause dysentery in a manner closely resembling that of *Shigella*.[84] EHEC causes disease by elaboration of verotoxin; it causes watery diarrhea that then becomes bloody.[23] Several *E. coli* strains produce verotoxin, with the best known being *E. coli* 0157:H7, and several of these strains have been associated with the hemolytic-uremic syndrome.[85]

Illness from *E. coli* infections occurs predominantly in children in parts of the world where it is endemic. The susceptibility to illness of travelers of all ages to endemic areas indicates that exposure with subsequent immunoprotection is an important mechanism in the age-specific attack rates. However, developmental differences in *E. coli* attachment may also play a role in these attack rates.[33]

Several recent advances have added important new tools for diagnosing *E. coli* infections. Gene probes are now available to identify enterotoxigenic, enteroinvasive, and enteropathogenic *E. coli* strains.[12] Highly specific polyclonal or monoclonal antibodies to heat-labile and heat-stable enterotoxins, surface antigens, and fimbriae have provided simple, rapid diagnostic tests. A new direct assay of stool filtrates for toxin production appears to be sensitive and specific.[86]

Vibrio Species

V. cholerae 01 is the best-known species in this family of motile, gram-negative, curved bacilli because it remains endemic or hyperendemic in many countries in the developing world. However, *V. cholerae* 01 cases have also been reported in the southeastern United States in the past two decades.[87] Exposure to untreated, contaminated sewage and eating uncooked oysters and crabs have been implicated as risk factors in this environment.[88] Cholera has a range of manifestations from mild, self-limited illness to severe purging leading to vascular collapse and death.

Immune mechanisms appear to be important in the risk of infection from cholera. Illness occurs primarily in young people in endemic areas, and these infections confer protective immunity.[42]

The other species of *Vibrio* that can cause illness include non-01 *V. cholerae*, *V. parahaemolyticus*, *V. fluvialis*, *V. furnissii*, and *V. mimicus*.[89] Most *V. cholerae* 01, non-01 *V. cholerae*, and *V. mimicus* produce similar enterotoxins, which act on cyclic AMP in enterocytes to increase output of electrolytes and water. Some nontoxigenic strains of *V. cholerae* can also be pathogenic.[90] The noncholera vibrios can cause a spectrum of disease from self-limited gastroenteritis to soft-tissue infections, necrotizing wound infections, and fulminant bacteremias.[87]

Clostridium difficile

C. difficile is a gram-positive, anaerobic bacterium that has been identified as the cause of several forms of intestinal illness. The most important of these is antibiotic-associated

(pseudomembranous) colitis, which can be caused by use of all of the widely prescribed antibiotics.[37] The organism acts by producing both a cytotoxin and an enterotoxin. The specific mechanism by which the organism causes disease is unknown, but the enterotoxin, which also has cytotoxic effects, is thought to be of most importance.

Very striking age-related differences occur in *C. difficile* infections. *C. difficile* is commonly present in the bowel of normal neonates, and 10 to 50 percent of asymptomatic infants and young children can produce *C. difficile* toxin.[90] By age 1, less than 5 percent of infants excrete the organism and even fewer have toxin in the stool.[91] The reasons infants appear to be protected from the toxin are not known.

The development of pseudomembranous colitis is thought to occur when antibiotics alter the normal enteric flora, giving *C. difficile* the opportunity to increase its numbers.

The clinical illness caused by *C. difficile* ranges from pseudomembranous colitis to chronic mild diarrhea. The chronic forms of illness have at times been associated with a pseudomembrane.[92]

The diagnosis of *C. difficile* diarrhea has routinely been made by detecting cytotoxin in the fecal sample. A rapid method for detecting fecal toxin has recently been reported.[93]

Efforts are now being made to type *C. difficile* isolates by bacteriocin production, susceptibility to bacteriophage infection, and immunochemical analysis.[94,95] Serotyping of strains has indicated that the strains found in the stools of asymptomatic neonates or young children are different from those found in ill adults.[96] These findings indicate that antibiotic-associated colitis in adults is more likely due to recent acquisition of *C. difficile* than to reactivation of a focus that has remained latent since childhood.

Aeromonas

Aeromonas hydrophila and the closely related species (*A. sobria* and *A. caviae*) are gram-negative motile bacilli that inhabit fresh and salt water and cause diarrhea in humans and animals. The usual vehicle of infection is water, although sewage, animal feces, and many types of food have been implicated.[97] The pathogenic mechanism of *A. hydrophila* is believed to be the production of an enterotoxin similar to that of *E. coli*. Although the role of *A. hydrophila* in human disease has long been debated, recent studies have documented a higher rate of *A. hydrophila* in patients with diarrhea than in well controls.[98,99]

The signs and symptoms associated with *A. hydrophila* infection include fever, watery stools occasionally with occult blood, and abdominal cramps.[98] The usual course is self-limited watery diarrhea, but chronic watery diarrhea lasting up to 3 months has been reported.[99] Hematochezia appears to be less common, but a colitis-like picture has been reported.[99,100]

Plesiomonas

P. shigelloides is a gram-negative rod that shares many similarities with *A. hydrophila*, including isolation from water and membership in the family *Vibrionaceae*. The evidence

TABLE 2
Composition of Oral Rehydration Fluids
(in millimoles per liter)

Fluids	Glucose	Na	K	Base	Osm
Infalyte	111	50	20	HCO$_3$ 30	270
Pedialyte	140	45	20	Citrate 30	270
Reosol	111	50	20	Citrate 34	269
Rehydralyte	140	75	20	Citrate 30	310
WHO ORS	111	90	20	Citrate 30	310

for its virulence is less than for *A. hydrophila.* Preliminary studies in Japan and Thailand indicate that the organism may be more frequently isolated from persons with diarrhea than from those without.[100]

The mechanism of pathogenicity is not known but may be related to the production of an enterotoxin.[12] The diarrhea associated with *P. shigelloides* is usually mild and self-limited, but bloody stools and protracted episodes have been reported.[101]

P. shigelloides, like *A. hydrophila,* grows well on primary nonselective media such as *Salmonella-Shigella* and MacConkey agars. An oxidase test distinguishes them from Enterobacteriaceae.[12]

TREATMENT

Regardless of the nature of the infecting organism, the great majority of bacterial enteric pathogens cause self-limited losses of electrolytes and water. Less than 10 percent of all acute diarrheal episodes progress to a measurable degree of dehydration.[24] However, a thoughtful and simple approach to the replacement of these fluid and electrolyte losses is required, because no good predictors are available initially to determine which episodes will be self-limited and which will be severe. Ideally, a simple, inexpensive, and effective therapy would be initiated at home early in the course of the diarrhea to prevent the development of dehydration. Such an intervention would have obvious benefit in the developing world, where an estimated 4.6 million children die each year from diarrhea.[1] In the United States the morbidity and mortality from diarrhea are less but still account for a sizeable number of hospital admissions and infant deaths, especially in the disadvantaged portions of the population.[2,3]

General Therapy

The treatment of diarrhea includes two major components: the replacement of fluid and electrolyte losses and the early provision of adequate nutrition. Both of these treatments can be successfully accomplished orally.

Oral Rehydration Therapy

Orally administered fluid and electrolyte solutions have been used effectively throughout the world to treat children with acute diarrhea.[102] The physiologic basis for these solutions is the coupled transport of glucose (and other organic solutes) with sodium to achieve enhanced absorption of salt and water.[103] (See Chapter 40, Part 2.)

Several formulations have been widely used and studied, including oral rehydration salts (ORS), the complete solution recommended by the World Health Organization (WHO) and UNICEF, homemade sugar and salt solutions (SSS), and improved oral fluid therapy formulations, which contain additives to increase absorption and improve nutritional value.

By far the most widely and successfully used of these solutions has been the WHO/UNICEF ORS, which contain glucose (20 g per liter) and three salts: sodium chloride (3.5 g per liter), potassium chloride (1.5 g per liter), and either trisodium citrate (2.9 g per liter) or sodium bicarbonate (2.5 g per liter).[104] Clinical trials of ORS in health facilities and communities have consistently demonstrated their ability to rehydrate successfully 90 percent or more of patients with dehydration from all causes of acute diarrhea,[105] to reduce significantly case-fatality ratios,[105,106] to reduce greatly the cost of rehydration therapy compared to intravenous therapy,[107,108] and to be administered safely and effectively by family members with little or no formal education.[107] These salts are usually packaged in aluminum foil containers, which give them a long shelf-life even in hot, humid conditions. In the United States, several similar commercial solutions are

TABLE 3
Oral Rehydration Studies, United States

Study	Degree of Dehydration	ORT Sodium (mEq/L)	Percentage Success	ORT Complications
Santosham[109]	Mild–severe	90	98%	4%
		50	100%	0%
Tamer et al[110]	Mild–severe	75	94%	2%
		50		
Santosham et al[111]	<5%	90	97%	0%
		50	97%	0%
		30	100%	0%
Listernik et al[108]	Mild–moderate	60	87%	0%

also available (Table 2) which have proved to have an effectiveness similar to the WHO/UNICEF formulation when used in well-nourished children (Table 3).

For maximum benefit of the co-transport of electrolytes, sugar, and water, the ratio of carbohydrate to sodium should not exceed 2:1.[112] The use of solutions having this composition is recommended by WHO and the American Academy of Pediatrics for rehydration.[112] For the provision of maintenance fluids, the rehydration solution should be given with equal volumes of breast milk or free water because the sodium requirement is less. Alternatively, a solution with a lower sodium concentration can be given.

Currently, research efforts are focused on finding improved oral rehydration solutions that can overcome the important limitations of ORS and SSS. By improving the absorbability of ORS, these solutions would reduce stool frequency, volume, and duration, ideally would be easily and safely prepared at home, and offer nutritional benefits.[113] Two prototypes for these solutions have used either d-hexoses (and their more complex forms di-, tri-, oligo-, and polysaccharides) or neutral amino acids (and their di- and tripeptide forms).[114] In their purified form, these compounds are very expensive, but several natural foods including rice, wheat, and potatoes contain high concentrations of glucose polymers.[113]

Rice has received the most attention to date because it is a staple food in many cultures and is the best absorbed of these foods. Studies of rice ORT have demonstrated decreased stool volume, shorter duration of diarrhea, reduced ORT requirement, and comparable failure rates compared with standard ORT.[115–118]

Nutritional Therapy

The feeding component of therapy for diarrhea is essential because diarrhea can have a profoundly negative effect on the nutritional status and growth of children.[120] However, in many countries classical medical teaching and traditional practices have both often called for the withholding of food from children who have acute diarrhea; the validity of these practices is now being rigorously questioned.[120,121] The rationale for withholding food during an episode of diarrhea has been based on the concern for malabsorption, which can occur because of an altered intestinal mucosa or more rapid intestinal transit time.[121] Theoretical concerns have also been raised about a depleted bile acid pool or the possible effect of macromolecular antigen uptake by the damaged intestine, predisposing to intestinal allergy.[121] These potential problems, however, have never been demonstrated to be of practical importance in acute diarrhea.[121]

Recent studies indicate that feeding can have a direct beneficial effect on the outcome of acute diarrhea. Intestinal nutrient uptake is known to be an important factor for repair following intestinal injury,[122] and continued feeding is essential to reduce nutritional deficits that could lead to malnutrition.[121]

Feeding can also have a direct effect on the diarrheal episode. The duration of diarrhea is usually not prolonged,[123] and when combined with ORS, feeding can actually shorten the episode.[111,116–119,124] Studies of ORS and breast milk,[125] rice powder,[116–118] lactose-free formula,[111] lactose-containing diets,[124,126,127] and mixed diets[128] indicate that rehydration and feeding are usually tolerated during a diarrheal episode.

The most important benefit of feeding is to offer nutritional rehabilitation to the patient with diarrhea. Although some element of malabsorption is often associated with diarrhea, it is rarely complete, and sizeable percentages of dietary carbohydrate, fat, and protein are absorbed.[128] Even when stooling rates have increased with feeding, the duration of diarrhea is usually not prolonged and measurable nutritional benefits have been observed.[128,129] Nutritional rehabilitation and weight gain may be the most important outcome variables to measure in trials of feeding during diarrhea because of their impact on the health and well-being of the child.

Antimicrobial Therapy

Antimicrobial therapy for the enteric pathogens included in this chapter is listed in Table 4.

Since most episodes of diarrhea are self-limited, antimicrobials are not generally recommended. In fact, the use of antibiotics in infections like salmonellosis may actually lead to a prolonged carrier state and an increased risk of bacteriologic and symptomatic relapse.[130] However, antibiotics do have a role in cholera, shigellosis, and *C. difficile*–induced diseases, and antiparasitic agents have long been recommend-

TABLE 4
Antimicrobial Therapy for Enteric Infection

Organism	Recommended Therapeutic Agents	Comments
Campylobacter jejuni	Erythromycin	Usually self-limited; early therapy may slightly shorten the course (Bi 120)
Escherichia	Trimethoprim-sulfamethoxazole (TMP/SFX)	ETEC usually requires only oral rehydration therapy
Salmonella enteritidis	TMP/SFX, chloramphenicol	Only children less than 3 months of age routinely require antibiotic therapy
Salmonella typhi	TMP/SFX, chloramphenicol	
Shigella species	TMP/SFX	
Yersinia enterocolitica		Usually self-limited; no controlled trials proving efficacy of antibiotics
Vibrios	Tetracycline, chloramphenicol, aminoglycosides	
Clostridium difficile	Vancomycin, metronidazole, cholestyramine	Vancomycin is recommended for the most severe cases
Aeromonas hydrophila	TMP/SFX	Most episodes appear to be mild and self-limited
Plesiomonas shigelloides	TMP/SFX	Most episodes appear to be mild and self-limited

ed for symptomatic infection with *Giardia lamblia* and *Entamoeba histolytica*.[131] The diagnosis of these illnesses and proper use of antimicrobial agents imply evaluation by an experienced health care worker.

Antidiarrheal Agents

The three major categories of antidiarrheal drugs are antimotility, antisecretory, and adsorbent agents. They are intended to decrease the frequency and volume of diarrheal stools. In general these agents have been shown to have little impact on episodes of acute diarrhea, although consumers continue to pay millions of dollars each year for them.[132]

Antimotility agents are primarily opioids that work by inhibiting smooth muscle contractions.[133] In controlled trials, these agents have been shown to slow transit time and to shorten the duration of diarrhea.[133,134] However, they have little or no effect on total stool volume and can have important side effects, including nausea, vomiting, drowsiness, and ileus. These side effects are seen less often in the synthetic derivatives.

Antisecretory drugs attempt to decrease intestinal secretion, which is the major cause of watery stool. The two agents most completely studied and available, aspirin and bismuth subsalicylate, have been shown to have a modest clinical impact.[135] Often, however, such large volumes of drugs are required that they are of little practical use.[136]

Commonly used adsorbent agents like kaolin, pectin, and charcoal act by binding to bacterial toxins. They usually have little effect on stool weight and water content, although they may improve stool form.[132] Cholestyramine, an exchange resin that can bind bacterial toxins and bile acids, has been shown to reduce the duration of diarrhea but can cause acidosis, hyperchloremia, and intestinal obstruction in patients not properly rehydrated.[124] Young children are probably the least responsive patients.

PREVENTION

Strategies that may help prevent diarrhea include maternal education programs, encouragement of breast-feeding, improved personal and domestic hygiene, improved water supply and sanitation, and immunization programs.[137] As mentioned previously, early use of oral rehydration therapy is the most effective method to prevent dehydration, which is the most common cause of severe illness and death.

Maternal education should be expanded to include the education of all infant caretakers and should contain similar themes in developing and developed countries. These common themes include guidelines for personal hygiene and sanitation; food selection, preparation, and handling; and assessment and management of illness.[138]

Breast milk helps protect against diarrheal disease by providing a nutritionally excellent and relatively uncontaminated food source, containing immunologic and antimicrobial properties and factors that stimulate intestinal maturation.[142] These benefits are seen especially in children less than 1 year old in developed and developing countries.[140]

Programs to improve personal and domestic hygiene, water supplies, and sanitation were crucial to the rapid decline in the impact of diarrheal disease in developed countries at the turn of this century.[4,141] However, major financial and cultural obstacles continue to limit progress in these areas in less developed countries. The rapid population growth in these areas makes universal provision of potable water and improved standards of sanitation and hygiene unlikely in the foreseeable future.[141]

The final area of preventive intervention is immunoprophylaxis. Epidemiologic and serologic studies have confirmed that infants and children are most at risk for infections caused by bacterial enteric pathogens like enterotoxigenic *E. coli*, *Shigella*, *V. cholerae* 01, and *C. jejuni*.[142-146] The high attack rates of organisms like enterotoxigenic *E. coli* and *Shigella* in adult travelers to less developed countries is further evidence that specific acquired immunity occurs.[141]

Vaccines to a variety of bacterial enteric pathogens have been produced for many years, but their effectiveness has been limited. Currently, new vaccines against enterotoxigenic *E. coli*, *V. cholerae* 01, and *Shigella* are being studied.[141]

The current *E. coli* vaccines are derived from either nonliving antigens or attenuated live strains. The nonliving antigens include toxoids of the heat-labile and heat-stable toxins (LT/ST) and purified fimbriae to elicit both antitoxic and anticolonization immunity.[141] Live attenuated *E. coli* vaccines act by colonizing the proximal small intestine and stimulating an immune response.[147] To date, an effective *E. coli* vaccine is not available.

Live attenuated *Shigella* vaccines have been shown to produce immunity,[148] but their usefulness has been very limited because they require multiple oral doses. Recently a hybrid *Shigella sonnei–Salmonella typhi* attenuated vaccine strain has been shown to be effective in preliminary trials. This vaccine is made by the addition of the plasmid containing the genes that encode the production of *Shigella sonnei* O antigen into an attenuated *S. typhi* strain.[149]

The newest developments in cholera vaccines involve the preparation of nonenterotoxigenic strains by recombinant DNA techniques.[150] Because of the use of recombinant DNA techniques, these contain the critical antigens that may be involved in immunity, are genetically stable, and are potentially less expensive.[141]

SUMMARY

Bacterial enteric pathogens continue to be responsible for an important proportion of diarrheal illnesses throughout the world. Although illness can be caused by four mechanisms, dehydration from fluid and electrolyte losses is the final common acute result of most severe infections. All of the major pathogens (see Table 1) can cause a spectrum of disease from mild symptoms to severe dehydration regardless of their primary mechanism of action. The invasive and cytotoxin-producing organisms can cause colitis with severe blood loss.

Treatment involves replacement of fluid and electrolyte losses and provision of adequate nutrition. Both of these therapies can usually be given orally. Antibiotics have a limited role in most enteric bacterial infections, which are usually mild and self-limited. Antidiarrheal agents should have an even more limited role.

Prevention or at least a dramatic reduction in the incidence and severity of diarrhea is possible through the practice of high standards of personal hygiene and sanitation, the use of uncontaminated foods, and the provision of potable water. In the less developed world, where these standards are not likely to be achieved in the near future, the use of safe and effective vaccines may play a major role in prevention of disease.

REFERENCES

1. Snyder JD, Merson MH. The magnitude of the global problem of acute diarrheal disease: a review of active surveillance data. Bull WHO 1982; 60:605–613.
2. Hospital use by children in the United States and Canada. Comparative International Vital Health and Statistic Reports 1984; 5:1.
3. Ho MS, Glass RI, Pinsky PF. Diarrheal deaths in American children: are they preventable? JAMA 1988; 260:3281.
4. Levine MM, Edelman R. Acute diarrheal infections in infants. I. Epidemiology, treatment and prospects for immunoprophylaxis. Hosp Pract 1979; 14:89–100.
5. Communicable Disease Surveillance Center. Campylobacter infections, 1977–80. Br Med J 1981; 282:1484.
6. Uhnoo I, Wadell G, Svensson L, et al. Aetiology and epidemiology of acute gastroenteritis in Swedish children. J Infect 1986; 13:73.
7. Black RE, Brown KH, Becker S. Longitudinal studies of infectious diseases and physical growth in children in rural Bangladesh. II. Incidence of diarrhea and association with known pathogens. Am J Epidemiol 1982; 115:315–324.
8. Edelman R, Levine MM. Acute diarrheal infections in infants. II. Bacterial and viral causes. Hosp Pract 1980; 15:97–104.
9. Blaser MJ, Wells JG, Feldman RA, et al. Campylobacter enteritis in the United States: a multicenter study. Ann Intern Med 1983; 98:360.
10. Kendell EJC, Tanner E. Campylobacter enteritis in general practice. J Hyg 1982; 88:155.
11. Glass RI, Stoll BJ, Huq MI, et al. Epidemiological and clinical features of endemic Campylobacter jejuni infection in Bangladesh. J Infect Dis 1983; 148:292.
12. Rennels MB, Levine MM. Classical bacterial diarrhea: perspectives and update—Salmonella, Shigella, Escherichia coli, Aeromonas and Plesiomonas. Pediatr Infect Dis J 1986; 5:S91–S100.
13. Bishop WP, Ulshen MH. Bacterial gastroenteritis. Pediatr Clin North Am 1988; 35:69–87.
14. Stuart HC. Mortality among infants and children and progress in reduction of rates from certain causes. J Pediatr 1939; 15:266–276.
15. Pickering LK, Bartlett AV, Woodward WE. Acute infectious diarrhea among children in day care: epidemiology and control. Rev Infect Dis 1986; 8:539–547.
16. Steffen R. Epidemiologic studies of traveler's diarrhea, severe gastrointestinal infections, and cholera. Rev Infect Dis 1986; 8 (Suppl 2):S122.
17. Blaser MJ, Reller LB. Campylobacter enteritis. N Engl J Med 1981; 305:1444.
18. Elwell LD, Shipley PL. Plasmid-mediated factors associated with virulence of bacteria to animals. Ann Rev Microbiol 1980; 34:465.
19. Hill HR, Meier FA. Host defense factors in the gastrointestinal tract. Pediatr Infect Dis J 1986; 5:S144–S147.
20. Case records of the Massachusetts General Hospital. N Engl J Med 1985; 313:805–815.
21. Carpenter CC. Mechanisms of bacterial diarrheas. JAMA 1980; 68:313–316.
22. Wilkins TD. Role of Clostridium difficile toxins in disease. Gastroenterology 1987; 93:389.
23. Levine MM. Escherichia coli infections. N Engl J Med 1987; 313:445–447.
24. Levine MM, Losonsky G, Herrington D, et al. Pediatric diarrhea: the challenge of prevention. Pediatr Infect Dis J 1986; 5:S29–S43.
25. Hentges DJ. The protective function of indigenous intestinal flora. Pediatr Infect Dis J 1986; 5:S17–S20.
26. Holmberg SD, Osterholm MT, Senger KA, et al. Drug-resistant Salmonella from animals fed antimicrobials. N Engl J Med 1984; 311:617–622.
27. Hentges DJ. Role of the intestinal microflora in host defense against infection. In: Hentges DJ, ed. Human intestinal microflora in health and disease. New York: Academic Press, 1983:311.
28. Grand RJ, Watkins JB, Forti FM. Development of human gastrointestinal tract: a review. Gastroenterology 1976; 70:790–810.
29. Gianella RA, Broitman SA, Zamcheck N. Influence of gastric acidity on bacterial and parasitic enteric infections: a perspective. Ann Intern Med 1973; 78:271–276.
30. Shub MD, Pang KY, Swann DA, Walker WA. Age-related changes in chemical composition and physical properties of mucus glycoproteins from rat small intestine. Biochem J 1983; 215:405–411.
31. Snyder JD, Podolsky DK, Walker WA. The role of mucus in intestinal host defense: developmental differences in composition and binding to cholera toxin. Pediatr Res 1986; 20:249A.
32. Israel EJ, Walker WA. Development of intestinal mucosal barrier function to antigens and bacterial toxins. In: Mestecky J, McGhee JR, Bienstock J, Ogra PL, eds. Recent advances in mucosal immunology. New York: Plenum Publishers, 1987, 673–683.
33. Cohen MD, Guarino A, Shukla R, et al. Age-related differences in receptors for Escherichia coli heat stable enterotoxin in the small and large intestine of children. Gastroenterology 1988; 94:367–373.
34. Walker WA. Role of the mucosal barrier in toxin/microbial attachment to the gastrointestinal tract. Ciba Found Symp 1985; 112:34–56.
35. Cooper MD, Lawton AR. The development of the immune system. Sci Am 1974; 231:59–72.
36. Altemeier WA, Smith RT. Immunologic aspects of resistance in early life. Pediatr Clin North Am 1965; 12:663–686.
37. Blaser MJ. Bacterial gastrointestinal infections. Gastroenterol Ann 1986; 3:317–340.
38. Kist M, Keller KM, Niebling W, et al. Campylobacter coli septicemia associated with septic abortion. Infection 1984; 12:88.
39. Taylor DN, McDermott KT, Little JR, et al. Campylobacter enteritis from untreated water in the Rocky Mountains. Ann Intern Med 1983; 99:38.
40. Fennell CL, Totten PA, Quinn TC, et al. Characterization of Campylobacter-like organisms isolated from homosexual men. J Infect Dis 1984; 149:58.
41. Quinn TC, Goodell SE, Fennel C, et al. Infections with Campylobacter jejuni and Campylobacter-like organisms in homosexual men. Ann Intern Med 1984; 170:187.
42. Glass RI, Stoll BJ, Huq MI, et al. Epidemiological and clinical features of endemic Campylobacter jejuni infection in Bangladesh. J Infect Dis 1983; 148:292.
43. Speelman P, Struelens M. Detection of Campylobacter jejuni and other potential pathogens in traveler's diarrhea in Bangladesh. Scand J Gastroenterol 1983; 18:19.
44. Blaser MJ, Black RA, Duncan DJ, Amer J. Campylobacter jejuni-specific antibodies are elevated in healthy Bangladeshi children. J Clin Microbiol 1985; 21:164.
45. Pennie RA, Zunino JN, Rose Jr CE, Guerrant RL. Economical, simple method for production of the gaseous environment required for cultivation of Campylobacter jejuni. J Clin Microbiol 1984; 20:320.
46. Ho DD, Ault MJ, Ault MA, Murata GH. Campylobacter enteritis: early diagnosis with Gram's stain. Arch Intern Med 1982; 142:10.
47. Warren JR, Marshall BJ. Unidentified curved bacilli on gastric epithelium in active chronic gastritis. Lancet 1983; i:1273.
48. Dooley CP, Cohen H. The clinical significance of Campylobacter pylori. Ann Intern Med 1988; 108:70–79.
49. Graham DY, Klein PD, Opekun LC, Alpert LC, et al. Epidemiology of Campylobacter pyloridis infection. Gastroenterology 1987; 92:1411.
50. Marshall BJ, Warren JB. Unidentified curved bacilli in the stomach of patients with gastritis and peptic ulceration. Lancet 1984; i:1311.
51. Nelson JD. Etiology and epidemiology of diarrheal diseases in the United States. Am J Med 1985; 78(Suppl 6B):76.
52. Price AB, Levy J, Dolby JM, et al. Campylobacter pyloridis in peptic ulcer disease: microbiology, pathology, and scanning electron microscopy. Gut 1985; 26:1183.
53. Drumm D, Sherman P, Cutz E, Karmali M. Association of Campylobacter pylori on the gastric mucosa with antral gastritis in children. N Engl J Med 1987; 316:1557–1561.
54. Marshall BJ, Armstrong J, McGetchie D, et al. Attempt to fulfill Koch's postulates for pyloric Campylobacter. Med J Aust 1985; 142:436.
55. Morris A, Nicholson G. Ingestion of Campylobacter pyloridis causes gastritis and raised fasting gastric pH. Am J Gastroenterol 1987; 82:192.

56. Blaser MJ, Newman LS. Reviews of human salmonellosis. I. Infective dose. Rev Infect Dis 1982; 4:1096.

57. Seals JE, Parrott PL, McGowan JE, Feldman RA. Nursery salmonellosis: delayed recognition due to unusually long incubation period. Infect Control 1983; 4:205.

58. Centers for Disease Control. Human salmonella isolates—United States, 1982. JAMA 1983; 250:3030.

59. Taylor DN, Wachsmuth IK, Shangkuan Y-H, et al. Salmonellosis associated with marijuana. N Engl J Med 1982; 306:1249.

60. Riley LW, Cohen ML, Seals JER, et al. Importance of host factors in human salmonellosis caused by multiresistant strains. J Infect Dis 1984; 149:878.

61. Axon ATR, Poole D. Salmonellosis presenting with cholera-like diarrhoea. Lancet 1973; i:745.

62. Hyams JS, Durbin WA, Grand RJ. Salmonella bacteremia in the first year of life. J Pediatr 1980; 96:57.

63. Buchwald DS, Blaser MJ. A review of human salmonellosis. II. Duration of excretion following infection with non-typhi Salmonella. Rev Infect Dis 1984; 6:345.

64. Taylor DN, Pollard RA, Blake PA. Typhoid in the United States and risk of the international traveler. J Infect Dis 1983; 148:599.

65. Colon AR, Gross DR, Tamer MA. Typhoid fever in children. Pediatrics 1975; 56:606.

66. Levine MM. Bacillary dysentery: mechanisms and treatment. Med Clin North Am 1982; 66:623.

67. Keusch GT, Donohue-Rolfe A, Jacewicz M. *Shigella* toxin(s): description and role in diarrhea and dysentery. Pharmacol Ther 1982; 15:403.

68. Blaser MJ, Pollard RA, Feldman RA. Shigella infections in the United States, 1974–1980. J Infect Dis 1983; 147:771.

69. Sansonetti PJ, Kopecko DJ, Formal SB. Shigella sonnei plasmids: evidence that a large plasmid is necessary for virulence. Infect Immun 1981; 34:75.

70. Middlebrook JL, Dorland RB. Bacterial toxins: cellular mechanisms of action. Microb Rev 1984; 48:199.

71. Rennels MB, Levine MM. Classical bacterial diarrhea: perspectives and update—*Salmonella, Shigella, Escherichia coli, Aeromonas,* and *Plesiomonas.* Pediatr Infect Dis 1986; 5:S91.

72. Black RE, Brown KH, Becker S. Effects of diarrhea associated with specific enteropathogens on the growth of children in Bangladesh. Pediatrics 1984; 73:799.

73. Jadhar M, Verghese R, Bhat P. Clinical and microbiological features of shigellosis in 100 South Indian infants and children under 5 years. Indian J Pediatr 1966; 3:393.

74. Marks MI, Pai CH, Lafleur L, et al. *Yersinia enterocolitica* gastroenteritis: a prospective study of clinical, bacteriologic, and epidemiologic features. J Pediatr 1980; 96:26.

75. Snyder JD, Christianson E, Feldman RA. Human *Yersinia enterocolitica* infections in Wisconsin. Am J Med 1982; 72:768.

76. Tacket CO, Narain JP, Sattin R, et al. A multistate outbreak of infections caused by *Yersinia enterocolitica* transmitted by pasteurized milk. JAMA 1984; 251:483.

77. Black RE, Jackson RJ, Tsai T, Meavesky M, Shayegani M, Freley JC, MacLeod KIE, Wakclee AM. Epidemic *Yersinia enterocolitica* infection due to contaminated chocolate milk. N Engl J Med 1978; 298:76.

78. Marks MI, Pai CH, Lafleur L, Lackman L, Hammerberg O. *Yersinia enterocolitica* gastroenteritis: a prospective study of clinical, bacteriologic, and epidemiologic features. J Pediatr 1980; 96:26–31.

79. Ahoven P. Human yersiniosis in Finland. II. Clinical features. Ann Clin Res 1972; 4:39–48.

80. Schiemann DA. Synthesis of a selective agar medium for *Yersinia enterocolitica.* Can J Microbiol 1979; 25:1298.

81. Back E, Bomberg S, Wadstrom T. Enterotoxigenic *Escherichia coli* in Sweden. Infection 1977; 5:2.

82. Remis RS, MacDonald KL, Riley LW, et al. Sporadic cases of hemorrhagic colitis associated with *Escherichia coli* 0157:H7. Ann Intern Med 1984; 101:624.

83. Deneke CF, McGowan K, Larson AD, Gorbach SL. Attachment of human and pig (K88) enterotoxigenic *Escherichia coli* strains to either human or porcine small intestinal cells. Infect Immun 1984; 45:522.

84. Knutton S, Williams PH, Lloyd DR, et al. Ultrastructural study of adherence to and penetration of cultured cells by two invasive *Escherichia coli* strains isolated from infants with enteritis. Infect Immun 1984; 44:599.

85. Karmali MA, Petric M, Lim C, et al. The association between idiopathic hemolytic uremic syndrome and infection by verotoxin-producing *Escherichia coli.* J Infect Dis 1985; 151:755.

86. Pai CH, Gordon R, Simms HV, Bran LE. Sporadic cases of hemorrhagic colitis associated with *Escherichia coli* 0157:H7. Ann Intern Med 1985; 101:738.

87. Blake PA, Allegra D, Snyder JD. A possible endemic focus of cholera in the United States. N Engl J Med 1980; 302–305.

88. Morris JG, Black RE. Cholera and other vibrioses in the United States. N Engl J Med 1985; 312:343.

89. Hickman-Brenner FW, Brenner DJ, Steigerwalt AG, et al. *Vibrio fluvialis* and *Vibrio furnissii* isolated from a stool sample of one patient. J Clin Microbiol 1984; 20:125.

90. Ellis ME, Mandal BK, Dunbar EM, Bundell KR. *Clostridium difficile* and its cytotoxin in infants admitted to hospital with infectious gastroenteritis. Br Med J 1984; 288:523.

91. Jarvis WB, Feldman RA. *Clostridium difficile* and gastroenteritis: how strong is the association in children? Pediatr Infect Dis 1984; 3:4.

92. Schwarz RP, Ulshen MH. Pseudomembranous colitis presenting as mild, chronic diarrhea in childhood. J Pediatr Gastroenterol Nutr 1983; 2:570.

93. Chang TW, Gorbach SL. Rapid detection of *Clostridium difficile* by toxin detection. J Clin Microbiol 1982; 15:465.

94. Hawkins CC, Buggy BP, Fekety R, Schlaberg DR. Epidemiology of colitis induced by *Clostridium difficile* in hamsters: application of a bacteriophage and bacteriocin typing system. J Infect Dis 1984; 149:775.

95. Poxton IR, Aronsson B, Mollby R, et al. Immunochemical fingerprinting of *Clostridium difficile* strains isolated from an outbreak of antibiotic-associated colitis and diarrhoea. J Med Microbiol 1984; 17:317.

96. Delmee M, Homel M, Wauters G. Serogrouping of *Clostridium difficile* strains by slide agglutination. J Clin Microbiol 1985; 21:323.

97. Ashkenazi S, Danziger Y, Varsano I, et al. Treatment of *Campylobacter* gastroenteritis. Arch Dis Child 1987; 62:84.

98. Aggar WA, McCormick JD, Gurwith MJ. Clinical and microbiological features of *Aeromonas hydrophila*–associated diarrhea. J Clin Microbiol 1985; 21:909–913.

99. Gracey M, Burke V, Robinson J. Aeromonas-associated gastroenteritis. Lancet 1982; ii:1304–1306.

100. Holmberg SD, Farmer JJ. *Aeromonas hydrophila* and *Plesiomonas shigelloides* as causes of intestinal infections. Rev Infect Dis 1984; 6:633.

101. Rolston KVI, Hopfer RL. Diarrhea due to *Plesiomonas shigelloides* in cancer patients. J Clin Microbiol 1984; 20:597.

102. Gabr M. Keynote state of issues address. In: Proceedings: Second International Conference on Oral Rehydration Therapy. Washington, DC: Agency for International Development, 1985:9..

103. Hirschhorn N. The treatment of acute diarrhea in children: an historical and physiological perspective. Am J Child Nutr 1980; 33:637–638.

104. WHO/UNICEF. The management of diarrhea and the use of oral rehydration therapy. 2nd ed. Geneva: WHO, 1985.

105. Mahalanbis D, et al. Oral fluid therapy of cholera among Bangladesh refugees. John Hopkins Med J 1973; 132:197–205.

106. Rahaman MM, et al. Diarrheal mortality in two Bangladesh villages with and without community-based oral rehydration therapy. Lancet 1979; ii:809–812.

107. Shepard DS. Procedures for assessing the cost effectiveness of a diarrheal disease control program based on oral rehydration therapy. In: Proceedings of International Conference on Oral Rehydration Therapy. Washington, DC: Agency for International Development, 1983.

108. Listernik R, Ziesel E, David AT. Outpatient oral rehydration in the United States. Am J Dis Child 1985; 140:211–215.

109. Santosham M. Oral rehydration therapy of infantile diarrhea: a controlled study of well-nourished children hospitalized in the U.S. and Panama. N Engl J Med 1982; 306:1070–1076.

110. Tamer AM, Friedman LB, Maxwell SRW. Oral rehydration of infants in a large urban U.S. medical center. J Pediatr 1985; 107:14–19.

111. Santosham M, Foster S, Reid R. Role of soy-based, lactose-free formula during treatment of acute diarrhea. Pediatrics 1985; 76:292–298.

112. AAP Committee on Nutrition. Use of oral fluid therapy and post-treatment feeding following enteritis in children in a developed country. Pediatrics 1985; 75:358–361.

113. Mahalanabis D, Merson M. Development of an improved formula-

tion of oral rehydration salts (ORS) with anti-diarrhoeal and nutritional properties: a "super ORS". In: Holmgren J, Lindberg A, Mollby R, eds. Development of vaccines and drugs against diarrhoea. 11th Nobel Conference. Lund, Sweden: Studentlitteratur, 1986.

114. Schulz SG. Sodium-coupled solute transport by small intestine: a status report. Am J Physiol 1977; 233:E249–E254.

115. Patra FC, Mahalanabis D, Jalan KN. Stimulation of sodium and water absorption by sucrose in the rat small intestine. Acta Paediatr Scand 1982; 71:103–107.

116. Molla AM, Hossain M, Sarker SA, et al. Rice-powder electrolyte solution as oral therapy in diarrhoea due to *Vibrio cholerae* and *Escherichia coli*. Lancet 1982; i:1317–1319.

117. Patra FC, Mahalanabis D, Jalan KN, et al. Is oral rice electrolyte solution superior to glucose electrolyte solution in infantile diarrhoea? Arch Dis Child 1982; 57:910–912.

118. Molla AM, Ahmed M, Khatun M, Greenough WB III. Rice based ORS reduces stool output in acute diarrhoea. Bull WHO 1984; 63:751–756.

119. Chen LC, Scrimshaw NS, eds. Diarrhea and malnutrition: Interactions, mechanisms, and interventions. New York: Plenum Press, 1983.

120. Subcommittee on Nutrition and Diarrheal Disease Control, Committee on International Nutritional Programs, Nutritional Research Council. Nutritional management of acute diarrhea in infants and children. Washington, DC: National Academy Press, 1985.

121. Brown KH, MacLean WC Jr. Nutritional management of acute diarrhea: an appraisal of the alternatives. Pediatrics 1984; 73:119–125.

122. Knudsen KH, Bradley EM, Lecocq FR, et al. Effect of fasting and refeeding on the histology and disaccharidase activity of the human intestine. Gastroenterology 1968; 55:46.

123. Chung AW, Viscorova B. The effect of early oral feeding versus early oral starvation on the course of infantile diarrhea. J Pediatr 1948; 33:14–22.

124. Isolauri E, Vesikari E. Oral rehydration, rapid feeding, and cholestyramine for treatment of acute diarrhea. J Pediatr Gastroenterol Nutr 1985; 4:366–374.

125. Khin-Maung V, Nyunt-Nyunt-Wai, Myo-Khin, Mu-Mu-Khin, Tin U, Thane-Toe. Effect on clinical outcome of breast feeding during acute diarrhea. Br Med J 1985; 290:587–589.

126. Rees L, Brook CGD. Gradual reintroduction of full strength milk after acute gastroenteritis in children. Lancet 1979; i:770–771.

127. Mahalanbis D. Nitrogen balance during recovery from secretory diarrhea of cholera in children. Am J Clin Nutr 1981; 34:1548–1551.

128. Molla A, Molla AM, Sarker S, et al. Absorption of nutrients during diarrhea due to *V. cholerae, E. coli*, rotavirus and shigella. In: Chen LC, Scrimshaw HA, eds. Diarrhea and malnutrition: Interactions mechanisms and interventions. New York: Plenum Publishing, 1981.

129. Brown KH, Gastanaduy AS, Saavedra JM, et al. Effect of continued oral feeding on clinical and nutritional outcomes of acute diarrhea in children. J Pediatr 1988; 112:191–200.

130. Neslon JD, Kusmiesz H, Jackson LH, et al. Treatment of *Salmonella* gastroenteritis with ampicillin, amoxicillin, or placebo. Pediatrics 1980; 65:125–130.

131. Du Pont HL. Nonfluid therapy and selected chemoprophylaxis of acute diarrhea. Am J Med 1985; 78(6B):81–90.

132. Portnoy BL, Du Pont HL, Pruit D, et al. Antidiarrheal agents in the treatment of acute diarrhea in children. JAMA 1976; 236:844–846.

133. Du Pont HL, Hornick RB. Adverse effects of Lomotil therapy in shigellosis. JAMA 1973; 266:1525–1528.

134. Kassem AS, Madkour AA, Massoud BZ, et al. Loperamide in acute childhood diarrhoea: a double blind controlled trial. J Diarrhoeal Dis Res 1983; 1:10–16.

135. Burke V, Gracey M, Suharyons S. Reduction by aspirin of intestinal fluid loss in acute gastroenteritis. Lancet 1980; i:1329–1330.

136. Du Pont HL, Sullivan P, Pickering LK, et al. Symptomatic treatment of diarrhea with bismuth subsalicylate among students attending a Mexican university. Gastroenterology 1977; 73:715–718.

137. Feachem RG, Hogan RC, Merson MH. Diarrheal disease control: reviews of potential interventions. Bull WHO 1983; 61:637–640.

138. Mata LJ. The children of Santa Maria Cauque. A prospective field study of health and growth. Cambridge: MIT Press, 1978.

139. Feachem RG, Koblinsky MA. Interventions for the control of diarrhoeal diseases among young children: promotion of breast feeding. Bull WHO 1984; 62:271–291.

140. Paine R, Coble RJ. Breast-feeding and infant health in a rural U.S. community. Am J Dis Child 1982; 136:36–38.

141. Levine MM, Losonsky G, Herrington D, et al. Pediatric diarrhea: the challenge of prevention. Pediatr Infect Dis J 1986; 5:S29–S43.

142. Black RE, Merson MH, Rowe B, et al. Enterotoxigenic *Escherichia coli* diarrhoea: acquired immunity and transmission in an endemic area. Bull WHO 1981; 59:263–268.

143. Du Pont HL, Olarte J, Evans DG, et al. Comparative susceptibility of Latin American and the United States students to enteric pathogens. N Engl J Med 1976; 295:1520–1521.

144. Levine MM, Gangarosa EJ, Werner M, et al. Shigellosis in custodial institutions. III. Prospective clinical and bacteriologic surveillance of children vaccinated with oral attenuated shigella vaccines. J Pediatr 1974; 84:803–806.

145. Kapikian AZ, Wyatt RG, Greenberg HB, et al. Approaches to immunization of infants and young children against gastroenteritis due to rotavirus. Rev Infect Dis 1980; 2:459–469.

146. Black RE, Levine MM, Brown KH, et al. Immunity to *Campylobacter jejuni* in man. Campylobacter III. In: Pearson A, Skirrow M, Lior H, et al, eds. Proceedings: Third international workshop on *Campylobacter* infections. London: Public Health Laboratory Service, 1985, in press.

147. Levine MM, Kaper JB, Black RE, et al. New knowledge on pathogenesis of bacterial enteric infections as applied to vaccine development. Microbiol Rev 1983; 47:510–550.

148. Mel DM, Arsic BL, Radovanovic ML, et al. Live oral Shigella vaccine: vaccination schedule and the effect of booster dose. Acta Microbiol Acad Sci Hung 1974; 21:109–114.

149. Formal SB, Baron LS, Kopecko DJ, et al. Construction of a potential bivalent vaccine strain: introduction of *Shigella sonnei* form I antigen genes in the *galE Salmonella typhi* Ty21a typhoid vaccine strain. Infect Immun 1981; 34:746–750.

150. Kaper JB, Lockman H, Baldini MM, et al. Recombinant nontoxigenic *Vibrio cholerae* strains as attenuated cholera vaccine candidates. Nature 1984; 308:655–658.

Intestinal Viral Infections

Graeme L. Barnes, M.D., Ch.B., F.R.A.C.P.

The report in 1973 of reovirus-like particles in epithelial cells in small bowel biopsies from children with acute non-specific diarrhea[1] led to a cascade of clinical and laboratory studies that have established rotavirus as the leading enteric viral pathogen. This discovery has improved the identification rate of the causes of childhood enteritis in developed countries from 10 to 20 percent in the early 1970s to 40 to 70 percent in the 1980s. Specific types of adenovirus that preferentially attack the gastrointestinal (GI) tract now account for 7 to 17 percent of cases in developed countries.[2] Norwalk agent, a small round virus known since 1972 to cause epidemic vomiting in adults,[3] has now been described as a cause of outbreaks of vomiting and diarrhea in children at school camps[4] and as a cause of nosocomial infection in a children's hospital ward.[5] Probably these are not "new" viruses but newly discovered viruses. In 1943, Light and Hodes stored stool samples from children with acute infectious diarrhea when searching for the elusive cause. In 1975 after rotavirus had been discovered, Hodes tested these samples again and found rotavirus in several of them.[9] Several other "novel" viruses have been described in association with acute diarrhea, but cause and effect have yet to be established for most. Many of these candidates are still named after the locality in which they were discovered (Hawaii, Snow Mountain, Breda) or for their appearance on electron microscopy (astrovirus) (Table 1).

Viruses also account for up to 30 percent of cases of infectious diarrhea in children in developing countries. Rotavirus is one of the single most important pathogens, because of its frequency and because it is over-represented in more severe, dehydrating disease.[6] Development of a rotavirus vaccine is an objective of the World Health Organization Diarrheal Diseases Control Program, and several candidates are being tested.

Enteric viruses are thought to be spread mainly by person-to-person contact or contact with contaminated feces (the fecal-oral route). However, there is some evidence that transmission via contaminated water supplies may be important in developing countries.[7] Santosham and others studied an outbreak of rotavirus diarrhea in an American Indian population and concluded that the rapid spread of disease to all areas of the reservation could best be explained by respiratory transmission,[8] a suggestion supported by studies in mice using EDIM, a murine rotavirus strain.

Discovery of these agents in nearly all cases was the result of the application of new technology, especially electron microscopy, to diarrheal disease. Most enteric viruses have proved difficult to grow in the laboratory, and hence they eluded recognition by traditional tissue culture techniques. Electron microscopic identification of rotavirus has been replaced by less cumbersome enzyme immunoassay (EIA) antigen detection tests, which can be undertaken in large batches of stools. An EIA is being developed for Norwalk agent, and a similar test has been used for several years to detect enteric adenoviruses.

There is a large overlap between human and veterinary medicine in this field. Knowledge of animal enteric viruses has often preceded their discovery in humans. Animal studies

TABLE 1
Fecal Viruses That Appear to Have the Intestinal Mucosa as Their Main Target

Agent and Pathogenicity in Humans	Disease Pattern		Comment
	Endemic	Epidemic	
Definite			
Rotavirus	+		
Adenovirus 40,41	+		Respiratory adenoviruses may also cause diarrhea.
Norwalk and some other calici-like agents		+	Includes Hawaii, Montgomery County, and Snow Mountain agents.
Probable			
Astrovirus	+		
Calicivirus		+	
Calici-like SRSV		+	Includes Taunton, Amulree, Otofuke, and Sapporo agents.
Coronavirus	+		(TGEV, used in animal models of viral enteritis, is a coronavirus.)
SRV	?	+	Includes enteroviruses, parvovirus, parvo-like viruses (Ditchling, Paramatta, Wollan, and cockle agents).
Possible			
Minireovirus	+		
Toroviridae	?	?	Berne, Breda viruses: animal viruses that possibly affect humans.

SRV = small round virus; SRSV = small round structured virus; TGEV = transmissible gastroenteritis virus.

have provided much of the understanding of current pathologic and pathophysiologic sequelae of viral enteritis. There are significant differences between human and animal viruses which become especially relevant when cross-protection between strains of virus becomes a concern.

PATHOPHYSIOLOGY

In Norwalk agent infection and rotavirus infection, the villi become shortened, microvilli are damaged, and the lamina propria is infiltrated with inflammatory cells. Brush border enzymes including disaccharidases have been found to be reduced in adult volunteers with Norwalk agent–induced illness[10] and in children with natural rotavirus infection.[11]

Animal models have been developed to investigate the mechanisms of viral diarrhea. Hamilton and his colleagues in Toronto have undertaken experiments in piglets using transmissible gastroenteritis virus (TGEV), a specific coronavirus infection affecting the upper intestinal epithelium. In 1976 they showed that sodium transport failed to respond normally to glucose, when studied either in Ussing short-circuited chambers or in suspensions of enterocytes isolated selectively from jejunal villi.[12] Further studies indicated that mature villous epithelial cells were shed and that there were proliferation and accelerated migration of cells from the crypts[13] so that at the height of diarrhea, the epithelium was composed predominantly of immature virus-free cells that had migrated to the villi in a relatively undifferentiated state. Recent studies in isolated membrane vesicles have shown diminished activity of the high-affinity glucose-Na co-transporter and diminished Na gradient–dependent alanine absorption.[13a,b] Infection of the distal small bowel leads to the loss of "ileal salvage" of excess fluid sent downstream from the jejunum,[14] highlighting the importance of extent of disease in

the production of clinical symptoms. Studies using human rotavirus in the same animal showed identical structural and functional abnormalities, giving confidence that the TGEV model is a reliable system for investigating viral diarrhea in general (Fig. 1).[15]

Rapid histologic and functional recovery with the return of a normal differentiated epithelium can be expected within one to two epithelial cell turnover cycles (5 to 10 days) after virus excretion has ceased. Clinical management is directed, therefore, at making the most of residual water, electrolyte, and calorie absorption while promoting healing of the mucosa. The principles of treatment are addressed later in this book.

THE EFFECT OF MALNUTRITION

The impact of viral gastroenteritis has an added dimension if the child is malnourished. While susceptibility to infection may not be greatly different, animal studies suggest that the severity of infection is greater,[16] and there is evidence from both laboratory studies and clinical studies in malnourished children that recovery is delayed.[17]

A detailed study of the effects of chronic protein-calorie malnutrition on small intestinal repair after acute viral enteritis was reported by Butzner and co-workers in 1985.[18] Malnourished and normally fed gnotobiotic (germ-free) piglets were infected with TGEV. In control piglets, structural changes present in the intestine at 40 hours had virtually recovered by 4 days, but the changes persisted through 15 days in malnourished animals. Recovery of mucosal enzymes and of glucose-stimulated sodium absorption was also delayed in malnourished piglets, suggesting that malnutrition delays intestinal repair after viral injury and reinforcing the need for early and effective nutritional rehabilitation during diarrhea.

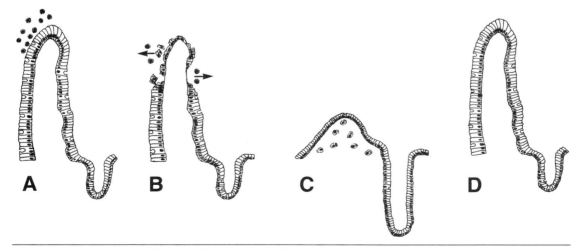

FIGURE 1 Postulated mechanism of rotavirus diarrhea. *A*, Mature enterocytes are infected. *B*, Virus multiplies in enterocytes, which are damaged and shed by 24 hours. *C*, Crypts hypertrophy by 42 hours, repopulating the surface with immature enterocytes. Villi are stunted. Inflammatory cells, predominantly plasma cells, appear in the lamina propria. Virus is no longer present. Disaccharidases, glucose absorption, glucose-stimulated sodium absorption at the brush border, and the sodium pump (Na+, K+-ATPase) at the basal lateral membrane are diminished. Thymidine kinase activity is increased. Cyclic AMP activity is not raised, and chloride secretion is not stimulated. *D*, Structure and function are normal by 15 days.

IMMUNODEFICIENCY

Virus infections of the GI tract are common in patients with immunodeficiency. One child with severe combined immunodeficiency chronically excreted five different viruses.[19] There are reports of prolonged excretion of rotavirus by such children; one group demonstrated changes in the strain of virus, suggesting that reinfection rather than prolonged infection was the problem.[20] Enteric viral infection is common after bone marrow transplantation[21] and as a complication of AIDS. Passive treatment with oral gamma globulin has been used in immunodeficiency[22] and also in premature newborn infants.[23]

ENTERIC VIRUSES THAT ARE NOT PRIMARY GUT PATHOGENS

This discussion focuses on viruses that cause gut disease by direct invasion of epithelial cells and mucosal damage. Some viruses replicate asymptomatically in the gut, produce a viremia, and attack distant target organs (e.g., poliovirus, hepatitis A). They will not be discussed further.

Another form of viral enteritis occurs when the gut is the target of viruses spread by the blood stream. In humans, cytomegalovirus is in this category; an increasing number of reports link this agent to infections of stomach, duodenum, ileum, colon, and rectum. Most but not all patients have an immune deficiency syndrome, especially AIDS. Associations with relapse of inflammatory bowel disease have been reported.

CURRENT STATUS OF ESTABLISHED AND CANDIDATE VIRAL PATHOGENS

Rotaviruses. These viruses are the single most important cause of diarrhea requiring admission to hospital during the first 6 to 24 months of life. Infection with these agents is common worldwide from birth to old age.[24] Most infections are asymptomatic or associated with mild symptoms. Attack rates for severe rotavirus diarrhea in young children are similar in developing and developed countries. The frequency and severity of rotavirus infection have been the justification for a vigorous search for an effective vaccine.

"Atypical" rotaviruses that lack the group A–specific common antigen have caused epidemics of severe diarrhea in adults and children in China and have recently been implicated there in an outbreak of diarrhea in newborn infants. Non–group A rotaviruses have now been reported from several countries, but they so far account for only 1 to 2 percent of rotavirus isolates.

Enteric Adenoviruses. These are now a well-recognized group of adenoviruses and have been assigned serotypes 40 and 41.[25] They cause approximately 7 to 17 percent of diarrheal disease in children admitted to hospital in developed countries.[2] Their importance in developing countries is not yet clear, primarily because of technical difficulties in identifying serotypes away from sophisticated laboratories. There is no reason to suppose that they will be any less important in the developing world than they are in developed countries.

Norwalk and Norwalk-like Agents (Hawaii, Montgomery County, Taunton, Amulree, Otofuke, Sapporo, and Snow Mountain Agents). These are calici-like viruses. They have been implicated in outbreaks of gastroenteritis occurring in families, schools, institutions, and communities, affecting adults, school-age children, family contacts, and some young children as well.[26] However, they do not appear to be important causes of severe endemic gastroenteritis in infants and young children in the United States. Antibody surveys suggest that Norwalk agent infects children earlier in life in Bangladesh and Ecuador, but the real incidence of symptoms caused by this group of viruses is not known.

Caliciviruses. There is some evidence that human caliciviruses (HCV) can cause outbreaks of diarrhea and vomiting in infants, adults, and the elderly. An electron microscopic survey of the causes of infantile gastroenteritis in North-West London showed that HCV accounts for about 5 percent of cases of identified viral diarrheas.[27] A distinction was made from Norwalk virus in that study, but Norwalk agent itself is thought by some to be a calicivirus.

Coronavirus. The role of coronavirus in both acute and chronic intestinal disease in humans is unclear.[28] Chronic excretion and an association with tropical sprue have discouraged human volunteer studies. Its accepted role in animal disease suggests that it will eventually become recognized as a cause of diarrhea in humans. Current evidence suggests that coronavirus does not play an important role in diarrhea in infants; it is seen more often in older children and young adults. TGEV of swine, which has been used as a model of human viral enteritis, is a member of this genus.

Other Small Viruses. Several other small viruses have been associated with human enteritis. Some are accepted pathogens in animals, but proof that they cause disease in humans is lacking.[29] They are shed generally in small numbers, so they are difficult to see and impossible to use as antigen for diagnostic testing. Lack of success in their cultivation has compounded the problem. *Astrovirus*, a small round virus (28 nm in diameter) with a starlike appearance on electron microscopy, was seen first in feces from children with acute diarrhea; a probable pathogen, its importance is difficult to establish, as it may be excreted with other known pathogens.[30] *Small round viruses* (SRV) and *small round structured viruses* (SRSV) are terms applied to other virus-like objects that are found in diarrheal stools and less frequently in normal stools and distinguished mainly by their surface structure. An association with disease is doubtful, and there is no information about their relative importance in children versus adults. *Berne* and *Breda viruses* constitute a new family of enveloped RNA viruses, the *Toroviridae*.[31] They are pleomorphic particles, 120 to 140 nm in diameter, found in diarrheal stools from calves and horses as well as human adults and children. Convincing evidence of pathogenicity in humans is lacking. In animals immature crypt cells as well as mature cells are infected; both colon and small bowel may be involved.

Cytomegalovirus (CMV). The significance of CMV as a cause of enteritis or colitis in humans is not clear. Reports link the virus to diarrhea in immunocompromised patients, but it seems an unlikely major cause of diarrhea in healthy children. It grows well in tissue culture, and, had it been common, it would have been found in the many studies undertaken before electron microscopy was used in the search for viral enteric pathogens. Anecdotal reports suggest that it may be a cause of colitis in infancy.

VIRAL ENTERITIDES

Human Rotavirus

Incidence

Infection is widespread throughout the world. Rotaviruses have been identified in stools from 10 to 40 percent of children admitted to hospital with acute diarrhea in developing countries and in 35 to 50 percent in developed countries. Severe infection occurs at a younger age in children in developing countries, where the majority of children admitted to hospital are 6 to 12 months old, compared with 12 to 18 months for children in developed countries.[24] All children can be expected to contact rotavirus by 5 years of age, and evidence is emerging that most will experience asymptomatic boosts in mucosal immunity to rotavirus several times each year. Rotavirus seems to be endemic in the community, and repeated contacts maintain a high level of protection against symptomatic disease after primary infection.

In temperate climates, severe rotavirus infections peak during the winter months, but cases are seen throughout the summer. In tropical areas, seasonal variations are less obvious. The attack rates for rotaviral diarrhea in children aged 6 to 24 months are 0.3 to 0.8 episode per child per year in both the developing and developed worlds.[24]

Neonatal rotavirus infection is common but often asymptomatic in healthy full-term infants, presumably owing to passive immunity from placental and breast milk antibodies. Premature or sick infants requiring special care are more likely to suffer symptomatic disease.[32] Clinical observations that unique strains of rotavirus often are responsible for endemic nursery infection have been supported by recent RNA-RNA hybridization experiments using nursery strains and strains from children with gastroenteritis.[33] The fourth genes of nursery strains were closely related to each other but not to the fourth genes of virulent community viruses.

Infection in children after 3 years of age is not usually severe, but it can necessitate admission to hospital. Rotaviruses have been identified in 5 percent of adults admitted to hospital in Thailand for severe diarrheal disease.

Most rotavirus infections are asymptomatic or associated with mild disease. Several studies from developing countries have reported similar rates of rotavirus isolation from both controls and diarrhea patients.[34,35] The balance among ingested dose of virus, mucosal immunity, breast-feeding, and sensitivity of detection methods probably influences these observations.

Outbreaks of diarrhea caused by "atypical" rotaviruses have been widespread in China, where they have affected adults, children, and newborn infants.[36] These "atypical" rotaviruses lack group A–specific common antigen, but they are morphologically identical to conventional human strains. So far they account for less than 1 percent of all severe rotavirus disease, but they have been identified in several parts of the world. If they become more common, current vaccine development strategies will need to be reconsidered.

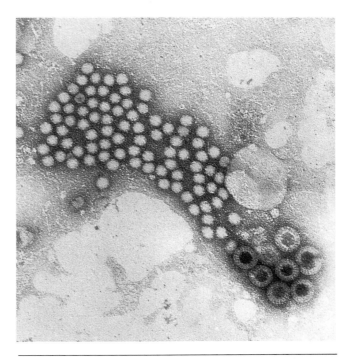

FIGURE 2 Electron microscopy of feces from an infant with acute diarrhea. The larger (70 nm diameter) particles are rotaviruses that have lost their electron-dense core. A group of smaller unidentified virus-like particles is seen here in association with rotavirus.

Virology

Rotaviruses are classified as a genus within the family *Reoviridae*.[37] The prefix "rota" refers to the wheel-like appearance of particles in feces seen by negative contrast electron microscopy (Fig. 2).

Complete particles, about 70 nm in diameter, exhibit a double-shelled capsid. Incomplete single-shelled particles are common but not infectious. Gel electrophoresis patterns separate rotaviruses into at least four major *groups* (A, B, C, and D). Neutralization assays directed at outer capsid glycoproteins classify rotaviruses into at least five *serotypes*. Complement fixation or IAHA assays detect inner capsid proteins, allowing classification of at least two *subgroups*.

Group A rotaviruses are most important to man. Strains within the group can be identified by gel electrophoretic pattern. Changes in electropherotype can be used to follow epidemiologic patterns in a given locality. Multiple electropherotypes exist simultaneously in most communities, but usually one or two are dominant in any one year in children admitted to hospital. Strains tend to remain dominant for 18 to 24 months and then disappear. Infections in nurseries have been associated with a single endemic electropherotype not identified among hospitalized children in the same community.[38] In one tertiary care nursery in the United States, where babies were transferred from a variety of community sources, several different electropherotypes were present.

The few epidemiologic studies available of serologic differences have concerned detection of subgroup I and II strains. Epidemiologic studies of serotypes rather than subgroups are needed to understand cross-protection (or lack of it) exhibit-

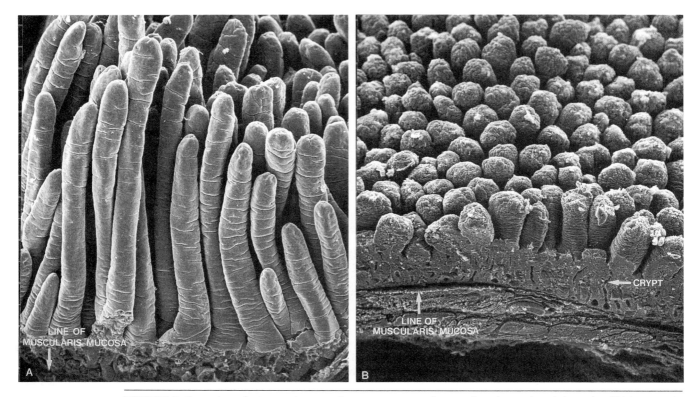

FIGURE 3 Scanning electron microscopic appearances of normal and rotavirus-infected calf jejunum. *A*, Jejunum from a normal conventionally reared calf, showing tall finger-like villi. *B*, Rotavirus-damaged intestine from a moribund calf. Rotavirus antigen was detected by immunoperoxidase staining of paraffin sections from adjacent tissue; most of the enterocytes on the surface of the stunted villi contained antigen. Note epithelial damage, decreased villous height, and increased crypt depth. (Courtesy of Dr. G.A. Hall, Institute for Animal Health, Compton, United Kingdom).

ed by antibodies raised by natural infection or vaccines. Animal studies suggest that there is not likely to be cross-protection between human rotaviruses of differing groups.

Pathophysiology

Rotavirus infects mature enterocytes on the apical half of the villi in the small bowel.[39] It does not infect the stomach, the colon, or other organs. Small bowel biopsies in children with nonspecific gastroenteritis led to the original recognition of rotavirus as a pathogen in humans[1] and demonstrated the severe histologic lesion it could cause (Fig. 3).[11]

Enterocytes are destroyed, villi become short, crypts deepen, and there is marked infiltration of the lamina propria by inflammatory cells. Diarrhea is caused by a combination of malabsorption and net fluid loss into the lumen of the small bowel due to a lack of mature absorptive cells (see Fig. 1). Stool sodium and chloride concentrations are generally in the range of 20 to 40 mmol per liter, compared with 80 to 120 mmol per liter found in cholera. Virus excretion precedes onset of diarrhea, and the height of the diarrhea may occur after virus shedding has ceased. Histologic recovery is rapid. Restoration of the duodenal mucosa to normal within 3 weeks was documented in the original group of children recognized to have this infection.[11] Fecal alpha$_1$-antitrypsin clearance

studies have shown a transient protein-losing enteropathy in the acute stage of the illness.[40] Changes in gut permeability with increased uptake of protein during the early phase of the infection have been shown.

Clinical Features

In severe cases, after an incubation period of 2 to 7 days, there is an abrupt onset of vomiting and fever.[41] Profuse watery diarrhea soon follows, leading to dehydration, acidosis, and electrolyte imbalance on occasions. In contrast to bacterial gastroenteritis, the stool fluid does not contain blood, white cells, or mucus. Abdominal cramps are much less frequent, but irritability and lethargy are often present. Respiratory symptoms have been reported in 20 to 40 percent of patients, but in several studies an equally high incidence has been found in controls. The temperature falls to normal quickly. Usually vomiting settles within 24 to 48 hours and diarrhea within 2 to 7 days.

Acute complications include hypernatremia or hyponatremia when water and electrolyte losses are discrepant. Febrile convulsions can occur as with any other cause of sudden high fever. Reye's syndrome, encephalitis, rectal bleeding, and intussusception have been described in association with rotavirus infection, but the evidence linking them as cause and effect is tenuous.

Depressed mucosal lactase activity is frequent,[11] but persisting lactose malabsorption is not common, as disaccharidase activities return to normal within a few days.

Treatment

Initial management is directed at correcting dehydration, acidosis, and electrolyte imbalance. The assessment of the degree of dehydration and treatment with oral or intravenous fluids are considered elsewhere. Early resumption of normal feeding is encouraged, especially in malnourished children, with special emphasis on breast-feeding. Even in children with lactose malabsorption, breast-feeding almost always can be continued. In a small group of infants lactose malabsorption can be a serious problem, requiring lactose-free feeding for days or even weeks. These cases, although rare, should not be overlooked in the appropriate enthusiasm for continued breast-feeding.

For the breast-fed infant with severe diarrhea, a combination of oral rehydration solution (ORS) and increasing volumes of breast milk can be offered. One regimen is to offer the infant 2 minutes of breast-feeding from each breast for each feed for the first 6 hours, followed by ORS. If this does not provoke more diarrhea, then the time on each breast can be increased, working back to full breast-feeding over 1 to 2 days. In older children early introduction of a balanced diet with starch-based solids (cracker biscuits, bread, rice) should be encouraged, as temporary mucosal damage leaves a much larger reserve of maltase and isomaltase than lactase. Small amounts of fruit juices can be given, but large volumes of sucrose-containing fluids should be avoided in the acute phase, and for babies these beverages should be diluted in half with water.

Drugs are contraindicated. Antibiotics have no place in viral diarrhea. Antiperistaltic agents may lead to pooling of fluid, which is effectively removed from the circulation and yet not revealed to the observer. Complications include respiratory depression, and deaths have occurred after atropine-like drugs. Antiemetics should be avoided. Vomiting is usually self-limiting and dystonic reactions to these drugs are common, especially in the dehydrated child.

Prevention

Improved sanitation and hygiene are unlikely to radically alter the incidence of rotavirus diarrhea in developing countries. Such measures have proved unsuccessful in North America and Europe, where the attack rates are similar to those in less developed parts of the world. The severity of illness and slow recovery in malnourished children, together with concerns that rotavirus infection may set the scene for bacterial overgrowth syndromes where fecal contamination of water supplies is common, have convinced the World Health Organization to encourage development of an oral rotavirus vaccine.[42] For practical reasons it will need to be compatible with oral poliovirus vaccine and preferably effective after one dose given to newborn infants. Several candidate vaccines have been through phase 1 and phase 2 trials. The first was a live attenuated vaccine derived from the NCDV strain of bovine rotavirus. Initial reports showed an 88 percent protection against clinically significant rotavirus

diarrhea during one epidemic season in Finland. However, subsequent trials in Gambia, Peru, and Rwanda showed it to be less effective. A second candidate is the live oral rhesus vaccine, which has shown early promise. It is more immunogenic that the bovine strain, but fever has been an early problem. Another approach is to develop genetic reassortants (rhesus-human hybrids) that express serotype antigens of serotypes 1, 2, and 4 and to use them in combination with the current serotype 3 rhesus rotavirus strain.

Passive prophylaxis has been tried in special situations. Human gamma globulin, given by mouth to newborn premature infants, has been shown to delay onset of excretion and to decrease the severity of rotavirus disease.[23] A similar approach has been tried in children with severe combined immunodeficiency, with some success in eradicating chronic infection.[22] Milk formula manufacturers are exploring the addition to their products of high-titer antirotavirus colostrum from immunized cows, to make the formula more acceptable when breast-feeding ceases.

Enteric Adenovirus

Incidence

Adenovirus serotypes 40 and 41 are recognized as the second most common cause of viral enteritis in children. They have been reported in 7 to 17 percent of cases in North America and in the United Kingdom.[2] In Brazil 2 percent of 746 children under 5 years of age with diarrhea shed enteric adenoviruses. In black South African children the figure was 6.5 percent, compared with 13.8 percent for rotavirus. There is no clear seasonal incidence. Serologic surveys have shown that more than one-third of children in England, New Zealand, Hong Kong, and Gambia have enteric adenovirus-specific antibodies.

Virology

The finding of large numbers of adenovirus particles in stools from children involved in an outbreak of diarrhea in 1974[43] and the inability to grow them in tissue culture led eventually to recognition of two specific adenovirus serotypes, 40 and 41, which preferentially infect the gut. Much is known about the structure of adenoviruses in general.[25] Serotypes 40 and 41 can be classified as a separate subgenus on the basis of the size of certain of the virion polypeptides. Mapping of the Ad 40 and Ad 41 genomes has proceeded to the point where probes can be used to identify these two serotypes.

The enteric adenoviruses differ from all other adenoviruses in that they fail to grow in human embryo kidney cells or in most heteroploid cell lines. They can be propagated for at least one cycle of replication in tertiary monkey kidney cells. Screening for enteric adenoviruses is usually initiated by a group-specific EIA, followed by a type-specific EIA based on absorbed reagents or monoclonal antibodies.

Pathophysiology

Virus particles are excreted in large quantities (up to 10^{11} particles per gram of stool), suggesting active multiplication in the GI tract. Particles have been recovered from small intestinal fluid of infected children.[25] The virus has been seen within the nucleus of small intestinal cells in a fatal case. In pigs the villi in the lower jejunum and ileum become stunted.[44] Ten to 20 percent of enterocytes are infected and show vacuolation of the cytoplasm, nuclear enlargement, and eventually cell rupture. The lamina propria is infiltrated with inflammatory cells. Viremia may occur, but the evidence for this is not definite.

Clinical Features

After an incubation period of 7 to 8 days, children infected by Ad 40 and Ad 41 suffer a clinically moderate disease with diarrhea and vomiting, but fever or respiratory symptoms are uncommon.[2] This is in contrast to gastroenteritis that can also be caused by established (nonenteric) adenoviruses, in which high fever and respiratory symptoms are common. Symptoms are similar for Ad 40 and Ad 41 except that Ad 41 affects older children (28 months versus 15 months in one study) and is associated with more abdominal pain and a more protracted course. The illness is generally similar to, but milder than, that associated with rotavirus infection.

Treatment and Prevention

As with other viral enteritis, there is no specific treatment. Management of dehydration and nutrition is required. No vaccine has been developed. Since this agent rarely causes severe diarrhea in children, development of a vaccine has a low priority.

Norwalk and Norwalk-like Agents

Incidence

Norwalk agent affects adults more than children.[26] A cross-sectional serum survey in Washington, DC, showed that Norwalk antibody was acquired gradually, beginning slowly in childhood and accelerating in adult years so that by the fifth decade of life, 50 percent of individuals possessed antibody. Antibody was not found in any infant under 3 years of age, and the incidence reached only 19 percent by 5 years. Norwalk antibody has been found in serum from most parts of the world with the exception of a highly isolated community of Ecuadoran Indians. Children in developing countries acquire antibody earlier in life than do children in the United States.

Disease caused by this group of agents has generally been in outbreaks in schools, camps, and institutions. Contaminated water supplies, shellfish, and infected food handlers have all been implicated as sources.

Virology

These viruses share certain characteristics that permit them to be grouped together.[26] Although the nucleic acid content has yet to be conclusively determined, there is now evidence that the virions contain RNA and that the virus structure is almost entirely assembled from a single polypeptide. These are features shared with caliciviruses, and Norwalk agent may

yet be classified as one of them. The sizes of the particles are reported to be 25 to 27 nm diameter or 30 to 35 nm. They have proved difficult to visualize on electron microscopy in the absence of specific antibody, so their exact surface structure is not certain. Norwalk and Montgomery County agents are antigenically related, but Hawaii agent is distinct. Other members of the group do not cross-react with Norwalk agent but may eventually prove to be part of the same genus.

Further progress is hampered by the inability to propagate these agents in vitro. Norwalk virus has been administered to numerous animals, but only chimpanzees have become infected. These laboratory difficulties mean that little is known about cross-protection between the various members of this group of agents. Human serology has depended upon radioimmunoassay and immune adherence hemagglutination assay in the past. A recently developed EIA will provide a means for more extensive testing in outbreaks of gastroenteritis.

Pathophysiology

The pathogenesis of Norwalk and Hawaii agent–induced illness has been studied in adult volunteers.[10] Virus has been detected in stool and in vomitus but has never been identified within the epithelial cells of the GI tract. There is broadening and blunting of the villi of the proximal small intestine. Microvilli appear shortened. Mononuclear cell infiltration and cytoplasmic vacuolization have been observed. The extent of small intestinal involvement is not known, but biopsies from stomach and colon are normal. Convalescent phase small intestine biopsies are normal. Brush border enzymes are decreased, and adenylate cyclase is normal.

Clinical Features

Nausea and vomiting occur in 80 percent or more of patients in outbreaks of Norwalk infection, and in volunteers.[10] Diarrhea and fever were present in less than 50 percent of volunteers, but abdominal cramps were common in both groups. Usually, illness is mild and self-limited and lasts 24 to 48 hours. A review of clinical associations of Norwalk-like virus in children reported that diarrhea was mild, vomiting frequent, and fever rare.[45] Mild fever occurred in only 3 of 28 patients. The agent was often found in association with other viral infectious agents.

Treatment

No specific treatment is available. Attention to hydration is required, and intravenous fluids may be needed if vomiting is persistent. Significant fluid loss from diarrhea is uncommon.

Prevention

No specific measures are yet available to prevent this infection. The virus is resistant to chlorine concentrations that are effective against other viruses. Simple hygienic measures, especially hand washing, when a family member is ill, should limit spread. Nosocomial infection in hospitalized children has been reported. Vaccine development has been proposed after a study of rotavirus and Norwalk virus infection in remote Panamanian islands.[46] A high level of protection by pre-existing humoral antibody was reported during a 7-year survey period. However, adult volunteer experiments have shown that even symptomatic infection has no protective effect 2 years later.[47] Six of 12 volunteers became ill at the fist challenge and developed antibody in serum. A second challenge after 24 months given to all 12 persons resulted in illness in the same six who were symptomatic the first time. A successful vaccine is unlikely to be developed in the near future.

Cytomegalovirus

Reports of the association of cytomegalovirus (CMV) with certain disorders of the stomach, small intestine, and colon are appearing with increasing frequency. Many are of patients with AIDS or other forms of immunodeficiency. Gastric ulcers,[48] gastritis,[49] and duodenitis[50] have been described in normal adults, adults with graft-versus-host disease, and adults after renal transplantation. One interesting report of CMV in association with hypertrophic gastropathy in four previously healthy children who presented with hypoproteinemia suggests that protein-losing enteropathy may be associated with this infection.[51] A child with AIDS and gastric outlet obstruction had CMV in the pyloric mucosa.[52] Enterocolitis, ileal perforation, and pneumatosis intestinalis have occurred in immunodeficient adults, but reports of small intestinal disease in children are sparse. Several papers describe colitis associated with CMV.[53,54] Not all patients were immunodeficient. Exacerbations of inflammatory bowel disease may be precipitated. A possible link with Hirschsprung's disease has been proposed.[55] Of three infants with CMV infection of the bowel, two had infected ganglion cells, one of whom had hypoganglionosis and the other colonic dysmotility. The third infant has classic short segment Hirschsprung's disease and colitis with CMV inclusions in vascular endothelium.

Treatment is supportive, with particular attention to underlying disease or drug therapy that may predispose to this infection. Immunosuppressive therapy may need to be reduced. New antiviral agents may have a role in the future.

REFERENCES

1. Bishop RF, Davidson GP, Holmes IH, Ruck BJ. Virus particles in epithelial cells of duodenal mucosa from children with acute non-bacterial gastroenteritis. Lancet 1973; ii:1281–1283.
2. Wadell G, Allard A, Johanson M, Svensson L, Uhnoo I. Enteric adenoviruses. In: Bock G, Whelan J, eds. Novel diarrhea viruses. Ciba Foundation Symposium 128. Chichester: John Wiley, 1987: 63.
3. Adler I, Zickl R. Winter vomiting disease. J Infect Dis 1969; 119:668–673.
4. Jenkins S, Horman JT, Israel E, Cukor G, Blacklow NR. An outbreak of Norwalk-related gastroenteritis at a boys' camp. Am J Dis Child 1985; 139:787–789.
5. Spender QW, Lewis D, Price EH. Norwalk like viruses: study of an outbreak. Arch Dis Child 1986; 61:142–147.
6. Shukry S, Zaki AM, DuPont HL, Shoukry I, el Tagi M, Hamed Z. Detection of enteropathogens in fatal and potentially fatal diarrhea in Cairo, Egypt. J Clin Microbiol 1986; 24:959–962.
7. Ramia S. Transmission of viral infections by the water route: implications for developing countries. Rev Infect Dis 1985; 7:180–188.

8. Santosham M, Yolken RH, Wyatt RG, Bertrando R, Black RE, Spira WM, Sack RB. Epidemiology of rotavirus diarrhea in a prospectively monitored American Indian population. J Infect Dis 1985; 152:778–783.
9. Hodes HL. American Pediatric Society presidential address. Pediatr Res 1976; 10:201.
10. Agus SG, Dolin R, Wyatt RG, Tousimis AJ, Northrup RS. Acute infectious non-bacterial gastroenteritis: intestinal histopathology. Histologic and enzymatic alterations during illness produced by the Norwalk agent in man. Ann Intern Med 1973; 79:18–25.
11. Davidson GP, Barnes GL. Structural and functional abnormalities of the small intestine in infants and young children with rotavirus enteritis. Acta Paediatr Scand 1979; 68:181–186.
12. McClung HJ, Butler DG, Kerzner B, Gall DG, Hamilton JR. Transmissible gastroenteritis. Mucosal ion transport in acute viral enteritis. Gastroenterology 1976; 70:1091–1095.
13. Shepherd RW, Butler DG, Cutz E, Gall DG, Hamilton JR. The mucosal lesion in viral enteritis. Extent and dynamics of the epithelial response to virus invasion in transmissible gastroenteritis of piglets. Gastroenterology 1979; 76:770–777.
13a. Rhoads JM, MacLeod RJ, Hamilton JR. Diminished brush border membrane Na-dependent L-alanine transport in acute viral enteritis in piglets. J Pediatr Gastroenterol Nutr 1989; 9:225–231.
13b. Rhoads JM, MacLeod RJ, Hamilton JR. Alanine enhances jejunal Na absorption in the presence of glucose: studies in normal piglets and in viral diarrhea. Pediatr Res 1986; 20:879–883.
14. Shepherd RW, Gall DG, Butler DG, Hamilton JR. Determinants of diarrhea in viral enteritis. The role of ion transport and epithelial changes in the ileum in transmissible gastroenteritis in piglets. Gastroenterology 1979; 76:20–24.
15. Davidson GP, Gall DG, Petric M, Butler DG, Hamilton JR. Human rotavirus enteritis induced in conventional piglets. Intestinal structure and transport. J Clin Invest 1977; 60:1402–1409.
16. Offer E, Riepenhoff-Talty M, Ogra PL. Effect of malnutrition on rotavirus infection in suckling mice: kinetics of early infection. Proc Soc Exp Biol Med 1985; 178:85–90.
17. Black RE, Brown KH, Becker S. Malnutrition is a determining factor in diarrheal duration but not incidence, among young children in a longitudinal study in rural Bangladesh. Am J Clin Nutr 1984; 39:87–94.
18. Butzner JD, Butler GD, Miniats OP, Hamilton JR. Impact of chronic protein-calorie malnutrition on small intestinal repair after acute viral enteritis: a study in piglets. Pediatr Res 1985; 19:476–481.
19. Chrystie IL, Booth IW, Kidd AH, Marshall WC, Banatvala JE. Multiple fecal virus excretion in immunodeficiency. Lancet 1982; i:282.
20. Eiden J, Losonsky GA, Johnson J, Yolken RH. Rotavirus RNA variation during chronic infection of immunocompromised children. Pediatr Infect Dis 1985; 4:632–637.
21. Yolken RH, Bishop CA, Townsend TR, Bolyard EA, Bartlett J, Santos GW, Saral R. Infectious gastroenteritis in bone marrow transplant recipients. N Engl J Med 1982; 306:1009–1012.
22. Losonsky GA, Johnson JP, Winkelstein JA, Yolken RH. Oral administration of human serum immunoglobulin in immunodeficient patients with viral gastroenteritis. A pharmacokinetic and functional analysis. J Clin Invest 1985; 76:2362–2367.
23. Barnes GL, Hewson PH, McLellan JA, Doyle LW, Knoches AML, Kitchen WH, Bishop RF. A randomised trial of oral gammaglobulin in low-birth-weight infants infected with rotavirus. Lancet 1982; i:1371–1373.
24. Bishop RF. Epidemiology of diarrheal disease caused by rotavirus. In: Holmgren J, Lindberg A, Mollby R, eds. Development of vaccines and drugs against diarrhea. 11th Nobel Conference. Lund: Studentlitteratur, 1986: 158.
25. Albert MJ. Enteric adenoviruses. Brief review. Arch Virol 1986; 88:1–17.
26. Kapikian AZ, Greenberg HB, Wyatt RG, Kalica AR, Chanock RM. The Norwalk group of viruses—agents associated with epidemic viral gastroenteritis. In: Tyrell DAJ, Kapikian AZ, eds. Virus infections of the gastrointestinal tract. New York: Marcel Dekker, 1982: 147.
27. Cubitt WD. The candidate caliciviruses. In: Bock G, Whelan J, eds. Novel diarrhoea viruses. Ciba Foundation Symposium 128. Chichester: John Wiley and Sons, 1987: 126.
28. Caul EO, Egglestone SI. Coronaviruses in humans. In: Tyrell DAJ, Kapikian AZ, eds. Virus infections of the gastrointestinal tract. New York: Marcel Dekker, 1982: 179.
29. Bishop RF. Other small virus-like particles in humans. In: Tyrell DAJ, Kapikian AZ, eds. Virus infections of the gastrointestinal tract. New York: Marcel Dekker, 1982: 195.

30. Nazer H. Rice S, Walker-Smith JA. Clinical associations of stool astrovirus in childhood. J Pediatr Gastroenterol Nutr 1982; 1:555–558.
31. Woode GN. Breda and Breda-like viruses: diagnosis, pathology and epidemiology. In: Bock G, Whelan J, eds. Novel diarrhoea viruses. Ciba Foundation Symposium 128. Chichester: John Wiley, 1987: 175.
32. Bishop RF, Cameron DJS, Veenstra AA, Barnes GL. Diarrhea and rotavirus infection associated with differing regimens for postnatal care of newborn babies. J Clin Microbiol 1979; 9:525–529.
33. Flores J, Midthun K, Hoshino Y, Green K, Gorziglia M, Kapikian AZ, Chanock RM. Conservation of the fourth gene among rotaviruses recovered from asymptomatic newborn infants and its possible role in attenuation. J Virol 1986; 60:972–979.
34. Simhon A, Mata L, Vives M, Rivera L, Vargas S, Ramjirez G, Lizano L, Gatarinella G, Azofeifa J. Low endemicity and low pathogenicity of rotaviruses among rural children in Cost Rica. J Infect Dis 1985; 152:1134–1142.
35. Barrjon-Romero BL, Barreda-Gonzjalez J, Doval-Ugalde R, Zermerno-Eguia LJ, Heurta-Perna M. Asymptomatic rotavirus infections in day care centers. J Clin Microbiol 1985; 22:116–118.
36. Wang SS, Cai RF, Chen J, Li RJ, Jiang RS. Etiologic studies of the 1983 and 1984 outbreaks of epidemic diarrhoea in Guangxi. Intervirology 1985; 24:140–146.
37. Holmes IH. Basic rotavirus virology in humans. In: Tyrell DAJ, Kapikian AZ, eds. Virus Infections of the Gastrointestinal Tract. New York: Marcel Dekker, 1982: 111.
38. Tufvesson B, Polberger S, Svanberg L, Sveger T. A prospective study of rotavirus infections in neonatal and maternity wards. Acta Paediatr Scand 1986; 75:211–215.
39. Pearson GR, McNulty MS, Logan EF. Pathological changes in the small intestine of neonatal calves naturally infected with reo-like virus (rotavirus). Vet Rec 1978; 102:454–458.
40. Sarker SA, Wahed MA, Rahaman MM, Alam AN, Islam A, Jahan F. Persistent protein losing enteropathy in post measles diarrhoea. Arch Dis Child 1986; 61:739–743.
41. Uhnoo I, Olding-Stenkvist E, Kreuger A. Clinical features of acute gastroenteritis associated with rotavirus, enteric adenoviruses and bacteria. Arch Dis Child 1986; 61:732–738.
42. Kapikian AZ, Hoshino Y, Flores J, Midthun K, Glass RI, Nakagomi O, Nakagomi T, Chanock RM, Potash L, Levine MM, Dolin R, Wright PF, Belshe RE, Anderson EL, Vesikari T, Gothefors L, Wadell G, Perex-Schael I. Alternative approaches to the development of a rotavirus vaccine. In: Holmgren J, Lindberg A, Mollby R, eds. Development of vaccines and drugs against diarrhea. Lund: Studentlitteratur, 1986: 192.
43. Flewett TH, Bryden AS, Davies H. Epidemic viral enteritis in a long-stay children's ward. Lancet 1975; i:4–5.
44. Hall GA. Comparative pathology of infection by novel diarrhoea viruses. In: Bock G, Whelan J, eds. Novel diarrhoea viruses. Ciba Foundation Symposium 128. Chichester: John Wiley, 1987: 192.
45. Storr J, Rice S, Phillips AD, Price E, Walker-Smith JA. Clinical associations of Norwalk-like virus in the stools of children. J Pediatr Gastroenterol Nutr 1986; 5:576–580.
46. Ryder RW, Singh N, Reeves WC, Kapikian AZ, Greenberg HB, Sack RB. Evidence of immunity induced by naturally acquired rotavirus and Norwalk virus infection on two remote Panamanian islands. J Infect Dis 1985; 151:99–105.
47. Parrino TA, Schreiber DS, Trier JS, Kapikian AZ, Blacklow NR. Clinical immunity in acute gastroenteritis caused by the Norwalk agent. N Engl J Med 1977; 297:86–89.
48. Andrade JdeS, Bambirra EA, Lima GF, Moreira EF, De Oliveira CA. Gastric cytomegalic inclusion bodies diagnosed by histologic examination of endoscopic biopsies in patients with gastric ulcer. Am J Clin Pathol 1983; 79:493–496.
49. Hochhauser L, Thompson G, Somers S. Opportunistic gastritis in graft-versus-host disease. J Can Assoc Radiol 1983; 34:316–318.
50. Kodama T, Fukuda S, Takino T, Omori Y, Oka T. Gastroduodenal cytomegalovirus infection after renal transplantation. Endoscopy 1985; 17:157–158.
51. Marks MP, Lanza MV, Kahlstrom EJ, Mikity V, Marks SC, Kvalstad RP. Pediatric hypertrophic gastropathy. AJR 1986; 147:1031–1034.
52. Victoria MS, Nangia BS, Jinkdrak K. Cytomegalovirus pyloric obstruction in a child with acquired immunodeficiency syndrome. Pediatr Infect Dis J 1985; 4:550–552.
53. Weber JN, Thom S, Barrison I, Unwin R, Forster S, Jeffries DJ, Boylston A, Pinching AJ. Cytomegalovirus colitis and oesophageal ulceration in the context of AIDS. Gut 1987; 28:482–487.
54. Berk T, Gordon SJ, Choi HY, Cooper HS. Cytomegalovirus infection of the colon: a possible role in exacerbations of inflammatory bowel disease. Am J Gastroenterol 1985; 80:355–360.
55. Dimmick JE, Bove KE. Cytomegalovirus infection of the bowel in infancy: pathogenetic and diagnostic significance. Pediatr Pathol 1984; 2:95–102.

PART **10**

Parasitic and Fungal Infections of the Digestive Tract

Michael J. G. Farthing, B.Sc., M.D., F.R.C.P.

Parasitic infections of the gastrointestinal (GI) tract occur worldwide and have a substantial morbidity and mortality. Prevalence is highest in the economically deprived regions of the world, notably in the tropics. Infants and young children are particularly susceptible to *Giardia lamblia, Ascaris lumbricoides,* and *Trichuris trichiura*; in addition to producing GI symptoms, these parasites may impair growth and development. There has been ambivalence as to the clinical relevance of many of these common intestinal parasitic infections in children, which appear to co-exist with their host without causing significant morbidity. The development of new drugs for the control of these infections has been slower than for many other infectious diseases, to some extent because much of the pharmaceutical industry has been focused on the profitable industrialized world.

These common infections do have a major impact on child health and clearly need to be considered as one of the objectives of any diarrhea control program. Several GI parasites have become relatively common in industrialized parts of the world as foreign travel and immigration have increased.

PARASITES OF THE SMALL INTESTINE

A variety of protozoa and helminths may infect the small intestine (Table 1); some can simultaneously colonize the large intestine as well, notably *Cryptosporidium* sp. and *Strongyloides stercoralis*, the latter as part of the hyperinfection syndrome.

Protozoa

Giardia lamblia

This flagellate protozoan exists as a motile trophozoite and as a chitin-walled cyst, the latter being the infective form of the parasite. The trophozoite has a smooth dorsal surface and a convex ventral surface occupied by the ventral disk (Fig. 1). This disk consists of contractile proteins that are thought to mediate attachment of the parasite to the intestinal epithelium. There is substantial heterogeneity among *Giardia* isolates as judged by isoenzyme and restriction fragment length polymorphism analysis.[1,2]

Epidemiology. *Giardia* is found in most countries of the world, prevalence being highest in the developing world, where rates can approach 30 percent, particularly in young children. Age-specific prevalence rates increase throughout infancy and childhood but fall toward adult levels during adolescence.[1] *Giardia* is transmitted by food and water and by direct person-to-person spread. Although it is unproven, there is compelling evidence to suggest that giardiasis is a zoonosis,[3] both wild and domestic animals acting as potential reservoirs of infection.

The mechanism by which *Giardia* causes diarrhea and malabsorption has not been determined.[2] Jejunal morphology may be normal, although partial and even total villous atrophy has been reported.[4,5] The presence of a mucosal in-

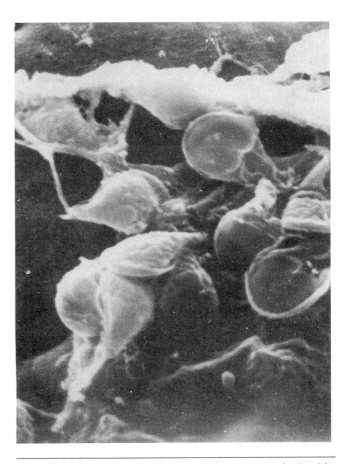

FIGURE 1 Scanning electron micrograph of *Giardia lamblia* trophozoites in mucus on human jejunal mucosa.

flammatory response, with an early increase in intraepithelial lymphocytes,[6,7] suggests that mucosal damage may be immunologically mediated. Interestingly, T-cell deficient nude mice fail to develop significant alterations in villous architecture during experimental infection, supporting the view that activated T cells may be responsible for the mucosal abnormality. Steatorrhea, however, can occur in the absence of significant histopathologic abnormality, suggesting that other factors such as bacterial overgrowth, bile salt uptake by *Giardia*, and inhibition of pancreatic lipase may be additional factors.[2]

Clinical Aspects. Adults and older children commonly carry *Giardia* without symptoms, but infection early in life is usually symptomatic. Acute infection often begins with watery diarrhea that persists and is associated with anorexia and abdominal distention. Untreated chronic diarrhea with steatorrhea ensues, and growth may be impaired.[8] Chronic giardiasis is associated with immunoglobulin deficiency,[9] which may be accompanied by diffuse nodular lymphoid hyperplasia involving the small and sometimes also the large intestine.[10]

Diagnosis. Identification of *Giardia* forms by microscopy of feces, duodenal fluid, or mucosal biopsy remains the gold standard for diagnosis. However, even after examination of multiple stool specimens, only 80 percent of positive individuals will be detected. A variety of approaches has been used

TABLE 1
Parasites of the Small Intestine

Protozoa
  *Giardia lamblia**
  Cryptosporidium sp.*
  *Isospora belli**
  Sarcocystis sp.*

Nematodes
  *Strongyloides stercoralis**
  *Capillaria philippinensis**
  *Trichinella spiralis**
  *Trichostrongylus orientalis**
  Ascaris lumbricoides
  Ankylostoma duodenale
  Necator americanus

Cestodes
  Taenia saginata
  Taenia solium
  Hymenolepis nana

Trematodes
  Fasciolopsis buski
  Heterophyes heterophyes
  Metagonimus yokogawai

* Parasites that can cause diarrhea and malabsorption.

to detect *Giardia* antigent in feces, and an ELISA has now been made commercially available. Measurement of specific anti-*Giardia* IgG antibody has not been helpful, but there is an early IgM response in acute giardiasis which can distinguish current from past infection.[11,12]

Treatment. The drugs of choice are nitroimidazole derivatives, namely metronidazole (30 mg per kilogram as a single dose on 3 consecutive days) or tinidizole (30 mg per kilogram as a single dose). Alternatives include mepacrine (2 mg per kilogram three times daily for 7 days) and furazolidone (1.25 mg per kilogram four times daily for 7 days). Adverse effects with nitroimidazole derivatives include anorexia, nausea, vomiting, and peripheral neuropathy. In addition to GI side effects, mepacrine causes yellowing of the skin and sclerae and blood dyscrasias.

Cryptosporidium Species

This is a coccidian parasite that takes up an intracellular but extracytosplasmic location in the host intestinal epithelial cell. Although recognized by veterinarians as an important cause of diarrhea in animals, the first human infection with *Cryptosporidium* was discovered in a 3-year-old immunocompetent child in 1976.[13] Subsequently, the majority of cases reported have occurred in immunocompromised individuals, particularly those with human immunodeficiency virus (HIV) infection.[14] The parasite can be found in the small and large intestines and reproduces both sexually and asexually. The ability to complete its life cycle within the human host is probably a major factor in persistent infection.[15,16]

Epidemiology. *Cryptosporidium* sp. is found throughout the developed and developing world, with prevalence rates of 10 percent or more in the latter. As with *Giardia*, asymptomatic carriage is well recognized. Infection is spread by water and by direct person-to-person transmission.[16] The mechanism by which this parasite produces acute watery diarrhea is unknown, although a variety of morphologic abnormalities have been described including disruption of the microvillous membrane (Fig. 2) and a spectrum of morphologic abnormalities from partial to subtotal villous atrophy. Specific virulence factors have not been identified.

Clinical Features. Acute infection in an immunocompetent individual usually has an incubation period of 1 to 7 days, followed by fever, abdominal discomfort, nausea, vomiting, and high-volume watery diarrhea. The illness may resolve within 2 days or continue for 2 to 3 weeks.[15] Dehydration occurs in children, and the illness tends to be more severe in the malnourished. Isaccs et al found that 7 of 213 children (3.2 percent) with chronic diarrhea in the United Kingdom had cryptosporidiosis.[17] Two had had symptoms for more than 4 months, with failure to thrive. Asymptomatic carriage is reported in children, particularly those in the developing world. Symptoms tend to be more severe and prolonged in the immunocompromised host and may contribute to the terminal illness of patients with AIDS.

Diagnosis. Oocysts can be detected in feces, duodenal fluid, and occasionally in sputum using a variety of stains, including trichrome, modified acid-fast stain, and auramine.[18] Cyst concentration techniques may be required. Serum antibody responses (IgG, IgM, and IgA) occur in cryptosporidiosis and may be useful in diagnosis.[19]

Treatment. Macrolide antibiotics such as erythromycin, spiramycin, and clindamycin fail to eradicate the parasite but do appear to reduce parasite numbers and, transiently, stool volume.[20] In patients with HIV infection, azidothymidine has been reported to reduce stool volume and eradicate the parasite.[21] Hyperimmune bovine colostrum has recently induced a remission in a 3-year-old child with hypogammaglobulinemia and cryptosporidiosis.[22] Treatment is otherwise supportive with oral glucose electrolyte solutions for dehydration, although in immunocompromised individuals parenteral fluids and total parenteral nutrition may be required.

Isospora belli and Sarcocystis Species

These intracellular coccidian parasites are rare in immunocompetent individuals but have been recognized in increasing numbers of patients with HIV infection and AIDS. Oocysts are ingested in contaminated food, namely undercooked beef and pork. Like *Cryptosporidium* sp., these parasites produce varying degrees of partial villous atrophy and an associated inflammatory response in the mucosa consisting of lymphocytes, plasma cells, and eosinophils.[23-25]

Although these parasites are carried without symptoms, children can develop profuse watery diarrhea and go on to a chronic malabsorptive state with steatorrhea and weight loss. Diagnosis is by the detection of oocysts in feces, duodenal

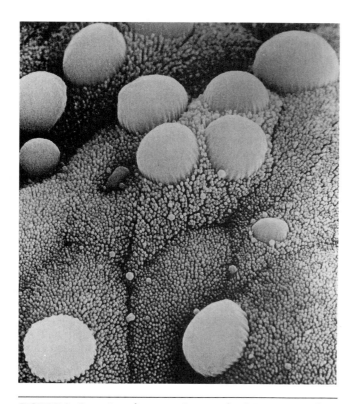

FIGURE 2 Scanning electron micrograph of *Cryptosporidium* sp. (Courtesy of Patricia Bland and David Burden, ARFC, Institute for Animal Disease Research, Compton.)

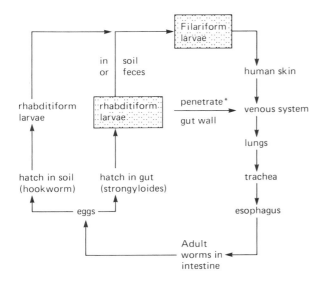

Life cycle of hookworm and *Strongyloides stercoralis*

* Only occurs extensively in hyperinfection syndrome

▨ Infective form of parasite

FIGURE 3 Life cycle of *Strongyloides stercoralis* and hookworm.

fluid, or jejunal mucosal biopsies.[25] Nitroimidazole derivatives, furazolidone, and trimethoprim-sulfamethoxazole are effective, but recurrence of infection is common. Treatment may need to be continued for many weeks.

Nematodes

Many helminths appear to be able to co-exist with their human host without causing a significant disturbance of intestinal function. Small intestinal nematodes may be considered as two groups—those that do and do not cause diarrhea (Table 1).

Strongyloides stercoralis

Adult worms live predominantly in the duodenum and jejunum, although occasionally there is extensive involvement of the whole gut. The life cycle is summarized in Figure 3. *S. stercoralis* is found in the tropics and subtropics and also in Eastern Europe, Italy, Australia, and the southern United States. An important group of individuals still carrying this parasite are ex-servicemen who served in Southeast Asia, particularly those on the Thai-Burma railroad.[26,27] Adult worms invade the intestinal mucosa (Fig. 4)) and produce an inflammatory response involving mononuclear cells and eosinophils. In addition, there may be varying degrees of partial villous atrophy.

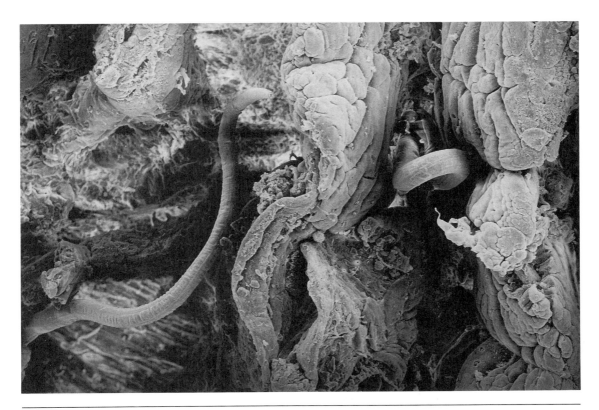

FIGURE 4 Scanning electron micrograph of *Strongyloides* adult worms invading intestinal mucosa. (Courtesy of Tim McHugh.)

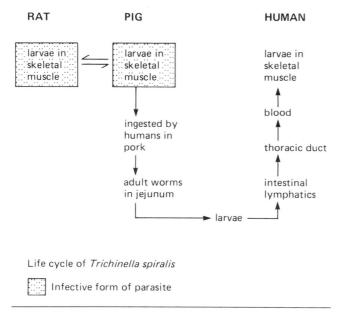

Life cycle of *Trichinella spiralis*

▦ Infective form of parasite

FIGURE 5 Life cycle of *Trichinella spiralis*.

Clinical Features. Penetration of the skin by filariform larvae often produces a local reaction, followed 1 week later by respiratory symptoms, including cough, wheeze, and transient pulmonary infiltrates as adolescent worms migrate through the airways. Diarrhea may follow 2 weeks later as the parasite colonizes the small intestine. Abdominal symptoms may pass unnoticed, but children may develop a "celiac-like" syndrome. Occasionally, severe infection is associated with protein-losing enteropathy[28,29] and intestinal obstruction.[30]

Autoinfection can occur in the same individual by invasion of either the colon or the perianal area, which results in a form of cutaneous larva migrans known as larva currens.

Diagnosis. Larvae or adult females can be detected in feces, duodenal fluid, sputum, or jejunal biopsies. Multiple stool specimens may need to be examined to find larvae, but negative stool examination does not exclude infection.[27] Serology is usually positive in up to 80 percent of patients.

Treatment. Thiabendazole, 25 mg per kilogram twice daily for 2 to 3 days, will eradicate the parasite from at least 80 percent of patients. Side effects are common and include nausea, dizziness, weakness, anorexia, vomiting, and headaches. Longer courses of therapy may be used in treatment failures, and alternative drugs include mebendazole, flubendazole, and albendazole.

Capillaria philippinensis

An important infection in Southeast Asia, particularly the Philippines and Thailand, this parasite causes severe diarrhea and malabsorption. Infection generally follows the ingestion of raw fish. After a 1- to 2-month incubation period, nonspecific abdominal symptoms may be noted, followed by severe watery diarrhea. In some cases this progresses to intestinal malabsorption with profound weight loss. If untreated, mortality approaches 10 percent.

Parasite forms (ova, larvae, and adult worms) can be detected in stool or intestinal biopsy specimens. Infection can be eradicated by mebendazole and thiabendazole, provided that treatment is continued for 3 to 4 weeks.[31]

Trichinella spiralis

T. spiralis occurs worldwide in communities that eat pork. Unlike other nematodes, *T. spiralis* requires two hosts to complete its life cycle (Fig. 5). Initially diarrhea and abdominal pain predominate, usually occurring several days after eating contaminated pork. After 1 to 2 weeks, infected individuals experience an acute febrile illness associated with periorbital edema, an erythematous rash, and severe muscular pains which may last for up to 6 weeks. Associated complications include pneumonitis, myocarditis, and encephalitis.[32,33]

Diagnosis can be confirmed by demonstrating larvae in skeletal muscle biopsies. Often there are eosinophilia and elevation of serum CPK and SGOT. Treatment is with thiabendazole, but in patients with disseminated infection, concomitant corticosteroid therapy is recommended to minimize allergic reactions.

Trichostrongylus orientalis

Found predominantly in the Far East, this small round worm infects those who ingest contaminated food or drink. Diarrhea occurs, but usually infection is asymptomatic. Ova can be detected in duodenal fluid or feces, and treatment is with thiabendazole.

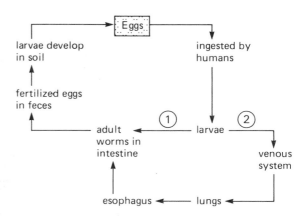

Life cycles of ① *Trichuris trichiura, Enterobius vermicularis*
② *Ascaris lumbricoides*

▦ Infective form of parasites

FIGURE 6 Life cycle of *Ascaris lumbricoides, Trichuris trichiura,* and *Enterobius vermicularis*.

Ascaris lumbricoides

Ascaris, one of the most common parasitic infections of humans, is the largest human intestinal nematode. It is found worldwide but is most evident in the developing world, where in very deprived communities prevalence may exceed 90 percent.[34] The life cycle is summarized in Figure 6.

Clinical Features. Most individuals with *Ascaris* infection are symptom-free, but during the pulmonary phase migrating larvae may produce cough with sputum, wheezing, fever, and eosinophilia. Heavy infections, particularly in children, may cause anorexia and abdominal cramps: some evidence suggests that the parasite may impair growth and development. Large worm burdens can produce intestinal obstruction, particularly in children. Worms may migrate into a variety of locations, including the pancreatic and biliary system, causing duct obstruction with jaundice and pancreatitis, obstruction of the appendix and appendicitis, volvulus, intussusception, intestinal perforation, and peritonitis.[34]

Diagnosis. Ova and adult worms may be detected in feces and larvae in sputum or gastric washings.

Treatment. Mebendazole, albendazole, and flubendazole are all effective. Other drugs including piperazine citrate, levamisole, and pyrantel pamoate may also be used. Intestinal obstruction from nematode infestation may require operative treatment, but anthelminthic drugs combined with intestinal suction and intravenous fluids often are tried first. Bile and pancreatic duct obstructions can be relieved endoscopically.

Ankylostoma duodenale and Necator americanus

A. duodenale (old world hookworm) is found in Africa, Asia, Australia, and parts of Southern Europe, whereas *N. americanus* predominates in Central and South America, together with some locations in Southeast Asia, the Pacific, and Nigeria. Morphologically the parasites are similar, with identical life cycles (see Fig. 3). Adult worms attach firmly to the small intestinal mucosa by a buccal capsule consisting of tooth or plate-like cutting organs. It is estimated that more than 500 million persons in the world are infected with these parasites.

Clinical Features. Filariform larvae penetrate the skin where a local inflammatory reaction may develop (ground itch). Pulmonary symptoms are less dramatic than those of *Ascaris*, but upper abdominal discomfort, mild diarrhea, and associated eosinophilia usually ensue. The dominant clinical response to infection is iron deficiency anemia, which is proportional to the worm load and to the amount of iron taken in the diet. Occasionally, heavy infection can result in protein-losing enteropathy and hypoproteinemia.

Diagnosis. Ova and rhabditiform larvae can be detected in stool and duodenal fluid.

Treatment. Mebendazole is effective against both species of the hookworm, but other drugs are also active, including albendazole, flubendazole, pyrantel embonate, and levamisole. Oral iron supplements should be given to treat iron deficiency anemia.

Cestodes (Tapeworms)

Four tapeworms are common human pathogens, namely *Taenia saginata, Taenia solium, Diphyllobothrium latum*, and *Hymenolepis nana*. These flatworms are similar structurally; their heads have suckers and in *T. solium*, there are hooks also. The head is joined by a short, slender neck to several segments called proglottids, which form the body of the worm. Nutrients are absorbed directly through the cuticle, as they do not possess an intestinal tract. These worms are hermaphrodites, with cross-fertilization occurring between proglottids. Adult worms reside in the intestinal tract, whereas larvae exist in tissues, particularly muscle; infection is transmitted to humans by the eating of infected tissues (Fig. 7).

Taenia saginata (Beef Tapeworm)

Most patients are symptom-free, although mild, vague abdominal discomfort and occasional diarrhea may occur. Occasionally adult worms obstruct the appendix or pancreatic duct, causing appendicitis and pancreatitis, respectively. Generally infection is apparent to the host only when proglottids are identified in the feces. Praziquantel, 10 mg per kilogram as a single dose, is the treatment of choice, although niclosamide, 2 g as a single chewed dose, is also effective. Infection can be avoided by thorough examination of beef for encysted larvae known as cysticerci, although freezing at −10°C for 5 days or cooking at 57°C for several minutes destroys them.

Taenia solium (Pork Tapeworm)

Clinical features and treatment of the adult worm infection are similar to those of *T. saginata*. However, a serious complication of *T. solium* occurs when infection with larvae results in their dissemination to many sites, including skeletal muscle, brain, subcutaneous tissue, the eye, and myocardi-

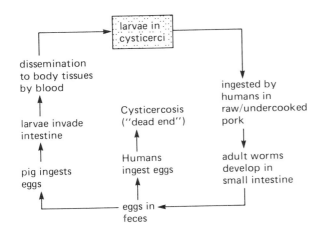

Life cycle of *Taenia solium*

☐ Infective form of the parasite

FIGURE 7 Life cycle of *Taenia solium* (pork tapeworm).

um, a condition known as cysticercosis. The cysts remain alive for many years but eventually produce a local inflammatory reaction and calcify. Cerebral involvement may present as epilepsy, as a space-occupying lesion, or as focal neurologic deficits. Ocular involvement produces retinitis, uveitis, conjunctivitis, or choroidal atrophy. Diagnosis can be established by biopsy of skin nodules, although calcified cysticerci usually can be detected radiographically. Encouraging results have been obtained with praziquantel in the treatment of cysticercosis. Surgery or photocoagulation may be required for retinal lesions.

Diphyllobothrium latum (Fish Tapeworm)

This tapeworm is found mainly in Scandinavia, the Baltic, Japan, and the Swiss lakes. Infection in humans occurs by eating raw or undercooked fish containing the infective plerocercoid form of the parasite. Infection is usually asymptomatic, although abdominal discomfort, vomiting, weight loss, and occasionally intestinal obstruction can occur. *D. latum* can cleave the vitamin B_{12}–intrinsic factor complex and consume 80 to 100 percent of dietary vitamin B_{12}. Megaloblastic anemia due to vitamin B_{12} deficiency is relatively uncommon although well recognized in Finland. Diagnosis and treatment are as for other tapeworms.

Hymenolepis nana (Dwarf Tapeworm)

This worm more frequently infects children than adults but has other natural hosts in rats and mice. Infection generally produces no symptoms, although very heavy infection may result in diarrhea and abdominal pain. Treatment is with praziquantel or niclosamide.

Trematodes

A large number of flukes infect the biliary and intestinal tract of humans, producing a broad spectrum of disease. *Fasciolopsis buski*, the largest human fluke (up to 7 cm in length), is found most often in the Far East.[35] It attaches to the proximal small intestine, causing ulceration, bleeding and occasionally abscesses. Although asymptomatic infection occurs,

heavy parasite burdens in undernourished children result in intermittent diarrhea, abdominal pain, and protein-losing enteropathy with hypoalbuminemia, edema, and ascites; progressive weight loss and even ileus may develop. Praziquantel is now the treatment of choice, although hexylresorcinol and tetrachloroethylene were used previously.

Heterophyes heterophyes and *Metagonimus yokogawai* are very small flukes found in the Far East. Natural hosts include dogs, cats, foxes, humans, and other fish-eating mammals. Infection may be asymptomatic, but heavy infections produce intermittent diarrhea and abdominal discomfort. Ova can be detected in feces, and treatment is the same as for *F. buski*.

PARASITES OF THE COLON AND RECTUM

Protozoa

Entamoeba histolytica and the ciliate, *Balantidium coli*, are the important protozoal pathogens of the large intestine (Table 2). However, it is now clear that *Cryptosporidium* sp. can infect the entire small and large intestine, and indeed the first case of human infection was diagnosed by rectal biopsy. *Giardia lamblia* is predominantly a small intestinal pathogen, but isolated reports in both humans and animals suggest that this parasite may occasionally cause colitis.

Entamoeba histolytica

This organism is found worldwide, but its prevalence is highest in developing countries. Up to 500 million individuals worldwide carry the parasite, with an annual mortality of approximately 75,000.[36] Amebiasis is relatively uncommon in infancy and childhood,[37] but when infection occurs morbidity and mortality tend to be high.

The parasite exists in two forms, the motile trophozoite and the cyst. In the infective form of *E. histolytica*, the cyst can exist for long periods outside the human host.[38] Cysts are spread in food and water and also by person-to-person contact.

Virulence varies between strains of *E. histolytica*, which can be distinguished by isoenzyme electrophoresis.[39] This finding may explain some of the clinical diversity of *E. histolytica* infection, which varies from asymptomatic carriage to severe invasive disease. The capacity of invasive parasites to kill colonic epithelial cells on contact appears to depend on cytotoxic proteins, including proteolytic and hydrolytic enzymes.[40]

Clinical Features. The term *amebiasis* covers a wide range of clinical syndromes from asymptomatic infection to amebic colitis and extraintestinal amebiasis, usually hepatic abscess. Most infected individuals throughout the world (80 to 90 percent) are asymptomatic carriers. Acute amebic dysentery produces symptoms similar to those of bacterial dysentery; in its most severe form it may progress to colonic dilatation and severe toxemia. This progression is particularly likely to occur in pregnancy, in the puerperium, and in malnourished infants and young children.[41] Chronic amebic colitis begins more insidiously, with cyclic remissions during which bowel function may return to normal or even to constipation. The pattern may mimic nonspecific inflam-

TABLE 2
Parasites of the Colon and Rectum

Protozoa
Entamoeba histolytica
Balantidium coli
Cryptosporidium sp.
Trypanosoma cruzi
Nematodes
Trichuris trichiura
Enterobius vermicularis
Anisakis
Oesophagostomum sp.
Angiostrongylus costaricensis
Trematodes
Schistosoma sp.

TABLE 3
Treatment of Amebiasis in Children

Intestinal amebiasis
    Metronidazole,
        50 mg/kg daily for 10 days,
        followed by diloxanide furoate,
        20 mg/kg daily for 10 days

Amebic liver abscess
    Metronidazole,
        50 mg/kg daily for 10 days

Asymptomatic cyst passer
    Diloxanide furoate,
        20 mg/kg daily for 10 days
        ± metronidazole

---

matory bowel disease such as Crohn's disease.[42] Constitutional upset is mild to moderate, although complications such as colonic stricture and fibrotic masses of granulation tissue known as an ameboma may occur.[43]

An amebic liver abscess can develop within days, months, or even years after the onset of amebic colitis, but in up to 50 percent of cases, there is no clear antecedent history of colonic involvement.[44] Nonspecific symptoms such as low-grade fever and weight loss may begin insidiously, or there may be an acute fulminant illness with localized hepatic pain or evidence of direct extension into pleural or pericardial cavities. Distant spread to lung, brain, and kidney occurs when the abscess ruptures into a hepatic vein.

Diagnosis. Demonstration of *E. histolytica* trophozoites and cysts in feces remains the mainstay of diagnosis. Examination of a fresh saline wet mount should reveal motile trophozoites containing ingested red blood cells. Nonpathogenic intestinal amebae are not erythrophagic. Trophozoites may be seen in rectal mucosal biopsy specimens or in slough from rectal ulcers. It is unusual to see trophozoites in pus from a liver abscess. Serology for IgG antibodies is positive in 70 to 80 percent of patients with amebic colitis and approaches 100 percent with amebic liver abscess.[45] The treatment of amebiasis in children is summarized in Table 3.

Balantidium coli

This trematode is the only ciliate that produces clinically significant infection in humans; it is restricted largely to communities in close proximity to pigs, the preferred host.[46-48] It occurs mainly in Papua New Guinea, the Philippines, and Central and South America. The cyst is the infective form, although the trophozoite can survive outside the human host for a week or more in moist conditions. Clinically, *B. coli* infection closely resembles amebiasis, and diagnosis is made by identification of the large motile trophozoite in feces. Cysts are seen relatively rarely. Tetracycline, 500 mg, four times daily for 10 days, is the usual treatment, but the parasite is also sensitive to ampicillin and metronidazole.

Trypanosoma cruzi (South American Trypanosomiasis, Chagas' Disease)

T. cruzi, a hemoflagellate, does not directly affect the GI tract. The primary infection generally occurs in early childhood, the parasite being transmitted through the bite of a blood-sucking vector insect of the Reduviidae. During the blood meal the infected form of the parasite is deposited with the insect's feces on the skin and rubbed into the bite wound or a mucous membrane susceptible to invasion such as the conjunctiva. The vast majority of initial illnesses pass unnoticed but in some cases there is marked fever, lymphadenopathy, and hepatosplenomegaly, and in severe infection there may be signs and symptoms of acute myocarditis. Death can occur as a result of this acute illness, but the individual may recover within a few weeks or months. The development of the "mega syndromes" occurs many years later, with more than 90 percent of symptomatic patients being 20 years of age or more. In Brazil, achalasia and megaesophagus occur in approximately 6 percent of seropositive patients, whereas megacolon appears to be less common, affecting only 1 percent. In Argentina and Chile, however, megacolon is more common than megaesophagus.

A medical approach to the management of these conditions is tried initially, but ultimately surgery is required.

Nematodes

The most common nematodes to infect the colon and rectum are *Trichuris trichiura* (whipworm) and *Enterobius vermicularis* (threadworm). In the hyperinfection syndrome *S. stercoralis* also colonizes the large intestine, producing ulceration and inflammatory changes after invasion and autoinfection.

Trichuris trichiura

This parasite is found worldwide, with a high prevalence in the developing world. In some particularly deprived communities, prevalence may be as high as 90 percent.[49-51] Infection is transmitted by ingestion of ova following maturation outside the host for several weeks (see Fig. 6). Colonization involves the distal ileum and cecum, although the entire colon may be involved.

Clinical Features. Light infections are often asymptomatic, but when larger numbers of parasites are present (greater than 20,000 ova per gram of feces), diarrhea with blood and mucus is characteristic.[52] Other symptoms include abdominal pain, anorexia, weight loss, tenesmus, and rectal prolapse. There is evidence to suggest that within endemic areas, some children are more susceptible than others to whipworm infection. There is now persuasive evidence to suggest that chronic heavy infection is an important contributor to impairment of the young patients' growth and development.[50,53]

Diagnosis. Typical barrel-shaped eggs can be detected in feces, and adult worms can be seen endoscopically attached to the colonic mucosa, often with ulceration and inflammatory changes.

Treatment. Mebendazole is now the treatment of choice, although it should not be used in children under the age of 2 years. Multiple courses may be necessary to clear infection.

Enterobius vermicularis

This parasite is found worldwide, although it is more prevalent in temperate and cold climates. Children are most often infected, but infection can spread rapidly between family

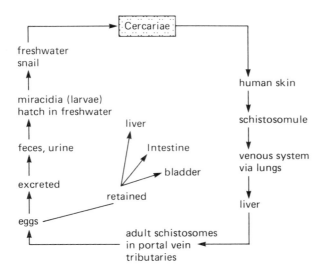

Life cycle of *Schistosoma sp.*

☐ Infective form of the parasite

FIGURE 8 Life cycle of *Schistosoma* sp.

members, those in residential institutions, and any group living in overcrowded circumstances. Infection is spread by direct transmission of ova from person to person or indirectly on clothing or house dust. The life cycle is summarized in Figure 6. Anal pruritus is usually the only symptom, occurring mainly at night when adult females lay their eggs in the perianal region. Symptoms of appendicitis may result from worms entering the lumen of the appendix; very occasionally adult worms migrate through the intestinal wall and are found in the genital tract, peritoneum, omentum, lung, urinary tract, liver, spleen, or kidney.[54-56]

Diagnosis. Ova can be detected in the perianal region by applying clear adhesive tape to the perianal skin and examining this microscopically. Ova may also be found under fingernails.

Treatment. Mebendazole is the drug of choice, although pyrantel pamoate and piperazine are also effective. It is wise to treat the entire family.

Other Nematodes

Anisakis, transmitted to humans by eating uncooked fish, is found in Japan, Holland, Scandinavia, and the Pacific coast of South America. Larvae attach to the gastric or intestinal mucosa, causing ulceration and occasionally perforation.[57-59] *Oesophagostomum* sp. infects mainly ruminants, primates, and pigs but occasionally causes human infection. The worm often penetrates the intestinal wall, resulting in multiple nodules along the intestine, some of which develop into paracolic abscesses requiring surgical drainage.

Angiostrongylus costaricensis was first described in Costa Rican children who suffered quite severe pain in the right iliac fossa, fever, and anorexia. An inflammatory mass involving cecum, appendix, and terminal ileum is characteris-

tic.[60] Inflammatory reaction is a result of intramural eggs that have been discharged from adult worms living in terminal mesenteric arterioles.

Trematodes

Schistosoma Species

Epidemiology. Schistosomiasis is one of the most important parasitic infections worldwide, with a high morbidity and mortality. More than 200 million individuals are infected with this parasite. Five species are known to cause intestinal disease in humans: *S. mansoni* (Africa, Central and South America, the Carribean, and the Middle East), *S. japonicum* (Japan, the Philippines, southeast China, and Taiwan), *S. haematobium* (Africa), *S. mekongi* (Southeast Asia), and *S. intercalatum* (Zaire and Gabon). Human infection is totally dependent on the intermediate host, the freshwater snail. The life cycle is summarized in Figure 8.

Clinical Features. Invasion of the skin by cercariae produces a local inflammatory response known as "swimmers' itch." Within a week there may be a generalized allergic response, with fever, urticaria, myalgia, general malaise, and associated eosinophilia. The acute phase of *S. japonicum* infection is known as Katayama fever. Hepatosplenomegaly also occurs in the early stages and in children is more marked in those with heavy parasite loads.[61] Intestinal symptoms of diarrhea, blood, and mucus can occur immediately but may be delayed for months or even years. Extensive colonic ulceration and polyp formation are characteristic of *S. mansoni* infections.[62] In severe cases there may be marked iron and protein loss. Stricture formation and intestinal obstruction are characteristic, as are localized granulomatous masses within the gut wall, known as bilharziomas.

S. japonicum can involve both small and large intestine and may be more severe than that due to *S. mansoni*. *S. japonicum* colitis, like extensive, longstanding ulcerative colitis, has premalignant potential.[63] *S. haematobium* produces rectal inflammation and bladder involvement. The inflammatory changes in the intestine in schistosomiasis are due entirely to an intense immune response to eggs deposited in the intestinal wall.

Diagnosis. Characteristic ova of each species can be detected in feces or in intestinal biopsies. Specific antibodies can be detected by ELISA in more than 95 percent of patients during the first few weeks of infection.

Treatment. Praziquantel given as a single dose (40 mg per kilogram for *S. mansoni*; 60 mg per kilogram in divided doses for *S. haematobium*) is probably the drug of choice. Oxamniquine is also effective.[64,65]

FUNGAL INFECTIONS

A child who is well, with intact host defense mechanisms, is not considered to be susceptible to fungal infections of the digestive tract. As immunosuppressive therapies become more aggressive and myelotoxic regimens more effective, opportunities increase for fungi to invade and establish themselves in humans. Patients disabled from chronic malnutrition and those exposed to intense antimicrobial infection are susceptible to these organisms too. Of course, the advent and spread of acquired immunodeficiency syndrome have produced a group of chronically immunosuppressed patients open to a wide range of organisms, including fungi. The digestive tract is not a preferred site of infection in cases of disseminated fungal infection, but certain species are capable of infecting the esophagus, the stomach, or the intestine.

A consequence of modern treatment and recently evolving patterns of disease, these opportunistic infections have been recognized only in recent years. No doubt additional GI fungal infections of significance will emerge and be recognized in the years to come.

Candidiasis

Candida species are 4- to 6-μm oval cells that reproduce by budding; there are at least 80 species, of which eight, including *C. albicans*, are of GI significance.

In disseminated candidiasis, widespread involvement of several organs occurs. The major risk factor leading to this very serious problem is neutropenia. The liver may be involved, in addition to heart, brain, kidney, lung, spleen, and eye.[66]

Esophagitis caused by *Candida* species is seen in immunosuppressed children and in those with hematologic malignancy. In such cases, oral thrush may be seen in as few as 20 percent of cases.[6] Treatment with nystatin usually is effective. Ketoconazole and fluconazole can be used, and in severe disease, particularly when oral medication cannot be taken, intravenous amphotericin B is used.

Candida is isolated from up to 15 percent of gastric ulcers, but no pathogenetic role for the organism in ulcer disease has been established.[68] *Candida* peritonitis with infection localized usually to the peritoneum is seen after bowel surgery and in patients undergoing chronic ambulatory peritoneal dialysis. *Candida* infection has been associated with acute watery diarrhea in newborn infants, although its causative role has not been clearly established in these babies.[69] *C. albicans* can invade the small and large intestine in terminally ill patients.

Aspergillosis

The mold of the genus *Aspergillus* reproduces by means of spores that germinate, resulting in hyphae, the form in which they are associated with disease. Most cases of invasive *Aspergillus* infection are seen in severely immunocompromised patients. In about 20 percent of such cases of invasive infection the small and large intestines are involved in addition to the esophagus and stomach.[70] Amphotericin B is the treatment of choice.

Zygomycosis

Zygomycetes are ubiquitous agents found in organic debris, on fruit, and in soil. They grow rapidly on any carbohydrate substrate. The terms *mucormycosis* and *phycomatosis* have been used in the past for these infections.

These agents can infect the subcutaneous and submucosal tissues in an immunocompetent host, but in the debilitated host they can cause an acute fulminant invasive infection.[71]

Intestinal zygomycosis is encountered in severely malnourished children and sometimes as a complication of severe chronic intestinal disease such as amebic colitis.[72] On occasion the infection can occur without apparent predisposition.

Coccidioidomycosis

Coccidioides is a dimorphic fungus endemic in the southwestern United States. Arthroconidia arising from mycelial growth cause infection when inhaled. Coccidioidomycosis is usually a pulmonary infection; spores can escape the chest during primary infection and with dissemination, on rare occasions, the terminal ileum and colon are involved.[73]

Acknowledgment

Dr. Farthing is a Wellcome Trust Senior Lecturer, and he gratefully acknowledges financial support by the Wellcome Trust.

REFERENCES

1. Farthing MJG, Giardiasis. In: Pounder RE, Chiodini PL, eds. Advanced Medicine 23. London: Bailliere Tindall, 1987:287.
2. Farthing MJG. Host-parasite interactions in human giardiasis. Q J Med 1989; 70:191–204.
3. Faubert GM. Evidence that giardiasis is a zoonosis. Parasitol Today 1988; 4:66–68.
4. Ament ME, Rubin CE. Relation of giardiasis to abnormal intestinal structure and function in gastrointestinal immunodeficiency syndrome. Gastroenterology 1972; 62:216–226.
5. Levinson JD, Nastro LJ. Giardiasis with total villous atrophy. Gastroenterology 1978; 74:271–275.
6. Wright SG, Tomkins AM. Quantification of the lymphocytic infiltrate in jejunal epithelium in giardiasis. Clin Exp Immunol 1977; 29:408–412.
7. Rosekrans PCM, Lindeman J, Meijer CJLM. Quantitative histological and immunohistochemical findings in jejunal biopsy specimens in giardiasis. Virchows Arch [A] 1981; 393:145–151.
8. Farthing MJG, Mata L, Urrutia JJ, Kronmal RA. Natural history of *Giardia* infection of infants and children in rural Guatemala and its impact on physical growth. Am J Clin Nutr 1986; 4:393–403.
9. Webster ADB. Giardiasis and immunodeficiency diseases. Trans R Soc Trop Med Hyg 1980; 74:440–448.
10. Webster ADB, Kenwright S, Ballard J, Shiner M, Slavin G, Levi AJ, Loewi G, Asherson GL. Nodular lymphoid hyperplasia of the bowel in primary hypogammaglobulinaemia: study of *in vivo* and *in vitro* lymphocyte function. Gut 1977; 18:364–372.
11. Farthing MJG, Goka AKJ. Immunology of giardiasis. In: Wright R, Hodgson HJ, eds. Clinical gastroenterology: immunological aspects of the gut and liver. 1987: 589–603.
12. Farthing MJG, Goka AKJ, Butcher PK, Arvind AS. Serodiagnosis of giardiasis. Serodiag Immunother 1987; 1:233–238.
13. Nime FA, Burek JD, Page DL, Holscher MA, Yardley JH. Acute enterocolitis in a human being infected with the protozoan Cryptosporidium. Gastroenterology 1976; 70:592–598.
14. Navin TR, Hardy AM. Cryptosporidiosis in patients with AIDS. J Infect Dis 1987; 55:150.
15. Tzipori S. Cryptosporidiosis in animals and humans. Microbiol Rev 1983; 47:84–96.
16. Tzipori S. Cryptosporidium: Notes on epidemiology and pathogenesis. Parasitol Today 1985; 1:159–165.

17. Isaacs D, Hunt GH, Phillips AD, Price EH, Raafat F, Walker-Smith JA. Cryptosporidiosis in immunocompetent children. J Clin Pathol 1985; 38:76–81.

18. Casemore DP, Armstrong M, Sands RL. Laboratory diagnosis of cryptosporidiosis. J Clin Pathol 1985; 38:1337–1341.

19. Casemore DP. The antibody response to Cryptosporidium: development of a serological test and its use in a study of immunologically normal persons. J Infect 1987; 14:125–134.

20. Portnoy D, Whiteside ME, Buckley E, McLeod CL. Treatment of intestinal cryptosporidiosis with spiramycin. Ann Intern Med 1984; 101:202–204.

21. Gazzard BG. HIV disease and the gastroenterologist. Gut 1988; 29:1497–1505.

22. Tzipori S, Roberton D, Chapman C. Remission of diarrhoea to cryptosporidiosis in an immunodeficient child treated with hyperimmune bovine colostrum. Br Med J 1986; 293:1276–1277.

23. Trier JS, Moxey PC, Schimmel EM, Robles E. Chronic intestinal coccidiosis in man: intestinal morphology and response to treatment. Gastroenterology 1974; 66:923–935.

24. DeHovitz JA, Pape JW, Boncy M, Johnson WD. Clinical manifestations and therapy of Isospora belli infection in patients with the acquired immunodeficiency syndrome. N Engl J Med 1986; 315:87–90.

25. Sturchler D. Parasitic diseases of the small intestinal tract. In: Gyr K, ed. Bailliere's clinical gastroenterology. London: Bailliere Tindall, 1987: 397.

26. Gill GV, Bell DR. Strongyloidiasis in ex prisoners of war in South East Asia. Br Med J 1980; 280:1319.

27. Pelletier LL, Gabre-Kidan T. Chronic strongyloidiasis in Vietnam veterans. Am J Med 1985; 78:139–140.

28. O'Brien W. Intestinal malabsorption in acute infection with Strongyloides stercoralis. Trans R Soc Trop Med Hyg 1975; 69:69–77.

29. Burke JA. Strongyloidiasis in childhood. Am J Dis Child 1978; 132:1130–1136.

30. Walker-Smith JA, McMillan B, Middleton AW, Robertson S, Hopcroft A. Strongyloidiasis causing small-bowel obstruction in an aboriginal infant. Med J Austral 1969; 2:1263–1265.

31. Cross JH, Basaca-Sevilla V. Intestinal capillariasis. In: Pawlowski ZS, ed. Clinical tropical medicine and communicable disease. London: Bailliere Tindall, 1987: 735.

32. Grove DI, Warren KS, Mahmoud AAF. Trichinosis. In: Warren KS, Mahmoud AAF, eds. Geographic medicine for the practitioner. Chicago: University of Chicago Press, 1978: 121.

33. Despommier D. Biology. In: Campbell WC, ed. Trichinella and trichinosis. New York: Plenum Press, 1983: 75.

34. Pawlowski ZS. Ascariasis. In: Pawlowski ZS, ed. Clinical tropical medicine and communicable diseases. London: Bailliere Tindall, 1987: 595.

35. Sadun EH, Maiphoom C. Studies on the epidemiology of the human intestinal fluke Fasciolopsis buski (Lankester) in Central Thailand. Am J Trop Med Hyg 1953; 2:1070–1075.

36. Guerrant RL. Amebiasis: introduction, current status and research questions. Rev Infect Dis 1986; 8:218–227.

37. Oyerinde JPO, Ogunbi O, Alonge AA. Age and sex distribution of infections with Entamoeba histolytica and Giardia intestinalis in the Lagos population. Int J Epidemiol 1977; 6:231–234.

38. Sepulveda B. Amebiasis: host-pathogen biology. Rev Infect Dis 1982; 4:836–842.

39. Sargeaunt PG, Williams JE. Electrophoretic isoenzyme patterns of the pathogenic and non-pathogenic intestinal amoebae of man. Trans R Soc Trop Med Hyg 1979; 73:225–227.

40. Gitler C, Mogyoros M, Calef E, Rosenberg I. Lethal recognition between Entamoeba histolytica and the host tissues. Trans R Soc Trop Med Hyg 1985; 79:581–586.

41. Lewis EA, Antia AU. Amoebic colitis: review of 295 cases. Trans R Soc Trop Med Hyg 1969; 63:633–638.

42. Sanderson IR, Walker-Smith JA. Indigenous amoebiasis: an important differential diagnosis of chronic inflammatory bowel disease. Br Med J 1984; 289:823.

43. Pittman FE, Pittman JC, El-Hashimi WK. Studies of Human Amebiasis. III Ameboma: A radiologic manifestation of amebic colitis. Dig Dis 1973; 18:1025–1031.

44. Merritt RJ, Coughlin E, Thomas DW, Jariwala L, Swanson V, Sinatra FR. Spectrum of amebiasis in children. Am J Dis Child 1982; 136:785–789.

45. Arvind AS, Shetty N, Farthing MJG. Serodiagnosis of amoebiasis. Serodiag Immunotherapy 1988; 2:79–84.

46. Arean VM, Koppisch E. Balantidiasis, a review and report of cases. Am J Pathol 1956; 32:1089–1115.

47. Walzer PD, Judson FN, Murphy KB, Healy GR, English DK, Schultz MG. Balantidiasis outbreak in Truk. Am J Trop Med Hyg 1973; 22:33–41.

48. Baskerville L. Balantidium colitis. Report of a case. Am J Dig Dis 1970; 15:727–731.

49. Harland PSEG. Trichuriasis in Africa and the Caribbean. In: Walker-Smith JA, McNeish S, eds. Diarrhoea and malnutrition in childhood. London: Butterworths, 1986: 85.

50. Cooper ES, Bundy DAP. Trichuris in St. Lucia. In: Walker-Smith JA, McNeish, AS, eds. Diarrhoea and malnutrition in childhood. London: Butterworths, 1986: 91.

51. Chanco PP, Vidad JY. A review of trichuriasis, its incidence, pathogenicity and treatment. Drugs 1978; 15(Suppl 1):87–93.

52. Wong HB, Tan KH. Severe whipworm infestation in children. Sing Med J 1961; 2:34–37.

53. De Carneri I, Garofano M, Grass L. Investigation of the part played by Trichuris infections in delayed mental and physical development of children in Northern Italy. Riv Parassitol 1967; 28:103–122.

54. Chandrasoma DT, Mendis KN. Enterobius vermicularis in ectopic sites. Am J Trop Med Hyg 1977; 26:644–649.

55. Neafie RC, Connor DH, Meyers WM. Enterobiasis. In: Binford CH, Connor DH, eds. Pathology of tropical and extraordinary diseases. Vol 2. Washington, DC: Armed Forces Institute of Pathology, 1976: 457.

56. McDonald GSA, Hourihane DO'B. Ectopic Enterobius vermicularis. Gut 1972; 13:621–626.

57. Yokogawa M, Yoshimura H. Clinicopathologic studies on larval anisakiasis in Japan. Am J Trop Med Hyg 1967; 16:723–728.

58. Pinkus GS, Coolidge C, Little MD. Am J Med 1975; 59:114–120.

59. Hadidjaja P, Ilahude HD, Mahfudin H, Burhanuddin, Hutomo M. Larvae of anisakidae in marine fish of coastal waters near Jakarta, Indonesia. Am J Trop Med Hyg 1978; 27:51–54.

60. Loria-Cortes R, Lobo-Sanahuja JF. Clinical abdominal angiostrongylosis. A study of 116 children with intestinal eosinophilic granuloma caused by Angiostrongylus costaricensis. Am J Trop Med Hyg 1980; 29:538–544.

61. Strickland GT, Merritt W, El-Sahly A, Abdel-Wahab F. Clinical characteristics and response to therapy in Egyptian children heavily infected with Schistosoma mansoni. J Infect Dis 1982; 146:20–29.

62. Smith JH, Said MN, Kelada AS. Studies on schistosomal rectal and colonic polyposis. Am J Trop Med Hyg 1977; 26:80–84.

63. Chen, Chang, Chuang, Chen, Wang, Tang, Chou. Colorectal cancer and schistosomiasis. Lancet 1981; i:971–973.

64. Van den Bossche H. Chemotherapy of parasitic infections. Nature 1978; 273:626–630.

65. Pearson RD, Guerrant RL. Praziquantel: a major advance in anthelminthic therapy. Ann Intern Med 1983; 99:195–198.

66. Myerwitz RL, Pazin GJ, Allen CM. Disseminated candidiasis. Changes in incidence, underlying diseases and pathology. Am J Clin Pathol 1977; 48:29.

67. Holt H. Candida infection of the esophagus. Gut 1986; 9:227.

68. Minoli G, Terruzzi V, Ferrara A, et al. A prospective study on Candida as a gastric opportunistic germ. Digestion 1982; 25:30.

69. Kumar V, Chandrasekaran R, Kumar L. Candida diarrhea. Lancet 1976; i:752.

70. Young RC, Bennet JE, Vogel CL, et al. Aspergillosis: the spectrum of the disease in 98 patients. Medicine 1970; 49:147.

71. Rinaldi MG. Zygomycosis Infect. Dis Clin North Am 1988; 3:19.

72. Neame P, Raynor D. Mucormycosis—a report of twenty-two cases. Arch Pathol 1960; 70:261.

73. Weisman IM, Moreno AJ, Parker AL, et al. Gastrointestinal dissemination of coccidiomycosis. Am J Gastroenterol 1986; 81:589.

PART 11

Gastrointestinal Allergy

Martin Stern, M.D.

DEFINITION AND FREQUENCY

Gastrointestinal (GI) allergic reactions to food components have been reported since ancient times.[1] With the introduction of cow's milk feeding during infancy in the beginning of our century, cow's milk allergy in infants has become a major pediatric problem that has been covered extensively by recent books and reviews.[2-4] In addition, both the frequency and the public awareness of allergies to other food components have been rising. In this situation, clear-cut definitions are needed to overcome the much-cited state of "controversy and confusion" in the field of GI food allergy. Collaboration of allergologists and gastroenterologists has led to definitions that are not oversimplified, and at the same time practical[5,6]:

The term *food intolerance* designates any form of a reproducible adverse reaction to a certain food. It may be caused by different pathogenetic mechanisms.

The term *food idiosyncrasy*, although infrequently used, has been coined for intolerance reactions caused by toxic or biochemical mechanisms (such as primary lactose malabsorption, favism, or adverse reactions to salicylate, tartrazine, and sulfur dioxide).

The term *food allergy* is restricted to clinical reactions to food components that are caused by pathologic immune reactions. These reactions are observed in different organ systems—mainly the skin, the respiratory tract, and the GI tract.

Only the term *food allergy* will be further dealt with in this discussion. Immediate and delayed-onset patterns have been established clinically and pathogenetically.[6]

It is essential to keep to these definitions in order to make a rational approach possible with regard to diagnosis and therapy. Only by a well-defined approach can public anxiety about possible hazardous effects of ubiquitous food components be diminished rather than enhanced. Many "ill-defined" syndromes of alleged food allergy[7] still await confirmation and will be omitted here. There is no clear borderline between these syndromes and allergic forms of Munchausen syndrome by proxy[8] on one hand and mere food aversions on the other. Parents' perceptions of their children's complaints tend toward food intolerances, particularly in families with a higher level of education.[9]

Owing to different diagnostic criteria, data on the relative frequency of food allergy are conflicting. Reported prevalence of cow's milk allergy, for example, spans 0.3 to 7.5 percent.[2,10] If one includes atopic symptoms, the figure may even reach 30 to 47 percent.[11] In a prospective Scandinavian study using strict diagnostic criteria,[12] a prevalence of 1.9 percent was found. This figure appears to come close to the real frequency in an unselected population. Extensive epidemiologic studies, however, are still missing.

The natural history of food allergy exhibits transience in many children and persistence of symptoms throughout childhood in a minority of cases.[13-15] Thus, by the third year of life, most children are able to tolerate the food component to which an allergic reaction was first shown. This points to a dynamic view of the problem and brings maturational aspects of the GI mucosal barrier system into sight. Observations in infants, showing clinical symptoms and GI damage by cow's milk allergy decreasing in the last decade,[16] indicate that environmental factors that have been changing in the last few years obviously also play a role in the development of GI food allergy.

GASTROINTESTINAL MUCOSAL IMMUNITY

Macromolecular Absorption

The concept of a GI mucosal barrier system against penetration of foreign antigens, e.g., from microbes or food proteins, helps to clarify immunophysiologic and immunopathologic GI functions.[17] Briefly, the gut lumen contains macromolecules that are partly absorbed intact. By confrontation with a nonspecific and a specific immunologic barrier system, these molecules are "handled" and modified. Normally, oral tolerance of the absorbed antigen is induced, but in some cases, a harmful local mucosal immune reaction may lead to GI allergy.

Potential antigens can pass the enterocyte level by different routes, as animal models have shown[17,18] (Table 1). Microfold "M" cells overlying Peyer's patches are specialized for antigen uptake, thus providing a short route from the gut lumen to immunocompetent cells of the gut-associated lymphoid tissue (GALT). Enterocytes are also capable of antigen uptake via endocytosis and exocytosis, subjecting the macromolecules to lysosomal digestion. In the animal model, immaturity causes increased antigen entry through the gut.[19] This information has stimulated research into maturational aspects of macromolecular uptake and of the mucosal barrier system.

TABLE 1
Routes of Macromolecular Passage

M cells overlying Peyer's patches
Enterocytes (endocytosis/exocytosis)
Intercellular gaps

TABLE 2
Elements of the Gastrointestinal Mucosal
Barrier

A. Nonspecific
    Proteolysis (stomach, pancreas)
    Motility, secretion (gut)
    Mucus, glycocalyx (gut)
    Microvillous membrane (MVM)
    Enterocyte level: Lysosomes

B. Specific
    Gut-associated lymphoid tissue (GALT)
    Secretory immunoglobulin A (sIgA)
    Macrophages, mast cells, immunoglobulin-producing cells,
        intraepithelial lymphocytes, helper-suppressor T cells

---

In the human, macromolecular absorption has recently been shown by direct methods. It was found in healthy adults[20] but was increased in premature[21-23] and in malnourished[24] infants. Different food protein antigens were shown to cross the mucosal barrier to a different degree during postnatal maturation.[23] Thus, antigen molecular specificity appears to play a role in differential uptake, and findings regarding some molecules may not be applicable to others.

Nonspecific Gut Mucosal Barrier: Antigen Handling

Different mechanisms interact to form a nonspecific and a specific part of the mucosal barrier system (Table 2).[17] Nonspecific degradative mechanisms decrease the antigen load with which the gut surface is confronted. There is evidence[25] showing that in young animals intolerant to soy, more soy antigens survive intraluminal digestion than in con-

trols. This may indicate a pathophysiologic mechanism. In a recent series of experiments,[26-28] it was shown in rats that different mechanisms of antigen handling such as antigen binding, breakdown, and uptake are interrelated. Different cow's milk proteins were handled in a different way, in that some proteins (bovine serum albumin, BSA) were left almost intact, whereas others (beta-lactoglobulin, beta-LG) were completely degraded very rapidly. There was less degradation in very young rats.[27] Immaturity in experimental animals led to increased binding of cow's milk antigens to microvillous membranes.[28] As a consequence of these findings, immature experimental animals are confronted with more intact food antigen that is bound to the enterocyte surface. Biophysical investigations of the microvillous membrane structure[29] and biochemical investigations of the intestinal mucous composition[30] have shown maturational differences during early postnatal development that may well contribute to the functional changes in antigen handling.

From an immunologic viewpoint, food protein antigen handling may lead to different results: complete degradation destroying all immunogenic epitopes or incomplete degradation that either renders the molecules less immunogenic or uncovers new antigenic sites of the original molecule.[31-33] Alternatively, incomplete degradation may generate new tolerogenic moieties.[34,35] The specificity of the resulting reaction thus is determined on the molecular level of the antigen and on the reaction level of the individual confronted with this antigen.

Specific Gut Mucosal Barrier: Local Secretory Immune Response (Fig. 1)

The elements of GALT (Table 2) are capable of mounting a local immune response separate from the systemic immune system, triggered by different stimuli such as macromolecules

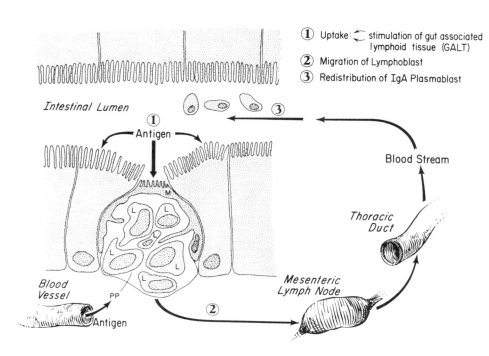

① Uptake: ⊂ stimulation of gut associated lymphoid tissue (GALT)
② Migration of Lymphoblast
③ Redistribution of IgA Plasmablast

Intestinal Lumen

Blood Vessel

FIGURE 1 IgA plasma cell cycle. Schematic representation of the cell cycle for IgA-producing plasma cells populating the intestinal mucosa. Lymphocytes (L) within gut-associated lymphoid tissues (GALT), primarily Peyer's patches (PP) of the ileum, are stimulated by antigens entering from the intestinal lumen (1) via specialized epithelium (M cells), across conventional absorptive cells, or from the systemic circulation. Lymphoblasts migrate to mesenteric nodes for further maturation (2) and then enter the systemic circulation as plasmablasts to redistribute along intestinal mucosal surfaces (3) and produce secretory IgA antibodies in response to intestinally absorbed antigens. Symbols in figure: (1) uptake of luminal and systemic antigen by gut-associated lymphoid tissue (GALT); (2) migration of lymphoblast; and (3) redistribution of IgA plasmablast to submucosal sites. (From Stern and Walker.[3])

from food. This local immune response involves the formation and secretion of secretory immunoglobulin A (sIgA) to the mucosal surface.[36-38] Immune exclusion and immune elimination of possibly harmful foreign substances from the gut lumen are accomplished by this response. Antibody-dependent mucous secretion[17,30] shows a linkage of non-specific and specific elements of the GI barrier. The local immune response is subject to complex regulation on the cellular level, the result of this response being either formation of secretory antibodies to the antigen ingested or cell-mediated immunity or tolerance[39-41] to the respective antigen. Oral tolerance depends on different regulatory factors, such as age at first antigen presentation, and on molecular specificity of the ingested substance (see above). Tolerance is an example of a mature local immune response, opposed to priming, which takes place in immature individuals.[39]

Postnatal maturation affects the local immune response considerably. In the first few weeks of life, human infants are not capable of an adequate mature response, since different elements of the specific mucosal barrier are not fully developed at birth.[37,42] Postnatal encounter with microbes and food proteins triggers development of local immunity, particularly the sIgA response, in humans. In premature infants, antibody production to food proteins was not observed before the thirty-fifth week of gestational age.[43] GI mucosal immunity basically is a physiologic phenomenon. Several factors, e.g., disturbances of the nonspecific or the specific part of the GI barrier system or defects in maturation and immune regulation, may interact to produce a local immune response that is harmful, resulting in GI allergy.

NATURE OF FOOD ANTIGENS (Table 3)

Cow's Milk Proteins

Cow's milk proteins are the predominant first foreign proteins given to young infants in most developed countries. Presumably this is the reason why allergy to cow's milk proteins is by far the most frequent food allergy in infancy. In later age groups, many other allergens, such as peanuts or hen's egg white, are becoming more important. When single cow's milk proteins are compared as to their clinical significance in eliciting an allergic response,[44] the major whey protein, beta-lactoglobulin (LG), a dimeric protein with a molecular weight of 36,000, ranges first. Casein, which is in fact a mixture of similar protein molecules with a molecular weight around 24,000, comes next. In addition to antigenic function, some caseins contain peptides with an opioid effect on the small intestine (e.g., beta-casomorphins). All the other cow's milk proteins (more than 25 are known) can act as allergens, too. In most cases of cow's milk allergy, more than one allergen is involved. Secondary reactions to primarily uninvolved food antigens ("bystander antigens") also occur.

Not many food allergens have been identified as exactly as the proteins of cow's milk, except for the major codfish antigen, which could be obtained in crystalline pure form.[45] As few as 16 amino acids appear to be sufficient in the codfish model to obtain allergenicity. Beyond the fact that most food allergens are proteins, molecular biochemical understanding of allergen composition and specificity is still very

TABLE 3
Food Antigens

A. Cow's Milk Proteins
Caseins
Whey proteins: beta-lactoglobulin, alpha-lactalbumin, bovine serum albumin, bovine immunoglobulins

B. Soy Proteins
2S-globulin, soy trypsin inhibitor, soy lectin

C. Others
Hen's egg white, ovalbumin
Fish, crustaceans, shrimp
Beef, pork
Peanuts and other legumes, beans, peas
Nuts and seeds, cocoa, chocolate
Citrus fruits, apple, strawberries
Wheat and other cereals
Spices, yeast
"Hidden ingredients" (mostly nonprotein)

---

incomplete.[46] Much remains to be learned about antibody-binding specificity (IgG, IgE) of food antigen epitopes and about the molecular mechanisms of triggering an immune response.

As was found for intraluminal and lysosomal food antigen handling and degradation,[26,31,32] food antigens are also modified by food technologic processing such as heat treatment, homogenization, and spray-drying.[47,48] In fact, new antigens may be revealed by these processes, and thus processed cow's milk may be more allergenic than raw milk.[48] In general, complex protein antigens are more likely to be destroyed by food processing, and thus controversial data do exist.[47] After ingestion of cow's milk formula, it must be expected that there will be confrontation with a wide variety of single proteins and proteolytic degradation products that bear allergenic as well as tolerogenic potential.

Human breast milk has recently been shown by direct methods to contain foreign food proteins (from cow's milk, egg, wheat, and peanut). These proteins are able to elicit an allergic response with different GI and dermal manifestations in the breast-fed infant.[49-51] Thus, breast-fed infants may be primed with foreign food proteins. A lack of specific maternal antifood protein secretory IgA was found to play a permissive role in the development of food allergic disease in the infants.[50] These facts are making the identification of the relevant food antigen in breast-fed infants very difficult. Maternal diet has to be taken into account in that respect.

Soy

Soy proteins have long been known to cause GI lesions similar to the ones produced by cow's milk in young infants.[52] The enteropathy in soy allergy is accompanied by changes in immunohistochemistry and morphometry, suggesting immune mechanisms for the development of the disease.[53] Soy allergy often develops as a secondary event after primary cow's milk allergy treated with a soy formula. Assumptions that soy is less allergenic than cow's milk cannot be substantiated. There is cross-reactivity between the legumes, soybeans, peas, and peanuts.

TABLE 4
Pathogenesis of Gastrointestinal Allergy:
Overview

A.	**Genetic predisposition, environmental factors**
B.	**Type I reaction:** Reaginic IgE antibodies, mast cell degranulation, mediators
C.	**Type III reaction:** Nonreaginic IgG antibodies, immune complexes
D.	**Type IV reaction:** Nonreaginic Cell-mediated immunity, T cells, lymphokines

In reaginic reactors, the soy component with the highest allergenic potency is a 2S-globulin,[54] again a relatively small food protein molecule. The potent allergen, soy trypsin inhibitor, has a molecular weight of 20,500.

Other Food Antigens

There are innumerable antigens in foods, most of which are encountered after early infancy. Major allergens are egg white and ovalbumin (a glycoprotein with a molecular weight of 44,000), peanuts, nuts, fish and meat of different sources, wheat, fruits (particularly citrus fruits), vegetables, and yeast.[55-57] Interestingly, there are cross-reactivities between birch pollen allergy (which is frequent in Scandinavia) and allergy to apple, carrot, and potato.[57] Wheat is known to be a strong allergen, wheat allergy and bakers' asthma being disease entities separate from celiac disease (see Chapter 27, Part 22), which is not an allergic disease in a strict sense.

Transfer RNA has been identified as a major allergen in shrimp allergy.[58] This is an example of a nonprotein allergen. Other nonprotein compounds such as dyes, preservatives, and antioxidants are often not shown in the food declaration. These "hidden ingredients"[59] can act as potent allergens as well.

PATHOGENESIS (Table 4 and Fig. 2)

Basis for Allergy Expression in the Newborn: Genetic Predisposition and Early Exposure

Immediate-type food allergy is genetically predetermined. In children with two atopic parents, the risk of developing skin reactions against foods is 58 percent.[60] Thus, atopy and food allergy are associated genetically. Genetic atopic predisposition is indicated by the capacity of the individuum to mount a pathologically high IgE response. The molecular basis of this (immune response genes?) has not yet been identified. Newborn screening by IgE determination in cord blood[61] is suitable to discriminate between high and low IgE responders. High IgE concentrations in cord blood (0.9 kU per liter or higher) correlate well (95 percent) with later specific IgE production and with the development of clinical symptoms.[62] Low IgE responses to foods were also found in healthy children.

Sensitization to egg white and cow's milk occurs in the first year of life. Clinical allergy to these allergens mostly ceases before school age, allergy to common inhalant allergens then becoming predominant.[62,63]

In addition to genetic influences on the development of food allergy, environmental factors such as early exposure to the antigen and duration of breast-feeding (quantity of exposure) apparently determine the occurrence of food allergy.[63,64] Small amounts of fed antigen eventually lead to sensitization, whereas larger amounts induce oral tolerance (see above). Intrauterine sensitization is possible, judged from immediate food allergic reactions on the first known extrauterine exposure and from signs of latent anaphylactic sensitization in low birth weight newborns.[65,66] Intrauterine sensitization may be accomplished either by placental transfer of minute quantities of food allergens or by the action of maternal antiidiotypic antibodies.[67] In contrast to IgG, IgE does not cross the human placenta. Other environmental factors influencing the development of GI food allergy, such as prior distur-

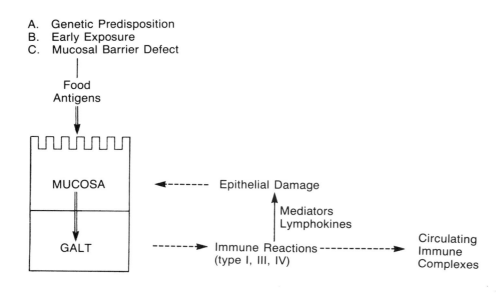

FIGURE 2 Immune pathogenesis of gastrointestinal allergy (schematic drawing). A–C, Predisposing factors (GALT = gut-associated lymphoid tissue). For further explanations, see text.

bances of the GI mucosal barrier by acute gastroenteritis,[68] are mostly hypothetic and await further proof.

Serum Food Antibodies

The formation of serum antibodies of IgG, IgA, or IgM class to food proteins is a physiologic phenomenon indicating exposure rather than sensitization to the respective food protein.[69] Serum food antibodies have been documented since the beginning of this century.[3] Antibody titers rise during the first few months of life and fall after infancy. Antibodies to different antigens such as the different cow's milk proteins, soy proteins, ovalbumin, and wheat proteins have been shown, depending on the foods introduced into the children's diet.[70] Although many healthy children show, for instance, cow's milk protein antibodies of IgG class in their sera, titers tend to be highest in cow's milk–allergic children.[71,72] This is particularly true for delayed reactions to the offending food protein. The situation is much clearer for immediate food-allergic reactions: Reaginic IgE food antibodies in high IgE responders play a significant role in pathogenesis of this type of food allergy[71] (see below).

The source of these food antibodies is in part the antibody-producing plasma cells of the small intestinal lamina propria, which have been demonstrated locally in food-allergic children.[73] Secretion of non-IgE antibodies into the intestinal lumen has been reported. It is increased by the action of GI hormones, such as pancreozymin and secretin.[74] Mesenteric lymph node and spleen antibody production accounts for the majority of food antibodies delivered into the serum. Most of these antibodies are not very disease-specific, since titers are also increased in nonallergic GI diseases such as inflammatory bowel disease or in liver disease. In these cases, food protein antibodies are an epiphenomenon of the GI mucosal lesion rather than its cause.

In food protein–induced enterocolitis, however, there is an altered immune response, in that children with a positive response on challenge with soy show an increase in IgA anti-soy antibodies and at the same time a decrease in IgM antibodies.[75] IgG and IgA antibody titers were elevated in the same group of patients compared to nonallergic controls. By antibody determination, it has recently been possible[76] to differentiate between cow's milk–allergic children with immediate reactions (less than 45 minutes after challenge) and late reactions (more than 20 hours after challenge), who had elevated IgE milk-specific antibodies in their sera, and children with intermediate reactions (1 to 20 hours after challenge), who had not. In the same paper, enzyme-linked immunosorbent assay (ELISA) IgG antibody levels were decreased after elimination of cow's milk in all patient groups, and there was no difference for IgA and IgM milk-specific antibodies when compared to controls. Subclass differentiation of IgG food antibodies has produced divergent data, some supporting a role for IgG4 antibodies in delayed skin reactions to milk[77] but others not substantiating a major role for these antibodies in producing allergic symptoms.[78]

In summary, serum food antibodies have been investigated extensively. No single antibody of any antigen or immunoglobulin specificity has been demonstrated to be solely responsible for a food-allergic reaction. Presumably, IgG and particularly IgE food antibodies take different parts in a complex pathogenetic chain of events that leads to the different forms of GI food allergy. Antibody determination has some diagnostic significance, but it does not replace the clinical approach to making the diagnosis.

Type I Hypersensitivity Reactions (Reaginic)

Different clinical patterns of food-allergic reactions are caused by different underlying immune mechanisms. By clinical and immunologic studies,[76,79] it has been possible to classify at least the main types of reactions, based on the classic definitions by Gell and Coombs (Table 4). Type I reaginic reactions, mediated by specific IgE antibodies to food allergens, have been identified as the main pathogenetic mechanism in immediate food allergic reactions. However, they are also found in late GI and eczematous reactions, in addition to cell-mediated type IV mechanisms.[71,79] In intermediate reactors to food allergens, type III mechanisms play a significant role. In contrast to the other groups, intermediate reactors do not exhibit positive skin prick tests to the offending food. Intermediate reactors in particular show GI reactions such as vomiting, diarrhea, and colic.[76]

In children with immediate onset of symptoms from the skin and GI tract after food challenge, there is a combination of family history of atopy, elevated total serum IgE, elevated specific IgE food antibodies measured by the radioallergosorbent technique (RAST), and positive skin prick tests with the food allergen that is not tolerated,[71,80,81] although the combined association is not an absolute one (total IgE: specificity 80 percent, sensitivity 94 percent, for immediate-type food allergy). The lack of IgE food antibodies does not exclude immediate-type food allergy.[81] Antibody titers do not reflect the degree of clinical sensitivity. In most of these children, follow-up showed an increasing tolerance to cow's milk, which was the main offending food allergen in this group. Age and antigen exposure were shown to influence development of specific IgE food and inhalant antibodies[62,63]: Humoral responses to foods and inhalants exhibit age differences that are important for the development of clinical symptoms, indicating a switch from food-allergic to inhalant reactions after toddler age (see above).

The RAST technique makes the investigation of countless allergens possible, including the commonly known food allergens (see Table 3), cross-reacting allergens such as birch pollen, and further allergens present in food such as molds and contaminants. It has to be kept in mind, however, that the finding of a specific IgE antibody alone does not necessarily mean a clinical allergic reaction to the specific allergen. GI proteolytic food antigen handling produces new antigens, also relevant for the formation of IgE antibodies shown by RAST.[32] When analyzed separately, single cow's milk proteins from whey and casein equally were shown to produce specific IgE antibodies in milk-allergic subjects. Different cow's milk substitutes (cow's milk formula) exhibited the same IgE reaction patterns, compared to cow's milk, whereas in vitro hydrolyzed casein formula did not react with the patients' sera.[82] Obviously, partial in vitro hydrolysis and milk processing are not able to destroy allergenicity of food proteins with regard to the production of a type I reaction involving formation of IgE antibodies.

When specific IgE food antibodies were compared to secretory IgA antibodies to the same food (apple) in adult patients allergic to birch with different reactivity to apple,[83] there was no difference in IgE antibodies found. However, it was found that the apple-sensitive patients lacked sIgA apple antibody in their saliva, compared to the apple-tolerant controls. This finding confirms the protective role of sIgA antibodies (specific mucosal barrier, see above) in food-allergic patients: The action of IgE antibodies (and production of clinical symptoms) may be prevented by sIgA even in the presence of high IgE titers.

Specific antifood IgE has been also found in intestinal washings of children with atopic dermatitis who were identified to be food allergic by challenge and who were serum RAST-negative for the food antigen not tolerated.[84] Along the same line, increased fecal IgE has been reported in allergic children,[85] indicating GI production and loss of IgE. Using immunohistochemical techniques in food-allergic children and adults,[86] lamina propria of the small intestinal mucosa was shown to contain increased numbers of IgE-containing cells. At the same time in the infants investigated, but not in the adults, partial villous atrophy and increased numbers of intraepithelial lymphocytes were found. This finding points to age-dependent differences in the pathogenetic mechanisms involved in food allergy. GI IgE production appears to be important for the development of food-allergic reactions, but it is not known how local GI and systemic production of IgE food antibodies is interrelated and how they are linked to the development of local morphologic and functional GI changes.

Not only in immediate reactors, but also in late reactors with atopic dermatitis, IgE food antibodies have been found in high titers.[87,88] This finding was paralleled by positive skin prick test results and by positive double-blind challenge reactions. One has to keep in mind, however, that atopic dermatitis and GI food allergy are separate disease entities that may show some overlap. It has been postulated[89] that IgE-containing immune complexes originating locally and circulating to the skin might be responsible for skin lesions in atopic eczema. These IgE complexes have been demonstrated in the blood in minute quantities. They are partially present in the form of double IgG-IgE complexes (anti-idiotypic IgG), but their pathogenetic role has not yet been proven.

Skin prick test results using food antigens have been shown to correlate well with mucosal provocation tests in immediate reactors, at least in older children and adults.[87,90,91] In addition, skin prick testing correlates well with RAST results. Correlation is good for some allergens, like fish, egg, pea, and peanut. It is much less reliable for cereal antigens. A negative skin prick test thus is an indicator against an immediate type I food-allergic reaction. A positive skin prick test is suggestive of type I allergy and has to be substantiated by clinical challenge, which remains the gold standard for diagnosis.[87]

The practical application of skin testing using food extracts in GI food allergy might indicate that the allergic reaction originates at the GI site of food encounter and is then propagated to distant sites like the skin, possibly by circulating IgE antibodies, or by circulating immune complexes. One

clearly has to differentiate between the gut as a vehicle of delivery of antigens to cause reactions in other organs (like the skin) and the gut as a target organ for food-allergic reactions. In fact, both gut functions might combine in clinical GI allergy.

Although IgE antibody production and skin testing have been widely investigated in type I food-allergic reactions, there remains much to be learned about the effector mechanisms bringing about allergic clinical effects. In analogy to other type I reactions such as drug-induced anaphylaxis, a decisive step is the binding of specific IgE antibodies to mast cells and basophils. After exposure to the specific food antigen, these cells bind the antigen by the ''bridging'' IgE molecule and are then able to release a variety of mediator substances. These substances are in turn able to influence capillary permeability, smooth muscle contractility, mucous secretion, and chemotaxis. Only single factors of this chain of events have been shown in food allergy. After intragastric provocation under endoscopic control,[92,93] immediate allergic reactions at the mucosal level (edema, erythema, petechial bleeding) were produced. At the same time, there were mast cell degranulation and histamine release shown directly. The reaction was most prominent in patients showing concomitant systemic reactions (urticaria, bronchospasm). Intragastric challenge results corresponded well to in vitro mast cell degranulation shown in small intestinal biopsy specimens incubated with food antigens such as egg white and cow's milk.[93]

High spontaneous release of histamine from peripheral leukocytes of food-allergic patients has been known for some time.[94] Plasma histamine levels increase after specific food challenges in food-allergic subjects,[95] and histamine may be released by peripheral leukocytes from egg-allergic patients after in vitro incubation with different egg antigens.[96] Similar techniques for diagnosis of food allergy have been tried (see below), but the results lack reproducibility and await further confirmation. The role of other mediators like prostaglandins and slow-reacting substance in the production of food-allergic reactions has been discussed.[97] Aspirin, a directly acting mast cell–degranulating agent, has been accused of producing a life-threatening reaction in food allergy,[98] showing that mediators are connected to the pathogenetic chain of events either directly or indirectly, producing and perhaps enforcing the same kind of result.

Type III Hypersensitivity Reactions (Nonreaginic)

Type II cytotoxic hypersensitivity has not been found in GI allergy. There is substantial evidence, however, for the existence of type III (Arthus type) reactions. Ultrastructural and immunohistochemical studies[99] have shown a sequence of pathogenetic events, timed exactly like a type III intermediate reaction: 6 hours after challenge, local increase in IgM and IgA plasma cells was observed (an increase in IgE cells which was also observed has been challenged by other groups on methodologic grounds). This was followed within 24 hours after challenge by local edema, endothelial reaction, basement membrane thickening, collagen fiber deposition, and infiltration with polymorphonuclear leukocytes. There was local deposition of IgG and complement C3 in the subepithelial connective tissue indicative of an immune complex reaction. At this point, there was some early enterocyte damage such as microvillous irregularity, increase in lysosomes, and mitochondrial swelling. Some of these findings, especially the local changes in IgM and IgA plasma cells, have been confirmed by others,[100] whereas other changes (on IgE cells and mast cells) have not. By later studies,[10] local immunoglobulin deposits at the basement membrane of the small intestine have been identified as antigen-antibody complexes containing bovine serum albumin and IgG, and sometimes complement.

In addition to local deposition, immune complexes containing food antigens (cow's milk and egg proteins) and immunoglobulins (IgG and IgE) have been demonstrated to circulate in the sera of food-allergic patients.[102-104] Data on complement binding (Clq and C3) by food antigen–containing immune complexes have been inconclusive up to now. The findings were not absolutely specific to food allergy, but the conclusion is justified from the data that normal individuals form IgA complexes,[89,105] whereas food-allergic patients form IgG and IgE, or even mixed, complexes. The latter complexes were particularly found in IgA-deficient patients.[105] Only in single cases[106] have these immune complexes in food allergy been shown to cause immune complex disease in organs distant to the gut, for instance glomerulopathy[106] or skin disease. Taken together with food antibody production (see above), type III immune complex reactions thus probably play an important role in the production of intermediate clinical allergic reactions to food antigens, although the information on single steps in this reaction chain is still incomplete.

Type IV Hypersensitivity Reactions (Nonreaginic)

Morphologic studies[107,108] point to the relevance of cell-mediated immune reactions in food allergy. The activity and relative number of intraepithelial lymphocytes are increased in cow's milk allergy. These lymphocytes, which bear T-cell characteristics, are the first line of cellular immunologic defense against small intestinal luminal antigen attack. They are in close proximity to the basal part of the surface enterocytes, indicating possible lymphoepithelial interaction. Intraepithelial lymphocytes were shown to react in number to challenge and to return to normal after elimination of the offending food antigen.[107] The changes were shown to correlate with villous-crypt cell kinetics in that high numbers of intraepithelial lymphocytes were connected with increased crypt mitotic activity and with decreased villous enterocyte height. Thus, there may be links between cell-mediated immunity and GI epithelial damage in food allergy.

Peripheral lymphocytes in food allergy exhibit altered (decreased) nonspecific lymphoblastic reactivity toward different mitogens.[109,110] It is not known if this finding represents a general defect in suppressor cell activity in food allergy postulated by some authors. More interestingly, there is specific lymphoblastic reactivity of peripheral lymphocytes in food allergy, as an indication for lymphocyte sensitization to specific food proteins such as beta-LG, casein, soy protein, and egg white.[109-111] The significance of these findings

remains to be elucidated. Not much is known about the functional specificity and sensitization of GALT lymphocytes involved in the GI response to food challenge.

Production of lymphokines by activated lymphocytes is a phenomenon well known from conditions other than food allergy.[112] Findings on the production of a cow's milk–specific leukocyte migration-inhibiting factor (an assumed lymphokine) in cow's milk allergy have led to conflicting results.[113] From animal models using GI parasitic infection and graft-versus-host reaction, a linkage between cell-mediated immune reactions and enterocyte damage has been postulated.[112] As assumed by these authors, the connecting link is an enterotropic lymphokine that brings about villous atrophy in experimental animals. Information on similar pathogenetic mechanisms in human food allergy is still lacking.

CLINICAL MANIFESTATIONS

A wide variety of symptoms has been ascribed to food allergy in children of different ages (Table 5). Most of these symptoms and symptom complexes (Table 5, A–D) have been proven to be allergic reactions to food components by double-blind, placebo-controlled elimination and challenge studies,[87] whereas others have not and merit a note of caution in this context (Table 5E). Since the gut functions not only as a target organ in GI allergy, but also as a vehicle for delivery of antigens to cause reactions in other organs (see above), it is conceivable that reactions in others organs, such as the skin and respiratory tract, and even the cardiovascular system in anaphylactic reactions, occur in GI food allergy. Frequently, combined reactions to the offending food are encountered on different organ levels. Depending on different criteria of selection and patients groups, different numbers

TABLE 5
Clinical Symptoms of Allergy

A.	**General** Anaphylaxis, shock, shock fragments
B.	**Gastrointestinal** Nausea, vomiting Diarrhea, malabsorption, failure to thrive Intestinal loss of blood, protein Abdominal pain, bloating
C.	**Respiratory** Sneezing, rhinorrhea Wheezing, cough Bronchospasm, dyspnea
D.	**Skin** Lip swelling, angioedema Itching, rash, urticaria Eczema
E.	**Others (?)** Joint swelling, pain Headache, apathy Irritability, hyperkinesis

are found in the literature as to the relative frequency of the organ reactions.[4,5,10,12] GI reactions are most common, with a frequency between 50 and 80 percent, followed by skin reactions between 20 and 40 percent and respiratory reactions between 10 and 25 percent. Systemic anaphylactic reactions (including shock fragments) occur in 15 percent. There is considerable overlap, and the reaction type may be changing, particularly with increasing age from infancy to adolescence. Thus, these figures are only rough estimates of the relative importance of the different organ reactions.

The clinical symptoms of GI food allergy may be sorted not only in terms of the organ systems affected but also in terms of the time a single reaction takes to develop after challenge. One may differentiate between immediate reactions (0 to 1 hour), intermediate reactions (1 to 24 hours), and late reactions (longer than 24 hours). This differentiation makes sense in pathogenetic terms, since different mechanisms are operative, both clinically and immunologically (see above).[6,76,79] For instance, GI reactions that lead to enteropathy, malabsorption, and failure to thrive are intermediate or late, whereas skin and respiratory reactions like angioedema and bronchospasm are immediate reactions. Again, there are examples for transience between the different types, and lumping all these reactions together as food allergy still appears justified.

General Manifestations: Anaphylaxis

Since the classic transfer experiments of Prausnitz and Küstner (who was allergic to cooked fish), it is known that reaginic antibodies that trigger a very potent immediate immune response, possibly leading to anaphylactic shock, can be formed after food sensitization. True immunologically mediated anaphylaxis has to be differentiated from anaphylactoid reactions that are triggered directly by non-immune mediator release, e.g., by aspirin.[98]

Anaphylactic shock induced by food ingestion has been observed at all ages but is most common during infancy. There are single reports that cow's milk antigens present in breast milk may induce anaphylaxis. More often, anaphylaxis occurs during challenge, which is then potentially lethal, for instance in food-allergic children with severe atopic eczema.[113] Fatal outcome certainly prohibits any deliberate challenge testing of children with a known anaphylactic reagibility to food components. Precautions taken before challenge (heparin lock, fluid administration) or subcutaneous adrenaline (1:1,000) injection immediately after an anaphylactic reaction is not necessarily effective in these cases.[113] Steroids and antihistamines are not effective immediately.

The degree of anaphylactic reactions may vary from lethal shock to minor symptoms, sometimes referred to as "shock fragments," such as urticarial rashes, lip and buccal swelling, and laryngeal and bronchial spasm. Most of the patients lose their anaphylactic reagibility with increasing age. Neither the severity of the reaction nor the natural history of an anaphylactic reaction can be predicted. It is recommended that patients carry with them isoprenaline/orciprenaline in the form of sublingual tablets or aerosol.

Gastrointestinal Manifestations

Food-Induced Enteropathy

Transient food intolerance of early childhood that disappears after the age of 2 or 3 years is the best-investigated form of GI manifestations of food allergy.[2–4,10,12,16,114,115] The most common prototype of this enteropathy is cow's milk–induced enteropathy, probably due to the fact that cow's milk usually is the first foreign protein introduced into an infant's diet. This type of enteropathy may also be induced by other food proteins, such as soy, egg, fish, rice, chicken, wheat. The reaction occurs in a delayed, nonimmediate way. Symptoms commonly seen are diarrhea, malabsorption, failure to thrive, vomiting, and abdominal pain. There may be intestinal loss of protein or even blood.

Morphologic studies of the small intestine in cow's milk–induced enteropathy have shown different degrees of villous atrophy with a nonhomogeneous, "patchy" distribution.[116] In severe cases, features indistinguishable from the lesion in celiac disease are found (flat mucosa, villous atrophy, crypt hyperplasia, cellular infiltration of lamina propria), but differentiation between the two conditions is possible by morphometry and crypt cell kinetics, by immunohistochemistry, and by the clinical course on differential challenge with cow's milk or gluten.[100,108,115] The enteropathy in cow's milk allergy is fully reversible after elimination of cow's milk. Since there are cases of cow's milk allergy with malabsorption but without severe enteropathy, a morphologic definition of the diagnosis based on small intestinal biopsy has not been generally accepted. This is also true for short-term challenge reactions controlled by small intestinal biopsy which produced equivocal results. The finding of a patchy enteropathy is by no means pathognomonic for any particular etiology.

The role of acute gastroenteritis predisposing to the subsequent development of cow's milk allergy has not been proven.[68] Secondarily, disaccharidase (lactase) deficiency occurs in cow's milk allergy owing to the intestinal surface lesion at the brush border level. This factor contributes to the perpetuation of symptoms and makes the differential diagnosis between cow's milk allergy and lactose intolerance difficult. Lactose intolerance therefore has to be excluded prior to challenge in order to make a definitive diagnosis of cow's milk allergy.

Eosinophilic Gastroenteropathy

Eosinophilic gastroenteropathy is a rare disorder distinct from food-induced enteropathy.[117] It is characterized by eosinophilic infiltration of the gastric and small intestinal mucosa. The features of protein-losing enteropathy (peripheral edema, ascites, wasting) are predominant, whereas generalized malabsorption (steatorrhea) is lacking. Iron-deficiency anemia due to GI blood loss is common. The onset is relatively late, compared to food allergy of infancy.

There is a positive family history of atopy, and there is evidence of IgE-mediated reactions to food components. Although food allergies, in particular IgE-mediated immune responses, have been found to play a role in eosinophilic gastroenteropathy, the condition often does not respond to elimination diets.[118] Multiple allergens, including inhalants, appear to be involved.[119] Corticosteroids have been found to be effective in uncontrolled studies.[118,119]

At present, there is no convincing explanation, in terms of pathogenetic mechanisms, of why some individuals exhibit a food-sensitive enteropathy whereas others exhibit eosinophilic gastroenteropathy with all the clinical differences described above.

Food-Induced Colitis

There is no solid evidence that inflammatory bowel disease (IBD, ulcerative colitis, Crohn's disease) is influenced by allergic reactions to foods. Circulating IgG antibodies to food antigens in IBD are certainly not sufficient to prove any primary pathogenetic significance of food allergy (see above). There is, however, a separate clinical entity of food-induced colitis.[120-122] Main clinical symptoms are chronic bloody diarrhea, anemia, and abdominal pain. Rectosigmoidoscopy reveals mucosal erythema and aphthous lesions, and histologically there is gross eosinophilic infiltration and focal ulceration. Food-induced colitis can be elicited by foreign food antigens present in breast milk[123] and by soy protein,[124] but it is mostly caused by cow's milk.

Two major clinical papers[121,122] clearly established the significance of food-allergic proctitis and colitis in children. All those children were less than 2 years of age, the symptoms (bloody diarrhea with mucous secretion, rectal bleeding) often starting before the age of 6 months. The onset of symptoms occurred shortly after introduction of cow's milk or other foreign food proteins. In most cases, there was a family history of allergy. There were peripheral blood eosinophilia, high total serum IgE levels, and high IgE food antibody titers. By endoscopic biopsy and histology, eosinophilic infiltration was shown, as well as local increase of IgE-containing lamina propria cells.[121,125] This type of colitis was relatively benign and responded well to elimination diet therapy. In a comparative study,[121] food-allergic colitis was found to be the major cause of colitis in infancy. It has to be noted, however, that, particularly in older patients,[125] eosinophilic colitis can be a precursor of ulcerative colitis. The main criteria for differentiation are increased IgE-containing cells and the prompt response of food-allergic patients to elimination diets. Single patients have been reported who showed allergic gastroenteropathy together with food-induced colitis. In rare cases,[126] necrotizing enterocolitis may be caused by a severe anaphylactic form of cow's milk allergy.

Other Gastrointestinal Manifestations

Besides small intestinal blood loss in food-induced enteropathy and eosinophilic gastroenteropathy and colonic blood loss in food-induced colitis of infancy, occult GI blood loss has been described to be a consequence of cow's milk feeding.[127] Children on pasteurized milk had positive guaiac stool tests without showing any sign of anemia.[127] In an older study, hypochromic microcytic anemia due to iron deficiency was reported in a similar series,[128] occurring reversibly during cow's milk feeding, possibly dependent on the ingestion of bovine serum proteins. Some of these children

also had hypoproteinemia and edema, and it may be that they had a mild form of allergic gastroenteropathy, but substantial evidence (morphologic study, double-blind elimination and challenge) was never acquired.

Edema of the ileum and small bowel occlusion have been shown by adequate means to be caused by cow's milk allergy.[129,130] This appears to be a rare event, however. Chronic aphthous oral ulcerations, gastroesophageal reflux,[131] and constipation have been ascribed to GI food allergy on very limited grounds.

Infantile colic has been found to be connected to cow's milk formula ingestion by a double-blind study.[132] There were no immunologic mechanisms identified, so that the definition of food allergy does not apply. Other studies indicating some significance of "food sensitivity" in abdominal migraine and in the irritable bowel syndrome[133,134] leave considerable doubt as to the definition of diagnosis, selection of patients, and specificity of food-related findings.

Clearly, there are important GI allergic reactions like enteropathy and colitis, undoubtedly caused by a reproducible immunologic reaction to food proteins. These defined manifestations respond extremely well to elimination of the offending food. It is essential, however, to maintain strict definitions and criteria for diagnostic purposes, in order not to mix up defined allergic reactions with ill-defined symptoms and reactions not proven to be allergic. Thus, many unnecessary and misleading diagnostic and therapeutic procedures can be avoided.

Nongastrointestinal Manifestations

Respiratory

Nonseasonal allergic rhinitis with sneezing, itching, mucosal congestion, and rhinorrhea is a typical example of an immediate reaction to food, occurring within minutes after a nasal provocation test.[4,135,136] Allergic rhinitis is the most common respiratory manifestation of food allergy. It may be complicated by chronic serous otitis media and sinusitis. Direct food exposure of the nasal mucosa appears to be more important than ingestion in triggering rhinitis. Skin tests are positive, and specific IgE antibodies to food proteins are found frequently. When allergic rhinitis is combined with lower respiratory tract disease, nasal provocation tests may be very helpful to check for activity of the disease and for single food antigen significance.[135]

Bronchial asthma due to food allergy often is underestimated, since history is mostly unhelpful: Symptoms occur gradually, with a delay of hours or even days after ingestion of the offending food.[4,137-139] The quantity of allergen needed to elicit the symptoms (bronchospasm, expiratory dyspnea, coughing) is higher than with allergic rhinitis. Severity and course of the disease are much more dangerous, still involving a risk of mortality, when there is lower respiratory tract disease. Food-allergic children with asthma tend to be older than children with predominant GI manifestations of food allergy. Skin test and RAST results for foods in these cases have only limited value, since they are often negative. Bronchial response after food ingestion challenge is the only reliable diagnostic criterion,[138,139] and it is the only acceptable basis for an elimination diet in asthmatic children reacting to food antigens. Oral disodium cromoglycate (DSCG) has been used in these children successfully, in addition to elimination diets.[138]

There is some doubt about the existence of a separate "Heiner's syndrome" with chronic rhinitis, otitis, wheezing, tachypnea, pulmonary infiltration, and hemosiderosis.[2,135] These symptoms were demonstrated together with GI blood loss and failure to thrive, and all the signs responded to elimination of cow's milk. Cow's milk precipitins were demonstrated in the patients' sera. The reaction was nonreaginic, but there was no double-blind proof of this chronic condition, and other groups failed to encounter similar patients.

Similar to primary GI manifestations of food allergy, respiratory manifestations (in particular lower respiratory tract disease) have to be challenge-proven under clinical conditions in order to establish a rational argument for elimination diet therapy. Respiratory manifestations of food allergy often occur in combination with other symptoms, particularly in the skin.

Skin

Lip swelling, angioedema, and urticarial rashes are facultative but frequent symptoms of food allergy, representing immediate reactions to the food ingested.[140] Food allergy has been identified to be the cause of chronic urticaria in a minority of patients.[141] In the patients with immediate skin reactions to food, solely specific IgE antibodies can be found in elevated titers, compared to patients with delayed reactions (atopic eczema), who at the same time had elevated IgG, IgA, and IgE food antibodies.[142] This finding indicates two types of immunologic reaction in skin manifestations of food allergy. Clinically, there is considerable overlap between the two, indicated by the development of acute urticaria in children with eczema, which is not infrequent during skin testing using food extracts.[143]

Atopic dermatitis (eczema) certainly is a very frequent (10 to 15 percent) multifactorial disease with a genetic predisposition (see above). It is characterized by an erythematous, papulovesicular rash that itches intensely and occurs at typical sites (head, flexural sides of extremities). Histologically, there is massive dermal edema (spongiosis) and round cell infiltration. Frequently, atopic dermatitis is combined with, and usually precedes, asthma and hay fever. Manifestations of atopic dermatitis peak during infancy. The disease usually disappears after 5 years, only 5 percent of the cases persisting into adulthood.[4,140] Food allergy is only one of the possible factors influencing atopic dermatitis.

Immediate food-allergic reactions, based on specific IgE reaginic antibodies, have been identified in atopic dermatitis but exhibit features distinct from acute skin reactions like urticaria.[4,142,144] Total serum IgE reaches much higher levels in atopic dermatitis than in asthma, hay fever, and urticaria. Food IgE antibody levels are much more elevated at the same time. Skin tests using foods are mostly positive[87] (see above), correlating very well with serologic findings. However, the actual role of reaginic antibodies in the pathogenesis of atopic dermatitis, which is clinically in part a delayed reaction, remains unclear.

Numerous food challenge and elimination studies of atopic patients in the past have not been done in a double-blind, placebo-controlled way and have led to very subjective results.[4] By applying strict criteria, recent studies have indeed made the case for an etiologic role of food antigens in some patients with atopic dermatitis.[145,146] It should be possible to identify these patients by a defined diagnostic approach before placing them on elimination diets.

Other Nongastrointestinal Manifestations

Inflammatory joint disease has recently been linked with cow's milk allergy based on blind, placebo-controlled challenge in a single adult patient.[147] There were no specific IgE antibodies, but there were marked increases in IgG, particularly IgG4 milk antibodies, and there were IgG-milk circulating immune complexes found. This fits very well with experimental data on immune complex disease (see above), but the data need to be confirmed by other groups before any conclusions can be drawn. At present, there is no scientific basis for dietary elimination therapy in rheumatoid disease.[4]

Another example of food-allergic immune complex disease may be immune complex glomerulopathy in a child with eosinophilic gastroenteropathy and the nephrotic syndrome.[148] Multiple immune complexes have been demonstrated (containing bovine serum albumin and casein), and the condition improved with diet and steroids. It is premature to draw any therapeutic conclusions from data like these.

A matter of considerable dispute is the possible involvement of central nervous symptoms in food-allergic reactions. Double-blind trials have shown that migraine[149-151] can be induced by many different foods, and an oligoantigenic diet was able to improve symptoms in many patients. There was no clearly proven immunologic effect of food components in these patients: Total serum IgE was normal and specific IgE antibodies to food were found in only some of the patients, in immune complex form.[150] Skin tests were invariably negative. There was no totally convincing exclusion of idiosyncratic reactions based on biochemical effects, e.g., of tyramine or phenolic compounds. The possibility of a direct histamine release remains open after these studies.[151] Nevertheless, further prospective studies on migraine and food allergy are eagerly awaited.

Even less well documented are studies of hyperactivity, hyperkinesis, and sleep disturbances, ascribed to food allergy.[152-155] The results are mainly anecdotal, and the consequences suggested are in part speculative. A mere placebo effect of the elimination diet was not excluded. The mechanisms by which the symptoms were produced could not be identified. Studies like this have led to considerable confu-

TABLE 6

Cow's Milk Allergy: Goldman's Diagnostic Criteria[156]

---

1. Symptoms subside after cow's milk elimination.
2. Symptoms relapse within 48 hours after challenge.
3. Three challenges produce equal relapses.

BUT

    Challenge in anaphylaxis is unethical.
    Multiple challenges are often impossible.
    Open challenge is subject to bias.
    Relapse after challenge may take more than 48 hours.

---

sion in parents and have lent support to irrational and irresponsible practices. There is no doubt that food substances may cause central nervous system alterations (e.g., by the action of opioid components or by vasopressor amines). However, there is no reason to assume food allergy in these cases or to institute any therapy guided by that assumption. Again, food allergy has to be proven by the appropriate diagnostic means before any sound therapeutic conclusion can be drawn.

DIAGNOSIS

Elimination and Challenge (Table 6)

The cornerstone of diagnosis in GI food allergy is a complete history and an unequivocal and reproducible reaction to elimination and challenge. Laboratory tests may help, particularly in children with immediate reactions, but by no means are substitutes for the clinical approach to establish the diagnosis (Table 7). Goldman's criteria (see Table 6)[156] for the diagnosis of cow's milk allergy have been abandoned for many reasons: They are too strict for routine use, they do not apply to anaphylactic reactions, they do not necessarily imply immunologic mechanisms, they are open to observers' and patients' bias, and they do not take into account reactions occurring after 48 hours (see Table 6).[4] A standard protocol for elimination and challenge testing has been modified, following most of the suggestions originally made by Powell[157]:

1. Challenges are done under close clinical control, on an inpatient basis. A known anaphylactic reaction precludes any challenge.
2. In suspected cow's milk allergy, lactose intolerance is excluded prior to challenge by appropriate means (e.g., by H_2 breath testing after an oral load of lactose, 2 g per kilogram).
3. Pretesting liquid food includes subsequent exposure of (a) an unaffected skin area and (b) the lips to one drop of the liquid (e.g., cow's milk). This is done to avoid possibly fatal anaphylactic reactions.[113] A heparin lock has to be installed, and the usual precautions (intravenous fluids, adrenaline, antihistamines, steroids) have to be prepared before challenge.
4. The oral challenge starts with small amounts (a few drops of liquid food). The child is carefully observed for the development of rashes, rhinorrhea, changes in respiratory rate, wheezing, vomiting, and diarrhea. A written challenge protocol has to be followed. If there is no obvious reaction, the challenge dose is increased in 5-ml steps at hourly intervals.
5. Four hours after challenge, oral feeding (usually hydrolysate formula in suspected cow's milk allergy) is resumed. If no reaction occurs, the challenge dose is increased to reach 10 ml per kilogram after 48 hours and full strength after 96 hours. The observation period is extended to 7 days. Stool samples are collected and examined for occult blood, pH, and carbohydrate (Clinitest method).

TABLE 7
Diagnostic Tests in Gastrointestinal Allergy

A. **Elimination and Challenge**
 Open/single-blind/double-blind (= gold standard)

B. **Skin Testing**
 Prick tests, defined standardized food antigens

C. **Immunologic Tests**
 Total serum IgE, intestinal IgE
 Serum IgE food antibodies (RAST)
 Serum IgG food antibodies (RIFT, ELISA)
 Circulating immune complexes, C1q binding
 Plasma histamine, basophil histamine release test
 Leukocyte migration inhibition test (LIF)

D. **Intestinal Biopsy and Malabsorption**
 Intragastral provocation under endoscopic control
 Small intestinal biopsy
 Rectosigmoidoscopy and biopsy
 Sugar absorption studies (e.g., xylose)

Challenge is done with defined foods.[158-161] Usually there is no need to use single food components (such as purified proteins), since there is no alternative practical consequence. A single well-documented reaction to challenge, in accordance with history, is sufficient for diagnosis. When doubts remain, double-blind, placebo-controlled challenge is done,[159] using challenge food hidden in some neutral tolerated food (younger children) or encapsulated dried food. This is the final gold standard of diagnosis (Table 7).

If there is no direct suspicion of a single food in clearly allergic reactions in older children, simple exclusion diets (e.g., lamb and rice) can be used in order to find the relevant allergen.[5] This approach has to be followed by definitive challenge studies. The widespread use of "rotating diets" in search of a suspected food allergy without subsequent challenging must be rejected sharply. Psychogenic factors, which are common in this field (see above), cannot be excluded, and misdiagnoses could reinforce aberrant behavior.[7,159,161]

Skin Tests

For diagnosis of GI food allergy, three criteria have to be fulfilled[158]: (1) identification of the allergen, (2) unequivocal reaction to elimination and challenge, and (3) identification of an immunologic mechanism involved. Numerous tests have been suggested to fulfill the last criterion and to support the diagnosis (Table 7). Skin tests have been widely used but can be accepted only with some criticism.[159,162] First, only the skin prick technique using defined and standardized food antigens is acceptable, since other techniques are known to cause nonspecific irritant or severe systemic reactions. Second, in children less than 3 years of age with delayed reactions, skin tests are often negative.

Generally, skin tests reliably indicate an immediate food sensitivity, results correlating well with family history and RAST findings (see above).[87,90,91] At least 80 percent of the IgE-mediated responders can be detected by skin prick testing.[4] In anaphylaxis, however, skin testing is replaced by

RAST. Usually, a "battery" of common antigens (egg, cow's milk, wheat, fish, soy, nuts, peanuts) is used in the initial evaluation.[87] A negative test result makes immediate reactions very unlikely, and further challenge studies can then be avoided. On the other hand, there are clinically insignificant skin prick test results with foods (false positives) which have to be identified by clinical challenge. These limitations considered, food skin prick testing is a valuable tool in immediately reacting patients.

Immunologic Tests

Owing to the many immune mechanisms involved in pathogenesis, different immunologic tests have been used for identification of allergic reactions. Only a very few of these tests can reliably be used to support the diagnosis (Table 7, C). Total serum IgE and specific IgE food antibodies, determined by RAST, are good predictors of an immediate reaction to any given food[71,81,163] and may even be used for identification of very young infants at risk to develop food allergy and atopy.[61,62] There are, however, many false positives, and there is considerable confusion over standardization and test reproducibility in commercial test kits for RAST.[164] One of the problems is different avidity of IgE antibodies to different food antigens. Generally, RAST is approximately as sensitive as skin prick testing, but it is much more expensive. It is recommended in anaphylactic reactors and in those with severe skin reactions to food. Possibly some of the problems inherent with RAST can be solved by application of enhanced ELISA[158] techniques to the clinical problem of food allergy diagnosis.

Serum IgG antibodies to common food antigens are a very frequent finding, indicating exposure rather than sensitization[69–72] By semiquantitative assay of IgG cow's milk antibodies (ELISA or red cell immunosorbent fluorescent technique, RIFT[72]), it is possible to differentiate between cow's milk–allergic subjects and controls. This is particularly true for intermediate and late reactors as opposed to immediate reactors.[76,79] Thus, there is some limited diagnostic value to semiquantitative IgG food antibody determination in children with nonimmediate food-allergic reactions. These children tend to show predominantly GI reactions.

Immune complexes containing food antigens and antibodies circulating in the serum have been investigated in food allergy.[103,104,165] Although the techniques applied are different (modified radioimmunoassay, Clq binding), results in food allergy appear promising, particularly in terms of identifying type III immune mechanisms. The diagnostic value of these data remains to be examined by other groups.

Mediator release in immediate reactors can be measured by plasma histamine determinations in food allergy[95] and by histamine measurement after incubation of peripheral basophil leukocytes in the presence of antigen.[96,166] This technique is time-consuming and costly. Results mostly accord with RAST and skin test results, degranulation depending on the presence of specific IgE antibodies. Recently, a simple and inexpensive basophil degranulation test has been advocated,[168] but results await confirmation by other groups.

Cell-mediated immune mechanisms like food antigen-specific lymphocyte sensitization, indicated by the production of a lymphokine, the leukocyte migration–inhibiting factor (LIF), have found some diagnostic interest.[109,113,167] Contrary to some enthusiastic results,[109,167] there are major drawbacks due to many false-positive findings,[113] to technical problems, and to high test costs.

There are many additional nonvalidated food allergy tests like leukocytotoxic testing, subcutaneous and sublingual provocation, and neutralization testing. These techniques have not been approved by the American Academy of Allergy and should be abandoned.[158] The case has to be made against establishing a variety of nonvalidated in vitro tests, with the aim to replace the conventional clinical diagnostic approach in food allergy. The same applies to paramedical approaches to establishing the diagnosis.

Intestinal Biopsy and Malabsorption

The GI tract has been investigated both morphologically and functionally, in order to establish diagnostic criteria in GI allergy. In general, reliability of clinical and immunologic methods has not been reached by gastroenterological methods in terms of clinical sensitivity and specificity.[4] Thus, a merely gastroenterological approach in GI allergy is not justified. It is very promising, however, to look at the connections between local immunologic events and epithelial lesions, even from the viewpoint of diagnosis.

One of the studies connecting both levels of investigation is the intragastric provocation under endoscopic control (IPEC), checked by morphology and mast cell degranulation assay.[92,93] Clinical and in vitro findings agree very well in food allergy,[93] and the procedure has been recommended for "doubtful cases." The study was restricted to immediate reactions. It is doubtful whether techniques like this can be widely applied in children, however.

Gastric biopsy is diagnostic in eosinophilic gastroenteropathy,[119] and small bowel biopsy has been widely applied to the study of children with food-induced enteropathy.[2–4,99,114–116] Owing to variability of the mucosal lesions found ("patchy enteropathy"), it has never been possible to establish a morphology-based definition of cow's milk allergy (see above). This is also true for biopsy evaluation after short-term challenge.[169] Morphometry[108] is of some help in descriptive pathology of food-allergic reactions. Immunohistochemically, it may be possible to identify food-allergic subjects by measuring IgE-containing mucosal plasma cells in partial villous atrophy.[86] This is another example of a connection between immunologic and morphologic observations.

For differential diagnosis of GI allergy (celiac disease, lymphangiectasia, microvillous atrophy, etc), small intestinal biopsy is an absolutely necessary tool, particularly in young infants with intermediate or late reactions.

In food-induced colitis, endoscopic colonic and rectal biopsy may be pathognomonic,[121,122] particularly when evaluated for IgE-containing mucosal plasma cells.[125] Thus, biopsy of the gastric, small intestinal, colonic, and rectal mucosa is an important diagnostic tool in GI allergy which adds substance to clinical and differential diagnoses.

Gut function tests, for instance sugar absorption tests, have been applied as noninvasive screening tests for malabsorption.[4,170] Initially, the blood xylose test was strongly advocat-

TABLE 8
Therapy for Gastrointestinal Allergy

A. Elimination Diet
   Infants
      Breast milk
      Hydrolysate formula (*casein*, soy, whey)
      Caveat: full soy formula
   Children
      Exclusion diet
      Elementary diet (rarely needed)
      Caveat: routine use of elimination diets

B. Drugs (Special indications: polyvalent allergy, respiratory symptoms)
   Disodium cromoglycate (DSCG, cromolyn) PO
   Ketotifen PO

ed even for diagnosis of cow's milk allergy in infants. Meanwhile, test accuracy has been questioned, and the test has been mostly abandoned, since there was no advantage of the test over clinical observation in evaluating a response to oral challenge with cow's milk. At present, there is no place for gut function tests in the diagnosis of GI allergy.

THERAPY

Allergen Elimination

After a definitive diagnosis of GI food allergy has been made, elimination of the food allergen identified is the therapy of choice (Table 8).[171,172] The indiscriminate routine use of elimination diets without firm diagnosis is a widespread malpractice, possibly causing malnutrition and symptoms of protein, calorie, and trace element deficiencies.[173]

In infants without secondary lactose intolerance, breast milk is given for therapy of cow's milk allergy, which is the most frequent food allergy in this age group. There is some concern about maternal diet during lactation, and mothers of highly reactive infants should be aware of the possibility of infant sensitization by minute quantities of foreign antigens in their breast milk (see below).[65]

For therapeutic use, highly specialized protein hydrolysate formula has been developed, containing hydrolysates from casein, whey and soy, medium chain triglycerides, and non-lactose carbohydrates.[174,175] From the viewpoint of molecular size of protein hydrolysis products and allergenicity, casein and soy hydrolysates are superior to whey products. Some highly sensitive infants have been reported to react to the remaining epitopes in whey hydrolysate formula. Most hydrolysates have a bitter taste but are tolerated when used consequently. Osmolality should be low, and there is some concern about the relatively high carbohydrate and low lipid composition of these formulae. Hydrolysate formula should be prescribed like a drug in therapy of food allergy. Full soy formula should not be considered first-choice therapy in food-allergic infants, since at least 20 percent of these children are known to develop secondary soy allergy.[53]

In older children, single foods can be avoided easily in many cases. One has to be aware of unlisted food components (e.g., milk proteins in margarine), and a dietician should be consulted in order to meet daily requirements (e.g., calcium in cow's milk–free diet[176]) (also see reference 176 for food lists and recipes). So-called oligoantigenic diets should be used only during the diagnostic approach, followed by food allergen challenge. Replacement of food by an elemental diet is only rarely needed. Nutritional needs of children under 12 are usually not met completely by an ordinary elemental formula designed for use in adults.[4,176] Establishing an effective and nutritionally satisfactory exclusion diet can be extremely difficult in the rare cases of polyvalent food allergy.

Fortunately, many food allergies disappear, since tolerance develops with increasing age, and elimination diets can be discontinued after a few years. Oral hyposensitization using food allergens has been proven to have no therapeutic effect. In mild cases, one should always keep in mind that the diet might be worse than the disease.

Drug Therapy

Reactions other than GI symptoms in food allergy (anaphylaxis, asthma, eczema) often have to be treated pharmacologically, in addition to elimination of the offending food.[4,5,158,171] General drug treatment of non-GI food allergy is beyond the scope of this chapter and will be omitted here. In cases of inadvertent food ingestion causing GI symptoms, antihistamines are used.

Results of the use of drugs in primary therapy of food allergy are inconclusive and have been reviewed elsewhere.[177,178] Oral DSCG (cromolyn, 4 × 100 mg per day) has been used in numerous older studies, which were mostly uncontrolled. It is not absorbed and may act by decreasing the uptake of food antigen at the gut level. There are some recent double-blind studies[179,180] demonstrating a positive therapeutic effect, particularly in food-allergic patients with atopic dermatitis,[179] but still there remain major criticism and contradicting results, particularly on the validation of symptoms.[158] It is well known from different controlled studies that DSCG can prevent respiratory symptoms and an asthmatic response to food challenge.[5,138]

Thus, oral DSCG may be useful in non-GI symptoms caused by food allergy. Its effectiveness in GI symptoms has not been proven. Application of DSCG in most cases is unnecessary and should be restricted to cases in which dietary control is not achieved.

Recently oral ketotifen has been recommended for use in GI allergy.[176,177,180] Well-controlled studies are lacking, however, and further evaluation of this drug is needed to produce conclusive evidence. The same applies to drugs like prostaglandin synthetase inhibitors (aspirin, indomethacin) that are known themselves to cause allergic symptoms occasionally and to other anti-inflammatory substances. Steroids certainly are indicated in eosinophilic gastroenteritis.[119]

PREVENTION

Early studies on the preventive effect of avoidance diets in infants have led to inconclusive data, some demonstrating postponement of allergic symptoms in breast-fed infants[181] and others prevention of atopic disease by breast-feeding[182]

TABLE 9
Prevention of Gastrointestinal Allergy

A. Identification of Infants at Risk (atopy/food allergy)
Family history of atopy
Cord blood IgE ≥ 0.9 kU/L

B. Dietary Prevention
Proven effect: Maternal diet during lactation
Possible effect: Late introduction of solid foods (>6 months)
　　Avoidance of cow's milk, egg (infancy)
No effect: Maternal diet during late pregnancy
Consequence: Exlcusive breast-feeding (4–6 months) in high-risk
　　infants (effect of hydrolysate formula not proven)

C. Caveat: Other Epidemiologic Factors
Parental smoking, pets, molds, mites

---

and by late introduction of solid foods (after 6 months).[183] Contrary findings were reported, and the topic remained controversial for some time.[184,185] Studies were extremely variable in design, size, and quality, and no firm conclusions could be drawn (for discussion see references 185 and 188).

Recently, well-designed controlled prospective studies on dietary prevention of food allergy and atopic disease have been initiated, most of which are still underway (Table 9). The major precondition for preventive studies is an adequate definition of infants at risk to develop food allergy or atopy. Epidemiologic studies have provided us with firm data on this (see Table 8,A; reference 60; see above). Based on clear-cut identification of infants at risk, these recent studies[186–191] have found new evidence, although some of the drawbacks of earlier studies do still apply. Thus, maternal diet during late pregnancy (when intrauterine sensitization may occur) has been found to be without effect on development of atopic sensitization and on the production of IgG and IgE antibodies to food in their infants.[189] During lactation, there was a beneficial effect of maternal food antigen avoidance while breast-feeding on the occurrence and severity of atopic eczema in the infants.[190] Contrary to earlier findings, one study[192] reported that artificially fed infants at risk to develop atopy exhibited a lower incidence of allergic symptoms than breast-fed controls before 18 months of age. There was no mention of maternal diet in this study. Long-term follow-up studies, including GI and non-GI manifestations of food allergy, have to be completed before final answers are available.

It has to be kept in mind, however, that there was no clear distinction made between food-allergic and atopic individuals in almost all of these studies. Moreover, exposure to other environmental factors like parental smoking, pets, and house dust allergens has not been controlled for. Dietary measures of allergen avoidance certainly are only a very limited approach to prevent atopic disease in general.

Protein hydrolysate formula has been used by some authors as a substitute for breast milk in allergy prevention,[187,188] but no preventive effect has been shown in infants. The widespread enthusiasm for hydrolysate formula for infants at risk to develop food allergy and atopy is enhanced by economic interests of some infant food producers, but it lacks backing by substantial and rational evidence. It should be warned against as long as there is no proof of preventive effects of hydrolysate formula. This specialized formula should be limited to therapeutic use.

The application of drugs like DSCG and ketotifen in prevention of food allergy has been reported in noninfant patients.[193,194] There is no clear-cut separation between symptom prevention and therapy in these studies, and major criticism applies, just as to therapy studies (see above). At present, no pharmacologic prevention of food allergy has been proven effective.

Gerrard's verdict that food allergy, at least cow's milk allergy in infants, "should in its turn become a historical curiosity"[2] does not appear to be timely in view of prevention studies cited, and GI food allergy probably will pose problems and questions for many more pediatric generations to come.

REFERENCES

1. Goldstein GB, Heiner DC. Clinical and immunological perspectives in food allergy. J Allergy Clin Immunol 1970; 46:270–291.
2. Bahna SL, Heiner DC. Allergies to milk. New York: Grune & Stratton, 1980.
3. Stern M, Walker WA. Food allergy and intolerance. Pediatr Clin North Am 1985; 32:471–492.
4. Brostoff J, Challacombe SJ. Food allergy and intolerance. London: Bailliere Tindall, 1987.
5. Lessof MH. Food intolerance and allergy—a review. Q J Med 1983; 52:111–119.
6. Ford RPK, Hill DJ, Hosking CS. Cow's milk hypersensitivity: immediate and delayed onset clinical patterns. Arch Dis Child 1983; 58:856–862.
7. May C. Defined versus ill-defined syndromes associated with food sensitivity. J Allergy Clin Immunol 1986; 78:144–148.
8. Warner JO, Hathaway MJ. Allergic form of Meadow's syndrome (Münchhausen by proxy). Arch Dis Child 1984; 59:151–156.
9. Rona RJ, Chinn S. Parents' perceptions of food intolerance in primary school chldren. Br Med J 1987; 294:863–866.
10. Gerrard JW, Mackenzie JWA, Goluboff N, Garson JZ, Maningas CS. Cow's milk allergy: prevalence and manifestations in an unselected series of newborns. Acta Paediatr Scand (suppl) 1973; 234:1–21.
11. Wood CB. How common is food allergy? Acta Paediatr Scand (suppl) 1986; 323:76–83.
12. Jakobsson I, Lindberg T. A prospective study of cow's milk protein intolerance in Swedish infants. Acta Paediatr Scand 1979; 68:853–859.
13. Businco L, Benincori N, Cantani A, Tacconi L, Picarazzi A. Chronic diarrhea due to cow's milk allergy. A 4 to 10 year follow-up study. Ann Allergy 1985; 55:844–847.
14. Bock SA. Prospective appraisal of complaints of adverse reactions to foods in children during the first 3 years of life. Pediatrics 1987; 79:683–688.
15. Eggleston PA. Prospective studies in the natural history of food allergy. Ann Allergy 1987; 59:179–182.
16. Verkasalo M, Kuitunen P, Savilahti E. Changing pattern of cow's milk intolerance. Acta Paediatr Scand 1981; 70:289–295.
17. Walker WA. Transmucosal passage of antigens. In: Schmidt E, Reinhardt MC, eds. Food allergy. New York: Raven Press, 1988: 15.
18. Owen RL. Sequential uptake of horseradish peroxidase by lymphoid follicle epithelium of Peyer's patches in the normal unobstructed mouse intestine: an ultrastructural study. Gastroenterology 1977; 72:440–451.
19. Udall JN, Pang K, Fritze L, Kleinman R, Walker WA. Development of gastrointestinal mucosal barrier. I. The effect of age on intestinal permeability to macromolecules. Pediatr Res 1981; 15:241–244.
20. Husby S, Jensenius JC, Svehag SE. Passage of undegraded dietary antigen into the blood of healthy adults. Scand J Immunol 1985; 22:83–92.
21. Roberton DM, Paganelli R, Dinwiddie R, Levinsky RJ. Milk antigen absorption in the preterm and term neonate. Arch Dis Child 1982; 57:369–372.
22. Jakobsson I, Lindberg T, Lothe L, Axelsson I, Benediktsson B. Human alpha-lactalbumin as a marker of macromolecular absorption. Gut 1986; 27:1029–1034.
23. Müller G, Bernsau I, Müller W, Weissbarth-Riedel E, Natzschka J, Rieger CHL. Cow milk protein antigens and antibodies in serum of

premature infants during the first 10 days of life. J Pediatr 1986; 109:869–873.

24. Heyman M, Boudraa G, Sarrut S, Giraud M, Evans L, Touhami M, Desjeux JF. Macromolecular transport in jejunal mucosa of children with severe malnutrition: a quantitative study. J Pediatr Gastroenterol Nutr 1984; 3:357–363.

25. Sissons JW, Thurston SM. Survival of dietary antigens in the digestive tract of calves intolerant to soyabean products. Res Vet Sci 1984; 37:242–246.

26. Stern M, Walker WA. Food proteins and gut mucosal barrier. I. Binding and uptake of cow's milk proteins by adult rat jejunum in vitro. Am J Physiol 1984; 246:G556–G562.

27. Stern M, Pang KY, Walker WA. Food proteins and gut mucosal barrier. II. Differential interaction of cow's milk proteins with the mucous coat and the surface membrane of adult and immature rat jejunum. Pediatr Res 1984; 18:1252–1256.

28. Stern M, Gellermann B. Food proteins and maturation of small intestinal microvillus membranes (MVM). I. Binding characteristics of cow's milk proteins and concanavalin A to MVM from newborn and adult rats. J Pediatr Gastroenterol Nutr 1988; 7:115–121.

29. Pang KY, Bresson JL, Walker WA. Development of the gastrointestinal mucosal barrier. Evidence for structural differences in microvillus membranes from newborn and adult rabbits. Biochim Biophys Acta 1983; 727:201–208.

30. Snyder JD, Walker WA. Structure and function of intestinal mucin: developmental aspects. Int Arch Allergy Appl Immunol 1987; 82:351–356.

31. Spies JR, Stevan MA, Stein WJ, Coulson EJ. The chemistry of allergens. XX. New antigens generated by pepsin hydrolysis of bovine milk proteins. J Allergy 1970; 45:208–219.

32. Schwartz HR, Nerurkar LS, Spies JR, Scanlon RT, Bellanti JA. Milk hypersensitivity: RAST studies using new antigens generated by pepsin hydrolysis of beta-lactoglobulin. Ann Allergy 1980; 45:242–245.

33. Faellstroem SP, Ahlstedt S, Carlsson B, Loennerdal B, Hanson LA. Serum antibodies against native, processed and digested cow's milk proteins in children with cow's milk protein intolerance. Clin Allergy 1986; 16:417–423.

34. Ferguson TA, Peters T, Reed R, Pesce AJ, Michael JG. Immunoregulatory properties of antigenic fragments from bovine serum albumin. Cell Immunol 1983; 78:1–12.

35. Bruce MG, Ferguson A. The influence of intestinal processing on the immunogenicity and molecular size of absorbed, circulating ovalbumin in mice. Immunology 1986; 59:295–300.

36. McNabb PC, Tomasi TB. Host defense mechanisms at mucosal surfaces. Ann Rev Microbiol 1981; 35:477–496.

37. Hanson LA, Ahlstedt S, Andersson B, Carlsson M, Cole ME, Cruz JR, Dahlgren U, Ericsson TH, Jalil F, Khan SR, Mellander L, Schneerson R, Svanborg Eden C, Söderström T, Wadsworth C. Mucosal immunity. Ann NY Acad Sci 1983; 409:1–21.

38. Bienenstock J, Befus AD. Some thoughts on the biologic role of immunoglobulin A. Gastroenterology 1983; 84:178–185.

39. Ferguson A, McI Mowat A, Strobel S. Abrogation of tolerance to fed antigen and induction of cell-mediated immunity in the gut-associated lymphoreticular tissues. Ann NY Acad Sci 1983; 406:486–497.

40. Weaver LT, Koritz TN, Coombs RRA. Tolerance to orally induced anaphylactic sensitization to cow's milk proteins and patency of the intestinal mucosa in the neonatal guinea pig. Int Arch Allergy Appl Immunol 1987; 83:220–222.

41. Wold AE, Dahlgren UIH, Ahlstedt S, Hanson LA. Lack of IgA antibody response in secretions of rat dams during long-term ovalbumin feeding. Int Arch Allergy Appl Immunol 1987; 84:332–338.

42. Perkkiö M, Savilahti E. Time of appearance of immunoglobulin-containing cells in the mucosa of the neonatal intestine. Pediatr Res 1980; 14:953–955.

43. Rieger CHL, Rothberg RM. Development of the capacity to produce specific antibody to an ingested food antigen in the premature infant. J Pediatr 1975; 87:515–518.

44. Lebenthal E. Cow's milk protein allergy. Pediatr Clin North Am 1975; 22:827–833.

45. Aas K. The biochemistry of food allergens. What is essential for future research. In: Schmidt E, Reinhardt MC, eds. Food allergy. New York: Raven Press (in press).

46. Taylor SL, Lemanske RF Jr, Bush RK, Busse WW. Food allergens: structure and immunologic properties. Ann Allergy 1987; 59:93–99.

47. Coombs RR, McLaughlan P. Allergenicity of food proteins and its possible modification. Ann Allergy 1984; 53:592–596.

48. Høst A, Samuelsson EG. Allergic reactions to raw, pasteurized, and homogenized/pasteurized cow milk: a comparison. A double-blind placebo-controlled study in milk allergic children. Allergy 1988; 43:113–118.

49. Cant A, Marsden RA, Kilshaw PJ. Egg and cow's milk hypersensitivity in exclusively breast fed infants with eczema, and detection of egg protein in breast milk. Br Med J 1985; 291:932–935.

50. Machtinger S, Moss R. Cow's milk allergy in breast-fed infants: the role of allergen and maternal secretory IgA antibody. J Allergy Clin Immunol 1986; 77:341–347.

51. Gerrard JW, Perelmutter L. IgE-mediated allergy to peanut, cow's milk, and egg in children with special reference to maternal diet. Ann Allergy 1986; 56:351–354.

52. Ament ME, Rubin CE. Soy protein—another cause of the flat intestinal lesion. Gastroenterology 1972; 62:227–234.

53. Perkkiö M, Savilahti E, Kuitunen P. Morphometric and immunohistochemical study of jejunal biopsies from children with intestinal soy allergy. Eur J Pediatr 1981; 137:63–69.

54. Shibasaki M, Suzuki S, Tajima S, Nemoto H, Kuroume T. Allergenicity of major components of soybean. Int Arch Allergy Appl Immunol 1980; 61:441–448.

55. Anet J, Back JF, Baker RS, Barnett D, Burley RW, Howden ME. Allergens in the white and yolk of hen's egg. A study of IgE binding by egg proteins. Int Arch Allergy Appl Immunol 1985; 77:364–371.

56. Fries JH. Peanuts: allergic and other untoward reactions. Ann Allergy 1982; 48:220–226.

57. Dreborg S, Foucard T. Allergy to apple, carrot and potato in children with birch pollen allergy. Allergy 1983; 38:167–172.

58. Nagpal S, Metcalfe DD, Rao PV. Identification of a shrimp-derived allergen as tRNA. J Immunol 1987; 138:4169–4174.

59. Miller JB. Hidden food ingredients, chemical food additives and incomplete food labels. Ann Allergy 1978; 41:93–98.

60. Kjellman NIM. Epidemiology of food allergy. In: Schmidt E, Reinhardt MC, eds. Food allergy. New York: Raven Press (in press).

61. Croner S, Kjellman NIM, Eriksson B, Roth A. IgE screening in 1701 newborn infants and the development of atopic disease during infancy. Arch Dis Child 1982; 57:364–368.

62. Hattevig G, Kjellman B, Björksten B. Clinical symptoms and IgE responses to common food proteins and inhalants in the first 7 years of life. Clin Allergy 1987; 17:571–578.

63. Rowntree S, Cogswell JJ, Platts-Mills TA, Mitchell EB. Development of IgE and IgG antibodies to food and inhalant antigens in children at risk of allergic disease. Arch Dis Child 1985; 60:727–735.

64. Stintzing G, Zetterstroem R. Cow's milk allergy, incidence and pathogenetic role of early exposure to cow's milk formula. Acta Paediatr Scand 1979; 68:383–387.

65. van Asperen PP, Kemp AS, Mellis CM. Immediate food hypersensitivity reactions on the first known exposure to the food. Arch Dis Child 1983; 58:253–256.

66. Lucas A, McLaughlan R, Coombs RR. Latent anaphylactic sensitization of infants of low birth weight to cow's milk proteins. Br Med J 1984; 289:1254–1256.

67. Cunningham-Rundles C. Isolation and analysis of anti-idiotypic antibodies from IgA-deficient sera. Ann NY Acad Sci 1983; 409:469–477.

68. Walker-Smith JA. Cow's milk intolerance as a cause of postenteritis diarrhoea. J Pediatr Gastroenterol Nutr 1982; 1:163–173.

69. Gunther M, Aschaffenburg R, Matthews RH, Parish WE, Coombs RRA. The levels of antibodies to the proteins of cow's milk in the serum of normal infants. Immunology 1960; 3:296–306.

70. May CD, Fomon SJ, Remigio L. Immunologic consequences of feeding infants with cow's milk and soy products. Acta Paediatr Scand 1982; 71:43–51.

71. Dannaeus A, Johansson SGO, Foucard T, Ohman S. Clinical and immunlogical aspects of food allergy in childhood. I. Estimation of IgG, IgA, and IgE antibodies to food antigens in children with food allergy and atopic dermatitis. Acta Paediatr Scand 1977; 66:31–37.

72. Stern M, Stupp W, Grüttner R. Cow's milk protein antibodies determined by immunofluorescence (RIFT) in cow's milk protein intolerance and in controls. Monatsschr Kinderheilkd 1982; 130:556–561.

73. Pearson JR, Kingston D, Shiner M. Antibody production to milk proteins in the jejunal mucosa of children with cow's milk protein intolerance. Pediatr Res 1983; 17:406–412.

74. Shah PC, Freier S, Park BH, Lee PC, Lebenthal E. Pancreozymin and secretin enhance duodenal fluid antibody levels to cow's milk proteins. Gastroenterology 1982; 83:916–921.

75. McDonald PJ, Goldblum RM, van Sickle GJ, Powell GK. Food protein-induced enterocolitis: altered antibody response to ingested antigen. Pediatr Res 1984; 18:751–755.

76. Firer MA, Hosking CS, Hill DJ. Humoral immune response to cow's milk in children with cow's milk allergy. Relationship to the time of clinical response to cow's milk challenge. Int Arch Allergy Appl Immunol 1987; 84:173–177.

77. Shakib F, Brown HM, Phelps A, Redhead R. Study of IgG sub-class antibodies in patients with milk intolerance. Clin Allergy 1986; 16:451–458.

78. Rowntree S, Platts-Mills TA, Cogswell JJ, Mitchell EB. A subclass IgG4-specific antigen-binding radioimmunoassay (RIA): comparison between IgG and IgG4 antibodies to food and inhaled antigens in adult atopic dermatitis after desensitization treatment and during development of antibody responses in children. J Allergy Clin Immunol 1987; 80:622–630.

79. Hill DJ, Firer MA, Shelton MJ, Hosking CS. Manifestations of milk allergy in infancy: clinical and immunologic findings. J Pediatr 1986; 109:270–276.

80. Dannaeus A, Johansson SGO. A follow-up study of infants with adverse reactions to cow's milk. I. Serum IgE, skin test reactions and RAST in relation to clincial course. Acta Paediatr Scand 1979; 68:377–382.

81. Björksten B, Ahlstedt S, Björksten F, Carlsson B, Fällström SP, Juntunen K, Kajosaari M, Kober A. Immunoglobulin E and immunoglobulin G4 antibodies to cow's milk in children with cow's milk allergy. Allergy 1983; 38:119–124.

82. Gjesing B, Osterballe O, Schwartz B, Wahn U, Lowenstein H. Allergen-specific IgE antibodies against antigenic components in cow milk and milk substitutes. Allergy 1986; 41:51–56.

83. Pastorello EA, Pravettoni V, Bigi A, Qualizza R, Vassellatti D, Schilke ML, Stocchi L, Tedeschi A, Ansaloni R, Zanussi C. IgE-mediated food allergy. Ann Allergy 1987; 59:82–89.

84. Marcucci F, Sensi LG, Bizzarri G. Specific IgE to food and inhalant allergens in intestinal washings of children affected by atopic eczema. Clin Allergy 1985; 15:345–354.

85. Kolmannskog S, Haneberg B. Immunoglobulin E in feces from children with allergy. Evidence of local production of IgE in the gut. Int Arch Allergy Appl Immunology 1985; 76:133–137.

86. Rosekrans PCM, Meijer CJLM, Cornelisse CJ, vdWal AM, Lindeman J. Use of morphometry and immunohistochemistry of small intestinal biopsy specimens in the diagnosis of food allergy. J Clin Pathol 1980; 33:125–130.

87. Sampson HA. IgE-mediated food intolerance. J Allergy Clin Immunol 1988; 81:495–504.

88. Amlot PL, Kemeny DM, Zachary C, Parkes P, Lessof MH. Oral allergy syndrome (OAS): symptoms of IgE-mediated hypersensitivity to foods. Clin Allergy 1987; 17:33–42.

89. Carini C, Brostoff J, Wraith DG. IgE complexes in food allergy. Ann Allergy 1987; 59:110–117.

90. Amlot PL, Urbanek R, Youlten LJ, Kemeny M, Lessof MH. Type I allergy to egg and milk proteins: comparison of skin prick tests with nasal, buccal, and gastric provocation tests. Int Arch Allergy Appl Immunol 1985; 77:171–173.

91. Atkins FM, Steinberg SS, Metcalfe DD. Evaluation of immediate adverse reactions to foods in adult patients. I. Correlation of demographic, laboratory, and prick skin test data with response to controlled oral food challenge. J Allergy Clin Immunol 1985; 75:348–355.

92. Reimann HJ, Ring J, Ultsch B, Wendt P. Intragastral provocation under endoscopic control (IPEC) in food allergy: mast cell and histamine changes in gastric mucosa. Clin Allergy 1985; 15:195–202.

93. Selbekk BH. A comparison between in vitro jejunal mast cell degranulation and intragastric challenge in patients with suspected food intolerance. Scand J Gastroenterol 1985; 20:299–303.

94. May CD. High spontaneous release of histamine in vitro from leukocytes of persons hypersensitive to food. J Allergy Clin Immunol 1976; 58:432–437.

95. Sampson HA, Jolie PL. Increased plasma histamine concentrations after food challenges in children with atopic dermatitis. N Engl J Med 1984; 311:372–376.

96. Clinton PM, Kemeny DM, Amlot P, Urbanek R, Lessof MH. Histamine release from peripheral blood leucocytes in egg-allergic patients. Clin Allergy 1986; 16:345–354.

97. Lessof MH, Anderson JB. Prostaglandins and other mediators in food intolerance. Clin Rev Allergy 1984; 2:79–93.

98. Cant AJ, Gibson P, Dancy M. Food hypersensitivity made life-threatening by ingestion of aspirin. Br Med J 1984; 288:755–756.

99. Shiner M. Ultrastructural features of allergic manifestations in the small intestine of children. Scand J Gastroenterol (suppl) 1981; 70:49–64.

100. Savilahti E. Immunochemical study of the malabsorption syndrome with cow's milk intolerance. Gut 1973; 14:491–501.

101. Bock SA, Remigio LK, Gordon B. Immunochemical localization of proteins in the intestinal mucosa of children with diarrhea. J Allergy Clin Immunol 1983; 72:262–268.

102. Frick OL. B-lactoglobulin in immune complexes in milk-sensitive children. J Allergy Clin Immunol 1982; 69:157.

103. Leary HL Jr, Halsey JF. An assay to measure antigen-specific immune complexes in food allergy. J Allergy Clin Immunol 1984; 74:190–195.

104. Paganelli R, Quinti I, D'Offizi GP, Papetti C, Carini C, Aiuti F. Immune complexes in food allergy: a critical reappraisal. Ann Allergy 1987; 59:157–161.

105. Cunningham-Rundles C, Brandeis WE, Good RH. Bovine antigens and the formation of circulating immune complexes in selective immunoglobulin A deficiency. J Clin Invest 1979; 64:272–279.

106. McCrory WW, Becker CG, Cunningham-Rundles C, Klein RF, Mouradian J, Reisman L. Immune complex glomerulopathy in a child with food hypersensitivity. Kidney Int 1986; 30:592–598.

107. Phillips AD, Rice SJ, France NE, Walker-Smith JA. Small intestinal intraepithelial lymphocyte levels in cow's milk protein intolerance. Gut 1979; 20:509–512.

108. Kosnai I, Kuitunen P, Savilahti E, Rapola J, Köhegyi J. Cell kinetics in the jejunal crypt epithelium in malabsorption syndrome with cow's milk protein intolerance and in coeliac disease. Gut 1980; 21:1041–1046.

109. Weil S, Kuperman O, Ilfeld D, Finelt M, Freier S. Nonspecific suppressor cell activity and lymphocyte response to beta-lactoglobulin in cow's milk protein hypersensitivity. J Pediatr Gastroenterol Nutr 1982; 1:389–393.

110. Fällström SP, Lindholm L, Ahlstedt S. Cow's milk protein intolerance in children is connected with impaired lymphoblastic responses to mitogens. Int Arch Allergy Appl Immunol 1983; 70:205–206.

111. Van Sickle GJ, Powell GK, McDonald PJ, Goldblum RM. Milk- and soy protein-induced enterocolitis: evidence for lymphocyte sensitization to specific food proteins. Gastroenterology 1985; 88:1915–1921.

112. Kay RA, Ferguson A. Intestinal T cells, mucosal cell-mediated immunity and their relevance to food allergic disease. Clin Rev Allergy 1984; 2:55–68.

113. David TJ. Anaphylactic shock during elimination diets for severe atopic eczema. Arch Dis Child 1984; 59:983–986.

114. Kuitunen P, Rapola J, Savilahti E, Visakorpi JK. Response of the jejunal mucosa to cow's milk in the malabsorption syndrome with cow's milk intolerance. A light and electron-microscopic study. Acta Paediatr Scand 1973; 62:585–595.

115. Walker-Smith J. Cow's milk protein intolerance. Transient food intolerance of infancy. Arch Dis Child 1975; 50:347–350.

116. Manuel PD, Walker-Smith JA, France NE. Patchy enteropathy in childhood. Gut 1979; 20:211–215.

117. Waldmann TA, Wochner RD, Laster L, Gordon RS. Allergic gastroenteropathy. A cause of excessive gastrointestinal protein loss. N Engl J Med 1967; 276:761–769.

118. Caldwell JH, Sharma HM, Hurtubise PE, Colwell DL. Eosinophilic gastroenteritis in extreme allergy. Immunopathological comparison with non-allergic gastrointestinal disease. Gastroenterology 1979; 77:560–564.

119. Katz AJ, Twarog FJ, Zeiger RS, Falchuk ZM. Milk-sensitive and eosinophilic gastroenteropathy: similar clinical features with contrasting mechanisms and clinical course. J Allergy Clin Immunol 1984; 74:72–78.

120. Gryboski JD, Burkle F, Hillman R. Milk-induced colitis in an infant. Pediatrics 1966; 38:299–302.

121. Jenkins HR, Pincott JR, Soothill JF, Milla PJ, Harries JT. Food allergy: the major cause of infantile colitis. Arch Dis Child 1984; 59:326–329.

122. Goldman H, Proujansky R. Allergic proctitis and gastroenteritis in

children. Clinical and mucosal biopsy features in 53 cases. Am J Surg Pathol 1986; 10:75–86.

123. Lake AM, Whitington PF, Hamilton SR. Dietary protein-induced colitis in breast-fed infants. J Pediatr 1982; 101:906–910.

124. Halpin TC, Byrne WJ, Ament ME. Colitis, persistent diarrhea, and soy protein intolerance. J Pediatr 1977; 91:404–407.

125. Rosekrans PCM, Meijer CJ, vd Wal AM, Lindeman J. Allergic proctitis, a clinical and immunopathological entity. Gut 1980; 21:1017-1-23.

126. de Peyer E, Walker-Smith JA. Cow's milk intolerance presenting as necrotizing enterocolitis. Helv Paediatr Acta 1977; 32:509–515.

127. Fomon SJ, Ziegler EE, Nelson SE, Edwards BB. Cow milk feeding in infancy: gastrointestinal blood loss and iron nutritional status. J Pediatr 1981; 98:541–545.

128. Wilson JF, Lahey ME, Heiner DC. Studies on iron metabolism. V. Further observations on cow's milk induced gastrointestinal bleeding in infants with iron-deficiency anemia. J Pediatr 1974; 84:335–344.

129. Pittschieler K. Cow's milk protein intolerance as a cause of small bowel occlusion. Helv Paediatr Acta 1986; 41:461–464.

130. Robertson D, Wright R. Oedema of the ileum: a possible manifestation of food allergy. Br Med J 1987; 294:350.

131. Forget P, Arends JW. Cow's milk protein allergy and gastro-oesophageal reflux. Eur J Pediatr 1985; 144:298–300.

132. Lothe L, Lindberg T, Jakobsson I. Cow's milk formula as a cause of infantile colic: a double-blind study. Pediatrics 1982; 70:7–10.

133. Bentley D, Katchburian A, Brostoff J. Abdominal migraine and food sensitivity in children. Clin Allergy 1984; 14:499–500.

134. Petitpierre M, Gumowski P, Girard JP. Irritable bowel syndrome and hypersensitivity to food. Ann Allergy 1985; 54:538–540.

135. Heiner DC. Respiratory diseases and food allergy. Ann Allergy 1984; 53:657–664.

136. Pastorello E, Ortolani C, Luraghi MT, Pravettoni V, Sillano V, Froldi M, Amabile G, Zanussi C. Evaluation of allergic etiology in perennial rhinitis. Ann Allergy 1985; 55:854–856.

137. Wilson NM. Food related asthma: a difference between two ethnic groups. Arch Dis Child 1985; 60:861–865.

138. Onorato J, Merland N, Terral C, Michel FB, Bousquet J. Placebo-controlled double-blind food challenge in asthma. J Allergy Clin Immunol 1986; 78:1139–1146.

139. Pelikan Z, Pelikan-Filipek M. Bronchial response to the food ingestion challenge. Ann Allergy 1987; 58:164–172.

140. Hannuksela M. Food allergy and skin diseases. Ann Allergy 1983; 51:269–271.

141. Juhlin L. Recurrent urticaria: clinical investigation of 330 patients. Br J Dermatol 1981; 104:369–381.

142. Firer MA, Hosking CS, Hill DJ. Cow's milk allergy and eczema: patterns of antibody response to cow's milk in allergic skin disease. Clin Allergy 1982; 12:385–390.

143. Salo OP, Maekinen-Kiljunen S, Juntunen K. Milk causes a rapid urticarial reaction on the skin of children with atopic dermatitis and milk allergy. Acta Derm Venereol 1986; 66:438–442.

144. Sampson HA. Role of immediate food hypersensitivity in the pathogenesis of atopic dermatitis. J Allergy Clin Immunol 1983; 71:473–480.

145. Sampson HA, McCaskill CC. Food hypersensitivity and atopic dermatitis: evaluation of 113 patients. J Pediatr 1985; 107:669–675.

146. Atherton DJ, Sewell M, Soothill JF, Wells RS, Chilvers CED. A double-blind controlled cross-over trial of an antigen avoidance diet in atopic eczema. Lancet 1978; i:401–403.

147. Panush RS, Stroud RM, Webster EM. Food-induced (allergic) arthritis. Inflammatory arthritis exacerbated by milk. Arthritis Rheum 1986; 29:220–226.

148. McCrory WW, Becker CG, Cunningham-Rundles C, Klein RF, Mouradian J, Reisman L. Immune complex glomerulopathy in a child with food hypersensitivity. Kidney Int 1986; 30:592–598.

149. Egger J, Carter C, Wilson J, Turner MW, Soothill JF. Is migraine food allergy? A double-blind controlled trial of oligo-antigenic diet treatment. Lancet 1983; ii:865–869.

150. Monro J, Carini C, Brostoff J. Migraine is a food-allergic disease. Lancet 1984; i:719–721.

151. Mansfield LE, Vaughan TR, Waller SF, Haverly RW, Ting S. Food allergy and adult migraine: double-blind and mediator confirmation of an allergic etiology. Ann Allergy 1985; 55:126–129.

152. Feingold B. Why your child is hyperactive. New York: Random House, 1975.

153. Lipton MA, Mayo JP. Diet and hyperkinesis—an update. J Am Diet Assoc 1983; 83:132–134.

154. Egger J, Carter CM, Graham PJ, Gumley D, Soothill JF. Controlled trial of oligoantigenic treatment in the hyperkinetic syndrome. Lancet 1985; i:540–545.

155. Kahn A, Rebuffat E, Blum D, Casimir G, Duchateau J, Mozin MJ, Jost R. Difficulty in initiating and maintaining sleep associated with cow's milk allergy in infants. Sleep 1987; 10:116–121.

156. Goldman AS, Anderson DW, Sellers WA, Saperstein S, Kniker WT, Halpern SR. Milk allergy. I. Oral challenge with milk and isolated milk proteins in allergic children. Pediatrics 1963; 32:425–443.

157. Powell GK. Milk- and soy-induced enterocolitis of infancy: clinical features and standardization of challenge. J Pediatr 1978; 93:553–560.

158. Atkins FM, Metcalfe DD. The diagnosis and treatment of food allergy. Ann Rev Nutr 1984; 4:233–255.

159. Bock SA. Food sensitivity: a critical review and practical approach. Am J Dis Child 1980; 134:973–982.

160. Leinhas JL, McCaskill CC, Sampson HA. Food allergy challenges: guidelines and implications. J Am Diet Assoc 1987; 87:604–608.

161. Metcalfe DD. A current practical approach to the diagnosis of suspected adverse reactions to foods. N Engl Reg Allergy Proc 1987; 8:22–26.

162. Hannuksela M. Diagnosis of dermatologic food allergy. Ann Allergy 1987; 59:153–156.

163. Johansson SG, Dannaeus A, Lilja G. The relevance of anti-food antibodies for the diagnosis of food allergy. Ann Allergy 1984; 53:665–672.

164. Sethi TJ, Lessof MH, Kemeny DM, Lambourn E, Tobin S, Bradley A. How reliable are commercial allergy tests? Lancet 1987; i:92–94.

165. McCarty EP, Frick OL. Food sensitivity: keys to diagnosis. J Pediatr 1983; 102:645–652.

166. Oehling A, Ona J, Trento H, Sanz ML, Dominguez MA. The diagnostic value of the histamine release test in food allergy. Allergol Immunopathol 1984; 12:439–448.

167. Khoshoo V, Bhan MK, Arora NK, Sood D, Kumar R, Stintzing G. Leucocyte migration inhibition in cow's milk protein intolerance. Acta Paediatr Scand 1986; 75:308–312.

168. Heycock E, Heatley RV, Shires SE, Littlewood JM. An in vitro test for cow's milk protein intolerance? Scand J Gastroenterol 1986; 21:1245–1249.

169. Berg NO, Jakobsson I, Lindberg T. Do pre- and postchallenge small intestinal biopsies help to diagnose cow's milk protein intolerance? Acta Paediatr Scand 1979; 68:657–661.

170. Ford RP, Barnes GL, Hill DJ. Gastrointestinal hypersensitivity to cow's milk protein: the diagnostic value of gut function tests. Aust Paediatr J 1986; 22:37–42.

171. Bahna SL. Management of food allergies. Ann Allergy 1984; 53:678–682.

172. Dannaeus A. Management of food allergy in infancy. Ann Allergy 1983; 51:303–306.

173. Editorial. How necessary are elimination diets in childhood? Br Med J 1980; i:138.

174. Pahud JJ, Schwarz K. Research and development of infant formulae with reduced allergenic properties. Ann Allergy 1984; 53:609–614.

175. Poulsen OM, Hau J. The two infant food formulae Pregestimil and Nutramigen used for feeding children allergic to cow's milk proteins. Allergy 1987; 42:158.

176. Francis DEM. Diets for sick children. Oxford: Blackwell, 1987.

177. Collins-Williams C. The role of pharmacologic agents in the prevention or treatment of allergic food disorders. Ann Allergy 1986; 57:53–60.

178. Sogn D. Medications and their use in the treatment of adverse reactions to foods. J Allergy Clin Immunol 1986; 78:238–243.

179. Businco L, Benincori N, Nini G, Businco E, Cantani A, De Angelis M. Double-blind crossover trial with oral sodium cromoglycate in children with atopic dermatitis due to food allergy. Ann Allergy 1986; 57:433–438.

180. Osvath P, Kelenhegyi K, Micskey E. Comparison of ketotifen and DSCG in treatment of food allergy in children. Allergol Immunopathol 1986; 14:515–518.

181. Halpern SR, Sellars WA, Johnson RB, Anderson DW, Saperstein S, Reisch JS. Development of childhood allergy in infants fed breast, soy or cow milk. J Allergy Clin Immunol 1973; 51:139–151.

182. Saarinen UM, Backman A, Kajosaari M, Siimes MA. Prolonged breast-feeding as prophylaxis for atopic disease. Lancet 1979; ii:163–166.

183. Kajosaari M, Saarinen UM. Prophylaxis of atopic disease by six months' total solid food elimination. Evaluation of 135 exclusively breast-fed infants of atopic families. Acta Paediatr Scand 1983; 72:411–414.

184. Kramer MS, Moroz B. Do breast-feeding and delayed introduction of solid foods protect against subsequent atopic eczema? J Pediatr 1981; 98:546–550.

185. Burr ML. Does infant feeding affect the risk of allergy? Arch Dis Child 1983; 58:561–565.

186. Bellanti JA. Prevention of food allergies. Ann Allergy 1984; 53:683–688.

187. Hamburger RN. Diagnosis of food allergies and intolerances in the study of prophylaxis and control groups in infants. Ann Allergy 1984; 53:673–677.

188. Zeiger RS, Heller S, Mellon M, O'Connor R, Hamburger RN. Effectiveness of dietary manipulation in the prevention of food allergy in infants. J Allergy Clin Immunol 1986; 78:224–238.

189. Lilja G, Dannaeus A, Fälth-Magnusson K, Graff-Lonnevig V, Johansson SGO, Kjellman NIM, Öman H. Immune response of the atopic woman and foetus: effects of high- and low-dose food allergen intake during late pregnancy. Clin Allergy 1988; 18:131–142.

190. Chandra RK, Puri S, Suraiya C, Cheema PS. Influence of maternal food antigen avoidance during pregnancy and lactation on incidence of atopic eczema in infants. Clin Allergy 1986; 16:563–569.

191. Hamburger RN, Casillas R, Johnson R, Mellon M, O'Connor RD, Zeiger R. Long-term studies in prevention of food allergy: patterns of IgG anti-cow's milk antibody responses. Ann Allergy 1987; 59:175–178.

192. Lindfors A, Enocksson E. Development of atopic disease after early administration of cow milk formula. Allergy 1988; 43:11–16.

193. Ortolani C, Pastorello E, Zanussi C. Prophylaxis of adverse reactions to foods. A double-blind study of oral sodium cromoglycate for the prophylaxis of adverse reactions to foods and additives. Ann Allergy 1983; 50:105–109.

194. Molkhou P, Dupont C. Ketotifen in prevention and therapy of food allergy. Ann Allergy 1987; 59:187–193.

PART
12

Pathogenesis of Intestinal Inflammation

Thomas T. MacDonald, B.Sc.(Hon.), Ph.D., M.R.C.Path.

Inflammation in the intestine, whether mediated by immunologic reactions, toxins, or infection, presents a major problem in children. The smaller size of children, especially neonates and infants, renders them more susceptible to the effects of intestinal water, electrolyte, or protein loss. Compromised colonic function can disrupt normal water and electrolyte economy, thus contributing to diarrhea. In addition, malabsorption in the small intestine secondary to inflammation can have severe nutritional consequences. As a general point, any condition that is associated with small intestinal villous atrophy and a reduction in the number of absorptive enterocytes causes reduction of brush border disaccharidases and peptidases, which may result in malabsorption.

Factors affecting the management of the pediatric patient are the deleterious effects of intestinal inflammation and malabsorption on their growth and development,[1] which can lead to delayed puberty and permanent short stature, as in the case of childhood Crohn's disease (for details, see elsewhere in this chapter). Growth failure is a problem in conditions of chronic intestinal inflammation such as inflammatory bowel disease rather than acute infectious diarrhea, which, although possibly more life-threatening, tends to have a relatively short course.

This discussion reviews the pathogenesis of intestinal inflammation in general, with particular reference to children and with a focus on the mechanisms of inflammation. For ease of discussion, the inflammatory process is subdivided into those with known causes, such as infection or food allergy, and idiopathic conditions such as lymphoid follicular hyperplasia, necrotizing enterocolitis, and inflammatory bowel disease. Details of the diagnosis and treatment in the particular inflammatory syndromes are covered in the relevant chapters elsewhere in the book.

PATHOGENESIS OF INTESTINAL INFLAMMATION IN FOOD ALLERGY

The term *food allergy* is used in this context to describe intestinal reactions to food in which an immune response can be shown to be the cause, or is highly likely to be the cause, of the intestinal inflammation.

IgE-Mediated Inflammation

Acute-onset reactions to many foods have been described, but the most common causes of IgE-mediated food allergies are cow's milk proteins and eggs. These disorders are usually transient in infancy but may persist throughout life. They are characteristically associated with elevated radioallergosorbent test (RAST) findings and positive skin-prick tests to the offending food antigens.[2] Clinically these acute-onset reactions are often associated with vomiting and abdominal pain as well as extraintestinal symptoms such as urticaria.[3] There is general agreement that the pathogenesis of this type of acute-onset reaction involves the cross-linking of IgE molecules on the mast cell surface in the mucosa by antigen. This results in rapid mast cell activation and the release of preformed mediators such as histamine, 5-hydroxytryptamine, eosinophil chemoattractants, proteoglycans, and tryptase and serine proteases.[4] In addition, the mast cell generates a number of mediators de novo after activation, such as prostaglandins, leukotrienes, and platelet-activating factor. These have multiple biologic effects, but in the gut most probably are important in causing smooth muscle contraction and increasing vascular and epithelial permeability. Recently two types of mast cells—mucosal mast cells and connective tissue mast cells—have been demonstrated in rodents. These differ in staining characteristics, size, response to secretagogues, and the type of proteoglycan they contain.[4] A current area of research is to determine whether such differences exist in man. Studies on primate and isolated human intestinal mast cells have shown that like rat mucosal mast cells, they do not release histamine when stimulated with the secretagogue 48/80. Thus, mast cell heterogeneity also probably exists in man.

The intestinal lesions caused by IgE-mediated reactions in humans have not been studied in detail, since it is obviously unethical to challenge and take a biopsy from an individual in whom the effect of the challenge is potentially life-threatening. However, in one study, food-allergic individuals were challenged on the gastric mucosa.[5] This caused swelling and erythema, mast cell degranulation was observed histologically, and histamine release was detected. Ultrastructural evidence of mast cell degranulation in jejunal biopsies after antigen challenge in the jejunum of two children with cow's milk allergy has also been obtained.[6] In rodents, experimental small intestinal IgE-mediated reactions can be easily elicited. These do not result in major changes in mucosal architecture[7]; however, there is extensive fluid leakage into the lumen, goblet cell discharge,[8] and, interestingly, increased uptake of bystander antigen.[9] Tissue

eosinophilia also develops, presumably owing to the eosinophil chemoattractant properties of mast cell products (Fig. 1).

Earlier reports described an increase in IgE-bearing cells in the intestine of infants with cow's milk protein intolerance[10]; however, it is difficult to distinguish between mast cells with surface IgE and IgE plasma cells. Since serum IgE can bind to mast cells in the mucosa, there is no a priori reason to expect IgE plasma cells in the mucosa to be increased in food allergy. Mast cell numbers are increased in celiac disease[11]; however, since IgE specific for gluten is not a feature of celiac disease, it is unlikely that IgE-mediated allergy is important in this condition. There is little information on mast cell density in the mucosa in other food allergies.

It is noteworthy that sensitization to cow's milk can occur in exclusively breast-fed infants via small amounts of cow's milk ingested by the mother and transmitted to the infant via breast milk.[12] The amount of antigen entering the infant gut to cause sensitization is very low, on the order of 1 to 5 pg per milliliter of milk.[120] After injection of 5 μg of iodinated bovine serum albumin (BSA) (10^7 counts per minute) into lactating mice, about 0.1 percent of the injected dose can be recovered from the stomach contents of individual pups 4 hours later.[118] Thirty-one percent of this radioactivity is trichloroacetic acid (TCA) precipitable, indicating that it is probably associated with intact BSA. In rats it is possible to elicit IgE responses with microgram amounts of antigen given orally.[13] Clearly every breast-fed infant must be exposed to small amounts of dietary maternal antigens in breast milk, but only in very rare cases does sensitization of the infant occur. Circulating maternal antibody may limit the transfer of antigen from the mother to the neonate,[118] but other factors in milk which may prevent sensitization to antigens to milk are poorly understood. Further details on gastrointestinal (GI) allergy are discussed elsewhere in this chapter.

FIGURE 1 Diagrammatic illustration of an IgE-mediated hypersensitivity reaction in the gut mucosa. On the left, mast cells in the lamina propria are coated with IgE. On the right, antigen has cross-linked the mast cell IgE, resulting in rapid mast cell degranulation. The mediators released cause fluid and protein leakage into the lumen due to increased epithelial permeability, the epithelial cells lift off the basement membrane, and eosinophils are attracted into the mucosa from the blood.

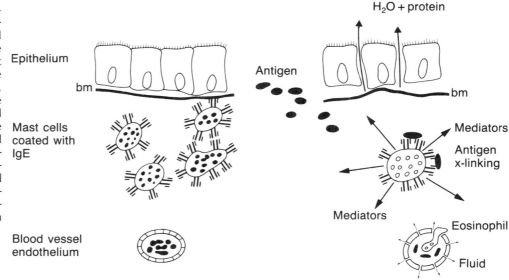

Immune Complex–Mediated Intestinal Damage

Serum antibodies to dietary antigens are common in normal children, especially infants,[14] and do not appear to be of any pathogenic significance. Children with celiac disease tend to have higher than normal antibody levels to gluten,[15] especially of the IgG1 and IgG3 isotypes[16]; however, their levels of antibodies to other foods are also raised.[17] Children with cow's milk protein intolerance also have increased serum antibodies to milk proteins.[3] Ultrastructural and immunofluorescent analysis of jejunal biopsies from children with cow's milk allergy challenged with milk has shown IgG and complement deposition in the lamina propria, suggestive of a local antigen-antibody reaction.[6] Ultrastructural changes also suggestive of immune complex formation have been described in the lamina propria of celiac children after gluten challenge.[18] In pigs, immune complex formation in the lamina propria results in a massive influx of neutrophils into the lumen, probably mediated by C3a and C5a, but there is little damage to intestinal structure.[19] Injection of preformed BSA immune complexes into rats causes rapid vascular congestion, mucosal edema, and necrosis, with some neutrophil infiltration.[20] However, the role such reactions play in the pathogenesis of intestinal inflammation in clinical food allergy is still unclear.[7] Of extreme interest is the description of celiac disease in a patient with hypogammaglobulinemia, which would indicate that anti-gliadin antibody is not necessary to develop the classic celiac flat mucosa.[21]

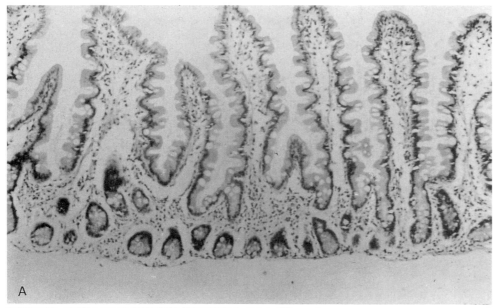

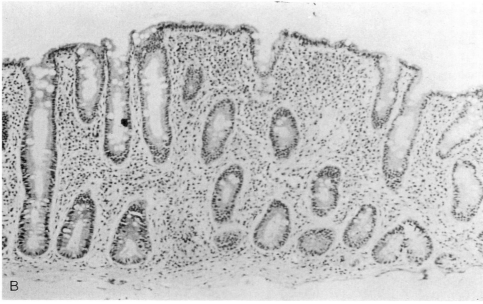

FIGURE 2 Histopathologic appearance of normal jejunal mucosa (*A*) and the flat jejunal mucosa of a child with untreated celiac disease (*B*). Note the increased lymphocytic infiltrate and the villous atrophy. The loss of surface area results in malabsorption. This morphologic appearance may be also be seen in severe giardiasis; however, in the latter there is little surface enterocyte damage (hematoxylin and eosin, original magnification ×100).

Cell-Mediated Immune Reactions to Food

Evidence is growing that cell-mediated immune reactions to food are important in food allergy.[22] Although peripheral blood lymphocytes from patients with food allergies show weak or negative reactions on challenge in vitro with specific antigen, the compartmental nature of the mucosal and systemic immune systems means that such negative results should not be overinterpreted. Late-onset enteropathy after milk ingestion and celiac disease have similar pathologic features, namely an increase in lymphocyte density in the epithelium and villous atrophy and crypt hypertrophy (Fig. 2). A major difference between these two conditions, however, is that celiac disease is a lifelong condition, whereas cow's milk protein enteropathy is a transient disease of children, usually infants.[3] The lesion in cow's milk protein enteropathy is usually less severe than that in celiac disease, and the mucosa is thinner than in celiac disease. A celiac-like mucosa is also found in patients with soy protein intolerance.[23]

The cellular infiltrate in the celiac mucosa has been extensively studied. There is an increase in plasma cells of all isotypes.[119] In untreated celiac disease there is an increase in the density of T cells in the lamina propria and the epithelium.[25] Gluten challenge causes a dose-dependent increase in intraepithelial lymphocytes[24]; however, the lymphocyte infiltrate is not accompanied by mucosal damage. This indicates that changes in epithelial lymphocyte numbers are secondary to immune reactions in the lamina propria. It is also unlikely that epithelial lymphocytes damage surface enterocytes in celiac disease, since there is also an increase in lymphocyte density in the hyperplastic crypts, but enterocyte morphology is unchanged.[37] Clinical relapse after commencement of a normal gluten-containing diet is quite variable, some children taking months to relapse.[3] Increased enterocyte HLA-DR expression suggests local production of interferon-gamma.[26] It is frequently forgotten that gluten sensitivity bears one of the hallmarks of an immune response, namely antigenic specificity. The strong association with HLA-DR3 and HLA-DQw2 is also suggestive of an immune-mediated reaction.[27] When cultured with gliadin in vitro, the lymphocytes in jejunal biopsies from celiac patients, but not controls, release lymphokines.[28] These data are summarized in Table 1.

One of the main problems in understanding celiac disease is that some patients with the characteristic HLA genotype can ingest gluten for many years before presenting clinically with overt celiac disease. This indicates that there must be some trigger that initiates the lesion. There is sequence homology between A-gliadin and adenovirus serotype 12, which has led to the suggestion that infection with this virus initiates an immune response that is perpetuated by antigens common to gluten and the virus.[29]

Perhaps the most compelling evidence that cell-mediated immunity to foods can cause intestinal damage comes from model systems. Cell-mediated immune reactions in mouse intestine cause villous atrophy and crypt cell hyperplasia.[30,31] Recent studies from the author's laboratory have extended these findings to human intestine. Taking the approach that if cell-mediated immune reactions can cause food allergy, then sensitization will have occurred *before* the patient presents with disease, we have focused on the effects of T-cell activa-

TABLE 1
Immunologic Basis for Celiac Disease

Antigen-specific disease
HLA-DR3 and DQw2 linked
Numerous T cells in the lesion
Increased HLA-DR expression on enterocytes
Antigen-specific lymphokine release from celiac biopsies
Increased anti-gliadin antibodies
Immunologic memory (T-cell response in the mucosa on challenge after years on gluten-free diet)

tion in human intestinal lamina propria.[32] Using explants of fetal human intestine cultured in vitro, the T cells present in the lamina propria can be activated directly by the addition of nontoxic lectins or monoclonal anti-CD3 antibody to the cultures. Within 72 hours this results in villous atrophy, crypt hypertrophy, and a dramatic increase in the rate of crypt cell proliferation (Fig. 3). These effects are inhibited by cyclosporin A, and the degree of tissue damage is related to the degree of mucosal T-cell activation.[32] In addition, T-cell activation results in interferon-gamma production, which causes increased epithelial HLA-DR expression.[33] Lamina propria T-cell activation also results in an increase in intraepithelial lymphocyte numbers, with most of the cells having the phenotype CD3+,4−,8−.[116]

These experiments formally demonstrate that activated T cells can cause a lesion in human intestine in organ culture, with many similarities to that seen in celiac disease and cow's milk protein enteropathy (Table 2), and it is highly likely that T cells produce these changes by releasing a factor mitogenic for crypt epithelial cells. However, it should be pointed out that one of the main features of celiac disease, namely surface enterocyte damage,[34] is not seen in the in vitro model system (Fig. 4).

Because the surface enterocyte is damaged in the flat mucosa of untreated celiac disease, attention has focused on the means by which damage to surface enterocytes can result in a mucosa with short villi and hyperplastic crypts. It should be pointed out that enterocyte damage is variable in untreated celiac disease.[35] Booth considered enterocyte damage to be a primary event in the pathogenesis of celiac disease, leading to increased epithelial cell loss, which in turn produced compensatory crypt cell hyperplasia.[36] It is noteworthy, however, that when partial villous atrophy appears in celiac disease, cow's milk protein enteropathy, and giardiasis, epithelial cell damage is not a prominent feature. In addition, even in a flat celiac mucosa, the enterocytes at the tops of the crypts are normal[37]; it is only when they migrate onto the surface that some of the epithelial cells become damaged. There is the possibility that enterocyte damage in celiac disease is a secondary phenomenon associated with changes in intestinal physiology and that the primary event in the pathogenesis of the flat mucosa is crypt hyperplasia. As long as mucosal thickness stays the same, crypt hyperplasia must result in villous atrophy. The two hypotheses to explain the cell-mediated genesis of a flat intestinal mucosa are shown in Figure 5, and the pathogenesis of food-sensitive enteropathy from sensitization to gut damage is shown in Figure 6.

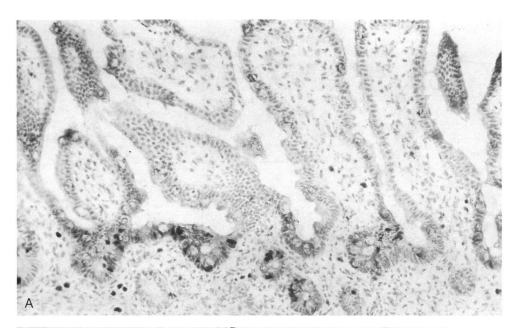

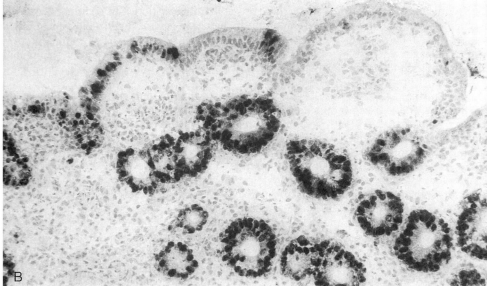

FIGURE 3 Appearance of jejunum from a 20-week-old fetus (*A*) and the appearance after 72 hours in explant culture in vitro in the presence of monoclonal anti-CD3 antibody to activate mucosal T cells (*B*).[32] Shown are frozen sections of fetal tissue stained by the immunoperoxidase method with a monoclonal antibody (Ki67) that identifies all dividing human cells.[32] In normal jejunum, cell division occurs in the crypts, with some in the lamina propria. Villi are long. After 3 days in culture with lamina propria T cells activated, there is villous atrophy and crypt cell hyperplasia (immunoperoxidase stain, original magnification ×100).

TABLE 2

Comparison Between the Lesion in Celiac Disease and T Cell–Mediated Enteropathy in Human Fetal Intestine in Organ Culture

Aspect of Mucosal Lesion	Celiac Disease	In Vitro Enteropathy
Villous atrophy	Yes	Yes
Crypt hyperplasia	Yes	Yes
Increased IEL density	Yes	Yes
Increased lamina propria T cells	Yes	Yes
Increased enterocyte HLA-DR expression	Yes	Yes
Increase in plasma cells	Yes	No
Enterocyte damage	Yes	No

Details of the changes in human intestine in the in vitro enteropathy model are taken from references 32, 33, and 116. There is no increase in plasma cells in the in vitro model, since there are no plasma cells and few B cells in fetal small intestine.[91]

IEL = intraepithelial lymphocyte.

Further evidence of a primary role for T cells in mediating villous atrophy and crypt hyperplasia comes from studies on patients with the T-cell tumor, malignant histiocytosis of the intestine (MHI).[38] In some, but not all, patients with this condition there is a history of gluten sensitivity. A hallmark of MHI is that in areas distant from the tumor mass the lesion is indistinguishable from untreated celiac disease. The major difference from celiac disease is that these patients are gluten refractory at the onset of the lymphoma. We interpret the flat mucosa in MHI to be a consequence of activated malignant T cells within the mucosa.

PATHOGENESIS OF INTESTINAL INFLAMMATION IN PARASITIC INFECTION

Although intestinal parasitic infection is less of a problem in the developed world, parasitic protozoa and helminths are endemic in the developing world. Since most intestinal para-

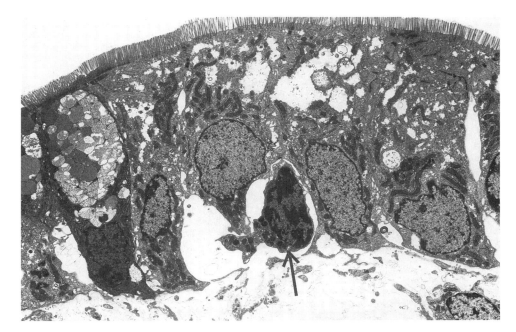

FIGURE 4 Electron microscopic appearance of surface epithelium in cultures of fetal human small intestine in which enteropathy has been induced by activating mucosal T cells. Note the normal microvillous structure and the epithelial goblet cell and columnar cells. A lymphocyte can also be seen in the epithelium (*arrow*) (×4,200).

CRYPT HYPERPLASIA SECONDARY TO ENTEROCYTE LOSS

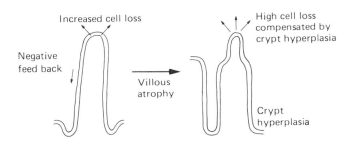

CRYPT HYPERPLASIA CAUSING THE FLAT MUCOSA

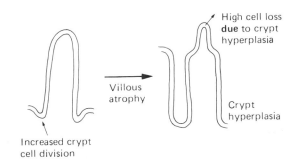

FIGURE 5 Diagrammatic illustration of two alternate mechanisms for the appearance of villous atrophy. The top panel depicts the conventional view, which is that crypt hyperplasia is secondary to increased loss of villous enterocytes. The lower panel illustrates the idea that crypt hyperplasia itself can produce an apparent villous atrophy. In the latter model, villous atrophy occurs because the crypts have moved up the side of the villus. As long as *total* mucosal thickness stays the same, crypt hypertrophy *must* produce villous atrophy.

sites are transmitted via contamination of food and water with fecal material, the lack of proper sanitary conditions is almost certainly the main cause of the high incidence of these infections. Because infants are more likely than older children or adults to ingest contaminated soil or water, there is a very high incidence of intestinal parasitic infection in infants. The pathogenesis and immune response to parasitic infections have been extensively studied in animal models, but there is relatively little information on the situation in humans. Although rodents infected with a parasitic nematode such as *Nippostrongylus brasiliensis* rapidly eliminate the worm from the intestine via a specific immune response,[39] the situation in humans is not clear and there is evidence that intestinal nematodes can survive for extended periods in the human intestine.[40]

Giardiasis

Giardia lamblia is a protozoan parasite with a world-wide prevalence which infects the upper small intestine. The trophozoite resides on the surface of the mucosa and is rarely invasive. Although most infections are subclinical and the host probably eliminates the infection from the upper small intestine by a specific IgA response,[41] chronic infection can occur in children and adults. In children chronic infection may be associated with growth failure, probably secondary to malabsorption.[42] The histologic appearance of the small bowel in patients with giardiasis can be normal; however, in more severe cases there may be crypt hyperplasia, villous atrophy, and an inflammatory infiltrate.[43] Enterocyte morphology is normal, although there may be shortening of the microvilli and disaccharidase levels may be low.[43] The lesion may be patchy. *Giardia* infection in mice has revealed that although the infection may not cause overt villous atrophy and crypt hypertrophy, the rate of epithelial cell turnover is dramatically increased.[44]

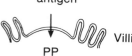

1. Sensitization to food proteins in Peyer's patches (PP)

2. Migration of activated T cells from PP to lamina propria

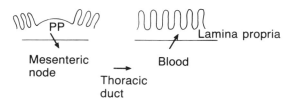

3. Sensitized T cells in lamina propria recognize antigen on the surface of lamina propria macrophages and dendritic cells

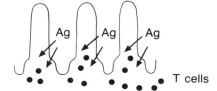

4a. Activated T cells release factors which increase crypt epithelial cell division and cause crypt hypertrophy

4b. Lamina propria T cell stimulation leads to cell division and increase in lamina propria T cells and IEL

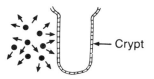

5. Crypt hypertrophy causes villous atrophy

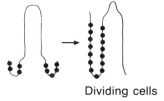

6. **Malabsorption:** caused by the replacement of mature villous enterocytes with less differentiated cells (lower enzyme levels) on the surface epithelium, as well as reduction in absorptive surface

FIGURE 6 Diagrammatic illustration of the sequence of events which results in the development of food-sensitive enteropathy. The following features are of importance. First, initial sensitization occurs in Peyer's patches. Second, disease occurs only if T cells in the lamina propria are re-exposed to antigen. Third, the target of the activated T cell is the crypt epithelial cell, which is induced to divide by the T-cell products.

Patients with defective cell-mediated immunity do not have an increased incidence of giardiasis; however, it can be a problem in common variable immunodeficiency, with up to 64 percent of patients affected.[45] These patients have no mucosal IgA plasma cells and prominent lymphoid nodules in their small intestine.[46] In severe cases these patients have a celiac-like flat mucosa, watery diarrhea, and weight loss. When *Giardia* is eliminated by chemotherapy the mucosa returns to normal.[43] It is tempting to speculate that it is the local T-cell response to *Giardia* antigens which is respon-

TABLE 3
Growth Retardation in Jamaican Children With Severe *Trichuris* Colitis

Patient	Age (yr)	Weight (kg)	Height (cm)	Height/Age (yr)	Height for Age (SDS)	Weight for Height (SDS)
1	7.07	13.7	102	4.03	−3.6	−1.7
2	5.12	11.3	94.5	3.2	−3.2	−2.1
3	4.5	9.3	94.5	2.96	−2.4	−3.2
4	8.85	15.3	106.2	4.88	−4.3	−1.5
5	4.05	13.06	90	2.45	−3.0	−0.3

Tanner-Whitehouse charts[115] are used for standard deviation scores (SDS). All children had *Trichuris* ova in their stools, and worms were identified in the stool after treatment with mibendazole at the Tropical Metabolism Research Unit, University of the West Indies, Kingston, Jamaica.

sible for the alterations in mucosal morphology and hence the disease. In the absence of IgA, parasite antigens could cross the epithelium to sensitize mucosal T cells. However, there is little evidence for T-cell response to *Giardia* other than the sometimes dramatic increase in intraepithelial lymphocytes during infection.[47]

Nematode Infections

Parasitic nematodes can occupy different microenvironments within the human GI tract. Roundworms such as *Ascaris* live in the lumen, *Trichinella spiralis* lives within the epithelium, hookworms live with their feeding parts buried in the mucosa, strongylids live in the mucosa, and *Trichuris trichiura* lives in the colon with its head buried under the epithelium. The exact impact of these parasites on human health is difficult to define, and there are very few hard clinical data on either the nature of the host protective immune response or the pathophysiology of infection. The decreasing level of infection with parasitic intestinal nematodes with increasing age can be taken as evidence of acquired immunity; however, this is also compatible with reduced exposure in adults due to behavioral changes and a reduction in worm burden due to loss of adult worms.[48] Examination of clinical material has demonstrated that nematode infection in the small intestine is associated with villous atrophy, crypt cell hyperplasia, and an increased inflammatory infiltrate.[49] The loss of absorptive surface results in malabsorption.

Direct damage to the intestine by nematodes undoubtedly contributes to the mucosal lesion, especially in hookworm and strongylid infection; however, there is evidence from animal studies that the immune response against the worms themselves, i.e., local hypersensitivity, can cause damage. Whereas infection of the small intestine of rats with *Nippostrongylus brasiliensis* causes villous atrophy, crypt cell hyperplasia, malabsorption, and diarrhea,[50] T cell–deficient rats show only minor changes in mucosal morphology.[51]

Trichuris trichiura Infection in Children

Recent studies on trichuriasis in children have given insight into the effect of parasite-induced colonic inflammation on the growth and development of children.

T. trichiura is a nematode parasite that inhabits the large intestine of man. Infection is acquired via the ingestion of oocysts in fecally contaminated soil. In the Carribbean, infestation is widespread in children.[52] Most cases are mild with no apparent symptoms, although heavy infections are associated with dysentery and severe stunting of growth (Table 3). The diarrheal stools of these infants contain blood and mucus, and rectal prolapse on defecation is common.[53] Many of the heavily infected, stunted children have finger clubbing. Wasting is not a feature of trichuriasis despite the shortness of stature. Following chemotherapeutic elimination of the parasite, there is pronounced catch-up growth.[54]

Since the colon, cecum, and terminal ileum can be visualized and biopsies taken during colonoscopy, we have been able to examine the mucosal lesions in children with severe trichuriasis (Fig. 7). Despite the heavy worm burdens, the colonic mucosa is remarkably normal, although there is a goblet cell hyperplasia, which may account for the heavily

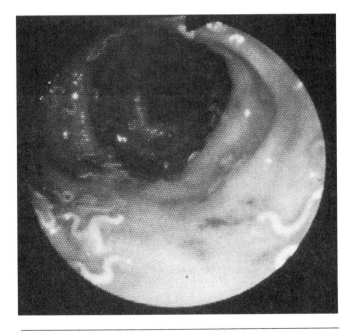

FIGURE 7 Endoscopic appearance of the nematode parasite *Trichuris trichiura* in the colon of a 6-year-old Jamaican child with severe *Trichuris* dysentery and stunting. White worms are clearly visible on the mucosa.

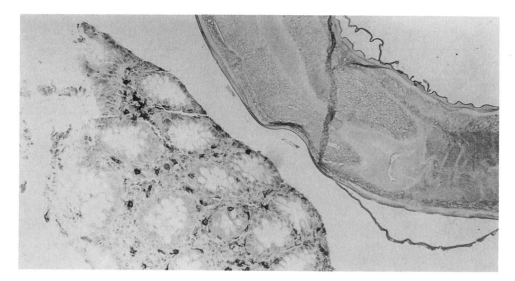

FIGURE 8 Immunohistochemical identification of IgE bound to mucosal mast cells in the colon of a child with *Trichuris* dysentery. Note the presence of the worm in the lumen. Sections were stained with monoclonal anti-IgE by the immunoperoxidase method. Staining is on the membrane of the cells and not intracellular, as would be expected of IgE plasma cells (immunoperoxidase stain, original magnification ×100).

mucoid stools. There is a prominent mucosal mast cell hyperplasia (Fig. 8) and macrophage infiltrate, but T-cell or neutrophil infiltrate is less pronounced. It is established that mast cell products can cause goblet cell secretion in rodents,[8] and this may also be the case in children with trichuriasis.

This particular parasite well illustrates the differences between experimental infection in rodents and the clinical situation; in the former, *Trichuris muris* infection is rapidly eliminated from the intestine via an acquired immune response,[55] whereas in humans there is no evidence that acquired immunity exists.[48] More details on parasite infections in children are described elsewhere in this chapter.

PATHOGENESIS OF INTESTINAL INFLAMMATION IN VIRAL AND BACTERIAL DISEASES OF THE INTESTINE

Space precludes a detailed examination of the pathogenesis of inflammation in particular diseases; however, several general points can be made. Organisms such as enterotoxigenic *Escherichia coli* or *Vibrio cholerae* produce few if any morphologic changes in the small intestine; however, the presence of numerous bacteria in the upper small bowel, which is normally relatively sterile, induces a nonspecific inflammatory infiltrate. On the other hand, organisms that invade and damage intestinal epithelial cells such as rotavirus or enteropathogenic *E. coli,* induce an inflammatory infiltrate and cause villous atrophy and crypt cell hyperplasia. This can cause secondary enzyme deficiencies of clinical importance such as postenteritis lactose intolerance.[3] Organisms that invade the lamina propria, such as *Shigella, Salmonella typhimurium,* and enteroinvasive *E. coli,* also provoke a profound local inflammatory response, which in the case of shigellosis classically results in neutrophil loss from the site of infection into the lumen and stool.

Finally there are bacteria that have a predilection to invade the Peyer's patches of the terminal ileum. These include *Yersinia enterocolitica, Salmonella typhi,* and even *Mycobacterium tuberculosis.* From animal studies it appears that these bacteria enter the Peyer's patches through specialized cells in the follicle epithelium, "M" cells, whose function is thought to be to sample luminal antigens.[56] In the Peyer's patches the bacteria multiply and form foci of inflammation. This can result in terminal ileitis indistinguishable clinically from Crohn's disease.

As mentioned above, the upper small bowel is relatively sterile. However, in a number of conditions such as malnutrition, immune deficiency, stagnant loop syndrome, achlorhydria, and short-gut syndrome, overgrowth of the small bowel with a predominantly coliform flora occurs.[3] This can result in steatorrhea and malabsorption. The mechanisms resulting in these clinical conditions are unclear, since the mucosal morphology in small bowel bacterial overgrowth is usually normal. However, in tropical sprue, small bowel overgrowth is accompanied by partial or total villous atrophy.[57]

Treatment with oral antibiotics can depress the population levels of the normal bacterial flora, allowing overgrowth of toxin-producing *Clostridium difficile* in the colon.[58] The toxins are cytopathic and cause severe colonic mucosal inflammation and pseudomembranous colitis. The bacterium never invades the mucosa, and the disease can be entirely explained by the effects of the toxins. Patients with *C. difficile* toxin–induced colitis usually have watery diarrhea; fever and hypoalbuminemia can also be a problem. Although *C. difficile* is found in 3 to 4 percent of normal adults and in up to 20 percent of hospital inpatients, infants commonly harbor toxin-producing *C. difficile* and have toxin in their stool with no apparent harmful effects.[59] At 6 to 8 months of age, the high carriage rates in children decrease and recovery rates become the same as for normal adults.

INTESTINAL INFLAMMATION OF UNKNOWN ORIGIN

Idiopathic inflammation of the intestine is more commonly seen in Europe and North America than in the developing world.[60] The most important of these conditions are the chronic inflammatory bowel diseases, ulcerative colitis, and

Crohn's disease. The age at onset of both of these conditions peaks around late adolescence[61]; thus, they are not uncommon disorders in teenagers. The incidence is lower in young children, but well-documented cases of Crohn's disease and ulcerative colitis have been observed in children 2 to 4 years of age, and ulcerative colitis in the neonate has also been described.[3] Crohn's disease is not seen in infants; if a biopsy in an infant of this age shows granulomas, the nitroblue tetrazolium (NBT) test for chronic granulomatous disease should be considered. Although the incidence of ulcerative colitis appears to have remained constant for the last few decades, there is evidence from a number of centers throughout the world that the incidence of Crohn's disease in adults has increased in recent years.[60] The incidence in children also appears to be increasing.[61] The etiology of inflammatory bowel disease (IBD) remains one of the major medical problems. Comprehensive reviews of IBD are available. Here the focus is on the pathogenesis of the intestinal lesion.

Crohn's Disease

Crohn's disease is characterized by transmural inflammation of any part of the GI tract, with fissures and a cobblestone appearance of the mucosa due to the skip lesions. The classic Crohn's lesion contains epithelioid granulomata, although they are not present in every case. Although the gross lesion is usually localized to the ileocecum, there is evidence that intestinal abnormalities occur throughout the length of the intestine.[63]

The agents or factors that precipitate Crohn's type lesions are unknown. Broadly speaking, opinion is divided into two camps—those who consider it to have an infectious etiology and those who consider it to be a disease of disordered immune regulation. The resemblance between the lesion in Crohn's disease and that of intestinal tuberculosis has led many investigators to propose that Crohn's disease is caused by a *Mycobacterium* species. There was recently a great deal of excitement generated by the observation that an organism, which turned out to be *Mycobacterium paratuberculosis*, was isolated from the intestine of two children with Crohn's disease.[64] This bacterium is the etiologic agent responsible for Johne's disease, a terminal ileitis of cattle histologically similar to Crohn's disease. Moreover, the organism caused a terminal ileitis in another species, goats, when fed in large amounts. Preliminary serologic evidence indicates that Crohn's patients have higher levels of antibodies to this bacterium than do controls,[65] but this has not been substantiated.[66] There is little doubt that *M. paratuberculosis* as well as numerous other mycobacterial species can occasionally be isolated from Crohn's patients, ulcerative colitis patients, and controls.[67] Enthusiasm for a mycobacterial origin of Crohn's disease must be tempered by the fact that antimycobacterial chemotherapy is ineffective in treating Crohn's disease. There is undoubtedly a host genetic component to the development of the disease. Immunosuppressive treatment, which would be expected to exacerbate mycobacterial infection, is the standard treatment for Crohn's disease. Finally, there is no epidemiologic evidence that Crohn's disease behaves like an infectious disease.

There is little evidence that other bacterial or viral agents are important in the development of Crohn's disease.

TABLE 4

Stigmata of Immunologic Reactions in the Intestine in Crohn's Disease

Aphthous ulceration overlying lymphoid follicles
Numerous ectopic lymphoid follicles in mucosa and submucosa
Granulomas in mesenteric lymph nodes and mucosa
Increased T cells and macrophages in lamina propria
Activated T cells in the diseased mucosa
Increase in lamina propria plasma cells, especially IgG
Increased expression of HLA-DR on epithelial cells
Remission induced by immunosuppressive drugs

Immunologic Basis for the Lesion in Crohn's Disease

The repeated failure to isolate a transmissible etiologic agent in Crohn's disease and the fact that the lesion in Crohn's disease appears to have an immunologic basis (Table 4) have led many workers to conclude that Crohn's disease is caused by an unregulated immune response to some as-yet-undefined enteric antigens. There must be some host component in the development of the lesion, since the incidence of IBD in the relatives of affected individuals is relatively high.[68] However, no genetic markers have been identified. The appearance of the Crohn's lesion strongly suggests that much of the mucosal damage is due to immune mechanisms. There is a dense lymphocytic infiltrate into the mucosa[69]; there is a great increase in plasma cell numbers, especially of the IgG isotype[70]; ectopic lymphoid follicles are seen; granuloma formation in the mucosa and draining mesenteric nodes are indicative of T-cell activation; and the increase in HLA-DR expression by enterocytes[71] is suggestive of local T cell–derived interferon-gamma production. The main problem with the immunologic hypothesis is that underlying abnormalities of immune regulation have not been convincingly demonstrated in Crohn's disease. It may well be that the assays used to study immunoregulation are inappropriate, so these negative findings should not be overinterpreted.

Circumstantial evidence that activated T cells are of importance in Crohn's disease comes from uncontrolled studies in which remission has been induced by treatment with cyclosporin A.[72]

The notion that luminal antigen plays a role in Crohn's disease is supported by studies in which remission can be induced by surgically induced bowel rest[73] or, alternatively, by parenteral nutrition or elemental diet.[74] In the latter, the parenteral nutrition or elemental diet undoubtedly improves the nutritional state of the patient, and it is interesting that these treatments also appear to resolve the level of intestinal inflammation, at least as determined by serum CRP and ESR.[74] It would be simplistic to assume that mucosal healing is entirely due to improved nutrition, and the mechanism by which this could occur is unknown.

A biologic relationship between inflammation and failure to thrive has recently been established with the discovery that cachectin and tumor necrosis factor alpha are the same molecules.[75] Cachectin is primarily a product of activated macrophages,[75] and it is noteworthy that in Crohn's disease there is a dense infiltrate of macrophages into the mucosa.[76] If these cells are producing cachectin, it could result in growth failure and weight loss in a child with Crohn's disease.

The end-point mediators of inflammation in diseased mucosa are prostanoids and leukotrienes. The levels of both of these groups of substances are increased in inflamed mucosa.[77,78]

Crohn's Disease in Children

Histopathologically Crohn's disease in children is the same as in adults. The special consideration for the pediatric patient is the effect of the intestinal inflammation on growth and development.[74] Steroid treatment can also inhibit growth. In a recent controlled trial,[74] it was shown that treatment with an elemental diet is as effective as steroids in inducing remission in children with Crohn's disease of the small intestine. Acceleration of linear growth was greater in the group treated with the elemental diet.

An advantage of investigating Crohn's disease in the pediatric patient is that it gives the opportunity to examine tissue closer to the onset of the disease. In adults with longstanding disease the initial lesion may be lost or obscured by the effects of inflammation, ulceration, tissue destruction, and repair. In the past, examination of resected tissue without gross disease has given clues to the genesis of the Crohn's ulcers and the transmural inflammation. Hadfield[79] considered that the earliest and most characteristic of the specific histologic lesions in Crohn's disease was lymphoid hyperplasia and giant cell formation in the lymph nodes of the submucosa. Later Rappaport et al[80] stated that "the available evidence suggests that the ulcer formation is not the primary lesion in regional enteritis but is preceded by lymphoid hyperplasia, formation of nodular granulomas, and submucosal edema." If in fact hyperplasia of the intestinal lymphoid follicles is a primary event or plays an important role in Crohn's disease, it is worthwhile considering the role that these structures play in the normal mucosal immune system. There is good evidence from animal studies that T cells in the Peyer's patches of the terminal ileum become sensitized to luminal antigens crossing the specialized lymphoepithelium overlying the follicle. These activated T cells then leave the Peyer's patch and migrate to the lamina propria, where they continue to proliferate only in the presence of the stimulating antigen.[81] Thus, it can be seen that cell-mediated lesions in the lamina propria can have their genesis in the Peyer's patches, an anatomically distant site. A clue that this may occur in Crohn's disease comes from studies of epithelial cell structure in areas of "normal" mucosa in Crohn's disease. Although most of the epithelium is normal, focal epithelial ulceration can be seen overlying granulomas.[80] Since the granulomas are probably the consequence of a T cell–mediated immune reaction and lamina propria T cells originate in the Peyer's patches, it would seem reasonable to assume, as did earlier workers, that the Peyer's patches may be the site of the primary lesion in Crohn's disease.

Studies from the author's laboratory further substantiate the notion that activated T cells are important in Crohn's disease. Using monoclonal anti-Tac antibody to identify activated T cells, we can show that Tac+ cells are present in large numbers in the lamina propria in active Crohn's disease in children (Fig. 9) but are absent from uninvolved mucosa in the same child.

A primary role for the lymphoid follicles in Crohn's disease is further substantiated by the endoscopic appearance of early Crohn's disease. One of the earliest signs is the presence of "punched-out" ulcers in the mucosa.[82] At biopsy these ulcers are seen to overlie lymphoid follicles (Fig. 10). Thus, in both the lymphoid follicles and the mucosa, epithelial damage and ulceration occur over zones of immune reactivity. It is also noteworthy that Crohn's disease is most

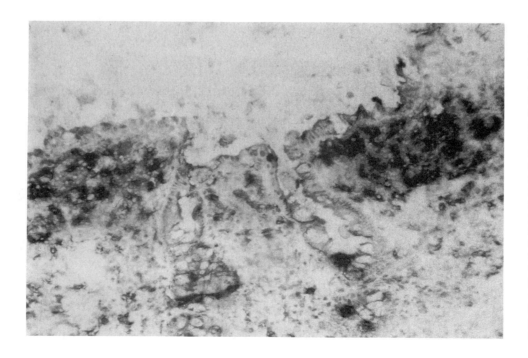

FIGURE 9 Activated T cells in the ileal lamina propria of a child with active Crohn's disease. Frozen sections were stained with anti–IL-2 receptor antibody (anti-Tac) by the immunoalkaline phosphatase method using fast red, since endogenous peroxidase in eosinophils in inflamed mucosa makes interpretation of immunoperoxidase-stained sections difficult. There are prominent subepithelial accumulations of Tac+ cells in the diseased mucosa. Serial sections stained with anti-CD3 reveal that most of the Tac+ cells are T cells. Tac+ cells are uncommon in normal small intestine (immunoalkaline phosphatase stain, original magnification ×100).

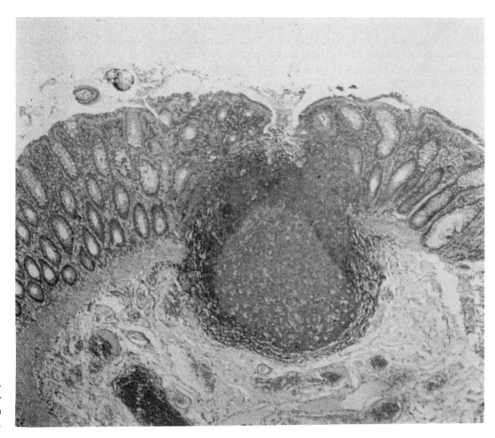

FIGURE 10 Aphthous ulcer overlying a colonic lymphoid follicle in a child with early Crohn's disease.

commonly seen in the terminal ileum, where Peyer's patches are most abundant. A hypothesis to explain Crohn's disease may be that individuals who develop the disease have an unregulated chronic hypersensitivity response in their gut-associated lymphoid follicles as well as in the lamina propria. The antigens in question are unknown, but there is no a priori reason to assume that different individuals respond to a common antigen.

There have been few immunologic studies on human Peyer's patches. Recently studies from the author's laboratory[117] have shown that Peyer's patches can be visualized in the terminal ileum of children during colonoscopy (Fig. 11). In vitro, Peyer's patch cells respond more vigorously to mitogens than do cells from the lamina propria.[117]

Ulcerative Colitis

The mucosal lesion in children with ulcerative colitis is similar to that of adults. The disease is restricted to the mucosa of the colon and rectum, although there may be backwash ileitis in severe cecal ulcerative colitis. The lesion is characterized by an acute inflammatory infiltrate, with numerous neutrophils in the lamina propria and epithelium, epithelial cell damage, crypt distortion, and goblet cell depletion. There is increased cell division in the crypts.[83]

No etiologic agent has been described for ulcerative colitis, and there is general acceptance that the condition is probably due to a colon-specific immunopathologic (perhaps

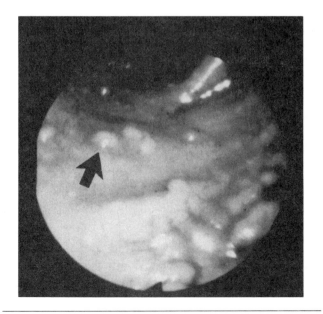

FIGURE 11 Endoscopic appearance of Peyer's patches visualized in the terminal ileum of a child during colonoscopy for suspected inflammatory bowel disease. Peyer's patches appear as raised areas of the mucosa (*arrow*).

autoimmune) reaction. In contrast to Crohn's disease, ulcerative colitis is cured by total colectomy. Thus, the lesion is organ-specific. Standard treatment is immunosuppressive therapy, which also suggests that the disease is due to an immune response.

It is well established that the sera of patients with ulcerative colitis contain antibodies that react with colonic epithelial cells.[84] This anticolon activity in the sera of some patients can be absorbed out using *E. coli* 014, which would suggest that colonic epithelial cells and *E. coli* 014 have antigens in common.[85] The anti-colon antibodies, however, are not cytotoxic for colonic epithelial cells, persist in patients for many years after colectomy, and are also at raised levels in Crohn's disease.[84] Thus, their role in the pathogenesis of ulcerative colitis is not clear.

Later studies focused on cytotoxicity, and it was shown that blood and mucosal cells from both ulcerative colitis and Crohn's disease patients are cytotoxic for autologous or allogeneic colonic enterocytes.[86] The effector cell in this system was not a T cell, and the target antigens were not identified. More recently work has been carried out to establish antigens unique to colonic epithelial cells which might serve as targets for autoimmune attack. Such glycoproteins have been identified,[87] and it has been shown that T cells from the gut mucosa of patients with ulcerative colitis and Crohn's disease can lyse target cells coated with the epithelial cell–associated antigens.[87] Table 5 summarizes the immunologic features of ulcerative colitis.

Lymphoid Follicular Hyperplasia (LFH)

This is a relatively rare condition in which children present with lower right quadrant pain, sometimes associated with diarrhea. At laparotomy, the terminal ileum is seen to be macroscopically enlarged and reddened.[88] Histologically there is hyperplasia of the Peyer's patches of the terminal ileum. These can become so hyperplastic that they obstruct the lumen. No infectious agent can be identified, so the antigenic stimulus for the profound lymphoid stimulation is unknown. It should be emphasized that, in contrast to adults, normal children have more abundant gut-associated lymphoid tissue than adults. LFH was once considered to be a prodrome of Crohn's disease; however, there is no evidence to suggest that this is true.

TABLE 5
Immunologic Features in Ulcerative Colitis

Organ-specific

Anti-colon antibodies in sera

Colon-specific antigens identified which can serve as targets for cellular cytotoxicity

Remission induced by immunosuppressive drugs

Acute inflammatory infiltrate in diseased colon

Autoimmune Enteropathy

This is a rare syndrome in which infants with intractable diarrhea have autoantibodies against intestinal epithelium.[89] It has not been shown that the autoantibodies cause tissue damage. The lesion is characteristically celiac-like, with severe villous atrophy and crypt cell hyperplasia and increased lymphocytes in the lamina propria. The disease usually presents several months after birth. Infants with this condition also have other autoantibodies such as anti-nuclear antibodies.

Elemental diet or total parenteral nutrition has no effect on the mucosal damage, but steroids may be effective. Failing that, the only possible treatment is maintenance therapy on total parenteral nutrition. In the presence of continuing high levels of anti–epithelial cell antibodies, the prognosis is poor.

Necrotizing Enterocolitis

This is a poorly understood condition of newborn infants in which there is a patchy or diffuse necrosis of the small or large intestine.[3] The disease is characterized by intramural hydrogen gas, which suggests that it may have a bacterial etiology. However, no pathogen or toxin has yet been identified. Hypoxia of the intestine may also be important in the development of this condition. Perforation and stenosis are secondary complications that may necessitate resection.

IMMATURITY OF THE INFANT INTESTINE

It is unlikely that immaturity of the intestine contributes to the development of Crohn's disease, since the disease does not appear until well after infancy. Immaturity of the intestine is also unlikely to be of importance in ulcerative colitis, since the disease seems to be due to an immune response itself. It is generally believed that necrotizing enterocolitis is associated with immaturity of the gut, since it occurs only in newborn infants.

Mucosal Immune System

The newborn infant has abundant serum IgG acquired transplacentally from the mother. However, the mucosal immune system is markedly deficient. T cells are found in human fetal gut from 14 weeks' gestation,[90] and by 19 weeks there are well-established Peyer's patches in the terminal ileum[9] (Fig. 12). Since there are no bacterial or dietary antigens to stimulate the mucosal IgA system, there are no IgA plasma cells in the intestinal lamina propria in the fetus.[92] At birth the mucosal immune system is stimulated by the bacteria that colonize the infant gut, germinal centers appear in the Peyer's patches,[93] and IgA plasma cells begin to appear by day 12.[92] This transient IgA deficiency at birth is probably of no consequence in the breast-fed baby, who receives abundant colostral IgA, but it may be a contributing factor to infection and to food hypersensitivity in the bottle-fed child.

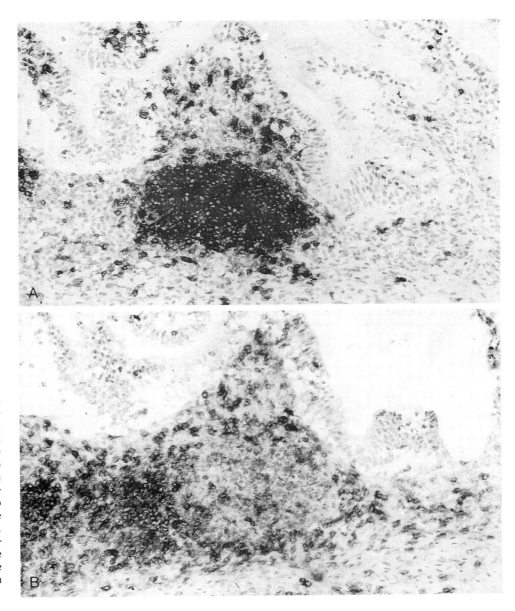

FIGURE 12 Serial frozen sections through a Peyer's patch in the ileum of a 20-week-old human fetus. Sections were stained with anti-CD35 (the C3b receptor) to identify B cells in a follicle and some macrophages (*A*) and with anti-CD5 to identify T cells in the T-cell zone adjacent to the B-cell follicle (*B*). Note also that in the fetus anti-CD5 also weakly stains follicle B cells (immunoperoxidase stain, original magnification ×100).

Colostral IgA can be detected in the serum of infants,[94] but it is unclear whether this is passively absorbed or is actively transported across the epithelium. Comparative studies of salivary IgA antibodies to *E. coli* O antigens in infants from birth to 6 months of age in Sweden and Pakistan have shown that in the latter, antibodies develop earlier and to a higher level than in the Swedish infants.[95] This is presumably a reflection of different socioeconomic conditions influencing bacterial contamination of the infant food.

Absorption of Antigens

The absorption of large numbers of macromolecules from the intestine may contribute to the development of intestinal allergy and hypersensitivity. In animals the postnatal intestine can absorb antigenically intact proteins in large quanti-

ties. In humans, however, this does not seem to be the case. In a study of serum beta-lactoglobulin (beta-LG) levels in infants fed a cow's milk formula, Roberton et al[96] found significant serum levels only in premature babies of less than 37 weeks' gestation. Thus, the decrease in the permeability of the epithelium to macromolecules in humans appears to occur before birth. Nevertheless, there is no doubt that antigens do cross the intestine of the child, since serum antibodies to BSA are present in virtually all milk-fed children. Recently Husby et al have measured the levels of ovalbumin and beta-LG in the serum of celiac children (on a gluten-free diet) and controls after challenge with gluten.[97] Comparable levels of antigen were detected in the serum 3 hours after feeding in both groups. Thus, it is unclear if challenge with gluten in celiacs results in increased permeability to other antigens. However, since gluten challenge of celiac children on a gluten-free diet may not induce intestinal damage for days or even weeks, it may be that intestinal permeability to other antigens is increased when the mucosa is flat. Interestingly, more infants given foods before 3 months of age have serum anti-food antibodies than infants given foods after 3 months of age. This indicates that the intestine is more permeable to food antigens in the first 3 months of life.[98]

Infectious gastroenteritis in man and animals leads to increased intestinal permeability to macromolecules, which might lead to sensitization and hypersensitivity.[99,100] However, since most children have gastroenteritis at some time in infancy, but only a minority develop food allergy, the relationship between increased permeability and food allergy is unclear.

Exposure to dietary antigens may influence the development of intestinal hypersensitivity, especially to wheat (reviewed in reference 3). In the late 1960s and early 1970s, the vogue in the United Kingdom was to administer wheat products at an early age. As a consequence of this early exposure, celiac disease presented at an early age. In addition, a condition of transient gluten intolerance was also observed, very similar to cow's milk protein enteropathy. After 1975 it was recommended that solid food not be introduced to the infant until after 4 to 6 months of age, and many infant foods are now gluten free. This has resulted in the presentation of celiac disease at a later age. More interestingly, the overall incidence of celiac disease also appears to be decreasing, although whether this is due to the time of gluten introduction or to other factors is unclear.

The concept of an immune and a nonimmune mucosal barrier to macromolecules has been advanced by Walker.[101] These work in concert to regulate absorption of antigens. The nonimmune factors include peristalsis, gastric acidity, and mucus. The main immune factor is the ability of secretory IgA to complex with antigen and thus prevent antigen absorption. This has been formally demonstrated in patients by Cunningham-Rundles and co-workers, who showed the presence of circulating immune complexes containing milk proteins in IgA-deficient patients after feeding milk.[102] The host homeostasis with the gut bacteria probably involves both immune and nonimmune factors. This is well illustrated by the studies of McLoughlin et al,[103] who showed that small bowel bacterial overgrowth occurred only in patients who had defective gastric acid, IgA deficiency, and truncal vagotomy. If any one of these parameters was normal, overgrowth did not occur.

Immaturity of the Gut in Relation to Infection

Young children are particularly susceptible to *E. coli* stable toxin–mediated diarrhea.[104] In a recent paper Cohen et al[105] measured the number of receptors on intestinal epithelial cells for *E. coli* enterotoxin in infants of different ages. It was clearly demonstrated that the number of enterotoxin receptors per cell was very much higher in infants than in older children. Since the function of the enterotoxin receptor on epithelial cells is not known, the reason for the decrease in the number of receptors with age remains to be established. However, it is clear that this obervation gives an explanation for the severe effects of *E. coli* enterotoxin in the young infant.[104]

FACTORS PREDISPOSING TO INTESTINAL INFLAMMATION

Congenital Abnormalities

Congenital abnormalities resulting in intestinal obstruction can produce the stagnant loop syndrome. This is due to stasis of intestinal contents which results in bacterial overgrowth of the small intestine. There is no morphologic change to the intestine, but there is steatorrhea and sugar and vitamin B_{12} malabsorption. It is not clear why there should be sugar malabsorption in the absence of intestinal damage, although it has been suggested that bacterial deconjugation of bile salts may be important.

The Beneficial Effect of Breast-Feeding

As well as the nutritional properties of breast milk (which are also present in infant formula milks), there are a number of factors that can protect the infant. These include the antibacterial molecules lactoferrin, lysozyme, and lactoperoxidase, but the most important factors present in breast milk and absent from cow's milk are immunologic. There are both lymphocytes and macrophages in breast milk and colostrum. These may contribute to host resistance in the intestine and cross the mucosal wall and provide some systemic immunity.

The high levels of IgA in colostrum (around 12 g per liter) are undoubtedly of greatest benefit to the newborn infant, especially in the developing world, where the chance of encountering a pathogen immediately after birth is high. The colostral IgA has specificities for antigens to which the mother has been exposed, so that, for example, antibodies against foods[106] and bacteria[107] are present. The IgA against bacterial and viral pathogens probably prevents intestinal infection by coating the pathogen and preventing adhesion to the mucosa. In this respect breast milk has been shown to reduce morbidity from diarrheal diseases.[108] IgA against food proteins may prevent food allergy by preventing antigen absorption and thus preventing sensitization. It has been suggested that atopy to food antigens is related to transient IgA deficiency.[109]

In a so-far-uncorroborated study from Scandinavia, it was shown that patients with Crohn's disease were breast fed a significantly shorter time than matched controls and that Crohn's patients were over-represented among those with a short period of breast-feeding.[110] Exactly how breast-feeding may protect against Crohn's disease, which develops many years later, is unclear.

Enterocyte HLA-DR Expression

In normal small intestine HLA-DR molecules are constitutively expressed by villous enterocytes.[111] Enterocytes in both man[112] and the rat[113] can present antigen to T cells in a major histocompatibility complex (MHC)–restricted fashion. Enterocyte HLA-DR first appears at about 20 weeks' gestation,[33] so it is unlikely that this is due to an immunologic stimulus. However, in inflamed bowel in celiac disease, inflammatory bowel disease, gastritis, autoimmune enteropa-

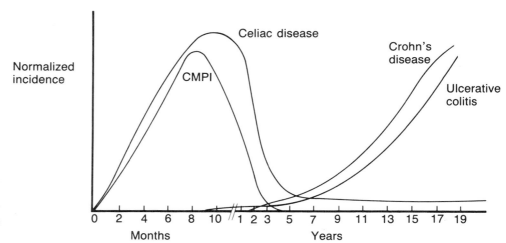

FIGURE 13 The age-related incidences of celiac disease, cow's milk protein intolerance (CMPI), Crohn's disease, and ulcerative colitis. Curves show the relative time of the appearance of these disorders and not the actual incidence.

thy, graft-versus-host disease, and parasite infection, enterocyte DR expression is increased and there is also expression on crypt epithelial cells. This increase is probably mediated by interferon-gamma[33] and is also probably nonspecific. There is the possibility that intestinal infection in the infant results in increased HLA-DR expression, which in turn could result in the presentation of self-antigens or food antigens to the immune system. A consequence of this might be food hypersensitivity or autoimmune disease. It has been proposed that increased DR expression may allow antigen presentation to activate suppressor cells, thus switching off harmful mucosal immune responses. However, since class II MHC molecules can bind antigen,[114] it seems more likely that increased DR in inflammatory situations plays a role in binding peptides and retaining them at the surface of the mucosa, thus preventing absorption of antigens.

The Effects of Antibiotics

Oral administration of clindamycin, ampicillin, and cephalosporins can dramatically reduce the levels of the normal intestinal flora. This allows the overgrowth and colonization of the intestine by *Clostridium difficile*, which can secrete toxins and cause pseudomembranous colitis. As mentioned above, many infants before the age of 6 to 8 months have the organism and toxin in their stools but have no sign of clinical disease.

Age of Onset of Inflammatory Disorders in Children

There is a great deal of variation in the onset of inflammatory disorders in the intestines of children. Celiac disease, for example, usually presents in the first 2 years of life,[3] but it can also present in much older children and adults. It is a subject of debate as to whether late-onset celiacs have celiac disease prior to diagnosis. Why some patients take so long to develop the disease is a mystery, but it does suggest a triggering event. However, since most patients present in infancy, this author feels that the trigger for the developing of the

disease is the development of a harmful immune response to gluten itself.

Cow's milk protein intolerance presents around 3 to 6 months of age, presumably as a consequence of antigenic exposure. The reason for the peak age at onset of inflammatory bowel disease in late adolescence and early adulthood is unknown. Figure 13 summarizes the age at onset of celiac disease, cow's milk protein intolerance, Crohn's disease, and ulcerative colitis.

SUMMARY AND CONCLUSIONS

Inflammation, by definition, is a result of the infiltration of inflammatory cells into the tissues. In a sense the gut is normally inflamed, since the mucosa is filled with plasma cells, T and B cells, mast cells, macrophages, and eosinophils. In fact, the gut-associated lymphoid tissue is by far the largest lymphoid compartment in the body, even in health. It is not surprising, therefore, since the gut is filled with lymphoid tissue and is also the interface betwen the external environment and the immune system, that most conditions of intestinal inflammation have a primary immunologic etiology. In many cases, such as food-sensitive enteropathy, treatment involves identifying the offending food antigen and eliminating it from the child's diet. There is little doubt that the adverse effects in most cases of food-sensitive enteropathy are immunologic in origin, but why milk-sensitive enteropathy is a transient disease of childhood whereas wheat-sensitive enteropathy is a lifelong affliction remains a puzzle.

In other conditions, such as parasite infection, there is evidence that it is not the parasite itself that causes intestinal damage, but the immune response generated against the parasite in the mucosa. However, there is in general a lack of clinical studies on host-parasite interactions in the human small intestine.

Finally, there are the idiopathic conditions in which there is profound intestinal inflammation but the trigger that precipitates the inflammation is unknown. Opinion is divided as to whether the trigger is an unidentified infectious agent or a disorder of the mucosal immune system.

The functions of digestion and absorption in the small bowel and water and ion resorption in the colon depend on the integrity of the epithelium. In celiac disease, for example, the malabsorption is entirely due to the loss of villous surface area and damage to the epithelial cells, as there is no primary defect in epithelial cells. Likewise in the colon in ulcerative colitis, diarrhea is due to impaired water absorption, since the colonic epithelium is damaged and mucus depleted. Immunosuppression in ulcerative colitis reduces intestinal inflammation, epithelial integrity is regained, and colonic function returns to normal. In contrast, in Crohn's disease, although immunosuppression can relieve ongoing inflammation in the mucosa, the nature of the lesion is such that the mucosa becomes fibrotic and scarred, leading to stenosis, and deep ulcers and fissures develop.

The major advances in understanding the pathogenesis of intestinal inflammation will probably come from an understanding of the ways in which mucosal immune responses alter epithelial cell structure, differentiation, and function.

REFERENCES

1. Kirschner BS, Voinchet O, Rosenberg IH. Growth retardation in inflammatory bowel disease. Gastroenterology 1978; 75:504–511.
2. Hill DJ, Firer MA, Shelton MJ, Hosking CS. Manifestations of milk allergy in infancy: clinical and immunologic findings. J Pediatr 1986; 109:270–276.
3. Walker-Smith JA. Diseases of the small intestine in childhood. 3rd ed. London: Butterworths, 1988.
4. Barrett KE, Metcalf DD. Mucosal mast cells and IgE. In: Heyworth MF, Jones AL, eds. Immunology of the gastrointestinal tract and liver. New York: Raven Press, 1988: 65.
5. Reimann HJ, Ring J, Ultsch B, Wendt P, Lorenz H, Schimdt U, Blumel G. Release of gastric histamine in patients with urticaria and food allergy. Agents Actions 1982; 12:111–113.
6. Shiner M, Ballard J, Smith ME. The small intestinal mucosa in cows milk allergy. Lancet 1975; i:136–140
7. Ferguson A. Models of intestinal hypersensitivity. Clin Gastroenterol 1976; 5:271–288.
8. Lake AM, Bloch KJ, Sinclair KJ, Walker WA. Anaphylactic release of intestinal goblet cell mucus. Immunology 1980; 39:657–665.
9. Turner MW, Boulton P, Shields JG, Strobel S, Gibson S, Miller HRP, Levinsky RJ. Intestinal hypersensitivity reactions in the rat. 1. Uptake of intact protein, permeability to sugars and their correlation with mucosal mast-cell activation. Immunology 1988; 63:119–124.
10. Kilby A, Walker-Smith JA, Wood CBS. Small mucosa in cows milk allergy. Lancet 1975; i:531.
11. Strobel S, Busuttil A, Ferguson A. Human intestinal mucosal mast cells: expanded population in untreated coeliac disease. Gut 1983; 24:222–227.
12. Lake AM, Whitington BPF, Hamilton JR. Dietary protein induced colitis in breast fed infants. J Pediatr 1982; 101:906–910.
13. Jarrett EEE. Stimuli for the production and control of IgE in rats. Immunol Rev 1978; 41:52–76.
14. Rothberg RM, Farr RS. Anti-bovine serum albumin and anti-alpha lactalbumin in the serum of children and adults. Pediatrics 1965; 35:571–588.
15. Kenrich KG, Walker-Smith JA. Immunoglobulins and dietary protein antibodies in childhood coeliac disease. Gut 1970; 11:635–640.
16. Husby S, Foged N, Oxelius VA, Svehag S-E. Serum IgG subclass antibodies to gliadin and other dietary antigens in children with coeliac disease. Clin Exp Immunol 1986; 64:526–535.
17. Ferguson A, Carswell F. Precipitins to dietary proteins in serum and upper intestinal secretions of coeliac children. Br Med 1972; 1:75–79.
18. Shiner M. Ultrastructural changes suggestive of immune reactions in the jejunal mucosa of coeliac children following gluten challenge. Gut 1973; 14:1–12.

19. Bellamy JEC, Nielsen NO. Immune-mediated emigration of neutrophils into the lumen of the small intestine. Infect Immun 1974; 9:615–619.
20. Kirkham SE, Bloch KJ, Bloch MB, Perry RP, Walker WA. Immune complex–induced enteropathy in the rat. 1. Clinical and histological features. Dig Dis Sci 1986; 31:737–743.
21. Webster ADB, Slavin G, Shiner M, Platts-Mills TAE, Asherson GL. Coeliac disease with severe hypogammaglobulinemia. Gut 1981; 22:153–157.
22. Ferguson A, MacDonald TT. Effects of local delayed hypersensitivity reactions on the small intestine. In: Ciba Foundation Symposium 46. Immunology of the gut. Elsevier-North Holland, 1977: 305.
23. Ament ME, Rubin CE. Soy protein—another cause of flat intestinal lesion. Gastroenterology 1972; 62:227–234.
24. Leigh RJ, Marsh MN, Crowe P, Kelly C, Garner V, Gordon D. Studies of intestinal lymphoid tissue. IX. Dose-dependent, gluten-induced lymphoid infiltration of coeliac jejunal epithelium. Scand J Gastroenterol 1985; 20:715–719.
25. Selby WS, Janossy G, Bofill M, Jewell DP. Lymphocyte subpopulations in the human small intestine. The findings in normal mucosa and in the mucosa of patients with adult coeliac disease. Clin Exp Immunol 1983; 52:219–228.
26. Arato A, Savilahti E, Taenio V-M, Vekasalo M, Klemola T. HLA-DR expression, natural killer cells and IgE containing cells in the jejunal mucosa of coeliac children. Gut 1987; 28:988–994.
27. Peterlin BM. Genetic aspects of gastrointestinal immunology. In: Heyworth MF, Jones AL, eds. Immunology of the gastrointestinal tract and liver. New York: Raven Press, 1980: 145.
28. Ferguson A, MacDonald TT, McClure JP, Holden RJ. Cell-mediated immunity to gliadin within the small intestinal mucosa in coeliac disease. Lancet 1975; i:895–901.
29. Kagnoff MF, Austin RK, Hubert JJ, Kasarda DD. Possible role for a human adenovirus in the pathogenesis of coeliac disease. J Exp Med 1984; 160:1544–1557.
30. MacDonald TT, Ferguson A. Hypersensitivity reactions in the small intestine. II. The effect of allograft rejection on mucosal architecture and lymphoid cell infiltrate. Gut 1976; 17:81–91.
31. MacDonald TT, Ferguson A. Hypersensitivity reactions in the small intestine. III: The effect of allograft rejection and graft-versus-host disease on epithelial cell kinetics. Cell Tissue Kinet 1977; 10:301–312.
32. MacDonald TT, Spencer JM. Evidence that activated mucosal T cells play a role in the pathogenesis of enteropathy in human small intestine. J Exp Med 1988; 167:1341–1349.
33. MacDonald TT, Weinel A, Spencer JM. HLA-DR expression in human fetal intestinal epithelium. Gut 1988; 29:1342–1348.
34. Yardley JH, Bayless TM, Norton JH, Hendrix TR. Celiac disease. A study of the jejunal epithelium before and after a gluten-free diet. N Engl J Med 1962; 267:1173–1179.
35. Araya M, Walker-Smith JA. Specificity of ultrastructural changes in small intestinal epithelium in early childhood. Arch Dis Child 1975; 50:844–855.
36. Booth CC. The enterocyte in coeliac disease. Br Med J 1970; 3:725–731.
37. Padykula HA, Strauss EW, Ladman AJ, Gardner FH. A morphologic and histochemical analysis of the human jejunal epithelium in nontropical sprue. Gastroenterology 1961; 40:735–765.
38. Isaacson PG, Spencer J, Connolly CE, Pollock DJ, Stein H, O'Connor NTJ, Bevan DH, Kirkham N, Wainscoat JS, Mason DY. Malignant histiocytosis of the intestine: a T-cell lymphoma. Lancet 1985; ii:688–691.
39. Jarrett EEE, Jarrett WFH, Urquart GM. Quantitative studies on the kinetics of establishment and expulsion on intestinal nematode populations in susceptible and immune hosts. Nippostrongylus brasiliensis in the rat. Parasitology 1968; 58:625–634.
40. Miller TA. Hookworm infection in man. Adv Parasitol 1979; 17:315–384.
41. Roberts-Thomson IC. Giardiasis: the role of immunological mechanisms to host-parasite relationships. In: Marsh MN, ed. Immunopathology of the small intestine. Chichester: John Wiley and Sons, 1987: 209.
42. Cole TJ, Parkin JM. Infection and its effect on the growth of young children: a comparison of Gambia and Uganda. Trans R Soc Trop Med Hyg 1977; 71:196–198.
43. Hoskins LC, Winawer SJ, Broitman SA, Gottlieb LS, Zamcheck N. Clinical giardiasis and intestinal malabsorption. Gastroenterology 1977; 53:265–279.
44. MacDonald TT, Ferguson A. Small intestinal architecture and protozoal infection in the mouse. Gastroenterology 1978; 74:496–500.

45. Webster ADB. Giardiasis and immunodeficiency diseases. Trans R Soc Trop Med Hyg 1980; 74:440–443.
46. Ament ME, Rubin CE. Relation of giardiasis to abnormal intestinal structure and function in gastrointestinal immunodeficiency syndromes. Gastroenterology 1972; 62:216–226.
47. Wright SG, Tompkins AM. Quantification of the lymphocytic infiltrate in jejunal epithelium in giardiasis. Clin Exp Immunol 1977; 29: 408–412.
48. Bundy DAP. Population ecology of intestinal helminth infections in human communities. Phil Trans R Soc 1988; 321:405.
49. Aziz MA, Siddiqui AR. Morphological and absorption studies of small intestine in hookworm disease (ancylostomiasis) in West Pakistan. Gastroenterology 1958; 55:242–250.
50. Symons LEA. Kinetics of the epithelial cells and morphology of villi and crypts in the jejunum of the rat infected by the nematode *Nippostrongylus brasiliensis*. Gastroenterology 1965; 49:158–168.
51. Ferguson A, Jarrett EEE. Hypersensitivity reactions in the small intestine. I. Thymus dependence of experimental "partial villous atrophy." Gut 1975; 16:114–117.
52. Bundy DAP, Cooper ES, Thompson DE, Anderson RM, Didier JM. Age-related prevalence and intensity of *Trichuris trichiura* infection in a St. Lucian community. Trans R Soc Trop Med Hyg 1987; 81:85–94.
53. Cooper ES,. Bundy DAP. Trichuriasis in St. Lucia. In: Walker-Smith JA, McNeish AS, eds. Diarrhoea and malnutrition in childhood. London: Butterworths, 1986: 91.
54. Cooper ES, Bundy DAP. Personal communication.
55. Wakelin D, Lee TDG. Immunobiology of Trichuris and Capillaria infection. In: Soulsby EJL, ed. Immune responses in parasite infections: Immunology, immunopathology and immunoprophylaxis. Vol 1, Nematodes. Boca Raton, FL: CRC Press, 1987: 61.
56. Owen RL. Sequential uptake of horseradish peroxidase by lymphoid follicle epithelium of Peyer's patches in the normal unobstructed mouse intestine: an ultrastructural study. Gastroenterology 1977; 72:440–451.
57. Mathan M, Mathan VI, Baker SJ. An electron-microscopic study of jejunal mucosal morphology in control subjects and in patients with tropical sprue in Southern India. Gastroenterology 1975; 68:17–32.
58. Bartlett JG. Pathogenesis and treatment of pseudomembranous enterocolitis. In: Branski D, Dinari G, Rozen P, Walker-Smith JA, eds. Frontiers of gastrointestinal research 13. Pediatric gastroenterology. Aspects of immunology and infections. Basel:Karger, 1986: 370.
59. Viscidi R, Willey S, Bartlett JG. Isolation rates and toxigenic potential of *Clostridium difficile* isolates from various patient populations. Gastroenterology 1981; 25:81:5–9.
60. Mayberry JF, Rhodes J. Epidemiological aspects of Crohn's disease: a review of the literature. Gut 1984; 25:886–899.
61. Rogers BH, Clark LM, Kirsner JB. The epidemiologic and demographic characteristics of inflammatory bowel disease. An analysis of a computerised file of 1,400 patients. J Chron Dis 1971; 24:743–748.
62. Lindquist BL, Jarnerot G, Wickbom G. Clinical and epidemiological aspects of Crohn's disease in children and adolescents. Scand J Gastroenterol 1984; 19:502–506.
63. Goodman MJ, Skinner JM, Truelove SC. Abnormalities in the apparently normal bowel mucosa in Crohn's disease. Lancet 1976; i:275–278.
64. Chiodini RJ, Van Kruininngen H, Thayer WR, Merkal RS, Coutu JA. Possible role of mycobacteria in inflammatory bowel disease. 1. An unclassified *Mycobacteria* species isolated from patients with Crohn's disease. Dig Dis Sci 1984; 29:1073–1079.
65. Thayer WR, Coutu JA, Chiodini RJ, Van Kruiningen HJ, Merkal RS. Possible role of Mycobacteria in inflammatory bowel disease. Mycobacterial antibodies in Crohn's disease. Dig Dis Sci 1984; 29:1080–1085.
66. Cho S-N, Brennan PJ, Yoshimura HH, Korelitz BI, Graham DY. Mycobacterial aetiology of Crohn's disease: serologic study using common mycobacterial antigens and a species-specific glycolipid from *Mycobacterium paratuberculosis*. Gut 1986; 27:1353–1356.
67. Graham DY, Markesich DC, Yoshimura HH. Mycobacteria and inflammatory bowel disease. Results of culture. Gastroenterology 1987; 92:436–442.
68. Lewkonia RM, McConnell RB. Familial inflammatory bowel disease—heredity or environment. Gut 1976; 17:235–243.
69. Selby WS, Janossy G, Bofill M, Jewell DP. Intestinal lymphocyte subpopulations in inflammatory bowel disease: an analysis by immunohistological and cell isolation techniques. Gut 1984; 25:32–40.
70. Kett R, Rognum TO, Brandtzaeg P. Mucosal subclass distribution of immunoglobulin G–producing cells is different in ulcerative colitis and Crohn's disease of the colon. Gastroenterology 1987; 93:919–924.
71. Selby WS, Janossy G, Mason DY, Jewell DP. Expression of HLA-DR antigens by colonic epithelium in inflammatory bowel disease. Clin Exp Immunol 1983; 53:614–618.
72. Allison MC, Pounder RE. Cyclosporin for Crohn's disease. Aliment Pharmacol Therap 1987; 1:39–43.
73. Burman JH, Thompson H, Cooke WT, Williams JA. The effects of diversion of intestinal contents on the progress of Crohn's disease of the large bowel. Gut 1971; 12:11–15.
74. Sanderson IR, Udeen S, Davies PSW, Savage MO, Walker-Smith JA. Remission induced by elemental diet in small bowel Crohn's disease. Arch Dis Child 1987; 61:123–127.
75. Old LJ. Tumor necrosis factor. Science 1985; 230:630–632..
76. Selby WS, Poulter LW, Hobbs S, Jewell DP, Janossy G. Heterogeneity of HLA-DR-positive histiocytes in human intestinal lamina propria: a combined histochemical and immunohistological analysis. J Clin Pathol 1983; 36:379–384.
77. Zifroni A, Treves AJ, Sachar DB, Rachmilewitz D. Prostanoid synthesis by cultured intestinal epithelial and mononuclear cells in inflammatory bowel disease. Gut 1983; 24:659–665.
78. Sharon P, Stenson WF. Enhanced synthesis of leukotriene B4 by colonic mucosa inflammatory bowel disease. Gastroenterology 1984; 86:453–460.
79. Hadfield G. The primary histological lesion of regional ileitis. Lancet 1939; ii:773–776.
80. Rappaport H, Burgoyne FH, Smetana HF. The pathology of regional enteritis. Milit Surg 1951; 109:463–502.
81. Guy-Grand D, Griscelli C, Vassalli P. The mouse gut T lymphocyte, a novel type of T cell. Nature, origin, and traffic in mice in normal and graft-verus-host conditions. J Exp Med 1978; 148:1661–1677.
82. Rickert RR, Carter HW. The "early" ulcerative lesion of Crohn's disease: correlative light- and scanning electron-microscopic studies. J Clin Gastroenterol 1980; 2:11–19.
83. Franklin WA, McDonald GB, Stein HO, Gatter KC, Jewell DP, Clark LC, Mason DY. Immunohistologic demonstration of abnormal colonic crypt cell kinetics in ulcerative colitis. Hum Pathol 1985; 16:1129–1132.
84. Langercrantz R, Hammarstrom S, Perlmann P, Gustafsson BE. Immunological studies in ulcerative colitis. III. Incidence of antibodies to colon-antigen in ulcerative colitis and other gastro-intestinal disease. Clin Exp Immunol 1966; 1:263–276.
85. Langercrantz R, Hammarstrom S, Perlmann P, Gustafsson BE. Immunologic studies in ulcerative colitis. IV. Origin of autoantibodies. J Exp Med 1968; 128:1339–1352.
86. Stobo JD, Tomasi TB, Huizenga KA, Spencer RJ, Shorter RG. In vitro studies of inflammatory bowel disease. Surface receptors of the mononuclear cell required to lyse allogeneic colonic epithelial cells. Gastroenterology 1976; 70:171–176.
87. Roche JK, Fiocchi C, Youngman K. Sensitization to epithelial antigens in chronic mucosal inflammatory disease. Characterisation of human intestinal mucosa-derived mononuclear cells reactive with purified epithelial cell-associated components in vitro. J Clin Invest 1985; 75:522–530.
88. Fieber SS, Schaefer HJ. Lymphoid hyperplasia of the terminal ileum. Gastroenterology 1966; 50:83–98.
89. Mirakian R, Richardson A, Milla PJ, Walker-Smith JA, Unsworth J, Savage MO, Bottazzo GF. Protracted diarrhoea of infancy: evidence in support of an autoimmune variant. Br Med J 1986; 293:1132–1136.
90. Spencer JM, Dillon SB, Isaacson PG, MacDonald TT. T cell subclasses in human fetal ileum. Clin Exp Immunol 1986; 65:553–558.
91. Spencer JM, MacDonald TT, Finn T, Isaacson PG. Development of Peyer's patches in human fetal terminal ileum. Clin Exp Immunol 1986; 64:536–543.
92. Perkkio M, Savilahti E. Time of appearance of immunoglobulin-containing cells in the mucosa of the neonatal intestine. Pediatr Res 1980; 14:953–955.
93. Bridges RL, Condie RM, Zak SJ, Good RA. The morphologic basis of antibody formation development during the neonatal period. J Lab Clin Med 1959; 53:331–357.
94. Ogra SS, Weintraub D, Ogra PL. Immunologic aspects of human colostrum and milk. III. Fate and absorption of cellular and soluble components in the gastrointestinal tract of the newborn. J Immunol 1977; 119:245–248.
95. Hanson LA, Carlsson B, Jalil F, Mellander L, Soderstrom T, Zaman S. Ontogeny of mucosal immunity. In: Branski D, Dinari G, Rozen P, Walker-Smith JA, eds. Frontiers of gastrointestinal research. 13. Pedi-

atric Gastroenterology. Aspects of Immunology and Infections. Basel: Karger, 1986: 1.

96. Roberton DM, Paganelli R, Dinwiddie R, Levinsky RJ. Milk antigen absorption in the preterm and term neonate. Arch Dis Child 1982; 57:369–372.

97. Husby S, Foged N, Host A, Svenhag S-E. Passage of dietary antigen into the blood of children with coeliac disease. Quantification and size distribution of absorbed antigens. Gut 1987;1 28:1062–1072.

98. Eastham EJ, Lichauco T, Grady MI, Walker WA. Antigenicity of infant formulas: role of immature intestine in protein permeability. J Pediatr 1978; 93:561–564.

99. Gruskay FL, Cook RE. The gastrointestinal absorption of unaltered protein in normal infants and in infants suffering from diarrhoea. Pediatrics 1955; 16:763–768.

100. Keljo DF, Butler DG, Hamilton JR. Altered jejunal permeability to macromolecules during viral enteritis in the piglet. Gastroenterology 1985; 88:998–1004.

101. Walker WA. Antigen handling by the small intestine. Clin Gastroenterol 1986; 15:1–20.

102. Cunningham-Rundles C, Brandeis WE, Good RA, Day NK. Milk precipitins, circulating immune complexes and IgA deficiency. Proc Natl Acad Sci USA 1978; 75:3387–3389.

103. McLoughlin GA, Hede JE, Temple JG, Bradley J, Chapman DM, McFarland J. The role of IgA in the prevention of bacterial colonisation of the jejunum of the vagotomised subject. Br J Surg 1978; 65:435–437.

104. Guerrant RL, Moore RA, Kirschenfeld PM, Sande MA. Role of toxigenic and invasive bacteria in acute diarrhea of childhood. N Engl J Med 1975; 293:567–573.

105. Cohen MB, Guarino A, Shukla R, Gianella RA. Age-related differences in receptors for *Escherichia coli* heat-stable enterotoxin in the small and large intestine of children. Gastroenterology 1988; 94:367–373.

106. McClelland DBL, MacDonald TT. Antibodies to cow's milk proteins in human colostrum. Lancet 1976; ii:1251–1252.

107. Glass RI, Svennerholm A-M, Stoll BJ, et al. Protection against cholera in breast-fed children by antibodies in breast milk. N Engl J Med 1983; 308:1389–1392.

108. Lepage P, Munyakazi C, Hennart P. Breast-feeding and infant mortality in children in Rwanda. Lancet 1981; ii:409–411.

109. Taylor B, Norman AP, Orgel HA, Stokes Cr, Turner MW, Soothill J. Transient IgA deficiency and the pathogenesis of infantile atopy. Lancet 1973; ii:111–113.

110. Bergstrand O, Hellers G. Breast-feeding during infancy in patients who later developed Crohn's disease. Scand J Gastroenterol 1983; 18:903–906.

111. Scott H, Solheim BG, Brandzaeg P, Thorsby E. HLA-DR-like antigens in the epithelium of the human small intestine. Scand J Immunol 1980; 12:77–82.

112. Mayer L, Shlien R. Evidence for function of Ia molecules on gut epithelial cells in man. J Exp Med 1987; 166:1471–1483.

113. Bland PW, Warren LG. Antigen presentation by epithelial cells of the rat small intestine. 1. Kinetics, antigen specificity and blocking an anti-Ia antisera. Immunology 1986; 58:1–7.

114. Guillet J-G, Lai M-Z, Briner TJ, Buus S, Sette A, Grey HM, Smith JA, Gefter ML. Immunological self, nonself discrimination. Science 1987; 235:865–870.

115. Tanner JM, Whitehouse RH, Cameron N, et al. Assessment of skeletal maturity and prediction of adult height. 2nd ed. London: Academic Press, 1983.

116. Monk TJ, Spencer J, Cerf-Bensussan N, MacDonald TT. Activation of mucosal T-cells *in situ* with anti-CD3 antibody: phenotype of the activated T cells and their distribution within the mucosal microenvironment. Clin Exp Immunol 1988; 74:216–222.

117. MacDonald TT, Spencer J, Viney JL, Williams CB, Walker-Smith JA. Selective biopsy of Peyer's patches during ileal endoscopy. Gastroenterology 1987; 93:1356–1362.

118. Harmatz PR, Bloch KJ, Kleinman RE, Walsh MK, Walker WA. Influence of circulating maternal antibody on the transfer of dietary antigen to neonatal mice via milk. Immunology 1986; 57:43–48.

119. Brandtzaeg P, Baklien K, Bjerke K, Rognum TO, Scott H, Valnes K. Nature and properties of the human gastrointestinal immune system. In: Miller K, Nicklin S, eds. Immunology of the gastrointestinal tract, Vol 1. Boca Raton, FL: CRC Press, 1987: 1.

120. Walker-Smith JA. Does breast feeding protect against atopic disease? In: Freed DLJ, ed. Health hazards of milk. London: Bailliere Tindall, 1984: 118.

PART **13**

Crohn's Disease

W. Daniel Jackson, M.D.
Richard J. Grand, M.D.

Since its earliest recognition as cases of nontuberculous ileitis in 1813 and its first nosologic characterization as a unique chronic inflammatory bowel disease, regional ileitis, by Crohn, Ginzburg, and Oppenheimer in 1932,[1] Crohn's disease has become more heterogeneous, including greater anatomic and histologic diversity. The return to the eponym Crohn's disease, now preferred to the earlier terms regional ileitis, regional enteritis, and granulomatous colitis, reflects the evolution of the concept with clinical experience. We now know that Crohn's disease can involve any region of the alimentary tract, is not unique in being regional, and does not require histologic presence of granulomas.[2,3] The pedi-

atric experience with Crohn's disease has been consistent with that in adults, with the major exception being the effects of the disease on growth and maturation in children and adolescents.

As currently understood, Crohn's disease is a chronic, transmural, inflammatory process that may affect any segments of the gastrointestinal (GI) tract from mouth to anus in a discontinuous fashion. The small bowel is involved in 90 percent of cases, particularly the distal ileum, which is involved in 70 percent of cases, usually in combination with colitis (ileocolitis), occurring in at least 50 percent of cases. Isolated colonic disease without clinical or radiologic evi-

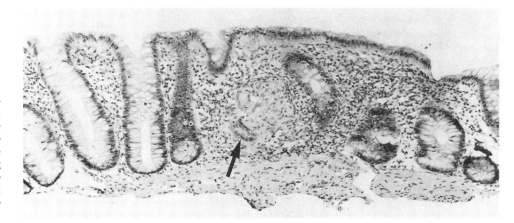

FIGURE 1 Colonic biopsy from an adolescent girl with active Crohn's disease. Note the distortion of the crypt architecture with a prominent noncaseating granuloma and giant cells (*arrow*) amid increased acute and chronic inflammation in the lamina propria.

dence of small bowel involvement occurs in 5 to 10 percent of cases.[4,5] Oral, esophageal, and gastric disease occurs less frequently and rarely without evidence of other bowel involvement. It is the upper GI involvement, particularly of the small bowel, that is responsible for many of the specific nutritional complications of Crohn's disease, and the colonic involvement that poses the greatest challenge for distinction from other infectious and inflammatory bowel diseases. Although Crohn's disease shares many features with ulcerative colitis, clinical, radiologic, and histologic patterns usually allow differentiation of the two disorders (see Table 1 in Part 14 of this chapter). Nevertheless, given the heterogeneity of presentation, the diagnosis of Crohn's disease cannot be excluded in any case of noninfectious colitis. This residual uncertainty has led to the use of the designation "indeterminate colitis" for those cases not fitting the typical patterns of either ulcerative colitis or Crohn's disease.[6,7] Therefore, this section should be read in conjunction with the following one on ulcerative colitis.

BASIS FOR DISEASE

Pathology

Unlike the findings in ulcerative colitis, the inflammation in Crohn's disease usually does not involve a continuous segment of bowel and often presents as discrete regions of inflammation, focal ulcerations (aphthae), or stricture with relatively intact intervening mucosa. As the disease progresses, in the 60 percent of cases involving the colon, right-sided inflammation predominates, with relative but rarely complete sparing of the rectum. Anal involvement, in the form of skin tags, anal fissures, abscesses, and fistulas, is prominent in Crohn's disease and occurs in approximately 25 percent of patients, often preceding intestinal symptoms. The most consistent feature of the inflammation is its transmural extension to all layers of the bowel wall and adventitia recognized grossly as mesenteric inflammation; fat encroachment on the antimesenteric serosal surface; stiffening of the small

FIGURE 2 High-power view of a large crypt abscess adjacent to a granuloma (*arrow*) in a patient with Crohn's disease.

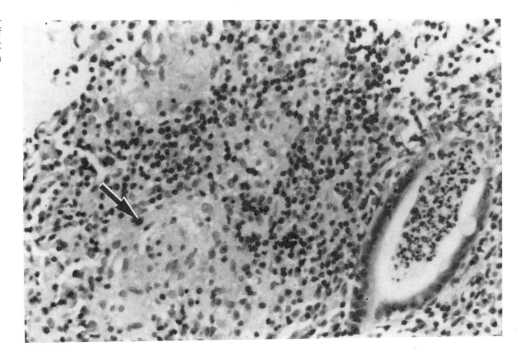

bowel loops due to fibrosis, adhesions, and stricture formation; and fistulae to other loops of bowel, bladder, vagina, or skin.[1,2]

The histology of the lesions in Crohn's disease reveals the transmural extent of the acute and chronic inflammation, often reaching the submucosa with edema, lymphoid aggregates, lymphatic dilatation, and fibrosis. The presence of fibrosis and histiocyte proliferation in the submucosa suggests Crohn's disease, although mucosal changes may resemble ulcerative or infectious colitis with cryptitis, crypt abscesses, and distortion of crypt architecture. Other areas of the bowel may be normal or may show only mild chronic inflammation. Noncaseating granulomas in the lamina propria or submucosa may be found in up to 50 percent of patients and, coupled with the transmural inflammation, disease distribution, and clinical presentation, provide the strongest support for the diagnosis of Crohn's disease (Figs. 1 and 2).[7,8]

Epidemiology

The incidence of Crohn's disease has risen to a plateau estimated in a Baltimore study at 3.5 new cases per 100,000 population per year, making Crohn's disease more common in pediatric practice than ulcerative colitis.[9] The epidemiology is similar to that of ulcerative colitis, with an increased prevalence among whites, especially in the Jewish population, approximately equal male and female representation, and a bimodal age of onset with peaks in the second and third, and fifth and sixth decades.[9,10] Cases of Crohn's disease in infants and young children occur less frequently (Table 1).[11] Chong et al reported from their experience of 106 children with chronic inflammatory bowel disease that two patients were infants with Crohn's disease. Most of the other infants had indeterminate mild colitis, two had allergic colitis, and one had suspected Behçet's disease.[12] However, the majority of pediatric cases are diagnosed between the ages of 10 and 16 years. Approximately 25 percent of all new cases in the population are less than 20 years of age.[10] Although there is an increased prevalence of Crohn's disease among first-degree relatives, no specific heritable pattern has been recognized.[13,14]

Etiology

As in ulcerative colitis, the etiology of Crohn's disease is unknown. The familial, racial, and ethnic clustering of Crohn's disease supports the concept of genetic predisposition to the disorder. Although there is no evidence for primary environmental causes, environmental influence may well act to promote disease in a genetically susceptible individual. Moreover, it is possible that there are different mechanisms responsible for an initial insult and for a chronic inflammatory response. Evidence for a multifactorial etiology and pathogenesis has mounted in several areas: genetics, environmental influences, mucosal integrity, and immunologic factors.

Genetic Basis

Clustering of cases according to family, race, and ethnicity supports the role of genetic factors in the disease. There is an increased prevalence of Crohn's disease in relatives; the frequency is greatest for those sharing the most genes with the patient, such as siblings and parents.[13] An estimated 21 percent of inflammatory bowel disease patients diagnosed as children have a family history of inflammatory bowel disease, with a strong concordance of disease, particularly for Crohn's disease.[10] Seven of eight monozygous pairs of twins reported with inflammatory bowel disease have been concordant for Crohn's disease.[15] As in ulcerative colitis, there is a greater prevalence of Crohn's disease among whites than nonwhites, although nonwhite incidence rates have sharply increased in the last decade. Rates of incidence of Crohn's disease are three to six times higher among the Jewish population.[9]

The association of ankylosing spondylitis with HLA-B27 and with inflammatory bowel disease has led to attempts to identify HLA-antigens associated with Crohn's disease. Such markers appear to be more prevalent in the Crohn's disease population than in ulcerative colitis or healthy controls,[16] but studies have not identified specific genotypes consistently associated with the disease. A similar situation holds for putative biochemical markers such as lysosomal enzymes.[15] Based on the epidemiologic data and the marker studies, it seems that there is no simple mendelian inheritance of inflammatory bowel disease.[17] Crohn's disease and ulcerative colitis are closely related disorders with a similar polygenic basis; their expression in the individual patient is probably modulated by environmental influences.

Environmental Influences

A number of putative infectious agents have been proposed and discounted in the etiology since Crohn's disease was first identified as an entity distinct from tuberculous ileitis. Because of opportunistic bacterial colonization of inflamed bowel mucosa, mere isolation of agents from tissue is insufficient to establish a role in etiology. Antibiotic treatment alone does not consistently alter the course of the disease. Stool cultures do not reveal a consistent pathogen, and there is no evidence for epidemic transmission or contagion.

An area of active research is the identification of a transmissible agent such as a virus or mycobacterium that can reproduce the disease in animal models. The mycobacterium hypothesis is appealing because of the involvement of the terminal ileum (resembling tuberculous ileitis) and the occurrence of granulomas in Crohn's disease. One study reports the isolation of an unclassified mycobacterium from tissue

TABLE 1
Ages at Onset of Symptoms in Inflammatory
Bowel Disease

Age at Onset (year)	Ulcerative Colitis (n = 465)	Crohn's Disease	
		(n = 166)	(n = 168)
0–9	2%[111]	—[112]	2%[112]
10–19	14%	19%	30%
20–29	24%	25%	38%
30–39	25%	16%	13%

Adapted from Motil and Grand.[63]

resected from patients with Crohn's disease which produced granulomatous ileitis when injected into rabbits. The mycobacterium was later isolated from the diseased animals.[18,19] *Mycobacterium linda,* isolated from the tissues of some patients, has been shown to produce nonspecific granulomatous mucosal inflammation when injected into goats.[20] Despite such studies, Koch's postulates have yet to be fulfilled for any microbiologic agent in man putatively linked to Crohn's disease.[21]

Other postulated environmental influences include psychosocial stressors, dietary factors such as cow's milk exposure, excessive consumption of refined carbohydrates or food additives, decreased intake of dietary fiber, and environmental toxins, including tobacco smoke. Most of these associations have been recognized epidemiologically and may simply reflect behavioral adaptations to the disease state rather than causes of the disease.[22] Although significant association of Crohn's disease with smoking tobacco has been identified in adults, the relevance to pediatric inflammatory bowel disease is unclear.

Epithelial Integrity

An impaired mucosal epithelial barrier, allowing increased and inappropriate antigenic exposure to the immune system, which may initiate or perpetuate an inflammatory response, has been proposed as a factor in the pathogenesis of inflammatory bowel disease.[23,24] Data suggest that mucosal integrity is impaired in Crohn's disease, leading to increased permeability to antigenic luminal proteins. Mucus secretions and composition may be altered. Reflecting the diminished barrier to luminal antigens are the frequent findings of elevated levels of antibodies specific for cow's milk protein,[25] enteric bacterial products,[26] and intestinal proteins in Crohn's disease patients.[27] Relevant to this issue is interest in the membranous (M) epithelial cells, which are believed to present macromolecules and organisms from the lumen to underlying gut-associated lymphoid tissue, predominant in the Peyer's patches of the ileum. To date, no specific abnormalities in M-cell structure or function have been related to Crohn's disease.[28] Whether impaired mucosal barrier function is more than a consequence of the inflammation of Crohn's disease and implicated in its etiology is unknown.

Immunologic Mechanisms

Defective or inappropriate immune responses have been factors proposed in the etiology, pathogenesis, and perpetuation of chronic inflammatory bowel disease. The histologic presence of an exuberant immune response and cell injury in the absence of specific exogenous agents, the favorable response to corticosteroids and immunosuppressive drugs, the variety of systemic complications, and extraintestinal manifestations (e.g., uveitis, arthritis) all suggest a major role of the immune system. Nevertheless, although abnormalities in each of the elements of the immune system have been recognized in patients with inflammatory bowel disease, none of these has been consistently observed or has proved to be specific to Crohn's disease or ulcerative colitis.

As discussed above, although Crohn's disease shares features with other inflammatory diseases with an immunogenetic basis, no consistent association has been demonstrated with a single HLA antigen. It is likely that the postulated immunogenetic abnormality is polygenic, a fact that may explain the heterogeneity of Crohn's disease involvement and presentation.[43]

Humoral immune function is intact in patients with inflammatory bowel disease; although antibodies against colonic mucosal cells have been detected in patients with Crohn's disease, they are not consistently observed, are relatively nonspecific, and are unlikely to be cytotoxic in vivo, and their levels do not correlate with clinical disease activity. Similar limitations have been encountered in allergic models of pathogenesis, despite findings of increased serum IgE levels and tissue mast cell activity in patients with Crohn's disease. Evidence for the role of immune complexes and complement-mediated injury is indirect, given the failure to identify such complexes in tissues or sera of patients with Crohn's disease.[43]

Altered local humoral immunity may be involved, according to one hypothesis. In the newborn period, a deficiency of secretory IgA or immature mucosal barrier function may allow increased exposure to macromolecules and sensitization to intestinal tissue antigens, bacteria, or food allergens, which may in turn induce an immune-mediated inflammatory response (such as seen in milk–induced or soy protein–induced colitis) or set the stage for the later induction of chronic inflammatory bowel disease. In the latter case, the hypothesis holds that the local gut-associated lymphoid tissue is sensitized to the antigens at various levels in the intestinal wall, forming the basis for a later activation of an antibody-dependent, cell-mediated, cytotoxic response after being triggered by exposure to cross-reacting antigens.[23] Although sensitized T cells and cytotoxic K cells have been detected in patients with active Crohn's disease, consistent with this hypothesis, the specificity of this phenomenon for inflammatory bowel disease and its presence as an etiologic factor prior to the development of inflammation have not been demonstrated.[43] Indeed, there is evidence that intestinal mononuclear cells in patients with inflammatory bowel disease are deficient in cytotoxic capability.[29,30]

It is clear from the above that most studies have been unable to identify an abnormality of the immune system which is specific in the pathogenesis of inflammatory bowel disease, consistently observed among patients, and unequivocally not the nonspecific consequence of chronic intestinal inflammation.

Many putative host factors may better be considered effects of the stresses of chronic illness or undernutrition accompanying the disease state. Agents implicated in the initiation of disease may not be necessary for the perpetuation of the chronic inflammatory response. That the etiology of inflammatory bowel disease has not been established despite great research effort may be a consequence of a multifactorial basis of disease.

CLINICAL FEATURES

Presentation

The presentation of Crohn's disease in children depends on the location and extent of inflammation. As in other diseases in pediatrics, the added dimension of growth and develop-

TABLE 2
Presenting Features in Crohn's Disease—
Children versus Adults

Clinical Finding	Numbers with Finding at Diagnosis		
	Combined (n = 175)	Adults (n = 140)	Children (n = 36)
Abdominal pain	52%	85%	82%
Diarrhea	25%	62%	88%
Weight loss	2%	50%	60%
Fever	—	41%	77%
Rectal bleeding	6%	13%	22%
Arthritis	2%	—	23%
Mass	2%	—	10%
Growth failure	—	—	30%

Adapted from Motil and Grand.[63]

ment must be considered in both diagnosis and treatment. In many cases, the onset is insidious, with nonspecific features of GI involvement or extraintestinal manifestations, such as growth failure, leading to delayed or incorrect diagnosis. One study reports an average delay of 13 months from onset of symptoms to diagnosis.[31] Diarrhea, abdominal pain (most frequently postprandial periumbilical cramping), fever, and weight loss are the most common presenting features and may reflect small bowel involvement. In patients with Crohn's disease, rectal bleeding, seen in 20 to 30 percent of cases, is much less common than in ulcerative colitis and generally signifies colonic involvement (Table 2). Three general patterns of clinical presentation based on anatomic involvement may be discerned but show considerable overlap (Table 3).[4,5]

Patients with the first pattern present with nonspecific extraintestinal manifestations and growth retardation. Clinically overt signs of GI involvement may not appear for years, although such inflammation may be extensive enough to cause early satiety, nausea, anorexia, and malabsorption syndromes. Over time, net energy and protein deficits are reflected in decreased weight-velocity, followed by decreased height-velocity and delayed sexual maturation. As a consequence of their nutritional, growth, and maturational problems, these patients may be referred to specialists in endocrinology for

TABLE 3
Crohn's Disease—Patterns of Presentation

Extraintestinal signs and growth retardation
Anorexia, malaise, fatigue
Delayed puberty and secondary sexual characteristics
Perianal disease, stomatitis, erythema nodosum
Anemia, hepatitis, renolithiasis, arthritis, clubbing

Upper gastrointestinal involvement
Nausea, vomiting, dyspepsia
Malabsorption, diarrhea
Mineral and vitamin deficiencies (Fe, Zn, Mg, folate, vitamin B_{12})
Abdominal mass, postprandial cramps

Colonic involvement
Diarrhea, urgency
Rectal bleeding, fecal leukocytes
Perianal fistulae, tags, abscess

assessment of short stature and hypogonadism or to psychiatrists for evaluation of anorexia nervosa. Certain extraintestinal features that may give clues to the presence of Crohn's disease include perianal disease, oral aphthae, erythema nodosum, large joint arthritis, uveitis, and digital clubbing. The blood smear may show anemia, and there may be an elevated white blood count and an inexplicably elevated erythrocyte sedimentation rate. Abdominal radiographs may show an unusual gas pattern with some small bowel dilatation. Understanding the challenge of recognition of this insidious mode of presentation leads to timely use of specific tests to confirm the diagnosis.

Another pattern of presentation is produced by small bowel involvement, which probably is responsible for much of the postprandial cramping, early satiety, nausea, and anorexia that patients report. Rarely, the esophagus or stomach may be affected. Gastroduodenal Crohn's disease may be insidious in onset or may present as peptic disease with symptoms of epigastric burning pain, nausea, and early satiety, often relieved by antacids or H_2 antagonists.[32] Radiologic appearance ranges from focal aphthae of the gastric antrum and prepyloric region to narrowing and edema of the gastric outlet on both sides of the pylorus.[32,33] Endoscopy reveals an erosive gastritis but with linear, serpiginous, or aphthous lesions.[32,34] Mucosal biopsies show nonspecific features, although some investigators have reported a remarkably high rate of granulomas on biopsies of the ulcer crater and edge.[32,35] Confidence that gastroduodenal abnormalities are due to Crohn's disease and not to peptic disease depends on the documented presence of Crohn's disease elsewhere in the GI tract, biopsy findings suggesting transmural involvement or granulomas, or "classic" endoscopic or radiologic appearance.[35] In some cases, steroid treatment of active disease elsewhere in the bowel may lead to resolution of proximal abnormalities.

With small intestinal involvement, diarrhea often occurs and, in the absence of colitis, most likely signifies a malabsorption syndrome or choleretic enteropathy due to ileal dysfunction. The malabsorption may be due to mucosal inflammation, partial obstruction leading to stasis and bacterial overgrowth, or enteroenteric or enterocolic fistulae. Estimates of the prevalence of malabsorption in children with Crohn's disease depend on the nutrient that is malabsorbed but range from 17 percent for lactose and 29 percent for fat to 70 percent for protein.[36] The frequency of lactose malabsorption is normal when adjusted for that expected for the ethnic distribution of Crohn's patients and may not be a consequence of small bowel inflammation.[37] However, the presence of lactose of xylose malabsorption indicates active proximal small bowel disease. Deficiencies of iron, folate, and vitamin B_{12} may be more pronounced in patients with small bowel disease, particularly those with terminal ileum involvement.[38,67]

Finally, colonic involvement may present as diarrhea, often associated with cramps and urgency to defecate following any distention of the inflamed colon by the fecal stream. Other signs of colitis may be indistinguishable from those seen in ulcerative colitis and include occult or overt rectal bleeding with mucus and an inflammatory exudate of neutrophils. Perianal disease is more frequent in Crohn's colitis than in ulcerative colitis and may be the only differentiating feature.

Involvement of the perineum may range from simple skin tags to painful perianal abscesses or relatively painless fissures and fistulae. A rare complication, marked dilatation of the colon with risk of perforation and sepsis, known as toxic megacolon, has been reported in Crohn's colitis, and the management is the same as outlined for toxic megacolon complicating severe ulcerative colitis (see Part 14 of this chapter). The rare presentation as acute abdomen is discussed below.

With Crohn's disease, these three patterns of anatomic involvement overlap in a clinical presentation unique for each patient, so that clinical diagnosis alone usually is not possible or sufficient.

Extraintestinal Signs

The systemic nature of Crohn's disease is apparent in the range of potential involvement of extraintestinal organs. Arthritis and arthralgias may occur in up to 11 percent of Crohn's disease patients and usually present as either a seronegative monoarticular arthritis of a knee or ankle or a migratory polyarthritis. Arthritis is more common in Crohn's patients with colonic involvement, either colitis or ileocolitis, and seems to parallel disease activity, although occasionally it precedes overt GI signs. It is usually a nondestructive synovitis of one or more large joints without joint deformity or sequelae.[39,40] Sacroiliitis and ankylosing spondylitis are rare, occur predominantly in patients with the histocompatibility marker HLA-B27, and follow a course independent of intestinal disease activity. The joint manifestations of Crohn's disease cannot be distinguished from those associated with ulcerative colitis.[41]

Approximately 5 percent of patients develop cutaneous lesions of erythema nodosum, erythema multiforme, or pyoderma gangrenosum, usually correlating with disease activity, especially colitis. Erythema nodosum is more commonly found in Crohn's disease than in ulcerative colitis and subsides with control of the intestinal inflammation. Pyoderma gangrenosum is a severe deep ulceration of the skin, often preceded by minor trauma or associated with surgical incisions or stoma sites. It is more common in ulcerative colitis, occurring in 0.5 to 5 percent of ulcerative colitis patients and approximately 0.1 percent of Crohn's disease patients. Management requires control of the underlying bowel disease, often with the addition of metronidazole, topical cromolyn sulfate, and occasional skin grafting.[42]

Signs of liver disease, indicated by an elevated alkaline phosphatase, occur in 8 percent or more of Crohn's patients.[44] However, Crohn's disease rarely presents as liver disease in children.[45] Mild histologic abnormalities of steatosis and pericholangitis may be more common, occurring in up to 20 percent of adults with biochemical abnormalities. Liver involvement correlates with bowel disease activity but rarely progresses to cirrhosis, sclerosing cholangitis, or chronic active hepatitis.[46] Cholelithiasis, usually asymptomatic, may follow ileal dysfunction or resection that interrupts the enterohepatic circulation of bile acids, leading to the decreased cholesterol solubility characteristic of lithogenic bile.[47,48] Prolonged periods of bowel rest without meal-stimulated gallbladder contraction allow stasis of bile in the gallbladder, which contributes to sludge and stone formation.[49,50]

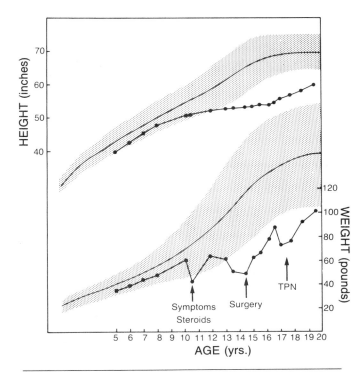

FIGURE 3 Growth curve of an adolescent with Crohn's disease. Note that the reduction in linear growth preceded the acute weight loss and onset of symptoms. Although growth finally accelerated after steroid treatment, limited surgical resection, and parenteral nutrition, premorbid percentiles were not achieved.

Urologic manifestations include calcium oxalate renal calculi due to the increased intestinal oxalate absorption and renal excretion accompanying steatorrhea in which fatty acids bind and limit Ca^{2+} cations available for forming the unabsorbable calcium oxalate salts. Renal calculi occur in approximately 5 percent of children with Crohn's disease, predominantly in those patients with ileal dysfunction.[39] Ureteral inflammation may develop from adjacent transmural bowel inflammation and lead to pyuria, obstruction, and infection. Hydroureter or hydronephrosis may result from renal stones, inflammation, or external compression from adjacent intestinal masses. Recurrent urinary tract infections and pneumaturia may herald enterovesical fistulae.[51]

Other signs of Crohn's disease include uveitis, acutely symptomatic in less than 3 percent and asymptomatic in up to 30 percent of patients[52]; aphthous stomatitis; osteoporosis[53]; anemias of chronic disease, iron deficiency, vitamin B_{12}, and folate deficiency; or zinc deficiency, implicated in taste dysfunction, acrodermatitis, poor healing, and growth failure.[5,54,55]

Undernutrition and Growth Failure

Since the first report of growth failure in a 15-year-old boy with Crohn's disease in 1937,[56] such observations have become more frequent, and growth failure is now recognized as a common feature, often preceding clinically overt GI disease.[57]

Weight loss occurs in up to 87 percent of children presenting with Crohn's disease and may average up to 5.7 kg in magnitude.[58] Often accompanying the weight loss are impaired linear growth, retarded bone development and mineralization, and delayed sexual maturation. These changes initially may be subtle and often precede overt bowel disease by months to years (Fig. 3), best recognized as a reduction in growth velocity over a 6-month to 1-year period. Other criteria of growth failure are a decrease of one standard deviation in height percentile and significant bone age retardation.[64] Most of these effects seem to be due to undernutrition, since they can be reversed by nutritional supplementation of energy and protein.[59,60]

The etiology of undernutrition in inflammatory bowel disease is multifactorial (Table 4). In the majority of patients with growth failure, dietary energy intake is less than the average requirement for age and may be due to anorexia from altered taste, early satiety, or meal-related cramps or diarrhea.[60] The associations between symptoms and eating established during active disease are difficult to extinguish, even after remission of inflammation is achieved. Small bowel involvement is often complicated by malabsorption with abnormal xylose absorption (16 percent), bile salt losses and steatorrhea (29 percent), and increased enteric protein excretion (70 percent).[61] Lactose intolerance occurs in approximately 17 to 20 percent of patients, reflecting the level of intolerance in the general population.[37] The malabsorption may be a consequence of mucosal inflammation or small bowel bacterial overgrowth. There may be hypoalbuminemia (50 percent), hypomagnesemia, hypocalcemia, fat-soluble vitamin losses, and iron, folate, vitamin B_{12}, and zinc deficiencies. Nutrient requirements are increased by the metabolic demands of fever and inflammation,[62] losses through fistulae, and demands for repletion of lean body mass and fat deficits. These nutrient needs are added to those normally imposed by growth, especially critical in adolescence. Such deficits in energy and protein may be insidious, yet a deficit of as little as 100 kcal per day becomes clinically apparent when integrated daily over several months.[63,64]

Most endocrine tests are normal in patients with growth retardation and short stature associated with Crohn's disease. Although bone age may be delayed and somatomedin C levels

depressed, both respond to nutritional therapy, and pituitary, thyroid, adrenal, and growth hormone studies are normal (for further details, see Chapter 2).[65] Similarly, arrested sexual maturation, with delayed puberty and menarche, responds to nutritional therapy and control of the disease. The relationship between nutritional deficits, linear growth retardation, and skeletal and sexual maturation has not been defined.

Growth failure may occur in the presence or absence of steroid therapy. Although there is evidence that corticosteroids may suppress linear growth, their use in controlling Crohn's disease often permits growth to resume at normal rates.[66] Whether or not accelerated or "catch-up" growth sufficient to reach the premorbid growth percentiles is possible during high-dose steroid treatment is unclear (Fig. 3). In some patients, disease activity may be controlled by alternate-day low-dose steroid treatment without significant adverse effects on growth.[66]

Over time, the patient with longstanding disease may adapt to a state of chronic undernutrition and become a "nutritional dwarf," characterized by height stunted below expected percentiles, appropriate weight for height, and normal to subnormal linear growth velocity. The consequences of untreated chronic undernutrition in a child with Crohn's disease are poor disease control, increased complications, delayed puberty, and permanent short stature.[57,67]

Complications

The major intestinal complications of Crohn's disease are due to the transmural nature of the inflammation, extending from mucosa to serosa. Contiguous loops of bowel or other organs may be enveloped in inflammation. Adhesions, strictures, and abscesses may develop, with risk of obstruction or bacterial overgrowth. Fistulae may form to any abdominal or pelvic structure and should be suspected to underlie any chronic draining ulcer or sinus. Fistulae may be enterocutaneous, enteroenteric, enterocolic, perirectal, labial, enterovaginal, and enterovesical. These fistulae may pose a nutritional hazard, being conduits for major losses of protein and other nutrients. Perianal disease occurs in 25 to 50 percent of patients with Crohn's disease, most often in the context of colonic inflammation. Skin tags, anal fissures, and perianal or perirectal fistulae or abscesses may precede other signs of intestinal Crohn's disease or develop during an exacerbation of colitis. Although often minor in appearance, these lesions can create severe discomfort and be quite refractory to treatment. Massive hemorrhage and toxic megacolon, which are potential complications of ulcerative colitis, occur only rarely in Crohn's disease.[68,69]

The risk of malignancy of all types appears to be increased in patients with longstanding Crohn's disease, estimated as much as 20 times greater than normal for patients with Crohn's disease diagnosed before the age of 21 years. Nevertheless, the incidence of small bowel carcinoma is extremely low, and the rates of colonic carcinoma are much lower than in ulcerative colitis. The association of colonic mucosal dysplasia with carcinoma in Crohn's disease is not sufficiently established to recommend prophylactic colectomy, although surveillance colonoscopy and biopsies are prudent in patients with longstanding colitis.[4,63,68,70]

TABLE 4
Causes of Malnutrition in Inflammatory Bowel
Disease

Inadequate intake	Excessive intestinal losses
Anorexia	Protein-losing enteropathy
Altered taste	Hematochezia
Abdominal pain	Bile salt–losing enteropathy
Malabsorption	Increased requirements
Protein	Fever
Carbohydrate (lactose)	Fistulae
Fat	Repletion
Minerals (Ca, Mg, Fe, Zn)	Growth
Vitamins (folate, B, A, D, K)	Hormonal imbalances
Bacterial overgrowth	Somatomedins
Drug inhibition (folate)	Insulin
Drug inhibition (folate)	
Ileal dysfunction	

Adapted from Motil and Grand.[63]

TABLE 5
Evaluation of the Child with Inflammatory
Bowel Disease

History
   Appetite, activity level, school attendance
   Nocturnal symptoms
   Bowel frequency, consistency, melena, mucus
   Family history
   Growth records
   Medications, antibiotics

Three-day diet record

Physical examination
   Height, weight, orthostatic vital signs
   Bone age, arm anthropometry, Tanner stage
   Loss of subcutaneous fat, muscle wasting, edema, pallor
   Oral lesions, rash, clubbing, arthritis, hepatomegaly, perianal signs

Laboratory tests
   CBC and differential, reticulocyte and platelet counts, prothrombin time,
      sedimentation rate, urinalysis
   Stool guaiac, leukocytes, and fat
   Serum total protein, albumin, transferrin, immunoglobulins
   Serum electrolytes, calcium, magnesium, phosphate, alkaline phosphatase
   Serum folate, vitamins A, E, D, and B_{12}, iron, zinc
   Stool bacterial culture, parasite examination, *C. difficile* toxin assay

Special tests
   Schilling's test
   Xylose absorption
   72-hour fecal fat, fecal alpha-antitrypsin
   Lactose breath test

Radiographic and endoscopic studies
   Upper GI and small bowel series, enteroclysis
   Air-contrast barium enema
   Computed tomography, ultrasonography
   Indium-111 leukocyte scan
   Colonoscopy with biopsies
   Bone age

Adapted from Motil and Grand.[63]

DIAGNOSIS

The diagnosis of Crohn's disease is based on clinical presentation, radiologic findings, mucosal appearance and histology, as well as exclusion of alternative etiologies. A complete history should be obtained, with attention to family history, exposure to infectious agents or antibiotic treatment, extra-

intestinal manifestations, and retardation in growth rate or in sexual development. Physical examination should include assessment of hydration, nutritional status, signs of peritoneal inflammation, and signs of chronic systemic disease. Features suggestive of Crohn's disease are stomatitis, perianal skin tags or inflammation, and clubbing. The presence of fever, orthostatic hypotension, tachycardia, and abdominal tenderness, distention, and mass should be considered indications for possible admission to the hospital (Table 5).[4,5,58,63]

Laboratory Evaluation

A complete blood count detects leukocytosis and identifies anemia. The erythrocyte sedimentation rate is elevated in over two-thirds of patients and may be useful as a marker of inflammatory activity. Serum total protein and albumin may be low as a consequence of severe undernutrition and enteric protein losses (Table 6). Serum magnesium, iron, and plasma zinc may be low owing to poor intake coupled with cumulative losses from sloughed intestinal epithelial cells or bleeding. Ileal dysfunction may be revealed by low vitamin B_{12} and fat-soluble vitamin levels. Urinalysis may reveal pyuria. Fresh stool should be obtained for examination of blood, leukocytes, and parasites and cultured for infectious

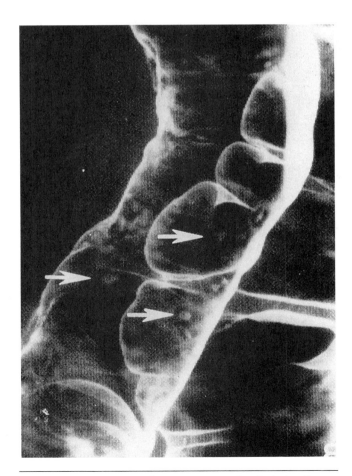

FIGURE 4 Air-contrast barium enema in Crohn's disease demonstrating aphthae (*arrows*) in the colon.

TABLE 6
Laboratory Abnormalities Found in
Inflammatory Bowel Disease

Value	Limits	Ulcerative Colitis (n = 22)	Crohn's Disease (n = 52)
Erythrocyte sedimentation rate	>20 mm/hr	90%	67%
Hematocrit	<33%	38%	50%
Leukocytosis	>10,000/mm^3	33%	28%
Iron	<50 μg/dl	68%	55%
Albumin	<3.3 g/dl	46%	45%
Folate	<3.6 ng/dl	34%	44%

Adapted from Motil and Grand.[63]

pathogens. In addition to screening for routine pathogens, microbiologic studies should include culture for *Yersinia enterocolitica*, isolation of toxigenic strains of *Escherichia coli*, and assay for *Clostridium difficile* toxin. Serologic titers may help exclude *Entamoeba histolytica*. The presence of pathogens may not exclude the existence of underlying Crohn's disease, but the infections must be treated first.[63]

Radiology

Radiographs of the chest and abdomen, both upright and supine, help evaluate the extent of bowel dilatation and exclude ileus, intestinal obstruction, or pneumoperitoneum, signifying perforation. If colitis is suspected and sigmoidoscopy is unavailable, a barium enema with air contrast to reveal mucosal detail may identify characteristic aphthous lesions and show cecal deformity, segmental involvement, or right-sided predominance (Figs. 4 and 5). However, in the presence of active disease, barium enema should be postponed to avoid

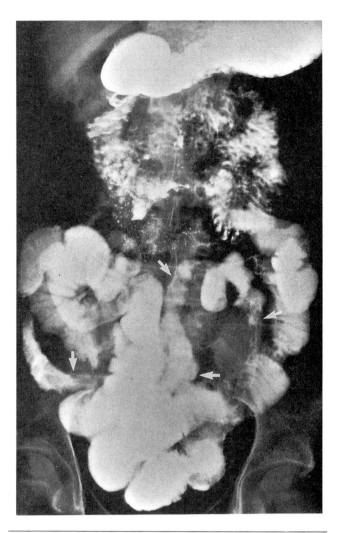

FIGURE 6 Small bowel follow-through of an upper gastro-intestinal series in a 16-year-old girl after treatment with prednisone for Crohn's disease presenting initially with marked small bowel obstruction and growth failure. Note the separation of bowel loops and the long S-shaped segment of constricted nodular terminal ileum (*arrows*). The cecum is elevated, suggesting a contracted ascending colon. Despite the narrowed lumen, there is no obstruction.

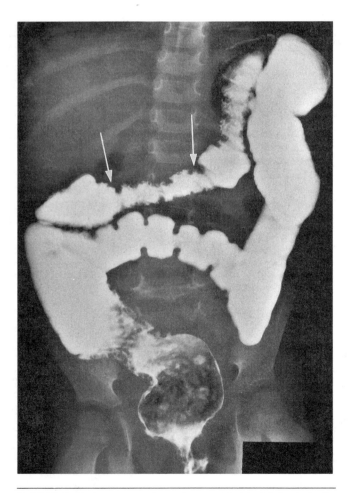

FIGURE 5 Barium enema in an 8-year-old girl with Crohn's disease, revealing segmental colitis involving discrete regions of the transverse colon (*between arrows*). Note the irregular mucosal margins consistent with active ulceration and edema. The rectum, shown with residual stool, was spared.

exacerbation of colitis. An upper GI series with small bowel follow-through or enteroclysis and careful fluoroscopic study of the terminal ileum is essential to define the small bowel involvement affecting more than 90 percent of Crohn's disease patients (Fig. 6). The terminal ileum or other loops may be relatively rigid, constricted, and nodular, with fixed deformities despite fluoroscopic manipulation, features due to the transmural nature of the inflammation in Crohn's disease (Fig. 7). Partial obstruction may be indicated by prestenotic dilatation. This appearance may be contrasted with that of the "backwash" ileitis seen in ulcerative colitis, in which mucosal detail is effaced and dilatation occurs without signs of bowel wall thickening. An abdominal mass, persistent focal tenderness, fever, or obstruction should be evaluated by ultrasonography or computed tomography (CT) to exclude abscess or lymphoma.[70] In situations in which Crohn's disease is

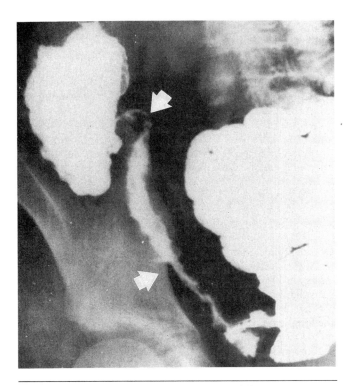

FIGURE 7 Spot film of a terminal ileum with long stenotic segments consistent with Crohn's disease. Note the straightening and separation of this segment from adjacent loops of bowel due to transmural inflammation and serosal fat.

suspected but difficult to demonstrate or in which complications are suspected, CT often can demonstrate the bowel wall thickening, fat wrapping, or abscess (Fig. 8).[71] Despite their value in assessment of disease extent, screening for complications, and diagnosis, radiographic findings have correlat-

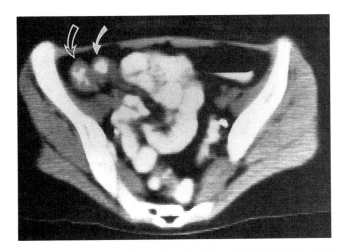

FIGURE 8 Axial computed tomogram of the lower abdomen of a 12-year-old girl with Crohn's ileocolitis. Arrows indicate thickened bowel wall of terminal ileum (*solid arrow*) and cecum (*open arrow*). Note the thickened mesentery. No abscesses or fistulae were demonstrated.

ed poorly with clinical disease activity or response to treatment in adults.[33,74] Indium-111–labeled autologous leukocytes have been advocated as a method to discover and monitor occult disease activity, including measures of disease extent and abscesses.[72] This technique has had limited application in children.[73]

Endoscopy

Colonoscopy with multiple biopsies of the colon and terminal ileum is the most sensitive and specific test for evaluating Crohn's disease (see discussions elsewhere in this book).[75,76] As reflected in its pathology, the lesions of Crohn's disease may appear as discrete ulcerations or aphthae of the mucosa, often with a central exudate and corona of erythema. Rectal or colonic strictures may be encountered. Intervening areas may be normal in both appearance and histologic characteristics. In the cases with colonic involvement (greater than 60 percent), disease tends to be more active in the proximal colon and cecum, although pancolitis is common. Despite the presence of perianal disease, the rectum is often spared. Since the histology of regions that appear grossly to be normal may show signs of nonspecific chronic inflammation, biopsies must be obtained from multiple sites regardless of gross endoscopic appearance. Suction rectal biopsies are helpful in differentiating among various causes of colitis.[77] Histologic features suggestive of chronicity are fibrosis, mononuclear and plasma cell infiltration, granulomas, and architectural distortion, including branching and drop-out of crypts. Endoscopy to explore the esophagus, stomach, and duodenum is indicated when involvement is suspected on clinical or radiologic grounds.[63,32]

Differential Diagnosis

Crohn's disease appears in many forms, which makes a challenge both of its diagnosis and of its differentiation from other entities. The presence of signs of inflammation—as fever, abdominal cramps or tenderness, extraintestinal lesions, or elevated sedimentation rate—often differentiates inflammatory causes of growth failure from endocrine or psychogenic syndromes such as growth hormone deficiency, hypopituitarism, and anorexia nervosa. Symptoms of abdominal pain, tenesmus, or nausea, signs of colitis on stool examination, barium study or colonoscopy with biopsy, or the presence of oral aphthae or perianal disease localize the inflammation to the GI tract. The presence of extracolonic disease or granulomas on biopsy favors Crohn's disease over ulcerative colitis, although in the absence of such features, Crohn's disease cannot be excluded. In some cases, Crohn's colitis clinically and histologically may be indistinguishable from ulcerative colitis until extracolonic or histologic features appear. Occasionally, evidence confirming Crohn's disease does not appear until inflammation develops in the ileostomy or ileoanal pouch of the patient who has had a colectomy for what was presumed to be ulcerative colitis.

Although Crohn's disease rarely presents as acute abdomen, a severe exacerbation of ileocolitis may produce right lower quadrant tenderness, ileus, mass, and fever with leukocytosis and an elevated erythrocyte sedimentation rate. In fact, acute appendicitis may herald or complicate Crohn's disease, which is recognized at laparotomy as unexpected ileocolonic involvement.[80,81] Toxic dilatation of an inflamed colon, complete or partial obstruction, stricture or edema causing obstruction, or fistula may present with tenderness or abdominal distention. Usually, however, signs of peritonitis are lacking, and acute symptoms occur in a chronic or subacute context. A careful history, with review of growth and extraintestinal signs, may suggest underlying inflammatory bowel disease. Nevertheless, regardless of etiology, signs of peritonitis or hemodynamic compromise warrant immediate surgical consultation.

In practice, chronic GI disorders are common in pediatric patients, with up to 10 percent of children between the ages of 7 and 11 years seeking medical attention for the complaint of recurrent abdominal pain, usually periumbilical in location.[78] The periumbilical nature of the pain is nonspecific and not pathognomonic for functional abdominal pain, since it is characteristic of most children presenting with inflammatory bowel disease.[79] In uncomplicated recurrent abdominal pain, discomfort due to stool retention, lactose intolerance, peptic disease, urinary tract infection, or psychosocial etiologies should be considered and eliminated. Henoch-Schönlein purpura may present with episodic abdominal and joint pain prior to specific signs of rash or hematuria. Nocturnal symptoms of pain or urgency, disturbed upper GI function indicated by nausea, vomiting, distention, or anorexia, or systemic signs of fever, weight loss, or extraintestinal inflammation point to possible inflammatory bowel disease. Unless there are signs of inflammation or growth disturbance, extensive evaluation for inflammatory bowel disease is unwarranted. Nevertheless, patients with this clinical pattern should be reevaluated at regular intervals to establish a correct diagnosis as soon as possible.

Rectal bleeding is more common in ulcerative colitis than in Crohn's disease and has many etiologies in addition to colitis, such as Meckel's diverticulum, hemolytic-uremic syndrome, intestinal polyps, and hemorrhoids. Anal fissures secondary to constipation usually present without signs of colitis, chronic perianal inflammation, or skin tags.[63]

Pathogens such as *C. difficile, Y. enterocolitica,* and *E. histolytica* must be excluded, along with the customary *Salmonella, Shigella,* and *Campylobacter* cultured in the setting of enterocolitis. These agents are often overlooked in the initial evaluation and may produce a chronic inflammatory picture resembling Crohn's ileocolitis. Tuberculosis,[82] *Yersinia,*[83] and lymphoma[84] may involve the small bowel, predominantly the terminal ileum, which is rich in lymphoid tissue and may resemble Crohn's disease clinically and radiographically. *Yersinia* may present with extraintestinal features or erythema nodosum and arthritis. Parasites such as *E. histolytica,*[85] *Giardia lamblia,* and *Cryptosporidium* may present as chronic abdominal pain and weight loss, suggesting chronic inflammatory bowel disease.

The patient with acquired immunodeficiency syndrome (AIDS) may present with weight loss, enterocolitis, a variety of skin rashes, and anal lesions that may suggest Crohn's disease. The enterocolitis may be due to a number of agents, including cytomegalovirus, *Cryptosporidium,* and *Mycobacterium avium-intracellulare.* The anal lesions may be con-

dylomata acuminata with proctitis due to *Chlamydia* or herpes simplex virus. Esophageal and gastric ulceration may also be encountered in these patients. AIDS should be considered in all patients with this presentation, especially if the patient has adenopathy and splenomegaly or is in a high-risk category (e.g., intravenous drug abuse, hepatitis B surface antigenemia, homosexuality).[86]

In contrast to most other rheumatologic diseases of childhood, the arthritis of Crohn's disease is usually asymmetric, involving large joints of the lower extremities without deformity, and nonspecific, found in other causes of colitis such as ulcerative colitis and *Yersinia.*[40]

TREATMENT

Optimal management of the patient with Crohn's disease usually requires a combination of nutritional support, judicious use of pharmacologic agents, and appropriate surgical consultation.

Since no pharmacologic regimen has been proven to alter the long-term outcome of Crohn's disease, the goals of treatment are to minimize the morbidity of disease exacerbations without introducing iatrogenic morbidity. No large-scale controlled trials of medical therapy have been performed in children below the age of 15 years. Most of the guidelines that follow are derived from studies of adults and modified by our experience.

Pharmacologic Therapy

Corticosteroids can effect short-term remissions of active small bowel disease in 70 percent of patients (Table 7). Unfortunately, symptoms may recur with reduction of the dosage such that 70 percent suffer relapse within 1 year. Continuous low-dose treatment does not seem to prevent relapse, but higher-dose alternate-day steroid dosage may allow control of symptoms with a minimum of side effects and a lower risk of growth retardation. Indications for steroid therapy are limited to (1) control of symptoms refractory to other agents, (2)

TABLE 7
Pharmacologic Therapy of Crohn's Disease

Acute exacerbation
 Methylprednisolone or prednisone: 1–2 mg/kg/day divided b.i.d., taper to 1 mg/kg/day q.d. and then to q.o.d. over 4–6 weeks depending on clinical response. When remission is achieved, taper and discontinue.

Remission
 Sulfasalazine: 50–75 mg/kg/day divided b.i.d. to q.i.d. (maximum 3–4 g/day)
 Folate supplement: 1 mg q.d.
 Asacol: 400-mg tablets; 0.8 to 4.8 g/day divided b.i.d. to t.i.d.
 Pentasa: 250 mg

Perianal disease or fistula
 Metronidazole: 15 mg/kg/day divided q8h (800 mg maximum)

Refractory disease
 Azathioprine: 2 mg/kg/day divided b.i.d.
 6-Mercaptopurine: 1.5 mg/kg/day divided b.i.d.

---

extensive active small bowel disease, (3) severe or persistent systemic and extraintestinal complications, and (4) postoperative recurrences.

In active disease, induction of remission is achieved with a dosage of 2 mg per kilogram per day of prednisone or methylprednisolone (up to 60 mg per day). Parenteral divided-dose administration is required for severe disease requiring hospitalization, later converted to twice daily or single daily oral prednisone as the patient responds to treatment. Upon continued clinical improvement, the alternate-day dosage is then tapered after 3 to 4 weeks by 2.5-mg to 5-mg weekly decrements over another 4 to 6 weeks. After tapering to an alternate-day regimen, the steroids are gradually discontinued as allowed by the patient's symptoms. In rare cases, higher doses of steroids have been required to. achieve control of disease.[63,66]

Potential morbidity of high-dose steroid therapy includes adrenal suppression, hypertension, osteoporosis, glaucoma, cataracts, masking of infectious intra-abdominal or joint disease, pseudotumor cerebri, hirsutism, cutaneous striae, diabetes, dysphoria, depression or hyperactivity, and altered body composition. An alternate-day regimen may minimize these effects and should be used when possible. The effects on growth are equivocal, since disease activity itself may cause growth retardation. Some patient resume normal growth velocity only after steroid suppression of their disease activity. These patients may require chronic low-dose alternate-day steroid therapy. Other patients, whose disease is quiescent, may show catch-up growth velocity only after steroid withdrawal. A general principle is to use enough corticosteroid to suppress disease activity rapidly and then to decrease the dose to a level adequate to control disease activity and allow growth and full function. The efficacy of steroids in preventing relapses over long-term treatment has not been proved.

In up to 75 percent of patients who cannot be managed without high-dose or prolonged corticosteroids, who are at risk for complications of steroid therapy, or who have disease that is too extensive for surgical removal, immunosuppressive agents (azathioprine, 6-mercaptopurine) are useful in maintaining remission and allowing reduction in steroid dosage. Azathioprine or 6-mercaptopurine seems to be particularly effective in cases with refractory perianal involvement or fistulae. Azathioprine is an S-substituted 6-mercaptopurine metabolized to 6-mercaptopurine in vivo (the latter is believed to be the active agent). The mechanism of action is incompletely defined, although cytotoxic and suppressive effects on natural killer cells and T lymphocytes have been identified. Although bone marrow suppression, pancreatitis, and opportunistic infection are potential risks, current evidence from clinical trials suggests that these complications are rare and can be weighed against the known morbidity of chronic steroid treatment. Lymphoid malignancy is an extraordinarily rare complication of immunosuppressive therapy.[87,88]

Although they may be efficacious as adjunctive therapy in mild to moderate active disease, azathioprine or 6-mercapto-purine optimally is begun during a state of relative remission prior to reduction or discontinuation of steroids, since full efficacy requires a mean of 3 months' treatment. Doses are gradually increased over 5 days to a full dosage of 2 mg

per kilogram per day in two doses for azathioprine and 1.5 mg per kilogram per day in two doses for 6-mercaptopurine, its active metabolite. Leukocyte count, serum transaminases, and amylase are monitored weekly for 1 month, then monthly. Mild leukopenia is an index of drug efficacy and may be reversible without changing the dose of medication. The duration of therapy is indefinite. Experience in adults suggests that the dose may be safely reduced after 1 year of remission to 1 mg per kilogram and continued for prolonged periods.[88] Given the limited pediatric experience with immunosuppressive agents, their use optimally should occur within an established protocol with the informed consent of the patient or parents.

Cyclosporine A, another immunosuppressive agent that has had dramatic efficacy in preventing organ transplant rejection, is being used in refractory cases of severe ulcerative colitis and Crohn's disease, including anecdotal use in a few children. It acts to suppress specific components of cell-mediated immunity, including cytotoxic lymphocytes, interleukin production, and plasma cell antibody production. These effects are apparently reversible. Its advantages over azathioprine (or 6-MP) are its less generalized immunosuppression and its more rapid onset of action, making it potentially safer and more effective in modifying the course of acute illness, possibly preventing surgery. Double-blind clinical trials in adults are underway and are proposed for children.[58,88]

Sulfasalazine, 50 to 75 mg per kilogram per day (maximum 3 to 4 g per day), is useful in the management of Crohn's colitis. In conjunction with steroid treatment, it is better than placebo in ileocolitis.[89,90,92,93] Although the National Cooperative Crohn's Disease Study did not prove it effective in preventing relapse. or in treating small bowel disease, others have found it useful in some cases of small bowel involvement, especially at higher doses than standard for colitis, and advocate it as a chronic regimen.[58,63,66,90,91] Sulfasalazine usually is introduced gradually according to patient tolerance. It often can be renewed after dosage reduction because of side effects of headache, nausea, vomiting, or bloody diarrhea. Neutropenia and oligospermia are reversible side effects, but the former can progress to profound agranulocytosis and is dangerous to the patient with a central venous catheter and inflamed bowel. Folate malabsorption due to competitive inhibition of absorption is treated with 1-mg daily supplements.[63]

Since the side effects of sulfasalazine are due primarily to the sulfapyridine moiety and the anti-inflammatory effects are due to the topical activity of the relatively poorly absorbed 5-amino-salicylate moiety,[93] alternative preparations of 5-aminosalicylic acid have been created to prevent proximal GI absorption (Asacol, Pentasa, Dipentum). These drugs are currently undergoing clinical trials of efficacy. Since Asacol and Pentasa, unlike sulfasalazine or Dipentum, do not require colonic bacteria to release the active agent, they potentially are active in the small intestine, and evidence is accruing for their usefulness in small intestinal Crohn's disease as well as Crohn's colitis.[93,94]

Metronidazole is an antimicrobial agent active against anaerobes, including *Bacteroides*, which is helpful in patients with Crohn's colitis unresponsive to sulfasalazine or with complications of perianal disease or small intestinal bacterial overgrowth. Potential morbidity includes an Antabuse-like effect, reversible peripheral neuropathy, usually presenting as lower limb paresthesias with chronic usage, and a putative increased risk of malignancy. The recommended dosage of 15 mg per kilogram per day in three doses (800 mg maximum daily dose) should be achieved gradually and continued until remission is achieved for up to 6 months. Long-term maintenance therapy at half the initial dose has been continued in some adult patients. In pediatric patients with Crohn's disease, metronidazole is usually used as an adjunct to sulfasalazine or steroids and rarely as primary or single therapy.[92,95,96]

Antimotility agents such as loperamide (0.1 mg per kilogram two or three times per day; maximum dose 4 to 6 mg) may be used to prolong intestinal transit time and facilitate fluid absorption, providing relief from diarrhea at night and at social functions. These agents should be used with caution and discontinued for symptoms of camping, distention, or fever. Agents that bind bile acids, such as cholestyramine, may be useful in reducing the choleretic diarrhea that follows ileal dysfunction or resection.[5,63]

Nutritional Therapy

Given the limitations and morbidity of some forms of medical treatment and the nutritional impact of Crohn's disease, it is appropriate that increased emphasis has been placed on nutritional rehabilitation and therapy as a way of altering the course of Crohn's disease (Table 8) (see elsewhere in this book for details). Optimal prospective management in patients with inflammatory bowel disease should include regular assess-

TABLE 8
Indications for Nutritional Therapy in Inflammatory Bowel Disease

Primary therapy for disease activity
Newly diagnosed inflammatory bowel disease
Chronic disease unresponsive to medical management
Short bowel syndrome
Closure of fistulae
Small bowel obstruction
Ostomy care

Supportive therapy for disease activity
Inoperable diffuse disease
Preoperative nutritional rehabilitation

Drug-nutrient interactions
Sulfasalazine-folate

Abnormalities of specific laboratory test
Anemia (microcytic, macrocytic)
Hypoproteinemia
Fat malabsorption
Lactose intolerance
Serum mineral deficiencies (Fe, Ca, Mg, K$^+$)
Serum vitamin deficiencies (folate, B$_{12}$, A, D)
Prolonged prothrombin time (vitamin K)
Depressed alkaline phosphatase (Zn)

Complications of inflammatory bowel disease
Malnutrition
Growth failure

Adapted from Grand.[64]

TABLE 9
Nutritional Therapy of Inflammatory Bowel Disease

Well-balanced, high-protein and high-energy diet
  ± Low residue
  ± Lactose-free
  ± Low-fat, medium-chain triglycerides, and cholestyramine supplemented

Enteral supplementation (140–150% of Recommended Daily Allowances for height-age)
  Continuous or intermittent nasogastric tube feeding
  Feeding gastrostomy, continuous or intermittent

Total parenteral nutrition (140–150% of Recommended Daily Allowances for height-age)
  Peripheral
  Central

Minerals and Vitamins	
Therapeutic	
Iron	
Ferrous sulfate (20% Fe)	6 mg elemental Fe/kg/day,
Ferrous gluconate (11.5% Fe)	divided in 3 oral doses
Iron dextran, intramuscular (Imferon)	Follow directions on package insert
Calcium	1200 mg/day
Magnesium	200–400 mg elemental magnesium/day intravenously
Zinc sulfate (22% Zn)	50–100 mg elemental zinc/day divided in 3 oral doses
Vitamin B$_{12}$	1 mg at 3-month intervals (subcutaneously or intramuscularly)
Vitamin D	400 U/day
Folate	1 mg daily
Supplemental	
Multivitamins with minerals (daily)	

Adapted from Motil and Grand.[63]

ment of growth and nutritional status. Data to follow are height by stadiometer, body weight, triceps skin-fold thickness, midarm muscle circumference, and serum levels of protein, albumin, and transferrin. A reduction in growth velocity over a 6-month interval may presage or reflect an exacerbation of Crohn's disease activity. Maintenance of optimal nutritional status with aggressive support of energy and protein intake may prolong remission or allow reduced corticosteroid treatment. The goals of nutritional therapy in Crohn's disease must include (1) recovery of metabolic homeostasis by correcting specific nutrient deficits and replacing ongoing losses; (2) provision of sufficient energy and protein for positive nitrogen balance (protein-synthesis) and healing; and (3) promotion of catch-up growth toward premorbid percentiles. One of the goals of nutritional therapy is to permit the progression to puberty. Consideration of Tanner stage and bone age is critical to gauge the potential for catch-up in linear growth by nutritional supplementation prior to pubertal epiphyseal closure.[64]

Deficiences in iron, folate, or vitamin B$_{12}$ should be corrected with appropriate supplements (Table 9). Magnesium depletion, better reflected by low urinary excretion after a challenge dose than by plasma concentration, should be corrected by parenteral magnesium sulfate. Low plasma zinc levels suggest low dietary intake, redistribution to circulating hepatic pools as a consequence of chronic inflammation, or depletion due to active mucosal inflammation and enteric losses. Treatment consists of supplements of zinc sulfate, 220 mg daily. Oral protein and calorie supplements are prescribed to make up deficits revealed by 3-day diet-diary analysis of voluntary intake. Guidelines for supplementation are to provide at least 140 percent of the recommended daily allowance (RDA) for height-age for both energy and protein intake. A low-residue diet is prudent in case of symptomatic stricture or narrowing by edema of the intestinal lumen.[67]

Continuous nocturnal nasogastric infusions through a soft Silastic catheter may be necessary in those patients who cannot voluntarily increase their intake. An elemental formula may be necessary if there is significant malabsorption. In severe or complicated Crohn's disease in which enteral feeding is not possible or bowel rest is desired, parenteral nutrition via a central venous catheter is necessary to achieve nutritional goals.[67]

Various degrees of bowel rest have been advocated in the treatment of refractory disease or fistulae. Complete bowel rest or exclusion of enteral nutrients has not been proved to reduce inflammation, although symptoms may be relieved owing to reduced stool weight, luminal distention, and peristalsis, particularly in cases of partial obstruction or severe colitis. Prospective trials have indicated that bowel rest adds little to the benefits of improved nutrition by total parenteral nutrition.[97] There is evidence from animal research that enteral or luminal nutrients are important to the maintenance of the intestinal epithelium, independent of general nutritional status. Villous atrophy and decrease in mucosal weight and protein content were observed in rats maintained on total parenteral nutrition. Although atrophy has not been demonstrated in humans, reversible reductions in brush border disaccharidases and peptidase activity have been reported in adults in similar conditions.[98] Unknown are the effects of diminished meal-related pancreatic, biliary, and gastric exocrine and endocrine secretions, which may stimulate epithelial growth, on the healing of inflamed bowel.

Elemental diets, formulae that are completely absorbed in the small intestine with virtually no residue, have been advocated as primary therapy for Crohn's disease to both induce and sustain remission. The therapeutic basis hypothesized includes (1) reduced antigenic stimulation; (2) altered bowel flora; and (3) altered intestinal secretions. The elemental formula (e.g., Vivonex) almost invariably must be administered by nasogastric feeding tube or in flavored form during the day, and maintenance over a long term may be difficult. In relatively small trials, its efficacy in inducing remission has been comparable to that of steroids, but the periods of remission are short. The major indications for an elemental diet are (1) malabsorption, (2) stricture, and (3) disease activity refractory to medical therapy.[99-102]

Weighing against the potential benefits of the partial bowel rest of elemental diet therapy or complete bowel rest with total parenteral nutrition in cases of colitis is evidence that some residue in the diet may be essential for optimal colonic epithelial nutrition. Fiber, nonabsorbed dietary carbohydrate in the form of pectin, guar, oat bran (all soluble fibers), or certain starches provide substrates for fermentation by colonic bacteria. Among the products of fermentation are short-chain fatty acids (e.g., propionate, acetate, and butyrate), which are preferred substrates for the colonic epithelium.[103] Interest

is growing in the clinical use of instilled short-chain fatty acids in the setting of diversion colitis in which dramatic healing has been demonstrated.[104] Healing of experimental colitis in rats has been attributed to effects of fermentable fiber.[105] These data suggest a potential application of fermentable dietary fiber or instilled short-chain fatty acids in inflammatory bowel disease.

The optimal nutritional therapy serves as an adjunct to medical therapy in controlling symptoms and inducing remission. As noted, short-term remissions have been achieved solely by aggressive nutritional support, either elemental, enteral, or parenteral. After nutritional rehabilitation and disease remission have been achieved, efforts should continue to ensure catch-up growth rates of at least 0.5 cm per month and 1 kilogram per month toward premorbid percentiles.[64,67]

Surgery

Unlike ulcerative colitis, in which disease is limited to the colon and can be cured to total colectomy, there is no definitive surgical solution to Crohn's disease. For this reason, as well as the high incidence of complications requiring repeat operation, surgery is reserved for the acute and chronic complications of Crohn's disease refractory to medical or nutritional therapy. Nevertheless, prolonged remissions may occur after resection.[106] Specific indications for operation include intestinal obstruction, fistula, abscess, uncontrolled hemorrhage, toxic megacolon, perforation, and growth failure in the setting of localized disease.[107,110] Percutaneous ultrasound- or CT-guided drainage of abscesses is an option, but without surgical resection recurrence is frequent.[108] Local resection is more successful in isolated small bowel disease than in the presence of colitis. Intractable colitis is managed by total proctocolectomy or colectomy with ileorectal anastomosis if the rectum is spared. The endorectal pull-through operation used for intractable ulcerative colitis should never be used for Crohn's disease, owing to the risk of postoperative perianal disease, including fistulae and abscesses. Perianal abscesses often need drainage with probing or contrast injection to exclude underlying fistulae; proctectomy is rarely required to control perianal disease; anal tags should not be excised.[64,110]

PROSPECTIVE MANAGEMENT AND PROGNOSIS

Crohn's disease is a chronic incurable disease requiring careful surveillance, patient education, and expert management by a team consisting of the pediatrician, gastroenterologist, nutritionist, psychiatrist or psychologist, social worker, and nurse. An alliance with a pediatric surgeon familiar with inflammatory bowel disease is essential for management of potential complications. The success of long-term management will be determined in part by the degree to which the patient and family understand and participate in the treatment.

Approaches to the psychological adjustment to Crohn's disease are dependent on the developmental status of the child and family dynamics. Young children are approached differently than adolescents, common issues being separation anxiety, body image, privacy, sexuality, and autonomy. Anxiety is enhanced by uncertainty of diagnosis. The child and family are often comforted after their unspoken suspicions of underlying cancer or AIDS are confronted and dispelled. Equivocation about the diagnosis of inflammatory bowel disease should be minimized. Presentation as a diagnosis of exclusion of infectious etiologies may not be as reassuring as pointing out the chronic features and other clinical evidence that make Crohn's disease the unique diagnosis. Invasive procedures may be made less traumatic by rehearsal in play therapy by a trained therapist. Compliance with treatment and prompt attention to early signs of relapse may be enhanced by careful patient and family education about the rationale and advantages of therapy and early intervention. Knowledge of or association with other successful patients with Crohn's disease and comparison with other children with chronic diseases such as asthma or diabetes may put the child's own experience in context.

Nutritional status and growth, sexual maturation, psychosocial adjustment to disease, and compliance with therapy should be monitored as carefully as one monitors the clinical signs and symptoms of disease activity. Frequency of follow-up depends on the course of disease activity, but intervals should be no greater than 6 months. Most children with Crohn's disease can expect to live full, productive lives with good general health. Mortality is low although morbidity is high, especially in patients with colonic involvement. Fertility is unaffected in Crohn's disease unless there is malnutrition or inflammatory damage to reproductive organs. Disease activity often remains stable or improved during pregnancy, although an exacerbation may follow delivery. There seems to be no increased risk to the fetus.[4] Although the incidence of colorectal carcinoma is increased over normal in Crohn's disease, the risk is poorly defined and is too low to warrant prophylactic colectomy.[64]

The management of Crohn's disease in children is complex and requires adaptation of the patient to the lifelong unpredictable nature of this disease and the morbidity of chronic medication and hospital visits, as well as to the demands of adolescent development. A willingness to become active in the management of his or her condition and to work with the team involved in each case is probably the patient's best prognostic feature.

SUMMARY AND CONCLUSIONS

Crohn's disease in children is varied in its presentation, regions and severity of GI involvement, and response to therapy. This heterogeneity is reflected in its etiology, which is probably multifactorial with significant environmental modulators of disease expression and activity. Children uniquely face the risk of impaired growth and development due to the chronic nutritional insults of Crohn's disease. In addition, the risks of chronic medication and the emotional burdens on family and patient are significant and cumulative. Those who care for children with Crohn's disease must integrate pharmacologic, nutritional, and psychosocial therapies for optimal outcomes.

REFERENCES

1. Crohn BB, Ginzburg L, Oppenheimer GD. Regional enteritis: a pathologic and clinical entity. JAMA 1932; 99:1323.
2. Crohn BB. Granulomatous disease of the large and small bowel, a historical survey. Gastroenterology 1967; 52:767.
3. Donaldson RM. Crohn's disease. In: Sleisinger MH, Fordtran JS, eds. Gastrointestinal disease. 3rd ed. Philadelphia: WB Saunders, 1983; 1088.
4. Kelts DG, Grand RJ. Inflammatory bowel disease in children and adolescents. Curr Probl Pediatr 1980; 10:5.
5. Motil K, Grand RJ, Ulcerative colitis and Crohn's disease in children. Pediatr Rev 1987; 9:109.
6. Price AB. Overlap in the spectrum of nonspecific inflammatory bowel disease. "Colitis indeterminate." J Clin Pathol 1978; 31:567.
7. Riddel RH. Pathology of idiopathic inflammatory bowel disease. In: Kirsner JB, Shorter RG, eds. Inflammatory bowel disease. 3rd ed. Philadelphia: Lea and Febiger, 1988:329.
8. Price AB, Morson BC. Inflammatory bowel disease: the surgical pathology of Crohn's disease and ulcerative colitis. Hum Pathol 1975; 6:7.
9. Calkins BM, Lilienfeld AM, Garland CF, Mendeloff AI. Trends in incidence rates of ulcerative colitis and Crohn's disease. Dig Dis Sci 1984; 29:913.
10. Mendeloff AI. The epidemiology of inflammatory bowel disease. Clin Gastroenterol 1980; 9:258.
11. Miller RC, Jackson M, Larson E. Regional enteritis in early infancy. Am J Dis Child 1971; 122:301–311.
12. Chong SKF, Blackshaw AJ, Morson BC, Williams CB, Walker-Smith JA. Prospective study of colitis in infancy and early childhood. J Pediatr Gastroenterol Nutr 1986; 5:352.
13. Lashner BA, Evans AA, Kirsner JB. Prevalence and incidence of inflammatory bowel disease in family members. Gastroenterology 1986; 91:396.
14. Mayberry JF, Rhodes J, Newcombe RG. Familial prevalence of inflammatory bowel disease in relatives of patients with Crohn's disease. Br Med J 1980; 1:84.
15. McConnell RB. Genetic aspects of idiopathic inflammatory bowel disease. In: Kisner JB, Shorter RG, eds. Inflammatory bowel disease. 3rd ed. Philadelphia: Lea and Febiger, 1988:87.
16. Smolen JS, et al. HLA antigens in inflammatory bowel disease. Gastroenterology 1982; 82:34.
17. Lewkonia RM, McConnell RB. Familial inflammatory bowel disease—heredity or environment. Gut 1976; 17:235.
18. Chiodini RJ, VanKruiningen HJ, Thayer WR, et al. Possible role of mycobacteria in inflammatory bowel disease. Dig Dis Sci 1984; 29:1073.
19. Gitnick G. Is Crohn's disease a mycobacterial disease after all? Dig Dis Sci 1984; 29:1086.
20. VanKruiningen HJ, Chiodini RJ, Thayer WR, et al. Experimental disease in infant goats induced by a mycobacterium isolated from a patient with Crohn's disease. Dig Dis Sci 1986; 31:1351.
21. Gorbach SL. Intestinal microflora in inflammatory bowel disease—implications for etiology. In: Kirsner JB, Shorter RG, eds. Inflammatory bowel disease. 3rd ed. Philadelphia: Lea and Febiger, 1988; 51.
22. Mendeloff AI, Calkins BM. The epidemiology of idiopathic inflammatory bowel disease. In: Kirsner JB, Shorter RG, eds. Inflammatory bowel disease. 3rd ed. Philadelphia: Lea and Febiger, 1988; 3.
23. Shorter RG, Huizenga KA, Spencer RJ. A working hypothesis for the etiology and pathogenesis of nonspecific inflammatory bowel disease. Am J Dig Dis 1972; 17:1024.
24. Walker WA, Isselbacher KJ. Uptake and transport of macromolecules by the intestine: possible role in clinical disorders. Gastroenterology 1974; 67:531–550.
25. Knoflach P, et al. Serum antibodies to cow's milk proteins in ulcerative colitis and Crohn's disease. Gastroenterology 1987; 92:479.
26. Blaser MJ, Miller RA, et al. Patients with active Crohn's disease have elevated antibodies to antigens of seven enteric bacterial pathogens. Gastroenterology 1984; 87:888.
27. Carlsson HE, Lagererantz R, Perlmann P. Immunologic studies in ulcerative colitis. VIII. Antibodies to colon antigens in patients with ulcerative colitis, Crohn's disease, and other diseases. Scand J Gastroenterol 1977; 12:707.

28. Wolf JL. The membranous epithelial (M) cell: a portal of antigen entry. In: Kirsner JB, Shorter KG, eds. Inflammatory bowel disease, Philadelphia: Lea and Febiger, 1988:75.

29. MacDermott PP, Bragdon MJ, Kodner IJ, Bertovitch MJ. Deficient cell-mediated cytotoxicity and hyporesponsiveness to interferon and mitogenic lectin activation by inflammatory bowel disease peripheral blood and intestinal mononuclear cells. Gastroenterology 1986; 90:6–11.

30. Gibson PR, Jewell DP. Local immune mechanism in inflammatory bowel disease and colorectal carcinoma. Gastroenterology 1986; 90:12–19.

31. Burbidge FJ, Huang S, Bayless TM. Clinical manifestations of Crohn's disease in children and adolescents. Pediatrics 1975; 55:866.

32. Rutgeerts P. Onette E, Vantrappan G, Geboes K, Broeckaert L, Talloen L. Crohn's disease of the stomach and duodenum: a clinical study with emphasis on the value of endoscopy and endoscopic biopsies. Endoscopy 1980; 12:288–294.

33. Goldberg HI, Caruthers SB, Nelson JA, Singleton JW. Radiographic findings of the National Cooperative Crohn's Disease study. Gastroenterology 1979; 77:925–937.

34. Danzi JT, Farmer RG, Sullivan BH, Rankin GB. Endoscopic features of gastroduodenal Crohn's disease. Gastroenterology 1976; 70:9–13.

35. Korelitz BI, et al. Crohn's disease in endoscopic biopsies of the gastric antrum and duodenum. Am J Gastroenterol 1981; 76:103.

36. Beeken WL. Absorptive defects in young people with regional enteritis. Pediatrics 1974; 52:69.

37. Kirschner BS, DeFavaro MV, Jenson W. Lactose malabsorption in children and adolescents with inflammatory bowel disease. Gastroenterology 1981; 8:829.

38. Jeejeebhoy KN, Ostro MJ. Nutritional consequences and therapy in inflammatory bowel disease. In: Kirsner JB, Shorter KG, Inflammatory bowel disease. Philadelphia: Lea and Febiger, 1988:513.

39. Gryboski JD, Spiro HD. Prognosis in children with Crohn's disease. Gastroenterology 1978; 74:807.

40. Lindsley CB, Schaller JG. Arthritis associated with inflammatory bowel disease. J Pediatr 1974; 84:6.

41. Palumbo J, Ward LC, Sauer WG, Sendamore HH. Musculoskeletal manifestations of inflammatory bowel disease. Mayo Clin Proc 1973; 48:411–416.

42. Klein JD, Biller JA, Leape L, Grand RJ. Pyoderma gangrenosum occurring at multiple incision sites. Gastroenterology 1987; 92:810–813.

43. Elson CO. The immunology of inflammatory bowel disease. In: Kirsner JB, Shorter KG, eds. Inflammatory bowel disease. 3rd ed. Philadelphia: Lea and Febiger, 1988:97.

44. Dew MJ, Thompson H, Allen RN. The spectrum of hepatic dysfunction in inflammatory bowel disease. J Med 1979; 48:113.

45. Kane W, Miller K, Sharp HL. Inflammatory bowel disease presenting as liver disease during childhood. J Pediatr 1980; 97:775.

46. Eade MN, Cooke WT, Brooke BN, Thompson H. Liver disease in Crohn's colitis: a study of 21 consecutive patients having colectomy. Ann Intern Med 1971; 74:518.

47. Cohen S, Kaplan M, Gottlieb L, Patterson J. Liver disease and gallstones in regional enteritis. Gastroenterology 1971; 60:237.

48. Heaton KW, Read AE: Gallstones in patients with disorders of the terminal ileum and disturbed bile salt metabolism. Br Med J 1969; 3:494.

49. Roslyn JJ, et al. Increased risk of gallstones in children receiving total parenteral nutrition. Pediatrics 1983; 71:784.

50. Holzbach RT. Gallbladder stasis: consequence of longterm parenteral hyperalimentation and risk factor for cholelilthiasis. Gastroenterology 1983; 84:1055.

51. Greenstein AJ, Janowitz MD, Sachar DB. The extraintestinal complications of Crohn's disease and ulcerative colitis: a study of 700 patients. Medicine 1976; 55:401.

52. Daum F, et al. Asymptomatic transient uveitis in children with inflammatory bowel disease. Am J Dis Child 1979; 133:170.

53. Jackson WD, Dawson-Hughes B, Grand RJ. Effects of Crohn's disease on bone mineral density in children. (Abstract) Gastroenterology 1988; 94:A203.

54. McClain C, Sontour C, Zieve L. Zinc deficiency: a complication of Crohn's disease. Gastroenterology 1980; 78:272.

55. Solomons NW, Rosenfeld RL, Jacob RA, et al. Growth retardation and zinc nutrition. Pediatr Res 1976; 20:923–927.

56. Snapper J, Gruen J, Foyer A. Observations sur l'ileite regionale. Proceedings of the Second International Congress of Gastroenterology. Brussels, 1937, pp 935–937.

57. Kirschner BS, Voincher O, Rosenberg IH. Growth retardation in inflammatory bowel disease. Gastroenterology 1978; 75:5048.

58. Kirschner BS. Crohn's disease in children and adolescents. In: Bayless TM, ed. Current management of inflammatory bowel disease. Toronto: BC Decker, 1989: 244.

59. Kirschner BS, Klich JR, Kalman SS, et al. Reversal of growth retardation in Crohn's disease with therapy emphasizing oral nutritional restitution. Gastroenterology 1981; 80:10–15.

60. Kelts DG, et al. Nutritional basis of growth failure in children and adolescents with growth failure. Gastroenterology 1979; 76:720.

61. Beeton WL, Bush HJ, Sylvester DL. Intestinal protein loss in Crohn's disease. Gastroenterology 1972; 62:207–215.

62. Beisel WR, Wannemacher RW, Neufeld HA. Relation of fever to energy expenditure. In: Kinney JM, Leuse E, eds. Assessment of energy metabolism in health and disease. Columbus, OH: Ross Laboratories, 1980:144.

63. Motil KJ, Grand RJ. Ulcerative colitis and Crohn's disease in children. In: Kirsner JB, Shorter RG, eds. Inflammatory bowel disease. 3rd ed. Philadelphia: Lea and Febiger, 1988: 227.

64. Grand RJ. Growth in children and adolescents. In: Bayless TM, ed. Current management of inflammatory bowel disease, Toronto: BC Decker, 1989:237.

65. Kirschner BS, Sutton MM. Somatomedin levels in growth-impaired children and adolescents with chronic inflammatory bowel disease. Gastroenterology 1986; 91:830.

66. Whitington PF, Barnes HV, Bayless TM. Medical management of Crohn's disease in adolescence. Gastroenterology 1977; 72:1338–1344.

67. Motil K, Grand RJ. Nutritional management of inflammatory bowel disease. Pediatr Clin North Am 1985; 32:447.

68. Bernstein L. Complications of inflammatory bowel disease. Pract Gastroenterol 11:35; 1987.

69. Markowitz J, Daum F, Aiges M, et al. Perianal disease in children and adolescents with Crohn's disease. Gastroenterology 1984; 86:829.

70. Winthrop JD, et al. Ulcerative and granulomatous colitis in children. Radiology 1985; 154:657.

71. Gore RM, et al. CT findings in ulcerative, granulomatous and indeterminate colitis. AJR 1984; 143:279.

72. Savery-Mutti S, et al. [111]Indium autologous leukocytes in inflammatory bowel disease. Gut 1983; 24:293.

73. Gordon I, Vivian G. Radiolabelled leukocytes: a new diagnostic test in occult infection/inflammation. Arch Dis Child 1984; 59:62.

74. Dobbins WO: Gastroduodenal Crohn's disease. In: Bayless TM, ed. Current management of inflammatory bowel disease, Toronto: BC Decker 1989: 218.

75. Williams CB, et al. Total colonoscopy in childhood. Arch Dis Child 1982; 57:49.

76. Hassal E, Barclay GN, Ament ME. Colonoscopy in childhood. Pediatrics 1984; 73:594.

77. Surawicz CM, Belic L. Rectal biopsy helps to distinguish acute self-limited colitis from idiopathic inflammatory bowel disease. Gastroenterology 1984; 86:104–113.

78. Apley J. The child with abdominal pains. 2nd ed. Oxford: Blackwell, 1975.

79. Grand RJ. Personal communication.

80. Fonkalsrud EW, Ament ME, Fleisher D. Management of the appendix in young patients with Crohn's disease. Arch Surg 1982; 117:11.

81. Yang SS, et al. Primary Crohn's disease of the appendix: report of 14 cases and review of the literature. Ann Surg 1979; 189:334.

82. Bhargava D, et al. Diagnosis of ileocecal and colonic tuberculosis by colonoscopy. Endoscopy 1985; 31:68.

83. VanTrappen G, et al. Yersinia enteritis and enterocolitis. Gastroenterology 1977; 72:220.

84. Sartoris DJ, Harell GS, Anderson MF, Zboralske FF. Small-bowel lymphoma and regional enteritis of the duodenum: radiographic similarities. Radiology 1984; 152:291.

85. Crowson T, Hines C. Amebiasis diagnosed by colonoscopy. Gastrointest Endosc 1978; 24:254.

86. Cone L. Update on AIDS. Dis Colon 1986; 29:60–64.

87. Verhave M, Winter HS, Grand RJ. Efficacy and safety of azathioprine

in children with inflammatory bowel disease. (Abstract) Gastroenterology 1987; 92:A1682.

88. Korelitz BI. Immunosuppressive therapy. In: Bayless TM, ed. Current management of inflammatory bowel disease. Philadelphia: BC Decker, 1989:252.

89. Van Hees PAM, Van Lier HJJ, et al. Effect of sulfasalazine in patients with active Crohn's disease: a controlled double-blind study. Gut 1981; 22:404–409.

90. Summers RW, Switz DM, et al. National Cooperative Crohn's Disease study: results of drug treatment. Gastroenterology 1979; 77:847–869.

91. Wenckert A, Kristensen M, et al. The longterm prophylactic effect of salazosulphapyridine (Salazopyrine^R) in primarily resected patients with Crohn's disease. Scand J Gastroenterol 1978; 13:161–167.

92. Ursing BO, et al. A comparative study of metronidazole and sulfasalazine for active Crohn's disease. The cooperative Crohn's disease study in Sweden. II. Result. Gastroenterology 1982; 83:550–562.

93. Klotz U, Maier K, Fischer C, Heinkel K. Therapeutic efficacy of sulfasalazine and its metabolites in patients with ulcerative colitis and Crohn's disease. N Engl J Med 1980; 303:1499–1502.

94. Riley SA, Mani V, et al. Comparison of delayed-release 5 amino alicylic acid (mesalamine) and sulfasalzine as maintenance treatment for patients with ulcerative colitis. Gastroenterology 1988; 94:1383–1389.

95. Hildebrand H, Berg NO, Hoevels J, Ursing B. Treatment of Crohn's disease with metronidazole in childhood and adolescence. Gastroenterol Clin Biol 1980; 21:19–25.

96. Ursing B. Metronidazole therapy. In: Bayless TM, Current management of inflammatory bowel disease. Toronto: BC Decker, 1989.

97. Greenberg GR, Fleming CR, Jeejeebhoy KN, et al. Controlled trial of bowel rest and nutritional support in the management of Crohn's disease. Gastroenterology 1985; 88:1405(A).

98. Guedon C, Schmitz J, Lerebours F, et al. Decreased brush border hydrolase activities without gross morphologic changes in human intestinal mucosa after prolonged total parenteral nutrition of adults. Gastroenterology 1986; 40:373–378.

99. O'Morain C, Segal AW, Levi AJ. Elemental diet as primary treatment of acute Crohn's disease: a controlled trial. Br Med J 1984; 288:1859–1862.

100. Sanderson IR, Udeen S, Davies PS, et al. Remission induced by elemen-

tal diet in small bowel Crohn's disease. Arch Dis Child 1987; 62:123–127.

101. Seidman EG, Bouthillia L, Weber AM, et al. Elemental diet vs prednisone as primary treatment of Crohn's disease. Gastroenterology 1986; 90:1625.

102. Sabbah S, Seidman EG. Dietary management of Crohn's disease in children and adolescents. In: Bayless TM. Current management of inflammatory bowel disease, Philadelphia: BC Decker, 1989:230.

103. Sakata T. Stimulatory effect of short chain fatty acids on epithelial cell proliferation in rat intestine: a possible explanation for trophic effects of fermentable fibre, gut microbes and luminal trophic factors. Br J Nutr 1987; 58:95–103.

104. Harig JM, Soergel KH, Komorowski RA, Wood CM. Treatment of diversion colitis with short chain fatty acid irrigation. N Engl J Med 1989; 320:23–28.

105. Rolandelli R, et al. Comparison of parenteral nutrition and enteral feeding with pectin in experimental colitis in the rat. Am J Clin Nutr 1988; 47:715–721.

106. Homer DR, Grand RJ, Colodny AH. Growth, course and prognosis after surgery for Crohn's colitis. Pediatrics 1977; 59:717.

107. Glotzer DJ. Indications for operation on inflammatory bowel disease—a surgeon's opinion. In: Kirsner JB, Shorter RG, eds. Inflammatory bowel disease. 3rd ed. Philadelphia: Lea and Febiger, 1988: 549.

108. Van Sonnenberg E, Mueller PR, Ferucci JT. Percutaneous drainage of 250 abdominal abscesses and fluid collections. I. Results, failures and complications. Radiology 1984; 151:337–341.

109. Gryboski J, Spiro HD. Prognosis in children with Crohn's disease. Gastroenterology 1978; 74:87.

110. Greenberger N. Indications for surgery in inflammatory bowel disease: a gastroenterologist's opinion. In: Kirsner JB, Shorter RG, eds. Inflammatory bowel disease, 3rd ed. Philadelphia: Lea and Febiger, 1988:529.

111. Goligher JC, et al. Ulcerative colitis. Baltimore: Williams & Wilkins, 1968.

112. Kyle J. Crohn's disease. New York: Appleton-Century-Crofts, 1972.

113. Banks BM, Zetzel L, Richter HS. Morbidity and mortality in regional enteritis: report of 168 cases. Am J Dig Dis 1969; 14:369.

PART
14

Ulcerative Colitis

W. Daniel Jackson, M.D.
Richard J. Grand, M.D.

Ulcerative colitis is a chronic relapsing inflammatory disease of the colonic and rectal mucosa of unknown etiology. It was first described in 1875 by Wilks and Moxon as an inflammatory bowel disease distinct from infectious colitis.[1] After the description of a transmural inflammatory disease of the small intestine, regional ileitis, by Crohn et al in 1932,[2,3] similar cases of transmural disease of the colon were recognized as distinct from ulcerative colitis. Cases of isolated colonic involvement in the absence of small bowel disease had features recognized in Crohn's disease. In 1960,

criteria differentiating ulcerative colitis from Crohn's colitis were established.[4] Experience has subsequently eroded some of the clinical, colonoscopic, and histologic distinctions between the two diseases, although many of the distinguishing features remain accurate. Given the lack of specific diagnostic features of ulcerative colitis to allow exclusion of the diagnosis of Crohn's disease of the colon, as many as 15 percent of cases of inflammatory bowel disease presenting as colitis remain indeterminate.[5] Similarity between the features of Crohn's disease and ulcerative colitis suggests a common basis of disease etiology and pathogenesis. Therefore, this discussion should be read in conjunction with the preceding part of this chapter.

BASIS OF DISEASE

Pathology

By definition, the inflammation in ulcerative colitis is limited to the colon and rectum. Table 1 contrasts the patterns of pathologic involvement in ulcerative colitis and Crohn's disease. Based on these patterns, a distinction between the two entities can be made provisionally in most cases. The distal colon is most severely affected, and the rectum is involved in the majority of patients with ulcerative colitis. Inflammation is limited primarily to the mucosa and consists of continuous involvement along the length of the bowel with varying degrees of ulceration, hemorrhage, edema, and regenerating epithelium. Although considered to be limited to the colon, inflammation may extend uninterrupted to the cecum and up to 25 cm into the terminal ileum as "backwash" ileitis, generally not associated with clinical small bowel disease. In severe disease in which the mucosal epithelium has been destroyed, inflammation may extend through the submucosa down to the muscularis. Intervening areas of regenerating granulation tissue and residual epithelium may form islands of tissue termed pseudopolyps. Thickening of the bowel wall and fibrosis are rare, although shortening of the colon and focal colonic strictures may occur in longstanding disease.[6]

The histology of the mucosa in ulcerative colitis lesions demonstrates continuous acute and chronic inflammation with mucosal and submucosal infiltration by polymorphonuclear leukocytes and mononuclear cells, rarely extending to the muscularis. The colonic crypts show the most characteristic changes. Cryptitis and crypt abscesses characterize acute inflammation, which may lead to chronic changes of crypt distortion with branching and drop out, diminished goblet mucous cells, and Paneth cell metaplasia. No granulomas and little fibrosis are present.[6]

Etiology

As with Crohn's disease, the cause of ulcerative colitis is unknown. Much of the research into the etiology of inflammatory bowel disease is reviewed under Crohn's Disease (see preceding part of this chapter). No infectious agent has been found, although the lesions resemble changes seen with infectious colitis.[7] There is evidence of an autoimmune process in serum antibodies to colonic mucosa, immune complex complement activation, and lymphocytes directed against colonic epithelium, but these phenomena are not consistently observed and do not correlate with disease activity. The therapeutic efficacy of glucocorticoids in controlling the activity of ulcerative colitis may be due to effects of suppression of immunologically mediated inflammation.[8] The association of ulcerative colitis with a high familial prevalence of atopic diseases and extraintestinal manifestations of erythema nodosum, arthritis, uveitis, and vasculitis supports the concept of immunologic factors in the pathogenesis. However, data are currently insufficient to determine whether immune mechanisms have a primary or secondary role.[8] There is insufficient evidence of an allergic etiology for ulcerative colitis. Although allergic colitis occurs, it is rarely seen after infancy and is usually transient.[9] No specific dietary practices have been unequivocally implicated as causes or risk factors. No data support a psychosomatic etiology in terms of stress, personality type, or psychiatric illness, although emotional and other psychosocial factors may affect the presentation and course of the disease.[10,11]

TABLE 1
Comparative Features of Ulcerative Colitis and Crohn's Disease

Site of Disease	Ulcerative Colitis	Crohn's Disease
Upper gastrointestinal tract	0%	20%
Ileum alone	0%	19%
Ileum and colon	Backwash ileitis	52%
Colon	90% (distal colon predominant)	9% (proximal colon predominant)
Rectum	Approximately 100%	50%
Perianal region	Rare	25%
Radiology	Continuous involvement, foreshortening, loss of haustra, irregular mucosal margins, normal terminal ileum	Segmental involvement, skip regions, mural thickening, stenotic separate loops, abnormal terminal ileum
Sigmoidoscopy	Hemorrhagic mucosa, diffuse continuous inflammation, pseudopolyps	Patchy involvement, skip regions, relative rectal sparing, focal aphthae, linear ulcers
Histology	Mucosal and submucosal inflammation, cryptitis, crypt abscess, distortion of architecture	Transmural inflammation, non-caseating granulomas, prominent lymphoid tissue, preserved goblet cells, fibrosis

Adapted from Jackson and Grand.[74]

Epidemiology

The incidence of ulcerative colitis increased gradually in the pediatric population until 1978 but since then has been relatively stable worldwide. The incidence in the general population ranges from 3.9 to 7.3 cases per 100,000, with the prevalence ranging from 41.1 to 79.9 cases per 100,000 population.[12,13]

In the 10- to 19-year-old age group, the incidence has been estimated at 2.3 cases per 100,000 age-specific population. Although no specific heritable patterns exist, 15 to 40 percent of patients may have other family members with inflammatory bowel disease, with an incidence approximately 10 times greater when there is a positive family history.[14-16]

The disease is more prevalent among the white population, and its representation is greater among those of Jewish heritage. Ulcerative colitis occurs more commonly in Northern Europe and North America, with an urban predominance. Males and females are represented equally. The distribution of age of onset is bimodal, peaks occurring in the second and third decades and again in the fifth and sixth decades. Between 15 and 40 percent of all patients with ulcerative colitis present before age 20 years, with peak onset in adolescence.[13] The disease is rare in individuals under 2 years of age, although infants with ulcerative colitis have been reported (see Table 1 in preceding part of this chapter).[17] Most cases of infantile colitis are due to cow's milk or soy protein allergy and are transient.[9]

CLINICAL FEATURES

Presentation

There are at least four patterns of presentation of ulcerative colitis differing by the extent of mucosal inflammation and systemic disturbance (Table 2). Extraintestinal manifestations of disease may be the presenting features and precede the manifestations of overt colitis. The first signs of disease may be growth failure characterized by decreased linear growth velocity.[18,19] Most studies have attributed growth deficiency to subtle chronic dietary caloric deficits caused by relative anorexia associated with gastrointestinal (GI) distress.[20-22] Increased metabolic demands from inflammation and exudative losses have been suspected but have not been proved.[23] Nondestructive arthritis involving peripheral large joints may precede the onset of intestinal symptoms.[24] The skin lesions of erythema nodosum erupt on the extensor surfaces of the arms and legs, often prior to recognition of colitis. The erythrocyte sedimentation rate, C-reactive protein, or orosomucoid (alpha$_1$ acid glycoprotein) may be elevated, suggesting a systemic reaction to an inflammatory process. Stool examination may reveal occult blood and leukocytes due to the underlying colitis. Some series report up to 25 percent of patients with elevated serum alkaline phosphatase levels. In our experience, this is extremely uncommon and, when present, reflects the presence of true primary liver disease. Of adult patients with biochemical abnormalities, 15 to 19 percent have steatosis on liver biopsies. Less commonly, patients have presented with or have developed later complications of sclerosing cholangitis or chronic active hepatitis.[25,26]

Ulcerative colitis most commonly presents with the insidious onset of diarrhea, later associated with hematochezia, usually without systemic signs of fever, weight loss, or hypoalbuminemia. In these patients, disease is often confined to the distal colon and rectum, the physical examination is normal without abdominal tenderness, and the course remains mild with intermittent exacerbations.

Approximately 30 percent of cases have moderate signs of systemic illness and present with bloody diarrhea, cramps often associated with urgency to defecate, anorexia and weight loss, malaise, mild anemia, and low-grade or intermittent fever. Colicky pain, urgency, and tenderness suggest dysmotility due to inflammation. Physical examination may reveal abdominal tenderness, and stool analysis shows varying amounts of blood and leukocytes.

Severe colitis occurs in approximately 10 percent of patients and is characterized by more than six bloody stools per day, significant anemia, hypoalbuminemia, fever, tachycardia, and weight loss. The abdomen may be diffusely tender or distended. A subgroup of patients may not respond to medical therapy and may require early colectomy. Criteria for recognizing these patients have been proposed and are discussed later in the section on surgery.[27]

Although exceptions exist, the severity of clinical presentation correlates roughly with the anatomic extent of disease involvement, ranging from mild proctitis to fulminant pancolitis. In addition, over time, disease often does not extend much beyond the borders of its initial involvement. The tempo and course of disease activity are often related to the intensity of its onset in most cases.

Complications

The most serious complication of ulcerative colitis is toxic megacolon. Although reported to occur in up to 5 percent of ulcerative colitis patients, it is relatively rarely encountered in our pediatric experience. Toxic megacolon is a medical and surgical emergency. As suggested by its name, dilatation of the diseased colon is accompanied by fever, ab-

TABLE 2
Ulcerative Colitis—Patterns of Presentation

Prodromal (<5%)
Growth failure, arthropathy, erythema nodosum, occult fecal blood, elevated erythrocyte sedimentation rate, nonspecific abdominal pain or altered bowel pattern

Mild disease (50%–60%)
Diarrhea, mild rectal bleeding, abdominal pain
No systemic disturbance

Moderate disease (30%)
Bloody diarrhea, cramps, urgency, abdominal tenderness
Systemic disturbance: anorexia, weight loss, mild fever, mild anemia

Severe disease (10%)
More than six bloody stools per day, abdominal tenderness with or without distention, tachycardia, fever, weight loss, significant anemia, leukocytosis, and hypoalbuminemia.

Adapted from Motil and Grand[11] and Jackson and Grand.[74]

dominal distension, and tenderness, and, depending on the tempo of presentation, tachycardia, hypokalemia, hypoalbuminemia, and dehydration. Flat and upright abdominal radiographs showing dilatation of the colon, often the transverse colon, differentiate toxic megacolon from other causes of acute abdomen (Fig. 1). A leukocytosis with a predominance of immature neutrophils or anemia may be present. Hypomagnesemia is likely and may contribute to colonic dysfunction. It is important to consider that some of these signs, particularly fever and tenderness, may be masked by high-dose steroid treatment. A high index of suspicion is prudent regarding any change in clinical appearance, including attention to reduction in stool frequency, which may reflect colonic dysmotility rather than clinical improvement. The patient with toxic megacolon is at risk of colonic perforation, gram-negative sepsis, and massive hemorrhage.[28,29,31]

The pathogenesis of toxic megacolon is probably multifactorial and includes disturbed motility due to extension of inflammation or inflammatory mediators to the muscularis mucosae and myenteric plexus, hypokalemia and hypomagnesemia impairing neuron and muscle fiber function, and edema from low oncotic pressure due to hypoproteinemia. Disrupted mucosal integrity may allow entry of bacteria to submucosal tissues, leading to necrosis and peritonitis. Absorptive function of the mucosa is also impaired, resulting in increased luminal fluid volume and electrolyte losses.[28,29]

Risk factors for toxic megacolon include drugs that impair motility, such as anticholinergic agents, narcotic analgesics, or antidiarrheal agents such as loperamide. Barium enemas and instrumentation (e.g., colonoscopy) in acute colitis have precipitated toxic megacolon, presumably from overdistention of the bowel wall. Metabolic abnormalities, such as hypokalemia, hypomagnesemia, or hypoproteinemia, impair

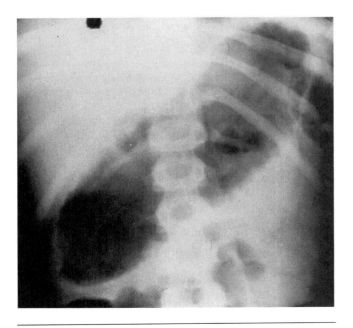

FIGURE 1 Massive dilatation of the transverse colon in a patient with fulminant ulcerative colitis developing acute abdominal distention.

colonic epithelial integrity and motor function and are frequently found in patients with toxic megacolon.[28,29]

Effective monitoring requires serial physical examination and periodic (every 8 to 12 hours) supine and upright radiographs to assess colonic caliber and exclude the presence of intra-abdominal free air indicative of perforation. Radiographic findings include colonic distention with loss of normal haustra and signs of edema. Once the disorder is recognized, optimal management mandates prompt surgical consultation and should include stool bacterial culture with assay for *Clostridium difficile* toxin and treatment with broad-spectrum antibiotics and high-dose steroids. A nasogastric tube or, if necessary, a long tube into the distal intestine decompresses the colon and minimizes further fluid accumulation. Fluid and electrolyte homeostasis should be restored with normal saline, albumin, and blood. If not previously initiated, parenteral hyperalimentation should begin in anticipation of a prolonged period of restricted enteral intake. Since most distention occurs in the anteriorly located transverse colon, positioning the patient prone with or without a rectal tube may facilitate colonic decompression. Patients who fail to respond to these aggressive medical measures and have persistence of toxic dilatation for longer that 48 hours, perforation, or ongoing hemorrhage require emergency colectomy.[28,29]

In longstanding ulcerative colitis, a colonic stricture may occur. Although in adults this may be due to carcinoma, in the pediatric age group, benign postinflammatory fibrotic strictures are most likely. These strictures usually are transient and respond to medical treatment.[28,30] Intra-abdominal and hepatic abscesses occur less commonly than in Crohn's disease, except after perforation or colectomy.[28] The increased risk of dysplasia and carcinoma in longstanding ulcerative colitis is described later in this discussion.[32-34]

Arthritis occurs in approximately 25 percent of patients and often correlates with disease activity. Less commonly, arthritis is the presenting feature. The arthritis of inflammatory bowel disease usually presents as a migratory polyarthritis or as a seronegative nondestructive synovitis of one or more large joints (knee or ankle) without joint deformity or other sequelae. Sacroiliitis and ankylosing spondylitis are rare, occur predominantly in patients with the histocompatibility marker HLA-B27, and follow a course independent of intestinal disease activity. The joint manifestations of ulcerative colitis are similar to those appearing less commonly in Crohn's disease.[23,24]

Pyoderma gangrenosum is a progressive deep ulceration of the skin that complicates healing of surgical incisions, stoma sites, or minor trauma. It occurs more commonly in ulcerative colitis patients than in Crohn's disease patients, often presenting during an exacerbation or on reduction of the steroid dosage. Although metronidazole and topical cromolyn sulfate have proved helpful, it is usually refractory to management until the underlying bowel disease is controlled. Skin grafting may be required for large lesions.[23,71]

DIAGNOSIS

The diagnosis of ulcerative colitis is based on clinical presentation, radiologic findings, mucosal appearance, and histology, as well as exclusion of other known etiologies of colitis. A complete history should be obtained, with attention to family history, exposure to infectious agents or antibiotic treatment, retardation in growth or sexual development, and extraintestinal manifestations. Physical examination should include assessment of hydration, nutritional status, and systemic and extraintestinal signs of chronic disease. The presence of fever, orthostatic hypotension, tachycardia, abdominal tenderness, distention, and masses indicates severe disease and the need for hospitalization.[27]

Laboratory Evaluation

A complete blood count detects leukocytosis or anemia. The erythrocyte sedimentation rate is elevated in approximately 70 percent of patients and is a marker of inflammatory activity.[35] Electrolyte disturbances are uncommon except when dehydration is present, but serum protein and albumin concentration may be low. Poor intake or losses from colonic inflammation and bleeding may cause low serum iron and magnesium levels. Stool should be examined for blood, leukocytes, and ova and parasites. Culture of fresh stool excludes *Salmonella, Shigella, Campylobacter,* toxigenic *Escherichia coli,* and *Yersinia.* Serologic titers may help exclude *Entamoeba histolytica.* The colitis due to the cytopathic toxin of *C. difficile* may resemble the lesions in ulcerative colitis or may complicate underlying inflammatory bowel disease. *C. difficile* enterocolitis is more prevalent in patients with ulcerative colitis than in the general population. Assay for *C. difficile* toxin should be obtained in all patients regardless of prior antibiotic treatment.[36,37] The identification of pathogens mandates specific treatment but does not exclude the diagnosis of ulcerative colitis.

Radiology

Chest and abdominal radiographs, both upright and supine, are used to evaluate the extent of colonic dilatation and help diagnose obstruction due to stricture and pneumoperitoneum from perforation. These films form a baseline for later comparisons. A barium enema should never be performed in patients with acute, active colitis because of the risk of precipitating toxic dilation. Single-contrast barium enema is rarely performed except in young children but helps in assessing the character and extent of colonic disease. In mild to moderate colitis without dilatation, an air-contrast barium enema may reveal enough mucosal detail to detect ulcerations. Even without air contrast, barium enema may reveal the chronic changes of foreshortening, loss of haustra, pseudopolyps, and strictures as well as spasm (Figs. 2 and 3). Unless defined on barium enema by reflux of contrast into the terminal ileum, an upper GI barium series and small bowel follow-through with fluoroscopic study of the terminal ileum are necessary to define small bowel involvement. A late film during the upper GI series to study the right colon may uncover colonic involvement. This technique is safer than a barium enema, although lack of colonic distention may make interpretation difficult. In Crohn's colitis, the ileum may be stiffened, nodular, and contracted, whereas in the backwash ileitis of ulcerative colitis, the ileum is dilated and

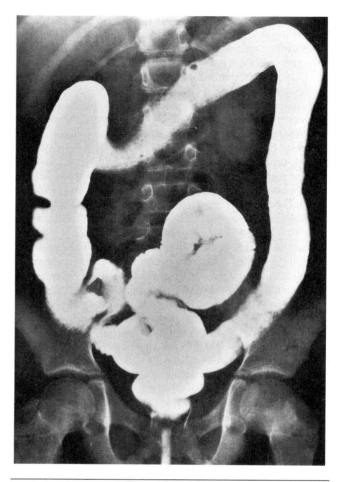

FIGURE 2 Single-contrast barium enema in a 10-year-old boy with ulcerative colitis. There is continuous involvement of the entire colon with reflux of barium into the terminal ileum through a normal ileocecal valve. The small caliber, shortening, and loss of haustra of the transverse and distal colon indicate longstanding disease. The irregular mucosal margins of the cecum and transverse colon suggest active ulceration. The poor coating and dilatation of the terminal ileum may represent backwash ileitis. There are no strictures or signs of obstruction.

mucosal detail is effaced. In ulcerative colitis, there should be no other signs of small bowel involvement.[38] In moderately to severely ill patients with bowel dilatation, extensive bleeding, persistent fever, or abdominal mass, abdominal ultrasonography or computed tomography may identify an intra-abdominal abscess,[39] the presence of which suggests Crohn's disease. Although ^{111}In-labeled leukocytes may define the extent of disease or locate an occult abscess in adults, the radiation dose is significant and the technique has been used rarely in pediatrics.[40,41]

Endoscopy

Flexible sigmoidoscopic or colonoscopic inspection of the colon and ileum, in conjunction with mucosal biopsies, provides the most sensitive and specific evaluation of intestinal inflammation and, in may cases, may make barium contrast

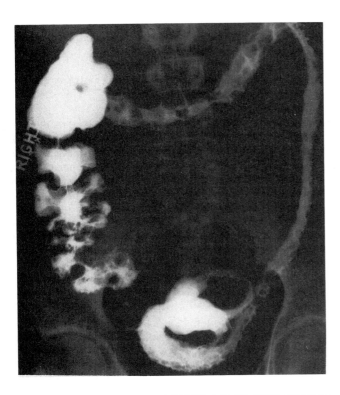

FIGURE 3 Barium enema demonstrating continuous involvement of colonic mucosa with edema and ulceration causing thumbprinting and spiculation of mucosal margins. Note the contracted lumen of the transverse and descending colon distal to the distorted and dilated ascending colon.

studies unnecessary. The development of flexible, small-caliber endoscopes has allowed colonoscopic evaluation of pediatric patients of all ages, including infants. Colonoscopy is indicated in the diagnostic evaluation when sigmoidoscopy and distal biopsies are normal or equivocal. In longstanding disease, colonoscopy allows surveillance of the entire colon for dysplasia. Colonoscopy is contraindicated in severe colitis because of the risks of perforation and hemorrhage, and the induction of toxic megacolon. A limited proctosigmoidoscopy often suffices to establish the diagnosis in most cases of active disease. Excessive bowel distention with air insufflation should be avoided, and the examination should be halted upon encountering areas of severe inflammation with mucosal atrophy and pseudopolyps or stricture.[42,43]

Active disease is characterized by diffuse continuous involvement of the mucosa with edema, erythema, and spontaneous or induced friability. Extensive erosions may be seen in the acute stages. In severe disease, the residual islands of relatively intact or regenerating mucosa or granulation tissue may appear polypoid above the atrophic surrounding mucosa. With active disease, mucosal edema causes a diminished vascular pattern, whereas with inactive disease, mucosal atrophy may reveal a granular mucosa with a prominent vascular pattern. In ulcerative colitis, proctitis is usually present and, although the entire colon may be involved, the distal colon usually is affected more severely.

In contrast, segmental or right-sided colonic inflammation with rectal sparing suggests Crohn's disease, and small bowel involvement should be sought on upper GI series with small bowel follow-through. In contrast to the left-sided or distal predilection of ulcerative colitis, Crohn's colitis tends to be more severe in the right or proximal colon, sparing the rectum in approximately half of the cases. The mucosa in Crohn's colitis appears less friable, and early involvement may present as discontinuous regions of erythema and edema. The aphthous lesions of Crohn's disease may be recognized as small discrete oval ulcers with erythematous coronas. Progression of Crohn's disease may lead to deep linear or serpiginous ulceration creating a cobblestone effect, to be distinguished from the pseudopolyp formations of ulcerative colitis. Ironically, ulcerations are more indicative of Crohn's disease than of ulcerative colitis.

During colonoscopy, biopsies should be obtained at all levels explored, regardless of gross endoscopic appearance, in order to increase the sensitivity and specificity of diagnosis. Biopsy of the terminal ileum is useful in distinguishing between Crohn's disease and ulcerative colitis. Histology often reveals insidious microscopic evidence of acute cryptitis or chronic changes such as crypt architectural distortion not apparent to the endoscopist. In cases in which limited rigid proctosigmoidoscopy is done, suction rectal biopsies using a Rubin tube produce excellent specimens for diagnosis.[44,50]

Sedation of patients is mandatory for extended examination by flexible sigmoidoscopy or colonoscopy. The combination of an anxiolytic-amnestic agent (benzodiazepines such as midazolam, 0.05 to 0.1 mg per kilogram, or diazepam 0.1 to 0.3 mg per kilogram) and a narcotic analgesic (meperidine 1 to 3 mg per kilogram) is synergistic in sedation and minimizes the dose of either drug. A reliable intravenous access should be maintained throughout the procedure. The drugs are administered incrementally until the desired level of sedation is achieved, not exceeding a predetermined maximum dose. Patients should be attended by a nurse in addition to the person assisting the endoscopist. Vital signs should be monitored frequently, including continuous heart rate and oxygen saturation with pulse oximetry. Naloxone, epinephrine, and diphenhydramine should be available for management of drug reactions, as well as oxygen and complete supplies for cardiopulmonary resuscitation.

Differential Diagnosis

A number of GI disorders that may mimic ulcerative colitis are prominent in the pediatric population. Up to 10 percent of children, particularly at ages 7 to 11 years, may seek medical attention for the complaint of recurrent abdominal pain, usually periumbilical in location.[45] In most of these children, extensive evaluation for inflammatory bowel disease is unnecessary unless there are associated features of fever, diarrhea, growth or nutritional disturbance, or other extraintestinal manifestations, or laboratory evidence of inflammatory disease or disorders. However, the periumbilical location of abdominal pain is not specific and should not be considered pathognomonic for functional abdominal pain, since it also is characteristic of most children presenting with inflammatory bowel disease.[46] Constipation, lactose intolerance, urinary tract infection, pregnancy, pelvic inflammatory disease, peptic disease, or psychosocial distress may cause recurrent abdominal pain and should be considered.

Rectal bleeding may be due to Meckel's diverticulum, hemolytic-uremic syndrome, polyposis, hemorrhoids, or anal fissures. The bleeding from Meckel's diverticulum is usually painless, copious, and without fecal leukocytes. Hemolytic-uremic syndrome can often be excluded by inspection of the blood smear and measuring the blood urea nitrogen.[47] Polyps may be detected by sigmoidoscopy or barium enema. Fissures may be secondary to constipation or may be among the perianal manifestations of Crohn's disease, particularly if inflammation is prominent.

Colitis, characterized by fecal leukocytes accompanying the bleeding and sigmoidoscopic evidence of inflammation, may be caused by infection or allergy.[48] Infection with *Salmonella, Shigella, Campylobacter, Yersinia, Aeromonas,* certain toxigenic strains of *E. coli,* and *E. histolytica* may resemble ulcerative colitis and should be excluded. *C. difficile* pseudomembranous colitis may present even in the absence of a history of antibiotic treatment and seems to be prevalent in patients with inflammatory bowel disease.[37,38] Since only approximately 50 percent of cases of acute self-limited (presumably infectious) colitis have positive cultures, and because of the delay in treatment pending results of microbiologic studies, endoscopic and pathologic diagnostic features have been sought.

Sigmoidoscopic appearance rarely can distinguish between acute infection and ulcerative colitis, although attempts have been made to define histologic criteria for distinction. Acute inflammatory changes of cryptitis and crypt abscesses with neutrophilic infiltration are seen in both entities. Signs of chronicity favor ulcerative colitis, such as round cell inflammation (lymphocytes, monocytes) and architectural distortion (branched crypts, reduced goblet cell numbers).[50,69,70] Even when a pathogen such as *Salmonella typhi, Edwardsiella tarda,* or *C. difficile* is identified, a chronic course consistent with ulcerative colitis may ensue after elimination of the pathogen with appropriate antibiotics. There is a greater incidence of *Salmonella* in stools of patients with ulcerative colitis, 3 to 5 percent versus 0.2 percent in the general population, suggesting either an increased host susceptibility or another predisposing factor.[7,49]

Food proteins, usually bovine milk or soy protein in infancy, may produce an allergic colitis distinguishable from ulcerative colitis only by histology, which reveals a predominant eosinophilic infiltration of the mucosa. Except for rare eosinophilic gastroenteritis, such a response occurs only in infancy and responds promptly to exclusion of the allergenic protein.[8]

Confident differentiation of ulcerative colitis from Crohn's colitis is impossible unless evidence of small bowel or gastroduodenal involvement, or extensive transmural or granulomatous inflammation can be demonstrated. There seem to be no clinical features unique to ulcerative colitis that cannot be found in the spectrum of Crohn's disease.[5,9,17,68] Endoscopic and histologic features favoring the provisional diagnosis of ulcerative colitis have been discussed and are contrasted in Table 1.

Prior to the onset of overt GI manifestations of ulcerative colitis, the patient may be followed for prodromal growth

retardation[20] or extraintestinal disease. For example, extraintestinal signs of ulcerative colitis may be mistaken for primary endocrine disorders, rheumatologic diseases, or anorexia nervosa.

THERAPY

Because ulcerative colitis is confined to the colon, total proctocolectomy is curative. However, because of the potential complications of surgery and the difficulties in adapting to an ileostomy and life without a colon, medical management is attempted initially, with surgery reserved for failure to respond, severe complications, chronic steroid dependence, or excessive risk of carcinoma in longstanding disease.

The goals of medical therapy of ulcerative colitis in children are the control of symptoms and the prevention of relapses. Choice of therapy depends upon the severity of the inflammation. Mild cases of colitis unaccompanied by systemic signs can be managed on an outpatient basis with rest, a low-residue diet, and the gradual introduction of sulfasalazine (Table 3). Response to treatment is expected within 2 weeks, with reduction in stool frequency, bleeding, and cramps. Subsequently, activity and diet may be liberalized as tolerated.

Moderate disease, in which colitis is accompanied by systemic signs, requires hospitalization for proper evaluation, observation for complications, and initiation of management. In addition to bedrest and a low-residue diet, corticosteroids are given. Sulfasalazine may be used as an adjunct, although additional benefits during acute management have not been proved in disease of moderate or greater activity. Hypoalbuminemia and anemia may require transfusion to optimize recovery. Failure to respond to this regimen often leads to a trial of bowel rest with nutritional support by elemental formula or parenteral nutrition. Recent evidence from studies of diversion colitis and the results of clinical trials in adults suggests that exclusion of enteral nutrients is of unproved ef-

TABLE 3
Pharmacologic Therapy of Ulcerative Colitis

Severe-moderate colitis
Methylprednisolone or prednisone: 1–2 mg/kg/day divided b.i.d. for 2 weeks; taper to 1–2 mg/kg/day q.d. and then to q.o.d. over 4–6 weeks depending on clinical response. When clinical remission is achieved, taper to discontinue.
Sulfasalazine: 50–75 mg/kg/day divided b.i.d. to q.i.d., initiated gradually during steroid taper by daily 250-mg increments until the full dose is achieved (maximum 3–4 g/day)
Folic acid supplementation: 1 mg q.d.

Mild or localized distal colitis
Sulfasalazine: 40–50 mg/kg/day divided b.i.d. to q.i.d.
Folic acid: 1 mg q.d.
Hydrocortisone enemas or foam
5-ASA (Dipentum, Pentasa, Asacol)

Refractory disease
Azathioprine: 2 mg/kg/day
6-Mercaptopurine: 1.5 mg/kg/day

Preventive maintenance
Sulfasalazine: 40–50 mg/kg/day divided b.i.d. to q.i.d.
5-ASA (Dipentum, Pentasa, Asacol)
Folic acid: 1 mg q.d.

ficacy unless mandated by symptoms and may indeed be detrimental to the colonic mucosa.[72,73] An extensive discussion of nutritional therapy considerations may be found in the preceding part of this chapter.

Severe disease with copious bloody diarrhea, weight loss, fever, abdominal tenderness or distention, leukocytosis, anemia, and hypoalbuminemia indicates loss of homeostasis and should be treated as an emergency with hospitalization and surgical consultation. A subgroup of these patients eventually requires colectomy for failure to respond to medical therapy or for the emergence of life-threatening complications such as toxic megacolon, hemorrhage, or perforation.[10] Central venous access is helpful in management of these cases and often is required to provide adequate parenteral nutritional support should bowel rest become necessary. Anemia and hypoalbuminemia should be corrected with blood and albumin transfusions. Dehydration and electrolyte disturbances should be anticipated and reversed. Magnesium is essential to colonic function and is often depleted, a fact reflected in continued low urinary magnesium excretion after a parenteral challenge dose of magnesium sulfate, even in the presence of normal serum magnesium levels. After blood cultures have been drawn and stool obtained for bacterial culture, parasite examination, and *C. difficile* toxin assay, broad-spectrum antibiotic coverage should begin. Intravenous adrenocorticotropic hormone (ACTH) or high-dose steroid treatment is essential. Intravenous ACTH has shown a statistically significant advantage in attaining remissions in exacerbations of ulcerative colitis only when there has been no recent steroid treatment.[51] Serial abdominal films should be obtained for surveillance of complications, which may be masked by steroid treatment. Computed tomography or ultrasound examination to exclude abscesses is indicated in patients who fail to respond to treatment. Most patients failing to respond to maximal medical regimen within 2 weeks ultimately require colectomy. Prolongation of medical treatment and postponement of surgery in these cases increase the risk of complications due to immunosuppression, steroid therapy, central venous catheters, transfusions, and hospitalization.[27]

Pharmacologic Agents

Sulfasalazine and steroids are the principal therapeutic agents for ulcerative colitis. Sulfasalazine has proved efficacious in the control of mild disease and in the reduction of the frequency of relapses once disease remission has been obtained. Sulfasalazine (salicylazosulfapyridine) is an azo-bonded combination of 5-aminosalicylate and sulfapyridine. The parent compound is split by colonic flora into the two constituents. The 5-aminosalicylate is poorly absorbed and is considered to be the active anti-inflammatory moiety, presumably through inhibition of mucosal prostaglandin synthesis. Among effects attributed to 5-aminosalicylic acid are inhibition of lipoxygenase activity, which mediates migration of polymorphonuclear leukocytes, inhibition of prostaglandin E_2 synthesis, reduction in the levels of thromboxane B_2 and 6-keto-prostaglandin F_1, and antisecretory effects.

The sulfapyridine is absorbed and excreted in the urine and is responsible for the side effects of allergy, hemolytic ane-

mia, rash, headaches, and nausea that are relatively common, often dose-dependent, and transient.[52] Neutropenia and oligospermia have been reported as complications of sulfasalazine therapy and are considered reversible. Ironically, cases of exacerbation of colitis have been reported.[53] The principal role of the azo-bonded sulfapyridine seems to be to prevent small intestinal absorption of the salicylate, since little of the parent compound is transported across the intestinal mucosa.

Alternative unabsorbable salicylate preparations have been formulated to avoid the sulfapyridine complications. These agents include a diazo-bonded dimer of 5-aminosalicylic acid (Dipentum), split by colonic bacteria to yield active drug, and other forms of 5-aminosalicylic acid (Asacol or Pentasa) incorporated into a pH-sensitive matrix that releases the active drug in the basic environment of the distal small bowel and colon.

Children at risk for glucose-6-phosphodiesterase deficiency should be screened prior to sulfasalazine treatment. Given the potential for intolerance, the dosage of sulfasalazine is gradually increased over 1 week from 10 mg per kilogram daily to a dosage of 40 to 50 mg per kilogram up to a maximum of 75 mg per kilogram in two to four divided doses. Symptoms and blood counts should be monitored closely. Because sulfasalazine impairs folate absorption, 1-mg daily folate supplements are usually provided.[2,3]

Corticosteroids are effective in the control of moderate to severe ulcerative colitis. In this context, steroids do not seem to adversely affect surgical outcome, if surgery becomes necessary. Treatment is begun with a relatively high dosage of prednisone or methylprednisolone (1 to 2 mg per kilogram per day) in two doses and sustained until disease is controlled, usually within 2 weeks, and then maintained in a single daily dose for another 2 to 4 weeks. Subsequently, with adjunctive use of sulfasalazine, the dose is tapered gradually by 5-mg decrements weekly to an alternate-day dosage of 1 mg per kilogram, followed by gradual withdrawal. If exacerbation of disease activity prevents complete withdrawal of steroids, chronic alternate-day steroid therapy may be necessary. Although the alternate-day steroid regimen causes less adrenal suppression and less severe side effects of hirsutism and altered body composition, patients remain at increased risk for osteoporosis, hypertension, and diabetes.[52] Effects on growth are equivocal, since disease activity itself may cause growth retardation. Some patients resume normal growth velocity only after steroid suppression of their disease activity. Other patients whose disease remains in remission may show catch-up growth velocity only after steroid withdrawal.[11,20]

Topical, nonsystemic corticosteroid therapy may be possible when disease is limited to the distal colon and rectum. Recent studies have confirmed the efficacy of 5-aminosalicylic acid enemas in the control of left-sided or distal colitis and in the maintenance of remission.[54] Hydrocortisone enemas have been used in an attempt to reduce the dose of systemic steroids necessary to control disease and may reach the transverse colon.[55] Rectal steroid foam is a more comfortable form of treatment for rectosigmoid disease. Nonabsorbable topical steroid enemas are currently undergoing clinical trials.[57]

Immunosuppressive agents are being administered increasingly as adjuncts to steroid therapy. Azathioprine and its active metabolite, 6-mercaptopurine, are appropriate agents in cases of ulcerative colitis refractory to or chronically dependent on steroid therapy. The major risks are consequences of immunosuppression and bone marrow suppression, including leukopenia and opportunistic infection. Lymphoproliferative malignancy, previously thought to be a complication of these agents, is extremely rare.[58,59]

Another immunosuppressive agent, cyclosporine, has been used in a few cases of fulminant colitis in children to prevent or delay surgery. Unfortunately, relapse is prompt following discontinuation of therapy, and chronic maintenance may be required. In addition to the potential complications of immunosuppression, cyclosporine commonly produces renal toxicity and hypertension. Its role in future therapeutic approaches is promising but unclear. Details of these agents are discussed in the preceding part of this chapter. As with prolonged steroid treatment, the potential benefits and risks of these agents must be weighed against the curative benefits and surgical risks of colectomy.[59]

Nutritional Therapy

The goals of nutritional therapy are to establish metabolic homeostasis by correcting nutrient deficits and replacing ongoing losses, to provide sufficient energy and protein for positive nitrogen balance or net protein synthesis, and to promote catch-up growth toward premorbid percentiles. The provision of adequate nutrients is essential for optimal healing. In ulcerative colitis, in which malabsorption is unlikely and increased metabolic demands are small or unproven, the undernutrition is caused by a reduced voluntary intake of calories and protein. On the basis of diet diary analysis of current intake, oral protein and calorie supplements are prescribed to make up calorie and protein deficits. Guidelines for supplementation are to provide at least 140 percent of the recommended daily allowance for height-age for both energy and protein. Continuous nocturnal nasogastric infusions of enteral formula through a soft Silastic catheter may be necessary in those who cannot voluntarily increase their intake. For severe disease, when bowel rest is desired as an adjunct to medical treatment, parenteral nutrition through a central venous catheter can achieve nutritional goals. Nutritional support in patients with ulcerative colitis is less likely to help establish a remission than in patients with Crohn's disease. Nevertheless, correction of nutrient deficiencies and maintenance of adequate nutritional status is of value in preventing deterioration of the patient's medical condition and in preparing the patient for surgery.[11,22,60]

Surgery

Surgery is indicated when medical and nutritional therapies fail to control the disease or to prevent significant physical and emotional morbidity. Although, in most cases, medical management is successful in controlling ulcerative colitis and prolonged remissions are possible, a cure can be obtained only through surgical excision.

Indications for colectomy in acute ulcerative colitis include uncontrolled hemorrhage; severe colitis failing to respond within 2 weeks to intensive treatment, including cor-

ticosteroids, antibiotics, bowel rest, and nutritional support; and complications of toxic megacolon, stricture, or perforation. Elective colectomy is indicated in patients with (1) prolonged steroid dependence or steroid-induced complications due to treatment of chronic active disease, (2) retardation of growth and sexual maturation despite nutritional support, and (3) longstanding disease or epithelial dysplasia of rectal or colonic mucosa, increasing the risk of carcinoma. The morbidity and mortality of elective colectomy in a patient whose disease activity is controlled and whose nutritional status has been optimized are much less than those in the acutely ill patient, in whom the risk of mortality can be up to 23 percent and the prospect of postoperative complications higher.[14,19]

There are several surgical options. A subtotal colectomy is usually performed, leaving a rectal stump as a blind Hartmann pouch and creating a terminal ileostomy. If the rectal disease cannot be controlled or ileostomy is preferred, complete proctectomy should be then performed electively. The risks of extraintestinal complications and carcinoma remain as long as there is residual diseased mucosa. If the disease in the rectal segment can be controlled with a combination of topical and systemic steroids, it is possible to perform a careful and complete rectal mucosectomy, preserving the pelvic nerves and the rectal musculature and sphincters through which the ileum may be pulled and anastomosed to the anus.[61,62] A variety of pouches may be constructed to create a reservoir to aid in continence. The J-pouch is currently recommended.[62] Inflammation of the neorectum or ileal pouch, termed pouchitis, suggests the presence of stasis, possible Crohn's disease, or residual diseased mucosa due to incomplete dissection of the rectal mucosa prior to ileal pull-through. Metronidazole has been the most effective agent in the treatment of pouchitis.[63] With the ileoanal pull-through and the use of antimotility agents such as loperamide, the patient often can have complete continence with relatively few bowel movements per day. Perianal irritation is treated topically with sitz baths, careful hygiene, and cholestyramine ointment, which may absorb irritating bile acids.

PROSPECTIVE MANAGEMENT AND PROGNOSIS

Ulcerative colitis is a chronic disease requiring careful surveillance, patient education, and expert management by a team consisting of the pediatrician, gastroenterologist, nutritionist, psychiatrist or psychologist, social worker, and nurse. An alliance with a pediatric surgeon familiar with inflammatory bowel disease is essential for management of potential complications. Since the success of management depends on the degree to which the patient and family understand and participate in the treatment, they must be educated about the disease and incorporated as members of the team, often a major challenge for the physician. Support groups and organizations such as the National Foundation for Ileitis and Colitis are indispensable not only in dissemenating information but also in providing a community to counter the isolation that often attends the diagnosis of a chronic disease. Nutrition and growth, sexual maturation, psychosocial adjustment to disease, and compliance with therapy should all be monitored as carefully as one monitors the clinical signs and symptoms of disease activity outlined in earlier paragraphs.

The frequency of follow-up depends on the course of disease activity, but intervals should be no greater than 6 months. Most children have the potential for a full, active life with good general health. Ten percent of patients experience only their presenting episode of colitis but must be followed carefully because of the risk of cancer in later life. Twenty percent of patients have intermittent symptoms, 50 percent have chronic disease, and the remaining 20 percent have chronically active, incapacitating disease.[14] The physician should always be alert for signs of the upper GI, perianal, or ileal pouch involvement that may unmask Crohn's disease.

The risk of colonic carcinoma in pediatric-onset ulcerative colitis increases dramatically to an estimated 10 percent per decade after the first 10 years of disease, depending on extent of involvement.[33,34,64] Because the risk is cumulative, patients with persistent symptoms and pancolitis of early onset in youth are at greatest risk. The risk of carcinoma appears to be less in patients with left-sided colitis or proctitis.[65] Most tumors arise in the distal colon and rectum and are probably preceded by histologic signs of epithelial dysplasia.[66] Histologic evidence of dysplasia in patients with longstanding disease is a definitive indication for proctocolectomy. Younger patients developing carcinoma may have a poorer prognosis.[67]

Sigmoidoscopy and rectal biopsy to detect dysplasia or polyps have been recommended every 6 months for patients with disease duration greater than 10 years, in conjunction with annual colonoscopy. However, such surveillance is costly, fallible, and not without morbidity. Moreover, the efficacy of surveillance in preventing lethal cancer is unproved. These considerations have led some to advocate prophylactic colectomy in patients with longstanding disease beginning in childhood or adolescence. More study is needed to determine the optimal management of carcinoma risk.[32]

The advent of steroids has dramatically altered the prognosis for medical management of ulcerative colitis, with fewer patients requiring surgery to control the disease. The majority of patients are able to resume full activities, including school and athletics. Ulcerative colitis has no specific effect on fertility and poses no risk to the fetus. However, poor nutritional status and use of medications such as 6-mercaptopurine and azathioprine are risk factors for pregnancy. Sulfasalazine may produce reversible oligospermia. If presenting during pregnancy, ulcerative colitis may be more severe. Approximately 30 to 50 percent of patients with pre-existing disease may experience exacerbations during pregnancy.[11,14]

Despite the successes of medical management, currently there is no medical cure. The medications used to control the disease have potential morbidity, and the risk of colonic carcinoma is significant and cumulative, warranting careful surveillance. Confronting a chronic disease, with frequent medical visits and frustrating relapses, or the prospects of surgery in childhood and adolescence, is a tremendous emotional burden for the patient and family, requiring ongoing psychosocial support. Colectomy both cures the disease and eliminates the risk of colorectal carcinoma but presents its own risks of potential morbidity, discomfort, and mortality.

All of these factors must be considered and reconciled by the patient, family, and medical team in the long-term management of children with ulcerative colitis.

SUMMARY AND CONCLUSIONS

Ulcerative colitis in children presents the clinician with a succession of challenges both for medical management and for long-term patient care. The diagnosis of ulcerative colitis following initial differentiation from self-limited infectious colitis is attended by a variable uncertainty owing to the difficulties in confidently excluding Crohn's disease. Medical management entails optimizing growth and development by ensuring adequate nutrient intake and appropriate use of anti-inflammatory agents to control exacerbations and prolong remissions. Ultimately the risks of long-term medical management and carcinoma must be confronted and weighed against the prospects for surgical cure by colectomy.

REFERENCES

1. Wilks S, Moxon W. Lectures on pathological anatomy. 2nd ed. London: J and A Churchill, 1875.
2. Crohn BB, Ginzburg L, Oppenheimer GD. Regional enteritis: a pathologic and clinical entity. JAMA 1932; 99:1323.
3. Crohn BB. Granulomatous disease of the large and small bowel, a historical survey. Gastroenterology 1967; 52:767.
4. Lockhart-Mummery H, Morson B. Crohn's disease (regional enteritis) of the large intestine and its distinction from ulcerative colitis. Gut 1960; 1:87.
5. Kirsner JB. Problems in the differentiation of ulcerative colitis from Crohn's disease of the colon: the need for repeated diagnostic evaluation. Gastroenterology 1975; 68:187.
6. Price AB, Morson BC. Inflammatory bowel disease: the surgical pathology of Crohn's disease and ulcerative colitis. Hum Pathol 1975; 6:7.
7. Lindeman RJ, Weinstein L, Levitan R, Patterson JF. Ulcerative colitis and intestinal salmonellosis. Am J Med Sci 1967; 106:856.
8. Elson CO. The immunology of inflammatory bowel disease. In: Kirsner JB, Shorter RG, eds. Inflammatory bowel disease, 3rd ed. Philadelphia: Lea & Febiger, 1988: 97.
9. Powell G. Milk and soy-induced enterocolitis of infancy. J Pediatr 1978; 93:553.
10. Drossman DA. Psychosocial aspects of ulcerative colitis and Crohn's disease. In: Kirsner JB, Shorter RG, eds. Inflammatory bowel disease. 3rd ed. Philadelphia: Lea & Febiger, 1988: 209.
11. Motil K, Grand R. Ulcerative colitis and Crohn's disease in children. Pediatr Rev 1987; 9:109.
12. Calkins BM, Lilienfeld AM, Garland CF, Mendeloff AI. Trends in incidence rates of ulcerative colitis and Crohn's disease. Dig Dis Sci 1984; 29:913.
13. Mendeloff AI. The epidemiology of inflammatory bowel disease. Clin Gastroenterol 1980; 9:258.
14. Kelts DG, Grand RJ. Inflammatory bowel disease in children and adolescents. Curr Probl Pediatr 1980; 10:5.
15. Farmer RG, Michener WM, Mortimer EA. Studies of family history among patients with inflammatory bowel disease. Clin Gastroenterol 1980; 9:271.
16. Lashner BA, Evans AA, Kirsner JB. Prevalence and incidence of inflammatory bowel disease in family members. Gastroenterology 1986; 91:1396.
17. Chong SKF, Blackshaw AJ, Morson BC, Williams CB, Walker-Smith JA. Prospective study of colitis in infancy and early childhood. J Pediatr Gastroenterol Nutr 1986; 5:352.
18. Berger M, Gribetz D, Korelitz BI. Growth retardation in children with ulcerative colitis: the effect of medical and surgical therapy. Pediatrics 1975; 55:459.

19. Motil KJ, Grand RJ, Davis-Kraft E. The epidemiology of growth failure in children and adolescents with inflammatory bowel disease. Gastroenterology 1983; 84:1254.
20. Kirschner BS, Voinchet O, Rosenberg IH. Growth retardation in children with inflammatory bowel disease. Gastroenterology 1978; 75:504.
21. McCaffery TD, et al. Severe growth retardation in children with inflammatory bowel disease. Pediatrics 1970; 45:386.
22. Motil KJ, Grand RJ. Nutritional management of inflammatory bowel disease. Pediatr Clin North Am 1985; 32:44.
23. Motil KJ, Grand RJ. Ulcerative colitis and Crohn's disease in children. In: Kirsner JB, Shorter RG, eds. Inflammatory bowel disease. 3rd ed. Philadelphia: Lea & Febiger, 1988: 227.
24. Lindsley CB, Schaller JG. Arthritis associated with inflammatory bowel disease. J Pediatr 1974; 84:6.
25. Dew MJ, Thompson H, Allen RN. The spectrum of hepatic dysfunction in inflammatory bowel disease. J Med 1979; 48:113.
26. Kane W, Miller K, Sharp HL. Inflammatory bowel disease presenting as liver disease during childhood. J Pediatr 1980; 97:775.
27. Werlin SL, Grand RJ. Severe colitis in children and adolescents. Diagnosis, course and treatment. Gastroenterology 1977; 73:838.
28. Huizenga KA, Schroeder KW. Gastrointestinal complications of ulcerative colitis and Crohn's disease. In: Kirsner JB, Shorter RG, eds. Inflammatory bowel disease. 3rd ed. Philadelphia: Lea & Febiger, 1988: 269.
29. Binder SC, Patterson JF, Glotzer DJ. Toxic megacolon in ulcerative colitis. Gastroenterology 1974; 66:1088.
30. Goulston SJM, McGovern VJ. The nature of benign strictures in ulcerative colitis. N Engl J Med 1969; 281:290.
31. Jalan KN, et al. An experience of ulcerative colitis. I. Toxic dilatation in 55 cases. Gastroenterology 1969; 57:68.
32. Collins RH, Feldman M, Fordtran JS. Colon cancer, dysplasia, and surveillance in patients with ulcerative colitis. (Review) N Engl J Med 1987; 316:1654.
33. Kewenter J. Ulcerative colitis: dysplasia and cancer risk. In: Bayless TM, ed. Current management of inflammatory bowel disease. Philadelphia: BC Decker, 1989: 146.
34. Devroede GJ, et al. Cancer risk and life expectancy of children with ulcerative colitis. N Engl J Med 1971; 285:17.
35. Gryboski J, Hillemeier C. Inflammatory bowel disease in children. Med Clin North Am 1980; 64:1185.
36. Trnka YM, LaMont JT. Association of Clostridium difficile toxin with symptomatic relapse of chronic inflammatory bowel disease. Gastroenterology 1981; 80:693.
37. Meyers S, et al. Occurrence of Clostridium difficile toxin during the course of inflammatory bowel disease. Gastroenterology 1981; 80:697.
38. Winthrop JD, et al. Ulcerative and granulomatous colitis in children. Radiology 1985; 154:657.
39. Gore RM, et al. CT findings in ulcerative, granulomatous, and indeterminate colitis. AJR 1984; 143:279.
40. Savery-Muttu S, et al. ¹¹¹Indium autologous leukocytes in inflammatory bowel disease. Gut 1983; 24:293.
41. Gordon I, Vivian G. Radiolabelled leukocytes: a new diagnostic tool in occult infection/inflammation. Arch Dis Child 1984; 59:62.
42. Williams CB, et al. Total colonoscopy in childhood. Arch Dis Child 1982; 57:49.
43. Hassall E, Barclay GN, Ament ME. Colonoscopy in childhood. Pediatrics 1984; 73:594.
44. Goodman MJ, Kirsner JB, Riddell RH. Usefulness of rectal biopsy in inflammatory bowel disease. Gastroenterology 1977; 72:952.
45. Apley J. The child with abdominal pains. 2nd ed. Oxford: Blackwell, 1975.
46. Grand RJ. Personal communication.
47. Bemer W. The hemolytic-uremic syndrome: initial clinical presentation mimicking ulcerative colitis. J Pediatr 1972; 81:275.
48. Harris JC, Dupont HL, Hornick RB. Fecal leukocytes in diarrheal illness. Ann Intern Med 1972; 76:697.
49. Dronfield MN, Fletcher J, Langman MJS. Coincident Salmonella injections and ulcerative colitis: problems of recognition and management. Br Med J 1974; 1:99.
50. Surawicz C, Belic L. Rectal biopsy helps to distinguish acute self-limited colitis from idiopathic inflammatory bowel disease. Gastroenterology 1984; 86:104.
51. Myers S, et al. Corticotropin versus hydrocortisone in the intravenous treatment of ulcerative colitis. A prospective, randomized, double blind clinical trial. Gastroenterology 1983; 85:351.
52. Goldstein PD, Alpers DH, Keating JP. Sulfapyridine metabolites in children with inflammatory bowel disease receiving sulfasalazine. J Pediatr 1979; 95:638.
53. Werlin SL, Grand RG. Bloody diarrhea—a new complication of sulfasalazine. J Pediatr 1978; 92:450.
54. Sutherland LR, Martin F, Greer S, et al. 5-Aminosalicylic acid enema in the treatment of distal ulcerative colitis, proctosigmoiditis, and proctitis. Gastroenterology 1987; 92:1894.
55. Truelove SC. Treatment of ulcerative colitis with local hydrocortisone hemisuccinate sodium. A report on a controlled therapeutic trial. Br Med J 1958; 2:1072.
56. Farthing MJG, Rutland MD, Clark ML. Retrograde spread of hydrocortisone containing foam given intrarectally in ulcerative colitis. Br Med J 1979; 2:822.
57. Hanauer SB, Kirsner JB, Barrett WE. The treatment of left-sided ulcerative colitis with tixocortol pivalate (TP). Gastroenterology 1986; 90:1449.
58. Verhave M, Winter HS, Grand RJ. Efficacy and safety of azathioprine in children with inflammatory bowel disease. (Abstract) Gastroenterology 1987; 92:1682.
59. Korelitz BI. Immunosuppressive therapy. In: Bayless TM, ed. Current management of inflammatory bowel disease. Philadelphia: BC Decker, 1989: 252.
60. Jeejeebhoy KN, Ostro MJ. Nutritional consequences and therapy in inflammatory bowel disease. In: Kirsner JB, Shorter RG, eds. Inflammatory bowel disease. Philadelphia: Lea & Febiger, 1988: 513.
61. Martin LW. Total colectomy and mucosal proctectomy with preservation of continence in ulcerative colitis. Ann Surg 1977; 186:477.
62. Fonkalsrud EW. Endorectal ileal pull-through operation in children. In: Bayless TM, ed. Current management in inflammatory bowel disease. Philadelphia: BC Decker, 1989: 133.
63. Cohen Z. Pouch inflammation following reservoir procedures. In: Bayless TM, eds. Current management in inflammatory bowel disease. Philadelphia: BC Decker, 1989: 137.
64. Lennard-Jones JE, et al. Cancer in colitis: an assessment of the individual risk by clinical and histologic criteria. Gastroenterology 1977; 73:1280.
65. Butt JH, Lennard-Jones JE, Ritchie JK. A practical approach to the risk of cancer in inflammatory bowel disease. Med Clin North Am 1980; 64:1203.
66. Morson BC, Dawson IMP. Gastrointestinal pathology. Oxford: Blackwell, 1979.
67. Hulten L, Kewenter J, Aaren C, Ojerskog B. Clinical and morphological characteristics of colitis, carcinoma and colorectal carcinoma in young people. Scand J Gastroenterol 1979; 14:673.
68. Tedesco FS. Differential diagnosis of ulcerative colitis and ileocolitis and other specific inflammatory diseases of the bowel. Med Clin North Am 1980; 64:1173.
69. Kumar NB, Nostrant TT, Appleman HD. The histopathologic spectrum of acute self-limited colitis (acute infectious-type colitis). Am J Surg Pathol 1982; 6:523.
70. Nostrant TT, Kamar NB, Appleman HD. Histopathology differentiates acute self-limited colitis from ulcerative colitis. Gastroenterology 1987; 92:318.
71. Klein JD, Biller JA, Leape L, Grand RJ. Pyoderma gangrenosum occurring at multiple incision sites. Gastroenterology 1987; 92:810–813.
72. Harig JM, Soergel KH, Komorowski RA, Wood CM. Treatment of diversion colitis with short chain fatty acid irrigation. N Engl J Med 1989; 320:23–28.
73. Rolandelli R, et al. Comparison of parenteral nutrition and enteral feeding with pectin in experimental colitis in the rat. Am J Clin Nutr 1988; 47:715–721.
74. Jackson D, Grand RJ. Ulcerative colitis. In: Oski F, ed. Principles and practice of pediatrics. Philadelphia: JB Lippincott, 1990: 1702.

PART **15**

Pseudomembranous Colitis

George Triadafilopoulos, M.D., D.Sc., F.A.C.P., F.A.C.G.
J. Thomas LaMont, M.D.

Pediatric pseudomembranous colitis is an unusual but frequently severe diarrheal disease characterized by the presence on the colonic mucosa of discrete yellow plaques or pseudomembranes composed of inflammatory exudate.[1] Most cases are related to exposure to antibiotics and subsequent colonization with *Clostridium difficile,* the major cause of this condition. Pseudomembranous colitis can occur at any age, although it is more common in adults than in children.[2] It is very rare in neonates and infants, although cases have been reported both with and without previous antibiotic therapy. The diagnosis should be considered in any pediatric patient with diarrhea during or after antibiotic therapy.

ETIOLOGY

Pseudomembranous colitis was first described in 1893 by Finney.[3] Subsequent reports made an association between pseudomembranous colitis and intestinal obstruction, sepsis, shock, and intestinal ischemia. With the introduction of chloramphenicol, tetracyclines, and neomycin in the early 1950s, a direct association of pseudomembranous colitis with antibiotic therapy was suggested. Initially, *Staphylococcus aureus* was proposed as the likely pathogen based upon stool cultures of toxigenic strains and a favorable therapeutic response to oral vancomycin.[4,5] However, after the introduction of lincomycin and clindamycin in the early 1970s, *S. aureus* was not considered relevant as an etiologic factor. *C. difficile* was first isolated in 1935 by Hall and O'Toole from the stools of healthy neonates.[6] Although culture supernatants of this organism were extremely toxic to laboratory animals, the organism was not considered pathogenic in humans. A major breakthrough occurred in 1977 when Larson et al[7] described a heat-labile toxin in the stool of a 12-year-old girl who developed pseudomembranous colitis after treatment with oral penicillin. The stool toxin caused human embryonic lung fibroblasts to undergo rounding and detachment from the culture surface. In 1978 *C. difficile* was identified as the source of the stool toxin in patients with antibiotic-associated colitis.[8] Subsequently, *C. difficile* and its toxin have been isolated in over 95 percent of cases of pseudomembranous colitis in adults and children.[9,10]

C. difficile is a gram-positive obligate anaerobic bacillus that grows on selective media in yellow circular colonies.[11] Nearly all strains produce toxins A and B in vitro. Identification of the organism from stool requires meticulous anaerobic techniques not generally available in most hospital microbiology laboratories. Stools of children or symptomatic adults with pseudomembranous colitis generally contain 10^3 to 10^7 *C. difficile* bacteria per gram wet weight, but im-

proper storage, freezing, or air exposure may diminish recovery.[12]

C. difficile produces two protein exotoxins, A and B, which have different physicochemical, biologic, and antigenic properties. Toxin A (enterotoxin) causes fluid secretion and inflammation when injected into animal ileal loops.[13] Toxin B (cytotoxin) is responsible for the characteristic rounding of fibroblasts in tissue culture.[14]

Toxin A (molecular weight 229,000) is heat- and acid-labile and protease-sensitive (Table 1). It is a potent enterotoxin causing secretion of fluid, increased vascular permeability, and epithelial necrosis when injected into rabbit ileal loops.[15] Highly purified toxin B in equimolar concentrations has no effect in animal intestine. Toxin A is also cytopathic to tissue culture cells, but it is far less potent than toxin B in the fibroblast assay. Toxin A causes release of prostaglandin E_2 and leukotriene B_4 from rabbit ileum and increases chemotaxis and stimulates intracellular calcium release in human neutrophils.[16] These observations suggest that toxin A may be more important in causing clinical disease, whereas toxin B may serve as a convenient marker of *C. difficile* enteric infection.[17] However, immunization experiments with toxoids A and B in hamsters suggest that antibodies to both toxins are necessary to protect against antibiotic-associated colitis.[18]

Toxin B, the cytotoxin, has a molecular weight of 50,000 to 250,000, is a heat- and acid-labile protein, and is sensitive to proteases.[19] It is lethal when injected intraperitoneally in

TABLE 1
Characteristics of *Clostridium difficile* Toxins

	Toxin A	Toxin B
Classification	Enterotoxin	Cytotoxin
Molecular weight	229,000	50,000–250,000
Characteristics	Heat- and acid-labile protein	Heat- and acid-labile protein
	Protease sensitive	Protease sensitive
Effects in experimental animals	Hemorrhagic enteritis	
	Mouse lethality	Mouse lethality
	Increased vascular permeability	
	Fluid secretion	
Mechanism	Stimulation of neutrophil chemotaxis	Actin disaggregation
	Intracellular Ca^{2+} release	

mice but has no effect on intestinal permeability or fluid secretion in rabbit ileal loops.[20,21] Toxin B exerts its effect on cell shape by disaggregating actin and disrupting the cytoskeleton.[14,22]

PATHOGENESIS

Role of Antibiotics. Pseudomembranous colitis develops as a result of colonization and toxin production by *C. difficile* in the colon after the normal microflora has been altered by antibiotic therapy.[23] The exact mechanism of this sequence is poorly understood, mainly because of the complexity of the normal fecal flora. The human colon is populated by 10^{10} to 10^{12} bacteria per gram of feces, most of them anaerobes. These compete with each other for nutrients and for attachment sites on the epithelial surface and presumably prevent colonization by *C. difficile*.[24]

Nearly all antibiotics have been associated with pseudomembranous colitis. Ampicillin, a widely used drug in pediatrics, is responsible for most cases in children.[25] Although clindamycin is frequently associated with pseudomembranous colitis in adults, it accounts for diarrhea and colitis much less frequently in children. Other antibiotics incriminated in pseudomembranous colitis include amoxicillin, penicillin, cephalothin, cefaclor, and, rarely, erythromycin, in spite of the extensive use of that drug in children (Table 2). Aminoglycosides, vancomycin, and antimycobacterial, antifungal, and antiparasitic agents have not been implicated in pseudomembranous colitis. The route of antibiotic administration is not a factor in pathogenesis,[26] and even agents with in vitro bactericidal activity against *C. difficile* may commonly trigger the infection.[27,28] For example, ampicillin and vancomycin are equally active against toxigenic *C. difficile* in vitro, yet ampicillin is a frequently incriminated agent in pediatric pseudomembranous colitis while vancomycin is used as an effective treatment for the disease.

Host Factors in *C. difficile* Infection. Enteric disease does not develop in all individuals who harbor toxigenic *C. difficile* in their gastrointestinal tract.[29] Variations in severity of the disease may relate to bacterial virulence factors of different strains of the organism or to variations in host defense mechanisms (Table 3).

TABLE 2
Antibiotics Associated with Pseudomembranous Colitis in Children

Common	Ampicillin
	Amoxicillin
Less common	Cephalosporins
	Clindamycin
	Penicillin
	Erythromycin
Rare	Tetracyclines
	Trimethoprim-sulfamethoxazole
	Aminoglycosides
	Metronidazole

TABLE 3
Pathogenesis of Pseudomembranous Colitis in Children

Defensive Factors	Offensive Factors
Gastric acid	Number of organisms
Chemotaxis	Altered gut microbial flora
Intestinal immunity	
Intestinal motility	Antibiotic use
Receptor availability	

Gastric acidity is an important defense factor against ingested *C. difficile* because low intragastric pH not only limits survival of ingested spores but also inactivates ingested toxins. Intestinal mucus provides a nonspecific physical barrier against bacterial proliferation and mucosal colonization. Normal intestinal peristaltic activity is important, as some patients with *C. difficile*– associated intestinal disease have other diseases or receive anti-diarrheal medications that reduce intestinal motility.[30] The mucosal and systemic immune systems provide a more complex defense mechanism against *C. difficile*. The immune response may be antitoxic, antibacterial, or both and may originate from the mucosal immune system or from the circulation. Antibodies to toxins A and B are present in the majority of older children and adults[31] (Fig 1). It is not clear at present whether serum toxin-neutralizing antibody protects against *C. difficile*–associated disease.

The intestinal epithelial cell has specific membrane receptors for various bacterial toxins.[32] Susceptibility to *C. difficile* toxins could be related to the presence or availability of receptors on the brush border membrane.[33] *C. difficile* toxin A binds to brush border membrane receptors of rabbit intestine,[34] and presumably such receptors are found in human intestine. Receptors for *Escherichia coli* heat-stable enterotoxin are reported to decrease[35] and those for *Shigella* enterotoxin to increase[36] with maturation of the intestine. By analogy with *Shigella* toxin, *C. difficile* toxin receptors may be absent or inaccessible in the human infant, thus explaining the apparent resistance to disease in infancy (see below).

Neutrophil activation and chemotaxis may alter the expression of bacterial diseases. *C. difficile* toxin A is a potent chemotactic agent for human neutrophils and causes severe inflammatory enteritis in rabbit ileal loops.[37] The possible role of inflammatory mediators, such as prostaglandins and leukotrienes, in the secretory and inflammatory process induced by toxin A is not yet well defined.[38,39] While *C. difficile* toxin B does not cause intestinal morphologic damage directly, it is a lethal toxin if the gut mucosa has been subjected to trauma or to toxin A.[40,41]

CARRIER STATE IN INFANCY

C. difficile and toxin B have been identified in the feces of up to 70 percent of healthy neonates and infants[42–44] in concentrations similar to those found in adults with pseudomembranous colitis.[45] Possible explanations for this asymptomatic carrier state in human infants include (1) ab-

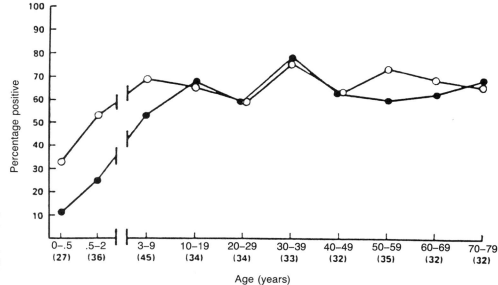

FIGURE 1 Age-related prevalence of antibodies to *C. difficile* toxin A (*closed circles*) and B (*open circles*) in 340 patients. The numbers in parentheses represent the number of individuals in each age group. (From Viscidi et al[31]; with permission of The University of Chicago Press, © 1983.)

sence of disease-producing enterotoxin A despite the presence of the "marker" cytotoxin B, (2) the protective effects of maternally derived antitoxin(s), (3) developmental absence of epithelial cell receptors for toxin, and (4) blunted inflammatory response to the toxin. At present the apparent resistance of newborns to this pathogen and its toxins remains unexplained.

EPIDEMIOLOGY

C. difficile is acquired from the environment, probably in the form of spores.[46] The organism has been isolated from the home environment[47] (Table 4) and the environment of hospitalized patients with the disease as well as from the hands and stools of asymptomatic family members and hospital personnel.[48] Infant carriers may in turn be exogenous sources of *C. difficile* for adults who are receiving antibiotics.[49] The isolation frequency of *C. difficile* inversely correlates with age.[50] The organism is present in the stool of up to 70 percent of healthy infants, in about 3 percent of asymptomatic children older than 1 year, and in only 2 percent or less of healthy adults[51-53] (Table 5). Some investigators have isolated *C. difficile* and cytotoxin significantly more often from the intestinal tract of formula-fed than breast-fed infants,[54] whereas others have failed to confirm such an association.[25,45]

As with other enteric pathogens, *C. difficile* may cause epidemic diarrhea in daycare centers. In one study,[55] *C. difficile* was introduced into a daycare center via an asymptomatic carrier. Within 5 weeks this child and five others developed diarrhea from *C. difficile*. Only two of these children had received antibiotics. Electrophoretic evaluation of the *C. difficile* isolated from these children suggested that they were identical. Similar outbreaks occurring in hospitalized adults also suggest that person-to-person spread of the same strain is responsible.[56] Interestingly, nurses, nurses' aides, and physicians have not been identified as carriers in hospital outbreaks.

TABLE 4
Distribution of *Clostridium difficile* Isolates Taken from Two Home Environments

Sites Cultured	No. Positive/No. Sampled (%)	
	Case-Associated Home	Control Home
Bathroom		
Floors	2/15 (13)	0/15
Sink cabinet	6/15 (40)	0/15
Inside toilet cover	1/10 (10)	0/10
Bedrooms		
Floors	1/15 (7)	0/10
Bookcase	1/4 (25)	0/5
Linens	0/10	0/5
Toys	0/15	0/7
Living room		
Crib	0/10	NA
Utility room		
Floor	1/10 (10)	0/5
Freezer door	1/5 (20)	0/5
Soiled clothing	0/5	0/5
Yard		
Soil	2/2 (100)	0/1
Tap water*	0/2	0/1
TOTAL	15/123 (12.2)[†]	0/84[†]

NA = not applicable.
* Samples taken from kitchen (100 ml per sample).
† $P < 0.001$.
From Kim et al[47]; with permission of The University of Chicago Press, © 1981.

TABLE 5
C. difficile Cytotoxicity Assay and *C. difficile* Isolation Rates in Stools of Different Populations*

Category	Percentage Culture	Percentage Assay
Healthy infants	15–70%	25–60%
Healthy children older than 1 year and adults	0–3%	0%
Antibiotic-associated colitis	60%	30%
Antibiotic-associated diarrhea without colitis	0–20%	15–25%
Patients with pseudomembranous colitis	95%	95–100%
Patients with inflammatory bowel disease in relapse		5–25%

* Compiled from references 25, 28, 42, 43, 50, 53, 69, and 72.

PATHOLOGY

The histologic features of pseudomembranous colitis can be divided into three types: Type 1, the earliest phase, consists of focal epithelial necrosis and exudation of fibrin and polymorphonuclear cells into the lumen. In type 2, the lesions consist of the typical dome-shaped plaque of fibrin, mucin, cellular debris, and neutrophils (summit lesion). The intervening mucosa between plaques is normal, creating a distinctive patchy distribution of the lesions (Fig. 2). Type 3 lesions are most advanced and show complete necrosis of the mucosa with a covering of cellular inflammatory debris. In the resolving or healing phase complete reconstitution of the mucosa occurs, but residual glandular irregularity may be seen.[57]

CLINICAL MANIFESTATIONS

The occasional severe or fatal case of *C. difficile* infection in children makes accurate and timely diagnosis a real challenge for the pediatrician. Pseudomembranous colitis represents only one end of a wide spectrum of conditions in children that can be associated with *C. difficile* infection, ranging from the asymptomatic carrier state to fulminant colitis.[58,59] As in adults, the manifestations of *C. difficile* infection in the pediatric population may be quite variable, ranging from acute self-limited diarrhea to toxic megacolon (Table 6).

Pseudomembranous Colitis in Children. The clinical syndrome of pseudomembranous colitis in children is characterized by the acute onset of profuse diarrhea and crampy abdominal pain that begin during the first week of antibiotic therapy. Diarrhea is frequent and may be associated with a sensation of incomplete evacuation (tenesmus), nausea, and vomiting.[60] High fever (38 to 40°C), chills, dehydration, hypotension, and shock may occur. Clinical examination reveals abdominal distention, diffuse or localized abdominal tenderness, and guarding in severe cases. Frank hematochezia is rare, but fecal leukocytes and occult gastrointestinal bleeding are commonly found on stool examination. Electrolyte imbalances, particularly hyponatremia and hypokalemia, are sometimes seen, whereas metabolic acidosis and hypoproteinemia occur only in prolonged illness.[61] Peripheral leukocytosis, occasionally up to 60,000 per cubic millimeter, with left shift is frequent. The diagnosis is confirmed on bedside flexible sigmoidoscopic examination, which re-

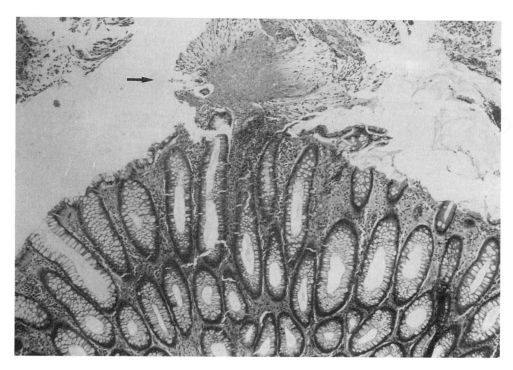

FIGURE 2 "Summit lesion." Colonic biopsy showing focal necrosis of the crypts, loss of surface epithelium, and inflammatory exudation. The pseudomembrane (*arrow*) is made up of fibrin, mucus, and inflammatory and necrotic cells. The surrounding mucosa is intact (hematoxylin and eosin, ×125).

TABLE 6
Clinical Features of Pseudomembranous Colitis in Children

Very common	Diarrhea
Common	Abdominal colic
	Fever
	Leukocytosis
	Dehydration
	Hypoalbuminemia
Uncommon	Bloody diarrhea
	Vomiting
Rare	Intestinal perforation
	Ascites
	Jaundice
	Toxic megacolon

veals the characteristic yellow-white raised plaques, approximately 2 to 4 mm in diameter, scattered over the mucosal surface (Fig. 3). These pseudomembranes may at times become confluent, giving the appearance of a shaggy white or tan membrane covering the mucosa. Petechiae and friability of the mucosa may be present.

Fulminant *C. difficile* Colitis. In fulminant *C. difficile* colitis, transmural extension of the inflammatory process results in microperforation of the bowel with localized peritonitis. In severe cases, the colon loses its muscular tone and begins to dilate, resulting in toxic megacolon (Fig. 4). Without timely treatment, fulminant colitis may rapidly lead to free perforation, generalized peritonitis, septicemia, renal failure, and death.[62] Fulminant *C. difficile* colitis may begin suddenly in

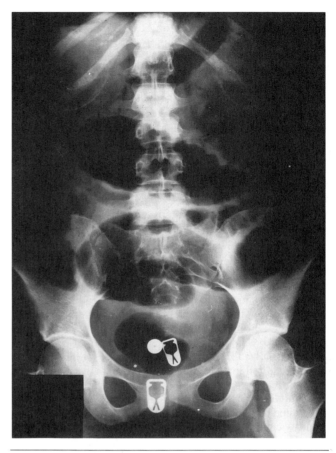

FIGURE 4 Plain abdominal radiograph of toxic megacolon in pseudomembranous colitis showing colonic dilatation, edema, and increased thickness of the colonic wall. (Courtesy of Philip Kramer, M.D.)

a child who is previously well or may develop during established infection. The patient appears toxic and may complain of steady localized pain, which contrasts with the crampy, intermittent pain of milder disease. Fever, tachycardia, localized tenderness, guarding, abdominal distention, decreased bowel sounds, and signs of profound toxemia are present. As acute toxic dilatation and paralytic ileus develop, diarrhea may diminish or cease.[63] Plain abdominal films show dilated loops of small bowel, air-fluid levels, and megacolon with edema and increased thickness of the colonic wall. Fulminant *C. difficile* colitis should be considered in children and adolescents who develop toxic megacolon, localized peritonitis, or paralytic ileus during or following antibiotic treatment. Early sigmoidoscopy and stool examination for *C. difficile* and its toxin may obviate a laparotomy. Fulminant *C. difficile* may also be an elusive cause of postoperative diarrhea and sepsis after all types of surgery.[64] In these cases, severe colonic distention, edema, and intestinal fluid sequestration cause prolonged ileus, difficulties in weaning from respiratory support, or unexplained fever and hypovolemia. Unsuspected and untreated fulminant pseudomembranous colitis leads to fatal outcome as a result of clostridial mucosal invasion, spore production, cytotoxemia, and terminal disseminated

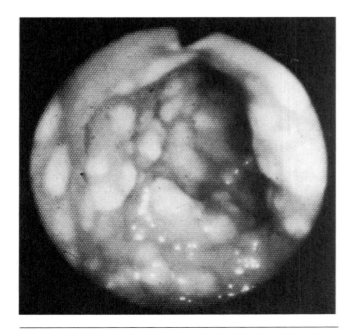

FIGURE 3 Endoscopic appearance of pseudomembranes. Endoscopic view of *C. difficile* colitis showing typical focal pseudomembranes scattered over the rectal mucosa.

coagulopathy and glomerulopathy.[65] Early treatment depends chiefly on specific antimicrobial therapy against C. difficile and its toxins and prompt recognition and correction of hypovolemia, hypoproteinemia, and acidosis. In addition, since the increased intestinal mucosal permeability to normal colonic microflora may lead to generalized sepsis, broad-spectrum antibiotic therapy is necessary in severe cases.[66] The prominent degree of exudative enteropathy may require replacement with plasma or salt-free human albumin.

Antibiotic-Associated Colitis without Pseudomembranes. The clinical features of antibiotic-associated colitis without pseudomembranes are milder than those seen with pseudomembranous colitis.[67] The disease usually begins insidiously, with anorexia, inability to tolerate feedings, tenesmus, lower abdominal cramps, and mucous diarrhea. Malaise, fever, abdominal tenderness, leukocytosis, hypoalbuminemia, and dehydration may be present. Sigmoidoscopy reveals diffuse or patchy colitis but without typical pseudomembranes. Sparing of the rectum with involvement of the more proximal parts of the colon may also occur.[68] Colonoscopy is much more likely to reveal pseudomembranes and other mucosal abnormalities than is proctosigmoidoscopy. In one study, pseudomembranes were present in 31 percent by proctoscopy alone, but in 85 percent when the entire colon was visualized by colonoscopy. However, colonoscopy is seldom required for clinical diagnosis except in complex and recurrent cases.

Antibiotic-Associated Diarrhea without Colitis. An acute self-limited diarrheal syndrome with mild abdominal pain frequently occurs in infants and children who receive antibiotics.[69] The diarrhea is mild, without systemic findings, and subsides when antibiotics are stopped. In only 20 percent of these cases of antibiotic-associated diarrhea without colitis are C. difficile and its toxin found in the stool; in the remainder the cause of diarrhea is not clear.[70]

Chronic C. difficile Diarrhea. Chronic C. difficile diarrhea associated with failure to thrive may be seen in the pediatric population[71] but apparently not in adults. This chronic diarrhea without classic symptoms of colitis may occur in both infants of few weeks of age and older children, particularly those who have previously received antibiotics. Diarrhea usually contains mucus, is associated with abdominal cramps, and commonly leads to dehydration and growth failure. Fever and rectal bleeding are rare. The diarrhea may last for months before the diagnosis is made. At examination, the patients lack definitive evidence of colitis, such as bloody stools, fecal leukocytes, or abnormal proctoscopic findings. C. difficile cytotoxin determination in the stool is diagnostic. Therapy is mandatory not only for symptomatic relief but also to prevent the potential for progression from diarrhea to frank colitis.

C. difficile Colitis Complicating Inflammatory Bowel Disease. C. difficile infection can occasionally occur in patients with ulcerative colitis or Crohn's disease, even without the prior use of antibiotics.[72-74] A 5 to 25 percent incidence of cytotoxin positivity has been reported in inflammatory bowel disease patients with relapse, mostly following antibiotic exposure.[75] The clinical symptoms of severe diarrhea, rectal bleeding, abdominal pain, and fever are easily confused with a recurrence of the chronic inflammatory bowel disease. Pseudomembranes do not occur in patients with C. difficile

infection co-existing with ulcerative colitis. It is recommended that stool cultures for enteric pathogens and toxin assay for C. difficile be obtained on all children with inflammatory bowel disease during acute relapses.[76]

Nonantibiotic C. difficile Colitis. C. difficile infection without prior antibiotic therapy is very rare but can occur in both children and adults. In a study of C. difficile infection in a daycare center (average age 11 months), less than 50 percent of cases were associated with antibiotic therapy. Patients undergoing chemotherapy may have altered bowel flora that predisposes to C. difficile infection,[77] whereas neutropenic patients may have impaired defense mechanisms against C. difficile toxins.[78] In addition, patients who are treated for malignancies, particularly hematologic, require many courses and combinations of antibiotics together with frequent and prolonged hospitalizations. Such treatment makes them liable to acquire hospital strains of C. difficile. C. difficile infection related to cancer chemotherapy has a presentation typical of antibiotic-associated diarrhea. Some, however, may present with atypical features such as abdominal pain, distention, and only minimal diarrhea that is commonly ascribed to cancer chemotherapy. C. difficile bacteremia, toxic necrotizing ileocecitis, intestinal perforation, ascites, jaundice, thrombotic glomerulopathy, and coagulopathy have been described in severely neutropenic patients treated for acute leukemia or lymphoma, but many of them had also received wide-spectrum antibiotics.[79,80] Because pseudomembranes are usually absent on sigmoidoscopy, the diagnosis may be missed and early death may occur. Therefore, toxin assay for C. difficile should be obtained in all patients treated with chemotherapy who develop abdominal symptoms.

Other Syndromes of Pediatric C. difficile Infection. Neonatal necrotizing enterocolitis (NEC), a potentially lethal disease of premature infants, has been attributed to intestinal ischemia, but its occurrence in outbreaks has suggested an infectious etiology. Although C. difficile cytotoxin may be present in some patients with neonatal NEC, infection with this organism is not the cause of the disease.[81-83] Toxin concentrations are uniformly low in NEC and generally do not differ from those found in healthy neonates.[84-86] Patients with cystic fibrosis would likely be at high risk for developing C. difficile infection, since they are hospitalized and receive antibiotics frequently throughout their lives. Nevertheless, C. difficile infection is unusual in patients with cystic fibrosis.[87] Epithelial cell–associated factors that prevent binding or action of toxin, as well as organism and host factors related to C. difficile, may be important. Cystic fibrosis patients have significantly higher colonization rates with Enterococcus, Lactobacillus, Pseudomonas, and Staphylococcus organisms that have a demonstrable inhibitory effect on C. difficile.[88] This may explain the relative paucity of cases in this group of patients.

C. difficile has been incriminated in the pathogenesis of enterocolitis of Hirschsprung's disease in children under 3 years of age, while in older children other clostridia may be involved.[89-91] For that reason, oral or rectal vancomycin has been used in the treatment of enterocolitis in Hirschsprung's disease.[92] A role for C. difficile has been proposed in some cases of infantile gastroenteritis,[93] failure to thrive,[94] sudden infant death syndrome,[95] and infant botulism but has been difficult to define. Nevertheless, until further studies are completed, children with diarrhea or other symptoms of enteritis whose stools contain *C. difficile* cytotoxin should be treated with oral vancomycin or metronidazole.

LABORATORY DIAGNOSIS

Fecal *C. difficile* Cytotoxin Assay. The tissue culture assay for toxin B in stool filtrates is currently the principal diagnostic tool for *C. difficile*–associated pseudomembranous colitis and diarrhea in both children and adults (Fig. 5)[96] Cytotoxin can be detected by this assay in about 95 percent of patients with documented pseudomembranes. It is also found in 25 to 40 percent of patients with antibiotic-associated diarrhea in whom pseudomembranes cannot be demonstrated in the rectum or sigmoid,[97] although they are occasionally present more proximally in the colon.[98] The presence of fecal cytotoxin in adults is almost invariably associated with diarrhea; however, in infants, fecal cytotoxin may be detected in asymptomatic carriers.[99,100] No correlation exists between cytotoxin titers and severity of the underlying bowel disease.[101,102] A provisional positive result may be obtained within 6 hours, although 24 to 48 hours are needed for confirmation. An enzyme-linked immunosorbent assay (ELISA) capable of detecting *C. difficile* toxin A has recently been reported but is not sufficiently specific for clinical use.[103] A new latex agglutination test for detection of *C. difficile* toxin A has recently been marketed.[104] The test is useful for rapid screening, since results are available in 30 minutes, but a positive test should be confirmed by cytotoxicity assay.

C. difficile **Stool Culture.** A positive culture for *C. difficile* using semiselective media suggests an etiologic association in patients with antibiotic-associated diarrhea.[105] However, this should be interpreted with caution if stool cytotoxin is absent because increased asymptomatic carriage of *C. difficile* occurs in infants and young children and may occur following antibiotics.

Stool Examination for Leukocytes. Examination of stool for leukocytes utilizing methylene blue stain is a rapid and convenient screening test for the presence of infectious colitis. The test is positive in approximately 50 percent of patients with *C. difficile* enteritis.[106] In addition, this test is not sensitive, as fecal leukocytes may be absent in cases of *C. difficile* diarrhea without colitis.

Sigmoidoscopy and Biopsy. Proctosigmoidoscopy is not mandatory for the diagnosis of pseudomembranous colitis but in some patients may provide useful information. The characteristic pseudomembranes are present in the rectum and sigmoid colon in approximately one-third of patients.[107] In the absence of pseudomembranes local changes include nonspecific colitis or mucosal edema. Mucosal biopsy is useful in confirming the diagnosis and excluding co-existent chronic inflammatory bowel disease.

Colonoscopy. This examination may be diagnostic in cases of *C. difficile* colitis with rectal sparing,[98] but it is considered by some to be potentially dangerous, since instrumentation may predispose to toxic megacolon or perforation.

Plain Abdominal Radiography. Plain films of the abdomen may show dilated loops of bowel with air-fluid levels, accumulation of peritoneal fluid, mucosal edema, and thumbprinting of the colon, but these features are not specific.[108] The main indication for plain abdominal radiography is to detect toxic megacolon in fulminant cases of *C. difficile* colitis.

Barium Radiography. Barium studies may show edematous bowel with mucosal ulcerations and scalloping. Air-

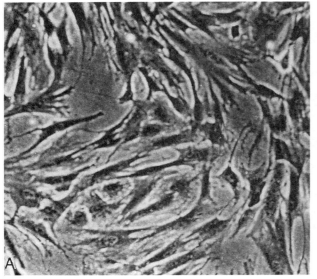
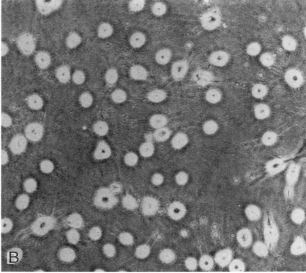

FIGURE 5 *C. difficile* cytotoxicity assay. *A*, Normal fibroblast monolayer. *B*, Characteristic cytopathic effect consisting of rounding and separation of cells in culture after application of stool containing *C. difficile* toxin B. This effect can be neutralized by preincubation of the stool sample with *C. difficile* antitoxin.

contrast examinations further suggest the presence of pseudomembranes but are generally not specific, are potentially dangerous, and are not recommended.[109]

DIFFERENTIAL DIAGNOSIS

C. difficile infection needs to be considered in any child presenting with diarrhea during or after antibiotic therapy. Other infectious diarrheas, such as those caused by *Salmonella, Shigella, Campylobacter, Yersinia, E. coli,* and cytomegalovirus, may present with similar symptomatology.[110] Initial presentation of idiopathic inflammatory bowel disease, such as ulcerative colitis and Crohn's disease, should be considered, but both of these diseases tend to be chronic in nature. Co-occurrence of *C. difficile* infection in patients with inflammatory bowel disease must be excluded. The vasculitides, such as Henoch-Schönlein purpura and the hemolytic uremic syndrome, are associated with hematologic, dermatologic, and renal abnormalities that provide clues to the diagnosis. In infants less than 6 months of age, necrotizing enterocolitis, Hirschsprung's disease, and cow's milk or soy protein intolerance more likely cause bloody, mucoid diarrhea (Table 7).

TREATMENT

Specific Therapy. The primary goal of therapy is to eliminate *C. difficile* and its toxins from the feces and to allow restoration of the normal colonic flora. A variety of specific and effective antimicrobials are available. The agent of choice in pseudomembranous colitis is oral metronidazole, 5 to 7 mg per kilogram three times a day for 10 days. Metronidazole appears uniformly bactericidal against *C. difficile,* and it is curative in more than 95 percent of cases. Metronidazole is the cheapest form of therapy with established efficacy, it has rare therapeutic failures, and relapse rates are 15 percent, similar to those of vancomycin.[111,112] An additional advantage of metronidazole is its potential for intravenous use in patients with ileus, which might prevent passage of oral drug to the colon.

Vancomycin was previously considered the antibiotic of

TABLE 7
Differential Diagnosis of Antibiotic-Associated Colitis in Children

Infectious colitis
Necrotizing enterocolitis
Chronic inflammatory bowel disease
Hirschsprung's disease
Hemolytic uremic syndrome with colitis
Henoch-Schönlein purpura
Cow's milk protein enterocolitis
AIDS enteropathy

choice in pseudomembranous colitis, but because of its high cost it is now recommended as a second-line agent.[113] The currently recommended dosage is 20 to 60 mg per kilogram per day (0.5 to 2 g per day) by month in four divided doses for 10 days. Vancomycin has no systemic toxicity, as it is not significantly absorbed after oral administration, is highly active against *C. difficile* in vitro, and has an initial response rate comparable to that of metronidazole.[111]

Oral bacitracin (20,000 U every 6 hours) is an inexpensive alternative to metronidazole treatment of *C. difficile* diarrhea and colitis, but no studies have been reported in children.[114] The agent is significantly less effective than vancomycin in clearing *C. difficile* from the stools, but its clinical response and relapse rates are similar. Bacitracin is not readily available in many hospital pharmacies, and this has limited its use.

General Measures. Discontinuation of the antibiotic therapy that preceded the *C. difficile* infection is generally recommended and often results in complete recovery without the use of metronidazole or vancomycin. This is often all that is necessary in mildly ill children without underlying diseases.[115] Adequate fluid and electrolyte replacement is important, especially in infants, as fluid losses may be great. Patients with documented pseudomembranes and others in whom *C. difficile* is considered the most likely pathogen are nursed in isolation, and enteric precautions are taken to reduce the risk of cross-infection for the duration of the illness.[116] Frequent evaluation of abdominal findings is important, as surgical intervention may be required in fulminant cases. Antiperistaltic agents, such as diphenoxylate (Lomotil), loperamide (Imodium), or codeine, are not recommended, since they may allow the pathogen to proliferate and prevent clearance of toxin. It has been suggested that antidiarrheal agents may prolong or exacerbate symptoms and predispose to toxic megacolon.[117] Anion-binding resins such as cholestyramine have also been used to treat pseudomembranous colitis in children.[118] Cholestyramine binds to clostridial toxins in vitro, but there are no controlled clinical studies to support their use as a primary therapy. There are no data to support the use of corticosteroids in pseudomembranous colitis, although these agents have been used in pediatric patients with pseudomembranous colitis.[119] Attempts to re-establish the normal flora with the use of lactobacilli preparations such as Lactinex and the use of fecal enemas have not been carefully studied.[120]

After institution of metronidazole or vancomycin therapy, diarrhea resolves in 3 to 5 days, and clearance of the organism and its toxins from stools occurs within the first week.[107,113] Fever and systemic manifestations resolve within the first 48 hours. Upon completion of therapy, endoscopy reveals complete resolution of pseudomembranes. Treatment of any underlying disease even with antibiotics should be continued. The pediatrician should always be alert for the development of complications of *C. difficile* infection such as ileus, toxic megacolon, or intestinal perforation and peritonitis. The cytotoxicity assay may remain positive in up to 30 percent of cases, even with clinical resolution; it does not imply failure of therapy and is not a predictor of clinical relapse.[121] As an isolated finding, a positive cytotoxicity assay does not constitute an indication for continuation or reinstitution of treatment.

RELAPSE

Despite the efficacy of metronidazole or vancomycin therapy in pseudomembranous colitis, relapses occur in up to 15 percent of cases and cannot be accurately predicted or prevented.[122] Patients with relapse usually have an initial good response to therapy and then, within several days to weeks, redevelop diarrhea, fever, or abdominal pain in association with the presence of cytotoxin in the stool. The persistence of *C. difficile* or its cytotoxin after a course of therapy in an asymptomatic patient does not by itself indicate a clinically significant relapse and does not require therapy. *C. difficile* may persist in spore form during therapy and convert to a vegetative form following cessation of therapy.[123] *C. difficile* reinfection and antibiotic resistance do not appear to be factors in relapse.[124,125] Treatment of *C. difficile* relapse is the same as for the initial disease, and most patients respond well to a second course of therapy.[126] A second relapse may occur in up to one-third of cases. For patients with multiple relapses, switching from one agent to another (metronidazole versus vancomycin) and continuing therapy for up to 3 weeks may be useful.[127] Combination of vancomycin with rifampin or a 2-week course of vancomycin followed by a 2- to 3-week course of cholestyramine to allow re-establishment of bowel flora has also been successful.[128] The efficacy of *Lactobacillus* preparations or fecal enemas to restore the normal flora has not been demonstrated.[129]

PREVENTION

The judicious use of antibiotics in children and adolescents can reduce the incidence of pseudomembranous colitis. Prophylactic vancomycin therapy for patients on antibiotics who are at risk for *C. difficile* infection is not recommended. *C. difficile* contamination of the hospital environment is common, particularly in areas of the hospital where patients with known infection have been treated. Persistence of *C. difficile* spores in a hospital room has been demonstrated for up to 40 days after discharge of a patient with a documented case. Therefore, thorough cleansing of hospital rooms after discharge of a known case is especially important. Hospital spread can possibly be limited by isolation of known cases to single rooms, careful handling of feces and soiled linen, and handwashing after examination of patients.[130]

REFERENCES

1. Trnka YM, LaMont JT. *Clostridium difficile* colitis. Adv Intern Med 1984; 29:85–107.
2. Buts JP, Weber AM, Roy CC, Morin C. Pseudomembranous enterocolitis in childhood. Gastroenterology 1977; 73:823–827.
3. Finney JMT. Gastroenterostomy for cicatrizing ulcer of the pylorus. Bull Johns Hopkins Hosp 1893; 4:53–55.
4. Hummel RP, Altemeier WA, Hill EO. Iatrogenic staphylococcal enterocolitis. Ann Surg 1964; 138:551–560.
5. Kahn MY, Hall WH. Staphylococcal enterocolitis: treatment with oral vancomycin. Ann Intern Med 1966; 65:1–8.
6. Hall IC, O'Toole E. Intestinal flora in newborn infants with description of a new pathogenic anaerobe, *Bacillus difficilis*. Am J Dis Child 1935; 49:390–402.
7. Larson HE, Parry FV, Price AB, et al. Underdescribed toxin in pseudomembranous colitis. Br Med J 1977; 1:1246–1248.
8. Larson HE, Price AB, Honour P, Boriello SP. *Clostridium difficile* and the aetiology of pseudomembranous colitis. Lancet 1978; i:1062–1066.
9. Bartlett FG, Moon N, Chang TW, et al. The role of *Clostridium difficile* in antibiotic-associated pseudomembranous colitis. Gastroenterology 1978; 75:778–782.
10. Viscidi RP, Bartlett JG. Antibiotic-associated pseudomembranous colitis in children. Pediatrics 1981; 67:381–386.
11. George WL, Sutter VL, Citron O, et al. Selective and differential medium for isolation of *Clostridium difficile*. J Clin Microbiol 1979; 9:214–219.
12. Wilson KH, Kennedy MJ, Fekety FR. Use of sodium taurocholate to enhance spore recovery on a medium selective for *Clostridium difficile*. J Clin Microbiol 1982; 15:443–446.
13. Mitchell TJ, Ketley JM, Haslam SC, et al. Effect of toxin A and B of *Clostridium difficile* on rabbit ileum and colon. Gut 1986; 27:78–85.
14. Pothoulakis C, Barone LM, Ely R, et al. Purification and properties of *Clostridium difficile* cytotoxin B. J Biol Chem 1986; 261:1316–1321.
15. Triadafilopoulos G, Pothoulakis C, O'Brien MJ, LaMont JT. Differential effects of *Clostridium difficile* toxins A and B on rabbit ileum. Gastroenterology 1987; 93:273–279.
16. Pothoulakis C, Sullivan R, Melnick DA, et al. *Clostridium difficile* toxin A stimulates intracellular calcium release and chemotactic response in human granulocytes. J Clin Invest 1988; 81:1741–1745.
17. Wilkins TD. Role of *Clostridium difficile* toxins in disease. Gastroenterology 1987; 93:389–391.
18. Kim P-H, Iaconis FP, Rolfe RD. Immunization of adult hamsters against *Clostridium difficile*-associated ileocecitis and transfer of protection to infant hamsters. Infect Immun 1987; 55:2984–2992.
19. Sullivan NM, Pellet S, Wilkins TD. Purification and characterization of toxins A and B of *Clostridium difficile*. Infect Immun 1982; 35:1032–1040.
20. Lyerly DM, Lockwood PE, Richardson SH, Wilkins TD. Biological activities of toxins A and B of *Clostridium difficile*. Infect Immun 1985; 35:1147–1150.
21. Pothoulakis C, Triadafilopoulos G, Clark M, et al. *Clostridium difficile* cytotoxin inhibits protein synthesis in fibroblasts and intestinal mucosa. Gastroenterology 1986; 91:1147–1153.
22. Wedel N, Toselli P, Pothoulakis C, et al. Ultrastructural effects of *Clostridium difficile* toxin B on smooth muscle cells and fibroblasts. Exp Cell Res 1983; 148:413–422.
23. George WL. Antimicrobial agent–associated colitis and diarrhea: historical background and clinical aspects. Rev Infect Dis 1984; 6(suppl):208–213.
24. Fekety R, Kim K-H, Batts DH, et al. Studies on the epidemiology of antibiotic-associated *Clostridium difficile* colitis. Am J Clin Nutr 1980; 33:2527–2532.
25. Viscidi R, Willey S, Bartlett JG. Isolation rates and toxigenic potential of *Clostridium difficile* isolates from various patient populations. Gastroenterology 1981; 81:5–9.
26. Bolton RP, Thomas DF. Pseudomembranous colitis in children and adults. Br J Hosp Med 1986; 35:37–42.
27. George WL. Antimicrobial agent–associated colitis and diarrhea. West J Med 1980; 133:115–123.
28. Bartlett J. Antibiotic-associated pseudomembranous colitis. Rev Infect Dis 1979; 1:530–539.
29. Vesicari T, Isolauri E, Maaki M, Groonroos P. *Clostridium difficile* in young children. Association with antibiotic usage. Acta Paediatr Scand 1984; 73:86–91.
30. Church JM, Fazio VW. A role of colonic stasis in the pathogenesis of disease related to *Clostridium difficile*. Dis Colon Rectum 1986; 29:804–809.
31. Viscidi R, Laughon BF, Yolken R, et al. Serum antibody response to toxins A and B of *Clostridium difficile*. J Infect Dis 1983; 148:93–100.
32. Freter R. Association of enterotoxigenic bacteria with the mucosa of the small intestine: mechanisms and pathogenic implications. In: Ouchterlony O, Holmgren J, eds. Cholera and related diarrheas. Basel: Karger, 1980: 155.
33. Krivan HC, Clark GF, Smith DF, Wilkins TD. Cell surface binding site for *Clostridium difficile* enterotoxin: evidence for a glycoconjugate containing the sequence Gal 1-3Gal 1-4GlcNAc. Infect Immun 1986; 53:573–581.

34. Pothoulakis C, McAndrew P, LaMont JT. Specific binding of radio-labelled *Clostridium difficile* toxin A on rabbit intestinal brush borders (BB) and cultured rat basophilic leukemia (RBL) cells. Gastroenterology 1988; 94:338.

35. Cohen MB, Guarino A, Shukla R, Gianella RA. Age-related differences in receptors for *Escherichia coli* heat-stable enterotoxin in the small and large intestine of children. Gastroenterology 1988; 94:367–373.

36. Mobassaleh M, Donohue-Rolfe A, Montgomery RK. Functional characterization of age dependent binding of Shigella toxin to rabbit intestinal microvillous membranes (MVM). Gastroenterology 1986; 90:1555.

37. Hughes S, Warhurst G, Turnberg LA, et al. *Clostridium difficile* toxin-induced intestinal secretion in rabbit ileum in vitro. Gut 1983; 24:94–98.

38. Triadafilopoulos G, Pothoulakis C, LaMont JT. *In vivo* production of leukotriene B$_4$ and prostaglandin E$_2$ in experimental *C. difficile* colitis. Am J Gastroenterol 1987; 82:950.

39. Triadafilopoulos G, Pothoulakis C, Weiss R, et al. Comparative study of *Clostridium difficile* toxin A and cholera toxin in rabbit ileum. Gastroenterology 1989; 97:1186–1192.

40. Arnon S, Mills D, Day P, Hendrickson R, Sullivan N, Wilkins T. Rapid death of infant rhesus monkeys injected with *Clostridium difficile* toxins A and B: physiologic and pathologic basis. J Pediatr 1984; 104:34–40.

41. Lyerly DM, Saum KE, MacDonald DK, et al. Effects of *Clostridium difficile* toxins given intragastrically to animals. Infect Immun 1985; 47:349–352.

42. Larson HE, Barclay FE, Honour P, Hill ID. Epidemiology of *Clostridium difficile* in infants. J Infect Dis 1982; 146:727–733.

43. Rietra PJGM, Slaterus KW, Zanen HC, Meuwissen SGM. Clostridial toxin in faeces of healthy infants. Lancet 1978; i:319.

44. Thompson CM, Gilligan PH, Fisher MC, Long SS. *Clostridium difficile* cytotoxin in a pediatric population. Am J Dis Child 1983; 137:271–274.

45. Stark PL, Lee A, Parsonage BD. Colonization of the large bowel by *Clostridium difficile* in healthy infants: quantitative study. Infect Immun 1982; 35:895–899.

46. Mulligan ME, George WL, Rolfe RD, et al. Epidemiological aspects of *Clostridium difficile*-induced diarrhea or colitis. Am J Clin Nutr 1981; 33:2533–2538.

47. Kim K-H, Fekety R, Batts DH, et al. Isolation of *Clostridium difficile* from the environment and contacts of patients with antibiotic-associated colitis. J Infect Dis 1981; 143:42–50.

48. Fekety R, Kim K-H, Brown D, et al. Epidemiology of antibiotic-associated colitis. Isolation of *Clostridium difficile* from the hospital environment. Am J Med 1981; 70:906–908.

49. Merida V, Moerman J, Colaert J, Lemmens P, Vandepitte J. Significance of *Clostridium difficile* and its cytotoxin in children. Eur J Pediatr 1986; 144:494–496.

50. Mulligan ME. Epidemiology of *Clostridium difficile*-induced intestinal disease. Rev Infect Dis 1984; 6(suppl):222–228.

51. Holst E, Helin I, Mardh P-A. Recovery of *Clostridium difficile* from children. Scand J Infect Dis 1981; 13:41–45.

52. Welch DF, Marks MI. Is *Clostridium difficile* pathogenic in infants? J Pediatr 1982; 100:393–395.

53. Gilligan PH, McCarthy LR, Genta VM. Relative frequency of *Clostridium difficile* in patients with diarrheal disease. J Clin Microbiol 1981; 14:26–31.

54. Cooperstock MS, Steffen E, Yolken R, et al. *Clostridium difficile* in normal infants and sudden death syndrome: an association with infant formula feeding. Pediatrics 1982; 70:91–95.

55. Kim K-H, DuPont HL, Pickering LK. Outbreaks of diarrhea associated with *Clostridium difficile* and its toxin in day care centers: evidence of person-to-person spread. J Pediatr 1983; 102:376–382.

56. Editorial. *Clostridium difficile*—a neglected pathogen in chronic-care wards? Lancet 1986; i:790–791.

57. Price AB, Davies DR. Pseudomembranous colitis. J Clin Pathol 1977; 30:1–12.

58. Lishman AH, Al-Jumaili IJ, Record CO. Spectrum of antibiotic-associated diarrhea. Gut 1981; 22:34–37.

59. Pothoulakis C, Triadafilopoulos G, LaMont JT. Antibiotic-associated colitis. Compr Therapy 1985; 11(12):68–73.

60. Beesley J, Eastman EJ, Jackson RH, Nelson R. Clindamycin associated pseudomembranous colitis. Acta Pediatr Scand 1981; 70:129–130.

61. Ecker JA, Williams RG, McKirkpatrick JE. Pseudomembranous enterocolitis—an unwelcome gastrointestinal complication of antibiotic therapy. Am J Gastroenterol 1970; 54:214–228.

62. Genta VM, Gilligan PH, McCarthy LR. *Clostridium difficile* peritonitis in a neonate: a case report. Arch Pathol Lab Med 1984; 108:82–83.

63. Werlin SL, Grand RJ. Severe colitis in children and adolescents: diagnosis, course and treatment. Gastroenterology 1977; 73:828–832.

64. Talbot RW, Walker RC, Beart RW. Changing epidemiology, diagnosis and treatment of *Clostridium difficile* toxin-associated colitis. Br J Surg 1986; 73:457–460.

65. Qualman SJ, Petric M, Karmali MA, Smith CR, Hamilton SR. The pathophysiology of fatal clostridial infection in pediatric pseudomembranous colitis; in press.

66. Fee HJ, Kearny JP, Ament ME, et al. Fatal outcome in a child with pseudomembranous colitis. J Pediatr Surg 1975; 10:959–963.

67. Christie DL, Ament ME. Ampicillin-associated colitis. J Pediatr 1975; 87:657–658.

68. Tedesco FJ, Corless JK, Brownstein RE. Rectal sparing in antibiotic-associated pseudomembranous colitis; a prospective study. Gastroenterology 1983; 83:1259–1260.

69. Gilligan PH, McCarthy LR, Genta VM. Relative frequency of *Clostridium difficile* in patients with diarrheal disease. J Clin Microbiol 1981; 14:26–31.

70. Tedesco FJ, Barton RW, Alpers DH. Clindamycin-associated colitis. Ann Intern Med 1974; 81:429–433.

71. Sutphen JL, Grand RJ, Flores A, Chang TW, Bartlett JG. Chronic diarrhea associated with *Clostridium difficile* in children. Am J Dis Child 1983; 137:275–278.

72. Trnka YM, LaMont JT. Association of *Clostridium difficile* toxin with symptomatic relapse of chronic inflammatory bowel disease. Gastroenterology 1981; 80:693–696.

73. Hyams JS, McLaughlin JC. Lack of relationship between *Clostridium difficile* toxin and inflammatory bowel disease in children. J Clin Gastroenterol 1985; 7:387–390.

74. Meyers S, Mayer L, Bottone E, et al. Occurrence of *Clostridium difficile* toxin during the course of inflammatory bowel disease. Gastroenterology 1981; 80:693–696.

75. Greenfield C, Ramirez-Aguilar JR, Pounder RE, et al. *Clostridium difficile* and inflammatory bowel disease. Gut 1983; 24:713–717.

76. Cudmore MA, Silva J Jr, Fekety R, et al. *Clostridium difficile* colitis associated with cancer chemotherapy. Arch Intern Med 1982; 142:333–335.

77. Rampling A, Warren RE, Bevan PC, et al. *Clostridium difficile* in haematological malignancy. J Clin Pathol 1985; 38:445–451.

78. Milligan DW, Kelly JK. Pseudomembranous colitis in a leukaemia unit: a report of five fatal cases. J Clin Pathol 1979; 32:1237–1243.

79. Fainstein V, Bodey GP, Fekety R. Relapsing pseudomembranous colitis associated with cancer chemotherapy. J Infect Dis 1981; 143:865.

80. Dosik GM, Luna M, Valdivieso M, et al. Necrotizing colitis in patients with cancer. Am J Med 1979; 67:646–656.

81. Han VK, Sayed H, Chance GW, Brabyn DG, Shaheed WA. An outbreak of *Clostridium difficile* necrotizing enterocolitis: a case for oral vancomycin therapy? Pediatrics 1983; 71:935–941.

82. Blakey JL, Lubitz L, Campell NT, Gillam GM, Bishop RF, Barnes GL. Enteric colonization in sporadic neonatal necrotizing enterocolitis. J Pediatr Gastroenterol Nutr 1985; 4:591–595.

83. Sherertz RJ, Sarubbi FA. The prevalence of *Clostridium difficile* and toxin in a nursery population: a comparison between patients with necrotizing enterocolitis and an asymptomatic group. J Pediatr 1982; 100:435–439.

84. Matthew OP, Bhatia JS, Richardson CJ. An outbreak of *Clostridium difficile* necrotizing enterocolitis. (Letter) Pediatrics 1984; 73:265–266.

85. Lishman AH, Al Jumaili IJ, Elshibli E, Hey E, Record CO. *Clostridium difficile* isolation in neonates in a special care unit. Lack of correlation with necrotizing enterocolitis. Scand J Gastroenterol 1984; 19:441–444.

86. Thomas DF, Fernie DS, Bayston R, Spitz L. Clostridial toxins in neonatal necrotizing enterocolitis. Arch Dis Child 1984; 59:270–272.

87. Peach SL, Borriello SP, Gaya H, Barclay FE, Welch AR. Asymptomatic carriage of *Clostridium difficile* in patients with cystic fibrosis. J Clin Pathol 1986; 39:1013–1018.

88. Welkon CJ, Long SS, Thompson CM Jr, Gilligan PH. *Clostridium difficile* in patients with cystic fibrosis. Am J Dis Child 1985; 139:805–808.

89. Brearly S, Armstrong GR, Nairn R, Gornall P, Currie AB, Buick RG, Corkery JJ. Pseudomembranous colitis: a lethal complication of Hirschsprung's disease unrelated to antibiotic usage. J Pediatr Surg 1987; 22:257–259.

90. Thomas DFM, Fernie DS, Bayston R, Spitz L, Nixon HH. Enterocolitis in Hirschsprung's disease: a controlled study of the etiologic role of *Clostridium difficile*. J Pediatr Surg 1986; 21:22–25.

91. Thomas DFM, Fernie DS, Malone M, et al. Association between *Clostridium difficile* and enterocolitis in Hirschsprung's disease. Lancet 1982; i:78–79.

92. Cooperstock MS. *Clostridium difficile*, enterocolitis and Hirschsprung's disease. (Letter) Lancet 1982; i:800.

93. Jarvis WR, Feldman RA. *Clostridium difficile* and gastroenteritis: how strong is the association in children? Pediatr Infect Dis 1984; 3:4–6.

94. Thompson CM, Gilligan PH, Fisher MC, et al. *Clostridium difficile* cytotoxin in a pediatric population. Am J Dis Child 1983; 137:271–274.

95. Cooperstock M, Steffen E, Yolkin R, et al. *Clostridium difficile* in normal infants and in sudden infant death syndrome: a relationship with infant formula feedings. Pediatrics; in press.

96. Brook I, Avery G, Glasgow A. *Clostridium difficile* in paediatric infections. J Infect 1982; 4:253–257.

97. Lashner BA, Todorczuk J, Sahm DF, et al. *Clostridium difficile* culture-positive toxin-negative diarrhea. Am J Gastroenterol 1986; 81:940–943.

98. Tedesco FJ. Antibiotic-associated pseudomembranous colitis with negative proctosigmoidoscopy examination. Gastroenterology 1979; 77:295–297.

99. Luzzi I, Caprioli A, Falbo V, Guarino A, Capano G, Alessio M, Malamisura B, Gianfrilli P. Detection of clostridial toxins in stools from children with diarrhea. J Med Microbiol 1986; 22:29–31.

100. Mardh PA, Helin I, Colleen M, et al. *Clostridium difficile* toxin in fecal specimens of healthy children and children with diarrhea. Acta Pediatr Scand 1982; 71:275–278.

101. Mollby R, Aronsson B, Nord CE. Pathogenesis and diagnosis of *Clostridium difficile* enterocolitis. Scand J Infect Dis 1985; 46:47–56.

102. Rolfe RD. Diagnosis of *Clostridium difficile*–associated intestinal disease. Crit Rev Clin Lab Sci 1986; 24:235–261.

103. Walker RC, Ruane PJ, Rosenblatt JE, et al. Comparison of culture, cytotoxicity assays, and enzyme-linked immunosorbent assay for toxin A and B in the diagnosis of *Clostridium difficile*–related enteric disease. Diagn Microbiol Infect Dis 1986; 5:61–69.

104. Peterson LR, Holter JJ, Shanholtzer CJ, et al. Detection of *Clostridium difficile* toxins A (enterotoxin) and B (cytotoxin) in clinical specimens. Evaluation of a latex agglutination test. Am J Clin Pathol 1986; 86:208–211.

105. Ryan RW. Considerations in the laboratory diagnosis of antibiotic-associated gastroenteritis. Diagn Microbiol Infect Dis 1986; 4:79S–86S.

106. Bolton RP, Thomas DF. Pseudomembranous colitis in children and adults. Br J Hosp Med 1986; 35:37–42.

107. Tedesco FJ. Pseudomembranous colitis. Pathogenesis and therapy. Med Clin North Am 1982; 66:655–664.

108. Templeton JL. Toxic megacolon complicating pseudomembranous colitis. Br J Surg 1983; 70:48.

109. Stanley RJ, Melson GL, Tedesco FJ. The spectrum of radiographic findings in antibiotic-related pseudomembranous colitis. Radiology 1984; 111:519–524.

110. Brown R, Tedesco FJ, Assad RT, Rao R. Yersinia colitis masquerading as pseudomembranous colitis. Dig Dis Sci 1986; 31:548–551.

111. Teasley DG, Gerding DN, Olson MM, et al. Prospective randomized trial of metronidazole versus vancomycin for *Clostridium difficile*–associated diarrhea and colitis. Lancet 1983; i:1043–1046.

112. Cherry RD, Portnoy D, Fabbari M, et al. Metronidazole: an alternate therapy for antibiotic-associated colitis. Gastroenterology 1982; 82:849–851.

113. Keighley MRB, Burdon DW, Arabi Y, et al. A randomized controlled trial of vancomycin for pseudomembranous colitis and postoperative diarrhea. Br Med J 1978; 2:1667–1669.

114. Young GP, Ward PB, Bayley N et al. Antibiotic-associated colitis due to *Clostridium difficile*: double-blind comparison of vancomycin with bacitracin. Gastroenterology; 89:1038–1045.

115. Bartlett JG. Treatment of *Clostridium difficile* colitis. (Editorial) Gastroenterology 1985; 89:1192–1195.

116. Communicable Disease Center. Guidelines for isolation precautions in hospitals. Infect Control 1983; 4:267–268.

117. Novak E, Lee JG, Seckman CE, et al. Unfavorable effect of atropine-diphenoxylate (Lomotil) therapy in clindamycin-caused diarrhea. JAMA 1976; 235:1451–1454.

118. Kreutzer EW, Milligan FD. Treatment of antibiotic-associated pseudomembranous colitis with cholestyramine resin. Johns Hopkins Med J 1978; 143:67–72.

119. Danemann HA. Corticosteroids for pseudomembranous colitis. (Letter) JAMA 1975; 234:151.

120. Bowden TA Jr, Mansberger AR Jr, Lykins LE. Pseudomembranous enterocolitis: mechanism for restoring floral homeostasis. Am Surg 1981; 47:178–183.

121. Bartlett JG, Tedesco FJ, Shull S, et al. Symptomatic relapse after oral vancomycin therapy of antibiotic-associated pseudomembranous colitis. Gastroenterology 1980; 78:431–434.

122. George WL, Volpicelli NA, Stiner DB, et al. Relapse of pseudomembranous colitis after vancomycin therapy. N Engl J Med 1979; 301:414–415.

123. Walters BAJ, Roberts R, Stafford R, et al. Relapse of antibiotic-associated colitis: endogenous persistence of *Clostridium difficile* during vancomycin therapy. Gut 1983; 24:206–212.

124. Vesicari T, Maaki M, Baer M, Groonroos P. Pseudomembranous colitis with recurring diarrhea and prolonged persistence of *Clostridium difficile* in a 10-year-old girl. Acta Paediatr Scand 1984; 73:135–137.

125. Tabaqchali S, Holland D, O'Farrell S, et al. Typing scheme for *Clostridium difficile*: its application in clinical and epidemiological studies. Lancet 1984; i:935–938.

126. Tedesco FJ. Treatment of recurrent antibiotic-associated pseudomembranous colitis. Am J Gastroenterol 1982; 77:220–221.

127. Holmes R, Byrne WJ. Relapsing pseudomembranous colitis. J Pediatr Gastroenterol Nutr 1986; 5:314–315.

128. Buggy BP, Fekety R, Silva J Jr. Therapy of relapsing *Clostridium difficile* associated diarrhea and colitis with the combination of vancomycin and rifampin. J Clin Gastroenterol 1987; 9:155–159.

129. Schwan A, Sjolin S, Trottestam U, et al. Relapsing *Clostridium difficile* enterocolitis cured by rectal infusion of homologous feces. Lancet 1983; ii:845.

130. O'Connor RA, Kelly CP, Walsh TN, Weir DG. Hospital outbreaks of *Clostridium difficile*. Lancet 1986; ii:350.

131. McFarland LV, Mulligan ME, Kwok RYY, Stamm WE. Nosocomial acquisition of *C. difficile* infection. N Engl J Med 1989; 320:204–209.

PART 16

Miscellaneous Intestinal Inflammatory Disorders

Barbara S. Kirschner, M.D.

EOSINOPHILIC GASTROENTEROPATHY

Eosinophilic gastroenteropathy (EG) is a chronic, relapsing disorder in which eosinophils constitute the predominant cell type in the inflammatory infiltrate of the gastrointestinal (GI) tract. The entity was described first by Kaijser in 1937.[1] Subsequently, patterns of clinical presentation were correlated with the extent of the eosinophilic infiltration (diffuse versus circumscribed) by Ureles et al[2] and the depth of the eosinophilic reaction (mucosal, muscular, and serosal) by Klein et al.[3]

In some cases in which specific foods clearly precipitate symptoms, this condition may be difficult to distinguish from the allergic gastroenteropathy described by Waldman et al.[4] However, at least 50 percent of patients with EG have no personal or family history of atopy, and often dietary restriction does not cause resolution of symptoms.[5-8] Furthermore, allergic gastroenteropathy is characterized by mucosal injury (partial or subtotal villous atrophy) rather than tissue eosinophilia.[9-13]

Epidemiology

EG is rare, with a peak incidence in the second and third decades.[14] Katz et al described 12 children with GI symptoms and blood and tissue eosinophilia.[7] These patients could be divided into two groups, those with milk-sensitive enteropathy and those with EG. The first group, infants with allergic histories who developed GI symptoms at about 5 months of age and improved with milk elimination, had IgG milk antibodies but not raised total IgE or IgE milk antibodies. The second group was older, averaging 4 years of age, with chronic symptoms including growth failure that did not respond to dietary manipulation. These children had signs of systemic allergy (asthma, rhinitis, urticaria) and elevated serum total IgE and IgE milk-specific antibodies. Intermittent use of corticosteroids was necessary to control the disease in the latter group. Others have noted that EG affects school-aged children (6 to 14 years) more frequently than infants and young children.[8,15]

Eosinophilic infiltration of the mucosa is associated with abdominal pain, peripheral edema resulting from protein-losing enteropathy, and hematochezia when the colon is diseased.[3-4,7-8,14-17] Several reports of EG in children have observed that the small bowel, especially the jejunum, is the most commonly involved site.[8,15] In children, inflammation of the submucosa and muscularis may be prominent, especially in the antral region, and frequently causes obstructive symptoms.[8,15] Serosal infiltration is the least common form and may be accompanied by eosinophilic ascites.[15,18]

Formula or food intolerance, especially to cow's milk protein,[4,19-20] soy protein,[9] or beef,[5] may be associated with eosinophilic infiltration of the mucosa. Even breast-milk colitis may be associated with increased eosinophils in the rectal biopsies.[21-22] Infectious agents such as *Giardia lamblia*, the roundworm *Eustoma rotundatum*, and cytomegalovirus have been implicated as possible agents that trigger an eosinophilic response, although further substantiation of this area is needed.[8,23] Oral medications such as gold have been observed to cause EG.[24]

Pathogenesis

The etiologic basis of EG is unknown. The prevalence of allergic histories varies widely in different series, from nil to greater than 70 percent.[4,6-8,23] Although food sensitivity may play a role in some patients, the inciting factor is undetermined in most.

Total IgE has been reported to be elevated in some patients and normal in others.[6-8,18,25-26] Serum immunoglobulin E (IgE) levels demonstrate variable responses to food challenge, suggesting that both IgE-mediated and IgE-independent mechanisms may be important in different patients with EG.[6-7] Caldwell et al noted that jejunal biopsy specimens from allergic patients with EG had increased IgE immunofluorescence, whereas nonallergic patients had increased IgA and IgM.[6]

Instillation into the jejunum of foods thought to provoke symptoms in specific patients has caused tissue eosinophilia in some[3,27] but not in others.[3,5] When specific food intolerances are identified, peripheral blood and tissue eosinophilia and elevated serum IgE may resolve with elimination of the offending dietary substance.[4,7] In most instances, management requires corticosteroids.[2-3,6-7,14-16,18,19] Some authors have reported beneficial results with disodium cromoglycate,[8,24] whereas others have observed no improvement in clinical symptoms with this medication.[25,26]

Clinical Manifestations

Gastrointestinal Symptoms. The most common GI symptoms of EG are vomiting (50 percent), abdominal pain (40 percent), and growth failure (35 to 100 percent). Gastroduodenal or small bowel edema and cellular infiltration of the submucosa and muscularis may cause obstructive symptoms. When the appendiceal wall is diffusely infiltrated with eosinophils, symptoms resemble those of acute appendicitis.[28] Rare GI complications include ileal perforation and colonic stricture.[15] Diarrhea may be associated with rectal bleeding

(23 percent), especially in infants.[7-8,15-18] Ascites containing large numbers of eosinophils accompanies serosal inflammation. Circumscribed polypoid lesions with heavy eosinophilic inflammation in the antrum or small intestine also may cause obstructive symptoms or intussusception.[15]

Peripheral Edema. Edema of the extremities and periorbital regions may develop in children with EG and hypoproteinemia. Hypoalbuminemia, present in 33 to 100 percent of children, results from protein-losing enteropathy.[4,7-8,16]

Laboratory Findings. Peripheral blood eosinophilia occurs in 70 to 100 percent of children with EG.[4,7-8,16-19] Increased bone marrow precursors may be observed in the absence of increased circulating eosinophils.[8] Elevated serum food-specific IgE antibodies occur in some patients, although their specificity and meaning are uncertain.[7,25] Iron deficiency is common, especially in children with enteric blood loss.[4,6,8] Intestinal absorptive function as assessed by D-xylose excretion and fecal fat determinations in a few pediatric patients has been normal.[4,6]

Diagnosis

The diagnosis of EG is strongly suggested when the characteristic symptoms are accompanied by blood eosinophilia. Further supportive evidence may come from a careful dietary history that elicits a temporal relationship between ingestion of specific foods and the onset of symptoms.

Total serum protein and albumin and circulating IgE levels should be measured. Specific food-related IgE antibodies may be helpful in some patients but are often not found even in cases of documented reactions to specific foods, especially cow's milk protein.

Radiographic studies may demonstrate narrowing and nodularity of the antrum and/or duodenum or thickened mucosal folds in the small bowel. Intestinal dilatation and flocculation of barium occur in some cases.

Endoscopic examination of the stomach and duodenum is often contributory, since it may show nodularity, erythema, friability, erosions, and ulceration in affected areas.[3,8,16,28] Decreased vascular pattern, friability, and erosions have also been observed in EG involving the colon.[8]

Proof of diagnosis depends on finding excessive eosinophils in biopsy or resected tissue specimens, assuming that other causes of eosinophilic infiltrates such as lymphoma, Crohn's disease, parasitism, vasculitis (especially polyarteritis nodosa), chronic granulomatous disease, and the hypereosinophilic disorder, Job's syndrome, have been excluded. Hoefer et al noted that lymphadenopathy and inflammation of the omentum and mesentery may be present in EG, but isolated ileal involvement and "fat-wrapping" (characteristic of Crohn's disease) are absent.[15] Gastric biopsies may demonstrate EG more consistently than intestinal biopsies, because the intensity of the latter infiltrate varies even within the same individual.[7]

Management

When specific foods provoke the characteristic symptoms, dietary elimination may resolve GI symptoms and the associated blood and tissue eosinophilia.[4,7] When symptoms persist, corticosteroids (1.0 to 2.0 mg per kilogram per day) and possibly oral disodium cromoglycate (20 to 50 mg four times daily) control symptoms in most children,[4,7-8,18,26] but some relapse when these medications are discontinued. Low dose (5 to 10 mg) or alternate-day corticosteroids are needed in some cases for long-term control.[7-8,18]

Occasionally bowel resection or gastroenterostomy has been performed in children with gastric outlet or small bowel obstruction,[3,8,15,26-28] but most of these complications were reported prior to the use of corticosteroid therapy.[15]

HEMOLYTIC UREMIC SYNDROME

The hemolytic uremic syndrome (HUS), first described by Gasser et al in 1955,[29] is defined as the development of microangiopathic hemolytic anemia, thrombocytopenia, and renal insufficiency in a previously healthy person. Now several forms of this syndrome, varying in their etiology, age at diagnosis, and prognosis, are recognized.[30-33] A prodrome of GI symptoms averaging 3 to 16 days precedes the development of the HUS in 90 to 100 percent of children.[34-36]

Epidemiology

Characteristically, the HUS occurs in children less than 5 years of age.[34-36] It is endemic in Argentina, southern Africa, and the western United States, and epidemics have occurred in many other parts of the world. Tarr and Hickman observed a fourfold increase in incidence in King County, Washington, from 0.63 to 2.81 cases per 100,000 children younger than 15 years between 1971 and 1980.[36]

An epidemic form occurring in the summer, associated with the abrupt onset of diarrhea,[34,36] has a good prognosis, with an expected mortality under 6 percent.[36] A sporadic form in older children has neither seasonal influence nor obvious prodrome and has a higher mortality.[33] Siblings who develop HUS during infancy more than one year apart are thought to have an autosomal recessive trait that predisposes them to HUS and a mortality rate of 68 percent.[30-32]

Enteric infections with various organisms have been associated with the development of HUS. These include *Shigella, Salmonella, Campylobacter, Yersinia*, and enteroviruses.[34,37]

Recent evidence shows that most cases of HUS in the Pacific Northwest (58 percent) were preceded by enteric infection with *Escherichia coli* 0157:H7.[38] Over a 2-year period, the organism was isolated from stools of nine patients with HUS in British Columbia's Children's Hospital, an incidence far in excess of the incidence in all stools submitted for routine diagnosis, 1.9 percent.[39] This 0157:H7 serotype was originally described as a cause of hemorrhagic colitis.[40] Subsequently, isolated cases of HUS were reported following outbreaks of gastroenteritis (both bloody and nonbloody) with *E. coli* 0157:H7.[38,41] All isolates of this serotype produce a toxin cytotoxic for Vero and HeLa cells in tissue culture (verotoxin) and have been sensitive to ampicillin and amoxicillin.[39] Some studies have shown a similarity of this toxin to Shiga toxin. Dissemination of the organism has been reported to occur through contaminated food (hamburger) as well as via person-to-person spread in a daycare center.[38] Thus, *E. coli* 0157:H7 appears to cause a spectrum of disease including diarrhea, hemorrhagic colitis, and HUS. The factors that determine which disease entity develops in an individual child are unknown, but geographic and genetic influences have been suggested.

Pathogenesis

The central lesion in HUS is vascular endothelial damage. Endothelial cells show swelling and separation from the basement membrane with widening of the subendothelial space.[42] Glomerular involvement occurs in the classic form in young children, whereas arteriolar lesions with intimal and subintimal edema, proliferation, and necrosis are more common in older children.[33,42]

The precipitating cause of this vascular injury is unknown. There may be a relationship between the verotoxin produced by *E. coli* 0157:H7 in epidemic HUS and endothelial damage.[38-41] Alternatively, perturbations in endothelial prostacyclin metabolism are postulated to be important in sporadic HUS.[42] Prostacyclin (PGI_2), a potent inhibitor of platelet aggregation, is normally produced in endothelial cells, and studies have suggested that PGI_2 deficiency, the presence of an inhibitor of PGI_2 production, or rapid degradation of PGI_2 occurs in patients with HUS.[42]

The vascular injury induces microangiopathic hemolytic anemia, thrombocytopenia, and local deposits of fibrin microthrombi. Ischemic changes result in focal or generalized renal cortical necrosis as well as damage to other organs (colon, liver, myocardium, brain, and adrenals).[42,43]

Clinical Manifestations

Gastrointestinal Signs. GI disease occurs in 90 to 100 percent of children with HUS. In most instances (70 to 80 percent), bloody diarrhea precedes the recognition of HUS by 3 to 16 days.[34-36] Other children have a prodrome of abdominal pain, nonbloody diarrhea, and/or vomiting. Resolution of the GI symptoms usually begins prior to the onset of renal insufficiency, with hematochezia clearing first, followed by improvement in the diarrhea and abdominal pain. Occasional patients have thrombosis of vessels in the muscularis and serosa, resulting in necrosis and perforation of the colon.[44]

Sigmoidoscopic appearance is characterized by hyperemia, edema, and petechiae, sometimes in association with ulceration.[44,45] Berman reported that the gross endoscopic appearance was indistinguishable from that of chronic nonspecific ulcerative colitis.[45] However, rectal biopsies in these children showed only edema and submucosal hemorrhage with scant inflammation.

Barium enema examinations may demonstrate focal or diffuse bowel wall edema, thumbprinting, filling defects, mucosal irregularity, fine marginal spiculations, colonic spasm, or colonic dilatation (Fig. 1).[44,45] Initially the findings may mimic chronic inflammatory bowel disease until the full syndrome becomes apparent.

Hemolytic Anemia. Microangiopathic hemolytic anemia with fragmented erythrocytes is present on peripheral blood

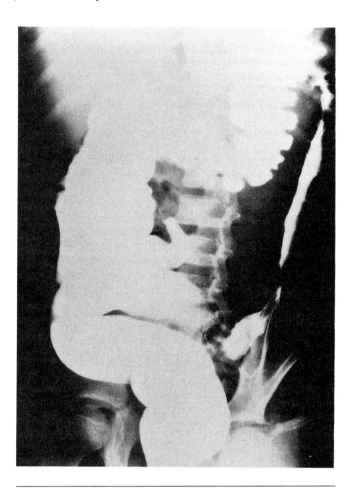

FIGURE 1 Barium enema in a 6-year-old child with hemolytic uremic syndrome. Extensive spasm and narrowing of the descending colon are illustrated during the period of bloody diarrhea. Gastrointestinal symptoms resolved 1 week later but were followed by the onset of acute renal failure.

smears in all children with HUS. It usually occurs suddenly within 1 to 2 days, resulting in a mean hemoglobin concentration of 6.1 g per deciliter.[35] Transfusions are required in 64 percent of children.

Thrombocytopenia. Thrombocytopenia (platelet count under 150,000 per cubic millimeter) occurs in 92 percent of children with HUS. As mentioned above, platelet aggregation defects may occur in the presence of normal platelet counts. Other tests of coagulation status, including prothrombin time and partial thromboplastin time, are normal.[34,35,42]

Renal Insufficiency. Although all children with HUS are azotemic (mean peak blood urea nitrogen of 95 mg per deciliter), the severity of the renal impairment is variable. Oliguria (less than 15 ml urine per kilogram body weight per day) and anuria (less than 25 ml urine per day) each occur in 32 percent of affected children.[35] One-third of children have no documented oliguria. Resulting hypertension may require peritoneal dialysis or may resolve following spontaneous diuresis. Recovery time for normalization of creatinine clearance averages 3.7 months and corresponds to the duration of the preceding oliguria. Chronic renal insufficiency persists in approximately 9.5 percent of children.[35]

Liver Disease. Elevations of hepatic enzymes (two- to 20-fold above normal) for serum glutamic-oxaloacetic transaminase (SGOT), serum glutamic-pyruvic transaminase (SGPT), gamma-glutamyl transpeptidase (GGTP), alkaline phosphatase, and 5' nucleotidase have been observed in most patients in whom these tests were done.[44,46] The transient hepatocellular injury may be caused by focal hepatic hypoxia.

Diagnosis

HUS in childhood usually occurs in a previously healthy child who develops diarrhea (generally bloody) and abdominal pain followed by the acute onset of hemolytic anemia, thrombocytopenia, and renal insufficiency. Initially, the gastrointestinal manifestations may be mimicked by intussusception, enteric infection, or inflammatory bowel disease (especially ulcerative colitis), which can be excluded by appropriate radiologic, bacteriologic, and histologic studies. Stool specimens should be obtained for enteric pathogens, including *E. coli* 0157:H7. This serotype metabolizes sorbitol slowly; therefore, *E. coli* strains with this characteristic can be sent to state laboratories for confirmation. Hematologic and renal findings are discussed above.

Treatment

Severe GI symptoms require hospitalization and intravenous fluids during the prodromal period prior to the development of the HUS. Since *E. coli* 0157:H7 is sensitive to ampicillin and amoxicillin, some authors suggest treating all cases with one of these antibiotics.[39] Butler et al observed that the administration of ampicillin to children with ampicillin-resistant strains of *Shigella dysenteriae I* was associated with a greater incidence of HUS than occurred in non–antibiotic treated children infected with the same organism. They also postulated that the risk of HUS might be reduced if children were treated early with appropriate antibiotics.[47] Recently, Tarr et al cautioned against the empiric use of antibiotics for *E. coli* 0157:H7 colitis until the risks and benefits have been analyzed by controlled clinical trials.[48] These authors expressed concern that the incidence of HUS might be increased through proliferation of *E. coli* 0157:H7, or the release of cytotoxins through bacterial lysis or "sublethal damage." Rarely, surgical intervention may be necessitated by bowel necrosis.[44]

The primary therapy is directed toward the renal insufficiency, hypertension, fluid balance, and hemolytic anemia. Peritoneal dialysis is employed as necessary.[34,35,49]

There is no direct evidence that anticoagulant therapy is beneficial.[32,50] Plasma transfusions, plasmapheresis, or exchange transfusion has been reported to improve the anemia, thrombocytopenia, and renal insufficiency in some children with HUS and may be considered in patients demonstrating a poor response to supportive therapy.[49-51] Prostacyclin levels that were low prior to plasma therapy become normal following the plasmapheresis.[52] The possible future role of antitoxin directed against the verotoxin remains to be investigated.[33]

HENOCH-SCHÖNLEIN PURPURA

Henoch-Schönlein purpura (HSP), a multisystem vasculitic disorder, primarily affects children under 7 years of age. Schönlein described an association of arthritis with purpura in 1837.[53] The clinical syndrome, subsequently extended to include abdominal pain and GI bleeding by Henoch in 1874,[54] is characterized by urticarial or purpuric skin lesions, colicky abdominal pain, sometimes with hematochezia, and arthralgias or arthritis and hematuria, which may be accompanied by proteinuria. Symptoms persist for an average of 3.9 weeks, although recurrences are common, occurring in 40 percent of patients.[55]

Epidemiology

In a review of 131 children with HSP, more than 75 percent were less than 7 years of age.[55] Seasonal variation was noted, with one-third of cases occurring during the spring. An upper respiratory infection or fever occurred within 1 to 3 weeks prior to the development of symptoms of HSP in 90 percent of children. Recently, a cluster of 20 cases was identified in Connecticut, of whom 10 were from Hartford County,[56] but no etiologic agent has been identified. Although the disorder has been known as anaphylactoid purpura, family and personal allergic histories do not appear to be more frequent than expected for a comparable age group.[55]

Pathogenesis

The cause of HSP is unknown: clinical observations suggest that infectious agents (including beta-hemolytic streptococci, varicella, and other viruses and mycoplasma) or medications (particularly penicillins) may trigger an immune response, leading to IgA immune complex deposition in blood vessel walls in susceptible hosts.[55-57] Activation of the alternate complement pathway may generate chemotactic factors and polymorphonuclear infiltration.[57]

Microscopic findings show perivascular infiltrates of polymorphonuclear leukocytes, lymphocytes, and occasional histiocytes around small blood vessels in the skin and GI tract, as well as IgA deposits in capillary walls and the dermal-epidermal junction. Intimal proliferation and thrombosis have been described in cerebral vessels in children with seizures.[55] Vasculitis results in edema and hemorrhage in various organs, including the intestine, pancreas, gallbladder, lung, myocardium, testis, and cerebral cortex.[55,58-62] In glomeruli there are diffuse polymorphonuclear infiltrates or hyalinization with thickening of the basement membrane of Bowman's capsule.

Clinical Manifestations

Skin Involvement. Skin lesions occur in 97 to 100 percent of children with HSP.[55,63] The initial rash usually is an urticarial eruption on the extensor surfaces of the legs, buttocks, and arms, which changes to red, nonblanching macules. Children under 2 years of age may present with scalp, facial, or extremity edema, while older children often show petechiae, especially on the lower extremities. Edema of the lower extremities is more common in children less than 3 years of age and is often seen in combination with facial or scalp swellings.

Gastrointestinal Involvement. GI symptoms are common, occurring in 65 to 90 percent of children.[55,63,64] Colicky abdominal pain, often associated with vomiting, results from submucosal edema and hemorrhage. Abdominal pain develops within 8 days of the rash in 75 percent of pediatric patients, although intervals as long as 150 days between GI symptoms and skin findings have been observed.[63] Hypoproteinemia may develop secondary to protein-losing enteropathy. Obvious GI bleeding (melena or hematochezia) occurs in 25 percent of children and hematemesis in approximately 10 percent. Children with abdominal pain frequently show tenderness to direct palpation (75 percent), but rebound tenderness is uncommon (9 percent).[63] Stools are guaiac-positive in 50 percent of children. Rare intestinal complications include intussusception (2 to 3 percent), perforation, pancreatitis, and cholecystitis.[55,58-62] When intussusception develops, it is seen in children 5 to 7 years of age; early surgical intervention markedly reduces mortality.[55,64,65] In one series of children who underwent exploratory laparotomy, excessive amounts of peritoneal fluid were observed.[58] Rarely, small bowel obstruction may develop from late-onset stricture formation.[66] Relapses of GI symptoms have been reported 7 years after the initial episode.[60]

Endoscopic examination may demonstrate coalescing purpuric lesions, especially in the descending duodenum, gastritis, or punctate erythematous and ulcerative changes in the colon.[65,67] Tomomasa et al described endoscopic findings in nine children with HSP.[67] No esophageal abnormalities were observed. Gastric changes in two children consisted of diffuse mucosal edema, patchy erythema, and multiple erosions. Diffuse severe erythema with erosions was noted in the duodenal bulb (two patients) and the second portion of the duodenum (three children). Rectosigmoid examination in six children demonstrated shallow ulcers in two, but studies were normal in the other four. Endoscopic biopsies revealed polymorphonuclear infiltrates in the lamina propria, predominantly around blood vessels.

Radiologic studies of the small bowel and colon show "thumbprinting" (Fig. 2), representing submucosal edema and hemorrhage, spasm, ulceration, and pseudotumor,[59] usually in the jejunum and ileum (Fig. 3), but the colon may be affected. Similar findings are seen in lymphoproliferative disorders, other hemorrhagic conditions (hemophilia, leukemia), scleroderma, and Crohn's disease.[59]

Joint Involvement. Arthritis and arthralgias, usually oligoarticular (93 percent) and nonmigratory, occur in 65 percent of children with HSP.[63] Ankles and knees are involved more than the upper extremities.

Renal Manifestations. Hematuria (gross or microscopic) seen in approximately 40 percent of all children with HSP,[55] is reported in 70 percent of children with GI disease.[64] Two-thirds of children with hematuria also develop proteinuria. Renal lesions are more frequent in older children than in those

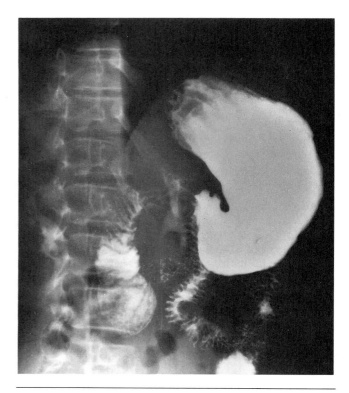

FIGURE 2 Upper gastrointestinal series demonstrating thickened folds and "thumbprinting" due to submucosal edema of the proximal jejunum in a 14-year-old girl with recurrent episodes of colicky abdominal pain.

less than 2 years of age and usually follow skin and GI involvement.[55] Serious complications include hypertension (sometimes leading to hypertensive encephalopathy) and renal failure. Glomerular lesions include glomerular proliferation, hyalinization, and IgA deposits in the mesangium. Autopsy studies of the kidneys demonstrate endothelial thickening, thrombosis, and medial necrosis of small renal arteries. In Europe HSP accounts for 15 percent of children receiving dialysis for renal failure.[68]

Diagnosis

The diagnosis of HSP rests on the presence of characteristic clinical features with supporting laboratory, endoscopic, and radiologic studies as indicated. Peripheral blood counts show leukocytosis (10,000 to 20,000 per cubic millimeter) with left shift in one-half of the children. Erythrocyte sedimentation is elevated (greater than 20 mm per hour) in 75 percent of children. Urinalyses may not demonstrate hematuria or proteinuria until several weeks after the initial presentation. The presence of microscopic blood should be checked in stool specimens. Endoscopic and radiologic studies may be helpful in equivocal cases, as seen when abdominal pain develops prior to skin or renal involvement.

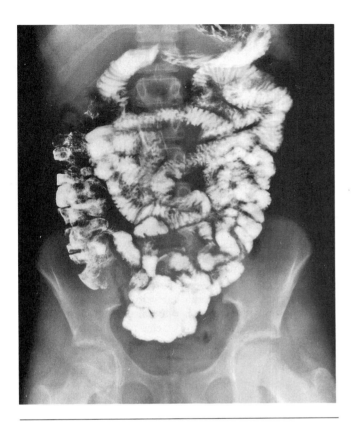

FIGURE 3 Upper gastrointestinal and small bowel follow-through demonstrating extensive thickening of mucosal folds in the descending duodenum and entire jejunum in a 10-year-old boy with recurrent vomiting and scattered skin lesions on the buttocks and lower extremities.

Management

Therapeutic intervention for HSP is directed usually at specific complications, such as severe abdominal pain, hypertension, renal insufficiency, and GI or cerebral hemorrhage. The efficacy of many recommended medical approaches has not been studied in controlled clinical trials.

Gastrointestinal Disease. Children with severe abdominal pain should be admitted to the hospital because of the potential risk of intussusception, hemorrhage, or perforation. Supportive care with intravenous fluids and nasogastric suction is helpful in comforting severely symptomatic children. The role of corticosteroid medications in treating the GI manifestations of HSP is controversial. Allen had the impression that abdominal pain resolved in the majority of children following steroid therapy (50 percent within 72 hours).[55] Tapering these medications was followed in some patients by clinical relapse that improved with reinstitution of steroids. Furthermore, no intussusception occurred in the steroid-treated patients. Rosenblum and Winter retrospectively compared the hospital course of 48 children with HSP, 58 percent of whom were treated with prednisone (1 to 2 mg per kilogram per day) and 42 percent of whom did not receive corticosteroids.[63] Abdominal pain resolved within 24 hours

in 44 percent of the steroid-treated group but in only 14 percent of the non–steroid-treated group. At 48 hours, resolution was 65 percent in the steroid and 45 percent in the other group, although this difference was not statistically different. By 72 hours after admission, resolution of pain was similar in both groups (75 percent). The report concluded that corticosteroid administration may hasten resolution of abdominal pain but that controlled trials should be undertaken. Relapse is frequent in HSP, with 40 percent of children developing symptoms as late as 7 years after the initial episode.[55,60]

Surgical treatment is required rarely for massive gastric hemorrhage, intussusception, intestinal perforation, or cholecystitis.[55,58,60,62] Careful and repeated physical examinations are necessary to identify early signs of these complications.

Renal Disease. The management of the renal complications of HSP will not be discussed, but clearly, blood pressure and renal output must be carefully monitored. Urine samples should be analyzed regularly for hematuria and proteinuria. Antihypertensive medications, fluid restriction, and dialysis may be necessary. Corticosteroids do not affect the course of renal disease, although immunosuppressive medications have improved renal function in some patients.[69]

BEHÇET'S DISEASE

Behçet's disease is a multisystem vasculitic disorder reported first in 1937.[70] The original description included aphthous stomatitis, genital ulcers, and uveitis. Since there are no pathologic or laboratory findings that definitively establish the diagnosis, several clinical criteria have been proposed.[71,72] Although the disease affects predominantly young adults in Japan, the Mediterranean region, and the Middle East, pediatric cases have been described.[73-75] Genetic predisposition is suggested by the observation that specific histocompatibility haplotypes predominate in some forms of the disease, but these are not found in all population groups.[76] Immunologic processes are thought to be causally related to the vasculitis, and thus current forms of therapy utilize immunosuppressive medications. The clinical presentation of Behçet's disease may closely resemble Crohn's disease, but the presence of genital ulcers, very severe oral ulceration, and neurologic complications aids in differentiating the two conditions.[75,77]

Epidemiologic Aspects

The prevalence of Behçet's disease varies greatly among different countries. It is most common in Japan (10 per 100,000) compared with England (0.6 per 100,000) and the United States (0.3 per 100,000).[72] The incidence appears to have increased between 1958 and 1977 in Japan. Presentation prior to the onset of puberty is unusual.[78] In one series of 297 patients, only 34 had symptoms prior to 19 years of age, with the youngest being 13 years old.[78] Recently, Ammann et al described six children whose onset of symptoms of Behçet's disease began at 2 months to 11 years of age.[74] While the majority of adult patients are male (70 percent), half of the pediatric patients are female.[74,75]

Familial cases are uncommon, but isolated instances involving parents with affected children have been described.[79] A transient form of Behçet's disease may occur in neonates born to mothers with the disease.[80]

Pathogenesis

The cause of Behçet's disease is unknown, although several areas of research suggest that immunologic and genetic factors contribute to the development of this disorder.[81] In addition, some authors have suggested that infection with herpes simplex virus type I may be etiologically important.

The primary histopathologic lesion consists of vasculitis that affects predominantly small vessels. Initially, there is endothelial proliferation and infiltration with mononuclear cells, which is followed by a polymorphonuclear response. The same vascular lesion may occur in large veins and cause thrombophlebitis as well as in large arteries, leading to gangrene or aneurysm formation. Studies have shown deposition of C3 and C9 in blood vessel walls and circulating immune complexes in patients with Behçet's disease. In the newborn form, transient circulating IgG immune complexes and reduced total hemolytic complement were measured, suggesting transplacental passage of immune complexes or autoantibodies.[80]

Lehner et al observed that specific HLA haplotypes are associated with some forms of Behçet's disease.[76] When compared with controls, HLA-B5 occurs more frequently in patients with ocular involvement, HLA-B27 is increased in those with arthritic symptoms, and HLA-B12 correlates with mucocutaneous signs.

Clinical Manifestations

Several classifications have been proposed to define the diagnostic criteria for Behçet's disease.[71,72] These consider the major manifestations (buccal ulceration, genital ulceration, uveitis, and skin lesions) as well as less frequent signs (GI lesions, thrombophlebitis, arthritis, central nervous system lesions, and family history).

Oral Ulcers. Painful recurrent oral ulcers are the most common feature of Behçet's disease. They persist for 7 to 14 days, subside spontaneously, and recur several days to months later.[82] Since this finding may occur in up to 10 percent of the normal population, additional manifestations are necessary to establish the diagnosis of the disease.

Genital Ulcers. Ulcerations on the genitalia are reported in 93 to 98 percent of patients of patients with Behçet's disease.[75,82] Their gross appearance and clinical course are similar to those of the oral ulcers.

Skin Lesions. The cutaneous manifestations of Behçet's disease are varied and include folliculitis, erythema nodosum, acne, vesicles, pustules, and other nonspecific lesions.[82] The formation of a sterile pustule at the site of needle trauma (Behçetin reaction) occurs in some patients.

Ocular Involvement. The signs of ocular disease are iritis with hypopyon and posterior uveitis. Visual impairment is usually bilateral and may result in optic nerve atrophy, glaucoma, and cataracts. This manifestation is less common in Western countries than in Japan and Turkey, where it is a major cause of blindness. Approximately 21 percent of pediatric patients have ocular involvement.[75]

Gastrointestinal Disease. The frequency of GI involvement in patients with Behçet's disease varies widely in different series and perhaps in different regions. Yazici et al reported that no patient had GI signs of Behçet's disease in their review of 297 patients from Turkey.[78] Japanese authors have observed intestinal symptoms in at least 15 percent of patients with Behçet's disease.[83] The most frequent complaints are abdominal pain, vomiting, flatulence, diarrhea, and constipation. Radiologic examinations demonstrate thickened mucosal folds, pseudopolyps, deformity of bowel loops, ulcerations, and fistulae.[75] Ulcerations are localized or diffuse, with the majority (76 percent) occurring in the ileocecal region.[84] Extension to the serosal surface may result in perforation. Recurrence is often at the site of anastomosis, and 44 percent of surgically treated cases require reoperation.[84] Rare cases of esophageal involvement have been reported.

The differentiation of Behçet's disease from chronic nonspecific ulcerative colitis and especially Crohn's disease depends on the character of the intestinal endoscopic and radiologic findings as well as the associated extraintestinal manifestations. At times, establishing the correct diagnosis may be complicated by the presence of Behçet's disease and ulcerative colitis or Crohn's disease in the same family.[77] Baba et al noted that the ileocecal location and the depth of the ulcers in Behçet's disease distinguish this disease from chronic ulcerative colitis.[83] In comparison with Crohn's disease there was less inflammation in the area surrounding the ulcer, and granulomas were not seen.[83,84] Fistula formation has been reported in Behçet's disease.[75,82] Several authors have emphasized that the recurrent genital ulcers and central nervous system signs seen in Behçet's disease are rarely found in ulcerative colitis or Crohn's disease.[77]

Vascular Disease. The vasculitic process described above can affect both arterial and venous systems. Small vessel disease accounts for many systemic signs, but large vessel involvement may result in severe complications. Recurrent superficial thrombophlebitis, vena cava thrombosis, and arterial occlusions leading to infarction and hemorrhage from rupture of aneurysmal dilatations have been reported.

Arthritis. Chronic nonmigratory seronegative polyarthritis affecting the knees, ankles, elbows, and wrists occurs in up to 50 percent of patients with Behçet's disease. The course tends to be nondestructive with rare radiologic evidence of bone erosion, although synovial thickening and effusion may occur.[82]

Neurologic Manifestations. Neurologic involvement is reported in 1 to 20 percent of patients with Behçet's disease. Episodes may be transient or progressive and include pyramidal signs, organic confusional states leading to dementia, meningoencephalitis, cranial nerve palsies, pseudotumor cerebri, and seizures.[81] There may be mild pleocytosis with or without an elevation of protein in the cerebrospinal fluid.

Diagnosis

There are no pathognomonic features of Behçet's disease, so the diagnosis depends upon the presence of characteristic clinical findings. The Mason and Barnes criteria described in 1969 require three major and two minor criteria (described above under Clinical Manifestations).[71] O'Duffy subsequently proposed that the diagnosis be based upon the presence of three of the following: recurrent oral ulcers, recurrent genital ulcers, uveitis, cutaneous vasculitis, synovitis, meningocephalitis, and cutaneous hyperreactivity to minor trauma.[72]

Management

Corticosteroid medications form the mainstay of treatment for Behçet's disease.[85] Relief of symptoms initially occurs in most patients, but recurrences are common. Local preparations are usually effective for genital ulcers, while oral or intravenous administration is required for uveitis, intestinal lesions, and neurologic manifestations. Immunosuppressive agents such as azathioprine, chlorambucil (combined with prednisone, 1.0 mg per kilogram per day), or cyclosporine (10 mg per kilogram per day) have been effective in patients with severe disease who did not respond to steroids or who required reduction in steroid dosage.[85,86] Two children with oral, genital, and intestinal ulceration that did not improve with steroid therapy achieved long-term control following treatment with chlorambucil.[74] Short-term improvement in GI symptoms was observed in a child treated with colchicine.[75]

Intestinal resection may be necessary for complications of intestinal disease, such as hemorrhage or perforation. Several groups observed that perforations are often multiple and more likely to occur in Behçet's disease than in Crohn's disease, presumably because the deep ulcers in Behçet's disease are surrounded by less inflammation and bowel wall thickening.[83,84]

REFERENCES

1. Kaijser R. Sur Kerintnis der allergischen affectionen des Verdauungs-Kanals von standprunkt des chirugen aus. Arch Klin Chirurg 1937; 188:36–64.
2. Ureles Al, Alschibaja T, Lodico D, Stabins SJ. Idiopathic eosinophilic infiltration of the gastrointestinal tract, diffuse and circumscribed. A proposed classification and review of the literature, with two additional cases. Am J Med 1961; 30:899–909.
3. Klein NC, Hargrove RL, Sleisinger MH, Jeffries GH. Eosinophilic gastroenteritis. Medicine 1970; 49:299–319.
4. Waldman TA, Wochner RD, Laster L, Gordon RS Jr. Allergic gastroenteropathy—a cause of excessive gastrointestinal protein loss. N Engl J Med 1967; 276:761–769.
5. Leinbach GE, Rubin CE. Eosinophilic gastroenteritis: a simple reaction to food antigens? Gastroenterology 1970; 59:874–889.
6. Caldwell JH, Sharma HM, Hurtubise PE, Colwell DL. Eosinophilic gastroenteritis in extreme allergy—immunopathological comparison with nonallergic gastrointestinal disease. Gastroenterology 1979; 77:560–564.
7. Katz AJ, Twarog FJ, Zeiger RS, Falchuk ZM. Milk-sensitive and eosinophilic gastroenteropathy: similar clinical features with contrasting mechanisms and clinical course. J Allergy Clin Immunol 1984; 74:72–78.
8. Whitington PF, Whitington GL. Eosinophilic gastroenteropathy in childhood. J Pediatr Gastroenterol Nutr 1988; 7:379–385.
9. Ament ME, Rubin CE. Soy protein—another cause of the flat intestinal lesion. Gastroenterology 1972; 62:227–234.
10. Fontaine JL, Navarro J. Small intestinal biopsy in cow's milk protein allergy. Arch Dis Child 1975; 50:357–362.
11. Perkkio M, Savilahti E, Kuitunen P. Morphometric and immunohistochemical study of jejunal biopsies from children with intestinal soy allergy. Eur J Pediatr 1981; 137:63–69.
12. Iyngkaran N, Abidin Z, Meng LL, Yadav M. Egg-protein-induced villous atrophy. J Pediatr Gastroenterol Nutr 1982; 1:29–33.
13. Maluenda C, Phillips AD, Briddon A, Walker-Smith JA. Quantitative analysis of small intestinal mucosa in cow's milk–sensitive enteropathy. J Pediatr Gastroenterol Nutr 1984; 3:349–356.
14. Kaplan SM, Goldstein F, Kowlessar D. Eosinophilic gastroenteritis—report of a case with malabsorption and protein-losing enteropathy. Gastroenterology 1970; 58:540–545.
15. Hoefer RA, Ziegler MM, Koop CE, Schnaufer L. Surgical manifestations of eosinophilic gastroenteritis in the pediatric patient. J Pediatr Surg 1977; 12:955–962.
16. Katz AJ, Goldman H, Grand RJ. Gastric mucosal biopsy in eosinophilic (allergic) gastroenteritis. Gastroenterology 1977; 73:705–709.
17. Sherman MP, Cox KL. Neonatal eosinophilic colitis. J Pediatr 1982; 100:587–588.
18. Trounce JQ, Tanner MS. Eosinophilic gastroenteritis. Arch Dis Child 1985; 60:1186–1188.
19. Kosnai I, Kuitanen P, Savilahti E, Sipponen P. Mast cells and eosinophils in the jejunal mucosa of patients with intestinal cow's milk allergy and celiac disease of childhood. J Pediatr Gastroenterol Nutr 1984; 3:368–372.
20. Shiner M, Ballard J, Smith ME. The small-intestinal mucosa in cow's milk allergy. Lancet 1975; i:136–140.
21. Lake AH, Whitington PF, Hamilton SR. Dietary protein–induced colitis in breast-fed infants. J Pediatr 1982; 101:906–910.
22. Lifschitz CH, Hawkins HK, Guerra C, Byrd N. Anaphylactic shock due to cow's milk protein hypersensitivity in a breast-fed infant. J Pediatr Gastroenterol Nutr 1988; 7:141–144.
23. Blackshaw AJ, Levinson DA. Eosinophilic infiltrates of the gastrointestinal tract. J Clin Pathol 1986; 39:1–7.
24. Martin DM, Goldman JA, Gilliam J, Nasrallah SM. Gold-induced eosinophilic enterocolitis: response to oral cromolyn sodium. Gastroenterology 1981; 80:1567–1570.
25. Elkon KB, Sher R, Seftel HC. Immunological studies of eosinophilic gastro-enteritis and treatment with disodium cromoglycate and beclomethasone dipropionate. S Afr Med J 1977; 52:838–841.
26. Colon AR, Soekin LF, Stern WR, Lessinger VS, Hefter LG, Hodin E. Eosinophilic gastroenteritis. J Pediatr Gastroenterol Nutr 1983; 2:187–189.
27. Greenberger NJ, Tannenbaum JI, Ruppert RD. Protein losing enteropathy associated with gastrointestinal allergy. Am J Med 1967; 43:777–784.
28. Jona JZ, Belin RP, Burke JA. Eosinophilic infiltration of the gastrointestinal tract in children. Am J Dis Child 1976; 130:1136–1139.
29. Gasser CE, Gautier E, Steck A, Sibernmann RE, Ochslin R. Hamolytischuramisches Syndrome: bilaterale Nierenrindennekrosen bei akuten erworbenen hamolytischen Anemien. Schweiz Med Wochenschr 1955; 85:905–909.
30. Kaplan BS, Chesney RW, Drummond KN. Hemolytic uremic syndrome in families. N Engl J Med 1975; 292:1090–1093.
31. Kaplan BS, Drummond KN. The hemolytic-uremic syndrome is a syndrome. N Engl J Med 1978; 298:964–966.
32. Feldhoff C, Pistor K, Bachmann H, Horacek U, Olbing H. Hemolytic uremic syndrome in 3 siblings. Nephrol Clin 1984; 22:44–46.
33. Drummond KN. Hemolytic uremic syndrome—then and now. N Engl J Med 1985; 312:116–118.
34. Lieberman E. Hemolytic-uremic syndrome. J Pediatr 1972; 80:1–16.
35. Tune BH, Leavitt TJ, Gribble TJ. A hemolytic-uremic syndrome in California: a review of 28 nonheparinized cases with long-term follow-up. J Pediatr 1973; 82:304–310.
36. Tarr PI, Hickman RO. Hemolytic uremic syndrome epidemiology: a population-based study in King County, Washington, 1971 to 1980. Pediatrics 1987; 80:41–45.
37. Koster F, Levin J, Walker L, Tung KSK, Gilman RH, Rahaman MM, Hajid A, Islam S, Williams RC. Hemolytic-uremic syndrome after shigellosis. Relation to endotoxemia and circulating immune complexes. N Engl J Med 1978; 298:927–933.

38. Neill MA, Tarr PI, Clausen CR, Christie DL, Hickman RO. *Escherichia coli* 0157:H7 as a predominant pathogen associated with the hemolytic uremic syndrome: a prospective study in the Pacific Northwest. Pediatrics 1987; 80:37-40.

39. Gransden WR, Damm S, Anderson JD, Carter JE, Lion H. Further evidence associating hemolytic uremic syndrome with infection by verotoxin-producing *Escherichia coli* 0157:H7. J Infect Dis 1986; 154:522-524.

40. Karmali MA, Petric M, Lim C, Fleming PC, Steele BT. *Escherichia coli* cytotoxin, haemolytic-uremic syndrome, and haemorrhagic colitis. Lancet 1983; ii:1299-1300.

41. Spika JS, Parsons JE, Nordenberg D, Wells JG, Gunn RA, Blake PA. Hemolytic uremic syndrome and diarrhea associated with *Escherichia coli* 0157:H7 in a day care center. J Pediatr 1986; 109:287-291.

42. Levin M, Barratt TM. Haemolytic uraemic syndrome. Arch Dis Child 1984; 59:397-400.

43. Upaphyaya K, Barwick K, Fishaut M, Kasqarian M, Siegel NJ. The importance of non-renal involvement in hemolytic-uremic syndrome. Pediatrics 1980; 65:115-120.

44. Whitington PF, Friedman AL, Chesney RW. Gastrointestinal disease in the hemolytic-uremic syndrome. Gastroenterology 1979; 76:728-733.

45. Berman W Jr. The hemolytic-uremic syndrome: initial clinical presentation mimicking ulcerative colitis. J Pediatr 1972; 81:275-278.

46. Van Rhijn A, Donckerwolcke, Kuijten RH, Van der Heiden C. Liver damage in the hemolytic uremic syndrome. Helv Paediat Acta 1977; 32:77-81.

47. Butler T, Islam MR, Azad MAK, Jones PA. Risk factors for development of hemolytic uremic syndrome during shigellosis. J Pediatr 1987; 110:894-897.

48. Tarr PI, Neill MA, Christie DL, Anderson DE. *Escherichia coli* 0157:H7 hemorrhagic colitis. N Engl J Med 1988; 318:1697.

49. Siegler RL. Management of hemolytic-uremic syndrome. J Pediatr 1988; 112:1014-1020.

50. Misani R, Appiani AC, Edefonti A, Gotti E, Bettinelli A, Giani M, Rossi E, Remuzzi G, Mecca G. Haemolytic uraemic syndrome: therapeutic effect of plasma infusion. Br Med J 1982; 285:1304-1306.

51. Rizzoni G, Claris-Appiani A, Edefonti A, Facchin P, Franchini F, Gusmano R, Imbasciati E, Paranello L, Perfumo F, Remuzzi G. Plasma infusion for hemolytic-uremic syndrome in children: results of a multicenter controlled trial. J Pediatr 1988; 112:284-290.

52. Gillor A, Bulla H, Roth B, Bussman K, Schror K, Tekook A, Gladtke E. Plasmapheresis as a therapeutic measure in hemolytic-uremic syndrome in children. Klin Wochenschr 1983; 61:363-367.

53. Schönlein JL. Allgemeine und specielle pathologie und Therapie, Vol 2. 3rd ed. Wurzburg: Herisau, 1837: 48.

54. Henoch EH. Veber ein eigenthumliche form von Purpura. Berl Klin Wochenschr 1874; 1:641-643.

55. Allen DM, Diamond LK, Howell DA. Anaphylactoid purpura in children (Schönlein-Henoch syndrome). Am J Dis Child 1960; 99:147-168.

56. Rasoulpour M, Cartter M, Tolentino N, Mshar P, Hadler JL. Henoch-Schönlein purpura—Connecticut. MMW 1988; 37:121-122.

57. Fauci AS, Haynes BF, Katz P. The spectrum of vasculitis. Clinical, pathologic, immunologic, and therapeutic consideration. Ann Intern Med 1978; 89:660-676.

58. Balf CL. The alimentary lesion in anaphylactoid purpura. Arch Dis Child 1951; 26:20-27.

59. Rodriquez-Erdmann F, Levitan R. Gastrointestinal and roentgenological manifestations of Henock-Schönlein purpura. Gastroenterology 1968; 54:260-264.

60. Scully RE, Galdabini JJ, McNeely BU. Clinicopathological exercises. N Engl J Med 1980; 302:853-858.

61. Branski D, Gross V, Gross-Kieselstein E, Roll D, Abrahamov A. Pancreatitis as a complication of Henoch-Schönlein purpura. J Pediatr Gastroenterol 1982; 1:275-276.

62. Clark JH, Fitzgerald JF. Hemorrhagic complications of Henoch-Schönlein syndrome. J Pediatr Gastroenterol Nutr 1985; 4:311-314.

63. Rosenblum ND, Winter HS. Steroid effects on the course of abdominal pain in children with Henoch-Schönlein purpura. Pediatrics 1987; 79:1018-1021.

64. Feldt RH, Stickler GB. The gastrointestinal manifestations of anaphylactoid purpura in children. Proc Staff Meet Mayo Clin 1962; 37:465-473.

65. Goldman LP, Lindenberg RL. Henoch-Schönlein purpura. Gastrointestinal manifestations with endoscopic correlation. Am J Gastroenterol 1981; 75:357-360.

66. Lombaard KA, Shah PC, Thrasher TV, Grill BB. Ileal stricture as a late complication of Henoch-Schönlein purpura. Pediatrics 1986; 77:396-398.

67. Tomomosa T, Hsa JY, Itoh K, Kuroume T. Endoscopic findings in pediatric patients with Henoch-Schönlein purpura and gastrointestinal symptoms. J Pediatr Gastroenterol Nutr 1987; 6:725-729.

68. Meadow R. Schönlein-Henoch syndrome. Arch Dis Child 1979; 54:822-824.

69. Goldbloom RB, Drummond KN. Anaphylactoid purpura with massive gastrointestinal hemorrhage and glomerulonephritis. An unusual case treated successfully with azathioprine and corticosteroids. Am J Dis Child 1968; 166:97-102.

70. Behçet H. Uber rezidivierende aphthose, durch ein Virus verursachte Geschwure am Mund, am Auge und an den Genitalien. Dermatol Wochenschr 1937; 105:1152-1157.

71. Mason RM, Barnes CG. Behçet's syndrome with arthritis. Ann Rheum Dis 1969; 28:95-102.

72. O'Duffy JD. Summary of international symposium on Behçet's disease. J Rheum 1978; 5:229-233.

73. Mundy TM, Miller JJ III. Behçet's disease presenting as chronic aphthous stomatitis in a child. Pediatrics 1978; 62:205-208.

74. Ammann AJ, Johnson A, Fyfe GA, Leonards R, Wara DW, Cowan MJ. Behçet syndrome. J Pediatr 1985; 107:41-43.

75. Stringer DA, Cleghorn GJ, Durie PR, Daneman A, Hamilton JR. Behçet's syndrome involving the gastrointestinal tract—a diagnostic dilemma in childhood. Pediatr Radiol 1986; 16:131-134.

76. Lehner T, Batchelor JR, Challacombe SJ, Kennedy L. An immunogenetic basis for tissue involvement in Behçet's syndrome. Immunology 1979; 37:895-900.

77. Yim CW, White RH. Behçet's syndrome in a family with inflammatory bowel disease. Arch Intern Med 1985; 145:1047-1050.

78. Yazici H, Tuzun Y, Pazarli H, Yurdakul S, Ozyazgan Y, Ozdogan H, Serdaroglu S, Ersanli M, Ulku BY, Muftuoglu AU. Influence of age of onset and patient's sex on the prevalence and severity of Behçet's syndrome. Ann Rheum Dis 1984; 43:783-789.

79. Gonzalez T, Gantes M, Bustabad S. HLA haplotypes in familial Behçet's disease. J Rheum 1984; 11:405-406.

80. Lewis MA, Priestley BL. Transient neonatal Behçet's disease. Arch Dis Child 1986; 61:805-806.

81. James DG. Behçet's syndrome. N Engl J Med 1979; 301:431-432.

82. Chajek T, Fainaru M. Behçet's disease. Report of 41 cases and a review of the literature. Medicine 1975; 54:179-196.

83. Baba S, Maruta M, Ando K, Teramoto T, Endo I. Intestinal Behçet's disease: report of five cases. Dis Colon Rectum 1976; 19:428-440.

84. Kasahara Y, Tanaka S, Nishino M, Unemura H, Shiraha S, Kuyama T. Intestinal involvement in Behçet's disease: Review of 136 surgical cases in the Japanese literature. Dis Colon Rectum 1981; 24:103-106.

85. Jorizzo JL. Behçet's disease: an update based on the 1985 international conference in London. Arch Dermatol 1986; 122:556-558.

86. Nussenblatt RB, Palestine AG, Chan C-C, Mochizuki M, Yancey K. Effectiveness of cyclosporin therapy for Behçet's disease. Arthritis Rheum 1985; 28:671-679.

PART 17

Necrotizing Enterocolitis

Esther J. Israel, M.D.

Neonatal necrotizing enterocolitis (NEC) is a disease of the immature mucosal barrier, occurring almost exclusively in the neonatal period. It is an enigmatic process in that little is truly known regarding its etiology, its presentation is often insidious, and a specific treatment regimen is not known to be curative. This discussion reviews the purported pathogenic factors and clinical course of NEC, outlining diagnostic and management approaches that have been helpful in lowering the mortality rate from 70 percent to 20 to 40 percent. Finally, a description of preventative measures is presented with a focus on the immature intestinal mucosal barrier as a primary target.

DEFINITION

A precise definition of NEC is difficult in that the pathogenesis is unknown and the clinical presentation can be varied, from acute and fulminant to insidious. The definition, by default, therefore, is based primarily on pathologic criteria, although one pathognomonic radiographic finding does exist, that of pneumatosis intestinalis. NEC is best defined as a disease of focal or diffuse ulceration and necrosis of the gastrointestinal (GI) tract, primarily the distal small bowel and colon, although the upper tract may be affected.

HISTORY

The first case of NEC, in a 2-day-old premature infant with vomiting and abdominal distention secondary to inflammation and perforation of the ileum, was reported in 1891 by Genersich.[1] The first series of patients was reported by von Willi in 1944[2] in the German literature, 62 patients with "malignant enteritis." The disease has gained increasing recognition in the English literature since the 1960s, with many comprehensive reports[3,4] indicating both a true increase in incidence and an increased awareness of the disease. This increase in incidence is in large part the result of the increased survival of infants of lower gestational age.

EPIDEMIOLOGY

NEC affects predominantly premature infants in the neonatal intensive care unit (NICU), although approximately 10 to 20 percent of affected neonates are term infants.[5,6] The incidence of the disease is 1 to 2 cases per 1,000 live births and 2.5 percent of all infants in neonatal intensive care units. There is no racial, seasonal, geographic, or sexual predilection. The age at onset of NEC is variable, occurring either early (first 10 days of life) or late. Some cases have been reported to occur as late as 10 weeks of age.[6] In infants less than 1,500 g at birth there does not appear to be any difference in potential risk factors in the early group versus the late group, except parenteral alimentation, which is more common in the late-onset group, suggesting that early feeding may be a risk factor.[7] This is not borne out, however, in other studies. In fact, there are no identifiable risk factors in infants of low birth weight, save their prematurity.[8] In full-term infants, relative gut immaturity may play a lesser role in NEC. Risk factors identified in this group (Table 1) include cyanotic congenital heart disease,[9] polycythemia, exchange transfusions, umbilical catheters, perinatal asphyxia, maternal pre-eclampsia, and smallness for gestational age,[10] which suggest mucosal injury and ischemia as important factors.

PATHOLOGY

The most common sites of GI tract involvement are the distal ileum and ascending colon, although lesions have been noted throughout. The earliest pathologic lesion includes superficial mucosal ulceration and submucosal edema and hemorrhage.[11,12] There is little infiltration of acute inflammatory cells early on. The mucosal process progresses to coagulative, transmural necrosis, leading to perforation. In some cases, intramural gas is noted as bubbles or gaseous strips in the submucosa and subserosa. If the disease does not progress to complete transmural disease and perforation, healing occurs by epithelialization and fibroblast proliferation, and granulation tissue is laid down. Strictures may then be noted.

PATHOGENESIS

No single etiologic factor has been found to be responsible for the disease in all patients. The pathogenesis is most like-

TABLE 1
Risk Factors for Necrotizing Enterocolitis

Premature	Full-Term
Lower gestational age	Cyanotic congenital heart disease
	Polycythemia
	Exchange transfusions
	Umbilical catheters
	Perinatal asphyxia
	Maternal pre-eclampsia
	Small for gestational age

ly related to numerous factors, some playing a more important role than others in any individual patient. There appear to be three major precipitating factors that act either individually or in concert to produce the lesion, particularly in the setting of the premature infant (Fig. 1). They are enteral feeding, infection, and intestinal ischemia.

Enteral Feeding. Milk feeding is a nearly universal observation among patients with NEC. The disease has been reported infrequently in infants who have never been fed enterally. Out of 537 infants in a compilation of six studies, only 7 percent had never been fed enterally. The pathogenic role for oral feeding has been studied. It appears that oral alimentation provides a substrate for the bacteria, which are then allowed to proliferate and contribute to the disease. The composition, rate of feeding, and age at onset of feeding in relation to the development of NEC have all been studied. Hyperosmolar feeding predisposes to NEC by directly damaging the intestinal mucosa and thereby disturbing the barrier or altering intestinal perfusion.[14] In a prospective investigation of low birth weight infants, 25 percent of infants fed a standard cow's milk formula developed NEC, as compared with 87.5 percent who were fed an elemental formula of high osmolality (650 mOsm per liter).[15] Present-day formulations address this problem, and care should be exercised in the administration of oral drugs to infants (some elixirs are hypertonic). There is evidence to suggest that formula feedings, compared with breast feeding, predispose to NEC. Breast milk contains many factors that potentially could mature the intestinal barrier and protect against the development of NEC. These include specific immunocompetent factors such as antibodies and cells such as lymphocytes and macrophages. The work of Pitt et al[16] in a rodent model of NEC demonstrates the role of maternal milk macrophages. Other nonspecific factors (complement, lysozyme, lactoferrin, growth factors) in breast milk may work either directly or indirectly to prevent the onset of NEC.

Ischemia. Touloukian et al[17] postulated that the pathologic findings observed in NEC were preceded by intestinal ischemia induced by a redistribution of the cardiac output, with decreased intestinal mucosal blood flow during an hypoxic episode. He and others have used this as a basis for animal models replicating NEC.[16-20] This shunting of blood is similar to the "diving reflex" in aquatic mammals. An overshooting of this mechanism could occur in infants with transient asphyxia, causing ischemic changes that may lead to necrosis. However, when NEC patients are compared with control infants matched for gestational age, very few risk factors that might cause ischemia are identified[9] more frequently in the NEC population.

Hyperviscosity and NEC were first related by Leake et al in 1975,[21] and studies in newborn dogs have substantiated this association.[22] Wilson, in a study of predisposing conditions to NEC in full-term infants, found polycythemia to be the most commonly recognized antecedent condition.[23] Recently, however, it has become apparent that the relationship of NEC to hyperviscosity may be related more to iatrogenesis than to the polycythemia. The management of the hyperviscosity syndrome with partial exchange transfusion[24,25] appears to play an important role in the development of NEC in term and premature infants. The risk of NEC secondary to partial exchange transfusion may be minimized with the use of a commercial plasma substitute (as opposed to fresh frozen plasma) and the use of peripheral vessels rather than umbilical vessels for the infusion and withdrawal.[26] If need be, an umbilical vein may be used for withdrawal. The suggested rate of infusion and withdrawal is 5 cc per kilogram per 3 minutes.[27]

Bacteria. The mucosal and systemic invasion of enteric bacteria is well recognized as playing an important role in the pathogenesis and evolution of NEC. However, the histopathology of the disease, which is relatively devoid of an acute inflammatory response, suggests that the bacterial proliferation and invasion are allowed to occur secondary to the already compromised intestinal mucosal barrier. Epidemiologic observations support a role for microbial organisms in that clustered cases have been observed in most neonatal intensive care units.[28,29] The role of milk leukocytes in the protection against experimental NEC supports the implication of bacteria in the pathogenesis of NEC.[16] The efficacy of feeding an IgA-IgG supplement to premature infants in preventing NEC[30] also points to the involvement of organisms in the disease process. A careful study in one NICU[31] showed that the organisms involved in NEC were normal bowel flora, gram-negative organisms (*Escherichia coli*, particularly) that entered the peritoneum and blood stream, most likely through an altered gut mucosa. Alteration of the virulence of the flora during antimicrobial therapy has also been suggested as one of the mechanisms responsible for the in-

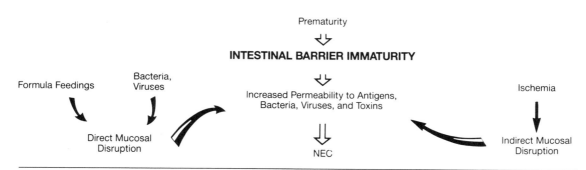

FIGURE 1 A proposed pathogenic framework for necrotizing enterocolitis, a disease of the immature mucosal barrier.

vasiveness of the disease.[32] Another theory proposes that the cleanliness and physical isolation of the NICU environment along with liberal use of antibiotics favor the development of NEC by allowing only a few competitive organisms to multiply without interference.[33] Other studies have substantiated this finding of the involvement of seemingly ordinary gut bacteria (*E. coli, Klebsiella, Staphylococcus epidermidis*[34]), whereas other investigators have noted associations with high-grade enteropathogens such as *Clostridium, Enterobacter, Pseudomonas, Salmonella*, rotavirus,[35] and enteroviruses.

Host Factors. There is one risk factor that appears to be important in all the epidemiologic studies of NEC, and that is the prematurity factor. Eighty to 90 percent of the infants with NEC are of low birth weight,[5,6] and the disease is even more frequently noted and more severe in the infants with the earliest postconceptual age.[36] This finding has led to the theory that NEC is a disease of the immature intestinal barrier.[37] The aforementioned three factors of enteral feeding, ischemia, and infectious organisms work together on the already compromised intestinal host defenses by further increasing mucosal permeability to enteric bacteria, toxins, and antigens (Fig.1). It is well recognized that numerous components of the intestinal host defense system undergo maturational changes through the prenatal and perinatal period.[38] Basal acid output is low at birth and is even lower in the preterm population.[39] Some protease levels are also quite low in the neonatal period,[40] and intestinal motility is apparently slower in the prenatal and perinatal period,[41,42] potentially contributing to overgrowth of bacteria. The mucosal surface, comprising mucus and the microvillous membrane, acts as a physical barrier to the influx of bacteria and their toxins as well as other antigens in the mature host, and it is well recognized that immaturity of this surface in neonatal animals results in increased uptake.[43,44] The state of this component of the barrier in the human premature infant has not been well studied as yet. The concentration of IgA in saliva,[45] stool,[46] and serum[47] of newborn animals and humans is low, and there is consistent impairment of cellular immunity in low birth weight infants,[48] with a reduced number of intestinal T lymphocytes, among other things. In a large, multicenter, collaborative trial using antenatal corticosteroids, a significantly decreased incidence of NEC was noted in infants treated with steroids.[49] Corticosteroids are one of the growth factors implicated in the physiologic maturation of the intestinal barrier and have been used pharmacologically in animal studies to mature many components of the microvillous surface[50,51] and the intact barrier to uptake of antigens.[52]

CLINICAL FEATURES

The clinical course of NEC may vary from a slow, indolent process to a fulminant one with progression to death in a few hours. The classic triad of symptoms includes abdominal distention, bilious vomiting, and blood in the stools. Few patients present in this classic manner, rather showing less specific signs indicative of generalized sepsis (Table 2). The diagnosis of NEC is suspected when the GI signs and symptoms predominate. Not every patient has every sign, and the

TABLE 2
Presenting Signs of Necrotizing Enterocolitis

Lethargy
Temperature instability
Apnea
Shock
Disseminated intravascular coagulation
Ileus
Clinitest-positive stools
Heme-positive stools or vomitus

signs vary in the time of their appearance, according to the severity of the disease process. The diagnosis of NEC is confirmed radiologically on the basis of pneumatosis intestinalis (air within the wall of the intestine) (Figs. 2 and 3) or air in the hepatic portal venous system (Fig. 3). Pneumatosis is often subtle, and much energy is expended in the NICU debating its presence, but it is one of the only pathognomonic signs of NEC. Other radiologic signs of NEC are listed in Table 3. Intestinal distention with multiple dilated loops of small bowel is most commonly seen, with separation of the loops suggesting mural edema. Pneumoperitoneum and intraabdominal fluid are very serious signs, requiring immediate intervention. It would be advantageous to have other objective tests performed to confirm the diagnosis of NEC, perhaps earlier in the course so that management may be instituted early. Recently other laboratory measurements have been suggested to aid in resolving this diagnostic dilemma. Reduced substance[53] and alpha$_1$-antitrypsin levels[54] in the stool have been suggested as early signs of the disease. A large increase in urine specific gravity at the onset of NEC has also been noted.[55] Metrizamide GI series have been found to be useful in neonates suspected of having NEC,[56] as has portal vein ultrasonography.[57] Although these tests may be helpful, they have not replaced the clinical presentation and plain abdominal radiography in the diagnostic evaluation. Bell and his co-workers[58] designed a set of diagnostic criteria which has since been modified[59] and is probably the most helpful tool in effecting some uniformity in therapeutic decision-making (Table 4). The advancing course of NEC is accompanied by signs of clinical decompensation—silencing of hyperactive bowel sound, worsening signs of sepsis with apnea, and increasing metabolic acidosis and hypotension. The fluids and electrolytes become increasingly hard to manage, and the hematologic system becomes more deranged, with decreased platelets and disseminated intravascular coagulation. Bowel necrosis generally accompanies this clinical deterioration.

TABLE 3
Radiologic Findings of Necrotizing Enterocolitis

Intestinal dilatation
Pneumatosis intestinalis
Intrahepatic air
Pneumoperitoneum
Intra-abdominal fluid

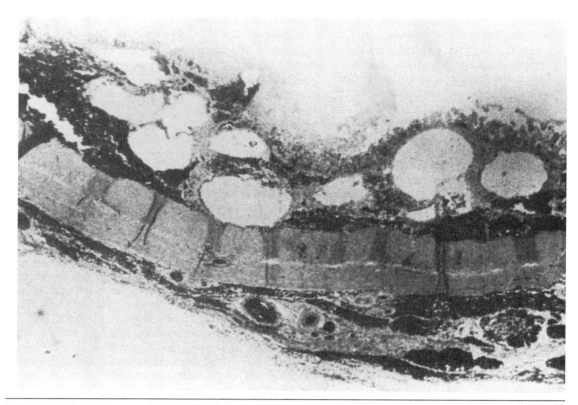

FIGURE 2 Photomicrograph of involved intestine in an advanced lesion showing mucosal necrosis and ulcerations, submucosal hemorrhage, and intramural air (pneumatosis). (From Santulli et al[78]; with permission of Pediatrics, © 1975.)

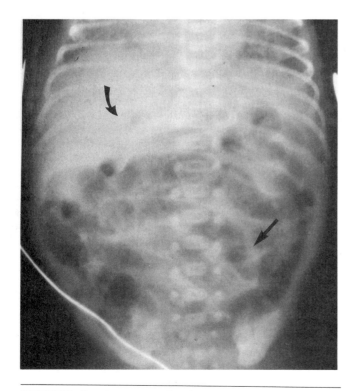

FIGURE 3 Roentgenogram showing pneumatosis (*lower arrow*) as linear intramural collections of air and portal venous air (*upper arrow*).

TABLE 4
Staging Criteria for the Management of Necrotizing Enterocolitis

Stage I (suspect)
  a. Any one or more historical factors producing perinatal stress.
  b. Systemic manifestations—temperature instability, lethargy, apnea, bradycardia.
  c. Gastrointestinal manifestations—poor feeding, increasing pregavage residuals, emesis (may be bilious or test positive for occult blood), mild abdominal distention, occult blood in stool (no fissure).
  d. Abdominal radiographs show distention with mild ileus.

Stage II (definite)
  a. Any one or more historical factors.
  b. Above signs and symptoms plus persistent occult or gross gastrointestinal bleeding; marked abdominal distention.
  c. Abdominal radiographs show significant intestinal distention with ileus; small bowel separation (edema in bowel wall or peritoneal fluid), unchanging or persistent "rigid" bowel loops, pneumatosis intestinalis, portal vein gas.

Stage III (advanced)
  a. Any one or more historical factors.
  b. Above signs and symptoms plus deterioration of vital signs, evidence of septic shock or marked gastrointestinal hemorrhage.
  c. Abdominal radiographs may show pneumoperitoneum in addition to others listed in II c.

From Bell et al. [58]

TREATMENT

The management of a patient with NEC is largely supportive. As soon as the diagnosis is suspected, certain measures are undertaken to prevent the progression of the disease (Table 5). All oral feedings are withheld, and a nasogastric tube is placed and suction applied. Intravenous access is assured to provide fluids and electrolytes as well as nutrition while the patient is NPO. The duration of oral intake restriction depends on the confirmation of the diagnosis of NEC, which is dictated by the radiographs as well as the clinical status. Many patients who do not go beyond stage 1 (see Table 4) and resolve their symptoms and signs with these measures are fed at 48 to 72 hours. If the period of enteral restriction appears to be longer (2 weeks if the patient reaches stage 2), strong consideration should be given to placement of a central venous catheter for the provision of total parenteral nutrition. The reinstitution of feedings after "true" NEC is generally done in a very slow and cautious manner with an elemental formulation to allow for optimal absorption of all nutrients and to avoid further potential injury to the intestinal mucosa.

Since bacteria have been implicated in the pathogenesis of NEC and because the presentation is frequently one of a septic infant, cultures of blood, stool, urine, and cerebrospinal fluid are obtained and broad-spectrum parenteral antibiotics are given. Antibiotic regimens that have been used include clindamycin and gentamicin,[44] ampicillin and kanamycin,[44] a combination of penicillin, gentamicin, and metronidazole or clindamycin,[60,61] and cefotaxime and vancomycin.[62] The routine inclusion of antianaerobic antimicrobial agents does not appear to be indicated from control studies.[61] In addition, it is unclear whether anticoagulase-negative *Staphylococcus* coverage with vancomycin is necessary in the initial stages,[62-64] unless obtained from culture or recognized to be endemic in a particular nursery. It is important to know the prevailing flora of the infants in the NICU as well as the current NEC bacteriology, since NEC cases cluster and the predominant organism also clusters. Infectious disease control measures are also instituted.[61] Enteric antibiotics have been used in the acute stages of the disease as well as prophylactically but overall are not considered to be helpful[65-69] and are rarely used.

An abdominal radiograph is obtained, to look for the pathognomonic signs of NEC, and is repeated every 6 hours to assess the progression of the disease. Cross-table lateral radiographs are a helpful adjunct to the anteroposterior view of the abdomen to evaluate the existence of pneumoperitone-um, a sign of intestinal perforation and the sole absolute indication for surgery. If the clinical course settles down, the radiographs may be spaced further apart.

A complete blood count with platelet count is obtained, particularly to look for thrombocytopenia and neutropenia, which are common in the more critically ill infants. Platelets are transfused if the count drops below 25,000, particularly in the face of active GI bleeding. The use of white cell transfusions remains controversial and has not been shown to be efficacious in altering outcome.

Strict attention must be given to the fluid and electrolyte status of the infant, since large "third-space" losses may occur with inflammation and edema of the intestine, and most infants require at least one and one-half to two times maintenance fluids. Large volumes of crystalloid and/or blood may be necessary to maintain perfusion and blood pressure. Severe metabolic acidosis may occur secondary to poor perfusion and is often difficult to manage in the more advanced stages. In the event of unremitting hypotension, inotropic agents may be utilized.

Ventilatory support may be necessary, particularly in the presence of severe apnea.

Surgery is reserved for those patients who do not respond to the medical management outlined above. The indications for surgery include pneumoperitoneum and cellulitis of the anterior abdominal wall, suggesting peritonitis and gangrenous bowel. Additionally, when metabolic acidosis appears to be irreversible with lack of response to bicarbonate infusions and/or respiratory failure is progressive, surgery is indicated. The classic operative strategy has been a relatively conservative one with resection of grossly gangrenous bowel and proximal enterostomy.[70] Fecal diversion and intestinal decompression were thought to be important factors in the management of NEC, particularly in patients with widespread gangrene.[71,72] The difficulties inherent in the management of jejunal stomas in neonates (see below), however, have led some surgeons to reconsider the role of primary anastomosis for selected infants with circumscribed disease[73-75] such as discrete intestinal perforations. When stomas are placed, the time of closure with anastomosis is generally dictated by stomal dysfunction from prolapse or stenosis, with associated weight loss and fluid and electrolyte imbalances.[76] In principle, one would prefer to perform the reanastomosis after good weight gain has been attained.[77]

The treatment of NEC is primarily supportive, and surgery is performed if necessary. Once the disease process is initiated, it takes its own course with the above support measures. The frontier of research, therefore, is at the prevention level rather than the treatment level.

TABLE 5
Initial Medical Management of Necrotizing
Enterocolitis

1. Nil per os
2. Nasogastric tube
3. Parenteral antibiotics
4. Fluid and electrolyte management
5. Frequent vital signs (including abdominal girth)
6. Serial abdominal radiographs
7. Serial platelet counts

PROGNOSIS

Morbidity and mortality from NEC have improved dramatically since the original descriptions. Whereas 22 percent of the infants survived in Santulli's study encompassing 1955 to 1974,[78] a mortality rate of 20 to 40 percent is now being seen.[5,6,59,79] Mortality is directly related to the presence of bacteremia and low birth weight.[79] The decrease in the mortality rate noted over the years is due to earlier diagnosis combined with intensive medical and surgical therapy. Morbidity related to the long-term effects of the disease on the GI tract is seen in 10 to 30 percent of affected children.[81] Most of the morbidity seen in these children, however, is more related to the associated prematurity and the degree of perinatal stress. Acute and more chronic complications related to the GI tract do exist (Table 6).

Strictures of the intestines are the most common sequelae of NEC, occurring in 20 to 36 percent of survivors of medical and surgical management.[82,83] These stenoses are noted primarily in the colon (the left side in particular) and are not necessarily symptomatic. Some spontaneously resolve,[82,83] whereas others require surgical resection secondary to symptoms of intestinal obstruction. If abdominal distention and obstipation are noted, immediate intestinal decompression and radiographic evaluation are performed. Recurrent bloody stools have also been attributed to the strictures, with microscopic evidence of remaining active enterocolitis at the site. Dilatation with a balloon catheter has been successfully employed in infants with strictures distal to their enterostomies, allowing for a less invasive surgical procedure upon closure.[84] Some investigators suggest routine investigation for stenoses with a barium enema on all NEC patients prior to leaving the nursery,[82] although some strictures have been noted as long as 6 months after the insult. This would serve to identify a population at risk, although intervention is not suggested solely on the basis of a narrowing seen on a radiologic study. A more conservative approach involves contrast studies once symptoms are manifest.

Short gut syndrome is seen in a small number of the surgically treated infants when large parts of gangrenous small intestine are resected. A conservative approach to surgery when a significant amount of the small bowel is affected involves proximal enterostomy placement without resection acutely and a return to the operating room 1 week later to assess the damage to the intestine. This approach diminishes the incidence of short gut. Survival after extensive resection does occur. If more than 70 percent of the intestine is removed, serious nutritional consequences prevail. Preservation of the terminal ileum and the ileocecal valve appear to be factors important to the survival of the infants. The predilection of NEC for this area of the GI tract sometimes makes this difficult. The use of total parenteral nutrition until adaptation of the intestine occurs is a prime therapeutic maneuver for short gut. However, cholestasis and the other problems with long-term total parenteral nutrition supervene.

TABLE 6
Gastrointestinal Complications of Necrotizing Enterocolitis

Intestinal or colonic strictures
Enterocolic fistulae
Fluid and electrolyte imbalances
Malabsorption
Cholestasis
Anastomotic leaks and stenosis after surgery
Short gut syndrome after surgery

Complications in the postoperative period secondary to enterostomy losses include fluid and electrolyte imbalances as well as nutritional deficiencies, particularly in the event of a superimposed viral enteritis.[85] Early enterostomy closure and reanastomosis avoid these difficulties.[86] Malabsorption secondary to the mucosal injury with subsequent failure to thrive may be avoided by feeding elemental formulas during the healing phase. Overall, the prognosis for those infants surviving the acute stage of NEC is good.[82,87,88]

PREVENTION

The management of the disease has classically been directed primarily at supportive care, and surgery is performed if clinical deterioration appears irreversible or perforation occurs. There is, however, no specific treatment for the disease. The frontier of research, therefore, has been directed at prevention of disease onset. From a pathophysiologic approach, attempts at modifying one of the precipitating factors should help to modify or prevent the disease process. With this basis of management, it appears that NEC might be ameliorated if bowel ischemia, bacterial proliferation, effects of oral feeding, or gut immaturity were eliminated or decreased. Since the ischemic episodes are beyond control after the obstetrician and pediatrician have made all efforts to avoid perinatal ischemia, efforts have focused on the latter three factors in an attempt to reduce the enteric antigenic load.

Feeding. Much effort has been directed toward modifying feeding regimens to prevent NEC, with attention given to osmolarity, volume, and timing of feeds. Although enteral substrate may be important to the development of NEC, and some studies have suggested delays in feeding,[89] the timing of initiation of feeding does not appear to contribute significantly to the process.[90,91] The provision of dilute, enteral calories early on is not contraindicated in the premature infant. Moreover, "slow" versus fast increases in the volume of feedings have not been shown to result in a difference in incidence of NEC,[92] although experience dictates a very slow regimen for increases in feeding.[93] Feedings with maternal milk are considered preferable because of the factors found in breast milk, which are potentially anti-infective and intestinal maturation-promoting.

Bacterial Proliferation. The use of prophylactic antibiotics has been studied[66-69] and is generally not thought to be effective. Supplementation of formula with an IgA-IgG preparation in low birth weight babies (in whom mucosal sIgA is suboptimal),[45,46] has recently been shown to prevent the development of NEC in these babies.[30] The presumption is that this antibody preparation prevents colonization and penetration of bacteria, reinforcing the importance of bacterial colonization and infestation as a pathogenic factor in the disease.

Host Maturation. Another approach to the prophylaxis of NEC is to enhance the immature intestinal barrier so that the other predisposing factors might not cause as much harm in the face of a more mature host. The effectiveness of host defense enhancement has been demonstrated for breast milk macrophages[16] in the rodent model of NEC. The inverse association of NEC with birth weight and maternal toxemia[94] suggests that the stress of the toxemia results in a maturation of the host defense system, thus decreasing the incidence of NEC. In fact, corticosteroids have been shown to be effective in preventing the occurrence of NEC in an animal model[95] as well as in humans.[40] Corticosteroids as well as other hormones and growth factors are important agents in the maturation of many components of the intestine,[96] including the intestinal barrier.[97] Specifically, cortisone acetate has been shown to mature the sequence of glycoconjugate development on the intestinal surface of the suckling rat necessary for bacterial attachment and colonization to occur.[97,98] Most recently, corticosteroids have limited the bacterial colonization of the intact neonatal rat intestine,[95,99] reinforcing the interplay of the factors of host maturity and bacterial colonization in the pathogenesis of NEC (see Fig. 1).

Further investigation into the factors that govern the maturation of the host defense system and the interactions of feeding and bacteria with this system may yield valuable information regarding the management of this enigmatic disease.

REFERENCES

1. Genersich A. Bauchfellentzundung beim Neugebornen in Folge von Perforation des Ileums. Virchows Arch [A] 1891; 126:485–494.
2. Von Willi H. Ueber eine bosartige Enteritis bei Sauglingen der ersten Trimenons. Ann Pediatr 1944; 162:87–112.
3. Frantz ID, L'Hevreux P, Engel RR, Hunt CE. Necrotizing enterocolitis. J Pediatr 1975; 86:259–263.
4. Touloukian RJ, Berdon WE, Amoury RA, Santulli TV. Surgical experience with necrotizing enterocolitis in the infant. J Pediatr Surg 1967; 2:389–397.
5. Brown EG, Sweet AY. Neonatal necrotizing enterocolitis. Pediatr Clin North Am 1982; 29:1149–1170.
6. Wilson R, Kanto WP, McCarthy BJ, et al. Epidemiologic characteristics of necrotizing enterocolitis: a population-based study. Am J Epidemiol 1981; 114:880–887.
7. Stoll RJ, Kanto WP, Glass RI, et al. Epidemiology of necrotizing enterocolitis in a case control study. J Pediatr 1980; 96:447–451.
8. Wilson R, Kanto WP, McCarthy BJ, Feldman RA. Age at onset of necrotizing enterocolitis: risk factors in small infants. Am J Dis Child 1982; 136:814–816.
9. Kliegman RM, Hack M, Jones P, Fanaroff AA. Epidemiologic study of necrotizing enterocolitis among low-birth-weight infants: absence of identifiable risk factors. J Pediatr 1982; 100:440–444.
10. Polin RA, Pollack PF, Barlow B, et al. Necrotizing enterocolitis in term infants. J Pediatr 1976; 89:460–462.
11. Wiswell TE, Robertson CR, Jones TA, Tuttle DJ. Necrotizing enterocolitis in full-term infants: a case-control study. Am J Dis Child 1988; 142:532–535.
12. Benirschke K. Neonatal enterocolitis. Am J Dis Child 1973; 126:15–22.
13. Rodin AE, Nichols MM, Hsu FL. Necrotizing enterocolitis occurring in full term infants at birth. Arch Pathol 1973; 96:335–338.
14. DeLemos RA, Roger JH, McLaughlin GW. Experimental production of necrotizing enterocolitis in newborn goats. Pediatr Res 1974; 8:380–383.
15. Book LS, Herbst JJ, Atherton SO, Jung AL. Necrotizing enterocolitis in low-birth-weight infants fed an elemental formula. J Pediatr 1975; 87:602–605.
16. Pitt J, Barlow B, Heird WC. Protection against experimental necrotizing enterocolitis by maternal milk. I. Role of milk leukocytes. Pediatr Res 1977; 11:906–909.
17. Touloukian RJ, Posch JN, Spencer R. The pathogenesis of ischemic gastroenterocolitis of the neonate: selective gut mucosal ischemia in asphyxiated neonatal piglets. J Pediatr Surg 1972; 7:194–205.
18. Barlow B, Santulli TV, Heird WC, Pitt J, Blanc WA, Schullinger JN. An experimental study of acute neonatal enterocolitis—the importance of breast milk. J Pediatr Surg 1974; 9:587–594.
19. Krasna IH, Howell C, Vega A, Ziegler IM, Koop CE. A mouse model for the study of necrotizing enterocolitis. J Pediatr Surg 1986; 21:26–29.
20. Harrison MW, Connell RS, Campbell JR, Web MC. Microcirculatory changes in the gastrointestinal tract of the hypoxic puppy: an electron microscope study. J Pediatr Surg 1975; 10:599–608.
21. Leake RD, Thanopoulos B, Nieberg R. Hyperviscosity syndrome associated with necrotizing enterocolitis. Am J Dis Child 1975; 129:1192–1194.
22. Leblanc MH, D'Cruz C, Pat K. NEC can be caused by polycythemic hyperviscosity in the newborn dog. J Pediatr 1984; 105:804–809.
23. Wilson R, Porillo M, Schmidt E, Feldman RA, Kanto WP. Risk factors for NEC in infants weighing more than 2,000 grams at birth: a case-control study. Pediatrics 1983; 71:19–22.
24. Black VD, Rumack CM, Lubchenco LO, Koops BL. Gastrointestinal injury in polycythemic infants. Pediatrics 1985; 76:225–231.
25. Wiswell TE, Cornish JD, Northam RS. Neonatal polycythemia: frequency of clinical manifestations and other associated findings. Pediatrics 1986; 78:26–30.
26. Hein HA, Lathrop SS. Partial exchange transfusion in term, polycythemic neonates: absence of association with severe gastrointestinal injury. Pediatrics 1987; 80:75–78.
27. Aranda JV and Sweet AY. Alterations in blood pressure during exchange transfusion. Arch Dis Child 1977; 52:545–548.
28. Book LS, Overall JC, Herbst JJ, Epstein B, Jung AL. Clustering of necrotizing enterocolitis: interruption by infection-control measures. N Engl J Med 1977; 297:984–986.
29. Moomjian AS, Peckham GJ, Fox WW, Pereira GR, Schaberg DA. Necrotizing enterocolitis—endemic vs epidemic form. Pediatr Res 1978; 12:530A.
30. Eibl MM, Wolf HM, Furnkranz H, Rosenkranz A. Prevention of necrotizing enterocolitis in low-birth-weight infants by IgA-IgG feeding. N Engl J Med 1988; 319:1–7.
31. Virnig NL, Reynolds JW. Epidemiological aspects of neonatal necrotizing enterocolitis. Am J Dis Child 1974; 128:186–190.
32. Bell MJ, Shackelford PG, Feigin RD, Ternberg JL, Brotherton T. Alterations in gastrointestinal microflora during antimicrobial therapy for NEC. Pediatrics 1979; 63:425–428.
33. Lawrence G, Bates J, Gaul A. Pathogenesis of neonatal necrotizing enterocolitis. Lancet 1982; i:137–139.
34. Scheifele DW, Bjornson GL, Dyer RA, Dimmick JE. Delta-like toxin produced by coagulase negative staphylococci is associated with neonatal necrotizing enterocolitis. Infect Immun 1987; 55:2268–2273.
35. Rotbart HA, Nelson WL, Glode MP, Triffon TC, et al. Neonatal rotavirus-associated necrotizing enterocolitis: case control study and prospective surveillance during an outbreak. J Pediatr 1988; 112:87–93.
36. Gaynes RP, Palmer S, Martone WJ, et al. The role of host factors in an outbreak of NEC. Am J Dis Child 1984; 138:118–120.
37. Lake AM, Walker WA. Neonatal necrotizing enterocolitis: a disease of altered host defense. Clin Gastroenterol 1977; 6:463.
38. Israel EJ, Walker WA. Host defense development in gut and related disorders. Pediatr Clin North Am 1988; 25:1–15.
39. Hyman PE, Clarke DD, Everett SL, et al. Gastric acid secretory function in preterm infants. J Pediatr 1985; 106:467–471.
40. Lebenthal E, Lee PC. Development of functional response in human exocrine pancreas. Pediatrics 1980; 66:56–60.
41. Morriss FJ, Moore M, Weisbrodt NW, et al. Ontogenic development of gastrointestinal motility. IV. Duodenal contractions in preterm infants. Pediatrics 1986; 78:1106–1109.
42. McLain CR. Amniography studies of the gastrointestinal motility of the human fetus. Am J Obstet Gynecol 1963; 86:1079–1087.
43. Udall JN, Pang KY, Fritze, et al. Development of the gastrointestinal mucosal barrier I. The effect of age on intestinal permeability to macromolecules. Pediatr Res 1981; 15:241–244.
44. Israel EJ, Pang KY, Harmatz PR, Walker WA. Structural and functional maturation of rat gastrointestinal barrier with thyroxine. Am J Physiol 1987; 252:G762–G767.
45. Selner JC, Merrill DA, Calman HN. Salivary immunoglobulins and albumin: development during the newborn period. J Pediatr 1968; 72:685–691.
46. Hanelberg B, Aarskog D. Human fecal immunoglobulins in healthy infants and children, and in some disease affecting the intestinal tract of the immune system. Clin Immunol 1975; 22:210–212.
47. Allensmith M, McClellan BH, Buterworth M, et al. The development of immunoglobulin levels in man. J Pediatr 1968; 72:276–281.
48. Chandra RK. Development of gastrointestinal tract cellular immunity during the perinatal period. In: Lebenthal E, ed. Textbook of gastroenterology and nutrition in infancy. New York: Raven Press, 1981.

49. Bauer CR, Morrison JC, Poole K, et al. A decreased incidence of necrotizing enterocolitis after prenatal glucocorticoid therapy. Pediatrics 1984; 73:682–688.

50. Pang KY, Newman AP, Udall JN, et al. Development of the gastrointestinal mucosal barrier. VII: In utero maturation of the microvillus surface by cortisone. Am J Physiol 1985; 249:G85–G89.

51. Chu SW, Ely IG, Walker WA. Age and cortisone alter host responsiveness to cholera toxin in the developing gut. Am J Physiol 1989; 256:G220–G225.

52. Israel EJ, Pang KY, Harmatz PR, Walker WA. Development of mucosal barrier function: thyroxine regulation of macromolecular uptake from the intestine of the rat. Pediatr Res 1986; 20:189A.

53. Book LS, Herbst JJ, Jung AL. Carbohydrate malabsorption in necrotizing enterocolitis. Pediatrics 1976; 57:201–204.

54. Shulman RJ, Buffone G, Wise L. Enteric protein loss in necrotizing enterocolitis as measured by fecal alpha$_1$-antitrypsin excretion. J Pediatr 1985; 107:287–289.

55. Stine MJ, Harris H. Urine specific gravity as an indicator of neonatal necrotizing enterocolitis. Pediatrics 1986; 78:1173.

56. Keller MS, Chawla HS. Neonatal metrizamide gastrointestinal series in suspected necrotizing enterocolitis. Am J Dis Child 1985; 139:713–716.

57. Lindley S, Mollitt DL, Seibert JJ, Golladay ES. Portal vein ultrasonography in the early diagnosis of necrotizing enterocolitis. J Pediatr Surg 1986; 21:530–532.

58. Bell MJ, Ternberg JL, Feigin RD, et al. Neonatal necrotizing enterocolitis: therapeutic decisions based upon clinical staging. Ann Surg 1978; 187:1–7.

59. Walsh M, Kliegman RM. Necrotizing enterocolitis: treatment based on staging criteria. Pediatr Clin North Am 1986; 33:179–201.

60. Yu VYH, Joseph R, Bajuk B, et al. Necrotizing enterocolitis in very low birthweight infants—a four year experience. Aust Pediatr J 1984; 20:29–33.

61. Faix RG, Polley TZ, Grasela TH. A randomized, controlled trial of parenteral clindamycin in neonatal necrotizing enterocolitis. J Pediatr 1988; 112:271–277.

62. Scheifele DW, Ginter GL, Olsen E, et al. Comparison of two antibiotic regimens for neonatal necrotizing enterocolitis. J Antimicrob Chemother 1987; 20:421–429.

63. Mollitt DL, Tepas JJ, Talbert JL. The role of coagulase-negative staphylococcus in neonatal necrotizing enterocolitis. J Pediatr Surg 1988; 23:60–63.

64. Scheifele DW, Bjornson GL, Dyer TA, Dimmick JE. Delta-like toxin produced by coagulase-negative staphylococci is associated with neonatal necrotizing enterocolitis. Infect Immun 1987; 55:2268–2273.

65. Rotbart H, Levin M. How contagious is necrotizing enterocolitis? J Pediatr Infect Dis 1983; 2:406–413.

65a. Bell MJ, Kosloske AM, Benton C, Matin LW. Neonatal necrotizing enterocolitis: prevention of perforation. J Pediatr Surg 1973; 8:601–604.

66. Egan EA, Mantilla G, Nelson RM, Eitzman DV. A prospective controlled trial of oral kanamycin in the prevention of neonatal necrotizing enterocolitis. J Pediatr 1976; 89:467–470.

67. Graylack LJ, Scanlon JW. Oral gentamicin therapy in the prevention of neonatal necrotizing enterocolitis. Am J Dis Child 1978; 132:1192–1194.

68. Hansen TN, Ritter DA, Speer ME, et al. A randomized controlled study of oral gentamicin in the treatment of neonatal necrotizing enterocolitis. J Pediatr 1980; 97:836–839.

69. Boyle R, Nelson JS, Stonestreet BS, et al. Alterations in stool flora resulting from oral kanamycin prophylaxis of necrotizing enterocolitis. J Pediatr 1978; 93:857–859.

70. Martin LW. Neonatal necrotizing enterocolitis: surgical considerations. In: Report of the 68th Ross Conference on Pediatric Research. Columbus, Ross Laboratories, 1975, pp 91–92.

71. Martin LW, Neblett WW. Early operation with intestinal diversion for necrotizing enterocolitis. J Pediatr Surg 1981; 16:252–255.

72. Cooper A, Ross AJ, O'Neill JA, Schnaufer L. Resection with primary anastomosis for necrotizing enterocolitis: a contrasting view. J Pediatr Surg 1988; 23:64–68.

73. Kiesewetter WB, Taghizadeh F, Bower RJ. Necrotizing enterocolitis: is there a place for resection and primary anastomosis? J Pediatr Surg 1979; 14:361–363.

74. Harberg FJ, McGil CW, Saleem MM, et al. Resection with primary anastomosis for necrotizing enterocolitis. J Pediatr Surg 1983; 18:743–746.

75. Sparnon AR, Kiely EM. Resection with primary anastomosis for necrotizing enterocolitis. Pediatr Surg Int 1987; 2:101–104.

76. Cogbill TH, Millikan JS. Reconstitution of intestinal continuity after resection for neonatal necrotizing enterocolitis. Surg Gynecol Obstet 1985; 160:330–334.

77. Kosloske AM. Necrotizing enterocolitis in the neonate. Surg Gynecol Obstet 1979; 148:259–260.

78. Santulli TV, Schullinger JN, Heird WC, et al. Acute necrotizing enterocolitis in infancy: a review of 64 cases. Pediatrics 1975; 55:376–387.

79. Kliegman RM, Fanaroff AA. Neonatal necrotizing enterocolitis: a nine year experience. II. Outcome assessment. Am J Dis Child 1981; 135:608–611.

80. Schullinger JN, Mollitt DL, Vinocur CD, et al. Neonatal necrotizing enterocolitis. Survival, management and complications: a 25-year study. Am J Dis Child 1981; 135:612–614.

81. Stevenson DK, Kerner JA, Malachowski N, Sunshine P. Late morbidity among survivors of necrotizing enterocolitis. Pediatrics 1980; 66:925–927.

82. Schwartz MZ, Hayden CK, Richardson CJ, et al. A prospective evaluation of intestinal stenosis following necrotizing enterocolitis. J Pediatr Surg 1982; 17:764–770.

83. Tonkin ILD, Bjelland JC, Hunter JC, et al. Spontaneous resolution of colonic strictures caused by necrotizing enterocolitis: therapeutic implications. AJR 1978; 130:1077–1081.

84. Ball WS, Kosloske AM, Jewell PF, et al. Balloon catheter dilatation of focal intestinal strictures following necrotizing enterocolitis. J Pediatr Surg 1985; 20:637–639.

85. Yolken R, Franklin C. Gastrointestinal adenovirus: an important cause of morbidity in patients with necrotizing enterocolitis and gastrointestinal surgery. Pediatr Infect Dis 1985; 4:42–44.

86. Rothstein FC, Halpin TC, Kliegman RM, et al. Importance of early ileostomy closure to prevent chronic salt and water losses after necrotizing enterocolitis. Pediatrics 1982; 70:249–253.

87. Hack M, Gordon D, Jones P, Fanaroff A. Necrotizing enterocolitis in the VLBW: An encouraging follow up report. Pediatr Res 1981; 15:534.

88. Abassi S, Pereira GR, Johnson L, et al. Long term assessment of growth, nutritional status, and gastrointestinal function in survivors of NEC. J Pediatr 1984; 104:550–553.

89. McCormack CJ, Emmens RW, Putnam TC. Evaluation of factors in high risk neonatal necrotizing enterocolitis. J Pediatr Surg 1987; 22:488–491.

90. LaGamma EF, Ostertag SG, Birenbaum H. Failure of delayed oral feedings to prevent necrotizing enterocolitis. Results of study in very-low-birth-weight neonates. Am J Dis Child 1985; 139:385–389.

91. Ostertag SG, LaGamma EF, Reisen CE, Ferrentino FL. Early enteral feeding does not affect the incidence of necrotizing enterocolitis. Pediatrics 1986; 77:275–280.

92. Book LS, Herbst JJ, Jung AL. Comparison of fast- and slow-feeding rate schedules to the development of necrotizing enterocolitis. J Pediatr 1976; 89:463–466.

93. Brown EG, Sweet AY. Preventing necrotizing enterocolitis in neonates. JAMA 1978; 240:2452–2454.

94. Kanto WP, Wilson R, Preart GL, et al. Perinatal events and necrotizing enterocolitis in premature infants. Am J Dis Child 1987; 141:167–169.

95. Israel EJ, Schiffrin EJ, Carter EA, et al. Corticosteroids as prophylaxis against necrotizing enterocolitis. Pediatr Res 1989; 25:219A.

96. Henning SJ. Development of gastrointestinal function. Viewpoints Dig Dis 1987; 19:1–4.

97. Israel EJ, Walker WA. Development of intestinal mucosal barrier function to antigens and bacterial toxins. In: Mestecky J, McGhee JR, eds. Recent advances in mucosal immunology. New York: Plenum, 1987:673.

98. Mahmood A, Torres-Pinedo R. Effect of hormone administration on sialylation and fucosylation of intestinal microvillus membranes of suckling rats. Pediatr Res 1985; 19:899–902.

99. Schiffrin EJ, Israel EJ, Carter EA, et al. Influence of prenatal mucosal barrier maturation on bacterial colonization in the newborn. Gastroenterology 1989; 96:A448.

PART 18

Genetically Determined Disaccharidase Deficiencies

Salvatore Auricchio, M.D.

An accurate description of diarrhea due to sugar intolerance was already given in 1921 by John Howland,[1] but only in the last 30 years has it been clarified that both secondary and primary, genetically determined, disaccharidase deficiencies may lead to malabsorption and intolerance of the corresponding disaccharides(s).*

Holzel et al[2] were the first to report, in 1959, children with intolerance to lactose, presumably due to congenital deficiency of intestinal lactase activity. The most common form of genetically determined disaccharidase deficiency, primary adult type hypolactasia, was described in 1963 in Europe[3] and in the United States[4] in populations having a high frequency of persistent high lactase activity in adult life.[5]

Hereditary sucrose malabsorption was described by Weijers et al[6] in 1960. Shortly thereafter, isomaltose malabsorption was demonstrated in this condition[7-9] due to absence or severe reduction of isomaltase activity.[10-13]

---

*In this chapter the term *disaccharidase* is used also to indicate enzymes in those cases in which oligosaccharides or glycosides other than disaccharides were used as substrates.

The identification of the genetic defects of intestinal disaccharidases stimulated an intensive and fruitful research on structure and biosynthesis of these brush border hydrolases[14-16]; this knowledge, along with the recent cDNA cloning of sucrase-isomaltase[17] and of lactase-phlorizin-hydrolase,[17a] is the basis for a better understanding of the molecular biology of genetically determined disaccharidase deficiencies.[18-21]

DISACCHARIDASES

Structure and Biosynthesis

Four disaccharidases are brush border enzymes: three are alpha-glucosidases (sucrase-isomaltase, maltase-glucoamylase, and trehalase) and one is a beta-glycosidase (lactase-glycosyl ceramidase or lactase-phlorizin hydrolase). Sucrase-isomaltase and maltase-glucoamylase are heterodimer complexes, each being composed of two similar but not identical subunits. Each subunit consists of a single,

TABLE 1
Molecular Forms of the Small-Intestinal Heterodimeric Glycosidases During Biosynthesis*

| Enzyme | Species | $10^{-3} \times M_r$ of: | | Mature Form[†] ($10^{-3} \times M_r$) | Transport Time (Min) |
		Primary Translation Product, Nonglycosylated Form	Transient Form		
Sucrase-isomaltase complex	Rabbit	200	230	275[‡] (120 + 140[‡,§,‖])	
	Pig	225	240	265 (140 + 150)	60–90
	Humans	210	217	231 (145 + 151)	
Maltase-glucoamylase (glucoamylase complex)	Pig	200	225	245 (125 + 135)	60–90
Lactase-phlorizin hydrolase (β-glycosidase complex)	Pig	210	225	245 (160)[#]	60–90
	Humans	200	214	262 (156)[#]	

*Most apparent M_r values listed were estimated from SDS-PAGE. They thus occasionally differ somewhat from those calculated from hydrodynamic parameters.

†Values in parentheses indicate the M_r of proteolytically cleaved mature forms.

‡Strong indication for anchoring via the N-terminal regions is available (i.e., change in the N-terminal amino acid residue during proteolytic solubilization and/or sizeable hydrophobic sequence in the N-terminal region), although not necessarily for the species indicated in the second column.

§Evidence for the nonparticipation of the C-terminal regions in the anchoring is available.

‖The M_r of the unglycosylated pro-sucrase-isomaltase, as deduced from cDNA cloning and sequencing, is 203,000.

#The proteolytic processing leading to the two final subunits takes place intracellularly.

From Semenza and Auricchio.[21]

glycosylated polypeptide chain with an apparent molecular weight in the 120 to 160 kDa range (Table 1).

The sucrase-isomaltase complex is anchored to the microvillous membrane of the enterocyte via the isomaltase subunit: the anchoring segment is located not far from the N-terminus, and most of the protein mass of isomaltase, inclusive of the C-terminus, and sucrase protrudes out the luminal side of the membrane. The sucrase subunit interacts with brush border membrane solely via isomaltase[14-16] (Fig. 1). The glucoamylase complex has a similar position in the membrane.[22-24]

As for the beta-glycosidase (lactose-phlorizin hydrolase), its subunit composition seems to be different, the final "beta-glycosidase complex" being composed of a single type of polypeptide chain and the two enzyme activities being associated with different domains of it.[17a] Recent cloning of sucrase-isomaltase cDNA from rabbit has confirmed Semenza's hypothesis[25-27] that sucrase-isomaltase complex is synthesized as a single precursor starting from the N-terminus of isomaltase. An optimal alignment of the two subunits reveals a high degree of homology between the isomaltase and sucrase portions (41 percent amino acid identity), indicating that sucrase-isomaltase evolved by partial gene duplication. The N-terminal, isomaltase region of human sucrase-isomaltase has extensive overall homology with rabbit sucrase-isomaltase.[28]

The gene encoding the human enzyme has been localized in chromosome 3.[28,29] The one-chain high molecular weight polypeptide precursor of sucrase-isomaltase is found first in the microsomal fraction and in the Golgi apparatus and then in the brush border of the enterocyte.[30-35] The precursor is transferred to the brush border membrane, where it is split into sucrase and isomaltase subunits, probably by pancreatic proteases. The maltase-glucoamylase component is also synthesized in pig intestine as a single gigantic polypeptide chain of 240 kDa, then cleaved into its two subunits by pancreatic

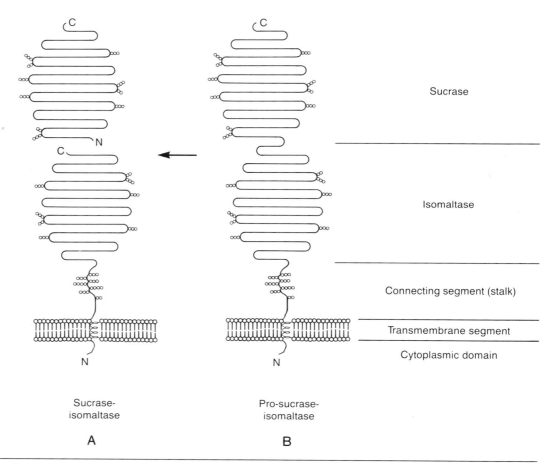

FIGURE 1 Positioning of sucrase-isomaltase (A) and of pro-sucrase-isomaltase (B) in the small intestinal brush border membrane. The (unspecified) interactions within and between the sucrase and isomaltase domains (or subunits, respectively) are not indicated. ooo = sugar chains. The sucrase-isomaltase complex (SI) of the small intestinal brush border membrane accounts for approximately 9 to 10 percent of the intrinsic protein. The isomaltase subunit alone interacts with the membrane directly, via a highly hydrophobic segment at its N-terminal region. The sucrase subunit is attached to the membrane solely via its interactions with the isomaltase subunit. The sucrase-isomaltase complex is synthesized as a single, very long (203 kDa) polypeptide chain (pro-SI), carrying the two sites of sucrase and isomaltase in an already enzymatically active form, with the isomaltase portion corresponding to the N-terminal part of pro-SI. Pro-SI is processed into final SI by pancreatic proteases. (From Semenza[15]; © 1986 by Annual Reviews Inc.)

proteases,[22-24] whereas in rat intestine the synthesis of a single protein of 145 kDa has been demonstrated by in vitro translation.[36]

The beta-glycosidase complex follows a different biosynthetic pattern from that of sucrase-isomaltase, as the polypeptide precursor[17a] probably undergoes more complex post-translational proteolytic events due to intrinsic enterocyte peptidases.[37-40] The glycosylation is apparently similar for all disaccharidase complexes[41] and includes two main steps, the co-translational acquisition of glucan units of a high mannose type at the endoplasmic reticulum and subsequent trimming and complex glycosylation in the Golgi apparatus (Figs. 2 and 3).

Two high molecular weight forms of the sucrase-isomaltase precursor, which rapidly incorporates labeled mannose, have been demonstrated in microsomes of the rat enterocyte.[34] The smaller of the two forms contains the core carbohydrate structure (the mannose-rich oligosaccharide sequence), thereby representing an incomplete glycosylated precursor of the enzyme moving from the rough endoplasmic reticulum to the Golgi apparatus. The other and larger form, apparently containing sialic acid as a terminal sugar residue, is probably the mature precursor, reglycosylated in the Golgi apparatus and destined for the plasma membrane. Similar results have been obtained in the pig[42,43] also for glucoamylase and lactase, and in humans.[20,38,44]

During its passage through the Golgi complex, intestinal brush border hydrolases are also glycosylated with O-linked oligosaccharides.[45,46] Actually, a mucin-type *O*-glycosidic linkage of the oligosaccharide chains is suggested by the presence in the disaccharidases of substantial amounts of *N*-acetylgalactosamine and blood group specificity as well[47-49] (Fig. 2). Sucrase-isomaltase, purified from rat intestinal microvillous membranes, contains a large proportion of asparagine-linked oligosaccharides, mainly of the complex type, with only a small amount of the high mannose type and a significant proportion of high molecular weight glycopeptides, which probably contain at least some *O*-glycosidically linked carbohydrate.[49]

The trehalase differs from the other brush border glycosidases in several respects. It is composed of a single type of polypeptide chain, considerably smaller than those of other glycosidases (Table 1)[50,51] and most likely anchored to the brush border membrane via phosphatidylinositol.[52]

Control

The activity and the structure of the disaccharidases are modulated by various mechanisms through the multistep process of synthesis and migration of the enzyme up to the brush border membrane and are influenced by various fac-

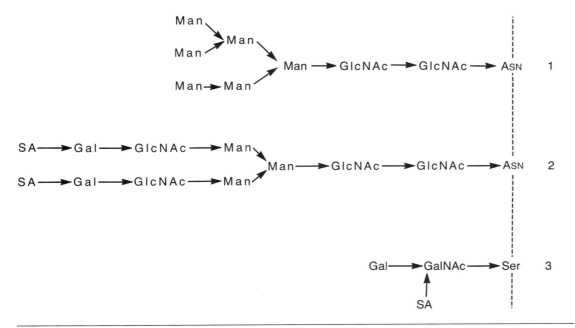

FIGURE 2 Two classes of linkage between the oligosaccharide chains and the polypeptide chains are present in glycoproteins. In the *N*-glycosidic linkage, high mannose (1) and complex (2) or hybrid-type oligosaccharide chains are *N*-glycosidically linked to an asparagine residue of the polypeptide. The mucin type *O*-glycosidic linkage is characterized by a linkage between an *N*-acetyl galactosamine residue and a serine or threonine residue on the polypeptide (3). Human blood group substances belong to this class of glycoproteins. A single glycoprotein may contain both simple and complex oligosaccharide chains, or it may contain both complex *N*-linked chains and *O*-linked chains. (Asn = asparagine; Ser = serine; GlcNAc = *N*-acetyl-D-glucosamine; GalNAc = *N*-acetyl-D-galactosamine; Man = mannose; Gal = galactose; SA = sialic acid.) (From Hannover and Lennarz[346].)

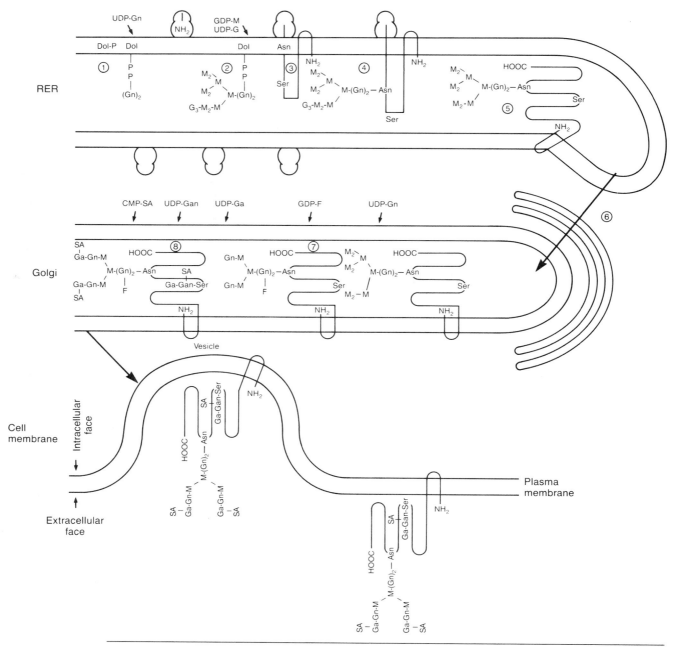

FIGURE 3 Proposed pathway for the synthesis and processing of *N*- and *O*-linked membrane glycoproteins. Abbreviations: Dol-P = dicholphosphate; M = mannose; G = glucose; F = fucose; Gn = *N*-acetylglucosamine; SA = sialic acid; Ga = galactose; Gan = *N*-acetyl galactosamine; RER = rough endoplasmic reticulum. Concomitant with the assembly of the oligosaccharide lipid and its saccharide unit facing the lumen of the endoplasmic reticulum (steps 1 and 2), the membrane protein destined to be both *N*- and *O*-glycosylated at asparagine (Asn) and serine (Ser) sites, respectively, is inserted through the endoplasmic reticulum (step 3). As the polypeptide elongation proceeds to a point where the asparagine residue is accessible to the luminal face of the RER, transfer of the oligosaccharide chain to the polypeptide occurs (step 4). All glucose residues are removed from the oligosaccharide chain; the protein in the RER is essentially complete if it is destined to be a glycoprotein containing a simple polymannose chain (step 5). The next stages involve migration of the glycoprotein to the Golgi complex (step 6) where the oligosaccharide chains of glycoproteins destined to have complex chains are modified by mannosidase removal of mannose residues and addition of *N*-acetyl glucosamine and fucosyl residues (step 7). In the final stage the capping sugars are added to complete the complex-type chain (step 8). Presumably concurrently *O*-linked chain assembly occurs by addition of *N*-acetyl galactosamine to a serine residue in the polypeptide followed by addition of galactose and sialic acid. Subsequent steps for secretory proteins involve packaging of the protein in secretory granules and the fusion of these granules in the plasma membrane, leading to deposition of the glycoprotein outside the cell surface. In the case of membrane proteins, as shown in the figure, the same mechanism probably operates, except that the polypeptide ends up as an integral component of the plasma membrane with its carbohydrate facing the external surface of the cell. (Modified from Hannover and Lennarz[346].)

tors, such as age of the animal, degree of differentiation of the cell along the villus, and its proximal versus distal location in the intestine. Studies on control mechanisms of disaccharidase activity at the gene level have been done on sucrase-isomaltase during development. Both in rabbits and humans, sucrase-isomaltase is most likely controlled at the transcriptional level, as the enzyme activities have a high correlation coefficient with the level of sucrase-isomaltase mRNA.[53-54]

Changes in glycosylation may also control the activity of the disaccharidases by affecting both enzyme activity[55] and rate of transport of the protein from the intracellular to brush border membrane location. The disaccharidases of the fetal intestine are structurally different from their corresponding adult enzymes, and this difference often relates to a different carbohydrate structure.[56,57] It has also been suggested that the decline of rat lactase at weaning may be related to changes of the glycosylation of the protein (see Development).

The disaccharidase structure and hence activity are also controlled by enterocyte life span and by degradation due to proteolytic (intraluminal) enzymes. Disaccharidase activities are low or absent in crypt cells and increase gradually as the cells migrate up to the tip of the villi. Brush border enzymes are continuously synthesized along the crypt-villus axis.[58] The turnover of brush border enzymes is in fact much faster than cell turnover.[59,60] The location of the onset of synthesis and the rate of turnover might condition the levels of enzyme activity along the crypt-villus axis. In the human small intestine, lactase, sucrase, and glucoamylase are most active near the middle region of the villi. A decrease in activity, particularly of sucrase, was found at the top of the villi.[61] This might be due to an increased digestion rate caused by pancreatic enzymes.[62] In addition, variations in the structure of microvillar disaccharidases may occur along the intestine[63] and the villus during the life cycle of the enterocyte.[64] The rat brush border sucrase-isomaltase complex

does not turn over as a unit, but its subunits appear to be degraded at differential rates, and at least part of the carbohydrate moiety may be degraded more rapidly than the protein component.[65] The sucrase-isomaltase complex loses its sucrase subunit on the top of the villus[66] and in the distal part of the intestine.[67] In the human intestine, lactase-glycosyl ceramidase and sucrase-isomaltase attain their highest level in jejunum, and activity decreases toward the proximal and distal ends of the small intestine, whereas glucoamylase increases along the distal ileum.[68,69]

Several factors, such as dietary components and hormones, may alter the activity of brush border enzymes by varying their synthesis or degradation rate and probably also regulate their structure. The hormonal and dietary control of the levels of intestinal brush border enzymes during various developmental stages and during adult life is complex and far from being understood.[70-72]

Role in Normal Digestion

Table 2 summarizes the substrate specificities of the brush border disaccharidases. The enzymatic activities of the beta-glycosidase, lactase, and glycosyl ceramidase are involved in the digestion of the milk nutrients, lactose and glycosyl ceramides.[73] The enzymatic activities of the two alpha-glycosidase complexes, on the contrary, are involved in the digestion of plant carbohydrates, sucrose and starch, which appear in the diet of most humans after weaning.

In the average western diet, starch provides approximately 50 percent of absorbable carbohydrates, but disaccharides (mainly sucrose and lactose) are also important nutrients. In starch two types of polysaccharides are present, amylose and amylopectin. Amylose has a linear structure and is made up of alpha-1,4-linked glucose units. Amylopectin has a branched structure; the majority of the glucose residues are connected

TABLE 2
Types of Major Intestinal Disaccharidases: Representative Data on the
Substrate Specificities*

Glucoamylase-(maltase)-1 + Glucoamylase-(maltase)-2 = **the glucoamylase complex** (EC 3.2.1.20) = (the "heat-stable" maltases)
  The two subunits have similar, but probably not quite identical substrate specificities. They split 1,4-α-glucopyranosidic bonds from the nonreducing ends of amylose, amylopectin, glycogen, and straight-chain 1,4-α-glucopyranosyl oligomers, including maltose. Minor 1,6-α-glucopyranosidase activity.

Sucrase-(maltase) (EC 3.2.1.48) + Isomaltase-(maltase) (EC 3.2.1.10) = **the sucrase-isomaltase complex** = (the "heat-labile" maltases)
  Both subunits split maltose, maltotriose, maltitol (Semenza and Balthazar, unpublished), α-F-glucopyranoside and (less well) aryl-α-glucopyranosides. In addition, the sucrase subunit splits sucrose and turanose; the isomaltase subunit splits the 1,6-α-glucopyranosyl bonds in isomaltose, isomaltulose (palatinose), panose, and a number of branched limit α-dextrins.

Trehalase (EC 3.2.1.28)
  α,α^1-Trehalose, 6,6'dideoxy-α,α^1-trehalose, α- and β-F-glucopyranoside (tested on renal trehalase)

Lactase (EC 3.2.1.23) + Glycosyl ceramidase (EC 3.2.1.45-46) (= phlorizin hydrolase, EC 3.2.1.62) = **the β-glycosidase complex**
  A number of β-glycosides: α- and β-lactose, 3-(β-D-galactosido)-D-glucose, 6-β-D-galactosido)-D-glucose, aryl-β-galactopyranosides, aryl-β-glucopyranosides, methyl-β-galactopyranoside. The "lactase" subunit preferentially splits β-glycosides with hydrophilic aglycones (typically lactose, but also cellobiose, cellotriose, and -tetraose, and also, but much less, cellulose, whereas the "glycosyl ceramidase" subunit preferentially splits β-glycosides with a large, hydrophobic aglycone (typically, galactosyl- and glycosyl-β-ceramides, phlorizin, and other aryl-β-glycosides).

*From Semenza and Auricchio.[21]

by 1,4-alpha-glucosidic bonds (the linear chains), and the branch points are made by 1,6-alpha-glucosidic linkages. In the digestive tract, starch is hydrolyzed to glucose by salivary and pancreatic alpha-amylases, the latter being present in solution in the intestinal lumen (but also adsorbed at the surface of brush border membrane), plus the alpha-glucosidases of intestinal mucosa. The final (limit) products resulting from amylose hydrolysis by alpha-amylase in vitro are maltose and maltotriose[74]; those from amylopectin are glucose (in small amounts), maltose, maltotriose, and branched dextrins (Fig. 4).[75-79]

In humans older than 1 year, the alpha-amylase activity of duodenal juice after a test meal is very high. The amylopectin of a test meal, consisting of more than 5,000 glucose units, is digested at the end of the duodenum into oligosaccharides composed of an average of three glucose units.[80] The major components of this carbohydrate mixture are maltose, maltotriose, and branched dextrins with both alpha-1,4 and one or more alpha-1,6 branching links (isomaltose is not produced in the digestion of starch by alpha-amylase).[80] Maltose, maltotriose, and at least some of these branched dextrins must be considered as limit products of the alpha-amylolysis in vivo, which are completely hydrolyzed into glucose by the combined action of the glucoamylase and the sucrase-isomaltase complexes (Fig. 5).[81-83]

Although intraluminal hydrolysis of free starch does proceed rapidly in vivo, the starch in most staple foods (wheat, corn, oats, potatoes) may escape complete digestion and absorption in the small intestine and thus reach the colon. After an oral load of 100 g of flour from different sources, the percentage of starch not absorbed by the healthy small bowel has been estimated to be 5 to 20 percent. The type of starch and the protein content of the flour appear to be important[84-88] (see also Disaccharide Malabsorption and Intolerance; Disaccharidase Deficiency).

Sucrase hydrolyzes maltose, maltotriose, and sucrose; isomaltase hydrolyzes maltose, isomaltose, and the 1,6-alpha-glucopyranosyl bonds occurring in alpha-amylase limit dextrins. The sucrase-isomaltase complex also hydrolyzes alpha-glucosides, with up to six glucose residues.[81] The maltase-glucoamylase complex hydrolyzes to glucose not only maltose and maltotriose, but also starch, glycogen, and related oligosaccharides from their nonreducing ends. This enzyme has very little, if any, isomaltase activity.[82,83,89-91] The human enzyme[92] has maximal affinity for a medium-sized (n = 9) 1,4-alpha-glucan, decreasing with changes in the length of the polysaccharide chain.

The sucrase-isomaltase complex accounts for all of the sucrase activity of the brush border membrane, for almost all or all of the isomaltase (1,6-alpha-oligosaccharidase) activity, and for about 80 percent of the maltase activities. In contrast, the maltase-glucoamylase complex accounts for a small percentage (if any) of the isomaltase activity, for about 20 percent of the maltase activity, and for all of the glucoamylase activity.

The digestion of branched alpha-amylase dextrins is of major importance from a nutritional point of view, since these dextrins account for approximately 25 percent of starch. The hydrolysis by brush border alpha-glucosidases of the shorter alpha-limit dextrins arising from branched regions of starch is shown in Figure 5.

In contrast to the hydrolysis of other oligosaccharides, that of lactose is the rate-limiting step for the absorption of this sugar.[93] Even in apparently normal individuals mucosal lactase activity is the lowest of all disaccharidases. The monosaccharides arising from the hydrolysis of lactose never appear in significant amounts at the luminal side of the brush border, indicating that the transport system(s) for its component monosaccharides, glucose and galactose, is (are) capable of completely absorbing the hydrolysis products presented to it.[94]

Development

In Mammals. At birth, the only disaccharidase activities present in the brush border membranes of most mammals are those of the beta-glucosidase and the maltase-

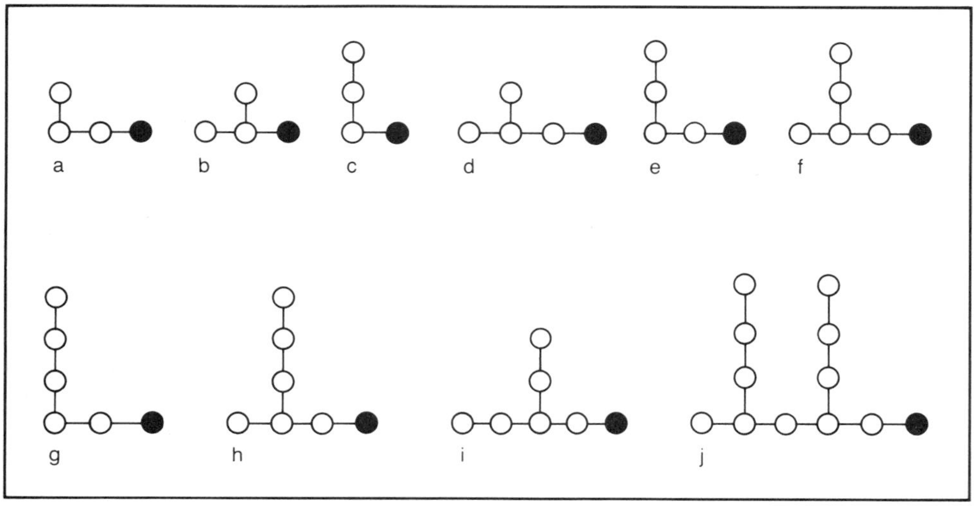

FIGURE 4 Branched limit dextrins from the alpha-amylolysis of amylopectin in vitro. Open circle = nonreducing glucose unit; closed circle = reducing glucose unit; thin bond = 1,4-alpha-glucopyranosidic bond; thick bond = 1,6-alpha-glucopyranosidic bond. (From Auricchio et al.[347] Reproduced with permission of S. Karger AG, Basel.)

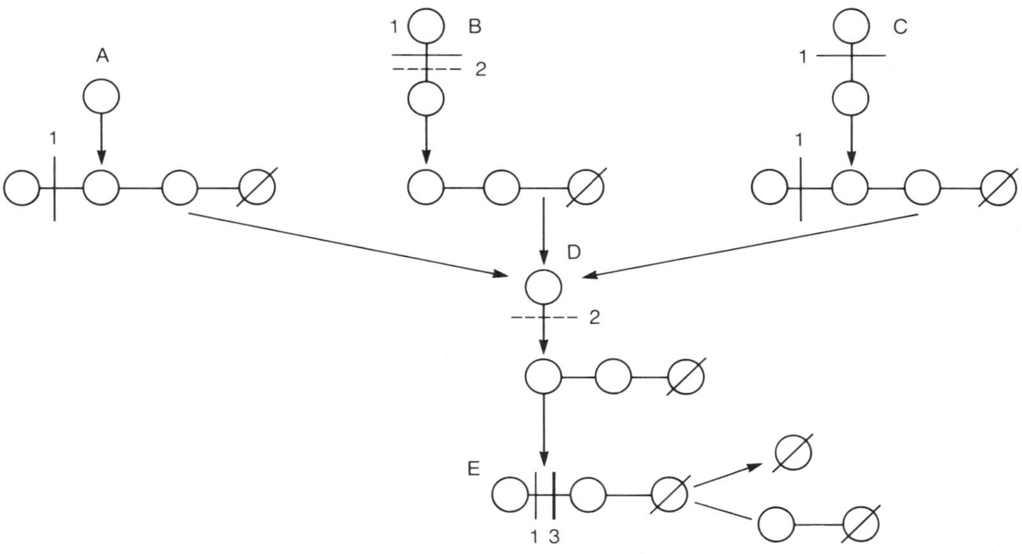

FIGURE 5 Hydrolysis by glucoamylase and by the sucrase-isomaltase complex of the shortest limit dextrins from exhaustive digestion of starch by alpha-amylase. Open circle = nonreducing glucose unit: open circle with slash = reducing glucose unit; bond = 1,4-alpha-glucopyranosidic bond; arrow = 1,6-alpha-glucopyranosidic bond. *A* is 6-alpha-D-glucopyranosyl-maltotetraose; *B* is 6-alpha-D-maltopyranosyl-maltotriose; *C* is 6-alpha-D-maltopyranosyl-maltotetraose; *D* is 6-alpha-D-glucopyranosyl-maltotriose; *E* is maltotriose. 1 (*thin bond*) = bond hydrolyzed by glucoamylase; 2 (*broken bond*) = bond hydrolyzed by isomaltase; 3 (*thick bond*) = bond hydrolyzed by sucrase. Hence, glucoamylase hydrolyzes the pentasaccharides (*A* and *B*) and hexasaccharide (*C*) to the tetrasaccharide (*D*). Isomaltase is also able to split *B* into *D*. The further degradation of *D* is accomplished mainly by the sucrase-isomaltase complex, with the isomaltase (and very slowly the sucrase) subunit converting *D* into glucose and maltotriose and the sucrase subunit (assisted by glucoamylase) converting maltotriose into maltose and glucose. (From Auricchio.[348])

glucoamylase. The sucrase-isomaltase activities develop later during extrauterine life in the rat[95] and rabbit[96] from days 15 to 18 to approximately days 25 to 30, i.e., at the time of weaning, when an active sucrase-isomaltase complex first appears in crypt cells and then progresses gradually to a uniform distribution along the villus.[97-99] At the same time lactase activity begins to decline; its level in adulthood is 10 percent or less of that at birth.

Initiation of the postnatal ontogenetic events in the (rat) gastrointestinal (GI) tract is probably determined by a genetic program,[100,101] whereas the terminal phase of intestinal development seems to be influenced by environmental factors such as nutrients and hormones.[102-104] Many findings in the literature argue against adaptation to dietary lactose as a controlling factor in decreasing lactase levels at weaning.[105-109]

The development of alpha-glucosidase activities is subjected to hormonal control. Cortisone-like steroids,[99,110-112] thyroxine,[110] insulin,[113] and epidermal growth factor[114] can induce their precocious appearance in the rat, rabbit, and mouse. A combined effect of glucocorticoids and thyroxine on the maturational patterns of lactase was demonstrated.[115-117] Thyroxine accelerates the decline of lactase activity,[118] and thyroidectomy at 6 days in the suckling rat results in persistence of high lactase activity.[117] Organ culture of fetal and neonatal small intestinal explants has also been used as a model to study the effect of hormones, growth factors, and nutrients on the development and regulation of brush border disaccharidases.[119-126]

In Humans. The developmental pattern of disaccharidases is different in humans from that in other mammals. Humans may retain high lactase activity in adulthood and develop alpha-glucosidase activities, inclusive of the glucoamylase, during fetal life.[127,128] Humans are therefore able to digest at birth not only lactose, but also disaccharides from plant sources.

Lactase activity appears in the small intestine during the third month of gestation. Mucosal enzyme activity rises gradually between the eighth and thirty-fourth weeks of gestation and then more rapidly until term. In neonates at term, lactase levels are two to four times higher than those found in infants between 2 and 11 months of age.[128-132]

The intestine of the 28- to 30-week-old preterm newborn shows some immaturity from both the morphologic and the functional point of view. However, there is evidence of accelerated morphologic and functional maturation of the intestine of the preterm newborn during extrauterine life.[127,128] Within the first week of life, preterm infants show a rapid postnatal rise in lactase activity.[128,133] Furthermore, most premature infants do not seem to suffer from lactose intolerance. Although incomplete lactose absorption in the small bowel occurs in preterm and term infants, adequate colonic salvage of malabsorbed carbohydrates is actually achieved by colonic flora.[134-139]

Alpha-glucosidase activities throughout fetal life are comparable to those of the adult intestine, with a marked increase at term.[128-132] In full-term newborns, the high level of glucoamylase activity[127] suggests that, at this age, the intestine can hydrolyze glucose polymers.[140] Alpha-amylase activity in the duodenal lumen does not reach normal adult levels until well after birth.[141,142] As a consequence of the low levels of alpha-amylase activity in duodenal juice, in most infants younger than 6 months of age, the duodenal hydrolysis of amylopectin is incomplete as compared with that in older infants.[80] Nevertheless, young infants may absorb limited amounts of starch and glucose polymers.[143-146] At this age intestinal glucoamylase, together with salivary amylase, which retains a significant amount of its activity in the intestine, may represent alternative pathways for glucose polymer hydrolysis during the period of pancreatic amylase deficiency.[147] Furthermore, in the young infant the colonic flora undoubtedly plays a significant role in salvaging unabsorbed starch and glucose polymers.

DISACCHARIDE MALABSORPTION AND INTOLERANCE; DISACCHARIDASE DEFICIENCY

The largest fraction of dietary disaccharides (and starch) is normally hydrolyzed and absorbed in the proximal portion of the small intestine. If they are not, their presence in the intestinal lumen in large quantities provides an osmotic load that stimulates peristalsis. Ileal flow rates may then exceed the critical levels, above which the right colon propels fluid onward,[148-150] resulting in the passage of frequent fluid stools, The unabsorbed sugar may in part be excreted unchanged in the feces and in part undergo bacterial degradation in the large intestine, causing fermentative diarrhea.

Sugar malabsorption is the failure to normally digest and absorb carbohydrates, with or without signs of clinical intolerance. Sugar intolerance refers to abdominal symptoms that result from sugar malabsorption such as flatulence, borborygmus, abdominal distention, pain, and diarrhea. *Intolerance* and *malabsorption* should thus not be used as synonyms.

Whether sugar malabsorption produces symptoms[151-154] depends not only on the intestinal digestive and absorptive capacity, but also on additional factors, such as the quantity of the ingested sugar, the rate of gastric emptying, the response of the small intestine to the osmotic load, the metabolic activity of colonic bacteria, and the absorptive capacities of the colon, principally for water and short-chain fatty acids.[155]

Unabsorbed carbohydrates, when present in the distal small intestine, inhibit gastric emptying and accelerate small intestinal transit, because of decreased water and sodium absorption.[156-161] All these factors, together with reduced digestion of the disaccharide, combine to reduce monosaccharide absorption, with consequent little or no increase in plasma levels of insulin, C-peptide, and gastric inhibitory peptide (GIP).[156,162] Accelerated duodenal-ileal transit may also contribute to the malabsorption of unrelated nutrients, such as starch or fat.[87,163,164]

Colonic bacterial flora salvage some of dietary carbohydrates not digested and absorbed by the small bowel through fermentation to gases (hydrogen, methane, and carbon dioxide) or to lactic, acetic, propionic, and butyric acids. These acids are readily absorbed from and/or metabolized by the colon.[165,166]

In normal adults it has been calculated that the colon may salvage up to 20 to 25 g of lactose and up to 50 g of starch[167-170] without changing the stool content of volatile fatty acids and lactic acid or its bacterial mass.[151,156] After the first year of life, children are able to absorb almost completely 170 g per square meter of body surface of cooked wheat or potato starch. Adaptation of the colonic flora to a dietary carbohydrate load may further increase this salvaging capacity.[171-173] Osmotic diarrhea occurs when this capacity is either reduced (i.e., by treatment with antibiotics)[174] or exceeded owing to the excessive amount of unhydrolyzed carbohydrate and of short-chain fatty acids and lactic acid generated within the colon.

In young infants with carbohydrate malabsorption, passage of carbohydrate content through the small intestine and colon is normally more rapid than in adults and the diarrhea is more severe. In adults abdominal discomfort and borborygmus may occur without diarrhea, principally because of a smaller dietary load of sugar in relation to body weight as well as a greater time for reabsorption within the colon.

We should also distinguish between disaccharide malabsorption and disaccharidase deficiency: the latter is diagnosed by the measurement of disaccharidase activity in homogenates of small intestinal biopsies obtained only from the proximal small intestine and therefore gives little information on the ability of the total bowel mucosa to hydrolyze the disaccharide. Whether the disaccharidase deficiency may lead to carbohydrate malabsorption depends on the severity of the deficiency and on the length of the gut involved.

Diagnosis of Carbohydrate Malabsorption and Carbohydrate Intolerance

Oral tolerance tests are used routinely for the diagnosis of carbohydrate malabsorption. Their interpretation is based on the extent of the blood glucose increase following oral administration of the sugar, on the appearance of gases (mainly hydrogen) in the expired air, or on the presence in feces of the malabsorbed carbohydrates and/or of their fermentation products by the colonic flora. (The amount of sugar administered in the oral tolerance tests is usually much larger than that present in a meal: 2 g of sugar per kilogram of body weight, maximum 50 g.) The first two tests measure the capacity of the small bowel to normally digest and absorb a carbohydrate load, the third one in addition provides information on the efficiency of colonic mechanisms to compensate for small bowel failure.

After sucrose and lactose tolerance testing, a peak rise in serum glucose of less than 20 to 25 mg per deciliter (during the first 90 minutes) is diagnostic of sugar malabsorption.[175,176] Accuracy of the test is improved if capillary and not venous blood is sampled.[177] The rise in blood glucose following administration of the disaccharide is best compared with that observed after administration of the component monosaccharides.[175,176] Both false-positive and false-negative results are reported in children with either lactose or sucrose oral tolerance testing in 20 to 30 percent of cases.[178] It is imperative that the child have no diarrhea at the time of the test.

The blood glucose increase following oral administration of a sugar provides no information, however, as to whether the sugar has been absorbed completely or not. Incomplete absorption can be deduced only by measuring parameters directly related to the carbohydrates reaching the colon; the carbohydrates will be degraded there by the resident microflora, thus releasing hydrogen that is carried via the circulation to be excreted in expired breath.

Indeed, measurement of the increase in breath hydrogen after a sugar load (the breath hydrogen test) is the most reliable and also the least invasive procedure for measuring carbohydrate malabsorption even in children.[179-182] A peak rise in breath hydrogen greater than 20 or 10[182,183] parts per million over the fasting baseline value after ingestion of a carbohydrate load or a carbohydrate-containing meal indicates sugar malabsorption. No antibiotic should be given before or during the test. False-negative hydrogen breath tests due to a colonic bacterial flora unable to produce hydrogen from unabsorbed carbohydrates amount to 2 to 9 percent.[184-186] Excretion of hydrogen in breath after a test meal may be quantitated by comparing it with hydrogen excretion after a dose of lactulose, which is assumed to be malabsorbed completely. This method has been recently validated in vivo in humans.[151] When the colon fails to compensate fully for the carbohydrate malabsorption in the small intestine, the sugars themselves and the products of their bacterial breakdown (such as lactic acid or volatile fatty acids) appear in the liquid stool.

Malabsorbed carbohydrates can be detected in feces as reducing substances,[1] by chromatographic methods, or by measuring fecal excretion of 13C-enriched sugars.[146,187]

The diagnosis of carbohydrate intolerance in an individual patient requires the demonstration that the symptoms are dependent on the presence in foods of the offending disaccharide.

Diagnosis of Disaccharidase Deficiency

The general principle for the assay of the disaccharidase activities in total homogenates of proximal small intestinal biopsies is the determination by either D-glucose-oxidase[188,189] or D-glucose-dehydrogenase[190] of the glucose released from the substrate.

Disaccharidases may also be measured by quantitative immunoelectrophoresis of proteins from single, unfractioned, small intestinal biopsies against a specific brush border protein antiserum.[191] A 30 percent variation in disaccharidase activities between assays performed on simultaneously biopsied specimens from the same area of distal duodenum in the same individual has been reported.[192]

The enzymatic activities are usually expressed either as units per gram of wet mucosa or as units per gram of protein (1 gram of mucosa wet weight contains approximately 100 mg of protein). There are no advantages in one way of expressing the results compared to the other. "Normal" enzymatic values are usually defined as those of the histologically normal small intestinal mucosa.[193-195] Disaccharidase "deficiency" is defined as the reduction of enzyme activity(ies) to levels lower than the normal mean plus at least two standard deviations.[195,196]

CONGENITAL SUCRASE-ISOMALTASE DEFICIENCY

Molecular Defect

Congenital sucrase-isomaltase deficiency is characterized by complete or almost complete lack of sucrase activity, a decrease of maltase activity to about one-third of the normal level, and a very marked reduction of isomaltase activity.[10] The residual maltase activity is mainly or totally due to the maltase-glucoamylase complex. The disease is a heterogeneous condition: Whereas all patients lack sucrase, some have only traces of isomaltase and others have reduced but still conspicuous isomaltase activity.[10,197-202] Glucoamylase activity is normal in most patients,[202] but reduction in the amount[197,199-201] and/or change in the sedimentation properties[203] of the enzyme have been observed in some cases.

Many steps in the complex chain of events coding for the expression of the enzyme on the brush border membrane and the regulation of a gigantic polypeptide chain such as the sucrase-isomaltase may be affected by a mutation. Interference may therefore derive with the synthesis, the membrane insertion, the glycosylation, the homing to the brush border membrane, the digestion by proteases of the enzyme, causing the lack of or appearance of an abnormal sucrase-isomaltase molecule. The possibility that in congenital sucrase-isomaltase deficiency the glucoamylase complex may also be affected indicates a relationship in the biologic regulations of the two alpha-glucosidase heterodimeric complexes.

Early observations have demonstrated the absence of sucrase-isomaltase activity and of the corresponding protein bands in gel electrophoresis of brush border membranes,[199-201,204] with the presence of a cross-reacting protein in the enterocytes of many of these patients.[197,199,205] The most recent studies in fact suggest that in many cases the disease is due to defective homing of pro-sucrase-isomaltase on the way to the brush border membrane.

Experimental models relevant to this problem have been elaborated in the last years, giving origin to a vast literature on the subject. Cellular mutations may influence processing and intracellular transport of glycoproteins.[206,207] On the other side, inhibitors of the biosynthesis and the processing of oligosaccharide chains[208] have demonstrated that normal glycosylation of disaccharidases is necessary for sorting of the enzymes in the brush border membrane. Tunicamycin, an antibiotic that inhibits *N*-linked high mannose glycosylation of proteins, greatly reduced the expression on brush border membrane of the disaccharidases in pig small intestine, and the newly synthesized enzymes were degraded intracellularly.[209]

Monensin, which interferes with complex glycosylation of lactase in the Golgi membranes, affects the further transport of the enzyme to the microvillous membrane in humans.[39] Similar studies have been done on other hydrolases of the kidney microvillous membrane.[210] It is also well known that there is a correlation of glycosylation forms with position in amino acid sequence of secreted and membrane glycoproteins,[211] so that a single substitution of amino acid may interfere with the processing and intracellular transport of disaccharidases. Finally disaccharidase transport from the rough endoplasmic reticulum to the Golgi apparatus and to the brush border membrane is slower than for other brush border hydrolases; this absorption suggests that the major disaccharidases have a complex biosynthetic mechanism on the way to the brush border membrane, possibly mediated by selective transport receptors.[212]

Defective homing of pro-sucrase-isomaltase between Golgi and brush border membranes was first reported by Hauri's group in one case of congenital sucrase-isomaltase deficiency, with reduced but still fairly high isomaltase activity[18]; at electron microscopy anti-sucrase-isomaltase antibodies revealed the presence of an antigen in the Golgi membranes. As other brush border hydrolases were normal, this observation may indicate a mutation in pro-sucrase-isomaltase which selectively hampers (by whatever mechanism) its homing to the brush border membrane. This conclusion is strengthened by pulse-labeled experiments using monoclonal antibodies which revealed the high mannose form only.[19,20] Indeed, the high-mannose form of pro-sucrase-isomaltase has reduced enzymatic activity as compared to the fully processed form, at least in the pig,[55] and, in patients with defective homing, is reported to be more easily degraded.[20]

More recently it has been confirmed that the disease is in most cases probably due to minor alterations of the protein (point mutations?), leading to transport-incompetent and functionally altered sucrase-isomaltase. By studying intestinal biopsies of eight patients by means of monoclonal antibodies to sucrase-isomaltase, it has in fact been demonstrated that all patients expressed the high-mannose enzyme, but its maturation and intracellular transport were blocked at different stages along the biosynthetic pathway. Three phenotypes were found: one in which the enzyme accumulated in the endoplasmic reticulum, one in which the enzyme was arrested and degraded in the Golgi apparatus, and one in which altered sucrase-isomaltase was transported to the brush border but was also missorted to other organelles.[19] (For a discussion of other potentially possible molecular defects see reference 21.)

Pathogenesis of Starch Malabsorption

On ingestion of starch, infants and young children with congenital sucrase-isomaltase deficiency get fermentative diarrhea of a considerably milder degree than upon ingestion of sucrose.[7,8] Intraluminal alpha-amylolysis of amylopectin is normal in these patients.[202]

Starch malabsorption is a consequence of deficient enzymatic activities of the sucrase-isomaltase complex which are involved in starch digestion—that is, the maltase, oligo 1,4-, and 1,6-glucosidase. This enzymatic defect impairs the mucosa's ability to digest the end and intermediary products of alpha-amylolysis of starch such as maltose, maltotriose, and low and high molecular weight branched dextrins. Nevertheless, the residual capacity of the mucosa to hydrolyze the alpha-1,4 glucanes arising from alpha-amylolysis, mainly due to glucoamylase complex, is still sufficient to ensure their adequate digestion.

The fact that in young patients starch is better tolerated than sucrose is attributable to a low content in 1,6-alpha-glucosyl

bonds of starches; to the reduced, but not necessarily absent, 1,6-alpha-glucosidase ("isomaltase") activity in these patients; to the salvaging role of colonic flora; and to a sufficient residual capacity to hydrolyze 1,4-alpha-glucopyranosidic bonds. In patients during the first few months of life the starch malabsorption is more severe than in older subjects, as a consequence of the physiologically incomplete intraluminal hydrolysis of the polysaccharide.[80]

Inheritance and Incidence

The disease occurs in families and is inherited as an autosomal recessive trait.[213] In small intestinal biopsies of heterozygotes, sucrase and isomaltase levels are intermediate between those of the patients and those of normal controls, with an abnormal sucrase-to-lactase ratio (in subjects with persistent high lactase activity in adult life[214]). Hereditary sucrase-isomaltase deficiency is probably rare in most human populations, as only some 200 cases have been reported up to 1984.[215]

Welsh et al found a 2 percent frequency of heterozygotes in a large series of small intestinal biopsies from white American subjects.[214] The disease is more common among the Eskimos of Greenland and Canada and in Canadian Indians, the reported incidence of homozygotes varying between 4 and 10 percent.[216-218] Owing to a certain selection in sampling, the true prevalence of the disease is certainly lower than the reported value.[219] The high frequency of the disease in some populations could be the result either of their high degree of inbreeding or of an unidentified biologic advantage produced by the mutation in populations who do not traditionally eat foods containing sucrose. Such advantage might be related to some role of sucrase-isomaltase other than its digestive function. An example of this possibility is the notion that, in the rabbit, the sucrase-isomaltase complex may serve as an intestinal receptor for an enteropathogenic *Escherichia coli*.[220]

Clinical Presentation

Symptoms appear when sucrose or starch-dextrins are added to the diet. Breast-fed infants or bottle-fed infants receiving lactose-containing formulas only remain well. Some milk formulas contain sucrose so that artificially fed infants can ingest sucrose from birth. The clinical manifestations in infants are watery osmotic-fermentative diarrhea, which may lead to dehydration and malnutrition and even to occasional vomiting and mild steatorrhea. Failure to thrive and other symptoms are severe in the young child. However, if sucrose ingestion is minimal or delayed until 6 months or later, stools may first appear soft with only a small fluid content that soaks into the diaper. There is a tendency to spontaneous improvement of symptoms with age; in particular, the starch tolerance improves after the first years of life.[221] The symptoms eventually persisting in adult life may be limited to some increase in bowel frequency and to minor abdominal distention, although episodes of diarrhea associated with large sucrose intake may still occur. In spite of this spontaneous favorable evolution, it is important that this condition be diagnosed as early as possible, so that the normal development of the child can be ensured by removal of sucrose from the diet.[222] Clinical patterns of various severity may be present in different members of the same family. In biopsy-proven cases of congenital sucrase-isomaltase deficiency, even a persistent challenge with large daily amounts of sucrose may fail to alter the stools, presumably because of a good colonic absorption.[1]

The diagnosis can be missed in children with chronic diarrhea,[222] particularly in older children with a mild clinical presentation and normal growth and development.[223] In adults the disease is a possible cause of refractory diarrhea or GI complaints.[224] Many adults with this disorder have symptoms dating back to childhood, but occasionally the symptoms may have appeared as late as at the time of puberty.[225-228]

Diagnostic Evaluation

The diagnosis is based on the demonstration of osmotic-fermentative diarrhea, with increased fecal excretion of lactic acid, elicited by sucrose and starch dextrins in the diet. A sucrose tolerance test will produce a flat blood glucose curve, with acid watery diarrhea and the presence of sucrose in the feces, whereas the absorption of a mixture of glucose and fructose is normal. The sucrose hydrogen breath test demonstrates excessive hydrogen excretion in the breath.[181,229,230] In only one study of a previously diagnosed patient did a sucrose tolerance test not show an abnormal breath hydrogen level.[231] The final diagnosis should be made, however, by demonstrating the absence of sucrase and isomaltase in small intestinal biopsies of the distal duodenum or proximal jejunum. The mucosa is normal histologically, and lactase levels should be within normal limits in those populations without a high incidence of late-onset hypolactasia.

In congenital sucrase-isomaltase deficiency, sucrase activity is absent or nearly so, isomaltase activity is either absent or heavily reduced, and maltase activity is severely reduced[10] when compared to normal alpha-glucosidase activities. In most cases, glucoamylase activity is normal. In the assay of glucoamylase with glycogen or high molecular weight soluble starch used as the substrates, it is necessary to inactivate (e.g., with chelating agents) pancreatic alpha-amylase, which is adsorbed on the small intestinal mucosa; if maltose is used as the substrate, the sucrase-isomaltase complex must first be heat-inactivated.[232,233]

Treatment

Most patients require dietary treatment, which should be more rigid in childhood than in adult life. Treatment in the first year of life consists in the elimination of sucrose, glucose polymers, and starch from the diet; symptoms subside within a few days. In infancy, care should be taken regarding the carbohydrate content of commercial milk preparations and also of medications such as cough or sedative syrups. Adult patients become expert in adjusting their own diet to the necessary degree of sucrose restriction. Restriction of starch intake is usually unnecessary after 2 to 3 years of age, although excessive amounts should be avoided.

Replacement therapy with sucrase or invertase has been attempted, but sucrose restriction is simpler and less expensive. Patients with congenital sucrase-isomaltase deficiency who intentionally or unintentionally consume sucrose can ameliorate the sucrose malabsorption by subsequently ingesting a small amount of viable yeast cells, preferably on a full stomach.[234] The possibility that dietary fructose increases the sucrase activity in these patients and may therefore be considered as a form of therapy[235] has not been confirmed.[236]

PRIMARY ADULT-TYPE HYPOLACTASIA

Molecular Defect

Human "primary adult-type hypolactasia" is to be compared most probably with the physiologic decline of lactase activity in adult mammals, whereas the "mutated" man with persistent lactase activity should be considered to have persistence of the enzyme into adulthood, as occurs in Caucasians and other human populations. The reason for the low lactase activity in adult mammals may be the synthesis of a defective protein and/or decreased synthesis of a normal protein.

The rate of incorporation of leucine into lactase (relative to the total microvillar protein synthesized) is found to be much lower in adult than in baby rats,[237] suggesting that the decline of lactase activity after weaning is due to a decreased rate of synthesis. The comparison of the intracellular forms of lactase protein in the suckling and adult rat has, on the contrary, suggested that different processing of the protein controls the enzyme activity at different ages.[238] Whereas a major molecular form corresponding to active lactase (170 kDa) is present in the brush border membrane of the suckling rat, a high molecular form corresponding to inactive lactase (300 kDa) is abundant in the intracellular membranes of the adult and faintly present in the suckling. This 300-kDa polypeptide exhibits a high mannose and fucose content. These results have been interpreted as suggesting that the post-weaning decline of lactase activity in rat is associated with changes at the level of lactase protein glycosylation, these changes causing the intracellular accumulation of inactive lactase protein in a high-mannosylated and fucosylated form. It may be hypothesized that the molecule is only weakly transferred to the cell surface and is degraded inside the cell by endogenous protease(s).

The level of lactase activity at weaning may also be regulated by the enterocytic life span. Parallel to the appearance and increase of sucrase activity and the decline of lactase activity taking place at the time of weaning in mammals, the life span of the enterocyte also decreases.[237,239-242] The correlation between the decline of intestinal lactase and the shortened life span of enterocytes is so close[241,242] that the former has been suggested to derive from the latter. In the adult rat membrane lactase appears fairly late in the life of the enterocyte, i.e., when the cell has already proceeded halfway along the length of the villus. In baby rats membrane lactase appears soon after the enterocyte has left the crypt.[97,98] One may in fact speculate that the biosynthetic pathway for lactase may develop later than that of the other disaccharidases during the life cycle of the enterocyte.

Recently it has been reported[243] that in the rat an early fall in lactase activity, between 15 and 23 days of postnatal life, is associated with a shortening of the time available for lactase expression in brush border membranes. A later fall, between 23 and 46 days of life, is due to a decreased rate of synthesis of the enzyme.

The intracellular biosynthesis of lactase has also been studied in suckling and adult rats, by comparing in vivo precursor forms of brush border lactase. The results of the studies on infant rats are consistent with the initial intracellular synthesis of a high molecular weight precursor form of the enzyme with subsequent transfer to brush border sites,[244] thus confirming the results of studies on intestinal explants maintained in culture.[40] Contrary to the results obtained from the suckling rat, the adult rat has multiple forms of lactase in the endoplasmic reticulum and Golgi apparatus which are subsequently transferred to the brush border with little or no post-translational change.[245] In conclusion, studies comparing infant and adult rat lactase suggest that the intestinal mucosa is endowed with a complex system of control, which influences the lactase gene expression with age.

With regard to the human lactase specifically, there is some experimental evidence suggesting that the difference between high and low lactase activity in the adult intestine may be due to differences in the regulation of biosynthesis and/or of degradation of beta-glycosidase. The beta-glycosidase present in the small intestine of subjects presenting with primary adult-type hypolactasia seems in fact to be identical to that present in adults with high lactase activity: It has the same electrophoretic mobility,[246] the same immunologic properties,[246,247] and the same specific lactase[246,247] and phlorizin hydrolase activities.[247,248] These findings are compatible with the hypothesis that lactase persistence in the adult human may be due to a continued synthesis of the infant enzyme, which normally switches off at weaning. On the other side the hypolactasia state might be caused in humans by a block in the transfer of lactase protein from the intracellular site to the microvillous membranes. Studies on the biosynthesis and maturation of human lactase-phlorizin hydrolase in the intestinal mucosa of adults with hypolactasia as well as a detailed comparison of the structure of the various intracellular forms of the enzyme in lactose absorbers compared with lactose malabsorbers will probably help in our understanding the molecular basis of the mutation leading to persistent high lactase activity in some human populations.

Finally, an increased proteolytic degradation may further decrease the lactase both in the postweaning experimental animal and in the human primary adult type of hypolactasia.[249]

Inheritance and Incidence

There are two physiologic human lactase phenotypes after the first years of life, one with high and the other with low lactase activity.[250] The variability of lactase activity represents a genetic polymorphism.[251]

In the great majority of the world's human populations intestinal lactase declines to about 5 to 10 percent of the level

at birth during childhood and adolescence, in a manner analogous to the ontogenetic events occurring in other mammals. Primary adult-type hypolactasia is the most common form of genetically determined disaccharidase deficiency. In some healthy subjects this decline of lactase activity does not occur, and lactase activity and lactose digestion capacity remain high throughout life. The two human phenotypes have been called lactose absorbers and lactose malabsorbers, "high lactose digestion capacity" and "low lactose digestion capacity,"[251] or "non–lactose digestors" and "lactose digestors."[252] The postweaning decline in lactase levels in an individual is not influenced significantly by dietary intake of milk and will occur even if high levels of milk intake are sustained. A genetic basis for the two adult lactase phenotypes was demonstrated when the classic methods of segregation analysis were applied to a large number of families.[253–255] Lactose malabsorbers are homozygous for a recessive autosomal allele, causing the physiologic postweaning decline of lactase activity, whereas lactose absorbers are either heterozygous or homozygous for a dominant allele, preventing the normal postweaning decline of lactase. The three genotypes may also be demonstrated by the trimodal distribution of sucrase/lactase or maltase/lactase activity ratios in intestinal biopsies.[256,257] Additional proof of monogenic inheritance of the lactase phenotypes is represented by the complete concordance of the lactase phenotype among monozygotic twins.[258]

The lactose malabsorber is a highly predominant phenotype in the native populations of Australia and Oceania, East and Southeast Asia, tropical Africa, and the Americas. Predominance of the lactose absorber phenotype is found in two separate groups of populations: (1) central and northern European and (2) nomadic, milk-dependent populations in the arid zones of North Africa and Arabia. Intermediate frequencies of the lactase phenotypes are found in populations originating from mixtures between peoples with high and low frequencies of adult-type hypolactasia. (For a review on the worldwide lactase phenotypes distribution, see reference 251.)

A natural selection in favor of the human phenotype with persistence of high lactase activity is considered a likely cause of the high prevalence of lactase persistence in some populations. According to the "culture historical hypothesis,"[259] the "selective advantage would only develop among peoples, whether farmers or pastoralists, who had a plentiful milk supply, who did not process their milk into products that were low in lactose and for whom milk provided essential nutrients that could not be readily obtained in the other food available." Such environmental conditions, described as "milk dependence," have probably not been present in Europe; it has therefore been supposed that European lactase persistence developed independently of that in nomadic pastoralists.[260,261]

Clinical Presentation

Subjects with primary adult hypolactasia usually reported no feeding problems during infancy, as the enzyme deficiency is not present at birth. The time of onset of the decline may vary among ethnic groups: by age 3 years in blacks and Mexicans and later in northern European and American white groups.[262–268] Prevalence of malabsorption increases with age, with a substantial percentage of individuals demonstrating abnormal tests only as teenagers.[265,266] It is likely that steadily declining lactase levels into and throughout adolescence account for the frequent onset of lactose intolerance in teenagers and young adults.[269-273]

Shortly after drinking milk, lactose malabsorbers usually suffer from abdominal discomfort, bloating, borborygmus, and sometimes loose bowel movements. Children more usually have loose, fluid stools as well as abdominal symptoms.[274-277] The clinical effects of lactose ingestion are related to dose, with a wide variation in response among individuals.[275,278] Many healthy subjects with low lactase activity experience no or only minimal symptoms with ordinary amounts of milk or other lactose-containing foods. The relationship of symptoms to milk ingestion may even go unrecognized by some patients. The conventional lactose load used in tolerance testing, 50 g, produces symptoms in 70 to 90 percent of malabsorbers, whereas 10 to 15 g of lactose or half a pint of milk will produce abdominal symptoms in only 30 to 60 percent.[153,278,279]

Lactose intolerance due to lactase deficiency should be considered as the possible cause of GI complaints in a number of patients with "idiopathic" diarrhea, the irritable bowel syndrome, and recurrent abdominal pain and also in children.[280] A coincident lactose intolerance may modify the pattern of clinical presentation of GI or other disease and a period on a lactose-free diet may often be of diagnostic value in patients with abdominal complaints.[281]

Intolerance to lactose may also have nutritional consequences. Most lactose intolerants drink less milk than do lactose tolerants,[153,282] this causing a decreased intake of calcium. As a matter of fact, an increased incidence of intestinal lactase deficiency has been reported in osteoporotic subjects,[283,284] which has been attributed to the avoidance of dairy products because of symptoms induced by lactose malabsorption and/or to the deleterious effect of lactose malabsorption on calcium absorption.[261,285-288]

It is not clear whether consumption of moderate quantities of milk may be dangerous to lactose malabsorbers. It may induce loss of calories and nutrients in feces, but this probably becomes a problem only if the overall intake is only marginally adequate.[289,290] As intestinal lactase activity in communities with a high prevalence of lactose malabsorbers usually declines by the age of 3 to 5 years, this raises important questions about the opportunity to provide lactose-containing diets for such groups, particularly in populations in which undernutrition and infectious diarrheas are common causes of secondary forms of lactase deficiency as well.[290-292] Treatment of malnourished children with milk may provoke diarrhea, thus interfering with nutritional rehabilitation. In many populations with a high prevalence of lactose malabsorbers, the consumption of products in which lactose is digested and fermented to lactic acid, such as in yogurt, cultured buttermilk, and curds, is widespread and traditional and causes no ill effects.

There is also no answer to the opposite question, i.e., regarding whether consumption of a lactose-rich diet in adult life may be dangerous in subjects with persistent high lactase activity. Simoons[293] has noted a high incidence of senile cataracts in some groups of people who consume large quantities of milk and lactose-rich dairy products and who in addition have a high frequency of persistent lactase activity in

adult life. Furthermore, a high frequency of lactose absorbers has been found among adults with idiopathic senile and presenile cataracts, when compared with controls, in a population with a high prevalence of primary adult-type hypolactasia[294]; this suggests that adults able to absorb galactose from a lactose-containing diet are especially susceptible to cataract formation.

Diagnostic Evaluation

Primary adult-type hypolactasia should be suspected if GI symptoms, especially abdominal pain, are related to milk ingestion. The diagnosis of lactose intolerance relies first of all on objective measurements of the clinical effects of the withdrawal and reintroduction of lactose. If the symptoms are due solely to lactose intolerance, response to a lactose-poor diet is excellent. Partial resolution of symptoms may suggest a coincidental problem of lactose malabsorption with another disorder, most often irritable bowel syndrome.[281] When GI symptoms occur after ingestion of cow's milk, they are not necessarily due to adult-type hypolactasia; they may relate to a secondary lactase deficiency due to some GI disease or to malabsorption of the monosaccharides deriving from the intestinal hydrolysis of lactose (glucose and galactose) or to allergic reaction to cow's milk protein[295,296] or to some other cause.[297]

The diagnoses of lactose malabsorption and lactase deficiency need the appropriate tests, i.e., oral tolerance test and an assay for lactase in a jejunal biopsy specimen (see above). It is in fact well known that the clinical intolerance to lactose may correlate poorly with the levels of intestinal lactase activity[298] or with the results of oral tolerance test or of the breath hydrogen test.[299,300]

The lactose tolerance test with blood glucose determination has been reported to give particularly poor results in children.[178] A more reliable method appears to be the lactose-ethanol tolerance test with blood or urinary galactose determination.[301-304] The lactose breath hydrogen test gives the best discrimination between lactose absorbers and malabsorbers.[262] Detection of reducing substances in feces using copper sulfate tablets (Clinitest)[305] is useful as a screening test for lactose malabsorption in infants on a milk-containing diet or after an oral load, but is relatively unreliable in the newborn period and in adults.

Isolated lactase deficiency (with normal alpha-disaccharidase activities) should be demonstrated in an intestinal biopsy specimen by measuring the lactase activity in the presence of *p*-chloromercury benzoate, so that only the relevant brush border enzyme is measured.[306] Alternatively, brush border lactase can be selectively determined by using cellobiose as the substrate,[307] which is not hydrolyzed by the other beta-galactosidases present in the cell homogenate. It has been agreed to consider as diagnostic for primary adult-type hypolactasia those levels of lactase activity which are less than 8 units per gram of protein or 0.7 unit per gram wet weight.[262,308] The maltase/lactase or sucrase/lactase ratios are superior to simple measurement of lactase activity in resolving the two distinct groups of adults with high and low lactase activity.[250]

Treatment

In most cases it is sufficient to avoid foods rich in lactose (fresh milk, powdered milk, and milk puddings), whereas foods containing small amounts of lactose are usually well tolerated. Some individuals with hypolactasia can even drink small amounts of milk without symptoms.

Evidence is accumulating that lactose-intolerant individuals are able to tolerate some fermented milks. In cultured or culture-containing milks the lactose content is reduced substantially during fermentation, and the cultured organisms, by virtue of being rich in lactase, are able to participate in the hydrolysis of ingested lactose.[309,311] Lactose malabsorbers tolerate yogurt better than unfermented milk,[309-315] whereas pasteurization of yogurt eliminates enhanced digestion of lactose, presumably by reducing lactase activity.[311,313] Furthermore, the calcium in the yogurt is absorbed normally by lactose malabsorbers, which makes it for them an excellent source of dietary calcium.[316]

In contrast to yogurt, which is a fermented product, sweet acidophilus milk is unfermented, made by adding a high concentration of viable *Lactobacillus acidophilus* cells to cold milk. Improved utilization of lactose in sweet acidophilus milk has been reported,[317] particularly after sonication,[314] which probably releases the lactase activity from the cells. Pretreatment of milk with beta-galactosidase derived from yeasts and fungi[318,319] makes it well tolerated by subjects with hypolactasia. Lactose digestion may also be facilitated in vivo during its passage through the GI tract by adding beta-galactosidases directly to milk at the moment of consumption. The success of this enzyme replacement therapy has been demonstrated in adults[320-325] and in children.[326-328]

CONGENITAL LACTASE DEFICIENCY

Congenital lactase deficiency is very rare.[329-332] The largest group of patients with this disorder is recorded from Finland, where 16 cases have been recently described.[333] Not more than 40 cases have been reported altogether.

It may be difficult to differentiate this entity from secondary lactase deficiency, i.e., following acute gastroenteritis. A long follow-up may in fact be required to be certain that those thought to have congenital (primary) lactase deficiency do not in fact have the temporary secondary disorder.[332]

A severe diarrhea starts during the first hours or days of life, with dehydration, malnutrition, and large amounts of lactose in the feces. On a lactose-free diet diarrhea stops and the children show good growth. Diarrhea returns promptly when lactose is added again to the diet. In the 16 patients of Savilathi et al there were four pairs of siblings and an equal sex distribution; the disease appears to have an autosomal recessive inheritance mode.[333] On a lactose-free diet, jejunal biopsies are morphologically normal; lactase activity is the only disaccharidase affected. This enzyme was originally thought to be totally absent in this disease,[334-336] but most probably lactase is present, albeit at trace levels,[333] much lower than in "adult-type" hypolactasia.

This congenital lactase deficiency should not be confused with the severe infantile lactose intolerance, first described by Durand.[337] In the latter disease the critically ill infant suffers from vomiting and failure to thrive on a lactose-containing diet, with lactosuria, aminoaciduria, and acidosis.[338-340] Cataracts also may be present.[338,339,341] This disorder is not a mucosal enzyme deficiency, because substantial evidence exists that jejunal lactase activity is normal; it is probably due to an abnormal permeability to the disaccharide of the gastric mucosa.[340]

TREHALASE DEFICIENCY

Trehalose is a disaccharide that occurs mainly in insects and in mushrooms.[342] Young mushrooms are the only dietary source in humans.

Isolated trehalose malabsorption was reported for the first time in an elderly woman[343] and in a family.[344] In the latter case, a 24-year-old man presented with diarrhea and vomiting after ingestion of a large amount of edible mushrooms. Peroral biopsies of the patient and of his father showed lack of trehalase activity: the blood sugar curves after trehalose oral tolerance test were flat, but not after other sugars, and diarrhea also occurred with pure trehalose. The genetic nature of the trehalase deficiency has been suggested, with an autosomal recessive type of inheritance.[344]

Trehalase deficiency is likely to go undetected, as ingestion of foods containing trehalose is not common; therefore, its real frequency is unknown. Studies on disaccharidase activities in intestinal biopsies suggest that this defect in adult white Americans is rare,[214] whereas it is highly frequent (10 to 15 percent) in Greenland Eskimos.[215,345]

Note: The complete primary structure of the beta-glycosidase complex (lactase-phlorizin hydrolase) and of its pre-pro form has recently been established.[349] The long pre-pro lactase phlorizin hydrolase (1,927 amino acid residues in human enzyme; 1,926 amino acids in rabbit homologue) comprises five domains: (1) a cleaved signal sequence of 19 amino acids; (2) a larger "pro" portion of 847 amino acids (in the rabbit), none of which appears in the mature brush border lactase-phlorizin hydrolase; (3) the mature enzyme, which contains both catalytic sites in a single polypeptide chain; (4) a membrane-spanning hydrophobic segment near the C-terminus, which serves as the membrane anchor; and (5) a short hydrophilic segment at the C-terminus, which must be cytosolic. Pre-pro-lactase-phlorizin hydrolase, therefore, differs in several respects from the alpha-glucosidase complexes: its mode of anchoring to the membrane is different; accordingly, its mode of biosynthesis is also different. Of the 1,900-odd amino acid residues of pre-pro-phlorizin hydrolase, not more than 60 percent at the C-terminal end appears as the "final" enzyme in the brush border membrane. The destiny and role, if any, of the "pro" portion (847 amino acids) are still unclear.

Furthermore, the levels of lactase mRNA have been measured in the small intestine: they first decline during weaning in rats and rabbits, paralleling the decrease of the enzyme itself. However, they rise again later, while lactase activity remains at low levels[350]: in the small intestine of the adult animal one finds high levels of lactase mRNA accompanied by very low levels of lactase activity. It is possible, therefore, that the decline of this enzyme in the adult animal is due to post-transcriptional events. Similarly, in humans no clear difference at the mRNA level was found between adults with hypolactasia and adults with persisting high lactase activity, a result that also indicates a post-transcriptional control of lactase expression.[350]

REFERENCES

1. Anderson CH, Gracey H. Disorders of carbohydrate digestion and absorption. In: Anderson CM, Burke V, Gracey M. Pediatric gastroenterology. 2nd ed. London: Blackwell Scientific, 1987: 353.
2. Holzel A, Schwarz V, Sutcliffe W. Defective lactose absorption causing malnutrition in infancy. Lancet 1959; i:1126–1128.
3. Auricchio S, Rubino A, Landolt M, Semenza G, Prader A. Isolated intestinal lactase deficiency in the adult. Lancet 1963; ii:324–326.
4. Dahlqvist A, Hammond JD, Crane RK, Dunphy JV, Littman A. Intestinal lactase deficiency and lactose intolerance in adults: preliminary reports. Gastroenterology 1963; 45:488–491.
5. Simoons FJ. The geographic hypothesis and lactose malabsorption. A weighing of the evidence. Dig Dis 1980; 23:963–980.
6. Weijers HA, Van de Kamer JH, Mossel DAA, Dick WK. Diarrhoea caused by deficiency of sugar splitting enzymes. Lancet 1960; 2:296–297.
7. Auricchio S, Prader A, Mürset G, Witt G. Saccharoseintoleranz: Dürchfall infolge hereditären Mangels an intestinaler Saccharaseaktivität. Helv Paediatr Acta 1961; 16:483–505.
8. Auricchio S, Dahlqvist A, Mürset G, Prader A. Isomaltose intolerance causing decreased ability to utilize dietary starch. J Pediatr 1963; 62:165–176.
9. Prader A, Auricchio S, Mürset G. Dürchfall infolge hereditaren Mangels an intestinaler Saccharaseaktivität (Saccharoseintoleranz). Schweiz Med Wochenschr 1961; 91:465–468.
10. Auricchio S, Rubino A, Prader A, Rey J, Jos J, Frézal J, Davidson M. Intestinal glycosidase activities in congenital malabsorption of disaccharides. J Pediatr 1965; 66:555–564.
11. Anderson CM, Messer M, Townley RRW, Freeman M, Robinson RJ. Intestinal isomaltase deficiency in patients with hereditary sucrose and starch intolerance. Lancet 1962; 2:556–557.
12. Anderson CM, Messer M, Townley RRW, Freeman M. Intestinal sucrase and isomaltase deficiency in two siblings. Pediatrics 1963; 31:1002–1010.
13. Burgess EA, Levin B, Mahalanabis D, Tonge RE. Hereditary sucrose intolerance. Levels of sucrase activity in jejunal mucosa. Arch Dis Child 1964; 39:431–438.
14. Semenza G. A unifying concept in the phylogenesis, biosynthesis, membrane insertion and physiopathology of sucrase-isomaltase and other brush border proteins. In: Alvarado F, van Os CH, eds. Ion gradient-coupled transport. Amsterdam: Elsevier, 1986: 41.
15. Semenza G. Anchoring and biosynthesis of stalked brush border membrane proteins: glycosidases and peptidases of enterocytes and renal tubuli. Annu Rev Cell Biol 1986; 2:255–313.
16. Spiess M, Hunziker W, Lodish HF, Semenza G. Molecular cell biology of brush border hydrolases: sucrase isomaltase and γ-glutamyl transpeptidase. In: Kenny AJ, Turner AJ, eds. Ectozymes. Amsterdam: Elsevier, 1987: 87.
17. Hunziker W, Spiess M, Semenza G, Lodish H. The sucrase-isomaltase complex: primary structure, membrane orientation and evolution of a stalked intrinsic brush border protein. Cell 1986; 46:227–234.
17a. Mantei N, Villa M, Enzler T, Wacker H, Boll W, James P, Hunziker W, Semenza G. Complete primary structure of human and rabbit lactase-phlorizin hydrolase: implications for biosynthesis membrane anchoring and evolution of the enzyme. EMBO J 1988; I:2705.
18. Hauri HP, Roth J, Sterchi EE, Lentze MJ. Transport to cell surface of intestinal sucrase-isomaltase is blocked in the Golgi apparatus in a patient with congenital sucrase-isomaltase deficiency. Proc Natl Acad Sci USA 1985; 82:4423–4427.
19. Naim HY, Sterchi E, Roth J, Hauri HP. Congenital sucrase-isomaltase deficiency in man. Evidence for different mutations interfering with the intracellular transport of sucrase-isomaltase. (Abstract) Experientia 1988; 44:64.
20. Lloyd ML, Olsen WA. A study of the molecular pathology of sucrase-isomaltase deficiency. A defect in the intracellular processing of the enzyme. N Engl J Med 1987; 316:438–442.
21. Semenza G, Auricchio S. Small intestinal disaccharidases. In: Scriver CR, Beaudet AL, Sly WS, Valle D. The metabolic basis of inherited disease. 6th ed. Montreal: in press.
22. Lee L, Forstner G. Hydrophobic binding domains of rat intestinal maltase-glucoamylase. Biochem Cell Biol 1986; 64:182–187.
23. Hu C, Spiess M, Semenza G. The mode of anchoring and precursor forms of sucrase-isomaltase and maltase-glucoamylase in chicken intestinal brush border membrane. Phylogenetic implications. Biochim Biophys Acta 1987; 896:275–286.
24. Norén O, Sjöström H, Cowell G, Tranum-Jensen J, Hansen OC, Welinder KG. Pig intestinal microvillar maltase-glucoamylase. Structure and membrane insertion. J Biol Chem 1986; 261:12306–12310.
25. Semenza G. The sucrase-isomaltase complex, a large dimeric amphipatic protein from the small intestinal brush border membrane: emerging structure-function relationships. In: Ahlberg P, Sundelöf LO, eds. Structure and dynamics of chemistry. Simp 500th Jubilee Univ. Uppsala, Sweden, 1977: 226.
26. Semenza G. Mode of insertion of the sucrase-isomaltase complex in the intestinal brush border membrane: implications for the biosynthesis of this stalked intrinsic membrane protein. In: Elliot K, Whelan WJ, eds. Development of mammalian absorptive processes. Ciba Found Symp 1979; 179:133–144.
27. Semenza G. The mode of anchoring of sucrase-isomaltase to the small intestinal brush border membrane and its biosynthetic implications. In: Rapaport S, Schewe T, eds. Proc. 12th FEBS meeting, Dresden. New York: Pergamon, 1978; 53:21–28.
28. Green F, Edwards Y, Hauri HP, Povey S, Ho MW, Pinto M, Swallow D. Isolation of cDNA probe for a human jejunal brush border hydrolase, sucrase-isomaltase and assignment of the gene locus to the chromosome 3. Gene 1987; 57:101–110.
29. West LF, Davis MB, Green FR, Lindenaim RH, Swallow DM. Regional assignment of the gene coding for human sucrase-isomaltase (SI) to chromosome 3q 25–26. Ann Hum Genet 1988; 52:57–61.
30. Danielsen EM. Biosynthesis of intestinal microvillar proteins. Pulse-chase labelling studies on aminopeptidase N and sucrase-isomaltase. Biochem J 1982; 204:639–645.
31. Danielsen EM, Sjöström H, Norén O, Bro B, Dabelsteen E. Biosynthesis of intestinal microvillar proteins. Characterization of intestinal explants in organ culture and evidence of the existence of proforms of the microvillar enzymes. Biochem J 1982; 202:647–654.
32. Hauri H, Quaroni A, Isselbacher KJ. Biogenesis of intestinal plasma membrane: posttranslational route and cleavage of sucrase-isomaltase. Proc Natl Acad Sci USA 1979; 76:5183–5186.
33. Wacker H, Yanssi R, Sonderegger P, Dokow H, Gersha P, Hauri HP, Christen P, Semenza G. Cell-free synthesis of the one-chain precursor of a major intrinsic protein complex of the small intestinal brush border membrane (pro sucrase-isomaltase). FEBS Lett 1981; 136:329–332.
34. Grand RJ, Montgomery RK, Perez A. Synthesis and intracellular processing of sucrase-isomaltase in rat jejunum. Gastroenterology 1985; 38:531–538.
35. Semenza G. Anchoring and biosynthesis of a major intrinsic plasma membrane protein: the sucrase-isomaltase complex of the small intestine brush border. In: Martonosi A, ed. The enzymes of biological membranes. 2nd ed. New York: Plenum Press, 1987: 331.
36. Alpers DH, Holms D, Seetharam S, May VL, Strauss AW. In vitro translation of intestinal sucrase-isomaltase and glucoamylase. Biochem Biophys Res Commun 1986; 134:37–43.
37. Bolton H, Ho M, Potter J, King T, Furth A, Griffiths B, Swallow D, Dovey S. Immunochemical characterization of lactase in subcellular fractions of human jejunal enterocytes. Biochem Soc Transact 1985; 13:97–98.

38. Skovbjerg H, Danielsen EM, Norén O, Sjöström M. Evidence for biosynthesis of lactase-phlorizin hydrolase as a single chain high-molecular weight precursor. Biochim Biophys Acta 1984; 798:247–251.

39. Naim HY, Sterchi EE, Lentze MJ. Biosynthesis and maturation of lactase-phlorizin hydrolase in the human small intestinal epithelial cells. Biochem J 1987; 241:427–434.

40. Buller HA, Montgomery KR, Sasak WV, Grand RJ. Biosynthesis, glycosylation, and intracellular transport of intestinal lactase-phlorizin hydrolase in rat. J Biol Chem 1987; 262:17206–17211.

41. Roth J. Subcellular organization of glycosylation in mammalian cells. Biochim Biophys Acta 1987; 906:405–436.

42. Danielsen EM, Sjöström H, Norén O. Biosynthesis of intestinal microvillar proteins. Putative precursor forms of microvillus aminopeptidase and sucrase-isomaltase isolated from Ca^{2+}-precipitated enterocyte membranes. FEBS Lett 1981; 127:129–132.

43. Danielsen EM, Skovbjerg H, Norén O, Sjöström H. Biosynthesis of intestinal microvillar proteins. Nature of precursor forms of microvillar enzymes from Ca^{2+} precipitated enterocyte membranes. FEBS Lett 1981; 132:197–200.

44. Hauri HP, Sterchi EE, Bienz D, Fransen JAM, Marxer A. Expression and intracellular transport of microvillus membrane hydrolases in human intestinal epithelial cells. J Cell Biol 1985; 101:838–851.

45. Maroux S, Feracci H, Corvel JP, Benajaba A. Aminopeptidase and proteolipids of intestinal brush border. In: Brush border membranes. Ciba Found Symp 1983; 95:39–49.

46. Green F, Greenwell P, Griffiths B, Dickson L, Swallow D. The ABH and Lewis antigens of human intestinal hydrolases. Biochem Soc Transact 1987; 15:401–402.

47. Kelly JJ, Alpers D. Blood groups antigenicity of purified human intestinal disaccharidases. J Biol Chem 1973; 248:8216–8221.

48. Triadou H, Audran E, Rousset M, Zweibaum A, Orhol R. Relationship between the secretor status and the expression of ABH blood group antigenic determinants in human intestinal brush border membrane hydrolases. Biochim Biophys Acta 1983; 761:231–236.

49. Herscovics A, Quaroni A, Bugge B, Kirsck K. Partial characterization of the carbohydrate units of rat intestinal sucrase-isomaltase. Biochem J 1981; 197:511–514.

50. Galand G. Purification and characterization of kidney and intestinal brush border membrane trehalase from the rabbit. Biochim Biophys Acta 1984; 789:10–15.

51. Yokota K, Nishi J, Takesue Y. Purification and characterization of amphiphilic trehalase from rabbit small intestine. Biochim Biophys Acta 1986; 881:405–414.

52. Takesue Y, Yokota K, Nishi Y, Taguki R, Ikesawa H. Solubilization of trehalase from rabbit renal and intestinal brush border membranes by a phosphoinositol-specific phospholipase C. FEBS Lett 1986; 201:5–8.

53. Sebastio G, Hunziker V, Ballabio A, Auricchio S, Semenza G. On the primary site of control in the spontaneous development of small-intestinal sucrase-isomaltase after birth: FEBS Lett 1987; 208:460–464.

54. Sebastio G, Hunziker V, O'Neill B, Malo C, Ménard D, Auricchio S, Semenza G. The biosynthesis of intestinal sucrase-isomaltase in human embryo is most likely controlled at the level of transcription. Biochem Biophys Res Commun 1987; 149:803–839.

55. Sjöström H, Norén O, Danielsen EM. The enzymatic activity of "high-mannose" glycosylated forms on intestinal microvillar hydrolases. J Pediatr Gastroenterol Nutr 1985; 4:980–983.

56. Auricchio S, Caporale C, Santamaria F, Skovbjerg H. Fetal forms of oligoaminopeptidase, dipeptidylaminopeptidase IV, and sucrase in human intestine and meconium. J Pediatr Gastroenterol Nutr 1984; 3:28–36.

57. Auricchio S, Sebastio G. Development of disaccharidases. In: Lebenthal E, ed. Textbook of gastroenterology and nutrition in early childhood. 2nd ed. New York: Raven Press, in press.

58. Neu J, Luida KV, Tsuboi KK, Sunshine P. Developmental characteristics of disaccharidases and epithelial migration rate along the crypt to villous in the rat small intestine. (Abstract) Pediatr Res 1979; 13: 405.

59. James WPT, Alpers DH, Gerber JE, Isselbacher KJ. The turnover of disaccharidases and brush border proteins in rat intestine. Biochim Biophys Acta 1971; 230:194–203.

60. Olsen WA, Korsmo H. The intestinal brush border membrane in diabetes. Studies of sucrose-isomaltose metabolism in rats with steptozotocin diabetes. J Clin Invest 1977; 60:181–188.

61. Skovbjerg H. Immunoelectrophoretic studies on human small intestinal brush border proteins. Relation between enzyme activity and immuno-reactive enzyme along the villous crypt axis. Biochem J 1981; 193:887–890.

62. Riby JE, Kretchmer N. Participation of pancreatic enzymes in the degradation of intestinal sucrase-isomaltase. J Pediatr Gastroenterol Nutr 1985; 4:971–979.

63. Cousineau J, Green JR. Isolation and characterization of the proximal and distal forms of lactase-phlorizin hydrolase from the small intestine of suckling rats. Biochim Biophys Acta 1980; 615:147–157.

64. Wilson JR, Dworaczyk DA, Weiser MM. Intestinal epithelial cell differentiation. Related changes in glycosyltransferase activities in rats. Biochim Biophys Acta 1984; 797:369–376.

65. Ahnen DJ, Santiago HA, Yoshioka C, Gray GM. Intestinal sucrase-α dextrinase: differential degradation of its protein and carbohydrate components in vivo. (Abstract) Gastroenterology 1982; 82:1006.

66. Sjöström H, Norén O, Danielsen EM, Skovbjerg H. Structure of microvillar enzymes in different phases of their life cycle. In: Brush Border Membranes. Ciba Found Symp 1983; 95:50–72.

67. Goda T, Koldovsky O. Evidence of degradation process of sucrase-isomaltase in jejunum of adult rats. Biochem J 1985; 229:751–758.

68. Skovbjerg H. Immunoelectrophoretic studies on human small intestinal brush border proteins. The longitudinal distribution of peptidases and disaccharidases. Clin Chim Acta 1981; 112:205–212.

69. Triadou N, Bataille J, Schmitz J. Longitudinal study of the human intestinal brush border membrane proteins. Distribution of the main disaccharidases and peptidases. Gastroenterology 1983; 85:1326–1332.

70. Henning SJ. Ontogeny of enzymes in the small intestine. Annu Rev Physiol 1985; 47:231–254.

71. Kedinger M, Haffen K, Simon-Hassman P. Control mechanisms in the ontogenesis of villus cells. In: Desnuelle P, Sjöström H, Norén O, eds. Molecular and cellular biology of digestion. Amsterdam: Elsevier, 1986: 323.

72. Koldowsky O. Developmental, dietary and hormonal control of intestinal disaccharidases in mammals (including man). In: Randle PJ, Steiner DF, Whelan WJ, eds. Carbohydrate metabolism and its disorders, Vol 3. London: Academic Press, 1981: 418.

73. Leese HJ, Semenza G. On the identity between the small-intestinal enzymes phlorizin-hydrolase and glycosylceramidase. J Biol Chem 1973; 248:8170–8173.

74. Whelan WJ, Roberts PJP. The mechanism of carbohydrate action. Part II, Alfa-amylolysis of linear substrates. J Chem Soc 1953; 19:28–35.

75. Whelan WJ. The action patterns of α-amylases. Die Stärke 1960; 12:358–361.

76. Roberts PJP, Whelan WJ. The mechanism of carbohydrase action. 5. Action of human salivary α-amylase on amylopectin and glycogen. Biochem J 1960; 76:246–253.

77. Bines J, Whelan WJ. The mechanism of carbohydrase action. 6. Structure of a salivary α-amylase limit dextrin from amylopectin. Biochem J 1960; 76:253–257.

78. Heller J, Schramm M. α-amylase limit dextrins of high molecular weight obtained from glycogen. Biochim Biophys Acta 1964; 81:96–103.

79. Nordin PH, French D. 1-Phenyl-flavazole derivates of starch dextrins. J Am Chem Soc 1958; 80:1445–1452.

80. Auricchio S, Della Pietra D, Vegnente A. Studies on intestinal digestion of starch in man. II. Intestinal hydrolysis of amylopectin in infants and children. Pediatrics 1967; 39:853–862.

81. Gray GM, Lally BC, Conklin KA. Action of intestinal sucrase-isomaltase and its free monomers on an α-limit dextrin. J Biol Chem 1979; 254:6038–6043.

82. Taravel FR, Datema R, Woloszczuk W, Marshall JJ, Whelan WJ. Purification and characterization of a pig intestinal α-limit dextrinase. Eur J Biochem 1983; 130:147–153.

83. Rodriguez IR, Taravel FR, Whelan WJ. Characterization and function of pig intestinal sucrase isomaltase and its separate subunits. Eur J Biochem 1984; 143:575–582.

84. Anderson IH, Levine AS, Levitt MD. Incomplete absorption of the carbohydrate in all purpose wheat flour. N Engl J Med 1981; 304:891–892.

85. Levine AS, Levitt MD. Malabsorption of starch moiety of oats, corn and potatoes. (Abstract) Gastroenterology 1981; 80: 1209.

86. Stephen AM, Haddad AC, Philips SF. Passage of carbohydrate into the colon. Gastroenterology 1983; 85:589–595.

87. Chapman RW, Sillery JK, Graham MM, Saunders DR. Absorption of starch by healthy ileostomates: effect of transit time and carbohydrate load. Am J Clin Nutr 1985; 41:1244–1248.

88. Goddard MS, Young G, Marcus R. The effect of amylose content on insulin and glucose responses to ingested rice. Am J Clin Nutr 1984; 39:388–398.

89. Sörensen SH, Norén O, Sjöström H, Danielsen EM. Amphiphilic pig intestinal microvillus maltase/glucoamylase. Structure and specificity. Eur J Biochem 1982; 126:559–568.

90. Dahlqvist A. Specificity of the human intestinal disaccharidases and implications for hereditary disaccharide intolerance. J Clin Invest 1961; 41:463–468.

91. Auricchio S, Semenza G, Rubino A. Multiplicity of human intestinal disaccharidases II. Characterization of the individual maltases. Biochim Biophys Acta 1965: 96:498–507.

92. Kelly JJ, Alpers DH. Properties of human intestinal glucoamylase. Biochim Biophys Acta 1973; 315:113–120.

93. Dawson DJ, Lobley RW, Burrows PC, Miller W, Holmes R. Lactose digestion by human jejunal biopsies: the relationship between hydrolysis and absorption. Gut 1986; 27:521–527.

94. Gray GM, Santiago N. Disaccharide absorption in normal and diseased human intestine. Gastroenterology 1966; 51:489–494.

95. Rubino A, Zimbalatti F, Auricchio S. Intestinal disaccharidase activities in adult and suckling rats. Biochim Biophys Acta 1964; 92:305–311.

96. Dubs R, Gitzelman R, Steinmann B, Lindenmann J. Catalytically inactive sucrase antigen of rabbit small intestine: the enzyme precursor. Helv Paediat Acta 1975; 30:89–102.

97. Simon PM, Kedinger M, Raul F, Grenier JF, Haffen K. Developmental pattern of rat intestinal brush border enzymatic proteins along the villous crypt axis. Biochem J 1979; 178:407–413.

98. Boyle JT, Kokonos M, Koldowsky O. Developmental profile of jejunal lactase and sucrase activity along the villous crypt in the rat. (Abstract) Pediatr Res 1982; 16:157.

99. Doell RG, Kretchmer N. Intestinal invertase: precocious development of activity after injection of hydrocortisone. Science 1964; 143:42–44.

100. Lee PC, Lebenthal E. Early weaning and precocious development of small intestine in rats: genetic, dietary or hormonal control. Pediatr Res 1983; 17:645–650.

101. Yeh KJ, Halt PR. Ontogenic timing mechanism initiates the expression of rat intestinal sucrase activity. Gastroenterology 1986; 90:520–526.

102. Henning SJ. Postnatal development: coordination of feeding, digestion and metabolism. Am J Physiol 1981; 241:G199–G214.

103. Henning SJ. Ontogeny of enzymes in the small intestine. Annu Rev Physiol 1985; 47:231–254.

104. Klein RM, McKenzie JC. The role of cell renewal in the ontogeny of the intestine. I. Cell proliferation patterns in adult, fetal and neonatal intestine. J Pediatr Gastroenterol Nutr 1983; 2:204–228.

105. Leichter J. Effect of dietary lactose on intestinal lactase activity in young rats. J Nutr 1973; 103:392–396.

106. Ferguson A, Gerskovitch VP, Russell RI. Pre and post-weaning disaccharidase patterns in isografts of fetal mouse intestine. Gastroenterology 1973; 64:292–297.

107. Bolin TD, Pirola RC, Davis AE. Adaptation of intestinal lactase in the rat. Gastroenterology 1969; 57:406–409.

108. Bolin TD, Mckern A, Davis AE. The effect of diet on lactase activity in the rat. Gastroenterology 1971; 60:432–437.

109. Montgomery RK, Sybicki MA, Grand RJ. Autonomous biochemical and morphological differentiation in the fetal rat intestine transplanted at 17 and 2 days of gestation. Dev Biol 1981; 87:76–84.

110. Malo CH, Ménard D. Hormonal control of intestinal glucoamylase activity in suckling and adult mice. Comp Biochem Physiol 1980; 65B:169–172.

111. Kedinger M, Simon PM, Raul F, Grenier JF, Haffen K. The effect of dexamethasone on the development of rat intestinal brush border enzymes in organ culture. Dev Biol 1980; 74:9–21.

112. Beaulieu JF, Calvert R. Influence of dexamethasone on the maturation of fetal mouse intestinal mucosa in organ culture. Comp Biochem Physiol 1985; 82A:91–95.

113. Ménard D, Malo CH, Calvert R. Insulin accelerates the development of intestinal brush border hydrolytic activities of suckling mice. Dev Biol 1981; 85:150–155.

114. Malo C, Ménard D. Influence of epidermal growth factor on the development of suckling mouse intestinal mucosa. Gastroenterology 1982; 83:28–35.

115. Moog FJ. The functional differentiation of the small intestine. II. The differentiation of alkaline phosphomonoesterase in the duodenum of the mouse. J Exp Zool 1951; 118:187–205.

116. Moog FJ. The functional differentiation of the small intestine. III. The influence of the pituitary-adrenal system on the differentiation of phosphatase in the duodenum of the suckling mice. J Exp Zool 1953; 124:329–346.

117. Yeh KJ, Moog F. Intestinal lactase activity in the suckling rat: influence of hypophysectomy and thyroidectomy. Science 1974; 183:77–79.

118. Malo CH, Ménard D. Opposite effects of one and three injections of cortisone or tyroxine on intestinal lactase activity in suckling mice. Experientia 1979; 35:493–494.

119. Kedinger M, Simon-Assman PM, Haffen K. Control mechanisms in the ontogenesis of villous cells. In: Desnuelle P, Norén O, Sjöström H, eds. Molecular and cellular biology of digestion. Amsterdam: Elsevier, 1986: 315.

120. Arsenault P, Ménard D. Comparative study of the effect of hydrocortisone and thyroxine on suckling mouse small intestine in organ culture. Comp Biochem Physiol 1984; 77A:721–725.

121. Beaulieu JF, Calvert R. Effect of dexamethasone on the fetal mouse small intestine in organ culture. Anat Rec 1984; 210:61–71.

122. Simon-Assman PM, Kedinger M, Grenier JF, Haffen K. Control of brush border enzymes by dexamethasone in the fetal rat intestine cultured in vitro. J Pediatr Gastroenterol Nutr 1982; 1:257–265.

123. Simon PM, Kedinger M, Raul F, Grenier JF, Haffen K. Organ culture of suckling rat intestine: comparative study of various hormones on brush border enzymes. In Vitro 1982; 18:339–346.

124. Raul F, Kedinger M, Simon PM, Granier JF, Haffen K. Comparative in vivo and in vitro effect of mono- and disaccharides on intestinal brush border enzyme activities in suckling rats. Biol Neonate 1981; 39:200–207.

125. Ménard D, Arsenault P, Gallo-Payet N. Epidermal growth factor does not act as a primary cue for inducing developmental changes in suckling mouse jejunum. J Pediatr Gastroenterol Nutr 1986; 5:949–955.

126. Arsenault P, Ménard D. Insulin influences the maturation and proliferation of suckling mouse intestinal mucosa in serum free organ culture. Biol Neonate 1984; 46:229–236.

127. Raul F, Lacroix B, Aprahamian M. Longitudinal distribution of brush border hydrolases and morphological maturation in the intestine of the preterm infant. Early Hum Dev 1986; 13:225–234.

128. Auricchio S, Rubino A, Muerset G. Intesinal glycosidase activities in the human embryo, fetus and newborn. Pediatrics 1965; 35:944–954.

129. Antonovicz I, Chang SK, Grand RJ. Development and distribution of lysosomal enzymes and disaccharidases in human fetal intestine. Gastroenterology 1974; 67:51–58.

130. Antonovicz I, Lebenthal E. Development pattern of small intestinal enterokinase and disaccharidase activity in the human fetus. Gastroenterology 1977; 72:1299–1303.

131. Dahlqvist A, Lindberg T. Fetal development of the small intestinal disaccharidase and alkaline phosphatase activities in the human. Biol Neonate 1965; 9:24–32.

132. Jirsova V, Koldovsky O, Heringova A, Uher J, Jodl J. Development of invertase activity in the intestines of human fetuses: appearance of jejunoileal differences. Biol Neonate 1968; 13:143–146.

133. Mayne A, Hughes CA, Sule D, Brown GA, McNeish AS. Development of intestinal disaccharidases in preterm infants, Lancet 1983; ii:622–623.

134. MacLean WC Jr, Fink BB. Lactose malabsorption by premature infants: magnitude and clinical significance. J Pediatr 1980; 97:383–388.

135. MacLean WC, Fink BB, Schoeller DA, Wong W, Klein PD. Lactose assimilation by full-term infants: relation of (13C) and H2 breath test with fecal (13C) excretion. Pediatr Res 1983; 17:629–633.

136. Lifshitz CH, O'Brian Smith E, Garza C. Delayed complete functional lactase sufficiency in breast-fed infants. J Pediatr Gastroenterol Nutr 1983; 2:478–482.

137. Chiles C, Watkins JB, Barr RG, Tsaj PY, Goldman DA. Lactose utilization in the newborn: role of colonic flora. (Abstract) Pediatr Res 1979; 13:365.

138. Bond JH, Currier BE, Buchwald H, Levitt MD. Colonic conservation of malabsorbed carbohydrate. Gastroenterology 1980; 78:444–447.

139. Kein CL, Liechty EA, Myerberg DZ, Mullett MD. Dietary carbohydrate assimilation in the premature infant: evidence for a nutritionally significant bacterial ecosystem in the colon. Clin Nutr 1987; 46:456–460.

140. Lebenthal E, Lee PC, Heitlinger LA. Impact of development of the

gastrointestinal tract on infant feeding. J Pediatr 1983; 102:1-9.

141. Lebenthal E, Lee PC. Development of functional response in human exocrine pancreas. Pediatrics 1980; 66:556-560.

142. Zoppi G, Andreotti G, Pajno-Ferrara F, Njai DM, Gaburro D. Exocrine pancreas function in premature and fullterm neonates. Pediatr Res 1972; 6:880-886.

143. De Vizia B, Ciccimarra F, De Cicco N, Auricchio S. Digestibility of starches in infants and children. J Pediatr 1975; 86:50-55.

144. Senterre J. Net absorption of starch in low birth weight infants. Acta Paediatr Scand 1980; 69:653-657.

145. Shulman RJ, Wong WW, Irving CS, Nichols BL, Klein PD. Utilization of dietary cereal by young infants. J Pediatr 1983; 103:23-28.

146. Klein PD, Klein ER. Application of stable isotopes to pediatric nutrition and gastroenterology: measurement of nutrient absorption and digestion using 13C. J Pediatr Gastroenterol Nutr 1985; 4:9-19.

147. Hodge C, Lebenthal E, Lee PC, Topper W. Amylase in the saliva and in the gastric aspirates of premature infants: its potential role in glucose polymers hydrolysis. Pediatr Res 1983; 17:998-1001.

148. Chauve A, Devroede G, Bastin E. Intraluminal pressures during perfusion of the human colon in situ. Gastroenterology 1976; 70:336-340.

149. Debongnie JC, Philips FS. Capacity of the human colon to absorb fluid. Gastroenterology 1978; 74:698-704.

150. Palma R, Vidon N, Bernier JJ. Maximal capacity for fluid absorption in human bowel. Dig Dis Sci 1981; 26:929-933.

151. Flourie B, Florent C, Jouany JP, Thivend P, Etanchaud F, Rambaud JC. Colonic metabolism of wheat starch in healthy humans. Gastroenterology 1985; 90:111-119.

152. Welsh JD. Isolated lactase deficiency in humans: reports on 100 patients. Medicine (Balt) 1970; 49:257-277.

153. Bayless TM, Rothfeld B, Massa C, Wise L, Paige D, Bedine MS. Lactose and milk intolerance: clinical implications. N Engl J Med 1975; 292:1156-1159.

154. Ringrose RE, Preiser H, Welsh JD. Sucrase-isomaltase (palatinase) deficiency diagnosed during adulthood. Dig Dis Sci 1980; 25:384-387.

155. Ravich WJ, Bayless TM. Carbohydrate absorption and malabsorption. Clin Gastroenterol 1983; 12:335-356.

156. Layer P, Zinsmeister AR, Di Magno E. Effect of decreasing intraluminal amylase activity on starch digestion and postprandial gastrointestinal function in humans. Gastroenterology 1986; 91:41-48.

157. Launiala K. The effect of unabsorbed sucrose and mannitol on small intestinal flow rate and mean transit time. Scand J Gastroenterol 1968; 3:665-671.

158. Launiala K. The effect of unabsorbed sucrose- or mannitol-induced accelerated transit on absorption in the human small intestine. Scand J Gastroenterol 1969; 4:25-34.

159. Goda T, Bustamante S, Edmond J, Grimes J, Koldowsky O. Precocious increase of sucrase activity by carbohydrates in the small intestine of suckling rats. II. Role of digestibility of sugars, osmolarity, and stomach evacuation in producing diarrhea. J Pediatr Gastroenterol Nutr 1985; 4:634-639.

160. Caspary WF, Kalish H. Effect of α-glucosehydrolase inhibition on intestinal absorption of sucrose, water, and sodium in man. Gut 1979; 20:750-755.

161. Azpiroz F, Malagelada JR. Luminal nutrients in the proximal and distal small intestine elicit gastric relaxation. Dig Dis Sci 1984; 29:564-567.

162. Jenkins DFA, Taylor RH, Goff WD. Scope and specificity of acarbose in slowing carbohydrate absorption in man. Diabetes 1981; 31:951-957.

163. Holgate AM, Read NW. Relationship between small bowel transit time and absorption of a solid meal. Dig Dis Sci 1983; 28:812-816.

164. Auricchio S, Ciccimarra F, De Vizia B. Starch malabsorption. XIII International Congress of Pediatrics Wien Osterreich 29 Aug-4 Sept 1971 Separatum, pp 139-150.

165. Cummings JH, Englyst HN. Fermentation in the human large intestine and the available substrates. Am J Clin Nutr 1987; 45:1243-1255.

166. Cummings JH, Pomare EW, Branch WJ, Naylor CPE, Macfarlane GT. Short chain fatty acids in human large intestine, portal, hepatic and venous blood. Gut 1987; 28:1221-1227.

167. Newcomer AD, McGill DB, Thomas PM, Hofmann AF. Tolerance to lactose among lactase deficient American Indians. Gastroenterology 1978; 74:44-50.

168. Saunders DR, Wiggins HS. Conservation of mannitol, lactulose and raffinose by the human colon. Am J Physiol 1981; 241:G387-G391.

169. Wolevar TMS, Cohen Z, Thompson LU, Thorne MJ, Jenkins MJA,

170. Prokipchuk EJ, Jenkins DJA. Ileal loss of available carbohydrate in man: comparison of a breath hydrogen method with direct measurement using a human ileostomy model. Am J Gastroenterol 1986; 81:115-122.

170. Levitt MN, Hirsh P, Fetzer CA, Sheahan M, Levine AS. H2 excretion after ingestion of complex carbohydrates. Gastroenterology 1987; 92:383-389.

171. Argenzio RA, Southworth M. Sites of organic acid production and absorption in gastrointestinal tract in the pig. Am J Physiol 1975; 228:454-459.

172. Orskov ER, Frase C, Mason WC, Mann SO. Influence of starch digestion in the large intestine of sheep on caecal fermentation, caecal microflora and faecal nitrogen excretion. Br J Nutr 1970; 24:671-676.

173. Florent CH, Flourie B, Leblond A, Rautureau M, Bernier JJ, Rambaud JC. Influence of chronic lactulose ingestion on the colonic metabolism of lactulose in man (an in vivo study). J Clin Invest 1985; 75:608-613.

174. Bhatia J, Prihoda AR, Richardson CJ. Parenteral antibiotics and carbohydrate intolerance in term neonates. Am J Dis Child 1986; 149:111-115.

175. Haemmerli UP, Kistler WJ, Ammann T, Marthaler T, Semenza G, Auricchio S, Prader A. Acquired milk intolerance in the adult caused by lactose malabsorption due to a selective deficiency of intestinal lactase activity. Am J Med 1965; 38:7-15.

176. Weijers HA, Van de Kamer JH, Dicke WH, Ijsseling J. Diarrhoea caused by deficiency of sugar-splitting enzymes. Acta Paediatr 1961; 50:55-59.

177. McGill DB, Newcomer AD. Comparison of venous and capillary blood samples in lactose tolerance testing. Gastroenterology 1967; 53:371-374.

178. Krasilnikoff PA, Gudmann-Høyer E, Moltke HH. Diagnostic value of disaccharide tolerance tests in children. Acta Paediatr Scand 1975; 64:693-698.

179. Fernandes J, Vos CE, Douwes AC, Slotema E, Degenhart HJ. Respiratory hydrogen excretion as a parameter for lactose malabsorption in children. Am J Clin Nutr 1978; 31:597-602.

180. Maffei HVL, Metz G, Bampoe V, Shiner M, Herman S, Brooke CGD. Lactose intolerance, detected by breath hydrogen test in infants and children with chronic diarrhoea. Arch Dis Child 1977; 52:766-771.

181. Perman JA, Barr RG, Watkins JB. Sucrose malabsorption in children: non invasive diagnosis by interval breath hydrogen determination. J Pediatr 1978; 93:17-22.

182. Robb TA, Davidson GP. Advances in breath hydrogen quantitation in paediatrics: sample collection and normalization to constant oxygen and nitrogen levels. Clin Chim Acta 1981; 111:281-285.

183. Kerlin P, Phillips SF. Differential transit of liquids and solid residue through the ileum of man. Am J Physiol 1983; 245:G38-G43.

184. Douwes AC, Schaap C, Van der KeiVan Moorsel JM. Hydrogen breath test in schoolchildren. Arch Dis Child 1985; 60:333-337.

185. Levitt MD, Donaldson RM. Use of respiratory hydrogen to detect carbohydrate malabsorption. J Lab Clin Med 1970; 75:937-945.

186. Bjorneklett A, Jenssen E. Relationship between hydrogen (H2) and methane (CH4) in man. Scand J Gastroenterol 1982; 17:985-992.

187. Shulman RJ, Kerzner B, Sloan HR, Boutton TW, Wong WW, Nichols BL, Klein PD. Absorption and oxidation of glucose polymers of different lengths in young infants. Pediatr Res 1986; 20:740-743.

188. Dahlqvist A. Method for assay of intestinal disaccharidases. Anal Biochem 1964; 7:18-25.

189. Auricchio S, Rubino A, Tosi R, Semenza G, Landolt M, Kistler HJ, Prader A. Disaccharidase activities in human intestinal mucosa. Enzymol Biol Clin 1963; 3:193-208.

190. Banauch D, Brummer W, Ebeling W, Metz H, Rindfrey M, Lang H. Eine Glucose-Dehydrogenase fur die Glucose-Bestimmung in Korperflussigkeiten. Z Klin Chem Klin Biochem 1975; 13:101-107.

191. Skovbjerg H, Sjöström A, Norén O, Gudmond-Høyer E. Immunoelectrophoretic studies on human small intestinal brush border proteins. A quantitative study from single, small intestinal biopsies. Clin Chim Acta 1979; 92:315-322.

192. Jönsson KA, Bodemar G, Tagesson C, Whalan A. Variation of disaccharidases activities in duodenal biopsy specimens. Scand J Gastroenterol 1986; 21:51-54.

193. Niessen KH, Schmidt K, Bruggmann G. Disaccharidasen der Dünndarmschleimhaut bei Säuglingen und Kindern. Z Gastroenterol 1975; 13:565-572.

194. McMichael WB, Webb J, Dowson AM. Jejunal disaccharidases and

some observations on the cause of lactase deficiency. Br Med J 1966; 2:1037–1041.

195. Calvin RT, Klish WJ, Nichols BL. Disaccharidase activities, jejunal morphology and carbohydrate tolerance in children with chronic diarrhea. J Pediatr Gastroenterol Nutr 1985; 4:949–953.

196. Eggermont E, Carchon H, Eeckels R. Centile values of small intestinal mucosal enzymatic activities in Caucasian children. Pediatr Res 1981; 15:1205A.

197. Hadorn B, Green JR, Sterchi EE, Hauri HP. Biochemical mechanism in congenital enzyme deficiencies of the small intestine. Clin Gastroenterol 1981; 10:671–698.

198. Freiburghaus AU, Schmitz J, Schindler M, Rotthauwe HW, Kuitunen P, Launiala K, Hadorn B. Protein patterns of brush border fragments in congenital lactose malabsorption and in specific hypolactasia of the adult. N Engl J Med 1976; 294:1031–1032.

199. Schmitz J, Bresson JL, Triadou N, Bataille J, Rey J. Analyse en electrophorèse sur gel de polyacrylamide des proteines de la membrane microvillositaire et d'une fraction cytoplasmique dans 8 cas de intolérance congénitale au saccharose. Gastroenterol Clin Biol 1980; 4:251–256.

200. Skovbjerg H, Krasilnikoff PA. Maltase-glucoamylase and residual isomaltase in sucrose intolerant patients. J Pediatr Gastroenterol Nutr 1986; 3:365–369.

201. Skovbjerg H, Krasilnikoff PA. Immunoelectrophoretic studies on human small intestinal brush border protein. The residual isomaltase in sucrose intolerant patients. Pediatr Res 1981; 15:214–218.

202. Auricchio S, Ciccimarra F, Moauro L, Rey F, Jos J, Rey J. Intraluminal and mucosal starch digestion in congenital deficiency of intestinal sucrase and isomaltase activities. Pediatr Res 1972; 6:832–839.

203. Eggermont E, Hers HG. The sedimentation properties of the intestinal α-glucosidases of normal human subjects and of patients with sucrose intolerance. Eur J Biochem 1969; 9:488–492.

204. Preiser H, Ménard D, Crane RK, Cerda JJ. Deletion of enzyme protein from brush border membrane in sucrase-isomaltase deficiency. Biochim Biophys Acta 1974; 363:279–284.

205. Triadou A, Audran E, Dellon A, Schmitz J. Heterogeneity of the defect affecting sucrase-isomaltase intracellular processing in congenital sucrose intolerance (CSI). In: Alvars F, Van Os CH, eds. Ion gradient coupled transport. IHSERM Symposium no. 26. Amsterdam:Elsevier, 1986: 367.

206. Tufaro F, Snider MD, McKnight SL. Identification and characterization of a mouse cell mutant defective in intracellular transport of glycoproteins. J Cell Biol 1987; 105:647–657.

207. Tartakof AM. Mutations that influence the secretory path in animal cells. Biochem J 1983; 216:1–9.

208. Elbein AD. Inhibitors of the biosynthesis and processing of N-linked oligosaccharide chains. Annu Rev Biochem 1987; 56:497–534.

209. Danielsen EM, Cowell GM. Biosynthesis of intestinal microvillar proteins. FEBS Lett 1984; 166:28–32.

210. Stewart JR, Kenny AJ. Proteins of the kidney microvillar membrane. Effects of monensine, vinblatine, swansonine and glucosamine on the processing and assembly of endopeptidase 24.11 and dyeptidylpeptidase IV in pig kidney slices. Biochem J 1984; 224:559–568.

211. Pollack L, Atkinson PH. Correlation of glycosylation forms with position in amino acid sequence. J Cell Biol 1983; 97:293–300.

212. Danielsen EM, Cowell GM. Biosynthesis of intestinal microvillar proteins. The intracellular transport of aminopeptidase N and sucrase-isomaltase occurs at different rates pre-Golgi but at the same rate post-Golgi. FEBS Lett 1985; 190:69–72.

213. Kerry KR, Townley RRW. Genetic aspects of intestinal sucrase-isomaltase deficiency. Aust Paediatr J 1965; 1:223–226.

214. Welsh JD, Poley JR, Bathia M, Stevenson DE. Intestinal disaccharidase activities in relation to age, race, and mucosal damage. Gastroenterology 1978; 75:847–855.

215. Gudmand-Høyer E, Krasilnikoff PA, Skovbjerg H. Sucrose-isomaltose malabsorption. In: Draper H, ed. Advances in Nutritional Research, Vol 6. New York: Plenum Press, 1984: 233.

216. Ellestead-Sayed JJ, Haworth JC, Hildes JA. Disaccharide consumption and malabsorption in Canadian Indians. Am J Clin Nutr 1977; 30:698–703.

217. Ellestead-Sayed JJ, Haworth JC, Hildes JA. Disaccharide malabsorption and dietary patterns in two Canadian Eskimo communities. Am J Clin Nutr 1978; 31:1473–1478.

218. Gudmand-Høyer E. Sucrose malabsorption in children: a report of thirty-one Greenlanders. J Pediatr Gastroenterol Nutr 1985; 4:873–877.

219. Hoegerman SF, Hoegerman G. Gene frequency of sucrase-isomaltase deficiency. N Engl J Med 1976; 295:284.

220. Cheney CP, Boedeker EC. Evidence that the sucrase-isomaltase complex may serve as an intestinal receptor for an enteropathogenic Escherichia coli (Abstract). Gastroenterology 1982; 82:1032.

221. Prader A, Auricchio S. Defects of intestinal disaccharide absorption. Annu Rev Med 1965;

222. Gudmand-Høyer E, Krasilnikoff PA. The effect of sucrose malabsorption on the growth pattern in children. Scand J Gastroenterol 1977; 12:103–107.

223. Antonovicz I, Lloyd JD, Khaw KT, Shwachman H. Congenital sucrase-isomaltase deficiency. Observation over a period of 6 years. Pediatrics 1972; 49:847–853.

224. Sonntag WM, Brill ML, Troyer WE, Welsh JD, Semenza G, Prader A. Sucrose-isomaltose malabsorption in an adult female. Gastroenterology 1964; 47:18–25.

225. Neale G, Clark M, Levin B. Intestinal sucrase deficiency presenting as sucrose intolerance in adult life. Br Med J 1965; 2:1223–1225.

226. Starnes CW, Welsh JD. Intestinal sucrase-isomaltase deficiency and renal calculi. N Engl J Med 1970; 202:1023–1024.

227. Jansen W, Que Cs, Veeger W. Primary combined saccharase and isomaltase deficiency. Arch Intern Med 1972; 116:1125–1127.

228. Cooper BT, Scott J, Hopkins J, Peters TJ. Adult onset sucrase-isomaltase deficiency with secondary disaccharidase deficiency resulting from severe dietary carbohydrate restriction. Dig Dis Sci 1983; 28:473–477.

229. Metz G, Jenkins DJA, Newman AJ, Blendis LM. Breath hydrogen in hyposucrasia. Lancet 1976; i:119–120.

230. Douwes AC, Fernandes J, Jongbloed AA. Diagnostic value of sucrose tolerance test in children evaluated by breath hydrogen measurement. Acta Paediatr Scand 1980; 69:79–82.

231. Gardiner AJ, Tarlow MJ, Symonds J, Hutchison JGP, Shuterland IT. Failure of the hydrogen breath test to detect primary sugar malabsorption. Arch Dis Child 1981; 56:568–572.

232. Eggermont E. The hydrolysis of the naturally occurring α-glucosides by the human intestinal mucosa. Eur J Biochem 1969; 9:483–487.

233. Auricchio S, Ciccimarra F, Starace E, Vegnente A, Giliberti P, Provenzale L. Glucamylase activity of human intestinal mucosa. Rendiconti Gastroenterol 1971; 3:1–8.

234. Harms HK, Bertele-Harms RM, Bruer-Kleis D. Enzyme-substitution therapy with the yeast Saccharomyces cerevisiae in congenital sucrase-isomaltase deficiency. N Engl J Med 1987; 316:1306–1309.

235. Greene HC, Stifel FB, Herman RH. Dietary stimulation of sucrase in a patient with sucrase-isomaltase deficiency. Biochem Med 1972; 6:409–413.

236. Krasilnikoff PA, Skovbjerg H. Lack of stimulation of sucrase and isomaltase with fructose in children with sucrose-isomaltose malabsorption. (Abstract) Pediatr Res 1986; 20:702.

237. Jonas MM, Montgomery RK, Grand RJ. Intestinal lactase synthesis during postnatal development in the rat. Pediatr Res 1985; 19:956–962.

238. Nsi-Emvo E, Launay JF, Raul F. Is adult type hypolactasia in the intestine of mammals related to changes in the intracellular processing of lactase? Cell Mol Biol 1987; 33:335–344.

239. Buts JP, De Meyer R. Postnatal proximodistal development of the small bowel mucosal mass in growing rat. Biol Neonate 1981; 40:62–69.

240. Buts JP, De Meyer R. Intestinal development in the suckling rat: effect of weaning, diet composition and glucocorticoids on thymidine kinase activity and DNA synthesis. Pediatr Res 1984; 18:145–150.

241. Tsuboi KK, Kwong LK, Neu J, Sunshine P. A proposed mechanism of normal intestinal lactase decline in the postweaned mammal. Biochim Biophys Res Commun 1981; 101:645–652.

242. Tsuboi KK, Kwong LK, D'Arlingue AE, Stevenson DK, Kerner JA, Sunshine P. The nature of maturational decline of intestinal lactase activity. Biochim Biophys Acta 1985; 840:69–78.

243. Smith MW, James PS. Cellular origin of lactase decline in postweaned rats. Biochim Biophys Acta 1987; 905:503–506.

244. Castillo RO, Kwong LK, Sunshine P, Quan R, Gray GM. Precursor forms of rat small intestinal lactase. (Abstract) Pediatr Res 1987; 21:266.

245. Quan R, Tsuboi KK, Gray GM. Lactase in the adult rat: multiple intracellular and brush border forms. (Abstract) Gastroenterology 1987; 92:1585.

246. Skovbjerg H, Gudmand-Høyer E, Fenger HJ. Immunoelectrophoret-

ic studies on human small intestinal brush border proteins. The amount of lactase protein in adult-free hypolactasia. Gut 1980; 21:360–364.

247. Potter J, Ho MW, Bolton H, Furth AJ, Swallow DM, Griffith B. Human lactase and the molecular basis of lactase persistence. Biochem Gen 1985; 23:423–439.

248. Lorenz-Meyer H, Blum AL, Haemmerli HP, Semenza G. A second enzyme defect in acquired lactase deficiency. Lack of small-intestinal phlorizin-hydrolase. Eur J Clin Invest 1972; 2:326–331.

249. Seetharam B, Perrillo R, Alpers DH. Effect of pancreatic proteases on intestinal lactase activity. Gastroenterology 1980; 79:827–831.

250. Newcomer AD, McGill DB. Distribution of disaccharidase activity in the small bowel of normal and lactase-deficient subjects. Gastroenterology 1966; 51:481–488.

251. Flatz G. The genetic polymorphism of lactase activity in adult humans. In: Scriver CR, ed. The metabolic basis of inherited disease. 6th ed. Montreal: in press.

252. Ransome-Kuti O. Lactose intolerance—a review. Postgrad Med J (Suppl) 1977; 53:73–83.

253. Sahi T, Isokoski M, Jussila J, Launiala K, Pyörälä K. Recessive inheritance of adult-type lactose malabsorption. Lancet 1973; 2:823–828.

254. Lisker R, Gonzales B, Daltabuit M. Recessive inheritance of the adult type of intestinal lactase deficiency. Am J Hum Genet 1975; 27:662–667.

255. Ransome-Kuti O, Kretchmer M, Johnson JD, Gribble JT. A genetic study of lactose digestion in Nigerian families. Gastroenterology 1975; 58:431–436.

256. Ho MW, Povey S, Swallow D. Lactase polymorphism in adult British natives: Estimating allele frequencies by enzyme assays in autopsy samples. Am J Hum Genet 1982; 34:650–657.

257. Flatz G. Gene dosage effect on lactase activity demonstrated in vivo. J Hum Genet 1984; 36:306–310.

258. Metneki J, Cziezel A, Flatz SD, Flatz G. A study of lactose absorption capacity in twins. Hum Genet 1984; 67:296–332

259. Simoons FJ. Primary adult lactose intolerance and the milking habit: a problem in biological and cultural interrelations. II. A culture historical hypothesis. Am J Dig Dis 1970; 15:695–699.

260. Flatz G, Rotthauwe HW. Lactose nutrition and natural selection. Lancet 1973; ii:76–77.

261. Cochet B, Yung A, Griessen M, Bartholdi P, Schaller P, Donath A. Effects of lactose on intestinal calcium absorption in normal and lactase deficient subjects. Gastroenterology 1983; 84:935–940.

262. Forget P, Lambet J, Grandfils C, Dandrifosse G, Genbelle F. Lactase insufficiency revisited. J Pediatr Gastroenterol Nutr 1985; 4:868–873.

263. Cook GC. Lactase activity in newborn and infant Baganda. Br Med J 1967; 1:527–530.

264. Keusch GT, Troncale FJ, Miller LH, Promadhat V, Anderson PR. Acquired lactose malabsorption in Thai children. Pediatrics 1969; 43:540–545.

265. Sahi T, Isokoski M, Jussila L, Launiala K. Lactose malabsorption in Finnish children of school age. Acta Paediatr Scand 1972; 61:11–16.

266. Sahi T, Launiala K. Manifestation and occurrence of selective adult-type lactose malabsorption in Finnish teenagers. Am J Dig Dis 1978; 23:699–703.

267. Chang MH, Hsu HY, Chen CJ, Lee CH, Hsu JY. Lactose malabsorption and small intestinal lactase in normal Chinese children. J Pediatr Gastroenterol Nutr 1987; 6:369–372.

268. Maggi R, Sayagues B, Fernandez A, Romero B, Barusso P, Hernandez C, Magarinos M, Mendez G, Dilascio C, Martell M. Lactose malabsorption and intolerance in Uruguayan population by breath hydrogen test (H2). J Pediatr Gastroenterol Nutr 1987; 6:373–376.

269. Sahi T, Launiala K, Laitinen H. Hypolactasia in a fixed cohort of young Finnish adults: a follow-up study. Scand J Gastroenterol 1983; 18:865–870.

270. Paige DM. Lactose malabsorption in children: prevalence, symptoms, and nutritional considerations. In: Paige DM, Bayless TM, eds. Lactose digestion: clinical and nutrition implications. Baltimore: Johns Hopkins University Press, 1981; 151.

271. Newcomer AD, Thomas PT, McGill D, Hoffmann AF. Lactase deficiency: a common genetic trait of the American Indian. Gastroenterology 1977; 72:234–238.

272. Caskey DA, Payne-Bose D, Welsh JD, Gearhart HI, Nance RD, Morrison RD. Effect of age on lactose malabsorption in Oklahoma native Americans as determined by breath hydrogen analysis. Am J Dig Dis 1977; 22:113–116.

273. Roggero P, Offredi ML, Mosca F, Perazzani M, Mangiaterra B, Ghislanzoni P, Marenghi L, Careddu P. Lactose absorption and malabsorption in healthy Italian children: Do the quantity of malabsorbed sugar and the small bowel transit time play roles in symptoms productions? J Pediatr Gastroenterol Nutr 1985; 4:82–86.

274. Jussila J, Launiala K, Gorbatow O. Lactase deficiency and a lactose-free diet in patients with "unspecific abdominal complaints." Acta Med Scand 1969; 186:217–222.

275. Gudmand-Høyer E, Dahlqvist A, Jarnum S. The clinical significance of lactose malabsorption. Am J Gastroenterol 1970; 53:460–473.

276. Mitchell KJ, Bayless TM, Huang SS, Paige DM, Goodgame RW, Rothfeld B. Intolerance of a glass of milk in healthy teenagers. (Abstract) Gastroenterology 1973; 64:773.

277. Sahi T. Dietary lactose and aetiology of human small intestinal hypolactasia. Gut 1978; 19:1074–1086.

278. Bedine MS, Bayless TM. Intolerance of small amount of lactose by individuals with low lactase levels. Gastroenterology 1973; 65:735–743.

279. Jones DW, Latham MC, Kosikowski FW, Woodward G. Symptoms response to lactose-reduced milk in lactose-intolerant adults. Am J Clin Nutr 1976; 29:633–638.

280. Kneepkens CMF, Bijleveld CMA, Vonk RJ, Fernandes J. The daytime breath hydrogen profile in children with abdominal symptoms and diarrhoea. Acta Paediatr Scand 1986; 75:632–638.

281. Ferguson A. Diagnosis and treatment of lactose intolerance. Br Med J 1981; 283; 1423–1425.

282. Fowkes FGR, Ferguson A. Prevalence of self-diagnosed irritable bowel syndrome and cow's milk intolerance in white and non white doctors. Scott Med J 1980; 26:41–44.

283. Birge SJ Jr, Keutmann HT, Cuatrecasas P, Wheaton GD. Osteoporosis, intestinal lactase deficiency and low dietary calcium intake. N Engl J Med 1967; 276:445–448.

284. Newcomer AD, Hodgson SF, McGill DB, Thomas BJ. Lactase deficiency prevalence in osteoporosis. Ann Intern Med 1978; 39:218–220.

285. Condon JR, Nassim JR, Millard JC, Hilbe A, Stainthorpe EM. Calcium and phosphorus metabolism in relation to lactose tolerance. Lancet 1970; i:1027–1029.

286. Kocian J, Skala I, Bakos K. Calcium absorption from milk and lactose free milk in healthy subjects and patients with lactose intolerance. Digestion 1973; 9:317–324.

287. Editorial: Lactase deficiency in osteoporosis. Lancet 1979; i:86–87.

288. Editorial: Lactose malabsorption and lactose intolerance. Lancet 1979; ii:831–832.

289. Sahi T, Jussila J, Penttila IM, Sarna S, Isokoski M. Serum lipids and protein in lactose malabsorption. Am J Clin Nutr 1977; 30:476–481.

290. Simoons FJ, Johnsson JB, Kretchmer N. Perspective on milk-drinking and malabsorption of lactose. Pediatrics 1977; 59:98–109.

291. Flatz G, Rotthauwe HW. The human lactase polymorphism: physiology and genetics of lactose absorption and malabsorption. In: Steiberg AG, Bearne AG, eds. Progr Med Genet 1977; 2:205–249.

292. Seakins JM, Elliott RB, Quested CM, Matatumua A. Lactose malabsorption in Polynesian and white children in the south west Pacific studied by breath hydrogen technique. Br Med J 1987; 295:876–878.

293. Simoons FJ. A geographic approach to senile cataracts: possible links with milk consumption, lactase activity and galactose metabolism. Dig Dis Sci 1982; 27:257–264.

294. Rinaldi E, Albini L, Costagliola C, De Rosa G, Auricchio S. High frequency of lactose absorbers among adults with idiopathic senile and presenile cataract in a population with a high prevalence of primary adult lactose malabsorption. Lancet 1984; 1:357–361.

295. Jackson W. Clinical manifestations. In: Jackson W, ed. Proceedings of the first food allergy workshop. Oxford: Medical Education Service Ltd, 1980: 41.

296. Lessoff MH, Wraith DG, Merrett TG, Merrett J, Buisseret PD. Food allergy and intolerance in 100 patients—local and systemic effects. Q J Med 1980; 49:259–263.

297. Rosado JL, Allen LH, Solomons NW. Milk consumption, symptom response, and lactose digestion in milk intolerance. Am J Clin Nutr 1987; 45:1457–1460.

298. Dawson DJ, Newcomer AD, McGill DB. Lactose tolerance tests in adults with normal lactase activity. Gastroenterology 1966; 50:340–346.

299. Davidson GP, Robb TA. Value of breath hydrogen analysis in management of diarrheal illness in childhood: comparison with duodenal biopsy. J Pediatr Gastroenterol Nutr 1985; 4:381–384.

300. Lifshitz CH, Bautista A, Gapalachrishna GS, Stuff J, Garza C. Absorption and tolerance of lactose in infants recovering from diarrhea. J Pediatr Gastroenterol Nutr 1985; 4:942–946.

301. Fischer W. Zapf J. Zur erworbenen Laktoseintoleranz. Klin Wochenschr 1965; 43:1243–1246.

302. Isokoski M, Jussila J, Sarna S. A simple screening for lactose malabsorption. Gastroenterology 1972; 62:28–31.

303. Arola H, Koivula T, Isokoski M. One point urinary lactose-tolerance test. Lancet 1982; 1:676.

304. Arola H, Koivula T, Jokela H, Jauhiainen M, Keyrilainemo Visitelo A, Isokoski M. Strip test is reliable in common prevalences of hypolactasia. Scand J Gastroenterol 1987; 22:509–512.

305. Kerry KR, Anderson CM. A ward test for sugar in faeces. Lancet 1964; i:981–982.

306. Asp MG, Dahlqvist A. Human small-intestinal β-galactosidases specific assay of three different enzymes. Anal Biochem 1972; 47:527–538.

307. Tsuboi KK, Schwarz SN, Burrill PH, Kwong LK, Sunshine P. Sugar hydrolases of the infant rat intestine and their arrangement on the brush border membrane. Biochim Biophys Acta 1979; 554:234–242.

308. Newcomer AD, McGill DB. Disaccharidase activity in the small intestine: prevalence of lactase deficiency in 100 healthy subjects. Gastroenterology 1967; 53:881–889.

309. Gallagher CR, Molleson AL, Caldwell HJ. Lactose intolerance and fermentated dairy products. J Am Diet Assoc 1974; 65:418–419.

310. Kilara A, Shahani KM. Lactase activity of cultured and acidified dairy products. J Dairy Sci 1976; 59:2031–2035.

311. Gilliland SE, Kim HS. Effect of viable starter culture bacteria in yogurt on lactose utilization in humans. J Dairy Sci 1984; 67:1–6.

312. Kolars JC, Levitt MD, Aouji M, Savaiano DA. Yogurt an autodigesting source of lactase. N Engl J Med 1984; 310:1–3.

313. Savaiano DA, Abdelak Abou El Anouar DAG, Smith DE, Levitt MD. Lactose malabsorption from yogurt, pasteurized yogurt, sweet acidophilus milk, and cultured milk in lactase-deficient individuals. Am J Clin Nutr 1984; 40:1219–1223.

314. McDonough FE, Hitchins AD, Wong NP, Wells P, Godwell CE. Modification of sweet acidophilus milk to improve utilization by lactose-intolerant persons. Am J Clin Nutr 1987; 45:570–574.

315. Martini MC, Bollweg GL, Levitt MD, Savaiano DA. Lactose digestion by yogurt β-galactosidase: influence of Ph and microbiol cell integrity. Am J Clin Nutr 1987; 45:432–436.

316. Smith TM, Kolars JC, Savaiano DA. Absorption of calcium from milk and yogurt. Am J Clin Nutr 1985; 42:1197–1200.

317. Kim HS, Gilliland SE. *Lactobacillus acidophilus* as a dietary adjunct for milk to aid lactose digestion in humans. J Dairy Sci 1983; 66:959–966.

318. Kosokowski FV, Wierzbicki LE. Lactose hydrolysis of raw and pasteurized milks by *Saccharomyces lactis* lactase. J Dairy Sci 1973; 56:146–148.

319. Rand AG Jr. Enzyme technology and the development of lactose-hydrolyzed milk. In: Paige DM, Bayless TM, eds. Lactose digestion: clinical and nutritional implications. Baltimore: Johns Hopkins University Press, 1981: 219.

320. Mizote H, Terasaki S, Ryu T. Clinical study of lactose intolerance after gastrectomy. Kurume Med J 1978; 25:295–300.

321. Rosado JL, Salomons NW, Lisker R. Enzyme replacement therapy for primary adult lactase deficiency: effective reduction of lactose malabsorption and milk intolerance by direct addition of β-galactosidases to milk at mealtime. Gastroenterology 1984; 87:1072–1082.

322. Rosado JL, Deodhar AD, Bourges H. The effect of the digestion products of lactose (glucose and galactose) on its intraintestinal in vivo hydrolysis by exogenous microbial β-D-galactosidase. J Am Coll Nutr 1986; 5:281–290.

323. Solomons NW, Vasquez-Velasquez L, Guerrero AM. The relative contribution of exogenous β-galactosidase to intraluminal lactose digestion in lactase-deficient individuals. Am J Clin Nutr 1988; in press.

324. O'Keefe S. The use of lactase enzyme in feeding malnourished lactose intolerant patients. Presented at the XIII International Congress of Nutrition. Brighton, England, 1985; 190–191.

325. Moskovitz M, Curtis C, Gavaler J. Does oral enzyme replacement therapy reverse intestinal lactose malabsorption? Am J Gastroenterol 1987; 82:632–635.

326. Vega-Franco L, Jimenez E, Vega C. Absorcion facilitada de lactosa medieante β-galactosidasa del Aspergillus. Rev Mex Pediatr 1975; 44:137–147.

327. Barillas C, Solomons HW. Effective reduction of lactose maldigestion in preschool children by direct addition of β-galactosidases to milk at mealtime. Pediatrics 1987; 79:766–772.

328. Biller JA, King S, Rosenthal A, Grand RJ. Efficacy of lactase-treated milk for lactose-intolerant pediatric patients. J Pediatr 1987; 111:91–94.

329. Holzel A, Schwarz V, Sutcliffe KW. Defective lactose absorption causing malnutrition in infancy. Lancet 1959; i:1126–1128.

330. Lifshitz F. Congenital lactase deficiency. J Pediatr 1966; 69:229–237.

331. Launiala K, Kuitunen P, Visakorpi J. Disaccharidases and histology of duodenal mucosa in congenital lactose malabsorption. Acta Paediatr Scand 1966; 55:257–263.

332. Levin B, Abraham JM, Burgess EA, Wallis PG. Congenital lactose malabsorption. Arch Dis Child 1975; 45:173–177.

333. Savilathi E, Launiala K, Kuitunen P. Congenital lactase deficiency: a clinical study on 16 patients. Arch Dis Child 1983; 58:246–252.

334. Asp NG, Dahlqvist A. Intestinal β-galactosidases in adult low lactase activity and in congenital lactase deficiency. Enzyme 1974; 18:84–102.

335. Asp NG, Dahlqvist A, Kuitunen P, Launiala K, Visakorpi JK. Complete deficiency of brush border lactase in congenital lactase malabsorption. Lancet 1973; ii:329–330.

336. Dahlqvist A, Asp NG. Accurate assay of low intestinal lactase activity with a fluorimetric method. Anal Biochem 1971; 44:654–657.

337. Durand P. Lattosuria idiopatica in un paziente con diarrea cronica ed acidosi. Minerva Pediatr 1958; 1:706–709.

338. Russo G, Mollica F, Mazzone D, Santonocito B. Congenital lactose intolerance of gastrogen origin associated with cataracts. Acta Paediatr Scand 1974; 63:457–460.

339. Hirashima Y, Shinozuka S, Ieiri T, Matsuda I, Ono Y, Murata T. Lactose intolerance associated with cataracts. Eur J Pediatr 1979; 130:41–45.

340. Berg NU, Dahlqvist A, Lindberg T. A boy with severe infantile gastrogen lactose intolerance and acquired lactase deficiency. Acta Paediatr Scand 1979; 68:751–758.

341. Hoskova A, Sabacky J, Mrskos A, Pospisil R. Severe lactose intolerance with lactosuria and vomiting. Arch Dis Child 1980; 55:304–305.

342. Birch JB. Trehalose. Adv Carbohydr Chem 1963; 18:201–225.

343. Bergoz R. Trehalose malabsorption causing intolerance to mushrooms. Gastroenterology 1971; 5:909–912.

344. Madzarovova-Nohejilova J. Trehalase deficiency in a family. Gastroenterology 1973; 65:130–133.

345. McNair A, Cudmand-Hoyer E, Jarnum S, Orrild L. Sucrose malabsorption in Greenland. Br Med J 1972; 2:19–21.

346. Hannover AJ, Lennarz WJ. Transmembrane assembly of membrane and secretory glycoproteins. Arch Biochem Biophys 1981; 211:1–9.

347. Auricchio S, Ciccimarra F, Della Pietra D, Vegnente A. Intestinal hydrolysis of starch. Mod Probl Pediatr 1968; 11:22–31.

348. Auricchio S. Brush border enzymes. In: Anderson CM, Burke V, Gracey M, eds. Paediatric gastroenterology. 2nd ed. Carlton, Victoria, Australia: Blackwell Scientific, 1987: 185.

349. Mantei N, Villa M, Enzler T, Wacker H, Boll W, James P, Hunziker H, Semenza G. Complete primary structure of human and rabbit lactase-phlorizin hydrolase. Implications for biosynthesis, membrane anchoring and evolution of the enzyme. EMBO J 1988; 7:2705.

350. Sebastio G, Villa M, Sartorio R, Guzzetta V, Poggi V, Auricchio S, Boll W, Mantei N, Semenza G. Control of lactase in human adult-type hypolactasis and in weaning rabbits and rats. Am J Hum Genet 1989; 45:489.

PART 19

Congenital Transport Defects

Jehan-François Desjeux, M.D.

GLUCOSE AND GALACTOSE MALABSORPTION

Glucose and galactose malabsorption (GGM) is a rare congenital disease resulting from a selective defect in the intestinal glucose and galactose/Na$^+$ co-transport system. It is characterized by the neonatal onset of severe watery acidic diarrhea. In the past, it usually resulted in death within the first weeks of life. Now that the disease has been identified, children recover if glucose and galactose are withdrawn from the diet. In 1962, it was simultaneously described in France as an "intolerance to actively transported sugars" by Laplane et al[1] and in Sweden by Lindquist and Meeuwisse as a "chronic diarrhea caused by monosaccharide malabsorption."[2] Twenty-five years later, approximately 40 cases have been reported in families of European, North American, and Asian origin.[3-4]

Genetics

Twenty-seven of 39 cases reported were girls.[3] The high consanguinity rate and the fact that no vertical transmission has been found argue in favor of an autosomal recessive mode of inheritance.[5] Although the proportion of siblings affected (six of 16) may appear high, the true expression rate is masked by the small sample numbers, and the size of the family concerned cannot be used as an argument against this mode of inheritance. In addition, a high proportion of consanguinous mating implies that the mutant gene is highly infrequent.[3]

Attempts to detect heterozygotes with reduced intestinal glucose absorption have been made in three familial studies. Meeuwisse and Dahlqvist[6] found reduced intestinal glucose accumulation in the father of one child, while the results were normal in the mother. Elsas et al[7] demonstrated, in both parents of an affected child and also in a half-sister, that glucose accumulation dropped to a level intermediate between those of the controls and the proband. However, when we studied the father and mother of three children with GGM (one is reported in reference 3), they exhibited no clinical symptom of the disease. Hydrogen breath tests after glucose and galactose were normal. With 50 g fructose we observed abdominal pain and diarrhea, as well as an increased breath hydrogen concentration; however, this response was probably physiologic.[8] In one family, glucose accumulation in the intestine was normal. Further studies are required before we can draw firm conclusions on the mode of detection of heterozygotes. The recent finding of a cDNA probe for the co-transporter present on chromosome 22 is a major breakthrough in the molecular understanding of glucose absorption.[9]

Pathophysiology

In GGM, diarrhea is a consequence of selective malabsorption of glucose and galactose. This defect is situated in the glucose/Na$^+$ co-transport system in the brush border membrane, a conclusion reached by means of in vivo and in vitro studies.

In vivo intubation studies were performed under various technical conditions. Initially, Meeuwisse and Melin[10] compared the absorption of glucose and fructose after ingestion of a test meal containing the same concentrations of both sugars. Glucose was always absorbed more slowly than fructose. These authors also demonstrated that lactose, sucrose, and maltose were hydrolyzed in the patients tested. In the more recent experiments, the jejunum was perfused using either a double-lumen tube[11,12] or a four-lumen tube incorporating an occlusive balloon, in order to isolate effectively a 25-cm segment of bowel distal to the duodenojejunal junction.[13] This study was done in two adults and a 9-month-old child. The results were essentially the same and may be summarized as follows: (1) Glucose and galactose were poorly absorbed. At low concentrations of 5.6 mM or less, a small amount of glucose was secreted in the lumen. At high concentrations of up to 280 mM, glucose absorption was less than 10 percent of the control value. (2) In one patient[13] the normal basal potential difference of the jejunal mucosa did not respond to the addition of intraluminal glucose, a result that was in agreement with the absence of a functional Na$^+$, D-glucose co-transporter. (3) The jejunal mucosa secreted electrolytes and fluid, suggesting that under the prevailing experimental conditions, the combined glucose-sodium-water absorption process was defective.[13] (4) Sucrose was hydrolyzed and fructose absorbed, suggesting that malabsorption of glucose and galactose is a selective defect.

In vitro, the major characteristic of GGM is the lack of intracellular glucose or galactose accumulation against a concentration gradient (Table 1). In principle, the disappearance of active glucose and galactose transport may be due either to a reduced driving force, i.e., a less steep Na$^+$ electrochemical gradient, or to decreased permeability of the brush border membrane. However, there is no evidence for the first possibility, since when intracellular sodium was measured with isotopic tracers, it was found to be lower and not higher in patients with GGM than in controls, an observation that may in fact indicate a steeper Na$^+$ electrochemical gradient.[3]

Furthermore, the transport of other solutes such as alanine or leucine via Na$^+$-solute co-transporter is not altered.[3,14,15] The autoradiographic studies of Schneider et al[16] and Stirling et al[17] clearly indicate a defect in glucose binding at the brush border membrane. The diminished glucose influx across the luminal membrane on intact epithelium or isolat-

TABLE 1
Intracellular Substrate Concentration at Various Substrate Concentrations in
the Medium in Jejunal Biopsies from Children

		C:M Substrate	
Substrate	Concentration (mM)	Controls (n)	Glucose and Galactose Malabsorption (n)
Glucose (Glc)	10	3.84 ± 0.21 (34)	0.95 ± 0.12* (8)
Glc + phlor	10 + 0.5	2.99 ± 0.2 (7)	0.52 (1)
Galactose	10	1.54 ± 0.12 (6)	0.52 ± 0.11* (4)
Glucose	0.1	15.77 ± 1.55 (13)	2.98 ± 0.90* (4)
Galactose (Gala)	0.1	4.11 ± 0.33 (13)	ND
Gala + phlor	0.1 + 0.5	1.50 ± 0.70 (3)	ND
Xylose	10	1.10 ± 0.08 (13)	0.92 and 0.93
Alanine	0.8	13.33 ± 1.68 (4)	16.83 ± 3.54 (3)

*Significantly different from controls ($P < 0.001$).
NOTE: Results are expressed as intracellular over extracellular concentrations (C/M). n = number of determinations; ND = not determined; phlor = phlorizin.
The pieces of jejunum were placed in a beaker containing the oxygenated medium at 37 °C for 1 hour. The C:M ratio is the result of steady-state uptake from brush border and basolateral membranes. C:M > 1 represents uptake in excess of simple diffusion. (From Evans et al[3].)

ed brush border membrane vesicle[18] and the selective absence of short-circuit current stimulation by glucose further substantiate this possibility. Taken together, these experimental findings indicate that in GGM the functional activity of the Na^+, D-glucose co-transporter at the brush border membrane is either absent or reduced. Participation of mutarotase in sugar transport was suggested recently, and the absence of this enzyme has been demonstrated in one case of GGM.[19]

Diarrhea develops as a consequence of glucose and galactose malabsorption. However, the relationship between sugar malabsorption and diarrhea is complex, as indicated by the following observations.[20,21]

1. In GGM, glucose does not stimulate absorption but initiates a secretion of water and electrolytes in the jejunum, as demonstrated by in situ perfusion.[12,13] The water secretion present in the absence of perfused sugar was stimulated by the presence of glucose, galactose, maltose, sucrose, and lactose, but not by fructose.[13] Sodium, potassium, and chloride were always secreted together with water. However, the mechanism of this secretion is not clear, as the solutions perfused were made isotonic with plasma (300 mOsm per kilogram). Water secretion during perfusion of solutions containing sucrose was also demonstrated by Launiala[22] in a case of sucrase-isomaltase deficiency during perfusion of solutions containing sucrose. It was identical to that observed in normal children during perfusion of mannitol, a poorly absorbed sugar. Thus, water and electrolyte secretion is related to the presence of unabsorbed sugar in the intestinal lumen.

2. Fluid secretion in the lumen of the small intestine is accompanied by a reduction in the transit time of the perfused solution, probably secondary to the increased flow rate in the segment under study.[22]

3. Unusually large amounts of water, electrolytes, and glucose enter the colon. In contrast to the distal tubule, the colon is known not to reabsorb water under active regulation of hydraulic conductivity.[23] Consequently, the osmolality of fecal water is only slightly greater than that of plasma, and the colon must therefore adjust to acute loads of water and glucose by a mechanism other than hydraulic conductivity.

The consequences of acute loading of carbohydrates and water have been examined experimentally. Stool output was measured in healthy volunteers given an acute load of sugars poorly absorbed by the small intestine.[24] Diarrhea occurred when the load exceeded 120 to 220 mmol of mannitol, 73 to 146 mmol of lactulose, or 80 mmol of raffinose. Similarly, diarrhea occurred when water entered the colon at a flow rate of 6.3 ml per minute or more.[25] The significance of a colonic threshold for water and carbohydrate loading is to be found in the three major activities of the colon: motility, absorption, and intraluminal bacterial metabolism. As we know very little about these activities in the human newborn, we can only attempt to draw conclusions from studies performed at different ages. The magnitude and consequences of the osmotic load entering the adult colon in the form of glucose were examined by Bond and Levitt.[26] Carbohydrates may be broken into short-chain fatty acids by the bacteria that are active under anaerobic conditions prevailing in the lumen of the colon. The fatty acids not absorbed in their ionized form would then hold an equal number of milliequivalents of cations. Thus, failure to absorb only 10 g, or 55 mOsmol, of glucose in the small bowel could result in a 220-mOsm load in the colon, which is the isotonic equivalent of about 650 ml of fecal water.

In fact, the short-chain fatty acids in the colon are absorbed and oxidized by the bacteria, and most of the remaining fecal glucose is converted into a larger molecular form with limited osmotic activity. Thus, the colonic flora benefits the host by reducing the osmotic load of unabsorbed carbohydrate and by salvaging a large percentage of the calories of carbohydrate not absorbed in the small bowel.[26] When the colonic capacity to remove glucose is exceeded, it is the unabsorbed carbohydrate rather than the short-chain fatty acids that enhances the output of fecal water.[25]

The adaptation of colonic flora to chronic glucose loading might also explain the ability to tolerate larger amounts of dietary glucose as patients with GGM grow older. This adaptation was examined in adults given a chronic load of lactulose, a nonabsorbable sugar.[27] After 8 days of a daily load of 20 g, fecal water and carbohydrate output declined, whereas galactosidase activity, free fatty acid production, and other bacterial colonic activities increased. Thus, chronic lactulose loading improved the efficiency of the carbohydrate digestion by colonic flora. A similar adaptive mechanism was found in one patient with GGM who was given a moderate amount of glucose.[28]

In conclusion, the diarrhea observed in GGM is the direct consequence of glucose malabsorption in the small intestine. Glucose malabsorption and water and electrolyte secretion in the small intestine generate an acute loading of the colon that exceeds its threshold. With time, the control of the colonic threshold for water and glucose loading is the main compensatory mechanism that reduces diarrhea secondary to glucose malabsorption.

Clinical Features

The clinical features of the disease are so typical that it is not recommended to wait for the results of the laboratory tests to remove glucose and galactose from the diet.

The main and usually the only symptom consists of profuse watery diarrhea, which is acidic and contains sugar. In affected children receiving lactose, fecal sugar consists mainly of glucose and galactose, with only a small amount of lactose. For the equivalent amount of sugar given by mouth (2 g per kilogram body weight), fecal excretion of galactose is much higher than that of glucose.[10] Incidentally, as the low stool pH results from the bacterial metabolism of the sugar in the colon, fecal acidity can be eliminated by antibiotics.[16]

Characteristically, diarrhea develops within 4 days of birth. Occasionally, it may be noticed later, within 2 weeks, or it may be diagnosed in adults.[10,11,13] Diarrhea quickly leads to remarkably severe dehydration. Thus, in a series of 8 patients, body weight losses of 17 to 24 percent were reported.[3] Metabolic acidosis and hyperosmolar dehydration gradually develop with serum protein concentrations increasing up to 7.6 g per 100 ml and sodium concentrations of up to 173 mEq per liter.

Related gastrointestinal (GI) signs and symptoms are uncommon. Abdominal distention and vomiting have been noticed. Anorexia is unusual. Apart from signs of severe dehydration, physical examination is normal.

Intermittent or permanent glycosuria after fasting or after a glucose load is a frequent finding. Thus, the combination of reducing sugars in watery feces and slight glycosuria despite low blood sugar levels is highly suggestive of GGM.[10] Three of the four patients in whom glycosuria was not present were from the same family.[29,30] Renal glycosuria has been studied by five authors,[7,31-34] but their results are contradictory. However, in general, the alterations they found in the renal glucose threshold and maximal glucose reabsorption were only moderate.

Some of the laboratory tests carried out in order to exclude causes of diarrhea other than GGM have given conflicting results; thus, hypochromic anemia and moderate steatorrhea have been observed. Although normal values for xylose absorption are common in GGM, low or borderline values have sometimes been recorded. The histology of the biopsies taken after the diarrhea has stopped was normal under light and electron microscopy. The fact that disaccharidase activities of these biopsies were within the control range further indicates the integrity of the intestinal mucosa. During an episode of diarrhea, nonspecific alterations in both histologic appearance and disaccharidase activities are sometimes observed.[3,6,10,16]

The abnormality of carbohydrate metabolism is confined to glucose transport in the small intestine and the proximal renal tubule. Glucose entry into the erythrocytes is normal,[35] and so is fasting blood glucose. Whereas galactose and glucose disappear from plasma at normal rates after intravenous infusion,[31,32,36] oral sugar tolerance tests with glucose, galactose, and lactose yield flat blood glucose response curves. In contrast, blood glucose increases considerably after oral fructose loading. These results are the consequence of selective malabsorption of glucose and galactose. Although these tests are commonly performed, they are not very useful in identifying GGM for three reasons: (1) When glucose or galactose is given at the dose of 2 g per kilogram body weight, it usually produces watery diarrhea, but this response is not specific to GGM and may aggravate the clinical status. (2) Approximately 25 percent of normal children have a flat blood glucose curve. (3) Moreover, in GGM, not all response curves are flat. The increase in blood glucose within 1 hour may reach 2 mmol per liter.

Malabsorption of glucose and galactose is easily identified by the breath hydrogen test.[37] It is safe to perform the first test with a dose of 0.5 g per kilogram body weight of glucose. Breath hydrogen concentration exceeds 20 ppm within 3 hours of glucose or galactose oral loading[3,38] in most cases, but after several days of glucose feeding, breath hydrogen production may decrease.[28]

Diarrhea improves immediately when patients are placed on a fructose-based milk formula free of glucose and galactose. The diagnosis of GGM can be established later by measuring glucose transport in a piece of jejunal biopsy. In this disorder biopsy tissue does not accumulate glucose (and galactose) against a concentration gradient.[3] From the technical point of view, it is wise to use a low glucose concentration in the incubation solution (e.g., 0.1 mM), in the presence and absence of phlorizin, and to check that alanine or leucine is actively transported (Table 1).[3] It should be noted that in acquired monosaccharide malabsorption with a flat intestinal mucosa, the concentration power of the remaining epithelium is still 30 percent of that of the control intestine.[15,39] Alternatively, intestinal perfusion in situ has been used successfully to assess the diagnosis of GGM.[11-13] In that case, it is essential to use a well-defined methodology to obtain unequivocal results.[40-42]

As affected children grow older and their diet becomes more diversified, dietary restrictions are increasingly difficult to maintain, and both children and parents learn to "titrate" the symptoms according to carbohydrate tolerance. In older children and adults, tolerance to the offending carbohydrates improves,[3,10,11,43-45] although malabsorption of glucose and galactose in the small intestine remains unchanged. In most cases, growth and mental development have been normal when glucose and galactose were removed from the diet[3]; adults with GGM live relatively normal lives.[10,11,13]

Treatment

Treatment consists of immediate rehydration (oral rehydration solutions that contain glucose must be avoided) and of feeding a glucose- and galactose-free diet. In the first 3 months of life, a commercial glucose- and galactose-free formula such as Galactomine 19 from Nutricia, supplemented with iron and vitamins, may be given. Alternatively, a special formula may be prepared as follows (grams per liter): calcium caseinate 19 to 29, fructose 39 to 59, and corn oil 34, to which electrolytes, vitamins, iron, and oligoelements should be added.[32]

DISORDERS OF FAT ABSORPTION: ABETALIPOPROTEINEMIA, HYPOBETALIPOPROTEINEMIA

Abetalipoproteinemia and hypobetalipoproteinemia are inherited deficiency states of the plasma lipoproteins, which contain a protein called apolipoprotein B (apo B). These lipoproteins include chylomicrons; very low density lipoproteins (VLDL), which are transporters of triglycerides; and the end products of VLDL catabolism, the low-density lipoproteins (LDL), which are transporters of cholesterol. The plasma of the patients suffering from abetalipoproteinemia does not contain chylomicrons, VLDL, and LDL. This state results from mutations at two or more loci. The heterozygote carriers enjoy good health. Subjects who were heterozygous for a different disorder were found to have marked deficiency of LDL, a condition termed familial hypobetalipoproteinemia.

The clinical features were first described in 1950[46] in an 18-year-old Jewish girl presenting with atypical retinitis pigmentosa, malformed erythrocytes, and a "form of Friedreich's ataxia." Profound hypocholesterolemia was added to the syndrome complex, and, in 1960, total absence of LDL from plasma was noticed in similar patients.[47-50] (For a recent extensive review, see reference 51.)

Genetics

Abetalipoproteinemia has been reported from 12 countries. Patients have included Caucasians, blacks, Arabs, Orientals, and a Maori. It is a familial disease predominating in males (70 percent) and having an autosomal recessive mode of inheritance. Consanguinity has been found in almost 50 percent of pedigrees. Obligate heterozygotes for classic abetalipoproteinemia cannot be identified in the absence of an affected child in the family.

Familial hypobetalipoproteinemia is distinguished from abetalipoproteinemia on genetic grounds: Heterozygotes for familial hypobetalipoproteinemia have low plasma levels of cholesterol and LDL. Homozygotes with familial hypobetalipoproteinemia are phenotypically indistinguishable from patients with abetalipoproteinemia except for possibly milder neuromuscular impairment. In 1969, investigators in America and France reported the appearance of hypobetalipoproteinemia in three and two successive generations, respectively,[52,53] establishing both the familial nature of the disorder and an apparent autosomal dominant mode of inheritance. It seems likely that this disorder represents a different mutation or mutations.[51] A truncated species of apo B was recently identified in the plasma lipoproteins of members of a kindred with familial hypobetalipoproteinemia. It was due to a four-base pair deletion in the apo B gene.[54]

Abetalipoproteinemia

Pathophysiology

The usual mechanisms for transport of triglyceride from the intestine and liver are abolished, and chylomicrons, VLDL, and LDL are absent from the plasma. The defect is presumed to involve the synthesis of apo B or intracellular assembling of apo B with lipid. In order to explain the secondary manifestations of the disease involving different systems and organs, the hypothesis of some generalized defect in cell membranes has been put forward. Severe malabsorption in infancy with deficiency of fat-soluble vitamin E and other substances has also been proposed as a mechanism of this condition.

The intraluminal phase of fat digestion seems normal in abetalipoproteinemia. The triglyceride in the affected cells does not appear to receive the normal apoprotein coating; it is not normally transported to the Golgi zone through the endoplasmic reticulum and does not serve as a lipoprotein precursor. The missing protein presumably is apo B, which is not detectable in the intestinal mucosa in abetalipoproteinemia.[55] The mucosal cells in abetalipoproteinemia absorb long-chain fatty acids and normally re-esterify them with glycerol. Presumably the triglycerides are hydrolyzed and the fatty acids transported in the portal venous system bound to albumin. Such a mechanism must account for the fact that steatorrhea in abetalipoproteinemia is relatively mild. The fatty liver in abetalipoproteinemia is due to the accumulation of triglycerides.

Neuromuscular changes in abetalipoproteinemia probably are due to abnormal lipid peroxidation of the highly unsaturated phosphatides of myelin, secondary to prolonged vitamin E deficiency. The serum level of vitamin E is very low.[56,57] Tocopherol absorption normally is greatest when it is administered with dietary fat, but the vitamin is also absorbed from food containing no lipids.[58] Enteric absorption of vitamin E and detectable blood levels can be achieved in abetalipoproteinemia only when very large quantities of fat-miscible preparations are ingested for prolonged periods.[59,60] Retinal changes in abetalipoproteinemia can be associated with the vitamin A malabsorption that accompanies the disease. Vitamin A absorption curves in abetalipoproteinemia are characteristically flat,[61–63] and low plasma concentrations are typical in untreated patients. When large supplements are given, levels rise to the normal range. Hypoprothrombinemia secondary to vitamin K malabsorption is also well documented in this disorder.[64]

Acanthocytes found in the peripheral blood in abetalipoproteinemia are the result of the reversal of phosphatidylcholine-to-sphingomyelin ratio (1:0.6 in abetalipoproteinemia and 1:3 in normal cells), while the totals of phospholipids and lipid are normal. LDL and their lipid-free apoprotein B are absent in the plasma of the affected subjects. The apoproteins A-I and A-II in abetalipoproteinemia are identical to their normal counterparts. The three C apolipoproteins common to VLDL and high-density lipoprotein (HDL) isolated from abetalipoproteinemia patients have the same amino acid composition as the controls.

Clinical Features

Because of its multisystem involvement, the clinical features of abetalipoproteinemia are highly diverse. GI symptoms appear early in life. Malodorous diarrhea develops during the first week of life in some infants. Others simply fail to thrive. Eventually, however, fat malabsorption is apparent. Some infants have vomiting and recurrent pulmonary infections. Neurologic lesions and ocular manifestations appear after 5 years or more. The neuromuscular manifestations are devastating. The earliest finding is the loss of stretch reflexes. The unusual severity and lack of sparing of the upper extremities warrant investigation of other possible causes, particularly selective loss of cell bodies in the spinal ganglions. Disturbances of proprioceptive pathways to the brain also occur early. Position and vibratory sensations are lost, and a positive Romberg's sign typical of sensory ataxia can be elicited in most subjects.

The age of onset of ocular abnormalities is highly variable, but retinitis pigmentosa has been a constant finding. Night blindness, nystagmus, and ophthalmoplegia are frequent. Blindness occurs if the macula is involved. Part if not all the symptoms are probably related to vitamin A deficiency.

The diagnosis is confirmed by the typical hematologic and small bowel biopsy findings. The proportion of acanthocytes is at least 50 to 70 percent. The acanthocyte is not unique to abetalipoproteinemia, but it is a simple test pointing to abnormality in plasma membrane lipid composition. In addition, mild to severe anemia with slightly elevated reticulocyte numbers is frequent. Autohemolysis is related to vitamin E deficiency.[56]

The basic feature of abetalipoproteinemia is found in the cytoplasm of jejunal epithelial cells where lipids are normally transported. Small bowel villi appear normal, but the enterocytes near the villous tip are filled with lipid droplets that distend the apical portion of the cell.

In the normal cell, triglycerides are surrounded by endoplasmic reticulum and Golgi apparatus, which contains clusters of chylomicrons. In abetalipoproteinemia large lipid droplets are free in the cytoplasm, and the cisternae of the Golgi apparatus are empty.[65] Tall et al[66] showed, through fluorescence antibody techniques, an absence of chylomicron apoprotein in the intestinal mucosa. Thus, the absence of apo B results in an inability of the cell to form chylomicrons and VLDL.

Abnormalities in the plasma are explained by the inability of the intestine to elaborate B protein–containing lipoproteins. Concentrations of all the major plasma lipids— cholesterol, triglycerides, and phospholipids—are reduced. Chylomicrons are absent after a fatty meal.[51]

Treatment

Restriction of intake of triglycerides containing long-chain fatty acids (C_{16} to C_{24}) relieves the GI manifestations in the infant and child with abetalipoproteinemia. Appropriate considerations should be given to the maintenance of the caloric balance in these patients, who suffer from malnutrition. In this respect, medium-chain triglycerides that are transported by a different mechanism can be useful. Fat-soluble vitamins A and K as well as linoleic acid should be provided in adequate doses. Vitamin E supplementation given by mouth at the very high dose of 100 mg per kilogram per day may limit the neurologic symptoms.[60] It is important to recognize affected children early, because early therapy may prevent early death and minimize the neurologic symptoms.

Familial Hypobetalipoproteinemia

It seems likely that this disorder, although chemically indistinguishable from typical abetalipoproteinemia, represents a different mutation or mutations.[51]

Clinical Features

In homozygotes, the GI findings mimic those of abetalipoproteinemia, including fat malabsorption and extensive neutral fat accumulation in enterocytes. In heterozygotes, fat absorption and intestinal mucosa are probably normal.[52,53,67,68] The neurologic manifestations and anal and ocular findings are moderate in homozygotes and probably absent in heterozygotes. All homozygotes reported had typical acanthocytes, whereas heterozygotes rarely have acanthocytes.

The main difference between familial hypobetalipoproteinemia and abetalipoproteinemia is that the heterozygotes of the former disease do not maintain a normal concentration of LDL[51]; they have a reduced synthesis of LDL with a normal catabolic rates.[69,70] Various forms of hypobetalipoproteinemia have been described,[71,72] indicating that the intestinal transport of triglyceride in the plasma of the enterocytes is under complex genetic control.

Treatment

Treatment is the same as for abetalipoproteinemia. Heterozygotes do not require treatment.

AMINO ACID TRANSPORT DEFECTS

Congenital defects of specific amino acid membrane transport systems are recognized in the epithelial cells of the small intestine and proximal tubule. The clinical consequences of these defects vary from abnormal amino acid profiles in the urine without clinical symptoms to severe life-threatening diseases.

Data suggesting an intestinal transport defect in cystinuria were available by the late nineteenth century, when diamines were detected in the urine of these patients,[73] the diamines being the result of colonic bacterial decarboxylation of malabsorbed amino acids.[74,75] More recently, Scriver and Rosenberg stimulated a comprehensive approach to the understanding of these genetic diseases.[76] Conversely, research on the nature of the transport defects has been at the origin of our understanding of many functional, genetic, nutritional, and therapeutic aspects of intestinal epithelium. For a recent review, see references 76 and 77.

Amino acid intestinal transport defects are identified by an increase in the selective urinary excretion of a group of amino acids (cystinuria, dibasic aminoaciduria, Hartnup disease, iminoglycinuria, and dicarboxylic aciduria) or a single amino acid (cystine, lysine, histidine, methionine, and tryptophan). These clinical observations have suggested that the intestinal and proximal tubule may share common transport systems, selective for a structure of amino acids and under genetic control.

Free amino acids in the intestinal lumen are taken up at the epithelial luminal membrane, where they are cotransported with Na against a concentration gradient. At the basolateral membrane they leave the cell by an Na-independent facilitated diffusion, which implies selective permeability but no other source of energy than the amino acid concentration gradient across the membrane.[78] Congenital amino acid transport defects result from reduced membrane permeability or an impaired transport system at one of the two membranes. For example, lysine permeability is reduced at the luminal membrane in cystinuria[79] and at the basolateral membrane in lysinuric protein intolerance.[80] Also, in cystinuria the luminal permeability for cystine is present, but the transport system is impaired (Fig. 1).[81]

It has long been thought that dietary proteins require complete hydrolysis to free amino acids before absorption but in Hartnup disease and in cystinuria the "affected" amino acids are absorbed in the form of homologous or mixed dipeptides.[82–87] These observations were interpreted as an indication of several transport pathways for the same group of amino acids. Apparently amino acid can be absorbed both free and in the form of dipeptide.[87] This dual mechanism is present at the luminal membrane but not at the basolateral membrane, where only free amino acids are transported in substantial amounts to the blood. Thus, the two membranes of the enterocytes and other epithelial cells display two different genetic controls of the transport systems. The transport systems present in the luminal membrane are typical of the epithelial

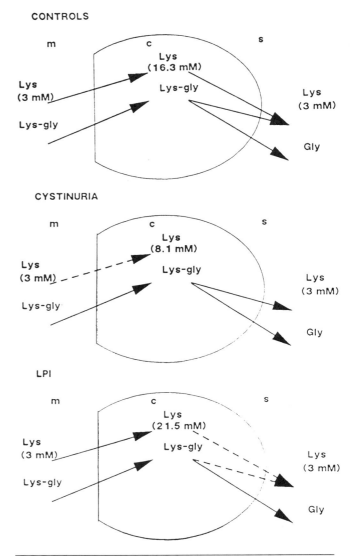

FIGURE 1 Genetic control of intestinal lysine transport. Dashed arrows represent defective transport system. Lysine is transported across the luminal membrane (mc) as free lysine or as a dipeptide (lys-gly), but only in free form across the basolateral membrane. In cystinuria, the free lysine system is defective without alteration of dipeptide transport, resulting in low intracellular lysine concentration (8.1 versus 16.3 mM in controls) and transepithelial absorption of lysine only from a dipeptide source. In lysinic protein intolerance (LPI), the defective intracellular system results in high intracellular lysine concentrations and transepithelial malabsorption of lysine in free form and as dipeptide. c = intestinal epithelial cells; m = mucosal side; s = serosal side.

cells, whereas those present in the basolateral membrane may be common with other nonepithelial cells.[88] For example, in cystinuria the defect is localized exclusively at the luminal membrane of the enterocytes and epithelial cells of the tubule, whereas in lysinuric protein intolerance the defect is localized at both the basolateral membrane of the epithelial cells and the plasma membrane of nonepithelial cells.[88] Also, differences in the properties of the two membranes may explain that the symptoms related to amino acid deficit are more important if the defect is at the basolateral membrane than at the luminal membrane.

Dibasic (or Diamino) Amino Acid Transport Defects

Lysine, arginine, ornithine, and cystine are the four amino acids found in the urine of cystinuric patients; the first three are characteristic of hyperdibasic aminoaciduria, and isolated cases of cystinuria or lysinuria have been reported. In addition, genetic heterogeneity may be present in the first two diseases, and the defects may not be identical in the kidney and the intestine. Therefore, genetic control for the transport of this group of amino acids must be at least at four different sites.

Cystinuria

Cystinuria is the most common congenital amino acid transport defect.[89]

Genetics. Cystinuria is inherited as an autosomal recessive trait. Homozygotes are encountered with a frequency of 1 in 10,000 to 1 in 15,000 in many ethnic groups. Cystine calculus represents 1 to 2 percent of all the calculi of the urinary tract. All homozygotes have identical urinary excretion patterns and abnormalities in renal clearance, but the pattern of intestinal transport defects and the amount of abnormal urinary excretion in heterozygotes suggest at least three different mutations.[90,91]

Pathophysiology. The pathophysiology of this disorder is not entirely understood.[89] At the level of the enterocytes the findings are as follows: (1) In vivo, the four amino acids are malabsorbed in the small intestine. (2) In the colon bacteria decarboxylate the amino acids, and the decarboxylated amino acids are reabsorbed and excreted in the urine. (3) When given as dipeptides the amino acids are absorbed into the blood. Thus, there is no significant amino acid deficit in this disease. In vitro, the uptake of the four amino acids is decreased as assessed by the intracellular steady-state concentration. (4) In vitro, the entry permeability across the luminal membrane is markedly reduced for lysine and presumably for arginine and ornithine.[79] (5) In contrast, the cystine entry permeability is not altered, but the exit permeability from the cytoplasm to the lumen is increased.[80] In summary, the defect is situated at the luminal membrane, but it is not possible to explain the results obtained so far with only one mutation.

Clinical Features. The symptoms observed in the disease are exclusively those of calculus in the urinary tract because of poor solubility of cystine at the usual urinary pH. There are no GI symptoms or signs.

Dibasic Aminoaciduria

Excessive excretion of lysine, arginine, and ornithine but not cystine has been described in different clinical diseases.

Lysinuric Protein Intolerance. Lysinuric protein intolerance (LPI) is characterized by renal dibasic aminoaciduria,

especially massive lysinuria, and inadequate formation of urea with hyperammonemia after protein ingestion. Since the first description of three patients by Perheentupa and Visakorpi[92] in 1965, more than 40 patients have been reported, most of them from Finland.[93]

Genetics. LPI is inherited as a autosomal recessive trait[94]; in Finland, one new case is diagnosed among 60,000 to 80,000 births. Heterozygotes are not detectable.

Pathophysiology. Most if not all symptoms can be explained by a selective intestinal and renal diamino acid transport defect leading to distortion of the urea cycle and hyperammonemia after amino nitrogen loading.[92] In vivo, the three amino acids—lysine, arginine, and ornithine—are malabsorbed by the small intestine and the kidney, given as free amino acids or dipeptides,[93,94] and the plasma concentrations of diamino acids are low. Entry of the amino acids across the luminal membrane of the epithelial cells is not impaired, but the exit permeability across the basolateral membrane to the blood is grossly impaired.[81] As a result, intracellular concentrations are increased. In addition, their transport may be impaired in hepatocytes.[97] Citrulline, a neutral amino acid participating in the urea cycle, is absorbed normally by the intestine.[98]

In the liver, the urea cycle transforms NH_4^+ liberated from deamination of glutamine into urea by means of three amino acids— citrulline, arginine, and ornithine. In LPI, one explanation for hyperammonemia after protein intake is a low availability of arginine and ornithine to the urea cycle in the liver.[92] Another possibility is a reversal of the urea cycle due to increased arginine and ornithine in the liver cells, if the genetic transport defect is also present in the liver.[97] Whatever the precise mechanism, it is clear that citrulline given intravenously or orally prevents the hyperammonemic and orotic aciduric responses to amino acid load. The production of orotic acid in the liver increases when the urea cycle is inhibited, so orotic aciduria is a useful clinical indicator of urea cycle function.[99] If the altered urea cycle is related to arginine and ornithine metabolism in LPI, the part played by the deficiency of lysine is still unclear in this disorder.

Clinical Features. Usually the disease appears after weaning as failure to thrive with anorexia, vomiting, and diarrhea.[93] Later features include protein aversion, growth retardation, hepatomegaly and splenomegaly, muscular weakness, osteoporosis, abnormalities of blood cells, elevation of serum activities of LDH, glutamyl transpeptidase (GPT), aldolase, ferritin, T_4 and thyroxine-binding globulin (TBG), and, occasionally, fragile hair. Forced feeding may lead to convulsions, coma, and mental retardation. The diagnostic chemical characteristics are increased urinary excretion with subnormal levels of the diamino acids and hyperammonemia and orotic aciduria after amino nitrogen intake.[93,99] In the absence of treatment LPI may lead to mental retardation and even death.

Treatment. Citrulline is the most valuable agent for treatment of LPI.[100,101] In a large series of 19 patients, citrulline (2 to 3 g daily) was offered with or without lysine to supplement an isocaloric diet. In addition, the patients were encouraged to increase their daily protein intake to 1.0 to 2.0 g per kilogram, according to age. This regimen led to improved protein nutrition, normalized orotic aciduria, catch-up growth, and improved liver histology. Although not curative, citrulline restores the urea cycle intermediates and protects the patients from hyperammonemia and its consequences. Additional lysine does not enhance the favorable effect but in some patients has provoked abdominal cramps and diarrhea.[101]

Other Hyperdibasic Aminoaciduria and Isolated Lysinuria. One patient with isolated hyperlysinuria and hyperammonemia had all the symptoms of LPI.[102] Three other patients, two with mental retardation, had increased urinary excretion of the three diamino acids without other symptoms.[103-105] Thus, the defect may be situated at the luminal membrane of the enterocytes.

Lowe's Syndrome. This syndrome is characterized by aminoaciduria, especially of lysine and arginine, with mental retardation, cataracts, hypotonia, renal disease, vitamin D–resistant rickets, and choreoathetosis. There is a partial intestinal defect of lysine and arginine absorption, but cystine absorption is normal.[106]

Neutral Amino Acid Transport Defects

Hartnup Disease

Hartnup disease is characterized by massive aminoaciduria involving a group of neutral monoamino-monocarboxylic amino acids that share a common transport system. For a general review, see reference 107.

Genetics. Hartnup disease is inherited as an autosomal recessive trait. The prevalence is one in 16,000 newborns. Heterozygotes have no clinical or biochemical abnormalities.

Pathophysiology. Symptoms are the consequences of selective intestinal malabsorption of free neutral amino acids. However, they are not only the consequence of amino acid deficiency, since neutral amino acids can be absorbed from dipeptides. The symptoms may be related to metabolites produced in the large intestine and toxic to the central nervous system. The intestinal malabsorption diminishes the amount of nicotinamide synthesized from tryptophan, thus causing pellagra-like manifestations.

Clinical Features. Hartnup disease is characterized by an intermittent red, scaling pellagra-like rash appearing after exposure to sunlight, by attacks of cerebellar ataxia, and occasionally by psychiatric changes ranging from emotional instability to delirium. Mental retardation is common. Increased urinary excretion of neutral amino acid is typical.

Treatment. In general patients have responded satisfactorily to prolonged oral administration of nicotinamide (50 to 150 mg daily) together with protein-enriched feeding.

Selective Methionine Malabsorption

Isolated defect of methionine absorption in the intestine and the kidney was reported in two male children with severe mental deficiency.[108] Silk postulated that the defect could be at the basolateral membrane.[77] Otherwise termed "Oasthouse urine disease," it is named for the peculiar odor of dried celery imparted to the urine containing beta-hydroxybutyric acid, a bacterial breakdown product of methionine. Clinical symptoms are white hair, edema, hypercapnia, mental retardation, and convulsions. In one patient treated with a methionine-free diet, diarrhea and convulsions subsided and mental state improved.

Isolated Tryptophan Malabsorption

Isolated tryptophan malabsorption in the intestine with normal renal excretion of amino acids was reported in two children with hypercalcemia and nephrocalcinosis.[109] The very high levels of tryptophan and its metabolic products in stools of these patients could be the consequence of a defect of mucosal uptake of peptide-bound and free tryptophan.[77] Otherwise termed "blue diaper syndrome," it is named for the bluish discoloration of the diapers, the urine containing indoles (indigotin) that are the bacterial breakdown of tryptophan. The mother of the children also excreted indoles in urine. Clinical symptoms are failure to thrive, recurrent unexplained fever, infections, irritability, and constipation.

Familial Iminoglycinuria

This disease is characterized by urinary excretion of proline, hydroxyproline, and glycine. Only some of the affected patients have impaired intestinal transport of these amino acids, leading to their accumulation in the stools. There is no treatment for this benign disorder.[110]

Dicarboxylic Aminoaciduria

Selective urinary excretion of glutamic and aspartic acids was reported in three children.[111,112] When associated with an intestinal transport defect, it may be revealed by fasting hypoglycemia.

Histidinuria

Isolated selective histidinuria with a mild defect of intestinal histidine transport was reported in children with moderate mental retardation or myoclonic attacks.

CONGENITAL CHLORIDE DIARRHEA

Congenital chloride diarrhea (CCD) is the consequence of a selective defect in intestinal Cl⁻ transport. An autosomal recessive disease characterized by life-long secretory diarrhea with high fecal Cl⁻ concentration, starting in utero, it usually resulted in severe lethal dehydration in the past; some infants survived with severe alkalosis, hypochloremia, hypokalemia, and retarded growth and development. CCD was first described by Gamble et al[113] and Darrow[114] in 1945, when each reported a child with "congenital alkalosis with diarrhea." Although patients have been reported in families of different countries,[115,116] most were born in Finland. The clinical features and the pathophysiology of the disease were extensively studied by Perheentupa and colleagues.[117-119]

Genetics

CCD is inherited as an autosomal recessive trait.[120] The gene appears to exist mainly in Finland but cases occur in most other populations, including most European countries, the United States, Canada, Argentina, India, and Japan. White, black, and Asiatic races are represented. Many patients may succumb, unrecognized. In Finland, where all deliveries take place in hospitals and the personnel in charge of newborn infants are well alerted to the possibility of CCD, one new case is now diagnosed among approximately 43,000 newborns.[121]

Pathophysiology

Diarrhea is a consequence of the selective malabsorption of Cl^-. This defect probably is situated at the Cl^-/HCO_3^- exchange transport system in the epithelium of the ileum and colon. This conclusion was reached from the following observations: (1) The most constant feature in CCD is the high water content of stools, with a high Cl^- and a low HCO_3^- concentration and a low pH. (2) Secretion of Cl^- by the stomach and renal Cl^- transport are normal.[115] (3) The transport of water, glucose, sodium, and bicarbonate is normal in the duodenum and jejunum[116] but abnormal in the ileum and colon, where the Cl^- concentration of the intestinal contents is supranormal only in these parts.[116,119] (4) In the ileum, perfusion studies indicated either impairment of Cl^- absorption and HCO_3^- secretion[122] or Cl^- secretion together with HCO_3^- absorption, while in the control situation, there is Cl^- absorption together with HCO_3^- secretion. Analysis of the flux as a function of the electrochemical gradient indicates that Cl^- and HCO_3^- are not transported actively, but active Na^+/H^+ exchange was observed. The simplest explanation for the ileal defect is an absence of Cl^-/HCO_3^- exchange.[115,116,121,122] In one piece of isolated ileum from a CCD patient, we found that theophylline stimulated a short-circuit current, thus suggesting that the electrogenic Cl^- secretion is still present. (5) In the colon, absence of Cl^-/HCO_3^- exchange was evident in three patients. No passive movements of these ions could be demonstrated, presumably because of the normally low permeability of the colonic epithelium. In the colon of the controls and the patients with CCD, Na^+ could be absorbed from concentrations as low as 20 mmol per liter, but in the absence of HCO_3^-, that is, in the situation normally prevailing in CCD, Na^+ absorption was reduced.[123,124]

Taken together, the high Cl^- content and acidic watery diarrhea observed in CCD can be interpreted as a consequence of a congenital defect of Cl^-/HCO_3^- exchange mechanism in the ileum and colon. The reduced HCO_3^- secretion results in acidity of intestinal contents and, presumably, in intracellular alkalinity and secondarily impairs Na^+ absorption by Na^+/H^+ exchange and therefore water reabsorption (see Chapter 21) (Fig. 2).

Clinical Features

The clinical features of the disease vary with the age of the child. Maternal polyhydramnios is a constant feature of CCD. Together with a lack of meconium and images of distended loops of ileum filled with fluid, it is an indication of the intrauterine onset of diarrhea. Prematurity is frequent. In amniotic fluid, electrolyte concentrations are normal.[117] Prenatal diagnosis might be possible in mothers with a previ-

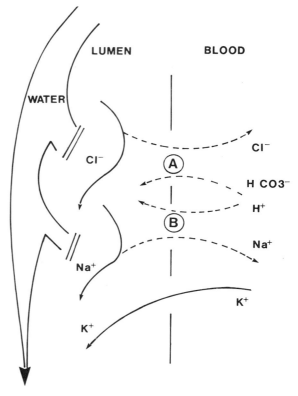

WATERY DIARRHEA

FIGURE 2 Ileal and colonic water and electrolyte transport in congenital chloride diarrhea. The primary defect is an absence of Cl^- absorption by Cl^-/HCO_3^- exchange (A). The acidity of the intestinal contents secondarily impairs Na^+ absorption by Na^+/H^+ exchange (B), which in turn stimulates K^+ secretion. In congenital Na^+ malabsorption, the primary defect is an absence of Na^+ absorption by Na^+/H^+ exchange (B). The alkalinization of the intestinal contents secondarily impairs Cl^- absorption by Cl^-/HCO_3^- exchanger (A). In both cases, the result is that water reabsorption is decreased as a consequence of decreased NaCl reabsorption.

ous child with CCD, but interruption of pregnancy is not recommended because the disease is treatable.

At birth the weights and lengths of patients with CCD are normal for gestational age.[117] The abdomen is usually large and distended, and intestinal contractions are visible. Loops of ileum and colon are dilated with air and fluid, and ascites is often present. The distended abdomen may lead to suspicion of lower intestinal obstruction, including Hirschsprung's disease; many patients with CCD are first seen by surgeons who may suspect volvulus.

Watery diarrhea is present from birth but often goes unnoticed because the fluid in the diaper is thought to be urine. Because of the diarrhea, dehydration develops rapidly and weight loss often amounts to 10 percent of the birth weight on the first day of life. Hyperbilirubinemia is common and is caused in part by the dehydration.

The first disturbances in electrolyte concentrations to develop are hyponatremia and hypochloremia with mild metabolic alkalosis. Stool volume is about 150 ml per 24 hours in the newborn patient, with median fecal electrolyte concentrations of Cl^-, Na^+, and K^+ of 120, 80, and 40 mmol per liter, respectively. If the child is dehydrated, the Cl^- concentration may be low, but after correction of water and electrolyte deficits it always exceeds 90 mmol per liter in stools. Thus, the diagnosis can be made within minutes in any hospital where Cl^- can be measured. A stool sample is easily obtained from the rectum with a soft catheter. This obviates contamination with urine, leading to falsely low values for fecal Cl^-. Hyponatremia is often present, and acidosis is compatible with CCD in the newborn.

Some infants survive for several months without diagnosis or adequate therapy. Since the diarrhea decreases with dehydration, the stool of these older patients may be soft and unformed instead of watery. Stool Cl^- concentration may be less than 100 mmol per liter; urine is, as a rule, Cl^--free, and the child has hypochloremia, hypokalemia, and metabolic alkalosis. The severity of this electrolyte disturbance depends on the salt intake and the effectiveness of the activation of the renin-aldosterone system, which invariably occurs.[125] These children may be in delicate balance with no reserves and may succumb to trivial intercurrent infections, which aggravate the diarrhea.

The basic feature of CCD is the high Cl^- concentration of the watery diarrhea. The median Cl^- concentration is 150 mmol per liter and after 3 months of age always exceeds the sum of the Na^+ and K^+ concentrations (the median concentration of these being 60 and 45 mmol per liter, respectively). Stool pH rises after the first months of life owing to increased NH_3 production.

Untreated patients show retarded growth and development, with mental and psychomotor retardation. Patients who are diagnosed late and who have had acute episodes of dehydration and anuria or chronic dehydration in the absence of continuous adequate substitution develop renal lesions resembling those seen in hypertensive disease.[117]

Treatment

Since the intestinal defect cannot be corrected, the only rational therapy is full and continuous replacement of the diarrheal losses of Cl^-, Na^+, and water. This treatment in fact maintains the diarrhea while preventing all its secondary consequences.[121] However, these sequelae are the only danger to the patient, and the patient learns to live a relatively undisturbed life on replacement therapy. The total dosage of the sum of NaCl and KCl should be adjusted to the minimum that maintains normal blood pH and small Cl^- loss in urine (more than 2 mmol per kilogram or 40 mmol per 24 hours, whichever is the smaller). The ratio of Na^+ to K^+ should be adjusted to maintain the serum concentration of both ions at about the middle of the normal range.

In the newborn patients, replacement therapy should be started as early as possible. To start therapy before dehydration has developed, the intravenous route is strongly recommended. For replacement of the continuing diarrheal loss, 6 to 8 mmol Cl^- per kilogram in 24 hours is needed, 1 to 2 mmol as KCl and the rest as NaCl.[125] Continuous

constant-rate infusion as an isomolar solution is recommended. In addition, the infant requires basal water and electrolyte maintenance and feeding, which can be given orally. With time a gradually increasing part of the replacement should be shifted from intravenous to oral route. A convenient solution consists of 0.7 percent (120 mmol per liter) NaCl + 0.3 percent (40 mmol per liter) KCl in water, the total dose being evenly divided among the infant's meals.

The average daily total Cl^- requirement has been 6 mmol per kilogram for the infant and young child and 3.3 mmol per kilogram for older patients. The average molar ratio of the Na^+/K^+ requirement has been 2:1 for patients under 3 years of age and 6:5 for older patients. Pertinent and valuable information on the management of these patients was recently presented by Holmberg.[121]

Prognosis

If the diagnosis is made early in the neonatal period and adequate therapy instituted immediately, the affected infant will show perfectly normal growth and development. Most children become continent for feces at the age of 3 to 4 years and undergo a completely normal social development.

CONGENITAL SODIUM DIARRHEA

Diarrhea related to congenital malabsorption of sodium was simultaneously described by two authors.[126,127] The ages of the patients, both girls, were 4 years and 9 years.

Of the three mechanisms of normal sodium absorption—uncoupled, coupled with organic solutes, and coupled in a 1:1 ratio with chloride—the last one is affected in this disease. Coupling with chloride is, in fact, the result of the presence of two separate exchange mechanisms, Na^+/H^+ and Cl^-/HCO_3^- counter-transports. In congenital sodium diarrhea the Na^+/H^+ exchange is defective in the jejunum, ileum, and colon. This defect was detected by both jejunal perfusion studies and studies on purified jejunal brush border membrane vesicles. In controls, the Na^+ uptake was seven times higher with an H^+ gradient (intravesicular pH 6.0, extravesicular pH 7.4) than without. In one patient, membrane vesicles showed very low Na^+ uptake in the presence of an H^+ gradient. Absorption of amino acids, glucose, and fatty acids was shown to be normal in these patients.

Babies who suffered from this condition were born from pregnancies complicated by maternal polyhydramnios; ultrasonography at the end of pregnancy showed the fetal abdomen to be distended by fluid-filled loops of intestine. Abdominal distention is present at birth, usually there is no meconium, and profuse watery diarrhea begins immediately after birth. This diarrhea is secretory in nature, and sodium content in the stools of these patients is very high, sometimes about 145 mEq per liter. However, in contrast to what is observed in congenital chloride diarrhea (CCD), chloride concentration in stool is lower than Na concentration and it further decreases after standard therapy for CCD. In addition, stool pH tends to be alkaline, in contrast to the low pH observed in CCD. As a result, patients present with metabolic acidosis that may be induced by standard chloride therapy for CCD. Orally administered sodium citrate and glucose electrolyte solution maintained normal growth of these two children, although the diarrhea continued. With treatment toilet training can be achieved, and the disease did not produce any social disadvantage.

PRIMARY HYPOMAGNESEMIA WITH SECONDARY HYPOCALCEMIA

Primary hypomagnesemia with secondary hypocalcemia (PHSH) is a congenital disease resulting from a selective defect in intestinal magnesium absorption. Since the first cases described,[128-130] approximately 20 cases have been reported.[131] It presents in early infancy with convulsions and tetany.

Genetics

A congenital etiology is suggested by the onset of illness in early infancy. PHSH is thought to be an autosomal recessive trait. The ratio of male to female affected is approximately 2:1. Most mothers have been healthy without complications during pregnancy, in contrast to the situation in transient neonatal hypomagnesemia with hypocalcemia. No vertical transmission has been found. Five cases suggestive of PHSH were noted in siblings of 21 patients.

Pathophysiology

Tetany and convulsions are refractory to calcium administration but responsive to magnesium injection. Also, in these cases less than 15 percent of ingested magnesium is absorbed, compared with 50 to 60 percent in control subjects. Milla et al[132] demonstrated in one patient a negative magnesium balance that could be accounted for by increased fecal losses and normal renal conservation while the calcium balance was normal. In this case, after oral magnesium therapy, magnesium balance became positive. Perfusion studies demonstrated net loss of magnesium into the intestinal lumen when low concentrations were perfused, whereas at high concentrations a net absorption was observed. They concluded that the primary abnormality is a defect in carrier-mediated transport of magnesium for low intraluminal concentrations of magnesium. These balance data support the existence of discrete and separate transport systems for magnesium and calcium.[133,134] The role of vitamin D in magnesium absorption has not been explored. The intracellular magnesium concentration of the striated muscles or red blood cells was reduced to 80 to 90 percent of that in the same tissues of control subjects.[130,135,136]

The origin of hypocalcemia in this disorder remains controversial.[131] It must be remembered that hypocalcemia is not specific to PHSH but that hypomagnesemia of various causes is frequently complicated by hypocalcemia.

Clinical Features

These patients appear normal in the first 10 days of life. Recurrent tetany with or without convulsions (and usually a diffuse EEG abnormality) is the main symptom. Some pa-

tients have loose stools (before magnesium therapy), edema, protein-losing enteropathy, and hydrocephaly.[132]

Serum calcium and magnesium levels are reduced; in most cases, the serum magnesium levels were far below 1 mEq per liter and the calcium less than 3.5 mEq per liter. The serum inorganic phosphate level varies, and potassium concentrations usually are normal.

As expected, the jejunal mucosa is normal under light and electron microscopy (moderately dilated endoplasmic reticulum),[131,137,138] and other absorptive functions are not altered (glucose, xylose, fat, vitamin A) in the absence of protein-losing enteropathy.

Treatment

Hypocalcemia is refractory to calcium injection but responsive to magnesium. Initially it is given intramuscularly in the form of magnesium sulfate (0.4 mmol per kilogram daily) with oral calcium gluconate (13 mmol per kilogram daily), calciferol (40,000 units daily), and phenytoin (7.5 mg per kilogram daily). Then oral magnesium alone in the form of magnesium chloride has to be given daily. The daily magnesium dose required to maintain normal magnesium and calcium plasma concentrations was 25 to 150 mEq per day, with a median of 35 mEq per day.[131]

The prognosis is good except for loose stools that might be related to the nature or dose of the magnesium given for maintenance treatment.

ACRODERMATITIS ENTEROPATHICA

Acrodermatitis enteropathica (AE) is an autosomal recessive disorder resulting from a selective defect in the intestinal absorption of zinc. It is characterized by acral and orificial skin lesions and diarrhea. If untreated it may be fatal in early childhood. Described first by Brandt in 1936,[139] the fundamental importance of zinc in this disease and in nutrition was first recognized by Moynahan in 1973.[140] For a recent extensive review, see reference 141.

Genetics

AE is familial and inherited as an autosomal recessive trait. Other siblings are affected in nearly two-thirds of reported cases, and a history of parenteral consanguinity may be obtained. Females are affected slightly more often than males.[142]

Pathophysiology

Zinc is involved in nucleic acid metabolism and protein synthesis, and it is a component of many human enzymes, explaining the diversity of symptoms and their severity.

The symptoms observed in AE are the consequences of zinc depletion, which can also be found in several other clinical situations including protein-energy malnutrition, nutritional zinc deficiency, and a defect of mammary zinc secretion.[143,144]

In AE, zinc deficiency can be explained entirely by an intestinal defect. Net absorption of zinc is low as whole body retention of orally administered ^{65}Zn is reduced.[145] In addition, balance studies in untreated patients indicate net zinc secretion. However, the nature of the intestinal defect remains uncertain.

The defect may be at the enterocyte level. In AE, nonspecific histologic abnormalities, including partial villous atrophy, have been demonstrated in several cases.[146,147] These changes are not constant and appear to be the result of zinc deficiency, since they are not found in treated cases.[147] Atherton et al[148] studied 10-minute ^{65}Zn accumulation by jejunal mucosal biopsies of three patients with AE on zinc therapy and after treatment had been withdrawn. In both situations, they found a marked reduction in zinc uptake compared with controls: The mean tissue/medium gradient of ^{65}Zn for the control subjects was 7.5 ($\pm$0.8), compared with 1.7 ($\pm$0.2) for the patients. The tissues accumulated glucose normally. They concluded that there is defective uptake of zinc in AE. The same conclusion was reached by Hambidge and Walravens[141] after finding that the zinc content of a jejunal biopsy from an AE patient was lower than that of controls.

In fact, the absorption of zinc and other trace metals is more complex than the absorption of minerals transported in great quantities like Na^+, Cl^-, or HCO_3^-. Trace metals are bound in the intestinal lumen, within the cell, and in the plasma to proteins that may interact with the membrane transporters. For example, in Menkes' disease high copper levels in the enterocytes may be the consequence of abnormal high binding to intracytoplasmic specific proteins. In AE, the low intracellular zinc content suggests abnormal membrane transport, but it does not exclude an abnormal relationship with zinc-binding ligands (ZBL). Delay in the clinical onset of the disease until after weaning in the breast-fed infant, together with substantial improvement achieved by treatment with human milk, is often interpreted as an indication that the ZBL present in human milk is a substitute for a defective ZBL in the duodenal juice of these patients.[141]

An intriguing finding is the presence of abnormal lysosome-like structures in the Paneth cells of AE patients,[149] although these abnormalities do seem to disappear with treatment.[154] These cells are unusual in that they show a positive histochemical staining for zinc, and it has been postulated that these cells have a role in zinc metabolism. As Paneth cells have many similarities to pancreatic acinar cells,[150] it would be interesting to investigate the presence of ZBL in these cells.

Finally, oral zinc therapy results in rapid and complete remission. This observation suggests that at high luminal concentration zinc is absorbed in AE.[151] In addition, this observation suggests that the defect is present only at the absorptive step, as clinical symptoms rapidly improve with zinc therapy, in contrast to Menkes' disease, in which copper administration is not effective.

Clinical Features

The symptoms that are the consequences of a severe zinc deficiency state[152,153] are delayed until after weaning in breast-fed infants.

A skin rash is the most dramatic and constant clinical feature. It consists of scaling erythematous eruptions that tend to be bullous or pustular and occur around the mouth and anus. The rash shows affinity for interdigital areas and ap-

pears symmetrically over buttocks, hands, feet, and elbows. With time it may involve more of the face and become plaque-like. Other areas of epithelial involvement are represented as partial or total alopecia, dystrophic nails, photophobia, conjunctivitis, and glossitis. Diarrhea beginning during or shortly after the onset of skin lesions may be severe, and steatorrhea is common. Psychologic and behavioral abnormalities are prominent, with irritability, lethargy, anorexia, and depression occurring even during relatively mild stages of the disease. Intellectual capacity is not impaired. The infants are extremely susceptible to infection, and more than half have secondary monilial infection. Failure to gain weight is easily explained by anorexia, malabsorption, infection, and possibly zinc deficiency.

A low plasma zinc in association with the typical clinical findings is diagnostic. The plasma zinc level is usually less than 6 mmol per liter and is frequently less than 3 mmol per liter (control range 10 to 17 mmol per liter). Urine zinc excretion rates are depressed. Neither erythrocyte nor hair zinc provides a sensitive index.[141] Neither prenatal diagnosis nor detection of heterozygotes is necessary because of the excellent prognosis with zinc therapy.

Treatment

Oral zinc therapy is logical and definitive.[141] It consists of 30 to 45 mg Zn^{2+} per day (or approximately 2 mg per kilogram of body weight per day in very young infants), the doses being adjusted to maintain normal plasma levels. The nature of the salt does not appear to be important for its efficacy, but it should not be administered with meals that could depress zinc absorption. If the patient is moribund it may be necessary to administer zinc intravenously initially. Plasma copper concentrations should be monitored periodically to ensure that zinc therapy is not compromising copper status.

Clinical improvement is obvious within the first weeks of therapy. The patient will recover entirely except for nail dystrophy. Before zinc treatment was devised, many patients died during late childhood. Untreated females who have survived and become pregnant have had children with a high incidence of congenital malformations.

MOLYBDENUM TRANSPORT DEFICIENCY

Molybdenum transport deficiency has been postulated by Duran et al,[155] who have reported a child with severe neurologic abnormalities, lens dislocation, and dysmorphic features of the head, who had evidence of both xanthine oxidase and sulfite oxidase deficiency.

MENKES' (STEELY-HAIR) DISEASE

Menkes' disease is a congenital disease resulting from a selective defect in intestinal copper absorption leading to copper deficiency. The same defect that prevents copper absorption and causes copper to accumulate in mucosal cells is also present in most other cells of the body, including cultured fibroblasts. The severity of the disease is explained by defective synthesis of copper enzymes.

The clinical features, neuropathology, and X-linked inheritance were clearly described in the first report by Menkes in 1962.[156] Hunt's discovery[157-159] of similar disturbances of copper metabolism in the X-linked mottled mutants in mice provided an animal model that appears to be homologous with the human disease. The clinical features and the pathophysiology of the disease have been studied extensively by Danks.[160]

Genetics

Menkes' disease is inherited as an X-linked recessive trait.[161] Female heterozygotes may present mosaic skin, depigmentation, patchy sun tanning, pili torti, or abnormal cell culture (skin biopsy) results. Measurement of placental copper levels seems to be a good method of diagnosing heterozygotes when females are born into affected families.[162] Full manifestations of the disease have been described in one Japanese girl, the sister of a severely affected male.[163] The incidence is presumably in the range of 1 in 50,000 to 1 in 100,000.

Genetic heterogeneity has been suspected from the observations of a mildly affected boy,[164] an X-linked form of cutis laxa with reduced level of the copper enzyme lysyl oxidase,[165] and an X-linked copper malabsorption with incomplete clinical features.[166]

Pathophysiology

Selective copper intestinal malabsorption is only part of a more general disturbance of copper transport in many tissues, as indicated by the poor results obtained with parenteral copper delivery. Copper metabolism has been studied in the patients and also in mottled mutant mice[167] and in fibroblast cells from patients and affected mice. The apparent paradox of the disease is that the fibroblasts accumulate five times more copper than normal yet show reduced levels of copper enzymes lysyl oxidase, cytochrome oxidase, and superoxide dismutase.[168-172] Thus, the basic cellular defect seems to cause copper to accumulate to abnormal levels in a form or location that renders it inaccessible for the synthesis of copper enzymes.[167]

In the intestine, copper malabsorption is associated with an increase in copper content (50 to 90 μg per gram dry weight in the duodenal mucosa of Menkes' disease versus 7 to 29 in controls). This copper accumulation is expressed also in cultured fibroblasts, but there is normal initial influx and efflux of copper,[173] excessive retention of radiocopper after 24-hour exposure, diminished release of the isotope during further incubation in free medium, inability to grow in low copper medium, and increased susceptibility to toxic effects of added copper. Therefore, it seems likely that the basic defect in Menkes' disease involves a step in intracellular rather than membrane transport.[173]

The clinical manifestations result from low copper enzyme activity including defective disulfide bonds in keratin in the hair,[161,174] tyrosinase deficiency expressed in depigmentation,[175] and lysyl oxidase deficiency expressed in defective elastin formation and responsible for the severe arterial disease.[172] The severe neurologic lesions may be related to decreased dopamine beta-hydroxylase, cytochrome oxidase, and superoxide dismutase activities.[158,159]

Clinical Features

The key components of the clinical syndrome are abnormal hair, progressive cerebral degeneration, hypopigmentation, bone changes, arterial rupture and thrombosis, and hypothermia.[161,167,176]

Cord copper and ceruloplasmin are normal at birth and do not decrease until after the first 2 weeks of life. Male infants are affected; frequently they are premature with neonatal hypothermia and hyperbilirubinemia. Between 1 and 2 months the infant becomes lethargic and feeds poorly. Seizures may develop early. Motor development usually does not progress beyond a smile. The muscle tone may be flaccid or increased, but deep tendon reflexes are increased and bilateral ankle clonus is present.

Two clinical findings help identify Menkes' disease: (1) The hair becomes tangled, lusterless, and grayish or ivory colored, with a stubble of broken hair palpable over the occiput and temporal regions where the hair rubs on the sheets. Pili torti are found microscopically. (2) The facies are characteristic, with pudgy cheeks and abnormal eyebrows, recognizable even in babies who have no hair.[160]

GI manifestations are vomiting and diarrhea, possibly accompanied by protein-losing enteropathy.[177] Deterioration is progressive until the patient is unresponsive and requires tube feedings. These infants are particulary susceptible to respiratory infection.

Diagnosis can be made by 2 weeks of age when serum copper and ceruloplasmin levels are very low. The liver content of copper is grossly reduced, and duodenal biopsy specimens show greatly increased copper content.[178] Oral ^{64}Cu is poorly absorbed. The disturbances of copper handling in cultured cells constitute the most definitive test for the disease.[169,171,179]

Treatment

Parenteral copper administered up to 600 ng per kilogram per week may restore serum copper levels, but no form of treatment has yet proved to be truly effective.

DISORDERS OF VITAMIN B$_{12}$ TRANSPORT

Several disorders of vitamin B$_{12}$ transport result from the absence or malfunction of proteins bound to vitamin B$_{12}$ to transport it from food to its metabolic targets. Normally the binding of alimentary vitamin B$_{12}$ to proteins is disrupted by the chlorhydropeptic activity of the stomach.[180] The cobalamins thus liberated are bound to two proteins in gastric juice, intrinsic factor (IF) and the ligands (R). These ligands are found also in saliva, tears, white blood cells, and serum, where they are called transcobalamin I and III (TCI and TCIII). The affinity of R for B$_{12}$ is greater than that of IF, but IF has a specificity for the nucleus of B$_{12}$. Bound to R, B$_{12}$ is not absorbed. Pancreatic enzymes must first split the complex R-B$_{12}$ before B$_{12}$ can bond to new molecules of IF.[181-183] Vitamin B$_{12}$ must be presented to the terminal ileum in the complex form IF-B$_{12}$ to be absorbed by a selective mechanism that transports B$_{12}$ into the portal vein, IF remaining in the intestinal lumen. TCIII is then the protein required to deliver vitamin B$_{12}$ to the bone marrow and other target tissues. The origin of TCIII remains uncertain, macrophages, intestinal cells, hepatocytes, and granulocytes being the candidates; TCII is required to transport vitamin B_{12} entering the ileal enterocyte into portal blood.[184] In utero both vitamin B_{12} and its transport protein TCII are derived from the mother. TCI binds most of the circulating B_{12} but does not appear to have other specific physiologic functions. Within the cells, vitamin B_{12} is the co-enzyme of apoenzymes implicated in the control of basic cellular processes, i.e., the synthesis of methionine from homocysteine (methionine synthetase) and the conversion of methylmalonic acid to succinic acid (methylmalonyl-CoA mutase).[185]

Congenital vitamin B_{12} transport defects include absence or malfunction of IF, intestinal malabsorption (congenital pancreatic insufficiency and ileal malabsorption), and absence or malfunction in TCII. (For recent reviews see references 186 and 187.) As a result, the main clinical feature of vitamin B_{12} deficiency is megaloblastic anemia.

Vitamin B_{12} Malabsorption of Gastric Origin

Congenital Intrinsic Factor Deficiency or Malfunction

This disorder, a vitamin B_{12} malabsorption of gastric origin, is characterized by severe macrocytic and megaloblastic anemia; it may be associated with neuropathy with loss of reflexes and impaired vibration sense, particularly in children who have been given folic acid.[187]

The serum vitamin B_{12} level is abnormally low in all untreated patients. Absorption of the vitamin is grossly impaired, and the defect might be corrected by repeating the absorption test with an extraneous source of intrinsic factor. However, lack of correction of the defect in the presence of IF has been observed.[188] The characteristic finding is a selective absence of IF without any other gastric abnormality. No antibodies against parietal cell or IF have been detected in these cases.[189]

Usually first symptoms develop between 9 months and 2 years; occasionally the rapid onset of anemia is not seen until the second decade of life.[190,191] The transfer of maternal vitamin B_{12} to the child may explain this delay of symptoms. In one case of a 13-year-old boy, the IF was present, reacted with an antiserum against normal IF, but did not promote the intestinal absorption of vitamin B_{12}.[192] In healthy parents of children with IF deficiency, gastric secretion has been found to be "low normal."[193,194]

The treatment is vitamin B_{12} replacement by injection, i.e., hydroxycobalamin 250 μg monthly or 1 mg per 2 or 3 months, for the rest of the patient's life. It is essential to start early and convince the family to adhere strictly to this treatment, as delayed therapy or relapses may cause permanent brain damage.[194]

Addisonian Pernicious Anemia

This disease may begin in the second decade of life with all the characteristics of the pernicious anemia found in adults, including gastric atrophy, achlorhydria, and low or absent IF.[195] It may be associated with IgA deficiency that is not corrected after vitamin B_{12} therapy.[196] There is a genetic determinant, but its precise role remains uncertain.

Vitamin B_{12} Malabsorption of Intestinal Origin

Congenital defects in exocrine pancreatic secretion are frequently associated with vitamin B_{12} malabsorption, but severe anemia is not a common finding. These patients are treated with pancreatic extracts.[181,182,197]

Congenital Selective Vitamin B_{12} Malabsorption

According to Chanarin,[194] this congenital disease with proteinuria was described by Imerslund[198] and Gräsbeck et al[199] and possibly earlier by Davis et al[200] and Najman et al.[201] The least common familial intestinal disorder, this disease is inherited as an autosomal recessive trait, both sexes being equally affected, and often several siblings of the same family have the disorder. Consanguinity is frequent, and clusters for disease are present in Scandinavia and among Moroccan families.[198,202]

The nature of the selective ileal defect remains unknown. The proposed mechanism, a defective vitamin B_{12} receptor at the luminal membrane of the enterocytes, seems to have been ruled out in one patient studied by Mackenzie et al.[203] They found that the homogenate of ileal biopsies from the terminal ileum could bind the B_{12}-IF complex. Another clue is the presence of proteinuria. It might indicate that this disease is due to selective protein malabsorption in intestinal and renal epithelium.

Severe vitamin B_{12} deficiency is revealed within the first two decades, frequently in the first 2 years of life, by megaloblastic anemia. There may be a history of several episodes of relapse with severe anemia. The clinical manifestations include pallor, weakness, irritability, loss of appetite often associated with vomiting, fever, glossitis, and constipation. Sometimes mild jaundice is noted as well as purpura and diarrhea. Liver and spleen may be enlarged. There may be evidence of diminished vibration sense, extensor plantars, and mental retardation.

Hematologic findings include anemia, low white cell and platelet count, increased mean corpuscular volume, severe megaloblastic anemia, and megaloblastic hematopoiesis; serum and red cell folate levels are normal. GI findings include normal gastric secretions and normal intestinal absorption of fat, glucose, xylose, vitamin A, starch, and carotene. There is impaired absorption of vitamin B_{12} which is not improved in the presence of IF; this selective intestinal defect is associated with the presence of IF and TCII. Although not a constant finding, the presence of proteinuria has been frequently reported in the absence of renal insufficiency.

The treatment and the prognosis are essentially the same as in IF deficiency.

Vitamin B_{12} Deficiency by Transport Protein (Transcobalamin II) Deficiency

Congenital Deficit in Transcobalamin II

This deficit is responsible for very severe neonatal megaloblastic anemia.[194,204-206] Untreated children die early in infancy. This is a familial disease in which both sexes are affected.

The clinical features include failure to thrive and frequently diarrhea and vomiting. On examination the infant is pale and apathetic. The tongue may be red and inflamed, with shallow mouth ulcers. The blood shows severe anemia, leukopenia, thrombocytopenia, significant macrocytosis, and hypersegmented neutrophils. Malabsorption syndrome, neurologic disorders, and immunodeficiency are common findings.[205]

Although there is vitamin B_{12} deficiency, the level of vitamin B_{12} in serum is normal and bound to TCI with little functional activity. By contrast, the vitamin B_{12} content of tissues would be expected to be very low.[194] There is total absence of vitamin B_{12} transport protein TCII in serum or plasma of affected children and half the normal level in both parents and heterozygous siblings.

In addition, vitamin B_{12} intestinal absorption is impaired, perhaps reflecting the inability to produce TCII in the ileal enterocytes and thus to transport vitamin B_{12} out of the cell to the portal blood.[194]

Treatment consists of injection of large doses of vitamin B_{12}, i.e., 1 mg hydroxycobalamin twice weekly. The prognosis seems to be strongly dependent on the adherence to this treatment for life.

Transcobalamin II Malfunction

Two cases of megaloblastic anemia with normal vitamin B_{12} plasma levels were reported in two adult women who had had anemia in infancy that responded to high doses of vitamin B_{12}. In the first case, TCII (TCII Cardeza) was present in normal quantity and could bind vitamin B_{12}; however, it was unable to promote vitamin B_{12} entry into the cells.[207] In the second case, TCII (TCII Denver) was present by immunoassay, but it could not bind vitamin B_{12}.[208]

CONGENITAL FOLATE MALABSORPTION

Congenital folate malabsorption, described in only seven patients, may be the consequence of a selective defect in intestinal and blood-brain barrier folate transport.

Genetics

The occurrence of the disorder in two siblings, consanguinity in three families,[209-216] and one father with an intermediate response to serum folate after oral loading have suggested an autosomal recessive inheritance.

Pathophysiology

Loading tests with folic acid and its derivatives lead to the conclusion that the folate deficiency is caused by a defect in folate transport across the gut and the blood-brain barrier. It would be interesting to look for the presence of the 56-kDa protein in the brush border membranes; this recently discovered protein is a component of the folate transport system in intestinal cells.[217]

Clinical Features

All seven patients reported so far have been girls.[209-216] As pointed out by Rowe, the clinical features are not identical in all cases, but the main constant feature is severe megaloblastic anemia that may begin by the age of 3 months.[218] Neurologic symptoms include ataxia, convulsions, mental retardation, and intracranial calcification. The third group of symptoms may be present in the first week of life and includes mouth ulcers, stomatitis, glossitis, failure to thrive, and diarrhea.

There are no intestinal abnormalities (morphologic appearance and absorption of fat, sugars, or vitamin A). Low folate levels in serum and CSF reflect folate deficiency; serum levels may be low before tissue stores are depleted, as indicated by normal red blood cell folate content. The bone marrow shows a lag in maturation of erythrocytic and granulocytic precursors.

Loading tests with oral folic acid (5 mg) are not followed by an increase in folic acid concentration in serum or cerebrospinal fluid,[209] but this loading test could be useful to detect heterozygotes. In contrast, plasma clearance of folic acid is normal following intravenous injection in affected subjects.

Treatment

The megaloblastic anemia responds to folic acid given parenterally (15 mg per day for a week and then every 3 to 4 weeks) or orally at a dose of 10 to 40 mg per day. Neurologic symptoms respond poorly. In fact, they may be exacerbated by oral folic acid. In one patient oral treatment using methionine (60 mg per kilogram daily) associated with vitamin B_{12} (20 mg per kilogram) and folic acid (2 mg per kilogram) resulted in the disappearance of the convulsions.[209]

FAMILIAL RICKETS AND OSTEOMALACIA

Rickets and osteomalacia may be the consequence of several congenital metabolic errors. The two main types, vitamin D-dependent rickets and familial hypophosphatemic rickets, are subdivided according to the nature of the primary defect or clinical and biologic findings. For a recent review, see Rasmussen and Anast.[219]

In any form of rickets at least two factors determine severity of the bone lesions: the amount of specific vitamin D metabolite(s) available and the calcium × phosphate ion product (or more likely the phosphate concentration per se).[219] The two known causes of rickets are deficiency of vitamin D and deficiency of phosphate. As the mucosa of the small intestine is the target of vitamin D metabolites and the site of phosphate absorption, the intestine participates in the pathophysiology of this group of diseases.

Genetics

These diseases are inherited with autosomal recessive transmission except for familial hypophosphatemic rickets, which is inherited as an X-linked dominant trait.

Pathophysiology

The absorption of both calcium and phosphate is greatly reduced in all forms of vitamin D deficiency. The major hormonal factor in the regulation of their absorption is 1,25-$(OH)_2$ vitamin D_3.[220-224] The main site of action is at the calcium or phosphate influx across the luminal membrane.

The primary defects of vitamin D–dependent rickets are either low activity of 1-alpha-hydroxylase, the enzyme responsible for the conversion of 25-(OH)D to 1,25(OH)$_2$D in type I and the abnormal function in the 1,25-$(OH)_2$D target tissues, such as intestinal mucosa and bone, in type II. In type I the clinical and biochemical manifestations are completely reversible following treatment with vitamin D; the dose of vitamin D is 10 to 300 times the normal requirement to maintain healing. This does not mean, however, that vitamin D is not absorbed by the intestine, as the serum 25-(OH)D levels were normal in untreated patients and elevated in patients receiving therapeutic doses of vitamin D_3 or 25-(OH)D_3.[225-227] In type II, the high level of circulating 1,25-$(OH)_2$D suggests an abnormality in the target tissues, including intestine, bone, and keratinocytes from human epidermis.[228] The most likely candidate for a defect is the cytosol receptor as reported in androgen-resistant patients.[229] The occurrence of alopecia in some families with the type II defect points to the possible physiologic activity of 1,25-$(OH)_2$D in skin.

Familial hypophosphatemic rickets is thought to be the consequence of a decrease in tubular reabsorption of phosphate and tubular synthesis of 1,25-$(OH)_2D_3$ in response to a normal hypophosphatemic stimulus. Apparently in this disease the defect in phosphate transport is found in the renal tubule but not in the intestinal mucosa. In the kidney, the defect is on the parathyroid hormone (PTH)-sensitive component of phosphate transport,[230] which may be controlled by a gene on the X chromosome. The PTH-insensitive component, possibly controlled by an autosomal gene, remains present.[231,232] Administration of 1,25-$(OH)_2$D does not restore plasma phosphate concentration to normal or correct the renal tubular defect. In the intestine, there is phosphate malabsorption, and 1,25-$(OH)_2$D in small doses induces a marked increase in the rate of intestinal phosphate absorption.[233,234] In addition, phosphate uptake was found normal in jejunal biopsies from hypophosphatemic subjects.[235] Thus, no selective phosphate transport defect has been found in the intestinal mucosa, and phosphate intestinal malabsorption can be interpreted to be a consequence of altered vitamin D metabolism.

Clinical Features

Vitamin D–dependent rickets type II is the only congenital rickets in which a primary defect may exist in the intestinal mucosa, among other possible targets for vitamin D metabolites.[236-242]

The clinical features characteristic of vitamin D–dependent rickets include hypotonia, muscle weakness, growth failure, convulsions, and the deformities of the extremities of the bone. The biochemical findings include hypocalcemia, hypophosphatemia, elevated serum alkaline phosphatase activity, elevated serum immunoreactive parathyroid hormone, and increased urinary excretion of amino acids and cyclic AMP.

The main feature of this type of rickets is that the circulating levels of 1,25-$(OH)_2$D are elevated rather than depressed,[243] an indication of end-organ refractoriness to this metabolite. This hypothesis is further supported by the occurrence of rickets at birth, in contrast to the situation in vitamin D–deficient or vitamin D–dependent rickets type I, in which no evidence of rickets at birth has been reported. However, the disease can be recognized in late childhood or in adult life. The second important feature is the presence of alopecia totalis, with no abnormal lymphocytic infiltration in the biopsy of the scalp.[237] It may be noted at birth or between 6 and 9 months of age at the time that rickets is diagnosed.[237,239,240] It is not a constant finding,[241,242] and it is not clear whether vitamin D–dependent rickets type II with and without alopecia are the same disease.

This difference may reflect different degrees of sensitivity to 1,25-$(OH)_2$D and may have therapeutic consequences. In the form with alopecia, it appears that patients are resistant to pharmacologic doses of vitamin D preparations, 25-(OH)D_3, and 1,25- $(OH)_2D_3$. Improvement was observed in one patient who received phosphate supplements, in another who received calcium supplements and subsequently 24,25-$(OH)_2D_3$, and in a third who received 1-alpha-(OH)D_3.[219] It is possible that patients without alopecia are more responsive to vitamin D, 25-(OH)D, and possibly to 1,25-$(OH)_2$D, than patients with alopecia.[219]

PRIMARY BILE ACID MALABSORPTION

Two boys with congenital diarrhea due to primary bile acid malabsorption were reported.[244,245] There was no known family history of GI disease. However, in one father the bile salt enterohepatic circulation may have been impaired.

The fecal bile acid excretion rates were increased (960 and 991 mg per square meter per day) and similar to those observed in children with neonatal intestinal resection. The cholic and chenodeoxycholic acid kinetic studies documented rapid disappearance of the labeled bile acid from duodenal bile. Interruption of the bile salt enterohepatic circulation was further documented by the presence of a reduced intraluminal bile salt concentration and absence of increase of serum cholylglycine after a meal. In vitro uptake of taurocholate (0.1 to 10 mM) by the ileal epithelium of these two patients was reduced compared with controls. All these findings suggest that the congenital diarrhea observed in these two children may be the consequence of a defect of ileal bile acid transport.

Clinical Features

After uneventful gestation, diarrhea begins on the second day of life and persists despite multiple formula changes. Later, physical examination reveals anasarca, hepatomegaly, a rash on the buttocks, and failure to thrive. Stool output is increased, and the coefficient of fat absorption is less than 50 percent.

Extensive evaluations including morphologic studies of the intestinal epithelium, liver biopsy (moderate steatosis), lactose and glucose tolerance tests, pancreatic secretion, and vitamin B_{12} absorption are normal.

Treatment with medium-chain triglycerides, with reduction of long-chain triglyceride intake and zinc supplementation, is followed by reduced stool output, increased fat absorption, and improvement of nutritional status.

REFERENCES

1. Laplane R, Polonovski C, Etienne M, Debray P, Lods JC, Pissaro B. L'intolérance aux sucres à transfert intestinal actif. Ses rapports avec l'intolérance au lactose et le syndrome coeliaque. Arch Fr Pediatr 1962; 19:895–944.
2. Lindquist B, Meeuwisse GW. Chronic diarrhoea caused by monosaccharide malabsorption. Acta Paediatr 1962; 51:674–685.
3. Evans L, Grasset E, Heyman M, Dumontier AM, Beau JP, Desjeux JF. Congenital selective malabsorption of glucose and galactose. J Pediatr Gastroenterol Nutr 1985; 4:878–886.
4. Desjeux JF. Congenital selective Na^+, D-glucose cotransport defect leading to renal glycosuria and congenital selective intestinal malabsorption of glucose and galactose. In: Scriver CR, Beaudet AL, Sly WS, Valle D, eds. The metabolic basis of inherited disease. 6th ed. New York: McGraw-Hill, 1989: 2463.
5. Melin K, Meeuwisse GW. Glucose-galactose malabsorption. A genetic study. Acta Pediatr Scand (suppl) 1969; 188:19–24.
6. Meeuwisse GW, Dahlqvist A. Glucose-galactose malabsorption. A study which biopsy of the small mucosa. Acta Paediatr Scand 1968; 57:273–280.
7. Elsas LJ, Hillman RE, Paterson JH, Rosenberg LE. Renal and intestinal hexose transportin familial glucose-galactose malabsorption. J Clin Invest 1970; 49:576–585.
8. Ravich WJ, Bayless TM, Thomas M. Fructose: incomplete intestinal absorption in humans. Gastroenterology 1983; 84:26–29.
9. Hediger MA, Coady MJ, Ikeda TS, Wright EM. Expression cloning and cDNA sequencing of the Na^+/glucose co-transporter. Nature 1987; 330:379–381.
10. Meeuwisse GW, Melin K. Glucose-galactose malabsorption. A clinical study of 6 cases. Acta Paediatr Scand (suppl) 1969; 188:3–18.
11. Hughes WS, Senior JR. The glucose-galactose malabsorption syndrome in a 23-year-old woman. Gastroenterology 1975; 68:142–145.
12. Fairclough PD, Clark ML, Dawson AM, Silk DBA, Milla PJ, Harries JT. Absorption of glucose and maltose in congenital glucose-galactose malabsorption. Pediatr Res 1978; 12:1112–1114.
13. Phillips SF, McGill DB. Glucose-galactose malabsorption in an adult: perfusion studies of sugar, electrolyte, and water transport. Am J Dig Dis 1973; 18:1017–1024.
14. Eggermont E, Loeb H. Glucose-galactose intolerance. Lancet 1966; ii:343–344.
15. Desjeux JF, Sandler L, Sassier P, Lestradet H. Acquired and congenital disorders of intestinal transport of D-glucose in children. Rev Eur Etud Clin Biol 1971; 16:364–366.
16. Schneider AJ, Kinter WB, Stirling CE. Glucose-galactose malabsorption. Report of a case with autoradiographic studies of a mucosal biopsy. N Engl J Med 1966; 274:305–312.
17. Stirling CE, Schneider AJ, Wong MD, Kinter WB. Quantitative radioautography of sugar transport in intestinal biopsies from normal humans and a patient with glucose-galactose malabsorption. J Clin Invest 1972; 51:438–451.
18. Booth IW, Patel PB, Sule D, Brown GA, Beyreiss K. Demonstration of defective jejunal brush border Na^+-coupled glucose transport in congenital glucose-galactose malabsorption. Pediatr Res 1987; 22:98.
19. Keston AS, Meeuwisse G, Fredrikson B. Evidence for participation of mutarotase in sugar transport: absence of the enzyme in a case of glucose-galactose malabsorption. Biochem Biophys Res Commun 1982; 108:1574–1580.
20. Caspary WF. Diarrhoea associated with carbohydrate malabsorption. Clin Gastroenterol 1986; 15:631–655.
21. Gray GM. Intestinal disaccharidase deficiencies and glucose-galactose malabsorption. In: Stanbury JB, Wyngaarden JB, Fredrickson DS, eds. The metabolic basis of inherited disease. 4th ed. New York: McGraw-Hill, 1978: 1729.
22. Launiala K. The effect of unabsorbed sucrose and mannitol on the small intestinal flow rate and mean transit time. Scand J Gastroenterol 1968; 3:665–671.
23. Bridges RJ, Rummel W. Mechanistic basis of alterations in mucosal water and electrolyte transport. Clin Gastroenterol 1986; 15:491–506.
24. Saunders DR, Wiggins HS. Conservation of mannitol, lactulose and raffinose by the human colon. Am J Physiol 1981; 241 (Gastrointest Liver Physiol 4):G397–G402.
25. Palma R, Vidon N, Bernier JJ. Maximal capacity for fluid absorption in human bowel. Dig Dis Sci 1981; 26:929–934.
26. Bond JH, Levitt MD. Fate of soluble carbohydrate in the colon of rats and man. J Clin Invest 1976; 57:1158–1164.
27. Argenzio RA, Moon HW, Kemeny LJ, Whipp SC. Colonic compensation in transmissible gastroenteritis of swine. Gastroenterology 1984; 86:1510–1509.
28. Sarles J, Collard Y, Arnaud-Battandier F, Bresson JL, Schmitz J, Ricour C, Rey J. Fermentation acide et production d'hydrogène par la flore colique dans un cas de malabsorption du glucose et du galactose. Gastroenterol Clin Biol 1985; 9:848–849.
29. Dubois R, Loeb H, Eggermont E, Mainguet P. Etude clinique et biochimique d'un cas de malabsorption congénitale du glucose et du galactose. Helv Paediatr Acta 1966; 6:577–587.
30. Lebenthal E, Garti R, Mathoth Y, Cohen B, Katzenelson D. Glucose-galactose malabsorption in an Oriental-Iraqi Jewish family. J Pediatr 1971; 78:840–850.
31. Abraham JM, Levin B, Oberholzer VG, Russel A. Glucose-galactose malabsorption. Arch Dis Child 1967; 42:592–597.
32. Meeuwisse G. Glucose-galactose malabsorption. An inborn error of carrier-mediated transport. Vol. 7. Lund, Sweden: University of Lund, 1970.
33. Liu HY, Anderson GJ, Tsao MU, Moore BF, Giday Z. Tm glucose in a case of congenital intestinal and renal malabsorption of monosaccharides. Pediatr Res 1967; 1:386–394.
34. Beauvais P, Vaudour G, Desjeux JF, Le Balle JC, Birot JY, Brissaud HE. La malabsorption congénitale du glucose-galactose. Un nouveau cas avec l'étude in vitro de l'absorption intestinale et l'étude du TmG. Arch Fr Pediatr 1971; 28:573–591.
35. Meeuwisse GW. Glucose-galactose malabsorption: a study on the transfer of glucose across the red cell membrane. Scand J Clin Lab Invest 1970; 25:145–152.
36. Pruitt AW, Achord JL, Fales FW, Patterson JH. Glucose-galactose malabsorption complicated by monilial arthritis. Pediatrics 1969; 43:106–110.
37. Bond JH, Levitt MD. Investigation of small bowel transit time in man utilizing pulmonary hydrogen (H_2) measurement. J Lab Clin Med 1975; 85:546–555.
38. Douwes AC, Van Caillie M, Fernandes J, Bijleveld CMA, Desjeux JF. Interval breath hydrogen test in glucose-galactose malabsorption. Eur J Pediatr 1981; 137:273–276.
39. Desjeux JF, Sassier P, Tichet J, Sarrut S, Lestradet H. Sugar absorption by flat jejunal mucosa. Acta Paediatr Scand 1973; 62:531–537.
40. Modigliani R, Bernier JJ. Absorption of glucose, sodium, and water by the human jejunum studied by intestinal perfusion with a proximal occluding balloon and at variable flow rates. Gut 1971; 12:184–193.
41. Modigliani R, Rambaud JC, Bernier JJ. The method of intraluminal perfusion of the human small intestine. I. Principle and technique. Digestion 1973; 9:176–192.
42. Rey F, Drillet F, Schmitz J, Rey J. Influence of flow rate on the kinetics of the intestinal absorption of glucose and lysine in children. Gastroenterology 1974; 66:79–85.
43. Wimberley PD, Harries JT, Burgess EA. Congenital glucose-galactose malabsorption. Proc R Soc Med 1974; 67:755–756.
44. Anderson CM, Kerry KR, Townley RRW. An inborn defect of intestinal absorption of certain monosaccharides. Arch Dis Child 1965; 40:1–6.

45. Elsas LJ, Lambe DW. Familial glucose-galactose malabsorption: remission of glucose intolerance. J Pediatr 1973; 83:226–232.

46. Bassen FA, Kornzweig AL. Malformation of the erythrocytes in a case of atypical retinitis pigmentosa. Blood 1950; 5:381–392.

47. Salt HB, Wolff OH, Lloyd JK, Fosbrooke AS, Cameron AH, Hubble DV. On having no beta-lipoprotein: a syndrome comprising abetalipoproteinemia, acanthocytosis, and steatorrhea. Lancet 1960; ii:325–326.

48. Mabry CC, Di George AM, Auerbach VH. Studies concerning the defect in a patient with acanthocytosis. Clin Res 1960; 8:371–378.

49. Lamy M, Frezal J, Polonovski J, Rey J. L'absence congénitale de bétalipoprotéines. CR Soc Biol (Paris) 1960; 154:1974–1979.

50. Schwartz JF, Rowland LP, Eder H, Marks PA, Osserman EF, Hirschberg E, Anderson H. Bassen-Kornzweig syndrome: deficiency of serum beta-lipoprotein. Arch Neurol 1963; 8:438–442.

51. Herbert PN, Assmann G, Gotto AM Jr, Fredrikson DS. Familial lipoprotein deficiency: abetalipoproteinemia, hypobetalipoproteinemia, and Tangier disease. In: Stanbury JB, Wyngaarden JB, Fredrikson DS, Goldstein JL, Brown MS, eds. The metabolic basis of inherited disease. 5th ed. New York: McGraw-Hill, 1984:589.

52. Mars H, Lewis LA, Robertson AL Jr, Butkus A, Williams GH Jr. Familial hypo-β-lipoproteinemia: a genetic disorder of lipid metabolism with nervous system involvement. Am J Med 1969; 46:886–892.

53. Richet G, Durepaire H, Hartmann L, Ollier MP, Polonovski J, Maitrot B. Hypolipoproteinémie familiale asymptomatique prédominant sur les bêta-lipoprotéines. Presse Med 1969; 77:2045–2048.

54. Young SG, Northey ST, McCarthy BJ. Low plasma cholesterol levels caused by a short deletion in the apolipoprotein B gene. Science 1988; 241:591–593.

55. Glickman RM, Green PHR, Lels RS, Lux SE, Kilgore A. Immunofluorescence studies of apolipoprotein B in intestinal mucosa. Absence in abetalipoproteinemia. Gastroenterology 1979; 76:288–292.

56. Kayden HJ, Silber R. The role of vitamin E deficiency in the abnormal autohemolysis of acanthocytosis. Trans Assoc Am Physicians 1965;78:334–338.

57. Muller DPR, Harries JT, Lloyd JK. Vitamin E therapy in a-beta-lipoproteinemia. Arch Dis Child 1970; 45:715–801.

58. McCormick EC, Cornwell DG, Brown JB. Studies on the distribution of tocopherol in human serum lipoproteins. J Lipid Res 1960; 1:221–227.

59. Muller DP, Harries JT, Lloyd JK. The relative importance of the factors involved in the absorption of vitamin E in children. Gut 1974; 15:966–971.

60. Muller DP, Lloyd JK, Bird AC. Long-term management of abetalipoproteinemia. Possible role of vitamin E. Arch Dis Child 1977; 52:209–214.

61. Bach C, Polonovski J, Polonovski C, Leluc R, Jolly G, Moszer M. L'absence congénitale de β-lipoprotéines: une nouvelle observation. Arch Fr Pediatr 1967; 24:1093–1098.

62. Ways P, Reed CF, Hanahan DJ (technical assistance of Dong D, Palmer S, Murphy M, Roberts G). Red cell and plasma lipids in acanthocytosis. J Clin Invest 1963; 42:1248–1253.

63. Farquhar JW, Ways P. Abetalipoproteinemia. In: Stanbury JB, Wyngaarden JB, Fredrickson DS, eds. The metabolic basis of inherited disease. 2nd ed. New York: McGraw-Hill, 1966:509.

64. Ways PO, Parmentier CM, Kayden HJ, Jones JW, Saunders DR, Rubin CE. Studies on the absorptive defect for triglyceride in abetalipoproteinemia. J Clin Invest 1967; 46:35–40.

65. Dobbins WO III. An ultrastructural study of the intestinal mucosa in congenital betalipoprotein deficiency with particular emphasis upon the intestinal absorptive cell. Gastroenterology 1966; 50:195–201.

66. Tall AR, Green PH, Glickman RM, Riley JW. Metabolic fate of chylomicron phospholipids and apoproteins in the rat. J Clin Invest 1979; 64:977–989.

67. Cottrill C, Glueck CJ, Leuba V, Millet F, Puppione D, Brown WV. Familial homozygous hypobetalipoproteinemia. Metabolism 1974; 23:779–791.

68. Van Buchem FSP, Pol G, De Gier J, Böttcher CJF, Pries C. Congenital β-lipoprotein deficiency. Am J Med 1966; 40:794–799.

69. Levy RI, Langer T, Gotto AM, Fredrickson DS. Familial hypobetalipoproteinemia, a defect in lipoprotein synthesis. Clin Res 1970; 18:539–543.

70. Sigurdsson G, Nicoll A, Lewis B. Turnover of apolipoprotein-B in two subjects with familial hypobetalipoproteinemia. Metabolism 1977; 26:25–31.

71. Steinberg D, Grundy SM, Mok HYI, Turner JD, Weinstein JB, Brown WV, Albers JJ. Metabolic studies in an unusual case of asymptomatic familial hypobetalipoproteinemia with hypoalphalipoproteinemia and fasting chylomicronemia. J Clin Invest 1979; 64:292–301.

72. Malloy MJ, Kane JP, Hardman DA, Hamilton RL, Dalal KB. Normotriglyceridemic abetalipoproteinemia. Absence of the B-100 apolipoprotein. J Clin Invest 1981; 67:1441–1450.

73. Von Udransky L, Baumann E. Ueber das vorkomnaen von diaminen, sogenannten ptomainen, bei cystinurie. Z Physiol Chem 1889; 13:562–568.

74. Milne MD, Crawford MA, Girao CB, Loughridge LW. The metabolic disease in Hartnup disease. QJ Med 1960; 20:407–410.

75. Milne MD, Asatoor AM, Edwards KDG, Loughridge LW. The intestinal absorption defect in cystinuria. Gut 1961; 2:323–327.

76. Scriver CR, Rosenberg LE. Amino acid metabolism and its disorders. Philadelphia: WB Saunders, 1973.

77. Silk DBA. Disorders of nitrogen absorption. Clin Gastroenterol 1982; 11:47–72.

78. Danisi G, Tai YH, Curran PF. Mucosal and serosal fluxes of alanine in rabbit ileum. Biochim Biophys Acta 1976; 455:200–213.

79. Coicadan L, Heyman M, Grasset E, Desjeux JF. Cystinuria: reduced lysine permeability at the brush border of intestinal membrane cells. Pediatr Res 1980; 14:109–112.

80. Desjeux JF, Rajantie J, Simell O, Dumontier AM, Perheentupa J. Lysine fluxes across the jejunal epithelium in lysinuric protein intolerance. J Clin Invest 1980; 65:1382–1387.

81. Desjeux JF, Vonlanthen M, Dumontier AM, Simell O, Legrain M. Cystine fluxes across the isolated jejunal epithelium in cystinuria: increased efflux permeability at the luminal membrane. Pediatr Res 1987; 21:477–481.

82. Asatoor AM, Bandoh JK, Lant AF, Milne MD, Navab F. Intestinal absorption of carnosine and its constituent amino acids in man. Gut 1970; 11:250–254.

83. Asatoor AM, Cheng B, Edwards KDG, Lant AF, Matthews DM, Milne MD, Navab F, Richard AJ. Intestinal absorption of two dipeptides in Hartnup disease. Gut 1970; 11:380–387.

84. Asatoor AM, Harrison BDW, Milne MD, Prosser DI. Intestinal absorption of an arginine containing peptide in cystinuria. Gut 1972; 13:95–98.

85. Hellier MD, Holdsworth CD, Perrett D. Dibasic amino acid absorption in man. Gastroenterology 1973; 65:613–618.

86. Navab F, Asatoor AM. Studies on intestinal absorption of amino acids and a dipeptide in a case of Hartnup disease. Gut 1970; 11:373–379.

87. Silk DBA, Perrett D, Clark ML. Jejunal and ileal absorption of dibasic amino acids and an arginine containing dipeptide in cystinuria. Gastroenterology 1975; 68:1426–1432.

88. Smith DW, Scriver CR, Tenenhouse HS, Simell O. Lysinuric protein intolerance mutation is expressed in the plasma membrane of cultured skin fibroblasts. Proc Natl Acad Sci USA 1987; 84:7711–7715.

89. Segal S, Thier SO. Cystinuria. In: Stanbury JB, Wyngaarden JB, Fredrickson DS, Goldstein JL, Brown MS, eds. The metabolic basis of inherited disease. 5th ed. New York: McGraw-Hill, 1984; 1175.

90. Rosenberg LE, Downing S, Durant JL, Segal S. Cystinuria: biochemical evidence for three genetically distinct diseases. J Clin Invest 1966; 45:365–368.

91. Morin Cl, Thompson MW, Jackson SH, Sass-Kortsak A. Biochemical and genetic studies in cystinuria: observations on double heterozygotes of genotype I/II. J Clin Invest 1971; 50:1961–1976.

92. Perheentupa J, Visakorpi JK. Protein intolerance with deficient transport of basic amino acids; another inborn error of metabolism. Lancet 1965; ii:813–817.

93. Simell O, Perheentupa J, Rapola J, Visakorpi JK, Eskelinen LE. Lysinuric protein intolerance. Am J Med 1975; 59:229–240.

94. Norio R, Perheentupa J, Kekomäki M, Visakorpi JK. Lysinuric protein intolerance, an autosomal recessive disease; a genetic study of 10 Finnish families. Clin Genet 1971; 2:214–222.

95. Rajantie J, Simell O, Perheentupa J. Lysinuric protein intolerance. Basolateral transport defect in renal tubule. J Clin Invest 1981; 67:1078–1082.

96. Rajantie J, Simell O, Perheentupa J. Basolateral-membrane transport defect for lysine in lysinuric protein intolerance. Lancet 1980; 1:1219–1221.

97. Rajantie J, Simell O, Perheentupa J. "Basolateral" and mitochondrial membrane transport defect in the hepatocytes in lysinuric protein intolerance. Acta Paediatr Scand 1983; 72:65–70.

98. Rajantie J, Simell O, Perheentupa J. Intestinal absorption in lysinuric protein intolerance: impaired for diamino acids, normal for citrulline. Gut 1980; 21:519–524.

99. Rajantie J. Orotic aciduria in lysinuric protein intolerance: dependence on the urea cycle intermediates. Pediatr Res 1981; 15:115–119.

100. Awrich AE, Stackhouse WJ, Cantrell JE, Patterson JH, Rudman D. Hyperdibasic aminoaciduria, hyperammonemia, and growth retardation: treatment with arginine, lysine and citrulline. J Pediatr 1975; 87:731–738.

101. Rajantie J, Simell O, Rapola J, Perheentupa J. Lysinuric protein intolerance: a two-year trial of dietary supplementation therapy with citrulline and lysine. J Pediatr 1980; 97:927–932.

102. Brown JH, Fabre LF, Farrell GL, Adams ED. Hyperlysinuria with hyperammonemia: a new metabolic disorder. Am J Dis Child 1972; 124:127–132.

103. Whelan DT, Scriver CR. Hyperdibasic aminoaciduria: an inherited disorder of amino acid transport. Pediatr Res 1968; 2:525–527.

104. Kihara H, Valente M, Porter MT, Fluarty AL. Hyperdibasic aminoaciduria in a mentally retarded homozygote with a peculiar response to phenothiazines. Pediatrics 1973; 51:223–229.

105. Oyanagi K, Sogawa T, Minami R, Nakao T, Chiba T. The mechanism of hyperammonemia in congenital lysinuria. J Pediatr 1979; 94:255–257.

106. Lowe CV, May CD. Am J Dis Child 1951; 82:459–472.

107. Jepson JB. Hartnup disease. In: Stanbury JB, Wyngaarden JB, Fredrickson DS, eds. The metabolic basis of inherited disease. 4th ed. New York: McGraw-Hill, 1978: 1563.

108. Hooft CJ, Timmermans J, Snoeck J, Antener I, Van Den Hende C. Methionine malabsorption in a mentally defective child. Lancet 1964; ii:20–21.

109. Drummond KN, Michael AF, Ulstrom RA, Good RA. The blue diaper syndrome: familial hypercalcaemia and indocamuria. Am J Med 1965; 37:928–948.

110. Scriver CR. Familial iminoglycinuria. In: Stanbury JB, Wyngaarden JB, Fredrickson DS, Goldstein JL, Brown MS, eds. The metabolic basis of inherited disease. 5th ed. New York: McGraw-Hill, 1984: 1792.

111. Robitaille P, Melancon SB, Dallaire L, Lemieux B, Potier M. Proceedings: dicarboxylic aminoaciduria: a new metabolic disease involving the transport of glutamic and aspartic acids. J Urol Nephrol 1974; 81:715–716.

112. Melancon SB, Dallaire L, Lemieux B, Robitaille P, Potier M. Dicarboxylic aminoaciduria: an inborn error of amino acid conservation. J Pediatr 1977; 91:422–427.

113. Gamble JL, Fahey KR, Appleton J, Mac Lachlan E. Congenital alkalosis with diarrhea. J Pediatr 1945; 26:509–518.

114. Darrow DC. Congenital alkalosis with diarrhea. J Pediatr 1945; 26:149–152.

115. Pearson AJG, Sladen GE, Edmonds CJ. The pathophysiology of congenital chloridorrhea. Q J Med 1973; 42:453–466.

116. Turnberg LA. Abnormalities in intestinal electrolyte transport in congenital chloride diarrhea. Gut 1971; 12:544–551.

117. Holmberg C, Perheentupa J, Launiala K, Hallman N. Congenital chloride diarrhea: clinical analysis of 21 Finnish patients. Arch Dis Child 1977; 52:255–267.

118. Perheentupa J, Eklund J, Kojo N. Familial chloride diarrhoea (congenital alkalosis with diarrhoea). Acta Paediatr Scand (suppl) 1965; 159:119–120.

119. Launiala K, Perheentupa J, Pasternack A, Hallman N. Familial chloride diarrhea—chloride malabsorption. Mod Probl Paediatr 1968; 11:137–149.

120. Norio N, Perheentupa J, Launiala K, Hallman N. Congenital chloride diarrhea, an autosomal recessive disease. Genetic study of 14 Finnish and 12 other families. Clin Genet 1971; 2:182–192.

121. Holmberg C. Congenital chloride diarrhea. Clin Gastroenterol 1986; 15(3):583–602.

122. Bieberdorf FA, Gorden P, Fordtran JS. Pathogenesis of congenital alkalosis with diarrhea. J Clin Invest 1972; 51:1958–1968.

123. Holmberg C, Perheentupa J, Launiala K. Colonic electrolyte transport in health and in congenital chloride diarrhea. J Clin Invest 1975; 56:302–310.

124. Holmberg C. Electrolyte economy and its hormonal regulation in congenital chloride diarrhea. Pediatr Res 1978; 12:82–86.

125. Holmberg C, Perheentupa J. Congenital chloride diarrhea. Adv Int Med Pediatr 1982; 49:137–172.

126. Holmberg C. Perheentupa J. Congenital Na$^+$ diarrhea: a new type of secretory diarrhea. J Pediatr 1985; 106:56–61.

127. Booth IW, Murer H, Stange G, Fenton TR, Milla PJ. Defective jejunal brush border Na$^+$/H$^+$ exchange: a cause of congenital secretory diarrhea. Lancet 1985; i:1066–1069.

128. Paunier L, Radde IC, Kooh SW, Fraser D. Primary hypomagnesemia with secondary hypocalcemia. J Pediatrics 1965; 67:945(A).

129. Paunier L, Radde IC, Kooh SW, Cohen PE, Fraser D. Primary hypomagnesemia with secondary hypocalcemia in an infant. Pediatrics 1968; 41:385–402.

130. Salet J, Polonovski C, De Gouyon F, Pean G, Melekian B, Fournet JP, Aymard P, Raynaud C, Vincent J. Tetanie hypocalcémique récidivante par hypomagnésémie congénitale: une maladie métabolique nouvelle. Arch Fr Pediatr 1966; 23:749–768.

131. Yamamoto T, Kabata H, Yagi R, Takashima M, Itokawa Y. Primary hypomagnesemia with secondary hypocalcemia. Report of case and review of the world literature. Magnesium 1985; 4:153–164.

132. Milla P, Agget PJ, Wolff OH, Harries JT. Studies in primary hypomagnesemia: evidence for defective carrier-mediated small intestinal transport of magnesium. Gut 1979; 20:1028–1033.

133. Brannan PG, Vergne-Marini P, Pak CYC, Hull AR, Fordtran JS. Magnesium absorption in the human small intestine: results in normal subjects, patients with chronic renal disease, and patients with absorptive hypercalciuria. J Clin Invest 1976; 57:1412–1418.

134. O'Donnel JM, Smith MW. Uptake of calcium and magnesium by rat duodenal mucosa analysed by means of competing metals. J Physiol 1973; 229:733–749.

135. Ghazali S, Hallett RJ, Barrett TM. Hypomagnesemia in uremic infants. J Pediatr 1972; 81:747–750.

136. Paunier L, Sizonenko PC. Asymptomatic chronic hypomagnesemia and hypokalemia in a child: cell membrane disease? J Pediatr 1976; 88:51–55.

137. Nordio S, Donath A, Macagno F, Gatti R. Chronic hypomagnesemia with magnesium-dependent hypocalcemia. I. A new syndrome with intestinal magnesium malabsorption. Acta Paediatr Scand 1971; 60:441–448.

138. Stromme JH, Steen-Johnson J, Harnes K, Hofstad F, Brandtzaeg P. Familial hypomagnesemia—a follow-up examination of three patients after 9 to 12 years of treatment. Pediatr Res 1981; 15:1134–1139.

139. Brandt T. Dermatitis in children with disturbances of the general condition and absorption of food elements. Acta Dermatol Venereol 1936; 17:513–546.

140. Moynahan EJ. Le zinc et le poil dans l'acrodermatitis enteropathica. Bull Soc Fr Dermatol Syphylogr 1973; 80:541–543.

141. Hambidge KM, Walravens PA. Disorders of mineral metabolism. Clin Gastroenterol 1982; 11(1):87–117.

142. Gryboski J. Congenital disorders of absorption. In: Lebenthal E, ed. Textbook of gastroenterology and nutrition in infancy. New York: Raven Press, 1981: 931.

143. Aggett PJ, Atherton DJ, More J, Davey J, Delves HT, Harries JT. Symptomatic zinc deficiency in a breast-fed preterm infant. Arch Dis Child 1980; 55:547–550.

144. Zimmerman AW, Hambidge KM, Lepow ML, Greenberg TR, Stover ML, Casey CE. Acrodermatitis in breast-fed premature infants: evidence for a defect of mammary zinc secretion. Pediatrics 1982; 69:176–183.

145. Lombeck I, Schnipperring HG, Ritzl F, Feinendegen LE, Bremer HJ. Absorption of zinc in acrodermatitis enteropathica. Lancet 1975; i:855.

146. Rayhanzadeh S, Dantzig P. Acrodermatitis enteropathica, with pathological findings in jejunum and skin. Pediatrics 1974; 54:77–80.

147. Kelly R, Davidson GP, Townley RRW, Campbell PE. Reversible intestinal mucosal abnormality in acrodermatitis enteropathica. Arch Dis Child 1976; 51:219–222.

148. Atherton DJ, Muller DPR, Aggett PJ, Harries JT. A deficit in zinc uptake by jejunal biopsies in acrodermatitis enteropathica. Clin Sci 1979; 56:505–507.

149. Lombeck I, Von Bassewitz DB, Becker K, Tinschmann P, Kastner H. Ultrastructural findings in acrodermatitis enteropathica. Pediatr Res 1974; 8:82–88.

150. Sénégas-Balas F, Bastie MJ, Balas D. Histological variations of the duodenal mucosa in chronic human pancreatitis. Dig Dis Sci 1982; 27:917–922.

151. Casey CE, Hambidge KM, Walravens PA. Zinc binding in human duodenal secretions. J Pediatr 1979; 95:1008–1010.

152. Moynahan EJ. Acrodermatitis enteropathica. A lethal inherited human zinc-deficiency disorder. Lancet 1974; ii:399–400.

153. Neldner KH, Hambidge KM. Zinc therapy in acrodermatitis enteropathica. N Engl J Med 1975; 292:879–882.

154. Bohane TD, Cuts E, Hamilton JR, Gall DG. Acrodermatitis enteropathica, zinc, and the Paneth cell. Gastroenterology 1977; 73:587–592.

155. Duran M, Beemer FA, Heiden CVD, Korteland J, De Bree PK, Brink M, Wadman SK, Lombeck I. Combined deficiency of xanthine oxidase and sulfite oxidase: defect of molybdenum metabolism or transport. J Inherited Metab Dis 1978; 1:175–178.

156. Menkes JH, Alter M, Steigleder GK, Weakley DR, Sung JH. A sex-linked recessive disorder with retardation of growth, peculiar hair and focal cerebral and cerebellar degeneration. Pediatrics 1962; 29:764–768.

157. Hunt DM. Catecholamine biosynthesis and the activity of a number of copper-dependent enzymes in the copper-deficient mottled mouse mutants. Comp Biochem Physiol 1977; 57:79–83.

158. Hunt DM. Copper and neurological function. In: CIBA Foundation symposium 79: biological roles of copper. Amsterdam: Excerpta Medica, 1980.

159. Hunt DM. Primary defect in copper transport underlies mottled mutants in the mouse. Nature 1974; 249:852–854.

160. Danks DM. Hereditary disorders of copper metabolism in Wilson's disease and Menkes' disease. In: Stanbury J, Wyngaarden JB, Fredrickson DS, Goldstein JL, Brown MS, eds. The metabolic basis of inherited disease. 5th ed. New York: McGraw-Hill, 1984:1251.

161. Danks DM, Campbell PE, Stevens BJ, Mayne V, Cartwright E. Menkes' kinky hair syndrome: an inherited defect in copper absorption with widespread effects. Pediatrics 1972; 50:188–201.

162. Horn N, Jensen OA. Menkes' syndrome: subcellular distribution of copper determined by ultrastructural histochemical technique. Ultrastruct Pathol 1980; 1:237–242.

163. Iwakawa Y, Niwa T, Tomita M. Menkes' kinky-hair syndrome: report on an autopsy case and his female sibling with similar clinical manifestations. Brain Dev (Tokyo) 1979; 11:260.

164. Procopis P, Camakaris J, Danks DM. A mild form of Menkes' syndrome. J Pediatr 1981; 98:97–99.

165. Byers PH, Siegel RC, Holbrook KA, Narayanan AS, Bornstein P, Hall JG. An X-linked cutis laxa: defective cross-link formation in collagen due to decreased lysyl oxidase activity. N Engl J Med 1980; 303:61–65.

166. Haas RH, Robinson A, Evans K, Lascelles PT, Dubowitz V. An X-linked disease of the nervous system with disordered copper metabolism and features differing from Menkes' disease. Neurology (NY) 1981; 31:852–859.

167. Danks DM. Copper transport and utilisation in Menkes' syndrome and in mottled mice. Inorg Perspect Biol Med 1977; 1:73–87.

168. Goka TJ, Stevenson RE, Hefferan PM, Howell RR. Menkes' disease: a biochemical abnormality in cultured human fibroblasts. Proc Natl Acad Sci USA 1976; 73:604–606.

169. Camakaris J, Danks DM, Ackland L, Cartwright E, Borger P, Cotton RGH. Altered copper metabolism in cultured cells from human Menkes' syndrome and mottled mouse mutants. Biochem Genet 1980; 18:117–131.

170. Chan WY, Garnica AD, Rennert OM. Cell culture studies of Menkes kinky-hair syndrome. Clin Chim Acta 1978; 88:495–507.

171. Beratis NG, Price P, La Badie G, Hirschorn K. ^{64}Cu metabolism in Menkes' and normal cultured skin fibroblasts. Pediatr Res 1978; 12:699–702.

172. Royce PM, Camakaris J, Danks DM. Reduced lysyl oxidase activity in skin fibroblasts from patients with Menkes' syndrome. Biochem J 1980; 192:579–586.

173. Herd SM, Camakaris J, Christofferson R, Wookey P, Danks DM. Uptake and efflux of copper-64 in Menkes' disease and normal continuous lymphoid cell lines. Biochem J 1987; 247:341–347.

174. Danks DM, Stevens BJ, Campbell PE, Gillespie JM, Walker-Smith J, Blomfield J, Turner B. Menkes' kinky-hair syndrome. Lancet 1972; i:1100–1102.

175. Holstein TJ, Fung RQ, Quevedo WC, Bienjeki TC. Effects of altered copper metabolism induced by mottled alleles and diet on mouse tyrosinase. Proc Soc Exp Biol Med 1979; 162:264–268.

176. Grover WD, Johnson WC, Henkin RI. Clinical and biochemical aspects of trichopoliodystrophy. Ann Neurol 1979; 5:65–71.

177. Gryboski J. Congenital disorders of absorption. In: Lebenthal E, ed. Textbook of gastroenterology and nutrition in infancy. New York: Raven Press, 1981:931.

178. Danks DM, Cartwright E, Stevens BJ, Townley RRW. Menkes' kinky-hair disease: further definition of the defect in copper transport. Science 1973; 179:1140–1142.

179. Prins HW, Van Den Hamer CJA. Primary biochemical defect in copper metabolism in mice with a recessive X-linked mutation analogous to Menkes' disease in man. J Inorg Biochem 1979; 10:19–27.

180. Jones BP, Broomhead AF, Kwan YL, Grace CS. Incidence and clinical significance of protein-bound vitamin B$_{12}$ malabsorption. Eur J Haematol 1987; 38:131–138.

181. Allen RH, Seetharam B, Podel ER, Alpers DH. Effect of proteolytic enzymes on the binding of cobalamin to R protein and intrinsic factor. J Clin Invest 1978; 61:47–54.

182. Allen RH, Seetharam B, Allen NC, Podel ER, Alpers DH. Correction of cobalamin malabsorption in pancreatic insufficiency with a cobalamin analogue that binds with high affinity to R protein but not intrinsic factor. J Clin Invest 1978; 61:1628–1634.

183. Parmentier Y, Marcoullis G, Nicolas JP. The intraluminal transport of vitamin B$_{12}$ and the exocrine pancreatic insufficiency. Proc Soc Exp Biol Med 1979; 160:396–400.

184. Chanarin I, Muir M, Hughes AV, Hoffbrand A. Evidence for an intestinal origin of transcobalamin II during vitamin B$_{12}$ absorption. Br Med J 1978; 1:1453–1455.

185. Rosenberg LE. Disorders of propionate, methylmalonate, and cobalamin metabolism. In: Stanbury JB, Wyngaarden JB, Fredrickson DS, eds. The metabolic basis of inherited disease. 4th ed. New York: McGraw-Hill, 1978:411.

186. Zittoun J. Les anémies par carence et anomalie congénitale du métabolisme de la vitamine B$_{12}$ chez l'enfant. Ann Pediatr (Paris) 1982; 29:252–256.

187. Chanarin I. Disorders of vitamin absorption. Clin Gastroenterol 1982; 11:73–85.

188. Giorno JL, Dandine M, Gaudelus J, Nathanson M, Blanckaert D, Perelman R. Deficit congénital en facteur intrinsèque. Ann Pediatr (Paris) 1985; 32:277–280.

189. Miller DR, Bloom GE, Streiff RR, Lobuglio AF, Diamond LK. Juvenile congenital pernicious anemia. N Engl J Med 1966; 275:978–983.

190. Le Prise PY, Zittoun J, Roudier G, Richier JL. Anémie pernicieuse juvénile chez un garçon de 17 ans. Nouv Presse Med 1974; 3:2633–2634.

191. Harris Jones JN, Swain HT, Tudhok GR. Pernicious anemia without gastric atrophy and in presence of free hydrochloric acid; report of a case. Blood 1957; 12:461–465.

192. Katz M, Lee SK, Cooper BA. Vitamin B$_{12}$ malabsorption due to a biologically inert intrinsic factor. N Engl J Med 1972; 287:425–429.

193. Sutter M, Riedler G, Tönz O. Kindliche perniziöse Anämie bei kongenitalem Fehlen von intrinsic Factor und intermediärer Intrinsic-factor-sekretion bei den Eltern. Helv Paediatr Acta 1978; 33:267–274.

194. Chanarin I. The megaloblastic anemias. 2nd ed. Oxford: Blackwell, 1979.

195. Quinto MG, Leikin SL, Hung W. Pernicious anemia in a young girl associated with idiopathic hypoparathyroidism, familial Addison's disease and moniliasis. J Pediatr 1964; 64:241–246.

196. Spector JJ. Juvenile achlorhydric pernicious anemia with IgA deficiency: a family study. JAMA 1974; 228:334–336.

197. Matuchansky C, Rambaud JC, Modigliani R. Vitamin B$_{12}$ malabsorption in chronic pancreatitis. Gastroenterology 1974; 67:406–407.

198. Imerslund O. Idiopathic chronic megaloblastic anemia in children. Acta Paediatr Scand 1960; 49(suppl 119):1–115.

199. Gräsbeck R, Gordin R, Kantero I, Kuhlbäck B. Selective vitamin B$_{12}$ malabsorption anal proteinuria in young people: a syndrome. Acta Med Scand 1960; 167:289–296.

200. Davis RW, Christian RM, Ervin DM, Young LE. Pernicious anemia in childhood. Report of case in six year old girl responding to refined liver extract, folic acid and vitamin B$_{12}$ in successive relapses. Blood 1949; 4:1361–1366.

201. Najman E, Brasil B. Megaloblastische Anämie mit Relapsen ohne Achylia gastrica in Kinder salter. Ann Paediatr 1952; 178:47–59.

202. Ben-Bassat I, Feinstein A, Ramot B. Selective vitamin B$_{12}$ malabsorption with proteinuria in Israël. Isr J Med Sci 1969; 5:62–68.

203. Mackenzie IL, Donaldson RM Jr, Trier JS, Mathan VI. Ileal mucosa in familial selective vitamin B$_{12}$ malabsorption. N Engl J Med 1972; 286:1021–1025.

204. Hakami N, Neiman PE, Canellos GP, Lazerson J. Neonatal megalo-

blastic anemia due to inherited transcobalamin II deficiency in two siblings. N Engl J Med 1971; 285:1163–1170.

205. Hitzig WH, Dohmann U, Pluss HJ, Vischer D. Hereditary transcobalamin II deficiency: clinical findings in a new family. J Pediatr 1974; 85:622–628.

206. Burman JF, Mollin DL, Sourial NA, Sladden RA. Inherited lack of transcobalamin II in serum and megaloblastic anemia: a further patient. Br J Haematol 1979; 43:27–38.

207. Haurani FI, Hall CA, Rubin R. Megaloblastic anemia as a result of an abnormal transcobalamin II (Cardeza). J Clin Invest 1979; 64:1253–1259.

208. Seligman PA, Steiner LL, Allen RH. Studies of patient with megaloblastic anemia and abnormal transcobalamin II. N Engl J Med 1980; 303:1209–1212.

209. Corbeel L, Van Den Berghe G, Jaeken J, Van Tornout J, Eeckels R. Congenital folate malabsorption. Eur J Pediatr 1985; 143:284–290.

210. Luhby AL, Eagle FJ, Roth E, Cooperman JM. Relapsing megaloblastic anemia in an infant due to a specific defect in gastrointestinal absorption of folic acid. Am J Dis Child 1961; 102:482–483.

211. Lanzkowsky P, Erlandson ME, Bezan AI. Isolated defects of folic acid absorption associated with mental retardation and cerebral calcification. Blood 1969; 34:452–465.

212. Lanzkowshy P. Congenital malabsorption of folate. Am J Med 1970; 48:580–583.

213. Poncz M, Colman N, Herbert V, Schwartz E, Cohen AR. Therapy of congenital folate malabsorption. J Pediatr 1981; 98:76–79.

214. Poncz M, Colman N, Herbert C, Schwartz E, Cohen AR. Congenital folate malabsorption. J Pediatr 1981; 99:828–829.

215. Santiago-Borrero PJ, Santini R Jr, Perez-Santiago E, Maldonado N. Congenital isolated defect of folic acid absorption. J Pediatr 1973; 82:450–455.

216. Su PC. Congenital folate deficiency. N Engl J Med 1976; 294:1128.

217. Reisenauer AM. Affinity labeling of the intestinal folate binding protein. Gastroenterology 1988; 94:A372.

218. Rowe PB. Inherited disorders of folate metabolism. In: Stanbury JB, Wyngaarden JB, Fredrickson DS, Goldstein JL, Brown MS, eds. The metabolic basis of inherited disease. 5th ed. New York: McGraw-Hill, 1984:498.

219. Rasmussen H, Anast C. Familial hypophosphatemic rickets and vitamin D-dependent rickets. In: Stanbury JB, Wyngaarden JB, Fredrickson DS, Goldstein JL, Brown MS, eds. The metabolic basis of inherited disease. 5th ed. New York: McGraw-Hill, 1984:1743.

220. Frymoyer JW, Hodgkin W. Adult-onset vitamin D-resistant hypophosphatemic osteomalacia. J Bone Joint Surg 1977; 59:101–106.

221. Lawson DE, Fraser DR, Kodicek E, Morris HR, Williams DH. Identification of 1,25-dihydroxychole-calciferol, a new kidney hormone controlling calcium metabolism. Nature (London) 1971; 230:228–230.

222. Holick MF, Schnoes HK, DeLuca HF, Suda T, Cousins RJ. Isolation and identification of 1,25-dihydroxychole-calciferol: a metabolite of vitamin D active in intestine. Biochemistry 1971; 10:2799–2804.

223. Boyle IT, Miravet L, Gray RW, Holick MF, DeLuca HF. The response of intestinal calcium transport to 25-hydroxy-and 1,25-dihydroxyvitamin D_3 in nephrectomized rats. Endocrinology 1972; 90:605–608.

224. Garabedian M, Tanaka Y, Holick MF, DeLuca HF. Response of intestinal calcium transport and bone calcium mobilization to 1,25-dihydroxyvitamin D_3 in thyroparathyroidectomized rats. Endocrinology 1974; 94:1022–1027.

225. Fanconi A, Prader A. Pseudo-vitamin D-deficiency rickets. In: Burland WL, Barltrop D, eds. Mineral metabolism in pediatrics. Oxford: Blackwell, 1969:19.

226. Hamilton R, Harrison J, Fraser D, Radde I, Morecki R, Paunier L. The small intestine in vitamin D-dependent rickets. Pediatrics 1970; 45:364–372.

227. Balsan S, Garabedian M. 25-Hydroxychole-calciferol: a comparative study in deficiency rickets and different types of resistant rickets. J Clin Invest 1972; 51:749–759.

228. Feldman D, Chen T, Hirst M, Golston K, Karasek M, Cone C. Demonstration of 1,25-dihydroxyvitamin D_3 receptors in human skin biopsies. J Clin Endocrinol Metab 1980; 51:1463–1465.

229. Griffin JE, Wilson JD. The syndromes of androgen resistance. N Engl J Med 1980; 302:198–209.

230. Glorieux F, Scriver CT. Loss of a parathyroid hormone-sensitive compound of phosphate transport in X-linked hypophosphatemia. Science 1972; 175:99–1000.

231. Tenenhouse HS, Scriver CR, McInnes RR, Glorieux FH. Renal handling of phosphate in vivo and in vitro by the X-linked hypophosphatemic male mouse: evidence for a defect in the brush border membrane. Kidney Int 1978; 14:236–244.

232. Tenenhouse HS, Scriver CR. Renal brush border membrane adaptation to phosphorus deprivation in the Hyp/Y mouse. Nature 1979; 281:225–227.

233. Stearns G, Oelke MJ, Boyd JD. Mineral metabolism in late rickets. Am J Dis Child 1931; 42:88–92.

234. Chan JC, Lovinger RD, Mamunes P. Renal hypophosphatemic rickets: growth acceleration after long-term treatment with 1,25-dihydroxyvitamin D_3. Pediatrics 1980; 66:445–454.

235. Glorieux FH, Morin CL, Travers R, Delvin EE, Poirer R. Intestinal phosphate transport in familial hypophosphatemic rickets. Pediatr Res 1976; 10:691–696.

236. Balsan S, Garabedian M, Lieberherr M, Gueris J, Ulmann A. Serum 1,25-dihydroxyvitamin D concentrations in two different types of pseudo-deficiency rickets. In: Norman AW, Schaefer K, Herrath DV, Griboleit HG, Colburn JW, DeLuca HF, Mawer EB, Suda T, eds. Vitamin D basis research and its clinical application. Berlin: Walter de Gruyter, 1979:1143.

237. Rosen JF, Fleischman AR, Finberg L, Hamstra A, DeLuca HF. Rickets with alopecia: an inborn error of vitamin D metabolism. J Pediatr 1979; 94:729–735.

238. Liberman UA, Halabe A, Samuel R, Kauli R, Edelstein S, Weisman Y, Papapoulos SE, Fraher LJ, Clemens TL, O'Riordan JLH. End-organ resistance to 1,25-dihydroxychole-calciferol. Lancet 1980; i:504–506.

239. Sockalosky JJ, Ulstrom RA, DeLuca HF, Brown DM. Vitamin D-resistant rickets: end-organ unresponsiveness to 1,25 $(OH)_2D_3$. J Pediatr 1980; 96:701–703.

240. Tsuchiya Y, Nobutake M, Cho H, Kumagai M, Yasaka A, Suda T, Orimo H, Shiraki M. An unusual form of vitamin D-dependent rickets in a child: alopecia and marked end-organ hyposensitivity to biologically active vitamin D. J Clin Endocrinol Metab 1980; 51:685–690.

241. Marx SJ, Spiegel AM, Brown EM, Gardner DG, Downs RW Jr, Attie M, Hamstra AJ, DeLuca HF. A familial syndrome of decrease in sensitivity to 1,25-dihydroxyvitamin D. J Clin Endocrinol Metab 1978; 47:1303–1310.

242. Zerwekh JE, Glass K, Jowsey J, Charles YC. An unique form of osteomalacia associated with end-organ refractoriness to 1,25-dihydroxyvitamin D and apparent defective synthesis of 1,25-dihydroxyvitamin D. J Clin Endocrinol Metab 1979; 49:171–175.

243. Brooks MH, Bell NH, Love L, Stern PH, Orfei E, Queener SF, Hamstra AJ, DeLuca HF. Vitamin D-dependent rickets type II: resistance of target organs to 1,25-dihydroxyvitamin D. N Engl J Med 1978; 298:996–999.

244. Heubi JE, Balistreri WF, Partin JC. Refractory infantile diarrhea due to primary bile acid malabsorption. J Pediatr 1979; 94:546–551.

245. Heubi JE, Balistreri WF, Fondacaro JD, Partin JC, Schubert WK. Primary bile acid malabsorption: defective in vitro ileal active bile acid transport. Gastroenterology 1982; 83:804–811.

20

Bacterial Overgrowth

Gordon Forstner, M.D.
Philip Sherman, M.D.
Steven Lichtman, M.D.

Bacteria do not inhabit the upper small intestine and stomach in significant numbers, whereas in the colon concentrations of 100 billion organisms per milliliter are the norm. Colonic microflora will proliferate in the small intestine, however, whenever its intrinsic cleansing mechanisms are interrupted. Classically, colonic flora proliferate in the small intestine in areas of stasis. The clinical syndrome that results has been given a variety of names, i.e., stagnant loop, blind loop, contaminated small bowel, small bowel stasis, or small bowel bacterial overgrowth syndrome. In this discussion we will use the latter term, small bowel bacterial overgrowth (SBBO). The characteristic features of SBBO are (1) abnormal colonization of the upper small intestine by organisms that characteristically reside in the colon, (2) steatorrhea, and (3) anemia.

THE NORMAL INTESTINE

At birth the intestine is sterile, but soon after parturition orally ingested organisms begin to colonize the gut.[1] Commensal bacterial populations are not uniform in either number or type (Table 1). In the upper small intestine, aerobic bacteria typical of the oral cavity predominate. Their numbers do not exceed 10^5 organisms per milliliter. In the colon strict and facultative anerobes, adapted to growth within the fecal mass where bacterial metabolism quickly deprives the environment of oxygen, are most common. The total number of colonic bacteria per milliliter is at least one million times greater than that of the upper small intestine. Colonic species are listed in some detail in Table 1, but the list is nevertheless incomplete. There are at least 60 different bacterial species.[2] Many are in trace numbers, but under specific circumstances, some, like *Clostridium difficile*, proliferate and cause disease. The number of bacteria in the distal small intestine is greater than that of the proximal small intestine. Near the cecum there may be 10^8 organisms per milliliter and the composition of the flora is similar to that of the colon.

PRESERVATION OF THE NORMAL ENVIRONMENT

The relative sterility of the small intestine depends on a number of factors (Fig. 1) that act to reduce bacterial load and prevent colonization. They are conveniently divided into nonimmune and immune categories.

TABLE 1
Commensal Enteric Flora of the Normal
Intestinal Tract

Proximal small intestine
  <10^5 organisms per milliliter
  Aerobic, oral flora dominate
  Streptococcus, Lactobacillus, Neisseria

Distal small intestine
  >10^8 organism per milliliter
  Greater numbers of anaerobic and facultative anaerobic bacteria
  Bacteroides, Escherichia coli, Bifidobacterium

Colon
  >10^{10} organisms per milliliter
  Anaerobic and facultative anaerobic bacteria
  Bacteroides, Escherichia coli, Bifidobacterium, Clostridium

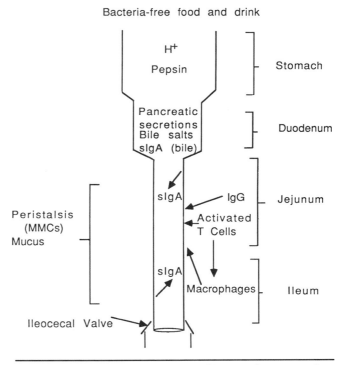

FIGURE 1 Prevention of small bowel bacterial overgrowth in health.

Nonimmune Antibacterial Factors

Gastric acidity acts an initial line of defense against ingested bacteria. Gastric juice with pH less than 4.0 is bactericidal for most organisms, although not immediately. In one experiment, bacteria instilled into the normal lumen of the stomach were killed within 15 minutes, but when instilled into the achlorhydric stomach they remained viable for at least 1 hour.[3] Chronic inhibition of gastric acid secretion by H_2 blockade has been shown to increase the number of gastric bacteria substantially.[4] The number of bacteria presented to the duodenum therefore depends on the number of organisms ingested and the length of their exposure to low pH.

Peristaltic propagation of luminal contents in a steady distal flow toward the colon is of major importance in reducing the growth of bacteria in the proximal intestine. Interdigestive migratory motor complexes (MMCs) are especially important in this role. Bacterial populations rise within hours when the complexes are ablated pharmacologically.[5]

Enzymatic digestion is probably of significance as well, since small numbers of bacteria might be expected to undergo normal digestive degradation. Pancreatic juice has antibacterial activity,[6] possibly because of its proteolytic and lipolytic enzymes, although other factors such as competitive binding and specific antibacterial activities cannot be ruled out. Bile acids and digestive secretions probably help to limit growth as well. Colonization requires access to preferential growth sites in stagnant niches such as the lumina of intestinal glands and membrane sites to which bacteria can bind. Just as importantly, it also requires a relatively large number of available bacteria to exploit these niches at any given instance. Intestinal secretions from the stomach, intestine, and pancreas are therefore a significant deterrent to growth due to their ability to dilute the bacterial mass.

Mucus is an example of an epithelial secretion with special properties that enable it to trap bacteria in an intraluminal location while moving organisms distally in bolus fashion. Mucus is composed of a variety of proteins and salts anchored within a viscous gel formed by a single carbohydrate-rich protein. Eighty percent of the mucus glycoprotein by weight is carbohydrate, and the protein itself is organized as a long thread of disulfide-bonded units, often amounting to a molecular weight of 5 to 10×10^6. These huge threads bind bacteria through specific lectin-like reactions with carbohydrate,[7] by hydrophobic interactions,[8] and probably through simple trapping. The carbohydrate serves as a nutrient for some bacteria, thus attracting them to a mobile colonization site that is continuously replaced. Huge numbers of organisms (Fig. 2) are found in the mucus coats of the colon[9] and stagnant loops,[10] whereas bacteria are relatively scarce on the underlying mucosa and glands, suggesting that mucus limits access of bacteria to the intestinal surface even in stagnant circumstances. This may explain why cellular damage is often minor in stagnant portions of the bowel even though bacterial counts are high.[11]

The *ileocecal valve* prevents retrograde colonization of the distal small bowel to a significant extent.[12] As noted in Table 1, the concentration gradient across the valve is not large, on the order of 100 times. In the absence of the valve, however, free reflux of right-sided liquid colonic content occurs and the total load of colonic bacteria exposed to the distal small intestine increases greatly.

Bacterial load also conditions intestinal colonization. Coprophagic animals, for example, harbor higher numbers of bacteria in the proximal small intestine than do humans, although colonic populations are equivalent. Poor environmental sanitation, particularly in warm climates, encourages ingestion of excessive numbers of bacteria and may increase the small intestinal bacterial count in this manner.

Immune Antibacterial Factors

Antibodies to indigenous intestinal bacteria develop early in life[13] and probably play an important role in controlling membrane colonization and mucosal penetration by bacteria and bacterial products. Antibodies to bacterial pilus proteins have been shown to inhibit binding to specific attachment sites on intestinal membranes.[14] *Combined immunodeficiency states*, notably AIDS, and combined B and T cell immunodeficiency predispose the upper intestine to opportunistic infestation by a variety of parasites. Loss of the capacity to secrete immunoglobulins into the intestinal lumen generally produces less dramatic effects, but upper intestinal colonization by specific parasites such as *Giardia lamblia* occurs frequently in hypogammaglobulinemia and secretory IgA (sIgA) deficiency. Specific IgG and IgA antibodies hasten the elimination of intestinal parasites such as *Giardia* and nematodes,[15] possibly by activating macrophages. The role that the immune system plays, if any, in modulating growth of intraluminal commensal bacteria in the intestine is less clear. There is evidence that agammaglobulinemic and hypogammaglobulinemic patients develop small intestinal bacterial overgrowth,[16-18] but it has been argued that other complications arising in these conditions, such as achlorhydria, are critically important. Dolby et al,[18] for example, compared three groups of patients, one with pernicious anemia, another with hypogammaglobulinemia and achlorhydria, and a third with hypogammaglobulinemia and normal gastric acidity. Bacterial overgrowth was found in the first two groups but not in the third. Although an impressive amount of sIgA enters the intestinal lumen in bile, direct transmucosal secretion is also important. Upper intestinal blind loops, produced experimentally in rats, produced and secreted sIgA with specificity for their colonic-type bacteria.[19] Antibodies secreted by the mucosa may help to prevent mucosal attachment by luminal bacteria. Secretory IgA may also enhance binding of certain bacteria to mucus.[20]

FACTORS PREDISPOSING TO THE DEVELOPMENT OF SMALL BOWEL BACTERIAL OVERGROWTH

A large number of specific clinical entities are reported to cause SBBO. Seemingly unrelated illnesses can, however, be grouped into four categories, depending on the mechanism by which the SBBO is produced. As summarized in Table 2, these include (1) anatomic abnormalities, (2) disorders of intestinal motility, (3) lesions that increase the number of

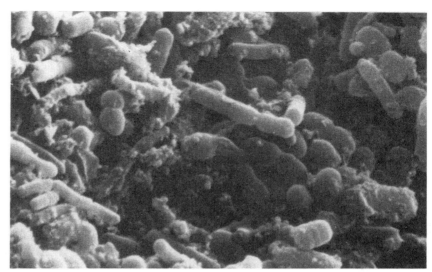

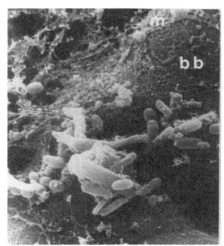

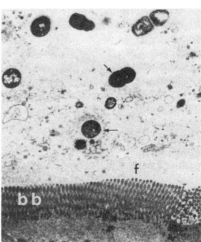

FIGURE 2 Association of bacteria with the mucous coat in small bowel bacterial overgrowth. *A,* Scanning electron micrograph of the unwashed small intestinal surface showing bacterial rods and chains embedded in multiple layers within the surface mucous coat. *B,* After gentle washing with saline, the brush border surface (bb) is exposed under strands of mucus (m). Bacteria remain bound to the mucous strands and not to the brush border. *C,* Transmission electron microscopy of an enterocyte with a layer corresponding to surface filaments (f) on the surface of the brush border (bb). Bacteria (*arrows*) are confined to the mucus outside the filamentous layer.

TABLE 2

Factors Predisposing to the Development of Small Bowel Bacterial Overgrowth

Anatomic abnormalities
  Diverticula, duplication
  Stricture, stenosis, web
  Blind loop

Motility disorders
  Pseudo-obstruction
  Absence of the migratory motor complexes
  Autonomic neuropathy (e.g., diabetes mellitus)
  Collagen vascular diseases (e.g., scleroderma)

Excessive bacterial load
  Achlorhydria
  Fistula
  Loss of the ileocecal valve

Abnormal host defenses
  Immunodeficiency
  Malnutrition
  Prematurity

bacteria presented to the upper small intestine, and (4) deficiencies of host defense.

Anatomic lesions include diverticula (Fig. 3), duplications, and mucosal strictures.[21] These lesions all interrupt normal gut motility and thereby provide a site of relative stasis for bacterial colonization and replication. Surgical procedures such as side-to-side anastomoses,[22] jejunoileal bypass,[23] and neoreservoirs[24] (Koch pouch, Ileal-anal anastomosis) may create areas of poorly drained bowel and SBBO. *Disruption of normal intestinal motor activity* causes intestinal stasis by interfering with peristaltic clearing function. Short-term disruption such as occurs with abdominal surgery is rarely a problem because, although SBBO develops, it rapidly clears with return of motor function. Severe clinical symptoms develop when motility is adversely affected on a more long-term basis. Idiopathic intestinal pseudo-obstruction syndrome is a frequent cause of symptomatic SBBO in children. Secondary causes of a disrupted motility pattern, such as progressive systemic scleroderma and diabetes mellitus with associated autonomic neuropathy, are more frequent consider-

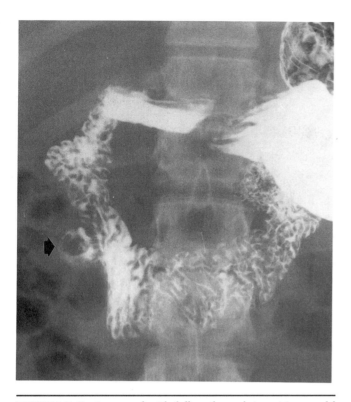

FIGURE 3 Barium meal with follow-through in a 13-year-old female demonstrates a diverticulum (*arrow*) of the duodenum. (Courtesy of Dr. David Stringer, Department of Radiology, The Hospital for Sick Children, Toronto.)

ations in adults. In the elderly, otherwise isolated absence of the MMC is associated with SBBO.[25] The MMC normally has an important "housekeeper" function, helping to keep the proximal small intestine relatively sterile.[26,27] Vantrappen et al[27] showed that 5 of 18 patients with clinically documented SBBO had an absent or disorderly MMC pattern. As activity of the MMC may not be fully developed in the immature gut,[28] the premature infant may be at particular risk. Motor abnormalities have subsequently been shown to occur in experimentally produced SBBO,[29] indicating that bacterial overgrowth can cause a motor abnormality independently and thus exacerbate the tendency to stasis. *An increased bacterial load* that overwhelms the normal host defenses can also result in SBBO. Coloenteric fistulae (Crohn's disease, surgical misadventures), loss of the ileocecal valve (postresection, e.g., in Crohn's disease or necrotizing enterocolitis), and loss of normal gastric output (autoimmune gastritis, malnutrition) may all permit entry into the small intestine of abnormally large numbers of bacteria and initiate SBBO even without appreciable early stasis. Poor sanitation, particularly in the absence of a clean water supply, may also lead to the habitual ingestion of such a large oral load of bacteria that gastric acidity is overwhelmed. *Abnormalities of host defense* such as, for example, the achlorhydria associated with hypogammaglobulinemia, are frequently associated with SBBO. Protein-calorie undernutrition is associated with SBBO in children[30-32] and causes loss of gastric acidity,[33,34] decreased mucin production,[35] and impaired cellular and humoral immune function.[36]

In many clinical settings, etiologic risk factors for SBBO overlap. For example, in underdeveloped countries it is difficult to separate the effects of an increased bacterial load due to poor hygenic conditions from the effects of co-existing protein-calorie undernutrition. In experimental animals, using the self-filling blind loop model of SBBO, we showed that malnutrition hastened the onset of deficiencies in mucosal hydrolase activities following intestinal stasis.[37] However, in the rat model protein-calorie deprivation without surgical intervention to induce intestinal stasis did not depress specific activities of brush border disaccharidases. Infants with the short bowel syndrome frequently have associated SBBO that complicates their clinical course and medical management. In this setting, SBBO is multifactorial, since it can be related to intestinal dysmotility, loss of the ileocecal valve, prior abdominal surgery, and associated malnutrition of the host. In some cases of postinfectious enteropathy, symptoms of chronic diarrhea appear to be related to associated SBBO.[38-41] Although the etiology of bacterial overgrowth in this setting is not clearly established, changes in gut motility, altered host defenses, and co-existing malnutrition may all be contributing factors. Inadequate preparation of food may also be a factor in some countries. For example, the red kidney bean contains a lectin, phytohemagglutinin, which is readily destroyed by heating but which can produce bacterial overgrowth in experimental animals when raw beans are fed to them.[42]

Pathophysiology

Excessive numbers of intraluminal bacteria alter intraluminal secretions and produce metabolic products, enzymes, and toxins that damage the mucosa and are absorbed. As a consequence, they produce intraluminal, mucosal, and systemic effects (Table 3) that greatly alter the performance of their human host.

Intraluminal Effects. Bacteria are metabolically active organisms, and it is not surprising that their nutritional demands conflict with those of the host when their numbers increase in a metabolically active area of the intestine. Not surprisingly, pathologic effects are maximal when overgrowth involves the upper small intestine. Intraluminal anaerobic

TABLE 3
Intraluminal Bacteria: Effects on Host

Intraluminal Effects	Mucosal Effects	Systemic Effects
Bile salt deconjugation 11α-Hydroxylation	Disaccharidase loss	Absorption of bacterial toxins, antigens
Bile salt depletion	Enterocyte damage Inflammation	Hepatic inflammation Immune complex formation
Lipid malabsorption	Protein loss	Cutaneous vasculitis
Vitamin B$_{12}$ malabsorption	Bleeding	Polyarthritis
Fermentation— short-chain fatty acids		
Release of proteases, toxins		

bacteria, particularly fecal strains, possess enzymes that deconjugate bile salts and convert their component cholic and chenodeoxycholic acids to the secondary bile acids deoxycholic and lithocholic.[43] The net result is to lower the concentration of bile salt in the duodenum and jejunum below the critical micellar concentration (CMC).[44,45] Above the CMC, much of the triglyceride and cholesterol in the lumen are present in mixed micelles containing hydrolyzed lipid products (fatty acids and mono- and diglycerides) and bile salts. Below the CMC, large liquid crystalline and insoluble emulsoid forms predominate. Since pancreatic lipase is water-soluble and must operate at a lipid-water interface, the great reduction in lipid surface area has disastrous consequences for fat digestion, and malabsorption of triglyceride, fat-soluble vitamins, and other lipid molecules results. Patchy histologic abnormalities, impaired uptake of lipolytic products, and slow chylomicron transport may also contribute to fat malabsorption.[46]

Intraluminal bacteria, particularly *Bacteroides* and coliforms, also utilize vitamin B_{12} and thus directly compete for dietary vitamin B_{12}, preventing its absorption. When radioactive vitamin B_{12} is administered to animals or patients with SBBO, most of the radioactivity subsequently recovered from the small bowel contents is bound to enteric microorganisms.[47,48] Once bound, the vitamin is unavailable to the hosts unless the bacteria die. Luminal bacteria also produce inactive cobamides that are not available to the affected host.[49] Vitamin B_{12} malabsorption not correctable by intrinsic factor may be the most consistent feature of clinically significant SBBO.[44]

Mucosal Effects. These are less dramatically expressed but in aggregate are equally deleterious. Although the bacteria that accumulate in SBBO do not produce classic enterotoxins,[50] they do produce enzymes[51,52] and metabolic products[53,54] that are potentially capable of injuring the mucosa. In experimental blind loops it has been shown that anaerobic bacteria elaborate proteases with elastase-like properties which remove or destroy glycoprotein enzymes on the brush border surface.[51,52] As a result, mucosal disaccharidase activities are reduced.[55] Monosaccharide transport may also be impaired, reflecting damage to the microvillous plasma membrane and the toxic effects of deconjugated bile salts.[53] Impaired transport of sodium and chloride has also been demonstrated.[56] In the self-filling blind loop, bacterial overgrowth produces a relatively mild morphologic lesion. Both villous height and crypt depth are increased.[57,58] Approximately 10 to 20 percent of the columnar cells in the upper half of the villi are swollen and vesiculated. Apical membrane microvilli of some, but not all enterocytes, are blunted, swollen, and budded. Damaged mitochondria and endoplasmic reticulum can be found. These experimental findings are in keeping with morphologic reports in humans,[59] which suggest that bacterial overgrowth causes a patchy mucosal lesion with segments of subtotal villous atrophy and a marked subepithelial inflammatory response. In infants, particularly, there is a well-established association between carbohydrate intolerance and small intestinal bacterial overgrowth.[37,60] Protein loss in the intestine may be sufficiently profound in both experimental animals[61] and humans[61,62] to cause hypoproteinemia. Chronic intestinal blood loss has also been documented[63] as a cause of anemia.

Systemic Effects. Bacterial products and antigens are absorbed through the damaged mucosa, causing systemic effects. One of us has recently shown that abnormalities in both hepatic function and liver architecture develop in the rat self-filling blind-loop model of bacterial overgrowth.[64] Immune responses are probably responsible for complaints of arthritis and dermatitis. Circulating immune complexes containing IgG, IgA, IgM, and complement have been detected during episodes of arthritis associated with SBBO caused by intestinal bypass surgery.[65,66] IgM, IgA, and C3 depositions in the reticular dermis have been demonstrated in association with necrosis of the upper dermis and adjacent vasculitis.[67,68]

CLINICAL FEATURES OF SMALL BOWEL BACTERIAL OVERGROWTH

Clinical symptoms (Table 4) occur in approximately one-third of all patients.[69,70] In those who are symptomatic, clinical effects range from mild inconvenience to complaints that are both chronic and disabling. In general, overgrowth of bacteria in the proximal small bowel results in greater disability than overgrowth in the distal small intestine. SBBO may occur at any age. Relative deficiencies in mucosal defenses in the immature host may place the very young at increased risk.

Diarrhea is a common complaint. Stools may be foul and greasy due to steatorrhea, or watery and explosive due to maldigestion of dietary carbohydrate. In children, growth failure may be an important additional clinical feature. Arrested weight velocity is usually the first feature to be noticed, but later a delay in height velocity and resultant short stature appear. Nutritional debilitation is multifactorial. Appetite is frequently diminished. Diets may be restricted in an attempt to decrease stool frequency. Maldigestion of fat, dietary carbohydrate,[53] and protein[62] and increased intestinal losses of endogenous proteins[61] also contribute.

Clinical evidence of vitamin deficiency is rarely seen. Usually, vitamin B_{12} deficiency is prevented in the pediatric population by adequate body stores of cobalamin. Iron deficiency anemia can occur, however, secondary to enteric iron loss.[63] Osteomalacia, rickets, and pellagra-like symptoms have been reported as a consequence of vitamin D

TABLE 4
Clinical Features of Small Bowel Bacterial Overgrowth

Classic	Systemic
Chronic diarrhea	Arthritis
Steatorrhea	Tenosynovitis
Anemia	Vesiculopustular rash
	Erythema nodosum
Others	Raynaud's phenomenon
Weight loss	Nephritis
Short stature	Hepatitis
Abdominal pain	Hepatic steatosis
Protein-losing enteropathy	
Hypoalbuminemia	
Osteomalacia	
Night blindness	
Ataxia	

malabsorption[71] and water-soluble B-vitamin[72] deficiency. Since luminal bacteria produce vitamin K and folic acid and these become available to the host, absorption may be enhanced. Serum folic acid may be elevated.[73]

Davidson et al[74] indicate that SBBO may be a significant cause of abdominal pain in young children due to secondary carbohydrate intolerance. Recurrent episodes of arthralgia, nondeforming polyarthritis, tenosynovitis, and cutaneous vasculitis (the arthritis-dermatitis syndrome) occur very commonly following intestinal bypass operations but have also been reported in other forms of SBBO.[67,75] The skin lesions are typically vesiculopustular or erythema nodosum–like. Paresthesias and Raynauds's phenomenon are common. Renal damage[72] and hepatic steatosis[77] have also been reported following jejunoileal bypass surgery and could conceivably appear in other forms of SBBO.

DIAGNOSIS OF SMALL BOWEL BACTERIAL OVERGROWTH

A well-directed medical history often provides important clues to suggest that a more detailed investigation related to the possibility of underlying bacterial contamination of the small intestine is warranted. A history of previous abdominal surgery should always be sought, because SBBO due to either alterations of intestinal motility or the creation of anatomic regions of intestinal stasis can occur as a long-term adverse complication of intestinal surgery. Specific surgical procedures that affect normal nonimmunologic host defenses may also predispose to small bowel bacterial overgrowth. For example, an interruption of the vagus nerve inhibits output of gastric acid and may result in an increase in the load of viable organisms that enter the proximal small intestine. Similarly, signs and symptoms suggestive of systemic disease— in particular, collagen vascular diseases—should be explored in a detailed history. Longstanding diabetes mellitus can result in alterations in intestinal motility due to an autonomic neuropathy. Although not uncommon in adults, small bowel bacterial overgrowth due to autonomic dysfunction is very unusual in children with diabetes mellitus. This age-related difference may simply relate to the duration of the underlying chronic disease.

Table 5 summarizes alternatives that are useful in establishing the diagnosis of clinically significant bacterial overgrowth. Not all patients with overgrowth of bacteria in the small bowel have clinical symptoms. Therefore, an initial evaluation should be directed at first determining if there is evidence of malabsorption of either fat or cobalamin (vitamin B_{12}). Serum levels of cobalamin are not, in general, a useful screening test for SBBO in children, since body stores of the vitamin are sufficient to maintain normal circulating levels for at least 5 years after the onset of cobalamin malabsorption in the gut. Elevated levels of folic acid may be useful as a screening test.

In the appropriate clinical setting, abnormal values of quantitative fecal fat excretion, Schilling's test with intrinsic factor, and folic acid indicate the need for more detailed investigations in order to establish the diagnosis of bacterial overgrowth. Although some physicians would simply proceed directly to an empiric course of antibiotic therapy, it should

TABLE 5
Diagnostic Tests for Small Bowel Bacterial Overgrowth

Screening
  Sudan stain of stool for neutral fat
  72-hour fecal fat
  Schilling's test with intrinsic factor
  Folic acid
  Barium meal with follow-through
Diagnostic
  A. Invasive
    Duodenal aspiration
      Culture
        Aerobic bacteria
        Anaerobic bacteria
        Exclude known enteropathogens
      Deconjugated bile salts
      Short-chain fatty acids

  B. Noninvasive
    Indicanuria
    Serum bile acids
    Breath tests

be emphasized that the clinical symptoms and abnormalities in screening laboratory tests are not specific to this diagnostic consideration.

A barium meal with follow-through should be performed in order to document the presence of intestinal strictures, diverticula, and delayed intestinal transit. Abnormalities in the radiologic study should prompt more extensive investigations. A normal barium meal study does not exclude the presence of clinically significant bacterial overgrowth in the small intesine. A biopsy of the duodenum should also be obtained, since the presenting symptoms of gluten-sensitive enteropathy in children can mimic SBBO. Patchy enteropathic changes with increased numbers of inflammatory cells are typical of SBBO.

Specific Diagnostic Tests

Quantitative culture of increased numbers of anaerobic bacteria in luminal fluid obtained from the proximal small intestine establishes the diagnosis of small bowel bacterial overgrowth. The presence of more than 10^5 colony-forming units of bacteria that are not typical residents of the oral cavity is an abnormal finding. Documentation of anaerobic colonic-type bacteria (in particular, *Bacteroides* species) is important, since normally these bacterial species do not reside in the mouth or stomach or colonize the upper small intestine. However, the culture of duodenal fluid as a diagnostic technique is not without its problems. Many hospitals do not have bacteriologic laboratories with the ability to culture fastidious strict anaerobes routinely. Fortunately, the presence of more than 10^5 colony-forming units of facultative anaerobic bacteria, such as *Escherichia coli* strains, is relatively good evidence of associated colonization by strict anaerobic bacteria. Quantitative duodenal cultures should therefore be performed even if one lacks anaerobic culture facilities.

Neither duodenal aspiration nor quantitative bacterial estimation is easily performed. A great deal of investigation has been focused, therefore, on establishing the utility of other diagnostic techniques. Two alternative tests that depend on the detection of bacterially derived products (unconjugated bile acids and short-chain fatty acids) may be performed on duodenal aspirates: (1) determination of conjugated and deconjugated bile acid profiles in duodenal fluid[78] and (2) assay of duodenal fluid for the presence of short-chain volatile fatty acids—i.e., acetic, propionic, butyric, isobutyric, valeric, and isovaleric.[79,80] Each test may be helpful if decidedly abnormal, but neither has been evaluated fully.

Duodenal aspiration is invasive, and sedation or physical restraint is usually required in children to permit the passage of an aspiration tube through the oral cavity into the upper small bowel. Since fluorography is often used to establish localization of the catheter tip, a small dose of radiation is frequently required. Noninvasive diagnostic methods are therefore attractive. Ideally, these noninvasive tests should demonstrate a high degree of sensitivity and specificity. Although the optimal, noninvasive diagnostic probe for use in children has not yet been defined, a number of options are available. Measurement of elevated urinary indican, produced by the conversion of dietary tryptophan to indican by intraluminal bacteria, is perhaps the simplest technique. Specificity is low, however, because indicanuria is not limited to bacterial overgrowth in the small intestine.[81] Provided that the technique is available, a relatively simply quantitative estimate of serum conjugated and free bile acids may be helpful. Total serum bile acids are often elevated in patients with SBBO, and almost all of the increase is represented by free bile acids, which are normally present in trace amounts.[82] Individual bile acid profiles show that deoxycholate is uniquely elevated, a finding that distinguishes SBBO from ileal resection, which is also associated with high serum levels of free bile acids.[82,83]

A number of studies have examined the utility of various breath tests as diagnostic tools (Table 6). Measurement of ^{14}C in expired air following oral ingestion of an appropriate substrate which is conjugated to the radioisotope appears to be an excellent alternative for noninvasive diagnostic purposes. ^{14}C-labeled bile acids, such as glycocholate, were the first substrates to be used.[84] Utilization of the substrate by luminal bacteria releases[14]C, which then equilibrates within the tissues of the host and is excreted from the lungs as [14]CO$_2$ in expired air. False-positive results may occur in patients with mucosal inflammation affecting the distal ileum. Several reports indicate that ^{14}C-labeled D-xylose is superior to ^{14}C-bile acid as substrate.[85,86] Unfortunately, the use of ^{14}C is not satisfactory for diagnostic purposes in children. The advent of stable radioisotopes, such as ^{13}C-substrate,[87] should permit the testing of oral D-xylose and glycocholate in children when suitable compounds become widely available.

The measurement of hydrogen levels in samples of expired air provides an alternative approach that is currently applicable to the pediatric population. Mammalian cells do not produce hydrogen, whereas many prokaryotic cells produce it as a by-product of substrate utilization. The commensal colonic microflora are generally excellent hydrogen producers. The hydrogen is absorbed and distributed throughout the body and subsequently expired in the breath. Provision of a nonabsorbable sugar, such as lactulose, supplies substrate to the colonic microbial flora and results in an increase in levels of expired hydrogen.[88] If a colonic type of microflora is present in the small intestine, an early hydrogen peak is observed following lactulose challenge (Fig. 4). Others have shown that absorbable carbohydrates, including lactose[89] and D-glucose,[90] may also be useful substrates in testing for SBBO.

Perman et al reported that elevations of the fasting level of breath H$_2$ in children correlate with the presence of small bowel bacterial overgrowth.[91] Previous meals containing

TABLE 6
Breath Tests for Use in the Diagnosis of Small Bacterial Overgrowth

1. **Radioisotopes**
   ^{14}C-glycocholate
   ^{14}C-D-xylose

2. **Stable radioisotopes**
   ^{13}C-conjugates

3. **Breath hydrogen**
   Fasting
   Lactulose
   Lactose
   Glucose

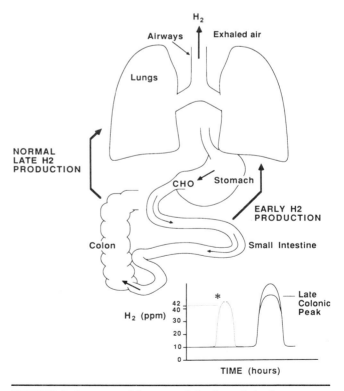

FIGURE 4 Conceptual framework for breath hydrogen testing. CHO denotes ingested carbohydrate. *An early peak and an elevated baseline of hydrogen measured in expired breath samples are both suggestive of small bowel bacterial contamination.

nonabsorbable carbohydrates[92-94] and endogenous glycoproteins[95] may elevate fasting breath H_2 and cause confusion in children. In children, however, a breath H_2 of greater than 42 parts per million was seen only with SBBO.[91]

Breath hydrogen testing is a convenient, widely available methodology for use in diagnosis of bacterial overgrowth. The technique has serious shortcomings, however, which limit its effectiveness. Douwes et al reported that 9.2 percent of 98 healthy school-age children who were tested were non–hydrogen producers.[96] Children with diarrhea and low fecal pH may have an altered intestinal flora that does not yield H_2 in expired air samples.[97-99] Concurrent use of medications, particularly antibiotics,[100] also affects bacterial fermentation of test sugars and may lower breath H_2 levels. A clear separation of "early" and "late" hydrogen peaks can be affected by the rate of gastric emptying and the intestinal transit time. In practice, two distinct peaks are often not documented.[101] Several recent reports indicate that the normal microbial flora of the oral cavity can also contribute to the early fermentation of the carbohydrate substrates and produce modest elevations in the levels of hydrogen in expired air.[102,103] Breath hydrogen tests require careful attention to technical details, which are sometimes difficult to reproduce. End-expiratory samples are most representative, but they are often difficult to obtain in toddlers and preschool-age children. Flow-through appliances that allow collection through a face mask are now available and appear to be more readily tolerated.[104,105] Storage of collected samples in appropriate, sealed containers is also critical for accurate results.[106,107]

To date, comparative studies in adults suggest that ^{14}C-D-xylose is the most appropriate substrate for use in breath testing.[85,101] The comparative sensitivity and specificity of other noninvasive diagnostic assays that are more suitable for use in children have not been clearly defined.

TREATMENT

Correction of the Underlying Disease

As illustrated in Table 2, there are multiple causes of SBBO, some of which are potentially treatable by surgery. Reports of surgical correction include an ileal carcinoid tumor causing obstruction,[108] a large Meckel's diverticulum,[109] and an ischemic jejunal stricture following blunt trauma to the abdomen.[110] Gastrointestinal, gastrocolic, and jejunocolic fistulae and intestinal strictures that occur following radiation or surgery or in Crohn's disease are also amenable to surgery. The fact that some cases of SBBO can be cured by surgical intervention emphasizes the importance of investigating each patient carefully for such lesions.

Other cases may be improved by treatment of the primary disease, as, for example, the use of steroids in patients with acute symptoms of Crohn's disease. When disordered motility is the primary problem, as in diabetes mellitus, scleroderma, and intestinal pseudo-obstruction, pharmacologic agents may occasionally be effective. Cisapride, a prokinetic agent,

may, for example, improve motility patterns in some patients with diabetes[111] and certain forms of intestinal pseudo-obstruction.[112]

Supportive Therapy

Careful attention should be given to ongoing nutritional and metabolic complications. Nutritional deficits should be anticipated and treated prophylactically. Energy intake may be limited by anorexia, abdominal pain, and malabsorption. Easily digestible nutritional supplements low in fat may be required to maintain normal growth and development. Medium-chain triglycerides have been advocated[46,108,113] and may be helpful. In intractable situations such as occur in the pseudo-obstruction syndromes, enteral nutrition with elemental formulae or parental nutrition should be employed to maintain growth, since the course of these diseases can be unpredictable, and marginal improvement may eventually allow an adequate oral intake.

Clinical evidence of vitamin deficiency is rare, but fat-soluble vitamin deficiencies have been reported in patients with SBBO, including a striking case of neurologic deterioration due to vitamin E deficiency,[114] night blindness due to vitamin A deficiency,[115] and osteomalacia due to vitamin D deficiency.[71,116] Patients with steatorrhea should receive fat-soluble vitamins. A good rule is to follow the recommendations for cystic fibrosis outlined in Chapter 29, Part 2. Vitamin B_{12} deficiency is rare in children because of the time required to deplete body stores. It is correctable by monthly injections of cyanocobalamin. Anemia may also require treatment with supplemental iron to correct iron deficiency secondary to enteric loss.[63] Treatment with iron may unmask a co-existent and unrecognized macrocytic anemia. B vitamins, vitamin K, and folic acid are normally not depleted by bacteria, which may indeed add to host supplies. Tabaqchali and Pallis[72] reported a very interesting case of nicotinamide deficiency, which developed in an elderly patient with multiple jejunal diverticula, steatorrhea, and severe protein malnutrition several weeks after apparently successful treatment with protein infusions and antibiotics. The sudden elimination of nicotinamide-producing bacteria in the upper intestine may have precipitated pellagra. The possibility of sudden loss of a vitamin source should be considered whenever evidence of deficiency appears during treatment.

Antibiotic Therapy

A variety of antibiotics have been used to treat SBBO successfully, but large studies comparing different antibiotics and protocols do not exist. The specific mechanisms by which antibiotics reverse different pathophysiologic events, such as disaccharide intolerance, protein-losing enteropathy, and steatorrhea, have not been entirely explained. Goldstein et al[117] stressed the importance of culturing intestinal contents in order to determine which antibiotic was most effective in treatment. They found that antibiotics effective against aerobes reduced both aerobic and obligate anaerobic bacterial counts. Aerobes lower oxygen tension and maintain low oxidation-reduction potentials (E_h), thereby allowing anaerobes to thrive. When broad-spectrum antibiotics are successful, they may often work by altering intestinal microecology so as to reduce the growth of a critical pathogen. Beeken and Kanich have also advocated the measurement of antibiotic sensitivities to plan treatment of SBBO in patients with Crohn's disease.[118] On the other hand, since no single organism is responsible for all of the abnormalities that occur in SBBO, others believe that isolation of organisms and testing for antibiotic sensitivity are not helpful.[113]

Table 7 summarizes a number of studies in which the antibiotic treatment of SBBO was evaluated by at least one objective parameter. Antibiotics have rarely been compared for effectiveness in the same group of patients. Barry et al[119] definitely showed, however, that metronidazole was superior to kanamycin in five patients with pseudo-obstruction. Total aerobic and anaerobic bacteria counts were reduced by treatment in four of five studies in which jejunal cultures were obtained. In the fifth study featuring metronidazole, only 1 of 12 patients had lower bacterial counts, although the drug seemed to be clinically effective in many cases. A similar discrepancy between bacterial counts and outcome was studied by Giannella et al[11] in rats with experimentally

produced SBBO treated with chloramphenicol. Although anaerobic counts were unchanged, *Bacteroides* virtually disappeared, suggesting that the effectiveness of antibiotics against that organism may be crucial. The antibiotic responses shown in Table 7 are generally consistent with the crucial role of anaerobes, particularly *Bacteroides*. Patients improved on tetracycline, metronidazole, trimethoprim-sulfamethoxazole, lincomycin, and broad-spectrum antibiotics, whereas kanamycin and neomycin, two antibiotics to which *Bacteroides* is generally resistant, were ineffective. *Bacteroides* also plays a crucial role in experimentally produced SBBO. Welkos et al[120] showed that kanamycin and penicillin lowered the number of aerobic bacteria in rats with self-filling blind loop but did not reverse vitamin B_{12} malabsorption. Metronidazole greatly diminished *Bacteroides* and corrected vitamin B_{12} malabsorption. Subsequently they showed that *Bacteroides* bound intrinsic factor–B_{12} complex in vitro much more avidly than five aerobic bacteria and seven other anaerobic bacteria.

These and other studies suggest that the most appropriate therapeutic approach is to choose an antibiotic that is effective against *Bacteroides*, such as tetracycline, metronidazole, chloramphenicol, or lincomycin. Of these four, metronidazole is the least likely to cause untoward side effects in chil-

TABLE 7
Results of Antibiotic Treatment of Small Bowel Bacterial Overgrowth

Underlying Cause	Number of Cases	Symptom or Laboratory Test	Antibiotic (No. Improved)	Intestinal Bacteria (No. Reduced)	Reference
Scleroderma	4	Stool fat	Tetr (3) (Kan, Neo, Sulf—fail)	ND	121
Jejunoileal bypass	5	Diarrhea, pain	Metr (5) (Kan—fail)	Anaerobic (5) Aerobic (0)	119
Billroth II	12	Diarrhea, pain, vomiting	Metr (6) Cotrimoxazole (1)	Total (1/3)	122
Pseudo-obstruction	1	Indoxyl sulfate excretion	Tetr (1) (Neo—fail)	ND	123
Postanastomosis	1	Stool fat	Tetr (1)	*E. coli* (1)	124
Billroth II	1	^{51}Cr clearance	Broad-spectrum (2)	Aerobic (2)	61
Pelvic radiation	1	Stool fat		Anaerobic (2)	
Jejunoileal bypass	12	Liver steatosis, diarrhea	Metr steatosis (12/12) diarrhea (9/12)	ND	77
None	9	Breath H_2, abdominal pain	Linc (4) Trimeth (2) Amox (1) Fluclox (1) Sulf (1)	ND	74
Malnutrition	14	Breath H_2, diarrhea	Metr (11)	ND	125
Mixed	18	Breath $^{14}CO_2$ (bile acid)	Tetr (12)	ND	26

Amox = amoxicillin; Fluclox = flucloxicillin; Kan = kanamycin; Linc = lincomycin; Metr = metronidazole; Neo = neomycin; Sulf = sulfisoxazole; Tetr = tetracycline; Trimeth = trimethoprim-sulfamethoxazole; ND = not determined.

dren and is probably the antibiotic of choice for initiating treatment. An initial course of 2 to 4 weeks may be followed by clinical improvement lasting many months. If relapse occurs, a second course of the same antibiotic for a longer period (4 to 8 weeks) may be tried. Relapse or persistence of steatorrhea, vitamin B_{12} malabsorption, or other complications may be amenable to relatively continuous antibiotic administration, accompanied by periodic alternation with broad-spectrum antibiotics such as trimethoprim-sulfamethoxazole or gentamicin. Chloramphenicol and lincomycin ought to be reserved for cases in which other antibiotics have failed.

REFERENCES

1. Long SS, Swenson RM. Development of anerobic fecal flora in healthy newborn infants. J Pediatr 1977; 91:298–301.
2. Drasar BS, Hill MJ. Human intestinal flora. London: Academic Press, 1974.
3. Giannella RA, Broitman SA, Zamcheck N. Influence of gastric acidity on bacterial and parasitic enteric infections: a perspective. Ann Intern Med 1973; 78:271–276.
4. Snepar R, Poporad GA, Romano JM, Kobasa WD, Kaye D. Effect of cimetidine and antacid on gastric microbial flora. Infect Immun 1982; 36:518–524.
5. Scott LD, Cahall DL. Influence of the interdigestive myoelectric complex on enteric flora in the rat. Gastroenterology 1982; 82:737–745.
6. Rubinstein E, Mark Z, Haspel J, Ben-Ari G, Dreznik Z, Mirelman D, Tadmor A. Antibacterial activity of the pancreatic fluid. Gastroenterology 1985; 88:927–932.
7. Drumm B, Roberton AM, Sherman PM. Inhibition of attachment of Escherichia coli RDEC-1 to intestinal microvillus membranes by rabbit ileal mucus and mucin in vitro. Infect Immun 1988; 56:2437–2442.
8. Drumm B, Neumann AW, Policova Z, Sherman PM. Bacterial cell surface hydrophobicity properties in the mediation of in vitro adhesion by the rabbit enteric pathogen Escherichia coli RDEC-1. J Clin Invest 1989; 84:1588–1594.
9. Baylis CE, Turner RJ. Examination of organisms associated with mucin in the colon by scanning electron microscopy. Micron 1982; 13:35–40.
10. Sherman P, Fleming N, Forstner J, Roomi N, Forstner G. Bacteria and the mucus blanket in experimental small bowel bacterial overgrowth. Am J Pathol 1987; 126:527–534.
11. Giannella RA, Rout WR, Toskes PP. Jejunal brush border injury and impaired sugar and amino acid uptake in the blind loop syndrome. Gastroenterology 1974; 67:965–974.
12. Griffen WO, Richardson JD, Medley ES. Prevention of small bowel contamination by the ileocecal valve. South Med J 1971; 64:1056–1059.
13. Crabbe PA, Bazin H, Eyssen H, Heremans JF. The normal microbial flora as a major stimulus for poliferation of plasma cells synthesizing IgA in the gut. Int Arch Allergy 1968; 34:362–375.
14. Beachey EH. Bacterial adherence: adhesin-receptor interactions mediating the attachment of bacteria to mucosal surfaces. J Infect Dis 1981; 143:325–345.
15. Kaplan BS, Uni S, Aikawa M, Mahmoud A. Effector mechanism of host resistance in murine giardiasis: specific IgG and IgA cell-mediated toxicity. J Immunol 1985; 134:1975–1981.
16. Borriello SP, Reed PJ, Dolby JM, Barclay FE, Webster ADB. Microbial and metabolic profile of achlorhydric stomach: comparison of pernicious anemia and hypogammaglobulinemia. J Clin Pathol 1985; 38:946–953.
17. Brown WR, Savage DC, Dubois RS, Alp MH, Mallory A, Kern F. Intestinal microflora of immunoglobulin deficient and normal human subjects. Gastroenterology 1972; 62:1143–1152.
18. Dolby JM, Webster ADB, Borriello SP, Barclay FE, Bartholomew BA, Hill MJ. Bacterial colonization and nitrite concentration in the achlorhydric stomachs of patients with primary hypogammaglobulinemia or classical pernicious anemia. Scand J Gastroenterol 1984; 19:105–110.
19. Lichtman S, Sherman P, Forstner G. Production of secretory immunoglobulin A in rat self-filling blind loops: local sIgA immune response to luminal bacterial flora. Gastroenterology 1986; 91:1495–1502.
20. Magnusson KE, Stjernstrom I. Mucosal barrier mechanisms: interplay between secretory IgA, IgG, and mucins on the surface properties and association of Salmonella with intestine and granulocytes. Immunology 1982; 45:239–247.
21. Bishop RF, Anderson CM. The bacterial flora of the stomach and small intestine in children with intestinal obstruction. Arch Dis Child 1960; 35:487–491.
22. Buchnall TE, Westall C. Ileocolic blind loops following side-to-side anastomoses. J R Soc Med 1980; 73:882–884.
23. Drenick EJ, Ament ME, Finegold SM, Corrodi P, Passaro E. Bypass enteropathy. Intestinal and systemic manifestations following small-bowel bypass. JAMA 1976; 236:269–272.
24. Kelly DG, Phillips SF, Kelly KA, Weinstein WM, Gilchrist MJR. Dysfunction of the continent ileostomy: clinical features and bacteriology. Gut 1983; 24:93–201.
25. Roberts SH, James O, Jarvis EH. Bacterial overgrowth syndrome without "blind loop": a cause for malnutrition in the elderly. Lancet 1977; ii:1193–1195.
26. Sarna SK. Cyclic motor activity; migratory motor complex: 1985. Gastroenterology 1985; 89:894–913.
27. Vantrappen G, Janssens J, Hellemans J, Ghoos Y. The interdigestive motor complex of normal subjects and patients with bacterial overgrowth of the small intestine. J Clin Invest 1977; 59:1158–1166.
28. Ruckebusch Y. Development of digestive motor complexes during perinatal life: mechanism and significance. J Pediatr Gastroenterol Nutr 1986; 5:523–526.
29. Justus PG, Fernandez A, Martin JL, King CE, Toskes P, Mathias JR. Altered myoelectric activity in the experimental blind loop syndrome. J Clin Invest 1983; 72:1064–1071.
30. Black RE, Brown KH, Becker S. Malnutrition is a determining factor in diarrheal duration, but not incidence, among young children in rural Bangladesh. Am J Clin Nutr 1984; 39:87–94.
31. Mata LJ, Jimenez F, Cordon M, Rosales R, Prera E, Schneider RE, Viteri F. Gastrointestinal flora of children with protein-calorie malnutrition. Am J Clin Nutr 1972; 25:1118–1126.
32. Heyworth B, Brown J. Jejunal microflora in malnourished Gambian children. Arch Dis Child 1975; 50:27–33.
33. Gracey M, Culity GJ, Suharjono S. The stomach in malnutrition. Arch Dis Child 1977; 52:325–327.
34. Gilman RH, Partanen R, Brown KH, Spira WM, Khanam S, Greenberg B, Bloom SR, Ali A. Decreased gastric acid secretion and bacterial colonization of the stomach in severely malnourished Bangladeshi children. Gastroenterology 1988; 94:1308–1314.
35. Sherman P, Forstner J, Roomi N, Khatri I, Forstner G. Mucin depletion in the intestine of malnourished rats. Am J Physiol 1985; 248:G418–G423.
36. Gross RL, Newberne PM. Role of nutrition in immunologic function. Physiol Rev 1980; 60:188–302.
37. Sherman P, Wesley A, Forstner G. Sequential disaccharides loss in rat intestinal blind loops: impact of malnutrition. Am J Physiol 1985; 248:G626–G632.
38. Challacombe DN, Richardson JM, Rowe B, Anderson CM. Bacterial microflora of the upper gastrointestinal tract in infants with protracted diarrhea. Arch Dis Child 1974; 49:270–277.
39. Hill ID, Mann MD, Moore L, Bowie MD. Duodenal microflora in infants with acute and persistent diarrhea. Arch Dis Child 1983; 58:330–334.
40. Penny ME, Harendra De Silva DG, McNeish AS. Bacterial contamination of the small intestine of infants with enteropathogenic Escherichia coli and other enteric infections: a factor in the aetiology of persistent diarrhea? Br Med J 1986; 292:1223–1226.
41. Househam KC, Mann MD, Mitchell J, Bowie MD. Duodenal microflora of infants with acute diarrheal disease. J Pediatr Gastroenterol Nutr 1986; 5:721–725.
42. Banwell JG, Boldt DH, Meyers J, Weber FL. Phytohemagglutinin derived from red kidney bean (Phaseolus vulgaris): a cause for intestinal malabsorption associated with bacterial overgrowth in the rat. Gastroenterology 1983; 84:506–515.
43. Hill MJ, Drasar BS. Degradation of bile salts by human intestinal bacteria. Gut 1986; 9:22–27.
44. Donaldson RM. Small bowel bacterial overgrowth. Adv Intern Med 1970; 16:191–212.
45. Kim YS, Spring N, Blum M, Terz J, Sherlock P. The role of altered bile acid metabolism in the steatorrhea of experimental blind loop. J Clin Invest 1966; 45:956–963.

46. King CE, Toskes PP. Small intestinal bacterial overgrowth. Gastroenterology 1979; 76:1035–1055.
47. Schonsby H, Hofstad T. The uptake of vitamin B₁₂ by the sediment of jejunal contents in patients with the blind-loop syndrome. Scand J Gastroenterol 1975; 10:305–309.
48. Giannella RA, Broitman SA, Zamcheck N. Vitamin B₁₂ uptake by intestinal microorganisms: mechanism and relevance to syndromes of intestinal bacterial overgrowth. J Clin Invest 1971; 50:1100–1107.
49. Brandt LJ, Bernstein LH, Wagle A. Production of vitamin B₁₂ analogues in patients with small-bowel bacterial overgrowth. Ann Intern Med 1977; 87:546–551.
50. Klipstein FA, Engert RF, Short HB. Enterotoxigenicity of colonising coliform bacteria in tropical sprue and blind-loop syndrome. Lancet 1978; ii:342–344.
51. Jonas A, Krishnan C, Forstner G. Pathogenesis of mucosal injury in the blind loop syndrome. Release of disaccharidases from brush border membranes by extracts of bacteria obtained from intestinal blind loops in rats. Gastroenterology 1978; 75:791–795.
52. Riepe SP, Goldstein J, Alpers DH. Effect of secreted Bacteroides proteases on human intestinal brush border hydrolases. J Clin Invest 1980; 66:314–322.
53. Gracey M, Burke V, Oshin A, Barker J, Glasgow EF. Bacteria, bile salts and intestinal monosaccharide malabsorption. Gut 1971; 12:683–692.
54. Prizont R, Whitehead JS, Kim YS. Short chain fatty acids in rats with jejunal blind loops. Gastroenterology 1975; 69:1254–1265.
55. Jonas A, Flanagan PR, Forstner GG. Pathogenesis of mucosal injury in the blind loop syndrome. Brush border enzyme activity and glycoprotein degradation. J Clin Invest 1977; 60:1321–1330.
56. Schulke JD, Fromm M, Menge H, Riecken EO. Impaired intestinal sodium and chloride transport in the blind loop syndrome of the rat. Gastroenterology 1987; 92:693–698.
57. Menge H, Kohn R, Dietermann KH, Lorenz-Meyer H, Riecken EO, Robinson JWL. Structural and functional alterations in the mucosa of self-filling intestinal blind loops in rats. Clin Sci 1979; 56:121–131.
58. Toskes PP, Giannella RA, Jervis HR, Rout WR, Takeuchi A. Small intestinal mucosal injury in the experimental blind loop syndrome. Gastroenterology 1975; 68:1193–1203.
59. Ament ME, Shimoda SS, Saunders DR, Rubin CE. Pathogenesis of steatorrhea in three cases of small intestinal stasis syndrome. Gastroenterology 1972; 63:728–747.
60. Burke V, Anderson CM. Sugar intolerance as a cause of protracted diarrhea following surgery of the gastrointestinal tract in neonates. Austr Pediatr J 1986; 2:219–227.
61. King CE, Toskes PP. Protein-losing enteropathy in the human and experimental rat blind loop syndrome. Gastroenterology 1981; 80:504–509.
62. Jones EA, Craigie A, Tavill AS, Franglen G, Rosenoer VM. Protein metabolism in the intestinal stagnant loop syndrome. Gut 1968; 9:466–469.
63. Giannella RA, Toskes PP. Gastrointestinal bleeding and iron absorption in the experimental blind loop syndrome. Am J Clin Nutr 1976; 29:754–757.
64. Lichtman SN, Sator RB, Schwab JH. Hepatic inflammation in small bowel bacterial overgrowth in rats. Gastroenterology 1988; 94:A263.
65. Rose E, Espinoza L, Osterland CK. Intestinal bypass arthritis: association with circulating immune complexes and HLAB27. J Rheumatol 1977; 4:129–134.
66. Clegg DO, Zone JJ, Samuelson CO, Ward JR. Circulating immune complexes containing secretory IgA in jejunoileal bypass disease. Ann Rheum Dis 1985; 44:239–244.
67. Klinkhoff AV, Stein H, Schlappner OL, Boyko W. Postgastrectomy blind loop syndrome and the arthritis-dermatitis syndrome. Arthritis Rheum 1985; 28:214–217.
68. Jorizzo JL, Apisarnthanarax P, Subrt P, Herbert AA, Henry JC, Raimer SS, Dinehart SM, Reinarz JA. Bowel bypass syndrome without bowel bypass. Arch Intern Med 1983; 143:457–461.
69. King CE, Toskes PP. Small intestinal bacterial overgrowth. Gastroenterology 1979; 76:1035–1055.
70. Bjorneklett A, Fausa O, Midtvedt T. Bacterial overgrowth in jejunal and ileal disease. Scand J Gastroenterol 1983; 18:289–298.
71. Schjonsby H. Osteomalacia in the stagnant loop syndrome. Acta Med Scand 1977; (Suppl) 603:39–41.
72. Tabaqchali S, Pallis C. Reversible nicotinamide deficiency encephalopathy in a patient with jejunal diverticulosis. Gut 1970; 11:1024–1028.
73. Hoffbrand AV, Tabaqchali S, Mollin DL. High serum folate levels in intestinal blind-loop syndrome. Lancet 1966; i:1339–1342.
74. Davidson GP, Robb TA, Kirubakaran CP. Bacterial contamination of the small intestine as an important cause of chronic diarrhea and abdominal pain: diagnosis by breath hydrogen test. Pediatrics 1984; 74:229–235.
75. Fairris GM, Ashworth J, Cotterill JA. A dermatosis associated with bacterial overgrowth in jejunal diverticula. Br J Dermatol 1985; 112:709–713.
76. Drenick EJ, Stanley TM, Border WA, Zawada ET, Dornfield LP, Upham T, Llach F. Renal damage with intestinal by-pass. Ann Intern Med 1978; 89:594–599.
77. Drenick EJ, Fisler J, Johnson D. Hepatic steatosis after intestinal bypass: prevention and reversal by metronidazole, irrespective of protein-calorie malnutrition. Gastroenterology 1982; 82:535–548.
78. Northfield TC, Drasar BS, Wright TJ. Value of small intestinal bile acid analysis in the diagnosis of the stagnant loop syndrome. Gut 1973; 14:341–347.
79. Chernov AJ, Doe WF, Gompertz D. Intrajejunal volatile fatty acids in the stagnant loop syndrome. Gut 1972; 13:103–106.
80. Hoverstad T, Bjorneklett A, Fausa O, Midtvedt T. Short-chain fatty acids in the small-bowel bacterial overgrowth syndrome. Scand J Gastroenterol 1985; 20:492–499.
81. Aarbakke J, Schjonsby H. Value of urinary simple phenol and indican determinations in the diagnosis of the stagnant loop syndrome. Scand J Gastroenterol 1976; 11:409–414.
82. Lewis B, Tabaqchali S, Panveliwalla D, Wootton IDP. Serum bile-acids in the stagnant-loop syndrome. Lancet 1969; i:219–220.
83. Setchell KDR, Harrison DL, Gilbert JM, Murphy GM. Serum unconjugated bile acids: qualitative and quantitative profiles in ileal resection and bacterial overgrowth. Clin Chim Acta 1985; 152:297–306.
84. Sherr HP, Sasaki Y, Newman A, Banwell JG, Wagner HN, Hendrix TR. Detection of bacterial deconjugation of bile acids by a convenient breath analysis technic. N Engl J Med 1971; 285:656–661.
85. King CE, Toskes PP, Giularter TR, Lorenz E, Welkos SL. Comparison of the one-gram D(¹⁴C)-xylose breath test to the (¹⁴C) bile acid breath test in patients with small-intestine bacterial overgrowth. Dig Dis Sci 1980; 25:53–58.
86. Schneider A, Novis B, Chen V, Leichtman G. Value of the ¹⁴C-D-xylose breath test in patients with intestinal bacterial overgrowth. Digestion 1985; 32:86–91.
87. Klein PD, Klein ER. Application of stable isotopes to pediatric nutrition and gastroenterology: mesurement of nutrient absorption and digestion using ¹³C. J Pediatr Gastroenterol Nutr 1985; 4:9–19.
88. Rhodes JM, Middleton P, Jewell DP. The lactulose hydrogen breath test as a diagnostic test for small bowel bacterial overgrowth. Scand J Gastroenterol 1979; 14:333–336.
89. Nose D, Kai H, Harada T, Ogawa M, Maki I, Tajuri H, Kanaya S, Kimura S, Shimizu K, Yabuuchi H. Breath hydrogen test in infants and children with blind loop syndrome. J Pediatr Gastroenterol Nutr 1984; 3:364–367.
90. Kerlin P, Wong L. Breath hydrogen testing in bacterial overgrowth of the small intestine. Gastroenterology 1988; 95:982–988.
91. Perman JA, Modler S, Barr RG, Rosenthal P. Fasting breath hydrogen concentration: normal values and clinical applications. Gastroenterology 1984; 87:1358–1363.
92. Anderson IH, Levine AS, Levitt MD. Incomplete absorption of the carbohydrate in all-purpose wheat flour. N Engl J Med 1981; 304:891–892.
93. Hanson CF, Winterfeldt EA. Dietary fiber effects on passage rate and breath hydrogen. Am J Clin Nutr 1985; 42:44–48.
94. Levitt MD, Hirsh P, Fetzer CA, Sheahan M, Levine AS. H₂ excretion after ingestion of complex carbohydrates. Gastroenterology 1987; 92:383–389.
95. Perman JA, Modler S. Glycoproteins as substrates for production of hydrogen and methane by colonic bacterial flora. Gastroenterology 1982; 83:388–393.
96. Douwes AC, Schaap C, Van Der Klein-Van Moorsel JM. Hydrogen breath test in school children. Arch Dis Child 1985; 60:333–337.
97. Perman JA, Modler S, Olson AC. Role of pH in production of hydrogen from carbohydrates by colonic bacterial flora. J Clin Invest 1981; 67:643–650.
98. Gardiner AJ, Tarlow MJ, Symonds J, Hutchinson JGP, Sutherland IT. Failure of the hydrogen breath test to detect primary sugar malabsorption. Arch Dis Child 1981; 56:368–372.

99. Moore D, Lichtman S, Durie P, Sherman P. Primary sucrase-isomaltase deficiency: importance of clinical judgement. Lancet 1985; ii:164–165.

100. Rao SSC, Edwards CA, Austen CJ, Bruce C, Read NW. Impaired colonic fermentation of carbohydrate after ampicillin. Gastroenterology 1988; 94:928–932.

101. King CE, Toskes PP. Comparison of the 1-gram (^{14}C) xylose, 10-gram lactulose-H$_2$, and 80-gram glucose-H$_2$ breath tests in patients with small intestine bacterial overgrowth. Gastroenterology 1986; 91:1447–1451.

102. Thompson DG, O'Brien DG, Hardie JM. Influence of the oropharyngeal microflora on the measurement of exhaled breath hydrogen. Gastroenterology 1986; 91:853–860.

103. Mastropaolo G, Rees WDW. Evaluation of the hydrogen breath test in man: definition and elimination of the early hydrogen peak. Gut 1987; 28:721–725.

104. Robb TA, Davidson GP. Advances in breath hydrogen quantitation in paediatrics: sample collection and normalization to constant oxygen and nitrogen levels. Clin Chim Acta 1981; 111:281–285.

105. Tadesse K, Leung DTY, Lau SP. A new method of expired gas collection for the measurement of breath hydrogen (H$_2$) in infants and small children. Acta Paediatr Scand 1988; 77:55–59.

106. Rumessen JJ, Gudmand-Hoyes E. Retention and variability of hydrogen (H$_2$) samples stored in plastic syringes. Scand J Clin Lab Invest 1987; 47:627–630.

107. Ellis CJ, Kneip J, Levitt MD. Storage of breath samples for H$_2$ analyses. Gastroenterology 1988; 94:822–824.

108. Banwell JG, Kistler LA, Giannella RA, Weber FL, Lieber A, Powell DE. Small intestinal bacterial overgrowth syndrome. Gastroenterology 1981; 80:834–845.

109. Savino JA. Malabsorption secondary to Meckel's diverticulum. Am J Surg 1982; 144:588–592.

110. Isaacs P, Rendall M, Hoskins EOL. Ischemic jejunal stenosis and blind loop syndrome after blunt abdominal trauma. J Clin Gastroenterol 1987; 9:96–98.

111. Feldman M, Smith HJ. Effect of Cisapride on gastric emptying of indigestible solids in patients with gastroparesis diabeticorum. Gastroenterology 1987; 92:171–174.

112. Hyman PE, McDiarmid SV, Napolitano J, Abrams CE, Tomomasa T. Antroduodenal motility in children with chronic intestinal pseudo-obstruction. J Pediatr 1988; 112:899–905.

113. Isaacs PET, Kim YS. Blind loop syndrome and small bowel bacterial contamination. Clin Gastroenterol 1983; 12:395–414.

114. Brin MF, Fetell MR, Green PHA, Kayden HJ, Hays AP, Behrens MM, Baker H. Blind loop syndrome, vitamin E malabsorption, and spinocerebellar degeneration. Neurology 1985; 35:338–342.

115. Levy NS, Toskes PP. Fundus albipunctatus and vitamin A deficiency. Am J Ophthalmol 1974; 78:926–929.

116. Manicourt DH, Orloff S. Osteomalacia complicating a blind loop syndrome from congenital megaesophagus-megaduodenum. J Rheumatol 1979; 6:57–64.

117. Goldstein F, Mandle RJ, Schaedler RW. The blind loop syndrome and its variants. Am J Gastroenterol 1973; 60:255–264.

118. Beeken WL, Kanich RE. Microbial flora of the upper bowel in Crohn's disease. Gastroenterology 1973; 65:390–397.

119. Barry RE, Chow AW, Billesdon J. Role of intestinal microflora in colonic pseudo-obstruction complicating jejunoileal bypass. Gut 1977; 18:356–359.

120. Welkos SL, Toskes PP, Baer H, Smith GW. Importance of anaerobic bacteria in the cobalamin malabsorption of the experimental rat blind loop syndrome. Gastroenterology 1981; 80:313–320.

121. Kahn IJ, Jeffries GH, Sleisenger MH. Malabsorption in intestinal scleroderma: correction by antibiotics. N Engl J Med 1966; 274:1339–1344.

122. Bjorneklett A, Fausa O, Midtvedt T. Small-bowel bacterial overgrowth in the postgastrectomy syndrome. Scand J Gastroenterol 1983; 18:277–287.

123. Pearson AJ, Brzechwa-Ajdukiewicz A, McCarthy CF. Intestinal pseudo-obstruction with bacterial overgrowth in the small intestine. Am J Dig Dis 1969; 14:200–205.

124. Donaldson RM. Studies on the pathogenesis of steatorrhea in the blind loop syndrome J Clin Invest 1965; 44:1815–1825.

125. Hammond-Gabbaden C, Heinkens GT, Jackson AA. Small bowel overgrowth in malnourished children as measured by breath hydrogen test. West Indian Med J 1985; 34:48–49.

PART **21**

Celiac Disease

John A. Walker-Smith, M.D.(Syd.), F.R.C.P.(Lon., Edin.), F.R.A.C.P.

The modern term *celiac disease* originated from a paper by Gee published in 1888, which he titled "the coeliac affection." He described this as "chronic indigestion which is met with in persons of all ages, yet is especially apt to affect children between one and five years old." Gee did not regard this condition as a newly recognized disorder but rather as a disease that had long ago been mentioned by ancient writers, notably Aretaeus the Cappadocian, who wrote in the first century AD.[2]

DEFINITION

Celiac disease may be defined as a disease of the proximal small intestine characterized by an abnormal small intestinal mucosa and associated with permanent intolerance to gluten. Removal of gluten from the diet leads to full clinical remission and restoration of the small intestinal mucosa to normal. Thus, celiac disease is a lifelong disorder affecting both children and adults which may present either in childhood or in adult life.

INCIDENCE AND GENETIC FACTORS

Environment factors obviously must influence the incidence of celiac disease because the disease cannot occur unless gluten is present in the child's diet. It is therefore most often found in places such as the British Isles, Europe, Australia, and North America, where wheat is a staple food. Indeed, most children diagnosed as having celiac disease have a European ethnic origin. There is a genetic explanation for this fact as well as an environmental one, because this disease either does not occur or is certainly very uncommon in blacks living in North America, South Africa, and Britain, nor does the condition appear yet to have been documented in the Chinese or Japanese.

Nelson et al[3] in Birmingham reported 17 Asian children with celiac disease whose parents originated from the Punjab or West Pakistan. Hitherto there had been few reports of celiac disease occurring in Asians, but, interestingly, there have been previous reports in children who came from the northern regions of the Indian subcontinent. There is now clear evidence of celiac disease in northern India.[3]

There are also reports of celiac disease in Arab children from Lebanon,[5] Iraq,[6] and Saudi Arabia.[7] In addition, Suliman[8] has described celiac disease in children from the Northern Sudan, the children being of mixed Arab and African origin. Thus, children with celiac disease may be encountered over a wide geographic region, but there seems to be a considerable variation in incidence from region to region. For example, there appears to be a wide variation in the incidence of celiac disease within Europe itself. The incidence of celiac disease in England was estimated to be between 1 in 2,000 and 1 in 6,000 in 1959.[9] By contrast, it has been shown that the incidence of celiac disease in the West of Ireland was 1 in 597 births.[10] When cases diagnosed in adults in whom the disease had not been recognized in childhood were considered, it was calculated that the overall incidence may be as high as 1 in 300. This latter report used small intestinal biopsy to make the diagnosis, whereas the earlier report did not, so the two studies are not exactly comparable. Nevertheless, the order of difference between the two reports appears to be highly significant. However, incidence figures based upon biopsy-confirmed cases are the only ones that can be relied upon. These range from the estimate of 1 in 300 in the West of Ireland,[10] 1 in 496 in eastern Austria,[11] 1 in 1,850 in Scotland,[12] 1 in 890 in Switzerland, [13] to 1 in 2,860 in Australia[14] and 1 in 6,500 in Sweden.[15]

There are at present no recognized differences in relation to the amount of gluten ingested or other environmental factors to explain regional differences in incidence between those countries in Europe with a lower and higher incidence of celiac disease. Thus, genetic factors must be invoked to explain this striking variation. There is, however, recent evidence that the incidence of celiac disease is falling, e.g., in County Galway a fall from 1.65 for 1,000 births to 0.73[16] and in Zurich from 1.4 to 0.44.[17] The reason for this is unknown, but an environmental factor is likely. Other evidence favors the importance of genetic factors in the etiology of celiac disease. This includes the observation that celiac disease may occur in more than one member of the same family (although most children with celiac disease have no such family history).[18] Two family studies have been reported in which all first-degree relatives of children with celiac disease had biopsies taken. In England, Rolles et al[19] found 4.5 percent of 89 first-degree relatives of 19 index children had celiac disease. In Sweden, Stenhammar et al[20] found that 2 percent of 100 first-degree relatives of 32 index cases had celiac disease. Celiac disease may also occur in twins. Studies in twins provide a rare opportunity to explore the relative importance of the respective roles of heredity and environment in the etiol-

ogy of celiac disease. A major problem in twin studies in children with celiac disease has been the difficulty in establishing zygosity to a high degree of probability. Fortunately, more recent studies have analyzed antigenic and biochemical genetic markers as well as the established methods such as shared placenta, physical characteristics, dermatoglyphics, and blood groups.

There are reports of concordance for celiac disease in monozygotic twins.[21-23] There are also reports of nonconcordance for monozygotic twins, once in adults[24] and several times in children.[25-27] The discordant twin reported by Walker-Smith has subsequently developed celiac disease established by serial biopsies related to gluten elimination and challenge.[25] This last observation raises the possibility that all children with discordance for celiac disease may in time develop the disease. However, this case study is also of exceptional importance because it shows that an environmental factor or factors, at present unknown, must be involved in the development of gluten sensitivity as well as an inherited predisposition. It also suggests that the small intestinal mucosa is normal until the disease manifests clinically. This observation has been confirmed by Maki et al.[29] Discordance of celiac disease in monozygotic twins has hitherto been regarded as strong evidence against the hypothesis that the disease is inherited as a dominant gene with incomplete penetrance.[30] In fact, Greenberg et al[31] have produced positive evidence in favor of recessive inheritance. At one time or another the familial occurrence of celiac disease has been explained on the basis of susceptibility to damage resulting from environmental factors being inherited by polygenic variation,[12] i.e., multifactorial inheritance or alternatively by a single major gene with reduced penetrance.

In another family study, Polanco et al[27] studied the effect of gluten supplementation in the healthy siblings of children with celiac disease, including nonconcordant monozygotic twins. In 13 children studied after 1 month, small bowel biopsy was normal. Thus, a high-gluten diet did not damage the mucosa. This argues against the view that excessive gluten intake is damaging for individuals who are genetically predisposed to celiac disease. The concept that there is a genetically determined susceptibility for the acquisition of celiac disease was established when an association with human leukocyte antigens (HLA) was demonstrated, particularly for HLA-B8.[32,33]

The HLA region on chromosome 6 codes for antigens expressed on the cell surface of lymphocytes and other tissues. Three series of class I (HLA-A, -B, and -C) and three series of class II (HLA-DR, -DQ, and -DP) antigens are now clearly defined. These antigens play important roles in the immune response of the host to foreign antigens. T lymphocytes responsible for cell-mediated immunity are activated by foreign antigens only when these are presented together with antigen-presenting cells that bear class II antigens, i.e., T helper cells (CD4). These cells recognize antigens usually together with class II antigens on the membrane of the presenting cell, e.g., the macrophage. However, suppressor-cytotoxic T cells (CD8) recognize antigens in the target cell, usually in association with class I antigens.

The highest gene frequencies for HLA-B8 occur in countries such Ireland, Britain, and Australia, where celiac disease occurs most often and where, in addition, wheat consumption is highest. There are two areas with HLA-B8 frequency over 15 percent—Northern and Central Europe and the northwest of the Indian subcontinent. When the HLA-B8 isolines are mapped out for Europe, it is clearly seen that north-west Europe has the highest incidence of HLA-B8. In fact, County Galway in Ireland has the highest recorded prevalence of HLA-B8.[34]

The frequency of HLA-B8 is higher in the Irish population than in any other country in Europe, paralleling the remarkably high incidence of celiac disease in Ireland. The incidence of HLA-B8 increases through Europe, moving in a northwesterly direction. Thus, the frequency of HLA-B8 in a racial group is a good marker for predisposition to celiac disease. However, it is clear that the gene controlling HLA-B8 or a closely linked gene could not be the only gene determining celiac disease, because many people with this histocompatibility gene do not have celiac disease. A stronger association has been shown with the class II antigens DR3 and DR7.[35,36] Tosi et al[37] suggested that the DQw2 antigen, a product of a gene separate from but closely linked to DR3 and DR7 genes, is primarily involved in the susceptibility to CD. These findings have been confirmed in 35 children with celiac disease in whom it was found that 98 percent were HLA DQw2.

As a proportion of patients with celiac disease do not have these antigens, it is likely that the genes that encode these antigens do not confer disease susceptibility per se but are markers for closely linked genes. There is also evidence that genes on other chromosomes may confer susceptibility. Recently the search for disease susceptibility has extended to detection and comparison of restriction fragment length polymorphisms (RFLP). This is a relatively common change in DNA sequence which destroys or creates a restriction enzyme recognition site. In anyone who is heterozygous for RFLP, one restriction band pattern corresponds to one chromosome and the other band pattern to the other of the chromosome pair. This allows one to track the transmission of a single chromosome region through a family. Hitman et al[39] found an increased frequency of the DR2 4.2-kb fragment in celiac disease, dermatitis herpetiformis, and diabetes mellitus. Their RFLP data, based on DR polymorphism, suggests that the disease susceptibility gene of this haplotype is in the DQ-DX subregion in patients with celiac disease. Others[40] have reported another fragment called 4.0-kb RsaI, which they found to be the most accurate means of identifying individuals at risk for developing celiac disease. It is possible that these fragments are derived directly from a celiac disease susceptibility gene. However, the identification of the disease susceptibility genes for celiac disease awaits elucidation.

The histocompatability antigen HLA-DR has been found in the normal enterocytes of the small intestinal mucosa in man.[41] Celiac disease HLA-DR has been found to extend down to the crypt enteroblasts.[42] In nine of 10 patients treated with a gluten-free diet there was normal expression of DR on gut epithelial cells. However, there is an abnormal induction of HLA-DR on the crypt enteroblasts of patients challenged with gluten within 2 hours.

PATHOGENESIS

Gluten is the protein found in the grain of wheat and some other cereals. Its harmful effect in children with celiac disease was first established by Dicke in Holland in 1950.[43] The gluten of rye, too, has been established to be toxic to such children, but there is uncertainty as to whether or not the gluten of barley and of oats is also toxic. Other cereals such as rice and corn are nontoxic to children with celiac disease.

Wheat gluten is the residue remaining after wheat starch has been extracted from the dough made from wheat flour. It is a large complex molecule that has been divided chemically into four heterogeneous classes of protein: gliadins, glutenins, albumins, and globulins. Gliadin is the alcohol-soluble glutamine- and proline-rich fraction of gluten, but it is itself a very complex protein.

Techniques such as starch-gel electrophoresis have shown that gliadin contains about 40 different components. Gliadins have been classified into groups of proteins called alpha, beta, gamma, and omega according to their relative electrophoretic mobility in gels. There is a similar antigenic structure for these individual gliadin subfractions.[44]

Most interest has centered on the alpha fraction. Evidence has been produced from in vivo studies that alpha-gliadin is damaging in celiac disease.[45] Ciclitira et al[46] have demonstrated that all four fractions induce jejunal mucosal damage 6 hours after intraduodenal challenge with 1 g of each of the four gliadin fractions. These latter studies were performed in only three adult treated patients. The total number of patients studied in this way is small, but their observations are remarkable for the rapidity of the mucosal changes. Severe damage was reported to occur after 6 hours.

Using an in vitro organ culture technique for testing toxicity, Jos and Charbonnier[47] have found that other fractions of gliadin, namely beta, gamma, and omega, are also damaging, although alpha and beta had the most severe effects.

As alpha-gliadin is present in variable amounts in different wheats, it is possible that some wheats are more toxic than others. Alpha-gliadin is itself still a complex protein, and just which fraction of it is toxic remains unknown. However, the amino acid sequence of A-gliadin, a component of alpha-gliadin, has now been determined.[48] A remarkable sequence homology has been found between A-gliadin and an early protein of adenovirus 12 (Ad12).[49] Furthermore, celiac patients have been shown to have circulating antibodies to Ad12; an incidence of 30.8 percent neutralizing antibody to Ad12 in children with celiac disease has been reported, compared to 12.8 percent in controls.[50] Others have not confirmed this intriguing observation.[51] The homology involves eight amino acids from a sequence of 12 amino acids that are identical between the two proteins. This observation has led to the suggestion that Ad12 infection may trigger celiac disease in a genetically predisposed individual. A synthetic dodecapeptide with amino acid residues 206 to 217, with sequence homology to Ad12, elicits cellular immune responses in the blood lymphocytes of celiac patients.[52]

It is possible that these sequences of amino acids are common to the other fractions of gluten and indeed may form a common determinant for all these damaging fractions of gliadin. However, the molecular configuration of a particular sequence may be more important. There are more beta turns in the damaging sequences of alpha-gliadin. These are known to be immunogenic. Another approach to the identification of the damaging fraction of gluten has been the use of enzymatic degradation of gluten or gliadin to determine the size of the damaging portion. When gluten is digested by fresh extracts of hog small intestinal mucosa and by crude papain, it is rendered nondamaging, although when it is digested by pepsin and trypsin it remains damaging. This observation has been taken as evidence that the damaging effect is due to a small peptide that is resistant to protein cleavage. Enzymatic degradation studies have suggested that the damaging fraction is an acidic polypeptide having a molecular weight below 1,500.

There are two main theories to account for the damaging effect of ingested gluten in patients with celiac disease. The first is a biochemical theory that there is a specific enzyme deficiency, and the second theory is that the fundamental cause of the disorder is immunologic.

EXPERIMENTAL APPROACHES

In order to test these theories, experimental approaches have had to be devised, but there are certain limitations to these. The only way the toxicity of a gliadin or a fraction of gliadin may be determined is by demonstrating damage to the small intestinal mucosa of patients with celiac disease, which imposes considerable limitations for research in this field. There are, however, two suitable methods now available.

First, there is in vivo testing,[45] in which a multiple hydraulic biopsy apparatus is introduced into the jejunum of a gluten-sensitive adult patient in remission, along with a third tube ending about 10 cm above the suction hole in the capsule. Down this tube, a solution of the material being tested may be passed, biopsies being taken sequentially afterwards. The results of using such a system have been referred to already. The limitations of this technique relate to the small number of patients studied and the variability in response to gluten from patient to patient. Clearly, some patients react much more quickly and more vigorously to gluten than do others.

Secondly, there is the technique of in vitro small intestinal organ culture.[53,54] This technique enables a small intestinal biopsy to be cultured for 24 to 48 hours and has proved to be a useful tool in investigating the pathogenesis of gluten toxicity in celiac disease. It has been shown that damaged surface absorptive cells in mucosal biopsies of patients with untreated celiac disease revert toward normal after only 24 hours of culture. This effect is inhibited if the mucosa is cultured in a medium containing gluten peptides. Various gluten fractions and subfractions have been investigated for their toxicity. The technique has been used with biopsy specimens from both adults and children and has been great virtue of permitting in vitro evaluation of mucosal function and metabolism. Although it has worked well in the laboratories of the authors referred to above, it has not proved to be reproducible by all workers.

BIOCHEMICAL THEORIES

Several biochemical theories have been put forward to account for the damaging effect of ingested gluten in celiac disease.

Peptidase Deficiency

The first biochemical theory proposed that a primary deficiency of an intestinal peptidase resulted in accumulation of a damaging peptide which caused epithelial cell and villous damage. In fact, many mucosal enzymes are deficient in the flat mucosa of active celiac disease. Thus, such mucosal dipeptidase deficiencies are not intrinsic to the mucosa of celiac patients but are secondary phenomena. Permanence of such a deficiency is a sine qua non for deficiency to be regarded as of primary etiologic significance.

Lectin Theory

A lectin is a hemagglutinating protein, which is a glycoprotein of nonimmune origin that, by its polyvalent nature, agglutinates cells and/or precipitates glycoconjugates.[55] Weiser and Douglas[56] considered the role of gliadin as a lectin. They suggested that the underlying defect in celiac disease is of glycoprotein synthesis or possibly of glycolipid synthesis, so that a sugar residue is exposed on the enterocyte surface; i.e., there is an alteration in cell surface membranes. This surface sugar residue reacts with wheat gluten in the manner of a lectin, analogous to the interaction of various plant lectins with other cell membranes, and results in epithelial cell damage.[57] The agglutinating properties of a crude gluten digest, purified gliadin fractions, and established plant lectins have been studied using mammalian erythrocytes, rat enterocytes, and normal and celiac human enterocytes as target systems.[58] Gliadin preparations failed to cause agglutination in any of the cells tested, although plant lectins, e.g., concanavalin A, wheat germ agglutinin, phytohemagglutinin, and peanut agglutinin, were all active cell agglutinins. It was concluded that the gliadin preparations studied were not true lectins.

Immunologic Abnormality

A great deal of work has been carried out demonstrating immunologic abnormalities in celiac disease. These include not only the demonstration of the presence of circulating antibodies to wheat fractions in the sera of patients with celiac disease but also antibodies to other dietary proteins.[59] This is a reversible phenomenon, as the antibodies disappear on a gluten-free diet pari passu with mucosal healing. The majority of circulating antibody against gliadin and casein in untreated adult patients is IgG3.[42] This observation is in keeping with the concept of a generalized increase in permeability of the small intestinal mucosa to macromolecules in celiac disease, secondary to small intestinal mucosal damage.

A factor of concern in interpreting abnormalities of antibody production in celiac disease is that these may not be specific for celiac disease.[60] For example, in one study the patterns of sera reacting to various cereal protein fractions were different in patients with celiac disease as compared to controls only by virtue of the height of the antibody titers.[61] Also, all individuals with HLA-B8 histocompatibility antigen, whether they had celiac disease or not, tended to have higher serum antibodies to a tryptic digest of gliadin than those without the antigen, although again higher levels were found in patients with celiac disease.[62] Abnormalities of the serum immunoglobulins, namely elevated IgA levels and depressed IgM levels, have also been demonstrated,[59] and these also appear to be secondary phenomena, as they are reversible on a gluten-free diet. The number of immunoglobulin-containing cells of the various immunoglobulin classes in small intestinal biopsy specimens has been investigated. Savilahti[63] compared the number of IgA- and IgM-containing cells in the lamina propria of biopsies taken from children with celiac disease and age-matched controls. He found that in the celiac group the number of IgA-containing cells was twice, and the number of IgM-containing cells 2.5 times, the level found in the control group. In some children, IgE cells may be increased. In any event, always in children but less often in adults with celiac disease, the mucosa returns to normal on a gluten-free diet, both morphologically and in relation to the numbers and distribution of the class of immunoglobulin-containing cells. One immunoglobulin abnormality that may on occasion be associated with celiac disease but is not reversed by a gluten-free diet is IgA deficiency. A higher incidence of celiac disease has been shown to occur in children with this immunologic disorder, as compared with children without it.

Rossipal[11] has tested cellular immunity in children with celiac disease using dinitrochlorobenzene (DNCB) and found that 53.8 percent of the children with untreated celiac disease had a negative DNCB test, compared with only 9 percent of the control group. Only 2.4 percent of children on a gluten-free diet from 2 months to 4 years had a negative DNCB test, so again this is a secondary phenomenon.

Further information concerning the immunopathogenesis of celiac disease has been provided by morphologic and immunologic studies of the small mucosa of celiac children in remission after challenge with gluten. Shmerling and Shiner[65] demonstrated that the first changes that occur in the small intestinal mucosa after gluten challenge are not in the epithelial cell itself but in the lamina propria. They used the electron microscope to study serial biopsies after gluten challenge and found that the first morphologic events occur in the basement membrane of the epithelial and endothelial cells, the endothelium of the small blood vessels, and the connective tissue fibrils, with infiltrating inflammatory cells. It was then shown that changes involving the deposition of immune complexes occur parallel with these ultrastructural abnormalities.[66] Using immunofluorescent techniques, they found evidence that antibody, mainly IgA, occurs in the basement membrane following gluten challenge in children previously on a gluten-free diet. In some children there was also deposition of complement. Evidence has also been found of complement deposition in the lamina propria after gluten challenge.[67] These two groups of workers have suggested

that an Arthus-type reaction (Gell and Coombs allergic reaction type III) may play an important role in the pathogenesis of celiac disease. The increased density of intraepithelial lymphocytes (IEL) compared with enterocytes in the small intestinal mucosa of children and adults with untreated celiac disease is a characteristic of most patients, but the high IEL count does not always parallel the overall severity of the mucosal lesion. The IEL level falls when the patient is placed on a gluten-free diet (Fig. 1).

There has been some controversy regarding the best way to quantitate the lymphocytes within the epithelium in untreated celiac disease. The usual way has been to relate the number of IELs to the number of villous epithelial cells. Thus, the number of such cells per 100 epithelial cells has been recorded. This measure gives an indicator of the density of the lymphocytes inside the epithelium. Marsh,[68] however, has related the number of lymphocytes in the epithelium to a constant square of muscularis mucosae. Using this technique, the absolute number of lymphocytes actually falls because of the dramatic reduction of villous surface area in celiac disease. Although this is of theoretic interest, it does not detract from the practical diagnostic value of the IEL count. Counted as a density, it is high in untreated celiac disease and falls on a gluten-free diet. Paradoxically, using Marsh's technique, the absolute numbers of villous IELs rise on a gluten-free diet. However, Marsh[69] has also shown that lymphocytes are

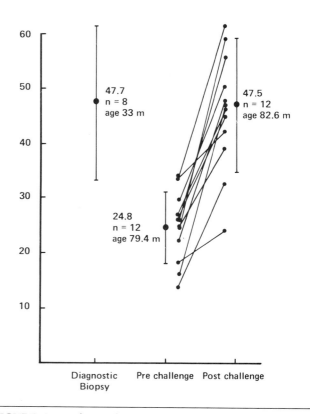

FIGURE 1 Numbers of intraepithelial lymphocytes per 100 epithelial cells in children with celiac disease at diagnosis, at prechallenge on a gluten-free diet, and after relapse following a positive challenge. (Courtesy of Alan Phillips, Queen Elizabeth Hospital for Children, London.)

increased in the crypts in celiac disease without any morphologic damage. The changes in IELs are not markers of mucosal damage per se.

By means of monoclonal antibodies, T cells can be defined by the presence or absence of surface antigens. These are now described by the cluster of differentiation classification, i.e., CD. IELs are morphologically and phenotypically diverse. Most express the pan–T-cell marker CD3, but a large proportion do not express CD5, a pan–T-cell marker in other tissues. Most express the CD8 antigen, usually associated with suppressor-cytotoxic function.[70] A small population of IELs are CD3+, 4−, 8−. Furthermore, about 20 percent of IELs are not T cells in that they do not express CD3 but do express CD7.[71] In patients with untreated celiac disease most IELs are CD8+. There is, however, a significant increase in CD3+, CD4−, and CD8− T cells in celiac disease, regardless of whether the patient is treated or untreated. However, CD3−, 7+ cells are markedly reduced in celiac disease. The cells that express CD3 but are subset (CD4 and CD8) negative are of special interest. They use the gamma/delta T-cell receptor (TCR) rather than alpha/beta. However, as yet, no unique function has been attributed to T cells using this TCR. The functional significance of these cells and their possible role in disease are at present unknown. Indeed, the significance of all these variations in surface markers of IELs in celiac disease remains unknown at present.

Thus, from this review it is clear that whatever the basic defect in celiac disease may prove to be, there can be no doubt that changes in immune status occur, involving both cellular and humoral mechanisms. These may be summarized as follows: When gluten is introduced into the diet of a patient with celiac disease, he or she becomes systemically immunized and develops humoral (IgG) antibodies and cell-mediated immunity (gluten-sensitized lymphocytes) to gluten antigens in addition to the usual secretory IgA response.[72] How central this is to the pathogenesis of celiac disease, is unclear. The final end-point of the pathogenetic process, of whatever sort, must be the enterocyte. The specificity of the target cell in this disease and the dependence of the disease process upon the presence of gluten suggest that if gluten-induced damage operates via an immunologic mechanism, then gluten or some fraction of it may bind to the enterocytes. This gluten binding then converts them into targets for cytotoxic effector cells or immunoglobulin and complement.[73] Rubin and his colleagues[74] as long ago as 1975 presented evidence that gluten does bind to the enterocyte in celiac disease, but so far this observation has not been confirmed by others.

On the evidence at present available, it does seem possible that an allergic reaction of the Gell and Coombs classification, types I, III, and IV, may occur within the lamina propria of the small intestinal mucosa and contribute to pathogenesis. Which of these allergic reactions is most likely to account for the pathology found in the small intestinal mucosa in untreated celiac disease? Animal models of the local effects of allergic reactions on the small intestinal mucosa may be helpful.[75] Type I or reaginic allergic reactions can be produced in a rat immunized and challenged with an intravenous dose of antigen.[76] The effect of such an immediate allergic reaction is the development within 5 or 10 minutes of microscopic edema, secretion of mucus, and increased blood flow. Histologically the mucosa may be entirely normal or just show some edema of the lamina propria and small subepithelial blebs. In a study of intraluminal antigen challenge of actively or passively immunized pigs to produce a type III or immune complex allergic reaction, a massive influx of polymorphs to the mucosa was shown but virtually no morphologic damage.[77] A variety of local cell-mediated reactions in the mucosa have been produced in animals, including graft-versus-host disease, rejection of transplanted allografts of intestine, and parasite infections in T-cell depleted hosts.[78-80] These models show that the earliest changes in these cell-mediated reactions are infiltration of lymphocytes into the lamina propria and into the epithelium. The crypts become hyperplastic, and crypt cell production rate is increased. Villi are shortened. These changes are probably mediated by lymphokines secreted by activated T cells. Thus, there is compelling morphologic evidence in these animal studies to suggest that cell-mediated immunity accounts for the mucosal changes in celiac disease.

These studies have recently been extended to show that activated T cells cause damage in human intestine. T cells in human fetal small intestine organ culture were activated in situ by pokeweed mitogen or anti-CD3 antibody.[81] This resulted in crypt epithelial cell hyperplasia and villous atrophy, i.e., the development of a small intestinal enteropathy with features resembling those of celiac disease except that the enterocyte remains normal.[82] All these changes could be inhibited by cyclosporin A, which is known to inhibit T cell–mediated reactions. Presumably in celiac disease, lymphocytes in the small intestinal mucosa which have been sensitized to gluten interact with gluten, which enters the mucosa from the gut lumen. This leads to activated T cells, which then produce mucosal damage.

However, evidence to support the notion that the lesion in celiac disease is a direct consequence of a T-cell response to gluten is still largely circumstantial. There is an increase in the number and density of T cells in the lamina propria and an increase in the number of crypt T cells in untreated celiac disease. Villous IELs in untreated celiac disease are larger than normal and have an increased mitotic index.[83] This is good morphologic evidence for their being activated. Many of the lamina propria T cells in untreated celiac disease are also IL-2 receptor positive, another indication that they are activated (T. MacDonald: personal communication). After T-cell activation the isoform of the CD45 leukocyte common antigen changes from the form recognized by CD45R monoclonal antibodies to the form recognized by the monoclonal antibody UCHL−1+. Normal IELs are UCHL+; however, normal lamina propria lymphocytes are a mixture of CD45R+ and UCHL−1+, indicating that they have been activated (D. Jones and J. Harvey: personal communication). Further evidence is that biopsies from untreated celiac patients release lymphokines when stimulated with gliadin in vitro.[84] In addition, the crypt epithelium in untreated celiac disease is HLA-DR+,[42] an effect considered to be due to the local production of interferon by activated T cells.[86]

PERMANENCY OF GLUTEN INTOLERANCE

Full recovery of the small intestinal mucosa to normal may occur in children on a gluten-free diet, yet there appears to be no natural recovery; i.e., the intolerance to gluten in children with celiac disease is permanent (see definition), although clinical manifestations of this may vary widely. However, this observation has been challenged by Schmitz et al,[88] who have described three children who originally had evidence of a gluten-sensitive enteropathy treated with a gluten-free diet. They all relapsed histologically after return to a gluten-containing diet. They remained well continuing on a normal diet, and later their mucosae were shown to have spontaneously improved, approaching normalcy. Subsequently an additional seven similar children have been described.[89] Whether these children have true celiac disease, i.e., by definition permanent gluten intolerance, and so will eventually relapse in adult life is not yet known. Indeed, these observations clearly open up an area of very interesting speculation. Are the cases described by Schmitz et al[88] really childhood celiac disease (i.e., cases of permanent gluten intolerance) or are they really cases of transient gluten intolerance? If the former is so, this suggests that small intestinal mucosal changes cannot continue to be regarded as the final arbiter for diagnosis of this disorder. This raises the possibility that an individual may indeed have celiac disease yet have mucosa that is normal at one period of life and becomes abnormal at a later date. The variable state of clinical expression of gluten intolerance is well known. A conceptual point of some importance is the notion that positive gluten challenge does not prove the permanence of a gluten intolerance but rather its persistence. It clearly remains possible that the expressivity of the disease may vary at different ages.[83] The experience of Schmitz et al is crucial in this regard. Will any or all of their patients eventually relapse?

The present uncertainties concern those children who have previously been gluten intolerant but apparently are now gluten tolerant. Will those children previously diagnosed as having transient gluten intolerance and those believed by Schmitz et al to have had natural recovery ultimately relapse? Only time will reveal this to us and so illuminate an increasingly complex situation for the small percentage of children who do not follow the conventional path of relapse with gluten challenge in a period of less than a year.

PATHOLOGY

Paulley[90] was the first to demonstrate an abnormal small intestinal mucosa in adults with celiac disease by examining mucosa obtained at laparotomy. Then Sakula and Shiner[91] in London reported, for the first time, observations of a small intestinal biopsy taken from a child with celiac disease, and they described the characteristic flat mucosa typical of celiac disease.

The fact that the most proximal part of the small intestine is the most abnormal accords with the concept of a noxious agent in the diet (namely, gluten) damaging the gut mucosa. Hydrolyzed gluten is harmless. By the time any ingested gluten that is not absorbed proximally reaches the ileum it has been completely hydrolyzed and so is no longer damaging to the bowel mucosa. Although the distal small intestinal mucosa is usually histologically normal in children with celiac disease, it too becomes abnormal when gluten is directly instilled into the ileum. Thus, the whole length of the small intestinal mucosa is sensitive to gluten.

Characteristically, the proximal small intestinal mucosa is flat, representing a considerable reduction in absorptive surface area. When such a mucosal biopsy is examined under the dissecting or stereomicroscope, it may be completely flat and featureless or it may have a flat mosaic appearance with irregular areas divided by grooves.

Fortunately, from a diagnostic point of view, the proximal small intestinal mucosa in untreated celiac disease is uniformly flat, so biopsy is a reliable way to obtain a representative section. However, when biopsies are examined after a gluten challenge, a patchy enteropathy may be seen,[92] and this may on occasion cause problems in assessment. Histologically, this flat mucosa has an appearance often known as subtotal villous atrophy but sometimes as total villous atrophy (Fig. 2). These are unsatisfactory terms because the mucosa is not truly atrophic; indeed, the crypts of Lieberkühn are lengthened. The simple term *flat mucosa* is preferable, although another term, *hyperplastic villous atrophy*, is acceptable.

There is also a variable cellular infiltration of the lamina propria with round cells. The surface epithelium is low, columnar, pseudostratified, or cuboidal. Booth[93] has suggested, using a hematologic analogy, that the surface epithelial cells lining the small intestinal mucosa be called enterocytes and the cells in the crypts enteroblasts. He described the surface epithelial cells in celiac disease as being microcytic enterocytes and the thickening of the enteroblastic layer as enteroblastic hyperplasia, with increased mitotic activity occurring in this layer to replace the abnormal enterocytes. The combined evidence of an elevated mitotic index, decreased cell cycle time, increased cell production rate, and increased mucosal cell loss rate in patients with celiac disease who have a flat small intestinal mucosa supports the concept of enteroblastic hyperplasia to account for this mucosal abnormality.

Some children diagnosed as having celiac disease have a proximal mucosa characterized under the dissecting microscope by short thick ridges, sometimes with a convoluted appearance and partial villous atrophy histologically. This appearance is certainly much less common than a flat mucosa in children with celiac disease, and it may occur in a variety of disorders of the small intestine other than celiac disease. It was found in four of 35 children with celiac disease, the diagnosis being proved by challenge. The severity of the biopsy findings is less important than the length of the small intestine affected. The precise length of abnormal gut mucosa appears to determine the severity of the clinical state.

Electron microscopic studies of small intestinal biopsies taken from children with celiac disease reveal abnormality of the enterocytes, which are patchy and of variable severity. Diminution of the size and number of the microvilli with branching is characteristic, as is evidence of epithelial cell damage, but such findings are not constant. There is also, sometimes, an increased deposition of collagen in the region of the basement membrane of the enterocyte, which may be thickened.

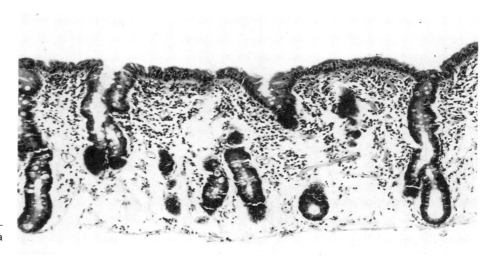

FIGURE 2 Histologic section of a flat mucosa.

CLINICAL FEATURES

Age of Onset

There is considerable variation in the age of onset of symptoms in celiac disease. Gee originally described symptoms as presenting most often between the ages of 1 and 5 years. This is true, but it may in fact present for the first time at any age from infancy to old age.

The trend toward an earlier introduction of cereals into the diet of infants in Britain in the 1970s was shown by Anderson et al[94] in Birmingham to be associated with a trend to an earlier age of presentation of children with celiac disease. They compared an 18-month period in 1950 to 1952 with a similar period of 1968 to 1969 and found a dramatic reduction in the age of presentation from 43.6 months to 9.3 months and a corresponding drop in the mean age of introduction of gluten-containing cereals into the diet from 9.4 to 3.4 months.

Since 1975, in Britain, this trend has been reversed. This follows the recommendations of the Department of Health and Social Security in their booklet "Present-day Practice in Infant Feeding". This booklet states that the introduction of any food to a baby's diet, other than milk, before the age of 4 to 6 months should be unnecessary. Furthermore, some products such as Farex, which formerly contained gluten, are now gluten-free, and there is an increasing trend to use rice cereal instead of wheat-containing products as weaning foods.

In fact, a review of 25 years of celiac disease at Queen Elizabeth Hospital for Children by Kelly et al[95] showed a significant rise in the age of presentation in the late 1970s and 1980s to an age even higher than that described in Birmingham in 1950 to 1962 (Fig. 3). In fact, in this analysis it seems that the number of children diagnosed as new cases between 1976 and 1985 is very similar to the number diagnosed at the hospital between 1960 and 1971. When the year of birth of this cohort of patients is examined, it is seen that children with celiac disease studied during this period were born most often in the late 1960s or early 1970s. Whether this observation does in fact solely relate to the age of introduction of gluten to the diet still remains to be established. This seems likely to be the case for bottle-fed infants. It is not the case, however, for breast-fed infants. Thus, the frequency of breast-feeding (now increasing once more) as well as the role of GI infection and other currently unknown environmental factors must all be taken into account. Other authors have described a decrease in incidence of celiac disease.[16,96,97] Whether this will now stabilize, as the Queen Elizabeth Hospital experience suggests, only time will tell.

There is usually a variable "latent interval" between the introduction of gluten into the diet and the development of clinical manifestations. The explanation for this interval remains unknown. In some children the interval may be months and in others years, but some infants may have symptoms as soon as gluten is added to their diet.

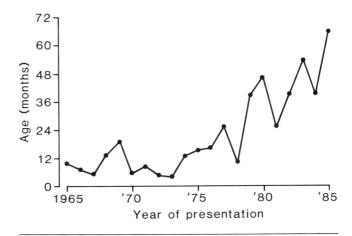

FIGURE 3 Age at presentation of celiac disease at Queen Elizabeth Hospital for Children, 1965 to 1985.

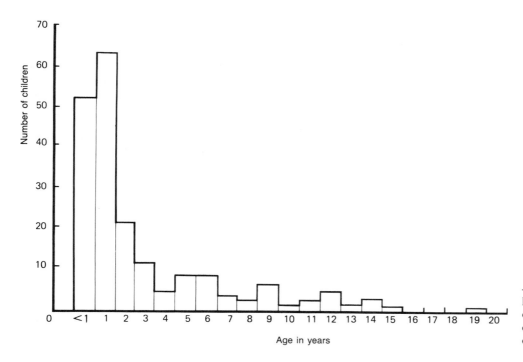

FIGURE 4 Age at first biopsy of 110 children with celiac disease seen at the Royal Alexandra Hospital, 1966 to 1972.

Once symptoms have appeared, there may be a delay in diagnosis, but with increased awareness of this condition and the ready availability of the technique of small intestinal biopsy in pediatric centers, this interval is becoming shorter. The age at diagnosis in 110 consecutive children with celiac disease diagnosed at the Royal Alexandra Hospital from 1966 to 1972 is illustrated in Figure 4 and in 192 children diagnosed at Queen Elizabeth Hospital from 1960 to 1985 in Figure 5. This indicates that while most cases are diagnosed in early childhood, the diagnosis may be made throughout the pediatric age spectrum.

CLINICAL PRESENTATION

The mode of presentation of celiac disease may be quite variable (Table 1). Diarrhea, which may be acute or insidious in onset, is the most common presenting symptom, and most children with celiac disease have a history of diarrhea. The stools are characteristically pale, loose, and very offensive and may resemble oatmeal porridge, as Gee described. The child may pass two or three such stools a day but often just one large, bulky stool. The child may also have recurrent attacks of more severe diarrhea, sometimes with the stools be-

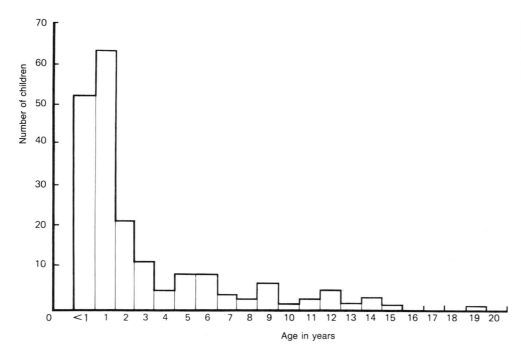

FIGURE 5 Age at first biopsy of 192 children with celiac disease seen at Queen Elizabeth Hospital, 1960 to 1985.

TABLE 1

Mode of Presentation of Celiac Disease in 52
Celiac Children at the Royal Alexandra Hospital

Diarrhea	32
Failure to thrive of no apparent cause	7
Vomiting	6
Weight loss	3
Anorexia	2
Short stature	1
Protuberant abdomen	1

coming watery. However, as has been recognized for some time, a few children with celiac disease may have constipation. These children may have a dilated colon, with constipation giving a clinical pattern that may be confused with that of Hirschsprung's disease. Failure to thrive is an important way in which celiac disease may present, and celiac disease needs to be considered in every child with this syndrome regardless of the presence of diarrhea. Other modes of presentation listed in Table 1 illustrate the broad spectrum of the clinical features of celiac disease. The symptoms present at the time of diagnosis in a group of children with celiac disease in Sydney are indicated in Table 2. Their great diversity is readily apparent.

Emotional symptoms are common in children with celiac disease, although they are not often the mode of presentation of this condition. Gibbons[98] drew attention to the fact that the child with celiac disease "is extremely irritable, fretful, capricious or peevish. Nothing seems to please him and altogether he is quite unlike himself."

The celiac child is often in a state of close dependence upon his mother, leading to a pronounced exacerbation of fretfulness and irritability when he is separated from her. This state is best described as "clingingness." In addition, the celiac

TABLE 2

Symptoms Present at Time of Diagnosis in 52
Celiac Children at the Royal Alexandra Hospital

Diarrhea	45
Abdominal distention	23
Vomiting	32
Lassitude	32
Weight loss	31
Irritability	30
Anorexia	25
Abdominal pain	23
Frequent respiratory infection	14
Failure to thrive	14
Sleep disturbance	9
Appetite increased	8
Acute edema	7
Muscle wasting	7
Pallor	7
Muscle weakness	4
Constipation	3
Mouth ulceration	2
Rectal prolapse	2
Skin infections	2

child is often emotionally withdrawn from his environment, and this withdrawal may even resemble autism. Not only may the child have these emotional symptoms, but his mother may become depressed, anxious, and abnormally preoccupied with her child.

Anorexia is classically said to be present in celiac children, but only about 50 percent may have this symptom and some children may in fact have an increased appetite. When specifically asked for, there is usually a history of abdominal distention, and some children complain of abdominal pain, although this is not usually severe. There is often a history of respiratory tract infections which may at first suggest cystic fibrosis as a diagnostic possibility. Although the classic appearance of a miserable child with a distended abdomen and wasted buttocks and shoulder girdles does still occur, abnormalities on physical examination of a child with celiac disease may be much less obvious. Indeed, some abdominal protuberance may be the only physical sign. Muscle wasting and loss of muscular power with hypotonia may be present, and the child may be delayed in his motor milestones. Measurements of height and weight are valuable, and the child's height and weight at diagnosis are often found to be below the tenth percentile and sometimes below the third. Nevertheless, single measurements may be within the normal range, and so isolated observations may not be useful diagnostically. Knowledge of earlier measurements of height and weight and the plotting of such observations on a percentile chart may prove very helpful diagnostically. Any child whose rate of weight gain has significantly slowed, especially when this is accompanied by a slowed rate of growth and GI symptoms, merits consideration for the diagnosis of celiac disease.

The most common modes of presentation for celiac disease may be divided as follows:

1. *Classic presentation at age 9 to 18 months.* There is gradual failure to gain weight or loss of weight after introduction of cereals, the child having been previously well. There is also anorexia and alteration in stools which are softer, paler, larger, and more frequent than usual. More than half of the 1972 to 1975 series at Queen Elizabeth Hospital fell into this category.
2. *Presentation in infants before 9 months.* Vomiting is frequent and may be projectile. Diarrhea may be severe, especially with intercurrent infections, not necessarily gastroenteritis. Abdominal distention may not be marked. This is now a less common age for presentation.
3. *Presentation with constipation.* These children are often very hypotonic, with marked abdominal distention.
4. *Presentation at older age.* Short stature, iron-resistant anemia, rickets, and personality problems all may occur.
5. *Presentation in Asian children in Britain.* They present later, often with iron-resistant anemia and rickets and/or short stature. Diarrhea is not a prominent feature.
6. *Presentation in asymptomatic siblings.* After a case is positively diagnosed, siblings should have clinical history and growth checked. If a suspicion of celiac disease arises, full blood count and serum folate and red cell folate measurements should be done. A biopsy should then be performed if there is evidence of a deficiency state or in addition if there is a gliadin antibody.

DIAGNOSIS

The diagnosis of celiac disease is based initially upon the demonstration of an abnormal small intestinal mucosa with features characteristic of celiac disease using the technique of small intestinal biopsy and then upon a clinical response to the withdrawal of gluten from the child's diet. A clinical response is demonstrated when there is significant weight gain and relief of symptoms. Some pediatricians would then consider the diagnosis of celiac disease to have been established.

However, reintroduction of gluten into the child's diet at a later date, when the small intestinal mucosa has been shown to return to normal, followed by mucosal deterioration with or without a clinical relapse is necessary before the diagnosis of celiac disease may be said to have been definitively established. Such a relapse in mucosal appearance may not occur for up to 2 years or exceptionally even longer after the reintroduction of gluten into the child's diet (Fig. 6). These diagnostic criteria for celiac disease are listed in Table 3.

These criteria in practice do not need to be fulfilled in every case diagnosed as celiac disease except in two particular situations: (1) A child previously diagnosed as suffering from celiac disease and having a gluten-free diet should be reinvestigated in order to fulfill these criteria if there is any doubt about the original diagnosis, particularly if the child was started on such a diet without a previous small intestinal biopsy. (2) The child was less than 2 years of age at the time of diagnosis. It must be appreciated that although a flat small intestinal mucosa is characteristic of celiac disease, there are other causes of such a mucosa (Table 4). In this age group there exists a syndrome of transient gluten intolerance. Nevertheless, in Western countries the great majority of children with a flat small intestinal mucosa who respond to a gluten-free diet do have celiac disease. However, in infants under the age of 2 years there is a chance that a flat small intestinal mucosa is due to causes other than celiac disease; hence, the ad-

TABLE 3
ESPGAN Diagnostic Criteria for Celiac Disease

Abnormal small intestinal mucosa (usually flat)
Clinical response to a gluten-free diet
Histologic response to a gluten-free diet
Histologic ± clinical relapse following gluten challenge

ESPGAN = European Society for Paediatric Gastroenterology and Nutrition.

vice is given to reinvestigate such children with serial biopsies related to elimination and challenge. These criteria are sometimes known as the Interlaken or ESPGAN criteria, as they arose from a meeting of the European Society for Paediatric Gastroenterology and Nutrition in Interlaken.[99] With some modifications, these criteria have stood the test of time and continue to be a valuable guide to diagnosis,[89] but there are now clearly some reservations, as the experience of Schmitz et al[88] makes clear. Such reinvestigation is justified in order to establish clearly the diagnosis of celiac disease when there is any doubt and so to justify the need for a lifetime of dietary restriction.

Technique for Diagnostic Gluten Challenge

This reinvestigation may be carried out in the following manner: A small intestinal biopsy is performed while the child is still on a gluten-free diet in order to demonstrate that the mucosa is in fact normal. If such a preliminary biopsy is abnormal, this suggests either that the child has celiac disease and is not keeping strictly to a gluten-free diet or that some other disease is present, so further investigations may be necessary. Usually, such a biopsy is normal when the child

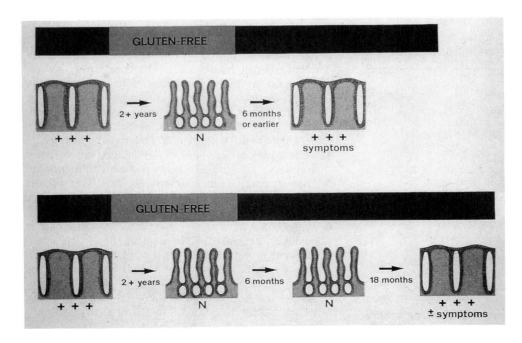

FIGURE 6 Diagrammatic representation of two patterns of response to a gluten challenge (dark portions of bands) of the small intestinal mucosa in children with celiac disease.

TABLE 4
Reported Causes of a Flat Small Intestinal
Mucosa in Childhood

Celiac disease, i.e., permanent gluten intolerance	
Transient gluten intolerance	Temporary
Cow's milk sensitive enteropathy	food-sensitive
Soy protein intolerance	enteropathies
Gastroenteritis and postenteritis syndromes	
Giardiasis	
Autoimmune enteropathy	
Acquired hypogammaglobulinemia	
Tropical sprue	
Protein-energy malnutrition	

has been on a gluten-free diet for 2 years or more. Earlier reinvestigation in a child with the typical features of celiac disease is not usually indicated. Once a normal mucosa has been demonstrated, the child is given a normal diet containing gluten, or gluten powder is added to his gluten-free diet. Gluten powder may be given to avoid the upset to a child produced by change from a diet already in use for some time. If the child does return to a "normal" diet, care must be taken to ensure that he does in fact eat gluten-containing foods. Whether gluten powder or normal diet is used, the amount of gluten should be in normal range of gluten intake appropriate to age (Table 5). A regular check by a dietitian of his daily wheat intake in grams per day is very useful. The author prefers such a return to a normal diet rather than the use of gluten powder.

Should significant symptoms ensue, a further biopsy is performed after an interval of a week following the return of such symptoms. If the mucosa is then abnormal, the diagnosis of celiac disease may be said to have been established; i.e., a histologic relapse has occurred on reintroduction of gluten to the diet. It is not necessary for the mucosa to be flat to diagnose such a relapse; the presence of significant mucosal abnormalities, such as increased plasma cells and lymphocytes in the lamina propria, abnormalities of the surface enterocytes, and especially a rise in the IEL count, is sufficient.

If symptoms fail to occur, small intestinal biopsy should be performed after 3 months' exposure to gluten, since histologic relapse may precede clinical relapse. If the mucosa is then still normal, the child is observed and kept on a normal diet, or a diet with added gluten, and another biopsy is performed if symptoms subsequently develop. If symptoms do not develop, a final biopsy is done after 2 years' exposure

TABLE 5
Wheat Protein Intake of a Normal Diet in
Children of Different Ages

Age (yr)	Wheat Protein (g/day)
Less than 1	Variable
1 to 3	5 to 10
3 to 6	7 to 12
6 to 9	10 to 15
9+	15 to 30

to gluten. If the mucosa is then abnormal, celiac disease is present; but if it is normal, celiac disease is considered most unlikely. The precise period of 2 years is somewhat arbitrary, and there are a few children reported in the literature to take longer than 2 years to relapse.

This entire procedure is complex and time-consuming for the child, his parents, and his professional attendants and so should not be undertaken unless really necessary. It is thus particularly important that a child not be treated with a gluten-free diet unless he has first had a small intestinal biopsy that demonstrates characteristic pathology. Failure to do this may lead to the performance some years later of these extensive investigations, only to show that the child did not have celiac disease and so did not need a gluten-free diet in the first place. This procedure of reinvestigation should really be needed only to establish the permanency or otherwise of the state of gluten intolerance in a child, previously shown to have an abnormal small intestinal mucosa and apparently to have responded clinically to the elimination of gluten from his diet, who was less than 1 year old at time of diagnosis.

REINVESTIGATION STUDIES

The practical application of such a diagnostic approach is now outlined. A study of 65 children previously diagnosed with celiac disease, using the technique just described as far as possible, was made at the Queen Elizabeth Hospital.[100] Two groups of children were included: (1) those who had an original diagnosis based upon an abnormal biopsy and a clinical response to a gluten-free diet (44 children) and (2) those in whom there was no original biopsy but a clinical response to a gluten-free diet (21 children).

Fifty gluten challenges were positive; i.e., there was evidence of histologic relapse after up to 2 years on a gluten-containing diet. Fifteen were negative; i.e., their mucosae were normal 2 or more years after a return to a normal gluten-containing diet. Looking specifically at the 37 children in this group who had an initial flat mucosa, six did not relapse after 2 years on a normal diet and are clinically well (i.e., 16 percent). This is a higher than the 3.6 percent reported by Shmerling[101] to the members of the European Society for Paediatric Gastroenterology but is in closer accord with findings of colleagues in Sweden, eight of 35, or 22 percent,[102] and in Finland, eight of 83, or 9 percent.[103] Figure 7 illustrates serial biopsies and weight gain with dietary gluten in a child with celiac disease.

Shmerling and Franckx[104] have described a long-term analysis of relapses following reintroduction of a gluten-containing diet in 91 children from a total of 314 children diagnosed in Zurich between 1960 and 1983. Most of those challenges were initiated by the patients themselves (68 percent). Seventy-one (81.4 percent) had a flat mucosa after return to a normal gluten-containing diet. In 11 (12 percent) the mucosa became abnormal but not flat, whereas six (6.6 percent) had a normal small intestinal mucosa after 2.24 to 6.92 years on a gluten-containing diet. The findings in the two latter groups are of especial interest. First, those who had deterioration of their mucosa but not a return to a flat appearance have had minimal progression of the lesion,

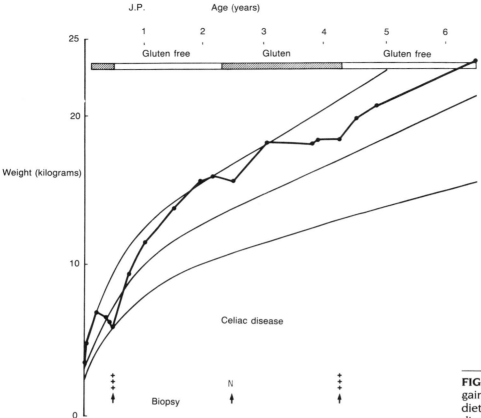

FIGURE 7 Serial biopsies and weight gain related to centile chart and to dietary gluten in a child with celiac disease.

although two of these had earlier in their lives a flat mucosa after a previous planned gluten challenge. These children have so far remained well on gluten, and the possibility remains of a natural recovery for childhood celiac disease, as suggested by Schmitz et al.[88] The last group who did not relapse are similar to those at Queen Elizabeth Hospital for Children diagnosed retrospectively as transient gluten intolerant (6.6 percent compared to 16 percent at QEH).

Whether these patients have had in reality transient gluten intolerance or whether they and the former group will both relapse later in adult life, only time will tell. It is of interest that these children were all originally diagnosed at an age of less than 2 years. It is in this group of children that formal gluten challenge is still recommended, although it is no longer routinely indicated for children who present after the age of 2 years.

Dose of Gluten

There have been until recently few hard data concerning the role of the dose of gluten in the pathogenesis of celiac disease. However, in one adult celiac patient Ciclitira and colleagues[46] have found dose-related effects. Gliadin 10 mg produced no mucosal damage upon biopsy, 100 mg minimal mucosal damage, 500 mg moderate damage, and 1,000 mg gross histologic damage after 3 hours of infusion.

INVESTIGATION OF A CHILD WITH CELIAC DISEASE

Investigation of a child with celiac disease at the time of initial diagnosis may reveal evidence of multiple deficiencies in absorption, e.g., steatorrhoea, hypoprothrombinemia, iron and folic acid deficiency anemia, low serum iron, low serum folate, and low red cell folate levels, a flat glucose tolerance test, and abnormal xylose absorption. Doubt has been cast upon the reliability of the xylose absorption test. In centers where small intestinal biopsy is available, a xylose test is no longer a routine diagnostic test, as it may occasionally give misleading results. It may remain a screening test for referral in centers where small intestinal biopsy is not available.

Gluten antibodies and other dietary protein antibodies may be found in children with untreated celiac disease. Detection of gluten antibodies has a more valuable diagnostic role than a 1-hour xylose test. However, this test by itself should not be relied on for diagnosis, because children with untreated celiac disease may have no circulating gluten antibodies, and gluten antibodies may occur in other enteropathies.[105] At Queen Elizabeth Hospital on the only occasions when gliadin antibody has been negative, reticulin antibodies have been positive.[106]

The percentage of children with untreated celiac disease who have such antibodies varies in different reports, chiefly related to the methods used. Antibodies of class IgA rather than IgG have greater specificity, but IgG antibodies are more sensitive. Circulating reticulin antibodies are often present, e.g., 85 per cent in one group of 22 children with celiac disease reported from the Queen Elizabeth Hospital.[98]

None of these investigations is abnormal in 100 percent of children who have celiac disease. So none of them is of value as a screening procedure, but some may be useful in establishing a baseline for future observations, and they may have a valuable role in investigating asymptomatic family members. However, the only diagnostic test for celiac disease at present is small intestinal biopsy while the child is eating a gluten-containing diet.

CLINICAL MANIFESTATIONS

Growth and Development Retardation

Severe growth retardation and delayed development, sometimes with delayed onset of puberty, were well known to the early observers of celiac disease. Gee[1] remarked in 1888 that "while the disease is active children cease to grow; even when it tends slowly to recovery, they are left frail and stunted." Growth retardation and delayed puberty continue to be important complications of celiac disease, albeit less common now, owing to earlier diagnosis and treatment. Prader and his colleagues[108,109] have shown that "catch-up growth" occurs once there has been a response to a gluten-free diet.

A diminished rise in the level of plasma growth hormone in response to hypoglycemia has been described. Hypothalamic hypofunction might be present in untreated celiac disease. Celiac disease may present with growth failure in the absence of GI symptoms and must be considered in the differential diagnosis of short stature.

Anemia in Celiac Disease

The incidence of anemia in children with celiac disease is variable. The most common type is a hypochromic microcytic anemia due to iron deficiency.

Only rarely does megaloblastic anemia occur in children with celiac disease.[110] Despite this, serum folate and red cell folate levels are usually reduced in children with untreated celiac disease. Not surprisingly, a red cell folate level has, therefore, been claimed to be useful as a screening test for celiac disease in childhood, but although a low level is usually found in children with celiac disease, it cannot be relied upon as a screening test, as an occasional child may have normal levels at the time of diagnosis. Folate levels rapidly rise on a gluten-free diet and tend to fall, albeit not always to a pathologic level, after a gluten challenge. Estimation of folate levels is thus a useful way to evaluate progress on a gluten-free diet of a child with celiac disease. The cause of these low levels is folic acid malabsorption, which has been well documented in adult studies. Malabsorption of dietary folate (pteroylpolyglutamate) has also been demonstrated.[111]

Hypoproteinemia

Hypoproteinemia is a common complication of celiac disease; for example, Hamilton et al[112] found hypoalbuminemia to be present in 12 of 37 children. There is good evidence from radioisotope studies that the hypoproteinemia found in children with celiac disease is due to protein-losing enteropathy. When there is severe hypoproteinemia the child may present with generalized edema mimicking the nephrotic syndrome. The edema is relieved by therapy with a gluten-free diet.

Hypoprothrombinemia

An abnormal prothrombin time due to malabsorption of vitamin K may occur in celiac disease. Some authorities recommend the estimation of prothrombin time and other parameters of coagulation before small intestinal biopsy is performed. Hypoprothrombinemia is rapidly corrected by intramuscular vitamin K.

Malignant Disease

The most serious complication of longstanding celiac disease is the development of malignancy. Gough et al[113] described three adults with celiac disease who developed lymphoma of the small bowel, apparently as a complication of celiac disease. Since then, there have been a number of reports of malignant disease occurring as sequelae to celiac disease. In Birmingham, the incidence of malignant disease was reviewed in 250 celiac disease patients diagnosed between 1941 and 1969 and lymphoma was found in 20 cases, GI cancer in 16, and some other malignancy in four.[114] Seventeen lymphomas have been described[115] in long-diagnosed adult patients with celiac disease. It thus appears to be principally a problem of adult life. However, there has now been one report of intestinal lymphoma occurring in a child in whom the diagnosis of celiac disease had been established by serial biopsies related to gluten elimination and challenge.[116] This first case was a 10-year-old North African child who had been diagnosed by biopsy as having celiac disease at the age of 10 years. Then, after the demonstration of a normal small intestinal mucosa on a gluten-free diet, she had a gluten challenge. Seven months later a malignant abdominal lymphoma was diagnosed. Despite chemotherapy she subsequently died. A brother also had been established to have celiac disease. Both children shared an unusual HLA phenotype for celiac disease, namely HLA antigens A2-B17/A29-B12. However, HLA antigens AW19 and B12 are linked to the development of malignant lymphoma,[117] which may have been significant in this case. Furthermore, Mediterranean lymphoma is more common in this ethnic group. This ethnic factor plus the fact that the disease affected others members of the family was suggested by Arnaud-Battandier and colleagues[116] to be significant to the risk of developing malignancy. The exceptional nature of this report in the literature is highlighted by the fact that in a questionnaire sent to members of the European Society for Paediatric Gastroenterology, out of 1,959 cases of celiac disease in children under 18 years of age, no case of lymphoma was reported.[101]

The lymphoma associated with enteropathy was formerly called malignant histiocytosis of the intestine. It is now clear that the malignant cell in these lymphomas is usually of T-cell origin.[117,118] Changes in subpopulations of IELs in enteropathy-associated T-cell lymphoma have been described. In fact, changes occur identical to those found with celiac disease, as described earlier in the discussion (Fig. 8). This does in fact suggest that this lymphoma is a complication of celiac disease.

In Birmingham, some protection has now been shown against this risk of malignancy in adults by the use of a gluten-free diet.[119] However, only long-term studies of individuals managed from childhood will reveal whether a gluten-free diet provides such protection for children.

The observation that activation of T cells in the lamina propria is induced by gluten in celiac disease and the observation that enteropathy-associated T-cell lymphoma is a complication of celiac disease are powerful arguments in favor of a strict gluten-free diet.

TREATMENT

Elimination of gluten from the child's diet usually leads to a dramatic and rapid clinical response, but this may sometimes be delayed. Weight gain and relief of emotional symptoms in the mother as well as the child usually occur first, before cessation of diarrhea and other signs of improvement. As time goes on weight gain in fact tends to increase somewhat beyond normal values for the child's age and height. This phase usually passes, and the child's weight then stabilizes along his correct percentile. Full catch-up growth occurs during the second year of treatment (Fig. 9).[120]

There is, however, some disagreement as to precisely what constitutes a gluten-free diet. All authorities are agreed that wheat and rye should be eliminated from the diet, but most also recommend elimination of barley and oats, although it is still not definitely established these two cereals are also damaging to children. Rice and maize (corn) are certainly not damaging to children with celiac disease. In practice, knowing just what is a gluten-free diet is difficult even in relation to wheat. The difficulty centers upon the use of foods based on wheat starch which are claimed to be gluten-free.

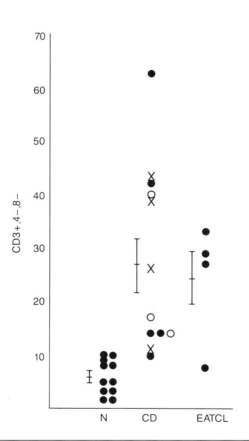

FIGURE 8 Percentage of intraepithelial lymphocytes CD3+, 4–, and 8– in celiac disease (CD), controls (histologically normal, N), and enteropathy-associated T-cell lymphoma (EATCL).

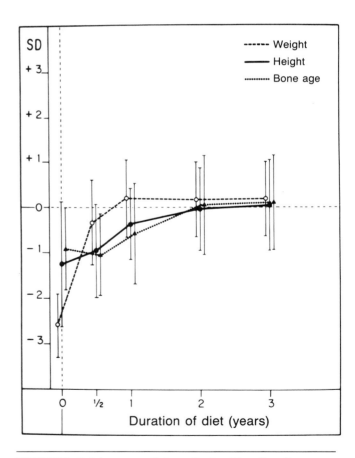

FIGURE 9 Catch-up growth in patients with celiac disease on a gluten-free diet. Mean (±SD) of differences from normal expressed as standard deviation (SD). n = 13. (From Barr et al,[126] with permission.)

Radioimmunoassays for wheat gliadin and some of its fractions have been used to determine the amount of gliadin in such foods.[35] In fact, such foods do contain very small amounts of gluten, estimated to be 7 mg (range, 5 to 13 mg) in one childhood study.[121] Although not producing observable morphologic damage in the small intestinal mucosa of adult and childhood celiac patients on an otherwise gluten-free diet, when regularly ingested these foods have been reported to induce symptomatic diarrhea in 40 percent of such patients who were tested[35]; the true significance of this observation is not clear.

Although secondary disaccharidase deficiency has clearly been demonstrated (by assay of small intestinal biopsies) to be present in virtually all children with celiac disease at the time of diagnosis, in only a few infants is clinical lactose intolerance present. In Zurich, a need for short-term dietary exclusion of dietary lactose occurred in only one of 319 children with celiac disease.[122] Only when there is evidence of such intolerance, e.g., an abnormal amount of reducing substances in the stool or diarrhea after a lactose load, is elimination of lactose from the diet indicated.

However, some infants do appear to be intolerant of cow's milk protein. This is suggested if symptoms first occurred with the introduction of milk to the child's diet before the child was exposed to gluten. When this happens, temporary avoidance of cow's milk may speed recovery. The need for the restriction of lactose or cow's milk protein is temporary, in contrast to the need for gluten restriction, which is permanent in individuals with celiac disease. The need for such permanent dietary restriction is based upon three principal premises: First, there is the fact that eventually the small intestinal mucosa will always become abnormal again when it is exposed to gluten, despite years of normalcy while on a gluten-free diet. Second, although such a mucosal relapse may not be followed at once by a clinical relapse, it may lead to slowing of growth and a failure to achieve full growth potential, or it may produce general malaise and lack of energy, often not perceived by the patient himself, except retrospectively when his gluten-free diet is reintroduced. Third, it is possible that long-term gluten restriction diminishes the risks of developing malignant disease as a complication of celiac disease. This has yet to be established. The patient with celiac disease and his parents should be advised that there is a permanent need for him to adhere strictly to his gluten-free diet. He should depart from it only on medical advice as part of a gluten challenge to reinvestigate his state of gluten tolerance, or to establish definitively the diagnosis of celiac disease. There are some who contest this view in teenagers and who recommend liberalization of gluten intake in asymptomatic patients who have completed their growth. It is also controversial whether asymptomatic siblings require treatment.

The child with celiac disease and his parents need careful support to provide them with up-to-date facts about a gluten-free diet. This may in part be given in Britain and other countries by the Celiac Societies, but regular attendance at a celiac clinic is the ideal. There, a specially trained dietitian is available to advise about a gluten-free diet and to discuss with the parents and child any problems they may have encountered with such a diet. At such a clinic the child's progress and general growth development can also be observed by the pediatrician. If they are unsatisfactory, this can then be investigated appropriately. However, such attendance once or twice a year should not undermine the general advice to the child that he is in every way a normal child as long as he continues strictly on his gluten-free diet.

CURRENT SITUATION IN CELIAC DISEASE

Celiac disease is currently defined in terms of an abnormal small intestinal mucosa responding to gluten elimination and challenge. However, it is now clear that the occasional patient may have the potentiality to develop clinical celiac disease at a later time despite a previous apparently normal small intestinal mucosal biopsy. Furthermore, a few children have been described who have had a small intestinal mucosa reacting to gluten who later recover spontaneously, at least for a time. Celiac disease has been regarded as a lifelong permanent disorder, but it is not known yet whether such children will in time invariably relapse. Clearly, the clinical expression of celiac disease is quite variable, as family studies make clear, and it also varies at different ages of life, being most severe clinically in early childhood, less severe in adolescence, and more severe again in adult life.

Immunologic mechanisms appear to be of paramount importance in pathogenesis, with the development of a cell-mediated immune reaction within the lamina propria of the small intestinal mucosa of critical importance; yet precisely how enterocyte damage occurs remains to be established. Which amino acid sequence in gliadin damages the small intestinal mucosa remains uncertain, but molecular configuration may be as important as the actual sequence. Finally, in terms of genetics, celiac disease is associated with an extended haplotype on chromosome 6, although not invariably. The susceptibility genes are not yet known. Thus, celiac disease still poses a formidable challenge to understanding of its pathogenesis, and much remains to be learned. Yet strict adherence to dietary gluten avoidance is remarkably effective treatment, causing surprisingly little inconvenience in most cases. An unresolved issue concerns the necessity for a long-term strict gluten-free diet to prevent malignancy, and enteropathy-associated T cell lymphoma in particular. The role of a low-gluten diet in asymptomatic teenagers who have completed their growth and the need for a gluten-free diet in asymptomatic family members remain contentious issues.

REFERENCES

1. Gee SJ. On the coeliac affection. St Bartholomew's Rep 1888; 24:17.
2. Dowd BD, Walker-Smith JA. Samuel Gee Arataeus and the coeliac affection. Br Med J 1974; 2:54.
3. Nelson R, McNeish AS, Anderson CM. Coeliac disease in children of Asian immigrants. Lancet 1973; 1:348.
4. Khoshoo V, Bhan MK, Jain R, Phillips AD, Walker-Smith JA, Unsworth DJ, Stintzing G. Coeliac disease as cause of protracted diarrhoea in Indian children. Lancet 1988; i:126–127.
5. Bitar JG, Salem AA, Nasr AT. Coeliac disease from the Middle East. Lebanese Med J 1970; 23:423.
6. Al-Hassany M. Coeliac disease in Iraqi children. J Trop Paediatr 1975; 21:178.

7. Nazer H, Sakati I. Coeliac disease in Saudi children. Proceedings of 4th Coeliac Symposium, 1990; in press.
8. Suliman GI. Coeliac disease in Sudanese children. Gut 1978; 19:121.
9. Carter C, Sheldon W, Walker C. The inheritance of coeliac disease. Ann Hum Genet 1959; 23:266.
10. Mylotte M, Egan-Mitchell B, McCarthy CF, McNicholl B. Incidence of coeliac disease in the West of Ireland. Br Med J 1973; 1:703.
11. Rossipal E. Investigation of the cellular immunity in infants and children with coeliac disease using the DNCB test. In: McNicholl B, McCarthy CF, Fottrell PE, eds. Perspectives in coeliac disease. Lancaster: MTP Press, 1978:377.
12. McCrae WM. Inheritance of coeliac disease. J Med Genet 1969; 6:129.
13. Shmerling DH, Leisinger D, Dradese A. On the familial occurrence of coeliac disease. Acta Paediatr Scand 1972; 61:501.
14. Shipman RT, Williams AL, Kay R, Townley RRW. A family study of coeliac disease. Aust NZ J Med 1975; 5:250.
15. Borgfors N, Selander P. The incidence of celiac disease in Sweden. Acta Paediatr Scand 1968; 57:260.
16. Stevens FM, Egan-Mitchell B, Cryan E, McCarthy CT, McNicholl B. Decreasing incidence of coeliac disease. Arch Dis Child 1987; 62:465–468.
17. McNicholl B. Discussion. In: McConnell RB, ed. Genetics of coeliac disease. Lancaster: MTP Press, 1981:52.
18. Gardner AJ, Mutton KJ, Walker-Smith JA. A family study of coeliac disease. Aust Paediatr J 1973; 9:18.
19. Rolles CJ, Kyaw-Myint TB, Sin W-K, Anderson CM. Family study of coeliac disease. Gut 1974; 15:18.
20. Stenhammar L, Brandt A, Wager MJ. A family study of coeliac disease. Acta Paediatr Scand 1982; 71:625–628.
21. Penna FJ, Mota JAC, Roquete MLV, Carvalho AST, Lemos ATO, Barbosa AJA, Leao E, Ferreira RAA, Castro LP. Coeliac disease in identical twins. Arch Dis Child 1970; 54:395.
22. Polanco I, Biemond I, Van Leeuwen A, et al. Gluten-sensitive enteropathy in Spain: genetic and environmental factors. In: McConnell RB, ed. Genetics of coeliac disease. Lancaster: MTP Press, 1981:211.
23. Shale DJ, Johnston DG, Haeer F, Roberts DF. Coeliac disease in monozygotic twins. Postgrad Med J 1982; 58:797–798.
24. Hoffman HN, Wollaeger EE, Greenberg E. Discordance for nontropical sprue (adult coeliac disease) and monozygotic twin pair. Gastroenterology 1966; 51:36–42.
25. Walker-Smith JA. Discordance for childhood coeliac disease in monozygotic twins. Gut 1973; 14:374.
26. McNeish AS, Nelson R. Coeliac disease in one of monozygotic twins. Clin Gastroenterol 1974; 3:143.
27. Polanco I, Mearin ML, Larrauri I, Biermonda, Wipkink-Bakkera, Denars. Effect of gluten supplementation in healthy siblings of children with coeliac disease. Gastroenterology 1987; 92:678–681.
28. Kamath KR, Dorney SFA. Is discordance for coeliac disease in monozygotic twins permanent? Pediatr Res 1983; 17:423.
29. Maki M, Koskimies S, Visakorpi J. Latent coeliac disease. 1990; in press.
30. Booth CC. The enterocyte in coeliac disease. Br Med J 1970; 4:14.
31. Greenberg DA, Hodge SE, Rutter JI. Evidence for recessive and against dominant inheritance at the HLA-'linked' locus in celiac disease. Am J Hum Genet 1982; 34:263–277.
32. Stokes PL, Asquith P, Holmes GKT, Mackintosh P, Cooke WT. Histocompatibility antigens associated with adult coeliac disease. Lancet 1972; ii:162.
33. Falchuk ZM, Rogentine GN, Strober W. Predominance of histocompatibility antigen HL-A8 in patient with gluten-sensitive enteropathy. J Clin Invest 1972; 51:1602.
34. McKenna R, Stevens FM, Bourke M, McNichols B, Albert ED, McCarthy CF. B-cell alloantigens associated with coeliac disease in the West of Ireland. In: McConnell RB, ed. Genetics of coeliac disease. Lancaster: MTP Press, 1981:181.
35. Keuning JJ, Pena AS, van Leeuwen A, van Hoof JP, van Rood R. HLA-DW3 associated with coeliac disease. Lancet 1976; i:506.
36. Betuel H, Gebuhrer L, Percebois H, Descos L, Minaire Y, Bertrand J. Association de la maladia coliaque de l'adulte avec HLA-DRW3 et -DRW7. Gastroenterol Clin Biol 1979; 3:605–606.
37. Tosi R, Visamara D, Tanigaki N, Ferrara GB, Cicimarra F, Buffalono W, Follo D, Auricchio S. Evidence that coeliac disease is associated with a DC locus allelic specificity. Clin Immunol Immunopathol 1983; 28:359–404.
38. Sachs JA, McCloskey D, Navarette C, Festenstein H, Elliot E, Walker-Smith JA, Griffiths CEM, Leonard JN, Fry L. Different HLA associated gene combinations contribute to susceptibility for coeliac disease and dermatitis herpetiformis. Gut 1986; 27:515–520.
39. Hitman GA, Niven MJ, Festenstein H, Cassell PG, Walker-Smith JA, Leonard JN, Fry L, Ciclitira P, Kumar P, Sachs JA. HLA Class NI alpha chain gene polymorphisms in patients with insulin dependent diabetes mellitus, dermatitis herpetiformis and coeliac disease. J Clin Invest 1987; 79:609–615.
40. Howell MD, Austin RK, Kelleher D, Neporn GF, Kagnoff MF. An HLA-D region restruction fragment length polymorphism associated with coeliac disease. J Exp Med 1986; 166:333–338.
41. Scott H, Ek J, Baklien K, Brandizaig P. Immunoglobulin producing cells injejunal mucosa of children with coeliac disease on a gluten-free diet and after gluten challenge. Scand J Gastroenterol 1980; 15:81.
42. Ciclitira PJ, Nelufer JM, Ellis HJ, Evans DJ. Gliadin IgG subclass antibodies in patients with coeliac disease. Int Arch Allergy Appl Immunol 1986; 80:258–261.
43. Dicke WK. Coeliakie: een onderzoek naar de nadelige invoileed van sommige graansoorte op de lijder aan coeliakie. Utrecht: M.D. Thesis, 1950.
44. Ciclitira PJ, Ellis HJ, Evans DJ, Lennox ES. Relation of antigenic structure of cereal proteins to their toxicity in coeliac patients. Br J Nutr 1985; 53:39–45.
45. Hekkens WT, Haex AJ, Willighagen RGL. In: Booth CC, Dowling H, eds. Coeliac disease. Edinburgh: Churchill Livingstone, 1970.
46. Ciclitira PJ, Evans DJ, Fagg NL, Lennox ES, Dowling RH. Clinical testing of gliadin fractions in coeliac patients. Clin Sci 1984; 66:357–364.
47. Jos J, Charbonnier L. In vitro toxicity of wheat gluten fractions and subfractions on coeliac intestinal mucosa. Acta Paediatr Belg 1976; 29:261.
48. Kasarda DD, Okita TW, Bernardin JE. Nucleic acid (cDNA) and amino acid sequences of a-type gliadins from wheat (*Triticum aestivum L*). Proc Natl Acad Sci USA 1984; 81:4712–4716.
49. Kagnoff MF, Austin RK, Hubert JJ, Kasarda DD. Possible role for a human advenovirus in the pathogenesis of coeliac disease. J Exp Med 1984; 160:1544–1557.
50. Kagnoff MF, Paterson YJ, Kumar PJ, Kasarda DP, Carbone FR, Unsworth DJ, Austin KR. Evidence for the role of a human intestinal adenovirus in the pathogenesis of coeliac disease. Gut 1987; 28:995–1001.
51. Howdle PD, Trejdosiewicz LK, Smart CJ, Blair GE. Evidence against the involvement of adenovirus in the pathogenesis of coeliac disease. Proceedings of 4th Coeliac Symposium, 1990; in press.
52. Karagiannis I, Jowell DP. Cellular hypersensitivity in coeliac disease. Immune responses of sensitized lymphocytes to a synthetic dodecapeptide sequence from A-gliadin 1988. Gastroenterol Int 1988; 1:427.
53. Browning TH, Trier JS. Organ culture of mucosal biopsies of human small intestine. J Clin Invest 1969; 48:1423.
54. Falchuk ZM, Katz AJ. Organ culture model of gluten-sensitive enteropathy. In: McNichol B, McCarthy CF, Fottrell PF, eds. Perspectives in coeliac disease. Third international coeliac symposium. Lancaster: MTP Press, 1978:65.
55. Goldstein IJ, Hughes RC, Monsigny M, Osawa T, Sharon N. What should be called a lectin? nature (London) 1980; 285–286.
56. Weiser MM, Douglas AP. Cell surface glycosyl-transferases of the enterocyte in coeliac disease. In: McCarthy CF, McNicholl B, eds. Perspectives in coeliac disease. Third international coeliac symposium. Lancaster: MTP Press, 1978:451.
57. Nicholson GL, Blaustein J. The interaction of Ricinus communis agglutinin with normal and tumor cell surfaces. Biochim Biophys Acta 1972; 66:543–547.
58. Colyer J, Farthing MJG, Kumar PJ, Clark ML, Ofannesia AD, Waldron NM. Reappraisal of the "lectin hypothesis" in the aetiopathogenesis of coeliac disease. Clin Sci 1986; 71:105–110.
59. Kenrick KG, Walker-Smith JA. Immunoglobulins and dietary protein antibodies in childhood coeliac disease. Gut 1970; 2:635.

60. Auricchio S, De Ritis G, De Vincenzi M, Silano V. Toxicity mechanisms of wheat and other cereals in celiac disease and related enteropathies. J Pediatr Gastroenterol Nutr 1985; 4:923–930.

61. Kieffer M, Frazier PJ, Daniels NWR, Coombs RRA. Wheat gliadin fractions and other cereal antigens reactive with antibodies in the sera of coeliac patients. Clin Exp Immunol 1982; 50:651–660.

62. Scott BB, Swinburne ML, Rajah SM. HL-As and the immune response to gluten. Lancet 1974; ii:374–377.

63. Savilahti E. Intestinal immunoglobulins in children with coeliac disease. Gut 1972; 13:958.

64. Kilby A, Walker-Smith J, Wood CBS. Small intestinal mucosa in cow's milk allergy. Lancet 1975; i:53.

65. Shmerling DH, Shiner M. The response of the intestinal mucosa to the intraduodenal instillation of gluten in patients with coeliac disease. In: Booth CC, Dowling RH, eds. Coeliac disease. Edinburgh: Churchill Livingstone, 1970:64.

66. Shiner M, Ballard J. Antigen-antibody reactions in the jejunal mucosa in childhood coeliac disease after gluten challenge. Lancet 1972; i:1202.

67. Doe WF, Henry K, Booth CC. Complement in coeliac disease. In: Hekkens WThJM, Pena AS, eds. Coeliac disease. Leiden: Stenfert Korese, 1974:189.

68. Marsh MN. Functional and structural aspects of epithelial lymphocyte, with implications for coeliac disease and tropical sprue. Scand J Gastroenterol (Suppl) 1985; 114:55–75.

69. Marsh MN, Hinde J. Morphometric analysis of small intestinal mucosa. III. The quantitation of crypt epithelial volumes and lymphoid cell infiltrates, with reference to coeliac sprue mucosae. Virchows Arch 1986; 409:11–22.

70. Selby WS, Janossy G, Jewell DP. Immunohistology characterisation of intraepithelial lymphocytes of the human gastrointestinal tract. Gut 1981; 22:169.

71. Spencer J, MacDonald TT, Walker-Smith JA, Ciclitira PJ, Walker-Smith JA. Changes in sub-populations of intraepithelial lymphocytes in coeliac disease and enteropathy associated T cell lymphoma (malignant histiocytosis of the intestine). Gut 1989:339–347.

72. Ferguson A. Coeliac disease and gastrointestinal food allergy. Immunological aspects of the liver and gastrointestinal tract. Lancaster: MTP Press, 1976.

73. Strober W. Gluten-sensitive enteropathy. Clin Gastroenterol 1976; 5:429–453.

74. Rubin W, Fauch AS, Sleisenger MH, Jeffries GH. Immunofluorescent studies in adult coeliac disease. J Clin Invest 1975; 44:475.

75. Ferguson A. Pathogenesis and mechanisms in the gastrointestinal tract. In: Proceedings of the First Fison Food Allergy Workshop. Oxford: Medicine Publishing Foundation, 1980: 23–28.

76. Bloch KJ, Bloch DB, Stearns M, Walker WA. Intestinal uptake of macromolecules. VI. Uptake of protein antigen in vivo in normal rats and in rats injected with Nippostrongylus brasiliensis or subjected to mild systemic anaphylaxis. Gastroenterology 1979; 77:1039.

77. Bellamy JEC, Nielsen NO. Immune-mediated emigration of neutrophils into the lumen of the small intestine. Infect Immunol 1974; 9:615.

78. MacDonald TT, Ferguson A. Hypersensitivity reactions in the small intestine. 2. Effects of allograft rejection on mucosal architecture and lymphoid cell infiltrate. Gut 1976; 17:81.

79. MacDonald TT, Ferguson A. Hypersensitivity reactions in small intestine. 3. The effects of allograft rejection and of graft-versus-host disease on epithelial cell kinetics. Cell Tissue Kinet 1977; 10:301.

80. Ferguson A, MacDonald TT. Effects of local delayed hypersensitivity on the small intestine. In: Immunology of the gut (Ciba Foundation Symposium No. 46). Amsterdam: Elsevier-North Holland, 1975:305.

81. MacDonald TT, Spencer J. Evidence that activated mucosal T-cells play a role in the pathogenesis of enteropathy in human small intestine. J Exp Med 1988; 167:1321–1349.

82. Ferreira RC, MacDonald TT. Changes in mucosal morphology and the rate of crypt cell renewal induced by a cell mediated immune response in human small intestine. 1990 Gastroenterology; in press.

83. Marsh MN. Studies of intestinal lymphoid tissue. III. Quantitative analyses of epithelial lymphocytes in the small intestine of human control subjects and of patients with coeliac sprue. Gastroenterology 1980; 79:481–492.

84. Ferguson A, MacDonald TT, McClure JP, Holden RJ. Cell-mediated immunity to gliadin within the small intestinal mucosa in coeliac disease. Lancet 1975; i:895–901.

85. Arnaud-Battandier F, Cerf-Bensussan N, Amesellem R, Schmitz J. Increased HLA-DR expression by enterocytes in children with coeliac disease. Gastroenterology 1986; 91:1206–1212.

86. MacDonald TT, Weinel A, Spencer JM. HLA-DR expression in human fetal intestinal epithelium. Gut 1988; 29:1342–1348.

87. Schmitz J, Jos J, Rey J. Transient mucosal atrophy in confirmed coeliac disease. McNicholl B, McCarthy CF, and Fottrell PE, eds. Perspectives in Coeliac Disease. Lancaster: MTP Press, 1978:259.

88. Schmitz J, Arnand-Battandier F, Jos J, Rey J. Long-term follow up of childhood coeliac disease (CD). Is there a "natural recovery"? Paediatr Res 1984; 18:1052.

89. McNeish AS, Harms, K, Rey J, Shmerling DH, Visakorpi J, Walker-Smith JA. Re-evaluation of diagnostic criteria for coeliac disease. Arch Dis Child 1979; 54:783.

90. Paulley JW. Observations on the aetiology of idiopathic steatorrhoea. Br J Med 1954; ii:1318.

91. Sakula J, Shiner M. Coeliac disease with atrophy of the small intestine mucosa. Lancet 1957; ii:876.

92. Manuel P, France NE, Walker-Smith JA. Patchy enteropathy. Gut 1979; 20:211–215.

93. Booth CC. Enteropoiesis: structural and functional relationships of the enterocyte. Postgrad Med J 1968; 44:12.

94. Anderson CM, Gracey M, Burke V. Coeliac disease. Some still controversial aspects. Arch Dis Child 1972; 47:292.

95. Kelly DA, Phillips AD, Elliot EJ, Dias JA, Walker-Smith JA. The rise and fall of coeliac disease 1960–1985. 1989; 64:1157–1160.

96. Littlewood JM, Crollick AJ, Richards IDG. Childhood coeliac disease is disappearing. Lancet 1980; 2:1935.

97. Dossetor JFB, Gibson AAM, McNeish AS. A recent reduction in the incidence of childhood coeliac disease in the west of Scotland. In: McConnell RB, ed. Genetics of coeliac disease. Lancaster: MTP Press, 1981:41.

98. Gibbons RA. The coeliac affection in children. Edinburgh Med J 1889; 35:321.

99. Meewisse GW. Diagnostic criteria in coeliac disease. Acta Paediatr Scand 1970; 59:461.

100. Walker-Smith JA, Kilby A, France NE. Reinvestigation of children previously diagnosed as coeliac disease. In: McNicholl B, McCarthy CF, Fottrell PF, eds. Perspectives in coeliac disease. Lancaster: MTP Press, 1978:267.

101. Shmerling DH. Questionnaire of the European Society for Paediatric Gastroenterology and Nutrition on Coeliac Disease. In: McNicholl B, McCarthy CF, Fottrell PF, eds. Perspectives in coeliac disease. Lancaster: MTP Press, 1978:245.

102. Lindberg T, Berg NP, Bonul FS, Jakobbson I. Liver damage in coeliac disease or other food intolerance in childhood. Lancet 1978: i;390.

103. Kuitnen P, Pelkonen P, Perkkio M, Savilahts E, Visakorpi K. Transient gluten intolerance. Acta Paediatr Belg 1977; 30:250.

104. Shmerling DH, Franckx J. Childhood coeliac disease: a long term analysis of relapses in 91 patients. J Paediatr Gastroenterol Nutr 1986; 5:565–569.

105. Unsworth DJ, Walker-Smith JA, Holborow EJ. Gliadin and reticulin antibodies in childhood coeliac disease. Lancet 1983; 1:874–875.

106. Dias J, Unsworth DJ, Walker-Smith JA. Antigliadin antibodies in screening for coeliac disease. Lancet 1987; ii:157.

107. Seah PP, Fry L, Holborow EJ, Rossiter MA, Doe WF, Magalhaes AF, Hoffbrand AV. Antireticulin antibody: incidence and diagnostic significance. Gut 1973; 4:113.

108. Prader A, Tanner JM, Von Harnack GA. Catch-up growth following illness or starvation. J Paediatr 1963; 62:646.

109. Prader A, Shmerling DH, Zachmann M, Biro Z. Catch-up growth in coeliac disease. Acta Paediatr Scand 1969; 58:311.

110. Dormandy KM, Waters AH, Mollin DL. Folic acid deficiency in coeliac disease. Lancet 1963; i:632.

111. Hoffbrandt AV, Douglas AP, Fry T, Stewart JS. Malabsorption of dietary folate (pteroylglutamates) in adult coeliac disease and dermatitis herpetiformis. Br Med J 1970; 4:85.

112. Hamilton JR, Lynch MJ, Reilly BJ. Active coeliac disease in childhood. Q J Med 1969; 38:135.
113. Gough KR, Read AE, Naish JM. Intestinal reticulosis as a complication of idiodpathic steatorrhoea. Gut 1962; 3:232.
114. Harris OD, Cooke WT, Thomson H, Waterhouse JAH. Malignancy in adult coeliac disease and idiopathic steatorrhoea. Am J Med 1967; 42:889.
115. Cooper BT, Holmes GKT, Cooke WT. Intestinal lymphoma associated with malabsorption. Lancet 1978; i:387.
116. Arnaud-Battandier F, Schmitz J, Ricour C, Rey J. Intestinal malignant lymphoma in a child with familial coeliac disease. J Paediatr Gastroenterol Nutr 1983; 2:320–325.
117. Isaacson PG, Spencer J, Connoly CE, et al. Malignant histiocytosis of the intestine: a T-cell lymphoma. Lancet 1985; 2:688–691.
118. Loughran TP, Kadin ME, Deeg HJ. T-cell intestinal lymphoma associated with coeliac sprue. Ann Intern Med 1986; 104:
119. Holmes GKT, Prior P, Lane MR, Pope D, Allan RN. Malignancy in coeliac disease—effect of a gluten free diet. Gut 1989; 30:333–339.
120. Barr DGD, Shmerling DH, Brader A. Catch-up growth in malnutrition, studies in coeliac disease after institution of gluten-free diet. Paediatr Res 1972; 6:521–527.
121. Ejderhamm J, Veress B, Strandvik B. The long term effect of continual ingestion of wheat starch containing gluten-free products in coeliac patients. Proceedings 4th Coeliac Symposium, 1990; in press.
122. Shmerling DH. Nutrition of infants with coeliac disease and with cystic fibrosis. In: Stern L, ed. Feeding the sick infant., Nestle Nutrition Workshop. Series Vol 11. New York: Raven Press, 1987:257.

PART 22

Idiopathic Villus Atrophy

Geoffrey P. Davidson, M.D., F.R.C.P.

In up to 30 percent of cases of prolonged severe diarrhea in infants, no specific cause can be identified.[1] In these idiopathic cases diarrhea often begins before 3 months of age and the outcome frequently is fatal.[2] In 1978, Davidson et al[3] described five infants who presented in the first few days of life with severe watery diarrhea, which was fatal in four cases. A similar illness in siblings of four patients suggested the possibility of an autosomal recessively inherited disorder. Candy et al[4] in 1981 described a similar illness in 24 patients from 10 families with an 87.5 percent mortality, and other reports of similar cases have been published.[5–8] Schmitz et al[7] suggested the term *congenital microvillus atrophy* to describe these patients, who develop a severe small intestinal lesion characterized by villus atrophy very early in life.

CONGENITAL MICROVILLUS ATROPHY

From birth or within the first week of life these patients have persistent watery diarrhea that persists in the absence of oral intake and requires parenteral nutrition for survival, as oral feeding results in increased stool output.

Genetics

The initial report suggested that this condition is inherited in an autosomal recessive manner based on the familial nature of the condition.[3] Two of the five children were products of a consanguineous marriage. Candy et al[4] reported consanguinity in 20 percent of the 10 families and supported an autosomal recessive inheritance of the condition. Others have also reported familial cases of fatal protracted

diarrhea.[6] Howard et al[9] suggested that in England the birth frequency of this condition may be half that of phenylketonuria.

Pathogenesis

The lesions observed in the jejunum of these patients is characterized by uniform hypoplastic villus atrophy with a loss of villus height without crypt hyperplasia, producing a thin mucosa but no inflammatory cell infiltrate in the lamina propria.[3] Severity of the lesion varies.[4] Marker perfusion studies of the proximal jejunum have shown a net secretory state with respect to Na^+ and water and a marked impairment of glucose-stimulated Na^+ transport.[3,4] Candy et al[4] found marked reduction in fructose and glucose absorption, decreased Na^+, K^+-ATPase, but normal adenylate cyclase activity. Vasoactive intestinal peptide, gastrin, glucagon, motilin, gastrin inhibitory peptide, and pancreatic polypeptide levels in serum have been found to be normal.[3] Prostaglandin levels have not been assayed, but prostaglandin synthetase inhibitors failed to influence stool volume, suggesting that prostaglandins do not have a major role in the pathogenesis of the diarrhea.[4] Electron microscopic studies reveal major abnormalities in the mucosal surface enterocytes which lack brush borders completely or possess shortened irregular microvilli (Fig. 1). The apical cytoplasm of the enterocyte contains a marked increase in electron-dense secretory granules of various sizes (Fig. 2). These granules seem to contain glycocalyx and brush border–related material. In some enterocytes intracellular cystic structures suggestive of invaginated brush borders are seen (Fig. 3). The crypt epithelium is well preserved, and other types of small intestinal epithelial

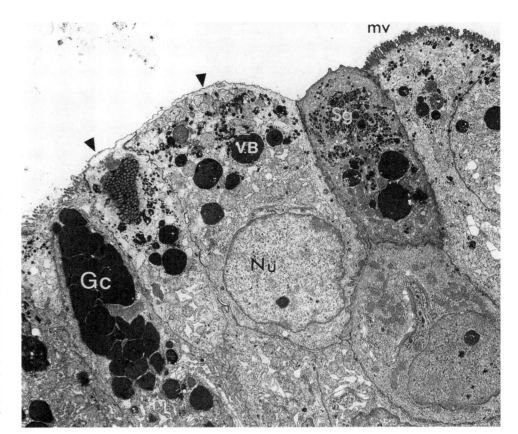

FIGURE 1 Low-magnification electron micrograph of surface enterocytes with absent brush border microvilli (*arrowheads*). One enterocyte (*upper right*) shows shortened apical microvilli (mv). The cytoplasm of enterocytes contains large osmiophilic vesicular bodies (VB) and numerous small secretory granules (sg), usually seen in crypt cells. The nucleus (Nu) is proximally placed but shows no abnormalities. A goblet cell (Gc) contains electron-dense mucous granules (owing to fixation in 2 percent osmium tetroxide) (×5,400). (From Davidson et al,[3] with permission.)

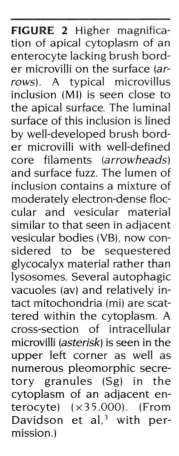

FIGURE 2 Higher magnification of apical cytoplasm of an enterocyte lacking brush border microvilli on the surface (*arrows*). A typical microvillus inclusion (MI) is seen close to the apical surface. The luminal surface of this inclusion is lined by well-developed brush border microvilli with well-defined core filaments (*arrowheads*) and surface fuzz. The lumen of inclusion contains a mixture of moderately electron-dense floccular and vesicular material similar to that seen in adjacent vesicular bodies (VB), now considered to be sequestered glycocalyx material rather than lysosomes. Several autophagic vacuoles (av) and relatively intact mitochondria (mi) are scattered within the cytoplasm. A cross-section of intracellular microvilli (*asterisk*) is seen in the upper left corner as well as numerous pleomorphic secretory granules (Sg) in the cytoplasm of an adjacent enterocyte) (×35,000). (From Davidson et al,[3] with permission.)

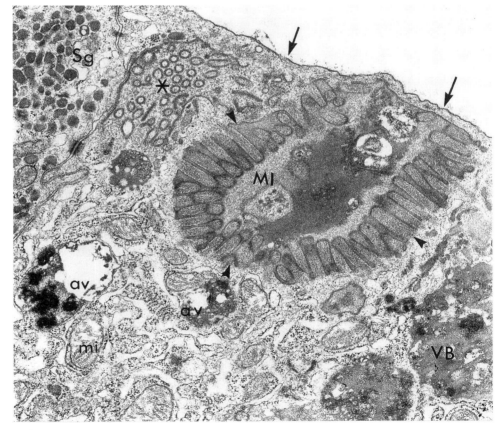

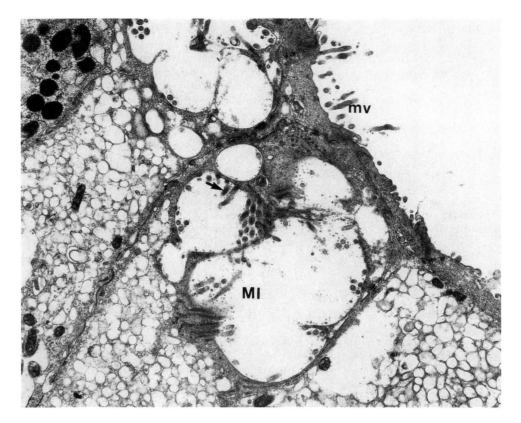

FIGURE 3 Electron micrograph of surface colonocytes from a rectal biopsy. The cytoplasm contains numerous electron-lucent vesicles and "multicystic" microvillus inclusions (MI) close to the apical surface. The lumen of inclusion is lined by clusters of irregular microvilli (*arrow*). Only sparse microvilli (mv) are seen on the apical surface (×20,000). (Courtesy of E. Cutz, M.D.)

cells including goblet cells, Paneth cells, and enteroendocrine cells show no obvious ultrastructural abnormalities. Phillips et al[8] have shown the presence of microvillus involutions and increased numbers of secretory granules in biopsy material from the colon, suggesting that both small and large intestines are involved.

Carruthers et al[10] suggested that the defect may be an abnormality of the enterocyte skeleton. In a polyacrylamide gel electrophoretic analysis of brush border proteins, they have shown a striking diminution of a 200 k molecular weight band as compared with normal controls. Decrease in this protein, which runs in electrophoresis in a position similar to that of skeletal muscle myosin, may mean that in these cases myosin fails to bind to the base of actin cables located in microvilli and anchored to the plasma membrane. The resultant perturbation of the membrane cytoskeleton at the terminal web could lead to transport derangements with subsequent microvillus involution formation. In human fetal intestinal organ culture, experiments with drugs designed to disturb the cytoskeleton tend to support the concept that an abnormality of the cytoskeleton is the basis of this disorder.[11]

Clinical Features

The major clinical manifestation of this disorder is the onset at birth or within the neonatal period of severe watery diarrhea associated with failure to thrive. Many infants are below their birth weight at diagnosis and gain weight only with the use of parenteral alimentation. Diarrhea persists until death in over 80 percent of cases.[3-8] Withholding oral intake and provision of adequate parenteral nutrition over prolonged periods fail to halt diarrhea. Fecal volume losses are massive, 100 to 800 ml per kilogram body weight per 24 hours with high electrolyte concentrations when no diet is given.

Candy et al[4] found extragastrointestinal or gastrointestinal-related abnormalities, absence of organ of Corti, premature fusion of skull sutures, bifid phalanges, renal dysplasia and hydronephrosis, absent corpus callosum, and vertebral and other skeletal abnormalities in 58 percent of patients. The most common gastrointestinal-related anomalies were hiatus and inguinal hernias, Meckel's diverticulum, universal mesentery and intra-abdominal adhesions, and calcification.

Laboratory Findings

A severe watery diarrhea with high stool electrolyte concentrations is the only constant finding in this condition. Most tests of small intestinal function, including fecal fat excretion, measurement of vitamin B_{12} absorption, intestinal protein loss, duodenal and rectal biopsies with mucosal morphometry, barium studies, intestinal perfusion studies, and intestinal mucosal disaccharidase assay, are abnormal. The majority of patients have severe steatorrhea and carbohydrate malabsorption. Gastrointestinal hormone levels and pancreatic function have been normal.

Studies of endocrine and immunologic function have revealed variable results, but abnormal data are difficult to interpret in malnourished infants. Candy et al[4] have suggested that in some cases there may be a primary immunologic defect.

Diagnosis

The most important clinical feature pointing to a diagnosis of congenital microvillus atrophy is severe persistent watery diarrhea unresponsive to withdrawal of oral diet and provision of adequate parenteral nutrition. The diarrhea is present at birth or soon after; in some cases, maternal polyhydramnios suggests diarrhea in utero.

The small intestinal mucosa usually shows features of villus atrophy without crypt hypertrophy. Examined by transmission electron microscopy, surface epithelial cells have shortened infrequent microvilli, increased lysosomal bodies, and membrane-bound bodies containing obvious microvilli. These microvillus inclusions are the major diagnostic feature. The crypt epithelium has increased numbers of secretory granules, but it is otherwise normal. Colonic epithelium is normal by light microscopy, but electron microscopic changes similar to the small intestinal abnormalities just described have been observed.[7]

Treatment

Many dietary manipulations, including exclusion of disaccharides, monosaccharides, cow's milk, soy protein, and gluten have been tried without benefit. In nearly all cases life can be sustained only by parenteral nutrition. A variety of therapeutic agents have been used without affecting the diarrhea. These include adrenocorticoids, oral broad-spectrum antibiotics, disodium cromoglycate, prostaglandin synthase inhibitors (e.g., aspirin, indomethacin), beta blockers, H_2 receptor blockers,[5] cholestyramine, and nonspecific antidiarrheal agents. Somatostatin,[7] berberine, and epidermal growth factor have produced partial improvement in some mucosal parameters but have not affected final outcome. Ileostomies have also been carried out in some cases with no beneficial effects.[2,6,7] Sandhu et al[12] reported that the opiate analogue loperamide reduced diarrhea in several infants with severe protracted diarrhea, but these patients may not have had congenital microvillus atrophy.

IDIOPATHIC ENTEROPATHY

This group of children with idiopathic severe protracted diarrhea differ from those with congenital microvillus atrophy in their later onset of symptoms, usually after the neonatal period, and absence of microvillus inclusions in their intestinal epithelial cells.

The severity of the lesion in this group of patients varies from normal to a completely flat mucosa. The clinical course varies, with some patients responding to dietary restriction whereas others require total parenteral nutrition and immunosuppressive therapy with prednisolone, azathioprine, or cyclophosphamide. The prognosis is also variable, from complete recovery to death. In some cases, the severe enteropathy may be related to an autoimmune disorder in which circulating autoantibodies to gut enterocytes are found.[13-16] Mirakian et al,[16] in a review of 25 patients with idiopathic protracted diarrhea, detected 14 with circulating enterocyte antibodies. These findings suggest that an autoimmune variant of protracted diarrhea exists. A persisting high titer of autoantibodies seems to indicate a poor prognosis in spite of aggressive treatment.

Carruthers et al[11] described an infant who was well until 2 months of age, when severe diarrhea which remitted with fasting began. The small and large intestinal mucosae show characteristic microvillus inclusions, but, unlike those with congenital microvillus atrophy, brush border protein analysis showed myosin to be present.

It is likely that a proportion of infants who fit this later-onset pattern of diarrhea suffered an acute infective insult that rendered their small intestine intolerant to foreign protein and/or bacterial colonization, resulting in diarrhea and malnutrition. Lloyd-Still et al[17] have described similar patients. The prognosis for complete recovery is quite good, although prolonged parenteral nutrition and use of highly specialized diets may be required.

In summary, idiopathic villus atrophy probably represents the final common pathway for a number of pathogenetic mechanisms affecting the gut mucosa. In a small percentage of cases, a defined etiology can be found. It may be anticipated that, in time, this group of severely ill infants will become better defined, the pathophysiologic mechanisms better understood, and treatment more successful.

REFERENCES

1. Larcher VF, Shepherd RW, Francis DEM, Harries JT. Protracted diarrhea in infancy. Analysis of 82 cases with particular reference to diagnosis and management.
2. Avery GB, Villavicencio O, Lilley JR, Randolph JG. Intractable diarrhea in early infancy. Pediatrics 1968; 41:712–722.
3. Davidson GP, Cutz E, Hamilton JR, Gall DG. Familial enteropathy: a syndrome of protracted diarrhea from birth, failure to thrive, and hypoplastic villus atrophy. Gastroenterology 1978; 75:783–790.
4. Candy DCA, Larcher CF, Cameron DJS, Norman AP, Tripp JH, Milla P, Pincott JR, Harries JT. Lethal familial protracted diarrhea. Arch Dis Child 1981; 56:15–23.
5. Fisher SE, Boyle JT, Holtzapple P. Chronic protracted diarrhea and jejunal atrophy in an infant. Dig Dis Sci 1981; 26:181–186.
6. Goutet JM, Boccon-Gibod L, Chatelet F, Ploussard JP, Navarro J, Polonovski C. Congenital and familial protracted diarrhea (PD) with enterocyte brush border abnormalities: Davidson's disease. Pediatr Res 1982; 16:1045.
7. Schmitz J, Ginies JL, Arnaud-Battandier F, Jos J, Desjeux JF, Triodou N, Ricour C, Rey J. Congenital microvillus atrophy: a rare cause of neonatal intractable diarrhea. Pediatr Res 1982; 16:1014.

8. Phillips AD, Jenkins P, Raafat F, Walker-Smith JA. Congenital microvillus atrophy: specific diagnostic features. Arch Dis Child 1985; 60:135–140.

9. Howard FM, Carter CO, Candy DCA, Harries JT. A family study of protracted diarrhea in infancy. J Med Genet 1981; 18:81–86.

10. Carruthers L, Phillips AD, Dourmashkin R, Walker-Smith JA. Biochemical abnormality in brush border membrane protein of a patient with congenital microvillus atrophy. J Pediatr Gastroenterol Nutr 1985; 4:1–6.

11. Carruthers L, Dourmashkin R, Phillips A. Disorders of the cytoskeleton of the enterocytes. Clin Gastroenterol 1986; 15:105–121.

12. Sandhu BK, Tripp JH, Milla PJ, Harries JT. Loperamide in severe protracted diarrhea. Arch Dis Child 1983; 58:39–43.

13. Fisher SE, Smith WI Jr, Rabin BS, Tomasi TB Jr, Lester R, Van Thiel DH. Secretory component and serum immunoglobulin A deficiencies with intestinal autoantibody formation and autoimmune disease: a family study. J Pediatr Gastroenterol Nutr 1982; 1:35–42.

14. Walker-Smith JA, Unsworth DJ, Hutchins J, Phillips AD, Holborow EG. Autoantibodies against gut epithelium in child with small intestinal enteropathy. Lancet 1982; i:566–567.

15. Savage MO, Mirakian R, Wozniak ER, Jenkins HR, Malone M, Phillips AD, Milla PJ, Bottazzo GF, Harries JT. Specific autoantibodies to gut epithelium in two infants with severe protracted diarrhea. J Pediatr Gastroenterol Nutr 1985; 4:187–195.

16. Mirakian R, Richardson A, Milla PJ, Walker-Smith JA, Unsworth J, Savage MO, Bottazzo GF. Protracted diarrhea of infancy: evidence in support of an autoimmune variant. Br Med J 1986; 293:1132–1136.

17. Lloyd-Still JD, Shwachman H, Filler RM. Protracted diarrhea of infancy. I. Clinical studies of 16 infants. Am J Dis Child 1973; 125:358–368.

PART **23**

The Gut in Malnutrition

Oscar Brunser, M.D.
Magdalena Araya, M.D.
Julio Espinoza, M.D.

Malnutrition has been associated with human history since the earliest ages. In developed countries the appearance of primary malnutrition is anecdotal and linked to high-risk groups, but in the Third World a variable proportion of the population suffers from malnutrition at some time during their lifetime, with infants being at greatest risk. Very few malnourished children die because of actual lack of food; in the majority of cases death is a consequence of an intercurrent ailment, often an infection, the evolution of which is favored by, among other things, associated immune defects.[1] In human malnutrition it becomes difficult to separate the consequences of nutrient deficiencies from those that appear in relation to the adverse conditions of the environment in which these children live and grow.[2]

In an attempt to isolate each of the variables that modulate the response of the small intestinal mucosa in malnutrition, models utilizing different animal species have been tested. The results obtained in these studies have resulted in a better understanding of many aspects of the responses of the small intestine to nutrient deprivation. Differences inherent in each of the species evaluated, added to the artificial isolation of the variables, yield results that may not be applicable to man.

Morphologic and histologic organization of an organ reflects a need to perform certain functions. In the case of the small intestine, digestion and transport of nutrients and maintainance of a functional barrier against molecules with antigenic capacity and microorganisms are important needs. The large surface presented to the lumen by the valvulae conniventes, the villi, and the microvilli makes the small intestinal mucosa especially suited for these purposes. A significant proportion of the metabolic needs of the intestinal mucosa are satisfied by nutrients present in the lumen.[3] It is logical that malnutrition might exert negative effects in most aspects of the structure and function of this organ. Although the mucosa also receives nutrients provided by the systemic circulation, the need for the luminal components is so important that even though total parenteral nutrition may restore the nutritional status of the body, it does not lead to normalization of many enzymatic activities in the small intestinal mucosa.[4]

MORPHOLOGY OF THE SMALL INTESTINE

The earliest descriptions of the intestine in autopsy studies of malnourished patients described the wall as thin and distended, with variable amounts of fluid in the lumen.[5,6] The advent of devices for peroral biopsy of the mucosa in the late 1950s opened the possibility for detailed microscopic studies of the human intestine mucosa. The first studies on the morphology of the small intestinal mucosa in malnutrition were carried out in East Africa on patients with kwashiorkor.[7,8] A lesion of variable severity was observed, resembling that of celiac disease, with a flattened surface, elongated crypts, damage to the surface epithelium with irregular nuclei, and infiltration with lymphocytes; cellularity of the lamina propria was increased, mainly by lymphocytes, plasma cells, eosinophils, and polymorphs. After 1 year, no significant changes were observed despite clinical improvement. In the light of knowledge available now, it is possible to postulate that these patients actually suffered from chronic environmental enteropathy due to repeated episodes of enteral infection, subclinical malnutrition, or specific nutrient deficiences, all of which prevented histologic restoration.

In a comparative study of patients with rather pure forms of marasmus and kwashiorkor carried out in Chile, a majority of patients with kwashiorkor had severe lesions, such as those already described in African children, but in cases of marasmus most patients had a normal mucosal architecture (Figs. 1 and 2), although the mucosa was thin with relatively low mitotic counts in the crypts of Lieberkühn.[9] Fine structural studies in marasmus revealed alterations of the microvilli of the brush border, which are short or sparse or branched. Large autophagosomes are present in the supranuclear cytoplasm, and their transition to residual bodies can be established. Deposits of collagen-like and finely fibrillar materials are visible immediately beneath the basal lamella, even merging with it in some areas. Fat droplets are embedded in this dense matrix frequently.[10] An interesting finding in this study is that not every cell is damaged equally and normal cells are seen. After 3 to 4 months of nutritional rehabilitation, the brush border improved, size of the residual bodies reduced, and dense deposits disappeared from the lamina propria below the basal lamella, with persistence of the collagen fibers. The appearance of large mitochondria with numerous cristae constituted a new finding that may reflect subclinical nutrient deficiencies associated with accelerated growth or the effect of some of the drugs used during treatment. Similar abnormalities have been reported in studies performed in Brazilian children[11]; plasma cells in the lamina propria had flattened, closely packed cisternae, suggesting that these cells were not synthesizing immunoglobulins normally.

In infants with kwashiorkor, severe alterations of mucosal

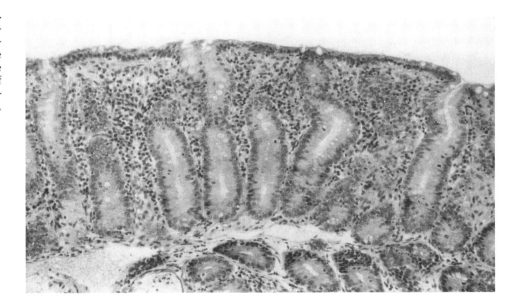

FIGURE 1 Flat mucosa in a patient with kwashiorkor. Crypts extend to the surface of the mucosa. There is damage to the surface epithelium. Cellularity of the lamina propria is also increased (hematoxylin and eosin, ×60).

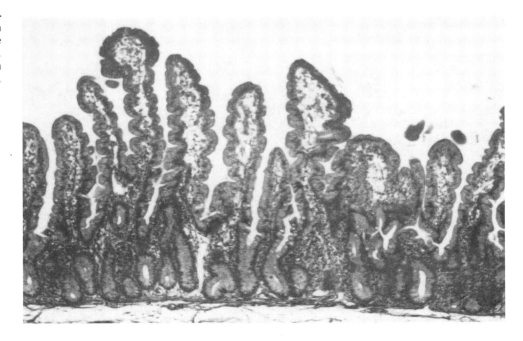

FIGURE 2 Jejunal mucosa from a patient with marasmus. The architecture is well preserved, with tall villi slightly irregular in shape (hematoxylin and eosin, ×35). (From Brunser et al.[60])

fine structure have been reported by Shiner and co-workers.[12] These abnormalities consist of increased numbers of polyribosomes, rounded mitochondria, short microvilli, autophagosomes, and sparseness of the basal lamella. In another study, epithelial cells contained lipids in the endoplasmic reticulum or the cytoplasm.[13] There was no fat in the Golgi apparatus or as chylomicrons in the intercellular space or in the lamina propria. Lipids persisted in the cells even after an 8-hour fast. The authors interpreted these accumulations of fat as evidence of the same derangements of lipoprotein synthesis that cause fat deposits in the hepatocytes. Adult protein malnutrition induces similar changes.

In experimental animal models of protein-energy malnutrition, some changes comparable to those observed in humans have been described. One of these changes is thinning of the basal lamella of the mature, absorptive epithelium in pigs (Fig. 3).[14] Severe lesions, characterized by flattening of the mucosa, have been reported,[15] but this finding has not been corroborated in other studies.[14,16]

The fact that similar changes appear at the light microscopic and the fine structural level in other conditions such as celiac disease, dermatitis herpetiformis, tropical sprue, and chronic environmental enteropathy suggests that the intestinal mucosa may have a rather limited range of morphologic responses to a variety of pathologic stimuli.[17]

CELL RENEWAL

The epithelium of the small intestine has one of the fastest turnover rates in the body; in humans this is about 5 days for the jejunum and 3 for the ileum.[18,19] The mitotic index (i.e., the percentage of mitotic figures identified in the crypts of Lieberkühn) in the epithelium of small intestinal mucosa is significantly decreased in severely marasmic patients.[9] With beginning nutritional rehabilitation (or weight gain), this index increases without reaching normal values. The mitotic index is moderately decreased in kwashiorkor.

A normal process of cell renewal permits the villi to maintain an epithelium that has its normal enzymatic complement. This process also leads to the rapid replacement of damaged cells that are shed and replaced by younger ones. It is possible that in marasmus, with its low mitotic index, the enterocytes lining the villi have exceeded their normal lifespan and that this is the reason why they contain autophagosomes and residual bodies. On the other hand, because the thickness of the mucosa is reduced, the decreased mitotic activity may end up providing a normal turnover rate for a reduced epithelial cell population.

Renewal of the absorptive cells of the small intestine has been studied in animal models. Species studied include fish fasted for 14 months and rats of various ages subjected to various dietary restrictions for different periods of time and starting at different ages. Starvation may not mirror what happens to marasmic malnutrition because it induces an acute stress reaction that mimics some of the results obtained with glucocorticoid injections.[20,21] Using starvation models in rats and mice, a reduced number of cells in the crypts, a reduced mitotic index, and slower cell migration rates have been demonstrated. The duration of the synthetic (S) and premitotic (G_2) phases of the cell cycle is increased.[22] Other studies have reported that the presynthetic phase (G_1) is also lengthened.[23] These data suggest that a decrease in the availability of energy slows the mitotic cycle. In models of protein malnutrition, cell migration along the villi and the rate of DNA synthesis are diminished also[16,24,25]; even the mitotic phase can be lengthened, suggesting that not only is adequate energy required but adequate amounts of protein are needed for normal cell renewal. During prolonged fasting in freshwater fish (*Cyprinus carpio*) the nuclei of some crypt cells become pyknotic, perhaps an indication that some cells die in situ. In parallel with these changes in crypt cell renewal, there is a decrease in thymidine kinase activity, indicating decreased DNA synthesis.[26]

Under normal circumstances total thickness of the intestinal mucosa and the proportion between depth of the crypts

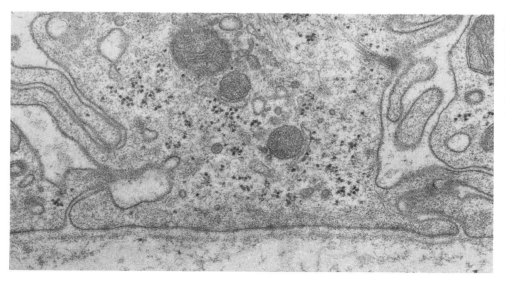

FIGURE 3 Base of epithelial cell from a Yorkshire pig with kwashiorkor. The basal lamella is attenuated and with breaches. Cytoplasmic organelles appear normal (×12,000). (From Brunser et al.[60])

and height of villi are kept within narrow limits, because there is a dynamic equilibrium between cell desquamation at the tip of the villi and cell renewal in the crypts. These two processes are independent and influenced separately by a number of factors.

Certain mechanisms that contribute to the control of cell renewal in the epithelium may be of importance in the genesis and maintenance of the changes observed in malnutrition. One of them is the action of hormones. Thyroxine and anterior pituitary hormones increase crypt cell proliferation; these hormones are reduced in infantile marasmus. Furthermore, the response to their specific secretory stimuli is also reduced. Glucocorticoids decrease cell proliferation in the crypts but accelerate their differentiation and the attainment of adult levels of enzymes in the brush border.[20]

Luminal contents also exert an effect on cell proliferation. Parenteral alimentation induces a decrease of mucosal weight and thickness, of DNA and protein, and of disaccharidase activity.[27] Proximal segments of the intestine were more affected than the ileum. The presence of unabsorbed nutrients in the intestinal lumen may stimulate local nutrition and trigger the release of hormones from the enteroendocrine system, some of which increase cell renewal rates. Thus, gastrin reverts the decrease of mitosis in the crypts of Lieberkühn induced by intravenous hyperalimentation.[28] Other hormones or neurotransmitters also have effects on cell proliferation: Low doses of serotonin stimulate mitosis, whereas large doses have the opposite effect. Norepinephrine and beta-blockers stimulate mitosis in the crypt and, on the contrary, epinephrine, proterenol, alpha-blockage by phentolamine, and sympathectomy decrease it. Probably increase in the cellular mass of the villi exerts a negative feedback on proliferative activity in the crypts. This response may be explained by the presence of peptides called chalones, which exert an inhibitory effect on cell reproduction. Maternal milk also contains polypeptides such as the epithelial growth factor (EGF), which increase DNA synthesis in cell cultures and may influence epithelial renewal in the small intestine.[29]

Pancreatic and biliary secretions have been shown to induce enlargement of the villi of the ileum when the duodenal papillae are transplanted distally.[30] The presence of a normal resident flora stimulates cell division in the crypts. In gnotobiotic animals the mucosa has long, slender, pointed villi with shallow crypts and reduced mitotic activity.[31,32] In malnourished children who were free of diarrhea and who had not received antibiotics, bacterial counts were abnormally high in the jejunal lumen; these organisms, predominantly aerobes, diminish to normal levels after adequate refeeding.[33]

Several of the above-mentioned factors are altered in malnutrition, and it becomes difficult to establish in what proportion each one of them contributes to the derangement of intestinal function in affected children. In addition, the stomach produces less acid and pepsin during severe malnutrition, and potentially pathogenic microorganisms have been cultured from its contents.[34] The concentration of conjugated bile acids in the small intestinal lumen is decreased, whereas that of their unconjugated homologues is increased.[35] In both marasmus and kwashiorkor the pancreas shows signs of histologic and fine structural damage as well as decreased enzymatic output and decreased response to specific stimuli.[36–39] Recovery of pancreatic function after malnutrition may require long periods on adequate diets.

ABSORPTION OF NUTRIENTS

In malnutrition small intestinal function is impaired, more severely so in kwashiorkor, in which malabsorption is the rule, than in marasmus. Usually sufficient absorptive capacity remains so that dietary therapy leads to disappearance of fatty liver, hypoproteinemia, and other indicators of specific nutrient deficiencies. In fact, weight gain and clinical improvement begin promptly when a diet adequate in both quality and quantity is provided. Severe fat malabsorption, described in the late 1950s in patients in Africa,[40] has been corroborated in other regions in the world.[41,42] In these patients, as in those with celiac disease, unsaturated fatty acids are absorbed more efficiently than saturated fat,[43] and nitrogen loss through the feces, some of it endogenous, is increased.[40] Amino acid transport, decreased in adults with long-term nutrient restriction,[44] may not be universal since mucosal biopsies from patients incubated in media containing lysine or alanine transported these amino acids in concentrations comparable to those of normal controls.[45] Dipeptide hydrolases studied in malnourished children were found to be decreased.[46]

Diarrhea in response to ingestion of carbohydrates is a frequent observation in patients with kwashiorkor. Decreased levels of disaccharidases have been described by several authors in different parts of the world.[47] Many of these findings originated from areas in which genetic, late-onset lactase deficiency occurs in the majority of the population, but evidence has accumulated that kwashiorkor either directly or indirectly induces disaccharidase deficiency, and that this is probably proportional to the severity of nutrient deprivation.[48] Monosaccharide absorption was studied using the marker-perfusion technique in Jamaican children. At low concentrations of glucose (2.5 percent), there were no differences between children with kwashiorkor and control children. Malabsorption became apparent at higher concentrations in the perfusate, when water was either not absorbed efficiently or was secreted into the lumen. As a result, luminal content was transported to lower segments of the intestine or even into the colon, where glucose was fermented by the bacterial flora.[49] Nevertheless, most infants with kwashiorkor tolerate isotonic sugar solutions if they are provided slowly. Tolerance to oral carbohydrates is also related to colonization of the upper segments of the small intestine by an abnormal flora. Coello-Ramírez and Lifshitz demonstrated that in malnourished patients with diarrhea, higher bacterial counts were associated with reduced capacity to digest and transport sugars.[50] In an experimental model in young rats, malnutrition made the intestinal mucosa more susceptible to the loss of disaccharidase activity associated with bacterial overgrowth.[51] The D-xylose test in blood has been used to screen for the presence of malabsorption in kwashiorkor, but there seems to be no correlation between histologic damage and blood levels of the sugar in a 1-hour test.[42]

There is evidence of malabsorption of other nutrients, such as vitamins A and B_{12} in patients with kwashiorkor.[42,52] The absorption of some inorganic substances, such as iodine, has been reported to be decreased in malnourished patients from Zaire.[53]

Information about changes in absorptive capacity in marasmic malnutrition is scarce. Transport of fat appears to be normal, and nitrogen excretion is only slightly increased. One-hour blood levels of D-xylose were decreased in some patients and normal in others. In Turkish patients, blood levels and urinary excretion of D-xylose were consistently low.[54] In numerous studies of transport in experimental models of malnutrition, results are quite variable. In some publications absorption seems to be enhanced while in others it seems to decrease. A possible explanation may be the different animal species, ages, degrees of malnutrition, and concentration of substrates infused at different speeds, which make few of these studies strictly comparable.[55] In a study of severely malnourished patients, it was shown that the transepithelial mucosa-to-serosa flux of the macromolecule horseradish peroxidase was three times higher during malnutrition than after nutritional rehabilitation.[56] Increased permeability to macromolecules has also been demonstrated in malnourished animals. In a model of malnutrition in rats, unconjugated bile salts increased the passage of horseradish peroxidase through the junctional complex of epithelial cells or into the intercellular spaces. The microscopic structure of junctional complexes appears normal under the electron microscope in infantile marasmus (Fig. 4), but it is tempting to speculate

that in malnourished children, in whom damage to the mucosa of the small intestine, an abnormal bacterial flora, and luminal concentrations of unconjugated bile salts have been demonstrated, the passage of macromolecules across the mucosa should be increased. The depressed capacity to mount an immune response in malnutrition probably explains why allergic reactions to proteins or other antigenic molecules in foodstuffs are seldom observed in malnourished patients.[57,58] Further evidence of damage to mucosal permeability is provided by studies in severely malnourished Gambian children, in whom the ratio of lactulose-mannitol excretion in the urine was increased in comparison to that of controls.[59]

The only way to rehabilitate malnourished children is by providing adequate amounts of nutrients, even if a certain proportion of them will not be absorbed. It is important to understand the nature and magnitude of the morphologic and functional derangements in the gut so that the remaining capacities of the digestive tract are utilized to the fullest extent and further damage to an already injured structure is avoided. Each patient responds in his particular way to nutrient deprivation; therefore, dietary management must be tailored to the individual's requirements and capabilities.

REFERENCES

1. Scrimshaw NS, Taylor CE, Gordon JE. Interactions of nutrition and infection. Geneva: World Health Organization, 1968.
2. Mata LJ. The children of Santa María Cauqué: a prospective field study of health and growth. Cambridge, MA: MIT Press, 1978.
3. Roediger WE. Metabolic basis of starvation diarrhoea: implications for treatment. Lancet 1986; i:1082–1084.
4. Heymsfield SB. Gastrointestinal anatomic and hormonal differences between enteral and parenteral feeding. In: Greene HL, ed. Enteral nutrition. Amsterdam: Excerpta Medica, 1984: 17.
5. Scrimshaw NS, Béhar M, Arroyave G, Tejada C, Viteri F. Kwashiorkor in children and its response to protein therapy. JAMA 1957; 164:555–558.
6. Dean RFA. Digestion in kwashiorkor. Mod Probl Paediatr 1957; 2:133–145.
7. Stanfield JP, Hith MSR, Tunnicliffe R. Intestinal biopsy in kwashiorkor. Lancet 1965; ii:519–523.
8. Burman D. The jejunal mucosa in kwashiorkor. Arch Dis Child 1965; 40:526–531.
9. Brunser O, Reid A, Mönckeberg F, Maccioni A, Contreras I. Jejunal biopsies in infant malnutrition: with special reference to mitotic index. Pediatrics 1966; 38:1605–1612.
10. Brunser O, Castillo C, Araya M. Fine structure of the small intestinal mucosa in infantile marasmic malnutrition. Gastroenterology 1976; 70:495–507.
11. Martins Campos JV, Fagundes Neto U, Patricio FRS, Wehba J, Carvalho AA, Shiner M. Jejunal mucosa in marasmic children. Clinical, pathological, and fine structural evaluation of the effect of protein-energy malnutrition and environmental contamination. Am J Clin Nutr 1979; 32:1575–1591.
12. Shiner M, Redmond AOB, Hansen JDL. The jejunal mucosa in protein-calorie malnutrition. A clinical, histological and ultrastructural study. Exp Mol Pathol 1973; 19:61–78.
13. Theron JJ, Wittman W, Prinsloo JG. The fine structure of the jejunum in kwashiorkor. Exp Mol Pathol 1979; 14:184–199.
14. Brunser O, Steckel A, Schlesinger L. Fine structure of the small intestinal mucosa in experimental malnutrition. (Abstract) Acta Paediatr Scand 1971; 61:498.
15. Platt BS, Heard CRC, Stewart RJC. The effect of protein-calorie deficiency on the gastrointestinal tract. In: Munro HN, ed. C.I.O.M.S. Symposium on the role of the gastrointestinal tract in protein metabolism. Oxford: Blackwell Scientific, 1964: 227.

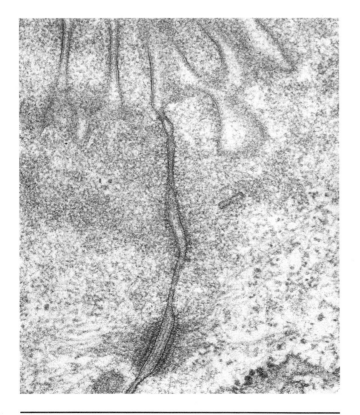

FIGURE 4 Junctional complex in human marasmic malnutrition. Structures appear normal from the morphologic point of view (×60,000). (From Brunser et al.[60])

16. Neutra MR, Maner JH, Mayoral LG. Effects of protein-calorie malnutrition on the jejunal mucosa of tetracycline-treated pigs. Am J Clin Nutr 1974; 27:287–295.

17. Brunser O, Araya M. Damage and repair of small intestinal mucosa in acute and chronic diarrhea. In: Lebenthal E, ed. Chronic diarrhea in children. New York: Nestle Nutrition, Vevey/Raven Press, 1984: 31.

18. Lipkin M, Sherlock P, Bell B. Cell proliferation kinetics in the gastrointestinal tract of man. II. Cell renewal in the stomach, ileum, colon and rectum. Gastroenterology 1963; 45:721–729.

19. MacDonald WC, Trier JS, Everett NB. Cell proliferation and migration in the stomach, duodenum and rectum of man: radioautographic studies. Gastroenterology 1964; 46:406–417.

20. Herbst JJ, Koldovsky O. Cell migration and cortisone induction of sucrase activity in jejunum and ileum. Biochem J 1972; 126:471–476.

21. Baker SS, Suthutvoravut U, Walker WA. Short-term malnutrition in neonatal rabbits. I. Brush border enzymes. J Pediatr Gastroenterol Nutr 1987; 6:961–966.

22. Hopper AF, Rose PM, Wannemacher RW. Cell population changes in the intestinal mucosa of protein-depleted or starved rats. II. Changes in cellular migration rates. J Cell Biol 1972; 53:225–230.

23. Wiebecke B, Heybovitz R, Löhrs U, Eder M. Der einfluss des hungers auf die profiterationskinetic der dünn-und dickdarmschleimhaut der maus. Virchow's Arch [B] 1969; 4:164–175.

24. Hopper AF, Wannemacher RW, McGovern PA. Cell population changes in the intestinal epithelium of the rat following starvation and protein-depletion. Proc Soc Exp Biol Med 1968; 128:695–698.

25. Rose PM, Hopper AF, Wannemacher RW. Cell population changes in the intestinal mucosa of protein depleted or starved rats. I. Changes in the mitotic cycle time. J Cell Biol 1971; 50:887–892.

26. Guiraldes E, Hamilton JR. Effect of chronic malnutrition on intestinal structure, epithelial renewal, and enzymes in suckling rats. Pediatr Res 1981; 15:930–934.

27. Johnson LR, Copeland EM, Dudrick SJ, Lichtenberg LM, Castro GA. Structural and hormonal alterations in the gastrointestinal tract of parenterally fed rats. Gastroenterology 1975; 68:1177–1183.

28. Johnson LR, Lichtenberg LM, Copeland EM, Dudrick SJ, Castro GA. Action of gastrin on gastrointestinal structure and function. Gastroenterology 1975; 68:1184–1193.

29. Gaull GE, Isaacs CE, Wright CE, Kruger L, Tallan HH. Growth modulators in human milk: implications for milk banking. In: Williams AF, Baum JD, eds. Human milk banking. New York: Nestle Nutrition, Vevey/Raven Press, 1984: 63.

30. Altmann GG. Influence of bile and pancreatic secretions on the size of the intestinal villi in the rat. Am J Anat 1971; 132:167–178.

31. Abrams GC, Bauer H, Sprinz H. Influence of the normal flora on mucosal morphology and cellular renewal in the ileum. A comparison of germ-free and conventional mice. Lab Invest 1963; 12:355–364.

32. Gordon HA, Bruckner-Kardoss E. Effect of normal microbial flora on intestinal surface area. Am J Physiol 1961; 210:175–182.

33. Mata LJ, Jimenez F, Cordón M, Rosales R, Prera E, Schneider RE, Viteri F. Gastrointestinal flora of children with protein-calorie malnutrition. Am J Clin Nutr 1972; 25:1118–1126.

34. Gilman RH, Partanen R, Brown KH, Spira WM, Khanam S, Greenberg B, Bloom SR, Ali A. Decreased gastric acid secretion and bacterial colonization of the stomach in severely malnourished Bangledeshi children. Gastroenterology 1988; 94:1308–1314.

35. Schneider RE, Viteri FE. Luminal events of lipid absorption in protein-calorie malnourished children: relationship with nutritional recovery and diarrhea. II. Alterations in bile acid content of duodenal aspirates. Am J Clin Nutr 1974; 27:788–796.

36. Blackburn WR, Vinijchaikul K. The pancreas in kwashiorkor. An electronmicroscopic study. Lab Invest 1969; 20:305–318.

37. Barbezat GO, Hansen JDL. The exocrine pancreas and protein-calorie malnutrition. Pediatrics 1968; 42:77–92.

38. Danús O, Urbina AM, Valenzuela I, Solimano G. The effect of refeeding on pancreatic function in marasmic infants. J Pediatr 1970; 77:334–337.

39. Durie PR, Forstner GG, Gaskin KJ, Weizman Z, Kopelman HR, Ellis L, Largman C. Elevated serum immunoreactive pancreatic cationic trypsinogen in acute malnutrition: evidence of pancreatic damage. J Pediatr 1985; 106:233–238.

40. Holemans K, Lambrechts A. Nitrogen metabolism and fat absorption in malnutrition and in kwashiorkor. J Nutr 1955; 56:477–494.

41. Reddy V. Absorption of fat in kwashiorkor. Indian J Med Res 1972; 60:628–631.

42. Viteri FE, Flores JM, Alvarado J, Behar M. Intestinal malabsorption in malnourished children before and during recovery. Relation between severity of protein deficiency and the malabsorption process. Am J Dig Dis 1973; 18:201–211.

43. Dutra de Oliveira JE, Rolando E. Fat absorption studies in malnourished children. Am J Clin Nutr 1964; 15:287–292.

44. Adibi SA, Allen ER. Impaired absorption rates of essential aminoacids induced by either dietary calorie or protein deprivation in man. Gastroenterology 1970; 59:404–413.

45. Woodd-Walker RB, Hansen JDL, Saunders SJ. The in vitro uptake of lysine and alanine by human jejunal mucosa in protein-calorie malnutrition in gastroenteritis and after neomycin. Acta Paediatr Scand 1972; 61:140–144.

46. Kumar V, Ghai OP, Chase HP. Intestinal dipeptide hydrolase activity in undernourished children. Arch Dis Child 1971; 46:801–804.

47. Bowie MD, Barbezat GO, Hansen JDL. Carbohydrate absorption in malnourished children. Am J Clin Nutr 1967; 20:89–93.

48. Römer H, Urbach R, Gómez MA, López A, Perozo-Ruggeri G, Vegas ME. Moderate and severe protein-energy malnutrition in childhood: effects on jejunal mucosal morphology and disaccharidase activities. J Pediatr Gastroenterol Nutr 1983; 2:459–464.

49. James WPT. Sugar absorption and intestinal motility in children when malnourished and after treatment. Clin Sci 1970; 39:305–318.

50. Coello-Ramírez P, Lifshitz F. Enteric microflora and carbohydrate intolerance in infants with diarrhea. Pediatrics 1972; 49:233–242.

51. Sherman P, Wesley A, Forstner G. Sequential disaccharidase loss in rat intestinal blind loops: impact of malnutrition. Am J Physiol 1985; 248:G626–G632.

52. Arroyave G, Viteri F, Behar M, Scrimshaw NS. Impairment of intestinal absorption of vitamin A palmitate in severe protein malnutrition (kwashiorkor). Am J Clin Nutr 1959; 7:185–190.

53. Ingenbleek Y, Beckers C. Evidence of intestinal malabsorption of iodine in protein-calorie malnutrition. Am J Clin Nutr 1973; 26:1323–1330.

54. Gürson GT, Saner G. D-Xylose test in the marasmic type of protein-calorie malnutrition. Helv Pediatr Acta 1969; 24:510–518.

55. Karasov WH, Diamond JM. Adaptation of intestinal nutrient transport. In: Johnson LR, ed. Physiology of the gastrointestinal tract. 2nd ed. New York: Raven Press, 1987: 1489.

56. Heyman M, Boudraa G, Sarrut S, Giraud M, Evans L, Touhami M, Desjeux JF. Macromolecular transport in jejunal mucosa of children with severe malnutrition: a quantitative study. J Pediatr Gastroenterol Nutr 1984; 3:357–363.

57. Enwonwu CO. Potential relevance of impaired histidine metabolism to the immunodeficiency in human protein-energy malnutrition. Nutr Res 1986; 6:337–348.

58. Stinnett JD. Nutrition and the immune response. Boca Raton, FL: CRC Press, 1983: 111.

59. Behrens RH, Lunn PG, Northrop CA, Hanlon PW, Neale G. Factors affecting the integrity of the intestinal mucosa of Gambian children. Am J Clin Nutr 1987; 45:1433–1441.

60. Brunser O, Araya M, Espinoza J. Gastrointestinal tract changes in the malnourished child. In: Suskind RM, Lewinter-Suskind, eds. The malnourished child. Vevey: Nestec Ltd; New York: Raven Press, 1990: 261.

PART 24

Secondary Enzyme Deficiencies

Fayez K. Ghishan, M.D.

Carbohydrates in the diet of infants, children, and adults provide a substantial portion of total calories ingested. Lactose in the milk is the main carbohydrate source for infants, whereas starch accounts for 60 percent of total carbohydrates in adults. Sucrose and lactose account for 30 and 10 percent, respectively.[1] Malabsorption of carbohydrates occurs secondary to congenital defects in the intestinal brush border enzymes involved in the hydrolysis of a specific carbohydrate[2–7] or secondary to an iatrogenic insult causing damage to the functional integrity of the small intestine.[8–11] Congenital defects in the hydrolysis of specific carbohydrates such as congenital lactase or sucrase-isomaltase deficiencies are rather rare and generally present at birth. Secondary enzyme deficiencies are common clinical problems worldwide and can present at any age secondary to various insults to the intestinal tract. Table 1 depicts a list of the known secondary enzyme defects.

PHYSIOLOGY OF CARBOHYDRATE DIGESTION AND ABSORPTION

Carbohydrates are divided as simple monosaccharides (glucose, fructose, and galactose), disaccharides (lactose, sucrose, maltose), or polysaccharides. Monosaccharides are the end result of hydrolysis of disaccharides and polysaccharides and are rarely found in the normal diet. Glucose and galactose are transported across the enterocyte by a carrier-mediated process requiring the inwardly directed sodium gradient which is maintained by the Na^+,K^+-ATPase pump located at the basolateral membrane of the enterocytes.[12] The exit across the basolateral membrane of the enterocyte occurs by a carrier-mediated process not requiring sodium.[13] Disaccharides are maltose (two glucose limits), lactose (galactose and glucose), and sucrose (glucose and fructose). These sugars are commonly found in the diet and are hydrolyzed by brush border enzymes such as maltase, sucrase, and lactose. The development of the disaccharidases is critical to the digestive process of the sugars, especially for premature infants.[14–17] Figure 1 depicts disaccharidase activities of jejunal mucosa of human fetuses in relationship to lunar months of

TABLE 1
Secondary Enzyme Deficiencies

Enterokinase deficiency
Disaccharide deficiencies
   Lactase deficiency
   Sucrase-isomaltase deficiency
Glucoamylase deficiency

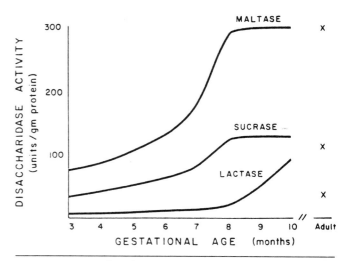

FIGURE 1 Disaccharidase activity of jejunal mucosa of human fetus in relation to lunar months of gestational age. (Modified from Auricchio S, et al. In: Younoszai MK. Gastrointestinal function during infancy, infant nutrition, 2nd ed. Philadelphia: WB Saunders, 1974.)

gestational age. Sucrase-isomaltase, maltase, and trehalase are alpha-glucosidases and attain maximal activity by the eighth lunar month of gestation. The activities of sucrase-isomaltase and maltase are greater than the activity of lactase.[14–16] Lactase activity, a beta-galactosidase, is low before 24 weeks of gestation and increases markedly toward term. It is estimated that preterm infants born before 32 weeks of gestation can hydrolyze only one-third the quantity of lactose hydrolyzed by full-term infants.[10] Lactase activity remains high in the small intestine of full-term babies and remains elevated throughout the infancy period. After the infancy period, in certain populations such as blacks, lactase activity declines so that by early childhood (6 to 10 years) lactose malabsorption becomes evident. This condition is termed primary late-onset lactase deficiency and affects a high percentage (80 percent) of certain populations such as Asians, Jews, blacks, and American Indians.[18–20]

Complex carbohydrates in the form of starches consist of polymers of glucose either in linkage between 1 and 4 carbons (amylose) or between 1 and 6 branch linkages (amylopectin). Starch digestion begins with the action of salivary and pancreatic amylases, which are specific for the internal 1-4 linkage, resulting in maltoses. Following luminal action of amylases, the residual units are in the form of maltose (two glucose units), maltotriose (three glucoses), and alpha-dextrins (a mixture of maltose and maltotriose in 1-6 linkage). These sugars are broken down by mucosal amylases.

Glucoamylase is one of those enzymes responsible for the digestion of glucose polymers (maltodextrine and corn syrup solids).

PATHOPHYSIOLOGY

Disaccharidase deficiencies are due to either a congenital defect or a late-onset genetically determined deficiency or secondary to small intestinal injury. Secondary enzyme deficiencies may involve one or more of the disaccharidases,[8–11] enterokinase[21] or glucoamylase,[22] depending on the severity of the injury. Disaccharidase deficiencies are the most commonly encountered entities following intestinal injury. Table 2 depicts the causes of secondary mucosal enzyme deficiencies. Because the disaccharidases are localized at the luminal surface of the enterocyte membranes, any insult, whether viral or immunologic, to the enterocyte results in a decrease in disaccharidase level. Moreover, it is clear from a number of studies that lactase deficiency is the most common, whereas glucoamylase and enterokinase deficiencies are exceedingly rare. The reasons for the frequent occurrence of lactase deficiency with intestinal injury are not well known. It is conceivable that because the activity of lactase is lower than that of other mucosal enzymes as well as because of the distal location of lactase on the villus tip, lactase may degrade earlier than other enzymes.[23] Alternatively, it appears that certain proteolytic enzymes preferentially attack lactase.[24] In support of this concept, pancreatic enzymes were reported to reduce lactase activity in intestinal biopsies to a greater extent than other disaccharidases when fed to patients with pancreatic insufficiency.[24] Malnutrition per se was suggested as a factor resulting in disaccharidase, deficiencies; however, animal models of malnutrition failed to show a decrease in mucosal enzyme activities.[25] It is possible that other factors working in conjunction with malnutrition may predispose to a decrease in disaccharidase activity. Malnutrition coupled with bacterial overgrowth in an animal model caused a more severe decrease in lactase activity, and the decrease was extended to include other disaccharidases such as maltase and sucrase.[26]

The end result of mucosal enzyme deficiencies is diarrhea, which can progress to malnutrition in susceptible infants. In the setting of disaccharidase deficiencies, the offending sugars are not hydrolyzed in the small intestine, thereby passing to the colon, where fermentation occurs, resulting in the production of organic acids such as lactic acid, which generates an osmotic load leading to secretion of fluid to the colonic lumen. Studies have shown that 42 to 75 percent of a lactose load is recovered in the ileum of a lactase-deficient individual, whereas only 8 to 10 percent may be present in a normal control.[27] Therefore, normally in 24 hours, the stool contains no more than 30 to 40 mg of lactic acid, whereas in lactase-deficient subjects, the level may reach more than 1,000 mg. The stool pH in such a situation is well below 5.5. The presence of such an osmotic load may lead to an increase in intestinal motility with increased transit time.[28] During the process of fermentation, H_2 gas is generated.[29] In normal men, approximately 84 to 90 percent of H_2 that is produced by fermentation of unabsorbed carbohydrate is eliminated with flatus. The remaining H_2 is excreted by the lungs. The factors that tend to minimize or maximize the degree of carbohydrate malabsorption clearly depend on the severity of the intestinal injury, the degree of decrease in disaccharidases, the ingested carbohydrate load, associated malnutrition, and the status of the immune system.[30–32] The major complication of continued ingestion of sugars that cannot be hydrolyzed is chronic diarrhea with continued losses of fluids, electrolytes, minerals, and trace elements. Such losses have been documented in animal models of osmotic diarrhea, especially during the suckling period.[33] Chronic diarrhea can lead to malnutrition with secondary bacterial overgrowth of the small intestine which may aggravate disaccharidase deficiency, thus resulting in a vicious circle of enzyme deficiencies → chronic diarrhea → malnutrition → enzyme deficiencies. Interruption of this cycle is essential to restore normal intestinal function.

In the case of enterokinase deficiency, an enzyme known to activate trypsinogen to trypsin, which catalyzes the other proteolytic enzymes, a predominantly protein maldigestion occurs. Congenital defects in enterokinase have been reported in nine patients. All the patients had diarrhea and failure to thrive with hypoproteinemia.[34] Secondary enterokinase deficiency has been reported in infants with mucosal injury secondary to chronic intractable diarrhea and cow's milk enteropathy but not in patients with celiac disease.[21] These observations cast doubt about the topographic localization of the enterokinase. In fact, Takano et al suggested that enterokinase is present in goblet cells and that the differential level of enterokinase activity in celiac disease versus small intestinal atrophy from chronic intractable diarrhea may be related to the degree of goblet cell depletion.[35]

Secondary glucoamylase deficiency has been described in patients with severe mucosal injury,[22] although theoretically it may lead to amylase maldigestion. Its clinical significance is minimal. Congenital glucoamylase deficiency has not been described.

TABLE 2
Small Intestinal Injuries Resulting in Secondary Deficiencies

---

Celiac disease
Bacterial overgrowth
Cow's milk enteropathy
Giardiasis
Rotavirus infection
Chronic protracted diarrhea
Protein-energy malnutrition
Crohn's disease of the small intestine
Short bowel syndrome
Drugs: neomycin, kanamycin, colchicine
Immunodeficiency syndromes
Radiation enteritis

CLINICAL ASPECTS OF SECONDARY ENZYME DEFICIENCIES

The most common carbohydrate malabsorption secondary to enzyme deficiencies is disaccharidase deficiency, which is generally seen with mucosal injury of the small intestine. The onset of symptoms can occur shortly after the injury. The degree of the deficiency is related to the extent of the villous injury. The symptoms depend on the load of the offending sugar and the extent of the deficiency. The symptoms include abdominal cramping, watery diarrhea, and bloating with flatulence. In younger infants, the symptoms may be more severe secondary to greater losses of water and electrolytes. In general, symptoms secondary to congenital defects in mucosal enzymes appear at birth with intolerance to breast milk or modified cow's milk formula containing the offending sugar. These infants appear healthy at birth. The diagnosis of disaccharidase deficiency is based on a number of clinical and laboratory parameters. A clinical history of mucosal injury such as celiac disease or chronic protracted diarrhea should alert the physician to the possibility of secondary enzyme deficiency. The laboratory investigation of secondary enzyme deficiency includes the following:

1. *Stool examination:* The stools are generally watery, with pH below 5.5 due to the presence of organic acids. Reducing substances can be detected easily by diluting one part of the stool with one part of watery and then adding one Clinitest tablet. An orange color is easily noted if sugars are present. The intensity of the color can be graded from 0.5 percent to 2 percent. It is important to note that sucrose is not a reducing substance; therefore, addition of 10 drops of 0.1 N HCl is recommended to hydrolyze the sucrose to glucose and galactose, followed by addition of the Clinitest tablet. Because of the presence of organic acids in the stools, its osmolality will be greater than the sum of $(Na^+ + K^+) \times 2$; however, in secretory diarrhea the stool osmolality equals the sum of $(Na^+ + K^+) \times 2$. Table 3 depicts the differential diagnosis between osmotic and secretory diarrhea.

2. *Oral tolerance tests:* This test is based on the observation that a rise in blood glucose is expected if a disaccharide is hydrolyzed within the intestine after its oral ingestion. In the event of an enzyme deficiency, the disaccharide is not hydrolyzed in the small intestine, resulting in less glucose to be transported, thus generating a flat serum glucose curve.

The suspected disaccharide is given at 2 mg per kilogram in a 10 percent solution after 6 hours of fasting. Blood glucose is measured at 0, 30, 60, 90, and 120 minutes. A rise of greater than 25 mg per deciliter over baseline is considered normal. The advantages of the oral tests relate to their simplicity and the ability to correlate clinical symptoms with results. The disadvantages are related to additional factors that may interfere with the results, such as delayed gastric emptying[36] and intestinal transit time. Increased peripheral utilization may also decrease the blood level of glucose, but this can be minimized by measurement of capillary blood glucose, since capillary glucose peak levels are higher than venous levels.[37] Moreover, it is important to note that 30 percent of normal healthy adults who tolerate lactose in their diet may have a flat glucose curve after lactose load. In a study comparing various indirect methods of detecting lactose deficiency, the oral lactose tolerance test had a 24 percent (6/25) false-negative rate and a 4 percent (1/25) false-positive rate.[38]

A precautionary note is essential when performing oral tolerance tests, especially in young infants with chronic diarrhea and malnutrition because of the potential for significant water and electrolyte losses in severe disaccharidase deficiency, resulting in significant dehydration and possible shock.

3. *Measurement of mucosal activity of disaccharidases:* Determination of the mucosal activity of disaccharidases has been used in the overall management of patients with disaccharide intolerance. However, the limitation of such an invasive approach and lack of correlation between symptoms and mucosal disaccharidase measurements make the determination of disaccharidase activity of limited value. Sampling errors because of partial and patchy mucosal injury are probably the major limiting factor in the utilization of disaccharidase activity.[39,40]

4. *Breath hydrogen tests:* This test is based on the observation that when malabsorbed carbohydrates reach the colon and are fermented by the colonic bacteria, H_2 gas is formed and approximately 10 to 15 percent is eliminated through the lungs.[29] Therefore, determination of H_2 concentration in breath samples might serve as a useful tool for the evaluation of carbohydrate malabsorption. The test has gained popularity because of its noninvasive nature; however, the test has certain limitations that need to be taken into account when interpreting the results of H_2 concentration in the breath.

The test is performed by administration of the test substrate (lactose or sucrose 2 g per kilogram orally after 8 hours of fasting). H_2 concentration in expired breath is determined at basal level and every 30 minutes for 4 hours. The end-expired tidal air is collected at the nose through a mask or a small nasal prong attached to a 50-ml syringe. The air may also be collected through a small intranasal tube positioned just below the base of the tongue in the posterior pharynx. Three to 5 ml of air is aspirated toward the end of each breath until approximately 30 ml have been collected.[41] H_2 concentrations in the samples are determined by gas-liquid chromatography. A portable machine is now available from Quintron Instrument Company (Milwaukee, WI).

Certain considerations need to be taken into account when performing a breath H_2 test. First the basal level of H_2 may be high in certain individuals, precluding accurate rise in H_2 following carbohydrate malabsorption. Second, the amount of carbohydrate reaching the colon may differ among patients; therefore, breath H_2 concentration may differ from one patient to another. Third, colonic pH may influence the production of H_2. In vitro studies have shown that optimal degradation of glucose, paralleled by release of H_2, occurred at pH 7.0 to 7.5. Inhibition of bacterial glucose metabolism and H_2 production occurred at acid pH.[43] The effect of pH on H_2 production from glucose metabolism was reproduced with lactose and sucrose.[43] Fourth, antibiotic use may alter

TABLE 3
Differential Diagnosis of Osmotic and Secretory Diarrhea

Stools	Osmotic Diarrhea	Secretory Diarrhea
Electrolytes	Na <70 mEq/liter	Na >70 mEq/liter
Osmolality	$> (Na^+ + K^+) \times 2$	$= (Na^+ + K^+) \times 2$
pH	<5	>6
Reducing substances	Positive	Negative
Volume	<200 ml/day	>200 mg/day

the bacterial flora and diminish H_2 production. Fifth, the presence of anaerobic bacteria in the small bowel may give a false-positive breath H_2. Finally, the absence of adequate H_2-producing colonic flora can give a false-negative breath hydrogen.[44]

DIFFERENTIAL DIAGNOSIS

Chronic diarrhea secondary to disaccharidase deficiency presents with osmotic diarrhea, which should be differentiated from secretory diarrhea. Table 3 depicts the main points of the differential diagnosis. Clinically, however, elimination of offending carbohydrate results in amelioration of symptoms, whereas in secretory diarrhea the patient continues to have diarrhea despite taking nothing by mouth. Secondary enzyme deficiencies can be differentiated from congenital enzyme defects by their late onset and a history of a preceding mucosal injury. The severity of underlying mucosal injury determines the nutritional and clinical status of the patient. For example, the diarrhea of a patient with celiac disease may not improve upon the elimination of lactose from their diet because of the underlying flat mucosa with malabsorption of various nutrients.

Table 4 depicts a schematic approach for differential diagnosis of chronic diarrhea and secondary enzyme deficiencies.

TABLE 4

Secondary Enzyme Deficiencies: Determination of the Offending Carbohydrate—Algorithm

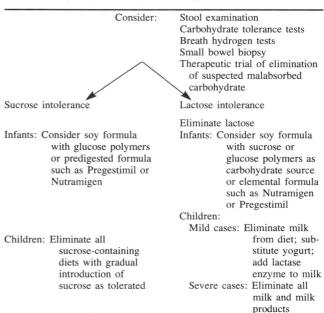

Consider: Stool examination
Carbohydrate tolerance tests
Breath hydrogen tests
Small bowel biopsy
Therapeutic trial of elimination of suspected malabsorbed carbohydrate

Sucrose intolerance

Infants: Consider soy formula with glucose polymers or predigested formula such as Pregestimil or Nutramigen

Children: Eliminate all sucrose-containing diets with gradual introduction of sucrose as tolerated

Lactose intolerance

Eliminate lactose
Infants: Consider soy formula with sucrose or glucose polymers as carbohydrate source or elemental formula such as Nutramigen or Pregestimil
Children:
Mild cases: Eliminate milk from diet; substitute yogurt; add lactase enzyme to milk
Severe cases: Eliminate all milk and milk products

CLINICAL COURSE

The clinical course of secondary enzyme deficiency depends largely on the extent and severity of the underlying disease. Every effort should be made to identify the primary intestinal insult and to institute therapy, coupled with elimination of the offending carbohydrate. Recovery in general may take days to weeks, depending on the underlying injury. Studies utilizing breath hydrogen tests in infants with rotavirus infection had shown an incidence of 30 to 50 percent lactose intolerance. The mean recovery was 2 to 4 weeks after the acute enteritis. However, in infants less than 6 months old, the average recovery time was 4 to 8 weeks.[45-46] The long-term prognosis is excellent if appropriate therapeutic modulates are utilized for the primary mucosal disease.

TREATMENT

Treatment of secondary disaccharidase deficiency includes elimination of the offending carbohydrate from the diet and therapy of the underlying mucosal injury. Table 4 depicts a practical approach to therapy of disaccharidase deficiency. In infants with disaccharidase deficiency, a dietary change to an elemental formula in which the carbohydrate source is glucose polymers is essential; however, it is clear that such a change also constitutes a change from unmodified milk protein to protein hydrolysate, thus making it different to differentiate whether the cause was lactose or the unmodified protein.

Secondary sucrose intolerance is seen only in severe cases of diarrhea. In contrast to lactase, sucrase can be induced by its substrate. Early reintroduction of sucrose, as tolerat-

ed, is desirable to induce sucrase activity. The management of sucrose intolerance in infants requires a dietary change to a formula containing glucose polymers. In older children, elimination of the offending disaccharide from the diet is advisable. In mild cases of lactase deficiency, yogurt can be substituted for milk, as it contains beta-galactosidase activity, which hydrolyzes lactose to glucose and galactose.[47,48] Lactase is also available as Lact-Aid (Sugar Low Company, Atlantic City, NJ) drops or tablets, which can be added to the milk, resulting in hydrolysis of lactose to glucose and galactose.

REFERENCES

1. Gray GM. Carbohydrate digestion and absorption. N Engl J Med 1975; 292:1225.
2. Antonowicz I, Lloyd-Still JD, Khaw KT. et al. Congenital sucrase-isomalton deficiency. Pediatrics 1972; 49:847.
3. Burgen EA, Levin B, Mahalanatis D. et al. Hereditary sucrase intolerance. Levels of sucrase activity in jejunal mucosa. Arch Dis Child 1964; 39:431.
4. Holzel A, Schwarz V, Stucliffe KW. Defective lactose absorption causing malnutrition in infancy. Lancet 1959;i:1126.
5. Auricchio S, Rubino A, Landholt M. et al. Isolated intestinal lactase deficiency in the adult. Lancet 1963; ii:324.
6. Savilahti E, Launiala K, Kuitunen L. Congenital lactase deficiency. A clinical study on 16 patients. Arch Dis Child 1983; 58:246.
7. Rossi E, Hadorn B. Congenital enzyme deficiencies of the small intestine: molecular basis and nutritional and therapeutic implications. J Pediatr Gastroenterol Nutr 1983; 2(suppl):S321.
8. Gracey M, Burke V. Sugar induced diarrhea in children. Arch Dis Child 1973; 48:331.
9. Harries JT. Disorders of carbohydrate absorption. Clin Gastroenterol 1982; 11:17.

10. Davidson GP, Goodwin D, Robb TA. Incidence and duration of lactose malabsorption in children hospitalized with acute enteritis: study in a well nourished urban population. J Pediatr 1984; 105:587.

11. Hyams JS, Krause PJ, Gleason PN. Lactose malabsorption following rotavirus injection in young children. J Pediatr 1981; 99:916.

12. Ghishan FK, Wilson FA. Developmental maturation of D-glucose transport by rat jejunal brush border membrane vesicles. Am J Physiol 1985; 248:G87–G91.

13. Wright EM, Van Os AC, Mircheff AC. Sugar uptake by intestinal basolateral membrane vesicles. Biochim Biophys Acta 1980; 597:112.

14. Antonowicz I, Lebenthal E. Developmental pattern of small intestinal enterokinase and disaccharidase activities in the human fetus. Gastroenterology 1977; 72:1299.

15. Auricchio S, Rubino A, Murset G. Intestinal glycosidase activities in the human embryo, fetus and newborn. Pediatrics 1965; 35:944.

16. Dahlquist A, Lindberg T. Fetal development of the small intestinal disaccharidase and alkaline phosphatase activities in the human. Biol Neonate 1966; 9:24.

17. Mobassaleh M, Montgomery RK, Biller JA, Grand R. Development of carbohydrate absorption in the fetus and neonate. Pediatrics 1985; 75(suppl):160.

18. Bayless TM, Rosenweig NS. A racial difference in incidence of lactase deficiency. JAMA 1966; 197:968.

19. Huany SS, Bayless TM. Milk and lactose intolerance in healthy orientals. Science 1966; 160:83.

20. Simoons FJ. The geographic hypothesis and lactose malabsorption. Am J Dig Dis 1978; 23:963.

21. Lebenthal E, Antonowicz I, Schwachman H. Enterokinase and trypsin activities in pancreatic insufficiency and disease of the small intestine. Gastroenterology 1976; 70:508.

22. Lebenthal E, Lee PC. Glucoamylase and disaccharidase activities in normal subjects and in patients with mucosal injury of the small intestine. J Pediatr 1980; 97:389.

23. Boyle JT, Celano P, Koldovsky O. Demonstration of a difference in expression of maximal lactase and sucrase activity along the villus in the adult rat jejunum. Gastroenterology 1980; 79:503.

24. Seetharam B, Pezzilo R, Alpers DH. Effect of pancreatic proteases on intestinal lactase activity. Gastroenterology 1980; 79:827.

25. Adams JL, Leichter. Effect of protein deficient diets with various amounts of carbohydrate on intestinal disaccharidase activities in the rat. J Nutr 1973; 103:1716.

26. Sherman P, Wesley A, Forstner G. Sequential disaccharidase loss in rat intestinal blind loops: impact of malnutrition. Am J Physiol 1985; 248:G626.

27. Bond JH, Levih MD. Quantitative measurement of lactose absorption. Gastroenterology 1976; 70:1058.

28. Launiala K. The effect of unabsorbed sucrose and mannitol on the small intestinal flow rate and mean transit time. Scand J Gastroenterol 1968; 39:665.

29. Levitt MD. Production and excretion of hydrogen gas in man. N Engl J Med 1969; 281:122.

30. Lifschitz F, Coello-/Ramirez P, Conteras-Gutierrez ML. The response of infants to carbohydrate oral loads after recovery from diarrhea. J Pediatr 1971; 79:612.

31. Brunser O, Reid A, Monckeberg RGF. Jejunal mucosa in infant malnutrition. Am J Clin Nutr 1968; 21:976.

32. Sriratanaban A, Thayer WR. Small intestinal disaccharidase activities in experimental iron and protein deficiency. Am J Clin Nutr 1971; 24:411.

33. Ghishan FK, Parker P, Helinek J. Intestinal maturation: effect of luminal osmolality on net mineral secretion. Pediatr Res 1981; 15:985.

34. Ghishan FK, Lee PC, Lebenthal E, Johnson P, Bradley CA, Greene HL. Isolated congenital enterokinase deficiency: recent findings and review of the literature. Gastroenterology 1983; 85:727–731.

35. Takano K, Suzuki T, Yasuda K. Immunohistochemical localization of enterokinase in the porcine intestine. Okajimas Folia Anat Jpn 1971; 48:15.

36. Kern F, Sutruthers JE. Intestinal lactase deficiency and lactose intolerance in adults. JAMA 1966; 195:927.

37. McGill DB, Newcomer AD. Comparison of venous and capillary blood samples in lactose tolerance testing. Gastroenterology 1967; 53:371.

38. Newcomer AD, McGill DB, Thomas PJ, Hofman AF. Prospective comparison of indirect methods for detecting lactase deficiency. N Engl J Med 1975; 293:1232.

39. Harrison M, Walker-Smith JA. Reinvestigation of lactose intolerant children: lack of correlation between continuing lactose intolerance and small intestinal morphology, disaccharidase activity and lactose tolerance tests. Gut 1977; 18:48.

40. Hyams JS, Stafford RJ, Grand RJ, Watkins JB. Correlation of lactose breath hydrogen test, intestinal morphology and lactose activity in young children. J Pediatr 1980; 97:609.

41. Barr RG, Perman JA, Schoeller DA, Watkins JB. Breath tests in pediatric gastrointestinal disorders—new diagnostic opportunities. Pediatrics 1978; 62:393.

42. Maffei HVL, Metz GL, Jenkins DJA. Hydrogen breath tests: adaptation of a simple technique to infants and children. Lancet 1976; 1:1110.

43. Perman JA, Modles S, Olson AC. role of pH in production of hydrogen from carbohydrates by colonic bacterial flora. J Clin Invest 1981; 67:643.

44. Lifschitz CH. Breath hydrogen testing in infants with diarrhea. In: Lifshitz F, ed. Carbohydrate intolerance in infants. New York: Dekker, 1987:31.

45. Hyams JS, Krause PJ, Gleason PA. Lactose malabsorption following rotavirus infection in young children. J Pediatr 1981; 99:916.

46. Davidson GP, Goodwin D, Robb T. Incidence and duration of lactose malabsorption in children hospitalized with acute enteritis: study in a well nourished urban population. J Pediatr 1984; 105:587.

47. Kolars JC, Levitt MD, Aouji M, Savaiano DA. Yogurt: an autodigesting source of lactose. N Engl J Med 1984; 310:1.

48. Payne DL, Welsh JD, Manion CV, Tsegaye A, Herd LD. Effectiveness of milk products in dietary management of lactose malabsorption. Am J Clin Nutr 1981; 34:2711.

Idiopathic Prolonged Diarrhea

Kenneth H. Brown, M.D.

Robert E. Black, M.D., M.P.H.

Idiopathic prolonged diarrhea (IPD) is a disorder of infancy and childhood characterized by diarrhea of abrupt onset that continues for more than 2 or 3 weeks. For the purpose of this review, diarrhea is defined as an increased frequency of bowel movements that are of reduced consistency or excessive water content. The etiology of IPD remains uncertain, although a number of contributory mechanisms have been postulated. Other terms, such as *persistent postenteritis diarrhea*, have been used to describe this syndrome, which begins after the newborn period, a feature that distinguishes it from most congenital abnormalities of the gastrointestinal (GI) tract. Other distinct illnesses, such as protein-sensitive enteropathy and so-called intractable diarrhea of early infancy are considered elsewhere in this text.

EPIDEMIOLOGY

Diarrhea of abrupt onset is most commonly caused by a specific enteric infection or exposure to enterotoxins.[1] These illnesses generally are short-lived, with a median duration of less than 1 week. The duration of diarrheal illnesses, however, follows a continuous unimodal distribution that is skewed to the right.[1-4] Thus, a small proportion of cases persist for a longer period, and the distinction between acute and prolonged episodes is somewhat arbitrary. Usually, a minimum of 2 or 3 weeks' duration has been used to define IPD.

The incidence of IPD is highest in situations in which enteric infections are common, suggesting a link between the two problems. Young children living in unsanitary conditions are at greatest risk of both acute diarrhea and IPD. Prospective, community-based epidemiologic studies in less-developed countries have found that between 2 and 20 percent of all diarrheal episodes last for more than 2 weeks, but nearly all resolve within 2 months.[1-4] Because children in less-developed countries may experience an average of up to 10 episodes of diarrhea during each of the first 3 years of life, their risk of IPD is correspondingly increased.[1-4]

Virulence factors inherent to individual infectious agents as well as specific host factors may influence the incidence of IPD. Because some organisms may be more likely to induce IPD, the epidemiology of these agents will influence the relative frequency of the syndrome. In Bangladesh, for example, *Shigella*-associated dysentery is particularly common, especially in older children; and these illnesses are more likely to become prolonged.[1] The incidence of IPD reflects to some extent the occurrence of *Shigella* infections in that setting. Other studies have implicated enteroadherent, enteropathogenic, or enterotoxigenic *Escherichia coli, Campylobacter jejuni, Aeromonas hydrophila, Giardia lamblia, Entamoeba histolytica,* and *Cryptosporidium* in prolonged diarrhea. As described below, these infectious agents may cause prolonged diarrhea either because the infection itself is persistent or because they induce complications that prolong the period of symptomatic disease. In some circumstances it may be impossible to assign a causal role to agents isolated from patients with IPD because the same organisms are found in an identical proportion of symptom-free individuals in the same area. *C. jejuni* and *G. lamblia* can be isolated from a sizable proportion of children with IPD in some settings, but a similar proportion of well children may also harbor these agents. Thus, the relationship between these enteric infections and IPD remains uncertain in those areas where the infections are endemic.

Risk factors for IPD appear to include the host's age, nutritional status, and immunologic competence, as well as dietary practices and other therapeutic interventions applied before or during acute diarrhea. The age of the child is related clearly to the incidence of all diarrhea and, in some studies, to the proportion of all episodes that become prolonged.[1-4] It is not known, however, exactly how age affects the risk of IPD. It is possible that age merely acts as a proxy for other important risk factors, such as nutritional status or immunologic development. The status of passively acquired immunologic protection, such as maternal IgG and breast milk IgA, is also age-dependent, as in the integrity of non-immunologic barriers to infection; such as gastric acidity.[5,6]

The duration of diarrhea in malnourished children, including illnesses associated with specific pathogens, is significantly more prolonged than in their better-nourished counterparts.[7] Experimental studies have identified similar negative relationships between nutritional status and diarrheal duration.[8] GI abnormalities that occur in malnourished children, like reduced concentrations of intestinal mucosal enzymes, pancreatic insufficiency, and bacterial colonization of the small intestine, may contribute to the severity of infection-induced malabsorption and the ultimate duration of illness.[9,10] Delayed renewal of the intestinal mucosa following infection in malnourished individuals and malnutrition-induced immunodeficiency may similarly prolong the duration of symptoms.[8,11]

Whether deficiencies of specific micronutrients affect the incidence of IPD is unknown, but those nutrients required for intestinal mucosal renewal or immunologic competence may be important. Increased incidence rates of diarrhea have been reported recently in children with vitamin A deficiency, but it is not known whether these children had episodes that were prolonged.[12] Deficiencies of folic acid and of nicotinic acid may result in prolonged diarrhea.[13,14] These or other micronutrients may be involved in the pathogenesis of IPD.

Suboptimal immunologic responses, whether secondary to young age, malnutrition, infection, or underlying congenital abnormalities, may increase the risk of IPD. Severely malnourished children have defects in cell-mediated and secretory immune responses.[11] Systemic infections, such as measles, can also reduce immunologic competence, even in well-nourished children. In community-based studies, children recovering from measles were found to have an increased incidence of diarrhea compared with children who had not had measles, and the duration of illness and the case-fatality rates were greater in the post-measles patients.[15] Children who did not respond to intradermally applied common antigens, indicating depressed cellular immune function, had more prolonged diarrheal episodes than those with greater responsiveness, even after controlling for nutritional status.[16]

Dietary factors, including actual feeding practices as well as the kind and amounts of specific foods consumed before and during diarrhea, also can affect the duration of diarrheal illness. Feeding practices may influence the child's exposure to enteropathogens and the duration of illnesses. For example, breast-fed children living in unhygienic environments are less likely to have diarrhea than their non–breast-fed counterparts, and the duration of illness tends to be reduced in breast-fed infants.[17,18]

Malabsorption of carbohydrates occurs often during and after acute diarrhea.[19] Continued feeding of incompletely absorbed carbohydrates can result in an osmotic diarrhea that prolongs the duration of the original illness. Other dietary components may likewise extend the duration of diarrhea, but available information does not permit an assessment of the frequency of these later complications. Protein-sensitive enteropathy, which may develop transiently in a small proportion of young infants with acute diarrhea, does not appear to be an important problem in older children. The relationship between acute diarrhea and the development of protein sensitivity is unknown, but increased permeability of the mucosa to macromolecules has been reported during enteric infections. Plant lectins, another dietary component, have been used to induce prolonged diarrhea in experimental animal models,[21] but the role of lectins in naturally occurring human disease is not known.

Clearly, treatment of acute diarrhea may shorten or prolong the course of illness. Whereas appropriate antibiotic treatment of those enteric infections, such as cholera and shigellosis, that respond to antimicrobial therapy may reduce the length of disease, inappropriate therapy may prolong the illness. Drugs that produce pseudomembranous colitis by permitting the overgrowth of *Clostridium difficile,* for example, can induce prolonged diarrhea.[22] Likewise, antimotility drugs may prolong the course of dysentery.[23]

POSSIBLE MECHANISMS

IPD may result either from persistence of an initial infection, with its attendant injury to the intestinal mucosa, or from a series of other complications of the primary illness. The pathogenesis of the syndrome is not fully understood, but a number of hypothetical mechanisms have been proposed. It is difficult or in many cases impossible to distinguish between those factors that contribute to the occurrence of the disease and those that are complications. Probably IPD is a multifactorial disorder, although certain factors are undoubtedly of greater importance in individual patients.

Enteric infection may persist because certain organisms are particularly virulent or because the host is unable to eliminate the pathogen. Among the multiple enteric pathogens that can lead to IPD, various forms of pathogenic *E. coli* may play a prominent part. Enterotoxigenic *E. coli* has been associated with prolonged diarrhea in children in developing countries,[1] although it is unclear exactly what role they are playing. "Classic" enteropathogenic serotypes manifesting a variety of forms of adherence to tissue culture cells have been shown to cause small bowel pathology resulting in prolonged diarrhea in children.[24,25] The strains of enteroadherent *E. coli* may be of particular importance as causes of prolonged diarrhea. Likewise, in some areas *Shigella* spp. can cause prolonged dysenteric illnesses.[1]

As noted above, impaired host responses may occur in younger infants or may result from preceding infections or undernutrition. Whether or not the original infection persists, the mucosal damage induced by the infection may unleash a series of events that produce continued illness. Infection-induced maldigestion and malabsorption, as well as the secondary malnutrition that is the product of reduced intake and absorption of nutrients, can all contribute to the duration of illness.

Maldigestion of carbohydrates may occur when the intestinal mucosal surface area and/or the concentration of brush border carbohydrases is reduced by specific infectious agents. Not only can incompletely absorbed dietary carbohydrates increase the severity of diarrhea, but they may contribute to the colonization of the small intestine by colonic bacteria.[26] Maldigestion of fats may occur because of pancreatic or biliary insufficiency or because of mucosal injury.[27] Biliary insufficiency, in turn, may result from bacterial colonization of the small intestine or from interruption of the enterohepatic circulation due to ileal mucosal injury. Not only does steatorrhea increase the nutritional impact of the disease, but hydroxylated fatty acids produced by colonic bacteria from incompletely absorbed dietary fats can increase colonic mucosal secretion and the severity of diarrhea. Secondary malnutrition, resulting from malabsorption and illness-associated anorexia, may reduce the rate of intestinal mucosal renewal and recovery of pancreatic function and immune responses, thus perpetuating the syndrome.

CLINICAL AND LABORATORY FEATURES

The major clinical features of IPD are mild to moderately severe diarrhea and malabsorption. The stools, which are loose or watery, may contain mucus and blood if the initial infection produced a dysenteric illness. Evidence of carbohydrate malabsorption (fecal pH < 6.5, reducing substances) and/or steatorrhea (greasy, foul-smelling stools) may be present. Generally, once the illness has persisted for a sufficient length of time to be considered "prolonged," the rate of purging is not so severe as to produce clinically detectable dehydration. However, superimposed infections or carbohydrate intolerance may result in severe diarrhea and dehydration.

Children with IPD may be uncomfortable and irritable or may appear to be unaffected by the disease. Fever may or may not be present. Some, but not all, studies report partial anorexia among some patients. Nutrient intake may also be reduced by dietary manipulations imposed by the parents or recommended by medical personnel. Secondary malnutrition is a particularly worrisome complication of IPD, although it does not necessarily occur in all patients. Nevertheless, epidemiologic studies have shown that the generally negative effects of diarrhea on children's growth are especially severe among the subset of children who experience prolonged episodes of illness.[28] Clinical and laboratory evidences of malnutrition include reduced body mass and subcutaneous tissue by physical examination, anthropometric indicators of wasting (low weight for height, low subcutaneous fat reserves), and the usual clinical and biochemical indicators of individual nutrient deficiencies.

Microbiologic evaluation should include stool microscopic examination for leukocytes, ova, and parasites and stool culture for enteric pathogens. Intestinal intubation can be useful to identify pathogens in the small bowel. Laboratory tests, such as xylose absorption studies, carbohydrate tolerance tests, or breath hydrogen tests, and measurement of fecal fat excretion can be used to assess absorptive function but are of little diagnostic value with regard to the etiology of the illness. Intestinal biopsy is not required for diagnosis or treatment of this condition but may be useful to rule out other diseases.

The so-called downward spiral of infection, malnutrition, increased severity of infection, and death has been highlighted during field studies of diarrhea-associated mortality. Whereas it has been assumed previously that most diarrhea-related deaths are caused by dehydration, recent community-based studies have found that as many as half of these deaths may be related to IPD and malnutrition.[29] The importance of this syndrome cannot be overstated, particularly in less developed countries, where one-third to one-half of young children's deaths are related to diarrhea.

MANAGEMENT

Treatment of IPD requires attention to underlying infections, fluid and electrolyte abnormalities, intestinal malabsorption, and malnutrition (Table 1). A proportion of prolonged diarrheal episodes may be dysenteric. When *Shigella* spp., *C. jejuni,* or *E. histolytica* is isolated, appropriate antimicrobial therapy should be initiated, although the effectiveness of treatment for *Campylobacter* in patients with IPD remains uncertain.

In individual cases, nondysenteric prolonged diarrhea associated with pathogenic *E. coli* appears to respond to treatment with intravenous gentamicin or oral neomycin. One placebo-controlled trial of oral gentamicin (10 mg per kilogram per day) among American children with prolonged diarrhea found a significant overall reduction in the duration of illness in the antibiotic-treated group, especially in the subgroup of children with enteroadherent *E. coli*.[30] Thus, oral

TABLE 1
Common Complications of Idiopathic Prolonged Diarrhea and Their Possible Mechanisms

Complications	Possible Causal Mechanisms
Maldigestion	
Carbohydrate	Mucosal injury (infection)→reduced mucosal surface area and decreased concentrations of hydrolytic enzymes; possibly reduced stimulus to exocrine pancreas Secondary pancreatic insufficiency? (malnutrition)
Fat	Mucosal injury Biliary insufficiency (interruption of entero-hepatic circulation, small intestinal bacterial colonization) Secondary pancreatic insufficiency?
Malabsorption	Mucosal injury Abnormalities in intestinal transit?
Malnutrition	Anorexia Dietary deprivation Malabsorption

gentamicin may be effective, although perhaps only in those cases in which prolonged diarrhea is caused by a sensitive enteropathogenic or enteroadherent *E. coli*. Additional studies of the frequency of these particular infections and of the response to antibiotics of these and other agents associated with nondysenteric IPD are necessary before general recommendations on the use of antibiotics can be formulated.

High concentrations of anaerobic and facultative bacteria have been isolated from small bowel aspirates from children with IPD, but the pathophysiologic significance of these organisms is uncertain. Empiric therapy directed at these organisms has been suggested, but the therapeutic efficacy of this approach is unproven and cannot be generally recommended. *G. lamblia* may also be recovered from a subgroup of these patients. The specific role of this organism in the pathogenesis of IPD and the effectiveness of treatment are unknown. However, in nonendemic areas a therapeutic trial is indicated when *Giardia* is isolated from stool or intestinal aspirates of patients with IPD.

Deconjugation of bile acids may occur when small intestinal bacterial colonization complicates IPD. These deconjugated bile acids are not fully reabsorbed by the ileum and can stimulate mucosal secretion when they pass into the colon. Therefore, bile acid–binding agents like cholestyramine have been used to reduce fecal excretion in patients with IPD.[31] Bile acid–sequestering agents must be used only for limited periods of time, however, because they will exacerbate steatorrhea and may quickly deplete fat-soluble vitamin reserves.

Nutritional therapy must be provided to ameliorate the complications of malabsorption and, when necessary, to permit nutritional rehabilitation.[32] The amount of energy and nutrients absorbed should be adequate both to satisfy usual nutrient requirements and to permit recovery from any preexisting undernutrition. Special dietary sources might be required because of GI dysfunction during IPD.

Incomplete absorption of carbohydrates due to transient disaccharidase deficiency or reduced monosaccharide transport can be treated by reducing or eliminating the poorly absorbed carbohydrate from the diet. Malabsorption of lactose is most common, and controlled clinical trials have shown that hydrolysis of lactose by exogenous lactase will reduce the severity and duration of prolonged diarrhea.[33] Lactose-free diets would be expected to be similarly beneficial. For reasons that are not well understood, human milk seems to be relatively well tolerated by infants with diarrhea despite its high lactose content. In these extremely rare situations in which severe monosaccharide intolerance requires the removal of all carbohydrate from the diet, glucose must be provided intravenously to prevent hypoglycemia.[34]

The rather rare cases of severe malabsorption of fat can be managed by providing most of the dietary fat as medium-chain triglycerides. At least 3 percent of total dietary energy (calories) must be provided as essential fatty acids, however, to avoid symptoms of deficiency. The use of protein hydrolysates for proven or suspected protein sensitivity is discussed elsewhere. Despite the theoretic advantage of these products to reduce protein sensitivity, their high cost and increased osmolality make them undesirable for general use. Prolonged diarrhea of infancy can be treated with total parenteral nutrition, but even in severe cases, recent studies suggest that continued enteral feeding results in a shorter duration of illness.[35] Similarly, recent studies of the nutritional management of acute diarrhea have demonstrated that continued feeding is beneficial nutritionally and does not increase the risk of prolonged illness.[36,37]

Treatment of severe malnutrition and specific nutritional deficiency diseases is discussed elsewhere is more detail. Briefly, high-energy, nutrient-dense diets are advocated; a low-lactose diet is advised for patients in whom carbohydrate malabsorption is identified. Recently, staple foods have been employed rather than elemental diets in an effort to reduce dietary osmolality. More experience with these products is still required, but preliminary results suggest that they are well tolerated by children with IPD.

REFERENCES

1. Black RE, Brown KH, Becker S. et al. Longitudinal studies of infectious diseases and physical growth of children in rural Bangladesh. II. Incidence of diarrhea and association with known pathogens. Am J Epidemiol 1982; 115:315–324.
2. Lie K, Rukmono B, Oemijati S, Sahab K. Diarrhea among infants in a crowded area of Jakarta, Indonesia: a longitudinal study from birth to two years. Bull WHO 1966; 34:197–210.
3. Mata LJ. The children of Santa Maria Cauque: a prospective field study of health and growth. Cambridge, MA: MIT Press, 1978.
4. McAuliffe JF, Shields DS, de Sousa MA, Sakell J, Schorling J, Guerrant RL. Prolonged and recurring diarrhea in the northeast of Brazil: examination of cases from a community-based study. J Pediatr Gastroenterol Nutr 1986; 5:902–906.
5. Hong R. The immunologic system. In: Behrman RE, Vaughan VC, eds. Nelson's textbook of pediatrics. Philadelphia: WB Saunders, 1987; 455–461.
6. Grand RJ, Watkins JB, Torti FM. Development of the human gastrointestinal tract. Gastroenterology 1976; 70:790–810.
7. Black RE, Brown KH, Becker S. Malnutrition is a determining factor in diarrheal duration, but not incidence, among young children in a longitudinal study in rural Bangladesh. Am J Clin Nutr 1984; 37:87–94.
8. Butzner D, Butler DG, Miniats P, Hamilton JR. Impact of chronic protein-calorie malnutrition on small intestinal repair after acute viral gastroenteritis: a study in gnotobiotic piglets. Pediatr Res 1985; 19:476–481.
9. Suskind R. Gastrointestinal changes in the malnourished child. Pediatr Clin North Am 1975; 22:873–882.
10. Brunser O. Effects of malnutrition on intestinal structure and function in children. Clin Gastroenterol 1977; 6:341–353.
11. Suskind RM, ed. Malnutrition and the immune response. New York: Raven Press, 1977.
12. Sommer A, Katz J, Tarwotjo I. Increased risk of respiratory disease and diarrhea in children with preexisting mild vitamin A deficiency. Am J Clin Nutr 1984; 40:1090–1095.
13. Klipstein FA, Lipton SD, Schenk EA. Folate deficiency of the intestinal mucosa. Am J Clin Nutr 1973; 26:728–737.
14. Horwitt MK. Niacin. In: Goodhart RS, Shils ME, eds. Modern nutrition in health and disease. Philadelphia: Lea & Febiger, 1978.
15. Koster FT, Curlin GC, Aziz KMA, Haque, Azizul. Synergistic impact of measles and diarrhea in nutrition and mortality in Bangladesh. Bull WHO 1981; 59:901–908.
16. Koster FT, Palmer DL, Chakraborty J, Jackson T, Curlin G. Cellular immune competence and diarrheal morbidity in malnourished Bangladeshi children: a prospective field study. Am J Clin Nutr 1987; 45:115–120.
17. Khin-Maung-U, Nyunt-Nyunt-Wai, Myo-Khin, Mu-Mu-Khin, Tin-U, Thane-Toe. Effect on clinical outcome of breastfeeding during acute diarrhea. Br Med J 1985; 290:587–589.
18. Brown KH, Black FE, Lopez de Romaña G, Creed de Kanashiro H. Infant feeding practices and their relationship with diarrheal and other diseases in Huascar (Lima), Peru, Pediatrics 1989; 83:31–40.
19. Subcommittee on Nutrition and Diarrheal Diseases Control. Nutritional management of acute diarrhea in infants and children. Washington, DC: National Research Council, 1985.
20. Walker WA, Isselbacher KJ. Uptake and transport of macromolecules by the intestine. Gastroenterology 1974; 67:531–550.
21. Banwell JG, Boldt DH, Meyers J, Webus FL Jr. Phytohemagglutinin derived from red kidney bean (*Phaseolus vulgaris*): a cause for intestinal malabsorption associated with bacterial overgrowth in the rat. Gastroenterology 1983; 84:506–515.
22. Bartlett JG. Antibiotic associated pseudomembranous colitis. Rev Infect Dis 1979; 1:123–131.
23. Dupont HL, Hornick RB. Adverse effects of lomotil therapy in shigellosis. JAMA 1973; 226:1525–1528.
24. Ulshen MH, Rollo JL. Pathogenesis of *Escherichia coli* gastroenteritis in man—another mechanism. N Engl J Med 1980; 302:99–101.
25. Levine MM, Edelman R. Enteropathogenic *Escherichia coli* of classic serotypes associated with infant diarrhea: epidemiology and pathogenesis. Epidemiol Rev 1984; 6:31–51.
26. Coello-Ramirez P, Lifshitz F, Zuniga V. Enteric microflora and carbohydrate intolerance in infants with diarrhea. Pediatrics 1972; 49:233–242.
27. Jonas A, Avigad S, Diver-Haber A, Katznelson D. Disturbed fat absorption following infectious gastroenteritis in children. J Pediatr 1979; 95:366–372.
28. Black RE, Brown KH, Becker S. Effects of diarrhea associated with specific enteropathogens on the growth of children in rural Bangladesh. Pediatrics 1984; 73:799–805.
29. Bhan ML, Arora NK, Ghai OP. et al. Major factors in diarrhoea related mortality among rural children. Indian J Med Res 1986; 83:9–12.
30. Craft JC, Welborn CA, Holt EA, Ragon-Garcia C, Halsey NA, Daum RS. Oral gentamicin for treatment of persistent diarrhea due to enteroadhesive E. coli (EAEC). Interscience Conference on Antimicrobial Agents and Chemotherapy, New Orleans, 1986.
31. Hill ID, Mann MD, Househam KC, Bowie MD. Use of oral gentamicin, metronidazole, and cholestyramine in the treatment of severe persistent diarrhea in infants. Pediatrics 1986; 77:477–481.
32. MacLean WC Jr, Lopez de Romaña G, Massa E, Graham GG. Nutritional management of chronic diarrhea and malnutrition: primary reliance on oral feeding. J Pediatr 1980; 97:316–323.
33. Penny ME, Paredes P, Brown KH. Clinical and nutritional consequences of lactose feeding during persistent postenteritis diarrhea. Pediatrics 1989; 84:835–844.
34. Lifshitz F, Coello-Ramirez P, Gutierrez-Topete G. Monosaccharide intolerance and hypoglycemia in infants with diarrhea. J Pediatr 1970; 77:604–612.
35. Orenstein SR. Enteral versus parenteral therapy for intractable diarrhea of infancy: a prospective, randomized trial. J Pediatr 1986; 109:277–286.
36. Santosham M, Foster S, Reid R, et al. Role of soy-based, lactose-free formula during treatment of acute diarrhea. Pediatrics 1985; 76:292–298.
37. Brown KH, Gastañaduy, Saavedva JM, et al. Effect of continued oral feeding on clinical and nutritional outcomes of acute diarrhea in children. J Pediatr 1988; 112:191–200.

PART 26

Munchausen Syndrome by Proxy

Jay A. Perman, M.D.

"We may teach, and I believe should teach, that mothers are always right; but at the same time we must recognize that when mothers are wrong they can be terribly wrong."[1]

Hospitals can be a strong and dangerous addiction.[2]

In 1951 Richard Asher described a bizarre entity characterized by the deliberate falsification of one's medical history to secure extensive medical investigation, invasive procedures and operations, and prolonged or recurrent therapies.[3] He labeled the entity *Munchausen syndrome* after a famous eighteenth century German baron known for his outrageous and utterly false stories. Adults and older children fitting this syndrome subsequently became frequently recognized and reported,[4,5] but the critical relevance of this entity to the pediatrician emerged in 1977 when Meadow reported two cases of Munchausen syndrome *by proxy*.[1] Rather than falsification by the patients themselves, the parents falsified the medical history of these young children, resulting in prolonged investigation and treatment of the children for nonexistent illnesses. Munchausen syndrome by proxy (MSP) has now been widely reported as a form of child abuse in which the physician unwittingly participates in the abuse. Since gastrointestinal (GI) bleeding, diarrhea, and vomiting are common forms in which MSP presents, the pediatric gastroenterologist is likely to be drawn into such cases. Accordingly, the features, basis, means of recognition, and management of the disorder are presented in this discussion.

FEATURES

MSP usually occurs in children from early infancy to 7 years of age.[2] Cases have been reported in older children who participate in the falsification of the history by the parent in an attempt to protect the parent. GI manifestations of MSP are listed in Table 1 together with non-GI symptoms that may occur concomitantly. Children with MSP may present with persistent or recurrent symptoms and signs, but evaluation consistently indicates a discrepancy between the presentation and the child's general health. The symptoms and signs do not make sense, and the specialist usually says, "I have never seen a case like this one."

GI diagnoses in children subsequently shown to have MSP are listed in Table 2. The nature of the disorders diagnosed in these children, e.g., cystic fibrosis, supports the notion that the perpetrating parent is extremely cunning. Symptoms and signs are generally absent in the absence of the involved parent, who is almost exclusively the mother. Paternal involvement is extremely rare, and the father has usually been

TABLE 1

Symptoms and Signs of Munchausen Syndrome by Proxy

Gastrointestinal
- Hematemesis
- Rectal bleeding
- Vomiting, sometimes feculent
- Diarrhea
- Biochemical derangement

Other
- Allergies
- Hematuria
- Urinary tract infection
- Recurrent apnea, respiratory depression, or cardiorespiratory arrest
- Mental status changes
- Seizures
- Ataxia
- Recurrent coma
- Near-miss sudden infant death syndrome
- Sepsis; joint and soft tissue infections
- Diabetes or hypoglycemia
- Dehydration; hypernatremia
- Upper respiratory tract bleeding

reported to keep a low profile during his child's illnesses. In one reported case, the perpetrator was a baby sitter who herself had a history of Munchausen syndrome.[6]

The mother generally refuses to leave the hospital environment. Therefore it is not surprising that treatments given to

TABLE 2

Gastrointestinal Diagnoses in Patients with Munchausen Syndrome by Proxy

Diagnosis	Mechanisms of Deception
Intractable diarrhea	Laxatives[10]
Colitis	Laxatives[11]
Seizures/apnea secondary to gastroesophageal reflux	Asphyxiation[12]
Rectovesical fistula	Alteration of urine specimens[1]
Unexplained GI hemorrhage	Withdrawal of patient's blood from Broviac catheter[13]; exogenous sources of blood, usually the mother's[14]
Cystic fibrosis	Alteration of sweat tests and fecal fat analyses[15]
Unexplained vomiting with or without altered sensorium	Emetics[8]; sodium administration[1]
Failure to thrive	Withholding food[16]

a child prior to the recognition of MSP often are poorly tolerated because of sabotage of the therapy by the parent. For example, intravenous lines do not stay in, or oral medications are reported to the nurses as having been vomited. Despite all of this turmoil the mother is generally less worried about the child's condition than are the medical personnel.

The mother often has had previous nursing training. In a series of 19 cases reported by Meadow,[2] eight of the mothers had received nursing training and a ninth was a receptionist for a pediatrician. Mothers frequently had a previous history of falsification of symptoms and signs consistent with an illness similar to the child's and often had a history of previous psychiatric interventions.[2] The mother is seen as very pleasant, co-operative, and appreciative of the care given the child and often forms a close relationship with the staff. This relationship often causes disbelief in a diagnosis of MSP by hospital staff, leading to resistance in confronting the perpetrating parent.

IMPACT ON THE PHYSICIAN AND MEDICAL STAFF

There is a great deal of reluctance on the part of the caretakers to accept a diagnosis of MSP, and the possibility of this diagnosis therefore comes to be accepted late in the course of the child's management. The delay in acceptance stems from a reluctance to judge as deceptive a parent who has bonded strongly to the staff and from damage to the self-esteem of the managing physicians and nurses. No one likes to admit that he or she has been misled, has made the wrong diagnosis, and, most painfully, has inflicted inappropriate and often harmful treatment on the child.

BASIS OF THE DISORDER

It is possible that MSP is one end of a spectrum of maladaptive behaviors seen in parents who provide an embellished history for one reason or another. Parents may exaggerate details of the medical history because they find that it results in more prompt attention to or better care of their child by medical personnel. Parents who find some gain in placing extraordinary and unreasonable restrictions on their child's diet or activity may exaggerate or falsify history to obtain physician approval for their actions and thus also become a part of the spectrum of MSP. Often in full-blown cases, the mother's actions are prompted by her desire to form a closer relationship with her husband or by her need for distraction from family or household problems. Mothers are drawn to MSP by the excitement of the medical environment and occasionally by the challenge of matching wits with the medical specialist.[2]

RECOGNIZING THE MSP DISORDER; RECOMMENDED PROCEDURES IN SUSPECTED CASES

A common-sense approach is suggested in suspected cases of MSP. It is best for the managing physician to investigate the possibility of MSP rather than for social services or other agencies to do so.[7] The physician is in a better position to confirm the diagnosis because he is perceived by the parent to be caring and is trusted. This approach allows for a more detailed and inoffensive investigation and, it is hoped, forms the basis for the pediatrician to pursue the successful resolution of the problem.

Initially, the history should be carefully evaluated for a temporal relationship between symptoms and signs and the presence of the suspected parent. If the child is in hospital, the nursing staff should be asked if symptoms and signs have always been reported by the parent rather than directly observed by the staff. (Ideally, nurses should record what is directly observed versus what is reported by parents in all patients, not just those with suspected MSP.) The family history should be investigated, particularly with regard to falsification of the mother's education, employment record, and health history. Illnesses similar to the child's in the mother's history should be sought. The child should then be separated from the parent to determine whether the signs and symptoms persist in her absence. It should be remembered that an episode of real illness in the parent's absence does not rule out fabrication.

When MSP is suspected, the nurse should be instructed to immediately take custody of all biologic specimens. Biologic specimens obtained when the child is symptomatic should be saved for further investigation, e.g., toxicologic. In patients with diarrhea, laxative abuse should be considered. Phenolphthalein is a commonly used laxative in cases of MSP, and its presence is indicated by the development of a pink color if stool is alkalinized to pH 8.5. Stool levels of magnesium and sulfate may also be useful in detecting laxatives.[8] The reliability of apparent findings should be established; e.g., is the blood really the child's? A video camera approach to confirming the diagnosis has been used by some.[9] All findings should be carefully documented in the medical record.

MANAGEMENT OF MSP

Direct confrontation of the offending parent by the managing physician is usually the initial step of choice. I find it highly effective to tell the parent that what she is doing is now known and that the physician is going to help. Meadow has recommended this course of action as well.[7] Psychiatric consultation should be obtained for the perpetrating parent if at all possible. Compliance with state law usually dictates that the child protective service agency be contacted. Decisions regarding removing the child from the home must ultimately be made by attorneys representing the state agency, and insufficient information exists regarding predictors for which children would be safe if left in the home.

PROGNOSIS

It is important to remember that MSP may result in permanent handicap or death if not recognized early and managed effectively. Children who have suffered from MSP may at older ages fabricate their own histories, and they may believe themselves to be dysfunctional and disabled.[2]

REFERENCES

1. Meadow R. Munchausen syndrome by proxy. The hinterland of child abuse. Lancet 1977; ii:343–345.
2. Meadow R. Munchausen syndrome by proxy. Arch Dis Child 1982; 57:92–98.
3. Asher R. Munchausen's syndrome. Lancet 1951; i:339–341.
4. Sneed RC, Bell RF. The Dauphin of Munchausen: factitious passage of renal stones in a child. Pediatrics 1976; 58:127–130.
5. Reich P, Lazarus JM, Kelly MJ, Rogers MP. Factitious feculent urine in an adolescent boy. JAMA 1977; 238:420–421.
6. Richardson GF. Munchausen syndrome by proxy. Am Fam Physician 1987; 36:119–123.
7. Meadow R. Management of Munchausen syndrome by proxy. Arch Dis Child 1985; 60:385–393.
8. Jones JG, Butler HL, Hamilton B, Perdue JD, Stern HP, Woody RC. Munchausen syndrome by proxy. Child Abuse Negl 1986; 10:33–40.
9. Epstein MA, Markowitz RL, Gallo DM, Holmes JW, Gryboski JD. Munchausen syndrome by proxy: considerations in diagnosis and confirmation by video surveillance. Pediatrics 1987; 80:220–224.
10. Fleisher D, Ament ME. Diarrhea, red diapers, and child abuse. Clin Pediatr 1977; 17:820–824.
11. Ackerman NB, Strobel CT. Polle syndrome: chronic diarrhea in Munchausen's child. Gastroenterology 1981; 81:1140–1142.
12. Geelhoed GC, Pember PJ. SIDS, seizures or 'sophageal reflux. Another manifestation of Munchausen syndrome by proxy. Med J Aust 1985; 143:357–358.
13. Malatack JJ, Wiener ES, Gartner JC, Zitelli BJ, Brunetti E. Munchausen syndrome by proxy: a new complication of central venous catheterization. Pediatrics 1985; 75:523–525.
14. Kurlansky L, Lukoff JY, Zinkham WH, Brody JP, Kessler RW. Munchausen syndrome by proxy: definition of factitious bleeding in an infant by ^{51}Cr labeling or erythrocytes. Pediatrics 1979; 63:228–231.
15. Orenstein DM, Wasserman AL. Munchausen syndrome by proxy simulating cystic fibrosis. Pediatrics 1986; 78:621–624.
16. Zitelli BJ, Seltman MF, Shannon RM. Munchausen's syndrome by proxy and its professional participants. Am J Dis Child 1987; 141:1099–1102.

P A R T

27

Intestinal Polyps

Harland S. Winter, M.D.

A polyp of the gastrointestinal (GI) tract is a grossly visible protrusion from the mucosal surface. Most polyps are asymptomatic and go unrecognized, but in those individuals in whom they are detected, there are three major clinical presentations: bleeding, abdominal pain, and intestinal obstruction. Intestinal blood loss results from the protrusion of the polyp into the lumen. Both trauma from passing stool and ischemia as the polyp outgrows its blood supply may cause the surface of the polyp to ulcerate and eventually bleed. Abdominal pain may occur when the polyp serves as the lead point of an intussusception or when it stretches the bowel wall by mechanically dragging the bowel distally with active peristalsis. If the polyp grows large enough, it can obstruct the lumen of the bowel. This mode of presentation is most unusual in the pediatric population.

Polyps may be classified into neoplastic and non-neoplastic types. Neoplastic types are benign or malignant adenomas; and non-neoplastic polyps are inflammatory (also called juvenile) or hamartomatous. Because the classification of a patient with a polyp is a clinical-pathologic one, the histologic description of the polyp is critical to the establishment of a correct diagnosis. The reliability of colonoscopic biopsies in determining the histologic type of polyp has been evaluated by comparing the classification derived from grasp biopsies to that derived from examining the entire polyp. Approximately 25 percent of abnormalities that are seen when the polyp is evaluated microscopically are missed by the grasp biopsies.[1] Thus, polypectomy is necessary for the establishment of an accurate diagnosis.

The juvenile polyp, which is the type found in more than 90 percent of the pediatric population,[2] is primarily an acquired lesion, although there are families in whom a predisposition for inflammatory polyps exists. The most common polyposis syndromes—familial polyposis coli, Gardner's and Peutz-Jeghers—are inherited in an autosomal dominant pattern, although penetrance in Peutz-Jeghers, for example, may be variable. A detailed discussion of the genetics of the polyposis syndromes is presented in the clinical section of this discussion.

PATHOGENIC MECHANISMS

Neoplastic polyps are most often encountered in the adult population but can, on rare occasions, be found in younger patients. In the adult population, the evolution of an adenocarcinoma is an important question, and the pathophysiology and the relationship between adenomatous and malignant polyps have been extensively studied. An adenoma is composed of immature cells whose rate of proliferation exceeds the requirements needed for replacement of the crypt. Because of nonuniform growth of the polyp, the surface of an adenoma is frequently lobulated, giving it the appearance of a raspberry. As the polyp grows in size, it tends to become more dysplastic. Thus, the size of the adenoma correlates with the risk of its containing invasive malignancy.[3] Adenomatous polyps less than 1 cm in size have a less than 2 percent incidence of containing carcinoma, whereas patients with an adenoma more than 1 cm in diameter have a risk of colorectal carcinoma that is 2.7 times that of the general population.[4]

The histologic features of nuclear irregularity and increased mitotic activity are found in all adenomas. The degree of cellular atypia determines the degree of dysplasia. A single polyp may contain areas with differing degrees of dysplasia. Ex-

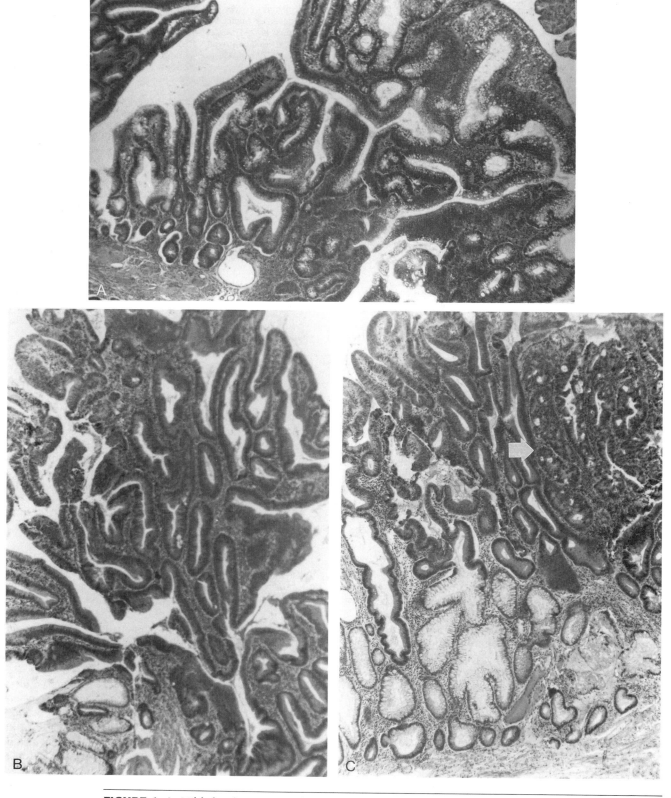

FIGURE 1 *A,* Mild dysplasia. *B,* Moderate dysplasia. *C,* Severe dysplasia.

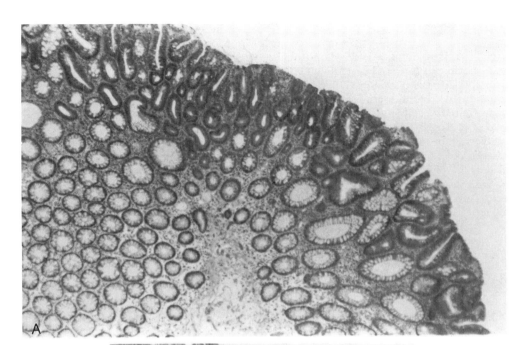

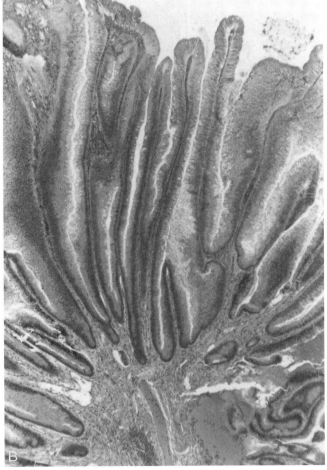

FIGURE 2 Adenoma: *A*, Tubular type. *B*, Villous type.

amples of mild and moderate dysplasia are shown in Figure 1 along with severe dysplasia.

In the normal colonic crypt, epithelial cell proliferation is confined to the proliferative and transitional cell zones. The zone of mature epithelial cells normally is devoid of dividing cells. As an adenoma develops, epithelial cell proliferation extends to the mature cell zone. Initially, cells in the mucosa do not increase, as the rate of proliferation equals the rate of extrusion. However, as the rate of proliferation increases and the interactions between the epithelial cells change, cells stack up on each other and a polypoid lesion develops. As the process continues, villous structures appear that are associated with higher degrees of dysplasia. Adeno-

mas can be classified histologically as tubular, tubulovillous, or villous (Fig. 2). Most polyps less than 1 cm in size are of the tubular type, whereas larger polyps are most often the tubulovillous or villous type.[5]

Non-neoplastic polyps are either inflammatory or hamartomatous. Inflammatory polyps are composed of well-differentiated, mature epithelial cells without cellular atypia. Numerous terms including *retention, juvenile,* and *hyperplastic* are used to describe these benign polyps. The dome of an inflammatory polyp is characteristically smooth, but cysts within the head of the polyp may protrude from the surface, giving it a lobulated appearance and making it difficult to visually distinguish an inflammatory polyp from an adeno-

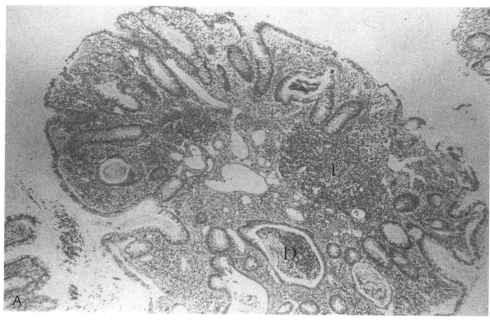

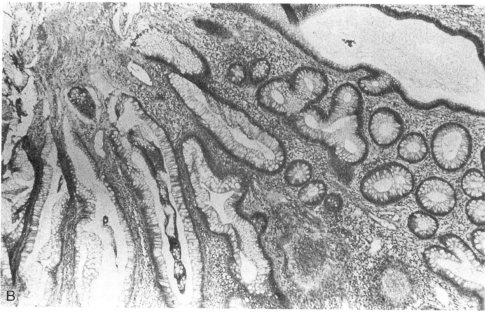

FIGURE 3 Photomicrographs of juvenile polyps revealing areas with *A,* lymphoid aggregates (L) and glandular dilatation (D), and *B,* epithelial proliferation.

ma. Because the cysts are filled with mucin, they have been termed *retention polyps*. Cystic change in an adenoma is rare.

In an inflammatory polyp, the migration from the base of the crypt is slower than normal,[6] suggesting that the mechanism of polyp formation is an abnormality of detachment of mature cells from the surface. In addition to the glandular proliferation seen in inflammatory polyps, varying degrees of acute or chronic inflammation and mesenchymal proliferation can be noted (Fig. 3). In some inflammatory polyps, areas of adenomatous change and dysplasia can be identified.[3]

The features that distinguish an inflammatory polyp from the hamartomatous type are depicted in Figure 4. In a hamartomatous polyp, multiple cell types including absorptive epithelial cells, goblet cells, argentaffin cells, and Paneth cells can be identified throughout the epithelium. The most characteristic finding, however, is the branching appearance produced by smooth muscle fibers of the mucuslaris mucosae mixed with bands of collagen. The basic mucosaccharides and the neutral mucins that are found in the epithelium of the polyp are qualitatively similar to those identified in normal mucosa.[7] This observation has caused some investigators to hypothesize that malignancies observed in the patients with hamartomatous polyposis syndromes arise de novo secondary to a genetic predisposition.[8] Nevertheless, at least one patient has been described in whom a metastasizing carcinoma arose from a jejunal hamartoma.[8]

CLINICAL FEATURES

The clinical features of patients with single or multiple intestinal polyps vary with the type of polyp as well as the age of presentation. Distinct clinical entities are frequently organized by histologic type of the polyp (Table 1).

Isolated Adenomas

With the exception of polyposis syndromes, neoplastic polyps are generally found in the adult population, in which it is generally accepted that adenomas are the precursors of adenocarcinoma of the colon.[9] Although there may be multifactorial genetic and environmental factors to explain the two- to threefold increase in colon cancer among first-degree relatives of patients with colon cancer, it appears that the inheritance of colonic adenomas and colorectal cancer is dominant.[10] From autopsy studies, the prevalence of adenomas ranges from 9.5 to 61 percent, with a mean of 29.5.[11] Thus, children with a parent or other first-degree relative who has colorectal adenocarcinoma or adenomas should receive appropriate genetic counseling and consider surveillance when they become adults. The presence of an adenoma in an individual under the age of 30 should raise the suspicion of a polyposis syndrome.

Isolated Inflammatory Polyp

Inflammatory or juvenile polyps are the most common type encountered in the pediatric population and can be found in 1 percent of pre-school or school-age children. The mean age in one study was 6 years,[1] but other studies have noted a slightly lower average age, with a peak in the 2 to 5 year range.[12,13] There is a male predominance. Painless hematochezia is the presenting symptom in approximately 90 percent of children, but other presenting problems include abdominal pain, prolapse of either the polyp or the rectum, pruritus, pain after defecation, passing mucus, diarrhea, or constipation.

Prior to the introduction of colonoscopy for children, most juvenile polyps were thought to be single and within the view

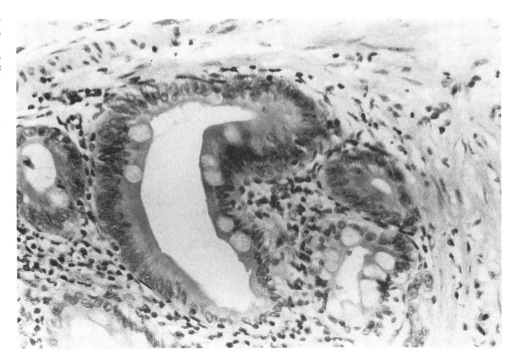

FIGURE 4 Histologic features of a hamartomatous polyp, demonstrating smooth muscle fibers associated with bands of collagen.

TABLE 1
Classification of Polyps

Adenomatous
Isolated polyp
Familial polyposis coli
Gardner's syndrome
Turcot's syndrome

Inflammatory
Isolated polyp
Juvenile polyposis coli
Generalized juvenile polyposis
Cronkhite-Canada syndrome

Hamartomatous
Peutz-Jeghers syndrome
Cowden's disease

of the sigmoidoscope. Recent studies have identified more than one polyp in more than 50 percent of children and have found that about 60 percent of the polyps are proximal to the rectosigmoid.[1,14] Inflammatory polyps have very low if any malignant potential. In children with juvenile polyps who were followed for slightly more than 6 years, no cases of malignant change were identified.[15] However, there have been isolated case reports of adenocarcinoma arising from a single juvenile polyp, which brings into question the reliability of this dictum.[16] Others have reported mixed juvenile polyps and adenomas in children less than 6 years of age.[17] If an adenomatous change is noted in a patient with one or two inflammatory polyps, the possibility of generalized juvenile polyposis should be considered.

Lymphoid polyps of the colon are usually in the rectum. They also have been called benign lymphomas, multiple lymphoid polyposis, benign giant follicular hyperplasia, and focal lymphoid hyperplasia.[18,19] They resemble inflammatory polyps with two characteristic exceptions: prominent lymphoid nodules and follicles with germinal centers containing stimulated lymphocytes and macrophages. Because these polypoid lesions need to be distinguished from lymphoid malignancies, the entire polyp should be removed for pathologic evaluation. There is a low incidence of recurrence and no evidence of subsequent problems.

Juvenile Polyposis Coli

Juvenile polyposis is a disorder characterized by multiple inflammatory polyps throughout the colon.[20] There are both a familial and a sporadic form of the disease. The clinical manifestations vary, with some patients developing life-threatening hemorrhage[21] and others remaining asymptomatic despite a large polyp burden. Painless rectal bleeding and rectal prolapse are the most common clinical features. Patients with a family history of juvenile polyps present at an older age (mean age 9.5 years) than do individuals who do not have a family history of juvenile polyposis coli (mean age 4.5 years).[20] This same pattern of presentation has been reported in individuals with familial polyposis coli. Those with a family history of familial polyposis coli first develop symptoms at an average age of 29 years, compared with those without a family history, in whom symptoms first develop

at an average age of 23 years.[20] Tho ... op symptoms in infancy often are the most ... anage.[22]

The clinical aspects of juvenile ... li closely resemble those of familial polyposi ... not permit reliable differentiation.[23] Table 2 lists features that may assist the clinician in making the distinction. Juvenile polyposis usually presents prior to adolescence and may become clinically evident before the age of 5 years. In contrast, familial polyposis coli rarely presents in childhood, but usually a diagnoisis is established by the age of 30 years. Painless hematochezia is the most common symptom in patients with juvenile polyposis coli, but failure to thrive and rectal prolapse are not unusual. Diarrhea is frequently the presenting symptom in patients with familial polyposis coli, but it may be accompanied by abdominal pain, anemia, melena, or intussusception. Despite the clinical presentation, because the clinical features of the two syndromes are so variable, a histologic diagnosis is necessary.

The malignant potential of juvenile polyposis is much less than that of familial polyposis coli. There have been reports of individuals with juvenile polyposis coli[24] who develop adenomatous changes in polyps 25 years following removal of multiple inflammatory colonic polyps.[25] Some may subsequently develop adenocarcinoma of the colon.[3,26]

The polyps in the Ruvalcaba-Myhre-Smith syndrome[27] are found in the colon and the tongue. Although described by some to be hamartomatous, Dr. Rodger Haggitt has found them to be typical inflammatory polyps. Other features of the syndrome include macrocephaly, mental retardation, abnormal facies, and pigmented macules on the shaft and glans of the penis.

Juvenile polyposis coli is distinguished from isolated juvenile polyp(s) by the number of polyps in the colon and from generalized juvenile polyposis by the location of the polyps. When the number of polyps exceeds 10, one must begin to consider that the patient has a syndrome rather than a sporadic disease. The implications for the individual are significant, as the cancer risk may increase with the number of polyps. At this time experience does not support an increased risk of GI malignancy for patients with either isolated juvenile polyposis or juvenile polyposis coli.[28]

Generalized Juvenile Polyposis

Generalized juvenile polyposis is closely related to juvenile polyposis coli, and the distinction is made by the location of the polyps. Juvenile polyposis coli refers to multiple

TABLE 2
Clinical Distinction Between Juvenile Polyposis Coli and Familial Polyposis Coli

	Juvenile Polyposis Coli	Familial Polyposis Coli
Type of polyp	Inflammatory	Adenomatous
Age of onset	Preadolescence	Variable, but by age 30 years
Symptoms before 5 years of age	Usual	Rare
First symptoms	Hematochezia	Diarrhea

juvenile polyps found only in the colon, whereas, in generalized juvenile polyposis, polyps are found throughout the GI tract.[29] This classification may be somewhat arbitrary, as the two conditions may be a continuum, with the generalized form having a greater clinical expression of polyposis.

The clinical features of generalized juvenile polyposis are similar to those described for juvenile polyposis coli. Symptoms may begin either in infancy[30] or in childhood. Finding inflammatory polyps in the stomach[31] or the small intestine distinguishes this syndrome from other related disorders. Because of the extensive polyposis and GI dysfunction, malabsorption and hemorrhage are potential problems. Intussusception, hypoalbuminemia, diarrhea, electrolyte abnormalities, failure to thrive, and clubbing are more common because of the extracolonic involvement.[32] Unlike juvenile polyposis coli, in which numerous associated conditions have been identified, only pulmonary arteriovenous malformations have been associated with generalized juvenile polyposis.[33]

The question of adenomatous change and adenocarcinoma of the GI tract is an important issue in patients with the generalized form of juvenile polyposis. Patients with the disorder as well as kindreds in which the disorder has been identified have an increased incidence of adenomata and adenocarcinoma of the stomach, duodenum, colon, and pancreas.[34] Patients and family members with this form of polyposis should have regular surveillance of these organs.

Familial Polyposis Coli

Familial polyposis coli is an autosomal dominant disorder in which about 20 percent of affected individuals do not have a family history.[35,36] The incidence in the general population is approximately 1 in 8,000 births. It is characterized by hundreds to thousands of adenomas of the colon (Fig. 5). Extraintestinal manifestations are generally associated with Gardner's syndrome, although many investigators do not consider these two disorders to be distinct genetic entities. The view linking the two disorders is supported by the epidemiologic observation that members of familial polyposis coli kindreds may have extracolonic manifestations. Isolated reports have linked hepatoblastoma and acute myelocytic leukemia to familial polyposis coli.[37]

The incidence of gastric and small intestinal lesions is significant in patients with multiple adenomas[38–40] but seems to be over 50 percent in both the United States and Japan.[41] In the stomach, fundic gland hyperplasia is the most frequently discovered lesion, but adenomata, adenocarcinoma, and microcarcinoid can be found. Adenomas also may exist throughout the small intestine.[42,43]

In contrast to juvenile polyposis coli, polyps usually do not become apparent until after puberty (Table 2); however, any child with a positive family history and GI symptoms should be evaluated with a proctosigmoidoscopy. Symptoms generally do not begin until 10 years following the development of polyps. Diarrhea is often the earliest symptom but may be associated with abdominal pain and/or hematochezia. If the condition is untreated, the risk of developing colonic cancer by the age of 55 years is almost 100 percent.

In addition to the clinical and pathologic diagnostic criteria, the biochemical marker, ornithine decarboxylase level, is elevated in the normal-appearing mucosa as well as in the adenomatous tissue in patients with familial polyposis coli.[44] This observation correlates with the finding that when normal-appearing mucosa from an individual with familial polyposis coli is radiolabeled with ^{3}H-thymidine, the proliferative zone extends to the surface.[39] The evidence of alterations in cellular metabolism is provided by the recent use of molecular probes. These reagents reveal that the adenomas contain a spectrum of altered proto-oncogenes that can be found prior to the development of overt malignancy.[45]

Gardner's Syndrome

Gardner's syndrome was described in 1950 by Gardner and Stephens, who reported nine cases of intestinal adenocarcinoma among descendants of one couple with a family history of bone and soft-tissue abnormalities.[46,47] This kindred was first brought to their attention by a medical student who was interested in the inheritance of malignancy. McKusick initially suggested that Gardner's syndrome, the triad of GI polyposis in conjunction with bone and soft-tissue tumors (Fig. 6), was distinct from intestinal polyposis coli.[48] However, the distinction between the two entities may not be so clear.

The major feature that separates these two conditions, both characterized by hundreds to thousands of colonic adenomas, of which 98 percent are less than 0.5 cm in diameter, is the presence of extracolonic manifestations in patients with Gardner's syndrome. Symptoms, with the exception of extracolonic manifestations, are identical to those found in familial polyposis coli. Polyps of the stomach and duodenum are common in Gardner's syndrome, occurring in 68 and 90 percent of affected individuals, respectively. [49–52] The most prevalent tumors of the gastric fundus are fundic gland hyperplasia. Adenomas can be found in the stomach, duodenum, and ileum, and some may evolve into adenocarcinoma.[53] Periampullary carcinoma of the duodenum, with an incidence as high as 12 percent,[54] is usually asymptomatic but may present with symptoms of necrotizing pancreatitis.[55] Lymphoid polyps of the ileum also exist and must be distinguished from the premalignant adenomatous variety. Other extraintestinal manifestations include benign osteomas of the frontal and mandibular bones, cortical thickening of the long bones and occasionally the ribs, epidermoid cysts[56] (most commonly on the legs, followed by the face, scalp and arms), supernumerary and impacted teeth, dental cysts, odontomas, benign fibrous tissue tumors (fibromas, lipomas, desmoids, mesenteric fibromatosis[57]), central nervous system tumor,[58] and papillary carcinoma of the thyroid.[59] It is only by careful review of the history of the kindred that a precise distinction between Gardner's syndrome and familial polyposis coli can be made.

The most important extraintestinal manifestation of Gardner's syndrome from a diagnostic viewpoint is the ocular feature of hypertrophy of retinal pigment epithelium, which can be identified in more than 90 percent of affected individuals and in individuals who are at risk to develop colonic polyposis.[60,61] The lesion has been seen in a 3-month-old infant

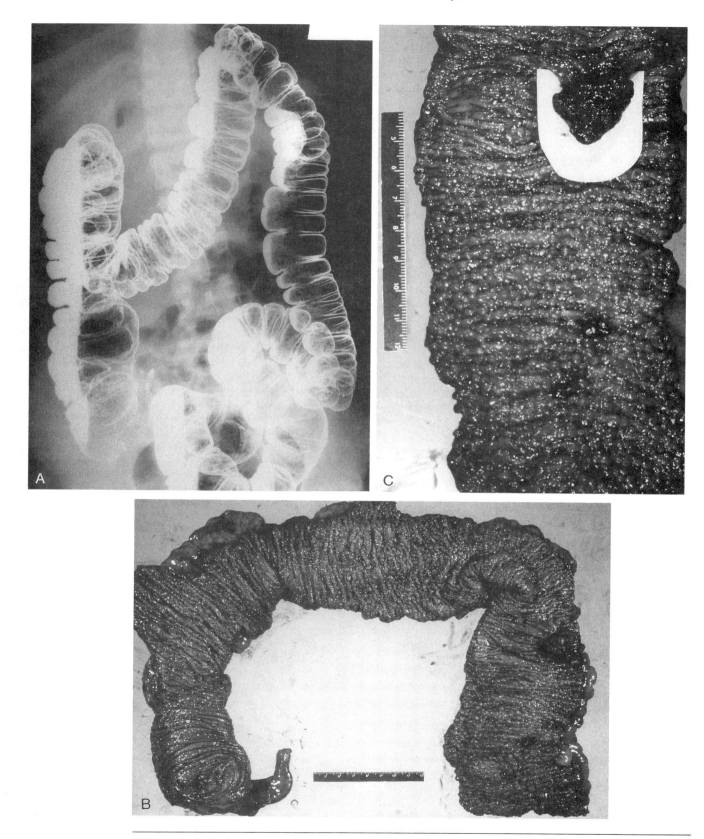

FIGURE 5 *A*, Barium enema of an adolescent with familial polyposis coli. *B*, Colectomy specimen showing the distribution of colonic polyps in familial polyposis coli. Appendix and cecum are on the left. *C*, Large polyp was present in descending colon, along with numerous smaller polyps. (Courtesy of Ed Matczak, Department of Pathology, The Children's Hospital, Boston.)

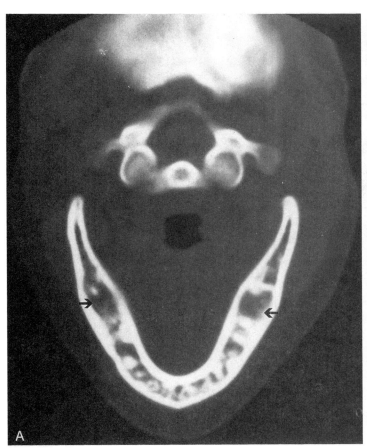
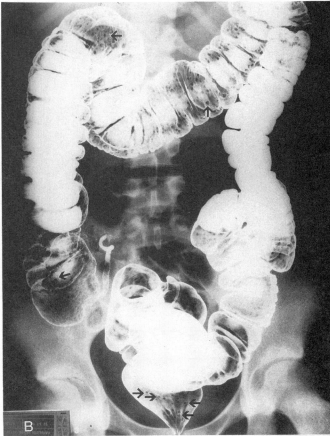

FIGURE 6 *A*, Computed tomography scan of mandible revealed bony defects (*arrows*). *B*, Barium enema with air contrast demonstrates small polyps in the rectum and throughout the colon (*arrows*).

prior to the expression of colonic polyposis. Family members who are at risk should have a careful retinal examination. In more than 75 percent of those with Gardner's syndrome, the lesions occur bilaterally.

There has been a clinical impression that the number of colonic polyps in Gardner's syndrome is less than the number found in familial polyposis coli. One reason for this apparent difference is that individuals with Gardner's syndrome are identified at an earlier age because of the extraintestinal manifestations. The range in age for the development of polyps is 4 to 72 years, and symptoms often appear a decade after polyps can be detected. On the average, colonic polyps occur around 25 years, with the average onset of symptoms around 33 years of age. Attempts have been made to identify individuals at risk for malignant change prior to the histologic change. This is of particular importance in the pediatric and adolescent population for whom the clinician may need to determine the timing of a colectomy. Unfortunately, no reliable markers exist that can predict when an epithelium will become malignant.[62]

Turcot's Syndrome

Turcot's syndrome is a rare autosomal recessive disorder in which adenomas of the colon are associated with brain tumors. Many of the reported patients have been adolescents.

Possibly because of the age of the patients, these individuals have a lower number of colonic polyps. However, they frequently become malignant before the patient is 30 years of age. Glioblastoma multiforme, a high-grade astrocytoma, is the most common tumor of the central nervous system, and it is found primarily in the cerebrum. Nevertheless, tumors also have been identified in the brain stem and the spinal cord. Medulloblastomas have been reported as well.[63] Any patient with a brain tumor and unexplained diarrhea should be evaluated for Turcot's syndrome, as the GI symptoms may be subtle.

Peutz-Jeghers Syndrome

Peutz-Jeghers syndrome is a condition inherited as an autosomal dominant and characterized by hamartomatous GI polyps and abnormal brown pigmentation of the lips, oral mucosa, and skin (Fig. 7). Polypoid lesions have also been found in the mucosa of the upper respiratory tract, trachea, gallbladder, and ureter.[6] The intestinal hamartomatous polyps range in size from 0.1 to 3.0 cm and, as discussed previously, have a lower incidence of malignant change than do adenomas. The glandular architecture tends to be disorganized, smooth muscle is present within the polyp, the glandular lumen is straight and lined with mature colonic epithelial cells, and mitoses appear normal (see Fig. 4).

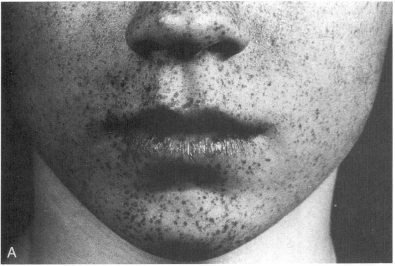

FIGURE 7   *A*, Facial features of Peutz-Jeghers syndrome, demonstrating pigmented lesions of the lips and face. *B*, Pigmented cutaneous lesion on the knee.

Abdominal pain due to mechanical blockage or intussusception is the most common symptom (Fig. 8). GI hemorrhage from ulceration or sloughing of a polyp may cause chronic iron deficiency anemia. Almost all patients have small intestinal polyps, but some also have polyps of the colon which may cause hematochezia. Adenocarcinoma of the colon has been reported.[64,65] Those in the stomach or duodenum may cause hematemesis from mucosal sloughing, but duodenal and jejunal adenocarcinoma and epithelioid leiomyosarcoma originating in a hamartomatous polyp have been described as well.[66,67] Most individuals do well over many decades without the development of carcinoma,[68] and the association with gastric and duodenal malignancy is about 3 percent.

A freckle-like pigmentation of the lips usually appears in childhood. This pigmentation of the lips is the most consistent dermatologic finding. It may not be as reliable in older patients because the freckles tend to fade with age. In contrast, lesions of the buccal mucosa, present in over 80 percent of individuals, are a more reliable sign in older individuals and may appear earlier in infancy than cutaneous lesions. Fewer than 5 percent of patients with polyposis do not have cutaneous pigmentary changes.

In addition to the intestinal polyps and dermatologic manifestations, between 5 and 12 percent of females develop sex cord tumors, of the ovary. Peutz-Jeghers syndrome has been associated with precocious puberty in girls and with feminizing gonadal tumors in boys.[69]

Cowden's Disease

Cowden's disease, or GI polyposis with orocutaneous hamartomas,[70] is an autosomal dominant disorder that usually presents between the ages of 10 and 30 years. Polyps can be found anywhere in the GI tract, including the esophagus.[71] They are hyperplastic with both prominent epithelial hyperplasia and multiple smooth muscle bundles between the glands extending toward the surface. The striking increase in connective tissue as well as the glandular hyperplasia characterize these polyps as hamartomatous. In addition, glycogenic acanthosis of the esophagus and ganglioneuromatosis of the colon have been reported.[72] Approximately one-third of patients with Cowden's disease have GI involvement, but many patients have not had extensive intestinal evalua-

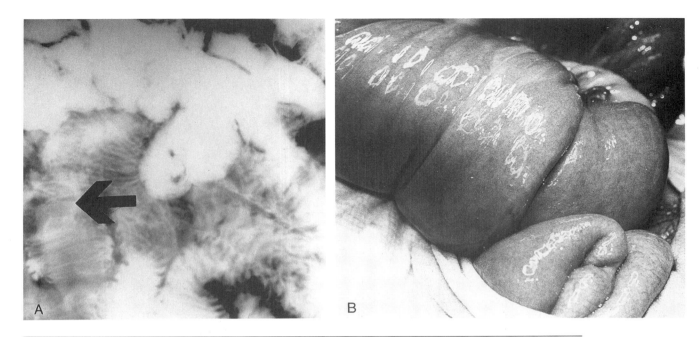

FIGURE 8 Small intestinal polyp in Peutz-Jeghers syndrome. *A*, Small bowel radiograph demonstrating jejunal polyp; this subsequently served as the lead point for recurrent intussusception. *B*, Intraoperative photograph of jejunojejunal intussusception in patient with Peutz-Jeghers syndrome. The larger diameter bowel contains the intussusception.

tion. Although there has been at least one report of adenocarcinoma of the colon in a patient with Cowden's disease,[73] there does not appear to be an increased incidence of GI malignancy.

Extraintestinal manifestations include orocutaneous hamartomas of the face, hands, mouth, lips, tongue, and nares.[74] Malignancies of the breast and thyroid seem to occur only in women. Breast cancer is found in 50 percent of the women, and thyroid disease, with a lower incidence of malignancy, occurs in two-thirds of patients.[75]

Cronkhite-Canada Syndrome

Cronkhite-Canada syndrome is rare in children; the average age of patients is 62 years. The clinical features include juvenile polyps of the stomach and the colon, chronic diarrhea with protein-losing enteropathy, alopecia, onychodystrophy, and brown macular lesions of the skin.[76] Alimentary tract polyps also can be found in the esophagus and the small intestine. Bacteriologic, chromosomal, and immunologic studies have failed to uncover a cause for the symptoms.[77] A family history of polyps or GI tract malignancy is usually not identified. Although the malabsorption may be severe and the clinical features progressive, spontaneous improvement and resolution have been reported.[78,79] The polyps were initially described as adenomatous, but more recent descriptions have shown that they are inflammatory.[80] Some may have features of hamartomatous polyps. GI malignancy is found in 15 percent of affected individuals.[81]

Table 3 summarizes the disorders involving intestinal polyps.

Miscellaneous

Colonic polyps have been associated with acromegaly,[82] acrochordons (skin tags),[83,84] ischemic colonic injury,[85] schistosomiasis,[86] and idiopathic ulcerative colitis.[87] The basal cell nevus syndrome has been implicated in association with multiple gastric hamartomatous polyps.[88]

TREATMENT

The treatment of intestinal polyps depends upon the type of polyp and the age at which it is detected. Small hyperplastic polyps can be identified in the colon in up to 34 percent of individuals examined in autopsy studies.[89-91] Recent studies in a group of asymptomatic adults with a rectosigmoid polyp that was less than 1 cm in diameter revealed that if the polyp was hyperplastic then the probability that a more proximal adenoma could be found was 29 percent. If the diminutive distal polyp was itself an adenoma, then the incidence of a more proximal adenoma was 33 percent.[92] What is missing are the data concerning the incidence of adenomas in asymptomatic individuals who do not have a small polyp in the distal colon. Thus, it is difficult to determine how reliable screening sigmoidoscopy will be for the early detection of adenomas. This issue is of major importance in the adult population but is rarely of clinical significance in the pediatric population. In families with a strong history of colon cancer and adenomas, education concerning therapy should begin in adolescence, when a screening sigmoidoscopy should be considered.

When a polyp is identified in a child, clinical data are frequently helpful in deciding whether or not one should sus-

TABLE 3
Disorders Involving Intestinal Polyps

	Isolated Juvenile Polyp	Juvenile Polyposis Coli	Generalized Juvenile Polyposis	Familial Polyposis Coli	Gardner's Syndrome	Turcot's Syndrome	Peutz-Jeghers Syndrome	Cowden's Disease	Cronkhite-Canada Syndrome
Type of polyp	Inflammatory	Inflammatory	Inflammatory ± adenomatous	Adenomatous	Adenomatous	Adenomatous	Hamartomatous	Hamartomatous	Inflammatory
Location	Colon	Colon	Esophagus, small intestine, colon, stomach	Colon	Colon, stomach, duodenum	Colon	Colon, stomach, small intestine, nose, bronchi, urinary tract	Esophagus, stomach, small intestine, colon	Esophagus, stomach, small intestine, colon
Heredity	None	Autosomal dominant	Autosomal dominant	Autosomal dominant	Autosomal dominant	Autosomal recessive	Autosomal dominant	Autosomal dominant	None
Present at birth	No	+	+	±	±	±	+	+	+
Malignancy potential	None	Possible	Probable	Definitely of colon	Definitely of colon, duodenal, adenocarcinoma, thyroid and adrenal carcinoma	Definitely of colon, thyroid cancer	2–3%, usually of duodenum	Breast and thyroid	Gastrointestinal cancer in 15% of adults
Extraintestinal manifestations	None	None	None	None	Osteomas of cranium, mandible, fibromata, abnormal dentition, lymphoid polyps, sebaceous or epidermoid cysts, mesenteric fibromatosis, lipomas, desmoid tumors		Sex cord tumors of the ovary, lesions of the endocervix	Congenital anomalies, thyroid tumors, breast hypertrophy and cancer	Alopecia, onychodystrophy, hyperpigmentation
Associated conditions	None	Malrotation, extra digit, undescended testes, mesenteric lymphangiomata, amyotonia congenita, hydrocephalus, hypertelorism	Pulmonary arteriovenous malformations	Hepatoblastoma, acute myelogenous leukemia	Periampullary carcinoma, bile duct cancer, papillary thyroid cancer	Brain tumors	Melanotic pigmentation of lips, buccal mucosa, skin	Orocutaneous hamartomas	
Incidence	1:100 pre-school and school-aged children	1:100,000	1:8000 of general population						

pect multiple polyps. Because in most school-aged children these polyps are inflammatory, one need not emergently remove them. Care should be taken to instruct the family to preserve in formalin any tissue that is passed. If there is rectal bleeding, the polyp can be removed endoscopically. The frequency with which these polyps slough is unknown, but it is not unreasonable to wait for a few months in an otherwise clinically stable patient to determine if the polyp has fallen from its stalk.

Endoscopic removal of a polyp[93] is a safe and effective therapy even in young children. Care should be taken to avoid bowel preparations that contain mannitol, as fatal colonic explosions have been reported.[94] The availability of CO_2 in the procedure room during a polypectomy diminishes the possibility of ignition of combustible gas during the removal of a polyp.

If the polyp is confirmed histologically to be of the inflammatory type, further evaluation is not needed unless one of the familial syndromes is suspected. In the child with juvenile polyposis coli or generalized juvenile polyposis, surveillance is the major issue. Because the reported number of these families is small, precise recommendations concerning repeated endoscopic evaluation do not exist. Early in the development of the polyps, the clinician should attempt to determine the rates at which the polyps are growing and new polyps are forming. Therefore, annual colonoscopy for a few years may be necessary. If there is little change, examinations can be performed less frequently. Large or growing polyps should be removed and examined microscopically. As the risk for malignancy is low, decisions about colectomy often depend upon symptoms such as rectal prolapse, pain with defecation, rectal bleeding, or recurrent and refractory protrusion of polyps from the rectum. With the improvements in surgical technique for endorectal pull-through, these children do not require permanent ileostomy.[95] Although there is never an optimal time for colectomy, adolescence should be avoided if at all possible.

In children with familial polyposis coli or Gardner's syndrome, the decision concerning colectomy is based upon the potential for the development of adenocarcinoma. Polyps may be noticed in adolescence but have been reported in infancy. In the affected individual, the timing of a colectomy is controversial. Some clinicians suggest that colectomy should be performed in young children as soon as the diagnosis is established,[96] whereas others recommend close clinical observation with colectomy either when all the polyps cannot be removed endoscopically or when severe atypia is identified.[97] One of the earliest reports of colonic carcinoma occurred in a child of 9 years. These decisions must be individualized; the risk of cancer must be balanced against the optimal time for colectomy. The child needs to be involved in this decision, especially if the surgery is planned to occur during adolescence. If there are less than 10 polyps in the colon and all can be removed at the time of colonoscopy, then repeat endoscopy should be performed every 6 months to evaluate the rate of recurrence and assess the grade of atypia in the adenomas.

Most patients with familial polyposis coli eventually have a colectomy. The distribution and the number of colonic polyps may vary greatly among individuals, and there are some surgeons who believe that for those family members with a small number of localized polyps, a limited resection may be sufficient. However, these patients still require continued surveillance. For those individuals in whom total colectomy is required, there are three surgical options. The abdominal colectomy with mucosal proctectomy and creation of a reservoir at the ileoanal anastomosis has become the operation of choice because of the preservation of the rectal sphincter mechanism. Unlike patients with ulcerative colitis, individuals with polyposis do not have the severe mucosal inflammation that may interfere with the creation of a reservoir. Results are usually favorable. Other surgical options include total abdominal colectomy with ileoanal anastomosis. This can be offered to those patients who have a limited number of rectal polyps that can be removed at the time of surgery. These individuals must have endoscopic evaluation of the remaining colonic tissue every 6 months. Another surgical option is a total proctocolectomy with creation of an ileostomy. This operation eliminates the possibility for development of colonic adenocarcimona, but these patients must still be evaluated for the possible occurrence of periampullary carcinoma, intra-abdominal desmoids, and mesenteric fibromatosis.

Currently, there is no medical therapy that is totally effective for the treatment of colonic polyps. Various agents have been tried, including vitamins A, C, and E, indomethacin, and calcium. The nonsteroidal anti-inflammatory drug sulindac has been shown to be effective in eliminating colonic polyps in some patients with familial polyposis coli.[98-100] The clinical role for this therapy remains to be clarified.

Jejunal polyps in Peutz-Jeghers syndrome may cause problems because of intestinal obstruction or recurrent intussusception of the small intestine. Surgical resection should be avoided, if possible, because the formation of adhesions may predispose to future obstruction. With the improvement in endoscopic equipment, small intestinal polyps can be removed intraluminally.[101] If the polyp cannot be reached with an endoscope, laparatomy may be beneficial to directly telescope the bowel over the instrument, permitting more extensive investigation. Polyps that cannot be reached by passing the endoscope through the mouth can be inserted through an enterotomy.[102] Broad-based polyps may still require resection of the bowel.

SUMMARY

Polyps in children are frequently a benign condition that does not carry a risk of chronic disease and surveillance. As the genetics of these disorders becomes better understood, clinicians may be able to predict with a higher degree of accuracy those individuals with multiple or atypical polyps who are at risk for more serious sequelae. At the present time, lacking molecular probes for these disorders, physicians must rely upon clinical and pathologic data to support their long-term treatment plan.

Acknowledgment

I would like to thank Donald Antonioli, M.D., not only for his critical review of this manuscript, but also for his teaching of gastrointestinal pathology.

REFERENCES

1. Livstone EM, Troncale FJ, Sheahan DG. Value of a single forceps biopsy of colonic polyps. Gastroenterology 1977; 73:1296–1298.
2. Mestre JR. The changing pattern of juvenile polyps. Am J Gastroenterol 1986; 81:312–314.
3. Lofti AM, Spencer RJ, Ilstrup DM, Melton JM III. Colorectal polyps and the risk of subsequent carcinoma. Mayo Clin Proc 1986; 61:337–343.
4. Grigioni WF, Alampi G, Martinelli G, Piccaluga A. Atypical juvenile polyposis. Histopathology 1981; 5:361–376.
5. Day DW, Morson BC. In: Morson BC, ed. The pathogenesis of colorectal cancer. Philadelphia: WB Saunders: 1978.
6. Hayashi T, Yatani R, Apostol J, Stemmermann GN. Pathogenesis of hyperplastic polyps of the colon: a hypothesis based upon ultrastructural and in vitro cell kinetics. Gastroenterology 1974; 66:347.
7. Estrada R, Spjut HJ. Hamartomatous polyps in Peutz-Jeghers syndrome: a light-, histochemical, and electron-microscopic study. Am J Surg Pathol 1983; 7:747–754.
8. Matuchansky C, Babin P, Coutrot S, Druart F, Barbier J, Maire P. Peutz-Jeghers syndrome with metastasizing carcinoma arising from jejunal hamartoma. Gastroenterology 1979; 77:1311–1315.
9. Shinya H, Wolff WI. Morphology, anatomic distribution and cancer potential of colonic polyps: an analysis of 7,000 polyps endoscopically removed. Ann Surg 1979; 190:679–683.
10. Burt RW, Bishop DT, Cannon LA, Dowdle MA, Lee RG, Skolnick MH. Dominant inheritance of adenomatous colonic polyps and colorectal cancer. N Engl J Med 1985; 312:1540–1544.
11. Dworkin BM, Winawer SJ. Neoplastic colonic polyps: a review. Curr Concepts Gastroenterol 1985; 9:3–9.
12. Mazier WP, Bowman HE, Sun KM, Muldoon JP. Juvenile polyps of the colon and rectum. Dis Col Rect 1974; 17:523–528.
13. Toccalino H, Guastavino E, de Pinni F, O'Donnell JC, Williams M. Juvenile polyps of the rectum and colon. Acta Paediatr Scand 1973; 62:337–340.
14. Douglas JR, Campbell CA, Salisbury DM, Walker-Smith JA, Williams CB. Colonoscopic polypectomy in children. Br Med J 1980; 281:1386–1387.
15. Roth SI, Helwig EB. Juvenile polyps of the colon and rectum. Cancer 1963; 16:468–479.
16. Liu TH, Chen MC, Tseng HC, Chou L, Lu C. Malignant change of juvenile polyp of colon. Chin Med J 1978; 4:434–439.
17. Cynamon HA, Milov DE, Andres JM. Diagnosis and management of colonic polyps. J Pediatr 1989; 114:593–596.
18. Byrne WJ, Jimenez JF, Euler AR, Golladay ES. Lymphoid polyps (focal lymphoid hyperplasia) of the colon in children. Pediatrics 1982; 69:598–600.
19. McNicholas T, Brereton RJ, Raafat F. Lymphoid polyps of the rectum. J Pediatr Gastroenterol Nutr 1985; 4:297–302.
20. Veale AMO, McColl I, Bussey HJR, Morson BC. Juvenile polyposis coli. J Med Genet 1966; 3:5.
21. Middleton P, Ferguson W, Exsanguinating uncontrollable lower gastrointestinal hemorrhage due to juvenile polyposis: report of a case. Dis Col Rect 1977; 20:690–694.
22. Sachatello CR, Hahn IS, Carrington CB. Juvenile gastrointestinal polyposis in a female infant: report of a case and review of the literature of a recently recognized syndrome. Surgery 1974; 75:107–113.
23. Grotsky HW, Rickert RR, Smith WD, Newsome JF. Familial juvenile polyposis coli: a clinical and pathologic study of a large kindred. Gastroenterology 1982; 82:494–501.
24. Sandler RS, Lipper S. Multiple adenomas in juvenile polyposis. Am J Gastroenterol 1981; 75:361–366.
25. Mills SE, Fechner RE. Unusual adenomatous polyps in juvenile polyposis coli. Am J Surg Pathol 1982; 6:177–183.
26. Rozen P, Baratz M. Familial juvenile colonic polyposis with associated colon cancer. Cancer 1982; 49:1500–1503.
27. Ruvalcaba RHH, Myhre S, Smith DW. Sotos syndrome with intestinal polyposis and pigmentary changes of the genitalia. Clin Genet 1980; 18:413–416.
28. Stemper TJ, Kent TH, Summers RW. Juvenile polyposis and gastrointestinal carcinoma: a study of a kindred. Ann Intern Med 1975; 83:639–646.
29. Sachatello CR, Pickren JW, Grace JT Jr. Generalized juvenile gastrointestinal polyposis: a hereditary syndrome. Gastroenterology 1970; 58:699–708.
30. Le Luyer B, Le Bihan M, Metayer P, Metayer J, Mallet E, de Menibus CH. Generalized juvenile polyposis in an infant: report of a case and successful management by endoscopy. J Pediatr Gastroenterol Nutr 1985; 4:128–134.
31. Watanabe A, Nagashima H, Motol M, Ogawa K. Familial juvenile polyposis of the stomach. Gastroenterology 1979; 77:148–151.
32. Grosfeld JL, West KW. Generalized juvenile polyposis coli: clinical management based on long-term observations. Arch Surg 1986; 121:530–534.
33. Cox KL, Frates Jr RC, Wong A, Gandhi G. Hereditary generalized juvenile polyposis associated with pulmonary arteriovenous malformation. Gastroenterology 1980; 78:1566–1570.
34. Beacham CH, Shields HM, Raffensperger EC, Enterline HT. Juvenile and adenomatous gastrointestinal polyposis. Dig Dis 1978; 23:1137–1143.
35. Murphy EA. Genetic aspects of multiple polyposis coli. Dis Colon Rectum 1983; 26:470–474.
36. Murphy EA, Krush AJ, Dietz M, Rhode CA. Hereditary polyposis coli. III. Genetic and evolutionary fitness. Am J Hum Genet 1980; 32:700–713.
37. Kingston JE, Herbert A, Draper GJ, Mann JR. Association between hepatoblastoma and polyposis coli. Arch Dis Child 1983; 58:959–962.
38. Kurtz RC, Sternberg SS, Miller HH, Decosse JJ. Upper gastrointestinal neoplasia in familial polyposis. Dig Dis Sci 1987; 32:459–465.
39. Yao T, Iida M, Ohsat K, Watanabe H, Omae T. Duodenal lesions in familial polyposis of the colon. Gastroenterology 1977; 73:1086–1092.
40. Iida M, Yao T, Watanabe H, Itoh H, Iwashita A. Fundic gland polyposis in patients without familial adenomatosis coli: its incidence and clinical features. Gastroenterology 1984; 86:1437–1442.
41. Boman BM, Levin B. Familial polyposis. Hosp Pract May 15, 1986; 155–170.
42. Watanabe H, Enjoji M, Yao T, Iida M, Ohsato K. Accompanying gastro-enteric lesions in familial adenomatosis coli. Acta Pathol Jpn 1977; 27:823–839.
43. Watanabe H, Enjoji M, Yao T, Ohsato K. Gastric lesions in familial adenomatosis coli: their incidence and histologic analysis. Hum Pathol 1978; 9:269–283.
44. Luk GD, Baylin SB. Ornithine decarboxylase as a biologic marker in familial colonic polyposis. N Engl J Med 1984; 311:80–83.
45. Meltzer SJ, Ahnen DJ, Battifora H, Yokota J, Cline MJ. Protooncogene abnormalities in colon cancers and adenomatous polyps. Gastroenterology 1987; 92:1174–1180.
46. Gardner EJ, Stephens FE. Cancer of the lower digestive tract in one family group. Am J Hum Genet 1950; 2:41–48.
47. Gardner EJ. A genetic and clinical study of intestinal polyposis, a predisposing factor for carcinoma of the colon and rectum. Am J Hum Genet 1951; 3:167–176.
48. McKusick VA. Genetic factors in intestinal polyposis. JAMA 1962; 182:271–277.
49. Ushio K, Sasagawa M, Doi H, Yamada T, Ichikawa H, Hojo K, Koyama Y, Sano R. Lesions associated with familial polyposis coli: studies of lesions of the stomach, duodenum, bones and teeth. Gastrointest Radiol 1976; 1:67–80.
50. Utsunomiya J, Maki T, Iwama T, Matsunaga Y, Ichikawa T, Shimomura T, Hamaguchi E, Aoki N. Gastric lesion of familial polyposis coli. Cancer 1974; 34:745–754.
51. Yao T, Iida M, Ohsato K, Watanabe H, Omae T. Duodenal lesions in familial polyposis of the colon. Gastroenterology 1977; 73:1086–1092.
52. Burt RW, Berenson MM, Lee RG, Tolman KG, Freston JW, Gardner EJ. Upper gastrointestinal polyps in Gardner's syndrome. Gastroenterology 1984; 86:295–301.
53. Coffey RJ Jr, Knight CD Jr, van Heerden JA, Weiland LH. Gastric adenocarcinoma complicating Gardner's syndrome in a North American woman. Gastroenterology 1985; 88:1263–1266.
54. Naylor EW, Lebenthal E. Gardner's syndrome: recent developments in research and management. Dig Dis Sci 1980; 25:945–959.
55. Burt RW, Rikkers LF, Gardner EJ, Lee RG, Tolman KG. Villous adenoma of the duodenal papilla presenting as necrotizing pancreatitis in a patient with Gardner's syndrome. Gastroenterology 1987; 92:532–535.

56. Hood AB, Krush AJ. Clinical and dermatologic aspects of the hereditary intestinal polyposes. Dis Colon Rectum 1983; 16:546–548.

57. Mathias JR, Smith WG. Mesenteric fibromatosis associated with familial polyposis. Dig Dis 1977; 22:741–744.

58. Binder MK, Zablen MA, Fleischer DE, Sue DY, Dwyer RM, Hanelin L. Colon polyps, sebaceous cysts, gastric polyps, and malignant brain tumor in a family. Dig Dis 1978; 23:460–466.

59. Butson ARC. Familial multiple polyposis coli with multiple associated tumors. Dis Colon Rectum 1983; 26:578–592.

60. Lewis RA, Crowder WE, Eierman LA, Nussbaum RL, Ferrell RE. The Gardner syndrome: significance of ocular features. Ophthalmology 1984; 91:916–925.

61. Traboulsi EI, Krush AJ, Gardner EJ, Booker SV, Offerhaus GJA, Yardley JH, Hamilton SR, Luk GD, Giardiello FM, Welsh SB, Hughes JP, Maumenee IH. Prevalence and importance of pigmented ocular fundus lesions in Gardner's syndrome. N Engl J Med 1987; 316:661–667.

62. Lev R, Lebenthal E, Rossi T, Lance P. Histochemical and morphological analysis of colonic epithelium from children with Gardner's syndrome and adults bearing adenomatous polyps. J Pediatr Gastroenterol Nutr 1987; 6:414–425.

63. Radin DR, Fortgang KC, Zee C-S, Mikity VG, Halls JM. Turcot syndrome: a case with spinal cord and colonic neoplasms. Am J Radiol 1984; 142:475–476.

64. Miller LJ, Bartholomew LG, Dozois RR, Dahlin DC. Adenocarcinoma of the rectum arising in a hamartomatous polyp in a patient with Peutz-Jeghers syndrome. Dig Dis Sci 1983; 28:1047–1051.

65. Tweedie JH, McCann BG. Peutz-Jeghers syndrome and metastasising colonic adenocarcinoma. Gut 1984; 25:1118–1123.

66. Patterson MJ, Kernen JA. Epithelioid leiomyosarcoma originating in a hamartomatous polyp from a patient with Peutz-Jeghers syndrome. Gastroenterology 1985; 88:1060–1064.

67. Lehur P-A, Madarnas P, Devroede G, Perey BJ, Menard DB, Hamade N. Peutz-Jeghers syndrome: association of duodenal and bilateral breast cancers in the same patient. Dig Dis Sci 1984; 29:178–182.

68. Long JA Jr, Dreyfuss JR. The Peutz-Jeghers syndrome: a 39-year clinical and radiographic follow-up report. N Engl J Med 1977; 297:1070.

69. Solh HM, Azoury RS. Najjar SS. Peutz-Jeghers syndrome associated with precocious puberty. J Pediatr 1983; 103:593–595.

70. Lloyd KM, Dennis M. Cowden's disease: a possible new syndrome complex with multiple system involvement. Ann Intern Med 1963; 58:136–142.

71. Weinstock JV, Kawanishi H. Gastrointestinal polyposis with orocutaneous hamartomas (Cowden's disease). Gastroenterology 1978; 74:890–895.

72. Lashner BA, Riddell RH, Winans CS. Ganglioneuromatosis of the colon and extensive glycogenic acanthosis in Cowden's disease. Dig Dis Sci 1986; 31:213–216.

73. Burnett JW, Goldner R, Calton GJ. Cowden's disease. Br J Dermatol 1975; 93:329–336.

74. Thyresson HN, Doyle JA. Cowden's disease (multiple hamartoma syndrome). Mayo Clin Proc 1981; 56:179–184.

75. Sogol PB, Sugawara M, Gordon E, Shellow WVR, Hernandez F, Hershman JM. Cowden's disease: familial goiter and skin hamartomas: a report of three cases. West J Med 1983; 139:324–328.

76. Nishiki M, Takasugi S, Kanao M, Okumichi T, Tamura T, Ezaki H. Cronkhite-Canada syndrome: a case report and analytical review of 37 other cases reported in Japan. Hiroshima J Med Sci 1984; 33:607–614.

77. Ali M, Weinstein J, Biempica L, Halpern A, Das KM. Cronkhite-Canada syndrome: report of a case with bacteriologic, immunologic presentation and new therapeutic strategy. Endoscopy 1985; 17:102–104.

78. Peart AG, Sivak MV Jr, Rankin GB, Kish LS, Steck WD. Spontaneous improvement of Cronkhite-Canada syndrome in a postpartum female. Dig Dis Sci 1984; 29:470–474.

79. Russell DMcR, Bhathal PS, St. John DJB. Complete remission in Cronkhite-Canada syndrome. Gastroenterology 1983; 85:180–185.

80. Rubin M, Tuthill RJ, Rosato EF, Cohen S. Cronkhite-Canada syndrome: report of an unusual case. Gastroenterology 1980; 79:737–741.

81. Daniel ES, Ludwig SL, Lewin K, et al. The Cronkite-Canada syndrome. Medicine 1982; 61:293–309.

82. Klein I, Parveen G, Gavaler JS, Vanthiel DH. Colonic polyps in patients with acromegaly. Ann Intern Med 1982; 97:27–30.

83. Leavitt J, Klein I, Kendricks F, Gavaler J, VanThiel DH. Skin tags: a cutaneous marker for colonic polyps. Ann Intern Med 1983; 98:928–930.

84. Luk GD, Colon Neoplasia Work Group. Colonic polyps and acrochordons (skin tags) do not correlate in familial colonic polyposis kindreds. Ann Intern Med 1986; 104:209–210.

85. Levine DS, Surawicz CM, Spencer GD, Rohrmann CA, Silverstein FE. Inflammatory polyposis two years after ischemic colon injury. Dig Dis Sci 1986; 31:1159–1167.

86. Hussein AMT, Medany S, el Magd AMA, Sherif SM. Multiple endoscopic polypectomies for schistosomal polyposis of the colon. Lancet 1983; i:673–674.

87. Forde KA, Gold RP, Holck S, Goldberg MD, Kaim PS. Giant pseudopolyposis in colitis with colonic intussusception. Gastroenterology 1978; 75:1142–1146.

88. Schwartz RA. Basal-cell-nervous syndrome and gastrointestinal polyposis. N Engl J Med 1978; 299:49.

89. Vatn WH, Stalsberg H. The prevalence of polyps of the large intestine in Oslo: an autopsy study. Cancer 1982; 49:819–825.

90. Williams AR, Balasooriya BA, Day DW. Polyps and cancer of the large bowel: a necropsy study in Liverpool. Gut 1982; 23:835–842.

91. Bombi JA. Polyps of the colon in Barcelona, Spain. An autopsy study. Cancer 1988; 83:120–122.

92. Achkar E, Carey W. Small polyps found during fiberoptic sigmoidoscopy in asymptomatic patients. Ann Intern Med 1988; 109(11):880–883.

93. Bess MA, Spencer RJ. Colonoscopic polypectomies. Mayo Clin Proc 1979; 54:32–34.

94. Taylor EW, Bentley S, Youngs D, Keighley MRB. Bowel preparation and the safety of colonoscopic polypectomy. Gastroenterology 1981; 81:1–4.

95. Dinari G, Nitzan M, Rosenbach Y, Dintsman M, Wolloch Y. Generalized gastrointestinal juvenile polyposis and its treatment. Am J Proctol Gastroenterol Colon Rect Surg 1983; Aug:5–8.

96. Leggett PL, Arensman RM, Falterman KW. Familial polyposis in children: early detection and preferred treatment. South Med J 1984; 77:462–464.

97. Boman BM, Levin B. Familial polyposis. Hosp Pract 1986; 21:155–170.

98. Waddell WR, Ganser GF, Cerise EJ, Loughry RW. Sulindac for polyposis of the colon. Am J Surg 1989; 157:175–179.

99. Jones IT, Jagelman DG, Fazio VW, Lavery IC, Wenkley FL, McGannon E. Desmoid tumors in familial polyposis coli. Ann Surg 1986; 204(1):94–97.

100. Gonzaga RA, Lima FR, Carneiros-Maciel J, Amarante-Junior M. Sulindac treatment for familial polyposis coli. (Letter) Lancet 1985; i:751.

101. Paterlini A, Huscher C, Salmi A. Jejunal endoscopic polypectomy in the Peutz-Jeghers syndrome. Endoscopy 1983; 15:270–271.

102. Mathus-Vliegen EMH, Tytgat GNJ. Peutz-Jeghers syndrome: clinical

PART 28

Appendicitis

Barry Shandling, M.B., Ch.B., F.R.C.S.(Eng.), FRCSC, F.A.C.S.

PATHOGENESIS

A recent historical review of appendicitis examines the disease from its earliest anatomic descriptions to its more recent history, especially in Europe and North America.[1] Appendectomy is the most common emergency operation in childhood, and appendicitis is found in all levels of society with equal incidence.[2] Occasionally one observes a strong family history of appendectomies,[3,4] and a definite familial incidence of the disease has been documented.[5] The lesion occurs most frequently in patients 15 to 24 years of age and least frequently in the age group 0 to 4 years. There is a slight male dominance, and the overall incidence of the condition is 140 per 100,000 according to the Central Bureau of Statistics.[6] The condition does occur in infancy,[7] even in newborn infants. A high-fiber diet results in a lower incidence of fecalith formation, and in societies with low dietary fiber intake there is a significantly higher incidence of appendicitis.[8-10] In addition to fecaliths, other potential etiologic agents include parasites; pips; chips of bone, metal, and wood; and a low water intake.[11] Various microorganisms have been incriminated; these include *Bacteroides fragilis*,[12] *Escherichia coli, Campylobacter fetus*,[13] *Streptococcus milleri*,[14] *Yersinia enterocolitica, Streptococcus pneumoniae*,[15] *Pasteurella multocida, Pseudomonas aeruginosa,* and *Schistosoma japonicum.*[16,17] There is no good evidence that pinworms (*Enterobius vermicularis*) are a cause of appendicitis.[18]

PATHOLOGY

Stasis, often the consequence of a fecalith or a small pebble of feces within the lumen, coupled with the infective contents of the appendix, leads to invasive inflammation within the wall of the appendix. This spreads to involve the seromuscular layers, with the formation of a fibrinous exudate on the serosal surface of the organ. Thrombosis of the appendicular artery ensues, which may lead to gangrene of the tip of the organ. The other site at which gangrene may develop is in the wall of the inflamed appendix immediately overlying a fecalith. Gangrene leads to the escape of the infective contents of the appendix through a perforation to result in either localized or generalized peritonitis. In the case of the former a periappendicular abscess results, walled off from the rest of the peritoneal cavity by the adjacent cecum, omentum, and ileal loops. There may be a fecalith floating free within such an abscess. Rarely there will be fibrous tissue present within the appendix, representing presumed previous attacks of appendicitis with resolution and scarring. Obstruction, the result of a tumor (argentaffinoma), may be the cause of inflammation. There are several reports of granulomatous appendicitis (Crohn's disease) with the inflammatory changes confined to that organ.[19-24] The presence of inflammation in the right lower quadrant and the fibrinous exudate may result in adhesions of contiguous loops of bowel leading to intestinal obstruction. In infancy and early childhood the omentum is not as large as in an older individual, and this may result in less efficient localization of the inflammation. Thus, perforation with peritonitis is said to ensue more rapidly in very young children.

CLINICAL FEATURES

Symptoms

Pain is a sine qua non of acute appendicitis. The duration of the pain is the single most important fact to elicit in the history of appendicitis.[25,26] Usually the preceding history is one of hours to 1 or 2 days. If the pain has been present for more than 72 hours, the diagnosis of appendicitis is less likely unless an appendicular abscess is present. Initially, before the serosa of the appendix is inflamed, pain is referred to the central abdominal periumbilical region. The pain may be colicky at first, because the organ is contracting repeatedly in a futile attempt to overcome the obstruction. Then the parietal peritoneum becomes inflamed as the disease progresses, and the pain becomes steady and localized to the right iliac fossa. Infrequently, if the appendix is in the pelvis, pain may be experienced in the labium majus or the scrotum[24] and testis or penis. There may be dysuria or even frequency of urination.

Vomiting occurs in 90 percent of cases. It is not marked nor persistent, and it has no effect on the pain. With the vomiting anorexia is common with or without nausea. Movement (such as the car trip to the hospital) usually aggravates the pain. There may be no alteration in bowel habit, but if the appendix is retroileal or pelvic in position diarrhea may have developed owing to the adjacent inflammation in the wall of the rectum or ileum. The child may walk with a stoop and be unable to fully extend the right hip, the consequence of inflammation in the psoas or iliopsoas muscles if there is a retrocecal or retroileal appendicitis. There may even be an associated headache.

Signs

The young patient tends to lie very still, the right hip slightly flexed, with an associated lumbar lordosis. Jiggling the examining table may result in a wince. If generalized peritonitis is present, the child is likely to move only the eyes. When there has been much vomiting in association with decreased fluid intake, clinical signs of dehydration are present, with diminished tissue turgor and eyeball tension, dryness of mucous membranes, and a decreased urinary output. In advanced cases the signs of shock with or without gram-negative sepsis are dramatic.

In the absence of perforation there is usually a low-grade pyrexia, varying from 37.5 to 38.5⁰ C. If there is a temperature above 39⁰ C in the absence of peritonitis, appendicitis is unlikely. With peritonitis the temperature may be very high or subnormal; the latter is an ominous finding.

When proceeding to palpation it is well to remember that a small child with a severe bellyache, brought usually for the first time to a large, busy emergency department, cannot understand why a stranger in a white coat is prodding at the painful belly, thus actually making it worse. The examiner must proceed gently and slowly. It is wise not to examine the child in silence but to carry on a two-way conversation. Questions should be asked of the patient which are calculated to make him think of the answer, which itself may require expanded explanation. The patient is asked to "puff out" the abdomen and then to "pull it in." With inflammation of the peritoneum, localized pain is felt, usually in the right lower quadrant. While the child is thus concentrating or talking, tentative palpation of the abdomen is begun, commencing furthest away from where the maximum tenderness is anticipated. Such diversionary tactics take the child's mind off the abdomen and minimize any tendency toward exaggeration of the signs.

Initial palpation is done using a stethoscope as a palpating device. Children are familiar with this instrument and know that it causes no pain. Proceeding to manual palpation, the hand is not lifted off the abdomen as in playing a piano. Rather, it is slid around on the abdomen without exerting pressure, so that the child becomes accustomed to its feel. All the while the examiner is looking not at the patient's abdomen but at the face. It is only thus that subtle degrees of tenderness can be noted and the patient spared unnecessary pain by having to declare discomfort instead of the examiner noting it sooner. If the examiner causes pain, voluntary guarding may ensue, thus rendering thorough abdominal palpation difficult or impossible.

The cardinal signs of unperforated appendicitis are three: constant, localized, and severe tenderness. The tenderness does not change in its location as the examination continues. Nor can there be tenderness other than in one localized area if the appendix has as yet not perforated. So slight a degree of tenderness as to be elicited only upon direct interrogation is not found in appendicitis. The tenderness is usually localized to McBurney's point, which is at the junction of the middle and lateral thirds of a line joining the umbilicus and the right anterior superior iliac spine. Involuntary guarding of the muscles of the abdominal wall over the site of maximal tenderness is usually found. Indeed, the total absence of guarding should be regarded as strong evidence against a diagnosis of appendicitis. If the inflamed appendix is adjacent to the right psoas muscle, the child may keep the right hip flexed and walk stooped over because of spasm of the psoas muscle—the so-called psoas sign. Sometimes palpation in the left lower quadrant results in pain in the right lower quadrant, presumably the consequence of cecal distention—Rovsing's sign.

I find that rectal examination, while traditionally insisted upon, contributes little to the diagnosis of appendicitis, which is usually made by examination of the abdomen. It is in cases of unusual location of the appendix that the finger in the rectum may be of value, as with pelvic appendicitis or abscess, or in girls who may have pelvic inflammatory disease. I never try to elicit rebound tenderness. If positive, the sudden cruel pain experienced by the child upon sudden release of pressure serves only to break down any confidence in the ability of the physician not to cause further discomfort. Furthermore, the sign is often positive when there is no appendicitis, probably more as a consequence of startling the child, and often negative in the presence of inflammation of the appendix.

LABORATORY FINDINGS

The white blood cell count is usually mildly elevated, up to about 15,000 per cubic millimeter,[26] with a shift to the left, but in infants counts of 20,000 per cubic millimeter or more are not unusual.[27,28] However, normal or subnormal counts are not rare and a leukocytosis is often seen in cases of viral enteritis, the most common condition to be differentiated from appendicitis. The only real reason to do a leukocyte count in appendicitis is to diagnose concomitant leukemia. Urinalysis is normal except when the inflamed appendix abuts on the right ureter or bladder. Under such circumstances there may be polymorphonuclear cells found in the urine.

INVESTIGATIONS

There is little indication for diagnostic imaging in appendicitis.[29] An abdominal film will show a (calcified) fecalith in 10 percent of cases. This finding, in a case of questionable appendicitis, is a very strong indication for operation. There may be a scoliosis to the right and a soft tissue mass. Recently claims have been made for the usefulness of barium enema in the diagnosis of appendicitis.[30-32] Absence of filling of the appendix, not in itself significant, together with edema of the cecum and/or ileum and a space-occupying lesion with distortion of the cecal wall may be seen.[33,34] Conversely, complete filling of the appendix rules out obstructive appendicitis. Recently a barium meal has been suggested as providing 95 percent accuracy in the diagnosis of appendicitis.

Ultrasonographic examination[35-38] of the abdomen may show a fecalith and may be useful in the diagnosis of an appendicular abscess; CT scan[39,40] may be used for the same purpose.

However, the diagnosis of appendicitis is made by the bedside. The finding of constant severe point tenderness in a patient with a short history of abdominal pain must lead the physician to conclude, other things being equal, that the child has appendicitis and that an operation is necessary.

DIFFERENTIAL DIAGNOSIS

When a patient with right lower quadrant pain and tenderness turns out not to have appendicitis, the most likely, but difficult to confirm, diagnosis is viral enteritis. Tenderness is less extreme and the fever may be higher. There may be mesenteric lymph node enlargement leading to the popular diagnosis of mesenteric adenitis, but I know of no convincing evidence of the existence of the latter condition as a specific disease entity. Many children with pain, with or without tenderness in the right lower quadrant, have constipation. A detailed history, absence of fever, significant rectal findings, and the gratifying response to the administration of an enema differentiate constipation from appendicitis. Urinary tract infection, perhaps in association with vesicoureteral reflux, should be suspected when urinalysis reveals a significant bacteriuria or pyuria or when there is loin tenderness. Smaller children with tonsillitis or pharyngitis may experience abdominal pain, but there is no point tenderness on abdominal examination. Older girls may develop pelvic inflammatory disease with diffuse lower abdominal pain and tenderness or hemorrhage or torsion of a right-sided ovarian cyst with significant rectal findings.[41]

Rare conditions that will require differentiation from appendicitis include primary peritonitis, pneumonia, Henoch-Schönlein purpura,[42] rheumatic fever, Crohn's disease, and external iliac adenitis secondary to an infective source on the leg, buttock, or perianal area. A patient with arrested hydrocephalus and an infected ventriculoperitoneal shunt may well have localized abdominal pain and tenderness. Here an ultrasonographic examination may show an encysted collection of cerebrospinal fluid. Such patients are almost never found to have appendicitis.

COMPLICATIONS

Untreated appendicitis may resolve, but usually it progresses to perforation with either the formation of a periappendicular abscess or the development of a generalized peritonitis. Subsequently the patient may develop other localized intraperitoneal suppuration with abscess and fistula formation in the pelvis,[43] elsewhere within the abdomen, or specifically in a subphrenic location.

When perforation occurs, an adynamic ileus usually complicates the clinical picture. Vomiting, at times feculent, abdominal distention, and constipation may mimic intestinal obstruction. Indeed, there may actually be intestinal obstruction present due to adhesion formation. With pelvic peritonitis obstruction to the lumen of the uterine tubes may result in diminished fertility or even sterility.[44] With overwhelming infection there may be portal pyemia and the development of pyelophlebitis.

TREATMENT

Acute appendicitis without perforation necessitates appendectomy. There is a growing body of surgeons who, because appendectomy involves opening contaminated bowel, administer one dose of antibiotics preoperatively.[45,46] Currently cefoxitin is the drug of choice in North America, although metronidazole may be as effective.[47,48] Both are given preoperatively by the intravenous route. The operation is usually done through a right lower quadrant muscle-splitting approach, and the mortality is very low. In a recent review three patients out of 8,738 died, and there was a 2.04 percent complication rate.[49] Because most children with appendici-

tis vomit and drink relatively little, it is important to rehydrate any patient who is dehydrated before rushing off to the operating room. A few hours spent getting the patient fit for surgery is far more important than proceeding directly to an operation, no matter what time of the day or night. When there is peritonitis with such severe dehydration that the patient requires 10 percent or more of his body weight as replacement fluid, it is best given as lactated Ringer's solution.

The treatment of a localized perforation with a periappendicular abscess is controversial, and while some surgeons proceed to appendectomy I prefer to treat these children nonoperatively with antibiotics and intravenous fluids. The abscess usually drains itself spontaneously into an adjacent loop of bowel, and the appendix can be removed electively 2 to 3 months later.[50]

In cases of unperforated appendicitis, the patient may be expected to be discharged on the third postoperative day.[51] It is wise to discharge the child only after a bowel movement has occurred, either spontaneously or following insertion of a suppository. When there has been peritonitis it will be necessary to decompress the alimentary tract by means of a nasogastric tube and administer intravenous fluids. Parenteral nutrition may be considered in severely depleted patients. If there is evidence of intraperitoneal suppuration, reliance should be placed in the first instance on antibiotic treatment. Drugs of choice are ampicillin, gentamicin, and either metronidazole or clindamycin. It is very rarely necessary to reoperate in the early postoperative period to drain such purulent collections. Indeed, foolhardy early reoperation may result in multiple fecal fistulae, intestinal obstruction, and further septicemia. Drainage is instituted nowadays by a radiologist skilled in interventional techniques, using a needle through which is inserted a fine catheter.

REFERENCES

1. Seal A. Appendicitis: a historical review. Can J Surg 1981; 24:427–433.
2. Poikolainen K, Saarinen M, Eskola J. Acute appendicitis not associated with social class among children. Int J Epidemiol 1985; 14:333–334.
3. Shperber Y, Halevy A, Oland J, Orda R. Familial retrocaecal appendicitis. J R Soc Med 1986; 79:405–406.
4. Brender JD, Marcuse EK, Koepsell TD, Hatch EI. Childhood appendicitis: factors associated with perforation. Pediatrics 1985; 76:301–306.
5. Brender JD, Marcuse EK, Weiss NS, Koepsell TD. Is childhood appendicitis familial? Am J Dis Child 1985; 139:338–340.
6. Sreide O. Appendicitis—a study of incidence, death rates and consumption of hospital resources. Postgrad Med J 1984; 60:341–345.
7. Bax NM, Pearse RG, Dommering N, Molenaar JC. Perforation of the appendix in the neonatal period. J Pediatr Surg 1980; 15:200–202.
8. Jones BA, Demetriades D, Segal I, Burkitt DP. The prevalence of appendiceal fecaliths in patients with and without appendicitis. A comparative study from Canada and South Africa. Ann Surg 1985; 202:80–82.
9. Brender JD, Weiss NS, Koepsell TD, Marcuse EK. Fiber intake and childhood appendicitis. Am J Public Health 1985; 75:399–400.
10. Segal I, Paterson A, Walker AR. Characteristics and occurrence of appendicitis in the black population in Johannesburg, South Africa. J Clin Gastroenterol 1986; 8:530–533.
11. Nelson M, Morris J, Barker DJ, Simmonds S. A case-control study of acute appendicitis and diet in children. J Epidemiol Community Health 1986; 40:316–318.
12. Tovar JA. Prevention of suppurative complications of appendiceal peritonitis (author's translation). Ann Esp Pediatr 1980; 13:513–522.

13. Van Spreeuwel JP, Lindeman J, Bax R, Elbers HJ, Sybrandy R, Meijer CJ. Campylobacter-associated appendicitis: prevalence and clinicopathologic features. Pathol Annu 1987; 1:55–65.

14. Madden NP, Hart CA. *Streptococcus milleri* in appendicitis in children. J Pediatr Surg 1985; 20:6–7.

15. Heltberg O, Korner B, Schouenborg P. Six cases of acute appendicitis with secondary peritonitis caused by *Streptococcus pneumoniae*. Eur J Clin Microbiol 1984; 3:141–143.

16. Onuigbo WI. Appendiceal schistosomiasis. Method of classifying oviposition and inflammation. Dis Colon Rectum 1985; 28:397–398.

17. Ricosse JH, Emeric R, Courbil LJ. Anatomopathological aspects of schistosomiasis. A study of 286 pathological specimens (author's translation). Med Trop 1980; 40:77–94.

18. Nutting SA, Murphy F, Inglis FG. Abdominal pain due to *Enterobius vermicularis*. Can J Surg 1980; 23:286–287.

19. Andersen JC. Crohn's disease limited to the vermiform appendix. Acta Chir Scand 1987; 153:441–446.

20. Timmcke AE. Granulomatous appendicitis: is it Crohn's disease? Report of a case and review of the literature. Am J Gastroenterol 1986; 81:283–287.

21. Allen DC, Biggart JD. Granulomatous disease in the vermiform appendix. J Clin Pathol 1983; 36:632–638.

22. Payan HM, Gilbert EF, Hafez R. Granulomatous appendicitis. Dis Colon Rectum 1981; 24:432–436.

23. Yang SS, Gibson P, McCaughey RS, Arcari FA, Bernstein J. Primary Crohn's disease of the appendix: report of 14 cases and review of the literature. Ann Surg 1979; 189:334–339.

24. Wilkins SA Jr, Holder LE, Raiker RV, Wilson TH Jr. Acute appendicitis presenting as acute left scrotal pain: diagnostic considerations. Urology 1985; 25:634–636.

25. Fujita W, Shigemoto H, Nishimoto T, Tsukiyama K, Ugaji Y. Acute appendicitis: a study on 118 patients. Nippon Geka Gakkai Zasshi 1985; 86:464–469.

26. Buchman TG, Zuidema GD. Reasons for delay of the diagnosis of acute appendicitis. Surg Gynecol Obstet 1984; 158:260–266.

27. Clavien PA, Junod P, Chapuis G. A prospective study of 776 cases of acute nontraumatic abdominal pain. Acute appendicitis and its diagnosis. Schweiz Med Worchenschr 1987; 117:1205–1212.

28. Lippert H, Detzner D. Preoperative examination findings in patients with a perforated appendix. Zentralbl Chir 1986; 111:801–806.

29. Kniskern JH, Eskin EM, Fletcher HS. Increasing accuracy in the diagnosis of acute appendicitis with modern diagnostic techniques. Am Surg 1986; 52:222–225.

30. Wild RE, Rutledge R, Herbst CA Jr. The use of barium enema in the evaluation of patients with possible appendicitis. Am Surg 1985; 51:474–476.

31. Picus D, Shackelford GD. Perforated appendix presenting with severe diarrhea. Findings on barium-enema examination. Radiology 1983; 149:141–143.

32. Garcia C, Rosenfield NS, Markowitz RI, Seashore JH, Touloukian RJ, Cicchetti DV. Appendicitis in children. Accuracy of the barium enema. Am J Dis Child 1987; 141:1309–1312.

33. Schisgall RM. Use of the barium swallow in the diagnosis of acute appendicitis. Am J Surg 1983; 146:663–667.

34. Erwin BC, Moskowitz PS, Shochat SJ, Zboralske FF. Roentgenographic features of acute nonobstructive appendicitis: a case report. Gastrointest Radiol 1985; 10:89–91.

35. Niekel RA, Lampmann LE. Graded compression sonography in acute appendicitis. ROFO 1986; 145:441–445.

36. Forel F, Filiatrault D, Grignon A. Ultrasonic demonstration of appendicolith. J Can Assoc Radiol 1983; 34:66–67.

37. Meiser G, Meissner K, Sattlegger P. Ultrasound study of "acute appendicitis": an elective procedure or obligation in general surgery. A prospective study. Ultraschall Med 1987; 8:197–202.

38. Puylaert JB, Rutgers PH, Lalisang RI, de Vries BC, van der Werf SD, D'Orr JP, Blok RA. A prospective study of ultrasonography in the diagnosis of appendicitis. N Engl J Med 1987; 317:666–669.

39. Barakos JA, Jeffrey RB Jr, Federle MP, Wing VW, Laing FC, Hightower DR. CT in the management of periappendiceal abscess. AJR 1986; 146:1161–1164.

40. Butsenko VN, Antoniuk SM, Shatalov AD, Mustafin SZ. Prevention and treatment of complications of acute appendicitis. Khirurgiia (Mosk) 1985; 9:103–105.

41. Bongard F, Landers DV, Lewis F. Differential diagnosis of appendicitis and pelvic inflammatory disease. A prospective analysis. Am J Surg 1985; 150:90–96.

42. Najem AZ, Barillo DJ, Spillert CR, Kerr JC, Lazaro EJ. Appendicitis versus pelvic inflammatory disease. A diagnostic dilemma. Am Surg 1985; 51:217–222.

43. Haas GP, Shumaker BP, Haas PA. Appendicovesical fistula. Urology 1984; 24:604–609.

44. Reiss HE. Effect of perforated appendicitis in girls on subsequent fertility. Br Med J 1984; 288:570.

45. Corder AP, Bates T, Prior JE, Harrison M, Donaldson PJ. Metronidazole v. cefoxitin in severe appendicitis—a trial to compare a single intraoperative dose of two antibiotics given intravenously. Postgrad Med J 1983; 59:720–723.

46. Coleman RJ, Blackwood JM, Swan KG. Role of antibiotic prophylaxis in surgery for nonperforated appendicitis. Am Surg 1987; 53:584–586.

47. Sirinek KR, Levine BA. Antimicrobial management of surgically treated gangrenous or perforated appendicitis: comparison of cefoxitin and clindamycin-gentamicin. Clin Ther 1987; 9:420–428.

48. Lose G, Holm B, Bauer T, Graversen P, Kristensen ES, Larsen E, Persson M, Skjoldborg H, Vennits B. Three days cefotoxin in perforated appendicitis. Ann Chir Gynaecol 1986; 75:270–273.

49. Cortesi N, Manenti A, Rossi A, Zanni C, Barberini G, Gibertini G. Acute appendicitis and its postoperative complications. Apropos of a series of 8738 cases. J Chir (Paris) 1985; 122:577–579.

50. Nunez D Jr, Huber JS, Yrizarry JM, Mendez G, Russell E. Nonsurgical drainage of appendiceal abscesses. AJR 1986; 146:587–589.

51. Birken GA, Schropp KP, Boles ET Jr, King DR. Discharge planning for children with perforated appendicitis. J Pediatr Surg 1986; 21:592–595.

Drug-Induced Bowel Injury

Brent Scott, M.D.C.M., FRCPC

Anecdotal evidence suggests that drug-induced gastrointestinal (GI) injury is relatively common, and a wide variety of medications have been implicated, but an accurate estimate of the incidence of adverse GI reactions to drugs is difficult to obtain. Data provided by the Division of Drug and Biological Product Experience of the United States Food and Drug Administration show that 18 percent of all adverse reactions reported to that agency in 1984 were related to the GI tract. The Boston Collaborative Drug Surveillance Program of 1970[2] found that adverse GI drug reactions developed in 4.8 percent of patients receiving medication in hospital.

Drugs induce intestinal injury or dysfunction through single or multiple mechanisms, whereas a single adverse effect can result from the use of any one of several classes of therapeutic agents. The more common adverse effects of therapeutic agents are listed in Table 1; this discussion covers those therapeutic agents that have been associated with each effect.

DRUG-INDUCED SUPPRESSION OF THE RATE OF CELL TURNOVER

Function of the GI tract is affected frequently during treatment of malignant disease with anti-neoplastic, cytotoxic, or chemotherapeutic agents. Many cytotoxic drugs with diverse modes of action are in current usage: alkylating agents (e.g., nitrogen mustard; cyclophosphamide; carmustine [BCNU] lomustine [CCNU], and methyl-CCNU of the nitrosourea family), antimetabolites (e.g., the folate antagonist, methotrexate; the pyrimidine analogues 5-fluorouracil, cytosine arabinoside, and 6-mercaptopurine), antibiotics (e.g., actinomycin D, daunomycin, and doxorubicin), the vinca alkaloids (e.g., vincristine and vinblastine), and miscellaneous others (e.g., steroids, cis-platinum, l-asparaginase, hydroxyurea, etc.). The specific adverse intestinal effects of each group, as discussed in recent reviews,[3-5] differ with each agent and vary tremendously from patient to patient. Current cytotoxic agents have a relatively narrow therapeutic index, and they do not discriminate between normal and diseased tissues. Often their adverse GI effects are potentiated by combination chemotherapy, prolonged or frequent administration, radiotherapy, and underlying malnutrition.

Nausea and Vomiting. Most patients treated with nitrogen mustard, streptozotocin, cis-platinum, or dacarbazine (DTIC) and many receiving the nitrosoureas, high-dose methotrexate, the antibiotic cytotoxics, and procarbazine or L-asparaginase will be affected.[3-5] In contrast, the vinca alkaloids produce only minimal nausea and vomiting. The mechanisms by which these chemotherapeutic agents stimu-late the chemoreceptor trigger zone and the vomiting center in the area postrema of the fourth ventricle are unknown.[6] Nausea and vomiting are best treated by prophylactic administration of powerful antiemetic compounds such as the phenothiazines or haloperidol.

Mucositis. Antineoplastic drugs arrest mitotic activity, often for several days, with the greatest impact being seen in those systems with relatively rapid cell turnover—bone marrow, GI crypt epithelium, and spermatogonia.[3-5,7] In the human small intestine, Trier found that mitotic activity decreased beginning as early as 2 hours and was minimal 21 hours after administration of a single bolus of methotrexate.[8,9] The mucosa was normal by light microscopy, but ultrastructural changes including swollen fragmented mitochondria and swollen Golgi apparatus and endoplasmic reticulum were apparent on electron microscopy. In response to most cytotoxic agents there is a phase of degeneration and progressive mucosal injury,[3-5] a mucositis that is focal while variable in severity. In the small bowel partial villous atrophy may occur, and superficial erosions, ulceration, and hemorrhage may develop throughout the intestine. Mucositis is most often the result of treatment with methotrexate, but it is seen with the use of 5-fluorouracil, actinomycin D, doxorubicin, cytosine arabinoside, bleomycin, and vinblastine. Typically these patients have abdominal pain, vomiting, ileus or diarrhea, melena or hematochezia, hypokalemia, and sometimes protein-losing enteropathy. Treatment is supportive. Regeneration begins within days of injury, and although inflammatory changes persist for 3 to 4 weeks, the gross changes in the mucosa are usually repaired within 14 days.[5]

Malabsorption. The effects of malignancy, radiotherapy, and cytotoxic drugs on intestinal structure and function have been reviewed.[3-5] Most of the work has been in animals, and only a limited number of studies have assessed the effect of chemotherapy on absorption in humans. Primary intestinal malignancies, small intestinal lymphoma in particular, may be associated with malabsorption. Anorexia, cachexia, and malnutrition either are presenting features or develop during the progression of most malignant disorders, and in these

TABLE 1
Adverse Effects of Drugs on the
Gastrointestinal Tract

Suppression of the rate of cell turnover
Malabsorption
Mucosal inflammation
Alteration of enteric flora
Intestinal pseudo-obstruction
Ischemia
Hemorrhage

patients severe malnutrition itself can impair digestion and absorption. Decreased xylose absorption and disaccharidase activity have been observed, often in association with the morphologic changes of partial villous atrophy.[10] Only slight elevation of fecal fat excretion has been documented.[11] Vitamin B_{12} and folate deficiency occurs, particularly in patients receiving prolonged therapy with folate antagonists (methotrexate alone or in combination with sulfa-containing antibiotics such as trimethoprim-sulfamethoxazole).[3-5]

Acute Intestinal Pseudo-obstruction. Colicky abdominal pain, adynamic ileus, and constipation occur frequently in patients receiving vincristine.[12] Symptoms develop within 3 days of treatment and usually resolve within 2 weeks with supportive management. The disorder, presumably the result of a toxic action of the drug on the enteric nervous system, can occur without signs or symptoms of peripheral nerve dysfunction.

Infection. Chemotherapy frequently results in bone marrow suppression, in addition to intestinal mucositis. Absolute leukopenia and the presence of diffuse intestinal ulceration favor local or generalize sepsis due to enteric organisms. The degree to which chemotherapy directly predisposes patients to opportunistic enteric infection is difficult to ascertain, since many patients are also receiving antibiotics and corticosteroids, and disorders like lymphoma and leukemia are themselves immunosuppressive. GI infections in the immunocompromised host are commonly caused by *Candida*, cytomegalovirus, and *Cryptosporidium*.[5]

Neutropenic Enterocolitis. This disorder (also called agranulocytic necrosis, necrotizing enteropathy, typhlitis, or the ileocecal syndrome) occurs in association with chemotherapy, particularly of the leukemias and lymphomas, but also with the use of cytotoxics and immunosuppressives in other neoplastic conditions and following organ transplantation.[5,13-15] Symptoms, which are nonspecific, include fever, nausea and vomiting, right lower quadrant abdominal pain, distention, diarrhea, and bloody stools and can mimic acute appendicitis. There is abdominal guarding, rebound tenderness, a fullness or mass in the right lower quadrant, and decreased bowel sounds. Intestinal gas is decreased in the right lower quadrant in abdominal films, and there may be marked distortion and edema of the cecum and ileum in a barium enema. The lesion is a diffuse patchy necrosis of the mucosa in the ileocecal region, accompanied by focal ulceration, hemorrhage, and infiltration with bacteria, fungi, and inflammatory cells. There is controversy over treatment; some recommend conservative supportive management, but because perforation often is a fatal event, others recommend early surgical resection.

Hemorrhage. GI hemorrhage is an uncommon complication of the thrombocytopenia induced by chemotherapy.[5]

DRUG-INDUCED MALABSORPTION

Many drugs have been associated with intestinal malabsorption.[1,5,16,17] They are listed in Table 2, where they are categorized according to the underlying mechanism. The severity and significance of drug-induced malabsorption depend upon a combination of risk factors including (a) underlying nutritional status of the patient, (b) nutritional quality of the diet

and use of supplements, (c) drug dosage, (d) frequency of administration of the drug, (e) duration of treatment, concurrent usage of several medications with similar additive or potentiating effect, and the presence of underlying disease which impairs nutrient intake, digestion, or absorption or increases nutrient loss or dietary requirements.[17] Drugs may impair absorptive processes by several mechanisms.

Adverse Intraluminal Reactions. Drugs may interact with nutrients in the gut lumen to adversely affect absorption by solubilization in a nonabsorbable vehicle; by formation of a gel, precipitate, or chelate that cannot be absorbed; or by competitive inhibition of receptor-mediated absorption.[17]

Nonabsorbable monosaccharide (mannitol), disaccharide (lactulose), hydrophilic dietary fiber, and magnesium salts are associated with obligate fecal water loss, an effect commonly exploited in laxative therapy. The potential for nonabsorbable mono- and disaccharides to produce explosive concentrations of hydrogen by fermentation in the colon makes these drugs inappropriate as preparations for intestinal surgery or endoscopy employing electrical cautery or coagulation.[18] Mineral oil, a nonabsorbable lipid, is another frequently utilized laxative agent. Chronic ingestion of mineral oil at or soon after mealtime is associated with wasting of the fat-soluble vitamins A, D, E, and K.[17] Aluminum and magnesium hydroxide abuse has been associated with depletion of phosphorus and calcium and osteomalacia.[19,20] Neomycin treatment in doses of 3 to 12 per day produces a malabsorption syndrome,[21-23] not only because of consequent mucosal injury but also because cationic amino groups of neomycin complex with anionic groups of intestinal micelles to form an insoluble precipitate resulting in enteric loss of bile salts, cholesterol, fatty acids, monoglycerides, and fat-soluble vitamins. Another antibiotic, tetracycline, probably impairs calcium absorption through chelation.[17] Chronic therapy with sulfasalazine in malnourished children with inflammatory bowel disease[23] or with trimethoprim-sulfamethoxazole in leukemic children who are also malnourished and are being treated with the folate antagonist methotrexate[3-5] has resulted in folate deficiency states. The sulfa moiety of sulfasalazine and trimethoprim-sulfamethoxazole has a chemical structure resembling that of folate and competes for absorption at the luminal receptor. Hypocholesterolemic agents like cholestyramine are prescribed for long periods in an effort to reduce mortality from the cardiovascular complications of hypercholesterolemia. Depletion of fat-soluble vitamins and folate has been reported in such patients,[25] resulting from adsorption of luminal bile acids by this powerful chelator and interference with lipid absorption. In animal models lipid also accumulates in the mucosa in response to these agents, causing interference with exit of the lipid from the epithelium.[26]

Increased Rate of Intestinal Transit. Read[27] has shown that the cathartics lactulose and magnesium sulfate and the prokinetic agent metoclopramide increase the rate of intestinal transit sufficiently that measurable deterioration in fat absorption occurs.

Mucosal Injury. Cytotoxic agents cause mucosal injury and affect absorption as discussed above. High doses of neomycin also have been associated with partial villous atrophy, increased mitotic activity, inflammation in the lamina propia, ballooned enterocytes with fragmented microvilli, and

TABLE 2
Drug-Induced Malabsorption

Drug	Action	Nutrient Malabsorbed
Adverse intraluminal reactions		
Mannitol	Intraluminal	Water and electrolytes
Lactulose	Osmotic effect	
Dietary fiber		
Magnesium salts		
Mineral oil	Dissolution into a nonabsorbable lipid	Vitamins A, D, E, and K
Aluminum and magnesium hydroxide	Intraluminal precipitation	Phosphate, calcium
Neomycin	Complexes with and precipitates micelles	Bile salts, cholesterol, fatty acids, monoglycerides, vitamins A, D, E, and K
Tetracycline	Precipitation	Calcium
Sulfonamides (trimethoprim-sulfamethoxazole, sulfasalazine)	Competition for absorption	Folate
Cholestyramine	Absorption of bile acids	Bile acids, lipid, vitamins A, B_{12}, D, E, and K, folate
Increased rate of intestinal transit		
Lactulose	Decreased time for absorption	Lipid
Magnesium sulfate		
Metoclopramide		
Mucosal injury		
Chemotherapy	Villous atrophy, immature, damaged enterocytes	Disaccharides, vitamin B_{12}, folate
Neomycin	Villous atrophy, damaged enterocytes	Disaccharides, D-xylose, vitamin B_{12}, folate
Colchicine	Mucosal injury	Disaccharides, D-xylose, sterols, bile acids, lipid, vitamins A, B_{12}, D, E, and K
Bisacodyl, danthron, phenolphthalein, senna, ricinoleic acid, cascara	Secretion, increased rate of transit, mucosal irritation	Water, potassium, protein-losing enteropathy
Impaired secretion and absorption		
H_2 antagonists	Impaired acid secretion and proteolysis	Vitamin B_{12}
Thiazides, ethacrynic acid	Block Na^+ absorption	Na^+, glucose, amino acids
Parenteral effects on nutrient metabolism		
Isoniazide, cimetidine	Hydroxylation of vitamin D	Calcium
Phenytoin	Promotes catabolism of vitamin D	Calcium
Corticosteroids	Multiple mechanisms	Calcium

swollen mitochondria and endoplasmic reticulum.[21–23] In addition to the steatorrhea and fat-soluble vitamin loss secondary to binding and precipitation of micelles, neomycin use can induce decreased D-xylose absorption, decreased lactase activity, and a partial blockade of vitamin B_{12} malabsorption.[16] Colchicine is used rarely to treat children; it inhibits microtubular function in mitosis and has been shown to damage the intestinal mucosa,[28,29] leading to decreased lactase activity and impaired absorption of sterols, bile acids, fat, fat-soluble vitamins, D-xylose, and vitamin B_{12}. Intestinal injury from several stimulant laxatives (bisacodyl, danthron, phenolphthalein, senna, ricinoleic acid, and cascara) may result in a syndrome of diarrhea, weakness, hypokalemia, and protein-losing enteropathy.[30]

Impaired Secretion and Absorption. Drugs can cause malabsorption by interfering with gastric, pancreatic, or biliary secretions and by blocking mucosal absorptive pathways.[17] The H_2 antagonists cimetidine and ranitidine inhibit gastric acid production. As a result, gastric digestion of protein is affected and there is a decrease in the release of protein-bound vitamin B_{12}, with less being available to bind with intrinsic factor. Chronic use of these agents has been associated with vitamin B_{12} deficiency.[31] The thiazide diuretics and ethacrynic acid inhibit active sodium absorption; they may interfere somewhat with sodium-dependent absorption of glucose and amino acids by the enterocyte,[1] but this effect is not of clinical significance.

Parenteral Effects on Nutrient Metabolism. Some drugs act parenterally to alter nutrient metabolism by inhibiting intermediary metabolism or by promoting catabolism.[17] Bone lesions may occur with the use of isoniazid or cimetidine, which inhibit hepatic and/or renal hydroxylation of vitamin

D, and of phenytoin, which alone or in combination with phenobarbitol promotes catabolism of active vitamin D metabolites.[32,33] The folic acid deficiency and megaloblastic anemia associated with chronic phenytoin therapy occurs because the drug induces enzymatic catabolism of folic acid.[17] Corticosteroids have a variety of effects on calcium metabolism, including decreased absorption.[17]

DRUG-INDUCED MUCOSAL ULCERATION

Medicines that have been implicated in erosive injury of the small or large bowel are listed in Table 3. Mucosal ulceration caused by chemotherapeutic agents, drug-induced intestinal ischemia, and antibiotic-induced pseudomembranous colitis are covered elsewhere in this discussion.

Small Intestine. It is a widely held clinical opinion that acetylsalicylic acid (ASA), other nonsteroidal anti-inflammatory drugs (NSAIDs), and corticosteroids are ulcerogenic in man.[34] Numerous anecdoctal reports support a causal association between the ingestion of these drugs and intestinal hemorrhage or perforation. Patients admitted to hospital with perforation of the bowel or hemorrhage from a point below the duodenum were reported to be more than twice as likely as controls to be taking NSAIDs.[35] In a prospective, blinded, placebo-controlled study of normal men, the acute administration of NSAIDs was associated with the development of erosive duodenitis.[36] However, some believe that a cause-and-effect relationship between NSAID ingestion and mucosal injury is not yet established with absolute certainty.[34,37] Certainly there is controversy over the true incidence and impact of the problem. The newer "slow-release" or enteric-coated formulations of ASA, which are designed to bypass the stomach, produce fewer gastric lesions, less gastric cell desquamation, less gastric bleeding, and less distress than regular ASA. These preparations can still irritate the intestinal mucosa, but it is not known if their effect is greater than that occasioned by the use of the non–enteric-coated preparations.[34]

Patients with rheumatoid arthritis take NSAIDs on a chronic basis. Asymptomatic duodenal erythema and erosions are found in roughly 5 percent of these patients.[34] Since a control group cannot be studied, it is not certain if there is a contribution of rheumatic disease itself to ulcerogenesis. Recently Nagaraj et al reported that very low birth weight infants who receive indomethacin therapy for closure of patent ductus arteriosus have a 10 percent incidence of small bowel perforation.[38]

Anecdotal reports suggest that corticosteroids have an increased association with gastroduodenal ulceration and perforation, the symptoms of which may be partially masked by the drug, thus leading to a dangerous delay in diagnosis.[34,39] A large study by Lewis et al[40] and a recent study by Conn and Blitzer,[41] which combined the data from 42 randomized trials involving a total of more than 5,000 subjects, did not show a significant association between corticosteroid usage and ulceration. However, Messer et al[42] analyzed the combined results of even more controlled trials and did find a significant increase in ulcer prevalence for the steroid-treated group compared with controls.

TABLE 3
Drug-Induced Mucosal Ulceration

Small Bowel	Colon
Chemotherapeutic agents*	Chemotherapeutic agents*
Drugs causing intestinal ischemia[†]	Drugs causing colonic ischemia[†]
Acetylsalicylic acid, other NSAIDs	Soap suds enema
Corticosteroids	Hydrogen peroxide enema
Ferrous salts	Gold therapy in rheumatoid arthritis
Potassium salts	Methyldopa
Clofazimine	Sulfasalazine

*See Drug-Induced Suppression of the Rate of Cell Turnover, in text.
†See Table 5.

Ferrous salts can cause ulceration, hemorrhage, and perforation if they come in prolonged contact with the intestinal mucosa in high concentration.[5] This situation seldom arises except in cases of accidental poisoning in which multiple capsules have been ingested.

Potassium salts are well-known causes of ulceration of the oral, esophageal, gastric, and intestinal mucosa when they are delivered in high concentration to a localized area. This problem was recognized by Lawrason et al,[43] who reported 484 instances of small intestinal ulceration-obstruction, of which 57 percent were associated with a history of taking potassium salts. Enteric-coated KCl preparations have caused intestinal ulceration, hemorrhage, obstruction, and even death.[44] In an effort to reduce the frequency of these GI complications, wax-matrix, slow-release KCl tablets and microencapsulated preparations were developed. These products have been considered safe, but cases of ulceration still occur, even with relatively low doses.[45,46] Delay in GI transit such as occurs with the concurrent use of anticholinergic therapy increases the risk of mucosal ulceration.[46]

Clofazimine is an antituberculosis drug that has been reported to cause granulomatous or eosinophilic enteritis leading to ulceration.[47]

Colon. Enemas are the most common cause of colonic inflammation. Nearly a third of patients receiving soap suds enemas experience immediate irritative effects and abnormal colonic function for days to months after their use.[48] The injury is caused by a direct detergent action of mucosa, related to the concentration of the enema. Proctosigmoidoscopic changes range from mild hyperemia, edema, and increased mucus production to hemorrhage with superficial or occasionally full-thickness necrosis of the bowel wall.[49] Three percent hydrogen peroxide enemas have caused acute hemorrhagic colitis, eventually resulting in death.[50] Hypertonic saline, Fleet, and bisacodyl enemas cause mild inflammation, mucin depletion, and edema; these changes usually resolve within a week of treatment.[5]

Enterocolitis is a recognized complication of gold therapy in the treatment of rheumatoid arthritis,[51] although only 26 patients have been reported with this complication. Most had received low total doses of gold salt, and few had other manifestations of gold toxicity (rash or neutropenia) before developing fulminant enterocolitis.

An acute reversible colitis associated with fever, rash, and eosinophilia has been reported with the use of methyldopa.[52]

An allergic or autoimmune etiology is suspected. Sulfasalazine-induced exacerbations of ulcerative colitis have also been observed.[53,54] The prompt return of colitis symptoms on rechallenge of these patients suggests a possible toxic effect, although the mechanism is not clear.

DRUG-INDUCED ALTERATION OF ENTERIC FLORA

The association of opportunistic enteric infection with the use of chemotherapy and antibiotics has been discussed earlier. Even the immunocompetent individual is at risk for opportunistic secondary superinfection during prolonged courses of broad-spectrum antibiotic coverage.

Antibiotic-Associated Pseudomembranous Colitis. Ampicillin and the cephalosporins are the agents most often causing antibiotic-associated pseudomembranous colitis (AAC),[55] but almost all antibiotics except vancomycin, bacitracin, and the parenteral aminoglycosides have been reported to cause the syndrome. The disorder may develop at any age, even after a single dose of orally or parenterally administered antibiotic; in one-third of cases it occurs up to 6 weeks after therapy is discontinued. Patients develop fever, abdominal cramps and tenderness, and diarrhea that is usually watery and voluminous but in 20 percent of cases may be bloody. The typical endoscopic appearance is a spectrum of mild erythema and edema to hemorrhagic colitis with multiple elevated white-yellow plaques 3 to 20 mm in diameter with normal intervening mucosa, "pseudomembranous colitis."[56] A normal proctosigmoidoscopic examination does not exclude the diagnosis, as one-third of cases may have rectal sparing. The diagnosis is conclusively established with the isolation of *Clostridium difficile* and a positive tissue culture assay for *C. difficile* cytotoxin. Cholestyramine can be used to bind enterotoxin, but the treatment of choice is oral vancomycin, with metronidazole being a good alternative.[57] Up to 50 percent of patients relapse within 3 to 10 days after therapy, and a second relapse can be expected in one-third of these individuals, for whom a prolonged tapering course of therapy has been effective.[57]

DRUG-INDUCED INTESTINAL PSEUDO-OBSTRUCTION

Intestinal pseudo-obstruction, including drug-induced ileus, is discussed elsewhere. Table 4 lists those drugs that have been implicated.[1,5] Anticholinergic medications prescribed as antispasmodics or as parasympatholytic agents for ulcer therapy in excessive dosage can block the "final common pathway" (muscarinic cholinergic) of intestinal smooth muscle excitation and induce ileus. Ganglionic blockers, once used in the treatment of hypertension, also cause ileus by blocking nicotinic cholinergic transmission between enteric neurons. Several classes of drugs have important anticholinergic effects: the tricyclic antidepressants, the phenothiazines, and benztropine and trihexyphenidyl used in the treatment of Parkinson's disease. The psychotropic drugs seem most likely to affect colonic motility and are associated frequent-

TABLE 4
Drug-Induced Intestinal Pseudo-obstruction

Anticholinergic agents	Verapamil
Ganglionic blockers	Cyclosporine
Tricyclic antidepressants	Narcotics
Phenothiazines	Cytotoxic agents (vincristine)
Benztropine/trihexyphenidyl	Anthraquinone purgatives
Clonidine	

ly with constipation. Constipation or frank intestinal pseudo-obstruction have been reported with the use of clonidine and verapamil. Transient ileus has been reported with the initiation of cyclosporine therapy. The narcotics are notorious for potentiating postoperative ileus and predisposing to constipation.

Two other classes of drugs cause intestinal pseudo-obstruction by damaging the myenteric plexus: the cytotoxic agents and the anthraquinone purgatives. The ileus caused by cytotoxics and vincristine has been covered earlier in this discussion. Long-term use or abuse of anthraquinone laxatives (e.g., cascara, senna) is associated with melanosis coli,[58] toxic damage to the myenteric plexus,[59,60] and an end-stage colon that is unable to contract effectively (the cathartic colon).[61]

DRUG-INDUCED INTESTINAL ISCHEMIA

Intestinal ischemia can result from or be potentiated by medications that result in arterial obstruction or constriction and those that cause a reduction in blood volume or pressure. Drugs causing arterial or venous thrombosis, intense arterial constriction, and hypovolemia or hypertension are listed in (Table 5).

Thrombosis. Several drugs have been associated with what is presumed to be an immunologically mediated or hypersensitivity angiitis.[5] The temporal association between administration of these drugs and onset of symptoms is quite variable. The reaction is dose-dependent. There is an inflammatory infiltrate in all three layers of the vessel wall and the

TABLE 5
Drug-Induced Intestinal Ischemia

Thrombosis	Arterial Spasm
Necrotizing vasculitis	Vasopressin
Organic arsenicals	Ergot
Gold salts	Methysergide maleate
Mercurials	
Bismuth	
Amphetamine	**Hypotension**
DDT	Diuretics
Penicillin	Antihypertensives (methyldopa,
Sulfonamides	hydralazine, ganglionic
Serum	blockers)
Oral contraceptive steroids	Digoxin
	Antiarrhythmics
	Alpha-adrenergic blockers

adjacent tissue. The endothelial lining of involved vessels is intact, and although edema may decrease blood flow, thrombosis is not a feature of the reaction. In contrast, a small group of drugs induce an immunologic reaction that *is* associated with necrotizing vasculitis and thrombosis (Table 5).[5]

The use of oral contraceptive steroids is associated with a relatively hypercoagulable state that predisposes to aterial and venous thrombosis, including superior and inferior mesenteric arterial obstruction. Hoyle et al[62] reported a study in which almost 50 percent of patients with ischemic small bowel symptoms associated with oral contraceptive therapy died of irreversible small intestinal infarction. Ischemic colitis has a better prognosis than small intestinal ischemia; in many cases it resolves with discontinuation of the drug and conservative management.[64,68] Oral contraceptive–induced ischemic colitis has caused clinical and endoscopic features that mimic Crohn's colitis,[64] and there is evidence to suggest that there may be an increased risk of Crohn's disease in oral contraceptive users.[65]

Arterial Spasm. Vasopressin is a potent vasoconstrictor that is infused intravenously or given directly into a specific artery to reduce hemorrhage. Unfortunately, both delivery routes may result occasionally in ischemic necrosis of extensive areas of the intestine.[66,67] Ergot alkaloids, used for migraine, can induce marked arterial spasm and in a few cases mesenteric artery spasm or intestinal ischemia leading to colitis and stricture formation.[5] Methysergide maleate, another medication occasionally used to treat migraine, has also been associated with mesenteric artery insufficiency.[5]

Hypotensive Agents. Aggressive use of diuretics and antihypertensive agents can lead to intestinal ischemia through hypovolemia and hypotension. The catecholamines, antiarrhythmics, and alpha-adrenergic blockers, used under various circumstances to maintain or modify cardiac rate, rhythm, and output, decrease intestinal blood flow as well.[68]

The ischemic effects of digoxin appear to be limited to the small intestine. Digitalis glycosides decrease splanchnic blood flow in patients with congestive heart failure, and stimulation of the renin-angiotensin system in this setting causes additional vascular constriction and impaired circulation. Usually patients develop abdominal pain, distention, vomiting, diarrhea, and melena in association with typical clinical features of digoxin toxicity. Digoxin-induced ischemia can result in hemorrhagic necrosis of the small intestine and death.[69]

DRUG-INDUCED INTESTINAL HEMORRHAGE

Thrombolytic agents have the potential for causing GI hemorrhage, but there are few case reports.[5] Hemorrhage with the use of antineoplastic agents is usually the result of mucosal ulceration and thrombocytopenia. Most drug-associated cases of GI hemorrhage occur as a complication of anticoagulant therapy.[1,5] Up to 40 percent of patients on anticoagulants experience some GI bleeding, but serious complications are infrequent.[5] In medical inpatients major GI tract complications occurred in only 1.2 percent of patients on heparin and 0.2 percent of those on warfarin.[70] Anticoagulant-related

hemorrhage within the GI tract most commonly takes the form of an intramural hematoma but may occur as a retroperitoneal hemorrhage or frank bleeding into the gut lumen.[5]

Intramural hematoma of the gut is rarely spontaneous; it is preceded by abdominal trauma in 67 to 75 percent of cases. Anticoagulants are implicated in 9 to 36 percent of these spontaneous cases.[71] The duodenum is the most common site of occurrence because its anatomic fixation renders it more susceptible to blunt trauma, stretch, and tears. Bleeding may result in colicky pain and partial or complete obstruction of the intestinal tract and biliary or pancreatic ducts. An ileus with vomiting and fullness, jaundice, or pancreatitis may result. Minor intraluminal bleeding occurs in about 25 percent of cases and major hemorrhage in 3.5 percent. Intussusception is a rare complication. On examination, a low-grade fever is common, and there is usually tenderness and guarding at the site of the lesion. In 40 to 76 percent of patients an enlarging mass may be palpable. The definitive diagnostic procedure is a barium upper GI series, which reveals the classic radiologic lesions of a "coiled spring" or "picket fence," representing edema of the valvulae conniventes.[71] Treatment requires reversal of anticoagulation with fresh frozen plasma and vitamin K, continuous nasogastric suction, and intravenous hydration. Most hematomas undergo spontaneous reabsorption, and symptoms resolve in 14 to 90 days. Surgical intervention is required only if medical therapy is unsuccessful or if there is continued major intraluminal bleeding.[71]

One-third of retroperitoneal hematomas are related to anticoagulant therapy.[72] Although most arise primarily in the retroperitoneum, injection of heparin into the thigh may occasionally result in hemorrhage into fascial compartments that communicate with the retroperitoneal space. Retroperitoneal blood may extend into the mesentery and reach the bowel wall directly or form a mass over which the bowel becomes stretched. Pain and symptoms of partial bowel obstruction result. Treatment is similar to that for intramural hemorrhage.

REFERENCES

1. Lewis JH. Gastrointestinal injury due to medicinal agents. Am J Gastroenterol 1986; 81:819–834.
2. Jick H, Miettinen OS, Shapiro S, et al. Comprehensive drug surveillance. JAMA 1970; 213:1455–1460.
3. Shaw MT, Spector MH, Ladman AJ. Effects of cancer, radiotherapy, and cytotoxic drugs on intestinal structure and function. Cancer Treat Rev 1979; 6:141–151.
4. Mitchell EP, Schein PS. Gastrointestinal toxicity of chemotherapeutic agents. Semin Oncol 1982; 9:52–64.
5. Riddell RH. The gastrointestinal tract. In: Riddell RH, ed. Pathology of drug-induced and toxic diseases. New York: Churchill Livingstone, 1982:515.
6. Harris JG. Nausea, vomiting and cancer treatment. Cancer 1978; 28:194–201.
7. Lipkin M. Proliferation and differentiation of gastrointestinal cells. Physiol Rev 1973; 53:891–915.
8. Trier JS. Morphologic alterations induced by methotrexate in the mucosa of the human proximal intestine. I. Serial observations by light microscopy. Gastroenterology 1962; 42:295–305.
9. Trier JS. Morphologic alterations induced by methotrexate in the mucosa of human proximal intestine. II. Electron microscopic observation. Gastroenterology 1962; 43:407–424.
10. Craft AW, Kay HEM, Lawson DM, et al. Methotrexate-induced malab-

sorption in children with acute lymphoblastic leukemia. Br Med J 1977; 4:1511–1512.

11. Smith FP, Kisner DL, Widerlite L, et al. Chemotherapeutic alterations of small intestinal morphology and function: a progress report. J Clin Gastroenterol 1979; 1:203–207.

12. Weiss H, Walker M, Wiernik P. Neurotoxicity of commonly used antineoplastic agents. N Engl J Med 1974; 291:75–81.

13. Sherman NJ, Williams K, Woolley MM. Surgical complications in patients with leukemia. J Pediatr Surg 1973; 8:235–244.

14. Wagner ML, Rosenberg HS, Fernbach DJ, Singleton EB. Typhlitis: a complication of leukemia in childhood. AJR 1970; 109:341–350.

15. Alt B, Glass NR, Sollinger H. Neutropenic enterocolitis in adults. Review of the literature and assessment of surgical intervention. Am J Surg 1985; 149:405–408.

16. Falloon WW. Drug production of intestinal malabsorption. NY State J Med 1970; 70:2189–2192.

17. Roe DA. Drug effects on nutrient absorption, transport, and metabolism. Drug Nutr Interact 1985; 4:117–135.

18. Bigard MA, Gaucher P, Lassalle C. Fatal colonscopic explosion during colonscopic polypectomy. Gastroenterology 1979; 77:1307–1310.

19. Spencer H, Kramer L. Antacid-induced calcium loss. Arch Intern Med 1983; 143:657–659.

20. Lotz M, Ney R, Bartter FC. Osteomalacia and debility resulting from phosphorus depletion. Trans Assoc Am Physicians 1964; 11:281–295.

21. Dobbins WO, Herrero BA, Mansbach CM. Morphologic alterations associated with neomycin induced malabsorption. Am J Med Sci 1968; 255:63–77.

22. Jacobson ED, Prior JT, Faloon WW. Malabsorption syndrome induced by neomycin: morphologic alterations in the jejunal mucosa. J Lab Clin Med 1960; 56:245–250.

23. Keusch GT, Troncale FJ, Plaut AG. Neomycin-induced malabsorption in a tropical population. Gastroenterology 1970; 58:197–202.

24. Franklin JL, Rosenberg IH. Impaired folic acid absorption in inflammatory bowel disease: effects of salicylazosulfapyridine (Azulfidine). Gastroenterology 1973; 64:517–525.

25. West RJ, Lloyd JK. The effect of cholestyramine on intestinal absorption. Gut 1975; 16:93–98.

26. Cassidy MM, Lightfoot FG, Grau L, et al. Lipid accumulation in jejunal and colonic mucosa following chronic cholestyramine (Questran) feeding. Dig Dis Sci 1985; 30:468–476.

27. Read NW. Speculations on the role of motility in the pathogenesis and treatment of diarrhea. Scand J Gastroenterol 1983; 18(suppl 84):45–63.

28. Race TF, Paes IC, Faloon WW. Intestinal malabsorption induced by oral colchicine. Comparison with neomycin and cathartic agents. Am J Med Sci 1970; 259:32–41.

29. Webb DI, Chodos RB, Mahar CQ, Falloon WW. Mechanisms of vitamin B_{12} malabsorption in patients receiving colchicine. N Engl J Med 1968; 279:845–850.

30. Tedesco FJ. Laxative use in constipation. Am J Gastroenterol 1985; 80:303–309.

31. Streeter AM, Goulston KJ, Bathur FA, et al. Cimetidine and malabsorption of cobalamin. Dig Dis Sci 1982; 27:13–16.

32. Hahn TJ, Avioli LV. Anticonvulsant-drug-induced mineral disorders. In: Roe DA, Campbell TC, eds. Drug and nutrients: the interactive effects. New York: Marcel Dekker, 1984:409.

33. Bengoa JM, Bolt MJG, Rosenberg IH. Hepatic vitamin D 25-hydroxylase inhibition by cimetidine and isoniazid. Gastroenterology (Abstract) 1983; 84:1363.

34. Domschke S, Domschke W. Gastroduodenal damage due to drugs, alcohol and smoking. Clin Gastroenterol 1984; 13:405–436.

35. Langman MJS, Morgan L, Worrall A. Use of anti-inflammatory drugs by patients admitted with small or large bowel perforation and hemorrhage. Br Med J 1985; 290:347–349.

36. Lanza F, Rack MF, Lynn M, et al. An endoscopic comparison of the effects of etodolac, indomethacin, ibuprofen, naproxen, and placebo and the gastrointestinal mucosa. J Rheumatol 1987; 14:338–341.

37. Katzka DA, Sunshine AG, Cohen S. The effect of nonsteroidal antiinflammatory drugs on upper gastrointestinal tract symptoms and mucosal integrity. J Clin Gastroenterol 1987; 9:142–148.

38. Nagaraj MS, Sandhu AS, Cook LN, et al. Gastrointestinal perforation following indomethacin therapy in very low birth weight infants. J Pediatr Surg 1981; 16:1003–1007.

39. Remine SG, McIlrath DC. Bowel perforation in steroid-treated patients. Ann Surg 1980; 192:581–586.

40. Lewis GP, Jusko WJ, Burke CW, Graves L. Prednisone side-effects and serum protein levels: a collaborative study. Lancet 1971; ii:778–780.

41. Conn HO, Blitzer BL. Non-association of adrenocorticosteroid therapy and peptic ulcer. N Engl J Med 1976; 294:473–479.

42. Messer J, Sacks HS, Reitman D, Chalmers TC. Corticosteroids do cause peptic ulceration (abstract). Gastroenterology 1982; 82:1130.

43. Lawrason FD, Alpert E, Mohr FL, McMahon FG. Ulcerative-obstructive lesions of the small intestine. JAMA 1965; 191:641–644.

44. Boley SJ, Allen AC, Schulz L, Schwartz S. Potassium-induced lesions of the small bowel. I. Clinical aspects. II. Pathology and pathogenesis. JAMA 1965; 193:997–1000, 1001–1006.

45. Weiss SM, Rutenberg HL, Paskin DL, Zeren HA. Gut lesions due to slow-release KC tablets. N Engl J Med 1977; 296:111–112.

46. McMahon FG, Akdamar K, Ryan JR, Ertan A. Upper gastrointestinal lesions after potassium chloride supplements: a controlled clinical trial. Lancet 1982; ii:1059–1061.

47. Riddell RH. The gastrointestinal tract. In: Riddell RH, ed. Pathology of drug-induced and toxic disease. New York: Churchill Livingstone, 1982:515.

48. Pike BF, Phillipi PJ, Lawson LH. Soap colitis. N Engl J Med 1971; 285:217–218.

49. Earnest DL. Other diseases of the colon and rectum. In: Sleisenger MH, Fordtran JS, eds. Gastrointestinal disease: pathophysiology, diagnosis, management. 3rd ed. Philadelphia: WB Saunders, 1983:1294.

50. Meyer CT, Brand M, Deluca VA, et al. Hydrogen peroxide colitis: a report of three patients. J Clin Gastroenterol 1981; 3:31–35.

51. Marcuard SP, Ehrinpreis MN, Fitter WF. Gold induced ulcerative proctitis: report and review of the literature. J Rheumatol 1987; 14:142–144.

52. Graham CF, Gallagher K, Jones JK. Acute colitis with methyldopa. N Engl J Med 1981; 304:1044–1046.

53. Schwartz AG, Targan SR, Saxon A, et al. Sulfasalazine-induced exacerbation of ulcerative colitis. N Engl J Med 1982; 306:409–412.

54. Adler RD. Sulfasalazine induced exacerbation of ulcerative colitis. N Engl J Med 1982; 307:315.

55. Bartlett JG. Anti-microbial agents implicated in Clostridium difficile toxin-associated diarrhea or colitis. Johns Hopkins Med J 1981; 149:6–9.

56. Gebhard RL, Gerding DN, Olson MM, et al. Clinical and endoscopic findings in patients early in the course of Clostridium difficile-associated pseudo-membranous colitis. Am J Med 1985; 78:45–48.

57. Bartlett JG. Treatment of Clostridium difficile colitis. Gastroenterology 1985; 89:1192–1195.

58. Wittoesch JH, Jackman RJ, McDonald JR. Melanosis coli: general review and study of 887 cases. Dis Colon Rectum 1958; 1:172–180.

59. Smith B. Pathologic changes in the colon produced by athraquinone purgatives. Dis Colon Rectum 1973; 16:455–458.

60. Steer HW, Colin-Jones DG. Melanosis coli: studies on the toxic effects of irritant purgatives. J Pathol 1975; 115:199–205.

61. Tedesco FJ. Laxative use in constipation. Am J Gastroenterol 1985; 80:303–309.

62. Hoyle M, Kennedy A, Prior AL, et al. Small bowel ischemia and infarction in young women taking oral contraceptives and progestational agents. Br J Surg 1977; 64:533–537.

63. Barcewicz PA, Welch JP. Ischemic colitis in young adult patients. Dis Colon Rectum 1980; 23:109–114.

64. Tedesco FJ, Volpicelli NA, Moore FS. Estrogen-associated and progesterone-associated colitis: a disorder with clinical and endoscopic features mimicking Crohn's colitis. Gastrointest Endosc 1982; 28:247–249.

65. Lesko SM, Kaufman DW, Rosenberg L, et al. Evidence of an increased risk of Crohn's disease in oral contraceptive users. Gastroenterology 1985; 89:1046–1049.

66. Renert WA, Button KF, Fuld SL, et al. Mesenteric venous thrombosis and small bowel infarction following infusion of vasopressin into the superior mesenteric artery. Radiology 1972; 102:299–302.

67. Joffe SN. Nonshunting procedures for control of variceal bleeding. Semin Liver Dis 1983; 3:235–250.

68. Granger DN, Richardson PDI, Kvietys PR, Mortillaro NA. Intestinal blood flow. Gastroenterology 1980; 78:837–863.

69. Lely AH, van Enter CHJ. Non-cardiac symptoms of digitalis intoxication. Am Heart J 1972; 83:149–152.

70. Jick H, Porter J. Drug-induced gastrointestinal bleeding. Lancet 1978; ii:87–89.

71. Birns MT, Katon RM, Keller F. Intramural hematoma of the small intestine presenting with major upper gastrointestinal hemorrhage. Gastroenterology 1979; 77:1094–1100.

72. Morrison FS, Wurzel HA. Retroperitoneal hemorrhage during heparin therapy. Am J Cardiol 1964; 13:329–332.

PART 30

Radiation Enteritis

Barry Z. Hirsch, M.D.
Ronald E. Kleinman, M.D.

Radiation therapy for intra-abdominal or pelvic malignancies can adversely affect almost every organ within the radiation field. Following delivery of radiation to the abdomen, the liver, kidneys, bone, skin, and the entire gastrointestinal (GI) tract are at risk of complications. In children, abdominal radiation is administered most often for Wilms' tumor with extension into the abdomen, pelvic rhabdomyosarcomas, and retroperitoneal soft tissue sarcomas. Before 1970 most radiotherapy equipment operated at 200 to 250 kV, providing therapy in the orthovoltage range. This resulted in high doses to the skin and a large amount of radiation damage to many organs. Modern equipment provides radiation in the megavoltage range (4 MeV or higher), which may be directly focused on the tumor, resulting in a smaller dose to the surrounding tissues and thus fewer complications.

In children the incidence of serious acute or chronic intestinal effects of radiation therapy is unknown. Of adult patients treated for abdominal or pelvic malignancies, 2.4 to 25 percent develop GI dysfunction.[1,2] Children appear to be at least as tolerant as adults to the acute effects of radiation, and the recovery of GI mucosa, oral mucosa, skin, and bone marrow in children appears to be more prompt in this age group.[3]

CLINICAL MANIFESTATIONS

The clinical presentations of radiation enteritis have been divided into three phases: early, delayed, and very late.[4] The early phase occurs during radiation therapy, the delayed phase months after completion of therapy, and the very late phase, which has been much better characterized in adults than in children, may occur years later.[4] In a study of 44 children who received total abdominal orthovoltage radiation, over two-thirds had vomiting and diarrhea during radiation therapy and in almost one-third of these, symptoms were characterized as severe.[4] Although the early phase effects were brief and self-limited, 11 percent of the children subsequently developed delayed symptoms, occurring within 2 months of therapy, consisting of vomiting, diarrhea, and abdominal distention with radiographic evidence of a small bowel obstruction.[4] These children were found to have intense adhesions and fibrosis at laparotomy.[4] The true incidence of delayed reactions may have been as high as 36 percent, since the reported incidence does not take into account children who died shortly after completing their course of radiation. All of the children who developed delayed reactions had been transiently symptomatic during the early phase. In contrast, 50 percent of adult patients who are acutely asymptomatic will develop late complications.[5]

The use of megavoltage therapy and focused radiation reduces the incidence of these complications significantly. At The Children's Hospital in Boston the incidence of small bowel obstructions in patients receiving para-aortic radiation for Hodgkin's disease is 2.5 percent.[6] Similarly, of 36 children with retroperitoneal rhabdomyosarcomas, only one small bowel fistula was reported.[7] It appears that while early-phase problems are quite common, delayed and very late complications are uncommon today.

When chemotherapy is administered concurrent with abdominal radiation there is a higher incidence of enteritis, the most serious adverse reactions occurring in the early and delayed phases. Actinomycin D, doxorubicin, bleomycin, and 5-fluorouracil are the most commonly implicated chemotherapeutics.[4,8-11] Previous abdominal surgery also increases the risk of enteritis following radiation therapy.[12] Adhesions resulting from surgery fix the normally mobile small bowel mesentery, thereby increasing the likelihood of radiation reaching a given area.[12] Additional risk factors for radiation-induced enteritis reported in adults include female sex, thin abdominal wall, previous pelvic inflammatory disease, and co-existing vasculitis (Table 1).[13-15]

PATHOPHYSIOLOGY

The pathophysiology of radiation-induced enteritis is thought to involve a combination of morphologic and vascular changes resulting in fat malabsorption, protein leakage into the intestinal lumen, and electrolyte disturbances (Table 2).[4,16,17] Patients frequently develop an enteropathy due to the malabsorption of bile acids.[18] Small bowel biopsies taken from patients with symptoms show villous blunting with dilatation of lymphatics and a moderately dense round cell infiltrate in the lamina propria (Fig. 1).[4] These abnormalities have been noted within the first 12 hours of radiation therapy.[18] Plasma cells predominate initially,[18] whereas lymphocytes are relatively rare owing to their sensitivity to

TABLE 1
Risk Factors for Radiation Enteritis

More than 3,500 cGy of radiation in the megavoltage range (much lower doses in the orthovoltage range)
Concurrent chemotherapy
Previous abdominal surgery
Thin abdominal wall
Vasculitis
Female sex

TABLE 2
Clinical Presentation of Radiation Enteritis

Protein-losing enteropathy
Malabsorptive syndromes
Electrolyte disturbances
Vomiting and diarrhea

radiation.[18] During the third and fourth weeks of therapy, polymorphonuclear leukocytes aggregate and form microabscesses.[18] Electron microscopy reveals shortened microvilli, enlarged nucleoli, dilated mitochondria and endoplasmic reticulum, and decreased cytoplasmic secretory granules.[18] In both children and adults these villous changes are completely reversible, returning to normal within 2 weeks of the completion of therapy (Fig. 2).[4,16-18] Late effects, such as strictures and fistulas, appear to result from damage to vascular or connective tissues of the small bowel.[12] Obliterative arteritis and fibrosis develop from radiation damage to the full thickness of the bowel wall.

The total dose of radiation is the most important factor in determining whether radiation enteritis will occur. Other important factors include the dose rate of the radiation, the overall treatment time, the size of each dose fraction, and the number of portals.[15] As we noted, previous surgery and concomitant chemotherapy also exacerbate the effects of a given dose of radiation. Most pediatric patients who undergo radiation therapy receive 1,500 to 3,000 centigrays (cGy) to the abdomen or pelvis.* Total body irradiation for bone marrow transplantation delivers from 1,200 to 1,500 cGy at a very low dose rate. Patients with Hodgkin's disease receive approximately 3,600 cGy, but this involves a highly limited field

---

*One cGy is equal to 1 rad and is the currently accepted convention for expressing units of absorbed radiation dose.

in the region of the para-aortic nodes. Pelvic rhabdomyosarcomas and retroperitoneal soft tissue sarcomas (Table 3) require between 4,500 and 6,000 cGy. Tolerance levels for abdominal radiation have been defined for adults. The TD/5/5 and TD/50/5 refer to the dose of radiation at which up to 5 percent or 50 percent of adults given a designated dose of radiation will develop intestinal damage within 5 years.[19] For the adult small bowel the TD/5/5 is 4,500 cGy and the TD/50/5 is 6,500 cGy.[19]

The diagnosis of radiation-induced enteritis is based on a typical clinical presentation with supporting radiographic findings or evidence of malabsorption. It can be difficult to distinguish radiation symptoms from those of tumor recurrence. Because no one symptom is pathognomonic, valuable diagnostic tests include upper GI contrast study with small bowel follow through, lactose hydrogen breath test, fecal fat collection, stool alpha$_1$-antitrypsin concentration and small bowel mucosal biopsy. Characteristic radiologic findings include abnormal mucosal folds, strictures, fistulas, or adhesions (Fig. 3).[20]

TREATMENT

Symptomatic treatment should be provided during the early phase. Diarrhea and colicky abdominal pain usually respond to antispasmodic agents and diminish with time after administration of radiation.[21] Low-fat, lactose-free diets have been found to be helpful,[22] and cholestyramine reduces the symptoms of ileitis and diarrhea.[23] Therapy for diarrhea, steatorrhea, lactose intolerance, malnutrition, obstruction, and nonspecific abdominal pain is more often necessary in the late phase when these symptoms are more pronounced and prolonged, than during the earlier phases, which are usually transient.[4,21] Nutritional support appears to be most important and sometimes requires elemental diets or even parenteral nutrition.[24] Sulfasalzine and corticosteroids have been used in combination with bowel rest and parenteral nutrition,

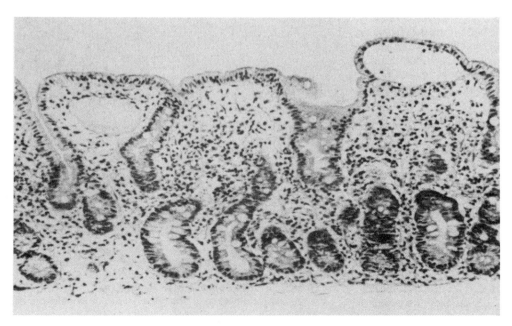

FIGURE 1 Histologic picture of the small bowel at the time of obstruction demonstrates severe villous blunting, distended lymphatics, and an abnormally dense mucosal round cell infiltrate. The normal columnar epithelium is lost, and only low cuboidal cells are present. Villi are shortened (hematoxylin and eosin, ×10). (From Donaldson, et al.[4])

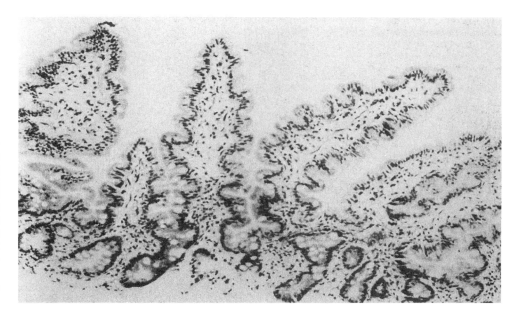

FIGURE 2 Histologic picture of the small bowel following dietary regimen, demonstrating replacement of mucosal villi and disappearance of the mucosal inflammatory infiltrate and distended lymphatics. The patient was treated with a specific diet for 13 months following biopsy seen in Figure 1 (hematoxylin and eosin, ×10). (From Donaldson, et al.[4])

TABLE 3
Tumors Requiring Significant Abdominal Radiation

Wilms' tumor
Pelvic rhabdomyosarcomas
Retroperitoneal soft tissue sarcomas

although neither therapy is clearly effective.[25] Radiation enteritis usually resolves after several months and rarely becomes chronic.[26] The indications for surgery include obstruction, perforations, and fistulas.[21] Bypass of the affected bowel appears to be the surgical treatment of choice.[27]

SUMMARY

In summary, in spite of new and improved techniques of administration, enteritis remains an adverse effect of radiation therapy to the abdomen. Early radiation enteritis is characterized by mucosal injury and malabsorption, whereas chronic injury leads to submucosal damage, resulting in bowel obstructions and fistulas. Early mucosal changes are largely reversible. For some patients with chronic symptoms nutritional support therapy may be necessary, occasionally in conjunction with abdominal surgery to bypass the affected bowel.

REFERENCES

1. Manson GR, Guernsey JM, Hanks GE, Nelson TS. Surgical therapy for radiation enteritis. Oncology 1968; 22:241.
2. Roswit B, Malsky SJ, Reid CB. Severe radiation injuries of the stomach, small intestine, colon and rectum. Am J Roentgenol 1963; 157:62.

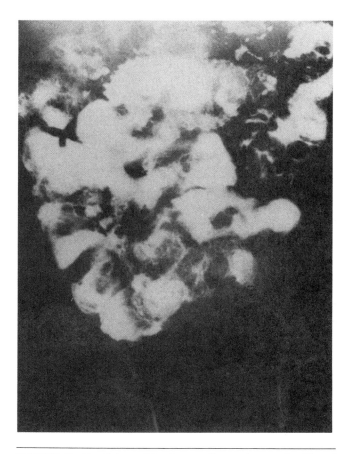

FIGURE 3 Small bowel barium radiograph reveals dilated small bowel with sharp angulations, thickened, straightened folds, and increased intraluminal secretions or fluid, with increased separation of small bowel loops. (From Donaldson, et al.[4])

3. Simone JV, Cassady JR, Filler RM. Cancers of childhood. In: DeVita VT, Hellman S., Kosenberg SA, eds. Cancer principles and practice of oncology. Philadelphia: JB Lippincott, 1982:1257.

4. Donaldson SS, Jundt S, Ricour C, Sarrazin D, Lemerle J, Schweisguth O. Radiation enteritis in children. A retrospective, clinicopathologic correlation, and dietary management. Cancer 1975; 35:1167–1178.

5. Kline JC, Buchler DA, Boone ML, et al. The relationship of reactions to complications in the radiation therapy of cancer of the cervix. Radiology 1972; 105:413.

6. March P, Tarbell NJ, Weinstein H, et al. Stage IA-IIA supradiaphragmatic Hodgkin's disease: prognostic factors in surgically staged patients treated with mantle and para-aortic irradiation. J Clin Oncol, in press.

7. Loughlin KR, Retik AB, Weinstein HT, et al. Genitourinary rhabdomyosarcoma in children. Submitted.

8. Roswit B, Malsky SJ, Reid CB. Severe radiation injuries of the stomach, small intestine, colon, and rectum. Am J Radiol 1972; 114:460–475.

9. Phillips TL. Chemical modifications of radiation effect. Cancer 1977; 39:987–999.

10. Stein RS. Radiation-recall enteritis after actinomycin-D and Adriamycin therapy. South Med J 1978; 71:960–961.

11. Phillips TL, Fu KK. Quantification of combined radiation therapy and chemotherapy effects on critical normal tissue. Cancer 1976; 37:1186.

12. Novak JM, Collins JT, Donowitz M, Farman J, Sheahan DG, Spiro HM. Effects of radiation on the human gastrointestinal tract. J Clin Gastroenterol 1979; 1:9–39.

13. Potish RA, Jones TK, Levitt SH. Factors predisposing to radiation-related small bowel damage. Radiology 1979; 132:479.

14. Potish RA. Prediction of radiation-related small bowel damage. Radiology 1980; 135:219.

15. Earnest DL, Trier JS. Radiation enteritis and colitis. In: Sleisenger MH, Fordtran JS, eds. Gastrointestinal disease. 3rd ed. Philadelphia: WB Saunders, 1983: 1259.

16. Tarpilla S. Morphological and functional response of human small intestine to ionizing irradiation. Scand J Gastroenterol (Suppl) 1971; 6:9–48.

17. Trier JS, Browning TH. Morphologic response of the mucosa of human small intestine to x-ray exposure. J Clin Invest 1966; 45:194–204.

18. Kinsella TJ, Bloomer WD. Tolerance of the intestine to radiation therapy. Surg Gynecol Obstet 1980; 151:273–284.

19. Rubin P, Casarette G. A direction for clinical radiation pathology. In: Vaeth JN, ed. Frontiers of radiation therapy and oncology, Vol 6. Baltimore: University Park Press, 1972: 1.

20. Mendelson RM, Nolan DJ. The radiological features of chronic radiation enteritis. Clin Radiol 1985; 36:141–148.

21. Zentler-Munro PL, Bessell EM. Medical management of radiation enteritis—an algorithmic guide. Clin Radiol 1987; 38:291–294.

22. Bounous G, Le Bei E, Shuster J, Gold P, Tahan WT, Bastin E. Dietary protection during radiation therapy. Strahlentherapie 1975; 149:476–483.

23. Chary S, Thompson DH. A clinical trial evaluating cholestyramine to prevent diarrhea in patients maintained on low fat diets during pelvic radiation therapy. Int J Radiat Oncol Biol Phys 1984; 10:1885–1890.

24. Beer WH, Fan A, Halstead CH. Clinical and nutritional implications of radiation enteritis. Am J Clin Nutr 1985; 41:85–91.

25. Loiudice TA, Lang JA. Treatment of radiation enteritis: a comparison study. Am J Gastroenterol 1983; 78:481–487.

26. Jaffe N, McNeese M, Mayfield JK, Riseborough EJ. Childhood urologic cancer therapy related sequelae and their impact on management. Cancer 1980; 45:1815–1822.

27. Wobbes T, Verschueren RCJ, Evert-Jan CL, Jansen W, Paping RHL. Surgical aspects of radiation enteritis of the small bowel. Dis Colon and Rectum 1984; 27:89–92.

PART **31**

Diverticular Disease
Barry Shandling, M.B., Ch.B., F.R.C.S.(Eng.), FRCSC, F.A.C.S.

Diverticulum is a Latin word meaning "wayside house of ill-repute." Few abnormalities in the human body are more aptly named, as the consequences of harboring such an appendage may be serious, even fatal.

In children, by far the most common diverticulum of the alimentary tract to become symptomatic is that named after Johann Friedrich Meckel, who described in 1809 what is now known as Meckel's diverticulum.[1-3] Other diverticula of the alimentary tract are rare.

MECKEL'S DIVERTICULUM

Pathogenesis

Early in intrauterine life the vitellointestinal duct connects the yolk sac and the intestine. By the sixth week of intrauterine life this canal is obliterated, and thus the fetal gut is separated from the yolk sac. If this separation does not occur or is incomplete, certain anatomic variations result that may cause major problems after birth. By far the most common of these is a diverticulum on the antimesenteric border of the ileum, about 50 to 75 cm proximal to the ileocecal sphincter. This diverticulum varies in length from 2 or 3 cm to 10 cm or more. It occurs in 2 to 3 percent of individuals. If the vitellointestinal duct becomes obliterated but not absorbed, a fibrous band extends from the tip of the Meckel's diverticulum to the back of the umbilicus. If obliteration is incomplete or partial, cystic masses may be encountered anywhere along the course of this band.[4] The vitellointestinal duct may remain completely patent. It is lined by typical ileal mucous membrane, which may have ectopic gastric and/or pancreatic tissue in its wall.[5]

If a fibrous band only is found, there may be ectopic tissue at the back of the umbilicus or in a cyst. The diverticulum itself mostly resembles ileal tissue, but it may have ectopic gastric and/or pancreatic tissue in its wall. Duodenal, jejunal, and colonic tissue may be found as well. It is such tissue that can give rise to symptoms. The diverticulum may have a base wider than its diameter or the diameter of the ileum, or the base may be narrow, giving rise to obstruction of the diverticulum.

In at least 30 percent of cases there is ectopic tissue in the mucosa, and the acid/pepsin secretion may cause ulcerations of the ileal mucosa within the diverticulum or even multiple small ulcers in the terminal ileum adjacent to the base of the diverticulum. These erosions may cause major alimentary hemorrhage. Less often a broad-based Meckel's diverticulum may invaginate into the ileum. Less frequently Meckel's diverticulum may become inflamed spontaneously or very rarely with the presence of a foreign body. Progression may lead to inflammation, perforation of the inflamed organ, peritonitis, and abscess formation.

Intestinal obstruction in association with Meckel's diverticulum develops in one of three ways. First, a fibrous band from the tip of the Meckel's diverticulum to the umbilicus may be the axis around which a loop of bowel twists, leading to a volvulus. Second, a band running alongside the diverticulum to the umbilicus, the remains of the vitellin artery, can give rise to obstruction based on a volvulus. Third, if the diverticulum becomes invaginated, it is propelled distally, dragging with it more ileum and forming an intussusception with the inside-out Meckel's diverticulum as the lead point.

If the vitellointestinal duct remains patent, the patient may discharge ileal contents and even flatus via the umbilicus.

When the Meckel's diverticulum enters an indirect inguinal hernial sac, this is known as a Littre's hernia. Under such circumstances there are signs and symptoms of a strangulated hernia without any evidence of obstruction.

Carcinoid tumors occurring in a Meckel's diverticulum have been documented.

Clinical Features

Hemorrhage

Usually hemorrhage is the result of peptic ulceration, and usually it occurs in children less than 2 years of age.[6] There is sudden, often repeated, painless blood loss with the passage per rectum of bright red or maroon-colored blood, mixed with the stool or quite independent of the passage of stool. There may be some crampy abdominal pain. The hemoglobin concentration may drop by 10 to 20 percent; but Meckel's diverticulum does not as a rule give rise to sudden exsanguinating hemorrhage. If the hemorrhage is a consequence of intussusception, there are typical red currant jelly stools with abdominal pain, vomiting, and a palpable abdominal mass.

Pain

Abdominal pain without the passage of blood may occur in association with Meckel's diverticulitis. Initially referred to the periumbilical central abdominal position, when inflammation of the parietal peritoneum is present or even perforation develops there are localized pain and tenderness. The clinical picture may be identical to that of appendicitis, and indeed it is usually misdiagnosed as such. Chronic recurrent, central abdominal pain, in the absence of any physical signs, may be due to a low-grade inflammation in the organ.

Abdominal pain of the type seen in patients with intestinal obstruction may also be due to a Meckel's diverticulum. Severe colicky periumbilical pain, accompanied by vomiting

of a bilious or a feculent nature, may be the result of a bowel obstruction. In infants and children who have not had a previous operation and who have no intussusception, the most common cause of intestinal obstruction is that associated with the remains of a Meckel's diverticulum.

Diagnosis

Until the advent of radiopharmaceuticals there was no way of diagnosing Meckel's diverticulum, for it cannot be demonstrated on contrast studies, either barium enema or upper gastrointestinal (GI) series. Technetium is excreted by the gastric mucosa; therefore, if there is ectopic gastric mucosa present it should be demonstrable by virtue of this excretion (Fig. 1). The Meckel's diverticulum is seen as a concentration of photons in addition to the bladder and stomach, usually in the right lower quadrant.[7] Nowadays with the addition of intravenous cimetidine, there is 95 percent accuracy with this method of diagnosis. False-positive findings are extremely

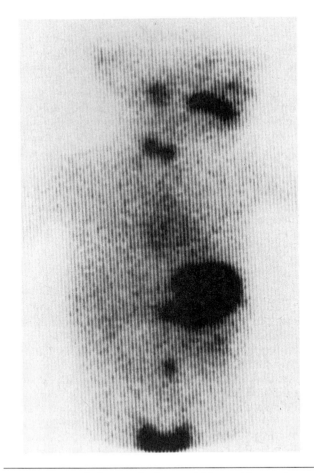

FIGURE 1 Meckel's scan in 2-year-old boy with massive rectal bleeding. Note normal uptake of radionuclide in salivary glands, thyroid, stomach, and bladder, as well as abnormal uptake by ectopic gastric mucosa in Meckel's diverticulum in midabdomen. At operation there was an ulcer in the intestinal mucosa at the neck of the diverticulum.

rare. Ectopic gastric mucosa, almost invariably present in a tubular duplication leading to rectal bleeding, is also demonstrable on a ^{99m}Tc scan. Approximately 2.5 sq cm of gastric mucosa is necessary in order to demonstrate the presence of a Meckel's diverticulum. With a history of abdominal pain and/or rectal bleeding and a positive Meckel's scan, usually in the absence of physical signs other than significant hemorrhage, a confident diagnosis can be made.

When a Meckel's diverticulum is present in conjunction with an enteric fistula opening at the umbilicus, a fistulogram is indicated. The dye enters the ileum via a patent vitellointestinal duct, leading in turn to a Meckel's diverticulum.

Treatment

Actually most diverticula are encountered in the course of an operation when the presence of a diverticulum is quite unexpected. Usually the operation has been undertaken for a mistaken diagnosis of appendicitis. The surgeon under such circumstances is all too pleased to find an alternative lesion, whether inflamed or not, and diverticulectomy should be undertaken. If a diverticulum is found in the presence of appendicitis I would recommend excision of the lesion, as appendectomy already constitutes a "clean-contaminated" procedure. The same indication applies to any operation involving breaching the wall of the intestinal tract. However, the resection is contraindicated in the case of a "clean" operation, such as a splenectomy or tumor resection.

When the diverticulum is incriminated as the cause of the bleeding and/or pain, then it should be resected. Usually resection of the anomaly is possible without the necessity for excising any adjacent ileum. However, if resection is undertaken for hemorrhage and if there is a suspicion of the presence of an ulcer in the ileum at or near the base of the diverticulum, then the questionable segment of small intestine must be excised together with the diverticulum and an end-to-end anastomosis done.

OTHER DIVERTICULA

Diverticula of the alimentary tract, although rare in childhood, may be found anywhere from the pharynx to the rectum.[8-12] They may be congenital or acquired. The most frequent site for congenital diverticula is the duodenum. If a diverticulum is found on the mesenteric side of the intestine it may well be a form of duplication,[5] but duplications do not occur on the antimesenteric border of the bowel.[10] A syndrome with a familial incidence has been reported consisting of cochleosaccular degeneration with hereditary deafness, absent gastric motility, progressive sensory neuropathy, and small bowel diverticulitis. Three sisters were thus affected.[11]

Acquired diverticula may be found in the esophagus at the anastomotic site after operation for esophageal atresia. Pulsion diverticula of the esophagus arise in the cricopharyngeal region. I have described one such case in a child with cutis laxa. Injuries to the esophagus, such as corrosive burns, may cause diverticula to develop in weakened portions of the wall of the gullet.[12] Diverticulosis of the appendix has been described in association with cystic fibrosis.[13] Side-to-side anastomoses are notorious for resulting in diverticula at the anastomotic sites after many years. Such diverticula are examples of pulsion diverticula and enlarge with the passage of time.

Diverticula of the intestinal tract may produce signs and symptoms in much the same way as a Meckel's diverticulum will, with diverticulitis, hemorrhage, and fistula formation. A huge diverticulum may result in obstruction or volvulus.[5]

Clinical Features

Clinical features are similar to those encountered with Meckel's diverticulum, except that inflammation and obstruction are more common than hemorrhage. Diverticula of the esophagus may give rise to dysphagia; others, more distally situated, may result in pain, hemorrhage, and peritonitis.

In the esophagus and duodenum the diagnosis can be established by means of barium and other contrast medium studies. As one proceeds distally through the small bowel, it becomes less likely that such studies will readily reveal the presence of the diverticula. Ultrasonographic demonstration of large saccular diverticula may be possible. Diverticulum of the colon, while not uncommon in adults, is extremely unusual in the pediatric age group. The condition is demonstrable by means of a barium enema.

Treatment

Diverticulosis per se probably requires no treatment unless symptomatic. Apart from hemorrhage, it is likely to be diverticulitis that will require surgical treatment. Operations for diverticula of the GI tract necessitate resection of the diverticulum, either alone or together with a small portion of the bowel from which it arises. Thus, either a repair of the wall of the bowel or end-to-end anastomosis after resection is necessary to restore the integrity of the alimentary canal.

REFERENCES

1. Vane DW, West KW, Grosfeld JL. Vitelline duct anomalies. Experience with 217 childhood cases. Arch Surg 1987; 122:542–547.
2. Le Neel JC, Heloury Y, Leborgne J, Horeau JM, Malvy P. Meckel's diverticulum. Is it necessary to search for it? Is it necessary to remove it? Appropos of 116 cases. J Chir (Paris) 1983; 120:233–237.
3. Van der Werken C, Sybrandy R. Meckel's diverticulum—an investigation based on pathological findings in 130 patients treated by surgery. Neth J Surg 1981; 33:123–126.
4. Moor KL. The developing human. Philadelphia: WB Saunders, 1977: 112.
5. Helin I, Flodmark P, Lindhagen T, Nettelblad SC, Rausing A. Occult bleeding from giant small-bowel diverticula. Acta Paediatr Scand 1983; 72:463–465.
6. Seagram CGF, Louch RE, Stephens CA, et al. Meckel's diverticulum: a 10 year review of 218 cases. Can J Surg 1968; 11:369–373.
7. Bergquist TH, Nolan NG, Stephens DH, et al. Specificity of ^{99m}Tc-pertechnetate in scintigraphic diagnosis of Meckel's diverticulum: review of 100 cases. J Nucl Med 17:465–469, 1976.
8. Tan EC, Tung KH, Tan L, Wee A. Diverticulitis of caecum and ascending colon in Singapore. J R Coll Surg Edinb 1984; 29:373–376.

9. Molander ML, Fries M. A solitary ileal diverticulum in a child. A case report. Z Kinderchir 1984; 39:67–68.
10. Nagar RC. Congenital jejunal diverticulum leading to diverticulitis and volvulus. J Indian Med Assoc 1981; 76:137–138.
11. Igarashi M, MacRae D, O-Uchi T, Alford BR. Cochleo-saccular degeneration in one of three sisters with hereditary deafness, absent gastric motility, small bowel diverticulitis and progressive sensory neuropathy. ORL J Otorhinolaryngol Relat Spec 1981; 43:4–16.
12. Peters ME, Crummy AB, Wojtowycz MM, Toussaint JB. Intramural esophageal pseudodiverticulosis. A report in a child with a sixteen-year follow up. Pediatr Radiol 1982; 12:262–263.
13. Au GDH. Diverticulosis of the vermiform appendix in patients with cystic fibrosis. Hum Pathol 1987; 1:75–79.

PART **32**

Intestinal Neoplasms

Alan M. Leichtner, M.D.

Although neoplasia is a major consideration in the differential diagnosis of significant gastrointestinal (GI) symptoms in the adult, the diagnosis of intestinal tumors in the pediatric age group is usually unexpected. Some familiarity with these rare tumors is advisable, however, because delay in diagnosis almost always adversely affects patient outcome.

Rather than provide an encyclopedic list of all forms of intestinal neoplasia, this discussion focuses on four areas in detail: carcinoma, lymphoma, leiomyoma and leiomyosarcoma, and carcinoid tumors of the intestine. These tumors constitute the bulk of intestinal neoplasia in the pediatric age group, and the clinical material presented should provide an approach that can be utilized in the diagnosis of very rare tumors as well. Where appropriate, comparison to corresponding tumors in adults is made. Various benign neoplasms occur in the intestine, including adenomas, leiomyomas, lipomas, hamartomas, and others, but only those of special relevance are considered.

CARCINOMA OF THE INTESTINE

Carcinoma of the Colon

Although there are fewer than 500 cases reported in the pediatric literature, carcinoma of the colon is the most common primary malignant solid tumor of the GI tract in childhood. In several large series of children with malignant tumors in various sites, approximately 1 percent of patients had colonic neoplasms.[1-3] The frequency of colon cancer increases with age and only between 1 and 4 percent of cases of carcinoma of the colon occur in individuals less than 30 years of age.[4] Nevertheless, colon cancer occurring in this age group demonstrates some unique features. Since the colon and rectum are the most frequent sites for carcinoma in the GI tract in childhood, most of the following discussion focuses on tumors at these sites.

Epidemiology

The overall incidence of carcinoma of the colon and rectum continues to increase, and in 1987 approximately 145,000 new cases were diagnosed in the United States.[5] The reported incidence of colorectal carcinoma is higher in developed countries in northwest Europe, the United Kingdom, Canada, and the United States and less frequent in Africa and Asia. Individuals from lower-risk areas who migrate to high-risk areas develop an incidence of colon carcinoma similar to that in the high-risk area.

Based on the Third National Cancer Survey, Odone estimated that the incidence of colon cancer in children under 20 years of age was 1.3 cases per million.[3] Most cases occurred in children between the ages of 10 and 19 years, who had an adjusted approximate incidence of 6.8 cases per million children. Even infants, however, can develop colon carcinoma; the youngest reported patient was only 9 months old at the time of diagnosis.[6]

A definite male predominance has been reported for carcinoma of the colon in children, with a male-to-female ratio of approximately 2:1.[7] Although in adults carcinomas of the colon and rectum are also more frequent in males than in females, the difference is not so pronounced.

Etiology

Much research has focused on attempts to identify environmental agents associated with the development of colon and rectal cancer. As recently summarized, the risk of colorectal carcinoma is associated with a diet high in calories, fat, and cholesterol and low in fiber.[8] One widely held hypothesis is that such a diet may result in increased delivery of bile acids into the colon with subsequent bacterial metabolism to putative carcinogenic agents. Conversely, a diet high in fiber may protect the colonic epithelium from such carcinogens. Exposure to radiation and chemicals such as organic solvents may also play an etiologic role. Ten of 13 adolescent patients presenting with colon carcinoma during a 2-year period had exposure to agricultural chemicals.[2]

A number of predisposing conditions confer a high risk for the development of colon carcinoma in certain individuals. These conditions are listed in Table 1. According to Lynch,[9] the total colon cancer burden can be roughly divided into four types: (1) sporadic, accounting for 70 to 80 per-

TABLE 1
Putative Conditions Predisposing to Colon Carcinoma

Diet high in calories, fat, and cholesterol and low in fiber
Exposure to radiation or chemicals
Inflammatory bowel disease: ulcerative colitis, Crohn's disease
Polyposis syndromes: Familial polyposis coli, Gardner's syndrome, juvenile polyposis, Peutz-Jeghers syndrome
Hereditary syndromes without polyposis: Lynch I, Lynch II, familial predisposition to adenoma formation
Previous ureterosigmoidostomy
Bacteremia or endocarditis secondary to *Streptococcus bovis*

cent of the total; (2) familial, representing patients with at least two first-degree relatives with a history of colon cancer but no definable genetic inheritance pattern, 10 to 20 percent; (3) hereditary cancer in patients with polyposis, less than 1 percent; and (4) hereditary nonpolyposis colon cancer, 5 to 6 percent. Colon cancer developing in patients with inflammatory bowel disease probably constitutes less than 1 percent of the total. Because of the relatively small number of cases reported in children, the incidence of predisposing conditions is not accurately defined. However, the specific incidence of pre-existing polyposis or colitis in children with colon cancer has been estimated to be approximately 10 percent, significantly higher than in the adult population.[10]

Cancer in patients with inflammatory bowel disease is a much-feared complication. The relative risk of colon cancer in patients with ulcerative colitis is probably increased by a factor of approximately 20-fold. The total duration of the colitis, but not an early age of onset, seems to be an important risk factor.[11] After the first 8 to 10 years of disease, the incidence of colorectal cancer increases by about 0.5 to 1 percent per year. Also a significant risk factor is the anatomic extent of the colitis, with patients having universal colitis at a higher risk than patients with solely left-sided disease.[11] Colorectal cancer associated with ulcerative colitis has several unique features, including an increased likelihood of multiple lesions, the ability to arise from flat mucosa rather than an adenoma, and the occurrence in a relatively younger population (mean age in the thirties).[12,13] The risk of developing colorectal cancer in patients with Crohn's disease is also increased, perhaps not to the same extent as in ulcerative colitis. The risk of developing small bowel cancer in Crohn's disease is, however, extremely increased.[14] Although in ulcerative colitis virtually all GI cancers occur at sites in the colon of active or past inflammation, one-third of cases of GI cancers in Crohn's disease occur in grossly normal segments of intestine. Therefore, the ability to detect cancer in Crohn's disease is diminished and the prognosis seems to be worse.[14]

Certain of the GI polyposis syndromes carry a high risk for the development of colon carcinoma. Most notable among these are familial polyposis coli and Gardner's syndrome. Both these autosomal dominant disorders are characterized by the presence of adenomas in the colon and to a lesser extent in the small intestine and stomach. The eventual risk of colon cancer approaches 100 percent. In a large series of af-

fected families, the risk for large bowel cancer in males with a polyposis syndrome was 1 percent by age 17 years, 50 percent by age 28 years, and 90 percent by age 45 years.[15] The latency period between the appearance of the adenomas and the development of cancer averages 10 years, although carcinoma of the colon in association with this syndrome has occurred as early as the first decade of life. As might be expected, the frequency of multiple lesions is more common in familial polyposis coli than in the general population with colon cancer and approaches 48 percent of cases.

The hamartomatous polyp syndromes have also been associated with a higher-than-normal risk for the development of colon cancer. Peutz-Jeghers syndrome has been reported to be complicated by the development of colon cancer in 2 to 3 percent of patients, although it is not clear whether this figure is higher than might be expected for normal individuals.[16] In juvenile polyposis, it does appear that the risk of colon cancer is increased and that the carcinoma probably arises in co-existing adenomas or mixed juvenile-adenomatous polyps.[17]

Autosomal dominant inheritance of the tendency to develop colon cancer can occur not only in association with polyposis syndromes such as familial polyposis coli and Gardner's syndrome, but also in the absence of polyposis. In fact, hereditary nonpolyposis colon cancer is approximately five times more common than familial polyposis–associated cancer.[18] Kindreds with hereditary nonpolyposis colon cancer can be divided into two syndromes: (1) Lynch syndrome I, or hereditary site-specific colon cancer, which is characterized by an increased incidence of cancer in the colon only, and (2) Lynch syndrome II, or the cancer family syndrome, which is also associated with an increased risk of extracolonic adenocarcinomas, including female genital, breast, and pancreatic cancers. The unique features of hereditary nonpolyposis colon cancer include a propensity for proximal lesions, an increased incidence of simultaneous and subsequent colon cancers, and a relatively early age of onset with a mean age of approximately 45 years.[18] Unfortunately, colon cancer may even develop in childhood; one member of a family with hereditary nonpolyposis colon cancer was diagnosed with adenocarcinoma of the colon at age 14.[19] The basic concept of the pathogenesis of sporadic colon cancer is that virtually all lesions arise in adenomas. Recently, it has been hypothesized that if one considers not just the incidence of colon cancer in families but also the incidence of the presumed precursor adenomas, heredity may play a role in a high percentage of cases of colon cancer previously thought to be sporadic.[20]

A very unusual yet intriguing predisposing condition for the development of adenocarcinoma of the colon is preceding ureterosigmoidostomy for exstrophy of the bladder (Fig. 1). In a series of 93 patients with ureterosigmoidostomies, 5 percent developed carcinoma of the colon at the level of the ureteral implants after a mean follow-up period of approximately 18 years.[21] Careful surveillance of these patients and consideration of colon resection are suggested. The factor in the urine predisposing to carcinogenesis has not yet been identified.

Although not yet reported in the pediatric age group, an association of bacteremia or bacterial endocarditis secondary to *Streptococcus bovis* and carcinoma of the colon has been

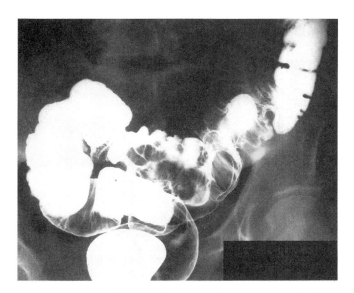

FIGURE 1 View of rectosigmoid colon during barium enema in a 33-year-old patient who had undergone uterosigmoidostomy in infancy for repair of bladder exstrophy. A polypoid tumor is seen in the sigmoid. (From the Teaching Collection, Department of Radiology, The Children's Hospital, Boston.)

noted in adults.[22] Subsequent reports have confirmed the need to consider the possibility of a co-existing malignancy in individuals with these infections. More research is required, however, before a role for *Streptococcus bovis* in the pathogenesis of colon carcinoma is established.

Pathology

Unlike adult patients, in the majority of whom lesions tend to be in the rectosigmoid area and thus in reach of the sigmoidoscope,[23] cancers of the colon in children tend to be more evenly distributed throughout the large intestine.[24] In fact, in a recent series, 50 percent of patients had a primary lesion in the right or transverse colon.[25]

Histologically, carcinomas of the large bowel in adults are usually moderately to well-differentiated adenocarcinomas. Several subtypes of adenocarcinoma are recognized, however, and include a mucinous or colloid variety, which is characterized by large collections of extracellular mucin (Fig. 2). In adults, this variety comprises up to 15 percent of colorectal carcinomas, and patients with mucinous tumors have a poorer 5-year survival than patients with nonmucinous tumors—34 percent and 53 percent, respectively.[26] In contrast to the situation in adult patients, the majority of children with colon carcinoma have this mucinous variant.[7,24,25]

Cancers of the colon and rectum grow locally by transmural invasion, eventually penetrating the bowel wall. Regional lymphatics and subsequently distant nodes become involved by tumor. The common sites of hematogenous spread include the liver, lungs, and vertebrae.

The most commonly employed scheme for classifying the progression of local and regional invasion by colonic cancers is a modification of the Dukes' system by Astler and Coller.[27] Tumors designated A are limited to the mucosa; B1

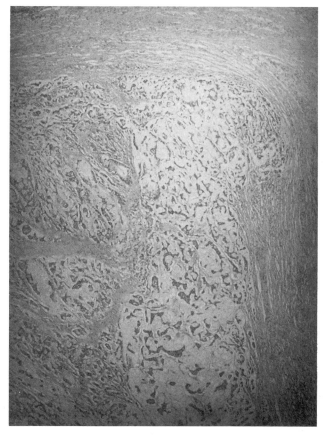

FIGURE 2 Mucinous carcinoma of the colon. The tumor cells seen infiltrating the wall of the colon are surrounded by abundant amounts of extracellular mucin. (Courtesy of Dr. Donald Antonioli.)

tumors have extended into but not through the muscularis propria; B2 tumors have penetrated the bowel wall but have not involved lymph nodes; C1 tumors are limited to the bowel wall but have involved lymph nodes; and C2 tumors have penetrated the bowel wall and involved lymph nodes. Distant metastases obligate placement in category D. Enker et al recently compiled data from a number of reports of colon cancer in younger patients and determined that 2.2 percent of patients had tumors classified as stage A, 16.2 percent as B, 47.6 percent as C, and 34 percent as D in this scheme. A total of 82 percent of patients had cancers that had progressed to full penetration of the bowel wall, lymph node involvement, or distant metastases. These percentages are significantly greater than the corresponding numbers in series of adult patients (Table 2).[28]

Clinical Features

The most common presenting symptom in children with carcinoma of the colon is abdominal pain, found in approximately 95 percent of patients. Vomiting, weight loss, rectal bleeding, and changes in bowel habit are also frequent symptoms. Classically, lesions of the right colon may become

TABLE 2
Comparison of Staging of Adult Versus Young
Patients with Colon Cancer

Stage	Adult	Young
A—Limited to mucosa		2.2%
	60%	
B—Through mucosa but no nodes involved		16.2%
C—Nodes involved		47.6%
	40%	
D—Distant metastases		34.0%

TABLE 4
Physical Findings of Children with Colon
Cancer

Symptom	Percentage of Patients
Mass	59
Distention	48
Emaciation	23
Tenderness	14
Anemia	14

quite large before causing symptoms of obstruction or bleeding. In contrast, more distal tumors frequently produce concentric narrowing of the lumen with resultant constipation and blood loss. As noted in Table 3, lesions of the left colon in childhood do indeed more frequently result in presenting symptoms of constipation and rectal bleeding than do right-sided lesions, although palpable abdominal masses were more frequently noted with the latter.[7] Overall, the presenting symptoms are somewhat different from those of adults, in whom abdominal pain is less common and changes in bowel habits and rectal bleeding are more frequent.[23]

As noted by Middelkamp, children presenting with carcinoma of the colon frequently have signs of acute large bowel obstruction. The physical findings at the time of initial presentation are shown in Table 4. Approximately 60 percent of patients had an abdominal mass, distention was noted in 50 percent, and approximately 15 percent had abdominal tenderness.[7]

Diagnosis

Although sigmoidoscopy may demonstrate a distal lesion, most lesions in children are more proximal and require colonoscopy or barium enema for diagnosis. For the detection of small lesions, colonoscopy is clearly more sensitive and provides the advantage of allowing biopsies to be obtained. In some children, evidence of a mass lesion or bowel obstruction may even be noted on a plain film of the abdomen. Ultrasonography, computed tomography, magnetic resonance imaging, and nuclear medicine studies may be useful in demonstrating metastatic disease.

The use of carcinoembryonic antigen (CEA) levels for the management of adult patients with colon cancer is well es-

tablished. However, little information is available about the use of this serologic marker in the pediatric population. Rao et al noted that 4 of 20 children with advanced colon cancer had normal CEA levels, and in 9 of 23 patients the test failed to correlate with progression or the presence of residual disease after surgery.[25] Clearly, the use of this and other serologic markers for disease activity in children must await further study.

The differential diagnosis of carcinoma of the colon includes tuberculosis of the bowel, inflammatory bowel disease, especially Crohn's disease, duplications and other benign causes of intestinal obstruction, and appendicitis. Other malignant tumors should be considered but are extremely rare.

Treatment

The primary mode of treatment for children with carcinoma of the colon is surgery. A wide resection of the involved segment of bowel with removal of the lymphatic drainage should be performed. In a recent series, however, complete resection was possible in only 40 percent of children.[25] Consideration should also be given to resection of the omentum in all patients and oophorectomy in female patients, as these are frequent sites of recurrence. Adjuvant chemotherapy or primary chemotherapy for patients with metastatic disease has unfortunately been of little benefit in younger patients with colon carcinoma. 5-Fluorouracil alone or in combination with other agents has most often been employed. The place of chemotherapy, radiation therapy, combination therapy, and newer therapeutic modalities in the treatment of colon cancer in this age group must await further study.

The prognosis for children with carcinoma of the colon is dismal. Andersson reported only a 2.5 percent 5-year survival,[24] although a few cases of apparent cure have been noted. The advanced stage of colon carcinoma in children at the time of diagnosis and the fact that many children present already with symptoms of a mass or intestinal obstruction suggest that diagnosis is often delayed. This may result from a number of factors. First, abdominal pain and other presenting symptoms are often vague in this age group and in those children with predisposing conditions, symptoms due to the tumor may be confused with those of the underlying disease. Secondly, the lesions are less likely to occur in the rectosigmoid colon and be detected by digital examination or sigmoidoscopy. Finally, as stated above, most colon carcinomas in children are of the mucinous variety, which tends to be very aggressive.

TABLE 3
Presenting Symptoms of Children with Colon
Cancer by Site of Tumor

Symptom	Site of Tumor	
	Right (%)	Left (%)
Pain	93	87
Vomiting	52	29
Constipation	17	32
Weight loss	21	19
Blood in stool	14	23
Mass	10	0

Conclusion

Although colon carcinoma is the most common primary GI tumor in childhood, it is unusual, and as a result, diagnosis is often delayed. Future efforts should focus on improved means of early diagnosis. In the approximately 10 percent of patients with a known underlying condition, regular surveillance should begin as soon as the risk of developing colon carcinoma becomes significant. For patients with inflammatory bowel disease, particularly ulcerative colitis, surveillance to detect dysplasia may aid in the diagnosis of carcinoma. For patients with Gardner's syndrome and familial polyposis coli, as well as those at risk for hereditary nonpolyposis colon cancer, consideration should be given to early prophylactic colectomy. Evaluation of the role of nonsurgical therapies in the treatment of children with established colon cancer will be aided by multicenter trials aimed at the younger population with this tumor.

Carcinoma of the Small Intestine

Even in the adult population, adenocarcinoma of the small intestine is exceedingly rare, although it does account for approximately one-half of malignant neoplasms of the small intestine.[29] These tumors are most commonly found in the proximal small intestine, particularly the duodenum. The cases of adenocarcinoma of the small intestine reported in childhood have occurred in association with the Peutz-Jeghers syndrome.[30] Other at-risk individuals include those with familial polyposis and Gardner's syndrome as well as patients with Crohn's disease of the small intestine. Although the youngest reported patient with adenocarcinoma of the small intestine complicating Crohn's disease was 21 years of age, her symptoms of inflammatory bowel disease began at age 10.[31] Of 36 cases collected by Nesbit, 28 occurred in the ileum and 11 occurred in previously bypassed bowel.[32] Unfortunately, the location of small intestinal adenocarcinomas makes surveillance of patients with Crohn's disease or a polyposis syndrome difficult. However, unusual pain, bleeding, or symptoms of obstruction necessitate consideration of this diagnosis.

LYMPHOMA

Primary small intestinal lymphoma accounts for 12.5 to 18 percent of all small bowel malignancies in Western Europe and North America.[33] Although the incidence of non-Hodgkin's lymphoma increases with age, there are striking differences between these tumors in adults and children with regard to such fundamental properties as histologic type, sites of occurrence, clinical behavior, and recommended treatment. Furthermore, important differences are also noted in GI lymphomas reported in Western and non-Western populations.

In adults, lymphomas of the digestive tract are virtually always of the non-Hodgkin's type.[34] Although primary digestive tract lymphomas are thought to constitute 2 to 5 percent of all non-Hodgkin's lymphomas, such calculations are complicated by the fact that it is sometimes difficult to determine whether disseminated abdominal tumors actually arose in the GI tract.[35,36] The stomach is the most common primary site for GI lymphoma, composing approximately 40 to 50 percent of cases. Of the remainder, 25 to 30 percent occur in the small intestine and about 10 to 20 percent occur in the colon.

The most common site for primary small intestinal lymphoma is the ileum. The majority of non-Hodgkin's lymphomas of the intestine are classified as diffuse large cell or histiocytic lymphomas. In contrast to the course in affected children, intestinal lymphomas in adults are relatively indolent. The most common symptoms are abdominal pain, weight loss, nausea, vomiting, and abdominal masses noted in approximately 52 percent.[37] Various combinations of surgery, radiotherapy, and chemotherapy have been used for treatment, and the overall 5-year survival is approximately 40 percent.[38]

The nature and behavior of lymphomas involving the GI tract in childhood are quite different and are the focus of the following discussion.

Epidemiology

Lymphoma is the third most common malignant neoplasm of children in the United States and accounts for 10 percent of all cancers diagnosed in children less than 15 years of age.[39] Thirty to 40 percent of children with non-Hodgkin's lymphoma present with abdominal tumors,[40] although primary involvement of the GI tract probably occurs in less than one-half of patients. The ratio of affected males to females is approximately 2 or 3 to 1.

Etiology and Pathogenesis

Although in most children with non-Hodgkin's lymphoma no pre-existing conditions are identified, there are a number of recognized predisposing factors. Several inherited or acquired immunodeficiency syndromes are associated with an increased risk for the development of both Hodgkin's and non-Hodgkin's lymphoma. These conditions include ataxia-telangiectasia, Wiscott-Aldrich syndrome, common variable agammaglobulinemia, X-linked agammaglobulinemia, severe combined immunodeficiency syndrome, and others. In the X-linked lymphoproliferative syndrome, Epstein-Barr virus (EBV) infection may be associated with fatal infectious mononucleosis or the development of B-cell lymphoma.[41]

Even more impressive epidemiologically is the association of EBV and Burkitt's lymphoma in Africa.[42] Only a minority of children with Burkitt's lymphoma in North America, however, carry EBV DNA in their cells. Although no specific infectious agent has been isolated, the high burden of intestinal pathogens found in non-Western countries is thought to result in the immunoproliferation that precedes the development of so-called Mediterranean lymphoma.

Certain drugs have also been implicated in the pathogenesis of non-Hodgkin's lymphoma. Transplant recipients are known to be at increased risk for the development of this malignancy as a result of immunosuppressive therapy. Furthermore, patients treated for Hodgkin's lymphoma have been reported to subsequently develop non-Hodgkin's lymphoma.

Much research has focused on investigation of the molecular pathogenesis of lymphoma and other tumors. In Burkitt's lymphoma, it is hypothesized that a chromosomal translocation occurs that may deregulate an oncogene and result in cellular proliferation. Similar mechanisms may play a role in other types of lymphoma. This subject has been recently reviewed by Magrath.[43]

Pathology

Much confusion surrounds the classification of the childhood lymphomas as a result of the use of many different schemes. Most lymphomas are diffuse rather than nodular (follicular) in childhood. The diffuse lymphomas can be divided into three main categories: (1) large-cell or histiocytic lymphomas (mostly B-cell and non-T, non-B neoplasms), (2) lymphoblastic (almost all T-cell), and (3) undifferentiated or small, noncleaved cell, which includes Burkitt's lymphoma (B-cell) (Table 5).[44]

Children who present with abdominal lymphoma usually have lymphomas of the undifferentiated type, and conversely the majority of undifferentiated lymphomas present as abdominal tumors. Rarely, there may be associated inguinal or iliac lymphadenopathy. Bone marrow involvement occurs in 20 to 40 percent of patients with undifferentiated lymphomas. Although initial involvement of the central nervous system is unusual, relapse in the meninges is a significant problem for children with advanced stage abdominal undifferentiated lymphomas.

Clinical Features

Children with abdominal lymphoma frequently present with abdominal pain, distention, a change of bowel habits, or nausea and vomiting. A right lower quadrant mass may be palpable. Occasionally, peritoneal signs may be present and suggest a "surgical abdomen." Most commonly, primary intestinal lymphomas involve the terminal ileum, cecum, or appendix and may result in ileocecal intussusception. With extensive involvement, ascites may be present and the diagnosis made by paracentesis.

Diagnosis

Diagnosis of non-Hodgkin's lymphoma requires biopsy for histopathologic examination; immunophenotyping and cytogenetics should also be included. With extensive disease,

a bone marrow aspirate and biopsy or cytocentrifugation and examination of ascitic fluid may prevent the need for laparotomy, which may delay therapy. On barium study, primary intestinal lymphoma with limited involvement of the abdominal structures may easily be confused with Crohn's disease, certain cases of appendicitis, and various benign lesions, including leiomyomas and duplications (Fig. 3). The classically cited barium study reveals an ileocecal intussusception due to an ileal tumor (Fig. 4).

Formal staging studies should be performed expeditiously in children, since progression of disease is rapid and therapy should be begun without delay. Investigations should include a chest radiograph, a nuclear medicine scan to assess bony involvement, computed tomography or magnetic resonance imaging of the abdomen, a spinal tap, and a bone marrow examination. A scheme for staging of Burkitt's lymphoma is shown in Table 6.[44] Of note is the fact that stage AR, in which greater than 90 percent of the tumor has been surgically resected, has a favorable prognosis similar to stages A and B, in which there is no abdominal tumor.[44,45]

Simple blood studies may reveal anemia or leukoerythroblastosis, which may indicate bone marrow involvement. Serum lactate dehydrogenase levels may correlate with the tumor burden. Other lymphocyte-derived factors are under investigation as possible prognostic markers.[43]

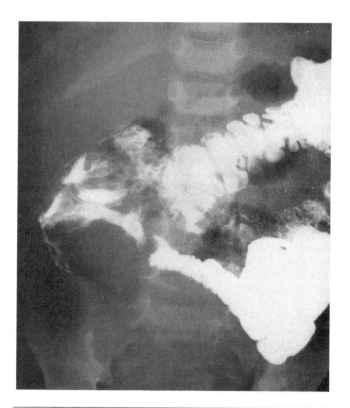

FIGURE 3 Contrast study of the small bowel in a 3-year-old boy with a 6-week history of abdominal discomfort and malaise. His mother had noted an abdominal mass when bathing him. The ileum is noted to be nodular and narrowed. At surgery, an ileal Burkitt's lymphoma was noted. (From the Teaching Collection, Department of Radiology, The Children's Hospital, Boston.)

TABLE 5
Modified Rappaport Classification of Childhood Non-Hodgkin's Lymphomas

---

Nodular

Diffuse
    Large cell (histiocytic)—mostly B-cell and non–T, non–B cell
    Lymphoblastic—almost all T-cell
    Undifferentiated (small, noncleaved)
        Burkitt—B-cell
        Non-Burkitt

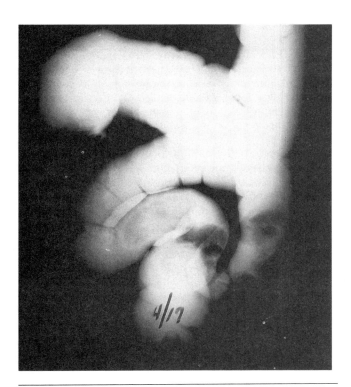

FIGURE 4 A barium enema in a 4-year-old boy with a 2-month history of abdominal pain. The barium column stops abruptly in the ascending colon at the site of an ileocecal intussusception. Laparotomy revealed a Burkitt's lymphoma of the ileocecal valve. (From the Teaching Collection, Department of Radiology, The Children's Hospital, Boston.)

Treatment

If evaluation does not reveal extensive abdominal involvement or ascites and the bone marrow studies are normal, the primary bowel lesion and associated mesentery should be resected and a primary anastomosis performed. Mesenteric nodes should be removed for pathologic study. Chemotherapy is central to all treatment plans. Most protocols include cyclophosphamide, methotrexate, vincristine, prednisone, and an anthracycline. Induction therapy is followed by maintenance

TABLE 6
Clinical Staging of Childhood Burkitt's Lymphoma

Stage	Site of Tumor
A	Single extra-abdominal site
B	Multiple extra-abdominal sites
C	Intra-abdominal tumor
D	Intra-abdominal tumor with involvement of multiple extra-abdominal sites
AR	Stage C, but with more than 90% of tumor surgically resected

treatment in all children, although those with localized or completely resected intra-abdominal disease require less intensive treatment. Central nervous system prophylaxis is generally indicated in all patients with advanced stage C or D disease but can be safely omitted in those with completely resected ileocecal primary tumors. As of this time, there is no role for radiation therapy, even in localized GI disease. All patients with a large tumor burden are at risk for rapid tumor lysis during the initial chemotherapy and resulting metabolic derangements. Therefore, these children should receive allopurinol, vigorous hydration, and urinary alkalinization. Hemodialysis may be required in children who are azotemic at presentation.

Prognosis

In patients with abdominal disease without bone marrow or central nervous system involvement, the expectancy of cure lies between 50 and 90 percent in all major protocols.[43] The presence of bone marrow involvement or CNS disease at the time of diagnosis confers a poor prognosis.

Non-Western or Mediterranean Lymphoma

Immunoproliferative small intestinal disease is a disorder characterized by the proliferation of immunoglobulin A–secreting B lymphocytes throughout the small intestine. In alpha-chain disease, this process is associated with detectable alpha heavy chains in the serum.[33] Most cases of alpha-chain disease have been reported from the Middle East and North America, although it occurs elsewhere when the socioeconomic status is low and hygiene poor. The current hypothesis is that malnutrition and repeated infectious diarrheas or parasitic infestations of the gut result in antigenetic stimulation and immunoproliferation. A diffuse infiltrate of plasma cells is noted throughout the lamina propria of the small intestine, and the villous structure may be distorted. Interestingly, alpha-chain disease generally occurs in individuals between 10 and 40 years of age but may occasionally be observed in young children. Most cases occur in males.

Patients with alpha-chain disease frequently present with malabsorption and a protein-losing enteropathy. The vast majority have chronic diarrhea, abdominal pain, and weight loss. In advanced disease, a large-cell, immunoblastic lymphoma develops and is frequently multifocal.

Early in the disease antibiotic medications may induce remission; with advanced lymphoma combinations of surgery, radiotherapy, and chemotherapy have been employed. Although long-term remissions have been recorded, the prognosis is quite poor.

A recent series of 37 Iraqi children with primary intestinal lymphoma provides information regarding the distribution of different kinds of lymphoma in a non-Western pediatric population. Eleven children had Mediterranean lymphoma, and the remaining 26 had lymphomas localized to the ileal or ileocecal region, half of which were characterized as Burkitt's lymphoma.[46]

Other Gastrointestinal Disease Predisposing to Lymphoma

Although not reported in children, lymphoma has been noted to occur with increased frequency in adult patients with celiac disease, especially in those above age 50 years.[47] Most of these tumors would be classified as large cell or histiocytic, non-Hodgkin's lymphomas. The tumor usually involves the small intestine but may occur in other extranodal tissues. The diagnosis is frequently delayed because of confusion of the symptoms with those resulting from poor control of the celiac disease. The prognosis in this setting is very poor. There is no evidence thus far to indicate that a gluten-free diet protects against the development of lymphoma in patients with celiac disease.[48]

Crohn's disease and ulcerative colitis are not only complicated by an increased incidence of adenocarcinoma but are also associated with a higher-than-predicted risk of lymphoma. In Crohn's disease the lymphoma is typically found in the ileum.[49] Although primary lymphoma of the colon is very uncommon, 24 cases of primary colonic lymphoma associated with ulcerative colitis have been reported, also suggesting an association between these disorders.[50]

Conclusions

As knowledge of the lymphocyte and other elements of the mucosal immune system increases, it is likely that the diagnosis and management of intestinal lymphoma of childhood will undergo rapid refinement. Already, molecular biologic techniques to detect chromosomal changes of malignant cells and distinguish lymphoma from benign cellular proliferation are being performed. These advances should permit further elucidation of the unique nature of lymphoma in the pediatric age group.

LEIOMYOSARCOMA

Although leiomyosarcomas represent approximately 20 percent of small bowel malignancies in adults,[51] they are rare in the pediatric age group. Soft-tissue sarcomas account for approximately 7 percent of all malignancies in childhood,[39] but less than 2 percent of them are leiomyosarcomas.[52] The three most extensive series of childhood leiomyosarcomas have included only 10 cases in each report.[53-55] Thirteen of 30 cases were gastrointestinal in origin, with 11 lesions occurring in the stomach and one each in the jejunum and cecum. As of 1983, only eight cases of colorectal leiomyosarcomas has been reported, including one tumor of the sigmoid colon in a 7-week-old infant.[56] In adults, the stomach is also the most common GI site for leiomyosarcomas. Skandalakis and Gray reported 45 percent of lesions to be in the stomach, 40 percent to be in the small or large intestine, and 15 percent to be in the esophagus.[57]

Of the leiomyosarcomas of the intestine in adults, approximately three-fourths occur in the small bowel and the remainder in the colon.[58] Angerpointner collected 15 cases of intestinal leiomyosarcoma in children as of 1981.[59] Approximately one-half of the lesions were reported in the small

bowel, one-half in the colon and rectum, and one case was noted in a Meckel's diverticulum.

Most GI leiomyosarcomas arise in the muscularis propria, with both submucosal and subserosal extension.[55] Ulceration of the overlying mucosa is commonly found. Typically, the tumors invade local structures directly, but metastasis to regional lymph nodes, liver, and lungs may occur. Differentiation of malignant lesions from benign leiomyomas may be difficult. In adults, mitotic counts appear to be the best predictor of malignant behavior of the tumor. In addition, size and local invasiveness seem to be important prognostic factors.[60] Although the paucity of cases prohibits the development of accurate diagnostic criteria for malignancy in childhood, mitotic counts and lesion size also appear to be important factors in this age group.[55]

The most frequent clinical feature in patients with leiomyosarcomas of the GI tract appears to be GI bleeding. Usually, the blood loss is occult and patients present with symptoms of anemia. Occasionally, however, acute GI hemorrhage may occur. Pain may result from either obstruction of the intestinal tract or metastasis. Two of 15 children with intestinal leiomyosarcoma presented with a jejuno-jejunal intussusception.[59] Occasionally, an abdominal mass may be palpable.

Barium contrast studies are useful in localizing leiomyosarcomas with significant intramural or submucosal growth (Fig. 5). Upper endoscopy and colonoscopy may help exclude other diagnoses and can permit histologic confirmation if

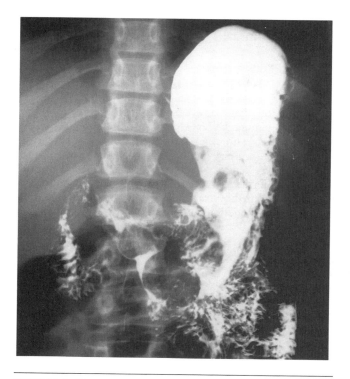

FIGURE 5 Upper gastrointestinal series in a 10-year-old girl with severe anemia and tarry stools. A large nodular leiomyosarcoma is seen in the gastric antrum. (From the Teaching Collection, Department of Radiology, The Children's Hospital, Boston.)

tumor has eroded through the mucosa. Ultrasonography, computed tomography, and magnetic resonance imaging of the abdomen may provide information regarding involvement of adjacent structures (Fig. 6).

The primary mode of therapy for GI leiomyosarcomas in childhood is complete resection of the tumor. Both adjuvant radiation and chemotherapy have been used for treatment of these tumors, but the role of these therapies, especially in the pediatric age group, remains to be determined. In adults, curative resection results in an overall survival rate of 63 percent at 5 years for patients with GI sarcomas, whereas patients who had only partial excision or biopsy survived a median of only 9 months.[60]

Stromal tumors of the GI tract, such as leiomyomas and leiomyosarcomas, are unusual but clinically important in the pediatric age group. Future research is necessary to clarify whether these tumors arise from myocytes or are really undifferentiated mesenchymal tumors and to better characterize their behavior so that diagnosis and therapy can be improved.

CARCINOID TUMORS

Carcinoid tumors are unusual in adults and rare in children. Although usually found incidentally in the appendix in a child undergoing appendectomy, these tumors may play a role in the pathogenesis of appendicitis in some children or even cause bowel obstruction when they occur in other parts of the intestine. The medically fascinating carcinoid syndrome, resulting from secretion of a variety of physiologically active substances, definitely can occur in the pediatric age group but has been reported only rarely.

Carcinoid tumors arise from the endocrine cells of the GI epithelium. These cells are now thought to be of endodermal derivation and are the source of a variety of GI peptides and hormones. Along with other endocrine tumors, carcinoids have been designated APUDomas because the cells of origin are capable of amine precursor uptake and decarboxylation.[61]

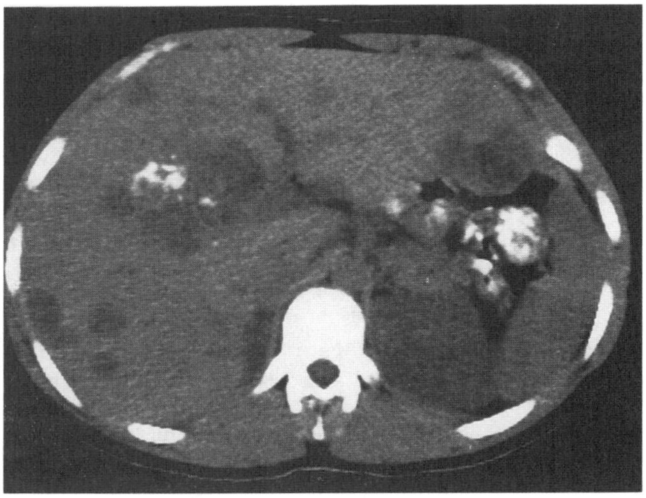

Incidence

In adults, carcinoid tumors probably account for only 1 or 2 percent of clinically evident GI neoplasms, although in a large autopsy series, carcinoids were found in 1.2 percent of individuals.[62] Approximately 40 percent of carcinoid tumors occur in the appendix, with the ileum (10 percent) and rectum (15 percent) also being common sites.[63] Carcinoid tumors have been occasionally found elsewhere in the GI tract, in the colon, stomach, duodenum, and esophagus, as well as in duplications and Meckel's diverticula. In addition, reported extraintestinal sites include the gallbladder and biliary tree, pancreas, gonads, thymus, and bronchial tree. Tumors of the ileum and stomach are not infrequently multicentric. Appendiceal carcinoids in women are reported to be more common and are diagnosed at a younger age than in men, perhaps because these tumors tend to be removed at incidental appendectomy during pelvic and gallbladder surgery.[64]

In children, almost all reported carcinoid tumors have been found in the appendix. A female predominance has also been noted in the series of appendiceal carcinoids in children, although in this age group the difference cannot be explained on the basis of a higher likelihood of having an incidental appendectomy during other surgery.[65,66] Other reported sites of carcinoid tumors in children are the small intestine,[67,68] a Meckel's diverticulum,[69] the stomach,[70] the colon,[71,72] the pancreas,[73] and GI duplications.[74,75]

FIGURE 6 A computed tomogram of the abdomen of the patient whose upper gastrointestinal series is shown in Figure 4. Multiple liver metastases are demonstrated. The largest is calcified. (From the Teaching Collection, Department of Radiology, The Children's Hospital, Boston.)

Pathology

Carcinoid tumors are composed of round or polygonal cells arranged in clusters or rosettes (Figs. 7 and 8). Those containing a high content of serotonin stain with silver in the argentaffin reaction, hence the previous designation of these tumors as argentaffinomas. Newer diagnostic techniques include electron microscopy[76] to identify characteristic membrane-bound secretory granules and immunohistologic staining for the protein chromogranin A.[77] Primary carcinoid tumors tend to be small and slow-growing. However, more than 75 percent of lesions larger than 2 cm in diameter have already metastasized when discovered.[78] In comparison to tumors at other sites, colonic and ileal tumors tend to metastasize more frequently. Common sites of metastatic spread include regional lymph nodes, the liver, the mesentery, and the peritoneum.

In a series of 30 patients in the pediatric age group with appendiceal carcinoids, tumors ranged between 0.1 and 2.5 cm in size, with most lesions being quite small. Although tumor invaded through the submucosa into the muscularis or deeper in 27 of 30 cases, only one tumor extended through the muscularis into the serosal fat, and there were no

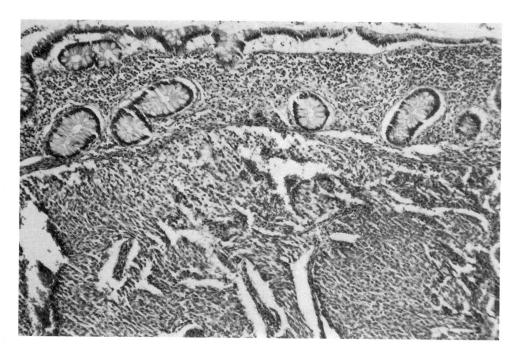

FIGURE 7 Appendiceal carcinoid. The mucosa of the appendix is seen at the top. Below, the remainder of the appendiceal wall is replaced by tumor cells. (Courtesy of Dr. Antonio Perez-Atayde.)

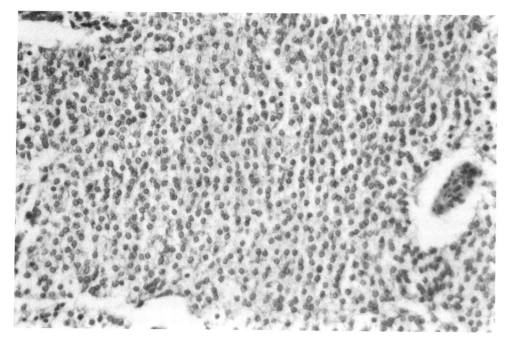

FIGURE 8 Higher-power view of the carcinoid tumor shown in Figure 7. Small, homogeneous tumor cells are arrayed in a trabecular pattern.

metastases.[65] In a second large series, infiltration of the serosa was noted in 9 or 25 children, with lymph node metastases in only one.[66]

Pathophysiology—The Carcinoid Syndrome

The endocrine cells in carcinoid tumors are able to release a number of substances with physiologic actions. These include 5-hydroxytryptamine (5-HT) or serotonin, 5-hydroxytryptophan (5-HTP), a variety of kinin peptides, histamine, catecholamines, and prostaglandins.

Tryptophan ingested in the diet is hydroxylated to 5-HTP and then converted to serotonin. Serotonin's major metabolite, 5-hydroxyindoleacetic acid (5-HIAA), is produced by the enzyme monoamine oxidase, either in the tumor or in the blood. The putative physiologic effects of serotonin include intestinal hypermotility and resulting diarrhea, fibrogenesis, such as seen at the tumor site or within the heart, bronchoconstriction, edema, and flushing.

Recent information suggests that a variety of other compounds including the bradykinins, prostaglandins, and calcitonin may play a role in the production of cutaneous flushing or other aspects of the carcinoid syndrome. In particular, the bradykinins have been demonstrated to have the capability to produce profound vasodilatation and may also induce fibrosis.

The carcinoid syndrome is usually associated with carcinoid tumors, typically ileal in location, which have extensive liver metastases. Presumably, primary tumors limited to sites drained via the portal system may produce physiologically active substances, but these are cleared by the liver before causing significant effects. However, primary ovarian and bronchial lesions may, because of their location, release mediators directly into the systemic circulation, resulting in symptoms of the carcinoid syndrome.

Less common manifestations of the carcinoid syndrome include ascites and arthralgias. Particularly devastating are valvular lesions of the right side of the heart which have been reported as complications of the syndrome. Presumably, fibrosis leads to stenosis and incompetence of the tricuspid and pulmonic valves, and, as a result, congestive heart failure may occur.

Clinical Features

Up to 60 percent of carcinoid tumors in some series of adult patients are asymptomatic and are found incidentally.[79] When symptoms do occur, most common are abdominal pain and sequelae of intestinal obstruction. GI bleeding is unusual. Less than 15 percent of patients present with symptoms suggestive of the carcinoid syndrome. Before the classic episodes of flushing occur, the patient may experience mild episodic symptoms that are not brought to the attention of his or her physician. Vasomotor episodes can be induced by exercise, the ingestion of alcohol and certain foods, emotion, changes in posture, abdominal palpation, and infusion of calcium and epinephrine.

While in adults most appendiceal carcinoids are found at incidental appendectomy, the vast majority of children present with signs or symptoms of acute appendicitis.[65,66] In fact, 60 percent of patients in one series and 83 percent of those in another actually had histologic evidence of appendicitis. Although cases have been reported in which the tumor clearly obstructs the appendiceal lumen, causing distention or secondary infection, in many others the tumor was located at the tip of the appendix and was believed not to play a role in production of appendicitis.

Documented cases of the carcinoid syndrome have been reported in children but are distinctly unusual. Biorck et al described a case of unusual cyanosis in a boy with pulmonary stenosis and tricuspid insufficiency in 1952.[67] Apparently this child had episodes of cyanosis, rash, and wheezing. The patient died after angiography and at autopsy was noted to have a malignant carcinoid of the jejunum with metastases to the liver. Although the authors could only speculate on a relationship between the carcinoid tumor and the patient's cardiac disease at that time, it now seems evident that the two conditions were related. In their review of carcinoid tumors in children, Field and co-workers reported a 15-year-old male with symptoms of the carcinoid syndrome.[80] More recently, Chow et al reported four children between the ages of 8 and 14 years old who had malignant (metastatic) carcinoid tumors but did not have the classic carcinoid syndrome.[68] Thus, although carcinoid tumors in children are

usually found in the appendix at the time of appendectomy, they can be found at other sites and produce significant morbidity and mortality as a result of metastasis, with or without the concurrent development of the carcinoid syndrome.

Diagnosis

In the absence of the carcinoid syndrome, diagnosis of a GI carcinoid is rarely made before surgery.[79] On physical examination, 10 to 15 percent of adult patients may have a palpable mass. In addition, individuals with carcinoid syndrome may have an abnormal funduscopic examination,[81] cutaneous telangiectasia and a purplish discoloration of the skin, auscultatory findings of right-sided valvular heart disease and congestive heart failure, and hepatomegaly.

The standard test for diagnosis of the carcinoid syndrome is the urine test for 5-HIAA. A qualitative or "spot" test is available which will detect this metabolite when 30 mg or more is excreted in a normal 24-hour urine volume. However, because many patients with serotonin-secreting carcinoid tumors have an increase in 5-HIAA excretion only to between 8 and 30 mg per 24 hours, a more sensitive quantitative test is advised. During the urine collection, the patient should not eat serotonin-rich foods such as bananas, pineapples, walnuts, and various other nuts and fruits. Also, several medicines, notably glyceryl guaiacolate, methenamine mandelate, and various phenothiazines may cause falsely positive or negative results.[76] Occasionally, it may be helpful to measure levels of serotonin in whole blood or in urinary collections. Gastric and bronchial carcinoids may secrete high levels of 5-HTP and histamine which can be quantitated in the urine. Even with extensive liver metastases, standard liver function tests may be remarkable only for mild elevation of the alkaline phosphatase or gamma-glutamyl transpeptidase.

Endoscopy and proctoscopy detect virtually all upper GI and rectal tumors, respectively.[79] Contrast radiographic studies are less sensitive for GI carcinoids and reveal lesions in only 25 percent or fewer of patients with these tumors. Ultrasonography and computed tomography of the abdomen may detect mass lesions and are helpful for evaluation of possible hepatic metastases. Angiography has also been demonstrated to be a sensitive technique for the detection of hepatic metastases.[82] Recently, the pheochromocytoma scanning agent ^{131}I-metaiodobenzylguanidine has been shown to be concentrated by carcinoid tumors and may eventually prove to be helpful in diagnosis.[83]

Treatment

The treatment of carcinoid tumors of the appendix has been recently reviewed, and simple appendectomy was judged sufficient for treatment of adult patients with apparently localized tumors, less than 2 cm in largest dimension.[84] For larger tumors, right hemicolectomy was recommended. A conservative approach for children is also supported by the available data. In the two previously mentioned large series of carcinoid tumors of the appendix in children, none of 55 patients treated with simple appendectomy showed recurrence after a mean follow-up of 12 to 13 years.[65,66] Small rectal lesions also may be treated by local excision alone. Clearly, however, more aggressive surgery is warranted for patients with carcinoid tumors with regional spread in whom involved nodes and areas of regional invasion should be removed.[85]

Treatment of patients with the carcinoid syndrome must be individualized. If the hepatic metastasis is resectable, the patient should undergo surgery. The primary ileal or colonic lesions, if they cause symptoms by virtue of obstruction of the bowel lumen, should be removed, although such surgery is very unlikely to be curative. The role of chemotherapy has been recently reviewed.[85,86] 5-Fluorouracil, streptozotocin, and a variety of other agents have been used singly and in combination, with rather poor results. Hepatic artery occlusion for treatment of hepatic metastasis may provide some relief of symptoms of the carcinoid syndrome but does not seem to improve survival.[85] As of this time, radiation therapy seems to be of little benefit.

Another aspect of the treatment of the carcinoid syndrome is the use of various agents to provide symptomatic relief by blocking the effects of serotonin and other active substances released by the tumor. This approach, although appealing as supportive therapy, is complicated by the fact that many specific details of the pathophysiology of the syndrome are unknown. Of demonstrated benefit is the combination of an H_1 histamine antagonist and an H_2 histamine antagonist in the treatment of symptoms of gastric carcinoid tumors. Recently, a long-acting analogue of somatostatin was shown to be of benefit in the treatment of the malignant carcinoid syndrome. It relieved flushing and diarrhea in 22 of 25 patients and led to a decrease in the urinary excretion of 5-HIAA by 50 percent or more in 18 of 25 patients. Whether this analogue is acting by inhibiting the release of amines or peptides from the tumor or by some other mechanism is not yet clear. Nevertheless, it seems to hold promise for control of symptoms in certain patients with the carcinoid syndrome.[87]

Prognosis

The prognosis for adults or children with small appendiceal or rectal carcinoid tumors is excellent. Although tumors in the colon and ileum carry the least favorable prognosis, the 5-year survival rate for patients with carcinoids in these sites is as high as 60 percent. Even patients with hepatic metastases and the carcinoid syndrome have lived 10 or more years after diagnosis because of the indolent nature of their tumors.

Conclusions

Most carcinoid tumors in children are found incidentally at the time of appendectomy and are cured by that procedure. Nevertheless, this diagnosis should be considered in children with abdominal masses or unusual episodic symptoms.

SUMMARY

To avoid misdiagnosis of GI tumors, the possibility of such lesions *must* be considered in all children with severe GI symptoms. A knowledge of disorders predisposing to the development of malignancy such as inflammatory bowel disease, familial polyposis, or immune deficiencies is essential for timely diagnosis of GI tumors in children and institution of surveillance programs for high-risk individuals entering adulthood. Both for diagnosis and management, a multidisciplinary approach involving experts from radiology, pathology, surgery, and oncology is critical. Significant advances in the care of these patients await the analysis of larger series of patients as well as progress in the basic science laboratory.

Acknowledgments

The author is grateful to Drs. Donald Antonioli and Howard Weinstein for their review of this chapter.

REFERENCES

1. Sessions RT, Riddell DH, Kaplan HJ, Foster JH. Carcinoma of the colon in the first two decades of life. Ann Surg 1965; 162:279–284.
2. Pratt CB, Rivera G, Shanks E, Johnson WW, Howarth C, Terrell W, Kumar APM. Colorectal carcinoma in adolescents: implications regarding etiology. Cancer 1977; 40:2464–2472.
3. Odone V, Chang L, Caces J, George SL, Pratt CB. The natural history of colorectal carcinoma in adolescents. Cancer 1982; 49:1716–1720.
4. Hoerner MT. Carcinoma of the colon and rectum in persons under twenty years of age. Am J Surg 1958; 96:47–53.
5. Silverberg E, Lubera J. Cancer statistics. Cancer 1987; 37:2–19.
6. Kern WH, White WC. Adenocarcinoma of the colon in a 9-month-old infant: report of a case. Cancer 1958; 11:855–857.
7. Middelkamp JN, Haffner H. Carcinoma of the colon in children. Pediatrics 1963; 32:558–571.
8. Soybel DI, Bliss DP, Wells SA Jr. Colon and rectal carcinoma. Curr Probl Cancer 1987; 11:257–356.
9. Lynch HT, Rozen P, Schuelke GS, Lynch JF. Hereditary colorectal cancer review: colonic polyposis and nonpolyposis colonic cancer (Lynch syndrome I and II) Surg Dig Dis 1984; 2:224–260.
10. Chabalko JJ, Fraumeni JF Jr. Colorectal cancer in children: epidemiologic aspects. Dis Colon Rectum 1975; 18:1–3.
11. Greenstein AJ, Sachar DB, Smith H, et al. Cancer in universal and left-sided ulcerative colitis. Factors determining risk. Gastroenterology 1979; 77:290–294.
12. Greenstein AJ, Slater G, Heimann TM, Sachar DB, Aufses AH. Comparison of multiple synchronous colorectal cancers in ulcerative colitis, familial polyposis coli, and de nova cancer. Ann Surg 1986; 203:123–128.
13. Greenstein AJ, Sachar DB, Pucillo A, et al. Cancer in universal and left-sided ulcerative colitis: clinical and pathological features. Mt. Sinai J Med 1979; 46:25–32.
14. Greenstein AJ, Sachar DB, Smith H, Janowitz HD, Aufses AH. Patterns of neoplasia in Crohn's disease and ulcerative colitis. Cancer 1980; 46:403–407.
15. Bassey HJR. Familial polyposis coli. Baltimore: Johns Hopkins University Press, 1975.
16. Burdich D, Prior JT. Peutz-Jeghers syndrome: a clinicopathological study of large family with a 27-year follow-up. Cancer 1982; 50:2139.
17. Stemper TJ, Kent TH, Summers RW. Juvenile polyposis and gastrointestinal carcinoma: a study of a kindred. Ann Intern Med 1975; 83:639.
18. Fitzgibbons RJ Jr, Lynch HT, Stanislav GV, Watson PA, Lanspa SJ, Marcus JN, Smyrk T, Kriegler MD, Lynch JF. Recognition and treatment of patients with hereditary nonpolyposis colon cancer (Lynch syndromes I and II). Ann Surg 1987; 206:289–294.
19. Aiges HW, Kahn E, Silverberg M, Darrm F. Adenocarcinoma of the colon in an adolescent with the family cancer syndrome. J Pediatr 1979; 94:632–633.
20. Cannon-Albright LA, Skolnick MH, Bishop T, Lee RG, Burt RW. Common inheritance of susceptibility to colonic adenomatous polyps and associated colorectal cancers. N Engl J Med 1988; 319:533–537.
21. Eraklis AJ, Folkman MJ. Adenocarcinoma at the site of ureterosigmoidostomies for exstrophy of the bladder. J Pediatr Surg 1978; 13:730–734.
22. Roses DF, Richman H, Localio SA. Bacterial endocarditis associated with colorectal carcinoma. Ann Surg 1974; 179:190–191.
23. Falterman KW, Hill CB, Markey JC, Fox JW, Cohn I Jr. Cancer of the colon, rectum, and anus: a review of 2313 cases. Cancer 1974; 34:951–959.

24. Anderson A, Bergdahl L. Carcinoma of the colon in children: a report of six new cases and a review of the literature. J Pediatr Surg 1976; 11:967–971.

25. Rao BN, Pratt CB, Fleming ID, Dilawari RA, Green AA, Austin BA. Colon carcinoma in children and adolescents: a review of 30 cases. Cancer 1985; 55:1322–1326.

26. Symonds DA, Vickery AL Jr. Mucinous carcinoma of the colon and rectum. Cancer 1976; 37:1891–1900.

27. Astler VB, Coller FA. The prognostic significance of direct extension of carcinoma of the colon and rectum. Ann Surg 1954; 139:846.

28. Enker WE, Paloyan E, Kirsner JB. Carcinoma of the colon in the adolescent: a report of survival and analysis of the literature. Am J Surg 1977; 133:737–741.

29. Zollinger RM Jr, Sternfeld WC, Schreiber H. Primary neoplasms of the small intestine. Am J Surg 1986; 151:654–658.

30. Cordts AE, Chakot JR. Jejunal carcinoma in a child. J Pediatr Surg 1983; 18:180–181.

31. Goldman LI, Bralow SP, Cox W, Peale AR. Adenocarcinoma of the small bowel complicating Crohn's disease. Cancer 1970; 26:1119–1125.

32. Nesbit RR, Elbadawi NA, Morton JH, Cooper RA Jr. Carcinoma of the small bowel. A complication of regional enteritis. Cancer 1976; 37:2948–2959.

33. Rambaud J-C. Small intestinal lymphomas and alpha-chain disease. Clin Gastroenterol 1983; 12:743–765.

34. Lewin KJ, Ranchod M, Dorfman RF. Lymphomas of the gastrointestinal tract. A study of 117 cases presenting with gastrointestinal disease. Cancer 1978; 42:693–707.

35. Herrmann R, Panahon AM, Barcos MP, Walsh D, Stutzman L. Gastrointestinal involvement in non-Hodgkin's lymphoma. Cancer 1980; 46:215–222.

36. Green JA, Dawson AA, Jones PF, Brunt PW. The presentation of gastrointestinal lymphoma. Br J Surg 1979; 66:798.

37. Fitch DD, Wilson JAP. Primary gastrointestinal lymphoma. S Med J 1985; 78:909–913.

38. Cooper BT, Read AE. Small intestinal lymphoma. World J Surg 1985; 9:930–937.

39. Young JL, Miller RW. Incidence of malignant tumors in US children. J Pediatr 1975; 86:254–258.

40. Wollner N, Burchewal JH, Lieberman PH, et al. Non-Hodgkin's lymphoma in children: a comparative study of two modalities of therapy. Cancer 1976; 37:123–134.

41. Purtillo DT, DeFlorio D, Hutt LM, et al. Variable phenotype expression of an X-linked lymphoproliferative syndrome. N Engl J Med 1977; 297:1077–1081.

42. Epstein MA, Achong BG, Barr YM. Virus particles in culture lymphoblasts from Burkitt's lymphoma. Lancet 1964; 1:702–703.

43. Magrath IT. Malignant non-Hodgkin's lymphoma. In: Pizzo PA, Poplack DG, eds. Principles and practices of pediatric oncology. Philadelphia: JB Lippincott, 1989: 415.

44. Link MP. Non-Hodgkin's lymphoma in children. Pediatr Clin North Am 1985; 32:699–720.

45. Magrath IT, Lwanga S, Carswell W, Harrison N. Surgical resection of tumor bulk in management of abdominal Burkitt's lymphoma. Br Med J 1974; 2:308–312.

46. Al-Bahrani Z, Al-Mondhiry H, Al-Saleem T, Zaini S. Primary intestinal lymphoma in Iraqi children. Oncology 1986; 43:243–250.

47. Cooper BT, Holmes GKT, Cooke WT. Lymphoma risk in coeliac disease of later life. Digestion 1982; 23:89–92.

48. Holmes GKT, Stokes PL, Sorahan TM, Prior P, Waterhouse JAH, Cooke WT. Coeliac disease, gluten-free diet, and malignancy. Gut 1976; 17:612–619.

49. Collins WJ. Malignant lymphoma complicating regional enteritis: case report and review of the literature. Am J Gastroenterol 1977; 68:177–181.

50. Bashiti HO, Kraus FT. Histiocytic lymphoma in chronic ulcerative colitis. Cancer 1980; 46:1695–1700.

51. Wilson JM, Melvin DB, Gray GF, Thorbjarnarson B. Primary malignancies of the small bowel: a report of 96 cases and review of the literature. Ann Surg 1974; 180:175–179.

52. Jenkin D, Sonley M. Soft-tissue sarcomas in the young. Medical treatment advances in perspective. Cancer 1980; 46:621–629.

53. Yannopoulos K, Stout AP. Smooth muscle tumors in children. Cancer 1962; 15:958–971.

54. Botting AJ, Soule EH, Brown AL Jr. Smooth muscle tumors in children. Cancer 1965; 18:711–720.

55. Lack EE. Leiomyosarcomas in childhood: a clinical and pathologic study of 10 cases. Pediatr Pathol 1986; 6:181–197.

56. Posen JA, Bar-Maor JA. Leiomyosarcoma of the colon in an infant: a case report and review of the literature. Cancer 1983; 52:1458–1461.

57. Skandalakis JE, Gray SW. Smooth-muscle tumors of the alimentary tract. In: Ariel IM, ed. Progress in clinical cancer. New York: Grune & Stratton, 1965: 692.

58. Akwari OE, Dozois RR, Weiland LH, Beahrs OH. Leiomyosarcoma of the small and large bowel. Cancer 1978; 42:1375–1384.

59. Angerpointner TA, Weitz H, Haas RJ, Hecker WC. Intestinal leiomyosarcoma in childhood: case report and review of the literature. J Pediatr Surg 1981; 16:491–495.

60. McGrath PC, Neifeld JP, Lawrence W Jr, Kay S, Horsley JS III, Parker GA. Gastrointestinal sarcomas: analysis of prognostic factors. Ann Surg 1987; 206:706–710.

61. Pearse AGE. The APUD concept and hormone production. Clin Endocrinol Metab 1980; 9:211–222.

62. Berge T, Linell F. Carcinoid tumors. Acta Pathol Microbiol Scand 1976; 84:322.

63. Godwin JD. Carcinoid tumors: an analysis of 2837 cases. Cancer 1975; 36:560–569.

64. Moertel CG, Dockerty MB, Judd ES. Carcinoid tumors of the vermiform appendix. Cancer 1968; 21:270–278.

65. Ryden SE, Drake RM, Franciosi RA. Carcinoid tumors of the appendix in children. Cancer 1975; 36:1538–1542.

66. Andersson A, Bergdahl L. Carcinoid tumors of the appendix in children: a report of 25 cases. Acta Chir Scand 1977; 143:173–175.

67. Biorck G, Axen O, Thorson A. Unusual cyanosis in a boy with congenital pulmonary stenosis and tricuspid insufficiency: fatal outcome after angiocardiography. Am Heart J 1965; 44:143–148.

68. Chow CW, Sane S, Campbell PE, Carter RF. Malignant carcinoid tumors in children. Cancer 1982; 49:802–811.

69. Hecks B, Kadinski S. Carcinoid tumor of a Meckel's diverticulum. Lancet 1922; ii:70.

70. Lutzow-Holm G. Carcinoid tumors of the stomach: two cases. Acta Chir Scand 1952; 104:193–200.

71. Suster G, Weinberg AG, Graivier L. Carcinoid tumor of the colon in a child. J Pediatr Surg 1977; 12:739–742.

72. LaFerla G, Baxter RA, Tavadia HB, Harper DR. Multiple colonic carcinoid tumours in a child. Br J Surg 1984; 71:843.

73. King MD, Young DG, Hann IM, Patrick WJA. Carcinoid syndrome: an unusual cause of diarrhoea. Arch Dis Child 1985; 60:269–271.

74. Rubin SZ, Mancer JFK, Stephens CA. Carcinoid in a rectal duplication: a unique pediatric surgical problem. Can J Surg 1981; 24:351–352.

75. Horie H, Iwasaki I, Takahashi H. Carcinoid in a gastrointestinal duplication. J Pediatr Surg 1986; 21:902–904.

76. Feldman JM. Carcinoid tumors and syndrome. Semin Oncol 1987; 14:237–246.

77. O'Connor DT, Deftos LJ. Secretion of chromogranin A by peptide-producing endocrine neoplasms. N Engl J Med 1986; 314:1145–1151.

78. Olney JR, Urdaneta LF, Al-Jurf AS, Jochimsen PR, Shirazi SS. Carcinoid tumors of the gastrointestinal tract. Am Surg 1985; 51:37–41.

79. Thompson GB, van Heerden JA, Martin JK Jr, Schutt AJ, Ilstrup DM, Carney JA. Carcinoid tumors of the gastrointestinal tract: presentation, management, and prognosis. Surgery 1985; 98:1054–1062.

80. Field JL, Adamson LF, Stoeckle HE. Review of carcinoids in children: functioning carcinoid in a 15-year-old male. Pediatrics 1962; 29:953–960.

81. Wong VG, Melman KL. Ophthalmic manifestations of the carcinoid flush. N Engl J Med 1967; 277:406.

82. Callatz C, Stage JG, Henriksen FW. Angiography in the diagnosis of the carcinoid syndrome. Scand J Gastroenterol 1979; 53:111–114.

83. McEwan AJ, Shapiro B, Sisson JC, Beierwaltes WH, Ackery DM. Radioiodobenzyl guanidine for the scintigraphic location and therapy of adrenergic tumors. Sem Nucl Med 1985; 15:132–153.

84. Moertel CG, Weiland LH, Nagorney DM, Dockerty MB. Carcinoid tumor of the appendix: treatment and prognosis. N Engl J Med 1987; 317:1699–1701.

85. Moertel CG. Treatment of the carcinoid tumor and the malignant carcinoid syndrome. J Clin Oncol 1983; 1:727–740.

86. Kvols LK, Buck M. Chemotherapy of endocrine malignancies: a review. Semin Oncol 1987; 14:343–353.

87. Kvols LK, Moertel CG, O'Connell MJ, Schutt AJ, Rubin J, Hahn RG. Treatment of the malignant carcinoid syndrome: evaluation of a long-acting somatostatin analogue. N Engl J Med 1986; 315:663–666.

PART 33

Motility Disorders

Brent Scott, M.D.C.M., FRCPC

PHYSIOLOGIC BACKGROUND

The small intestine and colon are specialized segments of a long convoluted tube into which liters of secretions and liquid and solid foods are delivered each day. Ingested nutrients are digested and absorbed, and about 200 ml of indigestible residue is excreted daily as semisolid stool. The secretory, absorptive, and motor events involved in normal digestion are highly co-ordinated functions under complex myogenic, neural, and hormonal regulation. Neither the specific functions (secretion, absorption, and motility) nor the regulatory mechanisms (myogenic, neural, and hormonal) act independently of one another. In this regard, alteration of secretion or absorption can provoke changes in motility, just as variation in intestinal motor activity and propulsion can affect absorption and secretion. Similarly, neural and hormonal signals modulate the intrinsic motor activity of intestinal smooth muscle, while intestinal motor activity in turn influences neural and hormonal output. This discussion reviews patterns of intestinal motor activity seen in health and disease and discusses the mechanisms, clinical features, and management of intestinal pseudo-obstruction.

Structural/Functional Relationships

Motor activity of the small intestine and colon is the result of the mechanical activity of the two perpendicularly oriented layers of smooth muscle in the muscularis externa: a thick inner circular layer and a thinner outer longitudinal layer. The longitudinal layer is continuous in the small intestine, but in the colon it is concentrated into three bands, or taeniae. A mesh-like ganglionated neural plexus is located throughout the length of the gut in the submucosa (Meissner's plexus) and between the circular and longitudinal layers (myenteric or Auerbach's plexus).

Intestinal smooth muscle cells are uninucleate, spindle-shaped, 500 to 700 μm in length at rest, and one-quarter of that when maximally contracted.[1] Numerous flask-shaped invaginations of the cell membrane (caveolae) are closely associated with the sarcoplasmic reticulum; like the transverse tubules of cardiac and skeletal muscle, they are probably involved in excitation-contraction coupling. Over much of the area of the cell surface not occupied by caveolae, electron-dense material adheres to the inner side of the cell membrane in irregularly distributed patches, or dense bands. The apposition of dense bands at adjacent points on smooth muscle cells constitutes an intermediate junction that is thought to serve as a mechanical coupling between cells. These bands serve as points of attachment for an irregular arrangement of thin (actin) and intermediate filaments, which together with the thicker myosin filaments constitute the major structural proteins of the contractile apparatus in smooth muscle.

Intestinal smooth muscle cells, arranged in branching bundles or fasciae limited by connective tissue, are functionally coupled so that contraction of all cells within the bundle occurs synchronously in response to excitatory stimulation. A second form of junction between smooth muscle cells, where the plasma membranes of adjacent cells fuse, is termed nexus or gap junction. Within these junctions numerous 2 to 3-nm channels serve as low-resistance intercellular pathways for conduction of ionic currents and spread of excitation or inhibition from cell to cell. Gap junctions are numerous in the circular muscle but infrequent in the longitudinal muscle layer of the intestines. Since this latter tissue exhibits synchronization of function, there must be other mechanisms or structures responsible for electrical coupling or communication between cells.

Contraction of gut smooth muscle, which depends on two major contractile proteins in the form of thin (actin) and thick (myosin) filaments,[2] is modulated by the level of free intracellular calcium. These proteins do not interact at resting levels of intracellular calcium less than 10^{-7} M; interaction occurs at higher concentrations and is maximal at levels above 10^{-5} M. When levels of free intracellular calcium are high, the ion combines with the calcium-receptor protein calmodulin, which is complexed with the regulatory protein myosin light chain kinase (MLCK). The binding of calcium to calmodulin activates MLCK, which mediates the interaction of ATP with myosin cross-bridges. Myosin cross-bridges detach from actin in the presence of ATP, which is hydrolyzed, forming ADP and a phosphorylated myosin cross-bridge. Phosphorylation of the myosin cross-bridge causes a conformational change and promotes interaction with actin. When the "activated" myosin cross-bridge attaches to actin, ADP and inorganic phosphate are released, the myosin cross-bridge changes its conformation, and there is a return to "ground" state. The return to ground state, while myosin is attached to actin, powers a sliding and shortening of the overlapping actin-myosin filaments.

Regulation of Intestinal Motor Activity

Neurohumoral Mechanisms. Intestinal smooth muscle is innervated by neurons in the myenteric plexus of the enteric nervous system (ENS).[3] The human ENS, which contains more than 10^8 neurons, roughly as many as are present in the spinal cord, is quite independent of central nervous system (CNS) control. It does receive modulatory input from the CNS via the sympathetic and parasympathetic divisions of the autonomic nervous system (ANS). The number of neurons within the ENS is immense compared to the number of these efferent autonomic fibers, and the vast majority of ganglion cells in the myenteric plexus are not directly innervated by axons of the ANS. The ENS is in fact capable of complex independent activity and has peripheral projections that actually modulate the output of the autonomic ganglia.

The myenteric plexus of the ENS contains integrative circuits that are responsive to input from sensory receptors, the CNS (via autonomic pathways), and intrinsic synaptic circuits that generate programmed or patterned motor activity (Fig. 1). There is great diversity of neurotransmitter release within ENS neurons, but acetylcholine (Ach) is the final common pathway for excitatory neural control of intestinal motility. Within the ENS, Ach acts as the excitatory neural transmitter between vagal fibers and intrinsic enteric neurons, between enteric neurons, and between enteric neurons and intestinal smooth muscle. The action of Ach on other neurons within enteric ganglia is mediated via nicotinic receptors, and its action on smooth muscle is mediated through muscarinic receptors. As a consequence, ganglionic blocking agents such as hexamethonium or muscarinic antagonists such as atropine abolish intestinal motility. Norepinephrine exerts a direct inhibitory effect on intestinal smooth muscle (mediated by beta-adrenergic receptors), but usually it causes indirect inhibition by decreasing Ach release. Even more powerful than adrenergic inhibition is the as-yet-unidentified nonadrenergic noncholinergic (NANC) neurotransmitter released by inhibitory neurons of the ENS. In contrast to the discrete neuromuscular junctions present in striated muscle, the myenteric neurons that innervate intestinal smooth muscle have expansions or varicosities along the length of the axon, each of which contains vesicles of neurotransmitter. When released, neurotransmitters diffuse across relatively wide spaces and influence many smooth muscle cells.

Scattered throughout the epithelial lining of the intestinal crypts and villi are specialized chromaffin, osmiophilic, and acidophilic cells that possess blood-mediated endocrine and/or local paracrine glandular properties.[4] These cells synthesize a variety of peptides and amines which are stored in secretory granules and released from the basal surface of the cell in response to stimuli, which include luminal substances that activate receptors on the apical surface of the cell and direct neural stimulation. Some display mainly endocrine effects (gastrin secretin, CCK, and glucagon) and others paracrine effects (somatostatin and bombesin). These substances exert a local effect not only on adjacent epithelial cells but also on nerve endings and smooth muscle fibers as they diffuse into the blood stream. Recently the same active substances found in gut endocrine cells have been identified in the secretory granules of neurons in the enteric and central nervous system, where they function as neurotransmitters. The neural and endocrine cells of the gut are two very closely integrated systems modulating digestive function.

Myogenic Mechanisms. Intestinal smooth muscle is an electrically excitable tissue that generates three types of membrane electrical potential: resting potential, slow wave potential, and the action or spike potential. Through altered smooth muscle membrane potential, various regulatory mechanisms exert control over intestinal motor activity.

The resting electrical potential difference of the smooth muscle membrane is a diffusion potential arising out of ionic gradients across the cell membrane and the selective permeability of that membrane for different ions.[5,6] The resting smooth muscle cell maintains an unequal distribution of ions across its membrane. The fluid inside (sarcoplasm) has a relatively high concentration of potassium and a low concentration of sodium and chloride, whereas in the extracellular fluid the relationship is reversed. This disequilibrium is maintained through the activity of energy-dependent ionic pumps, e.g., Na, K-ATPase located in the cell membrane. It is the natural tendency of ions to diffuse down their respective concentration gradients, the degree depending on the permeability of

FIGURE 1 A schematic model of the function of the myenteric plexus of the enteric nervous system.

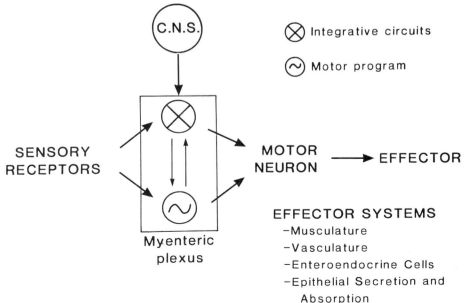

the cell membrane for that specific ionic species. Because the resting membrane is much more permeable to potassium than to sodium, potassium leaks out of the cell down its diffusion gradient, giving rise to an electric potential difference (inside negative). An equilibrium is achieved rapidly where the tendency of potassium to diffuse out of the cell and down its concentration gradient is balanced by an equal but opposite electric potential difference (the equilibrium potential) tending to draw potassium ions inward. The smooth muscle membrane varies resting membrane potential by selectively altering membrane permeability and allowing different ionic species to flow down their respective chemical gradients and create an equilibrium potential. The equilibrium potentials for potassium, sodium, and chloride are −91, +62, and −22 millivolts, respectively. When the membrane is permeable to more than one ionic species, membrane potential is weighted toward the equilibrium potential of the ion to which the membrane is most permeable.

Smooth muscle membrane potential, recorded from any site along the length of the small intestine, shows a slow rhythmic oscillation, termed the slow wave potential (Fig. 2A). This slow wave activity is not fully understood; it may result from oscillatory activity of a current-generating sodium pump or from cyclic changes in membrane permeability.[6] It has been widely held that slow wave activity originates in longitudinal muscle and is conducted to the circular layer, but recent data suggest that they might be generated in the interstitial cells of Cajal located between the muscular layers. Whatever the origin, slow wave activity is independent of neural tissue, and some functional or actual electric coupling exists between smooth muscle cells which permits coordinated oscillation of smooth muscle slow wave potential. The electric coupling is such that at any specific location, variation in slow wave potential is circumferentially synchronous or in phase, but slow wave frequency is not identical, nor is the oscillation simultaneous at all points along the bowel. There is an aborally decreasing gradient in small intestinal slow wave frequency. In man, the slow wave frequency is 11 cycles per minute in the duodenum[7] and 8 cycles per minute in the ileum.[8] The intact bowel can be described as an infinite number of overlapping contractile units. If actually transected into multiple segments, each piece of bowel is capable of generating a slow wave potential, and the frequency in each decreases as a function of distance from the pylorus.[9] In continuity the proximal segment of higher intrinsic slow wave frequency acts as a pacemaker and is able to influence adjacent segments with an inherently lower frequency to oscillate at the higher frequency. Eventually electric coupling between cells is insufficient to "drive" more distal segments to oscillate at a frequency greater than they generate intrinsically. As a result, in intact bowel there is a stepwise decrement in slow wave frequency, with successive frequency plateaus being separated by regions of waxing and waning of the slow wave frequency (Fig. 2B). The length of each of the frequency plateaus becomes progressively shorter in more caudal regions of the bowel. Within each plateau region the slow wave frequency is uniform; however, the oscillations do not occur simultaneously throughout the segment. There is a proximal-to-distal phase lag (Fig. 2C). Although the proximal segment of higher intrinsic frequency is able to influence the aboral segments to oscillate at the higher frequency, there

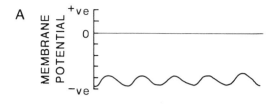

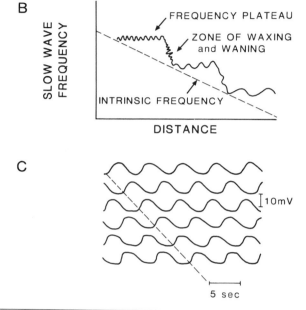

FIGURE 2 *A,* Schematic representation of the slow wave potential recorded with a suction electrode at a single location along the small intestine. *B,* A diagram illustrating the stepwise decrement in slow wave frequency with increasing distance along the intestine. Successive frequency plateaus are separated by regions of waxing and waning of the slow wave. The dashed line represents the intrinsic slow wave frequency that would be manifest at that point if the contractile unit were not being influenced by more proximal segments of high intrinsic frequency. (Adapted from Diamant and Bortoff.[9]) *C,* A diagrammatic representation of slow waves recorded simultaneously from six suction electrodes spaced several centimeters apart within a region of frequency plateau on the small intestine. There is a delay in onset of the slow wave which increases with distance (phase lag), and the slow wave appears to propagate aborally. (Adapted from Diamant and Bortoff.[9])

is a slight delay involved which increases with distance. As a result, if one records from closely spaced sites within a frequency plateau the slow wave appears to propagate aborally, much like the waveform propagated along a rope when the free end is moved up and down.

The third type of variation in smooth muscle membrane potential is the action or spike potential (Fig. 3), a rapid high-amplitude oscillation that has a one-to-one association with contraction.[10] Spike activity in small intestinal smooth muscle occurs only during the depolarized phase of the slow wave. In the presence of excitatory cholinergic activity and/or a low background level of inhibitory influences, there is a partial depolarization of smooth muscle membrane potential such that the additional depolarization during the oscillation of the slow wave potential achieves the level of depolarization necessary to initiate action potentials.[5] At that critical level of depolarization, the threshold potential, voltage-dependent calcium channels in the smooth muscle membrane open to increase membrane calcium permeability. Since the intracellular concentration of calcium is 10^{-7} M and the extracellular concentration is 10^{-3} M, there is an inward flux of calcium. As calcium ions move down their concentration gradient into the cell, there is a rapid depolarization of the membrane potential (the action potential) associated with intracellular accumulation of positively charged calcium ions. The increase in sarcoplasmic calcium concentration associated with the action potential mediates coupling of smooth muscle excitation-contraction. When excitatory cholinergic activity is absent and inhibitory influences predominate, there is hyperpolarization of the membrane, and the depolarization produced by oscillation of the slow wave potential is insufficient to reach threshold and initiate spike activity.

The myogenic basis for segmental or nonpropagating ring contractions and for propagating or peristaltic contractile activity can now be appreciated.[11] Events leading to localized small intestinal excitation (e.g., local distention with stimulation of stretch receptors, activation of myenteric neurons, and release of Ach) result in depolarization of the membrane and an increased level of local excitability. The additional decrease in membrane potential during slow wave depolarization is now sufficient to initiate action potentials. Because intestinal slow wave activity is circumferentially synchronous, spike discharge activity occurs simultaneously in a ring of smooth muscle and a single segmental contraction is observed. If local excitation is persistent, nonpropagated ring contractions occur at a maximum rate equal to the slow wave frequency at that site. When neurohumoral activity leads to an increased level of background excitability in smooth muscle over a longer small intestinal segment, spike potentials are generated over the length of that segment at a maximum frequency equal to the rate of oscillation of the slow wave potential. However, the slow wave potential in the segment exhibits a proximal-to-distal phase lag, and the slow wave, the superimposed spike potentials, and the associated circumferential ring contractions appear to migrate aborally (Fig. 4). In the proximal bowel, where the longest slow wave frequency plateaus occur, contractions migrate over long distances and propulsion of luminal contents is more rapid. In the terminal small intestine, where frequency plateaus are shortest, contractions migrate over markedly reduced distances.

The role of myoelectric activity in the control of colonic motor function is not as well understood as it is in the small intestine, and many concepts remain controversial.[12] Smooth muscle in the human colon does exhibit a slow wave variation in membrane potential and spike potential activity. Just as in the intestine, spikes occur only during the most depolarized phase of the slow wave potential, and for each oscillation with superimposed spikes there is an associated contraction. In human colon the slow wave is at least partly mediated by an inward calcium flux, and high amplitude slow wave activity may contribute to the development of muscle contractions. Myoelectric activity in the human colon is remarkable in other ways. There is no discernable myoelectric activity in colonic muscle in the absence of stretch, neural, or hormonal stimulation. In the colon both the frequency and amplitude of the slow wave are variable with time, and the frequency of the slow wave in circular muscle can be different from that in the longitudinal layer. Although slow wave activity in human colonic muscle can be exceedingly irregular, cholinergic stimulation in vitro changes irregular slow wave–spike complex activity to synchronous slow wave

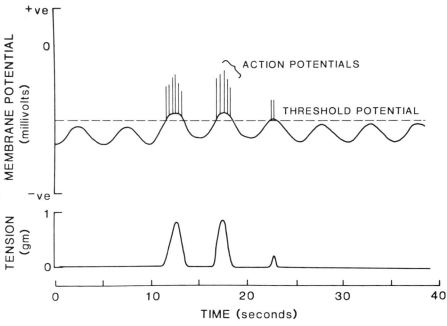

FIGURE 3 Diagrammatic representation of electric and mechanical activity recorded from a segment of intestine with a suction electrode and force transducer. In the presence of excitation and/or a low background level of inhibitory influences, the additional depolarization of the slow wave potential is such that the membrane potential exceeds the threshold and action potentials are generated. Bursts of action potential activity have a one-to-one association with contraction. Because action potentials occur only on the depolarization portion of slow waves, the maximal frequency at which contractions may occur is equal to the slow wave frequency.

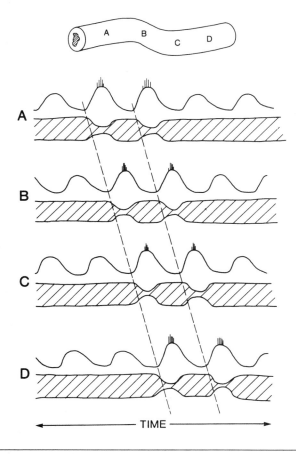

FIGURE 4 A diagrammatic representation of a segment of small intestine from which suction electrodes and intraluminal manometry catheters record myoelectric activity and intraluminal pressures at sites A, B, C, and D. When neurohormonal activity leads to an increased level of background excitability over this segment of intestine, slow wave depolarization is sufficient to generate bursts of spike potential activity. Because the slow wave exhibits a proximal to distal phase lag, the slow wave, the superimposed bursts of spike potentials, and the associated ring contractions propagate aborally.

activity with superimposed spike bursts. A similar stimulus-dependent phenomenon may account for the change from irregular nonpropagating contractions to regular propagating contractile activity in stimulated colon in vivo. Stimulated small intestine exhibits phasic contractile activity at 8 to 11 cycles per minute with full relaxation between slow wave–spike complexes, but stimulated human colonic muscle can develop slow wave–spike complex activity at frequencies above 20 cycles per minute which are associated with prolonged tonic contractions.

Integration of Mechanisms Controlling Intestinal Motility. Myoelectric characteristics intrinsic to intestinal smooth muscle—the slow wave and action potential— determine the temporal and spatial occurrence of contractile activity in a stimulated segment of bowel. However, neural and humoral influences determine whether contractions occur at all, into what patterns they are organized, and over what distances

they are propagated. Neural transmitters released by intrinsic nerves and circulating or locally released chemicals modulate the intrinsic behavior of the smooth muscle membrane potential over the length of the intestine to produce functional, coordinated patterns of contractile activity. Each overlapping contractile unit in the gut is associated with intrinsic or enteric neuronal circuitry capable of independently generating complex patterns of contractile activity. Integrative circuitry ensures that the function of each contractile unit is modified by input from adjacent contractile units, receptors within the intestinal mucosa, extrinsic nerves, and circulating or locally released hormones. The modulatory input from extrinsic nerves and circulating hormones reflects the central nervous and the endocrines systems' integration of an already enormous amount of sensory data from all other areas of the body and the environment.

PATTERNS OF CONTRACTILE ACTIVITY IN HEALTH AND DISEASE

Small Intestine

Intestinal Reflexes. One of the simplest organized patterns of contractions which can be elicited from the intestine is the myenteric or peristaltic reflex first described by Bayliss and Starling in 1899.[13] A distending bolus placed in the bowel initiates contraction above and relaxation below the point of stimulation. Neurons in the myenteric plexus hyperpolarize (inhibit) smooth muscle distal and depolarize (excite) smooth muscle proximal to the stimulus. The intestinal inhibitory reflex is another pattern of intestinal motor activity characterized by inhibition of intestinal contractions at all adjacent loci during marked distention of an area of bowel. This reflex appears to depend upon integrity of communication between extrinsic sympathetic nerves and the enteric nervous system.[14,15]

Migrating Myoelectric Complex. The migrating myoelectric (or motor) complex (MMC) is a recurrent band of excitatory myoelectric and associated contractile activity which propagates distally along the fasted gut from the lower esophageal sphincter to the ileocecal junction[16] (Fig. 5). The MMC, which occurs in most fasted mammals including man, is composed of four phases. Phase I is the period of motor quiescence, in which electric spike activity is absent and only slow waves are recorded. Phase II is an interval during which irregular spiking and associated contractile activity begin and become gradually more intense, with some but not all slow waves being associated with spike burst activity. Phase III is a period during which intense spike burst activity occurs on every slow wave and contractions occur at the intestinal slow wave frequency. Phase IV is a brief interval during which electric spike activity subsides rapidly, the complete cessation of spike and associated contractile activity marking the onset of Phase I of the next cycle of the MMC. The interval between the end of Phase III activity of successive cycles, the cycle period, is quite variable, but it averages roughly 100 minutes in the human.[17] Some complexes are initiated more distally in the jejunum and do not involve stomach or duodenum, and some fade out before traversing the whole length

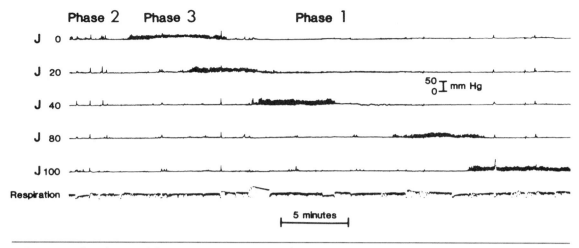

FIGURE 5 The phases of the migrating motor complex as seen in a recording of motility from the human jejunum. Distance of the recording orifice from the ligament of Treitz is shown to the left of each tracing. (From Kerlin and Phillips.[17])

of the intestine. An MMC may be initiated in the proximal gut before the preceding complex has reached the terminal ileum.[18] The MMC is propulsive of intraluminal contents and serves as an interdigestive "intestinal housekeeper,"[19] very efficiently propelling luminal contents ahead of the advancing front of Phase III activity.[20] Cyclic increases in gastric,[21] pancreatic,[21–24] biliary,[24–26] and intestinal[27] secretions are associated with the MMC and coupled with the propulsive motor pattern constitute an important intestinal defense mechanism preventing the intestinal injury and dysfunction associated with bacterial overgrowth.[28]

The mechanisms that regulate the MMC and control its initiation, cycling, aboral propagation, and association with rhythmic secretion remain controversial.[16] Experiments in dogs involving autotransplantation of the small intestine or resection and reanastomosis of segments of small bowel indicate that each area of the intestine can function independently to initiate all phases of the MMC.[29] Propagation of the MMC along a segment requires an intact ENS.[30] However, in the intact individual control of the MMC normally involves co-ordination of enteric neural activity with extrinsic neural (particularly vagal) and humoral (especially motilin) influences.

Fed Pattern. The ingestion of a meal interrupts the MMC and initiates a continuous pattern of irregular myoelectric spike and associated contractile activity.[16] This disruption is proportional to the amount and varies with the physical and chemical composition of the diet ingested. In man, ingestion of a mixed 450-Kcal meal results in disruption of the MMC for 3.5 hours.[28] In dogs, after ingestion of equicaloric amounts of peptides, glucose, or medium-chain triglycerides, the interruption of the MMC was respectively 165, 285, and 450 minutes.[31] After feeding, most contractions are segmental or migrate over short distances.[32] Intraluminal fat is associated with isolated contractile activity, carbohydrate or protein produce more sequential contractions, and a mixed meal is associated with even fewer isolated contractions and more sequential activity.[33] Intestinal flow is greatest distal to segments manifesting short periods of sequential contrac-

tions.[34] Progress is being made in the better identification of specific patterns of propulsive and nonpropulsive activity.[35]

Small intestinal transit time for the advancing front of a mixed 536-Kcal meal is about 4 hours.[36] There is a direct relationship between small bowel transit time and absorption. An increase in the length of time luminal contents are in contact with absorptive epithelium is associated with increased absorption of a meal.[37] Conversely, reduction of transit or contact time by administration of lactulose, metoclopramide, or magnesium sulfate results in a significant increase in ileal fat output.[37] Under normal circumstances, the digestion and absorption of the majority of dietary constituents is complete within the first 100 cm of intestine.[38] Under pathologic conditions the additional distal small bowel constitutes a valuable reserve of absorptive capacity. Two characteristics of ileal motility enhance its adaptive capacity. First, ileal transit time is normally slower than jejunal transit time, and, secondly, the presence of lipid or protein in the ileum enhances absorption by slowing transit through the intestine ("the ileal brake").[39]

Two-thirds of a meal will transit the intestine before return of MMCs, but after the first MMC intestinal clearance is more than 90 percent.[20] The mechanisms responsible for regulation of the fed pattern of intestinal motility is complex. Perfusion of isolated intestinal loops with glucose can induce a local fed pattern without interrupting MMCs,[40] suggesting that the ENS may mediate a local fed pattern without extrinsic neural or systemic hormonal influences. Probably hormones alone cannot initiate a fed pattern[41]; neural pathways are probably involved because in dogs the fed pattern is initiated in the isolated but extrinsically innervated intestinal loop after a meal. Furthermore, when the isolated loop is fed, both the loop and the unfed bowel in continuity show disruption of the fasting pattern.[42] The postprandial pattern depends upon stimulation of the ENS by intraluminal factors, upon intact extrinsic innervation, and probably upon hormonal modulation.[16]

MAPCs, RBAPs, Discrete Clusters of Contractions, Minute Rhythm. The migrating action potential complex

(MAPC) was first described by Mathias[43] as the myoelectric correlate of propulsive, aborally propagating ring contractions. Initially regarded as an abnormal pattern of motility which was induced by exposure of intestinal segments to bacterial pathogens or their toxins, the MAPC was considered a motor defense mechanism clearing unwanted substances from the intestinal lumen.[44] MAPCs have been induced in rabbit ileum by various agents and in the human intestine in response to ricinoleic acid, phenolphthalien, and secretory diarrhea.[45] The MAPC is similar to motor activity that has been termed minute rhythm,[37] laxative-induced pattern, or discrete clusters of aborally propagating contractions.[47,48] These terms describe a motor pattern characterized by a cluster of aborally migrating contractions. The myoelectric correlate of this activity is a discrete cluster of 3 to 15 slow waves with spike bursts superimposed on each depolarization and an aboral propagation velocity of about 60 cm per minute. This MAPC-like activity may be a basic propulsive motor pattern, which, in response to the stimulus of disease or injury, can be recruited to mediate enhanced propulsion. The MAPC occurs in intestinal segments in vitro[49] and appears to be mediated by an intrinsic reflex arc of the ENS.[50] Several pieces of evidence indicate that the MAPC is a primary motor response and not a secondary manifestation of increased intestinal secretion.[51,52]

Mathias described a second type of intestinal motor pattern in rabbit ileum exposed to invasive or toxigenic bacteria—repetitive burst of action potentials (RBAPs).[53-55] Defined as bursts of action potential activity of greater than 1.5 sec duration which might or might not be propagated, RBAPs were not associated with fluid movement. They occurred predominantly in response to invasive bacterial enteritis, and he postulated that the RBAP functioned as a "virulence factor" encouraging stasis and proliferation and facilitating tissue invasion. Motility has long been recognized as a major factor responsible for host defense and maintenance of normal gut microbial flora, and stasis is associated with bacterial overgrowth.[28] Furthermore, antidiarrheal therapy aggravates shigellosis and *C. difficile*, *Salmonella typhimurium*, and *Campylobacter jejuni* enteritis.[56-59] However, RBAP activity is not a specific feature of invasive bacterial enteritis, and in humans nonpropagating clusters of contractions are a feature of normal motility.[47] The functional significance of MAPC and RBAP in normal and disordered human intestinal motility awaits further clarification.

Intestinal Obstruction. Patients with partial mechanical small bowel obstruction have typical MMCs during fasting but when studied after feeding exhibit multiple discrete clusters of contractions separated by long quiescent periods.[47] Many are propagated aborally, and some are associated with crampy abdominal pain. Surgical relief of obstruction results in resolution of the abnormal postprandial contractile activity. Although this motor pattern never occurs in normal patients after a meal, it is a feature of normal fasted motility during Phase II. Thus, while discrete clustered contractions are a characteristic postprandial motor pattern in partial bowel obstruction, they are not unique or specific to obstruction. The mechanism of their regulation has not been studied.

Vomiting. The pattern of intestinal motility preceding emesis has been studied in dogs[60,61] and cats.[62] In dogs, emesis is preceded by disruption of the slow wave frequency, and retrograde propagation of a giant intestinal contraction from mid–small intestine to antrum, followed by a series of phasic contractions at all levels in the gut. In cats, emesis is preceded by a similar phenomenon, an aborally migrating burst of myoelectric spike potential activity. In both species the intestinal motor phase of emesis is abolished by atropine or vagotomy.

Functional Abdominal Pain. Central crampy abdominal pain is a frequent complaint of patients with functional bowel disorders. Clinicians have long hypothesized that this discomfort is due to disordered intestinal motility, but confirmation has been difficult to obtain. Kellow et al[63] recently compared intestinal motility in a group of adults with irritable bowel syndrome (IBS) to controls. All individuals exhibited MMCs when fasted and a fed pattern postprandially. During fasting IBS patients experienced a greater frequency of discrete clustered contractions than did controls; and the IBS patients but not controls experienced abdominal discomfort in association with these episodes. Even more striking was the relationship between pain and prolonged high-pressure contractions. These contractions are a normal feature of interdigestive and postprandial ileal motility in humans[8,64] and propel ileal contents through the high-pressure ileocecal sphincter zone into the cecum. Present in both controls and IBS patients, they were more frequent in the latter, and 61 percent of episodes in IBS patients were directly related to crampy discomfort, compared to 17 percent in controls. IBS patients also experienced discomfort during exaggerated prolonged tonic changes in ileal pressure that occurred postprandially. Thus, there appears to be a relationship between small intestinal motor patterns and crampy abdominal discomfort.

Colon

It is not clear precisely how myoelectric activity in the large bowel is regulated to slow the transit of colonic contents sufficiently to permit reabsorption of salt and water against concentration gradients[12,45,65] and excrete indigestible residue as formed stool. However, the gross patterns of contractions responsible for the flow of contents through the colon have been known for some time.

Segmentation. Transit through the colon is about 10 times slower than through the small bowel,[36] varying between 1 and 3 days. The ascending and sigmoid colon contribute significantly to this delay. Early radiologic studies[65] are consistent with more recent cineradiographic studies in humans[66] suggesting segmental ringlike contractions that may partially occlude the lumen and may be stationary or propagate slowly for short distances in an oral or aboral direction. Contractions propagating in an oral direction are more frequent in the cecum and ascending colon,[65] so transit through the proximal colon is slowed. In fact, food residues do not move through the colon in the order in which they leave the ileum.[67] The sigmoid colon appears to be specialized to obstruct the flow of feces. Generally less distensible and more tonically contracted than other segments of the large bowel,[68] it seems to be a zone of high tonic manometric pressure[69,70] exhibiting a greater frequency of retrograde peristaltic activity.[69]

Colonic Migrating Motor Complexes. In the transverse and descending colon distention appears more likely to stimulate aboral propagation of peristaltic contractions.[65] Sarna et al[71] have shown that in dogs these contractions may be grouped together in clusters termed colonic migrating motor complexes (CMMC) which migrate over short distances, usually in an aboral, but occasionally in an orad direction. The CMMC are thought to mix and transport luminal contents.

Mass Movement. A less frequent but very important pattern of colonic motor activity was first described in 1909 by Holzknecht, a German radiologist.[65,72] He observed a sudden shift of a column of feces over one third the length of the colon to an empty segment of similar length. Segmenting contractile activity disappeared in both the emptying and recipient segments prior to the shift of feces and returned shortly afterwards. Subsequent studies in humans using a variety of markers[73] and cineradiography[74] have all confirmed that colonic contents are transported distally in a series of infrequent massive shifts of colonic content. Mass movements tend to be more common during the waking hours, occurring only once or twice a day, often before defecation.[75] Infrequent large-amplitude caudad-migrating bands of contractions, termed giant migrating contractions,[76] have been associated with this mass movement.

Ingestion of food increases contractile activity in the colon[77,78] and the proportion of contractions which are propulsive.[68] In some people ingestion is associated with induction of mass movements and defecation.[68] This phenomenon has been termed the gastrocolic reflex, but Christensen[65] suggests the term be abandoned because the response may not be neural, the stimulus to its induction is not confined to the stomach, and the motor response to the stimuli is not restricted to the colon. In humans the response has no cephalic phase and it can occur after complete gastrectomy. There is good evidence for an intestinal phase, since the response occurs promptly after food, when amino acids or fatty acids are instilled into the duodenum. Since distal intestinal motility increases after eating, it is also likely that there is delivery of ileal contents into the colon and a colonic phase to the response.

Defecation. Defecation in the infant is a reflex response; in the older child and adult it is a controlled act occurring at a socially convenient time.[79] In many it becomes almost a conditioned response so that a regular bowel pattern is established at a fixed time each day.[80] The rectum can accommodate a gradual increase in volume,[81] but rapid rectal distention elicits a sensation of rectal fullness, contraction of the external anal sphincter and puborectal muscle, and relaxation of the internal anal sphincter. The external anal sphincter response probably is mediated through a spinal reflex, since it is absent in patients with low spinal injury,[82,83] whereas relaxation of the internal anal sphincter is mediated within the enteric neural plexus.[83-86] Reflex contraction of the external anal sphincter and puborectal muscle which occurs after rectal distention may prevent reflex defecation in the face of internal anal sphincter relaxation.[81] These contractions act as a brief "guarding reflex" that allows the sensitive anal mucosa to sample rectal contents so that we can determine whether evacuation of gas, liquid, or solid is occurring. When defecation does occur there is expulsion of feces from the rectum and, in at least some subjects, from part of the descending colon. The defecation response is under cortical control; but the lumbosacral cord can sustain the reflex, since it is re-established in patients who have had spinal cord injury above the lumbosacral level.

Motor Patterns Associated with Disease. It is not necessarily the quantity of contractions (hyper- or hypomotility) but the nature of their organization into patterns which determines colonic transit and clinical symptomatology.[37,45,65] For example, diarrhea can be the result of a decrease in the segmental and retrograde propagating contractile activity that normally slows transit and promotes absorption in the ascending colon, or it can be the result of an increased number of aborally propagating contractions. Clusters of large, aborally propagating contractions have been induced by laxatives, intracolonic infusion of fatty acids or bile acids, and fiber.[65] Similarly, constipation may be the result of hypomotility, as in the case of colonic ileus, or the result of increased segmenting contractile activity that inhibits colonic transit.

Hirschsprung's disease is characterized by a distal colonic segment of variable length in which there is an absence of ganglion cells in the enteric nervous system. The aganglionic segment is chronically contracted and aperistaltic, giving rise to symptoms of obstruction. Although the denervation is nonselective in nature (involves both excitatory and inhibitory neurons), the ultimate basis of the obstructing "spasm" seems to be the absence of enteric neural inhibition of tonic colonic contraction.[121]

Diverticular disease is characterized by herniations of the mucosa through the muscular wall of the colon at the site of penetration of blood vessels. Available data support the hypothesis of a myogenic lesion underlying diverticular disease.[12]

Functional colonic disorders characterized by pain, diarrhea, and constipation have been studied, but convincing evidence for specific motility abnormalities is lacking, partly because of the diversity of the syndromes, our lack of understanding of normal colonic motility, and inability to assess colonic motility in vivo.[65]

INTESTINAL PSEUDO-OBSTRUCTION

Intestinal pseudo-obstruction is a clinical syndrome characterized by GI obstruction in the absence of mechanical blockage of the lumen.[89-93] Pseudo-obstruction may result from any process that interferes with co-ordinated patterns of propulsive motor activity and normal intestinal transit. It may be acute and transient, in which case the term *paralytic ileus* is usually employed (Table 1), or it may be chronic in nature. It is useful to divide the chronic disorders into primary disorders of intestinal smooth muscle or the myenteric plexus and secondary systemic illnesses affecting GI neural and muscular function (Table 2).

Clinical Features

The clinical manifestations of acute intestinal pseudo-obstruction (paralytic ileus) and mechanical bowel obstruction are similar. Patients experience nausea, vomiting that

TABLE 1

Acute or Transient Intestinal
Pseudo-obstruction

---

1. Unrelieved mechanical obstruction
2. Postoperative
3. Drug toxicity
   a. Anticholinergic agents
   b. Phenothiazines
   c. Tricyclic antidepressants
   d. Narcotics
   e. Verapamil
   f. Cyclosporin
   g. Clonidine
   h. Ganglionic blockers
   i. Anti-Parkinsonian medications (benztropine, trihexyphenidyl)
4. Electrolyte imbalance
   a. Hypokalemia
5. Post-traumatic
   a. Shock
   b. Fracture of femur or pelvis
   c. CNS or spinal cord injury
6. Intra-abdominal inflammation (e.g., cholecystitis, pancreatitis, appendicitis, urinary tract infection)
7. Extra-abdominal inflammation (e.g., septicemia, pneumonia, meningitis)
8. Miscellaneous
   a. Irradiation
   b Chemotherapy
   c. Congestive heart failure, myocardial infarction

---

may be bile stained and exacerbated by ingestion of liquid or solids, crampy abdominal pain, and cessation of defecation.

The chronic intestinal pseudo-obstruction disorders may involve any or all segments of the GI tract, and symptoms reflect this heterogeneity.[89-93] Patients present with dysfunction of the esophagus, stomach, small intestine, and/or colon. Symptoms may be present at birth; they may begin during infancy, but in many they do not begin until later in life. Then the history may be one of insidious onset, intermittency, and slow progression to incapacitating illness over many years. Extensive involvement of the small intestine and colon leads to marked abdominal distention from accumulation of fluid and gas in distended bowel. The abdomen is hyper-resonant; loud borborygmi and a succussion splash may be heard. Patients often experience crampy abdominal pain that may be relieved by emesis or defecation and is occasionally so severe that they become dependent on analgesics. This dependence upon narcotics complicates assessment of their pain and may aggravate the problem of constipation. Vomiting may be copious and complicate management of fluid, electrolyte, and acid-base balance. Diarrhea is more common than constipation and can usually be attributed to bacterial overgrowth with steatorrhea and bile acid malabsorption. Reduced food intake and malabsorption result in weight loss, decreased adipose tissue stores, muscle wasting, hypoalbuminemia and edema, and specific nutrient deficiencies. Dysphagia is a relatively common feature when there is esophageal dysfunction; heartburn and esophagitis may develop if the antireflux mechanisms at the gastroesophageal junction are impaired. Symptoms of urinary retention point to a primary generalized visceral myopathy, since urinary tract involvement has

not yet been reported in individuals with visceral neuropathy or those disorders secondarily affecting intestinal smooth muscle. History and physical examination sometimes elicit symptoms and signs that suggest a specific syndrome of intestinal pseudo-obstruction or a systemic illness causing intestinal pseudo-obstruction.

Differential Diagnosis of Acute Paralytic Ileus

Although the symptoms and clinical presentation of mechanical obstruction and intestinal pseudo-obstruction may be similar, treatment is very different.[92] It is important that mechanical obstruction not be overlooked, as these patients may require surgical intervention. In contrast, surgery is to be avoided in intestinal pseudo-obstructive disorders in an effort to prevent future confusion over whether an exacerbation is related to pseudo-obstruction or to the development of adhesions. Since mechanical obstruction may cause proximal intestinal distention, activation of the intestinal inhibitory reflex, and a secondary generalized paralytic ileus, the distinction from pseudo-obstruction can be challenging.

The most common cause of acute intestinal pseudo-obstruction is transient postoperative ileus. Many factors can contribute to its development.[94] Anticholinergic drugs, given as preoperative medications, interfere with the "final common pathway" for stimulation of gut smooth muscle cells. Anesthetic agents themselves contribute little to postoperative ileus, and the duration of exposure and extent of manipulation of bowel during surgery have been shown not to correlate well with the duration of postoperative ileus. Normally contractile activity returns to the stomach in 3 to 4 hours, to the small bowel in 5 to 7 hours, to the proximal colon in 1 to 2 days, and to the distal colon in 2 to 3 days after abdominal surgery. Although the rate of contractile activity returns to normal at this time, effective organized propulsive activity does not return until later. The colon, which is most affected, exhibits delay of transit for up to 6 to 7 days after operation. Furthermore, the use of narcotic postoperative analgesia may contribute to slowed intestinal transit. Although paralytic ileus is presumably the result of unremitting activity of inhibitor neurons within the enteric nervous system, the exact mechanism of their activation remains unclear. Factors other than sympathetic inhibitory stimuli must be involved, since in human studies[95] there was no resolution with the use of alpha- and beta-adrenergic blocking drugs. It is interesting that neither morphine nor naloxone relieves postoperative ileus.

Drug-induced acute intestinal pseudo-obstruction is also relatively common.[89,91,93,96] Anticholinergic preparations prescribed as antispasmodics or as parasympatholytic agents in peptic ulcer therapy or ingested accidentally can block intestinal smooth muscle excitation. In large dosage phenothiazines are anticholinergic and antagonists of calmodulin, the calcium-binding protein involved in the mediation of excitation-contraction coupling. Phenothiazines can cause colonic pseudo-obstruction. High doses of tricyclic antidepressants also exert an anticholinergic effect and can induce a generalized ileus. The narcotics morphine and meperidine have long been recognized as factors contributing to prolonged postoperative ileus and constipation. Constipation has been

TABLE 2
Chronic Intestinal Pseudo-Obstruction*

I. Disorders of the Myenteric Plexus	II. Disorders of Intestinal Smooth Muscle
A. Primary	A. Primary
1. Developmental abnormalities	1. Familial visceral myopathy
a. Neuronal immaturity	a. Autosomal dominant
i. premature and term newborn infant	b. Autosomal recessive with ptosis and external
ii. syndrome of short small bowel, malrotation, and	ophthalmoplegia
pyloric hypertrophy	c. Autosomal recessive with dilatation of the entire GI tract
b. Aganglionosis	2. Sporadic visceral myopathies
i. segmental	a. Megalocystis-microcolon-intestinal hypoperistalsis
ii. Hirschsprung's disease	syndrome
iii. total colon and small bowel	B. Systemic disorders affecting visceral smooth muscle
c. Neuronal intestinal dysplasia	1. Muscular dystrophies
i. without extraintestinal manifestations	a. Myotonic
ii. with neurofibromatosis	b. Oculopharyngeal
iii. with multiple endocrine adenomatosis II	c. Duchenne
2. Familial visceral neuropathies	d. Facioscapulohumeral
a. Recessive with intranuclear inclusions	2. Endocrine
b. Recessive with mental retardation and calcification of	a. Hypothyroidism
the basal ganglia	3. Collagen vascular
c. Recessive with severe peripheral neuropathy, ptosis, and	a. Scleroderma
external ophthalmoplegia	b. Polymyositis
d. Dominant with none of the above	c. Systemic lupus erythematosus
3. Sporadic visceral neuropathies	4. Infiltrative disorders
4. Drug-induced visceral neuropathies	a. Amyloidosis
a. Chemotherapeutic agents	b. Lymphoma
b. Cathartic colon	
5. Severe idiopathic constipation	**III. Small Intestinal Diverticulosis**
B. Systemic disorders affecting the myenteric plexus	
1. Infectious	A. With myophathic changes
a. Chagas' disease (*Trypanosoma cruzi*)	1. Resembling visceral myopathy
b. Cytomegalovirus	2. Resembling scleroderma
2. Neurologic disorders	B. With neuropathic changes
a. Familial dysautonomia	1. Resembling visceral neuropathy with intranuclear inclusions
b. Shy-Drager syndrome	2. Secondary to Fabry's disease
c. Parkinson's disease	
3. Endocrine	
a. Diabetes mellitus	
b. Pheochromocytoma, intestinal ganglioneuromatosis	
4. Gastrointestinal	
a. Malabsorptive disorders	
b. Omphalocele, gastroschisis	
5. Paraneoplastic	
a. Small cell carcinoma of the lung	
b. metastatic carcinoid	

*Modified data from Krishnamurthy and Schuffler.[97]

reported with the use of the calcium channel blocker verapamil and with initiation of treatment with the immunosuppressive agent cyclosporine. The antihypertensive agent clonidine has also been reported to cause intestinal pseudo-obstruction, with symptoms referable primarily to the colon.

One of the common and reversible causes of transient intestinal pseudo-obstruction is severe electrolyte imbalance, particularly hypokalemia.

Ileus is frequently associated with post-traumatic shock, especially fracture of the femur or pelvis, and spinal cord injury. Within the abdomen acute inflammation of the gallbladder, pancreas, appendix, urinary tract, or peritoneum may be associated with a variable degree of ileus. Similarly, extra abdominal inflammation (generalized sepsis, pneumonia,

meningitis) or disorders of other organ systems (cranial injury, congestive heart failure, and myocardial infarction) have been associated with paralytic ileus. The use of abdominal irradiation and chemotherapy to treat neoplastic disease is also recognized to induce a variable degree of intestinal dysfunction, including symptoms of paralytic ileus.

Differential Diagnosis of Chronic Intestinal Pseudo-obstruction

Chronic intestinal pseudo-obstruction may be the result of a primary disorder of either intestinal smooth muscle or the enteric nervous system, or it may be associated with systemic disorders that secondarily affect the muscle or the myenteric plexus of the gut.[97] The classification in Table 2 has been adapted from the recent extensive review of the literature by Krishnamurthy and Schuffler.[97]

Primary Disorders of the Myenteric Plexus

Developmental Abnormalities of the Enteric Nervous System. The enteric ganglia are thought to develop from a craniocaudal migration and differentiation of precursor cells from the neural crest.[98] Differentiation, maturation, and development of neuronal and myoneural interconnections appear to depend upon the microenvironment of the developing gut.[98] The mechanisms responsible for developmental abnormalities of the ENS are not yet clear, but presumably events occur which disrupt the orderly process of fetal development. Short bowel, malrotation, atresia, and pyloric hypertrophy are developmental abnormalities of the GI tract which are frequently associated with enteric neural dysfunction.[97]

Poor feeding, vomiting, distention, and constipation are common in otherwise well premature infants. Manometric studies in these infants show immaturity of the normal fasted and fed motor patterns and progressive improvement with age.[99,99a] Histologic studies suggest immaturity of the population of enteric neurons.[97]

A familial syndrome characterized by short small bowel, malrotation, and pyloric hypertrophy[100,101] also shows the morphologic features of immaturity of the enteric neural plexus.[97]

The most common and most studied of the intestinal pseudo-obstructive disorders, Hirschsprung's disease, is characterized by aganglionosis or absence of the ENS for a variable distance proximal to the anorectal junction and is presumed to occur as a result of a failure of the normal craniocaudal migration of the precursors of the ENS.[97] Segmental aganglionosis has been described, but the mechanism is unclear. Complete aganglionosis of the colon and entire small intestine has also been reported.[102,103] Although there are case reports describing colonic dysfunction attributable to hypoganglionosis, the entity has not been well defined and quantitation of neurons or nerve fibers has not been done.[97]

Neuronal Intestinal Dysplasia. Intestinal neuronal dysplasia is characterized by marked proliferation of enteric neurons and nerve fibers for varying lengths of the colon and small intestine, associated with megacolon or symptoms of pseudo-obstruction.[97] The syndrome may occur in isolation but has been seen in association with neurofibromatosis and multiple endocrine adenomatosis type II.

Familial Visceral Neuropathies. Several familial disorders of the ENS have been described. Schuffler et al[104] were the first to describe a familial pseudo-obstructive disorder with apparent autosomal recessive inheritance and associated neurologic abnormalities: dysarthria, gait ataxia, absent tendon reflexes, impaired vibration and position sensation, and mild autonomic dysfunction.[104–106] The pupils and the esophageal smooth muscle of these patients showed denervation hypersensitivity. A significant reduction in the number of neurons in the myenteric plexus was evident in pathology specimens, and about one-third of the neurons in the enteric, central, peripheral, and autonomic nervous sys-

tems contained round eosinophilic intranuclear inclusions.

A second, probably autosomal recessive familial disorder of pseudo-obstruction, malabsorption, mental retardation, and calcification of the basal ganglia has been described in 4 of 16 siblings.[107]

Faber et al[108] recently reported yet another familial, recessively inherited neuropathic pseudo-obstructive disorder in patients of Jewish-Iranian ethnic background. These patients presented in the first two decades of life with symptoms of intestinal pseudo-obstruction, a severe progressive peripheral neuropathy, ptosis, and external ophthalmoplegia.

Two families have been reported with what appears to be a dominantly inherited intestinal pseudo-obstructive disorder without central autonomic or peripheral nervous system involvement.[109,110] Histologic assessment of tissue from these patients demonstrated degeneration and decreased numbers of neurons within the enteric ganglia.

Sporadic Visceral Neuropathies. Less than two dozen cases of sporadic (apparently nonfamilial) degenerative visceral neuropathy have been reported.[97] Schuffler has identified two distinct forms of the disorder on the basis of pathologic differences.[97]

Drug-Induced Visceral Neuropathies. Myenteric plexus lesions occur in patients and animals treated with the chemotherapeutic agents vincristine and daunorubicin.[111] Chronic ingestion of laxatives, particularly anthraquinone purgatives, can cause melanosis coli, or cathartic colon in humans and in animal studies,[112–114] characterized by a brown-black discoloration of the mucosa, degenerative changes in the neural plexus, and an atonic dilated dysfunctional colon. These lesions could represent a primary disorder that initially leads to constipation and laxative treatment; the visceral neuropathic changes in this disorder do resemble those in some cases of severe idiopathic constipation[115] and in primary colonic pseudo-obstruction[93] without laxative abuse.

Severe Idiopathic Constipation. A few patients with severe constipation have dysfunctional, elongated, and redundant colons.[115] Some of those who require colectomies for relief have a distinctive abnormality of their enteric neurons.

Systemic Disorders Affecting the Myenteric Plexus

Infectious Disorders. The South American parasite *Trypanosoma cruzi* causes Chagas' disease, which is characterized by achalasia-like esophageal dysfunction, intractable constipation and megacolon, or more generalized symptoms of intestinal pseudo-obstruction.[116] The parasite probably initiates an immune response that cross-reacts with neurons in the myenteric plexus. Intestinal pseudo-obstruction can result from cytomegalovirus infections involving the small intestinal myenteric plexus,[117] where viral particles can be seen in the neurons as intranuclear inclusions surrounded by a halo.

Neurologic Disorders. In familial dysautonomia or in primary orthostatic hypotension (Shy-Drager disease), intestinal motor dysfunction may be abnormal.[118] Parkinson's disease or its treatment has been associated with intestinal pseudo-obstruction.[96]

Endocrine Disorders. Intestinal motor dysfunction, primarily gastroparesis, a complication of long-term, poorly controlled insulin-dependent diabetes mellitus, probably results from autonomic neuropathy. Pseudo-obstructive symptoms have been reported also with pheochromocytoma and intestinal ganglioneuromatosis.[89-92]

Gastrointestinal Disorders. The basis for the abdominal distention, vomiting, and/or diarrhea in malabsorptive disorders such as celiac disease remains unclear. Infants with repaired omphalocele or gastroschisis are notoriously at risk for prolonged pseudo-obstructive symptoms. It has been suggested that the amniotic fluid is toxic to myenteric neurons, but this hypothesis has not been substantiated.[119]

Paraneoplastic Intestinal Pseudo-obstruction. Neoplastic disorders associated with pseudo-obstructive symptoms in adults include small cell carcinoma of the lung and metastatic carcinoid syndrome.[97]

Primary Disorders of Intestinal Smooth Muscle

Familial Visceral Myopathies. These rare disorders are characterized by degeneration, thinning, and fibrous replacement of smooth muscle in the GI tract, and in some the urinary tract.[120-131] Three types of familial visceral myopathy are recognized, each with a similar morphologic abnormality but differing genetic transmission and patterns of GI and bladder involvement.[97] Type 1 familial visceral myopathy with an autosomal dominant pattern of transmission is characterized by esophageal dilatation, megaduodenum, redundant colon, and megacystis.[120,121,123,125] Type 2 familial myopathy has an autosomal recessive pattern of transmission. These patients have ptosis, external ophthalmoplegia, and dilatation of the stomach and small intestine associated with numerous small intestinal diverticula but no megalocystis.[124,127-129] A third, and possibly autosomal recessive, type is reported in which there is marked dilatation of the entire GI tract from esophagus to rectum and no extraintestinal manifestations.[130]

Sporadic Visceral Myopathies. Primary visceral myopathy involving the entire GI tract and bladder has been reported sporadically.[97] It is not clear if in these cases the disorder is being transmitted by a recessive gene. Many are diagnosed in adulthood after lengthy progressive pseudo-obstructive symptoms, but Anuras et al[132] recently reported eight cases in children with severe and extensive dysfunction of the entire GI and urinary tracts. The microscopic appearance of the smooth muscle was relatively normal, and the underlying mechanism of smooth muscle dysfunction was not clear. Intestinal pseudo-obstruction has also been reported in infancy as a syndrome of megacystis–microcolon–intestinal hypoperistalsis.[133] The syndrome is similar to that in children reported by Anuras et al[132] in that they have gastric atony, small bowel atony, and megacystis but is different because of a high incidence in females, a small and malrotated colon, and stenotic segments in the distal small intestine, probably resulting from ischemia.

Systemic Disorders Affecting Visceral Smooth Muscle

Muscular Dystrophies. The GI manifestations of the muscular dystrophies have been reviewed recently.[134] Myotonic dystrophy is a dominantly inherited, slowly progressive my-

opathy involving skeletal muscle and smooth muscle. Pseudo-obstructive symptoms may predominate or even precede musculoskeletal features. Involvement of intestinal smooth muscle also occurs in oculopharyngeal muscular dystrophy, facioscapulohumeral muscular dystrophy, and Duchenne muscular dystrophy.

Endocrine Disorders. Patients with hypothyroidism frequently develop prolonged intestinal transit and constipation. The intestinal slow wave frequency is decreased in these patients. Dysfunction arises from myxedematous infiltrate between muscle fibers and the neural plexus, causing altered electric coupling between smooth muscle cells.[89]

Collagen Vascular Disorders. Scleroderma often involves intestinal smooth muscle; it is the most common cause of intestinal pseudo-obstruction in adults.[97] Intestinal involvement is similar but less frequent with polymyositis, and megaduodenum has been reported in systemic lupus erythematosus.

Infiltrative Disorders. Intestinal smooth muscle dysfunction may also result from the deposition and replacement of intestinal smooth muscle with amyloid or the infiltration of intestinal smooth muscle in lymphoma.[97]

Small Intestinal Diverticulosis

Krishnamurthy[135] recently reviewed the small intestinal diverticuloses, a heterogeneous group of disorders characterized by multiple diverticula in the small intestine. These diverticula result from structural abnormalities of either the smooth muscle or the myenteric plexus and are associated with a clinical picture of intestinal pseudo-obstruction. Two forms of myopathic involvement are described, one pathologically resembling primary visceral myopathy and another resembling scleroderma.[97] There are also two forms of neuropathic involvement, one resembling primary visceral myopathy with intranuclear inclusions and the second accumulation of glycolipid within myenteric neurons secondary to Fabry's disease.[97]

Diagnostic Approach and Management of Intestinal Pseudo-obstruction

In patients with symptoms or signs of impaired intestinal propulsion (dysphagia, nausea, vomiting, abdominal distention, or constipation), a primary goal of the history is to identify the cause.[89,93] Evidence of drug usage, urinary tract involvement, a systemic illness, or family history is particularly relevant. The patient with intestinal pseudo-obstruction also should be assessed for treatable secondary complications such as bacterial overgrowth with malabsorption and malnutrition.

There is no laboratory test that will diagnose intestinal pseudo-obstruction. Plain abdominal radiographs can indicate whether there is generalized ileus or the appearance of localized obstruction. Barium enema or an upper GI series and follow-through with water-soluble contrast medium may exclude mechanical obstruction of the colon and small bowel, respectively. Motor function of esophagus and stomach should be assessed. When smooth muscle function is disordered, one observes weakened contractility and increased diameter of the intestinal lumen, whereas damage to the myenteric plexus is characterized by stronger but unco-ordinated contractions and a smaller lumen.[91] Abdominal ultrasonography may be helpful in the assessment of the urinary tract.

Medications that might impair intestinal motility should be discontinued and tests performed to screen for underlying systemic disease. Thyroid function tests and anti-nuclear antibody, serum creatinine phosphokinase, and isoenzyme measurements are appropriate. When muscular dystrophy is suspected, a striated muscle biopsy may be necessary.

Manometric studies are much more sensitive than radiographic studies to evaluate motor disorders of the esophagus, small intestine, and rectum. Esophageal motility studies are particularly useful.[91] Patients with visceral myopathy have low-amplitude simultaneous or nonperistaltic swallow waves. In familial visceral neuropathy the esophagus exhibits marked spontaneous activity, supersensitivity to methacholine, and a failure of lower esophageal sphincter relaxation—features that resemble those seen in achalasia. Patients with esophageal involvement from scleroderma develop low-amplitude peristaltic swallow waves and decreased or absent lower esophageal sphincter pressure, all of which predispose to reflux esophagitis.[91] In small intestinal manometric studies performed in patients with intestinal pseudo-obstruction, the migrating myoelectric complex is sometimes absent during fasting.[28,91] The absence of normal intestinal motor function, and of the interdigestive housekeeper or MMC in particular, may predispose to bacterial overgrowth.[28] Rectal manometry to identify absence of the rectoanal inhibitory reflex is an important adjunctive test to the rectal mucosal biopsy in the diagnosis of Hirschsprung's disease.

Confirmation of a specific pathologic form of intestinal pseudo-obstruction during life requires surgical laparotomy and full-thickness biopsies of normal and abnormal areas of the gut,[97] except in Hirschsprung's disease, in which the absence of myenteric neurons can be inferred from the absence of submucosal neurons and hypertrophy of submucosal nerve trunks. Assessment of the myenteric plexus by conventional light microscopy requires thick (50 μm) sections, cut in the plane of the plexus and stained with silver,[111,136] to highlight the meshlike array of the ganglia and interconnecting nerve tracts.

It is generally recommended that laparotomy be avoided unless a definite therapeutic goal is entertained. Few pseudo-obstructive disorders are cured by surgical intervention; palliation may be achieved sometimes, but the outcome may be made worse by an operation. Ileostomy and colectomy in patients with severe obstructive colonic symptoms can result in massive ileal output with life-threatening fluid and electrolyte disorders.[93] Furthermore, postoperative adhesions can make the future evaluation of obstructive symptoms difficult in patients with underlying pseudo-obstruction.

There is no effective medical treatment for primary intestinal pseudo-obstruction. Cholinergic drugs such as bethanechol and neostigmine and prokinetic agents such as metoclopramide do not restore normal propulsive function.[91] It is not yet clear whether newer agents such as cisapride[137] are more efficacious. In a few systemic disorders of visceral smooth muscle or the myenteric plexus, treatment can lead to resolution of motor dysfunction—hypothyroidism and Chagas' disease. In most cases treatment is directed toward

managing abdominal pain, vomiting, and malnutrition.[91] Nutrient intake has been curtailed for a variety of reasons in these patients, and adequate intake is difficult to achieve, particularly since symptoms are often aggravated by food, and anorexia results. Bacterial overgrowth is associated with steatorrhea, fat-soluble vitamin malabsorption, and decreased absorption of the vitamin B_{12}–intrinsic factor complex. Mucosal damage may develop in association with stasis and contribute further to malabsorption. Achieving adequate caloric intake in such a clinical setting is made even more difficult by the fact that while lipid is the most calorically dense nutrient, it tends to cause slower gastric emptying and an aggravation of symptoms of early satiety, distention, and emesis. Excessive food fiber can be associated with the development of bezoars in the stomach or stagnant loops of intestine. Even without bezoar formation, symptoms of partial obstruction can sometimes be improved by a decrease in dietary fiber intake. In some patients liquid enteral feeds are useful as adjunctive therapy, but in patients with intractable symptoms total parenteral nutrition is often a requisite for repletion and maintenance of a satisfactory nutritional status. Antibiotics are used to treat bacterial overgrowth; however, they do not alter the natural course of the underlying illness and the persistence of pseudo-obstructive symptoms.

REFERENCES

1. Gabella G. Structure of muscles and nerves in the gastrointestinal tract. In: Johnson LR, ed. Physiology of the gastrointestinal tract. 2nd ed. New York: Raven Press, 1987: 335.
2. Hartshorne DJ. Biochemistry of the contractile process in smooth muscle. In: Johnson LR, ed. Physiology of the gastrointestinal tract. 2nd ed. New York: Raven Press, 1987: 423.
3. Wood JD. Physiology of the enteric nervous system. In: Johnson LR, ed. Physiology of the gastrointestinal tract. 2nd ed. New York: Raven Press, 1987: 67.
4. Solcia E, Capella C, Buffa R, et al. Endocrine cells of the digestive system. In: Johnson LR, ed. Physiology of the gastrointestinal tract. 2nd ed. New York: Raven Press, 1987: 111.
5. Bortoff A. Smooth muscle of the gastrointestinal tract. In: Christensen J, Wingate DL, eds. A guide to gastrointestinal motility. Bristol: John Wright and Son Ltd, 1983: 48.
6. Szurzewski JH. Electrical basis of gastrointestinal motility. In: Johnson LR, ed. Physiology of the gastrointestinal tract. 2nd ed. New York: Raven Press, 1987: 383.
7. Foulk WT. Code CF, Morlock CG, Bargen JA. A study of the motility patterns and the basic rhythm in the duodenum and upper part of the jejunum of human beings. Gastroenterology 1954; 26:601–611.
8. Code CF, Rogers AG, Schlegal J, Hightower NC, Bargen JA. Motility patterns in the termimal ileum: studies on 2 patients with ulcerative colitis and ileac stomas. Gastrenterology 1957; 32:651–665.
9. Diamant NE, Bortoff A. Nature of the intestinal slow-wave frequency gradient. Am J Physiol 1969; 216:301–307.
10. Daniel EE, Chapman KM. Electrical activity of the gastrointestinal tract as an indication of mechanical activity. Am J Dig Dis 1963; 8:54–102.
11. Bortoff A. Intestinal motility. N Engl J Med 1969; 280:1335–1337.
12. Huizinga JD. Electrophysiology of human colon motility in health and disease. Clin Gastroenterol 1986; 15:879–901.
13. Bayliss WM, Starling EH. The movements and innervation of the small intestine. J Physiol (Lond) 1899; 24:99–143.
14. Johansson B, Jonsson D, Ljung B. Tonic supraspinal mechanisms influencing the intestino-intestinal inhibitory reflex. Acta Physiol Scand 1967; 72:200–204.

15. Kreulen DL, Szurszewski JH. Reflex pathways in the abdominal prevertebral ganglia: evidence for a colo-colonic inhibitory reflex. J Physiol (Lond) 1979; 295:21–32.

16. Weisbrodt NW. Motility of the small intestine. In: Johnson LR, ed. Physiology of the gastrointestinal tract. 2nd ed. New York: Raven Press, 1987: 335.

17. Kerlin P, Philips S. Variability of motility of the ileum and jejunum in healthy humans. Gastroenterology 1982; 82:694–700.

18. Kellow JE, Borody TJ., Phillips SF, et al. Human interdigestive motility: variations in patterns from esophagus to colon. Gastroenterology 1986; 91:386–395.

19. Szurszewski JH. A migrating electrical complex of the canine small intestine. Am J Physiol 1969; 217:1757–1763.

20. Kerlin P. Zinsmeister A, Phillips S. Relationship to motility to flow of contents in the human small intestine. Gastroenterology 1982; 82:701–706.

21. Vantrappen GR. Peeters TL. Janssens J. The secretory component of the interdigestive motor complex in man. Scand J Gastroenterol 1979; 14:663–667.

22. Itoh A, Takahashi I, Nakaya M, Sukuzi T. Variation in canine exocrine pancreatic secretory activity during the interdigestive state. Am J Physiol 1986;241:G98–G103.

23. Konturek S, Thor PJ, Bilski J et al. Relationships between duodenal motility and pancreatic secretion in fasted and fed dogs. Am J Physiol 1986; 250:G570–G574.

24. Keane FB, DiMagno EP, Dozois RR, Go VLM. Relationships among canine interdigestive exocrine pancreatic and biliary flow, duodenal motor activity, plasma pancreatic polypeptide, and motilin. Gastroenterology 1980;78:310–316.

25. Peeters TL, Vantrappen G, Janssens J. Bile acid output and the interdigestive migrating motor complex in normals and in cholecystectomy patients. Gastroenterology 1980; 79:678–681.

26. Scott RB, Strasberg SM, El-Sharkawy T, Diamant NE. Regulation of the fasting entero-hepatic circulation of bile acids by the migrating myoelectric complex in dogs. J Clin Invest 1982; 71:644–654.

27. Greenwood B, Davison JS. The relationship between gastrointestinal motility and secretion. Am J Physiol 1987; 252:G1–G7.

28. Vantrappen G. Janssens J, Ghoos Y. The interdigestive motor complex of normal subjects and patients with bacterial overgrowth of the small intestine. J Clin Invest 1977; 59:1158–1166.

29. Sarna S, Condon RE, Cowles V. Enteric mechanisms of initiation of migrating myoelectric complexes. Gastroenterology 1983; 84:814–822.

30. Sarna S, Stoddard C, Belbeck L, McWade D. Intrinsic nervous control of migrating myoelectric complexes. Am J Physiol 1981; 241:G16–G22.

31. Schang JC, Danchel J, Sara P, et al. Specific effects of different food components on intestinal motility. Eur Surg Res 1978; 10:425–432.

32. Dusdieker NS, Summers RW. Longitudinal and circumferential spread of spike bursts in canine jejunum in vivo. Am J Physiol 1980; 239:G311–G318.

33. Eeckhout C, Vantrappen G, Peeters TL, Janssens J, DeWever I. Different meals produce different digestive motility patterns. Dig Dis Sci 1984; 29:219–224.

34. Summers RW, Dusdieker NS. Patterns of spike burst spread and flow in the canine small intestine. Gastroenterology 1981; 81:742–750.

35. Enrlein HJ, Schemann M, Siegle JL. Motor patterns of small intestine determined by closely spread extraluminal transducers and video fluoroscopy. Am J Physiol 1987; 253:G259–G267.

36. Read NW, Miles CA, Fisher D, et at. Transit of a meal through the stomach, small intestine, and colon in normal subjects and its role in the pathogenesis of diarrhea. Gastroenterology 1980; 79:1276–1282.

37. Read NW. Speculations on the role of motility in the pathogenesis and treatment of diarrhea. Scand J Gastroenterol 1983; 18(Suppl 84):45–63.

38. Borgstrom B, Dahlquist A, Lundh G, Sjovall S. Studies of intestinal digestion and absorption in the human. J Clin Invest 1957; 36:1521–1536.

39. Read NW, McFarlane A, Kinsman RI, et al. Effect of infusion of nutrient solutions into the ileum on gastrointestinal transit and plasma levels of neurotensin and enteroglucagon. Gastroenterology 1984; 86:274–280.

40. Eeckhout C, DeWever I, Vantrappen G, Hellemans J. Local disorganization of the interdigestive migrating motor complex (MMC) by perfusion of the thiry—Vella loop. Gastroenterology 1979; 76:1127.

41. Sarr MG, Kelly KA. Myoelectric activity of the autotransplanted canine jejunoileum. Gastroenterology 1981; 81:303–310.

42. Weisbrodt NW, Copeland EM, Thor PJ, Mukhopadhyay AK, Johnson LR, Nervous and humoral factors which influence the fasted and fed patterns of intestinal myoelectric activity. In: Vantrappen G, ed. Proceedings of the 5th International Symposium on Gastrointestinal Motility. Herentals, Belgium: Typoff Press, 1976:82.

43. Mathias JR, Carlson GM, DiMarino G, et al. Intestinal myoelectric activity in response to live Vibrio Cholerae and cholera toxin. J Clin Invest 1976; 58:91–96.

44. Mathias JR, Carlson GM, Martin JL, et al. Shigella dysenteriae I. Enterotoxin: proposed role in pathogenesis of shigellosis. Am J Physiol 1980; 239:G382–G386.

45. Read NW. Diarrhea motrice. Clin Gastroenterol 1986; 15:657–686.

46. Atchison WD, Stewart JJ, Bass P. A unique distribution of laxative-induced spike potentials from the small intestine of the dog. Dig Dis Sci 1978; 23:513–520.

47. Summers RW, Anuras S, Green J. Jejunal manometry in health partial intestinal obstruction and pseudo-obstruction. Gastroenterology 1983; 85:1290–1300.

48. Diamant SC, Scott RB, MAPCs—a feature of normal jejunal myoelectric activity in the rat. Can J Physiol Pharmacol 1987; 65:2269–2273.

49. Koch KL, Martin JL, Mathias JR. Mirgrating action—potential complexes in vitro in cholera-exposed rabbit ileum. Am J Physiol 1983; 244:G291–G294.

50. Mathias JR, Carlson GM, Dimarino AJ, et al. The effect of cholera toxin ileal myoelectric-activity: a neural-hormonal mechanism. In: Vantrappan G, ed. Proceedings of the 5th International Symposium on Gastrointestinal Motility. Herentals, Belgium, Typoff Press 1976: 219.

51. Mathias JR, Martin JL, Burns TW, Carlson GM, Shields RP. Ricinoleic acid effect on the electrical activity of the small intestine in rabbits. J Clin Invest 1978; 61:640–644.

52. Sinar DR, Burns TW. Migrating action potential complexes occur independent of fluid secretion from cholera toxin. Gastroenterology 1979; 76:1249.

53. Justus PG, Martin JL, Golberg DA, et al. Myoelectric effects of Clostridium difficile: motility—altering factors distinct from its cytotoxin and enterotoxin in rabbits. Gastroenterology 1985; 82:836–843.

54. Sninsky CA, Ramphal R, Gaskins DJ, et al. Alterations of myoelectric activity associated with Campylobacter jejuni and its cell-free filtrate in the small intestine of rabbits. Gastroenterology 1985; 89:337–344.

55. Burns TW, Mathias JR, Martin JL, et al. Alterations of myoelectric activity of small intestine by invasive Escherichia coli. Am J Physiol 1980; 238:G57–G62.

56. Kent Th, Formal SB, LaBrec EH. Acute enteritis due to Salmonella typhimurium in opium treated guinea pigs. Arch Pathol 1966; 81:501–508.

57. Dupont HL, Hornick MD. Adverse effects of Lomotil therapy in shigellosis. JAMA 1973; 226:1525–1528.

58. Novak E, Lee JG, Seckman CE, et al. Unfavorable effect of atropine-diphenoxylate (Lomotil) therapy in lincomycin-caused diarrhea. JAMA 1976; 235:1451–1454.

59. Nolan CM, Johnson KE, Coyle MB, Faler K. Campylobacter jejuni enteritis: efficacy of antimicrobial and antimotility drugs. Am J Gastroenterol 1983; 78:621–626.

60. Gregory RA. The nervous pathways of intestinal reflexes associated with nausea and vomiting. J Physiol (Lond) 1947; 106:95–103.

61. Lang IM, Marvig J, Sana SK, Condon RE. Gastrointestinal myoelectric correlates of vomiting in the dog. Am J Physiol 1986; 251:G830–G838.

62. Stewart JJ, Burks TF, Weisbrodt NW. Intestinal myoelectric activity after activation of central emetic mechanism. Am J Physiol 1977; 233:E131–E137.

63. Kellow JE, Phillips SF. Altered small bowel motility in irritable bowel syndrome is correlated with symptoms. Gastroenterology 1987; 92:1885–1893.

64. Quigley EMM, Borody TJ, Phillips SF, et al. Motility of the terminal ileum and ileocecal sphincter in healthy humans. Gastroenterology 1984; 87:857–866.

65. Christenson J. Motility of the colon. In: Johnson LR, ed. Physiology of the gastrointestinal tract. 2nd ed. New York: Raven Press, 1987; 665.

66. Ritchie JA. Movement of segmental constrictions in the human colon. Gut 1971; 12:350–355.

67. Wiggins HS, Cummings JH. Evidence for the mixing of residue in the human gut. Gut 1976; 17:1007–1011.

68. Ritchie JA. Colonic motor activity and bowel function. Part II: Dis-

tribution and incidence of motor activity at rest and after food and carbachol. Gut 1968; 9:502–511.

69. Baker WNW, Mann CV. The rectosigmoid junction zone: another sphincter? In: Thomas PA, Mann CV, eds. Alimentary sphincters and their disorders. London: MacMillan, 1981: 201.

70. Chowdhury AR, Dinoso VP, Lorber SH. Characterization of a hyperactive segment of the rectosigmoid junction. Gastroenterology 1976; 71:584–588.

71. Sarna SK, Condon RE, Cowles V. Colonic migrating and non-migrating motor complexes in dogs. Am J Physiol 1984; 246:G355–G360.

72. Holzknecht G. Die normale Peristaltik des Colon. Munch Med Wochenschr 1909; 56:2401–2403.

73. Holdstock DJ, Misiewicz JJ, Smith T, Rowlands EN. Populsion (mass movement) in the human colon and its relationship to meals and somatic activity. Gut 1970; 11:100–110.

74. Ritchie JA. Mass peristalsis in the human colon after contact with oxyphenisatin. Gut 1972; 13:211–219.

75. Horducci F, Bassotti G, Gaburri M, Morelli A. Circadian rhythms of human colonic motility. Dig Dis Sci 1985; 30:784.

76. Karaus M, Sarna SK. Giant migrating contractile during defecation in the dog colon. Gastroenterology 1987; 92:925–933.

77. Schang J-C, Devroede G. Fasting and postprandial myoelectrical spiking activity in the human sigmoid colon. Gastroenterology 1983; 85:1048–1053.

78. Sullivan MA, Cohen S, Snape WJ. Colonic myelectrical activity in irritable bowel syndrome: effect of eating and anticholine. N Engl J Med 1978; 298:878–883.

79. Read NW, Timms JM. Defecation and the pathophysiology of constipation. Clin Gastroenterol 1986; 15:937–965.

80. Preston DM. Normal bowel function and the pathophysiology of constipation. J Drug Res 1983; 8:1814–1821.

81. Ihre T. Studies on anal function in continent and incontinent patients. Scand J Gastroenterol 1974; 9 (Suppl):7–59.

82. Goligher JC, Hughes ESR. Sensibility of the rectum and colon: its role in the mechanism of anal continence. Lancet 1951; i:543–548.

83. Denny-Brown D, Robertson EG. An investigation of the nervous control of defecation. Brain 1935; 58:256–309.

84. Schuster MM, Hendrix TR, Mendeloff AI. The internal anal sphincter response: manometric studies on its normal physiology, neural pathways, and alteration in bowel disorders. J Clin Invest 1963; 42:196–207.

85. Meunier P, Mollard P. Control of the internal anal sphincter (manometric study with human subjects). Pflugers Arch 1977; 370:233–239.

86. Aaronson MJ, Freed MM, Burakoff R. Colonic myoelectric activity in persons with spinal cord injury. Dig Dis Sci 1985; 30:233–300.

87. Connell AM. The motility of the pelvic colon. I. Motilin in normals and in patients with asymptomatic duodenal ulcer. Gut 1961; 2:175–186.

88. Kubota M, Ito Y, Ikeda K. Membrane properties and innervation of smooth muscle cells in Hirschsprung's disease. Am J Phyiol 1983; 244:G406–G415.

89. Faulk DL, Anuras S, Christensen J. Chronic intestinal pseudo-obstruction. Gastroenterology 1978; 74:922–931.

90. Schuffler MD, Rohrmann CA, Chaffee RG, et al. Chronic intestinal pseudo-obstruction: a report of 27 cases and review of the literature. Medicine 1981; 60:173–196.

91. Schuffler MD. Chronic intestinal pseudo-obstruction syndromes. Med Clin North Am 1981; 65:1331–1358.

91a. Hyman PE, McDiarmid SV, Napolitano J, et al. Antroduodenal motility in children with chronic intestinal pseudo-obstruction. J Pediatr 1988; 112:899–905.

92. Snape WJ. Pseudo-obstruction and other obstructive disorders. Clin Gastroenterol 1982; 11:593–608.

93. Anuras S, Baker CRF. The colon in the pseudo-obstructive syndrome. Clin Gastroenterol 1986; 15:745–762.

94. Condon RE, Sarna SK. Motility after abdominal surgery. Clin Gastroenterol 1982; 11:609–620.

95. Heimbach DM, Crout JR. Treatment of paralytic ileus with adrenergic neural blocking drugs. Surgery 1971; 69:582–587.

96. Lewis JH. Gastrointestinal injury due to medicinal agents. Am J Gastroenterol 1986; 81:819–834.

97. Krishnamurthy S, Schuffler MD. Pathology of neuromuscular disorders of the small intestine and colon. Gastroenterology 1987; 93:610–639.

98. Gershon MF, Payette RF, Rothman TP. Development of the enteric nervous system. Fed Proc 1983; 42:1620–1625.

99. Bisset WM, Watt JB, Rivers RPA, Milla PJ. The motor response of the small intestine to milk feeds in preterm infants. Dig Dis Sci 1987; 32:903.

99a. Bisset WM, Watt JB, Rivers RPA, Milla PJ. Ontogeny of fasting small intestinal motor activity in the human infant. Gut 1988; 29:483–488.

100. Royer P, Ricour C, Nihoul-Fekete C, Pellerin D. Le syndrome familial de grele court avec malrotation intestinale et stenose hypertrophique du pylore chez le nourrisson. Arch Fr Pediatr 1974; 31:223–229.

101. Tanner MS, Smith B, Lloyd JK. Functional intestinal obstruction due to deficiency of argyrophilic neurones in the myenteric plexus. Familial syndrome presenting with short small bowel, malrotation, and pyloric hypertrophy. Arch Dis Child 1976; 51:837–841.

102. Hermann MM, Izant RJ, Bolande RP. Aganglionosis of the intestine in siblings. Surgery 1963; 53:664–669.

103. Boggs JD, Kidd JM. Congenital abnormalities of intestinal innervation. Absence of innervation of jejunum, ileum and colon in siblings. Pediatrics 1958; 21:261–265.

104. Schuffler MD, Bird TD, Sumi SM, et al. A familial neuronal disease presenting as intestinal pseudo-obstruction. Gastroenterology 1978; 75:889–898.

105. Patel H, Morman MG, Perry TL, Berry KE. Multiple system atrophy with neuronal intranuclear hyaline inclusions. Report of a case and review of the literature. J Neurol Sci 1985; 67:57–65.

106. Monoz-Garcia D, Ludwin SK. Adult-onset neuronal intranuclear hyaline inclusion disease. Neurology 1986; 36:785–790.

107. Cockel R, Hill EE, Rushton DI, et al. Familial steatorrhea with calcification of the basal ganglia and mental retardation. QJ Med 1973; 168:771–783.

108. Faber J, Fich A, Steinberg A, et al. Familial intestinal pseudo-obstruction dominated by a progressive neurologic disease at a young age. Gastroenterology 1987; 92:786–790.

109. Roy AD, Bharucha H, Nevin NC, et al. Idiopathic intestinal pseudo-obstruction: a familial visceral neuropathy. Clin Genet 1980; 18:290–297.

110. Mayer EA, Schuffler MD, Rotter JI, Hanna P, Mogard M. A familial visceral neuropathy with autosomal dominant transmission. Gastroenterology, in press.

111. Smith B. The neuropathology of the alimentary tract. London: Edward Arnold, 1972.

112. Wittoesch JH, Jackman RJ, McDonald JR. Melanosis: general review and a study of 887 cases. Dis Colon Rectum 1958; 1:172–180.

113. Smith B. Pathologic changes in the colon produced by anthraquinone purgatives. Dis Colon Rectum 1973; 16:455–458.

114. Riemann JF, Schmidt H, Zimmerman W. The fine structure of colonic submucosal nerves in patients with chronic laxative abuse. Scand J Gastroenterol 1980; 15:761–768.

115. Krishnamurthy S, Schuffler MD, Rohrmann CA, Pope CE II. Severe idiopathic constipation is associated with a distinctive abnormality of the myenteric plexus. Gastroenterology 1985; 88:26–34.

116. Earlam RJ. Gastrointestinal aspects of Chagas' disease. Dig Dis Sci 1972; 17:559–571.

117. Sonsino E, Mouy R, Foucaud P, et al. Intestinal pseudo-obstruction related to cytomegalovirus infection of myenteric plexus. N Engl J Med 1984; 311:196–197.

118. Shy GM, Drager GA. A neurological syndrome associated with orthostatic hypotension. Arch Neurol 1960; 15:761–768.

119. O'Neill JA, Grosfeld JL. Intestinal malfunction after antenatal exposure of viscera. Am J Surg 1974; 127:129–132.

120. Faulk DL, Anuras S, Gardner GD, et al. A familial visceral myopathy. Ann Intern Med 1978; 89:600–606.

121. Shaw A, Shaffer H, Teja K, et al. A perspective for pediatric surgeons: chronic idiopathic intestinal pseudo-obstruction. J Pediatr Surg 1979; 14:719–727.

122. Jacobs E, Ardichvili D, Perissino A, Gotignies P, Hanssens JF. A case of familial visceral myopathy with atrophy and fibrosis of the longitudinal muscle layer of the entire small bowel. Gastroenterology 1979; 77:745–750.

123. Schuffler MD, Pope CE. Studies of idiopathic intestinal pseudo-obstruction. II. Hereditary hollow visceral myopathy: family studies. Gastroenterology 1977; 73:339–344.

124. Anuras S, Mitros FA, Nowak TV, et al. A familial visceral myopathy with external ophthalmoplegia and autosomal recessive transmission. Gastroenterology 1983; 84:346–353.

125. Schuffler MD, Lowe MC, Bill AH. Studies of idiopathic intestinal pseudo-obstruction. I. Hereditary hollow visceral myopathy: clinical and pathological studies. Gastroenterology 1977; 73:327–338.

126. Mitros FA, Schuffler MD, Teja K, Auras S. Pathology of familial visceral myopathy. Hum Pathol 1982; 13:825–833.

127. Ionasescu V. Oculogastrointestinal muscular dystrophy. Am J Med Genet 1983; 15:103–112.

128. Ionasescu V, Thompson SH, Ionasescu R, et al. Inherited ophthalmoplegia with intestinal pseudo-obstruction. J Neurol Sci 1983; 59:215–228.

129. Ionasescu V, Thompson SH, Aschenbrener C, Anuras S, Risk WS. Late-onset oculogastrointestinal muscular dystrophy. Am J Med Genet 1984; 18:781–788.

130. Anuras S, Mitros, FA, Milano A, et al. A familial visceral myopathy with dilatation of the entire gastrointestinal tract. Gastroenterology 1986; 90:385–390.

131. Foucar E, Lindholm J, Anras S, et al. A kindred with dysplastic nevus syndrome associated with visceral myopathy and multiple basal cell carcinomas. Lab Invest 1985; 52:23A.

132. Anuras S, Mitros A, Soper RT, et al. Chronic intestinal pseudo-obstruction in young children. Gastroenterology 1986; 91:62–70.

133. Puri P, Lake BD, Gorman F, O'Donnell B, Nixon HH. Megacystis microcolon intestinal hypoperistalsis syndrome: a visceral myopathy. J Pediatr Surg 1983; 18:64–68.

134. Nowak RV, Ionesescu V, Anuras S. Gastrointestinal manifestations of the muscular dystrophies. Gastroenterology 1982; 82:800–810.

135. Krishnamurthy S, Kelly MM, Rohrmann CA, Schuffler MD. Jejunal diverticulosis: heterogeneous disorder caused by a variety of abnormalities of smooth muscle or myenteric plexus. Gastroenterology 1983; 85:538–547.

136. Schuffler MD, Jonak Z. Chronic idiopathic intestinal pseudo-obstruction caused by a degenerative disorder of the myenteric plexus. The use of Smith's method to define the neuropathology. Gastroenterology 1982; 82:476–486.

137. Camilleri M, Brown ML, Malagelada JR. Impaired transit of chyme in chronic intestinal pseudo-obstruction. Correction by Cisapride. Gastroenterology 1986; 91:619–626.

PART 34

The Gut in Systemic Endocrinopathies

Ross W. Shepherd, M.D., M.R.C.P., F.R.A.C.P.

The endocrine and nervous systems regulate homeostatic and metabolic activities of the human body, including those occurring in the gastrointestinal (GI) tract. These systems determine the pace of growth and development in the intestinal tract; they are essential for control of GI function, particularly in terms of motility, secretion, and to a lesser extent, absorption. Thus, it is not surprising that manifestations of disordered GI function are features of various endocrine disorders. Unfortunately, the pathophysiologic bases for these GI features of endocrinologic diseases are poorly understood.

DIABETES MELLITUS

The diabetic is susceptible to the same spectrum of GI disease as the general population. However, there are certain features of diabetes that are associated with specific disturbances of gut function, whereas other associations of diabetes with GI disease are related to genetic predisposition. The suggested mechanisms leading to GI disturbances in insulin-dependent diabetes include autonomic neuropathy, microangiopathy, hyperglycemia, electrolyte disturbances, and abnormalities in blood levels or release of insulin, glucagon, and other hormones such as GIP or motilin.[1] In young patients, the frequency of GI disturbances related to degenerative complications such as autonomic neuropathy and microangiopathy are less common than those associated with metabolic changes, gut hormone release, or genetic association.

Infant of Diabetic Mother

Perinatal mortality and morbidity increased in this group of infants related to the metabolic effects of hyperglycemia and hyperinsulinemia and an increased incidence of congenital anomalies from possible teratogenic effects.[2] The more closely controlled the metabolism of the diabetic pregnant patient, the greater is the potential for a normal infant.[1] A list of abnormalities, including GI defects, associated with increased morbidity and mortality in infants of diabetic mothers is given in Table 1. Congenital anomalies are the most frequent contributor to perinatal mortality of these patients. Perinatal mortality in the offspring of insulin dependent diabetics may be no different from that of nondiabetics after correction for deaths due to congenital anomalies,[3] but

TABLE 1 Abnormalities Causing Increased Morbidity in Infants of Diabetic Mothers

Macrosomia (birth injury, asphyxia)
Respiratory distress syndrome
Hypoglycemia, hypocalcemia, and hypomagnesemia
Hyperbilirubinemia and polycythemia
Cardiomyopathy
Congenital anomalies
CNS malformations
Congenital heart disease
Small left colon syndrome

recent tight control of the pregnant diabetic may diminish the frequency of these congenital malformations.[4] One such rare congenital defect of the GI tract is the neonatal small left colon syndrome.[5] The etiology of this deformity is obscure. Diagnosis can be difficult because of increased vomiting and abdominal distention in infants of diabetic mothers, but the lesion should be considered and excluded by radiologic studies if symptoms occur. With conservative management, the condition usually resolves during the neonatal period, but occasionally surgery is necessary.

Nonspecific Abdominal Pain

Children with diabetes in ketoacidosis often complain of abdominal pain, raising the possibility of co-existent appendicitis, pancreatitis, or an acute abdomen. Anorexia, nausea and vomiting can occur in up to 75 percent of patients in ketoacidosis.[6] Pancreatitis is particularly likely to be suspected because serum amylase concentrations may be elevated to very high levels,[7] but analysis of isoenzymes has shown that salivary and not pancreatic amylase is responsible for this rise in most cases. However, pancreatitis is rare in diabetic children,[8] and in most cases, the abdominal pain accompanying diabetic ketoacidosis in children resolves within 6 to 12 hours after the institution of fluid, electrolyte, and insulin therapy. A diabetic with ketoacidosis and abdominal pain should have the metabolic disorder treated and abdominal signs closely observed before any surgical intervention is contemplated. In some cases, nasogastric aspiration may be necessary for gastric stasis and/or gastritis.

Esophagogastric Disorders

Diabetes may cause motor disorders of the esophagus and stomach secondary to autonomic neuropathy and possibly altered gut hormone release,[1] but these disorders are rare in children. Impaired esophageal clearing, monilial esophagitis, and gastric atony have been described.[9] These problems may lead to erratic diabetic control with episodes of hyperglycemia interspersed with hypoglycemia. Conversely, symptoms and signs of gastric atony may be corrected by the institution of meticulous control. Gastric atony in childhood and adolescent diabetics is more likely to be related to the metabolic disorder than to a longstanding neuropathy, as in adults. True diabetic gastroparesis is a feature of severe longstanding insulin dependent diabetes, seen usually in adult patients with evidence of neuropathy. This entity presents with unexplained weight loss, anorexia, epigastric pain, bloating, and fullness. More severe cases have severe vomiting. A few cases may have gastric moniliasis or bacterial overgrowth. Diagnosis of this disorder is made by barium meal. Treatment is unsatisfactory, but improvement of symptoms can be obtained with metoclopramide or domperidone, and surgical drainage is unhelpful.[10] Diabetics seem to develop atrophic gastritis at a younger age than do healthy individuals,[11] but in most diabetics, basal acid output and maximal acid output in response to pentagastrin are normal and food-stimulated acid secretion is normal.[1] Gastric acid secretion can be impaired in response to hypoglycemia, which suggests

that vagal denervation is responsible. Immunologic mechanisms may contribute to this gastritis; there is an increased incidence of gastric parietal cell antibodies in young diabetics.

Diabetic Diarrhea

Diarrhea is a relatively common complaint among young diabetics, but the disabling form of autonomic diabetic diarrhea is most common in middle age. Diarrhea may be the presenting feature of diabetes in children, and physicians treating children with acute diarrhea, particularly if associated with marked weight loss and dehydration, should be aware of this possibility. The occurrence of polyuria and glycosuria should lead to the diagnosis of diabetes mellitus in this situation. In established diabetics, diarrhea may persist or alternate with episodes of constipation. The stools are often watery and may contain undigested food. Nocturnal diarrhea is not uncommon. Other causes of diarrhea should be excluded, in particular celiac disease, which is associated with diabetes (see Table 2 and discussion below). Other causes of diarrhea, particularly those associated with malabsorption, closely resemble classic diabetic diarrhea. Possible etiologic factors in the occurrence of true diabetic diarrhea include autonomic neuropathy, as evidenced by its association with other neuropathy abnormalities, abnormalities of motility,[1] GI bacterial overgrowth, and abnormalities of bile salt metabolism,[12,13] since tetracycline relieves diabetic diarrhea,[12] or altered gut hormone secretion.[1] In a rat model, intestinal secretion related to impaired adrenergic regulation of mucosal ion transport reversed by clonidine has been observed. Absorption of nutrients is unimpaired in true diabetic diarrhea, but rapid intestinal transit may result in poor absorption of medication, particularly if it is a "slow-release" form or when diabetic control is erratic. The treatment of diabetic diarrhea is empirical. Good diabetic control should be applied vigorously. Codeine phosphate[12] and clonidine have been associated with improvement. Tetracycline and cholestyramine may be helpful, particularly if there is an abnormality of bile salt metabolism or bacterial overgrowth.

Association with Celiac Disease

Diabetes mellitus and celiac disease frequently co-exist,[14] related to a common genetic predisposition.[15] Approximately 80 percent of patients with celiac disease and 54 percent of patients with juvenile-onset diabetes have the histocompatibility antigen HLA-B8. One or more of these immune response genes may be in linkage disequilibrium with HLA-B8 and HLA-DR3, and this may be the basis for the predisposition to both celiac disease and diabetes mellitus.[15] All diabetics with significant chronic diarrhea should have a small intestinal biopsy for the exclusion of celiac disease. Clinical clues to the presence of co-existing celiac disease are a family history of celiac disease, frequent swings from hypo- to hyperglycemia, abdominal pain that may or may not predate the onset of diabetes, and evidence of malabsorption with growth failure.[16] A comparison of diabetic diarrhea and diabetes associated with celiac disease is given in Table 2.

TABLE 2 Features Distinguishing Diabetic Diarrhea and Celiac Disease Associated with Diabetes

	Diabetic Diarrhea	Celiac Disease
Onset of symptoms	Established diabetic	Often precedes diabetes
Symptoms and signs	Abdominal pain rare Variable watery diarrhea No steatorrhea Growth failure uncommon	Abdominal pain Steatorrhea Growth failure
Diabetic control	Poor with degenerative complications	Unstable with swings of blood sugar
Jejunal biopsy	Normal	Villous atrophy
Response to gluten-free diet	None	Remission of gastrointestinal symptoms Improved diabetic control Resolution of villous atrophy

Treatment of celiac disease with a strict gluten-free diet should relieve symptoms and improve diabetic control, although daily insulin requirements may increase.[17]

HYPOPARATHYROIDISM AND PSEUDOHYPOPARATHYROIDISM

Hypoparathyroidism is characterized by symptoms of neuromuscular hyperactivity, hypocalcemia, hyperphosphatemia, and diminished circulating immunoreactive parathyroid hormone. This condition occurs in children either as a congenital absence of the glands (e.g., Di George's syndrome), as neonatal hypoparathyroidism in babies delivered of mothers who have primary hyperparathyroidism, and as an idiopathic autosomal recessive abnormality termed multiple endocrine deficiency – autoimmune candidiasis (MEDAC) syndrome or juvenile familial endocrinopathy–hypoparathyroidism – Addison's disease – mucocutaneous candidiasis (HAM) syndrome. The usual early symptoms of hypoparathyroidism are cramps, tetany, and steatorrhea. The mechanisms by which parathormone is involved in intestinal absorption are unknown, but symptoms of malabsorption may be the earliest manifestation of hypoparathyroidism. With vitamin D_2 therapy, diarrhea decreases, steatorrhea disappears, and other evidence of malabsorption improves. Diagnosis of hypoparathyroidism as a basis for such malabsorption may be established by measuring parahormone levels or by changes in urinary phosphate excretion after intravenous infusions of parahormone or calcium. It should be noted that magnesium deficiency must be ruled out in patients who present with malabsorption and findings of hypoparathyroidism, since functional hypoparathyroidism occurs in patients with severe and prolonged hypomagnesemia. In true hypoparathyroidism, administration of vitamin D and calcium will correct hypocalcemia and improve the fat absorption as well as other manifestations of the disease.[18]

Mild malabsorption has been reported in pseudoparathyroidism, the designation for several forms of lack of target cell responsiveness to parathyroid hormone, sometimes associated with Albright's heredity osteodystrophy. Parathormone in some way facilitates the effect of vitamin D upon calcium absorption by the intestinal tract, and in pseudo-hypoparathyroidism, the end organs, including the gut, are not responsive to parathormone. GI problems similar to but less severe than those found in hypoparathyroidism are found in pseudohypoparathyroidism, but plasma parathyroid hormone levels are high.

PITUITARY AND HYPOTHALAMIC DISORDERS

The anterior pituitary is crucial for normal growth, sexual maturation, and endocrine function. The hypothalamus regulates anterior pituitary function by synthesizing small peptides that either promote or inhibit pituitary hormone secretion. After synthesis by neurons in the hypothalamus, these factors or peptides enter the hypothalamic pituitary portal circulation and are carried to the anterior pituitary cells. The release of these factors is controlled in part by central nervous system neurotransmitters. In addition, the hypothalamus has been considered to contain both the satiety (ventromedial) and feeding (lateral) centers, which are important in appetite and satiety.

Pituitary hormones have important effects on the gut. Adrenocorticotropic hormone (ACTH) stimulates cortisol secretion and enhances brush border enzyme activity, and thyrotropin-stimulating hormone (TSH) causes thyroxine secretion with major effects on gut motility. Growth hormone (GH) causes intestinal villous growth and enhances absorption, but there is no good evidence for the gonadotropins having any physiologic effect on the gut. However, prolactin is required for milk production in association with estrogen, progesterone, and insulin. Suckling is a major stimulus to prolactin release,[20] and there is evidence that during lactation, prolactin stimulates intestinal mucosal growth and increased absorptive capacity.

Hypopituitarism

Most forms of hypopituitarism (Table 3) involve growth hormone deficiency, which can be either isolated or associated with other pituitary hormone deficiencies. Hypopituitarism presents at varying ages with a range of symptoms. Infants

TABLE 3
Causes of Hypopituitarism in Children

Pituitary disease
   Panhypopituitarism due to tumor, trauma, infection, or irradiation;
      familial syndromes or aplasia
   Isolated growth hormone deficiency

Hypothalamic disease (GRF deficiency)
   Midline developmental defects
   Birth trauma
   Histiocytosis
   Tumors
   ? Psychosocial deprivation

Disorders of growth hormone responsiveness
   Receptor abnormalities (Laron dwarfism, pygmy)
   Protein-calorie malnutrition

with intrauterine hypopituitarism may present at birth with hypoglycemia, prolonged jaundice, and, if male, micropenis and undescended testes. Growth failure is a major manifestation, often apparent by the end of the first year of life, with rates of linear growth less than 4 cm per year. Hypoglycemia is limited mainly to young children, occurring typically after fasting, due to deficiencies of the hormones that antagonize insulin. Hypopituitary short stature is proportionally normal for age, with a tendency to be overweight for height and with prominent subcutaneous deposits of abdominal fat and delayed bone age. When nutritional deficiency causes short stature, there is disproportion, decreased weight for height, reduced subcutaneous fat stores, and only marginally delayed bone age. Hypopituitarism in children is rarely associated with thyroid deficiency and diabetes insipidus. Adolescent patients with hypopituitarism have delayed puberty and may have symptoms of lethargy, anorexia, weight loss, and diarrhea. These symptoms are similar to those seen in some patients with anorexia nervosa and primary GI disease such as inflammatory bowel disease and celiac disease; diarrhea may be a feature in common with all of these conditions. In true hypopituitarism, most of the GI symptoms are reversed by hormonal replacement.

Diencephalic Syndrome

The diencephalic syndrome is a rare symptom complex occurring in young infants, usually around 2 to 6 months of age, caused by a glioma of the hypothalamus. The prominent features of the syndrome are the preservation of alertness and presence of euphoria associated with marked emaciation and inanition.[21] Vomiting is common but mild and does not account for the apparent emaciation. Examination of the optic fundi may reveal optic atrophy, but this finding may not be present and excessive tremor, urine output, and diaphoresis are variable. Acute peptic ulceration and consequent GI hemorrhage have been reported. Older children with hypothalamic tumors frequently present with growth retardation, obesity, and altered temperature control. Diagnosis is confirmed by CT scan; this evaluation should be considered in all children with severe emaciation and failure to thrive. Remarkable reversal of the emaciation can be seen after radiotherapy for the glioma.

HYPOADRENOCORTICISM

The adrenal cortex secretes glucocorticoids and mineralocorticoids. In the gut, glucocorticoids bind to specific cytoplasmic receptors on the enterocyte and the activated receptor-steroid complex is then translocated to the nucleus and causes new messenger RNA synthesis. The net effect is to increase the absorptive capacity of the small intestine and enhance brush border membrane digestive capacity without increasing the number of cells.[22] The dominant effect of disorders of the adrenal gland on the gut is related to abnormalities of aldosterone metabolism. Although the effect of increased aldosterone production in increasing sodium absorption in the colon is trivial compared to its effect in the kidney, lack of production of aldosterone and end-organ failure to respond to aldosterone are often associated with significant intestinal salt wasting in addition to urinary loss.[23] Thus, in salt-losing states associated with hypoadrenocorticism, the additional sites of salt loss may contribute to the episodes of dehydration and hypovolemia. It has been suggested that aldosterone is important in modulating the permeability of the colon to sodium, not only during electrolyte disturbances, but also under normal circumstances.[24]

The most common adrenal defect in steroid biosynthesis in children is congenital adrenal hyperplasia. The most common deficiency is 21-hydroxylase deficiency (90 percent of cases), which is inherited as an autosomal recessive defect and results in salt wasting, hyperkalemia, and metabolic acidosis. Young patients have a poor appetite and fail to gain weight. The excessive loss of sodium eventually results in severe water loss and marked dehydration. Cardiovascular collapse can occur. A similar clinical picture can be observed in pyloric stenosis, but the hypokalemic alkalosis that accompanies this disorder contrasts with the low sodium chloride and bicarbonate levels and elevated potassium levels occurring in congenital adrenal hyperplasia. Abnormalities of the external genitalia in girls and relative increase in urine output in the face of dehydration, as well as increased pigmentation, will remind the physician of the possibility of congenital adrenal hyperplasia.

Destruction of the adrenal cortex by hemorrhage, infection, invasion by tumors, or autoimmune processes results in Addison's disease, a combined glucocorticoid and mineralocorticoid deficiency, recognized clinically by hypoglycemia, anorexia, weakness, and a failure to respond to stress. The defects are associated with renal salt wasting, hyperkalemia, and metabolic acidosis. Some patients with Addison's disease have been reported to have steatorrhea with normal jejunal histology[25] which reverses with hormonal replacement therapy. As with congenital adrenal hyperplasia, the diagnosis of Addison's disease can be difficult to establish, because dehydration and similar GI symptoms occur frequently in young children. Low serum sodium and chloride levels are often observed in pediatric practice, including disorders of aldosterone metabolism. Elevated levels of serum potassium may be masked by prolonged infusion of glucose but can be the most helpful feature. An adrenal crisis should always be considered in the differential diagnosis of dehydration and GI illness.

THYROID DISEASES

Thyroid hormones influence growth and development, oxygen consumption, heat production, nerve function, and metabolism of lipids, carbohydrates, proteins, nucleic acids, vitamins, and inorganic irons. In addition, they have important effects on other hormonal actions. Thyroid hormones have a prominent effect on gut motility. Hyper- and hypothyroidism are both associated with numerous GI problems.

Congenital Hypothyroidism

Newborn screening for congenital hypothyroidism is routine in most developed countries, so the diagnosis is usually made prior to the onset of clinical symptoms. Where newborn screening is not in place, the characteristic facies, enlarged protruding tongue, developmental retardation, and GI problems related to constipation and feeding disorders should suggest the diagnosis. A history of prolonged neonatal jaundice, the occurrence of an umbilical hernia, and a hoarse cry provide further clues to this diagnosis.

Acquired Hypothyroidism

Hypothyroidism may develop at any age in previously normal persons. Routine neonatal sequential screening of young children with Down's syndrome is warranted because of a significant association with hypothyroidism. The onset is usually insidious. A high proportion of patients have circulating anti-thyroid antibodies, and in children this type of hypothyroidism is mostly the end result of an autoimmune process (Hashimoto's thyroiditis). In other cases, endemic factors, goitrogenic agents, and secondary causes for hypothyroidism may occur. The spectrum of hypothyroidism related to Hashimoto's thyroiditis includes goiter, thyrotoxicosis, nephritis, diabetes mellitus, and other associations, including an association with ulcerative colitis. Chronic hypothyroidism causes a range of GI symptoms, including constipation, rectal prolapse, ascites, and disordered motility of the esophagus, stomach, duodenum, and colon.[26]

HYPERTHYROIDISM

Hyperthyroidism in pediatric practice, although rare, occurs as neonatal thyrotoxicosis or juvenile Graves' disease, a consequence of diffuse thyroid hyperplasia. The most common GI symptoms of hyperthyroidism at all ages is diarrhea. The symptom is accompanied by the usual systemic symptoms of thyrotoxicosis, including marked weight loss, voracious appetite, eye manifestations, and hyperactive sympathetic nervous system. Increased GI motility has been documented,[27] which may account for the steatorrhea that has been observed in some cases. In an experimental model of hyperthyroidism,

it has been shown that small intestinal mucosal thickness, mucosal protein content, and brush border enzymes are increased.[28]

REFERENCES

1. Atkinson M, Hosking DJ. Gastrointestinal complications of diabetes mellitus. Clin Gastroenterol 1983; 12:633–650.
2. Pedersen J. The pregnant diabetic and her newborn: problems and management. Baltimore: Williams & Wilkins, 1977.
3. Fuhrmann K, Reiker H, Seminler K, et al. The effect of intensified conventional insulin therapy before and during pregnancy on the malformation rate of offspring of diabetic mothers. Exp Clin Endocrinol 1984; 88:173–179.
4. Miller E, Hare JW, Clogerty JP, et al. Elevated maternal haemoglobin A1 in early pregnancy and major congenital abnormalities of diabetic mothers. N Engl J Med 1981; 304:1331–1335.
5. Davis WS, Campbell JB. Neonatal small left colon syndrome. Am J Dis Child 1975; 129:1024–1028.
6. Munk P, Freedman MH, Levison H, et al. The effect of bicarbonate on oxygen transport in Juvenile diabetic ketoacidosis. J Pediatr 1974; 84:510–514.
7. Warshaw AL, Feller ER, Lee KH. On the cause of raised serum amylase in diabetic ketoacidosis. Lancet 1977; i:929–930.
8. Sperling MA. Diabetic ketoacidosis. Pediatr Clin North Am 1984; 31:591–610.
9. White NH, Waltman SR, Krupin T, Santiago JV. Reversal of neuropathic and gastrointestinal complications related to diabetes mellitus in adolescence with improved metabolic control. J Pediatr 1981; 99:41–45.
10. Malagelada JR, Rees WDW, Mazzotta LJ, Go VLW. Gastric motor abnormalities in diabetic and postvagotomy gastroparesis: effect of metoclopramide and bethanechol. Gastroenterology 1980; 78:286–293.
11. Katz LA, Spiro HM. Gastrointestinal manifestations of diabetes. N. Engl J Med 1966; 275:1350–1361.
12. Malins JM, French JM. Diabetic diarrhoea. QJ Med 1957; 26:467–480.
13. Scarpello JH, Hague RV, Cullen DR, Sladen GE. The ¹⁴C-glycocholate test in diabetic diarrhoea. Br Med J 1976; 2:673–675.
14. Walsh CH, Cooper BT, Wright AD, et al. Diabetes mellitus and coeliac disease: a clinical study. QJ Med 1978; 47:89–100.
15. Hitman GA, Niveen MJ, Festenstein H, Cassell PG, Awad J, et al. HLA class II alpha chain gene polymorphisms in patients with insulin-dependent diabetes mellitus, dermatitis herpetiformis and celiac disease. J Clin Invest 1987; 79:609–615.
16. Cacciari E, Salardi S, Volta V, et al. Prevalence and characteristics of coeliac disease in type I diabetes mellitus. Acta Paediatr Scand 1987; 76:671–672.
17. Thain ME, Hamilton JR, Ehrlich RM. Co-existence of diabetes mellitus and celiac disease. J Pediatr 1974; 85:527–530.
18. Lorenz R, Burr IM. Idiopathic hypoparathyroidism and steatorrhoea: a new aid in management. J Pediatr 1974: 85:522–525.
19. Russell RI. Hypoparathyroidism and malabsorption. Br Med J 1967; 3:781–782.
20. Muller E, Dowling RH. Prolactin and the small intestine: effect of hyperprolactinaemia on mucosal structure in the rat. Gut 1981; 22:558–565.
21. Markesbery WR, McDonald JV. Diencephalic syndrome. AM J Dis Child 1973; 125:123–125.
22. Scott J, Batt RM, Peters TJ. Enhancement of ileal adaptation by prednisolone after proximal small bowel resection in the rat. Gut 1979; 20:858–864.
23. Oberfield SE, Levine LS, Carey RM, Bejar R, New MI. Pseudohypoaldosteronism: multiple target organ unresponsiveness to mineralocorticoid hormone. J Clin Endocrinol 1979: 48:228–234.
24. Milla PJ. Disorders of electrolyte absorption. Clin Gastroenterol 1982; 11:43–44.
25. McBrien DJ, Jones RV, Creamer B. Steatorrhoea in Addison's disease. Lancet 1963; i:25–26.
26. Duret RL, Bastenie PA. Intestinal disorders in hypothyroidism. Clinical and manometric study. Am J Dig Dis 1971; 16:723–727.
27. Thomas FB, Caldwell JH, Greenberger NJ. Diarrhoea in thyrotoxicosis. Ann Intern Med 1973; 78:669–675.
28. Wiley ZD, Lavigne ME, Liu KM, MacGregor IL. The effect of hyperthyroidism on gastric emptying rates and pancreatic exocrine and biliary secretion in man. Am J Dig Dis 1978; 23:1003–1008.

PART 35

Secretory Tumors Affecting the Gut

David J. Keljo, M.D., Ph.D.

Amine precursor uptake and decarboxylation or "APUD" cells are postulated to be of neural crest origin and to have migrated during embryogenesis to a variety of organs, including pituitary, thyroid, parathyroid, adrenal medulla, lung, pancreas, and gut.[1,2] These cells are capable of making a variety of hormones and neurotransmitters including parathyroid hormone, calcitonin, somatostatin, insulin, glucagon, vasoactive intestinal peptide, pancreatic polypeptide, gastrin, and others. Sporadic tumors of these cells arise, secreting one, or more frequently, several hormones in pharmacologic quantities.[33] The clinical syndrome produced generally reflects the action of only one of the hormones. A number of these secretory tumors present with gastrointestinal (GI) symptoms. Gastrinoma (Zollinger- Ellison) syndrome and VIPoma (Verner-Morrison) syndrome have been well described in the pediatric age group, and these syndromes are discussed here in some detail. Somatostatinoma syndrome, glucagonoma syndrome, and carcinoid syndrome have been reported only in adults but are discussed briefly here on the assumption that they will eventually be recognized in childhood as well. Finally, some space is devoted to a discussion of the familial multiple endocrine neoplasia (MEN) syndromes. It is now clear that early recognition of MEN syndromes is important to long-term survival, and clues are often present in childhood. Some of these patients present with secretory tumors. Another very interesting group of these patients presents with feeding problems and constipation in infancy.

GASTRINOMA SYNDROME (ZOLLINGER-ELLISON SYNDROME)

In 1955, Zollinger and Ellison described a syndrome of peptic ulcerations in the jejunum associated with islet cell tumors of the pancreas.[4] They postulated that this represented secretion by the islet cells of a substance that stimulated gastric acid secretion. This factor was subsequently demonstrated to be gastrin.[5] The major features of the syndrome are now understood to be gastric acid hypersecretion, peptic ulceration, diarrhea, and steatorrhea.[6] All of these can be understood in terms of the actions of gastrin.

Pathogenesis

Gastric acid is secreted by the parietal (oxyntic) cells located in the glands of the gastric fundus and body.[7] Secretion is an active process (against a 1,000,000:1 gradient) mediated by the H^+, K^+-ATPase located in the luminal membrane of these cells.[8] Gastric acid secretion is stimulated in vivo by at least four secretagogues, including histamine, calcium, acetylcholine, and gastrin, but gastrin is the only "physiologic" stimulus.[9,10] Histamine stimulation of acid secretion appears to be mediated by cyclic AMP.[11] The mechanism by which gastrin acts has not been clearly delineated. Gastrin receptors have been described in membranes from oxyntic tissue, but not on parietal cells per se. Gastrin enhances cellular response to histamine, and gastrin action is blocked by histamine receptor blockers.[12] It is possible that gastrin action is mediated through histamine. In addition to the acute effect of gastrin on acid secretion, gastrin stimulates hypertrophy of the gastric mucosa, and it may cause hypertrophy of pancreatic islets.[13]

Under physiologic conditions, gastrin is secreted by "G" cells in the gastric antrum and in the duodenum.[14] Gastrin exists in two major molecular forms—G17 and G34.[15] G17 is several times more potent as a stimulus for gastric acid secretion and is found in greater quantity in the cell than is G34. While G34 is less active than G17 in stimulating acid secretion, G34 is cleared more slowly from the bloodstream and is normally present in greater quantity in the blood than is G17. An immunoassay that has greater affinity for G17 than G34 will most accurately determine gastrin activity, whereas one that has equal affinity for both will most accurately determine gastrin quantity.

Physiologic stimuli for gastrin release include the anticipation of a meal (the "cephalic phase," mostly vagally mediated), distention of the gastric fundus (also vagally mediated), and the presence of protein in the gastric contents (mediated by peptides and amino acids?).[14] Physiologic inhibitors of gastrin release include acid in gastric contents and possibly secretin.[16] Hallmarks of aberrant gastrin release are the stimulation by calcium and by secretin.[17]

In the Zollinger-Ellison syndrome, gastrin is secreted from an ectopic source in unregulated quantities. The features of the disease are the results of excessive acid secretion. Peptic ulcers in these patients resolve when acid secretion is reduced below 10 mEq per hour.[18] Acid is responsible for the diarrhea and steatorrhea seen in these patients as well, since these symptoms resolve with gastrectomy.[6] Mechanisms of diarrhea include acid-induced damage to the mucosa and rapid intestinal transit. Steatorrhea is the result of inactivation of pancreatic enzymes, precipitation of bile salts, and damage to the intestinal mucosa.

Clinical Features

The age of onset of reported cases of Zollinger-Ellison syndrome has been from 7 to 90 years of age.[6] The peak incidence is between 30 and 50 years of age.[6] Approximately one-third of adult patients with Zollinger-Ellison syndrome have the familial MEN type I syndrome, in which are found (in decreasing order of frequency) tumors of the parathyroids, pancreatic islets, and pituitary.[19] Gastrinoma as part of this syndrome has not yet been described in childhood. The incidence of peptic ulcer disease tends to be somewhat higher in the families of patients with the sporadic form of Zollinger-Ellison syndrome than in the population at large.[20]

The major clinical features of Zollinger-Ellison syndrome are summarized in Table 1.

The vast majority (93 percent) of patients have presented with signs of recurrent peptic ulcer disease.[20] While the presence of multiple ulcers in unusual sites (e.g., jejunum) has been considered the hallmark, in fact nearly three-quarters of the ulcers are solitary and located in the duodenal bulb.[20] Ulcers in gastrinoma patients have, however, been found in the esophagus, the fundus, the distal duodenum, the jejunum, and even the colon.[20] Approximately 7 percent of patients have presented simply with intractable diarrhea, without evidence of ulcer disease.[20] Many patients with gastrinoma have had steatorrhea.[6]

Clear-cut criteria for pursuing the possibility of Zollinger-Ellison syndrome in children have not been established. Clinical signs of ulcer disease in the pediatric population include abdominal pain (particularly pain that awakens the patient from sleep, pain associated with nonbilious vomiting, pain relieved by eating), signs of upper GI bleeding (hematemesis, melena, iron deficiency anemia), and signs of perforation (acute abdomen, unexplained persistent fever and abdominal pain).[21] Upper endoscopy is now a routine procedure that can be performed in a child of virtually any age to investigate the possibility of peptic ulcer disease. Because ulcers are uncommon in the pediatric age group, it has been suggested that all children with ulcer should be investigated for gastrin hypersecretion.[21] Certainly documented recurrent ulceration, multiple ulcers, ulcers in unusual places, unusually large ulcers, a family history of Zollinger-Ellison syndrome, or symptoms in a patient with a family history of MEN I should stimulate an evaluation. Chronic diarrhea with an abnormal small bowel biopsy, steatorrhea, and a negative work-up for infection, celiac disease, or allergy should lead to an evaluation for gastrinoma.

Diagnosis

The sign of gastrinoma is the unregulated and excessive secretion of gastrin. Diagnostic tests for gastrinoma are summarized in Table 2. The best screening test is a fasting serum gastrin level (which in children with at least an 8-hour fast

TABLE 1
Features of Gastrinomas (Zollinger-Ellison) Syndrome

Recurrent peptic ulcer disease	93%
Multiple or in unusual sites	(¼)
Solitary in duodenal bulb	(¾)
Intractable diarrhea	7%
Steatorrhea	?%

TABLE 2
Testing for Gastrinoma

1. Measurement of fasting serum gastrin level
2. Measurement of secretin stimulation test
3. Measurement of basal gastric acid secretion

Elevated fasting gastrin level or positive secretin stimulation test in setting of elevated basal acid secretion strongly suggests presence of gastrinoma.

should be less than 50 pg per milliliter.[22] An elevated serum gastrin level should be further investigated with a provocative test, the easiest and most specific of which is the secretin stimulation test.[23,24] For this test, 2 units per kilogram of pure secretin (Kabi Group, Inc. Greenwich, CT) are injected intravenously over 30 seconds. Blood samples are taken for gastrin measurement 5 minutes before injection, just before injection, and at 5-minute intervals for 30 minutes after injection. Secretin has no effect on the gastrin level in normal patients and patients with benign "G" cell hyperplasia but results in at least a doubling of the gastrin level in patients with gastrinoma (it usually increases by more than 220 pg per milliliter). Occasional false-negative results are seen. A negative result in a patient with recurrent ulcer disease should probably be investigated with a study of gastric acid secretion, using pentagastrin. Patients with gastrinoma typically have high basal acid secretion rates, greater than 15 mEq per hour.[24] Normal basal acid secretion in children has been estimated at 0.04 ± 0.01 mEq per kilogram per hour.[25] A positive secretin stimulation test or an elevated fasting gastrin level in association with an elevated basal acid secretion should trigger an intensive search for a gastrinoma.[24]

Localization of the Tumor

Gastrinomas are frequently very small (3 cm or less in size) and frequently multiple.[24] Most arise in the pancreas, but they can arise anywhere in the abdomen, particularly in the stomach or in the duodenum.[20] Solitary gastrinomas have been reported in children in the liver and in the kidney.[26,27] At least 60 percent of gastrinomas are malignant, and a large proportion have already metastasized to liver or lymph nodes by the time they are found.[20]

Imaging studies have been most useful in detecting gastrinomas. Abdominal sonography, while not terribly sensitive, is useful if positive. Careful abdominal computed tomography with intravenous and GI contrast will pick up about 70 percent of gastrinomas and more than 80 percent of liver metastases, with a very high (greater than 90 percent) degree of specificity.[28] The addition of selective abdominal arteriography does not increase the detection of primary tumors but does raise the efficiency of identification of liver metastases to nearly 100 percent.[29] The role of selective venous sampling of gastrin levels in detecting primary tumors is controversial. In certain hands it would seem to be exceedingly effective and in others not useful at all.[30,31] Intraoperative sonography may turn out to be useful.[32] Management options for gastrinoma are outlined in Table 3.

TABLE 3
Management of Gastrinoma

Cure: surgical resection

Palliation
  Selective vagotomy + H_2 blocker therapy
  Gastrectomy (if medical management fails)
  5-Fluorouracil and chlorozotocin (if tumor bulk is a problem)
  Parathyroidectomy (MEN I patients)

Surgical Management

The only hope for cure of gastrinoma is complete surgical resection. Because the tumors are so small, maximal preoperative efforts to localize them should be made. It is accepted that the surgery should be undertaken only by a surgeon experienced in dealing with gastrinomas. The nature of the necessary exploration has been described.[19,33] Even if a tumor has not been identified in preoperative studies, exploration is recommended except in patients with MEN I, in which the likelihood of cure is exceedingly low.[19] Overall, 65 percent of patients will be found at surgery to have a gastrinoma, 65 percent of these in the pancreas, 21 percent in the duodenum, and 14 percent elsewhere in the abdomen.[34] Aggressive resection of local lymph nodes and resectable metastases is recommended.[19] Some surgeons have found intraoperative sonography of the pancreas useful in detecting small pancreatic tumors.[32] Successful resection occurs in approximately 15 percent.[19] Some advocate doing a highly selective vagotomy at the time of surgery to reduce subsequent need for H_2 blockers.[35] Others advocate a total gastrectomy to prevent subsequent peptic ulcer morbidity.[19] The only way to demonstrate complete resection is by demonstrating that the serum gastrin level returns to normal.

Medical Management

H_2 blockers form the cornerstone of medical therapy for Zollinger-Ellison syndrome. It is essential that an adequate dose be used and that its effect be monitored. The object is to keep acid secretion rates below 10 mEq per hour.[34] Two or three times the usual dose may be required to achieve that result. Anticholinergics may provide additional help if vagotomy was not previously performed.

Prior to the availability of H_2 blockers, the only patients who survived were those who underwent total gastrectomy.[20,36] The rest succumbed to complications of peptic ulceration. It has been suggested that, at least in some cases, total gastrectomy has led to regression of the tumor.[36] It is claimed that the morbidity of total gastrectomy is not excessive in these patients.[19,33,36] Some argue that H_2 blockers are expensive and that patients, even when compliant, eventually become resistant to the H_2 blockers and even to H^+, K^+-ATPase inhibitors; they suggest that primary gastrectomy is not unreasonable.[19] Others feel that total gastrectomy should be reserved for failure of medical management.[34]

Chemotherapy

No one has been cured of gastrinoma by chemotherapy.[19,34] Significant tumor regression has been achieved with chlorozotocin and 5-fluorouracil (5-FU) at the cost of considerable side effects, and this therapy is probably best reserved for circumstances in which tumor bulk is causing significant symptoms.[34]

Outlook

The patients with the best outcome are those in whom no tumor is found, those with solitary resectable tumors, and those with MEN I. In these patients the 10-year survival is in excess of 80 percent. In patients with unresectable metastases at the time of diagnosis, the 5-year survival is only 20 to 40 percent.[19,34] The data in the pediatric age group are much more limited than in adults, but they indicate that the survivals in this group may be better.[37]

Summary

Early accurate diagnosis is the only hope for the long-term survival of patients with gastrinoma. Key features of the disease and its diagnosis and management include the following:

1. Gastrinomas are small, frequently multiple, frequently malignant tumors that arise in the abdomen.
2. Manifestations of gastrin hypersecretion are gastric acid hypersecretion, peptic ulceration, diarrhea, and steatorrhea.
3. Diagnosis is most commonly made by demonstration of an inappropriate rise in the serum gastrin level in response to secretin injection.
4. Total surgical resection of tumor and metastases is the only way to cure gastrinoma.
5. Selective vagotomy and aggressive H_2 blocker therapy will control the manifestations in most patients.
6. Total gastrectomy is the only other way to control the symptoms. This should probably be reserved for failure of medical management.
7. Chemotherapy with 5-FU and chlorozotocin may be palliative when tumor bulk becomes a problem.
8. When unresectable metastases are present, 20 to 40 percent of patients survive 5 years. With totally resectable tumors, or when patients have MEN I, 80 percent survive 10 years.

VIPOMA SYNDROME (VERNER-MORRISON SYNDROME; WATERY DIARRHEA SYNDROME; PANCREATIC CHOLERA)

In 1958, Verner and Morrison described a syndrome of refractory watery diarrhea and hypokalemia associated with islet cell tumors of the pancreas.[38] In 1970, Said and Mutt described a polypeptide isolated from small intestine which caused systemic vasodilation, hypotension, and hyperglycemia.[39] Bloom et al in 1973 demonstrated that patients with watery diarrhea syndrome (WDS) have markedly elevated serum levels of this vasoactive intestinal peptide (VIP).[40] This triggered a series of studies from a variety of laboratories which showed that the major features of WDS resulted from the actions of VIP.[41-47]

Pathogenesis

VIP is a 28 amino acid peptide widely distributed through the gut and the central nervous system.[48] Of the many neurotransmitter and hormonal agents impinging on the gut, only VIP and the prostaglandins have been shown to stimulate adenylate cyclase activity, hence secretion by the enterocytes.[49] It has been hypothesized that fluid secretion by the crypt enterocytes keeps gut contents fluid and carries mucosal immunoglobulins from their site of secretion in the crypts to the rest of the intestinal surface.[50] It may be that VIP is the physiologic regulator of this function.[50]

Intravenous infusion of VIP both in man and in animals stimulates cyclic AMP production by enterocytes, producing effects very similar to those of cholera toxin (Table 4).[41,44,47,49] In the villous enterocytes, the electroneutral coupled NaCl transport mechanism (which may facilitate much of the bulk flow of water and salt under physiologic conditions in vivo) is inhibited.[45,46,51] In crypt cells, luminal membrane permeability to chloride is increased, permitting an active secretion of chloride driven by a sodium-coupled cotransport process located in the basal lateral membrane.[45,46,51] The combination of the active secretion of chloride (water and sodium follow passively) by crypt cells with decreased passive absorption of water and salt by villous cells results in copious watery diarrhea, an isotonic solution of electrolytes.

Potassium absorption in the small bowel is a largely passive process and is reduced when bulk absorption of water and sodium is reduced.[51] Studies in patients with pancreatic cholera have indicated that most potassium losses in this disease are colonic.[42] VIP stimulation of adenyl cyclase activity in the colon has been shown to stimulate potassium secretion.[43] It has been suggested that aldosterone released in response to vascular volume contraction also stimulates potassium secretion by the colon, but this is unproven.[52] The results of increased potassium losses are hypokalemia and acidosis.

Vasodilatation, manifested by facial flushing, was one of the earliest reported effects of VIP and has been reproduced in man by infusion of VIP-producing blood levels seen in WDS.[39,47] Hyperglycemia has been reported in animals, has been seen in some patients with WDS, but has not been reproduced by VIP infusion.[47,53] Hypercalcemia has been reported in patients with VIPoma, but the mechanism is not known.[53]

Clinical Features

WDS has been reported in all age groups, and the clinical features are summarized in Table 5.[53-64] Virtually all patients have presented with watery diarrhea and hypokalemia. Several have presented with incontinence. Fecal losses while fasting have been at least 20 ml per kilogram per day and in most cases exceed 50 ml per kilogram per day.[65] Fecal osmolality is entirely accounted for as twice the sum of the concentrations of sodium and potassium. Steatorrhea is not a feature of the syndrome.[53] Hypochlorhydria is seen in about 70 percent of patients, hyperglycemia in 20 to 50 percent, and hypercalcemia in 20 to 50 percent. Flushing is present in about 20 percent and is frequently intermittent, indicating that hormone release by the tumor is also sporadic.[53]

In the pediatric age group, most of the VIPomas so far described are ganglioneuromas or ganglioneuroblastomas.[65] The tumors have been found in the neck, thorax, and suprarenal and pelvic areas. There is a single case report in the literature of a VIP-secreting pancreatic tumor (the more common VIPoma in the adult age group) in a 15-year-old girl.[64] A case of islet cell hyperplasia with associated VIP hypersecretion and villous atrophy has been reported, as has a case of villous atrophy with VIP hypersecretion with no tumor or hyperplasia found.[66,67] The relationship between the VIP and the villous atrophy in these cases is not clear.

Diagnosis

Diarrhea that persists during fasting in amounts greater than 20 ml per kilogram per day should raise a question of VIPoma. Table 6 lists a variety of causes of secretory diarrhea. Common causes would include infection (toxigenic *Escherichia coli*, cholera, *Salmonella*, *Clostridium difficile*) and laxative administration. Stool electrolytes, osmolality, and magnesium should be measured. If twice the sum of the sodium and potassium concentrations is significantly less than the osmolality, a search should be initiated for the osmotic agent (e.g., magnesium or lactulose). Stool should be

TABLE 4
Effect of Cyclic AMP on Intestinal Transport

1. Crypt cells: cyclic AMP enhances brush border membrane permability to chloride, resulting in chloride-driven secretion of electrolytes and water.
2. Villous cells: cyclic AMP reduces electroneutral Na/Cl co-transport, reducing absorption of electrolytes and water.
3. The net effect of #1 or #2 is copious secretion of water and electrolytes.
4. The sodium/glucose coupled co-transport pathway in villous cells is preserved, permitting oral rehydration with glucose/electrolyte solution.

TABLE 5
Features of Watery Diarrhea (VIPoma) Syndrome

Watery diarrhea	100%
Hypochlorhydria	70%
Hyperglycemia	20–50%
Hypercalcemia	20–50%
Flushing	20%

TABLE 6
Differential Diagnosis of Secretory Diarrhea

Infection with toxigenic organisms (e.g., *Escherichia coli*, cholera, *Salmonella, Clostridium difficile*)
Mucosal necrosis or atrophy
Surreptitious drug administration
   Laxatives
   Ipecac
Bile acid malabsorption
Congenital electrolyte transport defects
Hormone-secreting tumors
   VIP
   Prostaglandin E_2
   5-HIAA
   Serotonin

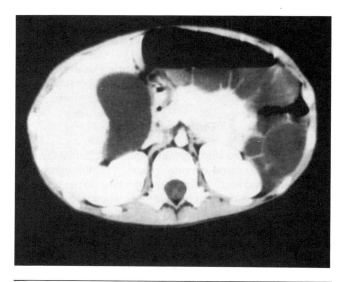

FIGURE 1 Abdominal CT scan of 5-year-old girl with watery diarrhea, showing pancreatic mass, excessive fluid in colon, and possible metastatic lesion in liver. Mass was VIPoma. (Courtesy of Alan Strickland, M.D.)

screened for phenolphthalein, senna, and other stimulant laxatives. If true secretory diarrhea is found, cultures should be obtained and a small bowel biopsy should be examined for adherent organisms. If vomiting is present, urine should be screened for emetine (N.B., this will not appear on routine toxic screens and must be specially ordered), as secretory diarrhea has been seen with Ipecac intoxication (personal observation). If all of the above does not yield a cause for secretory diarrhea, hormone-secreting tumors should be considered.

Secretory diarrhea is seen with VIPoma and with tumors secreting prostaglandin E_2, and it is important to measure both.[53,68] It must be remembered that diarrhea may also be a prominent feature of Zollinger-Ellison syndrome, and gastrin levels should be checked. Diarrhea is also a feature of carcinoid syndrome, and although symptomatic carcinoid has not yet been reported in childhood, if all else is normal, 5-hydroxyindoleacetic acid and serotonin levels should be measured.

It is important that hormone levels be measured in a reference laboratory with great experience in the area and that abnormal values be repeated. In one such laboratory, top normal fasting VIP is 170 pg per milliliter, and the lowest value found in a patient with VIPoma has been 225 pg per milliliter. The incidence of false-negative tests is not known.[53]

If blood tests support the diagnosis of VIPoma, a vigorous search must begin to locate the tumor, remembering that in childhood most of these tumors are ganglioneuromas or ganglioneuroblastomas and may be found anywhere from the pelvis to the neck.[53,65] Most tumors are localized by sonography or computed tomography (Fig. 1). Preoperative angiography is helpful.[53]

Since many of these tumors secrete a variety of hormones, preoperative screening with a broad panel of hormones including somatostatin, pancreatic polypeptide, insulin, and heliotropin should be done, as metastases may eventually secrete only one of these.[69]

Therapy

Surgery offers the only possible cure for VIPoma. It has been estimated that 70 percent of childhood VIPomas are resectable.[65,70] Preoperative stabilization of fluid and electrolyte balance is critical. Intraoperative ultrasonography may provide additional help in locating tumor not seen on preoperative imaging. It has been shown that with successful resection, VIP levels fall to normal within hours postoperatively.[61] Immune identification of the hormone in the resected tumor is also supportive evidence for the role of the tumor in the disease.

When resection has not been possible, management has been very difficult. Supportive therapy includes intravenous fluid and oral glucose electrolyte solution. A variety of agents have been used to reduce the diarrhea.[53] Prednisone has been effective for a period of time in a large number of patients in reducing the diarrhea, although it has no effect on the circulating level of VIP.[53,65] Somatostatin inhibits the release of VIP from pancreatic tumors, and the long-acting somatostatin analogue SMS 201-995 (Sandoz, East Hanover, NJ) has been very useful in controlling diarrhea from pancreatic VIPomas.[71,72] The role of SMS 201-995 in the treatment of VIPoma syndrome in childhood, in which most of the tumors are ganglioneuromas, has not yet been fully explored. Somatostatin has been used in one patient with a VIP-secreting neuroblastoma with reduction in VIP levels but without cessation of diarrhea.[73] Good control was obtained in an infant with an enlarged pancreas and elevated VIP levels.[74]

Streptozotocin and fluorouracil have been used with success in the treatment of pancreatic tumors.[75,76] Effectiveness of this regimen has not been tested in ganglioneuroblastomas.[65] Therapy of VIPoma is summarized in Table 7.

Outlook

In childhood VIPoma, in which 70 to 80 percent of the tumors are resectable, the outlook is excellent. When the tumor is not resectable, long-term symptomatic remissions may be obtainable with medication.

TABLE 7
Therapy of VIPoma

Cure: surgical resection
Palliation
Sandostatin
Prednisone
Streptozotocin
5-Fluorouracil
Supportive
IV fluids
Oral glucose/electrolyte solution
Total parenteral nutrition

Summary

With early diagnosis and meticulous surgery, most childhood VIPomas can be cured. Salient features of the disease and its diagnosis and management include the following:

1. VIPomas in childhood are most commonly ganglioneuromas, which may originate anywhere from the neck to the pelvis.
2. Pancreatic tumors secreting VIP occur rarely in children but are the most common VIP-secreting tumors in adults.
3. VIP hypersecretion causes secretory diarrhea, hypokalemia, hypochlorhydria, and flushing. Hyperglycemia and hypercalcemia are also sometimes seen with these tumors.
4. Diagnosis is made by demonstrating an elevated serum VIP level. Rare cases with identical symptoms have been reported to have normal VIP levels and elevated prostaglandin E_2 levels.
5. Total resection of the tumor and any metastases offers the only hope for cure. Seventy to 80 percent of the childhood tumors are resectable.
6. When resection has not been accomplished, long-term symptomatic remission has commonly been obtained with medication. The long-acting somatostatin analogue SMS 201-995 has been very useful for reduction of VIP secretion by pancreatic tumors. Efficacy in ganglioneuroblastoma has not been thoroughly evaluated. A variety of other agents, most notably prednisone, have been helpful in reducing the diarrhea.
7. 5-Fluorouracil and streptozotocin have been used palliatively for pancreatic tumors but have not been studied in ganglioneuromas.

SOMATOSTATINOMA

Somatostatin is a potent inhibitor of release of a variety of hormones, including gastrin, CCK, insulin, and secretin.[77] Symptoms of somatostatinoma therefore are diabetes, gallstones, steatorrhea, and hypochlorhydria. Somatostatinoma has not yet been recognized in a patient less than 20 years old.[69]

GLUCAGONOMA

Excessive secretion of glucagon induces a catabolic state, glucose intolerance, hypoaminoacidemia, and a characteristic dermatitis. The most striking features of glucagonoma syndrome are weight loss, a rash, and diabetes.[78-80] The rash begins as red scaly lesions on the extremities, in the creases, and about the mouth. These become bullous and finally crusty and confluent. Dystrophy of the nails and alopecia are also seen. All of these are probably manifestations of the severely catabolic state. Glucagonoma has not yet been described in a patient less than 20 years old. Diagnosis is suggested by diabetes and a characteristic rash and confirmed by glucagon level.

MULTIPLE ENDOCRINE NEOPLASIA SYNDROMES

Several familial groupings of multiple endocrine tumors have now been identified. They have been labeled according to the pattern of organ involvement as multiple endocrine neoplasia I (MEN I) (hyperparathyroidism, islet cell tumors of the pancreas, and nonfunctional adenomas of the pituitary), MEN IIA (medullary carcinoma of the thyroid, parathyroid hyperplasia, and pheochromocytoma), and MEN IIB (Multiple mucosal and alimentary tract neuromas, medullary carcinoma of the thyroid, and pheochromocytoma).[81]

Patients with MEN I comprise approximately one-sixth of all patients with hyperparathyroidism, one-third of all patients with Zollinger-Ellison syndrome, 4 percent of patients with insulinoma, and a small fraction of all patients with VIPoma syndrome, somatostatinoma syndrome, and glucagonoma syndrome.[81] The extent of involvement tends to increase with age. The parathyroid glands are most frequently involved. In one extensively studied kindred, the frequency of parathyroid involvement was essentially 0 percent at 15 years of age and 100 percent at 40 years of age.[82] In that kindred, hyperparathyroidism always preceded hypergastrinemia. Neither Zollinger-Ellison syndrome nor WDS has been reported in a patient with MEN I less than 20 years old, but it seems likely that they will appear. Annual screening of first-degree relatives of patients with MEN I has been recommended starting in the first decade of life.[83] This screening should include at least serum calcium, phosphorus, and gastrin, and other tests according to the family history. Pancreatic tumors in these patients tend to be multiple and are therefore rarely resectable. However, they are late to metastasize, and long survivals are the rule.[81] There is evidence that the hypergastrinemia is much ameliorated by parathyroidectomy.[84]

Patients with MEN II develop tumors of the thyroid (medullary carcinoma of the thyroid), adrenal medulla (pheochromocytoma), and sometimes parathyroid glands. MEN II has been divided into two subcategories depending on the presence (B) or absence (A) of mucosal and intestinal neuromas. MEN IIB (sometimes referred to in the literature as MEN III) is particularly important to gastroenterologists because children with this disorder frequently have marked feeding problems (poor suck), colic, and severe constipation in the first year of life.[86] Within the first few years of life, they develop unique nodules on their tongues and buccal

TABLE 8
Major Components of the Multiple
Endocrine Neoplasia (MEN) Syndrome

MEN I	Hyperparathyroidism Islet cell tumors of the pancreas Nonfunctional pituitary adenomas
MEN IIA	Medullary carcinoma of the thyroid Parathyroid hyperplasia Pheochromocytoma
MEN IIB (MEN III)	Multiple mucosal and alimentary tract neuromas Medullary carcinoma of the thyroid Pheochromocytoma

mucosae, as well as corneal neuromas.[85-87] Early diagnosis is critical because the form of medullary carcinoma of the thyroid seen in MEN IIB is particularly aggressive, and metastases may be found by 4 years of age.[85,87] Thyroidectomy at the first sign of calcitonin overproduction is indicated. With massive overproduction of calcitonin, diarrhea may be seen. Combined calcium and pentagastrin stimulation of calcitonin release has been the most sensitive test, and screening has been recommended on an annual basis from the first year of life.[88]

CARCINOID SYNDROME

While carcinoid tumors are seen in the pediatric age group, they are usually incidental findings at appendectomy.[89] Carcinoid syndrome has not yet been reported in a child. The tumors grow quite slowly, and symptoms do not generally occur until they are metastatic. Carcinoid syndrome appears to be mediated primarily by serotonin and bradykinin secreted by the tumor.[90] Symptoms include episodic flushing, facial swelling, palpitations, abdominal pain, and explosive diarrhea. Bradykinin and histamine are probably responsible for the flushing and palpitations. The mechanism of the diarrhea is not fully understood. Mesenteric fibrosis induced by serotonin can produce abdominal pain by compromising mesenteric vessels. Endocardial and cardiac valvular fibrosis is also likely caused by serotonin. Diagnosis is by measurement of urinary serotonin and 5-hydroxyindoleacetic acid and serum and platelet serotonin. Diet and medications can produce false-positive results. Cure is surgical. A number of drugs including steroids, methylsergide, periactin, and somatostatin analogue have been used to control the symptoms. Chemotherapy is palliative. Survivals are long.

REFERENCES

1. Pearse AGE. Peptides in brain and intestine. Nature 1976; 262:92–94.
2. Pearse AGE. The cytochemistry and ultrastructure of polypeptide hormone–producing cells of the APUD series and the embryologic, physiologic and pathologic implications of the concept. J Histochem Cytochem 1969; 17:303–313.
3. Larsson Lt, Grimelius L, Hakanson R, Rehfeld JF, Stadil F, Holst J, et al. Mixed endocrine pancreatic tumors producing several peptide hormones. Am J Pathol 1975; 79:271–284.
4. Zollinger RM, Ellison EH. Primary peptic ulcerations of the jejunum associated with islet cell tumors of the pancreas. Ann Surg 1955; 142:709–728.
5. Gregory RA, Grossman MI, Tracy HJ, Bentley PH. Nature of the gastric secretagogue in Zollinger-Ellison tumours. Lancet 1967; ii:543–544.
6. Isenberg JI, Walsh JH, Grossman MI. Zollinger-Ellison syndrome. Gastroenterology 1973; 65:140–165.
7. DiBona DR, Ito S, Berglindh T, Sachs G. Cellular site of gastric acid secretion. Proc Natl Acad Sci USA 1979; 76:6689–6693.
8. Forte JG, Machen TE, Obrink KJ. Mechanisms of gastric H+ and Cl− transport. Ann Rev Physiol 1980; 42:111–126.
9. Feldman M, Walsh JH, Wong HC, Richardson CT. Role of gastrin heptadecapeptide in the acid secretory response to amino acids in man. J Clin Invest 1978; 61:308–313.
10. Feldman M. Gastric secretion. In: Sleisenger MH, Fordtran JS, eds. Gastrointestinal disease. 3rd ed. Philadelphia: WB Saunders, 1983: 541.
11. Soll AH, Wollin A. Histamine and cyclic AMP in isolated canine parietal cells. Am J Physiol 1979; 237:E444–E450.
12. Richardson CT. Effect of H$_2$-receptor antagonists on gastric acid secretion and serum gastrin concentration. Gastroenterology 1978; 74:366–370.
13. Dembinski AB, Johnson LR. Growth of pancreas and gastrointestinal mucosa in antrectomized and gastrin-treated rats. Endocrinology 1979; 105:769–773.
14. Walsh JH, Isenberg JI, Ansfield J, Maxwell V. Clearance and acid-stimulating action of human big and little gastrins in duodenal ulcer subjects. J Clin Invest 1976; 57:1125–1131.
15. Calam J, Dockray GJ, Walker R, Tracy HJ, Owens D. Molecular forms of gastrin in peptic ulcer: comparison of serum and tissue concentrations of G17 and G34 in gastric and duodenal ulcer subjects. Eur J Clin Invest 1980; 10:241–247.
16. Isenberg JI, Walsh JH, Passaro EJ, Moore EW, Grossman MI. Unusual effect of secretin on serum gastrin, serum calcium, and gastric acid secretion in a patient with suspected Zollinger-Ellison syndrome. Gastroenterology 1972; 62:626–631.
17. Kolts BE, Herbst CA, McGuigan JE. Calcium and secretin-stimulated gastrin release in the Zollinger-Ellison syndrome. Ann Intern Med 1974; 81:758–762.
18. Jensen RT, Gardner JD, Raufman J, Pandol SJ, Doppman JL, Collen MJ. Zollinger-Ellison syndrome: current concepts and management. Ann Intern Med 1983; 98:59–75.
19. Zollinger RM. Gastrinoma: the Zollinger-Ellison syndrome. Semin Oncol 1987; 14:247–252.
20. Ellison EH, Wilson SD. The Zollinger-Ellison syndrome: reappraisal and evaluation of 260 registered cases. Ann Surg 1964; 160:512–530.
21. Murphy MS, Eastham EJ, Jimenez M, Nelson R, Jackson RH. Duodenal ulceration: review of 110 cases. Arch Dis Child 1987; 62:554–558.
22. Janik JS, Akbar AM, Burrington JD, Burke G. Serum gastrin levels in infants and children. Pediatrics 1977; 60:60–64.
23. McGuigan JE, Wolfe MM. Secretin injection test in the diagnosis of gastrinoma. Gastroenterology 1980; 79:1324–1331.
24. Jensen RT, Pandol SJ, Collen MJ, Raufman J, Gardner JD. Diagnosis and management of the Zollinger-Ellison syndrome. J Clin Gastroenterol 1983; 5(suppl 1):123–131.
25. Euler AR, Byrne WJ, Campbell MF. Basal and pentagastrin-stimulated gastric acid secretory rates in normal children and in those with peptic ulcer disease. J Pediatr 1983; 103:766–768.
26. Nord KS, Joshi V, Hann M, Khademi M, Saad S, Marquis J, et al. Zollinger-Ellison syndrome associated with a renal gastrinoma in a child. J Pediatr Gastroenterol Nutr 1986; 5:980–986.
27. Smith AL, Auldist AW. Successful surgical resection of an hepatic gastrinoma in a child. J Pediatr Gastroenterol Nutr 1984; 3:801–804.
28. Wank SA, Doppman JL, Miller DL, Collen MJ, Maton PN, Vinayek R, et al. Prospective study of the ability of computed axial tomography to localize gastrinomas in patients with Zollinger-Ellison syndrome. Gastroenterology 1987; 92:905–912.
29. Maton PN, Miller DL, Doppman JL, Collen MJ, Norton JA, Vinayek R, et al. Role of selective angiography in the management of patients with Zollinger-Ellison syndrome. Gastroenterology 1987; 92:913–918.
30. Cherner JA, Doppman JL, Norton JA, Miller DL, Krudy AG, Raufman J, et al. Selective venous sampling for gastrin to localize gastrinomas, a prospective assessment. Ann Intern Med 1986; 105:841–847.
31. Vinik AI, Thompson N. Controversies in the management of Zollinger-Ellison syndrome. Ann Intern Med 1986; 105:956–959.
32. Telander RL, Charboneau JW, Haymond MW. Intraoperative ultrasonography of the pancreas in children. J Pediatr Surg 1986; 21:262–266.
33. Thompson JC, Lewis BG, Wiener I, Townsend CM. The role of surgery in the Zollinger-Ellison syndrome. Ann Surg 1983; 197:594–607.
34. Jensen RT, Maton PN, Gardner JD. Current management of Zollinger-Ellison syndrome. Drugs 1986; 32:188–196.

35. Richardson CT, Peters MN, Feldman M, McClelland RN, Walsh JH Cooper KA, Willefore G, Dickerman RM, Fordtran JS. Treatment of Zollinger-Ellison syndrome with exploratory laparotomy, proximal gastric vagotomy and H₂-receptor antagonists. Gastroenterology 1985; 89:357–367.

36. Wilson SD, Ellison EH. Total gastric resection in children with the Zollinger-Ellison syndrome. Arch Surg 1965; 91:165–173.

37. Wilson SD. The role of surgery in children with the Zollinger-Ellison syndrome. Surgery 1982; 92:682–692.

38. Verner JV, Morrison AB. Islet cell tumor and a syndrome of refractory watery diarrhea and hypokalemia. Am J Med 1958; 25:374–380.

39. Said S, Mutt V. Peptide with broad biological activity: isolation from small intestine. Science 1970; 169:1217–1218.

40. Bloom SR, Polak JM, Pearse AGE. Vasoactive intestinal peptide and watery-diarrhoea syndrome. Lancet 1973; ii:14–16.

41. Schwartz CJ, Kimberg DV, Sheerin HE, Field M, Said SI. Vasoactive intestinal peptide stimulation of adenylate cyclase and active electrolyte secretion in intestinal mucosa. J Clin Invest 1974; 54:536–544.

42. Rambaud J, Modigliani R, Matuchansky C, Bloom S, Said S, Pessayre D, et al. Pancreatic cholera: studies on tumoral secretions and pathophysiology of diarrhea. Gastroenterology 1975; 69:110–122.

43. Racusen LC, Binder HJ. Alteration of large intestinal electrolyte transport by vasoactive intestinal polypeptide in the rat. Gastroenterology 1977; 73:790–796.

44. Krejs GJ, Barkley RM, Read NW, Fordtran JS. Intestinal secretion induced by vasoactive intestinal polypeptide. J Clin Invest 1978; 61:1337–1345.

45. Davis GR, Santa Ana CA, Morawski SG, Fordtran JS. Effect of vasoactive intestinal polypeptide on active and passive transport in the human jejunum. J Clin Invest 1981; 67:1687–1694.

46. Krejs GJ, Fordtran JS. Effect of VIP infusion on water and ion transport in the human jejunum. Gastroenterology 1980; 78:722–727.

47. Kane MG, O'Dorisio TM, Krejs GJ. Production of secretory diarrhea by intravenous infusion of vasoactive intestinal polypeptide. N Engl J Med 1983; 309:1482–1485.

48. Khalil T, Alinder G, Rayford PL. Vasoactive intestinal peptide. In: Thompson JC, Greeley GHJ, Rayford PL, Townsend CM, eds. Gastrointestinal endocrinology. 1st ed. New York: McGraw-Hill, 1987: 260.

49. Kimberg DV, Field M, Johnson J, Henderson A, Gershon E. Stimulation of intestinal mucosal adenyl cyclase by cholera enterotoxin and prostaglandins. J Clin Invest 1971; 50:1218–1230.

50. Field M, Chang EB. Pancreatic cholera. Is the diarrhea due to VIP? N Engl J Med 1983; 309:1513–1515.

51. Binder HJ. Absorption and secretion of water and electrolytes by small and large intestine. In: Sleisenger MH, Fordtran JS, eds. Gastrointestinal disease. 3rd ed. Philadelphia: WB Saunders, 1983: 822.

52. Levitan R, Ingelfinger FJ. Effect of D-aldosterone on salt and water absorption from the intact human colon. J Clin Invest 1965; 44:801–808.

53. Mekhjian HS, O'Dorisio TM. VIPoma syndrome. Semin Oncol 1987; 14:282–291.

54. Bloom SR, Long RG, Bryant MG, Mitchell SJ, Polak JM. Clinical biochemical and pathological studies on 62 VIPomas. Gastroenterology 1980; 78:1143.

55. Mitchell CH, Crast FW, Griffin R, Sunshine P. Intractable watery diarrhea, ganglioneuroblastoma, and vasoactive intestinal peptide. J Pediatr 1976; 89:593–595.

56. Jansen-Goemans A, Engelhardt J. Intractable diarrhea in a boy with vasoactive intestinal peptide-producing ganglioneuroblastoma. Pediatrics 1977; 59:710–716.

57. Iida Y, Nose O, Kai H, Okada A, Mori T, Lee P, et al. Watery diarrhoea with a vasoactive intestinal peptide-producing ganglioneuroblastoma. Arch Dis Child 1980; 55:929–936.

58. Carson DJ, Glasgow JFT, Ardill J. Watery diarrhoea and elevated vasoactive intestinal polypeptide associated with a massive neurofibroma in early childhood. J Royal Soc Med 1980; 73:69–72.

59. Kaplan SJ, Holbrook CT, McDaniel HG, Buntain WL, Crist WM. Vasoactive intestinal peptide secreting tumors of childhood. Am J Dis Child 1980; 134:21–24.

60. Hansen LP, Lund HT, Fahrenkrug J, Sogaard H. Vasoactive intestinal polypeptide (VIP)-producing ganglioneuroma in a child with chronic diarrhea. Acta Paediatr Scand 1980; 69:419–424.

61. Funato M, Fujimura M, Shimada S, Takeuchi T, Kozuki K, Iida Y. Rapid changes of serum vasoactive intestinal peptide after removal of gan-

62. Granot E, Deckelbaum RJ, Schiller M, Okon E, Goder K, Landau H, Bloom SR. Vasoactive intestinal peptide–secreting tumor appearing as growth failure. Am J Dis Child 1983; 137:1203–1204.

63. Socha J, Dobrzanska A, Rowecka K, Cichy W, Bierla J, Stodulski J, Wozniewicz B. Chronic diarrhea due to VIPoma in two children. J Pediatr Gastroenterol Nutr 1984; 3:143–148.

64. Brenner RW, Sank LI, Kerner MB, Schrager GO, Elguezabal A, Roth J. Resection of a VIPoma of the pancreas in a 15-year-old girl. J Pediatr Surg 1986; 21:983–985.

65. Long RG. Vasoactive intestinal polypeptide–secreting tumors (VIPomas) in childhood. J Pediatr Gastroenterol Nutr 1983; 122–126.

66. Ghishan FK, Soper RT, Nassif EG, Younoszai MK. Chronic diarrhea of infancy: nonbeta islet cell hyperplasia. Pediatrics 1979; 64:46–49.

67. Udall JN, Singer DB, Huang CTL, Nichols BL, Ferry GD. Watery diarrhea and hypokalemia associated with increased plasma vasoactive intestinal peptide in a child. J Pediatr 1976; 88:819–821.

68. Jaffe BM, Kopen DF, DeSchryver-Kecskemeti K, Gingerich RL, Greider M. Indomethacin-responsive pancreatic cholera. N Engl J Med 1977; 297:817–821.

69. Vinik AI, Strodel WE, Eckhauser FE, Moattari AR, Lloyd R. Somatostatinomas, PPomas, neurotensinomas. Semin Oncol 1987; 14:263–281.

70. Long RG, Bryant MG, Mitchell SJ, Adrian TE, Polak JM, Bloom SR. Clinicopathological study of pancreatic and ganglioneuroblastoma tumours secreting vasoactive intestinal polypeptide (VIPomas). Br Med J 1981; 282:1767–1770.

71. Santangelo WC, O'Dorisio TM, Kim JG, Severino G, Krejs GJ. Pancreatic cholera syndrome: effect of a synthetic somatostatin analog on intestinal water and ion transport. Ann Intern Med 1985; 103:363–367.

72. Wood SM, Kraenzlin MD, Adrian TE, Bloom SR. Treatment of patients with pancreatic endocrine tumours using a new long-acting somatostatin analogue: symptomatic and peptide responses. Gut 1985; 26:438–444.

73. Tiedemann K, Pritchard J, Long R, Bloom SR. Intractable diarrhoea in a patient with vasoactive intestinal peptide–secreting neuroblastoma: attempted control by somatostatin. Eur J Pediatr 1981; 137:217–219.

74. Smith SS, Shulman DI, O'Dorisio TM, McClenathan DT, Borgber JA, Bercu BB, Root AW. Watery diarrhea, hypokalemia, achlorhydria syndrome in an infant: effect of the long-acting somatostatin analogue SMS 201–995 on the disease and linear growth. J Pediatr Gastroenterol Nutr 1987; 6:710–716.

75. Moertel CG, Hanley JA, Johnson LA. Streptozocin alone compared with streptozocin plus fluorouracil in the treatment of advanced islet-cell carcinoma. N Engl J Med 1980; 303:1189–1194.

76. Kahn CR, Levy AG, Gardner JD, Miller JV, Gorden P, Schein PS. Pancreatic cholera: beneficial effect of treatment with streptozotocin. N Engl J Med 1975; 292:941–945.

77. Krejs GJ, Orci L, Conlon JM, Ravazzola M, Davis GR, Raskin P, et al. Somatostatinoma syndrome. N Engl J Med 1979; 301: 285–292.

78. McGavran MH, Unger RH, Recant L, Polk HC, Kilo C, Levin ME. A glucagon-secreting alpha-cell carcinoma of the pancreas. N Engl J Med 1966; 274:1408–1413.

79. Boden G. Insulinoma and glucagonoma. Semin Oncol 1987; 14:253–262.

80. Mallinson CN, Bloom SR, Warin AP, Salmon PR, Cox B. A glucagonoma syndrome. Lancet 1974; 2:1–5.

81. Brunt LM, Wells SA. The multiple endocrine neoplasia syndromes. Invest Radiol 1985; 20:916–927.

82. Marx SJ, Vinik AI, Santen RJ, Floyd JCJ, Mills JL, Green J 3rd. Multiple endocrine neoplasia type I: assessment of laboratory tests to screen for the gene in a large kindred. Medicine 1986; 65:226–241.

83. Humphrey GB, Pysher T, Holcombe J, Rowsey JJ, Burris TE, Lemerle J, et al. Overview of the multiple endocrine neoplasia syndromes in infancy and childhood. Cancer Treat Res 1983; 17:359–362.

84. Macleod AF, Ayers B, Young AE, Medd WE, Sonksen PH. Resolution of hypergastrinaelmia after parathyroidectomy in multiple endocrine neoplasia syndrome type I (MEN type I). Clin Endocrinol 1987; 26:693–698.

85. Jones BA, Sisson JC. Early diagnosis and thyroidectomy in multiple endocrine neoplasia, type 2b. J Pediatr 1983; 102:219–223.

86. Aine E, Aine L, Huupponen T, Salmi J, Miettinen P. Visible corneal nerve fibers and neuromas of the conjunctiva—a syndrome of type-3

multiple endocrine adenomatosis in two generations. Graefe's Arch Clin Exp Ophthalmol 1987; 225:213–216.

87. Norton JA, Froome LC, Farrell RE, Wells SA. Multiple endocrine neoplasia type IIb: the most aggressive form of medullary thyroid carcinoma. Surg Clin North Am 1979; 59:109–118.

88. Graham SM, Genel M, Touloukian RJ, Barwick KW, Gertner JM, Torony C. Provocative testing for occult medullary carcinoma of the

thyroid: findings in seven children with multiple endocrine neoplasia type IIa. J Pediatr Surg 1987; 22:501–503.

89. Grahame-Smith DG. Natural history and diagnosis of the carcinoid syndrome. Clin Gastroenterol 1974; 3:575–594.

90. Feldman JM. Carcinoid tumors and syndrome. Semin Oncol 1987; 14:237–246.

PART **36**

Protein-Losing Enteropathy

Roy Proujansky, M.D.

The loss of serum proteins across the gut mucosa can occur in association with a wide variety of gastrointestinal (GI) and non-GI disease states in the pediatric age patient. The effect on the patient is largely the result of the balance between excessive enteric protein loss and hepatic protein synthesis, protein distribution, and degradation in the rest of the body. We will review the relevant aspects of serum protein metabolism and the alterations that occur in a number of disease states.

NORMAL ALBUMIN METABOLISM

Albumin is a water-soluble molecule (molecular weight: 65,000) that functions to maintain the plasma oncotic pressure and as a transport protein for hormones, metals, ions, bilirubin, and a variety of other biologic molecules. Because of the nonselective nature of intestinal protein loss, the measurement of the serum albumin level has served clinically as an indicator of the degree to which abnormal loss may be occurring.

The maintenance of a steady-state serum albumin level is dependent on synthesis, breakdown, and tissue distribution. Albumin is synthesized in the liver at a rate of 120 to 200 mg per kilogram per day in the normal adult, with somewhat higher rates of albumin synthesis (180 to 300 mg per kilogram per day) occurring during the first year of life.[1] The predominant factor affecting albumin synthesis is nutrition. Food or protein deprivation is associated with a decrease in albumin synthesis of 50 percent within 24 hours. Amino acids, especially tryptophan, appear to be an essential nutritional requirement.[2,3] Hormonal influences also play a role, with cortisol and thyroid hormone acting to stimulate albumin synthesis. Experimentally, hypophysectomy and diabetes may be associated with decreased synthesis which correct with growth hormone or insulin replacement, respectively.[4,5]

Approximately one-third of total body albumin is located intravascularly. Extravascular albumin is distributed throughout the skin (30 to 40 percent of total extravascular pool), muscle, and viscera. An exchangeable pool of extravascular albumin exists, which can be mobilized to conserve serum albumin levels. The exchangeable pool size is 6 to 8 g per kilogram for children less than 1 year of age and 3 to 4 g per kilogram in the older child. Malnutrition may decrease the exchangeable pool to one-third normal size.

CONTRIBUTION OF THE GASTROINTESTINAL TRACT TO ALBUMIN METABOLISM

Between 6 and 10 percent of the plasma albumin pool is degraded normally in a 24-hour period. Loss into the GI tract accounts for less than 10 percent of albumin degradation in healthy subjects. In patients with protein-losing enteropathy, however, albumin catabolic rates average 43 percent higher than in healthy controls. Much of this albumin loss is at the expense of plasma albumin, having the net effect of increasing the fractional catabolic rate of the plasma pool by a factor of three. This is associated with a relatively modest increase in hepatic albumin synthesis (24 percent), suggesting a limited capacity of the liver to respond to these losses.[6,7]

The site of albumin loss at the mucosal surface is not well characterized. Postulated mechanisms of loss include diffusion between mucosal cells, rupture of lymphatics through the mucosal surface, and leakage of protein across ulcerated mucosa.[8] An immunofluorescent study in a canine model has demonstrated that in the setting of elevated intestinal venous pressure, transmucosal albumin flux occurred exclusively at the villous tip region. At normal venous pressures no loss was observed.[9] The sites of protein loss due to other mechanisms have not been characterized.

METHODS OF DIAGNOSIS OF ENTERIC PROTEIN LOSS

Methods for documenting the enteric loss of plasma proteins have evolved for the purpose of elucidating normal physiologic protein losses by this route as well as the alterations that occur in various disease states. Techniques employed for these studies fall into two categories: the injection of radiolabeled proteins or chemicals with the subsequent determination of radioactivity in enteric secretions or the direct determination of the presence of an endogenous protein in enteric secretions. Ideally, the molecule employed for these types of studies should distribute and be metabolized similarly to other plasma proteins. The molecule should not be selectively secreted, digested, or reabsorbed by the GI tract. If a radiolabel is employed, it should remain bound to its carrier and, if dissociated within the GI tract, it should not be reabsorbed.[10] To maximize its clinical utility, the technique employed should be safe and reproducible and should require a minimal amount of patient or laboratory effort for its performance.

Radiolabeled proteins that have been employed for the determination of enteric protein loss have included ^{131}I-albumin, ^{51}Cr-albumin, and [67]Cu-ceruloplasmin. Radioiodinated albumin was initially employed for a variety of physiologic studies of plasma protein distribution and metabolism and thus, initially, seemed to be a likely candidate for similar studies of enteric protein loss. However, free iodine is actively secreted by the salivary glands and gastric mucosa and reabsorbed in the intestine and is thus not suitable for these studies. ^{51}Cr-albumin has been used more extensively for studies of enteric protein loss because chromium is not actively reabsorbed or secreted into the intestine in appreciable quantities. The labeled albumin is given as an intravenous injection, and stools are collected for several days and assayed for radioactivity.[11,12] The use of ^{51}Cr-albumin has been somewhat limited in the pediatric population because of the need for a several-day stool collection, the requirement that stool not be contaminated by urine, the concern about the use of radioactive agents in the pediatric-age patient, and, in recent years, lack of availability of the radiopharmaceutical. ^{51}Cr-albumin is currently available on a limited basis in the United States. [67]Cu-ceruloplasmin has been found to give similar results to those obtained with ^{51}Cr-albumin, but its use has been limited by the cost of preparation and the brief half-life of [67]Cu.[10,13] Recently, ^{99m}Tc-labeled albumin has been utilized to visualize scintigraphically the sites of GI protein loss.[14]

Studies of enteric protein loss have also employed radiolabeled chemical agents believed to behave metabolically in a fashion similar to plasma proteins. ^{131}I-polyvinylpyrrolidone has been used for this purpose but has been faulted because of release of the iodine from the carrier molecule and variability in the molecular weights of the preparations employed.[15] ^{59}Fe-labeled iron-dextran has also been tried.[16] [51]CrCl_3 can be injected intravenously and can then bind to plasma proteins in vivo to give similar results to studies employing injected ^{51}Cr-albumin.[17]

In the last several years the measurement of fecal concentrations of alpha_1-antitrypsin (alpha_1-AT) has been used more routinely for the documentation of intestinal protein loss.[18,19] Alpha_1-AT has a molecular weight similar to that of albumin and is not actively secreted, absorbed, or digested by the GI tract. Alpha_1-AT can be detected in the stool following lyophilization, extraction by solubilization, and subsequent immunologic assay, with radial immunodiffusion appearing to be superior to immunonephelometry.[20] Stools

can be collected over several days and an alpha_1-AT clearance can be determined, or single stool specimens can be obtained and a fecal concentration of alpha_1-AT, expressed as milligrams per gram of stool, can be compared to control values. Variations in the extraction procedure employed have led to differences in the absolute values of alpha_1-AT concentration obtained by different investigators. Thus, control values may be different depending on the method employed.

Utilizing these techniques, the concentration of fecal alpha_1-AT has been found to correlate well with the presence of an enteric protein-losing state in children with various GI disorders.[21,22] This assay has been used as a reliable screening test and has also been shown to correlate with disease activity and the response to therapy. Alpha_1-AT clearance has been shown to correlate closely with determinations made by the intravenous [51]CrCl_3 technique.[23,24] Spot sample determinations of fecal alpha_1-AT concentration agree with measures of alpha_1-AT clearance done on more prolonged stool collections.[25,26] Thus, the lack of need for prolonged stool collections, along with the avoidance of radioisotopes, has made the alpha_1-AT assay very appealing for use in clinical pediatrics. Recent modifications of the technique have been suggested which will make the assay easier and less expensive to perform.[25,27]

While the fecal alpha_1-AT assay has been shown to be useful clinically, certain aspects of these assays need to be considered in the interpretation of assay results. Alpha_1-AT is degraded at a pH less than 3, and therefore the fecal alpha_1-AT assay is not reliable for the documentation of gastric protein loss. The presence of small amounts of blood loss into the GI tract will not appreciably alter the fecal alpha_1-AT concentration; however, gross hematochezia precludes the accurate determination of enteric protein loss by this method.[21] Fecal alpha_1-AT concentrations may also vary during infancy depending on the age of the patient and the type of feeding.[28,29] In spite of these considerations, the relative ease and reliability of the fecal alpha_1-AT assay are likely to result in its continued use clinically as the primary method for documenting enteric protein loss.

GASTROINTESTINAL DISEASES ASSOCIATED WITH ENTERIC PROTEIN LOSS

A number of disorders have been associated with excessive enteric protein loss in children. Using a pathophysiologic classification, these disorders can be divided into those due predominantly to excessive protein loss from intestinal lymphatics and those due to protein loss across an abnormal or inflamed mucosal surface (Table 1). An alternative classification scheme would be a more clinical approach distinguishing those disorders in which enteric protein loss is the major manifestation of the illness from those in which protein loss is present but is overshadowed by other clinical manifestations of these disorders. We will discuss those diseases that are characterized predominantly by a protein-losing state and will briefly review the contribution of enteric protein loss to the pathophysiology of disorders discussed at greater length in other sections of this book.

TABLE 1
Diseases Associated with Enteric Protein
Loss

Loss from intestinal lymphatics
  Primary intestinal lymphangiectasia
  Secondary intestinal lymphangiectasia
    Cardiac disease
      Constrictive pericarditis
      Congestive heart failure
      Cardiomyopathy
    Obstructed lymphatics
      Malrotation
      Lymphoma
      Tuberculosis
      Sarcoidosis
      Radiation therapy and chemotherapy
      Retroperitoneal fibrosis or tumor
      Arsenic poisoning

Loss from an abnormal or inflamed mucosal surface
  Ménétrier's disease
  Eosinophilic gastroenteritis
  Milk- and soy-induced enterocolitis
  Celiac disease
  Tropical sprue
  Ulcerative jejunitis
  Radiation enteritis
  Graft-versus-host disease
  Necrotizing enterocolitis
  Crohn's disease
  Ulcerative colitis
  Hirschsprung's disease
  Systemic lupus erythematosus
  Bacterial overgrowth
  Giardiasis
  Bacterial and parasitic infections
  Common variable immunodeficiency

Primary Intestinal Lymphangiectasia

Intestinal lymphangiectasia is a disorder characterized by diffuse or localized ectasia of the enteric lymphatics, often in association with lymphatic abnormalities elsewhere in the body.[10] The pathogenesis of these abnormal lymphatic structures is uncertain. Ectatic lymphatics may be located in the mucosa, submucosa, or subserosa, leading to loss of protein and lymphocytes into the gut or the peritoneal cavity. The mechanism of this lymphatic loss is believed to be from rupture of lymphatics across the mucosa with subsequent leakage of lymph into the bowel lumen. The resulting clinical picture is one of edema, which may be asymmetric, growth failure, and variable GI symptoms.

The presentation of primary intestinal lymphangiectasia may occur any time throughout infancy and childhood. GI symptoms, in decreasing order of frequency, include intermittent diarrhea, nausea, vomiting, and occasionally abdominal pain.[30] Steatorrhea may also occur. Edema may be symmetric and pitting if it is due to the presence of a hypoproteinemic state or, alternatively, may be asymmetric and nonpitting if it is due to an underlying lymphatic abnormality of the affected extremity. Lymphedema of an extremity may precede the onset of symptoms due to GI involvement. Lymphatic aberrations may also lead to the development of

a chylothorax or chylous ascites, which should be differentiated from pleural effusions or ascites resulting from hypoproteinemia. Primary intestinal lymphangiectasia may occur as an isolated abnormality or as part of a more generalized syndrome such as Noonan's syndrome or Klippel-Trenaunay-Weber syndrome.[31,32] Intestinal lymphangiectasia has also been noted to occur in families.[33]

In addition to the loss of albumin, patients with lymphangiectasia also frequently have reduced levels of immunoglobulins and a low circulating lymphocyte count due to the lymphatic loss. This may make differentiation from a primary immunodeficiency with GI disease somewhat difficult initially. Enteric lymphatic loss results in the predominant loss of T lymphocytes, leading to reduced delayed hypersensitivity skin test responses, prolonged homograft survival, and diminished blast transformation to mitogen stimulation in vitro.[34,35] Additional abnormalities that have been described include hyposplenism,[36] thymic hypoplasia,[37] and neutrophil dysfunction.[38] In spite of these abnormalities, patients with intestinal lymphangiectasia do not appear to have significant problems with infections.

The diagnosis of intestinal lymphangiectasia is suggested by the previously mentioned clinical findings and supported by the presence of hypoproteinemia and lymphocytopenia. Hypocalcemia is also occasionally present and may produce tetany. Steatorrhea may be demonstrable on a fecal fat collection, and fecal alpha$_1$-AT excretion may be increased. Barium studies may demonstrate thickening of the jejunal folds, fluid hypersecretion, and nodular or punctate lucencies in the mucosa of the small bowel.[30,39] Lymphangiography, which may be technically difficult to perform, has shown hypoplasia of the peripheral lymphatics in the injected limb, partial or complete absence of the thoracic duct, or, rarely, entry of contrast into the bowel lumen via mesenteric lymphatics.[10]

Biopsy of the small intestinal mucosa may demonstrate dilated lacteals associated with distortion of the villi (Fig. 1). However, because of the sometimes focal nature of the lymphatic abnormalities, capsule biopsy of the jejunal mucosa may miss the diagnostic lesion. Endoscopic abnormalities such as scattered white plaques or the presence of chyle-like substances covering the mucosa have been observed and have been useful for directing biopsies at the time of endoscopy.[40,41] The endoscopic and histologic findings are less obvious if the patient has been on a low-fat diet. Obviously, mucosal biopsy is not useful in patients with lymphangiectasia confined to deeper layers of the bowel wall.

The mainstay of treatment for intestinal lymphangiectasia is the use of a low-fat, high-protein, medium-chain (C 6:0 to C 12:0) triglyceride diet. Medium-chain triglycerides are not re-esterified within the intestinal cell and thus bypass the enteric lymphatics and directly enter the portal system. It is believed that the reduction in long-chain fats reduces lymphatic flow and pressure within the lymphatic system and decreases the amount of lymph leakage. This dietary approach can be implemented by the use of a specialized formula (Portagen) during infancy or the supplementation of a low-fat diet with medium-chain triglyceride oil in older children and adolescents. Utilizing this approach, several authors have reported favorable effects on hypoalbuminemia, GI symptoms,

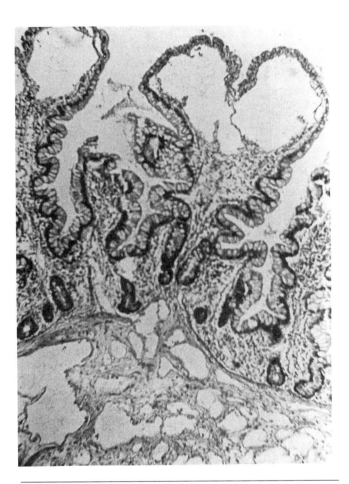

FIGURE 1 Microscopic view of intestinal biopsy demonstrating wide villi with dilated lacteals in the mucosa and enlarged submucosal lymphatics.

and growth.[30,42,43] This improvement may occur in spite of the ability to demonstrate ongoing protein loss. The need for dietary therapy is often permanent, although occasional spontaneous remissions do occur.

Not all patients respond completely to this dietary approach. Some patients require additional supplementation with calcium salts and water-soluble forms of fat-soluble vitamins.[44] Low gamma globulin levels may persist in some patients but are unlikely to require treatment because of the ability of patients with lymphangiectasia to generate specific antibodies.

Isolated reports have documented improvement in patients following localized resections of affected portions of the bowel or anastomosis of abnormal lymphatics to venous channels.[30,45] These approaches may be hampered by an inability to demonstrate radiographically such a localized lymphatic abnormality as well as the tendency for patients with the primary form of lymphangiectasia to have a more extensive lesion. Surgical shunts have been employed for patients with persistent chylothorax or chylous ascites with variable success.[46,47] The response of patients with congenital chylous ascites to treatment with total parenteral nutrition suggests the possible use of this modality to treat patients with intestinal lymphangiectasia resistant to other forms of therapy.[47]

Secondary Intestinal Lymphangiectasia

In addition to the occurrence of intestinal lymphangiectasia as a primary developmental abnormality, lymphangiectasia may occasionally be seen as a result of lymphatic obstruction or elevated lymphatic pressure. Cardiac lesions such as congestive heart failure[48] and constrictive pericarditis[49] act by increasing lymphatic pressure. Inflammatory processes that cause retroperitoneal lymph node enlargement[50] or fibrosis may lead to obstruction of enteric lymphatics. Chemotherapeutic agents or other toxic substances may directly damage the lymphatic structures.[51,52] Fleisher et al have described a few patients with a steroid-responsive acquired form of intestinal lymphangiectasia with elevated immunoglobulins and sedimentation rates suggesting an underlying inflammatory etiology.[53]

Ménétrier's Disease

Ménétrier's disease is a relatively rare disorder that is characterized by the presence of a marked protein-losing gastropathy associated with enlarged and thickened gastric folds in the fundus and the body of the stomach. Most patients have been less than the age of 10, and their illness has usually presented abruptly with the onset of vomiting, abdominal pain, and peripheral edema.[54] Laboratory findings often reveal a mild normochromic, normocytic anemia, eosinophilia, and hypoalbuminemia. Excessive protein loss has been demonstrated by the use of ^{51}Cr-albumin excretion.[54,55] The typical upper GI radiographic appearance has been thickened gastric folds in the fundus and body of the stomach, often with antral sparing (Fig. 2), and this has often been confirmed endoscopically.[56] Thickened folds have also been shown by ultrasonography.[55] Histologic examination of endoscopic or suction biopsies has shown a hypertrophic mucosa with elongated pits. Occasionally cystic or polypoid changes and an inflammatory infiltrate have been noted.[54] Several cases of Ménétrier's disease in childhood have been associated with histologic or serologic evidence of cytomegalovirus infection.[57-59]

The differential diagnosis of Ménétrier's disease in childhood is that of a protein-losing enteropathy associated with thickened GI folds. Eosinophilic gastroenteropathy may present in a similar fashion but usually involves the antrum and demonstrates a distinctive histologic picture on biopsy.[60] Gastric lymphoma and Zollinger-Ellison syndrome can produce similar clinical and radiographic pictures but are both very rare in the pediatric population.[56] Thickened gastric folds without discrete polyps have been noted on upper GI radiographs in the Peutz-Jeghers syndrome.[56]

Children with Ménétrier's disease most commonly have a self-limited illness without recurrence or sequelae. This is different from the adult form of the disease, which is a chronic disorder occurring in older patients (fourth through sixth de-

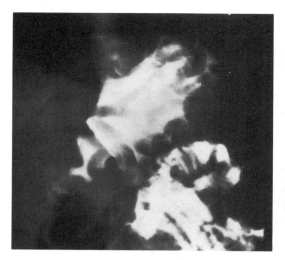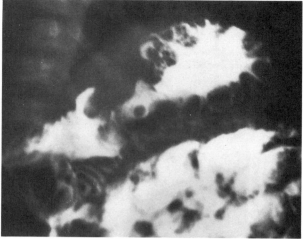

FIGURE 2   Upper gastrointestinal radiographs from a patient with Ménétrier's disease showing marked thickening of the gastric folds.

cades) and often requiring gastrectomy for control of disabling symptoms.[61] The chronic form of Ménétrier's disease has also been described in a family in which two of the members initially became symptomatic in childhood.[62] Fecal alpha₁-AT assay in an adult with Ménétrier's disease failed to demonstrate enteric protein loss in spite of an abnormal ^{51}Cr-albumin study.[63] Presumably this was due to inactivation of alpha₁-AT by gastric acid, as mentioned previously.

Enteric Protein Loss During the Course of Other Gastrointestinal Disorders

Intestinal lymphangiectasia and Ménétrier's disease are disorders that are somewhat uncommon but are characterized primarily by the manifestations of a protein-losing state. However, enteric protein loss is also a common occurrence in a number of diseases in which symptoms due to protein loss are overshadowed by other consequences of the disease process. We will briefly review the contribution of protein loss to a number of disorders that are discussed in greater detail elsewhere in this book.

Infections

GI protein loss during the course of infectious processes has not been extensively evaluated. Evidence for protein loss has been seen during the course of *Salmonella* infection,[8] giardiasis,[63] and other parasitic infestations.[64] Thomas et al found no difference in fecal alpha₁-AT excretion between control patients and infants with acute self-limited gastroenteritis.[21]

In addition to infectious processes, protein loss has also been associated with variations in the enteric flora. A correlation between *Clostridium difficile* colonization and fecal alpha₁-AT excretion has been detected in asymptomatic infants.[65] An increase in ^{51}Cr-albumin excretion has also been found in two patients with bacterial overgrowth of the small

bowel from blind-loop syndrome.[66] A decrease in protein loss was associated with prolonged antibiotic therapy in these patients.

Malabsorptive Disorders

A number of pediatric disorders that result in malabsorption of luminal nutrients have also been associated with enteric protein loss. Hypoalbuminemia is a common occurrence in the course of milk- and soy-sensitive enteritis in infants,[67] and enteric protein loss has been documented in this condition by ^{51}Cr-albumin and fecal alpha₁-AT excretion.[21,68] Marked enteric protein loss also occurs in the allergic and nonallergic forms of eosinophilic gastroenteritis.[69] A decrease in the degree of protein loss with treatment has been documented to occur in both of these conditions.

Active celiac disease has also been shown to result in increases in fecal alpha₁-AT.[21,22] Not only does this improve with treatment, but treated celiacs cannot be distinguished from normals on the basis of fecal alpha₁-AT excretion. These findings suggest the possibility of utilizing fecal alpha₁-AT excretion to monitor the response to gluten withdrawal as well as to monitor compliance of patients on a gluten-free diet.

Immunologic and Inflammatory Disorders

Inflammatory GI disorders have frequently been associated with some degree of protein loss. An elevated concentration of fecal alpha₁-AT has been detected in the stools of patients with probable necrotizing enterocolitis[70] and patients with graft-versus-host disease following bone marrow transplantation.[71] In each of these cases the possibility of using serial values to detect the onset and resolution of these conditions has been suggested.

Several studies have revealed the presence of GI protein loss in patients with idiopathic inflammatory bowel disease (ulcerative colitis and Crohn's disease).[21,26,72,73] Fecal alpha$_1$-AT excretion, fecal alpha$_1$-AT clearance, and ^{51}Cr-albumin excretion have all been found to be increased in patients with inflammatory bowel disease compared to controls. Fecal alpha$_1$-AT excretion has been shown to correlate with disease severity and, to some extent, with the degree of small bowel involvement but to correlate poorly with the Crohn's disease activity index.

Protein-losing enteropathy has been demonstrated in association with common variable immunodeficiency.[74] Thus, since hypogammaglobulinemia can be either the effect or the cause of a protein-losing state, one needs to exercise caution in discerning the etiology of hypogammaglobulinemia associated with hypoalbuminemia and enteric protein loss.

CONCLUSIONS

Protein-losing enteropathy occurs in the course of a number of GI disorders. Diseases whose manifestations are predominantly the result of the protein-losing state are relatively uncommon and can be differentiated on the basis of clinical, laboratory, radiographic, and endoscopic criteria. The increasing availability of clinically useful methods to document protein loss, such as the fecal alpha$_1$-AT assay, is likely to improve our ability to diagnose and treat these disorders.

REFERENCES

1. Rothschild MA, Oratz M, Schreiber SS. Albumin synthesis (first of two parts). N Engl J Med 1972; 286:748–757.
2. Hoffenberg R, Black E, Brock JF. Albumin and gamma-globulin tracer studies in protein depletion states. J Clin Invest 1966; 45:143–152.
3. Kirsch R, Frith L, Black E, Hoffenberg R. Regulation of albumin synthesis and catabolism by alteration of dietary protein. Nature 1968; 217:578–579.
4. Rothschild MA, Schreiber SS, Oratz M, McGee HL. The effects of adrenocortical hormones on albumin metabolism studied with albumin-I^{131}. J Clin Invest 1958; 37:1229–1235.
5. Rothschild MA, Bauman A, Yalow RS, Berson SA. The effect of large doses of desiccated thyroid on the distribution and metabolism of albumin-I^{131} in euthyroid subjects. J Clin Invest 1957; 36:422–428.
6. Rothschild MA, Oratz M, Schreiber SS. Albumin synthesis (second of two parts). N Engl J Med 1972; 286:816–821.
7. Wochner RD, Weissman SM, Waldmann TA, Houston D, Berlin NI. Direct measurement of the rates of synthesis of plasma proteins in control subjects and patients with gastrointestinal protein loss. J Clin Invest 1968; 47:971–982.
8. Jeffries GH, Holman HR, Sleisenger MH. Plasma proteins and the gastrointestinal tract. N Engl J Med 1962; 266:652–660.
9. Granger DN, Cook BH, Taylor AE. Structural locus of transmucosal albumin efflux in canine ileum. A fluorescent study. Gastroenterology 1976; 71:1023–1027.
10. Waldmann TA. Protein-losing enteropathy. Gastroenterology 1966; 50:422–443.
11. Waldmann TA. Gastrointestinal protein loss demonstrated by ^{51}Cr-labelled albumin. Lancet 1961; ii:121–123.
12. Waldmann TA, Wochner RD, Strober W. The role of the gastrointestinal tract in plasma protein metabolism. Am J Med 1969; 46:275–285.
13. Waldmann TA, Morell AG, Wochner RD, Sternlieb I. Quantitation of gastrointestinal protein loss with copper^{67}-labeled ceruloplasmin. J Clin Invest 1965; 44:1107.
14. Divgi CR, Lisann NM, Yeh SDJ, Benua RS. Technetium-99m albumin scintigraphy in the diagnosis of protein-losing enteropathy. J Nucl Med 1986; 27:1710–1712.
15. Gordon RS. Exudative enteropathy. Abnormal permeability of the gastrointestinal tract demonstrable with labelled polyvinylpyrrolidone. Lancet 1959; i:326–326.
16. Andersen SB, Jarnum S. Gastrointestinal protein loss measured with ^{59}Fe-labelled iron-dextran. Lancet 1966; i:1060–1062.
17. Van Tongeren JHM, Majoor CLH. Demonstration of protein-losing gastroenteropathy. The disappearance rate of ^{51}Cr from plasma and the binding of ^{51}Cr to different serum proteins. Clin Chim Acta 1966; 14:31–41.
18. Bernier JJ, Florent C, Desmazures C, Aymes C, L'Hirondel C. Diagnosis of protein-losing enteropathy by gastrointestinal clearance of alpha$_1$-antitrypsin. Lancet 1978; ii:763–764.
19. Crossley JR, Elliott RB. Simple method for diagnosing protein-losing enteropathies. Br Med J 1977; 1:428–429.
20. Buffone GJ, Shulman RJ. Characterization and evaluation of immunochemical methods for the measurement of fecal α_1-antitrypsin. Am J Clin Pathol 1985; 83:326–330.
21. Thomas DW, Sinatra FR, Merritt RJ. Random fecal alpha-1-antitrypsin concentration in children with gastrointestinal disease. Gastroenterology 1981; 80:776–782.
22. Dinari G, Rosenbach Y, Zahavi I, Sivan Y, Nitzan M. Random fecal α_1-antitrypsin excretion in children with intestinal disorders. Am J Dis Child 1984; 138:971–973.
23. Florent C, L'Hirondel C, Desmazures C, Aymes C, Bernier JJ. Intestinal clearance of α_1-antitrypsin. A sensitive method for the detection of protein-losing enteropathy. Gstroenterology 1981; 81:777–780.
24. Hill RE, Hercz A, Corey ML, Gilday DL, Hamilton JR. Fecal clearance of α_1-antitrypsin: a reliable measure of enteric protein loss in children. J Pediatr 1981; 99:416–418.
25. Maguzzu G, Jacono G, Di Pasquale G, Sferlazzas C, Tedeschi A, Santoro S, Conti Nibali S, Musso F, Balsamo V. Reliability and usefulness of random fecal α_1-antitrypsin concentration: further simplification of the method. J Pediatr Gastroenterol Nutr 1985; 4:402–407.
26. Thomas DW, Sinatra FR, Merritt RJ. Fecal α_1-antitrypsin excretion in young people with Crohn's disease. J Pediatr Gastroenterol Nutr 1983; 2:491–496.
27. Catassi C, Cardinali E, D'Angelo G, Coppa GV, Giorgi PL. Reliability of random fecal α_1-antitrypsin determination on nondried stools. J Pediatr 1986; 109:500–502.
28. Woodruff C, Fabacher D, Latham C. Fecal α_1-antitrypsin and infant feeding. J Pediatr 1985; 106:228–232.
29. Thomas DW, McGilligan KM, Carlson M, Azen SP, Eisenberg LD, Lieberman HM, Rissman EM. Fecal α_1-antitrypsin and hemoglobin excretion in healthy human milk-, formula-, or cow's milk-fed infants. Pediatrics 1986; 78:305–312.
30. Vardy PA, Lebenthal E, Shwachman H. Intestinal lymphangiectasia: a reappraisal. Pediatrics 1975; 55:842–851.
31. Vallet HL, Holtzapple PG, Eberlein WR, Yakovac WC, Moshang T, Bongiovanni AM. Noonan syndrome with intestinal lymphangiectasis. A metabolic and anatomic study. J Pediatr 1972; 80:269–274.
32. Jones KL. Smith's recognizable patterns of human malformation. 4th ed. Philadelphia: WB Saunders, 1988.
33. Shani M, Theodor E, Frand M, Goldman B. A family with protein-losing enteropathy. Gastroenterology 1974; 66:433–445.
34. Strober W, Wochner RD, Carbone PP, Waldmann TA. Intestinal lymphangiectasia: a protein-losing enteropathy with hypogammaglobulinemia, lymphocytopenia and impaired homograft rejection. J Clin Invest 1967; 46:1643–1656.
35. Weiden PL, Blaese RM, Strober W, Block JB, Waldmann TA. Impaired lymphocyte transformation in intestinal lymphangiectasia: evidence for at least two functionally distinct lymphocyte populations in man. J Clin Invest 1972; 51:1319–1325.
36. Foster PN, Bullen AW, Robertson DAF, Chalmers DM, Losowsky MS. Development of impaired splenic function in intestinal lymphangiectasia. Gut 1985; 26:861–864.
37. Sorensen RU, Halpin TC, Abramowsky CR, Hornick DL, Miller KM, Naylor P, Incefy GS. Intestinal lymphangiectasia and thymic hypoplasia. Clin Exp Immunol 1985; 59:217–226.
38. Bolton RP, Cotter KL, Losowsky MS. Impaired neutrophil function in intestinal lymphangiectasia. J Clin Pathol 1986; 39:876–880.
39. Shimkin PM, Waldmann TA, Krugman RL. Intestinal lymphangiectasia. Am J Roentgenol Radium Ther Nucl Med 1970; 110:827–841.
40. Asakura H, Miura S, Morishita T, Aiso S, Tanaka T, Kitahora T, Tsuchiya M, Enomoto Y, Watanabe Y. Endoscopic and histopathological study

on primary and secondary intestinal lymphangiectasia. Dig Dis Sci 1981; 26:312–320.

41. Hart MH, Vanderhoof JA, Antonson DL. Failure of blind small bowel biopsy in the diagnosis of intestinal lymphangiectasia. J Pediatr Gastroenterol Nutr 1987; 6:803–805.

42. Holt PR. Dietary treatment of protein loss in intestinal lymphangiectasia. Pediatrics 1964; 33:629–635.

43. Tift WL, Lloyd JK. Intestinal lymphangiectasia. Long-term results with MCT diet. Arch Dis Child 1975; 50:269–276.

44. Gutmann L, Shockcor W, Gutmann L, Kien CL. Vitamin E-deficient spinocerebellar syndrome due to intestinal lymphangiectasia. Neurology 1986; 36:554–556.

45. Mistilis SP, Skyring AP. Intestinal lymphangiectasia. Therapeutic effect of lymph venous anastomosis. Am J Med 1966; 40:634–641.

46. Lester LA, Rothberg RM, Krantman HJ, Shermeta DW. Intestinal lymphangiectasia and bilateral pleural effusions: effect of dietary therapy and surgical intervention on immunologic and pulmonary parameters. J Allergy Clin Immunol 1986; 78:891–897.

47. Cochran WJ, Klish WJ, Brown MR, Lyons JM, Curtis T. Chylous ascites in infants and children: a case report and literature review. J Pediatr Gastroenterol Nutr 1985; 4:668–673.

48. Davidson JD, Waldmann TA, Goodman DS, Gordon RS. Protein-losing gastroenteropathy in congestive heart-failure. Lancet 1961; i:899–902.

49. Nelson DL, Blaese RM, Strober W, Bruce RM, Waldmann TA. Constrictive pericarditis, intestinal lymphangiectasia, and reversible immunologic deficiency. J Pediatr 1975; 86:548–554.

50. Popovic OS, Brkic S, Bojic P, Kenic V, Jojic N, Djuric V, Djordjevic N. Sarcoidosis and protein losing enteropathy. Gastroenterology 1980; 78:119–125.

51. Kobayashi A, Ohbe Y. Protein-losing enteropathy associated with arsenic poisoning. Am J Dis Child 1971; 121:515–517.

52. Rao SSC, Dundas S, Holdsworth CD. Intestinal lymphangiectasia secondary to radiotherapy and chemotherapy. Dig Dis Sci 1987; 32:939–942.

53. Fleisher TA, Strober W, Muchmore AV, Broder S, Krawitt EL, Waldmann TA. Corticosteroid-responsive intestinal lymphangiectasia secondary to an inflammatory process. N Engl J Med 1979; 300:605–606.

54. Chouraqui JP, Roy CC, Brochu P, Gregoire H, Morin CL, Weber AM. Ménétrier's disease in children: report of a patient and review of sixteen other cases. Gastroenterology 1981; 80:1042–1047.

55. Bar-Ziv J, Barki Y, Weizman Z, Urkin J. Transient protein-losing gastropathy (Ménétrier's disease) in childhood. Pediatr Radiol 1988; 18:82–84.

56. Lachman RS, Martin DJ, Vawter GF: Thick gastric folds in childhood. AJR 1971; 112:83–92.

57. Leonidas JC, Beatty EC, Wenner HA. Ménétrier disease and

cytomegalovirus infection in childhood. Am J Dis Child 1973; 126:806–808.

58. Marks MP, Lanza MV, Kahlstrom EJ, Mikity V, Marks SC, Kvalstad RP: Pediatric hypertrophic gastropathy. AJR 1986; 147:1031–1034.

59. Coad NAG, Shah KJ. Ménétrier's disease in childhood associated with cytomegalovirus infection: a case report and review of the literature. Br J Radiol 1986; 59:615–620.

60. Katz AJ, Goldman H, Grand RJ. Gastric mucosal biopsy in eosinophilic (allergic) gastroenteritis. Gastroenterology 1977; 73:705–709.

61. Scharschmidt BF. The natural history of hypertrophic gastropathy (Ménétrier's disease). Am J Med 1977; 63:644–652.

62. Larsen B, Tarp U, Kristensen E. Familial giant hypertrophic gastritis (Ménétrier's disease). Gut 1987; 28:1517–1521.

63. Sherman P, Liebman WM. Apparent protein-losing enteropathy associated with giardiasis. Am J Dis Child 1980; 134:893–894.

64. Hoffman H, Hanekom C. Random faecal alpha-1-antitrypsin excretion in children with acute diarrhoea. J Trop Pediatr 1987; 33:299–301.

65. Cooperstock M, Riegle L, Fabacher D, Woodruff CW. Relationship between fecal α_1-antitrypsin and colonization with Clostridium difficile in asymptomatic infants. J Pediatr 1985; 107:257–259.

66. King CE, Toskes PP. Protein-losing enteropathy in the human and experimental rat blind-loop syndrome. Gastroenterology 1981; 80:504–509.

67. Powell GK. Milk- and soy-induced enterocolitis of infancy. J Pediatr 1978; 93:553–560.

68. Katz AJ, Twarog FJ, Zeiger RS, Falchuk ZM. Milk-sensitive and eosinophilic gastropathy: similar clinical features with contrasting mechanisms and clinical course. J Allergy Clin Immunol 1984; 74:72–78.

69. Waldmann TA, Wochner RD, Laster L, Gordon RS. Allergic gastroenteropathy. A cause of excessive gastrointestinal protein loss. N Engl J Med 1967; 276:761–769.

70. Shulman RJ, Buffone G, Wise L. Enteric protein loss in necrotizing enterocolitis as measured by fecal α_1-antitrypsin excretion. J Pediatr 1985; 107:287–289.

71. Weisdorf SA, Salati LM, Longsdorf JA, Ramsay NKC, Sharp HL. Graft-versus-host disease of the intestine: a protein losing enteropathy characterized by fecal α_1-antitrypsin. Gastroenterology 1983; 85:1076–1081.

72. Grill BB, Hillemeier AC, Gryboski JD. Fecal α_1-antitrypsin clearance in patients with inflammatory bowel disease. J Pediatr Gastroenterol Nutr 1984; 3:56–61.

73. Karbach U, Ewe K, Bodenstein H. Alpha$_1$-antitrypsin, a reliable endogenous marker for intestinal protein loss and its application in patients with Crohn's disease. Gut 1983; 24:718–723.

74. Ament ME, Ochs HD, Davis SD. Structure and function of the gastrointestinal tract in primary immunodeficiency syndromes. A study of 39 patients. Medicine 1973; 52:227–248.

PART

37

Idiopathic Constipation

Michael J. Pettei, M.D., Ph.D.
Murray Davidson, M.D.

Constipation is a poorly defined but common problem in the pediatric age group. It may be associated with significant functional disability and family discord. Although it is often easily remedied in the acute stage, the patient frequently presents long after the symptom initially appears when it may be more intractable. Difficulties with defecation are generally recognized as being common in infants and children.[1] It has been estimated that from 10 to 25 percent of children referred to pediatric gastroenterology practices are seen for disorders of defecation—attesting to the scope of the problem.[2,3] Chronic constipation with soiling is reported to make up 3 percent of referrals to teaching hospital clinics.[4,5] Despite the general pediatric consensus that difficulty with defecation is a common problem, it is amazing how few data are available about normal and abnormal stooling patterns.[6] Even the definition of constipation is poorly established and stirs controversy. It is difficult to define, in part, because interpretation of the normal defecation pattern is to some extent subjective and varies with the observer.

DEFINITION

Constipation is usually defined in terms of alterations in the frequency, size, consistency, or ease of passage of stool. The greatest amount of objective data has been gathered on the frequency of passage of stool, since it is difficult to quantify normal size, consistency, or ease of passage.[7] It has been established that most adults pass at least three stools per week.[8] Review of a number of studies in infants and children reveals an expected decline in the frequency of defecation with age. Nyhan[9] studied 800 infants evenly divided between breast and cow's milk formula feeding during the first week of life. The average number of daily stools rose from 1.4 on the day of birth to approximately four per day at 1 week of age. In babies, the gastrocolic reflex seems well-developed, with stools frequently passed during or just after a feeding. Weaver et al[10] studied 240 infants between 2 and 20 weeks of age, again evenly divided between breast and cow's milk formula feeding. Initially, breast-fed infants had more frequent bowel movements with a greater range in number, but by 16 weeks of age the mean frequency of defecation had declined to about two per day for both groups. Wolman[11] studied 1,000 cow's milk formula–fed infants between 1 and 12 months of age and noted a decline in average bowel action frequency from 2.7 to 1.7 bowel movements per day. Weaver and Steiner[12] studied 350 children 1 to 4 years old from a single general practice and found a decline from 1.6 bowel movements per day at 1 year old to 1.2 per day at 4 years. The normal range was fairly narrow, with only 4 percent of children at 1 year of age having more than three movements per day or less than one every other day. In adults, the average tends to be one movement per day, with a normal frequency between three stools per day and three stools per week.[8,13,14]

The transit time from the mouth to the anus is closely related to the frequency of bowel action. The decline in frequency of defecation with age correlates with increasing mean whole gut transit times: less than 10 hours in infants 1.5 months old,[15] 16 hours at 4 to 24 months old,[16] 26 hours in 3 to 13 year olds,[17] and 30 to 48 hours in adults.[18] The transit time is largely influenced by dietary fiber. The above studies on normal (i.e., average) defecation patterns were all carried out in Western, industrialized countries. The infants and children studied ate a predominantly low-fiber diet. Burkitt,[18] examining the contrasting pattern of gastrointestinal (GI) disease in Africa and Europe, noted the inverse relation between stool weight and transit time. Those eating a diet high in fiber produced large stools more often, compared to those on a low-fiber diet, who passed small stools infrequently. This appears to apply to children also.[12,19,20]

In summary, early life is the period of maximum defecation frequency, with more than four stools per day during the first week of life declining to 1.2 per day at 4 years of age. Thus by 4 years of age the adult pattern seems to be achieved,

with the norm tending to be a frequency of one bowel movement per day. These developmental patterns are illustrated in Figure 1. Despite these data defining "normal" stool frequency for age, constipation is still inadequately described since individuals who have stools in the "normal" range can have constipation as manifested by hard stools that are difficult to pass. Nevertheless, infants with no difficulty other than fewer numbers of stools than average seem to constitute a disproportionate percentage of those who later develop frank constipation.[21] This implies that recognition of the trend toward decreased stool frequency in the first years of life may lead to more timely intervention and possible avoidance of chronic constipation in later years.

NORMAL DEFECATION

The specialized anatomy and physiology of the anorectal region determine the combination of physical factors and reflexes that control defecation. Although far from complete, our knowledge of the interrelationship of the various autonomic and conscious controls over the sensory and motor components of the anorectal region has increased significantly in recent years.[22] The lumen of the rectum ends at the pelvic floor, where it passes through the levator ani muscles and continues as the anal canal. This canal is surrounded by the internal and external sphincters, which overlap each other considerably (Fig. 2). The distal continuation of the circular smooth muscle layer of the rectum becomes three to four times thicker to form the internal sphincter. The external sphincter is made up of striated muscle with various attachments and components at different levels. Both the internal and external sphincters have a resting tone that creates a high-pressure region in the anal canal. This zone represents a barrier to rectal pressure and is thought to be a mechanism for

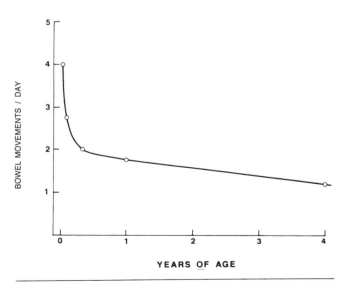

FIGURE 1 Developmental decline in average stool frequency. (Data averaged from references 9–12.)

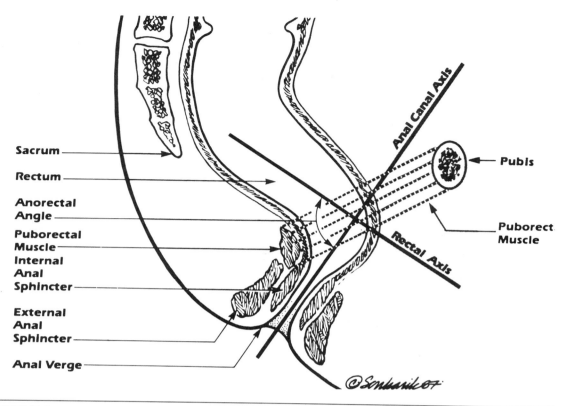

FIGURE 2 Anatomy of the anorectal region. (Adapted from Pettei[74].)

continence. Distention of the rectum by a bolus of stool from proximal bowel results in characteristic reflex relaxation (the rectosphincteric relaxation reflex) of the internal anal sphincter and simultaneous contraction of the striated external sphincter. This reflex relaxation of the upper anal canal allows rectal contents to come in contact with the highly sensory epithelium in the canal.[23] This helps distinguish the nature of the contents as solid, liquid, or gaseous, and the reflex contraction of the external sphincter maintains continence. Voluntary contraction of the external sphincter and puborectal muscles can extend the period of continence and presumably allow the rectum to accommodate the increased volume with a disappearance of the sense of urgency.

The axis of the rectum forms approximately a right angle with the axis of the anal canal and is created by the continuous tonic contraction of the striated puborectal muscle. This angle is present except when the hips are flexed more than 90 degrees or during defecation. This angulation is one of the most important mechanisms for fecal continence.

The stimulus to the initiation of defecation is distention of the rectum. This distention induces relaxation of the internal sphincter and contraction of the external sphincter. In adults, the subject takes up the squatting position for defecation. In doing so, the angulation between the rectum and the anal canal is straightened out. Increasing intra-abdominal pressure (the Valsalva maneuver) lowers the pelvic floor, with resulting increases in intrarectal pressure. Inhibition of the external sphincter permits expulsion of the fecal bolus.

Some aspects of the developmental processes affecting anorectal structure and function are known in the infant. Internal sphincter relaxation with rectal distention has been demonstrated in most term infants, but its presence in premature infants is unclear. The development of a normal reflex appears to depend on postnatal as well as gestational age. Holschneider et al[24] could consistently demonstrate normal reflexes only in infants older than 38 weeks' gestational age after they were 12 days old. Ito et al[25] first observed normal responses at 39 weeks. In contrast, Boston et al[26] reported normal responses down to 34 weeks' gestational age and Bowes and Kling[27] down to 27 weeks. Also of interest is a significantly higher maximal intraluminal pressure in the anal canal in infants less than 10 hours old, which may be related to the in utero absence of defecation.[16] Cyclic rhythmic contractions in the anal canal, similar to those found in Hirschsprung's disease, have been observed in some normal neonates.[26] For most of an infant's first year of life, defecation occurs by reflex action, since relaxation of the internal sphincter leads automatically to defecation. With time, the infant/toddler exerts more volitional control over bowel movements through the use of external sphincter and puborectal muscles and positional control. This is not synonymous with bowel training, which is the modification of defecation control to socially acceptable time and place.

PATHOGENESIS AND MECHANISMS

Failure of any portion of the mechanism for defecation results in difficulty with evacuation. Constipation is a symptom, not a disease, and as such is associated with many disorders. In the vast majority of children no associated abnormality is found, and the term *chronic functional (idiopathic) consti-*

pation is usually applied. There is no consensus regarding the pathophysiology of constipation— hence the term *idiopathic*. It seems probable that the mechanism underlying constipation may differ in patients of different ages and sexes. For example, the observation that severe, refractory constipation in young to middle-aged adults is almost entirely confined to women suggests that these patients share a common pathophysiology.[28] This may be the impaired delivery of stool to the rectum in these patients.[29] Given that there may be multiple mechanisms for constipation, our understanding is confounded by the fact that most studies are carried out on a range of patients of differing ages and sexes with differing severity of disease. This is not to mention differences in study methodology or outcome variables. Despite these problems, the clinical presentation of chronic retentive constipation is quite similar in referred children, and a current clinical model of chronic childhood constipation exists which entails a continuum of pathophysiology.

Genetic predisposition to chronic childhood constipation appears to be a major factor. Between 38 percent[4] and 65 percent[21] of children with constipation demonstrate a tendency toward constipation before 6 months of age. Another study found that in 40 percent constipation could be traced back to the first month of life,[30] before there are significant variations in diet or habits. In one study of twins, Bakwin and Davidson[31] found that concordance for constipation was six times greater among identical than among fraternal twins. Such a twin study is generally taken to indicate the importance of heredity over conditioning for a symptom. Recently, Gottlieb and Schuster,[32] utilizing another genetic technique (dermatoglyphic patterns), reported evidence for a congenital syndrome of early-onset constipation in an adult population. Since the history often dates to the first months of life, and there is frequently a positive family history,[21] genetic predisposition may play a role in a significant number of children with chronic constipation and encopresis. These studies and clinical experience suggest that just as patterns of growth and physical characteristics can be inherited, varied patterns of colonic motility also may be inherited. Constipation then could represent one extreme of a continuum of physiologic motility.

Waves of increased pressure in the rectum of constipated infants with colic have been shown to be similar to those in some adults with constipation or irritable bowel syndrome.[33] The increased ability of constipated children to absorb water in the distal colon has also been shown.[34] The infant with a tendency to constipation thus may have increased tonus in the distal colon associated with delay in stool passage and excessive drying of the intraluminal contents. The infant who passes one or two stools per day is usually not considered constipated even though these numbers represent a lower than average frequency (as previously detailed). However, between 6 and 12 months of age, as the number of stools per day decreases in the usual fashion, such an infant often begins to skip days and starts to eliminate small, dry scybala.

Between approximately 1 and 2 years of age, some children with a tendency toward constipation may develop a new set of problems related to fecal retention. In some, it develops gradually as a consequence of the decreasing stool frequency with increasing difficulty in passing the resultant excessively firm stools. In others, an acute episode of constipation

may occur associated with a change in diet (e.g., human to cow's milk), febrile illness, dehydration, bed rest, or failed attempts at toilet training. With increasing awareness that defecation is under voluntary control, a child may begin to withhold stool to avoid the pain of the severely constipated stools or associated anal fissures.

During this "stool-withholding" behavior, the child assumes a posture to avoid defecation. When the child experiences an urge to defecate, the toddler often retires to a corner of the room to hide or grip a piece of furniture for support, assumes an erect posture (the opposite of squatting), and holds the legs and gluteals stiffly together to help forcefully contract the external anal sphincter. Eventually, the rectum accommodates to its contents and the urge to defecate passes. This behavior initiates a vicious circle in which successively greater amounts of stool are retained in the rectum. The resulting larger bowel movement ultimately is passed with even greater pain, reinforcing the desire to withhold. Parents often erroneously interpret this behavior as extreme straining to pass stool. Persistence of this situation may lead to prolonged stretching of the rectal wall, which produces the state known as megarectum. Ultimately, the rectum reaches a maximal size and can accommodate no more stool. The force of the fecal mass shortens the anal canal and stool begins to leak to the outside. This condition of stool soiling unrelated to any organic defect is called encopresis.[35]

Encopresis

The term *encopresis* was first used in 1926 by Weissenberg to describe the fecal equivalent of enuresis.[36] Since that time there has been confusion concerning the definition of the term and the etiology of the condition it describes. Historically, encopresis was viewed as a mental disorder and is currently included in the *Diagnostic and Statistical Manual of Mental Disorders (DSM-III)*. Despite the large psychiatric literature on encopresis, no study has shown encopresis to be related to psychological trauma or stress; nevertheless, this became an almost universal assumption early-on.[37] In the psychiatric literature, encopresis has been recently defined as "uncontrolled defecation of emotional origin."[38]

However, Levine et al[39] found that medical intervention alone led to improvement without any symptom substitution. Abrahamian and Lloyd-Still[40] found that only 20 percent of patients with encopresis had significant psychological problems, and most of these started after the onset of encopresis. In contrast, there are a large number of recent studies delineating physiologic (principally manometric) abnormalities, which are outlined later.

Encopresis rarely begins before the age of 3. Levine found a mean age of 7 years, 4 months.[4] The overwhelming preponderance of males is persistently reported. Encopresis is reported to make up 3 percent of referrals to large teaching hospital clinics[4,5] and has been noted in 1.3 percent of those over 4[41] and 1 to 2 percent of 7 year olds.[42] The child often states that this "overflow" soiling occurs without the perceived urge to defecate and is involuntary. Parents often find this situation frustrating, and soiling frequently becomes a major issue of contention between parent and child. The parents often date the onset of their child's problem to the appearance of this soiling without knowledge of prior existing constipation. Rectal manometry suggests that the constantly stretched rectum of encopretic children exhibits decreased sensitivity to distention.[43] The child, therefore, has a lessened sense of rectal fullness with infrequent urge to defecate.

The term "psychogenic constipation" is still frequently applied to these children with chronic functional constipation in whom fecal retention and megarectum occur (for historical reasons outlined above). Although emotional and behavioral problems may be significantly associated with stool-withholding and soiling, appropriate therapy that corrects the physical problems often leads to resolution of the emotional tensions. This suggests that generalizations should not be made regarding psychological factors as the cause or effect of constipation and encopresis. By contrast, an uncommon state of nonorganic, nonretentive soiling exists which is often associated with serious psychiatric problems. There are, of course, numerous organic causes for fecal incontinence that by definition are not called encopresis.

Manometric Abnormalities

Certain techniques have been developed to investigate the pathophysiology of disorders involving the anal sphincters, rectum, and pelvic floor. These techniques can generally be grouped into four categories: anorectal manometry, electromyography, radiographic defecography, and rectal compliance. Of these, anorectal manometry is the methodology applied most frequently, at least in pediatrics. Over the last 10 years a large number of studies have documented abnormalities in children with chronic constipation and encopresis.

Anorectal manometry measures pressures and is a means of quantifying the function of the internal and external sphincters. There is no accepted standardized method for performing anal sphincter manometry, and this may account for some of the inconsistency that occurs from study to study. Different techniques have been used; the two most widely applied being fluid-filled open-tipped catheters and closed multiple balloon systems (Fig. 3). In the most common recording systems, fluid is perfused at a constant rate from the transducer (which measures pressure) to a small hole in the side of the probe. Pressures in the anorectal canal are usually measured at 1-cm intervals using a station pull-out technique or a continuous pull-out method. An inflatable balloon is attached to the end of the probe to ascertain the effects of rectal distention. The closed balloon recording system uses a rigid hollow support tube that is fitted with two balloons designed to straddle the internal and external sphincters. A catheter with a balloon is inserted through the hollow tube to reside in the rectum. This is a convenient method of detecting relative pressure changes in response to rectal distention. In both methods, the rectal balloon is inflated to ascertain the presence of the rectosphincteric reflex, that is, relaxation of the internal anal sphincter (IAS) and contraction of the external. The rectal balloon can also be used to ascertain rectal sensitivity: The threshold volume is the amount of rectal distention required to produce conscious awareness, and the critical volume is the amount required to initiate reflex IAS relaxation.

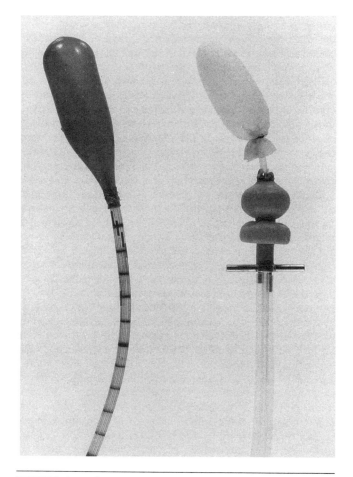

FIGURE 3 Catheters in use for anorectal manometry. *Left,* Open-tipped, water-perfused catheter with single rectal balloon. *Right,* Closed, triple-balloon recording system with external sphincter, internal sphincter, and rectal balloons.

Many investigators have reported various alterations in the manometric behavior of the anorectal segment in constipated and encopretic children. However, most studies are conflictory with regard to these alterations. Although qualitative results can be compared from series to series regardless of the instrumentation and techniques, lack of standardization prevents comparisons on a quantitative basis. The most consistent abnormality shown by manometry is an elevated threshold to perceive rectal distention.[43-47] This may correlate with the chronic rectal fullness of constipation and encopresis and the increased rectal size. Baseline anal canal pressure has been found to be increased,[30,44,45,48] similar to control[49,50] and low.[5,51] The differences in the anal resting tone in these studies could result from differences in the instruments used, the sites from which motor activity was recorded, or the severity and chronicity of the constipation. Several studies have reported abnormalities in the rectoanal inhibitory reflex. These include reduced relaxation[5,47,48,50] of the internal sphincter upon rectal distention and an increased minimum volume (critical volume) required to induce relaxation.[30,44,46,52] Some have demonstrated active contraction of the external anal sphincter during defecation in some constipated patients.[52,53] This was associated with a subset of constipated patients with an increased severity and poor response to treatment.[52]

It is important to remember that simply because certain manometric findings are associated with constipation in children does not assure these findings a role in the pathogenesis of this problem. In particular, it is unclear whether these abnormalities are primary or secondary to prolonged constipation. Although these types of studies give hope for a better understanding of the mechanism of prolonged constipation, the role of these abnormalities remains unclear. Any ultimate, future pathophysiologic understanding of chronic constipation must take into account the strong indications of genetic predisposition found in the onset in the first few months of life and family history and the evolving clinical model of transient constipation, voluntary withholding, fecal retention, and overflow soiling outlined previously.

Differential Diagnosis

Constipation is a symptom, not a disease, and as such it is associated with many disorders. A number of different classifications have been attempted. Table 1 classifies constipation caused by (1) delay of stool in reaching the distal colon, (2) excessively long retention in distal colon, and (3) difficulty in elimination from this segment. This listing allows for classification based on the presumed final common pathway. Table 2 lists some of the more common medications applicable

TABLE 2
Drugs Used in Children That May Cause Constipation

Antacids (calcium and aluminum compounds)
Anticholinergics (decongestants, antispasmodics)
Anticonvulsants
Antidepressive agents (phenothiazines)
Barium sulfate
Bismuth
Diuretics
Hematinics (especially iron)
Heavy metal ingestions (arsenic, lead, mercury)
Muscle paralyzers
Opiates

to pediatrics that may promote constipation, principally by hypomotility. The most frequently considered organic differential problem in patients with constipation is Hirschsprung's disease (congenital aganglionosis or congenital megacolon).

Hirschsprung's disease is a congenital anomaly of the GI tract characterized by the absence of the intramural ganglion cells of the submucosal and myenteric plexuses from the distal rectum to a variable length proximally. The defect occurs in about 1 in 5,000 live births and is four times more common in boys than girls. The disease is familial, with 7.2 percent of siblings of index cases affected. Those with long-segment disease are more likely to have a family history of Hirschsprung's disease, and males predominate only 2.8 to 1 over

TABLE 1
Conditions Associated with Constipation

I. Slowed gastrointestinal motility/prolonged gut transit time
  A. Generalized defects
    1. Hypothyroidism
    2. Hyperparathyroidism and other causes of hypercalcemia
    3. Hypokalemia, hyponatremia
    4. Lead ingestion
    5. Infant botulism
    6. Chronic intestinal pseudo-obstruction syndrome
    7. Drugs (see Table 2)
    8. Neuromuscular, such as those secondary to diabetes, lupus erythematosus, scleroderma, neurofibromatosis

  B. Isolated defects
    1. Hirschsprung's disease and Chagas' disease
    2. Abdominopelvic masses such as anterior sacral meningomyelocele, sacral teratoma, mesenteric nodal disease
    3. Malrotation, congenital intestinal bands, stenoses
    4. Acquired colonic strictures (IBD, NEC, infectious)
    5. Pyloric stenosis and other gastric emptying delays

II. Excessive distal colonic retention and drying
  A. Spastic constipation
  B. Malnutrition, underfeeding
  C. Low-fiber diet
  D. Dehydration and excessive urinary water losses, e.g., diuretics, diabetes

III. Difficulty with defecation
  A. Voluntary withholding
  B. Abnormalities in abdominal musculature (prune-belly syndrome, postgastroschisis, abdominal surgery)
  C. Disturbed neuromuscular innervation (spina bifida, meningomyelocele, spinal cord tumor, and paraplegia)
  D. Anorectal outlet obstructions (anal stenosis, stricture, postimperforate anus correction, anterior displaced anus, anal fissure)
  E. Hypotonia (Down's syndrome, cerebral palsy, myopathies)

females.[54] Association of congenital aganglionosis with Down's syndrome (trisomy 21) is 10 times more frequent than would be expected; about 2 percent of patients with congenital megacolon have Down's syndrome.[55] Developmentally, failure of the caudal migration of primordial ganglion cells from the neural crest results in an aganglionic segment. Thus, the aganglionic segment extends from the internal anal sphincter for a variable distance proximally. In approximately 75 percent of cases[56] the extent of involvement is the rectosigmoid colon, but in 6 to 21 percent of cases involvement extends to the cecum and rarely throughout the small bowel. The abnormal aganglionic segment is permanently contracted, causing dilation proximal to it. Absence of peristalsis in the aganglionic segment results in partial intestinal obstruction. Clinical findings and considerations for diagnosis are presented in the next section.

CLINICAL SIGNS AND SYMPTOMS OF CHRONIC CONSTIPATION

Symptoms associated with chronic constipation include intermittent abdominal pain, anorexia, abdominal distention, and excessive flatulence. Parents often describe a child with increasing irritability and decreasing appetite with the lack of a bowel movement and then a marked improvement in disposition and better appetite immediately after bowel movements. With encopresis, soiling characterized most typically by small amounts of soft stool is the most frequent finding. Often (10 percent of the time)[21] the initial complaint is an erroneous one of diarrhea. Both recurrent urinary tract infection[57] and enuresis[58] have been associated with encopresis and reported to improve upon resolution of the abnormal bowel habits. Often, the child with encopresis becomes socially ostracized, particularly by classmates, because of the obvious odors. This combined with the family discord leads to much social debility.

The diagnosis of chronic functional constipation and differentiation from the multiple organic causes listed rest principally on a detailed history and physical examination, with knowledge of the natural history of functional constipation. When taking a patient's history, special attention should be paid to stool frequency and size, the age of onset, dietary patterns, family history of constipation and functional bowel difficulties, evidence of whether the child perceives the urge to defecate, withholding behavior, the presence of soiling, and response to various therapeutic measures. The presence of specific associated findings such as vomiting, severe localized abdominal pain, persistent abdominal distention, and failure to thrive or weight loss should point to an organic cause. History should be directed with knowledge of the possible causes as listed in Table 1 and medications inquired into directly (Table 2). For example, in the breast-fed infant, questions and physical examination aimed at excluding infantile botulism need be considered; in the toddler, brief interrogation regarding pica (lead ingestion) should be undertaken.

The physical examination is particularly important for assessing the abdominal contents, anal tone and placement, sacral appearance and size, and contents of rectal ampulla as well as abdominal wall strength and neurologic status of the lower extremities. Abdominal distention is frequently not marked in patients with functional constipation, but fecal masses are often palpable above the pubic symphysis and in the left lower quadrants. Anorectal examination may reveal an ectopic anal opening, anal fissures, evidence of soiling, scybala, or the presence of a large amount of low-lying stool in a capacious rectum. Physical signs of underlying disorders include a patulous anus with neurologic disease, flat buttocks with sacral agenesis, and a pilonidal dimple with spina bifida occulta.[1] In anterior ectopic anus, the anal canal, surrounded by the internal anal sphincter, exits in the anterior perineal area, whereas the external anal sphincter remains distinct in its normal posterior location.[59] An external anal sphincter wink may be elicited in the usual location, posterior to the anal opening. In a separate condition, anteriorly located anus, a normal anal opening and associated sphincters are both displaced in the anterior perineum. This condition is associated with a posterior rectal shelf said to be etiologically related to constipation.[60]

Clinical Manifestations of Hirschsprung's Disease

The clinical symptoms of Hirschsprung's disease are those of partial bowel obstruction at the transition zone (the region where normal ganglionic bowel becomes abnormal aganglionic bowel). One report shows that 83 percent of those with Hirschsprung's disease develop difficulties with defecation in the first month of life, and 96 percent became symptomatic during the first year.[61] Typically, the infant, usually full-term and of average weight, has a delay in the passage of meconium. This is followed by abdominal distention, reluctance to eat, and finally bilious vomiting. Obstruction may lead to perforation. Older infants have constipation associated with abdominal distention and when symptomatic enough for hospitalization usually exhibit nonspecific signs of partial intestinal obstruction: failure to thrive, vomiting, abdominal distention, and intermittent diarrhea. On rectal examination the ampulla is found to be empty most of the time, although a high impaction may be palpable. Withdrawal of the examining finger often results in a gush of flatus and stool.

A severe form of enterocolitis associated with a mortality rate of about 33 percent[62] may develop most commonly in infants with Hirschsprung's disease. It can occur at any age either before or after operation but essentially never beyond 2 years. It is characterized by explosive, loose, heme-positive stools, fever, and prostration. In older children, the syndrome may feature persistent abdominal distention, recurrent fecal impaction, and obstipation. Intermittent bouts of partial intestinal obstruction, microcytic anemia, hypoalbuminemia, and failure to thrive are also associated.

Differentiation of Chronic Retentive Constipation from Hirschsprung's Disease

The most frequent organic differential problem in patients with constipation is Hirschsprung's disease (congenital megacolon). The conditions may almost always be distinguished, except in the newborn period, by significant differences in history and physical examination. Stool-withholding behavior indicates that stools are regularly being propelled to the rectum and renders unlikely the diagnosis of a problem more proximal (i.e., Hirschsprung's disease). Patients with Hirschsprung's disease rarely soil, since the retained stool is proximal to the rectum and involuntary passage of feces from an overfilled rectum is unlikely. On digital examination, the anal canal and rectum are almost always free of feces in the child with Hirschsprung's disease, whereas in the child with retentive constipation this region is usually packed with stool. Table 3 outlines these differences.

Procedures

When the patient with chronic constipation does not fit the developmental pattern outlined, does not present with the appropriate physical findings (especially with regard to Table 3), or is recalcitrant to therapy, then further evaluation should be considered. Attention should also be paid to the possibility of an underlying systemic or intestinal disease when constipation is of recent onset and is particularly severe. Investigations for Hirschsprung's disease include barium enema, rectal biopsy, and anorectal manometry, with definitive diagnosis ultimately taking place at the time of full-thickness colonic biopsy. The choice of study depends partly upon the experience of the available radiologic, pathologic, and manometric services as well as the presentation.

The barium enema study should be performed in an *unprepared* colon to better demonstrate the transition between the aganglionic distal segment, which is narrow or of normal caliber, and the proximal segment which is dilated (Fig. 4). This characteristic feature may not be demonstrable in the first weeks of life.[63] Even without a defined transition zone, reversal of the normal rectal/sigmoid ratio may be observed. In Hirschsprung's disease, the widest rectal diameter is usually smaller than the widest sigmoid diameter. In addition, late films taken 24 hours after barium administration show uniformly distributed retained barium in the colon.[64]

Since the diagnosis rests on histologic evidence of aganglionosis, rectal biopsy should be the most reliable method of diagnosis. Mucosal suction rectal biopsy is the procedure of choice, since it can be performed easily, requires no anesthesia, and carries minimal risk. If the depth of the biopsy is sufficient to show the presence of ganglia in the submucosal (Meissner's) plexus, classic Hirschsprung's disease is excluded. The absence of ganglia *accompanied* by hyperplastic neural elements in a biopsy of adequate depth and location is usually sufficient evidence for an operative approach.

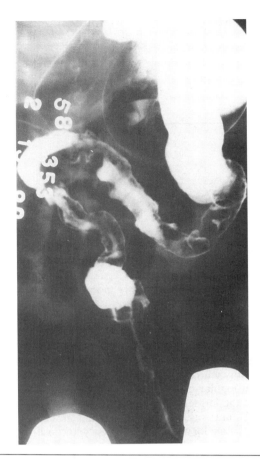

FIGURE 4 Barium enema study in Hirschsprung's disease. The transition from the narrow distal segment to the dilated proximal segment is observed.

Some have reported that application of acetylcholinesterase stains enhances the diagnostic features of the biopsy.[65,66] Care must be taken to obtain the biopsy at least 2.5 to 3.0 cm proximal to the dentate line, since there is a short naturally occurring aganglionic zone proximal to the dentate line.[67,68]

The most characteristic abnormality of function in Hirschsprung's disease is the failure of relaxation of the internal sphincter following rectal distention (the rectosphincteric relaxation reflex). This is the basis of the use of manometry as an excellent diagnostic tool for Hirschsprung's disease (Fig. 5); however, false-positive and false-negative tests may occur.[69] An entity known as ultra-short segment Hirschsprung's disease has been reported in which the only detectable abnormality is the lack of the rectosphincteric reflex. This entity may appear clinically similar to chronic retentive constipation[70] but is extremely rare.

PREVENTION AND TREATMENT OF CHRONIC IDIOPATHIC CONSTIPATION AND ENCOPRESIS

Therapy for constipation should take into account the particular developmental stage of the disorder. For patients with acute, simple constipation, dietary manipulations should be

TABLE 3
Clinical Comparison: Chronic Constipation versus Classic Hirschsprung's Disease

Signs and Symptoms	Constipation	Hirschsprung's Disease
Soiling	Common	Rare
Stool in ampulla	Common	Rare
Obstructive symptoms	Rare	Common
Large-caliber stools	Common	Rare
Stool-withholding behavior	Common	Rare
Enterocolitis	Never	Possible
Anorectal examination	Dilated ampulla	Narrow

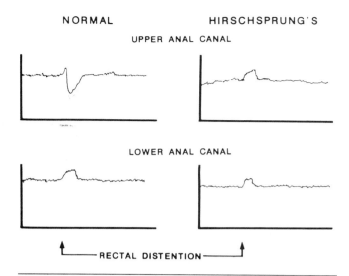

NORMAL   HIRSCHSPRUNG'S

UPPER ANAL CANAL

LOWER ANAL CANAL

←— RECTAL DISTENTION —→

FIGURE 5 Anorectal manometry in the diagnosis of Hirschsprung's disease (absence of the rectosphincteric relaxation reflex).

the mainstay of therapy. For example, infants usually have less difficulty with constipation ingesting breast milk or formula than regular cow's milk, owing to the higher lactose content of the former. In addition, infants who take laxative fruits (e.g., apricots, prunes, plums) and fibrous vegetables may compensate for an inherent tendency to constipation. For those with persistently firm stools, stool softness can be increased via colonic fermentation and gentle stimulation. Carbohydrate preparations such as dark corn syrup or malt soup extract (1 or 2 teaspoons two or three times daily), which are not fully digested and pass to the colon to undergo bacterial action, are preferable. Prudence must be exercised in using these agents in the first few months of life with colicky infants. Excessive gaseous distention from fermentation may make a constipated colicky infant more uncomfortable and irritable. For these, glycerin suppositories or rectal stimulation may be necessary for a short time. Reassurance should also be provided to the parent that the young infant may seem to be having difficulty with defecation, but the noises and grimaces may be normal if the stools are of normal consistency and frequency.

While overbearing preoccupation with bowel movements is not desirable, some attention is particularly necessary for the child with constipation between approximately 1 and 2 years of age. Benign neglect at this age can result in a pattern of chronic constipation which can result in stool-withholding behavior and eventually megarectum and encopresis. Thus, early attention to the possible need for laxative foods in the first year of life continues to be important. In the toddler, particular emphasis needs to be given to the avoidance of excessive dairy products and to the increased intake of high roughage foods. A number of different bran products can be tolerated at this age (e.g., bran cereals and bran muffins). However, toddlers often show quite tenacious dietary tendencies, and emphasis should be placed on finding a particular preference of the child that is beneficial and not letting the situation degenerate into a battle of wills be-

tween parent and child. The child almost always wins. In those who present with active stool-withholding behavior of short duration, therapy consisting of one to two cleansing enemas, followed by forced daily evacuation for several weeks with mild laxative or mineral oil therapy, is usually enough to reverse this pattern. Maintenance is achieved by dietary therapy, bowel training, or if necessary low-dose mineral oil or laxative therapy depending on the age of the child.

For children with chronic constipation who have progressed to an enlarged rectum and encopresis, treatment with a more regimented program is useful. Most are designed on the premise that maintaining the rectum empty of retained stool over time results in a decrease in rectal size and an increase of rectal sensitivity to distention.[21] Few controlled studies comparing different medication regimens exist.[71,72] Nevertheless, improvement has been reported in 90[21] to 95[73] percent of patients on such regimens. Before therapy is outlined, parents and patient should be educated to the natural history of encopresis with the removal of blame and to the observation that most soiling occurs involuntarily without the control of the child. Encouragement should be given that the most troublesome symptom, soiling, can usually be resolved quickly, although maintenance requires a prolonged effort.

The initial phase of therapy is disimpaction (Table 4).[74] This can be achieved effectively by the administration of a hypertonic phosphate enema (3 mg per kilogram) each morning and evening until the effluent contains no solid stool (usually two to six enemas). Since sodium (bi)phosphate enema abuse can result in hypernatremia or hyperphosphatemia, no more than two enemas each day for the initial 3 days should be advised without re-evaluation. They should be used in the individual without other significant medical problems (e.g., chronic heart failure or chronic renal failure) on an adequate fluid intake, and not in the very young child. Other cleanout regimens utilize suppositories, laxatives by mouth (bisacodyl), or rarely polyethylene glycol–electrolyte solution.[75] Rarely, the patient with severe, prolonged megarectum and hard impaction (fecaloma) may require multiple mineral oil enemas between phosphate enemas to achieve clean-out. Once an empty rectum is achieved, overflow soiling (encopresis) ceases.

The next phase of therapy is aimed at preventing the reaccumulation of retained feces and overcoming stool-withholding if present. Encopresis should not reoccur if rectal impactions are not permitted to reaccumulate. Prescription of a sufficient dose of stimulant or osmotic laxative (e.g., senna or lactulose) to "force" one to two stools daily should be sufficient. In those children in whom impressive megarectum has developed over years, this regimen often requires continuation on a prolonged basis. To achieve a faster solution to the problem, Davidson[21] introduced a high-dose mineral oil therapy (5 to 15 ml per kilogram divided into two doses per day) to induce multiple (four to six) bowel movements daily and achieve a more normal-sized rectum. This rigorous, high-dose mineral oil regimen is distasteful and difficult for most and thus has largely been abandoned. Forcible administration to an unwilling child should never be attempted for fear of aspiration.

The third stage of treatment is aimed at establishing regular bowel movements through the development of a conditioned response. Although evidence is sparse for advocating

TABLE 4
Treatment of Chronic Retentive Constipation

Colonic evacuation disimpaction
  Hypertonic phosphate enemas (3 ml/kg) twice daily until clear of solid stool (maximum
    of six without further examination)
  For some, medicated suppositories or oral laxatives (bisacodyl) can be substituted for enemas.
  For fecalomas, multiple mineral oil enemas between phosphate enemas

Prescription of laxative to "force" daily bowel movements
  Titration of dosage (senna, lactulose) to that necessary to achieve one or two bowel move-
    ments per day
  Rarely, high-dose mineral oil therapy (5–15 mg/kg b.i.d.) to achieve multiple movements
    (four to six times a day) to attain faster resolution of megarectum

Behavioral conditioning
  Sitting on the commode at the same time each day (after a meal) for 5 to 15 minutes
  Low-dose mineral oil therapy (30–60 ml q.h.s.) after laxative withdrawal to aid training
  High-fiber diet or administration of fiber supplement for older children (e.g., psyllium seed
    preparation)

---

regular bowel habits for normal individuals, the patient with chronic constipation should be encouraged to establish a routine. Conditioning to more frequent elimination assures softer stools and seems reasonable in children old enough to cooperate (e.g., over 3 to 4 years old). Advantage should be taken of the gastrocolic reflex by having the child sit on the commode for 5 to 15 minutes after a particular meal (usually breakfast) with proper foot support for leverage. For those on laxatives, the dosage should be gradually withdrawn over a few months while a regular bowel habit is formed. For those with more severe encopresis and megarectum, low-dose mineral oil therapy (30 to 60 ml at bedtime) may be needed upon laxative withdrawal to continue the bowel training. Concern about fat-soluble vitamin malabsorption with mineral oil has been lessened by the report of normal vitamin A and E status on mineral oil.[76] Concern about the development of dependency on laxatives is common, although there are few hard data to make a general conclusion. In the elderly, chronic use of laxatives was associated with the degeneration of ganglion cells of the myenteric plexus.[77]

For those who do not respond to the outlined regimen with a regular bowel habit, a more formalized behavior-modification program may be beneficial and, in particular, manometric biofeedback[78] may be useful. Parents should be cautioned to expect occasional bouts of acute constipation, which should be addressed promptly to avoid a recurrence of chronic problems. Children with *voluntary* fecal incontinence without megarectum or impaction (a distinct minority of less than 1 percent) are resistant to this regimen.[35] These children often have severe behavioral disorders and require psychiatric evaluation and treatment.

Prevention is always to be preferred over therapy. The attentive pediatrician with anticipatory guidance can do much to prevent the establishment of chronic constipation, stool-withholding, and encopresis. As already outlined, early recognition of these patterns with the institution of preventive dietary measures should abort the development of most of these behaviors. Once established, stool-withholding and encopresis do not respond to diet alone. Mention should be made of the benefits of adequate fluid ingestion, limited milk consumption, and the benefits of dietary fiber. Major changes in diet are usually unattainable and require adoption by the

family of a healthful diet with adequate fiber intake. Bran, in the form of a supplement, muffins, or a psyllium seed preparation can be used in the older child with spastic constipation.

SUMMARY AND CONCLUSIONS

Chronic idiopathic constipation and encopresis are common and often disabling problems in childhood. Our expanding knowledge of normal defecatory structure and function has extended our understanding of the traditional clinical behavioral model for the development of stool-withholding and encopresis. Despite this, much work remains to obtain a clearer understanding of the genesis and the optimal mode of therapy. Diagnosis rests almost completely on a thorough history and physical examination. Therapy can be effective, although in some cases prolonged. Manometry seems destined to play an increasing diagnostic and therapeutic (via biofeedback) role in the subgroup who respond poorly to traditional therapy. The primary care pediatrician can perform a major preventive function by anticipatory guidance and early dietary intervention. The diagnosis and treatment program can be provided by the pediatrician to most patients. The importance of attention to these disorders is confirmed by the amount of disordered family interaction and functional disability that can be promptly relieved by proper therapy.

REFERENCES

1. Fitzgerald JF. Difficulties with defecation and elimination in children. Clin Gastroenterol 1977; 6:283–297.
2. Fleisher PR. Diagnosis and treatment of disorders of defecation in children. Pediatr Ann 1976; 5:71–101.
3. Monar D, Taitz LS, Urwin OM, Wales JKH. Anorectal manometry results in defecation disorders. Arch Dis Child 1983; 58:257–261.
4. Levine MD. Children with encopresis: a descriptive analysis. Pediatrics 1975; 56:412–416.
5. Loening-Baucke V, Younoszai MK. Abnormal anal sphincter response in chronically constipated children. J Pediatr 1982; 100:213–218.
6. Schuster MM. Chronic constipation in children: the need for hard data about normal stools. J Pediatr Gastroenterol Nutr 1984; 3:336–337.
7. Weaver LT. Bowel habit from birth to old age. J Pediatr Gastroenterol Nutr 1988; 7:637–640.

8. Connell AM, Hilton C, Irvine G, et al. Variations of bowel habits in two population samples. Br Med J 1965; 2:1095–1099.

9. Nyhan WL. Stool frequency of normal infants in the first week of life. Pediatrics 1952; 10:414–425.

10. Weaver LT, Ewing G, Taylor LC. The bowel habit of milk-fed infants. J Pediatr Gastroenterol Nutr 1988; 7:568–571.

11. Wolman IJ. Intestinal motility in infancy and childhood. In: Wolman IJ, ed. Laboratory applications in clinical pediatrics. New York: McGraw-Hill, 1957: 696.

12. Weaver LT, Steiner H. The bowel habit of young children. Arch Dis Child 1984; 59:649–652.

13. Martelli H, DeVroede G, Arhan P, Duguay C, Dornic C, Faverdin C. Some parameters of large bowel function in normal man. Gastroenterology 1978; 75:612–618.

14. Drossman DA, Sandler RS, McKee DC, Lovitz AJ. Bowel patterns among subjects not seeking health care. Gastroenterology 1982; 83:529–534.

15. Foman SJ. Infant nutrition. Philadelphia: WB Saunders, 1974.

16. Triboulet H. Duree de la traversee chez l'enfant malade epreuve du carmin. Bull Soc Pediatr Paris 1909; 11:512–529.

17. Dimson SB. Carmine as an index of transit time in children with simple constipation. Arch Dis Child 1970; 45:232–235.

18. Burkitt DP, Walker ARP, Painter NS. Effect of dietary fibre on stools and transit-times, and its role in the causation of disease. Lancet 1972; ii:1408–1411.

19. Walker ARP, Walker BF. Bowel behavior in young black and white children. Arch Dis Child 1985; 60:967–970.

20. Burkitt D, Morley D, Walker A. Dietary fibre in under- and overnutrition in childhood. Arch Dis Child 1980; 55:803–807.

21. Davidson M, Kugler M, Bauer CH. Diagnosis and management in children with severe and protracted constipation and obstipation. J Pediatr 1963; 62:261–275.

22. Goldberg SM, Gordon PH, Nirvatrongs S. Essentials of anorectal surgery. Philadelphia: JB Lippincott, 1980: 1.

23. Duthie HL. Defecation and the anal sphincters. Clin Gastroenterol 1982; 11:121–131.

24. Holschneider AM, Kellner E, Streibl P, Sippell WG. The development of anorectal continence and its significance in the diagnosis of Hirschsprung's disease. J Pediatr Surg 1976; 11:151–156.

25. Ito Y, Donahoe PK, Hendren WH. Maturation of the rectoanal response in premature and perinatal infants. J Pediatr Surg 1977; 12:477–482.

26. Boston VE, Cywes S, Davies MRQ. Qualitative and quantitative evaluation of internal and sphincter function in the newborn. Gut 1977; 18:1036–1044.

27. Bowes KS, Kling S. Anorectal manometry in premature infants. J Pediatr Surg 1979; 14:533–535.

28. Preston DM, Lennard-Jones JE. Severe chronic constipation of young woman: idiopathic slow transit constipation. Gut 1986; 27:41–48.

29. Waldron D, Bowes KL, Kingma YJ, Cote KR. Colonic and anorectal motility in young women with severe idiopathic constipation. Gastroenterology 1988; 95:1388–1394.

30. Arhan P, Devroede G, Jehannin B, Faverdin C, Revillon Y, Lefevre D, Pellerin D. Idopathic disorders of fecal continence in children. Pediatrics 1983; 71:774–779.

31. Bakwin H, Davidson M. Constipation in twin. Am J Dis Child 1971; 121:179–181.

32. Gottlieb SH, Schuster MM. Dermatoglyphic (fingerprint) evidence for a congenital syndrome of early onset constipation and abdominal pain. Gastroenterology 1986; 91:428–432.

33. Jorup S. Colonic hyperperistalsis in neurolabile infants' studies in so-called dyspepsia in breast-fed infants. Acta Paediatr Scand 1952; 41(suppl 85):596–599.

34. Ziskind A, Gellis SS. Water intoxication following tap-water enemas. Am J Dis Child 1958; 96:699–704.

35. Fitzgerrald JF. Encopresis, soiling, constipation: What's to be done? Pediatrics 1975; 56:348–349.

36. Weissenberg S. Uber enkopresis. Kinderbeilk 1926; 40:674–677.

37. Stern HP, Prince MT, Stroh SE. Encopresis responsive to non-psychiatric interventions. Clin Pediatr 1988; 27:400–402.

38. Fisher SM. Encopresis. In: Noshpitz JD, ed. Basic handbook of child psychiatry. New York: Basic Books, 1979: 556.

39. Levine MD, Mazonson P, Bakow H. Behavioral symptom substitution in children cured of encopresis. Am J Dis Child 1980; 134:663–667.

40. Abrahamian FP, Lloyd-Still JD. Chronic constipation in childhood: a longitudinal study of 186 patients. J Pediatr Gastroenterol Nutr 1984; 3:460–467.

41. From birth to seven. Report from National Child Development Survey. London: 1972, p 399.

42. Levine MD. Encopresis: its potentiation, evaluation, and alleviation. Pediatr Clin North Am 1982; 29:315–330.

43. Meunier P, Mollard P, Marechal JM. Physiopathology of megarectum: the association of megarectum with encopresis. Gut 1976; 17:224–227.

44. Meunier P, Marechal JM, de Beaujeu MJ. Rectoanal pressures and rectal sensitivity studies in chronic childhood constipation. Gastroenterology 1979; 77:330–336.

45. Monar D, Taitz LS, Urwin OM, et al. Anorectal manometry results in defecation disorders. Arch Dis Child 1983; 58:257–261.

46. Cacchiatra S, Coremans G, Staiano A, et al. Gastrointestinal transit time and anorectal manometry in children with fecal soiling. J Pediatr Gastroenterol Nutr 1984; 3:545–550.

47. Loening-Baucke VA. Abnormal rectoanal function in children recovered from chronic constipation and encopresis. Gastroenterology 1984; 87:1299–1304.

48. Martelli H, Devroede G, Arhan P, Duguay C. Mechanisms of idiopathic constipation: outlet obstruction. Gastroenterology 1978; 75:623–631.

49. Bellman M. Studies on encopresis. Acta Pediatr Scand (Suppl) 1966; 1:170.

50. Behar J, Biancani P. Rectal function in patients with idiopathic chronic constipation. In: Romon C, ed. Gastrointestinal motility. Lancaster: MTP Press, 1984: 459.

51. Read NW, Timms JM, Barfield LJ, Donnelly TC, Bannister JJ. Impairment of defecation in young women with severe constipation. Gastroenterology 1986; 90:53–60.

52. Loening-Baucke VA, Cruikshank BM. Abnormal defecation dynamics in chronically constipated children with encopresis. J Pediatr 1986; 108:562–566.

53. Wald A, Chandra R, Chiponis D, Gabel S. Anorectal function and continence mechanisms in childhood encopresis. J Pediatr Gastroenterol Nutr 1986; 5:346–351.

54. Bugaighis AG, Lister J. Incidence of diabetes in families of patients with Hirschsprung's disease. J Pediatr Surg 1970; 5:620–621.

55. Passarge E. The genetics of Hirschsprung's disease. Evidence for heterogeneous etiology and a study of sixty-three families. N Engl J Med 1967; 276:138–143.

56. Kleinhaus S, Boley SJ, Sheran M, Sieber WK. Hirschsprung's disease: a survey of the members of the surgical section of the American Academy of Pediatrics. J Pediatr Surg 1979; 14:588–600.

57. Newmann PZ, deDomenico IJ, Nogrady MB. Constipation and urinary tract infection. Pediatrics 1973; 52:241–245.

58. O'Regan S, Yazbeck S, Hamberger B, Schick E. Constipation a commonly unrecognized cause of enuresis. Am J Dis Child 1986; 140:260–261.

59. Hatch TF. Encopresis and constipation in children. Pediatr Clin North Am 1988; 35:257–280.

60. Hendren WH. Constipation caused by anterior location of the anus and its surgical correction. J Pediatr Surg 1978; 13:505–512.

61. Tobon F, Schuster MM. Megacolon: special diagnostic and therapeutic features. Johns Hopkins Med J 1978; 135:91–105.

62. Bill AHJ, Chapman ND. The enterocolitis of Hirschsprung's disease. Am J Surg 1962; 103:70–74.

63. Pace JL. The age of appearance of the haustra of the human colon. J Anat 1971; 109:75.

64. Franken EA Jr. Gastrointestinal radiology in Pediatrics. Hagerstown, MD: Harper and Row, 1975: 323.

65. Trigg PH, Belin R, Haberkorn S, Long WJ, Nixon HH, Plaskes J, Spitz L, Willital GH. Experience with a cholinesterase histochemical technique for rectal suction biopsies in the diagnosis of Hirschsprung's disease. J Clin Pathol 1974; 27:207–213.

66. Toorman J, Bots G ThAM, Vio PMA. Acetylcholinesterase-activity in rectal mucosa of children with obstipation. Virchows Arch [A] 1977; 376:159–164.

67. Aldridge RT, Campbell PE. Ganglia cell distribution in the normal rectum and anal canal. A basis for the diagnosis of Hirschsprung's disease by anorectal biopsy. J Pediatr Surg 1968; 3:475–490.

68. Weinberg AG. The anorectal myenteric plexus; its relation to hypoganglionosis of the colon. Am J Clin Pathol 1970; 54:637.

69. Frenckner B. Anorectal manometry in the diagnosis of Hirschsprung's disease in infants. Acta Paediatr Scand 1978; 67:187.

70. Clayden GS, Lawson JON. Investigation and management of longstanding chronic constipation in childhood. Arch Dis Child 1976; 51:918–923.

71. Sondheimer, JM, Gervaise EP. Lubricant versus laxative in the treat-

ment of chronic functional constipation of children: a comparative study. J Pediatr Gastroenterol Nutr 1982; 1:223–226.

72. Perkin JM. Constipation in childhood: a controlled comparison between lactulose and standardized senna. Curr Med Res Opin 1977; 4:540–543.

73. Levine MD, Bakow H. Children with encopresis: a study of treatment outcome. Pediatrics 1976; 58:845–852.

74. Pettei MJ. Chronic constipation. Pediatr Ann 1987; 16:796–813.

75. Ingebo K, Heyman MB. Intestinal cleanout in children with encopresis and other intestinal disorders using a balanced polyethylene glycolelec-

trolyte solution. Gastroenterology 1987; 92:1446A.

76. Clark JH, Russel GJ, Fitzgerald JF. Serum beta-carotene, retinal and alpha-tocopherol levels during mineral oil therapy for constipation. Am J Dis Child 1987; 141:1210–1212.

77. Smith B. Effect of irritant purgatives on the myenteric plexus in man and the mouse. Gut 1968; 9:139–143.

78. Wald A. Chandra R, Gabel S, Chiponis D. Evaluation of biofeedback in childhood encopresis. J Pediatr Gastroenterol Nutr 1987; 6:554–558.

PART
38

Hirschsprung's Disease

Barbara S. Kirschner, M.D.

Congenital megacolon was reported first in 1888 by Hirschsprung, who observed dilatation and hypertrophy of the colon in two autopsied infants.[1] In 1920, Dalla Valle noted the absence of ganglion cells in the distal contracted segment.[2] A most important contribution to this field was made in 1948 by Swenson and Bill, who described the first successful definitive surgical procedure—resection of the aganglionic segment and reanastomosis.[3] Subsequently, attention has been directed toward developing methods that facilitate earlier diagnosis to reduce mortality and new surgical techniques to decrease postoperative complications.

EPIDEMIOLOGY

The best available epidemiologic information comes from a survey of 1196 patients conducted by the Surgical Section of the American Academy of Pediatrics in 1975–1976.[4] The disorder was diagnosed in 1:5000 live births and showed a male predominance of 3.8 to 1.0. Racial distribution was equal for Caucasian and black infants when corrected for the population at risk. A family history was noted in 7 percent of cases, except when the disease extended to the cecum; then the family prevalence increased to 21 percent.

Only 15 percent of infants are diagnosed within the first month of life, 64 percent by the third month, and 80 percent by 1 year,[4,5] but 8 percent may not be recognized until 3 to 12 years of age.[5] Diagnosis is relatively delayed in those with short-segment disease; 45 percent of these cases are not identified until 19 months to 7 years of age.[6] Among children with ultrashort-segment Hirschsprung's disease (5 cm or less), 81 percent are not diagnosed until 18 months to 14 years of age.[7] Most cases occur in full-term infants, with only 9.6 percent occurring in infants with birth weights under 6 pounds.[8]

The Hirschsprung's lesion is limited to the rectum and sigmoid in 75 percent of cases.[8,11] It includes the total colon in only 8 percent.[4] Several children with total colonic disease have also had aganglionosis of the ileum, jejunum, and duodenum.[9,10] Between 3 and 10 percent of cases of Down's syndrome may have Hirschsprung's disease.[8,12] In two large series of children with chronic constipation referred to medical centers to exclude Hirschsprung's disease, prevalence was 16 percent (24 of 150) and 23 percent (29 of 127),[5,13] but in medically treated children with protracted constipation prevalence was only 4 percent.[14]

PATHOGENESIS

Hirschsprung's disease results from the failure of craniocaudal migration of ganglion cell precursors along the GI tract during the fifth through twelfth weeks of gestation. The earlier in development that the arrest in migration occurs, the longer the aganglionic segment.[15] Absence of ganglion cells interrupts the expression of the inhibitory parasympathetic nerves in the myenteric plexus, thereby inhibiting relaxation of the contracted segment.[16] The preganglionic parasympathetic fibers are seen as long nerve trunks within the submucosal and intermuscular planes and also as thin fibers within the lamina propria and muscularis mucosae.[13,17] Their high acetylcholinesterase content provides a useful means for diagnosing Hirschsprung's disease, as will be discussed later. The aganglionic segment, internal sphincter, and anal canal remain constantly contracted, causing obstructive symptoms with proximal dilatation and hypertrophy of the colon. Intestinal ischemia may occur secondary to distention of the bowel wall and contribute to the development of enterocolitis, the leading cause of death in children with Hirschsprung's disease.[15]

CLINICAL MANIFESTATIONS

Presenting Symptoms

Swenson in a series of 501 children with Hirschsprung's disease reported that 94 percent failed to pass meconium in the first 24 hours and 57 percent in the first 48 hours after birth, in sharp contrast to normal infants, 94 percent of whom passed meconium in the first 24 hours of life.[8] Other symptoms included constipation (93 percent), vomiting (64 percent), diarrhea (26 percent), and perforation of the appendix or colon (3.4 percent). Inadequate nutrient intake and insufficient weight gain may occur. Fecal soiling, similar to that seen in functional megacolon, was noted in only 3 percent of cases and only in those older children with limited rectosigmoid involvement, a useful diagnostic point. Nissan and Bar-Maor did report fecal soiling in 13 percent of their group of 29 children with short-segment Hirschsprung's disease.[6] Fecal impactions recur frequently in these children. Kottmeier and Clatworthy observed rectal bleeding in 5 percent due to anal fissures.[18] Urinary retention with hydroureter and hydronephrosis may result from ureteral compression.

Physical Examination

Abdominal distention is seen in 83 percent of cases, an empty rectum on digital examination in 61 percent (especially those with long-segment disease), and rectal impaction in 7 percent (particularly in those with short-segment aganglionosis).[8] Rapid expulsion of stool often follows digital examination. When only children with short-segment disease are considered, retained feces in the rectum is noted in 93 percent.[6]

Enterocolitis is characterized by the presence of abdominal distention, explosive watery stools, fever, and, at times, hypovolemic shock. Bill and Chapman observed that 50 percent of their patients, one-third of whom died, had clinical signs of enterocolitis,[19] but in 13 percent of cases enterocolitis is not evident until the postoperative period. No specific bacterial pathogens have been implicated consistently in the etiology of the enterocolitis associated with Hirschsprung's disease.[14]

DIAGNOSIS

The importance of recognizing infants with Hirschsprung's disease early in their course is emphasized by the difference in mortality for those diagnosed without enterocolitis (4 percent) versus those with enterocolitis (33 percent).[20] Absence of gas in the pelvis on plain radiograph of the abdomen with the infant in the prone position suggests Hirschsprung's disease and a need for further studies. The limitations of each of the available methods for establishing the diagnosis must be appreciated.

Barium Enema

A single-contrast barium enema in the unprepared child is the standard method for localizing the transition zone between the contracted aganglionic segment and the dilated hypertrophied colon proximal to the aganglionic segment (see Color Plate IVC and D). The catheter without an inflated balloon should be placed just within the anal canal for barium administration to minimize the risk of failing to identify short-segment disease.[15]

Kottmeier and Clatworthy reported that barium enema was diagnostic in 81 percent, uncertain in 14 percent, and incor-

rect in 5 percent of their patients.[18] Swenson et al noted false-negative studies in 12 percent of their children, especially those less than 1 month of age or with disease limited to the rectum.[8] In 1986, Taxman et al still showed that while 80 percent of their patients had a transition zone radiologically apparent, 20 percent did not.[21] Delay in evacuation of barium is not a reliable sign of Hirschsprung's disease, as it is not present in 43 percent of patients. A rectal diameter narrower than the sigmoid colon is often seen in Hirschsprung's disease, an important diagnostic point, as children with severe functional megacolon have a dilated rectum that is larger than the more proximal colon.

Anal Manometry

In 1968, Tobon et al showed that balloon distention of the rectum was associated with contraction of the internal sphincter in 10 patients with Hirschsprung's disease in contrast to the expected normal relaxation.[16] This method detects approximately 95 percent of patients with aganglionosis, including infants less than 39 weeks and less than 2.7 kg,[6,13] although others have reported less accurate results in premature infants. Rosenberg and Vela described the use of a microtip pressure transducer to distinguish children with Hirschsprung's disease from those with chronic constipation.[22] They emphasized that sedation did not interfere with the internal sphincter response to balloon distention. Anal manometry is particularly useful in children with ultrashort-segment disease (5 cm or less) who may have normal barium enema studies and normal histochemical staining for acetylcholinesterase.[16]

Rectal Biopsy and Acetylcholinesterase

Recognition of the absence of ganglion cells in the myenteric (Auerbach's) plexus and submucous (Meissner's) plexus is the standard method for diagnosing Hirschsprung's disease. Aldridge and Campbell observed that normally the hypoganglionic zone extends an average of 3 mm above the pectinate line in premature infants and 8 mm in young children.[23] Hypertrophied nerves and stratified columnar epithelium were observed in this aganglionic zone. They recommend taking rectal biopsies for the diagnosis of Hirschsprung's disease 2 cm above the pectinate line in infants and 3 cm in older children to avoid errors caused by biopsies taken in the hypoganglionic zone. Subsequently, Campbell and Noblett observed that specimens taken at 2 to 3 cm were less often diagnostic than those taken at 3 to 4 cm above the pectinate line.[24] They cautioned against using enemas for preparation, since this causes mucosal edema, thereby reducing the amount of submucosa obtained with the biopsy capsule. Swenson reported that surgically obtained rectal biopsies were 98 percent reliable in diagnosing Hirschsprung's disease.[8] However, other authors have noted the absence of submucosa in 10 percent to 30 percent of their suction or forceps biopsy specimens.[25,26]

Histochemical stains of rectal suction or forceps biopsies for acetylcholinesterase have been more reliable in confirming Hirschsprung's disease than in recognizing the absence of ganglion cells.[13,26] Huntley et al described two patterns of acetylcholinesterase staining.[27] Their type A pattern consisting of prominently stained nerve fibers in the lamina propria and muscularis mucosae was diagnostic of Hirschsprung's disease. The type B pattern showed staining primarily in the muscularis mucosae and the immediately adjacent lamina propria. This pattern was seen in infants with Hirschsprung's disease who were less than 1 month of age but also gave false-positive results, occurring in three children with other conditions as well.

Differential Diagnosis

Rare cases are described with skip areas of aganglionosis, of degeneration of ganglion cells previously present, and of "spontaneous recovery" after the diagnosis with congenital colon aganglionosis.[12,28] Syndromes that must be distinguished from Hirschsprung's disease in the newborn period include meconium plug syndrome (some cases of which may be concomitant with Hirschsprung's disease), microcolon, hypothyroidism, sepsis, cystic fibrosis, and neuronal dysplasia.

The clinical and radiographic findings in infants with neuronal dysplasia are similar to those with Hirschsprung's disease.[12,29,30] Histologic features of hyperplasia of the submucous and myenteric plexuses, increased acetylcholinesterase staining, and giant ganglia may occur throughout the GI tract. Manometric studies may demonstrate failure of relaxation of the internal sphincter with rectal distention.[29]

In older children, additional conditions that mimic Hirschsprung's disease include functional megacolon,[14,18] constipation due to narcotics, anterior displacement of the anus,[31] and pseudo-obstruction syndrome.

MANAGEMENT

Medical Treatment

Only rarely have children with Hirschsprung's disease received medical therapy without subsequent surgery.[12] The role of medical intervention is to stabilize the child by restoring fluid and electrolyte balance, especially if enterocolitis is present, and to perform adequate evacuation of the colon with warm saline enemas through a rectal tube.[15] Broad-spectrum antibiotics should be used in patients with suspected enterocolitis. Older children should be given a clear liquid diet, antibiotics orally, and irrigation fluid in the colon.[32]

Surgical Treatment

In infants obstruction is relieved through the creation of a stoma proximal to the aganglionic segment. Definitive surgery is delayed usually until the child weighs approximately 20 pounds.[15] In older children, a preliminary colostomy may not be required, and definitive surgery may be performed after adequate irrigation of the colon.[15]

Four definitive surgical approaches have been used for Hirschsprung's disease. The Swenson procedure, resection of the aganglionic segment and reanastomosis, was described in 1948.[3] Subsequently it was modified[33] because of the high incidence of postoperative enterocolitis (15.6 percent), disrupted anastomosis (11 percent), and fecal incontinence (3.2 percent).[4] The Duhamel procedure, originally described in 1956 and later modified, connects the normal proximal colon to the posterior portion of the retained aganglionic rectum in a side-to-side fashion.[34] This technique provides contractions to propel feces through the sphincters without risking injury to the autonomic nerves.[15] In the Soave procedure reported in 1964,[35] the normal proximal ganglionic bowel is pulled through the muscular sleeve of the retained rectum, from which the aganglionic mucosa has been removed and anastomosed primarily (Boley) or secondarily (Soave). These two pull-through techniques were compared by Koltz, who noted a higher frequency of anal strictures and enterocolitis with the Soave procedure.[32] The pediatric surgical survey had similar results as well as a higher mortality with this operation (3.2 percent).[4] Fecal continence was present in 12 of 13 children with the Boley procedure followed for more than 3 years. The operation preferred by pediatric surgeons in the 1973–1974 survey was Boley, 39 percent, Duhamel, 30 percent, Swenson, 23 percent, and Soave, 8 percent.[4]

More limited operations have been described for children with short-segment and ultrashort-segment disease.[6,11,37] The anorectal myomectomy consists of cutting a strip 0.5 to 1.0 cm wide through the internal sphincter and varying lengths of rectal muscle (5 to 14 cm). The technique is used also in classic Hirschsprung's disease if a short aganglionic segment remains following a definitive procedure.[15]

REFERENCES

1. Hirschsprung H. Stuhltragheit neugeborener en Folge von Dilatation and Hypertrophie des Colons. Jahrb Kinderheilk 1888; 27:1–7.
2. Dalla Valle A. Ricerche istologiche di un cas di megacolon congenita. Pediatria (Napoli) 1920; 28:740–752.
3. Swenson O, Bill AH Jr. Resection of the rectum and rectosigmoid with preservation of the sphincter for benign spastic lesions producing megacolon. Surgery 1948; 24:212–220.
4. Kleinhaus S, Boley SJ, Sheran M, Sieber WK. Hirschsprung's disease. A survey of the members of the surgical section of the American Academy of Pediatrics. J Pediatr Surg 1979; 14:588–597.
5. Landman GB. A five-year chart review of children biopsied to rule out Hirschsprung's disease. Clin Pediatr 1987; 26:288–291.
6. Nissan S, Bar-Maor JA. Further experience in the diagnosis and surgical treatment of short segment Hirschsprung's disease and idiopathic megacolon. J Pediatr Surg 1971; 6:738–741.
7. Scobie WG, Mackinlay GA. Anorectal myectomy in treatment of ultrashort segment Hirschsprung's disease. Arch Dis Child 1977; 52:713–715.
8. Swenson O, Sherman JO, Fisher JH. Diagnosis of congenital megacolon: an analysis of 501 patients. J Pediatr Surg 1973; 8:587–594.
9. Descos B, Lachaux A, Louis D, Chopard LP, Gilly J, Chayvialle JA, Hermier M. Extended intestinal aganglionosis in siblings. J Pediatr Gastroenterol Nutr 1984; 3:641–643.
10. Saperstein L, Pollack J, Beck AR. Total intestinal aganglionosis. Mt Sinai J Med (NY) 1980; 47:72–73.
11. Poisson J, Devroede G. Severe chronic constipation as a surgical problem. Surg Clin North Am 1983; 63:193–217.
12. Martin LW, Torres AM. Hirschsprung's disease. Surg Clin North Am 1985; 65:1171–1180.

13. Morikawa Y, Donahoe PK, Hendren WH. Manometry and histochemistry in the diagnosis of Hirschsprung's disease. Pediatrics 1979; 63:865–871.
14. Davidson M, Kugler MM, Bauer CH. Diagnosis and management in children with severe and protracted constipation and obstipation. J Pediatr 1963; 62:261–275.
15. Lavery JC. The surgery of Hirschsprung's disease. Surg Clin North Am 1983; 63:161–175.
16. Tobon F, Reid NCR, Talbert JL, Schuster MM. Nonsurgical test for the diagnosis of Hirschsprung's disease. N Engl J Med 1968; 278:188–194.
17. Weinberg AG. Acetylcholinesterase and Hirschsprung's disease. J Pediatr Gastroenterol Nutr 1986; 5:837–843.
18. Kottmeier PK, Clatworthy WH. Aganglionic and functional megacolon in children—a diagnostic dilemma. Pediatrics 1965; 36:572–582.
19. Bill AH, Chapman ND. The enterocolitis of Hirschsprung's disease—its natural history and treatment. Am J Surg 1962; 103:70–74.
20. Swenson O, Davidson FZ. Similarities of mechanical intestinal obstruction and aganglionic megacolon in the newborn infant: a review of 64 cases. N Engl J Med 1960; 262:64–67.
21. Taxman TL, Yulish BS, Rothstein FC. How useful is the barium enema in the diagnosis of infantile Hirschsprung's disease? Am J Dis Child 1986; 140:881–884.
22. Rosenberg AJ, Vela AR. A new simplified technique for pediatric anorectal manometry. Pediatrics 1983; 71:240–245.
23. Aldridge RT, Campbell PE. Ganaglion cell distribution in the normal rectum and anal canal. A basis for the diagnosis of Hirschsprung's disease by anorectal biopsy. J Pediatr Surg 1968; 3:475–489.
24. Campbell PE, Noblett HR. Experience with rectal suction biopsy in the diagnosis of Hirschsprung's disease. J Pediatr Surg 1969; 4:410–415.
25. Dobbins WO, Bill AH Jr. Diagnosis of Hirschsprung's disease excluded by rectal suction biopsy. N Engl J Med 1965; 272:990–993.
26. Kekomaki M, Rapola J, Louhimo I. Diagnosis of Hirschsprung's disease. Acta Paediatr Scand 1979; 68:893–897.
27. Huntley CC, Shaffner L deS, Challa VR, Lyerly AD. Histochemical diagnosis of Hirschsprung disease. Pediatrics 1982; 69:755–761.
28. Weinberg RJ, Klish WJ, Smalley JR, Brown MR, Putnam TC. Acquired distal aganglionosis of the colon. J Pediatr 1982; 101:406–409.
29. Scharli AF, Meier-Ruge W. Localized and disseminated forms of neuronal dysplasia mimicking Hirschsprung's disease. J Pediatr Surg 1981; 16:164–170.
30. Saul RA, Sturner RA, Burger PC. Hyperplasia of myenteric plexus. Its association with early infantile megacolon and neurofibromatosis. Am J Dis Child 1982; 136:852–854.
31. Hendren WH. Constipation caused by anterior location of the anus and its surgical correction. J Pediatr Surg 1978; 13:505–512.
32. Klotz DH, Velcek FT, Kottmeier PH, Reappraisal of the endorectal pull-through operation for Hirschsprung's disease. J Pediatr Surg 1973; 8:595–600.
33. Swenson O. Partial internal sphincterotomy in the treatment of Hirschsprung's disease. Ann Surg 1964; 160:540–550.
34. Duhamel B. A new operation for the treatment of Hirschsprung's disease. Arch Dis Child 1960; 35:38–39.
35. Soave F. Hirschsprung's disease: a new surgical technique. Arch Dis Child 1964; 39:116–124.
36. Boley SJ. New modification of the surgical treatment of Hirschsprung's disease. Surgery 1964; 56:1015–1017.
37. Lynn HB, van Heerden JA. Rectal myectomy in Hirschsprung's disease. Arch Surg 1975; 110:991–994.

Index

Note: Page numbers followed by "f" refer to figures; those followed by "t" refer to tables.